Pharmacology

for Canadian Health Care Practice

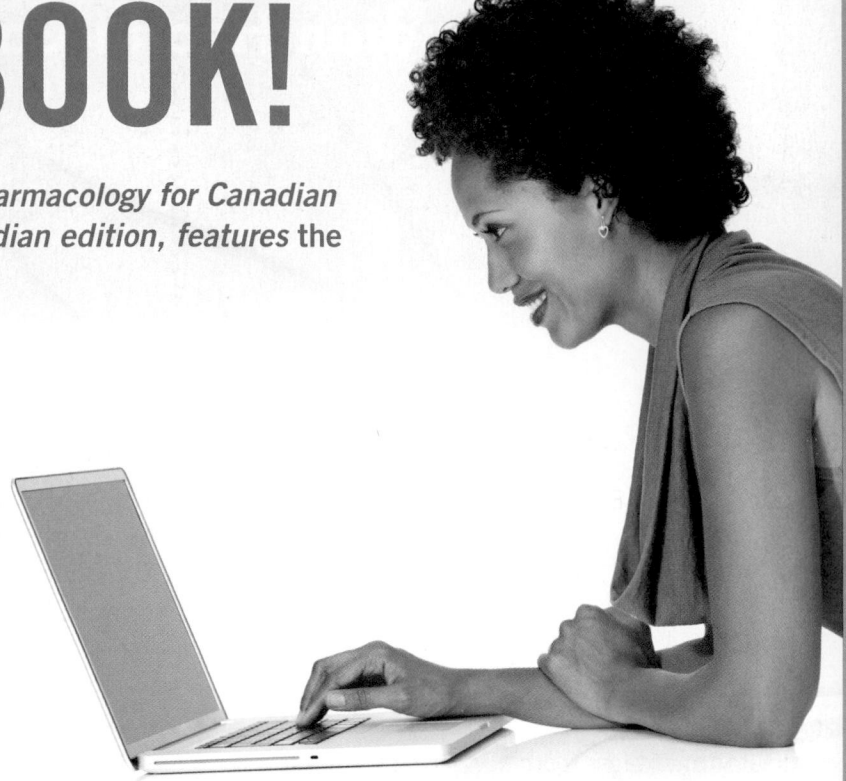

THIRD CANADIAN EDITION

Pharmacology
for Canadian Health Care Practice

Linda Lane Lilley, RN, PhD
Associate Professor Emeritus
School of Nursing
Old Dominion University
Norfolk, Virginia

Shelly Rainforth Collins, PharmD
Clinical Pharmacy Specialist
Coordinator of Clinical Pharmacy Services
Chesapeake Regional Medical Center
Chesapeake, Virginia
President
Drug Information Consultants
Chesapeake, Virginia

Julie S. Snyder, MSN, RN, BC
Adjunct Faculty
School of Nursing
Old Dominion University
Norfolk, Virginia

Beth Swart, RN, BScN, MES
Professor
Daphne Cockwell School of Nursing
Ryerson University
Toronto, Ontario

With Study Skills content by:
Diane Savoca
Coordinator of Student Transition
St. Louis Community College at Florissant Valley
St. Louis, Missouri

With special thanks to:
Franklin F. Gorospe IV, RN, BScN, MN
Instructor
Daphne Cockwell School of Nursing
Ryerson University
Toronto, Ontario
for his contribution to the third Canadian edition Study Skills
  content

ELSEVIER

ELSEVIER

Notices

Library and Archives Canada Cataloguing in Publication

Lilley, Linda Lane, author
  Pharmacology for Canadian health care practice / Linda Lilley, Shelly Rainforth Collins, Julie Snyder, Beth Swart.—Third Canadian edition.
Includes bibliographical references.
ISBN 978-1-927406-68-7 (paperback)
  1. Pharmacology—Textbooks. 2. Nursing—Canada—Textbooks. I. Collins, Shelly Rainforth, author II. Snyder, Julie S., author III. Swart, Beth, 1948-, author IV. Title.
RM301.L54 2016   615.1   C2016-900551-8

Vice President, Publishing: Ann Millar
Content Strategist: Roberta A. Spinosa-Millman
Content Development Specialist: Sandy Matos
Publishing Services Manager: Julie A. Eddy
Senior Project Manager: Marquita Parker
Copy Editor: Sherry Hinman
Proofreader: Michael Peebles
Cover Designer: Brett J. Miller, BJM Graphic Design and Communications
Design Direction: Amy Buxton
Cover Image: © Dmitry Yatsenko—Fotolia.com; © bitter. …—Fotolia.com
Typesetting and Assembly: Toppan Best-set Premedia Limited
Printing and Binding: Transcontinental

Elsevier Canada
555 Richmond Street West, Suite 1100, Toronto, ON, Canada M5V 3B1
Phone: 1-866-896-3331
Fax: 1-855-215-5738

Printed in Canada
1 2 3 4 5   20 19 18 17 16

Ebook ISBN: 978-1-77172-066-3

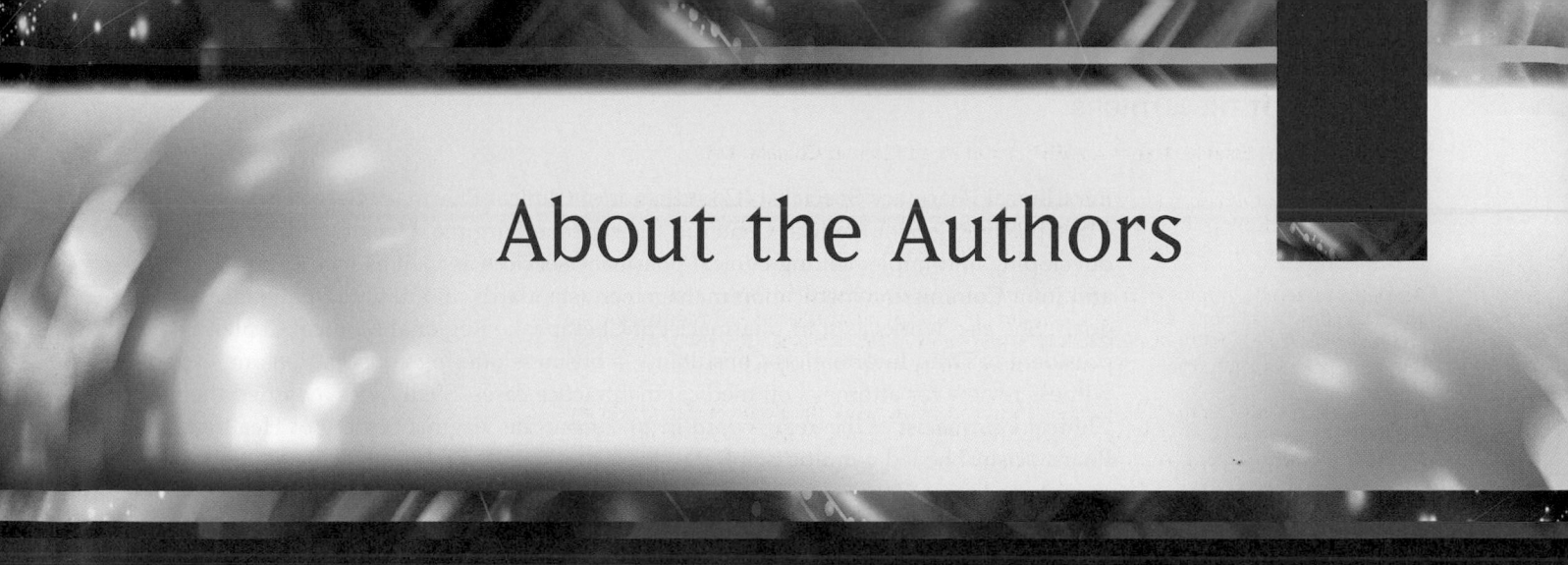

About the Authors

Linda Lane Lilley, RN, PhD

Linda Lilley received her diploma from Norfolk General School of Nursing, BSN from the University of Virginia, Master of Science (Nursing) from Old Dominion University, and PhD in Nursing from George Mason University. As an Associate Professor Emeritus and University Professor at Old Dominion University, her teaching experience in nursing education spans over 25 years, including almost 20 years at Old Dominion. Linda's teaching expertise includes drug therapy and the nursing process, adult nursing, physical assessment, fundamentals in nursing, oncology nursing, nursing theory, and trends in health care. The awarding of the University's most prestigious title of University Professor reflects her teaching excellence as a tenured faculty member. She has also been a two-time university nominee for the State Council of Higher Education in Virginia award for excellence in teaching, service, and scholarship. Linda received the 2012 Distinguished Nursing Alumni Award from Old Dominion University School of Nursing for her "continued work on the successful pharmacology textbook published by Elsevier" and to recognize her "extraordinary work and the impact [the book] has had on baccalaureate education." While at Old Dominion University, Linda mentored and taught undergraduate and graduate students as well as registered nurses returning for their BSN. Linda authored the MED ERRORS column for the *American Journal of Nursing* between 1994 and 1999 as well as numerous other peer-reviewed, published articles in professional nursing journals. Since retirement in 2005, Linda has continued to be active in nursing, serving as a member on dissertation committees with the College of Health Sciences and maintaining membership and involvement in numerous professional and academic organizations. Dr. Lilley has served as a consultant with school nurses in the city of Virginia Beach, a member on the City of Virginia Beach's Health Advisory Board, and currently a member of the City of Virginia Beach's Community Health Advisory Board and the Youth Community Action Team (YCAT). Linda also served as an appointed member on the national advisory panel on medication errors prevention with the U.S. Pharmacopeia in Rockville, Maryland. She continues to educate nursing students and professional nurses about drug therapy and the nursing process and speaks on the topics of drug therapy, safe medication use, humour and healing, and grief and loss.

Shelly Rainforth Collins, PharmD

Shelly Rainforth Collins received her Doctor of Pharmacy degree from the University of Nebraska College of Pharmacy in 1985, with High Distinction. She then completed a clinical pharmacy residency at Memorial Medical Center of Long Beach in Long Beach, California. She worked as a pediatric clinical pharmacist (neonatal specialist) at Memorial Medical Center before moving to Mobile, Alabama. She was the Assistant Director of Clinical Pharmacy Services at Mobile Infirmary Medical Center. She currently serves as the Clinical Pharmacy Specialist/Coordinator of Clinical Pharmacy Services at Chesapeake Regional Medical Center in Chesapeake, Virginia. Her practice focuses on developing and implementing clinical pharmacy services as well as medication safety and Joint Commission medication management standards and national patient safety goals. She also works as staff pharmacist at Chesapeake Regional Medical Center. She is president of Drug Information Consultants, a business offering consultation and expert witness review for attorneys on medical malpractice cases. Shelly was awarded the Clinical Pharmacist of the Year Award in 2007 from the Virginia Society of Healthsystem Pharmacists. She led a multidisciplinary team that won the Clinical Achievement of the Year Award from George Mason University School of Public Health in 2007 for promoting safety with narcotics in patients with sleep apnea; this program has also received national recognition. She was awarded the Service Excellence Award from Chesapeake Regional Medical Center. Shelly's professional affiliations include the American Society of Healthsystem Pharmacists and the Virginia Society of Healthsystem Pharmacists.

Julie S. Snyder, MSN, RN-BC

Julie Snyder received her diploma from Norfolk General Hospital School of Nursing and her BSN and MSN from Old Dominion University. After working in medical-surgical nursing, she worked in nursing staff development and community education. After 8 years, she transferred to the academic setting and has since taught fundamentals of nursing, pharmacology, physical assessment, gerontologic nursing, and adult medical-surgical nursing. She has been certified by the ANCC in Nursing Continuing Education and Staff Development and currently holds ANCC certification in Medical-Surgical Nursing. She is a member of Sigma Theta Tau International and was inducted into Phi Kappi Phi as Outstanding Alumni for Old Dominion University. She has worked for Elsevier as a reviewer and ancillary writer since 1997. Julie's professional service has included serving on the Virginia Nurses' Association Continuing Education Committee, serving as Educational Development Committee chair for the Epsilon Chi chapter of Sigma Theta Tau, serving as an item writer for the ANCC, working with a regional hospital educators' group, and serving as a consultant on various projects for local hospital education departments.

Beth Swart, RN, BScN, MES

Beth Swart, BScN, MES, is a professor in the School of Nursing, Ryerson University. She received her diploma in nursing from the Hospital for Sick Children School of Nursing, her BScN from the University of Toronto, and her MES from York University. For more than 40 years, Beth has taught nursing students at the baccalaureate level. She has also been a mentor to Masters students. Her areas of specialty are pathophysiology and epidemiology. Beth has also developed innovative Distance Education courses for RNs returning to university to pursue their degree. Research interests include differences in student learning between online and in-class teaching. Beth was for many years a board member of the Lambda-Pi Chapter-At-Large of Sigma Theta Tau International. She has served on the steering committee and the board of the National Immunization Education Initiative since 2003. In 2005, Beth received an award for teaching excellence in the faculty of Community Services. Beth has worked as a reviewer and author for Elsevier since 2004.

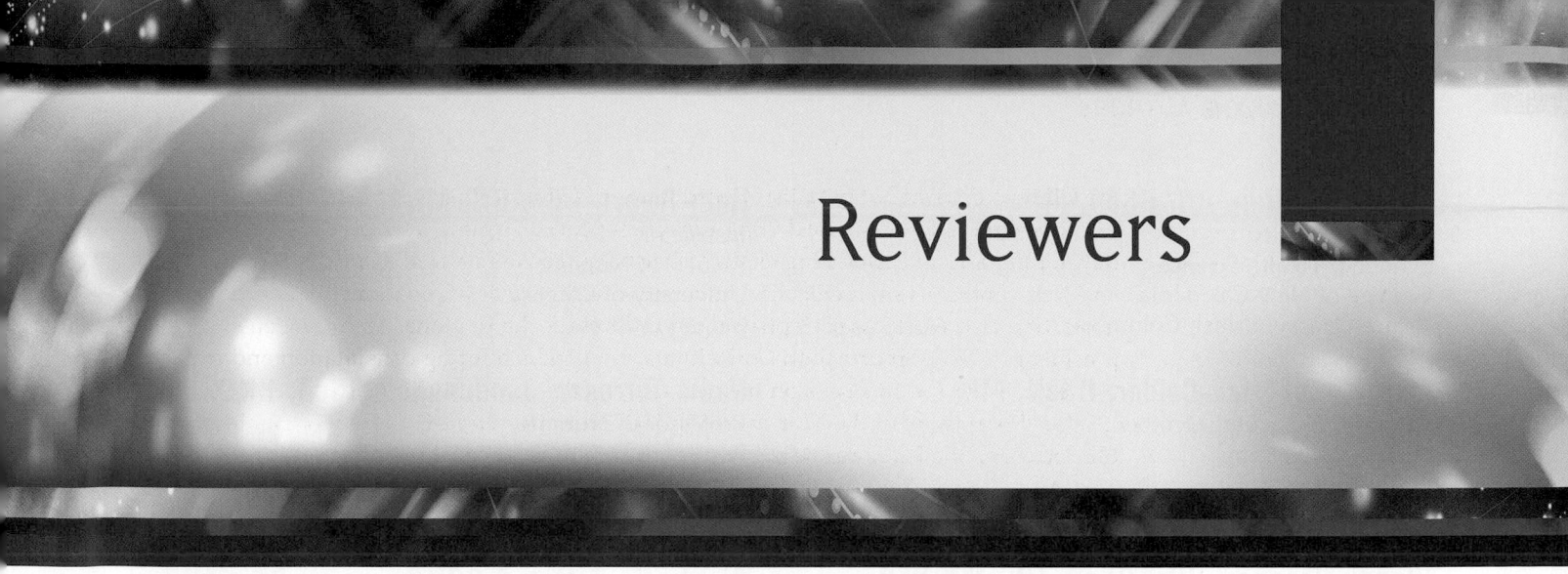

Reviewers

Marcia Brown, RN, BScN, MEd, CDE
Professor
York-Seneca Collaborative BScN Program
Faculty of Applied Arts & Health Sciences,
    King Campus
Seneca College of Applied Arts & Technology
King City, Ontario

Julie Duff Cloutier, RN, BScN, MSc
Assistant Professor
School of Nursing
Laurentian University
Sudbury, Ontario

Joan T. Crisp, RPN, RN, BSN, MEd
Nursing Faculty
Psychiatric Nursing Department
Douglas College
Coquitlam, British Columbia

Kerry Lynn Durnford, RN, MN
Nursing Faculty
Health and Human Services
Aurora College
Yellowknife, Northwest Territories

Kathryn Ellis, RN, BScN, MA (Ed.)
Professor
Centennial College Site
Centennial, Ryerson and George Brown Collaborative
    Nursing Degree Program
Toronto, Ontario

Paula Gauthier, RN, MSc
Learning Manager
Holland College
Charlottetown, Prince Edward Island

Wendy Gillespie, RN, MN
Instructor
Faculty of Nursing
University of Calgary
Calgary, Alberta

Marti Harder, RN, MSN
Department Head
Health Programs
Nicola Valley Institute of Technology
Merritt, British Columbia

Nicole Harder, RN, PhD
Assistant Professor
University of Manitoba
Winnipeg, Manitoba

Kristen Jones-Bonofiglio, RN, PhD
Assistant Professor
School of Nursing
Lakehead University
Thunder Bay, Ontario

Rupi Khaira, RN, PhD
Nursing Professor
School of Health Sciences
Seneca College of Applied Arts and Technology
King City, Ontario

Christina Kremer, BScPhm, CDE
Instructor
University of Ottawa Program
Algonquin College
Ottawa, Ontario

Brenda Lane, RN, BScN, DipAdEd, MN, CMSN(C)
Professor
Faculty of Health and Human Services
Vancouver Island University
Nanaimo, British Columbia

Nicole L'Italien, RN, BScN, MN
Nursing Faculty
School of Health Sciences
College of New Caledonia
Prince George, British Columbia

Lisa McKendrick-Calder, BScN, MN
Continuing Faculty Member
Faculty of Nursing
Grant Macewan University
Edmonton, Alberta

Wendy Neander, BSc, BScN, RN, MN PhD (cand.)
School of Nursing
University of Victoria
Victoria, British Columbia

Wanda Pierson, RN, BSN, MSN, MA, PhD
Faculty
School of Nursing
Langara College
Vancouver, British Columbia

Katherine Poser, RN, BScN, MNEd
Professor
School of Baccalaureate Nursing
St. Lawrence College
Kingston, Ontario

Faith Richardson, DNP, MSN/FNP, RN
Assistant Professor of Nursing
Trinity Western University School of Nursing
Langley, British Columbia

Saôde Savary, PhD
National Nursing Programs Director
The Eminata Group

Heather Scarlett-Ferguson, BSP, MEd, EdD (c)
Instructor
Health & Community Studies
MacEwan University
Edmonton, Alberta

Joy Shewchuk, RN, BSc, BSN, MSN
Professor, Nursing
Humber College
Toronto, Ontario

Ruth Swart, BSc, BN, MHS, EdD
Instructor
Faculty of Nursing
University of Calgary
Calgary, Alberta

Nadia Torresan-Doodnaught, BScN, RNC, MN
Professor of Nursing
Faculty of Health Sciences
Seneca College of Applied Arts & Technology
King City, Ontario

Stephanie Zettel, B.SC (Honours), BN, MN
Associate Professor
School of Nursing and Midwifery
Mount Royal University
Calgary, Alberta

With special thanks to PharmD reviewers:

Grace Frankel, BSc (Pharm), PharmD
Performance Based Assessment Coordinator & Pharmacy Practice Instructor
College of Pharmacy, Faculty of Health Sciences
Apotex Centre
University of Manitoba
Winnipeg, Manitoba

I fan Kuo, BSc (Pharm), ACPR, MSc, PharmD
Assistant Professor
College of Pharmacy, Faculty of Health Sciences
Apotex Centre
University of Manitoba
Winnipeg, Manitoba

Christine Leong, BSc (Gen), BSc (Pharm), PharmD
Assistant Professor
College of Pharmacy, Faculty of Health Sciences
Apotex Centre
University of Manitoba
Winnipeg, Manitoba

Christopher Louizos, BSc (Pharm), PharmD
Pharmacy Practice Instructor
College of Pharmacy, Faculty of Health Sciences
Apotex Centre
University of Manitoba
Winnipeg, Manitoba

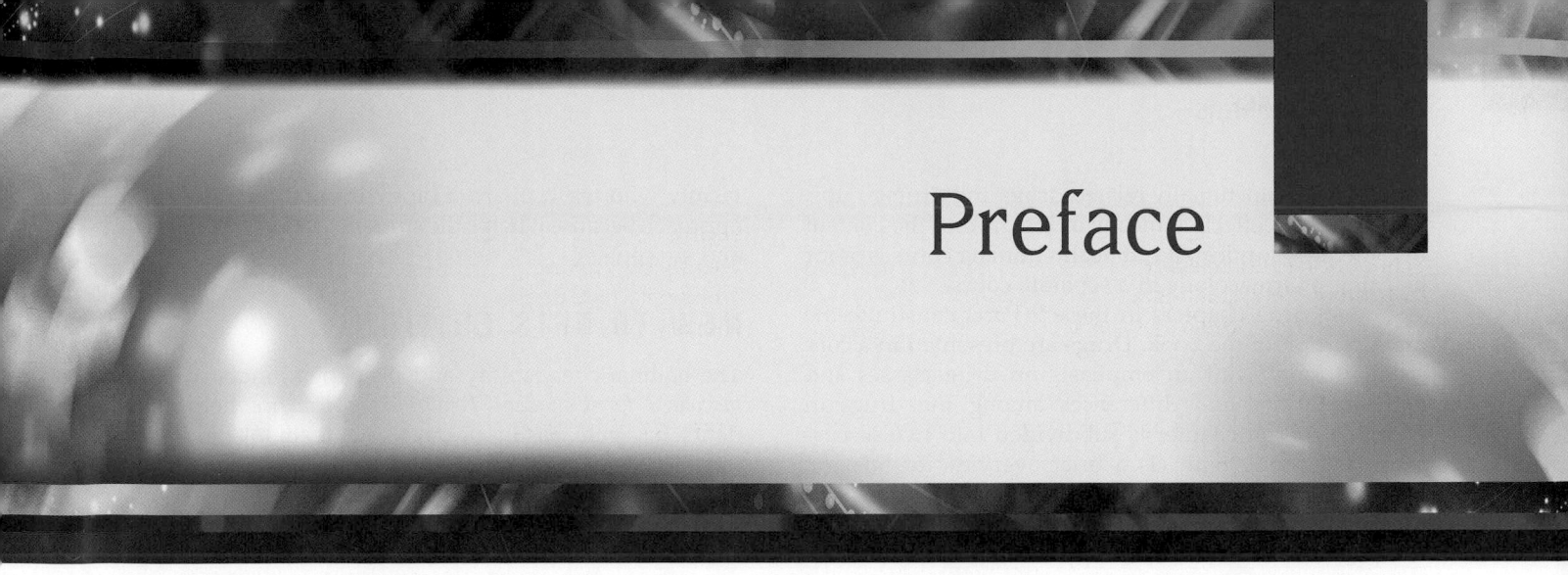

Preface

INTRODUCTION

The third edition of *Pharmacology for Canadian Health Care Practice* incorporates both the nursing process and evidence in practice as it is relevant to Canadian nursing. This text provides the most current and clinically relevant information in an appealing, understandable, and practical format. The clear writing style and full-colour design of *Pharmacology for Canadian Health Care Practice* are ideal for today's busy nursing student. The book not only presents drug information that the nursing student needs to know, but also provides information on what the professional nurse may encounter during drug administration in a variety of health care settings, including accounts of real-life medication errors and tips for avoiding those errors. Features that help set the book apart include:

- A focus on the role of prioritization in nursing care
- A strong focus on drug classes to help students acquire a better knowledge of how various drug classes work in the body, allowing them to apply this knowledge to individual drugs
- Canadian content relevant to Canadian students and educators that will strengthen their knowledge of the field
- Clinical practice guidelines produced or endorsed in Canada by national, provincial, or territorial medical or health organizations, or by professional societies, government agencies, or expert panels
- Ethnocultural examples that reflect the varied and complex ethnodemographic diversity of Canada
- Ease of readability to make this difficult content more understandable
- Integrated study skills content that helps students understand and learn the particularly demanding subject of pharmacology while also equipping them with tools that they can use in other courses and as lifelong learners who are building an evidence-based practice.

For this edition, the author team has focused even more closely on providing the most "need-to-know" information, enhancing readability, and emphasizing the nursing process and prioritization throughout. Many of the updates for this edition are in response to actual questions posed by students.

MARKET RESEARCH

To aid in the preparation of this text, nursing instructors from across Canada participated in extensive, detailed reviews of the Second Canadian Edition. These reviewers assessed changes that had occurred in the field of pharmacology since publication of the second edition and determined what was needed to better teach this subject to nursing students and how their evolving learning needs could be met.

This Canadian edition maintains the philosophy of making the challenging subject of pharmacology approachable and easy to understand. Additional concerns raised and enhancements suggested by educators and nursing students who served as reviewers or consultants throughout the manuscript's development, as well by the author and editors of this text, also have been addressed.

ORGANIZATION

This book includes 58 chapters presented in 10 parts, organized by body system. The 10 "concepts" chapters in Part 1 lay a solid foundation for the subsequent drug units and address the following topics:

- The nursing process and drug therapy
- Pharmacological principles
- Legal and ethical considerations
- Ethnocultural and lifespan considerations related to pharmacology
- Gene therapy and pharmacogenomics
- Preventing and responding to medication errors
- Patient education and drug therapy
- Over-the-counter drugs and natural health products
- Vitamins and minerals
- Drug administration techniques, including 100 drawings and photographs

Parts 2 through 10 present pharmacology and nursing management in a time-tested body systems and drug function framework. This approach facilitates learning by grouping functionally related drugs and drug groups. It provides an effective means of integrating the content into medical-surgical/adult health nursing courses or for teaching pharmacology in a separate course.

The 48 drug chapters in these 9 Parts constitute the main portion of the book. Drugs are presented in a consistent format with an emphasis on drug classes and key similarities and differences among the drugs in each class. Each chapter is subdivided into two discussions, beginning with (1) a brief overview of relevant anatomy, physiology, and pathophysiology and a complete discussion of pharmacology, followed by (2) a comprehensive yet succinct application of the nursing process.

Pharmacology is presented for each drug group in a consistent format:
- Mechanism of Action and Drug Effects
- Indications
- Contraindications
- Adverse Effects (often including Toxicity and Management of Overdose)
- Interactions
- Dosages

Drug class discussions conclude with specially highlighted Drug Profiles—brief narrative "capsules" of individual drugs in the class or group, including pharmacokinetics tables for each drug. Key drugs (prototypical drugs within a class) are identified throughout with a ▶▶ symbol for easy identification.

The pharmacology section is followed by a Nursing Process discussion that relates to the entire drug group. This nursing content is covered in the following, familiar nursing process format:
- Assessment
- Nursing Diagnoses
- Planning (including Goals and Expected Patient Outcomes)
- Implementation
- Evaluation

At the end of each Nursing Process section is a Patient Teaching Tips box that summarizes key points for nursing students and practicing nurses to include in the education of patients about their medications. These boxes focus on teaching how the drugs work, possible interactions, adverse effects, and other information related to the safe and effective use of the drug(s). The role of the nurse as patient educator and advocate continues to grow in importance in professional practice, so there is emphasis on this key content in each chapter in this edition.

Additionally, each Part begins with a Study Skills Tips section that presents a study skills topic and relates it to the unit being discussed. Topics include time management, note taking, studying, test taking, and others. This unique feature is intended to aid students who find pharmacology difficult and to provide a tool that may prove beneficial throughout their nursing school careers. This arrangement of content can be especially helpful to

faculty who teach pharmacology through an integrated approach because it helps the student identify key content and concepts.

NEW TO THIS EDITION

The hallmark readability and user-friendliness of *Pharmacology for Canadian Health Care Practice* helps students navigate easily through the textbook and thus the difficult subject of pharmacology and the nursing process.

The third edition of *Pharmacology for Canadian Health Care Practice* also features an enhanced focus on "need-to-know" content. The information on drug adverse effects has been streamlined to reflect only the most common and most serious adverse effects rather than listing all reported adverse effects. These adverse effects are also now listed in order of those most commonly seen. Another area that has been reduced for an optimized focus is that of drug dosages; only those dosages that are seen in most common indications are included in the text and tables. (For other dosages, the student should refer to an up-to-date drug handbook or drug reference.) This need-to-know approach to drug indications and adverse effects is crucial in helping the adult learner focus on the most essential content needed for safe drug administration.

Drugs included in the text are as up-to-date as possible. The availability of drugs changes frequently because manufacturers discontinue production or as a result of shortages.

The use of abbreviations has been limited to the most common abbreviations. While the use of abbreviations is not encouraged overall, abbreviations are still approved and used by agencies, and may also be part of the documentation method. The Institute of Safe Medication Practices (ISMP) Canada's "Do Not Use List" of abbreviations, symbols, and dose designations has been adhered to within this text.

It is important to remember that although this textbook provides all of the need-to-know *pharmacology* content that students will need for an entry level of practice, it is first and foremost a *nursing* textbook rather than a pharmacology textbook, with a strong emphasis on the nursing process and professional nursing practice. The section on implementation also offers all of the most essential information, followed by a section on the evaluation of therapeutic and adverse effects. These changes highlight the significance of the nursing process as a foundation in drug therapy while helping the student to make strong cognitive connections among nursing diagnoses, goals, and expected patient outcomes.

Pharmacology for Canadian Health Care Practice reflects the latest drug information and research through the following special boxes:
- Evidence in Practice
- Ethnocultural Implications

- Lab Values Related to Drug Therapy
- Legal and Ethical Principles
- Natural Health Products
- Preventing Medication Errors
- Special Populations: Adolescents
- Special Populations: Children
- Special Populations: The Older Adult
- Legal and Ethical Principles
- Pharmacokinetic Bridge to Nursing Process

The pharmacology and nursing content in each of the 58 chapters has been thoroughly revised and critically reviewed by nursing instructors, practising nurses, and PharmDs to reflect the latest drug information and nursing content. Key updates include:

- A more effectively organized classification of psychotherapeutic drugs in Chapter 17 into 3 subcategories: (1) anxiolytics, (2) mood stabilizers and antidepressants, and (3) antipsychotic drugs
- The most recent evidence-informed guidelines on management of diabetes in Chapter 33, with an emphasis on new diabetes drugs
- The most recent evidence in practice guidelines on the treatment of rheumatoid arthritis in Chapter 54
- Revision of Chapter 50 on immunosuppressant drugs to provide an emphasis on transplant therapy
- Revised Examination Review Questions at the end of each chapter, including alternate-item format and new dosage calculation questions

ADDITIONAL TEACHING AND LEARNING FEATURES

The book also includes a variety of innovative teaching and learning features that prepare the student for important content to be covered in each chapter and encourage review and reinforcement of that content. Chapter-opener features include the following:

- Learning objectives
- List of Evolve Resources available to students
- Summary of Drug Profiles in the chapter, with page number references
- Key terms with definitions and page number references (key terms being in **bold** type throughout the narrative to emphasize this essential terminology)

The following features appear at the end of each chapter.

- Patient Teaching Tips related to drug therapy
- Key Points boxes summarizing important chapter content
- Examination Review Questions, with answers provided upside-down at the bottom of the section for quick and easy review
- Critical Thinking activities

In addition to the special boxes listed previously, other special features that appear throughout the text include:

- Case Studies in every chapter, with answer guidelines provided on the Evolve website

- Dosages tables listing generic and trade names, pharmacological class, usual dosage ranges, and indications for the drugs

For a more comprehensive listing of the special features, please see the inside back cover of the book.

COLOUR

The use of colour continues to complement the text by making the book engaging for nursing students. Colour is used throughout to:

- Highlight important content
- Illustrate how drugs work in the body in numerous anatomic and drug process colour illustrations
- Improve the visual appearance of the content to make it more engaging and appealing to today's more visually sophisticated reader

The use of colour and other visual engagement devices in these ways significantly improves students' involvement and understanding of pharmacology.

SUPPLEMENTAL RESOURCES

A comprehensive ancillary package is available to students and instructors using *Pharmacology for Canadian Health Care Practice*. The following supplemental resources have been thoroughly revised for this edition and can significantly assist in the teaching and learning of pharmacology.

Study Guide

The student study guide—carefully aligned with the content and focus of the book—includes the following:

- Student Study Tips that reinforce the Study Skills in the text and provide a "how to" guide to applying test-taking strategies
- Worksheets for each chapter, with Examination Review questions (with application-based, alternate-item, and dosage calculation questions), critical thinking and application questions, and other activities
- Case Studies followed by related critical thinking questions
- An updated Overview of Dosage Calculations with helpful tips for calculating doses, sample drug labels, practice problems, and a quiz
- Answers to all questions (provided in the back of the book) to facilitate self study

Evolve Web Site

Located at http://evolve.elsevier.com/Canada/Lilley/pharmacology, the Evolve Web site for this book includes the following elements:

For Students

- More than 550 Review Questions for Exam Preparation
- Answers to Critical Thinking Activities from the book
- Printable Chapter Summaries for each chapter

- Answers to Case Studies from the book
- Audio Glossary
- Unfolding Case Studies

For Instructors

- **NEW** *TEACH for Nurses* Lesson Plans that focus on the most important content from each chapter and provide innovative strategies for student engagement and learning. These new Lesson Plans include strategies for integrating nursing curriculum standards, links to all relevant student and instructor resources, and an original instructor-only Case Study in each chapter.
- ExamView® Test Bank that features more than 800 examination–format test questions (including alternate-item questions) with text page references, rationales, and answers coded for NCLEX® Client Needs category, nursing process step, and cognitive level (Bloom's taxonomy). The robust ExamView® testing application, provided at no cost to faculty, allows instructors to create new tests; edit, add, and delete test questions; sort questions by NCLEX® Client Needs category, cognitive level, and nursing process step; and administer and grade tests online, with automated scoring and gradebook functionality.
- PowerPoint® Lecture Slides consisting of more than 2 100 customizable text slides for instructors to use in lectures. The presentations include Unfolding Case Studies and applicable illustrations from the book's Image Collection. Audience Response System Questions (three or more discussion-oriented questions per chapter for use with i>Clicker and other systems) are folded into these presentations.
- An Image Collection with over 250 full-colour images from the book for instructors to use in lectures
- Access to all student resources listed above

Elsevier eBooks

This exciting program is available to faculty who adopt a number of Elsevier texts, including *Pharmacology for Canadian Health Care Practice*. Elsevier eBooks is an integrated electronic study centre consisting of a collection of textbooks made available online. It is carefully designed to "extend" the textbook for an easier and more efficient teaching and learning experience. It includes study aids such as highlighting, e-note taking, and cut-and-paste capabilities. Even more importantly, it allows students and instructors to do a comprehensive search within the specific text or across a number of titles. Please check with your Elsevier Canada sales representative for more information.

ICONS AT A GLANCE

- CASE STUDY
- DRUG PROFILES
- ETHNOCULTURAL IMPLICATIONS
- EVIDENCE IN PRACTICE
- LAB VALUES RELATED TO DRUG THERAPY
- LEGAL & ETHICAL PRINCIPLES
- NATURAL HEALTH PRODUCTS
- PREVENTING MEDICATION ERRORS
- SPECIAL POPULATIONS: ADOLESCENTS
- SPECIAL POPULATIONS: CHILDREN
- SPECIAL POPULATIONS: OLDER ADULT

WE WELCOME YOUR FEEDBACK

We always welcome comments from instructors and students who use this book so that we may continue to make improvements and be responsive to your needs in future editions. Please send any comments you may have for us to the attention of the publisher at a.millar@elsevier.com.

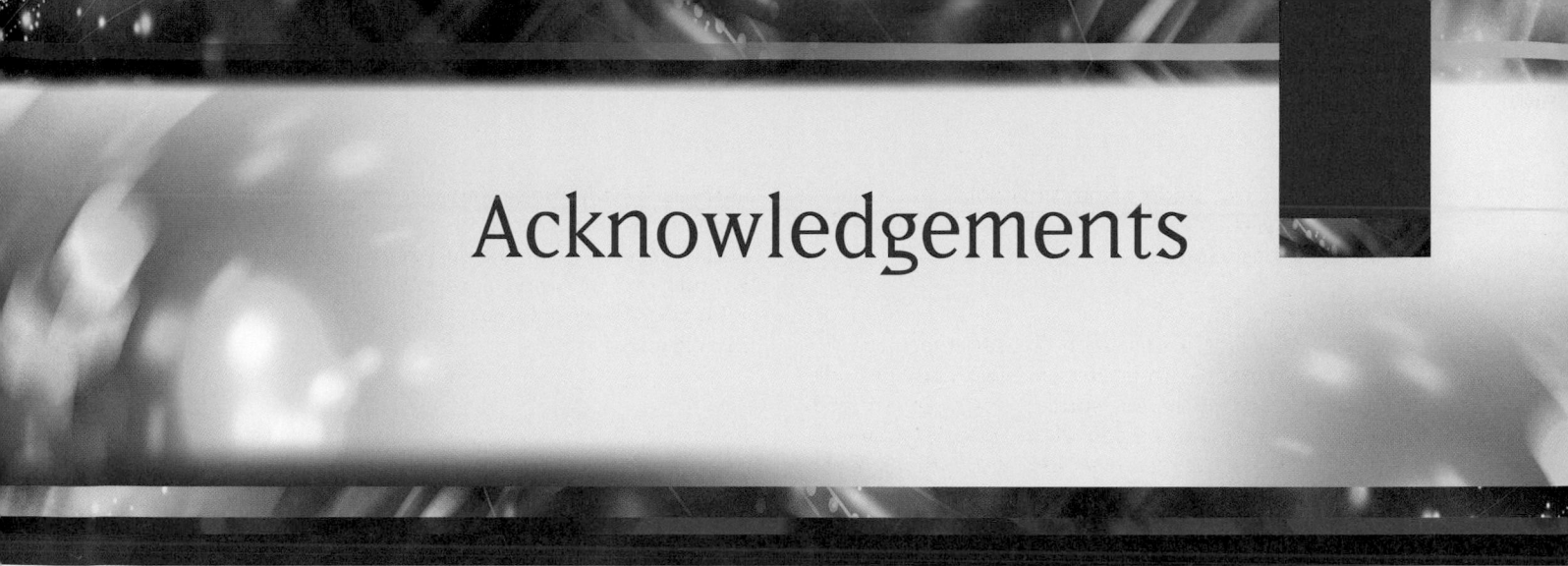

Acknowledgements

My part in this book would not have been possible without the original efforts of the American authors who conceptualized and wrote *Pharmacology and the Nursing Process*, which has shaped the content of *Pharmacology for Canadian Health Care Practice*. Linda Lane Lilley, RN, PhD; Scott Harrington, PharmD; Shelly Rainforth Collins, PharmD; and Julie S. Snyder, MSN, RN, BC, are to be commended for their thorough and expert handling of a vast and complex subject matter and for creating an excellent foundation over which the Canadian content could be easily laid.

I dedicate *Pharmacology for Canadian Health Care Practice* to my sons, Jeffrey I. and Derk, who continue to inspire me with their dedication, strength, and support; I could not have met the challenges of authoring this pharmacology textbook without their encouragement and understanding. To my students, both past and present, who are a never-ending source of inspiration and who constantly challenge me to make material relevant, fun, and interesting, I give heartfelt thanks for inspiring my writing in this book.

I could not have accomplished this project without the assistance of Roberta A. Spinosa-Millman, Managing Editor at Elsevier Canada, who encouraged, altered deadlines to fit my busy schedule, reminded me of deadlines, and supported me throughout the huge task of editing this book as a sole author. I want to thank Michael Anciado, BScN, Franklin Gorospe IV, RN, MN, and Dr. Charlotte Lee for their contributions to Chapters 11, 50, 52, and 53 respectively. Many individuals at Elsevier Canada are responsible for this Canadian edition. My thanks go to Ann Millar, Publisher; Sherry Hinman, Copy Editor; Sandy Matos, Content Development Specialist; and Marquita Parker, Senior Project Manager—St. Louis, for handling all the details involved in the final production of the book.

Thanks are due to the Canadian reviewers who reviewed content of this book and gave their invaluable comments, expertise, and editing suggestions on the draft manuscript. Thanks are also extended to Franklin Gorospe IV, for his work in revising the Study Skills Tips sections. As existing diseases and disorders and their treatments evolve, bringing with them new challenges and information in pharmacology, we will no doubt be looking forward to future editions of this textbook.

Beth Swart, RN, BScN, MES

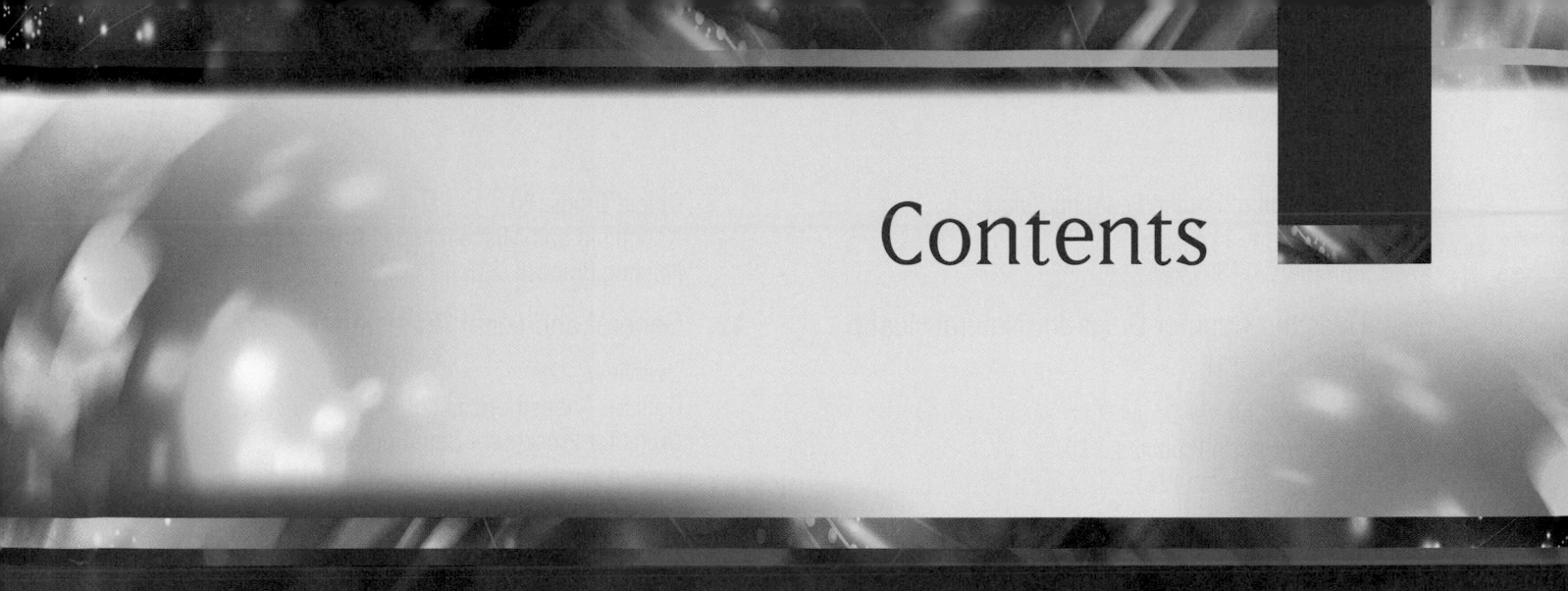

Contents

PART TWO

Drugs Affecting the Central Nervous System, 189

Study Skills Tips, 189

PART THREE

Drugs Affecting the Autonomic Nervous System, 375

Study Skills Tips, 375

PART FOUR

Drugs Affecting the Cardiovascular and Renal Systems, 431

Study Skills Tips, 431

PART FIVE

Drugs Affecting the Endocrine System, 599
Study Skills Tip, 599

PART TEN

Miscellaneous Therapeutics: Hematological, Dermatological, Ophthalmic, and Otic Drugs, 1025
Study Skills Tips, 1025

Pharmacology Basics

INTRODUCTION TO STUDY SKILLS CONCEPTS

"What should I study?"
"When is the best time for me to study?"
"How much of the material should I study?"
"How can I be effective in my studies?"

In the best of worlds, every student would have all the skills necessary to be effective in all academic areas. Unfortunately, one skill many students do not have is the ability to study effectively. Many students use a linear approach to studying and apply the same habitual study techniques regardless of topic areas. While those techniques might work well in some areas, others require a different approach. The purpose of this Study Skills Tips section is to introduce you to the steps to follow when learning text and maintaining focus on the appropriate material. This section also offers some specific examples for selected chapters in Part One to help you apply the study techniques and strategies discussed herein.

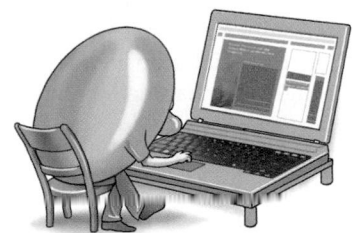

Extensive study skills—covering time management, note taking, mastering of the text, preparing and taking examinations, and development vocabulary—are presented in the *Study Guide* that accompanies this text.

These tools are important for any area of study but even more valuable when used in challenging technical areas such as nursing and pharmacology. The techniques described here and in the *Study Guide* will not necessarily make learning easy, but they will help you achieve your goals as a student.

Sleep plays an important role in memory and learning. A well-rested person can learn more easily and more thoroughly than a sleepy one. During sleep, the brain is not quiet; it replays the events of the day and seems to play an important role in making connections. During sleep, the brain turns recently acquired memories into long-term memories. It helps lock in the learning, likely one of its main biological functions.

UNDERLINING AND HIGHLIGHTING TEXT

Underlining or highlighting when reading is a helpful strategy. This approach has many functions for the student. It enables the student to go back to important sections of the reading, allows the student to control the pace of reading (prevents rushing). and helps the student reflect on the reading. There are some things to consider when using this approach. First, consider reading the material at least once before underlining or highlighting; far too often, students habitually underline or highlight a significant portion of the readings. Second, consider the objectives and chapter focus when underlining or highlighting—ask yourself, "Is this essential for learning the concept?" Often, students underline or highlight nonessential content. Third, consider why you are underlining or highlighting. Is it so you can go back to the selected text? If not, perhaps making text notations would be just as effective. Whether you fully or partially rely on this approach, remember that underlining or highlighting is a tool to facilitate your learning—do not allow it to distract you from your study techniques.

PURR

PURR is a handy mnemonic device that represents a four-step process to facilitate mastery of the material:
- *Prepare*
- *Understand*
- *Rehearse*
- *Review*

Using PURR is both challenging and rewarding. The challenge is that you are required to go through every chapter four times; this familiarizes you with the writing style of the author and enables you to objectively learn the materials presented and reflect on the concepts in a way that makes sense to you. The rewarding aspect of PURR is that it doesn't require you to actually *read* the chapter a minimum of four times; you only *go through* it four times. Only one of those times is a slow, careful, intensive reading; the other trips through the chapter are much quicker. The first time you go through the chapter should take only 5 to 10 minutes. Each time you go through the chapter, you process the information in distinctly different ways. The PURR approach will enhance your learning, and if you use it from the first reading on, you will find that it takes you less time than your previous approach.

Prepare

As with any complex process, reading the text is not something to dive into without thought and planning. *Pharmacology for Canadian Health Care Practice* is organized to help you learn the material, but you have to take advantage of what the authors have done to facilitate this learning. Preparing to read means setting goals and objectives for your own learning. The tools you need to help you do this are already in place; look at the opening pages of any chapter in the text and you will see a standard structure.

Every chapter begins with a title. Learn to use the title as the first step in preparing to learn. For instance, Chapter 3 is entitled "Legal and Ethical Considerations." The words in the title are specifically chosen to give you an idea of the topics covered in the chapter. Think about the title before you begin to read the chapter. Does it remind you of something? Are there any unfamiliar terms in it? If your answer is "no," that is great. If it is "yes," then you already have some focus for your reading because you know you will need to learn the unfamiliar terms and their meanings.

The next feature of every chapter is the objectives. Objectives are important for learning, and the authors have anticipated this. Think about objectives as your goal for reading the chapter. Read the objectives actively. Do not just look at the words; think about them. Ask yourself the following questions:
- What do I already know about this material?
- How do these objectives relate to earlier required readings?
- How do they relate to objectives the instructor has given?

The chapter objectives identify things you should be able to do after you have read the material. Do not wait until you have read the chapter to start trying to respond. *Preparing* means becoming engaged from the beginning. Studying the chapter objectives establishes a direction and purpose for your reading. This approach will enable you to maintain concentration and focus while you read.

Another feature in the opening pages of each chapter are the key terms. This is one of the most valuable tools the authors have provided. They know that there are many terms to learn, and the Key Terms section gives you a head start on learning them. Spend a few minutes on this section. Notice the terms that are also used in the chapter objectives. Go back and look at the objectives and think about what you have learned from the key terms. As you study them, look for shared root words, prefixes, or suffixes—words that share common elements usually also have a shared meaning. Learning the meaning of common word elements can simplify the whole process of learning vocabulary. Perhaps you remember in elementary school being told to "look for the little words in the big word." This is essentially the same technique that gives you a clue about the meaning of the concept—one that worked then and that will work now.

Now make a quick pass through the chapter or the assigned pages from the chapter. Look for anything that stands out in the chapter, such as boldfaced text, boxed material, and tables. These features provide a quick overview of the chapter, which will make the next steps in the PURR process much more effective and efficient.

The chapter headings show the major points to be covered. Study them and notice the major headings (topics) and the subordinate headings (subtopics). This is essentially a picture of the chapter, and using this picture is an essential step in preparing to read. As you read through the chapter headings, turn the topics and subtopics into a series of questions to answer when you finish reading. Think about the objectives and how the headings relate to them. Finally, in the headings devoted to specific classes of drugs, notice that there are elements that are common to all of them. The last two headings are always "Implementation" and "Evaluation." This tells you that you will be expected to know these two common elements at the end of every chapter. The minutes you spend preparing will pay off in a big way when you start to read. Think about it as going to an unfamiliar location. Preparing allows you to look at the map showing the route to your destination before you start travelling.

Preparing makes the whole approach to learning an active one. It may not make the chapters the most exciting reading you will ever do, but it will help you accomplish your personal learning objectives as well as those set by the authors.

On-the-Run Action. It is a good idea to do the prepare phase during "found" time. It should not take more than 5 to 10 minutes; time between classes, time spent waiting for the coffee to brew, or any other small block of time that usually just slips away can be used to accomplish this step.

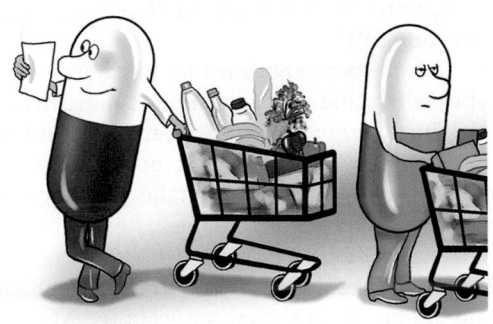

Understand

The time has now come to tackle the reading. Go to your desk, the library, or wherever you have chosen for dedicated and serious study. Reading the required pages is when all your preparation pays off. If you did the *prepare* step earlier in the day, it is not a bad idea to spend a minute or two going through the chapter features again to get your focus. As you read, remember the chapter objectives and notice the chapter headings in the body of the chapter. As you read, rephrase the chapter headings as questions to help keep yourself focused on the task at hand.

Because this is the first time you are really focusing on the concepts and details, this is not the time to do any text notations. Think as you read. Key terms are repeated, and their meanings are often expanded and clarified in the body of the text. Pay attention to these terms. Think about what they mean and how you would define them to someone else. Read for meaning; do not read just to get to the end—that is a passive action. Ask yourself questions. Analyze, respond, and react as you read. Find meaning in the words. Does it make sense? If it doesn't, ask yourself why.

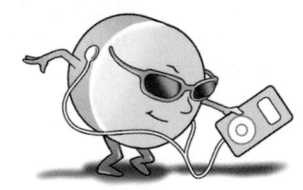

Often, there may be too many required pages to read with complete understanding in one session. If you find that your concentration is flagging or you do not remember what you read on the previous page, it is time to take a break. Finding yourself rushing through the material just to get to the end is also a sign that it is time to take a break. All too often, students have only one objective—to finish. You might be able to force yourself to continue reading, but you will not learn much. Often, this makes reading boring, long, and passive. Mark your place and take a 5- or 10-minute break. Take a walk, listen to music,

get a cold drink or a hot beverage, and then go back. When you come back to the reading, spend the first 3 or 4 minutes reviewing. Look back at the previous chapter heading and think about what you were reading before your break. The chapter can be broken down into many small reading sessions, but it is critical that you do not lose sight of the chapter as a whole. Spending these few minutes in review may seem like time that could be better spent continuing with the reading, but a brief review will save time in the long run.

There is no quick way to read a chapter. You will not find an "on-the-run action" for this step because it cannot be done in that way. *Understanding* requires your full, undivided attention. However, if you do the *prepare* step first, you will be surprised at how much more easily you get the reading done, and more importantly, how much more learning you achieve in the process.

Rehearse

Most study techniques involve some aspect of rereading, repeating, or regurgitating the concepts from the required reading. The PURR method uses *rehearse* as the third step in the process. It starts with consolidation of what you learned, establishing a basis for long-term memory. Rehearsal accomplishes two things. First, it helps you find out what you understood from the reading—knowing what you know is really important. It provides positive reinforcement that you are learning. Second, it identifies what you do not understand—this may be an even more important benefit. Knowing what you do not know before it appears on an examination is critical. It allows you to target specific areas of learning, making you more efficient in your studying.

How to Rehearse. Everything you do in the *prepare* and *understand* steps comes into play in the *rehearse* step. Rehearsal should begin with the features at the beginning of the chapter. Open the text to the beginning of the chapter. Start with the chapter title and begin to quiz yourself on what you have read. Compose three or four questions pertaining to the chapter title, and then try to answer them to your satisfaction. At this time, text notation is an excellent strategy. Text notation is the act of making notes that facilitate your ability to comprehend the material. Text notations are content material that helps you stay on track. For instance, answering the questions on a separate document allows you to stay on track with the chapter objectives. The questions you ask yourself should be both literal (asking for specific information presented in the chapter) and interpretive (testing your comprehension of concepts and relationships). An example of a literal question based on the Chapter 3 title might be, "What are the definitions of *ethnocultural*, *legal*, and *ethical*?" This question would help you determine whether you can satisfactorily define these terms in your own words. The process of asking and answering questions like these serves to move learning from short-term to long-term memory. Literal questions are important to help you grasp the factual information and terminology contained in the reading.

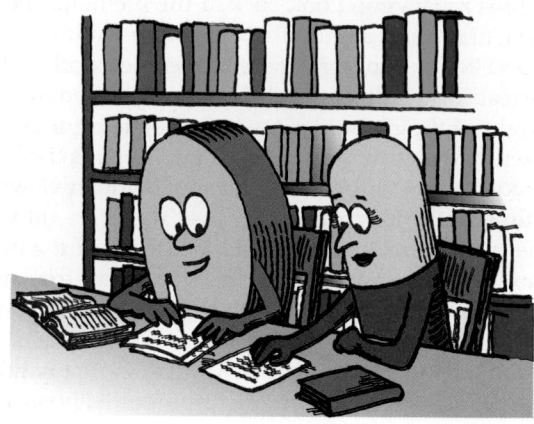

However, it is also necessary to ask questions that stimulate your thoughts about the concepts and the relationships between the facts and concepts presented in the chapter. An example of an interpretive question regarding the Chapter 3 title might be, "What are the most important ethnocultural, legal, and ethical concepts pertaining to the use of drugs?" Sometimes you will find that, even though the question is interpretive, the authors have anticipated the question and the text contains the direct answer to your question. Other times you will need to formulate your own response by pulling together bits and pieces of information from the entire readings.

Once you have exhausted the question potential for the chapter title, move on to the chapter objectives. Use the same process here. Rephrase the objectives as questions and try to answer them. Remember that the purpose of rehearsal is to reinforce what you have learned and to identify areas where you need to spend additional time (focused review).

Go to the Key Terms. Cover the definitions, and try to define each term in your own words. You can also cover the term, and on the basis of the definition, name the term. Do not just memorize the definition because you may find the information presented differently on an examination and then be unable to respond.

Now proceed to the chapter or assigned pages. The chapter headings are the main tools for rehearsal. Apply the same question-and-answer technique used for the title and objectives to test what you may already know about the chapter content. Turn the headings into questions and answer them. Look at the text for boldfaced and italicized items, lists, and other text conventions. These too can become the basis for questions. The tables and figures should also be used for this purpose. Keep in mind the importance of asking both literal and interpretive questions. Some of the questions you ask yourself should also tie different topic headings together. Ask yourself how topic A relates to topic B.

As you proceed through the chapter, do not worry if you cannot answer the questions you ask. As stated earlier, one of the goals of the rehearsal process is to

identify what you need to spend more time on. If you cannot respond to a particular question, put

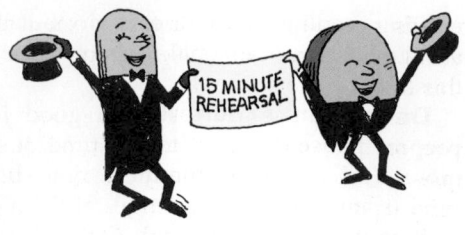

a mark in the margin at that place in the text to remind yourself to come back and spend more time on that material, but then move on. Rehearsal should be a relatively quick procedure. Once you become accustomed to the PURR method, it should take no more than 15 or 20 minutes to rehearse 15 pages after doing the *prepare* and *understand* steps.

As you reach the end of the chapter, skim the Implementation and Evaluation sections. Make sure that the relationship between these sections and the information in the rest of the chapter is clear. If you have questions or concerns, note them in the margins and ask your instructor to clarify those points. Although the objective is to master the chapter content as an independent learner, sometimes it is essential to ask questions of the instructor to facilitate the process.

When to Rehearse. Ideally, rehearsal should take place almost immediately after you finish reading the material. This enables you to complement the prepare and understand steps immediately while the material is still fresh in your mind. Take a 10- to 15-minute break, and then start the process. The longer the gap between reading and rehearsal, the more you will forget and the longer it will take to rehearse. If you are dividing the required readings into smaller segments, do the rehearsal for each segment before you begin reading the new material. This helps maintain the sense of continuity in the chapter. This may seem like a lot of work to do in a study session, but with practice, it will go quickly and you will be pleasantly surprised at the quality and quantity of your learning.

Review

Review is the fourth and final step in the PURR process, and it is an essential one. No matter how well you have learned material in the preceding steps, forgetting will always occur. Reviewing is the only way to store what you have learned in long-term memory. The good news is that, using the PURR model, you can review small segments of material and can do so relatively quickly.

How to Review. The basic review process is essentially the same as the rehearsal process, with some limited rereading as the only difference. When you cannot immediately answer a question, read the pertinent material again. *This does not mean you should read the entire chapter again.* Often, the answer to the question will pop into your mind after you have read only a few lines. When this happens, stop reading and go back to responding to your question. The idea is to reread only as much material as you need to make the answer clear. One or two words or one or two sentences may trigger personal recall, but it may also take two or three paragraphs for this to happen.

Frequency of Review. How many times should you review material in this way? The answer to this question depends on many factors, such as the difficulty of the material, the length of the required reading, and your own background. Only you can determine how often you need to review, but some guidelines will help you decide.

First, consider the difficulty of the material. If it is complex, contains many new terms and difficult concepts, and seems difficult to grasp, then you should review frequently. On the other hand, if the material is straightforward and you are able to relate it well to what you have already learned, then less frequent reviews will serve to keep the material in your memory. Second, consider how well the review went. If you had difficulty answering many questions to your satisfaction or had to do a lot of rereading, you should schedule another review soon (a day or two later at most).

Use the success of each review session to help you determine when to schedule another session. The review step is a means of monitoring the success of the learning process. If reviews go well, with limited need to reread, and you are able to give clear answers to your questions, then you can wait 4 or 5 days before reviewing this material again. A mediocre review, with more extensive rereading and poor answers, indicates that you should let only 2 or 3 days go by before reviewing the material again. And if the review goes poorly, you should plan to review the material again the next day. It is up to you to judge the success of each review and to decide how often you need to review. The nice thing about PURR is that it enables you to monitor your success and easily regulate the learning process.

Technique for Rehearsal and Review. Both rehearsal and review foster active learning, which helps you maintain interest in the material and strengthens your memory. For these benefits to occur, it is essential to review and rehearse orally. Simply talk aloud as you go through the material. Ask questions and give your answers out loud. This forces you to think about the material and helps you organize it and translate it into your own words. The object is not to memorize everything you have read but to understand and be able to explain it. Eventually you will need to answer questions on an examination. Framing questions as a part of the learning process is a way to anticipate examination questions. The more questions you ask yourself during study time, the more likely it is that some of the questions on the examination will be ones you have asked yourself. Furthermore, by rehearsing and reviewing orally, you will find it easier to recall the answers during the examination because you will actually be able to hear the rehearsed answers in your mind. Another advantage of rehearsing and reviewing orally is, as stated earlier, that it helps to identify what needs further

study. When your oral answer is fragmentary, contains many "uhs," and is disorganized, then you know you need to devote more time to learning that particular term, fact, or concept.

The PURR system may seem like a lot of work at first. Understandably, the idea of going through a chapter four times seems daunting. Add to this the need for several review sessions, and your first reaction might be, "This won't work" or "I don't have the time to do this." Don't take that attitude. This system does work. It cultivates interest, aids concentration, fosters mastery of the material, and ensures long-term retention, which is important not just for doing well on examinations but also for doing well as a nurse—the safe care of patients is at stake. The PURR system will work if you use it. It may take 3 or 4 weeks to get comfortable with it, but if you keep at it, pretty soon it will become a good habit. After a while, you will not be able to imagine studying in any other way.

Like all study systems, the PURR method is a model. It seems linear—P-U-R-R—but remember that it can be modified. The PURR method provides you with a starting framework for taking an active role in your study techniques. As you use it, you may discover ways of changing it that work better for you. That is great! Do not hesitate to make adjustments that better suit your learning style and strategies. Just remember as you start out that *preparation*, *understanding*, *rehearsal*, and *review* are solid learning principles and cannot be ignored.

Study skills tips are included on the two pages at the beginning of each part of this book. These hints are directly applied to the content found within the chapters in that part. Detailed information on specialized study skills—such as time management, note taking, examination preparation, and vocabulary building—can be found in the *Study Guide* that accompanies this text.

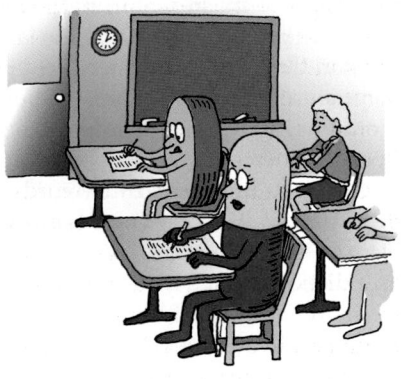

PHARMACOLOGY BASICS

Prepare

As you begin to work with individual chapters, consider how the first step in the PURR system can be used to help you set a purpose and become an active learner.

Chapter 1 Objectives

Consider Objective 1: "List the five phases of the nursing process." Now turn the objective into a question: What are the five phases of the nursing process?

Now move to Objective 2: "Identify the components of the assessment process for patients receiving medications, including the collection and analysis of subjective and objective data." Make it a question: What are the components of the assessment process for patients receiving medications, including the collection and analysis of subjective and objective data? You might recognize that this second question relates to Objective 1 because assessment is one phase of the nursing process. By putting Objective 2 into a question format, you expand on the focus of the first objective, and you start to focus on active learning with a clear purpose.

When you begin to read Chapter 1, you will discover that the five phases of the nursing process are repeated as topic headings—ASSESSMENT; NURSING DIAGNOSES—and you have the Objective 2 question on which to focus your reading. There are subheadings to guide you—ANALYSIS OF DATA. Begin now to develop the habit of applying this strategy to the objectives in every chapter assigned before you start to read. Remember to look at the chapter headings at this point as well. It is amazing how much you can learn by using the text structures provided.

Vocabulary Development

Turn to Chapter 2. Objective 1 makes an important point: "Define common terms used in pharmacology." Success depends heavily on knowledge of the terminology used in the field. The objective makes it clear that this chapter contains a number of terms that the author views as important to master. Starting particularly with Chapter 2, it is time to start mastering the language of this content. Look at the key terms. There are six terms that share the common element *pharmaco*. Although each of these six words has a different meaning, they all have something in common. *Pharmaco* is an example of a group word. No matter what prefixes, group words, or suffixes are added to it, part of the meaning of any word containing *pharmaco* will be "drug" or "medicine." Look up *pharmaco* in any dictionary and you will find "drug" or "medicine" as the definition. Although you probably already knew that, it is always beneficial when working on a new technique to start with something familiar. Look at four of the words that begin with *pharmaco*, and consider the final parts of the words:

dynamics   genetics   gnosy   kinetics

What do each of these word parts mean? The meaning of *pharmacodynamics* is simply the combination of the meaning of *pharmaco* and *dynamics*. The definition in the Key Terms begins, "The study of the biochemical and physiological interactions of drugs at their sites of

activity." You could simply memorize this definition, which would seem to accomplish

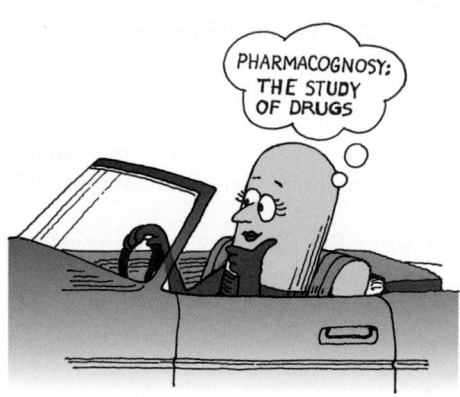

Objective 1. However, memorization does not always equal understanding. Try another approach. What does *dynamics* mean? Think about the word, and relate it to your own experience and background. It appears to deal with movement or action. After looking it up in the dictionary, all the meanings given seem to relate in some fashion to the idea of motion or action. A simplistic definition of *pharmacodynamics* would be "drugs in action." Certainly, this is not a technical or medical definition, but it contributes a great deal to an understanding of the definition provided in the Key Terms. This is the object of learning vocabulary. Do not memorize words without understanding. Apply a little thought, and relate the term and definition in a way that makes the meaning personal for you. When you do that, you will find that you understand the Key Terms definition better, and your ability to retain the meaning will be significantly improved. This means that the test item that asks you to select the definition for *pharmacodynamics* from a list of similar definitions will be much easier because you will remember action and movement and look for the choice that best represents that concept.

Apply this same strategy to *genetics*. You already know what genetics means. Now you must determine how to connect that to the meaning in the text. After you have the definitions of *gnosy* and *kinetics*, you can apply the same procedure. When you have done this with all four words, you will discover that you will not need to spend a lot of time trying to memorize esoteric definitions; you will have personalized the meanings. Those meanings will stay with you much more readily than those learned by rote memorization. And, by the way, do you know what *biochemical* and *physiological* mean? These terms are used in the Key Terms definition of *pharmacodynamics*. You need to know what they mean to fully understand the term *pharmacodynamics*.

Nursing Practice in Canada and Drug Therapy

Objectives

After reading this chapter, the successful student will be able to do the following:

1. List the five phases of the nursing process.
2. Identify the components of the assessment process for patients receiving medications, including the collection and analysis of subjective and objective data.
3. Discuss the process of formulating nursing diagnoses for patients receiving medications.
4. Identify goals and outcome criteria for patients receiving medications.
5. Discuss the evaluation process involved in the administration of medications and reflected in the goals and outcome criteria.
6. Develop a collaborative plan of care using the nursing process and the principles of medication administration.
7. List and briefly discuss the Ten Rights associated with safe medication administration.
8. Discuss the professional responsibility and standards of practice for the professional nurse as related to the medication administration process.

e-Learning Activities

Website
(http://evolve.elsevier.com/Canada/
Lilley/pharmacology/)

evolve

- Answer Key—Textbook Case Studies
- Answer Key—Critical Thinking Activities
- Chapter Summaries—Printable
- Review Questions for Exam Preparation
- Unfolding Case Studies

Key Terms

Adherence Active, voluntary, and collaborative involvement of the patient in the mutually acceptable prescribed course of treatment or therapeutic plan. (p. 10)

Critical thinking The ability to reason and think rationally in order to understand, solve problems, and make decisions; a major component of the nursing process, often considered the foundation on which to provide the best possible patient care, supported by current best evidence. (p. 8)

Goals Statements that are time-specific and describe generally what must be accomplished to address a specific nursing diagnosis. (p. 8)

Medication error Any preventable adverse drug event involving inappropriate medication use by a patient or health care provider. (p. 18)

Nonadherence An informed decision by a patient not to adhere to or follow a therapeutic plan or suggestion. (p. 11)

Nursing process An organizational framework for the practice of nursing that encompasses all steps taken by the nurse in caring for a patient: assessment, nursing diagnoses, planning (with goals and outcome criteria), implementation of the plan (with patient teaching), and evaluation. (p. 8)

Outcome criteria Descriptions of specific patient behaviours or responses that demonstrate the meeting or achievement of goals related to each nursing diagnosis. (p. 13)

Prescriber Any health care provider licensed by the appropriate regulatory body to prescribe medications. (p. 10)

OVERVIEW

The nursing practice environment in Canada is increasingly demanding, due in part to the increased acuity and complexity of patient care and the aging population. Nurses are expected to keep up to date with the rising use of intricate pharmacological therapies, including natural health products and over-the-counter drugs. In addition to rising costs, other factors such as professional shortages, advances in treatment modalities, and new technologies continue to challenge the health care system. In such an environment, knowledge of drugs, their adverse effects, and interactions is crucial for nurses to provide safe, ethical, competent care. Nurses are expected to be more accountable, with increased attention focused on safe medication practices. Evaluating and promoting therapeutic effects, as well as reducing the harm associated with adverse effects, adverse interactions, and drug toxicity, and making decisions about prn (*pro re nata* or "as needed") medications require excellent critical thinking and decision-making skills.

The **nursing process** is a well-established, research-supported framework for professional nursing practice. It is a flexible, adaptable, and adjustable five-step process consisting of assessment, nursing diagnoses, planning (including establishment of **goals** and outcome criteria), implementation (including patient education), and evaluation. As such, the nursing process ensures the delivery of thorough, individualized, and quality nursing care to patients. Through use of the nursing process combined with knowledge and skills, the professional nurse is able to develop effective solutions to meet patients' needs. The use of the nursing process is one way to organize nursing care and may be viewed as controversial in some educational and health care institutions that use other decision-making frameworks. Some view the nursing process as a repetitive tool developed prior to the technology era that may assist in developing an initial plan of care but is limited in assisting to make the detailed judgements and decision making required today. Others view it as the foundation of problem solving and believe it fits well with evidence-informed practice. However, it is still considered the major systematic framework for professional nursing practice.

Usually, the nursing process is discussed within nursing courses and in textbooks on the fundamentals of nursing practice, nursing theory, physical assessment, adult and pediatric nursing, and other nursing specialty areas. Because the nursing process is so important in the care of patients, the process in all of its five phases, along with evidence-informed practice examples, will be included in each chapter of this book as they relate to specific drug groups and classifications.

Critical thinking is one part of the nursing process and is often considered the foundation on which to provide the best possible patient care, supported by current best practice. *Clinical reasoning*, a more specific term, and *clinical judgement*, are key components of critical thinking in nursing. Clinical reasoning refers to the ways nurses analyze and understand patient care issues such as determining, preventing, and managing patient problems. A nurse who is proficient at clinical reasoning will be able to make timely and effective patient-centred decisions. Sound clinical reasoning is essential for preserving the standards of the nursing profession and promoting good patient outcomes. Clinical reasoning involves applying ideas to experience in order to arrive at a valid clinical judgement.

The elements of the nursing process address the physical, emotional, spiritual, sexual, financial, cultural, and cognitive aspects of a patient. Attention to these many aspects allows a more holistic approach to patient care. For example, a cardiologist may focus on cardiac functioning and pathology, a physiotherapist on movement, and a chaplain on the spiritual aspects of patient care. However, it is the professional nurse who thinks critically about processes and incorporates all of these aspects and points of information about the patient and then uses this information to develop and coordinate patient care. Therefore, the nursing process remains a central process and framework for nursing care. Box 1-1 provides guidelines for nursing care planning related to drug therapy and the nursing process.

ASSESSMENT

During the initial assessment phase of the nursing process, data are collected, reviewed, and analyzed. Performing a comprehensive assessment allows the nurse to formulate a nursing diagnosis related to the patient's needs—for the purposes of this textbook, specifically needs related to pharmacotherapy, of which one aspect is drug administration. Information about the patient may come from a variety of sources, including the patient; the patient's family, caregiver, or significant other; and the patient's chart. Methods of data collection include interviewing, direct and indirect questioning, observation, medical records review, head-to-toe physical examination, and nursing assessment. Data are categorized into objective and subjective data.

Subjective data include information obtained through a nursing history and shared through the spoken word

BOX 1-1	Guidelines for Nursing Care Planning

This sample presents useful information for developing a nursing process–focused care plan for patients receiving medications. Brief listings and discussions of what must be contained in each phase of the nursing process are included. This sample may be used as a template for formatting nursing care plans in a variety of patient care situations or settings.

Assessment

Subjective Data

Subjective data include all spoken information shared by the patient as part of taking a nursing history, such as concerns, problems, or stated needs (e.g., patient reports "dizziness, headache, vomiting, and feeling hot for 10 days").

Objective Data

Objective data include information available through the senses, such as what is seen, felt, heard, and smelled. Among the sources of data are the chart, laboratory test results, reports of diagnostic procedures, physical assessment results, and examination findings. Examples of specific data are age, height, weight, allergies, medication profile, and health history.

Nursing Diagnoses

Once the assessment phase has been completed, the nurse analyzes subjective and objective data about the patient and the drug and formulates nursing diagnoses. The following is an example of a nursing diagnosis statement: "Deficient knowledge related to lack of experience with medication regimen and Grade 2 reading level as an adult, as evidenced by inability to perform a return demonstration and inability to state adverse effects to report to the prescriber." This statement of the nursing diagnosis can be broken down into three parts, as follows:

- Part 1: "Deficient knowledge." This is the statement of the human response of the patient to illness, injury, medications, or significant change. This can be an actual response, an increased risk, or an opportunity to improve the patient's health status. The nursing diagnosis related to knowledge may be identified as either deficient or ready for enhanced (knowledge).
- Part 2: "Related to lack of experience with medication regimen and Grade 2 reading level as an adult." This portion of the statement identifies factors related to the response; it often includes multiple factors with some degree of connection between them. The nursing diagnosis statement does not necessarily claim that there is a cause-and-effect link between these factors and the response, only that there is a connection.
- Part 3: "As evidenced by inability to perform a return demonstration and inability to state adverse

effects to report to the prescriber." This statement lists clues, cues, evidence, or data that support the nurse's claim that the nursing diagnosis is accurate.

Nursing diagnoses are prioritized in order of criticality, based on patient needs or problems. The ABCs of care (airway, breathing, and circulation) are often used as a basis for prioritization. Prioritizing always begins with the most important, significant, or critical need of the patient. Nursing diagnoses that involve actual responses are always ranked above nursing diagnoses that involve only risks.

Planning: Goals and Expected Patient Outcome Criteria

The planning phase includes the identification of short-term and long-term goals and outcome criteria, provides time frames, and is patient oriented. Goals are objective, realistic, and measurable patient-centred statements with time frames, and are broad, whereas outcome criteria are more specific descriptions of patient goals.

Implementation

In the implementation phase, the nurse intervenes on behalf of the patient to address specific patient problems and needs. This is done through independent nursing actions; collaborative activities such as physiotherapy, occupational therapy, and music therapy; and implementation of medical orders. Family, significant others, and caregivers assist in carrying out this phase of the nursing care plan. Specific interventions that relate to particular drugs (e.g., giving a particular cardiac drug only after monitoring the patient's pulse and blood pressure), nonpharmacological interventions that enhance the therapeutic effects of medications, and patient education are major components of the implementation phase. See the previous text discussion of the nursing process for more information on nursing interventions.

Evaluation

Evaluation is the part of the nursing process that includes monitoring whether patient goals and outcome criteria related to the nursing diagnoses are met. Monitoring includes observing for therapeutic effects of drug treatment as well as for adverse effects and toxicity. Many indicators are used to monitor these aspects of drug therapy as well as the results of appropriately related nonpharmacological interventions. If the goals and outcome criteria are met, the nursing care plan may or may not be revised to include new nursing diagnoses; such changes are made only if appropriate. If goals and outcome criteria are not met, revisions are made to the entire nursing care plan with further evaluation.

by any reliable source, such as the patient, spouse, family member, significant other, or caregiver.

Objective data may be defined as any information gathered through the senses or that which is seen, heard, felt, or smelled. Objective data may also be obtained from a nursing physical assessment; past and present medical history; results of laboratory tests, diagnostic studies, or procedures; measurement of vital signs, weight, and height; and medication profile. Medication profiles include, but are not limited to, the following information: any and all drug use; use of home or folk remedies and natural health products or homeopathic treatments; intake of alcohol, tobacco, and caffeine; current or past history of illicit drug use; use of over-the-counter (OTC) medications (e.g., aspirin, acetaminophen, vitamins, laxatives, cold preparations, sinus medications, antacids, acid reducers, antidiarrheals, minerals, chemical elements); use of hormonal drugs (e.g., testosterone, estrogens, progestins, oral contraceptives); past and present health history and associated drug regimen(s); family history and racial, ethnic, or cultural attributes with attention to specific or different responses to medications as well as any unusual individual responses; and growth and developmental stage (e.g., Erikson's developmental tasks) and issues related to the patient's age and medication regimen. A holistic nursing assessment includes gathering of data about the whole individual, including physical and emotional realms, religious preference, health beliefs, sociocultural characteristics, race, ethnicity, lifestyle, stressors, socioeconomic status, education level, motor skills, cognitive ability, support systems, lifestyle, and use of any complementary and alternative therapies.

Assessment related to specific drugs is also important and involves the collection of specific information about prescribed, OTC, and natural health products or complementary and alternative therapeutic drug use, with attention to the drug's actions; signs and symptoms of allergic reaction; adverse effects; dosages and routes of administration; contraindications; drug incompatibilities; drug–drug, drug–food, and drug–laboratory test interactions; and toxicities and available antidotes. Nursing pharmacology textbooks provide a more nursing-specific knowledge base regarding drug therapy as related to the nursing process. Use of current references or those dated within the last 3 years is highly recommended. Examples of authoritative resources include the *Compendium of Pharmaceuticals and Specialties* (*CPS*; a subscription-based e-CPS is also available online), the drug manufacturer's insert, drug handbooks, and a licensed pharmacist. Some reliable online resources include Health Canada's Drug Product Database (http://www.hc-sc.gc.ca/dhp-mps/prodpharma/databasdon/index-eng.php), Objective Comparisons for Optimal Drug Therapy (http://www.rxfiles.ca/), and WebMD (http://www.WebMD.com). Other online resources are cited throughout this textbook.

Gather additional data about the patient and a given drug by asking yourself these simple questions: What is the patient's oral intake? Tolerance of fluids? Swallowing ability for pills, tablets, capsules, and liquids? If there is difficulty swallowing, what is the degree of difficulty and are there solutions to the problem, such as the use of thickening agents with fluids or the use of other dosage forms? What are the results of laboratory and other diagnostic tests related to organ functioning and drug therapy? What do kidney function studies (e.g., urea nitrogen, creatinine) show? What are the results of liver function tests (e.g., total protein, bilirubin, alkaline phosphatase, creatinine phosphokinase, other liver enzymes)? What are the patient's white blood cell and red blood cell counts? Hemoglobin and hematocrit levels? Current as well as past health status and presence of illness? What are the patient's experiences with use of any drug regimen? What has been the patient's relationship with health care providers or experiences with previous therapeutic regimens? What are current and past values for blood pressure, pulse rate, temperature, and respiratory rate? What medications is the patient currently taking, and how is the patient taking and tolerating them? Are there issues with **adherence** (implying collaboration and an active role between patients and their health care providers)? Has there been any use of traditional or folk medicines or remedies? What is the patient's understanding of the medication? Are there any age-related concerns? If patients are not reliable historians, family members, significant others, or caregivers may provide answers to these questions.

Once assessment of the patient and the drug has been completed, the specific prescription or medication order (from any **prescriber**) must be checked for the following six elements: (1) patient's name, (2) date the drug order was written, (3) name of drug(s), (4) drug dosage amount and frequency, (5) route of administration, and (6) prescriber's signature.

It is also important during the assessment to consider the traditional, nontraditional, expanded, and collaborative roles of the nurse. Physicians and dentists are no longer the only practitioners legally able to prescribe and write medication orders. Registered nurses do not order medications; they follow standard orders established by physicians. In some cases, depending on agency and provincial or territorial regulatory body, registered nurses can administer medications without a physician's order (e.g., registered nurses with an additional "certified practice"), according to agency-specific protocols, such as pyrexia protocols or bowel protocols, or certain classifications of drugs.

More recently, in some provinces (Ontario, British Columbia, and Alberta), the scope of practice for registered nurses was expanded to allow nurses the authority to dispense certain medications under certain circumstances. Dispensing involves preparing and transferring a medication for a patient or the patient's representative to be administered at a later date, for example, if a patient has a day pass and requires medication while absent or if a client is discharged from the emergency department and requires medication to be started. Dispensing entails ensuring that the medication is

CASE STUDY

The Nursing Process and Pharmacology

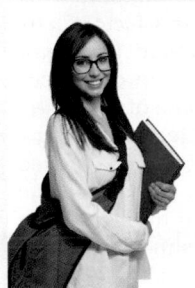

Katie, a 27-year-old teacher, is visiting the clinic today for a physical examination. She states that she and her husband want to "start a family," but she has not had a physical for several years. She was told when she was 22 years of age that she had "anemia" and was given iron tablets but states that she has not taken them for years. She said she "felt better" and did not think she needed them. She denies any use of tobacco or illegal drugs; she states that she may have a drink with dinner once or twice a month. She uses tea tree oil on her face twice a day to reduce acne breakouts. She denies using any other drugs.

1. During the physical assessment, what other questions does the nurse need to ask?
2. After laboratory work is performed, Katie is told she is slightly anemic. The prescriber recommends that she resume taking iron supplements as well as take folic acid. She is willing to try again and says that she is "all about doing what's right to stay healthy and become a mother." What nursing diagnoses would be appropriate at this time?
3. Katie is given a prescription that reads as follows: "ferrous fumarate 300 mg, PO for anemia." When she goes to the pharmacy, the pharmacist tells her that the prescription is incomplete. What is missing? What should be done?
4. After 4 weeks, Katie's latest laboratory results indicate that she still has anemia. However, Katie states, "I feel so much better that I'm planning to stop taking the iron tablets. I hate to take medicine." How should the nurse handle this?

_____

For answers, see http://evolve.elsevier.com/Canada/Lilley/pharmacology/

---

pharmaceutically and therapeutically appropriate for the intended use and that it will be used properly. It may also include accepting payment for a medication on behalf of a nurse's employer.

Nurse practitioners and physician assistants have the professional privilege of legally prescribing medications. As of 2016, there are 400 physician assistants (PAs) in Canada who support physicians in a variety of health care settings. The role for PAs began in Canada within the Canadian Forces Health Services 50 years ago, and physician assistants now practise in Manitoba, New Brunswick, Ontario and Alberta. Physician assistants are meant to extend the role of the physician; they work under the supervision of physicians and are not independent practitioners. PAs are regulated in Manitoba and New Brunswick through their respective College of Physicians and Surgeons; in Ontario, and Alberta, PAs practise by delegation under the _Medicine Act_ and the _Medical Act_, respectively. PAs are autonomous decision makers and perform a range of diagnostic and therapeutic services, including writing prescriptions. PAs must complete a two-year educational program that is accredited by the Canadian Medical Association (2015). Nurse practitioners (NPs) are registered nurses with an advanced degree who practise in the Extended Class. They have extra education and experience and are legally competent to diagnose, order and interpret diagnostic tests, prescribe medications, and perform procedures.

Analysis of Data

Once data about the patient and drug have been collected and reviewed, critically analyze and synthesize the information. Verify all information and document appropriately. It is at this point that the sum of the information about the patient and drug is used in the development of nursing diagnoses.

NURSING DIAGNOSES

Nursing diagnoses are developed by professional nurses and are used as a means of communicating and sharing information about the patient and the patient experience. Nursing diagnoses are the result of critical thinking, creativity, and analysis of the data collected about the patient and the drug. It is a clinical judgement about how a person responds to health conditions and life processes or vulnerability for that response. Nursing diagnoses related to drug therapy will most likely develop out of data associated with the following: deficient knowledge; risk of injury; **nonadherence**; various disturbances, deficits, excesses, or impairments in bodily functions; and other problems or concerns as related to drug therapy. The development and classification of nursing diagnoses has been carried out by the North American Nursing Diagnosis Association International (NANDA-I) (formerly NANDA). NANDA-I is the formal organization recognized by professional nursing groups (e.g., the Canadian Nurses Association [CNA] and the American Nurses Association) (NANDA International, 2014). NANDA-I is considered the major contributor to the development of nursing knowledge and the leading authority in the development and classification of nursing diagnoses. The purpose of NANDA-I is to increase the visibility of nursing's contribution to the care of patients and to further develop, refine, and classify the information and phenomena related to nurses and professional nursing practice. The use of a standardized language of nursing diagnoses documents the analysis, synthesis,

BOX 1-2 A Brief Look at NANDA and the Nursing Process

The North American Nursing Diagnosis Association International (NANDA-I) (formerly NANDA) fulfills the following roles: (1) increases the visibility of nursing's contribution to patient care, (2) develops, refines, and classifies information and phenomena related to professional nursing practice, (3) provides a working organization for the development of evidence-informed nursing diagnoses, and (4) supports the improvement of quality nursing care through evidence-informed practice and access to a global network of professional nurses. In 1987, NANDA and the American Nurses Association endorsed a framework for establishing nursing diagnoses, and in 1990, *Nursing Diagnoses* became the official journal of NANDA. In 2001 and 2003, NANDA modified and updated the listing of nursing diagnoses, but nursing diagnoses continued to be submitted for consideration by the ad hoc research committee of NANDA. This period resulted in changes such as replacement of the phrase *potential for* with *risk for*. The terms *impaired, deficient, ineffective, decreased, increased,* and *imbalanced* replaced the outdated terms *altered* and *alteration,* although the outdated terms may still be in use. In 2002, NANDA changed its name to NANDA-I ("I" for international) to reflect the organization's global reach. Every 2 years revisions are made to the nursing diagnoses, adding new and revised nursing diagnoses as well as retiring outdated ones. Most current is the *Nursing Diagnoses 2015–2017: Definitions and Classifications*, which provides more "linguistically

congruent diagnoses" (Herdman & Kamitsuru, 2014). The guide includes a total of 235 diagnoses supported by definitions, defining characteristics, related factors, and risk factors. There are 26 new diagnoses and 13 revised diagnosed based on global evidence. Seven diagnoses were removed. Changes were made to some of the definitions of nursing diagnoses, which impacted the risk and health promotion diagnoses. The word *risk* was removed from "risk" diagnoses and replaced with *vulnerable*; the health promotion diagnoses were altered to ensure that they are suitable for use across the health–illness continuum. Defining characteristics also were altered. There are 13 domains (spheres of knowledge) of diagnoses that are further divided into 47 classes (groupings that share common attributes). The new diagnoses include 14 risk diagnoses, one health promotion diagnosis, and 11 problem-focused diagnoses, in the area of: (1) cardiovascular function; (2) elimination; (3) emancipated decision making; (4) frailty in the elderly; (5) mobility; (6) mood and emotional regulation; (7) nutrition; (8) pain; (9) skin/tissue/mucous membrane function; (10) surgical recovery; and (11) thermoregulation. These domains are further divided into classes.

Herdman, T.H., & Kamitsuru, S. (Eds.) Nursing Diagnoses—Definitions and Classification 2015–2017. Copyright © 2014, 1994–2014 by NANDA International Inc. Used by arrangement with John Wiley & Sons Limited.

and accuracy required in making a nursing diagnosis and establishes nursing's contribution to cost-effective, efficient, quality health care. See Box 1-2 for more information about the 2015–2017 NANDA-I–approved nursing diagnoses.

More recently, a long-term project of the International Council of Nurses (ICN) to provide a unified language system was initiated. The International Classification for Nursing Practice (ICNP) is a framework that can be cross-mapped with other health care classification systems such as NANDA to create multidisciplinary health vocabularies or lexicons within information systems (ICN, 2014). The overall intent is that nursing diagnoses, nursing interventions, and nursing outcomes within the ICNP would be used in health care record documentation. The CNA has endorsed the ICNP as the standard for collecting nursing data. The objectives of the ICNP are as follows: (1) to establish a common language for describing nursing practice in order to improve communication among nurses and between nurses and others; (2) to describe the nursing care of people (individuals, families, and communities) in a variety of settings, both institutional and noninstitutional; (3) to enable comparison of nursing data across clinical populations, settings, geographic areas, and time; (4) to demonstrate or project trends in the provision of nursing treatments and care and the allocation of resources to patients according to

their needs based on nursing diagnoses; (5) to stimulate nursing research through links to data available in nursing information systems and health information systems; and (6) to provide data about nursing practice in order to influence health policymaking. "ICNP seeks to cover nursing diagnoses (which may also be used to represent nursing outcomes) and nursing interventions in entirety, accepting that this is a formative process and that nursing covers a broad range of health care and is not a clearly bounded discipline" (ICNP, 2013). There is a disparity in opinion across Canada about whether NANDA diagnoses, patient problems (actual or potential), nursing priorities, diagnostic reasoning, or clinical impression identification is the better approach.

Formulation of nursing diagnoses is usually a three-step process, with nursing diagnoses stated as follows: Part I of the statement is the human response of the patient to illness, injury, or significant change. This response can be an actual problem, an increased risk of developing a problem, or an opportunity or intent to increase the patient's health. Part II of the nursing diagnosis statement identifies the factor(s) related to the response, with more than one factor often named. The nursing diagnosis statement does not necessarily claim a cause-and-effect link between these factors and the response; it indicates only that there is a connection between them. Part III of the nursing diagnosis statement contains a listing of clues, cues, evidence, or other data that support the nurse's claim that this diagnosis is accurate. Tips for writing a nursing diagnosis include the following: begin with a statement of a human response; connect Part I of the statement or the human response with Part II—the cause—using the phrase *related to*; ensure that Parts I and II are not restatements of one another; include several factors in Part II of the statement, such as associated factors, if appropriate; select a cause for Part II of the statement that can be changed by nursing interventions; avoid negative wording or language; and, finally, list clues or cues that led to the nursing diagnosis in Part III of the statement, which may also include more defining characteristics (e.g., "as evidenced by").

The diagnoses most relevant to drug therapy will be used in this textbook. These nursing diagnoses, as well as all other phases of the nursing process, will be presented in the chapters to follow because of the framework of practice that the nursing process provides to all professional nurses; they are also used to organize the nursing sections of this textbook.

PLANNING

After data are collected and nursing diagnoses formulated, the planning phase begins; this phase includes identification of goals and outcome criteria. The major purposes of the planning phase are to prioritize the nursing diagnoses and specify goals and outcome criteria, including the time frame for their achievement. The planning phase provides time to obtain special equipment for interventions, review the possible procedures or techniques to be used, and gather information either for oneself (the nurse) or for the patient. This step leads to the provision of safe care if professional judgement is combined with the acquisition of knowledge about the patient and the medications to be given.

Goals and Expected Patient Outcome Criteria

Goals are objective, measurable, and realistic, with an established time period for achievement of the outcomes, which are specifically stated in the outcome criteria. Patient goals reflect expected and measurable changes in behaviour through nursing care and are developed in collaboration with the patient. Patient goals developed in the planning phase of the nursing process are behaviour based and may be categorized into physiological, psychological, spiritual, sexual, cognitive, motor, or other domains.

Outcome criteria are concrete descriptions of patient goals. They are patient focused, succinct, and well thought out. Outcome criteria also include expectations of behaviour indicating something that can be changed and with a specific time frame or deadline. The ultimate aim of these criteria is the safe and effective administration of medications. Outcome criteria also reflect each nursing diagnosis and serve as a guide to the implementation phase of the nursing process. Formulation of

outcome criteria begins with the analysis of the judgements made about patient data and subsequent nursing diagnoses and ends with the development of a nursing care plan. Outcome criteria provide a standard for measuring movement toward goals. In regard to medication administration, these outcomes may address special storage and handling techniques, administration procedures, equipment needed, drug interactions, adverse effects, and contraindications. In this textbook, specific time frames generally are not provided in each chapter's nursing process section because every patient care situation is individualized.

IMPLEMENTATION

Implementation is guided by the preceding phases of the nursing process (i.e., assessment, nursing diagnoses, and planning). Implementation requires constant communication and collaboration with the patient and members of the health care team involved in the patient's care, as well as any family members, significant other, or other caregivers. Implementation consists of initiation and completion of specific nursing actions by the nurse as defined by nursing diagnoses, goals, and outcome criteria. Nursing interventions or actions may be independent, collaborative, or dependent upon a prescriber's order. Statements of interventions include frequency, specific instructions, and any other pertinent information. With medication administration, the nurse needs to know and understand all of the information about the patient and about each medication prescribed (see assessment questions on p. 10). Implementation is based on the nurse's clinical judgement and knowledge. It also is important for the nurse to recognize that patients differ significantly in their attitude toward taking medications. The principles of informed consent and choice should underpin medication administration. It is critical for the nurse to explain the benefits and risks of a treatment in a way that the patient can grasp. Once patients understand the potential benefits and risks of therapy, they can make meaningful decisions.

Nurses are also advocates for all marginalized patients who face a diversity of issues related to equitable treatment and allocation of resources surrounding medications. Vulnerable and marginalized patients face lack of drug coverage, the inability to pay for prescriptions, and a multitude of other barriers that require health care members to provide facilitation and timely responses.

Nurses must also adhere to safe administration practices to prevent errors. Traditionally, in years past, nurses adhered to the Five Rights of medication administration: right drug, right dose, right time, right route, and right patient. However, these rights have been expanded to Ten Rights (summarized in Box 1-3). The Ten Rights are discussed in detail in the next sections of this chapter. The "rights" of medication administration have been identified as basic standards of care as related to drug therapy.

BOX 1-3 Ten Rights of Medication Administration

1. *Right Drug (or Right Medication):* Ensuring that the drug to be administered is the right medication that was ordered.
2. *Right Dose:* Ensuring that the dose ordered is correct for the patient's age and body parameters, and questioning doses that do not seem correct or are outside the patient's usual dose range.
3. *Right Time:* Ensuring that the drug is administered at the time ordered, at the right frequency, and according to institutional policy.
4. *Right Route:* Ensuring that the drug is administered by the route ordered as well as verifying that the route is safe and appropriate for the patient.
5. *Right Patient:* Ensuring that the drug is being administered to the patient it was intended for, by checking the drug order information against the patient's identification band.
6. *Right Reason:* Ensuring that the drug ordered is being given for the right reason, thus necessitating prior knowledge of the drug's actions and adverse effects.
7. *Right Documentation:* Ensuring that documentation of the medication administration is done after the drug has been administered, not before; moreover, ensuring that any unusual variances in time, dose, and drug reactions are properly recorded, as well as if the patient has refused the drug.
8. *Right Evaluation (or Right Assessment):* Ensuring that any special assessment requirements have been made prior to the drug administration, such as specific pulse rate and blood pressure readings and laboratory results; moreover, ensuring that appropriate monitoring of the patient has been done following drug administration and that follow-up measures are taken if the drug has not achieved its desired effect.
9. *Right Patient Education:* Ensuring that the patient has been given proper explanation of the drug being given, the reason for its administration, and what to expect in terms of the drug's effects and possible adverse effects.
10. *Right to Refuse:* Ensuring that the patient understands his right to refuse the drug being administered and to be informed of the potential consequences of refusal.

Nurses are required to practise under their provincial or territorial regulatory body's standards and agency policy, and these may vary. However, even the implementation of the Ten Rights does not reflect the complexity of the role of the professional nurse because they focus more on the individual patient than on the system as a whole or the entire medication administration process, beginning with the prescriber's order. Viewed from an individual patient focus, additional rights (or entitlements) must be considered when administering medications. These rights include the following:

- Patient safety, ensured by use of the correct procedures, equipment, and techniques of medication administration and documentation
- Individualized, holistic, accurate, and complete patient education
- Double-checking and constant analysis of the system (i.e., the process of drug administration, including all personnel involved, such as the prescriber, the nurse, the nursing unit, and the pharmacy department, as well as patient education)
- Proper drug storage
- Accurate calculation and preparation of the dose of medication and proper use of all types of medication delivery systems
- Careful checking of the transcription of medication orders
- Accurate use of the various routes of administration and awareness of the specific implications of their use
- Close consideration of special situations (e.g., patient difficulty in swallowing, use of a nasogastric tube, unconsciousness of the patient, advanced patient age)
- Implementation of all appropriate measures to prevent and report medication errors

Right Drug

Administration of the right drug begins with the registered nurse's valid licence to practise. Unregulated care providers (UCPs) may also assist with medication administration. Nurses may teach UCPs medication administration and documentation, but the nurse remains ultimately accountable for the process of medication administration. The registered nurse is responsible for checking all medication orders or prescriptions. Prepouring a medication and not administering it at the time of pouring, or having another nurse or student administer it, increases the risk of errors and confuses the line of accountability for the preparation of the medication. It is the nurse's responsibility and best practice to prepare medications as close as possible to the time they are to be administered, watch the patient take the medication, and not allow another individual to administer a medication for the nurse and sign it off. (NOTE: there are rare exceptions to this best practice such as preloading syringes for a mass immunization program or an urgent need for drugs during a cardiac arrest.) To ensure that the correct drug is given, the nurse must check the specific medication order against the medication label or profile three times before giving the medication. Conduct the first check of the right drug, drug name, and drug expiry date while preparing the medication for administration. At this time, consider whether the drug is appropriate for the patient and, if you are in doubt or believe an error is possible, contact the prescriber or pharmacist immediately (see Evidence in Practice Box on this page). Safety huddles are held on most acute care units, often with a pharmacist, to discuss new medications, changes to practice, or ways to manage errors. Usually a pharmacist is assigned to each unit to be available to answer questions. It is also appropriate at this time to note the drug's indication and be aware that a drug may have multiple indications, including off-label use and non–Health Canada-approved indications. In this textbook, each particular drug is discussed in the chapter that deals with its main indication, but those with multiple uses may also be cross-referenced in other chapters.

All medication orders or prescriptions are required by law to be signed by the prescriber involved in the patient's care. If a verbal order is given, the prescriber must sign the order within 24 hours or as per facility protocol. Verbal, telephone, or texting orders are often used in emergencies and time-sensitive patient care situations. Preprinted orders based on current evidence may also be available under certain circumstances. To be sure that the right drug is given, information about the patient and drug (see previous discussion of the assessment phase) must be obtained to make certain that all variables and data have been considered. Approved, current, authoritative references (see earlier discussion) are the reliable sources of information about prescribed drugs. Avoid relying upon the knowledge of peers as this is unsafe nursing practice. Remain current in your knowledge of generic (nonproprietary) drug names as well as trade names (proprietary name that is registered by a specific drug manufacturer); however, in clinical practice, only the drug's generic name is used, to reduce the risk of medication errors. A single drug often has numerous trade names, and drugs in different classes may have similarly spelled names, increasing the possibility of medication errors (see Preventing Medication Errors box). Therefore, when it comes to the "right drug" phase of the medication administration process, use the drug's generic name to help avoid a medication error and enhance patient safety. (See Chapter 2 for more information on the naming of drugs.)

If there are questions about a medication order at any time during the medication administration process, contact the prescriber for clarification. Never make any assumptions when it comes to drug administration, and, as previously emphasized in this chapter, confirm at least

 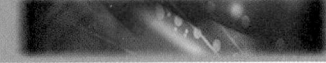

EVIDENCE IN PRACTICE

Patient Safety: Examining the Adequacy of the Five Rights of Medication Administration

Review

Patient safety is of utmost importance in health care today. For decades, the Five Rights (right drug, right patient, right dose, right route, right time) of medication administration have been the standard for safe medication practices; they are taught routinely in educational settings and implemented in practice. More recently, the Five Rights have been found to be lacking because of the focus on individual performance and the failure to include individual factors and system deficiencies. Patients are no longer passive recipients of care and are choosing to play increasingly greater roles in the process of care. As well, there has been a substantial increase in the number of medications available to treat patients and a distinct number of interrelated steps in administering medications.

Type of Evidence

In a Canadian study in 2010, the author critiqued the effectiveness of the Five Rights of medication administration, which had been developed primarily for use by nurses. The author examined the adequacy of the five Rs for nurses and for the increasing patient involvement in the medication administration process, while keeping patient safety in mind.

Results of the Study

The author discussed the impact of compromised medication administration, citing that approximately one in five adverse events occurs in hospitalized Canadian patients at the point of discharge home. Over 65% of these adverse events were medication adverse events and they were estimated to cost $750 million. Older adults are more vulnerable to medication adverse events; 1 in 11 older adults experience a preventable medication-related morbidity.

The author traced the history of the five Rs to a time when nurses were held accountable for any error in drug administration, and patients, families, and caregivers were the recipients of care, not participants in care. The limitations of this approach are discussed, as well as the drawbacks to simply continuing to add more rights. The author offers an ethical model that embraces patient-centred care called the expressive–collaborative model.

Link of Evidence to Nursing Practice

The five Rs are no longer sufficient for safe administration of medication; currently, 10 Rs are used, including a medication history and assessment, interpretation of assessment data, anticipating risks, providing patient education, and planning for evaluation of medication effectiveness as well as observing for potential interactions with other medications, food, or natural health products. Each of these clinical judgement actions requires vigilance and clinical reasoning. Medication administration is a complex, interrelated process involving many players and steps. Collaboration among all players, including the patient, caregiver, and family, is essential to safe, ethical, and competent care.

Source: Macdonald, M. (2010). Patient safety: Examining the adequacy of the 5 rights of medication administration. *Clinical Nurse Specialist, 24*(4), 196–201. doi:10.1097/NUR.0b013e3181e3605f

three times the right drug, right dose, right time, right route, right patient, and right reason—when removing the drug from the patient drawer or cabinet, when pouring the drug, and in many instances at the bedside, with the third check involving an identifier from the patient (this may not be required by all agencies) before giving the medication. You must adhere to the Ten Rights of medication administration according to the provincial or territorial regulatory body under which you are practising. With the increasing use of technology (such as texting, fax, email, cellphones) in health care to make communication between health care providers more "timely" and cost efficient, it is important to caution the nurse about the risks involved. The Information and Privacy Commissioner of Ontario (2009) reminds health care providers that "unauthorized access or disclosure of personal data can occur though loss or theft of a mobile communication device or through unauthorized interception during the wireless transmission of personal data. Without appropriate safeguards, storing personal data on a mobile computing device and transmitting it wirelessly can be like using an open filing cabinet in a waiting room." Recommendations for use of wireless technology include protected security features (e.g., data encryption, password protection, and device swiping). There may be specific agency policies for the transmission of patient information and documentation of the medical information or order transmitted, as well as procedures for the information becoming part of the permanent health record.

Right Dose

Whenever a medication is ordered, a dosage is identified from the prescriber's order. Always check the dose and confirm that it is appropriate to the patient's age and size. Check appropriate laboratory and diagnostic results such as potassium, creatinine, and ammonia levels. Also, check the prescribed dose against the available drug stocks and against the normal dosage range. Recheck all mathematical calculations, and pay careful attention to decimal points, the misplacement of which could lead to a tenfold or even greater overdose. Leading zeros, or zeros placed before a decimal point, are allowed, but in numbers less than 1, trailing zeros, or zeros following the decimal point, are to be avoided. For example, 0.2 mg is allowed but 2.0 milligrams is not acceptable because it

could easily be mistaken for 20 mg, especially with unclear penmanship. Patient variables (e.g., vital signs, age, gender, weight, height) require careful assessment because of the need for dosage adjustments in response to specific parameters. Children and older adult patients are more sensitive to medications than younger and middle-age adult patients; thus, use extra caution with drug dosage amounts for these patients.

Right Time

Each health care agency or institution has a policy regarding routine medication administration times; therefore, always check this policy. However, when giving a medication at the prescribed time, the nurse may be confronted with a conflict between the timing suggested by the physician and specific pharmacokinetic and pharmacodynamic (see Chapter 2) drug properties, concurrent drug therapy, dietary influences, laboratory or diagnostic testing, and specific patient variables. For example, the prescribed right time for administration of antihypertensive drugs may be four times a day, but for an active, professional 42-year-old male patient working 13 to 14 hours a day, taking a medication four times a day may not be feasible, and this regimen may lead to nonadherence and subsequent complications. Appropriate actions include contacting the prescriber and inquiring about the possibility of prescribing another drug with a different dosing frequency (e.g., once or twice daily).

For routine medication orders, nurses have long adhered to medication administration according to the 30-minute rule: no more than 30 minutes before or after the actual time specified in the prescriber's orders (i.e., if a medication is ordered to be given at 0900 hours every morning, the medication may be given anytime between 0830 and 0930 hours). According to the Institute for Safe Medication Practices (ISMP, 2011), such rigid rules lead to nurses taking shortcuts and subsequently making errors. The ISMP points out that "a one-size-fits-all, inflexible requirement to administer all scheduled medications within 30 minutes of the scheduled time is a precarious mandate, given that relatively few medications truly require exact timing of doses." The ISMP has recommended guidelines for the timely administration of drugs (see Box 1-4).

Medications designated to be given stat (immediately) must be administered within 30 minutes of the time the

---

 PREVENTING MEDICATION ERRORS

Right Dose?

The nurse is reviewing the orders for a newly admitted patient. One order reads: "Acetaminophen, 2 tablets PO, every 4 hours as needed for pain or fever."

The pharmacist calls to clarify this order, saying, "The dose is not clear." What does the pharmacist mean by this? The order says "2 tablets." Isn't that the dose?

NO! If you look up acetaminophen in a drug resource book, you will see that acetaminophen tablets are available in strengths of both 325 mg and 500 mg. The order is missing the "right dose" and needs to be clarified. *Never* assume the dose of a medication order.

BOX 1-4	Recommended Guidelines for Timely Administration of Medications

Type of Scheduled Medication	Goals for Timely Administration
Time-Critical Scheduled Medications Facility-defined time-critical medications* Including but not limited to medications with a dosing schedule more frequent than every 4 hours	Administer at the exact time indicated when necessary (e.g., rapid-acting insulin), otherwise within 30 minutes before or after the scheduled time.
Non–Time-Critical Scheduled Medications Daily, weekly, monthly medications	Administer within 2 hours before or after the scheduled time.
Medications prescribed more frequently than daily, but no more frequently than every 4 hours	Administer within 1 hour before or after the scheduled time.

*Limited number of drugs, where delayed or early administration of more than the 30 minutes may cause harm or subtherapeutic effect.
Adapted from Institute for Safe Medication Practices. (2011). "Guidelines for timely medication administration: Response to the CMS '30-minute rule.'" Retrieved from http://www.ismp.org/newsletters/acutecare/articles/20110113.asp. Used with permission from the Institute for Safe Medication Practices.

order is written. Assess and follow the hospital or facility policy and procedure for any other specific information concerning the 30-minutes-before-or-after rule. For medication orders with the annotation prn, the medication must be given at special times and under certain circumstances. For example, for an analgesic ordered every 4 hours prn for pain, after one dose of the medication, the patient reports pain. After assessment, intervention with another dose of analgesic would occur, but only 4 hours after the previous dose. In addition, because of the increasing incidence of medication errors related to the use of abbreviations, many prescribers are using the wording *as required* or *as needed* instead of the abbreviation *prn*. Military time is used when medication and other orders are written into a patient's chart (Figure 1-1).

Nursing judgement may lead to some variations in timing, and the nurse must document any change and the rationale for the change. If medications are ordered to be given once every day, twice daily, three times daily, or even four times daily, the times of administration may be changed if doing so is not harmful to the patient and if the medication or patient's condition does not require adherence to an exact schedule, but only if the change is approved by the prescriber. Never underestimate the effect of a change in the dosing or timing of medication because one missed dose of certain medications can be life threatening. Other factors must be considered in determining the right time, such as multiple-drug therapy, drug–drug or drug–food compatibility, scheduling of diagnostic tests, bioavailability of the drug (e.g., the need for consistent timing of doses around the clock to maintain blood levels), drug actions, and any biorhythm effects such as those that occur with steroids. It is also critical to patient safety to avoid using abbreviations for *any* component of a drug order (i.e., dose, time, and route).

Right Route

As previously stated, the nurse must know the particulars about each medication before administering it to

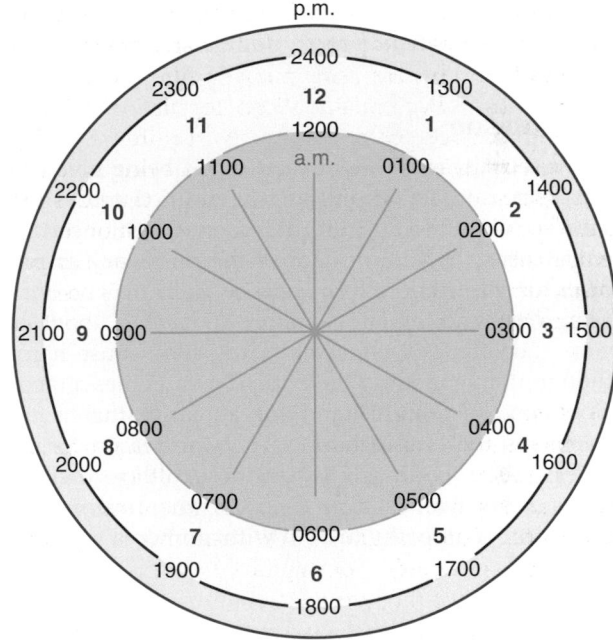

FIG. 1-1   The 24-hour clock. (From Sorrentino, S. A., & Remmert, L. N. (2012). Mosby's textbook for nursing assistants (8th ed., p. 69, Fig. 6-6). St Louis, MO: Mosby.)

ensure that the right drug, dose, and route are being used. A complete medication order includes the route for administration. If a medication order does not include the route, the nurse must ask the prescriber to clarify it. Never assume the route of administration.

Right Patient

Checking the patient's identity before giving each medication dose is critical to the patient's safety. Ask the patient to state his or her own name and then check the patient's identification band to confirm the patient's name, identification number, age, and allergies. With children, the parents or legal guardians are often the ones who identify the patient for the purposes of administration of prescribed medications. With newborns and labour and delivery situations, the mother and baby have identification bracelets with matching numbers, which must be checked before giving medications. With older adults or patients with altered sensorium or level of consciousness, asking them to state their names is neither realistic nor safe. Therefore, checking the identification band against the medication profile, medication order, or other treatment or service orders is crucial to avoid errors. Accreditation Canada (2013) has required organizational practices to improve the quality and safety of health services. One practice is to use at least two identifiers before providing care, treatment, or services to patients. Accreditation Canada identifies that the information obtained must be specific to the patient. Examples include a person-specific identification number such as a registration number; patient identification cards such as the health card with name, address, and date of birth; patient barcodes; double witnessing; or a patient wristband. The two identifiers may be in the same location, such as on a wristband. The patient's room number is not an acceptable identifier.

Right Reason

The nurse must ensure that the drug is being given for the right reason and clarify any medication orders that do not seem to fit within a right reason. When uncertain, always check the CPS or contact the pharmacy or prescriber for clarification. If the nurse administers an unfamiliar drug and remains unknowledgeable about its action and intended effect, the drug may cause harm, although unintended, to the patient. Sometimes a medication may be administered for a reason that is not obvious, as the classification is not the reason for the administration. For example, lactulose, although classified as a laxative, is also used for the treatment of hepatic encephalopathy to bind with ammonia to reduce toxic levels.

Right Documentation

Documentation of information related to medication administration is crucial to patient safety. Recording patient observations and nursing actions has always been an important ethical responsibility, but it has become a major medical–legal consideration as well. Because of its significance in professional nursing practice, correct documentation is becoming known as the "sixth right" of medication administration. Always assess the patient's chart for the presence of the following information: date and time of medication administration, name of medication, dose, route, and site of administration. Documentation of drug action may also be performed in the regularly scheduled assessments for any changes in symptoms the patient is experiencing, adverse effects, toxicity, and any other drug-related, physical or psychological symptoms.

Documentation must also reflect any improvement in the patient's condition, symptoms, or disease process as well as whether there has been no change or a lack of improvement. Not only must you document these observations, but you must also report them to the prescriber promptly, in keeping with your critical thinking and judgement. Document any teaching, as well as an assessment of the degree of understanding exhibited by the patient. Other information that needs documentation includes the following:

1. If a drug is *not* administered, with the reason why and any actions taken
2. Refusal of a medication with information about the reason for refusal, if possible. If a medication is refused, respect the patient's right (to refuse), determine the reason by assessing the patient's knowledge level as it pertains to refusing the drug, and document. Take appropriate action, including notifying the prescriber, and revise the nursing care plan. Never return unwrapped medication to a container, and discard according to agency policy; if wrapper remains intact, return medication to the pharmacy and revise the nursing care plan as needed.
3. Actual time of drug administration
4. Data regarding clinical observations and treatment of the patient if a medication error has occurred.

If there has been a medication error, complete an incident report with the entire event, surrounding circumstances, therapeutic response, adverse effects, and notification of the prescriber described in detail. However, do not record completion of an incident report in the medical chart. Always follow specific individual agency policies/protocols regarding medication errors and incident reporting.

Most provinces and territories are using or are moving to implement electronic health records. The electronic health record (EHR) is a collection of the personal health information of a patient that is stored electronically and kept under strict security. This information is accessible online from many separate, interoperable automated systems within an electronic network. It provides an online profile of a patient's drug prescription history. The system also informs of drug interactions.

Medication Errors

When the "rights" of drug administration are discussed, medication errors must be considered. Medication errors are a major problem for all in health care, regardless of the setting. The National Coordinating Council for Medication Error Reporting and Prevention (2015) defines a **medication error** as "any preventable event that may cause or lead to inappropriate medication use or patient harm while the medication is in the control of the health care professional, patient, or consumer. Such events may be related to professional practice, health care products, procedures, or systems, including prescribing, order communication, product labeling, packaging, and nomenclature, compounding, dispensing, distribution, administration, education, monitoring, and use" (http://www.nccmerp.org/aboutMedErrors.html). Both patient-related and system-related factors must always be considered when the medication administration process and the prevention of medication errors are being examined. See Chapter 6 for further discussion of medication errors and their prevention.

Evaluation

Evaluation occurs after the collaborative plan of care has been implemented. It is a systematic, ongoing, and dynamic part of the nursing process as related to drug therapy. It includes monitoring the fulfillment of goals and outcome criteria, as well as the patient's therapeutic response to the drug and its adverse effects and toxic effects. Documentation is also an important component of evaluation. The move to electronic health records (EHRs) and computer workstations that are located in patient rooms or wherever care is provided enables nurses to document point-of-care and real-time charting. Documentation must be accurate and present a clear and comprehensive picture of the patient's outcome criteria (see Legal and Ethical Principles).

Evaluation also includes monitoring the implementation of standards for nursing practice. Several standards are in place to help in the evaluation of outcomes of care, such as those established by nursing provincial and territorial governing bodies and the Canadian Council on Health Services Accreditation (CCHSA). Within the CCHSA, guidelines are established for nursing services, policies, and procedures. The CNA *Code of Ethics* (2008) and specific provincial/territory medication practice standards are also used in establishing and evaluating standards of care.

In summary, the nursing process is an ongoing and constantly evolving process (see Box 1-1). As it relates to drug therapy, the nursing process is the way in which the nurse gathers, analyzes, organizes, provides, and acts upon data about the patient within the context of prudent nursing care and standards of care. The nurse's ability to conduct astute assessments, formulate sound nursing diagnoses, establish goals and outcome criteria, correctly administer drugs, and continually evaluate patients' responses to drugs increases with additional experience and knowledge.

 LEGAL & ETHICAL PRINCIPLES

Nursing Documentation: Use of Technology

In many agencies, the transition to technology carries compelling implications for the nursing profession and the health care system. With the use of electronic health systems, handwriting is no longer needed, thus producing more legible and comprehensive patient records. Technology can take many forms, for example, computerized records, emails, faxes, texts, cellphones, tablets, and recordings. The use of technology carries a higher risk of breach of confidentiality. Nurses have an ethical responsibility to safeguard information obtained in the nurse–patient relationship. Therefore, certain precautions are required to protect privacy and maintain confidentiality:

- Do not disclose or allow access to any personal identification number or password. These are electronic signatures.
- Select a password that cannot be easily deciphered.
- Log off the system when you are not using it or when leaving the screen, to secure the computer and files.

- Protect patient data shown on screens with the use of a screen saver or "sleep," with the location of the device, or with the use of privacy screens.
- Maintain confidentiality of all electronic data, including print copies of any data.
- Make sure that all discarded print data that contains patient information is shredded.
- Access patient information only if it is essential to provide nursing care for that patient; doing so for purposes other than providing nursing care is a breach of confidentiality.

Source: College of Nurses of Ontario. (2009). Confidentiality and privacy—Personal health information. Retrieved from http://www.cno.org/Global/docs/prac/41069_privacy.pdf; College of Registered Nurses of British Columbia. (2013). Practice standard. Nursing documentation. Retrieved from https://www.crnbc.ca/standards/lists/standardresources/151nursingdocumentation.pdf

KEY POINTS

❖ The nursing process is an ongoing, constantly changing and evolving framework for professional nursing practice. It may be applied to all facets of nursing care, including medication administration.

❖ The phases of the nursing process include assessment; development of nursing diagnoses; planning, with establishment of goals and outcome criteria; implementation, including patient education; and evaluation.

❖ Nursing diagnoses are formulated based on objective and subjective data and help to drive the nursing care plan. Nursing diagnoses have been developed through a formal process, including NANDA-I and the International Classification for Nursing Practice and are constantly updated and revised. Safe, therapeutic, and effective medication administration is a major responsibility of professional nurses as they apply the nursing process to the care of their patients.

Continued

KEY POINTS—cont'd

❖ Nurses are responsible for safe and prudent decision making in the nursing care of their patients, including the provision of drug therapy; in accomplishing this task, they attend to the Ten Rights and adhere to legal and ethical standards related to medication administration and documentation. There are additional rights related to drug administration. These rights deserve worthy consideration before initiation of the medication administration process. Observance of all of these rights enhances patient safety and helps avoid medication errors.

EXAMINATION REVIEW QUESTIONS

1. An 86-year-old patient is being discharged to home on digoxin and has little information regarding the medication. Which statement best reflects a realistic outcome of patient teaching activities?
   a. The patient and patient's daughter will state the proper way to take the drug.
   b. The nurse will provide teaching about the drug's adverse effects.
   c. The patient will state all the symptoms of digoxin toxicity.
   d. The patient will call the prescriber if adverse effects occur.

2. A patient has a new prescription for a blood pressure medication that may cause him to feel dizzy during the first few days of therapy. Which is the best nursing diagnosis for this situation?
   a. Activity intolerance
   b. Risk for injury
   c. Disturbed body image
   d. Self-care deficit

3. A patient's chart includes an order that reads as follows: digoxin 0.025 mcg once daily at 0900 hours. Which action by the nurse is correct?
   a. The nurse gives the drug via the transdermal route.
   b. The nurse gives the drug orally.
   c. The nurse gives the drug intravenously.
   d. The nurse contacts the prescriber to clarify the dosage route.

4. The nurse is compiling a drug history for a patient. Which question from the nurse will obtain the most information from the patient?
   a. "Do you depend on sleeping pills to get to sleep?"
   b. "Do you have a family history of heart disease?"
   c. "When you have pain, what do you do to relieve it?"
   d. "What childhood diseases did you have?"

5. A 77-year-old male who has been diagnosed with an upper respiratory infection tells the nurse that he is allergic to penicillin. What is the most appropriate response by the nurse?
   a. "That is to be expected—lots of people are allergic to penicillin."
   b. "This allergy is not of major concern because the drug is given so commonly."
   c. "What type of reaction did you have when you took penicillin?"
   d. "Drug allergies don't usually occur in older individuals because they have built up resistance."

6. The nurse is preparing a care plan for a patient who has been newly diagnosed with type 2 diabetes mellitus. Put into correct order the steps of the nursing process, with 1 being the first step and 5 being the last step.
   a. Implementation
   b. Planning
   c. Assessment
   d. Evaluation
   e. Nursing diagnoses

7. The nurse is reviewing new medication orders that have been written for a newly admitted patient. Which orders will the nurse need to clarify? *Select all that apply.*
   a. Metformin (Glucophage®) 1000 mg PO twice a day
   b. Sitagliptin (Januvia®) 50 mg daily
   c. Simvastatin (Zocor®) 20 mg PO every evening
   d. Irbesartan (Avapro®) 300 mg PO once a day
   e. Docusate (Colace®) as needed for constipation

Answers: 1. a, 2. b, 3. d, 4. c, 5. c, 6. a = 4, b = 3, c = 1, d = 5, e = 2, 7. b, e

CRITICAL THINKING ACTIVITIES

1. What are the crucial responsibilities of the nurse when implementing drug therapy?

2. When medications were administered during the night shift, a patient refused to take his 0200 hours dose of an antibiotic, claiming that he had just taken it. What actions by the nurse would ensure sound decision making and maintain patient safety?

3. During a busy shift, the nurse notes that the chart of a newly admitted patient has a few orders for medications and diagnostic tests that were taken by telephone by another nurse. The nurse is on the way to the patient's room to do an assessment when the unit secretary says that one of the orders reads as follows: "furosemide, 20 mg, stat." What is the priority action by the nurse? How does the nurse go about giving this drug? Explain the best action to take in this situation.

CHAPTER 2

Pharmacological Principles

Objectives

After reading this chapter, the successful student will be able to do the following:

1. Define common terms used in pharmacology (see Key Terms).

2. Discuss the application of pharmaceutics, pharmacokinetics, and pharmacodynamics in drug therapy.

3. Explain the properties of various drug dosage forms and identify the advantages and disadvantages of the dose forms and drug delivery systems used in drug therapy.

4. Discuss the relevance of the four facets of pharmacokinetics (absorption, distribution, metabolism, excretion) to professional nursing practice, as related to drug therapy, for a variety of patients and health care settings.

5. Discuss the use of natural drug sources in the development of new drugs.

6. Describe evidence-informed nursing practice.

7. Discuss the role of evidence-informed practice as it relates to pharmacology and medication administration.

8. Develop a collaborative plan of care that takes into account general pharmacological principles in carrying out drug therapy.

e-Learning Activities

Website
(http://evolve.elsevier.com/Canada/Lilley/pharmacology/)

evolve

- Answer Key—Textbook Case Studies
- Answer Key—Critical Thinking Activities
- Chapter Summaries—Printable
- Review Questions for Exam Preparation
- Unfolding Case Studies

Key Terms

Additive effects Drug interactions in which the effect of a combination of two or more drugs with similar actions, administered at the same time, is the action of one plus the action of the other, with the total effect of both drugs being given (compare with *synergistic effects*). (p. 41)

Adverse drug event (ADE) Any undesirable occurrence related to administering or failing to administer a prescribed medication. (p. 41)

Adverse drug reaction (ADR) Any unexpected, unintended, undesired, or excessive response to a medication given at therapeutic dosages (compare with *adverse drug event*). (p. 42)

Adverse effects A general term for any undesirable effects that are a direct response to one or more drugs. (p. 40)

Agonists Drugs that bind to and stimulate the activity of one or more receptors in the body. (p. 38)

Allergic reaction An immunologic hypersensitivity reaction resulting from the unusual sensitivity of a patient to a particular medication; a type of adverse drug event. (p. 42)

Antagonists Drugs that bind to and inhibit the activity of one or more receptors in the body. Antagonists are also called *inhibitors*. (p. 38)

Antagonistic effects Drug interactions in which the effect of a combination of two or more drugs is less than the sum of the individual effects of the same drugs given alone; usually caused by an antagonizing (blocking or reducing) effect of one drug on another. (p. 41)

Bioavailability A measure of the fraction of drug administered dose that is delivered unchanged to the systemic circulation (from 0% to 100%). (p. 26)

Biotransformation One or more biochemical reactions involving a parent drug. (p. 34)

Blood–brain barrier The barrier system that restricts the passage of various chemicals and microscopic entities (e.g., bacteria, viruses) between the bloodstream and the central nervous system but allows for the passage of essential substances such as oxygen. (p. 34)

Chemical name The name that describes the chemical composition and molecular structure of a drug. (p. 24)

Contraindication Any condition, especially one related to a disease state or patient characteristic, including current or recent drug therapy, that renders a particular form of treatment improper or undesirable. (p. 39)

Cytochrome P450 The general name for a large class of enzymes that play a significant role in drug metabolism and drug interactions. (p. 34)

Dependence A state in which there is a compulsive or chronic need, as for a drug. (p. 40)

Dissolution The process by which solid forms of drugs disintegrate in the gastrointestinal tract and become soluble before they are absorbed into the circulation. (p. 25)

Drug Any chemical that affects the physiological processes of a living organism. (p. 23)

Drug actions The processes involved in the interaction between a drug and body cells (e.g., the action of a drug on a receptor protein); also referred to as *mechanisms of action*. (p. 24)

Drug classification A method of grouping drugs; may be based on structure or therapeutic use. (p. 24)

Drug effects The physiological reactions of the body to a drug. They can be therapeutic or toxic and describe how the body is affected as a whole by the drug. The terms *onset*, *peak*, and *duration* are used to describe drug effects (most often referring to therapeutic effects). (p. 37)

Drug-induced teratogenesis The development of congenital anomalies or defects in the developing fetus that are caused by the toxic effects of drugs. (p. 43)

Drug interaction Alteration of the pharmacological or pharmacokinetic activity of a given drug caused by the presence of one or more additional drugs; it is usually related to effects on the enzymes required for metabolism of the involved drugs. (p. 40)

Duration of action The length of time the concentration of a drug in the blood or tissues is sufficient to elicit a therapeutic response. (p. 37)

Enzymes Protein molecules that catalyze one or more of a variety of biochemical reactions, including those related to the body's physiological processes as well as those related to drug metabolism. (p. 38)

Evidence-informed practice (EIP) Continuous, interactive process involving the explicit, conscious, and judicious consideration of the best research evidence available to make collaborative decisions between the health care team and the patient and family when providing patient care. (p. 44)

First-pass effect The initial metabolism in the liver of a drug absorbed from the gastrointestinal tract before the drug reaches the systemic circulation through the bloodstream. (p. 26)

Generic name The name given to a drug approved by Health Canada; also called the *nonproprietary name* or the *official name*. The generic name is much shorter and simpler than the chemical name and is not protected by trademark. (p. 24)

Glucose-6-phosphate dehydrogenase (G6PD) deficiency A hereditary condition in which red blood cells break down when the body is exposed to certain drugs. (p. 42)

Half-life In pharmacokinetics, the time it takes for the blood level of a drug to be reduced by 50% (also called *elimination half-life*). (p. 36)

Idiosyncratic reaction An abnormal and unexpected response to a medication, other than an allergic reaction, that is peculiar to an individual patient. (p. 42)

Incompatibility The characteristic that causes two parenteral drugs or solutions to undergo a reaction when mixed or given together that results in the chemical deterioration of at least one of the drugs. (p. 41)

Intra-arterial Within an artery (e.g., intra-arterial injection). (p. 32)

Intra-articular Within a joint (e.g., intra-articular injection). (p. 32)

Intrathecal Within a sheath (e.g., the theca of the spinal cord), as in an intrathecal injection into the subarachnoid space. (p. 32)

Medication error (ME) Any preventable adverse drug event involving inappropriate medication use by a patient or health care professional; it may or may not cause patient harm. (p. 42)

Medication use process The prescribing, dispensing, and administering of medications and the monitoring of their effects. (p. 42)

Metabolite A chemical form of a drug that is the product of one or more biochemical (metabolic) reactions involving the parent drug. Active metabolites are those that have pharmacological activity of their own, even if the parent drug is inactive (see *prodrug*). Inactive metabolites lack pharmacological activity and are simply drug waste products awaiting excretion from the body (e.g., via the urinary, gastrointestinal, or respiratory tract). (p. 42)

Onset of action The time required for a drug to elicit a therapeutic response after dosing. (p. 37)

Parent drug The chemical form of a drug that is administered before it is metabolized by the body's biochemical reactions into its active or inactive metabolites. A parent drug that is not pharmacologically active is called a *prodrug*. A prodrug is then metabolized to pharmacologically active metabolites. (p. 26)

Peak effect The time required for a drug to reach its maximum therapeutic response in the body. (p. 37)

Peak level The maximum concentration of a drug in the body after administration, usually measured in a blood sample for therapeutic drug monitoring. (p. 37)

Pharmaceutics The science of preparing and dispensing drugs, including dosage form design (e.g., tablets, capsules, injections, patches, etc.). (p. 24)

Pharmacodynamics The study of the biochemical and physiological interactions of drugs at their sites of activity; it examines the properties of drugs and their pharmacological interactions with body protein receptors. (p. 24)

Pharmacoeconomics The study of economic factors impacting the cost of drug therapy. (p. 25)

Pharmacogenetics The study of the influence of genetic factors on drug response, including the nature of genetic aberrations that result in the absence, overabundance, or insufficiency of drug-metabolizing enzymes (also called *pharmacogenomics*; see Chapter 5). (p. 42)

Pharmacognosy The study of drugs that are obtained from natural plant and animal sources. (p. 25)

Pharmacokinetics The study of drug absorption, distribution, metabolism, and excretion (ADME) of drugs. (p. 24)

Pharmacology The broadest term for the study or science of drugs. (p. 23)

Pharmacotherapeutics The treatment of pathologic conditions through the use of drugs; also called *therapeutics*. (p. 24)

Prodrug An inactive drug dosage form that is converted to an active metabolite by various biochemical reactions once it is inside the body. (p. 34)

Receptor A molecular structure within or on the outer surface of a cell. Receptors bind specific substances (e.g., drug molecules), and one or more corresponding cellular effects (drug actions) occur as a result of this drug–receptor interaction. (p. 38)

Steady state The physiological state in which the amount of drug removed via elimination is equal to the amount of drug absorbed with each dose. (p. 37)

Substrates Substances (e.g., drugs or natural biochemicals in the body) on which enzymes act. (p. 35)

Synergistic effects Drug interactions in which the effect of a combination of two or more drugs with similar actions is greater than the sum of the individual effects of the same drugs given alone (compare with *additive effects*). (p. 41)

Therapeutic drug monitoring The process of measuring drug levels to identify a patient's drug exposure and to allow adjustment of dosages with the goals of maximizing therapeutic effects and minimizing toxicity. (p. 38)

Therapeutic effect The desired or intended effect of a particular medication. (p. 38)

Therapeutic index The ratio between the toxic and therapeutic concentrations of a drug. (p. 40)

Thin-film drug delivery Drug products that dissolve in the mouth and are absorbed through the oral mucosa. (p. 26)

Time-release technology A technique used in tablets and capsules such that drug molecules are released in the patient's gastrointestinal tract over an extended period of time. (p. 25)

Tolerance Reduced response to a drug after prolonged use. (p. 40)

Toxic The quality of being poisonous (i.e., injurious to health or dangerous to life). (p. 25)

Toxicity The condition of producing adverse bodily effects due to poisonous qualities. (p. 38)

Toxicology The study of poisons, including toxic drug effects, and applicable treatments. (p. 25)

Trade name The commercial name given to a drug product by its manufacturer; also called the *proprietary name*. (p. 24)

Trough level The lowest concentration of a drug reached in the body after it falls from its peak level, usually measured in a blood sample for therapeutic drug monitoring. (p. 37)

OVERVIEW

Any chemical that affects the physiological processes of a living organism can broadly be defined as a **drug.** The study or science of drugs is known as **pharmacology.** Pharmacology encompasses a variety of topics, including the following:
- Absorption
- Biochemical effects
- Biotransformation (metabolism)
- Distribution
- Drug history
- Drug origin
- Excretion
- Mechanisms of action
- Physical and chemical properties
- Physical effects
- Drug receptor mechanisms
- Therapeutic (beneficial) effects
- Toxic (harmful) effects

Pharmacology includes the following several sub-specialty areas: pharmaceutics, pharmacokinetics, pharmacodynamics, pharmacogenetics (pharmacogenomics), pharmacoeconomics, pharmacotherapeutics, pharmacognosy, and toxicology. Knowledge of these areas of pharmacology enables the nurse to better understand how drugs affect humans. Without understanding basic pharmacological principles, the nurse cannot fully appreciate the therapeutic benefits and potential toxicity of drugs.

Throughout the process of its development, a drug will acquire at least three different names. The **chemical name** describes the drug's chemical composition and molecular structure. The **generic name,** or nonproprietary name, is often much shorter and simpler than the chemical name. The generic name is used in most official drug compendiums to list drugs. The **trade name,** or proprietary name, is the drug's registered trademark and indicates that its commercial use is restricted to the owner of the patent for the drug (Figure 2-1). The patent owner is usually the manufacturer of the drug. Trade names are generally created by the manufacturer with marketability in mind. For this reason, they are usually shorter and easier to pronounce and remember than generic names. The patent life of a newly discovered drug molecule in Canada is 20 years. This is the length of time from patent approval until patent expiration. Because the research processes for new drug development normally require about 10 years, a drug manufacturer generally has the remaining 10 years for sales profits before patent expiration. A significant amount of these profits serves to offset the multimillion-dollar costs for research and development of the drug.

After the patent for a given drug expires, other manufacturers may legally begin to manufacture *generic* drugs with the same active ingredient. At this point, the drug price usually decreases substantially. Due to the high cost of drugs, many institutions have implemented programs in which one drug in a class of several drugs is chosen as the preferred agent, even though the drugs do not have the same active ingredients. This is called *therapeutic equivalence*. Before one drug can be therapeutically substituted for another, the drugs must have been proven to have the same therapeutic effect on the body.

Drugs are grouped together based on their similar properties. This is known as a **drug classification**. Drugs can be classified by their structure (e.g., β-adrenergic blockers) or by their therapeutic use (e.g., antibiotics, antihypertensives, antidepressants). Within the broad classification, each class may have subclasses; for example, penicillins are a subclass within the group of antibiotics, and β-adrenergic blockers are a subclass within the group of antihypertensives.

Three basic phases of pharmacology—*pharmaceutics, pharmacokinetics,* and *pharmacodynamics*—describe the relationship between the dose of a drug given to a patient and the activity of that drug in treating the patient's disorder. **Pharmaceutics** is the study of how various dosage forms influence the way in which the drug affects the body. **Pharmacodynamics,** on the other hand, is the study of what the drug does to the body.

Pharmacokinetics is the study of what the body does to the drug, involving the processes of absorption, distribution, metabolism, and excretion of drugs. Pharmacodynamics involves drug–receptor relationships. Figure 2-2 illustrates the three phases of drug activity, starting with the pharmaceutical phase, proceeding to the pharmacokinetic phase, and finishing with the pharmacodynamic phase.

Pharmacotherapeutics (also called *therapeutics*) focuses on the clinical use of drugs to prevent and treat diseases. It defines the principles of **drug actions**—the cellular processes that change in response to the presence of drug molecules. Some drug mechanisms of action are more clearly understood than others. Drugs are categorized into pharmacological classes according to their physiological functions (e.g., β-adrenergic blockers) and primary disease states treated (e.g., anticonvulsants, anti-infectives). Under the mandate of the Food and Drug Acts and Regulations, Health Canada regulates the approval and clinical use of all drugs, including the requirement of an expiration date on all drugs. This textbook focuses almost exclusively on current Health Canada–approved indications for the drugs discussed in each chapter and on drugs that are currently available in Canada at the time of this writing. Only Health Canada–approved indications are permitted to be described in the manufacturer's written information, or labelling, for a given drug product. At times, prescribers may elect to use drugs for non–Health Canada–approved indications. This use is known as *off-label prescribing* and often requires seasoned clinical judgement on the part of the prescriber. Evolving over time in clinical practice, previously off-label indications often become Health Canada–approved indications for a given drug.

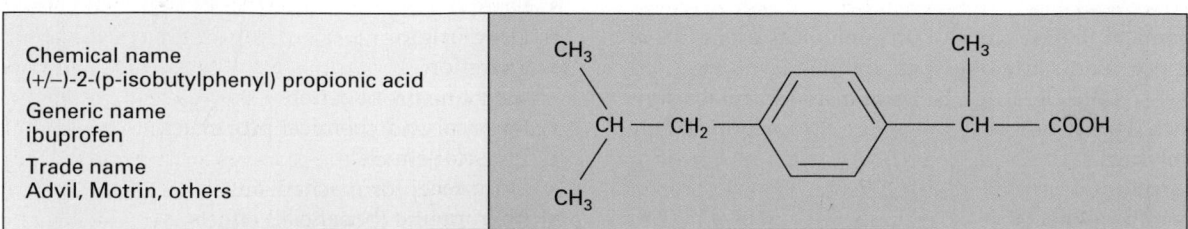

Chemical name
(+/−)-2-(p-isobutylphenyl) propionic acid

Generic name
ibuprofen

Trade name
Advil, Motrin, others

FIG. 2-1   Chemical structure of the common analgesic ibuprofen and the chemical, generic, and trade names for the drug.

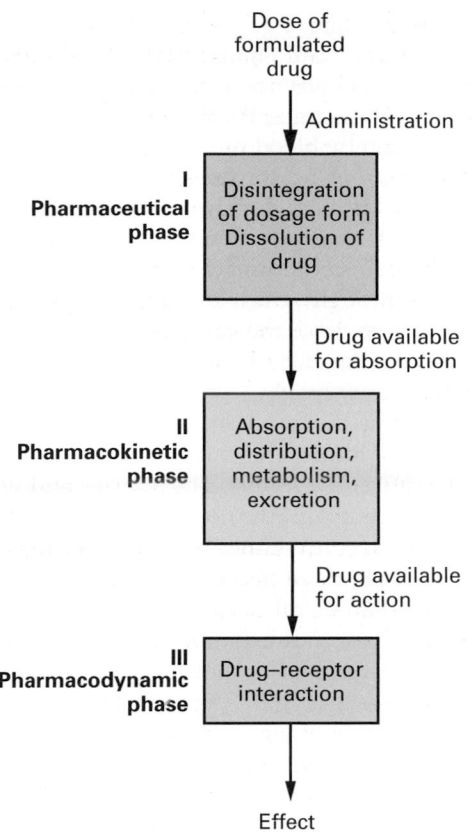

FIG. 2-2   Phases of drug activity. (From McKenry, L. M., Tessier, E., & Hogan, M. (2006). *Mosby's pharmacology in nursing* (22nd ed.). St. Louis: Mosby.)

The study of the adverse effects of drugs and other chemicals on living systems is known as **toxicology**. **Toxic** effects are often an extension of a drug's therapeutic action. Therefore, toxicology often involves overlapping principles of both pharmacotherapy and toxicology.

The study of natural (versus synthetic) drug sources (both plants and animals) is called **pharmacognosy**. **Pharmacoeconomics** focuses on the economic aspects of drug therapy.

In summary, pharmacology is a dynamic science that incorporates several different disciplines. Traditionally, chemistry has been seen as the primary basis of pharmacology, but pharmacology also relies heavily on physiology and biology.

PHARMACEUTICS

Different drug dosage forms have different pharmaceutical properties. Dosage form determines the rate at which drug **dissolution** (dissolving of solid dosage forms and their absorption [e.g., from gastrointestinal tract fluids]) occurs. A drug to be ingested orally may be in either a solid form (tablet, capsule, or powder) or a liquid form (solution or suspension). Table 2-1 lists various oral drug preparations and the relative rate at which they are absorbed. Oral drugs that are liquids (e.g., elixirs, syrups) are already dissolved and are usually absorbed more

TABLE 2-1	
Drug Absorption of Various Oral Preparations	
Liquids (e.g., elixirs, syrups)	Fastest
Suspension solutions	
Powders	
Capsules	
Tablets	
Coated tablets	
Enteric-coated tablets	Slowest

quickly than solid dosage forms. Enteric-coated tablets, by contrast, have a coating that prevents them from being broken down in the acidic pH environment of the stomach and therefore are not absorbed until they reach the more alkaline pH of the intestines. This pharmaceutical property results in slower dissolution and slower absorption.

Particle size within a tablet or capsule can make different dosage forms of the same drug dissolve at different rates, become absorbed at different rates, and thus have different times to onset of action. An example is the difference between micronized fenofibrate and nonmicronized fenofibrate. Micronized fenofibrate, for example, reaches a maximum concentration peak faster than does the nonmicronized formulation. Dosage form design for injectable drugs tends to be more straightforward than that for oral dosage forms. However, some injections are carefully formulated to reduce drug toxicity (e.g., liposomal amphotericin B).

Combination dosage forms contain multiple drugs in one dose. Examples of these combination forms include the cholesterol and antihypertensive medications atorvastatin calcium/amlodipine besylate tablets called Caduet and bacitracin zinc/neomycin sulphate/polymyxin B sulphate/hydrocortisone ointment (generic). There are numerous combination dosage forms; key examples are cited in the various chapters of this book.

A variety of dosage forms exist to provide both accurate and convenient drug delivery systems (Table 2-2). These delivery systems are designed to achieve a desired therapeutic response with minimal adverse effects. Many dosage forms have been developed to encourage patient adherence with the medication regime. **Time-release technology** is a technique used in tablets and capsules such that drug molecules are released in the patient's gastrointestinal tract over an extended period of time. Use of this technology allows drugs to be released continuously and more slowly into the blood stream. This results in prolonged drug absorption as well as duration of action. This is the opposite of immediate-release dosage forms, which release all of the active ingredients immediately upon dissolution in the gastrointestinal tract. Extended-release dosage forms are normally easily identified by various capital letter abbreviations attached to their names. Examples of this nomenclature are SR (slow release or sustained release), SA (sustained action), CR (controlled release), XL (extended length), and XT

TABLE	2-2

Dosage Forms

Route	Forms
Enteral	Tablets, capsules, oral soluble wafers, pills, time-release capsules, time-release tablets, enteric-coated tablets, elixirs, suspensions, solutions, lozenges or troches, caplets, rectal* suppositories, sublingual or buccal tablets
Parenteral	Injectable forms, solutions, suspensions, emulsions, powders for reconstitution
Topical	Aerosols, ointments, creams, pastes, powders, solutions, foams, gels, transdermal patches, inhalers, rectal*, and vaginal suppositories

*Note: Rectal enteral form is inserted into the rectum, while the topical rectal form is applied to the skin around the rectum.

(extended time). Continuous release is another example. Convenience of administration correlates strongly with patient adherence, because these forms often require fewer daily doses. Extended-release oral dosage forms must not be crushed, as this could cause accelerated release of drug from the dosage form and possible toxicity. Enteric-coated tablets also are not recommended for crushing. This would cause disruption of the tablet coating designed to protect the stomach lining from the local effects of the drug and prevent the drug from being prematurely disrupted by stomach acid. The ability to crush a tablet or open a capsule can facilitate drug administration when patients are unable or unwilling to swallow a tablet or capsule and also when medications need to be given through an enteral feeding tube. Capsules, powder, or liquid contents can often be added to soft foods such as applesauce or pudding, or dissolved in a beverage. Granules contained in capsules are usually for extended drug release and normally should not be crushed or chewed by the patient. However, they can often be swallowed when sprinkled on one of the soft foods. Consultation with a pharmacist, reading the product literature, or use of another suitable source is necessary if there is any question about whether a drug can be crushed or mixed with specific food or beverages.

An increasingly popular dosage form, **thin-film drug delivery**, refers to drug products that dissolve in the mouth and are absorbed through the oral mucosa. These include orally disintegrating tablets as well as thin wafers that also dissolve in the mouth when contact with liquid occurs. Depending on the specific drug product, the dosage form may dissolve on the tongue, under the tongue, or in the buccal (cheek) pocket.

The specific characteristics of various dosage forms have a large impact on how and to what extent the drug is absorbed. For a drug to work at a specific site in the body it must either be applied directly at that site in an active form or have a way of getting to that site. Oral dosage forms rely on gastric and intestinal enzymes and

pH environments to break down the medication into particles that are small enough to be absorbed into the circulation. Once absorbed through the mucosa of the stomach or intestines, the drug is then transported to the site of action by blood or lymph.

Many topically applied dosage forms work directly on the surface of the skin. Once the drug is applied, it is already in a form that allows it to act immediately. However, with other topical dosage forms, the skin acts as a barrier through which the drug must pass to get to the circulation; once there, the drug is then carried to the site of action (e.g., fentanyl transdermal patches for pain).

Dosage forms that are administered via injection are called *parenteral* forms. They must have certain characteristics to be safe and effective. The arteries and veins that carry drugs throughout the body can easily be damaged if the drug is too concentrated or corrosive. To be administered safely, the pH of injections must be similar to that of the blood. Parenteral dosage forms that are injected intravenously are immediately placed into solution in the bloodstream and do not have to be dissolved in the body. Therefore, 100% absorption is assumed to occur immediately upon intravenous or intra-arterial injection.

PHARMACOKINETICS

A drug's time to onset of action, time to peak effect, and duration of action are all characteristics defined by pharmacokinetics. Pharmacokinetics is the study of what happens to a drug from the time it is put into the body until the **parent drug** and all metabolites have left the body. Thus, the study of drug absorption, distribution, metabolism, and excretion represent the combined focus of pharmacokinetics.

Absorption

Absorption is the movement of a drug from its site of administration into the bloodstream for distribution to the tissues. **Bioavailability** describes the extent of drug absorption. For example, a drug that is absorbed from the intestine must first pass through the liver before it reaches the systemic circulation (Figure 2-3). If a large proportion of a drug is chemically changed into inactive metabolites in the liver, then a much smaller amount of drug will pass into the circulation (i.e., will be bioavailable). Such a drug is said to have a high **first-pass effect** (e.g., oral nitrates). First-pass effect reduces the bioavailability of drugs to less than 100%. Drugs administered by the intravenous route are 100% bioavailable because 100% of the drug reaches the systemic circulation. Drugs administered by mouth have reduced bioavailability (less than 100%) because a fraction of the drug reaches the systemic circulation. If two medications have the same bioavailability and same concentration of active ingredient, they are said to be bioequivalent (e.g., a brand-name drug and the same generic drug).

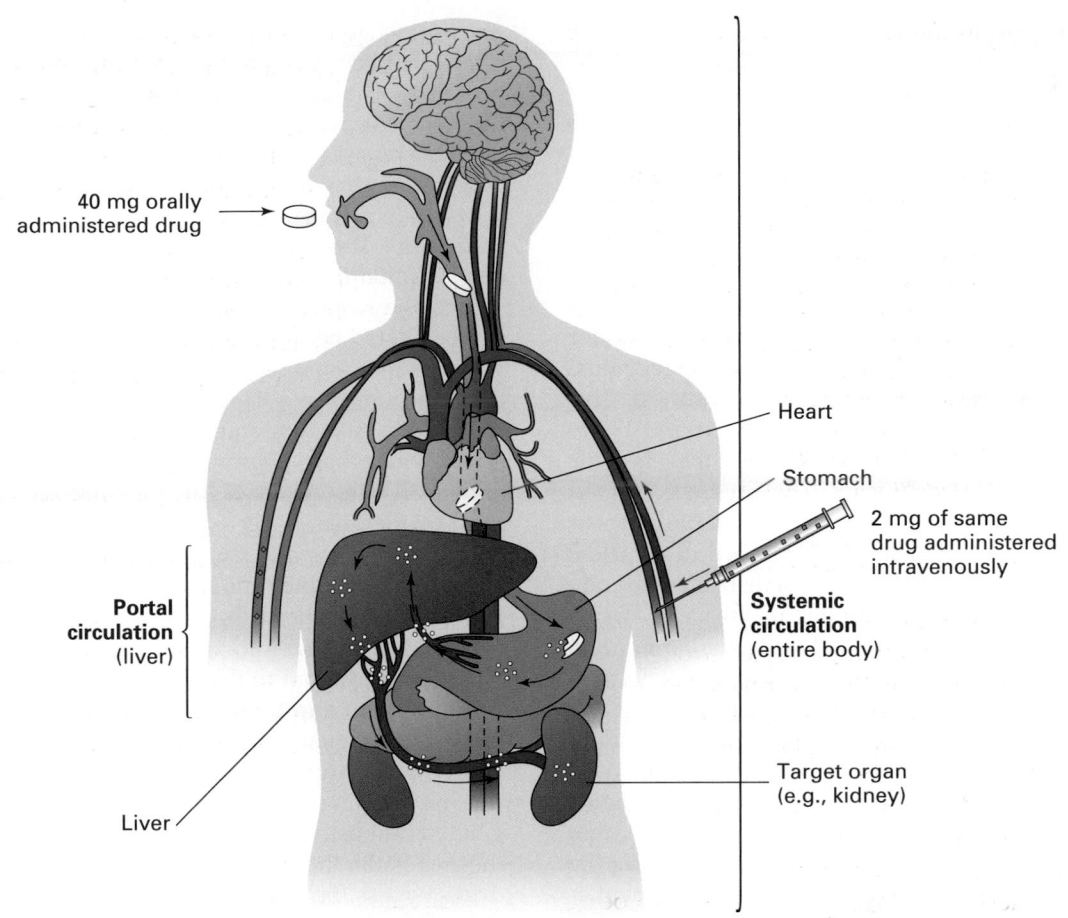

FIG. 2-3 First-pass effect of a drug by the liver before its systemic availability. (From McKenry, L. M., & Salerno, E. (1995). *Mosby's pharmacology in nursing* (19th ed.). St. Louis: Mosby.)

Various factors affect the rate of drug absorption. How a drug is administered, or its route of administration, affects the rate and extent of absorption of that drug. Although a number of dosage formulations are available for delivering medications, they can all be categorized into three basic routes of administration: enteral (gastrointestinal tract), parenteral, and topical.

Route

Enteral Route. In enteral drug administration, the drug is absorbed into the systemic circulation through the mucosa of the stomach or small or large intestine. The rate of absorption can be altered by many factors. Orally administered drugs are absorbed from the intestinal lumen into the mesenteric blood system and transported

---

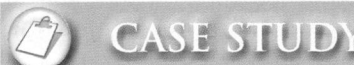

Nitroglycerin Therapy

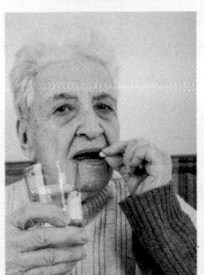

Four patients with angina are receiving a form of nitroglycerin, as follows:
  Charlotte, age 88, takes 10 mg four times a day to prevent angina.
  Dale, age 63, takes a form that delivers 0.2 mg/hr, also to prevent angina.
  Raissa, age 58, takes 0.4 mg only if needed for chest pain.
  Kenneth, age 62, is in the hospital with severe, unstable angina and is receiving 100 mcg/hr.

You may refer to the section on nitroglycerin in Chapter 24 or to a nursing drug handbook to answer these questions.

1. State the route or form of nitroglycerin that each patient is receiving. In addition, specify the generic name(s) and trade name(s) for each particular form.
2. For each patient, state the rationale for the route or form of drug that was chosen. Which forms have immediate action? Why would this be important?
3. Which form or forms are most affected by the first-pass effect? Explain your answer.

For answers see http://evolve.elsevier.com/Canada/Lilley/pharmacology/.

by the portal vein to the liver. Once the drug is in the liver, hepatic enzyme systems metabolize it, and the remaining active ingredients are passed into the general circulation. Enteric coating is designed to protect the stomach by having drug dissolution and absorption occur in the intestines. Taking an enteric-coated medication with a large amount of food may cause it to be dissolved by acidic stomach contents and thus reduce intestinal drug absorption and negate the coating's stomach-protective properties. Anticholinergic drugs slow gastrointestinal transit time (or the time it takes for substances in the stomach to be dissolved for eventual transport to and absorption from the intestines). This may reduce the amount of drug absorption and therapeutic effect for acid-susceptible drugs that become broken down by stomach acids. The presence of food may enhance the absorption of some fat-soluble drugs or of drugs that are more easily broken down in an acidic environment. If a large proportion of a drug is chemically processed into inactive metabolites in the liver, then a much less active drug will make it into circulation. Such a drug would have a high first-pass effect. Consequently, the oral dose has to be calculated to compensate for the lower bioavailability. For example, nitroglycerin administered orally undergoes rapid liver metabolism and as a result, has almost no pharmacological effect. If administered sublingually, the drug is absorbed into the system circulation via the rich supply of blood vessels under the tongue and is carried to its site of action prior to circulating through the liver.

The same drug given intravenously will bypass the liver altogether. This prevents the first-pass effect from taking place and therefore allows all of the drug to reach the circulation. For this reason, parenteral doses of drugs with a high first-pass effect are much smaller than enterally (orally) administered doses, yet they produce the same pharmacological response. See Table 2-3 for further discussion of the advantages, disadvantages, and nursing considerations related to the different routes of administration.

Many factors can alter the absorption of drugs, including acid changes within the stomach, absorption changes in the intestines, and the presence or absence of food and fluid. Various factors that affect the acidity of the stomach include the time of day; the age of the patient; and the presence and types of medications (e.g., H_2 blockers or proton pump inhibitors [see Chapter 39]), foods, or beverages. Enteric coating is designed to protect the stomach by having drug dissolution and absorption occur in the intestines. Taking an enteric-coated medication with a large amount of food may cause it to be dissolved by acidic stomach contents and thus reduce intestinal drug absorption and negate the coating's stomach-protective properties.

Anticholinergic drugs slow gastrointestinal transit time (or the time it takes for substances in the stomach to be dissolved for eventual transport to and absorption from the intestines). This may reduce the amount of drug

absorption and therapeutic effect for acid-susceptible drugs that become broken down by stomach acids. The presence of food may enhance the absorption of some fat-soluble drugs or of drugs that are more easily broken down in an acidic environment.

Drug absorption may also be altered in patients who have had portions of the small intestine removed because of disease. This condition is known as *short bowel syndrome*. Similarly, bariatric weight loss surgery reduces the size of the stomach. As a result, medication absorption can be altered because stomach contents are delivered to the intestines more rapidly than usual after such surgery. This phenomenon is called *gastric dumping*. Examples of drugs to be taken on an empty stomach and those to be taken with food are provided in Box 2-1. The stomach and small intestine are highly vascularized. When blood flow to the area is decreased, absorption may also be decreased. Sepsis and exercise are examples of circumstances under which blood flow to the gastrointestinal tract is often reduced. In both cases, blood tends to be routed to the heart and other vital organs. In exercise, blood is also routed to the skeletal muscles.

Sublingual and Buccal Routes. Drugs administered by the sublingual route are absorbed rapidly into the highly vascularized tissue under the tongue—the oral mucosa. Sublingual nitroglycerin is an example. Sublingually administered drugs are absorbed rapidly because the area under the tongue has a large blood supply. These drugs bypass the liver and yet are systemically bioavailable. The same applies for drugs administered by the buccal route (the oral mucosa between the cheek and the gum). Through these routes, drugs such as nitroglycerin are absorbed rapidly into the bloodstream and delivered rapidly to their site of action (e.g., coronary arteries).

BOX 2-1

Drugs to Be Taken on an Empty Stomach and With Food

Many medications are taken on an empty stomach with an adequate intake of fluid (180 to 240 mL of water). The nurse must give patients specific instructions regarding those medications *not* to be taken with food but on an empty stomach. Examples include alendronate sodium and risedronate sodium.

Medications that are generally taken with food include carbamazepine, iron and iron-containing products, hydralazine, lithium, propranolol, spironolactone, nonsteroidal anti-inflammatory drugs, and theophylline.

Macrolides and oral opioids are often taken with food (even though they are specified to be taken with a full glass of water and on an empty stomach) to minimize the gastrointestinal irritation associated with these drugs. If you are in doubt, consult with a licensed pharmacist or a current authoritative drug resource.

TABLE 2-3

Routes of Administration and Related Nursing Considerations

Route	Advantages	Disadvantages	Nursing Considerations
Intravenous (IV)	Provides rapid onset (drug delivered immediately to bloodstream); allows more direct control of drug level in blood; gives option of larger fluid volume, therefore diluting irritating drugs; avoids first-pass metabolism.	Higher cost; inconvenience (e.g., not self-administered); irreversibility of drug action in most cases and inability to retrieve medication; risk of fluid overload; greater likelihood of infection; possibility of embolism.	Continuous intravenous infusions require frequent monitoring to be sure that the correct volume and amount are administered and that the drug reaches safe, therapeutic blood levels. Intravenous drugs and solutions must be checked for compatibilities. Intravenous sites are to be monitored for redness, swelling, heat, and drainage—all indicative of complications, such as thrombophlebitis. If intermittent intravenous infusions are used, clearing or flushing of the line with normal saline before and after is generally indicated to keep the intravenous site patent and minimize incompatibilities.
Intramuscular (IM)	Intramuscular injections are good for poorly soluble drugs, which are often given in "depot" preparation form and are then absorbed over a prolonged period; onsets of action differ depending on route. IM route also provides a more immediate onset of action than PO for certain drugs prior to establishment of IV access (i.e., in the emergency department) or if the patient does not require IV access but is vomiting.	Discomfort of injection; inconvenience; bruising; slower onset of action compared to intravenous, although quicker than oral in most situations.	Using landmarks to identify correct intramuscular site is always required and recommended as a nursing standard of care. For adults, the intramuscular site of choice is the ventral gluteal muscle with use of a 38 mm (sometimes 25 mm in extremely thin or emaciated patients) and 20- to 25-gauge needle for aqueous solutions and 18- to 25-gauge needle for viscous or oil-based solutions. However, the deltoid muscle in the upper arm is the site of choice for vaccine administration in adults. Selection of the correct size of syringe and needle is key to safe administration by these routes and is based on thorough assessment of the patient as well as the characteristics of the drug.
Subcutaneous	Drugs given via the subcutaneous route are those that require slow, sustained absorption of a medication, such as insulin and low-molecular-weight heparin solutions. It is also often used in surgery and palliative care for slower absorption of pain medication and prolonged pain relief. The medication is injected under the epidermis into the fat and connective tissue beneath the dermis, where there is less blood flow and consequently a slower, steadier absorption rate compared with that of the intramuscular route.	Discomfort of injection; inconvenience; bruising; slower onset of action compared to intravenous/intramuscular, although quicker than oral in most situations. A wide variety of insulin pens and preloaded heparin syringes with tiny needles are available, enabling the 90-degree angle for injection. Subcutaneous injection into the abdomen should be to the right or left of and 5 cm away from the umbilicus to avoid the umbilical veins and the risk of bleeding.	Using landmarks to identify the correct subcutaneous site is always required and recommended as a nursing standard of care. Common sites for injection include the lateral and posterior aspects of the upper arm and under the greater trochanter of the femur in the thigh and abdominal area. Subcutaneous injections are recommended to be given at a 90-degree angle with a proper-size syringe and needle (4 to 8 mm); in emaciated or extremely thin patients, the subcutaneous angle is 45 degrees. Subcutaneous injections require a 26- to 30-gauge, 8 mm needle. Selection of correct size of syringe and needle is key to safe administration by the subcutaneous route and is based on thorough assessment of the patient as well as the characteristics of the drug.

Continued

TABLE 2-3

Routes of Administration and Related Nursing Considerations—cont'd

Route	Advantages	Disadvantages	Nursing Considerations
Oral	Usually easier, more convenient, and less expensive; safer than injection as dosing more likely to be reversible in cases of accidental ingestion (e.g., through induction of emesis, administration of activated charcoal).	Variable absorption; inactivation of some drugs by stomach acid or pH; problems with first-pass effect or presystemic metabolism; greater dependence of drug action on patient variables.	Enteral routes include oral administration and involve a variety of dosage forms (e.g., liquids, solutions, tablets, and enteric-coated pills or tablets). Some medications are recommended to be taken with food, while others are recommended not to be taken with food; it is also suggested that oral dosage forms of drugs be taken with a sufficient amount of fluid, such as 180 to 240 mL of water. Other factors to consider include other medicines being taken at the same time and concurrent use of dairy products or antacids. If oral forms are given via nasogastric tube or gastrostomy tube, tube placement in stomach must be assessed prior to giving the medication and the patient's head is to remain elevated; flushing the nasogastric tube with at least 30 to 60 mL of water before and after giving the drug is recommended to help maintain tube patency and prevent clogging; enteric-coated drugs cannot be crushed and administered via nasogastric tube, while capsules may be opened but granules are not to be crushed for administration.
Sublingual, buccal (subtypes of oral, but more parenteral than enteral)	Absorbed more rapidly from oral mucosa than oral route and leads to more rapid onset of action; avoids breakdown of drug by stomach acid; avoids first-pass metabolism because gastric absorption is bypassed.	Patient may swallow pill instead of keeping under tongue until dissolved; pills often smaller to handle. Salivary secretions are necessary for the absorption of sublingual medications.	Drugs given via the sublingual route are to be placed under the tongue; once dissolved, the drug may be swallowed. When using the buccal route, medication is placed between the cheek and gum. Both of these dosage forms are relatively nonirritating; the drug usually is without flavour and is water-soluble.

Route	Advantages	Disadvantages	Nursing Considerations
Rectal	Provides relatively rapid absorption; good alternative when oral route not feasible; useful for local or systemic drug delivery; usually leads to mixed first-pass and non–first-pass metabolism.	Possible discomfort and embarrassment to patient; often higher cost than oral route.	Absorption via this route is erratic and unpredictable, but it provides a safe alternative when nausea or vomiting prevents oral dosing of drugs. The patient must be placed on his left side so that the normal anatomy of the colon allows safe and effective insertion of the rectal dosage form. Suppositories are inserted using a gloved hand or gloved index finger and water-soluble lubricant. Drug must be administered exactly as ordered.
Topical	Delivers medication directly to affected area; decreases likelihood of systemic drug effects.	Sometimes awkward to self-administer (e.g., eye drops); can be messy; usually higher cost than oral route.	Most dermatologic drugs are given via topical route in form of a solution, ointment, spray, or drops. Maximal absorption of topical drugs is enhanced with skin that is clean and free of debris; if measurement of ointment is necessary—such as with topical nitroglycerin—application must be done carefully and per instructions (e.g., apply 2.5 cm of ointment). Gloves help minimize cross-contamination and prevent absorption of drug into the nurse's own skin. If the patient's skin is not intact, sterile technique is needed.
Transdermal (subtype of topical)	Provides relatively constant rate of drug absorption; one patch can last 1 to 7 days, depending on drug; avoids first-pass metabolism.	Rate of absorption can be affected by excessive perspiration and body temperature; patch may peel off; cost is higher; used patches must be disposed of safely; may cause skin irritation.	Transdermal drugs should be placed on alternating sites and on a clean, nonhairy, nonirritated area, and only after the previously applied patch has been removed and that area cleansed and dried. Transdermal drugs generally come in a single-dose, adhesive-backed drug application system.
Inhalational	Provides rapid absorption; drug delivered directly to lung tissues, where most of these drugs exert their actions.	Rate of absorption can be too rapid, increasing the risk of exaggerated drug effects; requires more patient education for self-administration; some patients may have difficulty with administration technique.	Inhaled medications are to be used exactly as prescribed and with clean equipment. Instructions need to be given to the patient/family/caregiver regarding medications to be used as well as the proper use, storage, and safe-keeping of inhalers, spacers, and nebulizers. Chapter 10 describes and shows how medications are inhaled.

Parenteral Route. The parenteral route is the fastest route by which a drug can be absorbed, followed by the enteral and the topical routes. *Parenteral* is a general term meaning any route of administration other than the gastrointestinal tract. It most commonly refers to injection. Intravenous injection delivers the drug directly into the circulation, where it is distributed with the blood throughout the body. Drugs given by intramuscular injection and subcutaneous injection are absorbed more slowly than those given intravenously. These drug formulations are usually absorbed over a period of several hours; however, some are specially formulated to be released over days, weeks, or months.

Drugs can be injected intradermally, subcutaneously, intravenously, intramuscularly, intrathecally, intraarticularly, or intra-arterially. Physicians and advanced practice nurses usually give **intra-arterial**, **intrathecal**, or **intra-articular** injections. Medications given by the parenteral route have the advantage of bypassing the first-pass effect of the liver. Parenteral administration offers an alternative route of delivery for those medications that cannot be given orally and poses fewer obstacles to absorption. However, drugs that are administered by the parenteral route must still be absorbed into cells and tissues before they can exert their pharmacological effect (see Table 2-3).

Subcutaneous, Intradermal, and Intramuscular Routes. Injections into the fatty subcutaneous tissues under the dermal layer of the skin are referred to as *subcutaneous* injections. Injections under the more superficial skin layers immediately underneath the epidermal layer of skin and into the dermal layer are known as *intradermal* injections. Injections given into the muscle beneath the subcutaneous fatty tissue are referred to as *intramuscular* injections. Muscles have a greater blood supply than the skin does; therefore, drugs injected intramuscularly are typically absorbed faster than drugs injected subcutaneously. Absorption from either of these sites may be increased by applying heat to the injection site or by massaging the site. Both methods increase blood flow to the area, thereby enhancing absorption. In contrast, the presence of cold, hypotension, or poor peripheral blood flow compromises the circulation, reducing drug activity by reducing drug delivery to the tissues. Most intramuscularly injected drugs are absorbed over several hours. However, specially formulated long-acting intramuscular dosage forms called *depot drugs* have been designed for slow absorption over a period of several days to a few months or longer. The intramuscular corticosteroid methylprednisolone acetate can provide anti-inflammatory effects for several weeks. The intramuscular contraceptive medroxyprogesterone acetate normally prevents pregnancy for 3 months per dose.

Topical Route. The topical route of drug administration involves application of medications to various body surfaces. Several topical drug delivery systems exist. Topically administered drugs can be applied to the skin, eyes, ears, nose, lungs, rectum, or vagina. Topical application delivers a uniform amount of drug over a longer period, but the effects of the drug are usually slower in their onset and more prolonged in their duration of action as compared with oral or parenteral administration. This can be a problem if the patient begins to experience adverse effects from the drug and a considerable amount of drug has already been absorbed. All topical routes of drug administration avoid first-pass effects of the liver, with the exception of rectal drug administration. Because the rectum is part of the gastrointestinal tract, some drug will be absorbed into the capillaries that feed the portal vein to the liver. However, some drugs will also be absorbed locally into the perirectal tissues. Therefore, rectally administered drugs are said to have a mixed first-pass and non–first-pass absorption and metabolism. Box 2-2 lists the drug routes and indicates whether they are associated with first-pass effects in the liver.

Ointments, gels, and creams are common types of topically administered drugs. Examples include sunscreens, antibiotics, and nitroglycerin ointment. The drawback to their use is that their systemic absorption is

 ## PREVENTING MEDICATION ERRORS

Does IV = PO?

The prescriber writes an order for "furosemide 80 mg IV STAT × 1 dose" for a patient who is short of breath because of pulmonary edema. When the nurse goes to give the drug, only the PO form is immediately available. Someone must go to the pharmacy to pick up the IV dose. Another nurse says, "Go ahead and give the pill. He needs it fast. It's all the same!" But is it?

Remember, the oral forms of medications must be processed through the gastrointestinal tract, be absorbed through the small intestine, and undergo the first-pass effect in the liver before the drug can reach the intended site of action. In contrast, IV forms are injected directly into the circulation and can act almost immediately because the first-pass effect is bypassed. The time until onset of action for the PO form is 30 to 60 minutes; for the IV form, this time is 5 minutes. This patient is in respiratory distress, and the immediate effect of the diuretic is desired. In addition, because of the first-pass effect, the available amount of orally administered drug that actually reaches the site of action would be less than the available amount of intravenously administered drug. Therefore, IV does NOT equal PO! Never change the route of administration of a medication; if questions come up, always check with the prescriber.

BOX 2-2

Drug Routes and First-Pass Effects

First-Pass Routes

Hepatic arterial
Oral
Portal venous
Rectal*

Non–First-Pass Routes

Aural (instilled into the ear)
Buccal
Inhaled
Intra-arterial
Intramuscular
Intranasal
Intraocular
Intravaginal
Intravenous
Subcutaneous
Sublingual
Transdermal

---

*Leads to both first-pass and non–first-pass effects.

often erratic and unreliable. Generally, these medications are commonly used for local effects rather than for systemic effects. Topically applied drugs can also be used in the treatment of illnesses of the eyes, ears, and sinuses. Eye, ear, and nose drops are administered primarily for local effects, whereas nasal sprays may be used for both systemic (e.g., sumatriptan for migraine headaches) and local (e.g., oxymetazoline for nasal sinus congestion). Vaginal medications may also be given for systemic effects (e.g., progestational hormone therapy with progesterone vaginal suppositories) but are more commonly used for local effects (e.g., treatment of vaginal infection with miconazole vaginal cream).

Transdermal Route. Transdermal drug delivery through adhesive drug patches is an elaborate topical route of drug administration that is commonly used for systemic drug effects. Some examples of drugs administered by this route are fentanyl (for pain), nitroglycerin (for angina), nicotine (for smoking cessation), estrogen (for menopausal symptoms), and rivastigmine (for Alzheimer's disease). Transdermal patches are usually designed to deliver a constant amount of drug per unit of time for a specified time period. For example, a nitroglycerin patch may deliver 0.2, 0.4 or 0.6 mg/hr over 24 hours, whereas a fentanyl patch may deliver 25 to 100 mcg/hr over a 72-hour period.

This route is suitable for patients who cannot tolerate oral administration and provides a convenient method for drug delivery.

Inhalation Route. Inhalation is another type of topical drug administration. Inhaled drugs are delivered to the lungs as micrometre-sized drug particles. This small drug size is necessary for the drug to be transported to the small, thin-walled air sacs (alveoli) within the lungs. Once the small particles of drug are in the alveoli, drug absorption is rapid via capillary contact. Many pulmonary and other types of diseases can be treated with such topically inhaled drugs. Examples of inhaled drugs are zanamivir, used for the prevention of influenza; salbutamol sulphate, used to treat bronchial constriction in individuals with asthma; and fluticasone propionate, used for its anti-inflammatory properties in patients with asthma and allergies.

Distribution

Distribution refers to the transport of a drug by the bloodstream to its site of action (Figure 2-4). Drugs are distributed first to those areas with extensive blood supply. Areas of rapid distribution include the heart, liver, kidneys, and brain. Areas of slower distribution include muscle, skin, and fat. Once a drug enters the circulating blood, it is distributed throughout the body. At this point, it is also starting to be eliminated by the organs that metabolize and excrete drugs—primarily the liver and kidneys. Only drug molecules that are not bound to plasma proteins can freely distribute to extravascular tissue (outside the blood vessels) to reach their site of action. Albumin is the most common blood protein and carries the majority of protein-bound drug molecules. (Figure 2-5). If a given drug binds to albumin, only a limited amount of the drug is *not* bound. This unbound portion is pharmacologically active and is considered "free" drug, whereas "bound" drug is pharmacologically inactive. Certain conditions that cause low albumin levels, such as extensive burns and malnourished states, result in a larger fraction of free (unbound and active) drug. This situation can raise the risk of drug toxicity.

When an individual is taking two medications that are highly protein bound, these medications may compete for binding sites on the albumin protein. Because of this competition, there is more free, unbound drug. This can lead to an unpredictable drug response called a *drug–drug interaction*. A drug–drug interaction occurs when the presence of one drug decreases or increases the action of another drug administered concurrently (i.e., given at the same time).

A theoretical volume, called the *volume of distribution*, is sometimes used to describe the various areas where drugs may be distributed. These areas, or *compartments*, may be the blood (*intravascular space*), total body water, body fat, or other body tissues and organs. Typically a drug that is highly water soluble (hydrophilic) will have a small volume of distribution and high blood concentrations. In contrast, fat-soluble drugs (lipophilic) have a large volume of distribution and low blood concentrations.

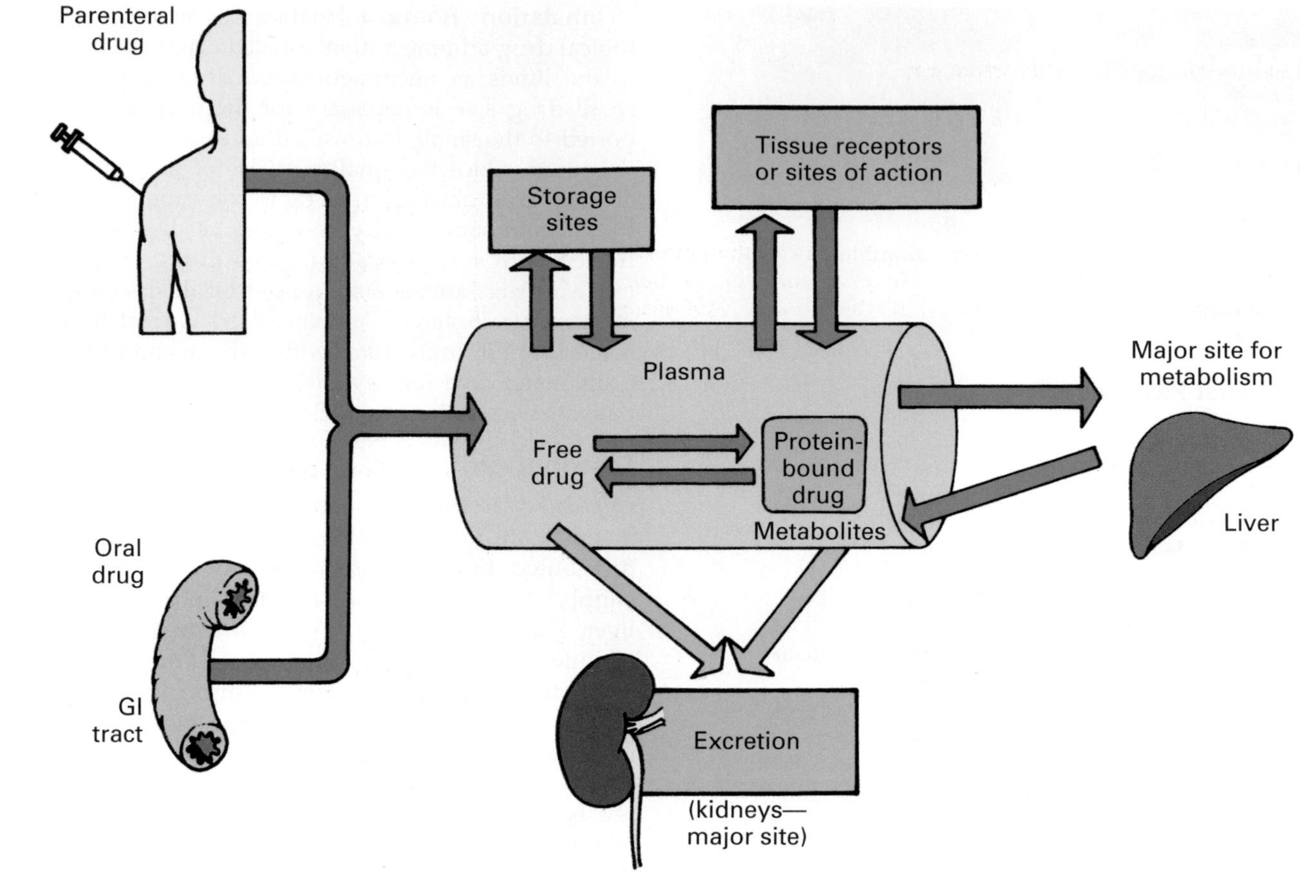

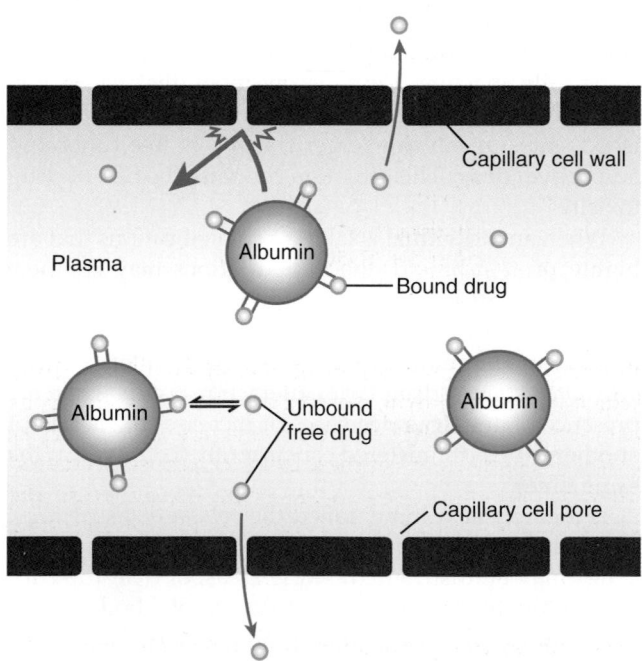

FIG. 2-4 Drug transport in the body.

There are some sites in the body into which it may be difficult to distribute a drug. These sites typically either have a poor blood supply (e.g., bone) or have physiological barriers that make it difficult for drugs to pass through (e.g., the brain due to the **blood–brain barrier**).

Metabolism

Metabolism is also referred to as **biotransformation**. It involves the biochemical alteration of a drug into any of the following: an inactive metabolite, a more soluble compound, a more potent metabolite (as in the conversion of an inactive **prodrug** to its active form), or a less active metabolite. Metabolism is the next step after absorption and distribution. The organ most responsible for the biotransformation or metabolism of drugs is the liver. Other metabolic tissues include the skeletal muscles, kidneys, lungs, plasma, and intestinal mucosa.

Hepatic metabolism involves the activity of a large class of enzymes, the **cytochrome P450** enzymes (or simply P450 enzymes), also known as *microsomal* enzymes. These enzymes control a variety of reactions that aid in the metabolism of medications. They are largely targeted against lipid-soluble (*nonpolar* [no charge]) drugs, (also known as *lipophilic* ["fat loving"]), which are typically difficult to eliminate. These include the majority of medications. Those medications with

FIG. 2-5 Protein binding of drugs. Albumin is the most prevalent protein in plasma and the most important of the proteins to which drugs bind. Only unbound (free) drug molecules can leave the vascular system. Bound molecules are too large to fit through the pores in the capillary wall.

TABLE 2-4

Mechanisms of Biotransformation

Type of Biotransformation	Mechanism	Result
Oxidation Reduction Hydrolysis	Chemical reactions	Increase polarity of chemical, making it more water soluble and more easily excretable. This often results in a loss of pharmacological activity. Forms a less toxic product with less activity
Conjugation (e.g., glucuronidation, glycination, sulfation methylation, alkylation)	Combination with another substance (e.g., glucuronide, glycine, sulphate, methyl groups, alkyl groups)	

TABLE 2-5

Common Liver Cytochrome P450 Enzymes and Corresponding Drug Substrates

Enzyme	Common Drug Substrates
1A2	amitriptyline, caffeine, theophylline, verapamil warfarin
2C9	diclofenac, glyburide, ibuprofen, losartan, rosiglitazone, tamoxifen
2C19	amitriptyline, diazepam, phenytoin, proton pump inhibitors, propranolol
2D6	amitryptyline, carvedilol, codeine, fentanyl, fluoxetine, haloperidol, hydrocodone, oxycodone, paroxetine, tricyclic antidepressants, risperidone, timolol
2E1	acetaminophen, ethanol
3A4	azole antifungals, amiodarone, atorvastatin, many chemotherapeutic drugs, diltiazem, ethinyl estradiol, indinavir, lidocaine, lovastatin, macrolides, progesterone, ritonavir, simvastatin, testosterone, verapamil

TABLE 2-6

Examples of Conditions and Drugs That Affect Drug Metabolism

Category	Example	Drug Metabolism Increased	Drug Metabolism Decreased
Diseases	Cardiovascular dysfunction		X
	Kidney insufficiency		X
Condition	Starvation		X
	Obstructive jaundice		X
	Genetic constitution		
	Fast acetylator	X	
	Slow acetylator		X
Drugs	Barbiturates	X	
	erythromycin (P450 inhibitor)		X
	ketoconazole (P450 inhibitor)		X
	phenytoin (P450 inducer)	X	
	rifampin (P450 inducer)	X	

water-soluble (*polar* or *hydrophilic* ["water loving"]) molecules may be more easily metabolized by simpler chemical reactions such as hydrolysis. Some of the chemical reactions by which the liver can metabolize drugs are listed in Table 2-4. Drug molecules that are the metabolic targets of specific enzymes are said to be **substrates** for those enzymes. Specific P450 enzymes are identified by standardized number and letter designations. Some of the most common P450 enzymes and their corresponding common drug substrates are listed in Table 2-5.

The biotransformation capabilities of the liver can vary considerably from patient to patient. Age can alter biotransformation (young or older adult patient) or if the patient has an unhealthy liver. The various factors that can alter the biotransformation include genetics, diseases, and the concurrent use of other medications (Table 2-6). Nurses must be alert to the various factors that can alter transformation with the accumulation of active metabolites and the risk for subsequent toxicity.

Many drugs can inhibit drug-metabolizing enzymes; these drugs are called *enzyme inhibitors*. Decreases or delays in drug metabolism result in the accumulation of

the drug and prolongation of the effects of the drug, which can lead to drug toxicity. In contrast, some drugs can stimulate drug metabolism and are called *enzyme inducers*. The presence of these drugs can cause decreased pharmacological effects. This often occurs with the repeated administration of certain drugs that stimulate the formation of new microsomal enzymes.

Excretion

Excretion is the elimination of drugs from the body. Whether they are parent compounds or active or inactive metabolites, all drugs must eventually be removed from the body. The primary organ responsible for this elimination is the kidney. Two other organs that play an important role in the excretion of drugs are the liver and

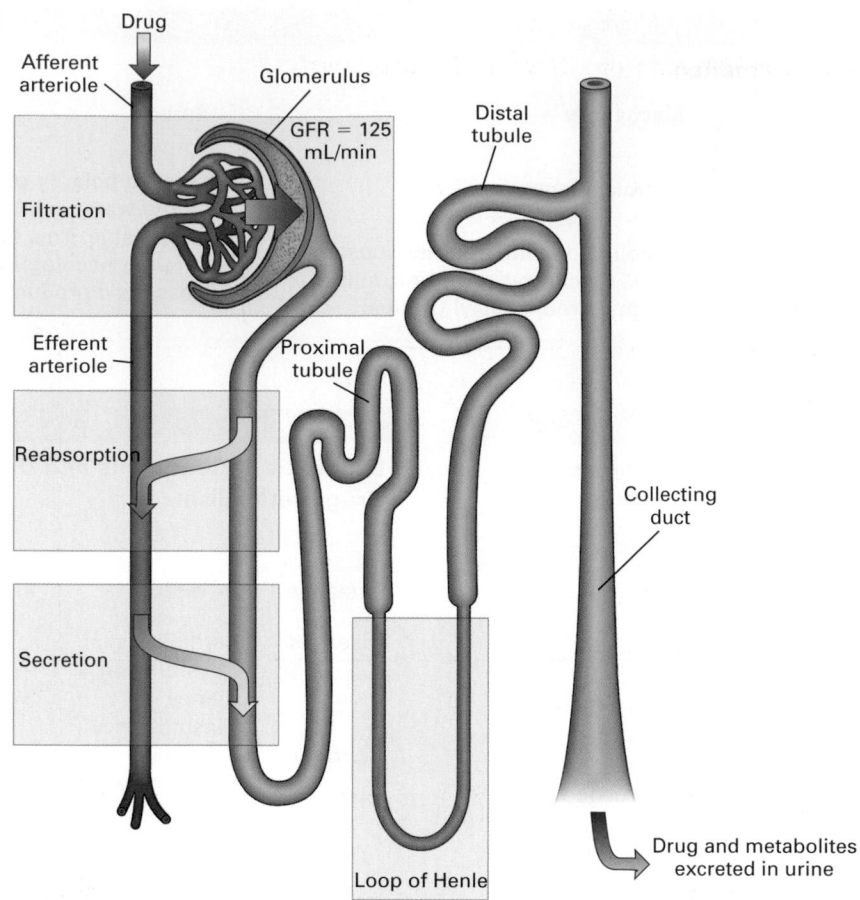

FIG. 2-6 Renal drug excretion. The primary processes involved in drug excretion and the approximate location where these processes take place in the kidney are illustrated. *GFR*, glomerular filtration rate.

the bowel. Most drugs are metabolized in the liver by various mechanisms. Therefore, by the time most drugs reach the kidneys, they have undergone extensive biotransformation, where the drug is converted to a less active form, and only a relatively small fraction of the original drug is excreted as the original compound. Other drugs may bypass hepatic metabolism and reach the kidneys in their original form. Drugs that have been metabolized by the liver become more polar and water-soluble. This change makes their elimination by the kidney much easier because the urinary tract is water-based. The kidneys are also capable of metabolizing various drugs, although usually to a lesser extent than the liver.

The actual act of kidney excretion is accomplished through glomerular filtration, active tubular reabsorption, and active tubular secretion. Free (unbound) water-soluble drugs and metabolites go through passive glomerular filtration. Many substances present in the nephrons go through active reabsorption and are taken back up into the circulation and transported away from the kidney. This process is an attempt by the body to retain needed substances. Some substances may also be secreted into the nephron from the vasculature surrounding it. The processes of filtration, reabsorption, and

secretion in urinary elimination are shown in Figure 2-6. Chronic kidney disease affects renal drug elimination. Certain drugs may require dosage adjustments (e.g., dose reductions or less frequent dosing) based on creatinine clearance or glomerular filtration rate.

The excretion of drugs by the intestines is another common route of elimination. This process is referred to as *biliary excretion*. Drugs eliminated by this route are taken up by the liver, released into the bile, and eliminated in the feces. Once certain drugs, such as fat-soluble drugs, are in the bile, they may be reabsorbed into the bloodstream, returned to the liver, and again secreted into the bile. This process is called *enterohepatic recirculation*. Enterohepatically recirculated drugs persist in the body for much longer periods. Less common routes of elimination are the lungs and the sweat, salivary, and mammary glands.

Half-Life

Another pharmacokinetic variable is the **half-life** of a drug. By definition, the half-life is the time required for serum drug levels to be reduced by one-half (50%) during the elimination phase. It is a measure of the rate at which the drug is eliminated from the body. For instance, if the peak level of a particular drug is 100 mg/L and the

TABLE 2-7

Example of a Drug Half-Life Viewed from Different Perspectives

Perspectives	Changing Values					
Hours after peak concentration	0	8	16	24	32	40
Drug concentration (mg/L)	100 (peak)	50	25	12.5	6.25	3.125 (trough)
Number of half-lives	0	1	2	3	4	5
Percentage of drug removed	0	50	75	88	94	97

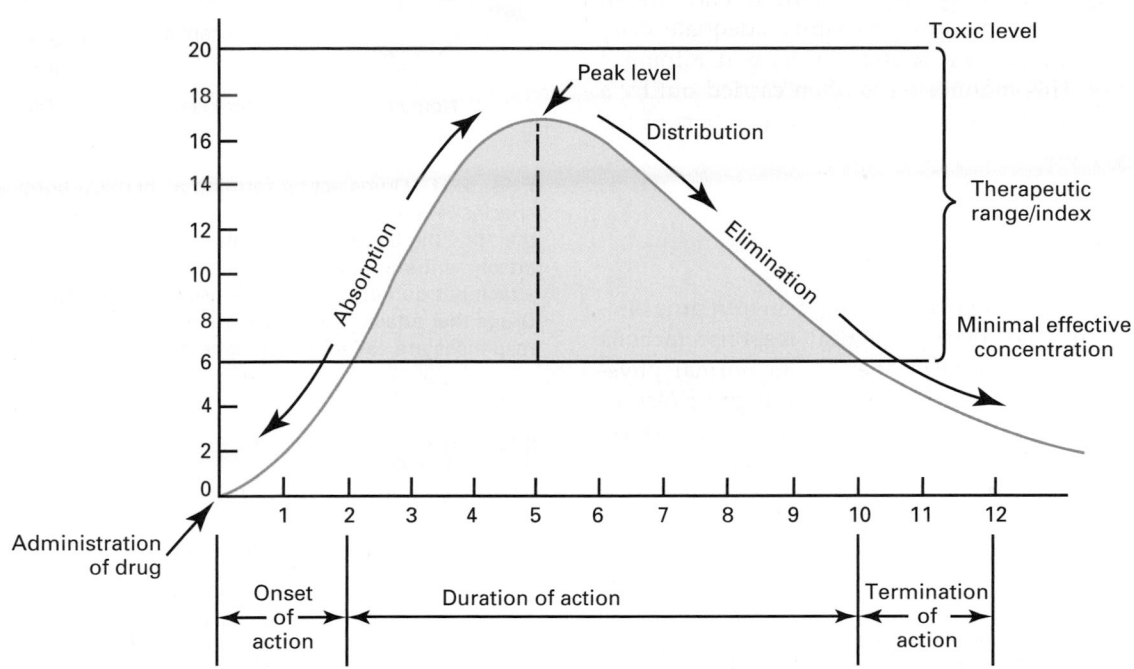

FIG. 2-7 Characteristics of drug effects and relationship to the therapeutic window. (From McKenry, L. M., Tessier, E., & Hogan, M. (2006). *Mosby's pharmacology in nursing* (22nd ed.). St. Louis: Mosby.)

measured drug level in 8 hours is 50 mg/L, then the estimated half-life for that drug is 8 hours. The concept of drug half-life viewed from several different perspectives is shown in Table 2-7.

After about five half-lives, most drugs are considered to be effectively removed from the body. At that time approximately 97% of the drug has been eliminated, and what little amount remains is too small to have either therapeutic or toxic effects.

The concept of half-life is clinically useful for determining when a steady state will be reached in a patient taking a particular drug. **Steady state** refers to the physiological state in which the amount of drug removed via elimination (e.g., kidney clearance) is equal to the amount of drug absorbed with each dose. This physiological plateau phenomenon typically occurs after four to five half-lives of administration of a drug. Therefore, if a drug has an extremely long half-life, it will take much longer for the drug to reach steady-state blood levels. Once steady-state blood levels have been reached, there are consistent levels of drug in the body that correlate with maximum therapeutic benefits.

Onset, Peak, and Duration

The pharmacokinetic terms *absorption*, *distribution*, *metabolism*, and *excretion* are all used to describe the movement of drugs through the body. The term *drug actions* refers to the processes involved in the interaction between a drug and a cell (e.g., a drug's action on a receptor). The terms *onset*, *peak*, *duration*, and *trough* are used to describe **drug effects**. *Peak* and *trough* are also used to describe drug concentrations, which are usually measured from blood samples.

A drug's **onset of action** is the time required for the drug to elicit a therapeutic response. A drug's **peak effect** is the time required for it to reach its maximal therapeutic response. Physiologically, this point corresponds to increasing drug concentrations at the site of action. The **duration of action** of a drug is the length of time that its concentration is sufficient (without more doses) to elicit a therapeutic response. These concepts are illustrated in Figure 2-7.

The length of time until the onset, peak of action, and duration of action play an important part in determining the **peak level** (highest blood level) and **trough level** (lowest blood level) of a drug. If the peak blood level is too high, then drug **toxicity** may occur. The toxicity may be mild, such as intensification of the effects of the given drug (e.g., excessive sedation resulting from overdose of a drug with sedative properties). However, it can also be severe (e.g., damage to vital organs due to excessive drug exposure). If the trough blood level is too low, then the drug may not be at therapeutic levels to produce a response. (A common example is antibiotic drug therapy with aminoglycoside antibiotics; see Chapter 44). In **therapeutic drug monitoring**, peak (highest) and trough (lowest) values are measured to verify adequate drug exposure, maximize therapeutic effects, and minimize drug toxicity. This monitoring is often carried out by a clinical pharmacist working with other members of the health care team.

PHARMACODYNAMICS

Pharmacodynamics is the relationship between drug concentrations and the pharmacological response (actions of the drug). Drug-induced changes in normal physiological functions are explained by the principles of pharmacodynamics. A positive change in a faulty physiological system is called a **therapeutic effect** of a drug. Such an effect is the goal of drug therapy. Understanding the pharmacodynamic characteristics of a drug can aid in assessing the drug's therapeutic effect.

Mechanism of Action

Drugs can produce actions (therapeutic effects) in several ways. The effects of a particular drug depend on the cells or tissue targeted by the drug. Once the drug is at the site of action, it can modify (increase or decrease) the rate at which that cell or tissue functions, or it can modify the strength of function of that cell or tissue. A drug cannot, however, cause a cell or tissue to perform a function that is not part of its natural physiology.

Drugs can exert their actions in three basic ways: through receptors, enzymes, and nonselective interactions. It should also be noted that not all mechanisms of action have been identified for all drugs. Thus, a drug may be said to have an unknown or unclear mechanism of action, even though it has observable therapeutic effects in the body.

Receptor Interactions

A **receptor** can be defined as a reactive site on the surface or inside of a cell. If the mechanism of action of a drug involves a receptor interaction, then the molecular structure of the drug is critical. Drug–receptor interaction is the joining of the drug molecule with a reactive site on the surface of a cell or tissue. Most commonly, this site is a protein structure within the cell membrane. Once a drug binds to and interacts with the receptor, a pharmacological response is produced (Figure 2-8). The degree to which a drug attaches and binds with a receptor is called its *affinity*. The drug with the best "fit" and

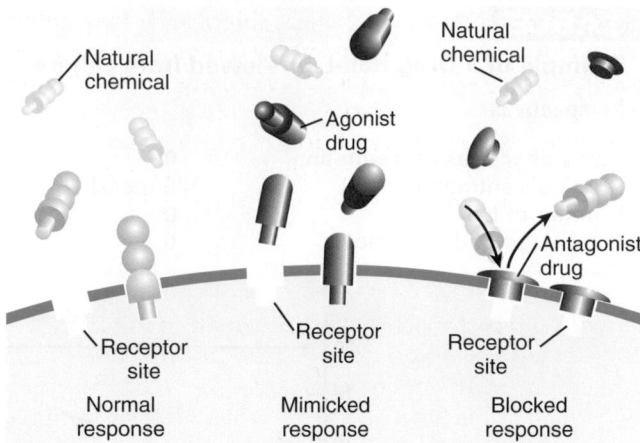

FIG. 2-8 Drugs act by forming a chemical bond with specific receptor sites, similar to a key and lock—the better the "fit," the better the response. Drugs with complete attachment and response are called **agonists**. Drugs that attach but do not elicit a response are called **antagonists**. Drugs that attach, elicit some response, and also block other responses are called *partial agonists* or *agonist–antagonists*.

TABLE 2-8

Drug–Receptor Interactions

Drug Type	Action
Agonist	Drug binds to the receptor; there is a response.
Partial agonist (agonist–antagonist)	Drug binds to the receptor; the response is diminished compared with the response elicited by an agonist.
Antagonist	Drug binds to the receptor; there is no response. Drug prevents binding of agonists.
Competitive antagonist	Drug competes with the agonist for binding to the receptor. If it binds, there is no response.
Noncompetitive antagonist	Drug combines with different parts of the receptor and inactivates it; agonist then has no effect.

strongest affinity for the receptor will elicit the greatest response from the cell or tissue. A drug becomes bound to the receptor through the formation of chemical bonds between the receptor on the cell and the active site on the drug molecule. Drugs interact with receptors in different ways, by either eliciting or blocking a physiological response. Table 2-8 describes the different types of drug–receptor interaction.

Enzyme Interactions

Enzymes are substances that catalyze nearly every biochemical reaction in a cell. Drugs can produce effects by interacting with these enzyme systems. For a drug to alter a physiological response in this way, it may either inhibit (more common) or enhance (less common) the action of a specific enzyme. This process is called *selective interaction*. Drug–enzyme interaction occurs when the drug chemically binds to an enzyme molecule in such a way that it alters (inhibits or enhances) the enzyme's interaction with its normal target molecules in the body.

Nonselective Interactions

Drugs with nonspecific mechanisms of action do not interact with receptors or enzymes. Instead, their main targets are cell membranes and various cellular processes such as metabolic activities. These drugs can either physically interfere with or chemically alter cellular structures or processes. Some cancer drugs and antibiotics have this mechanism of action. By incorporating themselves into the normal metabolic process, they cause a defect in the final product or state. This defect may be an improperly formed cell wall that results in cell death through cell lysis, or it may be the lack of a necessary energy substrate, which leads to cell starvation and death.

PHARMACOTHERAPEUTICS

Before drug therapy is initiated, an end point or expected outcome of therapy should be established. This desired therapeutic outcome is patient specific, established in collaboration with the patient, and if appropriate, determined with other members of the health care team. Outcomes need to be clearly defined and must be either measurable or observable by patient monitoring. Outcome goals must be realistic and prioritized so that drug therapy begins with interventions that are essential to the patient's well-being. Examples include curing a disease, eliminating or reducing a pre-existing symptom, arresting or slowing a disease process, preventing a disease or other unwanted condition, or otherwise improving quality of life.

Patient therapy assessment is the process by which a health care provider integrates knowledge of medical and drug-related facts with information about a specific patient's medical and social history. Items to be considered in the assessment are drugs currently used (prescription, over-the-counter, natural health products, and illicit drugs), pregnancy and breastfeeding status, and concurrent illnesses that could contraindicate initiation of a given medication. A **contraindication** for a medication is any patient condition, especially a disease state, that makes the use of the particular medication dangerous for the patient. Careful attention to this assessment process helps to ensure an optimal therapeutic plan. The implementation of a treatment plan can involve several types and combinations of therapies. The type of therapy can be categorized as acute, maintenance, supplemental (or replacement), palliative, supportive, prophylactic, or empirical.

Types of Therapy
Acute Therapy

Acute therapy often involves more intensive drug therapy and is implemented in patients who are acutely ill (those with a rapid onset of illness) or even critically ill. It is often needed to sustain life or treat disease. Examples are the administration of vasopressors to maintain blood pressure and cardiac output after open heart surgery, the use of volume expanders for a patient who is in shock, and intensive chemotherapy for a patient with newly diagnosed cancer.

Maintenance Therapy

Maintenance therapy typically does not eradicate problems the patient may already have but does prevent progression of a disease or condition. It is used for the treatment of chronic illnesses such as hypertension. In the latter case, maintenance therapy maintains the patient's blood pressure within target limits, which prevents certain end-organ damage. Another example of maintenance therapy is the use of oral contraceptives for birth control.

Supplemental Therapy

Supplemental (or replacement) therapy supplies the body with a substance needed to maintain normal function. This substance may be needed because it cannot be made by the body or because it is produced in insufficient quantity. Examples are the administration of insulin to patient with diabetes and of iron to patient with iron-deficiency anemia.

Palliative Therapy

The goal of palliative therapy is to make the patient as comfortable as possible. Palliative therapy focuses on providing patients with relief from the symptoms, pain, and stress of a serious illness. The goal is to improve quality of life for both the patient and the family. It is typically used in the end stages of an illness, when all attempts at curative therapy have failed; however, it can be provided along with curative treatment. Examples are the use of high-dose opioid analgesics to relieve pain in the final stages of cancer.

Supportive Therapy

Supportive therapy maintains the integrity of body functions while the patient is recovering from illness or trauma. Examples are provision of fluids and electrolytes to prevent dehydration in a patient with influenza who is vomiting and has diarrhea, and administration of fluids, volume expanders, or blood products to a patient who has lost blood during surgery.

Prophylactic Therapy and Empirical Therapy

Prophylactic therapy is drug therapy provided to prevent illness or other undesirable outcome during planned events. An example is the administration of disease-specific vaccines to individuals travelling to geographic areas where a given disease is known to be endemic.

Empirical therapy is based on clinical probabilities. It involves administration of a drug when a certain pathologic condition has an uncertain but high likelihood of occurrence based on the patient's initial presenting symptoms. A common example is use of antibiotics active against the organism most commonly associated with a specific infection before the results of the culture and sensitivity reports are available.

Monitoring

Once the appropriate therapy has been implemented, the effectiveness of that therapy—that is, the clinical response of the patient to the therapy—must be evaluated. Evaluating the clinical response requires familiarity with both the drug's intended therapeutic action (beneficial effects) and its unintended possible **adverse effects** (predictable adverse drug reactions). Examples of monitoring include observing for the therapeutic effect of reduced blood pressure following administration of antihypertensive drugs and observing for the toxic effect of leukopenia after administering antineoplastic (cancer chemotherapy) drugs. Another example is performing a pain assessment after giving pain medication. It should be noted that this text generally highlights only the most common adverse effects of a given drug, but it may have many other, less commonly reported adverse effects. Always keep in mind that patients may sometimes experience less common and less readily identifiable adverse drug effects. Consult comprehensive references, a pharmacist, or poison and drug information centre staff whenever there is uncertainty regarding adverse effects that a patient may be experiencing.

All drugs are potentially toxic and can have cumulative effects. Recognizing these toxic effects and knowing their manifestations are integral components of the monitoring process. A drug can accumulate when it is absorbed more quickly than it is eliminated or when it is administered before the previous dose has been metabolized or cleared from the body. Knowledge of the organs responsible for metabolizing and eliminating a drug, combined with knowledge of how a particular drug is metabolized and excreted, enables the nurse to anticipate problems and treat them appropriately if they occur.

Therapeutic Index

The ratio of a drug's toxic level to the level that provides therapeutic benefits is referred to as the drug's **therapeutic index.** The safety of a particular drug therapy is determined by this index. A low therapeutic index means that the difference between a therapeutically active dose and a toxic dose is small. This type of drug has a greater likelihood than other drugs of causing an adverse reaction, and therefore its use requires closer monitoring. Examples of such drugs are warfarin and digoxin. In contrast, a drug with a high therapeutic index, such as amoxicillin, is rarely associated with overdose events.

Drug Concentration

All drugs reach a certain concentration in the blood. Drug concentrations can be an important tool for evaluating the clinical response to drug therapy. Certain drug levels are associated with therapeutic responses, whereas other drug levels are associated with toxic effects. Toxic drug levels are typically seen when the body's normal mechanisms for metabolizing and excreting drugs are compromised. This commonly occurs when liver and kidney functions are impaired or when the liver or kidneys are immature (as in neonates). Dosage adjustments should be made in these patients to appropriately accommodate their impaired metabolism and excretion.

Patient's Condition

Another patient-specific factor to be considered is the patient's weight (e.g., obese or weakness or wasting of the body), presence of a critical illness, and the patient's concurrent diseases or other medical conditions. A patient's response to a drug may vary greatly depending on physiological and psychological demands. Disease of any kind, infection, cardiovascular function, and gastrointestinal function are just a few of the physiological elements that can alter a patient's therapeutic response. Stress, depression, and anxiety can also be important psychological factors affecting response.

Tolerance and Dependence

To provide optimal drug therapy, it is important to understand and differentiate between tolerance and dependence. **Tolerance** is a decreasing response to repeated drug doses. **Dependence** is a physiological or psychological need for a drug. Physical dependence is the physiological need for a drug to avoid physical withdrawal symptoms (e.g., tachycardia in a patient dependent on opioids). Psychological dependence, also known as *addiction*, is the obsessive desire for the effects of a drug. Addiction often involves the recreational use of drugs such as benzodiazepines, narcotics, and amphetamines but can also occur as a result of chronic persistent pain. See Chapter 18 for further discussion of dependence and addiction.

Interactions

Drugs may interact with other drugs, with foods, or with agents administered as part of laboratory tests. Knowledge of drug interactions is vital for the appropriate monitoring of drug therapy. The more drugs a patient receives, the more likely that a drug interaction will occur. This is especially true in older adults, who typically have an increased sensitivity to drug effects and are receiving several medications. In addition, over-the-counter medications and natural health products can interact significantly with prescribed medications. Food also can interact significantly with certain drugs. See Table 2-9 for the most common food and drug interactions.

Alteration of the action of one drug by another is referred to as **drug interaction.** A drug interaction can

TABLE 2-9

Examples of Drug Interactions and Their Effects on Pharmacokinetics

Pharmacokinetic Phase	Drug	Mechanism	Result
Absorption	Antacid with levofloxacin hemihydrate	Antacids bind to the levofloxacin hemihydrate, preventing adequate absorption	Decreased effectiveness of levofloxacin hemihydrate, resulting from decreased blood levels (harmful)
Distribution	warfarin with amiodarone	Both drugs compete for protein-binding sites	Higher levels of free (unbound) warfarin and amiodarone, which increases actions of both drugs (harmful)
Metabolism	erythromycin with cyclosporine	Both drugs compete for the same liver enzymes	Decreased metabolism of cyclosporine, possibly resulting in toxic levels of cyclosporine (harmful)
Excretion	amoxicillin with probenecid	Inhibits the secretion of amoxicillin into the kidneys	Elevates and prolongs the plasma levels of amoxicillin (can be beneficial)

either increase or decrease the actions of one or both of the involved drugs. Drug interactions can be either beneficial or harmful. Numerous drug interactions can occur and have been reported. Please note that only those drug interactions that are considered to be significant—with at least a good probability of occurring—or those that require dosage or therapy adjustment are discussed in this textbook. An authoritative resource may be used as a means of exploring all possible drug interactions.

Concurrently administered drugs may interact with each other and alter the pharmacokinetics of one another during any of the four phases of pharmacokinetics: absorption, distribution, metabolism, or excretion. Table 2-9 provides examples of drug interactions during each of these phases. Most commonly, drug interactions occur when there is competition between two drugs for metabolizing enzymes, such as the cytochrome P450 enzymes listed in Table 2-5. As a result, the speed of metabolism of one or both drugs may be enhanced or reduced. This change in metabolism of one or both drugs can lead to subtherapeutic or toxic drug actions.

Many terms are used to categorize drug interactions. When two drugs with similar actions are given together they can have **additive effects**. This means that the combined effects of the drugs combine such that if two drugs of similar action are administered at the same time, the action of one plus the action of the other results in the total effect of both drugs being given. This can be represented by 1 + 1 = 2 (summation of effects). Examples are the many combinations of analgesic products, such as acetylsalicylic acid and opioid combinations (acetylsalicylic acid and codeine) and acetaminophen and opioid combinations (acetaminophen and oxycodone). The total analgesic effect of both drugs results. Often drugs are used together for their additive effects so that smaller doses of each drug can be given.

Synergistic effects occur when the action of one drug enhances the action of another. The two drugs administered together interact in such a way that their combined effects are greater than the sum of the effects for each drug given alone (1 + 1 = greater than 2). The combination of hydrochlorothiazide with lisinopril for the treatment of hypertension is one example. It is important to remember that synergistic effects can also result in dangerous effects; for example, the combination of alcohol and acetaminophen may result in liver damage.

Antagonistic effects are said to occur when the combination of two drugs results in drug effects that are less than the sum of the effects for each drug given separately (1 + 1 = less than 2). An example of this type of interaction occurs when the antibiotic ciprofloxacin is given simultaneously with antacids, vitamins, iron, or dairy products. These drugs reduce the absorption of ciprofloxacin and lead to decreased effectiveness of the antibiotic.

Incompatibility is a term most commonly used to describe parenteral drugs. Drug incompatibility occurs when two parenteral drugs or solutions are mixed together and the result is a chemical deterioration of one or both of the drugs. The combination of two such drugs usually produces a precipitate, haziness, or colour change in the solution. Before administering any intravenous medication, the nurse must always inspect the bag for precipitate. If the solution appears cloudy or if visible flecks are seen, the bag must not be given to the patient and must be discarded. An example of incompatible drugs is the combination of parenteral furosemide and heparin sodium.

Adverse Drug Events

The recognition of the potential hazards and actual detrimental effects of medication use is a topic that continues to receive much attention in the literature. This focus has contributed to an increasing body of knowledge regarding this topic as well as the development of new terminology. Health care institutions are also under increasing pressure to develop effective strategies for preventing adverse effects of drugs.

Adverse drug event (ADE) is a broad term for any undesirable occurrence involving medications. A similarly broad term seen in the literature is *drug* *misadventure.* Patient outcomes associated with ADEs vary from no effects or mild discomfort to life-threatening complications, permanent disability, disfigurement, or death. ADEs can be preventable (see discussion of medication errors [MEs] later in Chapter 6) or nonpreventable. Fortunately, many ADEs result in no measurable patient harm. ADEs can be both external and internal. The most common causes of ADEs external to the patient are errors by caregivers (both professional and nonprofessional) and malfunctioning of equipment (e.g., intravenous infusion pumps). An ADE can be internal, or patient induced, such as when a patient fails to take medication as prescribed or drinks alcoholic beverages that he was advised not to consume while taking a given medication. An impending ADE that is noticed before it actually occurs is considered a potential ADE (and appropriate steps should be taken to avoid such a "near miss" in the future). A less common situation, but one still worth mentioning, is an adverse drug withdrawal event. This is an adverse outcome associated with discontinuation of drug therapy, such as hypertension caused by abruptly discontinuing blood pressure medication or return of infection caused by stopping antibiotic therapy too soon.

The two most common broad categories of ADEs are medication errors and adverse drug reactions. A **medication error (ME)** is a preventable situation in which there is a compromise in the Ten Rights of medication use: right patient, right drug, right time, right route, right dose, right documentation, right reason, right patient education, right to refuse, right assessment or right evaluation. MEs are more common than adverse drug reactions. MEs occur during the prescribing, dispensing, administering, or monitoring of drug therapy. These four phases are collectively known as the **medication use process.** See Chapter 6 for further discussion of MEs.

An **adverse drug reaction (ADR)** (see Chapter 6) is any reaction to a drug that is unexpected and undesirable and occurs at therapeutic drug dosages. ADRs may or may not be caused by MEs. ADRs may result in hospital admission, prolongation of hospital stay, change in drug therapy, initiation of supportive treatment, or complication of a patient's disease state. ADRs are caused by processes inside the patient's body. They may or may not be preventable, depending on the situation. Mild ADRs (e.g., drug adverse effects—see later in this chapter) usually do not require a change in the patient's drug therapy or other interventions. More severe ADRs, however, are likely to require changes to a patient's drug regimen. Severe ADRs can be permanently or significantly disabling, life threatening, or fatal. They may require or prolong hospitalization, lead to organ damage (e.g., to the liver, kidneys, bone marrow, skin), cause congenital anomalies, or require specific interventions to prevent permanent impairment or tissue damage.

ADRs that are specific to particular drug groups are discussed in the corresponding drug chapters in this book. Four general categories are discussed here: pharmacological reaction, hypersensitivity (allergic) reaction, idiosyncratic reaction, and drug interaction.

A pharmacological reaction is an extension of the drug's normal effects in the body. For example, a drug that is used to lower blood pressure in a patient causes a pharmacological ADR when it lowers the blood pressure to the point at which the patient becomes unconscious.

Pharmacological reactions that result in adverse effects are predictable, well-known ADRs resulting in minor or no changes in patient management. They have predictable frequency and intensity, and their occurrence is related to the dose. They also usually resolve with a change in dose or discontinuation of drug therapy.

An **allergic reaction** (also known as a *hypersensitivity reaction*) involves the patient's immune system. Immune system proteins known as *immunoglobulins* recognize the drug molecule, its **metabolite**(s), or another ingredient in a drug formulation as a dangerous foreign substance. At this point, an immune response may occur in which immunoglobulin proteins bind to the drug substance in an attempt to neutralize the drug. Various chemical mediators, such as histamine, as well as cytokines and other inflammatory substances (e.g., prostaglandins [Chapter 38]) usually are released during this process. This response can range from mild reactions such as skin erythema or mild rash to severe or even life-threatening reactions such as constriction of bronchial airways and tachycardia.

It can be assumed throughout this textbook that use of any drug is contraindicated if the patient has a known allergy to that specific drug product. Allergy information may be reported by patients as part of their history or may be observed by health care providers during a patient encounter. In either case, every effort must be made to document as fully as possible the name of the drug product and the degree and details of the adverse reaction that occurred—for example, "Penicillin; skin rash, pruritus" or "Penicillin; urticaria and anaphylactic shock requiring emergency intervention."

In more extreme cases of disease or injury (e.g., cancer, snakebite), it may be deemed reasonable to administer a given drug in spite of a reported allergic or other adverse reaction. In such cases, the patient will likely be premedicated with additional medications (e.g., acetaminophen [Tylenol®], diphenhydramine [Benadryl®], prednisone) in an attempt to control any adverse reactions that may occur.

An **idiosyncratic reaction** is not the result of a known pharmacological property of a drug or patient allergy but instead occurs unexpectedly in a particular patient. Such a reaction is a genetically determined abnormal response to ordinary doses of a drug. The study of such traits, which are solely revealed by drug administration, is called **pharmacogenetics** (see Chapter 5). Idiosyncratic drug reactions are usually caused by a deficiency or excess of drug-metabolizing enzymes. Many pharmacogenomic disorders exist, for example, **glucose-6-phosphate dehydrogenase (G6PD) deficiency.**

People who lack proper levels of G6PD have idiosyncratic reactions to a wide range of drugs (see Ethnocultural Implications box). There are more than 80 variations of the disease, and all produce some degree of drug-induced hemolysis.

The final type of ADR is due to drug interaction. As described earlier, drug interaction occurs when the simultaneous presence of two (or more) drugs in the body produces an unwanted effect. This unwanted effect can result when one drug either accentuates or reduces the effects of another drug. Some drug interactions are intentional and beneficial (see Table 2-9). However, most clinically significant drug interactions are harmful. Drug interactions specific to particular drugs are discussed in detail in the chapters dealing with those drugs.

Other Drug Effects

Other drug-related effects that must be considered during therapy are teratogenic, mutagenic, and carcinogenic effects. These can result in devastating patient outcomes and can be prevented in many instances by appropriate monitoring.

Teratogenic effects of drugs or other chemicals result in structural defects in the fetus. Compounds that produce such effects are called *teratogens*. Prenatal development involves a delicate program of interrelated embryological events. Any significant disruption in this process of embryogenesis can have a teratogenic effect. Drugs that are capable of crossing the placenta can cause **drug-induced teratogenesis**. Drugs administered during pregnancy can produce different types of congenital anomalies. The period during which the fetus is most vulnerable to teratogenic effects begins with the third week of development and usually ends after the third month. Chapter 4 describes the Health Canada safety classification for drugs used by pregnant women.

Mutagenic effects are permanent changes in the genetic composition of living organisms and consist of alterations in the chromosome structure, the number of chromosomes, or the genetic code of the deoxyribonucleic acid (DNA) molecule. Drugs that are capable of inducing mutations are called *mutagens*. Radiation, viruses, chemicals (e.g., industrial chemicals such as benzene), and drugs can all act as mutagenic agents in human beings. Drugs that affect genetic processes are active primarily during cell reproduction (mitosis).

Carcinogenic effects are the cancer-causing effects of drugs, other chemicals, radiation, and viruses. Agents that produce such effects are called *carcinogens*. Some exogenous causes of cancer are listed in Box 2-3.

PHARMACOGNOSY

Plants are an important and long-established resource of preparations used in medicine. *Pharmacognosy* involves the process of identifying medicinal plants and their ingredients, pharmacological effects, and therapeutic efficacy. Although many drugs in current use are synthetically derived, most were first isolated in nature. For example, almost all major groups of wild plants in Canada have edible members that are reported to have been used by indigenous people. Algae (e.g., seaweed), fungi (e.g., mushrooms), and roots are commonly used for their medicinal purposes. The four main sources for drugs are plants, animals, minerals, and laboratory synthesis. Plants provide many weak acids and weak bases (alkaloids) that are useful and potent drugs. Alkaloids are more common, including atropine (belladonna plant), caffeine (coffee bean), and nicotine (tobacco leaf). Animals are the source of many hormone drugs. Conjugated estrogens are derived from the urine of pregnant mares, hence the drug trade name Premarin. *Equine* is the term used

---

BOX 2-3
Exogenous Carcinogens

Dietary customs
Drug misuse
Carcinogenic drugs
Workplace chemicals
Radiation
Environmental pollution
Food-processing procedures
Food-production procedures
Oncogenic viruses
Smoking

 ## ETHNOCULTURAL IMPLICATIONS

Glucose-6-Phosphate Dehydrogenase Deficiency

Globally, glucose-6-phosphate dehydrogenase (G6PD) deficiency is the most common enzyme defect. It is found predominately in African, Middle Eastern, and South Asian populations. G6PD is an enzyme found in abundant amounts in the tissues of most individuals. It reduces the risk of hemolysis of red blood cells when they are exposed to oxidizing drugs such as acetylsalicylic acid. G6PD deficiency is inherited as an X-linked, recessive condition; consequently, the condition usually occurs in boys. Drugs to avoid in patients with G6PD deficiency are nitrofurantoin, primaquine, probenecid, and sulfonamides.

for any horse-derived drug. Insulin comes from two sources: pigs (porcine) and humans. Human insulin is now far more commonly used than animal insulins thanks to the use of recombinant DNA techniques. Heparin sodium is another commonly used drug that is derived from pigs (porcine heparin). Some common mineral sources of currently used drugs are salicylic acid, aluminum hydroxide, and sodium chloride.

PHARMACOECONOMICS

Pharmacoeconomics is the study of the economic factors influencing the cost of drug therapy. One example is performing a cost–benefit analysis of one antibiotic versus another when competing drugs are considered for inclusion in a hospital formulary. Such studies typically examine treatment outcomes data (e.g., how many patients recovered and how soon) in relation to the comparative total costs of treatment with the drugs in question.

TOXICOLOGY

The study of poisons and unwanted responses to both drugs and other chemicals is known as *toxicology*. Toxicology is the science of the adverse effects of chemicals on living organisms. Clinical toxicology deals specifically with the care of patients who have been poisoned. Poisoning can result from a variety of causes, ranging from drug overdose to ingestion of household cleaning agents to snakebite. Poison control centres are health care institutions equipped with sufficient personnel and information resources to recommend appropriate treatment for poisoning. They are usually staffed with specially trained pharmacists, nurses, and physicians who triage incoming calls and refer complex cases to clinical toxicologists.

Effective treatment for poisoning is based on a system of priorities, the first of which is to preserve the patient's vital functions by maintaining airway, ventilation, and circulation. The second priority is to prevent absorption of the toxic agent or speed its elimination from the body using one or more clinical methods available. Several common poisons and their specific antidotes are listed in Table 2-10.

EVIDENCE-INFORMED PRACTICE

In this information era, nurses encounter a plethora of health conditions and possible treatments, which include pharmacotherapeutics. In order to stay informed and current, **evidence-informed practice (EIP)**, also referred to as *evidence-based practice*, has emerged in the past 10 years as the "gold standard" for using current, valid, and relevant information when making clinical decisions. When applying EIP, results include more accurate diagnoses, effective and efficient interventions, and improved patient outcomes. Evidence derived from systematic reviews of randomized clinical trials (RCTs) is often considered the strongest level of evidence; however, descriptive and qualitative studies as well as expert opinions may be considered when making decisions. The development of clinical practice guidelines based on scientific evidence helps to integrate the best research evidence into practice. Within this textbook, Evidence in Practice boxes will be used to identify current, clinically relevant research evidence about specific prescription drugs as well as natural health products.

SUMMARY

A thorough understanding of pharmacological principles of pharmacokinetics, pharmacodynamics, pharmacotherapeutics, and toxicology is essential in drug therapy and for safe, quality nursing practice. Medications may be helpful in treating disease, but unless the nurse has an adequate, up-to-date knowledge base and clinical skills and engages in critical thinking and good decision making, any treatment may become harmful. Application of pharmacological principles enables the nurse to provide safe and effective drug therapy while always acting on behalf of the patient and respecting the patient's rights. Nursing considerations associated with various routes of drug administration are summarized in Table 2-3.

TABLE 2-10	
Common Causes of Poisoning and Their Antidotes	
Substance	**Antidote**
acetaminophen	acetylcysteine
Organophosphates (e.g., insecticides)	atropine
Tricyclic antidepressants, quinidine	sodium bicarbonate
Iron salts	deferoxamine
digoxin and other cardiac glycosides	digoxin antibodies
Ethylene glycol (e.g., automotive antifreeze solution), methanol	Ethanol (same as alcohol used for drinking), administered intravenously
Benzodiapenes	flumazenil
β-blockers	glucagon
Opiates, opioid drugs	naloxone
carbon monoxide (by inhalation)	Oxygen (at high concentrations), known as bariatric therapy

KEY POINTS

❖ The following definitions related to drug therapy are important to remember: *pharmacology*—the study or science of drugs; *pharmacokinetics*—the study of drug distribution among various body compartments after a drug has entered the body, including the phases of absorption, distribution, metabolism, and excretion; *pharmaceutics*—the science of dosage form design.

❖ The nurse's role in drug therapy and the nursing process is more than just memorizing the names of drugs, their uses, and associated interventions. It involves a thorough comprehension of all aspects of pharmaceutics, pharmacokinetics, and pharmacodynamics and the sound application of this

drug knowledge to a variety of clinical situations. Refer to Chapter 1 for more detailed discussion of drug therapy as it relates to the nursing process.

❖ Drug actions are related to the pharmacological, pharmaceutical, pharmacokinetic, and pharmacodynamic properties of a given medication, and each of these has a specific influence on the overall effects produced by the drug in a patient.

❖ Selection of the route of administration is based on patient variables and the specific characteristics of a drug.

❖ Nursing considerations vary depending on the drug as well as the route of administration.

EXAMINATION REVIEW QUESTIONS

1. An older woman took a prescription medicine to help her to sleep; however, she felt restless all night and did not sleep at all. The nurse recognizes that this woman has experienced which type of reaction or effect?
   a. Allergic reaction
   b. Idiosyncratic reaction
   c. Mutagenic effect
   d. Synergistic effect

2. While caring for a patient with cirrhosis or hepatitis, the nurse knows that abnormalities in which phase of pharmacokinetics may occur?
   a. Absorption
   b. Distribution
   c. Metabolism
   d. Excretion

3. A patient who has advanced cancer is receiving opioid medications around the clock to "keep him comfortable" as he nears the end of his life. Which term best describes this type of therapy?
   a. Palliative therapy
   b. Maintenance therapy
   c. Supportive therapy
   d. Supplemental therapy

4. The nurse is giving medications to a patient in heart failure. The intravenous route is chosen instead of the intramuscular route. Which patient factors most influences the decision about which route to use?
   a. Altered biliary function
   b. Increased glomerular filtration
   c. Reduced liver metabolism
   d. Diminished circulation

5. A patient has just received a prescription for an enteric-coated stool softener. When teaching the patient, the nurse should include which statement?
   a. "Take the tablet with 60 to 90 mL of orange juice."
   b. "Avoid taking all other medications with any enteric-coated tablet."
   c. "Crush the tablet before swallowing if you have problems with swallowing."
   d. "Be sure to swallow the tablet whole without chewing it."

6. Each statement describes a phase of pharmacokinetics. Put the statements in order, with 1 indicating the phase that occurs first and 4 indicating the phase that occurs last.
   a. Enzymes in the liver transform the drug into an inactive metabolite.
   b. Drug metabolites are secreted through passive glomerular filtration into the renal tubules.
   c. A drug binds to the plasma protein albumin and circulates through the body.
   d. A drug moves from the intestinal lumen into the mesenteric blood system.

7. A drug that delivers 500 mg has a half-life of 4 hours. How many milligrams of drug will remain in the body after 1 half-life?

Answers: 1. b, **2.** c, **3.** a, **4.** d, **5.** d, **6.** a = 3, b = 4, c = 2, d = 1, **7.** 250 mg

CRITICAL THINKING ACTIVITIES

1. A patient tells the nurse during the assessment that he experiences some "strange" problem with drug metabolism that he was born with, so he is not to take certain medications. What type of disorder is this patient referring to, and what are the problems it can cause in the patient when specific medications are taken? What is the nurse's priority action when a patient shares this information?

2. Charles is admitted to the trauma unit with multisystem injuries from an automobile accident. He arrived at the unit with multiple abnormal findings, including shock from blood loss, decreased cardiac output, and urinary output of less than 30 mL/hr. Which route of administration would you expect to be the best choice for this patient? Explain your answer.

3. You are administering medications to a patient who had an enteral tube inserted 2 days earlier for continuous feedings. As you review the medication list, you note that one drug is an enteric-coated tablet ordered to be given twice a day. What is the best action regarding giving this drug to this patient?

For answers see http://evolve.elsevier.com/Canada/Lilley/pharmacology/.

Legal and Ethical Considerations

Objectives

After reading this chapter, the successful student will be able to do the following:

1. Briefly discuss the important components of drug legislation at the provincial and federal levels.

2. Provide examples of how drug legislation impacts drug therapy, professional nursing practice, and the nursing process.

3. Discuss the various categories of controlled substances, and provide specific drug examples in each category.

4. Identify the process involved in the development of new drugs, including the investigational new drug application, the phases of investigational drug studies, and the process for obtaining informed consent.

5. Discuss the ethical principles of drug administration and how they apply to pharmacology and the nursing process.

6. Identify the principles involved in making an ethical decision.

7. Develop a collaborative care plan that addresses the legal and ethical care of patients, with a specific focus on drug therapy and the nursing process.

e-Learning Activities

Website
(http://evolve.elsevier.com/Canada/
Lilley/pharmacology/)

evolve

- Answer Key—Textbook Case Studies
- Answer Key—Critical Thinking Activities
- Chapter Summaries—Printable
- Review Questions for Exam Preparation
- Unfolding Case Studies

Key Terms

Bias Any systematic error in a measurement process. One common effort to avoid bias in research studies involves the use of blinded study designs. (p. 52)

Benzodiazepines and Other Targeted Substances Regulations Implemented in 2000, these regulations specify the requirements for producing, assembling, importing, exporting, selling, providing, transporting, delivering, or destroying benzodiazepines and other targeted substances. (p. 51)

Blinded investigational drug study A research design in which subjects in the study are purposely made unaware of whether the substance they are administered is the drug under study or a placebo. This method serves to minimize bias on the part of research subjects in

reporting their body's responses to investigational drugs. (p. 53)

Canada Health Act Canada's federal legislation for publicly funded health care insurance. (p. 54)

Controlled Drugs and Substances Act (CDSA) A Health Canada act that makes it a criminal offence to possess, traffic, produce, import, or export controlled substances. (p. 50)

Controlled substances Any drugs listed on one of the "schedules" of the *Controlled Drugs and Substances Act* (also a called *scheduled drug* if it is an item under the Food and Drug Regulations Part G). (p. 50)

Double-blind, investigated drug study A research design in which both the study investigator(s) and the subjects are purposely made unaware of whether the substance administered to a given subject is the drug under study or a placebo. This method minimizes bias on the part of both the investigator and the subject. (p. 53)

Drug Identification Number (DIN) A computer-generated number assigned by Health Canada placed on the label of prescription and over-the-counter drug products that have been evaluated by the Therapeutic Products Directorate (TPD) and approved for sale in Canada. (p. 52)

Ethics A set of principles, rights and responsibilities, and duties governing the moral values, beliefs, actions, and behaviours of human conduct and the rules and principles that ought to govern them. (p. 56)

Food and Drugs Act The main piece of drug legislation in Canada that protects consumers from contaminated, adulterated, and unsafe drugs and labelling practices; also addresses appropriate advertising and selling of drugs, foods, cosmetics, and therapeutic devices. (p. 49)

Food and Drug Regulations An adjunct to the *Food and Drugs Act*, these regulations clarify terms used in the Act and state the processes that companies must carry out to comply with the Act in terms of importing, preparing, treating, processing, labelling, advertising, and selling foods, drugs, cosmetics, natural health products including herbal products, and medical devices. (p. 49)

Informed consent Written permission obtained from a patient consenting to a specific procedure (e.g., receiving an investigational drug), after the patient has been given information regarding the procedure deemed necessary for him or her to make a sound or "informed" decision. (p. 52)

Investigational new drug (IND) A drug not yet approved for marketing by the Therapeutic Products Directorate of Health Canada but available for use in experiments to determine its safety and efficacy. (p. 52)

Investigational new drug application An application that must be submitted to the Therapeutic Products Directorate of Health Canada before a drug can be studied in humans. (p. 52)

Marihuana for Medical Purposes Regulations Regulations that define the manner in which access to marihuana (this is the Canadian spelling but *marijuana* is widely used) for medical purposes is permitted. (p. 51)

Malpractice A special type of negligence or the failure of a professional or individual with specialized education and training to act in a reasonable and prudent way. (p. 55)

Negligence The failure to act in a reasonable and prudent manner or failure of the nurse to give the care that a reasonably prudent (cautious) nurse would render or use under similar circumstances. (p. 55)

New drug submission The type of application that a drug manufacturer submits to the Therapeutic Products Directorate of Health Canada following successful completion of required human research studies. (p. 53)

Notice of Compliance A notification issued when Health Canada decides that a drug and its manufacturing process are safe and effective, allowing the pharmaceutical company to sell the product by prescription to the Canadian population. (p. 52)

Placebo An inactive (inert) substance (e.g., saline, distilled water, starch, sugar) that is not a drug but is formulated to resemble a drug for research purposes. (p. 52)

Precursor Control Regulations A scheme intended to allow Canada to fulfill its international obligations and meet its domestic needs with respect to the monitoring and control of precursor chemicals such as methamphetamine, γ-hydroxybutyrate (GHB), and other drugs listed in Schedules I, II, and III of the *Controlled Drugs and Substances Act*, across Canadian borders and within Canada. (p. 51)

Priority Review of Drug Submission A Health Canada policy that allows for earlier review of drug products for serious, life-threatening, or severely debilitating diseases or conditions for which there is no effective drug on the Canadian market. (p. 51)

Special Access Programme A program that allows health care providers to apply for access to drugs currently unavailable for sale in Canada. (p. 53)

LEGAL CONSIDERATIONS

Prescription drug use is vital to treating and preventing illness. However, due to safety reasons, its use is regulated and enforced by several different agencies, including Health Canada, the Royal Canadian Mounted Police, and individual provincial or territorial laws. Traditionally, only medical doctors and doctors of osteopathy had the privilege of prescribing medications. Dentists and podiatrists are also allowed to prescribe medications so long as it is within the scope of their practice. In some provinces or territories, other health care providers may also prescribe, including licensed physician's assistants and nurse practitioners.

As the number and complexity of prescriptions continue to increase and technology continually changes, so do the laws regarding their use. With the ever-changing role of the professional nurse and other members of the health care team and with the increasing pace of technologic advances, each role becomes more complex. Professional nurses have gained even more autonomy over their nursing practice. With this increasing autonomy comes greater liability and legal accountability; therefore, professional nurses must be aware and duly consider this responsibility as they practise. Specific laws and regulations are discussed later.

Canadian Drug and Related Legislation

Concerns over the sale and use of foods, drugs, cosmetics, and medical devices began in Canada long before such concerns arose in the United States. Canadian drug legislation began in 1875 when the Parliament of Canada passed an act to prevent the sale of adulterated foods, drinks, and drugs. Since that time, food and drugs have been controlled on a national basis. The Health Products Food Branch Inspectorate (HPFB) of Health Canada is the federal regulator responsible for the administration and enforcement of the *Food and Drugs Act* and **Food and Drug Regulations** and the *Controlled Drugs and Substances Act*, the two Acts that form the underlying foundation for the drug laws in Canada. The Therapeutic Products Directorate (TPD) is the Canadian federal authority that regulates these Acts. These Acts are designed to protect the Canadian consumer from potential health hazards and fraud or deception in the sale and use of foods, drugs, cosmetics, and medical devices.

The Personal Information Protection and Electronic Documents Act (PIPEDA) is federal law governing the collection, use, and disclosure of personal information. Several provinces and territories have legislation that deals specifically with the collection, use, and disclosure of personal health information by health care providers and health care organizations. For example, Ontario has the *Personal Health Information Protection Act* (PHIPA) of 2004, while British Columbia has the *Personal Health Information Access and Protection of Privacy Act* of 2008. Such acts require all health care providers, health insurance and life insurance companies, public health authorities, employers, and schools to maintain patient privacy regarding protected health information. Protected health information includes any individually identifying information such as patients' health conditions, account numbers, prescription numbers, medications, and payment information. Such information can be oral or recorded in any paper or electronic form. In 2013, a proposal was introduced to revise PHIPA to the *Electronic Personal Health Information Protection Act* (EPHIPA), intended to address the technological realities of electronic health records. The primary purpose of federal legislation is to ensure the safety and efficacy of new drugs and, in the case of privacy laws, to protect patient confidentiality.

Canadian Food and Drugs Act

The Canadian **Food and Drugs Act** is the primary piece of legislation governing foods, drugs, cosmetics, and medical devices in Canada. The Act has been amended several times since its inception in 1953. Table 3-1 summarizes these amendments. Schedule A of the Act lists the diseases for which treatments may not be promoted to the public. Sections 3(1) and 3(2) of the *Food and Drugs Act* prohibit any label claim or advertisement that is both directed to the general public and contains treatment, preventative, or cure claims for Schedule A diseases. Revisions to Schedule A came into force on June 1, 2008. The updated Schedule A generally includes life-threatening diseases such as cancer and acute forms of specific diseases. For example, "liver disease," which covers all liver diseases, disorders, and abnormalities, is now listed as "hepatitis," which is a more specific disease. The legend *Canadian Standard Drug*, or CSD, must appear on the inner and outer labels of the drug packaging to show that a drug meets the standards for which it is prescribed.

According to the Act, and to protect the consumer, drugs must comply with official prescribed standards stated in recognized pharmacopoeias and formularies listed in Schedule B of the Act. Recognized pharmacopoeias and formularies include the following:
- Pharmacopée française
- Pharmacopoeia Internationalis
- The British Pharmacopoeia
- The Canadian Formulary
- The National Formulary
- The Pharmaceutical Codex: Principles and Practices of Pharmaceuticals
- The United States Pharmacopoeia

Drugs listed in Schedule C are radiopharmaceuticals, and drugs listed in Schedule D include allergenic substances, immunizing agents (vaccines), insulin, anterior pituitary extracts, drugs obtained by recombinant DNA technology, and blood derivatives. The distribution of *drug samples*, defined as trial packages of medication, is also regulated, with the exception of the distribution under prescribed conditions to physicians, dentists, or pharmacists. All drugs that require a prescription are listed in Schedule F with the exception of narcotics and controlled drugs. Schedule F to the Food and Drug Regulations was replaced by a list of prescription drugs called the Prescription Drug List. The prescription status helps to ensure that consumers receive adequate risk and benefit information from a health care provider before taking the drug. The *Pr* symbol in the upper left quarter of the label—a black box with the letters *Pr* in white inside—identifies the product as a prescription drug. *The Food and Drugs Act* also regulates the information manufacturers may put on a drug label, including directions for use. A prescription may be refilled as often as indicated by the prescriber. Prescriptions are written (including facsimiles) or transmitted orally (via telephone to the pharmacist) by a qualified health care provider.

The **Food and Drug Regulations** are the current, consolidated regulations of the *Food and Drugs Act*. Parts G and J regulate controlled drugs and restricted drugs, respectively. Controlled drugs are dispensed only by prescription. A controlled drug must be marked with the symbol C in a clear manner and in a conspicuous colour and size, on the upper left quarter of the label. The proper

TABLE 3-1

Additions to the Food and Drugs Act

Schedule	Description
Schedules C and D	Drugs in these schedules must list where the drug was manufactured and the process and conditions of manufacturing.
Prescription Drug List	Replaces Schedule F. This is a list of medicinal ingredients in a drug that require a prescription. Excluded are drugs listed in the Controlled Drugs and Substances Act schedules that require a prescription.
Part G	These drugs, also known as *controlled drugs*, affect the central nervous system (CNS); labels on these drugs are marked *C.* Controlled drugs are categorized into three parts: Part I: designated controlled drugs with misuse potential that may be used for designated medical conditions outlined in Food and Drug Regulations. *Examples:* amphetamines, methylphenidate, pentobarbital, and preparations containing one controlled drug and one or more active noncontrolled drug Part II: controlled drugs with misuse potential prescribed for medical conditions. *Examples:* sedatives such as barbiturates and derivatives (secobarbital) and thiobarbiturates (pentothal sodium) Part III: controlled drugs with misuse potential. *Examples:* anabolic steroids (androstanolone), weight reduction drugs (anorexiants)
Narcotic Drugs and Preparations	Drugs with high-misuse potential. *Examples:* morphine, codeine more than 8 mg, amidones (methadone), coca and derivatives (cocaine), benzazocines (analgesics such as pentazocine), fentanyls
Part J	These are restricted drugs with high-misuse potential, dangerous physiological and psychological adverse effects, and no recognized medical use. *Examples:* lysergic acid diethylamide (LSD), mescaline (peyote), harmaline, psilocin and psilocybin (magic mushrooms)
Benzodiazepines and Other Targeted Substances Regulations	A "targeted substance" is either a controlled substance that is included in Schedule I or a product or compound that contains a controlled substance that is included in Schedule I. These are drugs with misuse potential. *Examples:* benzodiazepine tranquilizers such as diazepam, lorazepam, flumitrazepam, and zolpidem

name of the drug must also appear on the label and either precede or follow the brand name of the drug.

Controlled Drugs and Substances Act

The **Controlled Drugs and Substances Act (CDSA)** was passed in 1997, replacing the *Narcotic Control Act* and Parts III and IV of the *Food and Drugs Act*. The first *Narcotic Control Act*, passed in 1961, was enacted in response to the growing use and misuse of drugs in the middle and late 1960s. It replaced the previous Act, the *Canadian Opium and Narcotic Act of 1952*. The *Narcotic Control Act* and Parts III and IV of the *Food and Drugs Act* prohibited activities such as possession, possession for the purpose of trafficking, trafficking, importing and exporting, and cultivation of narcotics or controlled and restricted drugs.

The CDSA provides the requirements for the control and sale of narcotics, controlled drugs, and substances of misuse. **Controlled drugs** and substances for medical treatment may be legally obtained only with a prescription from a licensed medical practitioner. The letter N and the symbol ⟨C⟩ are printed on the label of all controlled drugs. The CDSA is based on eight schedules that list controlled drugs and substances based on

potential for misuse or harm or how easy they are to manufacture into illicit substances. A summary of Schedule I contains the most dangerous drugs, including opiates (opium, heroin, morphine, cocaine) and methamphetamine. Schedule II contains cannabis-related drugs, including marihuana and its derivatives. Schedule III contains the more dangerous drugs such as amphetamines and lysergic acid diethylamide (LSD). Schedule IV contains drugs such as barbiturates and anabolic steroids, which are dangerous but have therapeutic uses; a prescription is required for possession of drugs listed in Schedule IV. Schedules V and VI contain precursors required to produce controlled substances. Schedules VII and VIII contain amounts of cannabis and cannabis resin required for charge and sentencing purposes. The factors that determine the schedule under which a controlled substance should be placed are international requirements, the dependence potential and likelihood of abuse of the substance, the extent of its abuse in Canada, the danger it represents to the safety of the public, and the usefulness of the substance as a therapeutic agent. The Royal Canadian Mounted Police (RCMP) is responsible for enforcing the CDSA and related sections of the *Criminal Code* and exempts members of police forces from sections of the CDSA for the purpose of performing their duties.

The **Benzodiazepines and Other Targeted Substances Regulations** specify similar restrictions with regard to benzodiazepines, their salts and derivatives, and other targeted substances mentioned in Schedules I and II. The **Precursor Control Regulations**, introduced in 2003, address the need for the control of essential and precursor chemicals routinely used in clandestine labs for the production of methamphetamine, ecstasy, and other Schedule III drugs. The Marihuana Medical Access Program ended in March 2014; it was replaced with the Marihuana for Medical Purposes Regulations, which provide marihuana for medical use through licensed producers (Health Canada, 2015). A medical professional (initially a physician; a nurse practitioner will be able to prescribe in the future) prescribes dried medical marihuana using a government-approved form. Health Canada regulates only the producers of marihuana and is not involved in the decision-making process. Two important changes to the regulations took place in June 2015. First, the licensed regulators of marihuana for medical purposes is required upon request to supply reports every 4 months to provincial and territorial medical and nursing licensing bodies, providing information on how nurse practitioners and physicians are authorizing the use of marihuana. Second, the Supreme Court of Canada ruled that medical marihuana patients will be able to lawfully consume cannabis in other forms such as resins, oils, extractions, and edible marihuana, rather than being allowed to only smoke dried marihuana.

NEW DRUG DEVELOPMENT

The research into and development of new drugs is an ongoing process. The pharmaceutical industry is a multibillion-dollar industry. Pharmaceutical companies must continuously develop new and better drugs to maintain a competitive edge. The research required for the development of these new drugs may take several years. Hundreds of substances are isolated that never make it to market. Once a potentially beneficial drug has been identified, the pharmaceutical company must follow a regulated, systematic process before the drug can be sold on the open market. This highly sophisticated process is regulated and carefully monitored by Health Canada. The primary purpose of Health Canada's TPD is to protect the patient and ensure drug effectiveness.

This system of drug research and development is one of the most stringent in the world. It was developed out of concern for patient safety and drug efficacy. Much time, funding, and documentation are required to ensure that these two important objectives are met. Many drugs are marketed and used in foreign countries long before they get approval for use in Canada. Drug-related calamities are more likely to be avoided by this more stringent drug approval system. The thalidomide tragedy resulted from the use of a drug that was first marketed in Europe and then made available for distribution in Canada.

A balance must be achieved between making new lifesaving therapies available and protecting consumers from potential drug-induced adverse effects. In 2003, Canada introduced the Natural Health Products Regulations. These regulations cover natural health products such as vitamins and minerals, herbal remedies, homeopathic medicines, traditional medicines (e.g., traditional Chinese medicines), probiotics, and other products such as amino acids and essential fatty acids (e.g., omega-3). The manufacturers' primary obligation regarding such products is to not make "false or misleading" claims about their efficacy. For example, a product label may read "For depression," but cannot read "Known to cure depression." Reliable, objective information about these kinds of products is limited but is growing as more formal research studies are conducted. In 2008, Bill C-51 was drafted to complement and support the current policies for foods and health products, including natural health products. Consumer demand for alternative medicine products continues to drive this process. Patients must exercise caution in using such products and communicate regularly with their health care providers regarding their use.

Health Canada Drug Approval Process

The TPD of Health Canada is responsible for approving drugs for clinical safety and efficacy before they are brought to the market. There are stringent steps, each of which may take years, that must be completed before the drug can be approved. The TPD has made certain lifesaving investigational drug therapies available sooner than usual by offering a **priority review of drug submissions** process, also known as "fast-track" approval. Eligible submissions undergo a shorter review target of 180 days, compared to 300 days for non-priority submissions. Acquired immune deficiency syndrome (AIDS) was the first major public health crisis for which the TPD began granting expedited drug approval. This process allowed pharmaceutical manufacturers to shorten the approval process and allowed prescribers to give medications that showed promise during early Phase I and Phase II clinical trials to qualified patients with AIDS. In such cases, when a trial continues to show favourable results, the overall process of drug approval is hastened. The concept of expedited drug approval became controversial after the manufacturer recall of the anti-inflammatory drug rofecoxib (Vioxx) in 2004. This recall followed multiple case reports of severe cardiovascular events, including fatalities, associated with the use of this drug and concerns that the manufacturer withheld information about the drug's risks. This unfortunate example has reduced the number of drugs approved via the expedited approval process.

The drug approval process is quite complex and prolonged. It normally begins with preclinical testing phases, which include in vitro studies (using tissue samples and cell cultures) and animal studies. Clinical (human) studies follow the preclinical phase. There are four clinical phases (see below). The drug is put on the market after Phase III is completed if an **investigational new drug application** submitted by the manufacturer is approved by the TPD. Phase IV consists of postmarketing studies. The collective goal of these phases is to provide information on the safety, toxicity, efficacy, potency, bioavailability, and purity of the new drug. A **Notice of Compliance** is issued when Health Canada decides that the drug and the manufacturing process are safe and effective, allowing the pharmaceutical company to sell the product by prescription to the Canadian population. Once a drug is approved for sale, it is assigned a computer-generated **Drug Identification Number (DIN)** by Health Canada. The DIN is placed on the label of prescription and OTC drug products.

Preclinical Investigational Drug Studies

Current medical ethics still require that all new drugs undergo laboratory testing using both in vitro (cell or tissue) and animal studies before any testing in human subjects can be done. In vitro studies include testing of the response of various types of mammalian (including human) cells and tissues to different concentrations of the investigational drug. Various types of cells and tissues used for this purpose are collected from living or dead animal or human subjects (e.g., surgical or autopsy specimens). In vitro studies help researchers determine early on if a substance might be too toxic for human patients. Many prospective new drugs are ruled out for human use during this preclinical phase of drug testing. However, a small percentage of the many drugs tested in this manner are referred for further clinical testing in human subjects.

Four Clinical Phases of Investigational Drug Studies

Before any testing on humans begins, the subjects must provide informed consent, and the consent must be documented. **Informed consent** involves the careful explanation to the human test patient or research subject of the purpose of the study, the procedures to be used, the possible benefits, and the risks involved. This explanation is followed by written documentation on a consent form. The informed consent document, or consent form, must be written in language that is understood by the patient and must be dated and signed by the patient and at least one witness. Informed consent is always voluntary. By law, informed consent must be obtained more than a given number of days or hours before certain procedures are performed and must always be obtained when the patient is fully mentally competent. The informed consent process may be carried out by a nurse or other health care provider, depending on how a given study is designed.

Medical ethics dictate that participants in experimental drug studies be informed volunteers and not be coerced to participate in any way. Therefore, informed consent must be obtained from all patients (or their legal guardians) before they can be enrolled in an **investigational new drug (IND)** study. Some patients may have unrealistic expectations of the IND's usefulness. Often they have the misconception that because an investigational drug is new it must automatically be better than existing forms of therapy. Other volunteers may be reluctant to enter the study because they think they will be treated as "guinea pigs." Whatever the circumstances of the study, the research subjects must be informed of all potential hazards as well as the possible benefits of the new therapy. It must be stressed to all patients that involvement in IND studies is voluntary and that any individual can either decline to participate or quit the study at any time without affecting the delivery of any previously agreed-upon health care services.

Phase I

Phase I studies usually involve small numbers of healthy subjects (normally fewer than 100) rather than those who have the disease or ailment that the new drug is intended to treat. An exception might be a study involving a toxic drug used to treat a life-threatening illness. In this case, the only study subjects might be those who already have the illness and for whom other viable treatment options may not be available. The purpose of Phase I studies is to determine the potential adverse effects, the optimal dosage range, and the pharmacokinetics of the drug (i.e., absorption, distribution, metabolism, and excretion) and to determine if further testing is needed. Blood tests, urinalyses, assessments of vital signs, and specific monitoring tests are also performed. These trials usually last from a few days to a few weeks.

Phase II

Phase II studies involve larger numbers of volunteers (usually around 100 to 300) who have the disease or ailment that the drug is designed to diagnose or treat. Study participants are closely monitored for the drug's effectiveness and to identify any adverse effects. Therapeutic dosage ranges are refined during this phase. If no serious adverse effects occur, the study can progress to Phase III.

Phase III

Phase III studies involve larger numbers of patients (normally 1 000 to 3 000), who are followed by medical research centres and other types of health care facilities. The patients may be treated at the centre or may be spread over a wider geographic area. The purpose of this larger sample size is to provide information about infrequent or rare adverse effects that may not have been observed during previous smaller studies. To enhance objectivity, many studies are designed to incorporate a placebo. A **placebo** is an inert substance that is not a drug (e.g., normal saline), given to a portion of the research subjects to separate out the real benefits of the investigational drug from the apparent benefits arising out of researcher or subject **bias** regarding expected or desired results of the drug therapy. A study incorporating a placebo is called a *placebo-controlled study*. If the study subject does not know whether the drug being administered is a placebo or the investigational drug but the investigator does know, the study is referred to as a **blinded investigational drug study**. In most studies neither the research staff nor the subjects being tested know which subjects are being given the real drug and which are receiving the placebo. This further enhances the objectivity of the study results and is known as a **double-blind, investigated drug study** because both the researchers and the subjects are "blinded" to the actual identity of the substance administered to a given subject. Both the drug and placebo dosage forms given to patients often look identical, except for a secret code that appears on the medication itself or its container. At the completion of the study, this code is revealed or broken to determine which study patients received the drug and which were given the placebo. The code can also be broken before study completion by the principle investigator in the event of a clinical emergency that requires a determination of what individual patients received.

The three objectives of Phase III studies are to establish the drug's clinical effectiveness, safety, and dosage range. After Phase III is completed, Health Canada's TPD and Biologics and Genetic Therapies Directorate (BGTD) receive a report from the manufacturer, at which time the drug company submits a **new drug submission**. The approval of the application paves the way for the pharmaceutical company to market the new drug exclusively until the patent for the drug molecule expires. As mandated by the Canadian *Patent Act*, this is normally 20 years after discovery of the molecule and includes the 10- to 12-year period generally required to complete drug research. Therefore, a new drug manufacturer typically has 8 to 10 years after drug marketing to recoup research costs, which are usually in the hundreds of millions of dollars for a single drug.

Phase IV

Phase IV studies are postmarketing studies voluntarily conducted by pharmaceutical companies to obtain further proof of the therapeutic and adverse effects of the new drug. However, these studies may be mandated by Health Canada. Data from such studies are usually gathered for at least 2 years after the drug's release. Often these studies compare the safety and efficacy of the new drug with that of another drug in the same therapeutic category. An example would be a comparison of a new nonsteroidal anti-inflammatory drug with ibuprofen in the treatment of osteoarthritis. Some medications make it through all phases of clinical trials without causing any problems among study patients. However, when they are used in the larger general population, severe adverse effects may appear for the first time. If a pattern of severe reactions to a newly marketed drug begins to emerge, Health Canada may request that the manufacturer of the drug issue a voluntary recall. The drug can still be

prescribed; however, the prescriber must be made aware of the potential risk. If the drug manufacturer refuses to recall the medication, and if the number or severity of reactions reaches a certain level, then the Health Products and Food Branch Inspectorate of Health Canada may seek court action to condemn the product and allow it to be seized by legal authorities. Such an action, in effect, becomes an involuntary recall on behalf of the manufacturer. There are three designated classes of drug recall based on Health Canada's response to postmarketing data for a given drug:

- **Class I:** The most serious type of recall—use of the drug product carries a reasonable probability of serious adverse health effects or death.
- **Class II:** Less severe—use of the drug product may result in temporary or medically reversible health effects, but the probability of lasting major adverse health effects is low.
- **Class III:** Least severe—use of the drug product is not likely to result in any significant health problems.

Notification by Health Canada of a drug recall or drug warnings may be in the form of press releases, website announcements, or letters to health care providers. Health Canada's MedEffect website provides a voluntary program called MedEffect Canada, in which professionals and consumers are encouraged to report any adverse events seen with newly approved drugs. Recalls and Safety Alerts Database is a current comprehensive list of advisories, warnings, and recalls: http://www.hc-sc.gc.ca/dhp-mps/medeff/advisories-avis/index-eng.php. Drug information of this kind is continually evolving as new events are observed and reported by clinicians and patients. Recommended actions change with time, so use the most current information available along with sound clinical judgement.

Special Access Programme

The Health Canada **Special Access Programme** allows health care providers compassionate access to drugs unavailable for sale in Canada. The Special Access Programme is limited to those with serious or life-threatening conditions (e.g., intractable depression, epilepsy, transplant rejection, hemophilia and other blood disorders, terminal cancer, and AIDS) who may require experimental drugs for compassionate reasons or on an emergency basis when other conventional therapies have failed. New regulations were introduced in October 2013 that prevent special access to certain unauthorized controlled substances (e.g., products containing heroin, unauthorized forms of cocaine or other restricted drugs such as LSD, ecstasy, "magic mushrooms," and "bath salts.")

Patient Access to and Costs of Prescription Drugs

The twenty-first century in Canada has seen rapid growth in prescription drug use and costs. High drug expenses in Canada are a significant barrier for people to access prescription drugs outside of hospital. Law, Cheng, Dhalla, Heard, & Morgan (2013) found evidence that suggests that out-of-pocket expenses for drugs, occurring in one in ten Canadians, influence the decision to not adhere to prescription medications. Canadians affected are those with low incomes, those without drug benefits, and those in poor health.

Prescription drugs are not covered under the **Canada Health Act.** Patients must pay for a drug unless the drug is covered by a private drug plan or a federal, provincial, or territorial (F/P/T) drug plan. Most provincial plans provide for some costs of drugs to those who are poor, older adults, those with catastrophic drug costs, and people with certain conditions (e.g., cancer, HIV/AIDS). The federal government provides coverage for Indigenous peoples. Each Canadian province and territory has a formulary committee that decides which drugs are listed on its formulary and reimbursed by the drug benefit health plan, which have restricted access, and which are not covered. There is a wide variety of access to prescription drugs across the country—provincial and territorial drug plans vary in eligibility criteria, drugs covered, and financing. For example, most drugs are paid for patients over the age of 65; however they are required to pay dispensing fees (such fees vary among pharmacies based on the patient's drug coverage plan) and not all drugs are covered. For example, there may not be coverage if a trade name drug is prescribed rather than a generic drug. Provinces and territories base the decision to list a drug on a variety of factors such as effectiveness analyses, cost, government priorities, and patient advocacy. Some drugs may be restricted if they require special monitoring or if the cost is high.

Drug Advertising

Drug advertising in Canada is regulated by Health Canada. Direct-to-consumer advertising (such as ads in consumer magazines and on subways) is restricted to simply giving the names of prescription drugs, but these ads do not make claims for product effectiveness (this is not the case in the United States). Advertisements in professional health care journals contain claims and prescribing information. Advertising Standards Canada (ASC) and the Pharmaceutical Advertising Advisory Board (PAAB) review and clear advertisements according to standards set by the *Food and Drugs Act.* Although the clearance procedure is voluntary, most companies comply with the regulations.

LEGAL NURSING CONSIDERATIONS AND DRUG THERAPY

Provincial and territorial legislation dictates the boundaries for professional nursing practice. Nursing practice standards of care and nurse practice acts identify the definition of the scope and role of the professional nurse (Box 3-1). Nurse practice acts further define/identify: (1) the scope of nursing practice, (2) expanded nursing roles, (3) educational requirements for nurses, (4) stand-

---

BOX 3-1

Nurse Practice Acts

Nurse practice acts (NPAs) are regulatory laws that are instrumental in defining the scope of nursing practice and protect public health, safety, and welfare. Nursing practice in Canada is regulated by separate acts in each of the 10 provinces and 3 territories. These acts grant self-governance to the nursing profession, direct entry into nursing practice, define the scopes of practice, and identify disciplinary actions. NPAs are the most significant part of legislation in regard to professional nursing practice. Together, it is NPAs and common law that define nursing practice. Each province and territory has a website on which the NPAs are defined and outlined. For example, for nurses practising in New Brunswick or British Columbia, the websites are respectively: http://www.nanb.nb.ca/ and https://crnbc.ca/CRNBC/RegulationOfNurses/Pages/Default.aspx.

---

ards of care, (5) minimally safe nursing practice, and (6) differences between nursing and medical practice. In addition, provincial/territorial regulatory bodies of nursing define specific nursing practices such as guidelines concerning the administration of intravenous therapy. Additionally, guidelines from professional nursing groups (e.g., Canadian Nurses Association [CNA]), nursing specialty groups, institutional policies and procedures, and provincial/territorial hospital licensing laws all help to identify the legal boundaries of nursing practice. There is also case law or common law consisting of prior court rulings that affect professional nursing practice.

The CNA advances the practice and profession of nursing to improve health outcomes and strengthen Canada's health care system. The CNA is the national voice for nurses and has developed standards for nursing practice, policy statements, and similar resolutions. The standards describe the scope, function, and role of the nurse and establish clinical practice standards. Accreditation Canada requires that accredited hospitals fulfill certain standards in regard to nursing practice. One such requirement is that these institutions must have written policies and procedures. These policies and procedures are usually quite specific and are contained in policy and procedures manuals found on most nursing units, although many organizations now post their policies not only internally on the intranet but externally via the Internet. The nurse must know the policies and procedures of the employing institution because if the nurse is involved in a lawsuit, these policies and procedures are one of the standards by which the nurse will be measured. Nursing specialty organizations also define standards of care for nurses who are certified in specialty areas, such as oncology, surgical care, or critical care. Standards of care help to determine whether a nurse is acting appropriately when performing professional duties. It is critical to safe nursing practice to remain up to date on the ever-changing obligations and standards

BOX 3-2 Areas of Potential Liability for Nurses

Area	Examples Related to Drug Therapy and the Nursing Process
Failure to assess/evaluate	Failure to see significant changes in patient's condition after taking a medication; failure to report the changes in condition after medication; failure to take a complete medication history and nursing assessment/history; failure to monitor patient after medication administration
Failure to ensure safety	Lack of adequate monitoring; failure to identify patient allergies and other risk factors related to medication therapy; inappropriate drug administration technique; failure to implement appropriate nursing actions based on a lack of proper assessment of patient's condition
Medication errors	Failure to clarify unclear medication order; failure to identify and react to adverse drug reactions; failure to be familiar with medication prior to its administration; failure to maintain level of professional nursing skills for current practice; failure to identify patient's identity prior to drug administration; failure to document drug administration in medication profile

of practice and care. If standards of care are not met, the nurse becomes liable for **negligence** and **malpractice** (Box 3-2). Current nursing literature remains an authoritative resource for information on new standards of care. Provincial/territorial nursing associations have websites that include links to specific nurse practice acts and standards of care.

The legal–ethical dimensions of professional nursing care are also addressed in the legislation passed to amplify the guidelines contained in the Privacy Act (1983). The Privacy Act regulates how federal government institutions collect, use, and disclose personal information. Under these federal regulations (see p. 49), the privacy of patient information is protected, and standards are included for the handling of electronic data about patients (PIPEDA). PIPEDA also defines the rights and privileges of patients in order to protect privacy without diminishing access to quality health care. The assurance of privacy—even prior to establishment of the PIPEDA guidelines—was based on the principle of respect of an individual's right to determine when, to what extent, and under what circumstances private information can be shared or withheld from others, including family members. In addition, confidentiality must be preserved; that is, the individual identities of patients or research study participants are not to be linked to information they provide and cannot be publicly divulged. PIPEDA addresses the issues of confidentiality and privacy by prohibiting prescribers, nurses, and other health care providers from sharing with others any patient health care information, including laboratory results, diagnoses, and prognoses, without the patient's consent. Conflicting obligations arise when a patient wants to keep information away from insurance companies, and matters remain complicated and challenging in the era of improving technology and computerization of medical records. Health care facilities continue to work diligently, however, to adhere to PIPEDA guidelines and use special access codes to limit who can access information in computerized documents and charts.

In summary, federal and provincial or territorial legislation, standards of care, and nurse practice acts provide the legal framework for safe nursing practice, including drug therapy and medication administration. Further, as discussed in Chapter 1, the standard "Rights" of medication administration are yet another measure for ensuring safety and adherence to laws necessary for protecting the patient. Chapter 1 also discusses other patient rights that are part of the standards of practice of every licensed registered nurse and every student studying the art and science of nursing.

ETHICAL CONSIDERATIONS

Decisions in health care are seldom made independently of other people and are made with consideration of the patient, family, nurses, and other members of the health care team. All members of the health care team must make a concentrated effort to recognize and understand their own values and be considerate, nonjudgemental, and respectful of the values of others. The use of drug therapy has evolved from just administering whatever was prescribed to providing responsible drug therapy for the purpose of achieving defined outcomes that improve a patient's quality of life based on the nursing process.

Ethical principles are useful strategies for members of the health care team and include standards or truths on which ethical actions are made. Some of the most useful ethical principles in nursing and health care, specifically drug therapy, include autonomy, beneficence, nonmaleficence, justice, fidelity, and veracity (see Legal and Ethical Principles Box: Ethical Principles in Nursing and Health Care). However, day-to-day practice in nursing and health care pose many potential ethical conflicts. Each situation is different and requires compassionate and humane solutions. When answers to ethical dilemmas remain unclear and ethical conflict occurs, then the appropriate action must be based on ethical principles.

Ethical Nursing Considerations and Drug Therapy

Ethical nursing practice is based on basic ethical principles such as beneficence, autonomy, justice, fidelity, veracity, and confidentiality. The Canadian Nurses Association (CNA) *Code of Ethics for Registered Nurses* (2008) and the International Council of Nurses (ICN) *Code of Ethics for Nurses* (2012) serve as frameworks of practice for all nurses and as ethical guidelines for nursing care

LEGAL & ETHICAL PRINCIPLES

Ethical Principles in Nursing and Health Care

Element	Example
Providing safe, compassionate, competent, and ethical care	Nurses are attentive to the safety of people receiving care and to factors that may compromise their health. In short, it is a nurse's duty to do no harm. Nurses question and intervene to address unsafe, noncompassionate, unethical, or incompetent practice or conditions that interfere with their ability to provide safe, compassionate, competent, and ethical care to those to whom they are providing care, and they support others who do the same.
Maintaining privacy and confidentiality	Nurses acknowledge the importance of privacy and confidentiality and safeguard personal, family, and community information obtained in the context of a professional relationship.
Promoting justice	Nurses uphold principles of justice by safeguarding human rights, equity, and fairness and by promoting the public good.
Being accountable	Nurses are accountable for their actions and answerable for their practice. Nurses must maintain their fitness to practice.
Preserving dignity	Nurses have a nondiscriminatory and nonjudgemental approach to delivery of care.
Promoting and respecting informed decision making	Nurses support and advocate for their patients to promote informed decision making. Patients should be made aware of the choices and treatments available for their medical care and the potential outcomes of these choices and treatments and have their personal values considered in decisions about their medical care.
Promoting health and well-being	Nurses value health promotion and well-being and assisting patients to achieve their highest level of health.

Source: Based on Canadian Nurses Association. (2008). Code of ethics for registered nurses. Ottawa, ON: Retrieved from https://www.cna-aiic.ca/~/media/cna/page-content/pdf-fr/code-of-ethics-for-registered-nurses.pdf?la=en

LEGAL & ETHICAL PRINCIPLES

International Council of Nurses *Code of Ethics for Nurses*

The International Council of Nurses (ICN) first adopted *The ICN Code of Ethics for Nurses* in 1953; the Code has been revised several times since then, most recently in 2012. The 2012 revision is available in English, French, Spanish, and German. This Code is a globally accepted guide for ethical practice in nursing based on social values and needs. The preamble identifies the four fundamental responsibilities of nurses—promoting health, preventing illness, restoring health, and alleviating suffering—and points out that the need for nursing is universal. The Code makes it clear that inherent in professional nursing practice is respect for human rights, including the right to life, dignity, and the right to be treated with respect. Nursing care is respectful of and unrestricted by considerations of age, colour, creed, culture, disability or illness, sexual orientation, nationality, politics, race, or social status. Nurses render services to the individual, family, and community. The Code describes four principle elements that provide a framework for the standards of ethical conduct it defines: nurses and people, nurses and practice, nurses and the profession, and nurses and co-workers. The 2012 updated code reflects the current professional emphases on positive work environments and the use of evidence-informed practice. *The ICN Code of Ethics for Nurses* serves as a guide for action based on social values and needs and should be understood, internalized, and applied by nurses in all aspects of their work. Nurses can obtain assistance in translating these standards into conduct by discussing the Code with co-workers and collaborating with their national nurses' associations in the application of ethical standards in nursing practice, education, management, and research.

(see the Legal and Ethical Principles Box: International Council of Nurses *Code of Ethics for Nurses*).

Adherence to these ethical principles and codes of ethics ensures that the nurse is acting on behalf of the patient and with the patient's best interests. The professional nurse has the responsibility to provide safe nursing care to patients regardless of the setting, person, group, community, or family involved. Although it is not within the nurse's realm of ethical and professional responsibility to impose her values or standards on the patient, it *is* within the nurse's realm to provide information and to assist the patient in facing decisions regarding health care.

The nurse also has the right to refuse to participate in any treatment or aspect of a patient's care that violates the nurse's personal ethical principles. However, this must be done without abandoning the patient, and in some facilities the nurse may be transferred to another patient care assignment only if the transfer is approved by the nurse manager or nurse supervisor. The nurse must always remember, however, that the CNA *Code of Ethics for Registered Nurses* and professional responsibility and accountability require the nurse to provide non-judgemental nursing care from the start of the patient's treatment until the time of the patient's discharge. If transferring to a different assignment is not an option because of institutional policy and because of the increase in the acuteness of patients' conditions and the high patient-to-nurse workload, then the nurse must always act in the best interest of the patient while remaining an objective patient advocate.

It is always the nurse's responsibility to provide the highest quality nursing care and practice within the professional standards of care. The CNA *Code of Ethics for Registered Nurses*; *The ICN Code of Ethics for Nurses*; standards of nursing practice; federal, provincial, or territorial codes; ethical principles; and the previously mentioned legal principles and legislation are readily accessible and provide nurses with a sound, rational framework for professional nursing practice.

Another area of ethical consideration related to drug therapy and the nursing process is the use of placebos. A placebo is a drug dosage form (e.g., tablet or capsule) without any pharmacological activity due to a lack of active ingredients. However, there may be reported therapeutic responses, and placebos have been found to be beneficial in certain patients, such as those being treated for anxiety. Indeed, Raz et al. (2011) in an online survey of 606 physicians, including psychiatrists and nonpsychiatrists, 20% prescribed placebos regularly as part of routine clinical practice. Placebos are also administered frequently in experimental studies of new drugs to evaluate and measure the pharmacological effects of a new medicine compared with those of an inert placebo. Except in new drug studies, however, placebo use is considered to be unethical, creating mistrust among the nurse, the prescriber, and the patient. Many health care agencies limit the use of placebos to research only to avoid the possible mistrust. In Canada there are no specific formal guidelines on the use of placebo. If administration of a placebo is part of a research study or clinical trial, the informed consent process must be thorough and patients must be informed of their right to (1) leave the study at any time without any pressure or coercion to stay, (2) leave the study without consequences to medical care, (3) receive full and complete information about the study, and (4) be aware of all alternative options and receive information on all treatments, including placebo therapy, being administered in the study.

 CASE STUDY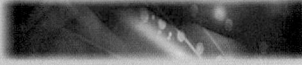

Clinical Drug Trial

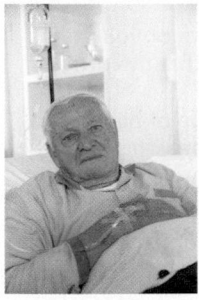 A patient on the cardiac telemetry unit, Claude, has had a serious heart condition for years and has been through every known protocol for treatment. The cardiologist has admitted him to a telemetry unit for observation during a trial of a new investigational drug. Claude exclaims, "I have high hopes for this drug. I've read about it on the Internet and the reports are wonderful. I can't wait to get better!"

1. What is the best way for the nurse to answer this statement?

The physician meets with Claude and the nurse to explain the medication and how the double-blind experimental drug study will work. The purpose of the medication and potential hazards of the therapy are described, as well as the laboratory tests that will be performed to measure the drug's effectiveness. The physician then asks the nurse to have Claude sign the consent form. When the nurse goes to get Claude's signature, he says, "I'll sign it, but I really didn't understand what that doctor told me about the placebo."

2. Should the nurse continue with getting the consent form signed? Explain your answer.

3. Claude tells the nurse, "How can I make sure I have the real drug and not the fake drug? I really want to see if it will help my situation." What is the nurse's best response?

4. After a week, Claude tells the nurse, "I don't see that this drug is helping me. In fact, I feel worse. But I'm afraid to tell the doctor that I want to stop the medicine. What do I do?" What is the nurse's best response?

For answers see http://evolve.elsevier.com/Canada/Lilley/pharmacology/.

KEY POINTS

❖ Various pieces of federal legislation, as well as provincial or territorial law, provincial or territorial practice acts, and institutional policies, have been established to help ensure the safety and efficacy of drug therapy and the nursing process.

❖ Privacy guidelines have increased awareness concerning patient confidentiality and privacy. It is important to understand the federal, provincial, or territorial legislation as it relates to drug therapy and the nursing process.

Continued

KEY POINTS—cont'd

❖ The *Food and Drugs Act* and the *Controlled Drugs and Substances Act* provide nurses and other health care providers with information on drugs that cause little to no dependence versus those associated with a high level of abuse and dependency.

❖ Always obtain informed consent as needed with complete understanding of your role and responsibilities as a patient advocate in obtaining such consent.

❖ In the IND research process, adhere to the study protocol while also acting as a patient advocate and honouring the patient's right to safe, quality nursing care.

❖ Adhere to legal guidelines, ethical principles, and the CNA *Code of Ethics for Registered Nurses* so your actions are based on a solid foundation.

❖ Placebo use remains controversial and if a placebo is ordered, question the prescriber about the specific rationale for its use.

EXAMINATION REVIEW QUESTIONS

1. Ahmed is undergoing major surgery and asks the nurse about a living will. He states, "I don't want anybody making decisions for me. And I don't want to prolong my life." Ahmed is demonstrating
   a. autonomy
   b. beneficence
   c. justice
   d. veracity

2. Jennifer is being counselled for possible participation in a clinical trial for a new medication. After she meets with the physician, the nurse is asked to obtain her signature on the consent forms. The nurse knows that this "informed consent" indicates which of the following?
   a. Once therapy has begun, the patient cannot withdraw from the clinical trial.
   b. The patient has been informed of all potential hazards and benefits of the therapy.
   c. The patient has received only the information that will help to make the clinical trial a success.
   d. No matter what happens, the patient will not be able to sue the researchers for damages.

3. A new drug has been approved for use and the drug manufacturer has made it available for sale. During the first 6 months, Health Canada receives reports of severe adverse effects that were not discovered during the testing and considers whether to withdraw the drug. This illustrates which phase of investigational drug studies?
   a. Phase I
   b. Phase II
   c. Phase III
   d. Phase IV

4. When discussing the laws on legal marihuana use in Canada with a patient, which facts does the nurse consider? (Select all that apply.)
   a. Marihuana is considered an illegal substance.
   b. Medical marihuana is produced via Health Canada–regulated producers.
   c. The Marihuana Medical Access Program governs the use of medical marihuana.
   d. Licensed regulators are required to provide quarterly reports upon request to provincial and territorial licensing bodies.
   e. Medical marihuana can legally be consumed in other forms.

5. The nurse is reviewing the four clinical phases of investigational drug studies. Place the four phases in the correct order of occurrence.
   a. Studies that are voluntarily conducted by pharmaceutical companies to obtain more information about the therapeutic and adverse effects of a drug
   b. Studies that involve small numbers of volunteers who have the disease or ailment that the drug is designed to diagnose or treat
   c. Studies that involve small numbers of healthy subjects who do not have the disease or ailment that the drug is intended to treat
   d. Studies that involve large numbers of patients who have the disease that the drug is intended to treat; these studies establish the drug's clinical effectiveness, safety, and dosage range

Answers: 1. a, 2. b, 3. d, 4. a, b, d, e. 5. a = 4, b = 2, c = 1, d = 3

CRITICAL THINKING ACTIVITIES

1. During a busy shift, the nurse is called to the telephone to speak to a family member of Sheila, who was admitted with pneumonia. The caller states, "I'm her grandson, and I want to know if the pneumonia she has is that contagious bug that's going around hospitals. Is she going to die?" Which guidelines will the nurse use to answer the family member?

2. The nurse is assessing a newly admitted 85-year-old woman. During the assessment, the nurse finds that the patient is wearing a copper ring around her left ankle. The ankle is swollen, with 3+ edema, and the copper ring is actually cutting into the skin. What is the nurse's priority action at this time?

3. Using the suggestions given in this chapter of your textbook, interview someone who is not in your ethnocultural group about cultural practices and drug therapy. Compare the person's practices with those of your family.

For answers see http://evolve.elsevier.com/Canada/Lilley/pharmacology/.

Patient-Focused Considerations

Objectives

After reading this chapter, the successful student will be able to do the following:

1. Discuss the influences of a patient's age on the effects of drugs and drug responses.

2. Summarize the impact of age-related physiological changes on pharmacokinetic aspects of drug therapy.

3. Explain how these age-related changes in pharmacokinetics influence various drug effects and drug responses across the lifespan.

4. Provide several examples of how age affects the absorption, distribution, metabolism, and excretion of drugs.

5. Identify drug-related concerns during pregnancy and lactation and provide an explanation of the physiological basis for these concerns.

6. Calculate a drug dose for a pediatric patient using the various formulas available.

7. Identify the importance of a body surface area nomogram for drug calculations in pediatric patients.

8. Discuss the various ethnocultural factors that may influence an individual's response to medications.

9. Identify various ethnocultural phenomena affecting health care and use of medications.

10. List the drugs more commonly associated with variations in response that are more commonly due to ethnocultural factors.

11. Develop a collaborative plan of care for drug therapy and the nursing process that takes into account lifespan and ethnocultural considerations.

e-Learning Activities

Website
(http://evolve.elsevier.com/Canada/Lilley/pharmacology/)

evolve

- Answer Key—Textbook Case Studies
- Answer Key—Critical Thinking Activities
- Chapter Summaries—Printable
- Review Questions for Exam Preparation
- Unfolding Case Studies

Key Terms

Active transport The active (energy-requiring) movement of a substance between different tissues via pumping mechanisms contained within cell membranes. (p. 60)

Culture The customary beliefs, social forms, and material traits of a racial, religious, or social group. (p. 69)

Diffusion The passive movement of a substance (e.g., a drug) between different tissues, from areas of higher concentration to areas of lower concentration. (Compare with *active transport*.) (p. 60)

Neonate A person younger than 1 month of age; newborn infant. (p. 61)

Nomogram A graphical tool for estimating drug dosages using various body measurements. (p. 63)

Older adult A person who is 65 years of age or older. (Note: Some sources consider older adults to be 50 to 55 years of age or older.) (p. 63)

Pediatric Pertaining to a person who is 18 years of age or younger. (Note: Some sources consider pediatric to be 12 years of age or younger.) (p. 61)

Polypharmacy The use of many different drugs concurrently in treating a patient who often has several health problems. (p. 66)

Race Descendants of a common ancestor; a tribe, family, or people believed to belong to the same lineage. (p. 69)

OVERVIEW

From the beginning to the end of life, the human body changes in many ways. These changes have a dramatic effect on the four phases of pharmacokinetics—drug absorption, distribution, metabolism, and excretion. Newborns, children, and older adults all have special needs. Drug therapy at the two ends of the spectrum of life is more likely to result in adverse effects and toxicity. This is especially true if certain basic principles are not understood and followed. Fortunately, response to drug therapy changes in a predictable manner in younger and older patients. Knowing the effect that age has on the pharmacokinetic characteristics of drugs helps predict these changes.

Most experience with drugs and pharmacology has been gained from the adult population. The majority of drug studies have focused on the population between 13 and 65 years of age. It has been estimated that approximately 75% of currently approved drugs lack Health Canada approval for pediatric use and therefore lack specific dosage guidelines for neonates and children (Rieder, Canadian Paediatric Society, & Drug Therapy and Hazardous Substances Committee, 2011). Fortunately, many excellent pediatric drug dosage books are available. Most drugs are effective in younger and older patients, but drugs often behave differently in patients at the opposite ends of the age spectrum. It is vitally important from the standpoint of safe and effective drug administration to understand what these differences are and how to adjust for them.

DRUG THERAPY DURING PREGNANCY

A fetus is exposed to many of the same substances as the mother, including any drugs that she takes—prescription, nonprescription, or illicit drugs. The first trimester of pregnancy is generally the period of greatest danger of drug-induced developmental defects.

Transfer of both drugs and nutrients to the fetus occurs primarily by **diffusion** across the placenta, although not all drugs cross the placenta. Recall from chemistry that diffusion is a passive process based on differences in concentration between different tissues. **Active transport** requires the expenditure of energy and often involves some sort of cell-surface protein pump. The factors that contribute to the safety or potential harm of drug therapy during pregnancy can be broadly broken down into three areas: drug properties, fetal gestational age, and maternal factors.

Drug properties that impact drug transfer to the fetus include the drug's chemistry, dosage, and concurrently administered drugs. Examples of relevant chemical properties include molecular weight, protein binding, lipid solubility, and chemical structure. Important drug dosage variables include dose and duration of therapy.

Fetal gestational age is an important factor in determining the potential for harmful drug effects to the fetus. The fetus is at the greatest risk for drug-induced developmental defects during the first trimester of pregnancy. During this period, the fetus undergoes rapid cell proliferation. Skeleton, muscles, limbs, and visceral organs are developing at their most rapid rate. Self-treatment of any minor illness is strongly discouraged anytime during pregnancy, but particularly during the first trimester. Gestational age is also important in determining when a drug can most easily cross the placenta to the fetus. During the last trimester, the greatest percentage of maternally absorbed drug gets to the fetus.

Maternal factors also play a role in determining drug effects on the fetus. Any change in the mother's physiology can affect the amount of drug to which the fetus may be exposed. Maternal kidney and liver functions affect drug metabolism and excretion. Impairment in either kidney or liver function may result in higher drug levels or prolonged drug exposure and thus increased fetal transfer. Maternal genotype may also affect how certain drugs are metabolized (pharmacogenetics). The lack of certain enzyme systems may result in adverse drug effects to the fetus when the mother is exposed to a drug that is normally metabolized by this enzyme.

Although exposure of the fetus to drugs is most detrimental during the first trimester, drug transfer to the fetus is more likely during the last trimester. This is the result of enhanced blood flow to the fetus, increased fetal surface area, and increased amount of free drug in the mother's circulation. There may be some specific situations when a drug may be used in one trimester but not in another.

It is important to use drugs judiciously during pregnancy; however, there are certain situations that require their use. Without drug therapy, maternal conditions such as hypertension, epilepsy, diabetes, and infection could seriously endanger both the mother and the fetus, and the potential for harm far outweighs the risks of appropriate drug therapy.

Motherisk, an international authority in maternal–fetal toxicology based at The Hospital for Sick Children, Toronto, Ontario, is a clinical, research, and teaching program. The Motherisk program provides evidence-informed research originating from primary literature and examines education on the safety or risk for the developing fetus to maternal exposure to drugs. The Motherisk program creates peer-reviewed statements derived from primary literature and examines fetal outcomes in addition to the risk–benefit profile of maternal treatment when evaluating the safety of medication use in pregnancy. The program provides expert counselling promoting the healthy development of the fetus and infants. The program recommends discussing the relative risks and benefits of any prescribed drug therapy and not taking over-the-counter (OTC) drugs or natural health products without consulting with the health care provider. Health care providers can go directly to evidence-informed research and education about the safety or risk for the developing fetus of maternal exposure to drugs and make clinical decisions based on risk or benefit information. Four help lines are available on the Motherisk website to give women and health care providers information on risk or safety of prescription and OTC drugs as well as natural health products. Their website with the hotline numbers is http://www.motherisk.org/women/index.jsp.

In 1979, in response to the thalidomide tragedy, the US Food and Drug Administration (FDA) implemented labelling requirements with the intent of providing evidence-informed information about the use of medication in pregnancy. In 2014, The FDA introduced a labelling rule that replaces the former product letter risk categories—A, B, C, D and X—with three detailed realistic subsections that describe the risks and benefits of prescription drugs and biologic medicines used by women who are pregnant and lactating. The three main categories include: pregnancy, lactation, and females and males of reproductive potential; the rule came into effect in June of 2015. Each section will include a detailed risk summary, clinical considerations section, and relevant data section. This information will guide heath care providers in decision making when prescribing for and counselling patients. The categories are described in Table 4-1. Over-the-counter drugs are not affected by the final rule.

DRUG THERAPY DURING BREASTFEEDING

Breastfed infants are at risk for exposure to drugs consumed by the mother. A wide variety of drugs easily cross from the mother's circulation into the breast milk and subsequently to the breastfeeding infant. Drug properties similar to those discussed in the previous section influence the exposure of infants to drugs via breastfeeding. The primary drug characteristics that increase the likelihood of drug transfer via breastfeeding include fat

TABLE	4-1

Pregnancy Safety Categories

Subsection	Description
Pregnancy	Provides information about the use of the drug in women who are pregnant (e.g., dose and potential risk to the developing fetus). Information about the existence of a pregnancy registry that collects and maintains data on how pregnant women are affected when they use the prescribed drug or biological product is also required.
Lactation	Provides information about the use of the drug while breastfeeding (e.g., amount of drug in breast milk and potential effects on the child being breastfed).
Females and Males of Reproductive Potential	Provides information about how a particular drug may affect pregnancy testing, contraception, and infertility. as it relates to the drug. This information has been included in labeling, but there was no consistent placement for it until now.

Note: Within the pregnancy and lactation subsections will be three subheadings: risk summary, clinical considerations, and data. These subheadings will provide more detailed information (e.g., human and animal data on the use of the drug, specific adverse reactions of concern for pregnant or breastfeeding women).
Source: U. S. Food and Drug Administration, (2016). Pregnancy and lactation labeling (drugs) final rule. Retrieved from http://www.fda.gov/Drugs/DevelopmentApprovalProcess/DevelopmentResources/Labeling/ucm093307.htm

solubility, low molecular weight, nonionization, and high concentration. Some drugs that are considered weak basic may accumulate in breast milk.

Fortunately, breast milk is not the primary route for maternal drug excretion. Drug levels in breast milk are usually lower than those in the maternal circulation. The actual amount of exposure depends largely on the volume of milk consumed. The ultimate decision as to whether a breastfeeding mother takes a particular drug depends on the risk–benefit ratio. The risks of drug transfer to the infant in relation to the benefits of continuing breastfeeding and the therapeutic benefits to the mother must be considered on a case-by-case basis.

CONSIDERATIONS FOR CHILDREN: NEONATAL AND PEDIATRIC PATIENTS

Pediatric patients are defined based on age. A **neonate** is defined as between birth and 1 month of age. An infant is between 1 and 12 months of age, a child is between 1 and 12 years of age, and an adolescent is between 13 and 19 years of age. The age ranges that correspond to the

SPECIAL POPULATIONS: CHILDREN

Pharmacokinetic Changes in Children

Absorption

- Gastric pH is less acidic because acid-producing cells in the stomach are immature until approximately 1 to 2 years of age.
- Gastric emptying is slowed because of slow or irregular peristalsis, which can result in a greater time difference between drug administration and plasma concentration. Drug absorption may potentially be increased.
- First-pass elimination by the liver is reduced because of the immaturity of the liver and reduced levels of microsomal enzymes.
- Reduced bile salt formation decreases bioavailability of lipophilic drugs.
- Intramuscular absorption is faster and irregular.

Distribution

- Total body water is 70 to 80% in full-term infants, 85% in premature newborns, and 64% in children 1 to 12 years of age, resulting in increased distribution and dilution of water-soluble drugs in these groups.
- Fat content is lower in young patients because of greater total body water.
- Protein binding is decreased because of decreased production of protein by the immature liver; lower protein binding can result in higher concentrations of free drugs in the body.

- More drugs enter the brain because of an immature blood–brain barrier. Consequently, some drugs will have an enhanced effect.

Metabolism

- Levels of microsomal enzymes are decreased because the immature liver has not yet started producing enough.
- Once liver enzymes are produced, older children may have increased metabolism and require higher doses or more frequent administration of medications (particularly pain medications).
- Many variables affect metabolism in premature infants, infants, and children, including the status of liver enzyme production, genetic differences, and substances to which the mother was exposed during pregnancy. For example, the neonatal liver is not yet developed sufficiently to be able to metabolize a large proportion of drug substrates.

Excretion

- Glomerular filtration rate and tubular secretion and resorption are all decreased in young patients because of kidney immaturity; drug excretion is decreased.
- Perfusion to the kidneys may be decreased, which results in reduced kidney function, concentrating ability, and excretion of drugs.

TABLE 4-2	
Classification of Young Patients	
Age Range	**Classification**
Younger than 38 wks gestation	Premature or preterm infant
Younger than 1 mo	Neonate or newborn infant
1 mo to younger than 1 yr	Infant
1 yr to younger than 12 yr	Child
13 yr to 19 yr	Adolescent

Note: The meaning of the term *pediatric* may vary with the individual drug and clinical situation. Often the maximum age for a pediatric patient may be identified as 16 years of age. Consult manufacturer's guidelines for specific dosing information.

various terms applied to pediatric patients are shown in Table 4-2.

Physiology and Pharmacokinetics

Pediatric pharmacotherapy focuses on the unique therapeutic needs of neonates, infants, children, and adolescents. Patients in these age groups offer challenges distinct from those of adult patients. Drugs behave differently in this population; for example, medications may not be absorbed, distributed, metabolized, or eliminated in the same manner as in adults, causing increased or decreased efficacy or safety. As well, pediatric patients handle drugs much differently from adult patients, based primarily on the immaturity of vital organs. In both neonates and older pediatric patients anatomical structures and physiological systems and functions are still in the process of developing. The Special Populations: Children box on this page lists those physiological factors that alter the pharmacokinetic properties of drugs in young patients.

Pharmacodynamics

Drug actions (or pharmacodynamics) are altered in young patients, and the maturity of various organs determines how drugs act in the body. Certain drugs may be more toxic, whereas others may be less toxic. The sensitivity of receptor sites may also vary with age; thus higher or lower dosages may be required depending on the drug. In addition, rapidly developing tissues may be more sensitive to certain drugs, and therefore smaller doses may be required. Because of this receptor sensitivity, certain drugs are generally contraindicated during the growth years. For instance, tetracycline may permanently discolour a young person's teeth; corticosteroids may suppress growth when given systemically (but not when delivered via asthma inhalers, for example); and quinolone antibiotics may damage cartilage.

Dosage Calculations for Pediatric Patients

Most drugs have not been sufficiently investigated to ensure their safety and effectiveness in children. In spite of this lack of research, there are numerous excellent pediatric dosage references. Because pediatric patients (especially premature infants and neonates) have small bodies and immature organs, they are particularly susceptible to drug interactions, toxicity, and unusual drug responses. Pediatric patients require different dosage calculations than adults do. Characteristics of pediatric patients that have a significant effect on dosage calculation include the following:

- The skin is thinner and more permeable.
- The stomach lacks acid to kill bacteria.
- The lungs have weaker mucous barriers.
- Body temperature is less well regulated and dehydration occurs easily.
- The liver and kidneys are immature and so drug metabolism and excretion are impaired.

Many formulas for pediatric dosage calculation have been used throughout the years. Formulas involving age, weight, and body surface area (BSA) are most commonly employed as the basis for calculations.

BSA-based formulas are the most accurate of the dosage formulas and are used primarily for calculating doses of chemotherapy and for high-risk infants such as preterm infants. The ratio of BSA varies with length. For the BSA method, the nurse needs the following information:

- Drug order with drug name, dose, route, time, and frequency
- Information regarding available dosage forms
- Pediatric patient's height in centimetres (cm) and weight in kilograms (kg)
- BSA **nomogram** for children (e.g., West nomogram [shown in Figure 4-1]; there are other modified formulations for determining BSA available)
- Recommended adult drug dosage

The West nomogram (see Figure 4-1) uses a child's height and weight to determine the child's BSA. This information is then inserted into the BSA formula to obtain a drug dosage for a specific pediatric patient. Online calculators that determine BSA using the West nomogram and other applications are widely available via the Internet.

Consider the following examples:

$$\frac{\text{BSA of child}}{\text{BSA of adult}} \times \text{adult dose} = \text{estimated child's dose}$$

$$\text{BSA of child (m}^2) \times \frac{\text{manufacturer's recommended dose}}{\text{m}^2} = \text{estimated child's dose}$$

The most commonly used method to calculate drug dosages is the body weight method. Most drug references recommend dosages based on milligrams per kilogram of body weight. Weight-based dosage calculators are available online. The following information is needed to calculate the pediatric dosage:

- Drug order (as discussed previously)
- Pediatric patient's weight in kilograms (1 kg = 2.2 pounds)
- Pediatric dosage as per manufacturer or drug formulary guidelines
- Information regarding available dosage forms

When using either of the previous methods, the nurse must do the following to ensure the correct pediatric dose:

- Determine the pediatric patient's weight in kilograms
- Use a current drug reference to determine the usual dosage range per 24 hours in milligrams (mg) per kilogram (kg)
- Determine the dose parameters by multiplying the weight by the minimum and maximum daily doses of the drug (the safe range)
- Determine the total amount of the drug to administer per dose and per day
- Compare the drug dosage prescribed with the calculated safe range
- If the drug dosage raises any concerns or varies from the safe range, contact the health care provider or prescriber immediately and do not give the drug

A common source of medication error and potential toxicity is confusing pounds with kilograms. Unless otherwise noted, the child's weight is to be given in kilograms, not pounds. Take great care to ensure that the correct weight is reported to the prescriber. In calculating pediatric dosages, the factor of organ maturity must always be considered along with BSA, age, and weight. When all of these physical developmental factors are considered, the likelihood of safe and effective drug administration is increased. Emotional developmental considerations must also be a part of the decision-making process in drug therapy with pediatric patients.

CONSIDERATIONS FOR OLDER ADULT PATIENTS

Due to the decline in organ function that occurs with advancing age, older adult patients handle drugs physiologically differently from adult patients. Drug therapy in older adults is more likely to result in adverse effects and toxicity.

An **older adult** is defined as one who is 65 years of age or older. The terms *elderly* and *older adult* have different meanings in different societies, so their definitions are somewhat arbitrary. In most developed countries, these terms refer to retirement age, which occurs around the age of 65. However, for research purposes, subgroups of older adults, such as the "younger old" (ages 65 to 75), the "older old" (ages 75 to 85), and "oldest old" (ages 85+) may be identified. It is also important to note that chronological age is not a precise marker for changes that

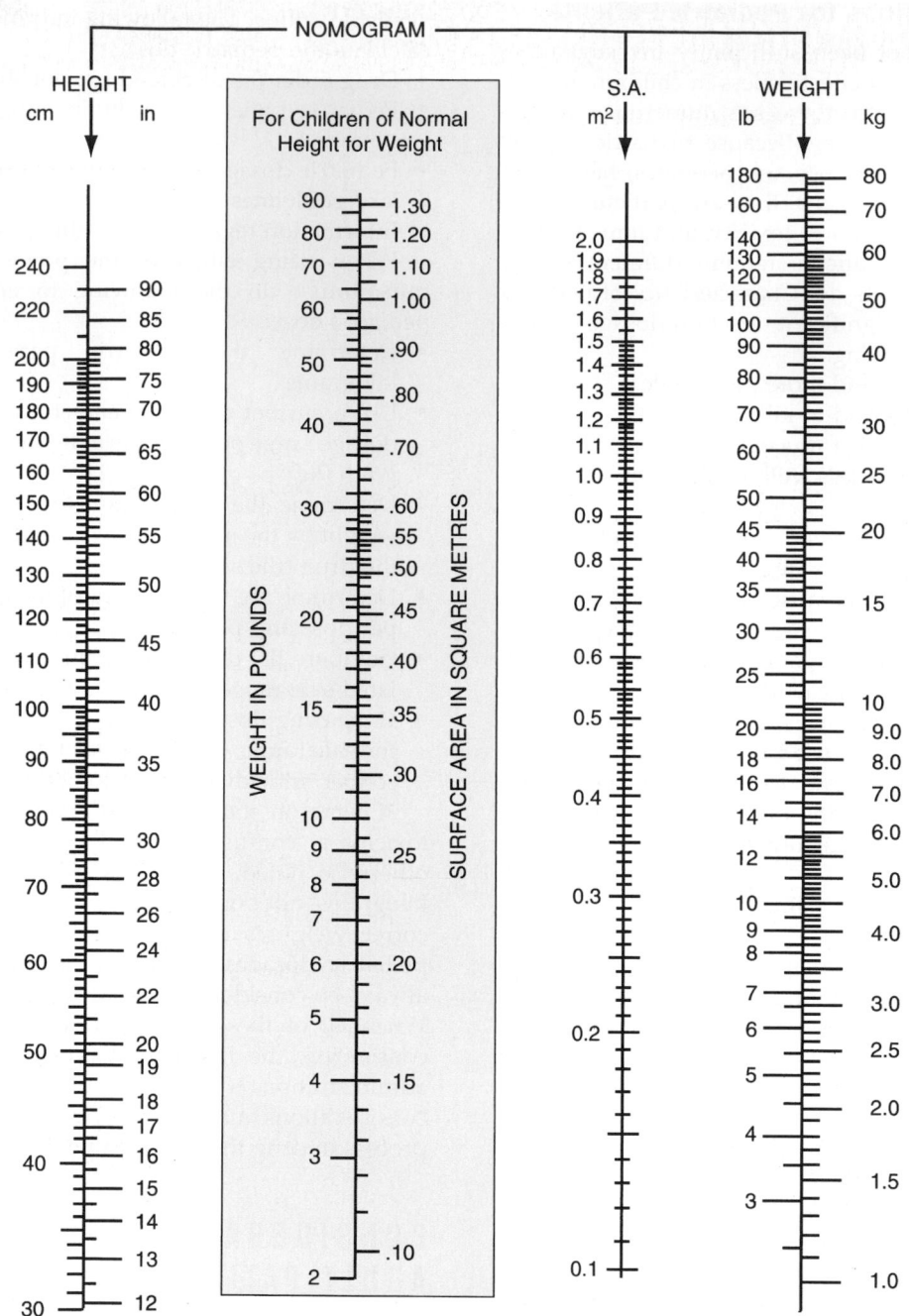

FIG. 4-1 West nomogram for infants and children. *S.A.*, surface area. (Modified from data by Boyd, E., & West, C. D. (2011). In R. M. Kliegman, B. Stanton, J. St. Geme, et al. (Eds.) *Nelson textbook of pediatrics* (19th ed.). Philadelphia: Saunders.)

accompany aging. There are dramatic variations in health status, levels of participation, and independence among older adults of the same age.

This segment of the population is growing at a dramatic pace (See Special Populations: Older Adults: Percentage of Population Older than 65 Years of Age). At the beginning of the twentieth century, older adults constituted a mere 5% of the total population in Canada.

At that time, more people died of infections than of degenerative, chronic illnesses such as heart disease, cancer, and diabetes. As medical and health care tech-

nology has advanced, so has the ability to prolong life. This has resulted in a growing population of older adults that is expected to continue for decades. In 2013, patients over 65 years of age made up 15.3% of the total population; this is expected to increase to 23% by 2030 (Public Health Agency of Canada, 2014). Older people aged 85 years and over make up the fastest growing age group in Canada. Life expectancy is currently approximately 81 years. These trends are expected to continue as new disease prevention and treatment methods are developed. However, in contrast,

SPECIAL POPULATIONS: OLDER ADULTS

Percentage of Population Older than 65 Years of Age

Year	Percentage Over Age 65
1900	5%
2001	12.6%
2021	18.5%
2031	22.8%
2061	25.5%

Source: Employment and Social Development Canada, 2015.

 ## SPECIAL POPULATIONS: OLDER ADULTS

Alzheimer's Disease in Canada

- Alzheimer's disease is fatal, progressive, and degenerative, affecting approximately 485 550 Canadians, and the figure is expected to double by 2031 (Alzheimer Society of Canada, 2015b).
- Advancing age is the most significant risk factor. Alzheimer's disease affects 5% of Canadians over the age of 65 and 25% of Canadians over the age of 85 (Duthley, 2013).
- Alzheimer's disease is the only cause of death among the top 10 in Canada that cannot be prevented, cured, or slowed. Death occurs about 3 to 9 years after diagnosis (Querforth & LaFerla, 2010).
- Family history and genetics are significant risk factors. Risk increases by 10 to 40% if a first-degree relative has Alzheimer's disease. The ApoE4 gene is the most important genetic risk factor.
- Gender also is a significant risk factor; 72% of those with Alzheimer's disease are women (Alzheimer Society of Canada, 2015a).
- Alzheimer's disease is characterized by the slow and initially insidious decline of memory and functional ability along with behavioural and personality changes.

- Hallmark abnormalities of Alzheimer's disease include deposits of the protein fragment beta-amyloid (plaques) and twisted strands of the protein tau (tangles) as well as evidence of nerve cell damage and death in the brain.
- New criteria and guidelines for diagnosing Alzheimer's recommend describing the disease in three stages. Studies are providing evidence that a preclinical stage where brain degeneration occurs may begin 10 years before the second stage, when clinical symptoms of mild cognitive impairment emerge. The third stage is dementia (The Lancet, 2013).
- Promising areas of research focused on early detection include biological markers such as low amyloid-β_{42} in cerebrospinal fluid and neuroimaging techniques. Such advances will facilitate the development of disease-modifying treatments, early diagnosis, and improve clinical care (Fraller, 2013).
- Currently, there is no pharmacological cure for Alzheimer's disease; however, there are several medications that may improve quality of life for those with Alzheimer's disease.

compared to the overall Canadian population, First Nations, Inuit, and Métis populations are younger and growing at a faster rate.

Issues in Clinical Drug Use in Older Adults

Older adults have considerable interindividual variability in health, disability, age-related changes, polymorbidity, and associated polypharmacy, making generalization of prescribing recommendations difficult. The older-adult population consumes a larger proportion of all medications than other population groups, taking between 20 and 40% of all prescription drugs and over 40% of OTC drugs. Older adults in Canada takes four times more OTC medications than any other age group (Canadian Institute for Health Information, 2014). At any given time, the average older adult takes four or five prescription drugs as well as two OTC medications, which can increase the risk of drug interactions. The most commonly used drug in older adults in Canada is a statin. Other commonly prescribed drugs for older adults include antihypertensives, β-blockers, diuretics, insulin, and potassium supplements. The most frequently used drugs are analgesics, laxatives, and nonsteroidal anti-inflammatory drugs (NSAIDs). Older adults, especially those of certain ethnicities, may use various folk remedies of unknown composition that are unfamiliar to their health care providers.

Not only do older adults consume a greater proportion of prescription and OTC medications, they commonly take multiple medications on a daily basis.

About 1 in 3 older adults takes more than 8 different drugs each day, with many taking 15 or more. In 2009, 63% of older adults had claims for 5 or more different drug classes, 23% had claims for 10 or more drug classes, and 30% of those older than 85 had claims for 10 or more drug classes (McPherson, Ji, Hunt, et al., 2012). One reason for the use of multiple medications is the occurrence of more chronic diseases, which now have even more drug options available for treatment. More than 80% of patients taking eight or more drugs have one or more chronic illnesses. More complicated medication regimens predispose older adults to self-medication errors, especially those with reduced visual acuity and manual dexterity. Such sensory and motor deficits can be particularly problematic when older adults split their own tablets. The practice of pill splitting occurs commonly for financial reasons because lower- and higher-strength tablets often have similar costs. Other factors that may contribute to medication errors in older adults include lack of adequate patient education and understanding of their drug regimens and use of multiple prescribers and multiple pharmacies. In this age of medical specialization, patients may see several prescribers for their many illnesses. It is therefore important for the patient to use only one pharmacy so that monitoring for drug interactions and duplicate therapy can occur.

Older adult patients are hospitalized frequently due to adverse drug reactions. Many people, including older adults, use natural health products, including herbal remedies and dietary supplements, which can interact with prescription drugs. The simultaneous use of multiple medications is called **polypharmacy**. The chance of a drug interaction is approximately 6% for a patient receiving two medications. The risk increases dramatically as the number of drugs the patient is taking increases. For a patient taking five medications, the chance of a drug interaction is 50%, and for those taking ten or more medications, the chance is 100%.

Some drugs may be given specifically to counteract the adverse effects of other drugs (e.g., a potassium supplement to counteract the potassium loss caused by certain diuretic medications). This is one example of what is known as the *prescribing cascade*. Often it is difficult to distinguish adverse drug effects from disease symptoms. Although such prescribing is sometimes appropriate, it also increases the potential for more adverse drug events (including drug interactions, hospitalization or prolonged hospital stays, hip fractures secondary to drug-induced falls, addiction risk, anorexia, confusion, urinary retention, and fatigue). Recognizing polypharmacy and taking steps to reduce it whenever possible by decreasing the number or dosages of drugs taken can significantly reduce the incidence of adverse outcomes. Various types of electronic health records, e-prescribing, computerized physician order entry, and electronic medication administration record (eMAR), as well as clinical decision support systems (used at the point of care to make evidence-informed decision) have the potential to reduce inappropriate prescribing and polypharmacy in older adults. Appropriate drug doses for older adult patients may sometimes be one-half to two-thirds of the standard adult dose. As a general rule, dosing for older adults should follow the advice, "Start low and go slow," which means to start with the lowest possible dose (often less than an average adult dose) and increase the dose slowly, based on patient response.

Another important issue is nonadherence with prescribed medication regimens. Drug nonadherence is reported to occur in roughly 40% of older adult patients and is associated with increased rates of hospitalization. Nonadherance is multifactorial and may include patient factors such as poor understanding of the disease, lack of involvement in the treatment decision-making process, ability to purchase medication, and suboptimal medical literacy; the occurrence of adverse effects; physician factors such as prescribing complex drug regimens and not explaining the benefits and adverse effects of a medication effectively; and health system factors such as an overtaxed health care system with inadequate time engaged with patients for proper assessment and understanding of the patients' needs (Brown & Bussell, 2011).

Physiological Changes

Physiological changes associated with aging affect the actions of many drugs. As the body ages, the functioning of several organ systems slowly declines. The collective physiological changes associated with the aging process have a major effect on the disposition and action of drugs. Table 4-3 lists some of the body systems most affected by the aging process.

The sensitivity of older adults to many drugs requires careful monitoring and dosage adjustment. The criteria for drug dosages in older adults must include consideration of body weight and organ functioning, with emphasis on liver, kidney, cardiovascular, and central nervous system function (similar to the criteria for pediatric dosages). With aging, there is a general decrease in body weight.

Changes in drug molecule receptors in the body can make a patient more or less sensitive to certain

TABLE	4-3

Physiological Changes in Older Adults

System	Physiological Change
Cardiovascular	↓ Cardiac output = ↓ absorption and distribution ↓ Blood flow = ↓ absorption and distribution
Gastrointestinal	↑ pH (alkaline gastric secretions) = altered absorption ↓ Peristalsis = delayed gastric emptying
Liver	↓ Enzyme production = ↓ metabolism ↓ Blood flow = ↓ metabolism
Kidney	↓ Blood flow = ↓ excretion ↓ Function = ↓ excretion ↓ Glomerular filtration rate = ↓ excretion

medications. For example, older adults commonly have increased sensitivity to central nervous system depressant medications (e.g., anxiolytics, tricyclic antidepressants) because of reduced integrity of the blood–brain barrier.

The most important organs from the standpoint of the breakdown and elimination of drugs are the liver and the kidneys. Measurement of kidney function is an essential element of care for older adults because it may evaluate effectiveness of drug therapies and allow for drug adjustments to prevent toxicity. Canadian guidelines to assess deteriorating kidney function and to stage kidney disease are based on the estimated glomerular filtration rate (eGFR) and the presence of albuminuria. *Albuminuria* is defined as a urine albumin-to-creatinine ratio greater than 2.0 mg/mmoL for men and greater than 2.8 mg/mmoL for women. Screening of the urine creatinine/albumin level should be incorporated into routine assessments for all older adults. The serum creatinine level in older adults may be lower because of the decline of muscle mass (creatinine is a by-product of muscle metabolism).

Liver function is assessed by testing the blood for liver enzymes such as aspartate aminotransferase (AST) and alanine aminotransferase (ALT). These laboratory values can help in assessing the ability to metabolize and eliminate medications and can aid in anticipating the risk of toxicity, drug accumulation, or both. Laboratory assessments need to be conducted at least annually, both for preventive health monitoring and for screening for possible toxic effects of drug therapy. Such assessments may be indicated more frequently (e.g., every 1, 3, or 6 months) in those patients requiring higher-risk drug regimens.

Pharmacokinetics

The pharmacokinetic phases of absorption, distribution, metabolism, and excretion (See Chapter 2) may be different in older adults from those in younger adults. Awareness of these differences helps the nurse ensure appropriate administration of drugs and monitoring of older adults. The Special Populations: Older Adults box: Pharmacokinetic Changes lists the four pharmacokinetic phases and summarizes how they are altered by the aging process.

Absorption

Absorption in older adults can be altered by many mechanisms. Advancing age results in reduced absorption of both dietary nutrients and drugs. Several physiological changes account for this reduction in absorption. Older adult patients have a gradual reduction in the ability of the stomach to produce hydrochloric acid, which results in a decrease in gastric acidity and may alter the absorption of some drugs. In addition, the combination of decreased cardiac output and advancing atherosclerosis results in a general reduction in the flow of blood to major organs, including the stomach. By 65 years of age, there is an approximately 50% reduction in blood flow to the gastrointestinal tract. Absorption, whether of nutrient or drug, is dependent on good blood supply to the stomach and intestines. The absorptive surface area of an older adult person's gastrointestinal tract is often reduced, thus decreasing drug absorption.

Gastrointestinal motility is important for moving substances out of the stomach and through the gastrointestinal tract. Muscle tone and motor activity in the gastrointestinal tract are reduced in older adults. This

---

 ## SPECIAL POPULATIONS: OLDER ADULTS

Pharmacokinetic Changes

Absorption

- Gastric pH is less acidic because of a gradual reduction in the production of hydrochloric acid in the stomach.
- Gastric emptying is slowed because of a decline in smooth muscle tone and motor activity.
- Movement throughout the gastrointestinal tract is slower because of decreased muscle tone and motor activity.
- Blood flow to the gastrointestinal tract is reduced by 40 to 50% because of decreased cardiac output and decreased perfusion.
- The absorptive surface area is decreased because the aging process blunts and flattens villi.

Distribution

- In adults 40 to 60 years of age, total body water is 55% in males and 47% in females; in those over 60 years of age, total body water is 52% in males and 46% in females.

- Fat content is increased because of decreased lean body mass.
- Protein (albumin) binding sites are reduced because of decreased production of proteins by the aging liver and reduced protein intake.

Metabolism

- The levels of microsomal enzymes are decreased because the capacity of the aging liver to produce them is reduced.
- Liver blood flow is reduced by approximately 1.5% per year after 25 years of age, which decreases liver metabolism.

Excretion

- Glomerular filtration rate is decreased by 40 to 50%, primarily because of decreased blood flow.
- The number of intact nephrons is decreased.

often results in constipation, for which older adults frequently take laxatives. The use of laxatives may accelerate gastrointestinal motility enough to actually reduce the absorption of drugs.

Distribution

The distribution of medications throughout the body is also different in older adults. There seems to be a gradual reduction in the total body water content with aging. Therefore, the concentrations of highly water-soluble (hydrophilic) drugs may be higher in older adults because they have less body water in which the drugs can be diluted. The composition of the body also changes with aging, with a decrease in lean muscle mass and an increase in body fat. In both men and women, there is an approximately 20% reduction in muscle mass between the ages of 25 and 65 years and a corresponding 20% increase in body fat. Fat-soluble or lipophilic drugs, such as hypnotics and sedatives, are primarily distributed to fatty tissues and may result in prolonged drug actions or toxicity.

Older adult patients may have reduced protein concentrations, due in part to reduced liver function. Reduced dietary intake or poor gastrointestinal protein absorption can cause nutritional deficiencies and reduced blood protein levels. Regardless of the cause, the result is a reduced number of protein-binding sites for highly protein-bound drugs. This change results in higher levels of unbound (active) drug in the blood.

Remember that only drugs that are not bound to proteins are active. Therefore, the effects of highly protein-bound drugs may be enhanced if their dosages are not adjusted to accommodate any reduced serum albumin concentrations. Some highly protein-bound drugs include warfarin and phenytoin.

Metabolism

Metabolism declines with advancing age. The transformation of active drugs into inactive metabolites is performed primarily by the liver. The liver loses mass with age and slowly loses its ability to metabolize drugs effectively due to reduced production of microsomal (cytochrome P450) enzymes. There is also a reduction in blood flow to the liver because of reduced cardiac output and atherosclerosis. A reduction in the hepatic blood flow of approximately 1.5% per year occurs after 25 years of age. All of these factors contribute to prolonging the half-life of many drugs (e.g., warfarin), which can potentially result in drug accumulation if serum drug levels are not closely monitored.

Excretion

Kidney function declines in roughly two-thirds of older adults. A reduction in the glomerular filtration rate of 40 to 50%, combined with a reduction in cardiac output leading to reduced kidney perfusion, can result in delayed drug excretion and therefore drug accumulation. This is especially true for drugs with a low therapeutic index such as digoxin. Kidney function needs to be monitored frequently. Appropriate dose and interval adjustments may be determined on the basis of results of kidney and liver function studies as well as the presence of therapeutic levels of the drug in the serum. If a decrease in kidney and liver function is known, the dosage is usually adjusted by the prescriber so that drug accumulation and toxicity may be minimized.

Problematic Medications for Older Adults

Certain classes of drugs are more likely to cause problems in older patients because of many of the physiological alterations and pharmacokinetic changes already discussed. Table 4-4 lists some of the more common medications that are problematic. Some drugs to be avoided in older adults have been identified by various professional organizations such as the Institute for Safe Medication Practices Canada, as well as by various other authoritative sources. Since the 1990s, an effective tool, the Beers Criteria, has been used to identify drugs that may be inappropriately prescribed, be ineffective, or cause adverse drug reactions in older adults (see the Evidence in Practice box on p. 70). The Beers Criteria are useful and help determine risk-associated situations for older adults and specific drugs that may be problematic.

TABLE	4-4

Medications and Conditions Requiring Special Considerations for Older Adults

Medication	Common Complications
ANALGESICS	
Opioids	Confusion, constipation, urinary retention, nausea, vomiting, respiratory depression, falls
Nonsteroidal anti-inflammatory drugs (NSAIDs)	Edema, nausea, gastric ulceration, bleeding, kidney toxicity
Anticholinergics and antihistamines	Blurred vision, dry mouth, constipation, confusion and sedation, urinary retention, tachycardia
Anticoagulants (heparin sodium, warfarin sodium)	Major and minor bleeding episodes, many drug interactions, dietary interactions
Antidepressants	Sedation and strong anticholinergic adverse effects (see above)
Antihypertensives	Nausea, orthostatic, hypotension, diarrhea, bradycardia, heart failure, impotence
Cardiac glycosides (e.g., digoxin)	Visual disorders, nausea, diarrhea, dysrhythmias, hallucinations, decreased appetite, weight loss

TABLE 4-4

Medications and Conditions Requiring Special Considerations for Older Adults—cont'd

Medication	Common Complications
CNS depressants (muscle relaxants, opioids)	Sedation, weakness, dry mouth, confusion, urinary retention, ataxia
Sedatives and hypnotics	Confusion, daytime sedation, ataxia, lethargy, increased risk of falls
Thiazide diuretics	Electrolyte imbalance, rashes, fatigue, leg cramps, dehydration

Condition	Drugs Requiring Special Caution and Monitoring
Bladder flow obstruction	Anticholinergics, antihistamines, decongestants, antidepressants
Clotting disorders	NSAIDs, aspirin, antiplatelet drugs
Chronic constipation	Calcium channel blockers, tricyclic antidepressants, anticholinergics
Chronic obstructive pulmonary disease	Long-acting sedatives and hypnotics, narcotics, β-blockers
Clotting disorders	NSAIDs, aspirin, antiplatelet drugs
Heart failure and hypertension	Sodium, decongestants, amphetamines, OTC cold products
Insomnia	Decongestants, bronchodilators, monoamine oxidase inhibitors
Parkinson's disease	Antipsychotics, phenothiazines
Syncope and falls	Sedatives, hypnotics, narcotics, central nervous system depressants, muscle relaxants, antidepressants, antihypertensives

ETHNOCULTURAL CONSIDERATIONS

Canada is a multiculturally diverse nation as evidenced by its constant and rapidly changing demographics, owing to persistent low fertility, strong immigration, and the number of descendants. Prior to the 1970s, 78.3% of immigration to Canada came from European countries (e.g., the United Kingdom, Italy, Germany, and the Netherlands). The influx of European-born immigrants has declined steadily.

In 2011, visible minority groups and immigrants comprised approximately 19% and 21% of the Canadian population, respectively. This number is expected to increase to between 29% and 32% by 2030 (Statistics Canada, 2014). By 2031, the South Asian and the Chinese population in Canada are projected to remain, as in 2006, the largest visible minority groups. In contrast, the Black and Filipino populations will grow at a slower pace. The Arab and West Asian populations, however, were projected to triple in numbers by 2013, making these groups the most rapidly growing group (Statistics Canada, 2014).

The Indigenous population is growing faster than the rest of the Canadian population, largely due to a younger population and high fertility. It is anticipated that this group will continue to grow in numbers to 2031.

Generation status adds to the diversity and complexity of the Canadian population. In 2011, the majority (81.5%) of first-generation Canadians, themselves immigrants, were of Chinese, East Indian, and English descent. The most frequently reported origins by the second generation, either alone or with other origins, were English, Canadian, and Scottish, while third generation were Canadian, English, or French (Statistics Canada, 2014). In addition, three in ten Canadians who are visible minorities are Canadian-born.

Such ethnocultural demographic shifts and changes significantly impact Canada's health care system and the delivery of care. The field of **ethnopharmacology** provides an expanding body of knowledge for understanding the specific impact of cultural factors on patient drug response. It is hampered, however, by the lack of clarity in terms such as **race, ethnicity,** and **culture.**

Race is based primarily upon genetically imparted physiognomical features, among which skin colour is a dominant, but not the sole, attribute. Nevertheless, it is possible for a person to be of mixed races, some of which, such as the mestizo of Latin America, have become recognized as evolved races in their own right. Furthermore, terminology may be ambiguous. Scholars may prefer to use the term *Caucasian* rather than *White*, but the former may not be well understood by many respondents. Other terminology evolves over time, such as the evolution in the United States of *African-American* from *Black* and earlier from *negro*. There may also be terminology in use in the common lexicon that is actually offensive to a group in question, for example, references to the Inuit as *Eskimo* or First Nations as *Indian* (Statistics Canada, 2012). The term *First Nations* originated in the 1970s to replace the offensive terminology *Indian*. In Canada, the term *Aboriginal* includes Inuit, First Nations, and Métis. The terms *Aboriginal* and *First Nations* are not interchangeable. The Inuit, meaning *people* in Inuktitut, the Inuit language, are a generally homogeneous indigenous people who live in Nunavut, the Northwest Territories, Northern Quebec and Northern Labrador. The Inuit population forms about 5% of all Aboriginal people in Canada. Métis are a distinct Aboriginal group with mixed ancestry as a result of intermarriage between Aboriginal women and European men. Métis culture draws on a blend of diverse cultural origins and is unique because of this.

EVIDENCE IN PRACTICE

Update on Application of the Beers Criteria for Prevention of Adverse Drug Events in Older Adults

Review

In 1991, a panel of experts led by Mark H. Beers, MD, identified a list of "potentially inappropriate medications" (PIM) for use in individuals 65 years of age and older. These criteria were intended for use with nursing home residents and then were expanded and revised to include all settings of geriatric care. The specific aim of the project was to predict adverse drug reactions (ADRs) in this age group. The Beers Criteria were updated in 1997 and 2002 and provided a listing of drugs and drug classes to be avoided in older adults. The criteria also identified disease states considered to be contraindications for some drugs. In 2005, research was conducted to confirm the relationship between PIM prescribing, as defined by Beers Criteria, and the occurrence of ADRs in older adult patients treated at outpatient clinics. In 2012, a list of medications was identified and classified into three categories: (1) potentially inappropriate medications and classes to avoid in older adults, (2) potentially inappropriate medications and classes to avoid in older adults with certain diseases and syndromes, and (3) medications to be used with caution in older adults. In 2015, The Beers Criteria expands the 2012 list with several drugs removed from the list and with some additions.

Type of Evidence

The 2015 Beers Criteria uses a more comprehensive, systematic review and grading of evidence than the previous 2012 updates. The quality of the criteria continued to include (1) application of an evidence-informed approach, (2) support of the American Geriatrics Society (AGS) in conjunction with an interdisciplinary panel of 13 experts in geriatric care and pharmacotherapy, (3) use of a time-tested method for developing care guidelines while using the Institute of Medicine's standards for evidence/transparency as an important benchmark, and (4) an extensive review of more than 6 700 high-quality research studies and clinical trials about prescription medications for this age group.

Results of the Study

Consistent with the 2012 AGS Beers Criteria, the 2015 criteria are intended to support clinical judgement. They include 40 potentially problematic medications or classes of medications. In addition, the 2015 Beers Criteria include: (1) separate guidance on avoiding 13 drug-drug combinations known to cause harm; (2), a specific list of 20 problematic medications to avoid or doses that need to be adjusted in older adults based on the patient's kidney function; and, (3) three new medications and two new "classes" of medications added to the list (e.g., proton pump inhibitors). New in 2015 are companion guides to assist the health care provider in using the guidelines as well as potential alternative suggestions to the use of high-risk medications in the older adult.

Link of Evidence to Nursing Practice

These criteria update drugs to avoid and use with caution in older adults. They also increase awareness of inappropriate medication use in this age group and may also be integrated into electronic health records. With the support of the AGS, the criteria will continue to develop over time and will continue to help improve the health of older adults. The criteria should be used as a starting point from which to develop a comprehensive process to improve medication appropriateness and safety.

Source: The American Geriatrics Society Beers Criteria Update Expert Panel. (2015). American Geriatrics Society updated Beers Criteria for potentially inappropriate medication use in older adults. *Journal of the American Geriatrics Society, 63* (11), 2227–2246. doi: 10.1111/jgs.13702

Métis people make up approximately 30% of the total Indigenous population. About 68% live in urban areas, with less than 3% living on reserves. First Nations people belong to over 50 distinct cultural groups or band associations such as Cree, Mi'kmaq, or Dene. Forty-seven percent of First Nations people live on reserves (Raphael, 2009).

It is impossible to know a patient's genotype by either physical appearance or health care history. Ethnocultural assessment needs to be part of the assessment phase of the nursing process. Acknowledgment and acceptance of the influences of a patient's cultural beliefs, values, and customs is necessary to promote optimal health and wellness. Some practices are discussed in the Ethnocultural Implications box on p. 71. It is important to emphasize that not every patient from the same country shares the same culture. Many countries encompass those of diverse ethnicities, languages, and religions. Even when a country is relatively homogenous in terms of ethnicity, socioeconomic, political, urban/rural, or regional differences may result in significant diversity, affecting every aspect of health. For this reason, each patient must be individually assessed regarding traditional beliefs and practices. Such assessment requires development of skills in intercultural communication. "Recipe book" approaches to assessment of patients from certain countries or of certain religions are not appropriate and pose risks to quality and safety of care. Religion also has important implications for both health and health care provision. Many lifestyle choices (e.g., diet, use of alcohol and tobacco) are affected by religious belief. Beliefs regarding female modesty, death and dying, reproductive health, hygiene, use of blood products, and other issues have important implications for many areas of health care provision. The increasing religious diversity of Canada strengthens the imperative for health organizations to develop responsive practice. It is important for health care providers to be aware of key areas affected by religious belief and practice in order to provide culturally responsive care. There is great diversity, not only within each of the world's religions, but also in individual faith and commitment to practice.

Ethnocultural Influences and Genetics on Drug Response

The concept of *polymorphism* is critical to an understanding of how the same drug may result in different responses in different individuals. For example, why does a patient of Chinese origin may require lower dosages of an antianxiety drug than a patient who is White? A patient who is Black may respond differently to antihypertensives from a patient who is White? **Drug polymorphism** refers to the effect of a patient's age, gender, size, body composition, and other characteristics on the pharmacokinetics of specific drugs. Factors contributing to drug polymorphism may be categorized into environmental

factors (e.g., diet and nutritional status), cultural factors, and genetic (inherited) factors.

Medication response depends greatly on the level of the patient's adherence with the therapy regimen. Yet adherence may vary depending on the patient's cultural beliefs, experiences with medications, personal expectations, family expectations and influence, and level of education. Adherence is not the only factor, however. Prescribers must also be aware that some patients use alternative natural health remedies that can inhibit or accelerate drug metabolism and therefore alter a drug's response.

Environmental and economic factors (e.g., diet) can contribute to drug response. For example, a diet high in fat has been documented to increase the absorption of the drug griseofulvin (an antifungal drug). Malnutrition with deficiencies in protein, vitamins, and minerals may modify the functioning of metabolic enzymes, which may alter the body's ability to absorb or eliminate a medication.

Historically, most clinical drug trials were conducted using White men, often university students, as research subjects. However, there are data that demonstrate the

ETHNOCULTURAL IMPLICATIONS

A Brief Review of Common Practices Among Canada's Major Cultural Groups

Cultural Group	Some Examples of Health Beliefs and Alternative Healers	Verbal and Nonverbal Communication; Touch/Time	Family	Biological Variations
Asian	May believe in traditional medicine; hot and cold foods; herbs/teas/soups; use of acupuncturist, acupressurist, and herbalist	High respect of others, especially of individuals in positions of authority Not usually comfortable with custom of shaking hands with those of opposite sex Present-oriented	Have close extended family ties; family needs more important than individual needs	Many drug interactions, lactose intolerance, thalassemia
Blacks of African descent	May practise folk medicine; employ "root doctors" as healers; spiritualist May use herbs, oils, and roots	Asking personal questions of someone met for the first time seen as intrusive and not proper Direct eye contact seen as rude Present-oriented	Have close extended family ties Women play important key role in making health care decisions	Keloid formation, sickle cell anemia, lactose intolerance
Indigenous	May believe in harmony with nature and ill spirits causing disease May use medicine man Rattles are shaken to call up the spirit of life when someone is ill	Speak in low tone of voice Light touch of a person's hand is preferred versus a firm handshake as a greeting Present-oriented	Have close extended family ties; emphasis on family	Lactose intolerance, cleft uvula problems

Note: Each patient is unique and has his or her own cultural attitudes, beliefs, values, customs, and norms and specific health practices which may or may not reflect some of the above examples.

impact of genetic factors on drug *pharmacokinetics* and drug *pharmacodynamics* or drug response (see Chapter 5). Some individuals of European and African descent are known to be *slow acetylators*. This means that their bodies attach acetyl groups to drug molecules at a relatively slow rate, which results in elevated drug concentrations. This situation may warrant lower drug dosages. A classic example of a drug whose metabolism is affected by this characteristic is the antituberculosis drug isoniazid. In contrast, some patients of Japanese and Inuit descent are more rapid acetylators and metabolize drugs more quickly, which predisposes them to subtherapeutic drug concentrations and may require higher drug dosages.

Levels of the cytochrome P450 enzymes (see Chapter 2) are also known to vary between ethnic groups. This variation has effects on the ability to metabolize many drugs. Most psychotropic drugs (see Chapter 17) are metabolized in the liver in a two-phase process. Cytochrome P450 enzymes often control Phase I of the hepatic metabolism of both antidepressants and antipsychotic drugs. This can affect plasma drug levels, and therefore the intensity of drug response, at different doses. Groups of Asian patients have been shown to be "poor metabolizers" of these drugs and often require lower dosages to achieve desired therapeutic effects. In contrast, White patients are more likely to be classified as "ultrarapid metabolizers" and may require higher drug dosages.

Variations are also reported between ethnic groups in the occurrence of adverse effects. For example, patients of African descent taking lithium may need to be monitored more closely than others for symptoms of drug toxicity, because serum drug levels may be higher than in White patients given the same dosage. Likewise, patients of Japanese and Taiwanese descent may require lower dosages of lithium. For the treatment of hypertension, thiazide diuretics appear to be more effective in Black people of African descent than in Whites. Several additional examples of racial and ethnic differences in drug response are outlined in the Ethnocultural Implications box below.

Individuals throughout the world share common views and beliefs regarding health practices and medication use. However, there are also specific ethnocultural influences, beliefs, and practices. Awareness of ethnocultural differences is critical for the care of patients because of the constantly changing Canadian demographic. As a result of these changes, attending to each patient's cultural background helps to ensure safe and high quality nursing care, including medication administration.

For example, some Black people of African descent have health beliefs and practices that include an emphasis on proper diet and rest; the use of herbal teas, laxatives, and protective bracelets; and the use of folk medicine, prayer, and the "laying on of hands." Reliance on various home remedies can also be an important component of their health practices. Some patients of Asian descent, especially Chinese patients, believe in the concepts of *yin* and *yang*. Yin and yang are opposing forces that lead to illness or health, depending on which force is dominant in the individual and whether the forces are balanced. Balance produces healthy states. Other common health practices of patients of Asian descent include use of acupuncture, herbal remedies, and heat. All such beliefs and practices need to be considered—especially when the patient values their use more highly than the use of medications. Many of these beliefs are strongly grounded in religion. The Asian and Pacific Island racial/ethnic group also includes people who are Thai, Vietnamese, Filipino, Korean, and Japanese, among others.

Indigenous peoples in Canada live in diverse geographical areas. They maintain a diverse variety of rituals, symbols, and practices, which may vary by region. Some may follow traditional religious practices exclusively or follow a mix of Christian and traditional practices, while others may choose new Indigenous practices.

ETHNOCULTURAL IMPLICATIONS

Examples of Varying Responses of Different Ethnocultural Groups to Major Drug Classes

Racial or Ethnic Group	Drug Classification	Response
Black of African Descent	Antihypertensive drugs	Black patients of African descent respond better to diuretics than to β-blockers and angiotensin-converting enzyme inhibitors; they respond less effectively to β-blockers and respond best to calcium channel blockers, especially diltiazem. They also respond less effectively to single-drug therapy.
Asian	Antipsychotic and antianxiety drugs	Asian patients require lower doses of certain drugs such as haloperidol and statins and also respond better to lower dosages of antidepressants. Chinese patients require lower dosages of antipsychotics. Japanese patients require lower dosages of antimanic drugs.

Note: The comparison group for all responses is patients who are White.

Their spirituality is deeply connected to the physical environment, including animals and plants, and life is seen as interconnected. Traditional medicines and practices remain an important part of the lives of Inuit, Métis and First Nations people in Canada. Some First Nations people follow the medicine wheel, which includes physical, emotional, intellectual, and spiritual aspects. These aspects are connected to Mother Earth. They believe in preserving harmony with nature or keeping a balance between the four aspects of the medicine wheel. When one area is not functioning well, the other three areas are affected. Illness results from a neglected or oppressed spirit. Many use a traditional Indigenous healer or sacred medicines. Medicine is distinguished from healing, which goes beyond mere treatment of sickness. Traditional healing includes a wide range of activities, from physical cures using herbal medicines and other remedies to the promotion of psychological and spiritual well-being using ceremony, counselling, and the accumulated wisdom of elders. The drum is considered a symbol of the living relationship between Indigenous people and the land. The traditional healer for this culture is not only the medicine man or woman but may also include a spiritualist and herbalist, among others. Healing occurs though a variety of methods including, the sweat lodge, healing lodges and circles, and the continuous journey toward Bimaadiziiwin or "the good life." "Smudging" is a common ceremony used to cleanse the body spiritually and physically. An herb such as sage or sweetgrass is burned and the smoke is rubbed or brushed over the body.

Ayurvedic and Unani are traditional healing methods commonly practised by South Asians that emphasize a balance between a person's behaviour, lifestyle, environment, and mind. For example, South Asians believe that the body's digestive forces maintain the bodily humours, and an imbalance in bodily humours leads to physical and psychological illnesses. Muslims believe that ill health occurs due to the will of Allah. It is important to remember that these beliefs vary from patient to patient; therefore, consult with the patient rather than assume that the patient holds certain beliefs because of belonging to a certain ethnic group.

Barriers to adequate health care for the ethnoculturally diverse Canadian patient population include language, poverty, access, pride, and beliefs regarding medical practices. Medications may have a different meaning to different cultures, as would any form of medical treatment. Therefore, before any medication is administered, complete a thorough ethnocultural assessment. This assessment includes questions in regard to the following:

- Languages spoken, written, and understood; need for an interpreter
- Health beliefs and practices
- Past uses of medicine
- Use of herbal treatments, folk remedies, home remedies, or natural health products
- Use of **over-the-counter (OTC) drugs**
- Usual responses to illness
- Responsiveness to medical treatment
- Religious practices and beliefs (e.g., many Christian Scientists believe in taking no medications at all)
- Support from the patient's ethnocultural community that may provide resources or assistance as needed, such as religious connections, leaders, family members, or friends
- Dietary habits

Ethnocultural Nursing Considerations and Drug Therapy

It is important to be knowledgeable about drugs that may elicit varied responses in culturally diverse patients or those from different racial or ethnic groups. Varied responses may include differences in therapeutic dosages and adverse effects, so that some patients may have therapeutic responses at lower dosages than are typically recommended. For example, in patients of Asian descent who take traditional antipsychotics, symptoms may be managed effectively at lower dosages than the usual recommended dosage range. Also, patients of Chinese descent require lower doses of antidepressants.

Another aspect of cultural care as it relates to drug therapy is the recognition that patterns of communication may differ based on a patient's race or ethnicity. Communication includes the use of language, tone, and volume of the voice, as well as spatial distancing, touch, eye contact, greetings, and naming format. It is important to assess and apply these aspects of cultural and racial or ethnic variations to patient care and to drug therapy and the nursing process. Precise instructions must be included in patient education about medication(s) and how to best and safely take them. Avoiding the use of contractions such as *can't*, *won't*, and *don't* is important with patients from other countries to prevent confusion. Instead, use of *cannot*, *will not*, and *do not* is recommended to improve understanding.

NURSING PROCESS

Assessment

Pediatric Considerations

Before any medication is administered to a pediatric patient, obtain a thorough health history and medication history with assistance from the parent, caregiver, or legal guardian. The following are areas to be included:

- Age
- Age-related concerns about organ functioning
- Allergies to drugs and food
- Baseline values for vital signs

- Physical assessment findings
- Height in centimetres and feet/inches
- Weight in kilograms and pounds
- Medical and medication history (including adverse drug reactions); current medication and related dosage forms and routes, and the patient's tolerance of the forms and routes
- Use of prescription and OTC medications in the home setting
- Level of growth and development and related developmental tasks
- Motor and cognitive responses and their age-appropriateness
- Age-related fears
- State of anxiety of the patient or family members or caregiver
- Usual method of medication administration, such as use of a calibrated spoon or needleless syringe
- Usual response to medications
- Resources available to the patient and family

The prescriber will determine the medication to be delivered. However, the nurse is responsible for detecting any errors in calculation of dosage, as well as for preparing the medication and administering the drug. The nurse needs to be aware that pediatric dosages are often less than 1 mL and require accurate medication dosage calculations that are checked several times. The Ten Rights of medication administration must be followed, of which correct dose is one right. In addition to an assessment of the patient, an assessment of the drug-related information is needed, focusing specifically on the drug's purpose, dosage ranges, routes of administration, cautions, and contraindications. Children are more sensitive than adults to medications because of their weight, height, physical condition, immature systems, and metabolism. As children grow older, their body surface areas and weights are still lower than those of adults, so extreme caution is continually needed when giving them medications. Immature organ and system development will influence pharmacokinetics and thus affect the way pediatric patients respond to drugs. Organ function may be determined through laboratory testing. The following studies may be ordered by the prescriber before beginning drug therapy as well as during and after drug therapy: liver and kidney function studies, red blood cell and white blood cell counts, and measurement of hemoglobin levels, hematocrit, and protein levels.

■ Older Adult Considerations

Assessment data to be gathered in older adults may include the following:

- Age
- Past and present medical history
- Allergies to drugs and food

- Dietary habits
- History of smoking and use of alcohol with notation of amount, frequency, and years of use
- Sensory, visual, hearing, cognitive, and motor-skill deficits
- Laboratory testing results, especially those that assess kidney and liver function
- List of all health-related care providers, including physicians, dentists, optometrists and ophthalmologists, podiatrists, alternative medicine health care practitioners such as osteopathic physicians, chiropractors, and nurse practitioners
- Listing of medications, past and present, including prescription drugs, OTC medications, and natural health products
- Existence of polypharmacy (the use of more than five medications)
- Self-medication practices
- Risk situations related to drug therapy as identified by the Beers Criteria (see Evidence in Practice box on p. 70)

The patient's insight into his or her own medical problems is a beneficial piece of information in developing a plan of care. It is also important for the nurse to realize that although older adults may be able to provide the required information themselves, many may be confused or poorly informed about their medications or health condition. In such cases, consult with a more reliable historian, such as a significant other, family member, or caregiver. Older adults may also have sensory deficits that require the nurse to speak slowly, loudly, and clearly, while facing the patient. Currently in Canada, drug information systems are now being used in about 50% of Canada's emergency rooms, and 3% of community pharmacies, resulting is safer use of medications and fewer adverse drug events. Access to electronic health care records for older adults is a significant step to improve the availability of information, quickly, and the quality and access to health care (Canada Health Infoway, 2013).

One way to collect data about the various medications or drugs being taken by older adults is to use the brown-bag technique to obtain that information from the patient or caregiver. This is an effective means of identifying various drugs that the patient is taking, regardless of the patient's age, and may be used in conjunction with a complete review of the patient's medical history or record. The brown-bag technique requires the patient or caregiver to place all medications used in a bag and bring them to the health care provider. All medications need to be brought in their original containers. A list of medications with generic names, dosages, routes of administration, and frequencies is then compiled and the list is then compared with what is prescribed and what the patient states is actually being taken. Medication reconciliation procedures are performed in health care facilities when assessing and tracking medications taken by the patient (see Chapter 6).

With older adults, thoroughly assess support systems and the patient's ability to take medications safely. Other data to collect include information about acute or chronic illnesses, nutritional problems, heart problems, respiratory illnesses, and gastrointestinal tract disorders. Laboratory tests that are often ordered for older adults include hemoglobin and hematocrit levels, red blood cell and white blood cell counts, serum electrolyte levels, protein and serum albumin levels, blood urea nitrogen level, serum and urine creatinine levels, and urine specific gravity.

■ Ethnocultural Considerations

A thorough ethnocultural assessment is needed for the provision of ethnoculturally competent nursing care. A variety of assessment tools and resources to incorporate into nursing care are provided in Box 4-1. However, various factors must be assessed and then applied to nursing care, specifically drug therapy and the nursing process. Some of the specific questions to consider about the patient's physical, mental, and spiritual health include the following:

■ Maintaining Health

- *For physical health:* Where are special foods and clothing items purchased? What types of health education are of the patient's ethnoculture? Where does the patient usually obtain information about health and illness? Folklore? Where are health services obtained? Who are the health care providers (e.g., physicians, nurse practitioners, community services, health departments, healers)?

BOX 4-1

Cultural Assessment Tools and Related Weblinks

- Several cultural assessment tools have been developed over the last decade. Madeline Leininger's Sunrise Model focuses on seven major areas of cultural assessment, including educational; economic; familial and social; political; technological; religious and philosophical; and cultural values, beliefs, and practices.
- Other comprehensive cultural assessment tools include those developed by Andrews and Bowls, 2008; Friedman, Bowden, and Jones, 2003; Giger and Davidhizar, 2002; and Purnell and Paulanka, 1998. Rani Srivastava's (2006) model, found in *The Healthcare Professional's Guide to Clinical Cultural Competence* (Healthcare Professional's Guides), contains further discussion on how populations are viewed by health care workers and not through the use of ethnocultural or religious labels.

- *For mental health:* What are examples of ethnoculturally specific activities for the mind and for maintaining mental health, as well as beliefs about reducing stress, rest, and relaxation?
- *For spiritual health:* What resources are used to meet spiritual needs?

■ Protecting Health

- *For physical health:* Where are special clothing and everyday essentials purchased? What are examples of the patient's symbolic clothing, if any?
- *For mental health:* Who within the family and community teaches the roles in the patient's specific ethnoculture? Are there rules about avoiding certain persons or places? Are there special activities that must be performed?
- *For spiritual health:* Who teaches spiritual practices and where can special protective symbolic objects such as crystals or amulets be purchased? Are they expensive and how available are they for the patient when needed?

■ Restoring Health

- *For physical health:* Where are special remedies purchased? Can individuals produce or grow their own remedies, herbs, and so on? How often are traditional and nontraditional services obtained? Is the process and medication ethnoculturally safe for this patient?
- *For mental health:* Who are the traditional and nontraditional resources for mental health? Are there ethnoculture-specific activities for coping with stress and illness?
- *For spiritual health:* How often and where are traditional and nontraditional spiritual leaders or healers accessed?

▨ Nursing Diagnoses: Age-Related

- Imbalanced nutrition, less than body requirements, related to the impact of age and drug therapy and possible adverse effects
- Deficient knowledge related to information about drugs and their adverse effects or about when to contact the prescriber
- Risk for injury related to adverse effects of medications or to the method of drug administration
- Risk for injury related to idiosyncratic reactions to drugs related to age-related drug sensitivity

▨ Planning

■ Goals

- Patient (caregiver, parent, or legal guardian) will state measures to enhance nutritional status due to age- and drug-related factors, as well as any adverse drug effects on everyday nutrition.

- Patient (caregiver, parent, or legal guardian) will state the importance of adhering to the prescribed drug therapy (or will take medication as prescribed with assistance).
- Patient will contact the prescriber when appropriate, such as when unusual effects occur during drug therapy.
- Patient (caregiver, parent, or legal guardian) will identify ways to minimize complications, adverse effects, reactions, and injury associated with the therapeutic medication regimen.

Expected Patient Outcomes

- Patient (caregiver, parent, or legal guardian) lists recommended caloric and protein intake as well as examples of all the major food groups with the assistance of nutritional consultation.
- Patient (caregiver, parent, or legal guardian) identifies when to contact the prescriber if nausea, vomiting, loss of appetite, diarrhea, constipation, or other problems arise during medication therapy.
- Patient (caregiver, parent, or legal guardian) states rationale for medication as well as importance in the timing, dosage, and duration of therapy and is able to identify what the specific medication looks like.
- Patient (caregiver, parent, or legal guardian) describes intended therapeutic effects of the medication(s), such as improvement in condition with decrease in symptoms and with limited adverse effects.
- Patient (caregiver, parent, or legal guardian) demonstrates safe method of self- or assisted medication administration, such as use of a week-long pill mechanism (e.g., blister pack or a dosette medication box) with day of week and associated times, and has all medications safely labelled.
- Patient (caregiver, parent, or legal guardian) follows instructions specific to the route of administration for the medication ordered, while also demonstrating (if appropriate) techniques, such as special application of an ointment as prescribed, measuring and taking liquid medication, and taking medication with proper food or fluids, for the duration of treatment.
- Patient (caregiver, parent, or legal guardian) lists the most frequent adverse effects and possible toxicity associated with medication regimen, while also stating when to contact the health care provider, such as occurrence of fever, pain, vomiting, rash, diarrhea, difficulty breathing, or worsening of the condition being treated.
- Patient (caregiver, parent, or legal guardian) reports safe medication administration upon return appointment after beginning prescribed therapy.
- Patient (caregiver, parent, or legal guardian) minimizes adverse effects and danger to self by taking medication(s) as prescribed, at the right time, with right dosing, and with attention to intake of proper amount of fluids (120 to 180 mL of water with oral

dosages) and with or without food, as indicated, while remaining aware of safety measures appropriate to specific drug regimen.

Implementation

It is always important to emphasize and practise the Ten Rights of medication administration (see Chapter 1) and follow the prescriber's order and medication instructions. Check all drugs three times against the Ten Rights and the prescriber's order before the drug is given to the patient. This usually applies in acute care and long-term care inpatient and outpatient situations. For pediatric patients, some specific nursing actions are as follows: (1) If needed, mix medications in a substance or fluid other than essential foods (e.g., milk, orange juice, cereal) because the child may develop a dislike for the essential food in the future. Instead, use a liquid or food item that may be used to make the medication(s) taste better such as sherbet or flavoured ice cream. Use this intervention only if the patient cannot swallow the dosage form or if the taste needs to be made more palatable. (2) Do not add drug(s) to fluid in a cup or bottle because the amount of drug consumed would then be impossible to calculate if the entire amount of fluid is not consumed. (3) Always document special techniques of drug administration so that others involved in the patient's care may benefit from the suggestion. For example, if the child takes an unpleasant-tasting pill, liquid, or tablet after eating a frozen Popsicle, then this information would be valuable to another caregiver. (4) Unless contraindicated, add small amounts of water or fluids to elixirs to enhance the child's tolerance of the medication. Remember that it is essential for the child to take the entire volume, so remain cautious with this practice and use only an amount of fluid mixture that you know the child will tolerate. (5) Avoid using the word *candy* in place of *drug* or *medication*. Medications must be called *medicines* and their dangers made known to children. Taking medications is not a game, and children must understand this for their own safety. (6) Keep all medications out of the reach of children of all ages. Be sure that parents and other family members in the same household understand this information and request child-protective lids or tops for their medications from the pharmacy. Childproof locks or closures may also be used on cabinets holding medications. (7) Inquire about how the child usually takes medication (e.g., preference of liquid versus pill or tablet dosage forms) and whether there are any methods from the family or caregiver that may be helpful. See Special Populations: Children box, on page 62, for recommendations and further information on medication administration beginning with infancy through adolescence. For more information about dosage calculations for medication administration in pediatric patients, visit the TestandCalc website, which provides examples and programs to help with pediatric drug dosage calculations (http://www.testandcalc.com).

Encourage older adult patients to take medications as directed and not to discontinue them or double up on doses unless recommended or ordered to do so by their health care provider or prescriber. The patient or caregiver must understand the treatment- and medication-related instructions, especially those related to safety measures such as keeping all medications out of the reach of children. Transdermal patches provide a different challenge in that if they fall off onto the floor or bedding, a child or infant in that environment may have accidental exposure to the effects of the medication. Serious adverse reactions have been reported concerning the accidental adhering of a transdermal patch to a child or infant while crawling or playing on the floor or carpet. Toxic and even fatal reactions may occur depending on the medication and dosage. Provide written and verbal instructions concerning the drug name, action, purpose, dose, time of administration, route, adverse effects, safety of administration, storage, interactions, and any cautions about or contraindications to its use. Remember that simple is always best. Always try to find ways to make the patient's therapeutic regimen easy to understand. Always be alert to polypharmacy, and be sure the patient or caregiver understands the dangers of multiple drug use. Patient education may prove to be helpful in preventing or minimizing problems associated with polypharmacy. If a nurse advocate or a nurse practitioner with prescription privileges has the opportunity to review the patient's chart, she or he must provide simplified written instructions outlining the purpose of the drug, how to best take the medication(s), and a list of drug interactions and adverse effects. Information must be provided in bold, large print. The Beers Criteria have proven helpful in promoting medication safety in older adults (see Evidence In Practice box on p. 77). These criteria provide a systematic way of identifying prescription medications that are potentially harmful to older adults. The prescriber and nurse must constantly remember that clinical judgement and knowledge base are important in making critical decisions about a patient's care and drug therapy. In addition, keeping abreast of evidence-informed nursing practice, such as the application of the Beers Criteria, is important for the nurse to remain current in clinical nursing practice. Specific guidelines for medication administration by different routes are presented in detail in Chapter 10.

In summary, drug therapy across the lifespan must be well thought out, with full consideration to the patient's age, gender, ethnocultural background, medical history, and medication profile. When all phases of the nursing process and the specific lifespan considerations discussed in this chapter are included, there is a better chance of decreasing adverse effects, reducing risks to the patient, and increasing drug safety.

Evaluation

When dealing with lifespan issues related to drug therapy, observation and monitoring for therapeutic effects as well as adverse effects are critical to safe and effective therapy. The nurse must know a patient's profile and history just as well as information about the drug. The drug's purpose, specific use in the patient, simply stated actions, dose, frequency of dosing, adverse effects, cautions, and contraindications need to be listed and kept available at all times . This information will allow more comprehensive monitoring of drug therapy, regardless of the age of the patient.

Nursing Diagnoses: Ethnocultural

- Sleep deprivation related to a lack of adherence to cultural practices for encouraging stress release and sleep induction
- Deficient knowledge (drug therapy) related to lack of experience and information about prescribed drug therapy

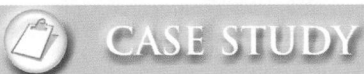

CASE STUDY

Polypharmacy and Older Adults

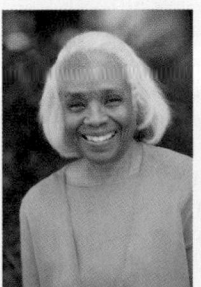

Rhonda, a 77-year-old retired librarian, sees several physician specialists for a variety of health problems. She uses the pharmacy at a large discount store but also has prescriptions filled at a nearby pharmacy, which she uses when she does not feel like going into the larger store. Her medication list is as follows:

Thiazide diuretic, prescribed for peripheral edema

Potassium tablets, prescribed to prevent hypokalemia
β blocker, prescribed for hypertension
Warfarin sodium, taken every evening because of a history of deep vein thrombosis

Thyroid replacement hormone for hypothyroidism
Multivitamin tablet for seniors

1. What medications may cause problems for Rhonda? Explain your answer.

2. What measures can be taken to reduce these problems?

Rhonda visits the pharmacy to pick up some medications for a cold. She has chosen a popular OTC decongestant, an antihistamine preparation, and a nonsteroidal anti-inflammatory drug for her "aches and pains."

3. Should she use these medications? If not, what advice would you give her about choosing OTC medications?

For answers see http://evolve.elsevier.com/Canada/Lilley/pharmacology/.

- Risk for injury related to adverse and unpredictable reaction to drug therapy due to racial or ethnic cultural factors

◩ Planning

◼ Goals

- Patient will state the need for assistance with non-pharmacological management of sleep deficit.
- Patient will request written and verbal education about medication therapy.
- Patient will state need for information about the influence of racial or ethnic cultural factors upon specific drug therapy with emphasis on safety measures.

◼ Expected Patient Outcomes

- Patient describes specific measures to enhance sleep patterns, such as regular sleep habits, decrease in caffeine, meditation, relaxation therapy, and journalling sleep patterns and noting those measures that enhance or take away sleep.
- Patient lists the various medication(s) with their therapeutic and adverse effects, dosage routes, and specific methods of adequate self-administration, drug interactions, and any other special considerations.
- Patient describes the impact of racial or ethnic influences (e.g., metabolic enzyme differences) on specific medications and the resulting potential for increase in adverse effects, toxicity, or increased or decreased effectiveness (medication therapy).

◩ Implementation

There are numerous interventions for implementation of ethnoculturally competent nursing care, but one important requirement is that nurses remain current in the knowledge of various ethnocultures and related activities and practices of daily living, health beliefs, as well as emotional and spiritual health practices and beliefs. Specifically, knowledge about medications that may elicit varied responses due to racial or ethnic variations is most important, along with application of concepts of culturally competent care and ethnopharmacology for each patient care situation.

Information of particular significance is the impact of cytochrome P450 liver enzymes on certain phases of drug metabolism (see previous discussion on p. 72). Specific examples of differences in certain cytochrome P450 enzymes can be found on p. 72. Consider additional factors, including the patient's verbal and nonverbal communication patterns; the patient's health belief systems; identification of health care providers or alternate healers; and the patient's interpretation of space, time, and touch. For example, cost may be a consideration in regard to adherence with the treatment regimen. Other lifestyle decisions (e.g., use of tobacco or alcohol) may also affect responses to drugs and must be considered during drug administration. In addition, a patient's ethnocultural background and associated socioeconomic status may create a situation that leads the patient to skip pills, split doses, and not obtain refills. This culture of poverty may be a causative factor in nonadherence and requires astute attention and individualized nursing actions.

◩ Evaluation

Ethnoculturally competent nursing care related to drug therapy may be evaluated through adherence (or nonadherence) to the medication regimen(s). Safe, effective, and therapeutic self-administration of drugs with minimal to no adverse or toxic effects will be present only when the patient is treated as an individual and has a thorough understanding of the medication regimen.

CASE STUDY

Otitis Media in a Child

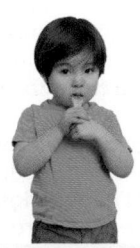

A parent brings her 2-year-old son, Bryson, to the community health clinic with reports of fussiness and tugging at his left ear for the past 48 hours. He has been coughing and has had a runny nose for 4 days that has been treated with saline nose sprays and use of a humidifier. He had a low-grade fever of 38.4°C axillary for the past 48 hours. It has now risen to 39°C. Bryson attends day care and both parents smoke cigarettes. Bryson's past medical history is significant for bilateral ear infections, with his last episode 5 months ago, which was treated with amoxicillin. His immunizations are up to date, including 13-valent pneumococcal conjugate vaccine. He is diagnosed with acute otitis media and prescribed amoxicillin and ibuprofen.

1. What characteristics of pediatric patients may have a significant effect on dosage calculation?
2. What pharmacokinetic factors may affect the administration of the ordered drugs for Bryson?
3. Bryson's mother is concerned that he has had a few episodes of otitis media. What health teaching would the nurse undertake with Bryson's mother?
4. Bryson weighs 11.5 kg. The recommended dose of amoxicillin to treat otitis media is 75 to 90 mg/kg/day divided bid. What dose range is appropriate for Bryson?

For answers see http://evolve.elsevier.com/Canada/Lilley/pharmacology/.

KEY POINTS

❖ There are many age-related pharmacokinetic effects that lead to dramatic differences in drug absorption, distribution, metabolism, and excretion in the young and older adults. At one end of the lifespan is the pediatric patient, and at the other end is older adult patients, both of whom are sensitive to the effects of drugs.

❖ For pediatrics, most common dosage calculations use the milligrams per kilogram formula related to age; however, BSA is also used for drug calculations, and organ maturity is considered. It is important for the nurse to know that many elements besides the mathematical calculation contribute to safe dosage calculations. Safety must remain the number one concern, with consideration of the Ten Rights of medication administration (see Chapter 1).

❖ The percentage of the population older than 65 years of age continues to grow, and polypharmacy remains a concern with the increasing number of older adult patients. For older adults, a current list of all medications and drug allergies must be on their person or with their family/caregiver at all times.

❖ The nurse's responsibility is to act as a patient advocate as well as to be informed about growth and developmental principles and the effects of various drugs during the lifespan and in various phases of illness.

❖ A variety of culturally based assessment tools are available for use in patient care and drug therapy.

❖ Drug therapy and subsequent patient responses may be affected by racial and ethnic variations in levels of specific enzymes and metabolic pathways of drugs.

EXAMINATION REVIEW QUESTIONS

1. The nurse is reviewing factors that influence pharmacokinetics in the neonatal pharmacokinetic factors in the neonatal patient. Which factor puts the neonatal patient at risk as related to drug therapy?
a. Immature renal system
b. Hyperperistalsis in the gastrointestinal tract
c. Irregular temperature regulation
d. Smaller circulatory capacity

2. The physiological differences in the pediatric patient compared with the adult patient affect the amount of drug needed to produce a therapeutic effect. The nurse is aware that one of the main differences is that infants have
a. increased protein in circulation.
b. fat composition less than 0.001%.
c. more muscular body composition.
d. water composition of approximately 75%.

3. While teaching 76-year-old Rahul about the adverse effects of his medications, the nurse encourages him to keep a journal of the adverse effects he experiences. This intervention is important for older adult patients because of which alterations in pharmacokinetics?
a. Increased kidney excretion of protein-bound drugs
b. More alkaline gastric pH, resulting in more adverse effects
c. Decreased blood flow to the liver, resulting in altered metabolism
d. Less adipose tissue to store fat-soluble drugs

4. The nurse is reviewing a list of medications taken by Huang, an 88-year-old patient. Huang says, "I get dizzy when I stand up." She also states that she has nearly fainted "a time or two" in the afternoons. Her systolic blood pressure drops 15 points when she stands up. Which type of medications may be responsible for these effects?
a. NSAIDs
b. Cardiac glycosides
c. Anticoagulants
d. Antihypertensives

5. A woman who is pregnant asks the nurse at the health care clinic how to know which drugs are safe to take during pregnancy. What is the nurse's best response?
a. "Continue to take any drugs previously prescribed by your health care provider as there are few studies to establish which drugs are safe to take during pregnancy."
b. "It is safe to continue taking the over-the-counter drugs that you are currently taking."
c. "It is advisable not to take any prescription or over-the-counter drugs while pregnant."
d. "It is best to consult with your health care provider about taking any prescription or over-the-counter drugs."

6. The nurse is preparing to administer an injection to a preschool-age child. Which approaches are appropriate for this age group? (Select all that apply.)
a. Explain to the child in advance about the injection.
b. Provide a brief, concrete explanation about the injection.
c. Encourage participation in the procedure.
d. Make use of magical thinking.
e. Provide comfort measures after the injection.

7. Yuri, a patient of Japanese descent, describes a family trait that manifests frequently—she says that members of her family often have "strong reactions" after taking certain medications, but her friends who are not of Japanese descent have no problems with the same dosages of the same medications.
a. Yuri may need lower dosages of the medications prescribed.
b. Yuri may need higher dosages of the medications prescribed.
c. Yuri should not receive these medications because of potential problems with metabolism.
d. These situations vary greatly, and Yuri's accounts may not indicate a valid cause for concern.

Continued

EXAMINATION REVIEW QUESTIONS—cont'd

8. Which factors does the nurse consider when evaluating polymorphism and medication administration? (Select all that apply.)
   a. Nutritional status
   b. Drug route
   c. Patient's ethnicity
   d. Cultural beliefs
   e. Patient's age

9. The nurse is preparing to give an oral dose of acetaminophen (Tylenol®) to a child who weighs 12 kg. The dose is 15 mg/kg. How many milligrams will the nurse administer for this dose?

Answers: 1. a, 2. d, 3. c, 4. d, 5. d, 6. b, d, e, 7. a, 8. a, d, e, 9. 180 mg

CRITICAL THINKING ACTIVITIES

1. A mother calls the clinic to ask how to give a tablet to her 4-year-old son. He is refusing to swallow it and will not chew it because it "tastes icky." The mother says she is ready to force her son to take this medication. What is the nurse's priority action?

2. A woman in her third trimester of pregnancy is having a checkup and asks for acetylsalicylic acid (ASA) for a headache. What is the nurse's best response?

3. A 22-year-old woman has brought her 16-month-old daughter to see the nurse practitioner because the toddler has symptoms of a sinus infection. After examining the toddler, the nurse practitioner writes a prescription for an antibiotic. The mother says, "Oh, I have tetracycline suspension at home that I took for an infection. Can't I just use that and save money?" What is the nurse's best answer?

For answers see http://evolve.elsevier.com/Canada/Lilley/pharmacology/.

CHAPTER 5

Gene Therapy and Pharmacogenomics

Objectives

After reading this chapter, the successful student will be able to do the following:

1. Identify the significance of the basic terms related to genetics and drug therapy.

2. Briefly discuss the major concepts of genetics as an evolving segment of health care, such as principles of genetic inheritance; deoxyribonucleic acid (DNA), ribonucleic acid (RNA), and their functioning; the relationship of DNA to protein synthesis; and the importance of amino acids.

3. Describe the basis of the Human Genome Project and its impact on the role of genetics in health care.

4. Discuss the gene therapies currently available.

5. Differentiate between the direct and indirect forms of gene therapy.

6. Identify the regulatory and ethical issues related to gene therapy as related to nursing and health care providers.

7. Briefly discuss pharmacogenomics and pharmacogenetics.

8. Discuss the evolving role of professional nurses as related to gene therapy.

e-Learning Activities

Website
(http://evolve.elsevier.com/Canada/
Lilley/pharmacology/)

evolve

- Answer Key—Textbook Case Studies
- Answer Key—Critical Thinking Activities
- Chapter Summaries—Printable
- Review Questions for Exam Preparation
- Unfolding Case Studies

Key Terms

Acquired disease Any disease triggered by external factors and not directly caused by a person's genes (e.g., an infectious disease, noncongenital cardiovascular diseases). (p. 83)

Alleles The two alternative forms of a gene that can occupy a specific locus (location) on a chromosome (see chromosome). (p. 83)

Chromatin A collective term for all of the chromosomal material within a given cell. (p. 83)

Chromosome Structures in the nuclei of cells that contain threads of deoxyribonucleic acid (DNA), which transmit genetic information, and that are associated with ribonucleic acid (RNA) molecules and synthesis of protein molecules. (p. 83)

Gene The biological unit of heredity; a segment of a DNA molecule that contains all of the molecular information required for the synthesis of a biological product such as an RNA molecule or an amino acid chain (protein molecule). (p. 83)

Gene therapy New therapeutic technologies that directly target human genes in the treatment or prevention of illness. (p. 84)

Genetic disease Any disorder caused by a genetic mechanism. (p. 83)

Genetic material   DNA or RNA molecules or portions of them. (p. 82)

Genetic polymorphisms   Variants that occur in the chromosomes of 1% or more of the general population (i.e., too frequently to be caused by a random recurrent mutation). (p. 86)

Genetic predisposition   The presence of certain factors in a person's genetic makeup, or genome (see next page), that increases the likelihood of developing one or more diseases. (p. 83)

Genetics   The study of the structure, function, and inheritance of genes. (p. 83)

Genome   The complete set of genetic material of any organism. It may be contained in multiple chromosomes (groups of DNA or RNA molecules) in higher organisms; in a single chromosome, as in bacteria; or in a single DNA or RNA molecule, as in viruses. (p. 84)

Genomics   The study of the structure and function of the genome, including DNA sequencing, mapping, and expression, and the way genes and their products work in both health and disease. (p. 84)

Genotype   The particular alleles present at a given site (locus) on the chromosomes of an organism that determine a specific genetic trait for that organism (compare phenotype). (p. 83)

Heredity   The characteristics and qualities that are genetically passed from one generation to the next through reproduction. (p. 83)

Inherited disease   Genetic disease that results from defective alleles passed from parents to offspring. (p. 83)

International Human Genome Project (IHGP)   A project by an international group of scientists to describe in detail the entire genome of a human being. (p. 84)

Nucleic acids   Molecules of DNA or RNA in the nucleus of every cell. DNA makes up the chromosomes and encodes the genes. (p. 82)

Personalized medicine   The use of molecular-level and genetic characterizations of both the disease process and the patient for the customization of drug therapy. (p. 86)

Pharmacogenetics   A general term for the study of the genetic basis for variations in the body's response to drugs, with a focus on variations related to a single gene. (p. 86)

Pharmacogenomics   A branch of pharmacogenetics (see earlier) that involves the survey of the entire genome to detect multigenic (multiple-gene) determinants of drug response. (p. 86)

Phenotype   The expression in the body of a genetic trait that results from a person's particular genotype (see earlier) for that trait. (p. 83)

Proteome   The entire set of proteins produced from the information encoded in an organism's genome. (p. 84)

Proteomics   The detailed study of the proteome, including all biological actions of proteins. (p. 84)

Recombinant DNA (rDNA)   DNA molecules that have been artificially synthesized or modified in a laboratory setting. (p. 85)

OVERVIEW

Genetic processes are a highly complex part of physiology and are far from being completely understood. Genetic research is one of the most active branches of science today, involving many types of health care providers, including nurses. Expected outcomes of this research include a deeper knowledge of the genetic influences on disease, along with the development of gene-based therapies. The practice of nursing requires an understanding of genetic concepts as well as genetically related health issues and therapeutic techniques. The goal of this chapter is to introduce some of the major concepts of this complex and emerging branch of health science. In 1996, in the United States, the National Coalition for Health Professional Education in Genetics (NCHPEG) was founded (http://www.nchpeg.org). The purpose of NCHPEG is to promote the education of health professionals and the public regarding advances in applied genetics.

Since the 1960s, published literature has described the role of nursing in genetics and genetic research. The Genetics Nursing Network was formed in 1984 and later became the International Society of Nurses in Genetics (ISONG). In 2005, the Canadian Nurses Association recognized the importance of knowledge of genetics in nursing, yet it is still not an official nursing specialty. The growing understanding of genetics is quickly creating demand for clinicians in all fields who can educate patients and provide clinical care that tailors health care services to each patient's inherent genetic makeup. This reality also calls for increasing the level of genetics education in nursing school curricula as well as continuing nursing education. Interestingly, the study of genetics has become commonplace in secondary and even primary education.

BASIC PRINCIPLES OF GENETIC INHERITANCE

Nucleic acids are biochemical compounds consisting of two types of molecules: deoxyribonucleic acid (DNA) and ribonucleic acid (RNA). DNA molecules make up the **genetic material** that is passed between all types of organisms during reproduction. In some viruses (e.g., human immunodeficiency virus [HIV]), it is actually

RNA molecules that pass the virus's genetic material between generations; however, this is an exception to the norm. A **chromosome** is a long strand of DNA contained in the nuclei of cells. DNA molecules, in turn, act as the template for the formation of RNA molecules, from which proteins are made. Humans normally have 23 pairs of chromosomes in each of their somatic cells. Somatic cells are the cells in the body other than the sex cells (sperm cells or egg cells), which have 23 single (unpaired) chromosomes. One pair of chromosomes in each cell is termed the sex chromosomes, which can be designated as either X or Y. The sex chromosomes are normally XX for females and XY for males. One member of each pair of chromosomes in somatic cells comes from the father's sperm cell and one from the mother's egg. **Alleles** are the alternative forms of a **gene** that can vary in regard to a specific genetic trait. Genetic traits can be desirable (e.g., lack of allergies) or undesirable (e.g., predisposition toward a specific disease). Alleles are dominant or recessive. Each person has two alleles for every gene-coded trait—one allele from the mother, the other from the father. An allele may be dominant or recessive for a given genetic trait. The particular combination of alleles, or **genotype**, for a given trait determines whether or not a person manifests that trait, or the person's **phenotype**. Genetic traits that are passed on differently to male and female offspring are said to be sex-linked traits because they are carried on either the X or Y chromosome. For example, hemophilia genes are carried by females but manifest as a bleeding disorder only in males. Hemophilia is an example of an **inherited disease;** that is, a disease caused by passage of a genetic defect from parents to offspring. A more general term is **genetic disease**, which is any disease caused by a genetic mechanism. Note, however, that not all genetic diseases are inherited. Chromosomal abnormalities (aberrations) can also occur spontaneously during embryonic development. In contrast, an **acquired disease** is any disease that develops in response to external factors and is not directly related to a person's genetic makeup. Genetics can play an indirect role in acquired disease, however. For example, atherosclerotic heart disease is often acquired in middle or later life. Many people have certain genes in their cells that increase the likelihood of this condition. This is known as a **genetic predisposition**. In some cases, a person may be able to offset a genetic predisposition through lifestyle choices, such as consuming a healthy diet and exercising to lessen the risk of developing heart disease.

Current literature differentiates "old genetics," which focused on single-gene inherited diseases such as hemophilia, from "new genetics." The new genetic perspective recognizes that common diseases, including Alzheimer's disease, cancer, and heart disease, are the product of complex relationships between genetic and environmental factors. These environmental factors, such as diet or toxic exposures, can initiate or worsen disease processes. Research into disease treatment is beginning to look at genetically tailored therapy.

DISCOVERY, STRUCTURE, AND FUNCTION OF DNA

Genetics is the study of the structure, function, and inheritance of genes. **Heredity** refers to the qualities that are genetically transferred from one generation to the next during reproduction.

A major turning point in the current understanding of genetics came in 1953, when Drs. James Watson and Francis Crick first reported the chemical structures of human genetic material and named the primary biochemical compound *deoxyribonucleic acid* (DNA). They later received a Nobel Prize for their discovery.

It is now recognized that DNA is the primary molecule in the body that serves to transfer genes from parents to offspring. It exists in the nucleus of all body cells as strands of chromosomes, collectively called **chromatin**. As described in Chapter 40, DNA molecules contain four different organic bases, each of which has its own alphabetical designation: *adenine (A), guanine (G), thymine (T),* and *cytosine (C)*. These bases are linked to a type of sugar molecule known as *deoxyribose*. In turn, these sugar molecules are linked to a "backbone" chain of phosphate molecules, which results in the classic double-helix structure of two side-by-side, spiral macromolecular chains. An important related biomolecule is *ribonucleic acid (RNA)*. RNA has a chemical structure similar to that of DNA, except that its sugar molecule is the compound *ribose* instead of deoxyribose, and it contains the base *uracil (U)* in place of thymine. RNA more commonly occurs as a single-stranded molecule, although in some genetic processes it can also be double stranded. In double-stranded structures, the base of each strand binds (via hydrogen bonds) to that of the other strand in the space between the two strands. This binding is based on complementary base pairing determined by the chemistry of the base molecules themselves. Specifically, adenine can bind only with thymine or uracil, whereas cytosine can bind only with guanine.

A nucleotide is the structural unit of DNA and consists of a single base and its attached sugar and phosphate molecules. A nucleoside is the base and attached sugar without the phosphate molecule. A relatively small sequence of nucleotides is called an *oligonucleotide* (the prefix *oligo-* means "a small number"). Certain new drug therapies involve synthetic analogues of both nucleosides and nucleotides (see Chapters 45, 49, 50, and 51). A related field is targeted drug therapy. Targeted drug therapy focuses on modifying the function of immune system cells (T cells and B cells) and biochemical mediators of immune response (cytokines). However, it is expected to focus on modifying specific genes as well. Current examples of targeted drug therapy are presented in Chapters 49, 50, 52, and 53. One of these drugs, the ophthalmic antiviral drug fomivirsen (not available in Canada), is an oligonucleotide with a chemical structure that is opposite (complementary) to that of a critical part of the messenger RNA (mRNA) of the cytomegalovirus.

For this reason, it is called an *antisense* oligonucleotide and it is the first of this new class of drugs. Other types of antisense oligonucleotide drugs are anticipated in the near future as one type of gene therapy.

An organism's entire DNA structure is its **genome**. This word is a combination of the terms *gene* and *chromosome*, and it refers to all the genes in an organism taken together. **Genomics** is the relatively new science of determining the location (mapping), structure (DNA base sequencing), identification (genotyping), and expression (phenotyping) of individual genes among the entire genome, and determining their functions in both health and disease processes.

Protein Synthesis

Protein molecules drive the functioning of all biochemical reactions. Protein synthesis is the primary function of DNA in human cells. There is a direct relationship between DNA nucleotide sequences and corresponding amino acid sequences. This relationship allows for precision in protein synthesis. Interestingly, it is estimated that only 2 to 3% of the human genome is involved in protein synthesis. Amino acid sequences control the shape of protein molecules, which ultimately affects their ability to function in the body. Mutations, undesired changes in DNA sequence, can affect the shape of protein molecules and impair or destroy their functioning.

In the cell nuclei, the double strands of DNA uncoil and separate, and a strand of mRNA forms on each strand through complementary base pairing, as described earlier in the chapter. This process is called *transcription* of the DNA. These mRNA molecules then detach from their corresponding DNA strands, leave the cell nucleus, and enter the cytoplasm, where they are then "read," or translated, by the ribosomes. Ribosomes are composed of a second type of RNA, known as *ribosomal RNA* (rRNA), as well as several accessory proteins. Individual sequences of three bases along the mRNA molecule serve to code for specific amino acid molecules. This translation process involves molecules of a third type of RNA, transfer RNA (tRNA). The tRNA molecules transport the corresponding amino acid molecules to the site of ribosomal translation along the mRNA strand in sequence, according to the three-base codes along the mRNA strand. This in turn results in the creation of chains of multiple amino acid molecules (polypeptide chains), which are known as *protein molecules*. The specificity of this code is important for proper protein synthesis and the process is similar for all living organisms—plant and animal.

There are countless specific amino acid sequences (polypeptides) that result in the synthesis of many thousands of types of protein molecules. Proteins include hormones, enzymes, immunoglobulins, and numerous other biochemical molecules that regulate processes throughout the body. They are involved in both healthy physiological processes and the pathophysiological processes of many diseases. Biomedical researchers continue to identify and describe many proteins that are part of disease processes. Manipulation of genetic material, as in gene therapy (see later in this chapter), can theoretically modify the synthesis of these proteins and therefore aid in the treatment of disease. This emerging science continues to give rise to novel terminology. The entire set of proteins produced by a genome is now known as the **proteome**. **Proteomics** is the study of the proteome, including protein expression, modification, localization, and function, as well as the protein–protein interactions that are part of biological processes. This science is expected to provide new drug therapies in the future. Furthermore, most clinically approved drugs interact with body proteins such as cell membrane receptors, hormones, and enzymes.

Human Genome Project

In 1990, an unprecedented genetic research project began, known as the **International Human Genome Project (IHGP)**. This project was a worldwide research initiative coordinated by the US Department of Energy and the National Institutes of Health (NIH). The project was completed in 2003, 2 years ahead of schedule. The goals of this project were to identify the estimated 30 000 genes—3 billion base pairs—in the DNA of an entire human genome. Additional goals included developing new tools for genetic data analysis and storage, transferring newly developed technologies to the private sector, and addressing the inherent ethical, legal, and social issues involved in genetic research and clinical practice. However, the ultimate goal was to develop improved prevention, treatment, and cures for disease. When the HGP began, there were 100 known human, disease-related genes. By its completion, there were 1 400.

GENE THERAPY

Background

Gene therapy is an experimental technique that uses genes to treat or prevent disease. It allows doctors to treat a disorder by inserting a gene into a patient's cells instead of using drugs or surgery. Researchers are testing several approaches to gene therapy, including the following:
- Replacing a mutated gene with a healthy copy of the gene
- Introducing a new gene into the body to help fight a disease
- Inactivating a mutated gene that is functioning improperly

Gene therapy research is based on the ongoing discovery of new details regarding cellular processes, including biochemical processes that occur at the molecular level. In addition, the increased understanding of allelic variation and its role in disease susceptibility can be used to guide attempts at preventive therapy based on a person's genotypic risk factors.

Although numerous gene therapy clinical trials have been approved by Health Canada, no gene therapy to date has been approved for routine treatment of disease. The goal of gene therapy is to transfer exogenous genes that will either provide a temporary substitute for, or initiate permanent changes in the patient's own genetic functioning to treat a given disease. Originally projected to provide treatment primarily for inherited genetic diseases, gene therapy techniques are now being researched for the treatment of acquired illnesses such as cancer, cardiovascular diseases, diabetes, infectious diseases, and substance misuse. In the future, in utero gene therapy may be used to prevent the development of serious diseases as part of the prenatal care for the unborn infant.

Description

During gene therapy, segments of DNA are injected into the patient's body in a process called *gene transfer*. These artificially produced DNA splices are also known as **recombinant DNA (rDNA)** and must usually be inserted into some kind of carrier or vector for the gene transfer process. Vectors currently being evaluated include spherical lipid compounds known as *liposomes*, free DNA splices known as *plasmids*, DNA conjugates in which DNA splices are linked (conjugated) to either protein or gold particles, and various types of viruses. Viruses are the most widely studied rDNA vectors thus far. One commonly used group of viruses is that of the adenoviruses, which includes human influenza viruses.

Limitations

Viruses used for gene transfer can also induce viral disease and be immunogenic in the human host. The proteins produced by such artificial methods can be immunogenic. Even in the absence of significant virus-induced disease, the positive effects (e.g., supplemented protein synthesis) may be only temporary, and further treatments may be required. As a result, viruses must be carefully chosen and modified in an effort to optimize therapeutic effects while minimizing undesirable adverse effects. The determination of an ideal gene transfer method remains a major challenge for gene therapy researchers. Figure 5-1 provides a clinical example of the potential use of gene therapy.

Current Application

One well-established, indirect form of gene therapy is called *rDNA technology*. It involves the use of rDNA vectors in the laboratory to make recombinant forms of drugs, especially biologic drugs such as hormones, vaccines, antitoxins, and monoclonal antibodies. The most common example is the use of the *Escherichia coli* bacterial genome to manufacture a recombinant form of human insulin. When the human insulin gene is inserted into the genome of bacterial cells, the resulting culture artificially generates human insulin on a large scale. Although this insulin must be isolated and purified from its bacterial culture source, the majority of the world's medical insulin supply has been produced by this method for well over a decade.

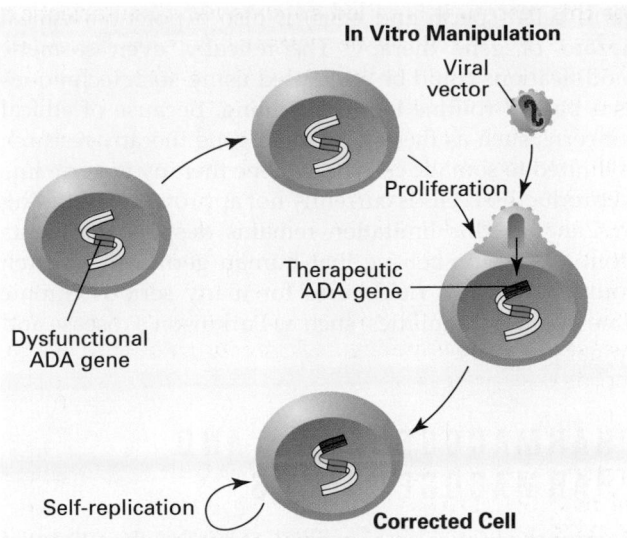

FIG. 5-1   Gene therapy for adenosine deaminase (ADA) deficiency attempts to correct this immunodeficiency state. The viral vector containing the therapeutic gene is inserted into the patient's lymphocytes. These cells can then make the ADA enzyme. (From Lewis, S. M., Dirksen, S. R., Heitkemper, M. M., et al. (2014). *Medical-surgical nursing in Canada: Assessment and management of clinical problems* (3rd ed.). (Canadian Eds. S. Goldsworthy, M. Barry, & D. Goodridge). Toronto, ON: Elsevier Mosby.)

Regulatory and Ethical Issues of Gene Therapy

Gene therapy research is inherently complex and can also carry great risks for its recipients. Thus, the issue of patient safety becomes significant. Research subjects who receive gene therapy often have a life-threatening illness, such as cancer, which may justify the risks involved. However, case reports of deaths in gene therapy trials have underscored these risks and raised awareness of patient safety. The Biologics and Genetic Therapies Directorate (BGTD) of Health Canada was assigned responsibility for oversight of gene therapy research in Canada. It reviews clinical trials involving human gene transfer. The Biologics and Genetic Therapies Directorate, Health Canada, must also review and approve all human clinical gene therapy trials, as it does with any type of drug therapy.

Any institution that conducts any type of research involving human subjects must have a research ethics board, whose purpose is to protect research subjects from unnecessary risks. An institutional biosafety committee is also required for gene therapy research. The role of this committee is to ensure compliance with the Medical Council of Canada (MCC)'s *Guidelines for the Handling of Recombinant DNA Molecules and Animal Viruses and Cells*.

A major ethical issue related to gene therapy techniques is that of eugenics. Eugenics is the intentional selection before birth of some genotypes that are considered more desirable than others. For similar reasons, the prospect of being able to manipulate genes in human germ cells (sperm and eggs) is also a potential ethical hazard of gene therapy. Theoretically, even cosmetic modifications could be attempted using such techniques as a part of routine family planning. Because of ethical concerns such as these, Canadian gene therapy research is limited to somatic cells only. Gene therapy in germ line (reproductive) cells is currently not approved for funding in Canada. This limitation remains despite arguments from those who believe that human germ cell research could potentially yield cures for many serious chronic illnesses and disabilities, such as Parkinson's disease and spinal paralysis.

PHARMACOGENETICS AND PHARMACOGENOMICS

Pharmacogenetics is a general term for the study of genetic variations in drug response and focuses on single-gene variations. A related science that pertains more directly to the HGP is **pharmacogenomics**. Pharmacogenomics is the combination of two scientific disciplines: pharmacology and genomics. Pharmacogenomics involves how genetics (genome) affect the body's response to drugs. Pharmacogenomics offer physicians the opportunity to individualize drug therapy based on a patient's genetic makeup, rather than giving the "standard" dose to all patients. The ultimate goal is to predict patient drug response and proactively tailor drug selection and dosages for optimal treatment outcomes. Warfarin sodium is an anticoagulant drug that is used to prevent blood clots (see Chapter 27). Research has shown that people with certain genetic variations (CYP2C9*2 or CYP2C9*3 alleles) are at increased risk of bleeding and require lower doses than those without the variation. In addition, variations in the gene that encodes *VKORC1* may make a patient more or less sensitive to warfarin sodium. This genetic variation occurs most frequently in the Asian population.

Individual differences in alleles that occur in at least 1% of the population are known as **genetic polymorphisms**. The word *polymorphism* literally means "many forms." Polymorphisms are considered too frequent to result from random genetic mutations. Polymorphisms that alter the amount or actions of drug-metabolizing enzymes can alter the body's reactions to medications. Known examples include those polymorphisms that affect the metabolism of certain antimalarial drugs, the antituberculosis drug isoniazid, and the variety of drugs that are metabolized by several subtypes of cytochrome enzymes. They can also alter the functioning of drug receptor proteins, cell membrane ion channels and drug transport proteins, and intracellular second messenger proteins (which carry out drug actions after a drug molecule binds to a cell membrane receptor).

Differences in cytochrome enzymes (see Chapter 2) are the best studied polymorphism effects thus far. Depending on their existing genes for these enzymes, patients can be genetically classified as "poor" or "rapid" metabolizers of CYP-metabolized drugs such as warfarin sodium, phenytoin, codeine sulphate, and quinidine. With warfarin sodium and phenytoin, a rapid metabolizer may require a higher dose of medication for the same effect, whereas a lower dose may be best for a poor metabolizer. With codeine sulphate, a poor metabolizer may actually need a higher dose to get the same analgesic effect that occurs when codeine sulphate is metabolized to morphine sulphate. In contrast, a rapid metabolizer may convert codeine sulphate to morphine sulphate too quickly, resulting in oversedation, and a lower dose may be sufficient. A similar situation is also likely to occur with quinidine. Because cytochrome enzymes are known to vary among racial and ethnic groups, the principle of "cultural safety" becomes one of the imperatives for routine gene-based drug dosing.

Studying both the genome of the patient and the genetics features of the pathology (e.g., tumour cells, infectious organisms) before treatment could allow for customized drug selection and dosing. Such analysis could permit the avoidance of drugs not likely to be effective as well as optimization of drug doses to minimize the risk of adverse drug effects. These applications of pharmacogenomics are examples of **personalized medicine**.

DNA Microarray Technology

Most drug dosage changes are still usually made on a trial-and-error basis by monitoring patient response. Researchers have developed an analytical tool known as a *high-density microarray*. This technology uses tiny microchip plates that contain thousands of microscopic DNA samples. A patient's blood can then be screened for thousands of corresponding DNA sequences that bind from the patient's blood sample to the sequences on the chip. This allows determination of the presence or absence of various genes, such as those related to drug metabolism. For example, the enzymes in the cytochrome system help metabolize from 25 to 30% of currently available drugs. Over 40 specific cytochrome genes have been identified thus far. The first DNA microchip for clinical use is the AmpliChip Microarray. It is used to screen blood samples for the individual's cytochrome enzyme profile. Although this type of genotypic profiling is not yet practical for widespread use, it will eventually become a standard in clinical practice.

Table 5-1 lists several other examples of current clinical applications of pharmacogenomics.

APPLICATION OF GENETIC PRINCIPLES RELATED TO DRUG THERAPY AND THE NURSING PROCESS

As noted previously, the recognition that genetic factors contribute, at some level, to most diseases continues to

TABLE 5-1

Clinical Applications of Pharmacogenomics

Genetic Technique	Application
Genotyping for presence of the CYP2D6 isoenzyme and CYP2D6 alleles, determining whether patients are poor, intermediate, extensive, or ultrarapid metabolizers related to these enzymes (under study)	*Psychiatry and general medicine:* Helps guide the prescribing of selected medications such as anticoagulants, immunosuppressants, antidepressants, antipsychotics, anticonvulsants, β-blockers, and antidysrhythmics
Genotyping for presence of the p-glycoprotein drug transport protein (under study)	*Cardiology, infectious diseases, oncology, and other practice areas:* Assists in drug selection and dosing for drugs such as digoxin, antiretrovirals, and antineoplastics
Genotyping for presence of thiopurine methyltransferase enzyme	*Oncology:* Used to temper toxicity through more careful dosing of the cancer drug 6-mercaptopurine in children with leukemia
Genotyping for variations in β-adrenergic receptors (under study)	*Pulmonology:* Determines which patients with asthma are more or less responsive to β-agonist therapy (e.g., albuterol) and which patients might benefit from other types of drug therapy
Genotyping for presence of the Philadelphia chromosome	*Oncology:* Identifies those patients with chronic myelogenous leukemia who may be stronger candidates for the cancer drug imatinib mesylate (Gleevec®)
Genotyping for presence of the *HER2/neu* proto-oncogene	*Oncology:* Identifies a subset of patients with breast cancer whose tumours express this gene, which indicates their suitability for treatment with the cancer drug trastuzumab (Herceptin®)
Viral genotyping of hepatitis C viruses (under study)	*Infectious diseases:* Can determine whether a particular infection warrants 26 versus 48 weeks of drug therapy (thereby reducing both costs and adverse drug effects)
Genotyping for the presence of factor V gene mutation	*Women's health:* Identifies women with a 7 to 100 times greater risk of thrombosis with oral contraceptive use compared to women without the mutation
Muscle biopsy test for patients with a family history of malignant hyperthermia	*Surgery:* Assesses the patient's risk of this adverse effect known to occur with administration of various inhalation anaesthetics and intraoperative paralyzing drugs
Genotyping for the presence of sodium channels associated with renin-angiotensin receptors and adrenal gland receptors	*Cardiology:* Allows refined antihypertensive drug selection
Race-based drug selection	*Cardiology:* Indicates use of the drug isosorbide dinitrate/hydralazine (BiDil®) for treatment of hypertension in patients of African descent due ultimately to genotypic variations in this patient population. This drug is not currently available in Canada.

CYP2D6, cytochrome enzyme subtype 2D6.

 CASE STUDY

Genetic Counselling

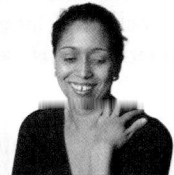

During the nurse's assessment of Darla, a newly admitted 38-year-old patient, Darla tells the nurse, "I'm allergic to codeine. Whenever I take it, it just knocks me out!" She tells the nurse that codeine does the same thing to all of her sisters.

The next day, the patient's oncologist comes in and explains the results of a genetic test that was performed on an outpatient basis. Darla agrees to allow the nurse to sit in on the conversation. The oncologist tells the patient that she has a type of gene that indicates that she has a strong chance of developing breast cancer within the next 5 years. The oncologist recommends that she undergo a bilateral mastectomy soon to avoid the possibility of developing breast cancer and suggests that she share this information with her sisters and her daughter, who is 18 years old. After the oncologist leaves, Darla tells the nurse, "I don't know what to do. I haven't talked to one of my sisters for years and I just know she won't believe me. I also don't want to worry my daughter. She is so young, and I'm sure she's too young to get cancer."

1. Does Darla have an actual allergy to codeine? What else could be happening?
2. Should the nurse tell Darla's sister and daughter? Explain your answer.
3. What is the best way for the nurse to handle this situation?

_____

For answers see http://evolve.elsevier.com/Canada/Lilley/pharmacology/.

grow. Thus, genetic influences on health, including the interaction of genetic and environmental (nongenetic) factors, will routinely affect nursing care delivery. In general, it is expected that in the next few years genetic research will move from the laboratory to more clinical practice settings.

Nurses in general practice settings will not be expected to perform in-depth genetic testing or counselling. Nurses—or other health care providers—with specialty certification in the field of genetics will conduct genetic testing and counselling. However, all nurses will need to have a working knowledge of relevant genetic principles. In this era of the "new genetics" paradigm, nurses are fully aware that nearly all diseases have a genetic component. Conditions such as myocardial infarction, cancer, mental illness, diabetes, and Alzheimer's disease are now viewed in a different light because of the known complex interactions between a number of factors, including the influence of one or more genes and a variety of environmental exposures for patients.

There are several other applicable skills regarding genetics for nurses in general practice settings. Assessment is the first step of the nursing process, and during the assessment the nurse may uncover factors that point to a risk for genetic disorders. During the initial assessment, the nurse obtains a patient's personal and family history. The family history is most effective if it covers at least three generations and includes the current and past health status of each family member. Assessment of factors possibly indicating an increased risk for genetic disorders is also important. A few examples of such factors are a higher incidence of a particular disease or disorder in the patient's family than in the general population; diagnosis of a disease in family members at an unusually young age; or diagnosis of a family member with an unusual form of cancer or with more than one type of cancer.

It is also important to inquire about any unusual reactions to a drug on the part of the patient, family members, significant others, and/or caregivers. An unusual or other than expected reaction to a drug in family members may point to a difference in the patient's ability to metabolize certain drugs. As indicated earlier in the chapter (as well as in Chapter 2), genetic factors may alter a patient's metabolism of a particular drug, resulting in either increased or decreased drug action. Every time a medication is administered, the patient's response to that drug must be assessed. Any unusual medication responses in a patient may point to a need for further investigation. Once a genetic variation is known, drug therapy may be adjusted accordingly.

As DNA chip technology becomes more affordable and accessible, it will be possible for patients to know in advance their relative risks for different diseases in later life. Genotype testing to identify a patient's drug-metabolizing enzymes will help prescribers better predict a patient's response to drug therapy.

Teaching about genetic testing and counselling may be another responsibility of the nurse. Patients will have questions and concerns about genetic testing and other issues. Nurses in general practice are not experts in genetic issues. However, the nurse may help with suggestions about genetic counselling, if appropriate. If genetic testing is ordered, the nurse may be a part of the testing process and will need to ensure that the informed decision making and consent procedure has been carried out correctly.

Maintaining privacy and confidentiality is of utmost importance during genetic testing and counselling. The patient is the one who decides whether to include or exclude any family members from the discussion and from knowledge of the results of the testing. Patients need to be reminded that undergoing the genetic test is not required and that they have the right to disclose or withhold test results from anyone. Nurses must protect against improper disclosure of information to other family members, friends of the family, other health care providers, and insurance providers. Nurses share the responsibility with other health care providers to protect patients and their families against the misuse of patients' genetic information.

Other responsibilities of the professional nurse may include development of clinical and social policy such as genetic nondiscrimination and prenatal testing policies, testing of genetic products for reliability, and tasks in genetic informatics to meet the challenge of sifting through a continually expanding body of knowledge.

SUMMARY

Increasing scientific understanding of genetic processes is expected to revolutionize modern health care in many ways. The artificial manipulation and transfer of genetic material, although not a standard treatment for disease, is the focus of over 300 human clinical gene therapy trials. The spectrum of diseases that may eventually be treatable by gene therapy includes inherited diseases that are present from birth, disabilities such as paralysis from spinal cord injuries, life-threatening illnesses such as cancer, and even chronic illnesses acquired later in life for which a person may have a genetic predisposition. The science of pharmacogenomics has already identified some of the genetic nuances in how different individuals' bodies metabolize drugs to their benefit or harm. Continued study in this area is expected to result in proactive customization of drug therapy to promote therapeutic benefits while minimizing or eliminating toxic effects. Genetic procedures and therapeutic techniques will likely become an increasing part of nursing practice as well as health care delivery in general. As the role and impact of genetics and genetically based drug therapy increase, so will their role in the nursing process.

KEY POINTS

❖ Genetic processes are a highly complex facet of human physiology, and genetics is becoming an integral part of health care that holds much promise in the form of new treatments for alterations in health.

❖ The Human Genome Project (HGP) described in detail the entire genome of a human individual.

❖ Basic genetic inheritance is carried by 23 pairs of chromosomes in each of the somatic cells; one pair of chromosomes in each cell is called the *sex*

chromosomes, identified as XX for females and XY for males.

❖ Applicable skills for general nurses include taking thorough patient, family, and drug histories; recognizing situations that may warrant further investigation through genetic testing; identifying resources for patients; maintaining confidentiality and privacy; and ensuring that informed consent is obtained for genetic testing and counselling.

EXAMINATION REVIEW QUESTIONS

1. Which is the most appropriate example of a product formed by an indirect form of gene therapy?
a. Stem cells
b. Insulin
c. Antigen substitution
d. Platelet inhibitors or stimulators

2. The nurse is explaining the general goal of gene therapy to a patient, which is to transfer exogenous genes to a patient for which result?
a. To change the patient's own genetic functioning to treat a given disease
b. To improve drug metabolism
c. To prevent genetic disorders in the patient's future children
d. To stimulate the growth of stem cells

3. What is the responsibility of research ethics boards?
a. Approving all forms of human clinical gene therapy
b. Identifying all major risks to the human subjects in a specific research protocol
c. Reviewing clinical trials involving human gene transfer
d. Analyzing genomes and determining whether they appear mutagenic

4. The presence of certain factors in a person's genetic makeup that increase the likelihood of eventually developing one or more diseases is known as
a. Genetic mutation
b. Genetic polymorphism
c. Genome predisposition
d. Genotype

5. The nurse is reviewing gene therapy. Which is a commonly studied adenovirus?
a. Hepatitis A and C virus
b. *Genovirum*
c. Human influenza virus
d. Pallodium

6. General responsibilities of the nurse regarding genetics may include which of these activities? (Select all that apply.)
a. Assessing the patient's personal and family history
b. Referring the patient to a genetic counsellor or other genetic specialist
c. Communicating the results of genetic tests to the patient and family
d. Maintaining privacy and confidentiality during the testing process
e. Answering questions about genetic test results

7. The nurse is assessing a patient for a possible increased risk for genetic disorders. Which of these, if present, may indicate an increased risk for a genetic disorder? (Select all that apply.)
a. Having a brother who died of a myocardial infarction at age 29
b. Having a family member diagnosed with more than one type of cancer
c. Having an uncle who was diagnosed with prostate cancer at age 73
d. A history of allergy to shellfish and iodine
e. Having a maternal grandmother, two maternal aunts, and a sister who were diagnosed with colon cancer

Answers: 1. b, 2. a, 3. b, 4. c, 5. c, 6. a, b, d, 7. a, b, e

CRITICAL THINKING ACTIVITIES

1. You are working on a medical–surgical unit as a newly graduated nurse. During an assessment, your patient states, "My doctor told me that I need to have genetic testing. I just don't understand. If they change my genes, then it will change the way I look!" What is the priority as you answer the patient's concerns?

2. An indirect form of gene therapy is already seen in contemporary health care practice. Explain this statement and provide examples.

3. Analyze the process for producing human insulin, and suggest a few theoretical examples of how this same process could be used in other areas of health care.

For answers see http://evolve.elsevier.com/Canada/Lilley/pharmacology/.

CHAPTER 6

Medication Errors: Preventing and Responding

Objectives

After reading this chapter, the successful student will be able to do the following:

1. Compare the following terms related to drug therapy in the context of professional nursing practice: adverse drug event, adverse drug reaction, allergic reaction, idiosyncratic reaction, medical error, and medication error.

2. Describe the most commonly encountered medication errors.

3. Develop a framework for professional nursing practice for prevention of medication errors.

4. Identify potential physical and emotional consequences of a medication error.

5. Discuss the impact of culture and age on the occurrence of medication errors.

6. Analyze the various ethical dilemmas related to professional nursing practice associated with medication errors.

7. Identify agencies concerned with prevention of and response to medication errors.

8. Discuss the possible consequences of medication errors for professional nurses and other members of the health care team.

e-Learning Activities

Website
(http://evolve.elsevier.com/Canada/
Lilley/pharmacology/)

evolve

- Answer Key—Textbook Case Studies
- Answer Key—Critical Thinking Activities
- Chapter Summaries—Printable
- Review Questions for Exam Preparation
- Unfolding Case Studies

Key Terms

Adverse drug event (ADE) Any undesirable occurrence related to administration of or failure to administer a prescribed medication. (p. 91)

Adverse drug reactions (ADRs) Unexpected, unintended, or excessive responses to medication given at therapeutic dosages (as opposed to overdose); one type of adverse drug event. (p. 91)

Allergic reaction An immunological hypersensitivity reaction resulting from an unusual sensitivity of a patient to a particular medication; a type of adverse drug event and a subtype of adverse drug reactions. (p. 91)

Idiosyncratic reaction Any abnormal and unexpected response to a medication, other than an allergic reaction, that is peculiar to an individual patient. (p. 91)

Malpractice Improper or unethical conduct or unreasonable lack of skill that results in harm and where compensation may be sought. All malpractice involves negligence. (p. 101)

Medical errors A broad term used to refer to any errors at any point of patient care that cause or have the potential to cause a patient harm. (p. 91)

Medication errors (MEs) Any preventable adverse drug events involving inappropriate medication use by a patient or health care provider; may or may not cause the patient harm. (p. 91)

Medication reconciliation   A procedure implemented by health care providers to maintain an accurate and up-to-date list of medications for all patients between all phases of health care delivery. (p. 99)

Negligence   Unintentional harm that results from conduct that does not meet a standard of care established by law. (p. 101)

GENERAL IMPACT OF ERRORS ON PATIENTS

Medical errors and medication errors (MEs) in particular have received much national attention. The study that brought medical errors to the public was the landmark study done in 1999 by the Institute of Medicine (IOM). According to this study, the number of patient deaths from medical errors in hospitals in the United States ranged from 44 000 to 98 000 annually, based on data from two large-scale studies. The IOM conducted a similar study in 2006 and found that medical errors harm at least 1.5 million people per year, including 117 000 hospitalizations at a cost of over $4 billion. A follow-up study in 2010 showed 25.1 "harms" per 100 admissions to the hospital. This study showed no significant change in rates of preventable errors since the IOM study. The landmark study of adverse events in Canadian hospitals undertaken in 2004 found that between 9 000 and 24 000 patients die each year because of adverse events or errors. Another Canadian study found that adverse drug–related events are responsible for 12% of emergency department visits. Of these, 68% were considered preventable (Zed, Abu-Laban, Balen, et al., 2008). A more recent report found that in 2007, 17% of—4.2 million—Canadians adults believed that a medical error had occurred to them when receiving health care in the previous 2 years (O'Hagan, MacKinnon, Persaud, et al., 2009). In this study, factors contributing to medical errors such as numerous prescriptions, a chronic condition, and insufficient time with the physician were cited.

Numerous health institutions have made prevention of medical errors a top priority. The most important change to recognize is that reporting of errors should not be punitive toward the reporter. In fact, all health care providers are encouraged to report errors. It has been shown that reporting of errors can prevent errors from occurring. Most errors occur as a "complex interplay of circumstances in the clinical environment" (Wilkins & Shields, 2008, p. ?) Increasingly, however, the literature reflects a shift in focus away from the individual nurse as the source of the ME to a consideration of the broader context. This concept has been taken a step further and has created "just culture." Just culture recognizes that systems are generally at fault when an error occurs, but that when professionals do not follow policies or have repeated errors, those professionals need remedial education and must be held accountable.

Medical errors can occur during all phases of health care delivery and involve all categories of health care providers. Some of the more common types of error include misdiagnosis, patient misidentification, lack of patient monitoring, wrong-site surgery, and MEs. Most studies have looked at medical errors occurring in hospitals; however, many serious MEs occur in the home. Errors occurring in homes can be quite harmful, as potent drugs once used only in hospitals are now being prescribed for outpatients. The majority of fatal errors at home involve the mixing of prescription drugs with alcohol or other drugs. Intangible losses resulting from adverse outcomes include patient dissatisfaction with, and loss of trust in, the health care system. This loss of trust, in turn, can lead to adverse health outcomes because patients are afraid to seek health services. This chapter focuses on the issues related to MEs and ways to prevent and respond to these errors.

MEDICATION ERRORS

An **adverse drug event (ADE)** is a general term that encompasses all types of clinical problems related to medication use. These errors include **medication errors (MEs)** and **adverse drug reactions (ADRs)**. The various subsets of ADEs and their interrelationships are illustrated in Figure 6-1. Adverse drug reactions are reactions that occur with the use of the particular drug. Two types of ADRs are **allergic reaction** (often predictable) and **idiosyncratic reaction** (usually unpredictable). MEs are a common cause of adverse health care outcomes and can range from having no significant effect to directly causing patient disability or death.

It is important to consider all of the steps involved in the medication use system when discussing MEs.

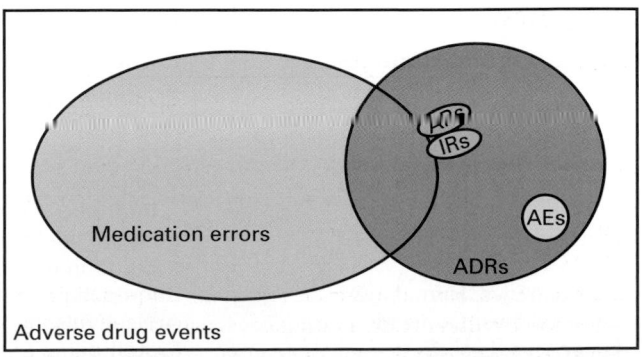

FIG. 6-1   Diagram illustrating the classes and subclasses of adverse drug events. *ADRs*, adverse drug reactions; *AEs*, adverse effects; *ARs*, allergic reactions; *IRs*, idiosyncratic reactions.

Identifying, responding to, and ultimately preventing MEs require an examination of the entire medication use process. Attention must be focused on all people and all steps involved in the medication use process, including the prescriber, the transcriber of the order, nurses, pharmacists, and any other ancillary staff involved. A systems approach takes the Tens Rights one step further and examines the entire health care system, the health care providers involved, and any other factor that has an impact on the error.

Drugs commonly involved in severe MEs include central nervous system drugs, anticoagulants, and chemotherapeutic drugs. "High-alert" medications have been identified as those that, because of their potentially toxic nature, require special care when prescribing, dispensing, or administering. High-alert medications are not necessarily involved in more errors than other drugs; however, the potential for patient harm is higher. The Institute for Safe Medication Practices' high-alert medications are listed in Table 6-1. MEs also result due to the large numbers of drugs with similarities in spelling or pronunciation (i.e., look-alike or sound-alike names). Several acronyms have been created to refer to these drugs, including SALAD (sound-alike, look-alike drugs) and LASA (look-alike, sound-alike). Mix-ups between such drugs are most dangerous when two drugs from different therapeutic classes have similar names. This can result in patient effects that are grossly different from those intended as part of the drug therapy. For a list of examples of commonly confused drug names, see Preventing Medication Errors: Institute for Safe Medication Practices: Examples of Look-Alike, Sound-Alike (LASA) Commonly Confused Drug Names below. More information on high-alert medications and SALADs can be found on the Institute for Safe Medication Practices Canada website at http://www.ismp-canada.org.

The application of TALLman lettering (combinations of uppercase and lowercase letters, rather than all uppercase or all lowercase lettering) is one of several techniques and strategies to differentiate similar drug names and optimize medication safety during all stages of the medication-use process. TALLman lettering creates a mental alert by changing the shape of words that look similar when seen in uppercase letters only. The Institute for Safe Medication Practices Canada, the Canadian Association of Provincial Cancer Agencies, and the International Medication Safety Network endorsed a list of sound-alike look-alike drug names used in oncology, where TALLman lettering is applied (e.g., VinCRIStine/VinBLAStine). For a full list of look-alike/sound-alike drug names with recommended TALLman lettering see http://www.ismp-canada.org.

It is widely recognized that most MEs result from weaknesses in the systems within health care organizations rather than from individual shortcomings. System weaknesses include failure to create a "just culture" or nonpunitive work atmosphere for reporting errors, excessive workload with minimal time for preventive education for staff, interruptions during medication preparation and administration, and lack of interdisciplinary communication and collaboration. All hospitals are required to analyze MEs and implement ways to prevent them. Nurses must take the time to report errors because without reporting, no changes can be made. When errors are reported, trends can be identified and processes can be changed to prevent the errors from occurring again.

ISSUES CONTRIBUTING TO ERRORS
Organizational Issues

Various strategies have been used to detect and document MEs in hospitals. MEs can occur at any step in the medication process: procuring, prescribing, transcribing,

 PREVENTING MEDICATION ERRORS

Institute for Safe Medication Practices: Examples of Look-Alike, Sound-Alike (LASA) Commonly Confused Drug Names

Names of Medications	Comments
carboplatin vs. cisplatin	Two different antineoplastic drugs
Celebrex® vs. Celexa® vs. Cerebyx	Anti-inflammatory drug versus antidepressant drug versus antiepileptic drug
dopamine vs. dobutamine	Vasopressor drugs of markedly different strengths; dobutamine is also a strong inotropic, affecting the heart
fentanyl vs. sufentanil	Both are injectable anaesthetics but with a significant difference in potency and duration of action
Humulin® vs. Humalog®	Short-acting versus rapid-acting insulin
Lamictal® vs. Lamisil®	Anticonvulsant/mood stabilizer versus antifungal drug
Losec® vs. Lasix®	Proton pump inhibitor versus diuretic
metronidazole vs. metformin	Antibiotic versus antidiabetic drug
Paxil® vs. Plavix®	Antidepressant versus antiplatelet drug
trazodone® vs. tramadol®	Antidepressant versus analgesic

TABLE 6-1

Examples of High-Alert Medications

Classes/Categories of Drugs

- Adrenergic agonists, IV (e.g., **EPINEPH**rine, phenylephrine, norepinephrine)
- Adrenergic antagonists, IV (e.g., propranolol, metoprolol, labetalol)
- anaesthetic agents, general, inhaled, and IV (e.g., propofol, ketamine)
- Antiarrhythmics, IV (e.g., lidocaine, amiodarone)
- Antithrombotic agents, including:
  anticoagulants (e.g., warfarin, low-molecular-weight heparin, IV unfractionated heparin)
  Factor Xa inhibitors (e.g., fondaparinux)
  Direct thrombin inhibitors (e.g., argatroban, bivalirudin, dabigatran etexilate, lepirudin)
  Thrombolytics (e.g., alteplase, reteplase, tenecteplase)
  Glycoprotein IIb/IIIa inhibitors (e.g., eptifibatide)
- Cardioplegic solutions
- Chemotherapeutic agents, parenteral and oral
- Dextrose, hypertonic, 20% or greater
- Dialysis solutions, peritoneal and hemodialysis
- Epidural or intrathecal medications
- Hypoglycemics, oral
- Inotropic medications, IV (e.g., digoxin, milrinone)
- Insulin, subcutaneous and IV
- Liposomal forms of drugs (e.g., liposomal amphotericin B) and conventional counterparts (e.g., amphotericin B deoxycholate)
- Moderate sedation agents, IV (e.g., dexmedetomidine, midazolam)
- Moderate sedation agents, oral, for children (e.g., chloral hydrate)
- narcotics/opioids
- IV
- Transdermal
- Oral (including liquid concentrates, immediate, and sustained-release formulations)
- Neuromuscular blocking agents (e.g., succinylcholine, rocuronium, vecuronium)
- Parenteral nutrition preparations
- Radiocontrast agents, IV
- Sterile water for injection, inhalation, and irrigation (excluding pour bottles) in containers of 100 mL or more
- Sodium chloride for injection, hypertonic, greater than 0.9% concentration

Specific Drugs

- epoprostenol (Flolan®), IV
- magnesium sulphate injection
- methotrexate, oral, non-oncologic use
- opium tincture
- oxytocin, IV
- nitroprusside sodium for injection
- potassium chloride for injection concentrate
- potassium phosphates injection
- promethazine, IV
- vasopressin, IV or intraosseous

ISMP List of High Alert Medications in Community/Ambulatory Health Care

Classes/Categories of Medications	Specific Medications
Antiretroviral agents (e.g., efavirenz, lami**VUD**ine, raltegravir, ritonavir, combination antiretroviral products)	car**BAM**azepine
Chemotherapeutic agents, oral (excluding hormonal agents) (e.g., cyclophosphamide, mercaptopurine, temozolomide)	chloral hydrate liquid, for sedation of children
Antihyperglycemic drugs, oral	heparin sodium, including unfractionated and low-molecular-weight heparin
Immunosuppressant agents (e.g., aza**THIO**prine, cyclo**SPORINE**, tacrolimus)	met**FORMIN**
Insulin, all formulations	methotrexate, non-oncological use
Opioids, all formulations	midazolam liquid, for sedation of children
Pediatric liquid medications that require measurement	propylthiouracil
Pregnancy category X drugs (e.g., bosentan, **ISO**tretinoin)	warfarin sodium

Source: Institute for Safe Medication Practices (2014). *ISMP List of High-Alert Medications in Acute Care Settings.* Retrieved from http://www.ismp.org/tools/institutionalhighAlert.asp; Used with permission from the Institute for Safe Medication Practices. ISMP List of High-Alert Medications in Community/Ambulatory Healthcare. Retrieved from http://www.ismp.org/communityRx/tools/highAlert-community.pdf. Used with permission from the Institute for Safe Medication Practices.

dispensing, administering, and monitoring. Prescribing faults and prescription errors are major problems among MEs. Most prescribing errors can be caught by the pharmacist before order entry or by nurses prior to administration. Administration is the next most common point in the process at which MEs occur, followed by dispensing errors and transcription errors. It is important for nurses to have good relationships with pharmacists, because the two professions, working together, can have a major impact in preventing MEs. Hospital pharmacists are usually available 24/7 and serve as great resources when the nurse has any question regarding drug therapy. In more rural areas, having a pharmacist or physician always available may not always be possible or feasible. In these circumstances, it is recommended that nurses work with the agency to develop policies and processes that outline what steps to take in the event of a potential ME. Patient involvement in patient safety is widely advocated. Patients who are involved and share in decision making in their health care have better outcomes when they take on the responsibility of asking questions and seeking more information when they need it. They learn more about their illnesses and the care provided, and they can advocate for their own safety at each health care encounter. Safer Healthcare Now! and the Canadian Patient Safety Institute function to raise awareness and promote best practices in patient safety. As part of the World Health Organization (WHO) and Pan American Health Organization initiative Patients for Patient Safety Canada advocates for patient-centred care and patient safety strategies to improve patient safety.

Effective use of technologies such as computerized prescriber order entry and bar coding of medication packages has also been shown to reduce MEs. In 2008, the Institute for Safe Medication Practices Canada and the Canadian Patient Safety Institute sponsored a round-table to discuss and seek consensus on a national initiative for pharmaceutical manufacturers related to the use of standardized bar codes for labelling pharmaceutical medications approved for use in Canada. By 2012, the GS1 global Automatic Identification and Data Capture application standard, a global bar code standard for pharmaceuticals, was adopted for Canada. In 2010, bar code verification was being used for only 8% of institutional beds and 33% of dispensing and compounding practices within hospital pharmacies in Canada (Institute for Safe Medication Practices Canada, 2013; Canadian Patient Safety Institute, 2013). Cost is a barrier to technological improvements in general. The cost of implementing current technology, including automated drug dispensing cabinets with electronic charting and computerized order entry, is often prohibitive, ranging from hundreds of thousands of dollars to millions. Nonetheless, these various technological advances have been shown to reduce MEs. For example, computerized order entry (also known as computerized physician order entry [CPOE]) eliminates handwriting and standardizes many prescribing functions. Bar coding of medications allows the nurse to use electronic devices for verification of correct medication at the patient's bedside. Computer programs are used in the pharmacy to screen for potential drug interactions. Despite all the benefits technology has to offer, workload issues (i.e., nursing staff shortage), inadequate education in the use of the equipment, or difficulties in mastering the use of complex technology can prevent the technology from eliminating errors as it was designed to do. Self-medication by patients (e.g., patient-controlled analgesia) has been shown to reduce errors, provided patients have adequate cognitive ability and mental alertness. The WHO has developed information about patient safety concerns, safety initiatives, and patient safety solutions (see Box 6-1).

Educational System Issues and Their Potential Impact on Medication Errors

All health care providers have an obligation to double-check any necessary medication information before proceeding. This includes stopping to check medication orders and being comfortable with one's knowledge of the drug *before* administering it. Numerous drug information guides are available for the nurse's use. Access to electronic references at the point of care are improving. Many institutions subscribe to online databases such as Lexicomp or UpTodate that provide quick and easy access to drug information.

Patient safety begins in the educational process, with nursing students and faculty members. Nurses are pivotal to the medication administration process and must therefore demonstrate safe and reliable practice. It is critically important for nurse educators to employ teaching strategies that address a just culture of safety, one that allows students to begin their careers with greater confidence and a healthy habit of self-monitoring. Commonly reported student nurse errors involve the following situations: unusual dosing times, medication administration record issues (unavailability of the record, failure to document doses given resulting in administration of extra doses, failure to review the record before medicating patients), administration of discontinued or "held" medications, failure to monitor vital signs or laboratory results, administration of oral liquids as injections, preparation of medications for multiple patients at the same time, and dispensing of medications in different doses from those ordered (e.g., tablets that need to be split in half).

Medication Errors and Related Sociological Factors

Effective communication among all members of the health care team contributes to improved patient care. Workplace bullying among nurses is becoming an increasing issue. Bullying is different from horizontal violence in that a real or perceived power differential between the initiator and recipient must be present (Einarsen, Hoel, Zapf, et al., 2011). Disruptive physician behaviour and workplace bullying, and a lack of

BOX 6-1	World Health Organization Initiatives about Medications and Health

The World Health Organization (WHO) posts information on its website regarding initiatives to promote patient safety in medication administration and other aspects of health care. As the WHO notes, no adverse event should ever occur anywhere in the world if the knowledge exists to prevent it from happening. Knowledge is of little use, however, if it is not applied in practice. The WHO Collaborating Center for Patient Safety Solutions has developed patient safety initiatives that can serve as a guide in redesigning the patient care process to prevent the inevitable errors from ever reaching patients. *Patient safety solutions* are defined by the WHO as any system design feature or intervention that has demonstrated the ability to prevent or mitigate patient harm arising from the health care process. Information about the first group of patient safety solutions (2008/2009) approved by the WHO center is available at http://www.ccforpatient safety.org. These patient safety concerns include avoiding confusion of medications with look-alike, sound-alike names; ensuring correct patient identification; enhancing communication during patient "handovers" between care units or care teams; ensuring performance of the correct procedure at the correct body site; maintaining control of concentrated electrolyte solutions; ensuring medication accuracy at transition points in care; avoiding catheter and tubing misconnections; and promoting single use of injection devices and improved hand hygiene to prevent health care–associated infections.

More information about patient safety and safety initiatives is provided in a national initiative—Safer Healthcare Now! (SHN). SHN is the flagship program of the Canadian Patient Safety Institute (CPSI). The overarching goal of the program is to reduce preventable injuries and deaths related to adverse events. They have identified four priority areas: infection prevention and control, medication safety, surgical care, and home care. Canadian Patient Safety Week is a national annual campaign launched by the CPSI to raise awareness of patient safety issues common to all health care organizations. For example, the 2013 message was "Don't hold back—Good healthcare starts with good communication." The theme was "Ask. Listen. Talk." and encouraged all health care providers, patients, and their families to ASK questions, LISTEN to the answers, and TALK openly about their concerns in order to improve patient safety. Patients for Patient Safety Canada is a patient-led program of the CPSI. These initiatives encourage patients to take a role in preventing health care errors by becoming more active, involved, and informed regarding all aspects of their health care. For more information on these programs, visit http://www.patientsafetyinstitute.ca/ or visit http://www.saferhealthcarenow.ca/.

institutional response to it, are significant factors affecting nurse job satisfaction and nursing staff retention, as well as the erosion of personal health and professional well-being. Disruptive behaviours can potentially result in communication breakdown and lack of collaboration among physicians, nurses, and other health care workers that can lead to medical errors, adverse events, and near misses, resulting in reduced patient care quality. It can also lead to recruitment and retention issues, impact workers' health and well-being, patient safety, organization outcomes, and societal outcomes.

Physician disruptive behaviour accounts for 5% of all cases taken before Canada's medical regulatory bodies (Canadian Medical Protective Association, 2013). The Canadian Medical Protective Association recommends that disruptive behaviour by physicians should be addressed by the health care institution where the conduct occurs. An adversarial approach should be avoided and a step-by-step approach followed, including: (1) early identification, (2) proactive intervention, (3) workplace assessment, and (4) remediation. This same approach should be used for workplace bullying.

Fortunately, communication between prescribers and other members of the health care team has improved over the years, with newer generations of prescribers. This is due in large part to more progressive approaches in medical education that emphasize a team orientation and zero tolerance to any form of violence. Such approaches recognize the ever-increasing complexities of health care delivery and the reality that no one team member can know every fact and provide for all patient care needs.

PREVENTING, RESPONDING TO, REPORTING, AND DOCUMENTING MEDICATION ERRORS: A NURSING PERSPECTIVE

Preventing Medication Errors

MEs are considered to be any preventable event that could lead to inappropriate medication use or harm. The major categories of ME according to the Canadian Medication Incident Reporting and Prevention System (2011) are (1) near miss or close call where an event could have resulted in unwanted consequences but did not, (2) no-harm event where an incident occurs but results in no injury to the patient, (3) ME that causes harm, and (4) critical incident resulting in serious harm. MEs may be prevented through a variety of strategies, including the following: (1) Multiple systems of checks and balances should be implemented to prevent MEs. (2) Prescribers should write legible orders that contain correct information, or orders should be written electronically if the technology is available. (3) Authoritative resources, such as pharmacists or current drug literature, should be consulted if there is any area of concern, beginning with the medication order and continuing throughout the entire medication administration process. (4) Nurses should always check the medication order three times before giving the drug and consult with authoritative resources (see Chapter 3) if any questions or concerns exist. Faculty members should not be the student's research source regarding medications, and the safe practice of using appropriate

resources should begin early in the educational process. (5) The rights of medication administration should be used consistently, which has been shown to substantially reduce the likelihood of a ME. See Preventing Medication Errors: How to Prevent Medication Errors below, for a more concise and detailed listing of ways to help prevent MEs. See Special Populations: Children on page 97 for a discussion of MEs in pediatric patients and special considerations for this age group.

PREVENTING MEDICATION ERRORS

How to Prevent Medication Errors

- As the first step to defend against errors, assess information about drug allergies, vital signs, and laboratory test results.
- Use two patient identifiers before giving medications.
- Never give medications that you have not drawn up or prepared yourself.
- Minimize the use of verbal and telephone orders. If verbal or telephone orders are used, be sure to repeat the order to confirm with the prescriber. Speak slowly and clearly, and spell the drug name aloud.
- List the reason for use of each drug and any educational materials on the medication administration record.
- Avoid abbreviations, medical shorthand, and acronyms because they can lead to confusion, miscommunication, and risk of error (see Legal & Ethical Principles: Use of Abbreviations, Symbols, and Dose Designations on page 99).
- Never assume anything about a drug order or prescription, including route. If a medication order is questioned for any reason (e.g., dose, drug, indication), never assume that the prescriber is correct. Always be the patient's advocate and investigate the matter until all ambiguities are resolved.
- Do not try to decipher illegibly written orders; instead, contact the prescriber for clarification. Illegible orders fall below applicable standards for quality medical care and endanger patient safety. If in doubt about any part of an order, always check with the prescriber. Compare the medication order against what is on hand by checking for the right drug, right dose, right time, right patient, and right route.
- *Never* use trailing zeros (e.g., 1.0 mg) in writing and/or transcribing medication orders. Use of trailing zeros is associated with increased occurrence of overdose. For example, "1.0 mg warfarin sodium" could be misread as "10 mg warfarin sodium," a 10-fold dose increase. Instead, use "1 mg" or even "one mg."
- Failure to use leading zeros can also lead to overdose. For example, .25 mg digoxin could be misread as 25 mg digoxin, a dose that is 100 times the dose ordered. Instead, write "0.25 mg."
- Carefully read all labels for accuracy, expiration dates, dilution requirements, and warnings.
- Remain current with new techniques of administration and new equipment.

- Encourage the use of generic names.
- Listen to and honour any concerns expressed by patients. If the patient voices a concern about being allergic to a medication or states that a pill is not what the patient usually takes, STOP, listen, and investigate.
- Strive to maintain your own health so you remain alert, and never be too busy to stop, learn, and inquire. In addition, engage in ongoing continuing education.
- Become a member of professional nursing organizations to network with other nursing students or professional nurses to advocate for improved working conditions and to stand up for the rights of nurses and patients.
- Know where to find the latest information on which dosage forms can be or should not be crushed or opened (e.g., capsules), and educate patients accordingly.
- Safeguard any medications that the patient had on admission or transfer so that additional doses are not given or taken by mistake. In such situations, safeguarding is accomplished by compiling a current medication history and resolving any discrepancies rather than ignoring them.
- Always verify new medication administration records if they have been rewritten or re-entered for any reason, and follow policies and procedures about this action.
- Make sure the weight of the patient is always recorded before carrying out a medication order, to help decrease dosage errors.
- Provide for mandatory recalculation of every drug dosage for high-risk drugs (e.g., highly toxic drugs), or high-risk patients (e.g., pediatric or older adults) because there is a narrow margin between therapeutic serum drug levels and toxic levels (e.g., for chemotherapeutic drugs or digitalis drugs, or in the presence of altered liver or kidney function in a patient).
- Always suspect an error whenever an adult dosage form is dispensed for a pediatric patient.
- Seek translators when appropriate—never guess what patients are trying to say.
- Educate patients to take an active role in ME prevention, both in the hospital setting and at home.
- Involve yourself politically in advocating for legislation that improves patient safety.

SPECIAL POPULATIONS: CHILDREN

Medication Errors

Of all the ways a pediatric patient may be harmed during medical treatment, MEs are the most common. As with older adult patients, when MEs occur, there is a higher risk of death in children. MEs involving inpatient pediatric patients occur frequently, estimated at a rate of 4.5 to 5.7 errors per 100 drugs used. The most common MEs in pediatrics are dosing errors. Research has begun to identify some of the groups of pediatric patients who are at highest risk of MEs (see Evidence in Practice box). These include the following patients: (1) those younger than 2 years of age, (2) those in intensive care units, specifically the neonatal intensive care unit, (3) those in the emergency department, where there is high patient turnover and there are diverse and unpredictable patient needs, (4) those receiving intravenous or chemotherapeutic drugs, immunosuppressive medications, lipid/total parenteral nutrition or opioids (Maaskant, Eskes, van Rijn-Bikker, et al., 2013), and (5) those whose weight has not been determined or recorded. The risk of harm is compounded when a high-alert medication is involved. The top five high-alert medications reported as causing harm or potential harm in Canadian pediatric health care settings are morphine sulphate potassium chloride, insulin, fentanyl, and salbutamol (Institute for Safe Medication Practices Canada, 2009). Mathematical dosage calculations for pediatric patients are also problematic. Once the drug has been ordered, in determination of the correct dosage, the problems of most concern include the following: (1) inability of the nurse to understand/perform the correct calculation or dilution, (2) infrequent use of calculations, and (3) decimal point misplacement, with potential overdosing or underdosing.

The following are some of the actions that can be taken to prevent pediatric MEs:

- Report all MEs, because this information is part of the practice of professional nursing and helps in identifying causes of ME.
- Know the drug thoroughly, including its on- and off-label uses, action, adverse effects, dosage ranges, routes of administration, high-alert drug status cautions (see Table 6-1), and contraindications (e.g., Is it recommended for use in pediatric patients?).
- Confirm information about the patient each and every time a dose is given, and check three times before giving the drug, by comparing the drug order with the patient's medication profile and verifying for the right drug, right dose, right time, right route, and right patient.
- Double-check and verify information on handwritten orders that may be incomplete, unclear, or illegible.
- Avoid verbal telephone orders in general. When they are unavoidable, always repeat them back to the prescriber over the telephone. Insist that the prescriber sign off any emergency in-person verbal orders before leaving the unit.
- Avoid distractions while giving medications.
- Communicate with everyone (e.g., parent, caregiver) involved in patient care.
- Make sure all orders are clear and understood when patients are handed over to other nurses with shift changes.
- Adopt standard concentrations of opioid solutions (high alert classification) intended for continuous intravenous infusion.
- Limit the number of concentrations and strengths of high-alert medications available on a unit.
- Use authoritative resources such as drug handbooks, Lexicomp, Pediatric & Neonatal Dosage Handbook, Compendium of Pharmaceuticals and Specialities, or information from the Health Canada Drug Product Database website (http://www.hc-sc.gc.ca/dhp-mps/prodpharma/databasdon/index-eng.php).

Responding to, Reporting, and Documenting Medication Errors

Responding to and reporting MEs are part of the professional responsibilities for which nurses are accountable. If a ME does occur, it must be reported, regardless of whether the error was made by a nursing student or a professional nurse. Follow facility policies and procedures for reporting and documenting the error closely and cautiously. Once the patient has been assessed and urgent safety issues have been addressed, report the error immediately to the appropriate prescriber and nursing management, for example, the nurse manager or supervisor. If the patient cannot be left alone due to deterioration of the patient's condition or the need for close monitoring after the ME, a fellow nurse or other qualified health care provider should remain with the patient and provide appropriate care while the prescriber is contacted.

Follow-up procedures or tests may be ordered or an antidote prescribed. These orders should be implemented as indicated by the prescriber. Remember that the nurse's highest priority at all times during the medication administration process and during a ME is the patient's physiological status and safety.

When a ME has occurred, complete all appropriate forms—including an incident report—as per the facility's policies and procedures, and provide appropriate documentation. Document the ME by providing only factual information about the error. Documentation should always be accurate, thorough, and objective. Avoid using judgemental words such as *error* in the documentation. Instead, chart factual information such as the medication that was administered, the actual dose given, and other details regarding the order (e.g., wrong patient, wrong route, wrong time). Also note any

EVIDENCE IN PRACTICE

Canadian Pediatric Adverse Events Study

Review

Numerous adult studies have been conducted to investigate the harm associated with adverse events. The Canadian Adverse Effects Study conducted by Baker and Norton and colleagues in 2004 highlighted the significance of hospital-related harm in the adult population. This landmark study found that 7.5% of adults admitted to hospital experience adverse events (AEs). This information provided the foundation for improved safety of health care delivery for adults. Although some recent epidemiological studies have contributed to the knowledge base of pediatric safety in acute care hospitals, the scope of the problem in this vulnerable population was limited. The lack of a comprehensive pediatric trigger tool limited the scope of the full burden of health care–associated harm.

Type of Evidence

This cross-sectional study used a retrospective chart review of 3 669 charts from April 2008 to March 2009 across four age groups: 0 to 28 days; 29 days to 1 year; older than 1 year to 5 years; and older than 5 years to 18 years). The validated Canadian Paediatric Trigger Tool was used to identify AEs in children admitted to 7 academic pediatric centres and 15 large community hospitals across 7 Canadian provinces. The purpose of the study was to determine the epidemiology (incidence and prevention) of AEs in the pediatric population.

Results of the Study

Two hundred and thirty-seven patients (9.2%) experienced an AE resulting in death, disability, prolonged hospital stay, or readmission. Children in the pediatric academic settings experienced more AEs (11.2%) than those in community hospitals (3.3%). More nonpreventable AEs occurred in the academic settings, while the incidence of preventable AEs was comparable in both settings.

The reason for hospitalization and the age of the patient also influenced the occurrence of an adverse event. Neonates aged 0 to 28 days were more likely to experience an adverse event. Neonates admitted to the intensive care unit for at least 1 day were 10 times more likely to experience an AE. Patients over the age of 28 days admitted to surgical units were two times as likely to experience an AE as those on medical units. Surgical errors were the most frequent overall. Children under 12 months of age experienced more AEs from medical procedures and clinical care. Children 12 months and older experienced more AEs from medication and diagnostic errors.

Errors in surgical units and intensive care units in academic settings were the most common overall compared to emergency services and maternal/obstetrical units in community settings.

Link of Evidence to Nursing Practice

This data informs health care providers that children hospitalized in health care settings across Canada are vulnerable to harm. Children cannot advocate for safe care, so health care providers and decision makers must be informed of the various dangers in pediatric health care delivery. The range and burden of health care–associated injuries established from this study is key to transformation of the system to make health care safer.

Sources: Canadian Patient Safety Institute. (2013). Canadian paediatric adverse events study. Retrieved from http://www .patientsafetyinstitute.ca/en/toolsResources/Research/commissioned Research/PaediatricAdverseEvents/Documents/CPSI_Canadian_ Paediatric_Adverse_Events_doc_March%205_2013_English_Final .pdf; Matlow, A. G., Baker, G. R., Flintoft, V., et al. (2012). Adverse events among children in Canadian hospitals: The Canadian Paediatric Adverse Events Study. *Canadian Medical Association Journal, 184*(13): E709–E718. doi:10.1503/cmaj.112153

observed changes in the patient's physical and mental status. In addition, document the fact that the prescriber was notified and any follow-up actions or orders that were implemented. Patient monitoring should be ongoing.

Most facilities require additional documentation when a ME occurs, consisting of an incident report or unusual occurrence report. Always follow facility policies and procedures or protocols in completing an incident report. Documentation should include only factual information about the error as well as all corrective actions taken. Complete any additional sections of the form to help with the investigation of the incident. Because these forms are forwarded to the facility's risk management department, this complete and factual information may help prevent errors in the future. Do not document on the patient's chart that an incident report was filled out, and do not keep a copy of the incident report; incident reports are not to be placed in the

patient's chart. The reporting of actual and suspected MEs should offer the option of anonymity. This may help to foster improved error reporting and safe medication practices. Internal, facility-based systems of error tracking may generate data to help customize policy and procedure development. All institutional pharmacy departments are required to have an adverse drug event monitoring program.

Nurses as well as health care facilities may also be involved in external reporting of MEs. There are nationwide confidential reporting programs that collect and disseminate safety information on a larger scale. One such program is the Canadian Medication Incident Reporting and Prevention System (http://www.ismp-canada.org/cmirps/), which collects incident reports of MEs. The Canada Vigilance Program is Health Canada's postmarket surveillance program that collects and assesses reports of suspected adverse reactions to health products marketed in Canada. The Health Canada

LEGAL & ETHICAL PRINCIPLES

Use of Abbreviations, Symbols, and Dose Designations

Medication errors often occur as a result of misinterpretation of abbreviations, symbols, and dose designations. The Institute for Safe Medication Practices Canada, Accreditation Canada, and the Canadian Patient Safety Institute support the elimination of dangerous abbreviations, symbols, and dose designations in health care to enhance the safety of Canadian patients and recommend that abbreviations be written out in full. As part of Accreditation Canada Required Organizational Practices, organizations are required to identify and implement a list of abbreviations, dose designations, and symbols that are not to be used in the organization. This list is inclusive of the following Institute for Safe

Medication Practices Canada "Do Not Use" chart on page 100.

Note: In Canada, the trend is now toward using "mcg" in practice, so it is important to note the difference between "mcg" and "mg" in orders.

It is the philosophy of the authors of this textbook to avoid abbreviations whenever possible.

Source: Adapted from Institute for Safe Medication Practices (2006). *List of error-prone abbreviations, symbols, and dose designations.* Retrieved from https://www.ismp-canada.org/download/ISMPCanadaListOfDangerousAbbreviations.pdf.

website (http://www.hc-sc.gc.ca/dhp-mps/medeff/vigilance-eng.php) is a valuable source of adverse reaction information. The Canada Vigilance Adverse Reaction Online Database (http://www.hc-sc.gc.ca/dhp-mps/medeff/databasdon/conditions_search-recherche-eng.php) is a nationwide database of adverse reactions since 1965. Adverse reaction reports are submitted by health care providers and consumers on a voluntary basis, online or by telephone. MedEffect e-Notice, provided by Health Canada, sends health product advisories and recalls and the *Health Product InfoWatch* and MedEffect content updates are available for free by email (http://www.hc-sc.gc.ca/dhp-mps/medeff/subscribe-abonnement/index-eng.php). ISMP Canada, Safer Heathcare Now!, and Accreditation Canada also provide useful information to health care providers aimed at safety enhancement.

Performing Medication Reconciliation

Communicating effectively about medications is a critical component of delivering safe care. **Medication reconciliation** (also called *MedRec*) is a formal process in which medications are "reconciled" at all points of entry and exit to and from a health care entity. Medication reconciliation requires a best possible medication history (BPMH) and entails a more systematic and comprehensive review of all the medications a patient is taking. The prescriber is then to assess those medications and decide if they are to be continued upon hospitalization. Medication reconciliation was designed to ensure that there are no discrepancies between what patients were taking at home and what they take in the hospital. Medication reconciliation should occur at entry into the facility, upon transfer from surgery, into or out of the intensive care unit, and at discharge.

Although this seems to be an easy process, numerous problems have been encountered since its inception in 2005. The first problem is that often patients do not know exactly what medications they are taking and may report, for example, that they take a "blue pill for blood

pressure." Sometimes the patient may have a list of medications but some of the medications were discontinued prior to admission, and often they fail to provide this vital piece of information. The patient or family may not be involved in the medication history–taking process. This can lead to the prescriber continuing a medicine based on faulty information. System and communication factors may also impact medication reconciliation, such as inadequate hospital policies for medication management upon transfer and lack of systems to verify that medications are properly documented, ordered, or transcribed. There may also be communication issues between physicians, about changes to medication orders or discrepancies, or poor communication between physicians and other team members. Hospitals throughout the country are working hard to figure out ways to avoid the problems described; this is an ongoing process. Medication reconciliation has been part of the Accreditation Canada program since 2006; however, due to the problems encountered, it scaled back its requirements in 2008 (available at http://www.accreditation.ca/sites/default/files/med-rec-en.pdf).

Medication reconciliation involves three steps:

1. Verification: Collection of the patient's medication information with a focus on medications currently used (including prescription drugs as well as over-the-counter medications and natural health products)
2. Clarification: Professional review of this information to ensure that all medications and dosages are appropriate for the patient
3. Reconciliation: Further investigation of any discrepancies and documentation of relevant communications and changes in medication orders

To ensure ongoing accuracy of medication use, the steps listed below should be repeated at each stage of health care delivery:

a. Admission
b. Status change (e.g., from critical to stable). It is the role of the health care provider to evaluate current

DO NOT USE

DANGEROUS ABBREVIATIONS, SYMBOLS AND DOSE DESIGNATIONS

The abbreviations, symbols, and dose designations found in this table have been reported as being frequently misinterpreted and involved in harmful medication errors. They should NEVER be used when communicating medication information.

Abbreviation	Intended Meaning	Problem	Correction
U	unit	Mistaken for "0" (zero), "4" (four), or cc.	Use "unit".
IU	international unit	Mistaken for "IV" (intravenous) or "10" (ten).	Use "unit".
Abbreviations for drug names		Misinterpreted because of similar abbreviations for multiple drugs; e.g., MS, MSO$_4$ (morphine sulphate), MgSO$_4$ (magnesium sulphate) may be confused for one another.	Do not abbreviate drug names.
QD QOD	Every day Every other day	QD and QOD have been mistaken for each other, or as 'qid'. The Q has also been misinterpreted as "2" (two).	Use "daily" and "every other day".
OD	Every day	Mistaken for "right eye" (OD = oculus dexter).	Use "daily".
OS, OD, OU	Left eye, right eye, both eyes	May be confused with one another.	Use "left eye", "right eye" or "both eyes".
D/C	Discharge	Interpreted as "discontinue whatever medications follow" (typically discharge medications).	Use "discharge".
cc	cubic centimetre	Mistaken for "u" (units).	Use "mL" or "millilitre".
µg	microgram	Mistaken for "mg" (milligram) resulting in one thousand-fold overdose.	Use "mcg".

Symbol	Intended Meaning	Potential Problem	Correction
@	at	Mistaken for "2" (two) or "5" (five).	Use "at".
> <	Greater than Less than	Mistaken for "7" (seven) or the letter "L". Confused with each other.	Use "greater than"/"more than" or "less than"/"lower than".

Dose Designation	Intended Meaning	Potential Problem	Correction
Trailing zero	Χ.0 mg	Decimal point is overlooked resulting in 10-fold dose error.	Never use a zero by itself after a decimal point. Use "Χ **mg**".
Lack of leading zero	. Χ mg	Decimal point is overlooked resulting in 10-fold dose error.	Always use a zero before a decimal point. Use "**0.**Χ mg".

Used with permission from Institute for Safe Medication Practices (2006).
Do Not Use, Dangerous abbreviations, symbols, and dose designations,
https://www.ismp-canada.org/download/ISMPCanadaListOfDangerousAbbreviations.pdf.

Report actual and potential medication errors to ISMP Canada via the web at https://www.ismp-canada.org/err_report.htm or by calling 1-866-54-ISMPC. ISMP Canada guarantees confidentiality of information received and respects the reporter's wishes as to the level of detail included in publications.

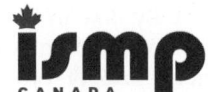

Institute for Safe Medication
Practices Canada
Institut pour l'utilisation sécuritaire
des médicaments du Canada

medications and specify in writing which medications are to be continued or discontinued with any status change, transfer, or discharge.

c. Patient transfer within or between facilities or health care provider teams

d. Discharge. (The latest medication list should be provided to the patient to take to the next health care provider, or this information should be otherwise forwarded to the health care provider; applicable confidentiality guidelines should be followed.)

Following are some applicable assessment and education tips regarding medication reconciliation:

1. Ask the patient open-ended questions and gradually move to yes–no questions to help determine specific medication information. (Details are important and sometimes even critical.)

2. Avoid the use of medical jargon unless it is clear that the patient understands and is comfortable with such language.

3. Prompt the patient to try to remember all applicable medications (e.g., patches, creams, eye drops, inhalers, professional samples, injections, natural health products). If the patient does provide a medication list, make a copy for the patient's chart.

4. Clarify unclear information to the extent possible (e.g., by talking with the home caregiver or the outpatient pharmacist who fills the patient's prescriptions, if needed).

5. Record the aforementioned information in the patient's chart as the first step in the medication reconciliation process.

6. Emphasize to the patient the importance of always maintaining a current and complete medication list and bringing it to each health care encounter (e.g., as a wallet card or other list). Many patients use their own computers for this. Also encourage patients to learn the names and current dosages of their medications.

OTHER ETHICAL ISSUES

Notification of Patients Regarding Errors

A landmark article published in the *Journal of Clinical Outcomes Management* in 2001 recognized the obligation of institutions and health care providers to provide full disclosure to patients when errors have occurred in their care. The article not only emphasized the ethical basis for this practice but also addressed the legal implications and was a starting point for understanding the issue of notification of patients about MEs. The Disclosure Working Group of the Canadian Patient Safety Institute (2011) recommended a just culture of disclosure. Apology legislation that has been introduced in eight Canadian provinces and one territory adds a legal component to meaningful apology and disclosure of a harmful event. The provinces and territory where this legislation exists provide statutory protection that any apology they make to a patient cannot be used against them in subsequent court proceedings as evidence to establish fault or liability. Critical to disclosure is honesty and transparency. Accreditation Canada includes disclosure in its Required Organizational Practice, which includes developing a formal, transparent organizational policy and process of disclosure to patients. This includes support for the patient, family, and health care worker. It is recommended that the term *error* be avoided in the context of disclosure because of the complex interplay of factors involved in patient safety incidents, as noted previously. The working group prefers the term *patient safety incident*. There are three types of patient safety incidents: (1) harmful incident (replaces preventable adverse incident) which results in harm to the patient; (2) near miss which did not reach the patient and results in no harm; and, (3) no-harm-incident which reaches the patient but no harm results. This terminology is an effort by the World Health Organization (2016) to standardize key concepts and to improve safety worldwide. Health care organizations offer needed financial support for reasonable expenses (e.g., travel expenses, temporary loss of wages) related to the disclosure process. As well, support is recommended for health care providers involved in the disclosure proceedings. The process of disclosure is outlined in the document available at http://www.patient safetyinstitute.ca/en/toolsResources/disclosure/ Documents/CPSI%20Canadian%20Disclosure%20 Guidelines.pdf.

Possible Consequences of Medication Errors for Nurses

The possible effects of MEs on patients range from no significant effect to permanent disability or even death in the most extreme cases. However, MEs may also affect health care providers, including nurses and student nurses, in a number of ways. An error that involves significant patient harm or death may take an emotional toll on the nurse involved in the error. Nurses may be named as defendants in malpractice litigation, with possibly serious financial consequences. In nursing, **negligence** is "conduct that does not meet a standard of care established by law" (Potter, Perry, Ross-Kerr et al., 2014, p. 9). It is characterized chiefly by inattention or thoughtlessness. Examples of negligent acts in nursing include MEs that result in injury, errors in instrument counts in surgical cases, and failure to monitor a client's condition adequately. **Malpractice** is improper or unethical conduct or unreasonable lack of skill that results in harm, and compensation may be sought. All malpractice involves negligence. Charges against health care workers are rare in Canada; however, as patients have become more knowledgeable about their rights, they are more likely to seek compensation for negligence.

Many nurses choose to carry personal malpractice insurance, also known as *professional liability protection*, although nurses working in publically funded institutional settings are usually covered by the institution's liability insurance policy. Nurses should obtain clear written documentation of any institutional coverage provided before deciding whether to carry individual malpractice insurance. The Canadian Nurses Protective Society (CNPS), established in 1988, is a not-for-profit society that offers legal advice, risk management services, legal assistance, and professional liability protection related to nursing practice to eligible nurses. These services are available to nurses who are members in a provincial or territorial professional organization or college (the sole exception is Quebec). Administrative responses to MEs vary from institution to institution. One possible response is a directive to the nurse involved to obtain continuing education or refresher training. Depending on the severity of the error, disciplinary action, including suspension or termination of employment, may also occur. However, hospitals have created a more proactive, open, and nonpunitive culture in the approach to MEs. Nurses who have violated regulations of the provincial or territorial standards of nursing practice may also be counselled or disciplined by the provincial or territorial regulatory bodies, which may suspend or permanently revoke their nursing licence. Student nurses are also held responsible and accountable for the quality of their clinical work. When in doubt about the correct course of action, students should consult with clinical instructors or more experienced staff nurses. If a student nurse realizes that an error has been committed, the student should notify the responsible clinical instruc-

tor immediately. The patient may require additional monitoring or medication, and the prescriber may also need to be notified. Although such events are preferably avoided, they can ultimately be useful, though stressful, learning experiences for the student nurse.

SUMMARY

The increasing complexity of nursing practice also increases the risk for MEs. Widely recognized and common causes of errors include misunderstanding of abbreviations, illegibility of prescriber handwriting, miscommunication during verbal or telephone orders, and confusing drug nomenclature. The structure of various organizational, educational, and sociological systems involved in health care delivery may also contribute directly or indirectly to the occurrence of MEs. Understanding these influences can help the nurse take proactive steps to improve these systems. Such actions can range from fostering improved communication with other health care team members, including students, to advocating politically for safer conditions for both patients and staff. The first priority when an error does occur is to protect the patient from further harm whenever possible. All errors should serve as red flags that warrant further reflection, detailed analysis, and future preventive actions on the part of nurses, other health care providers, and possibly even patients themselves.

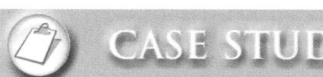

CASE STUDY

Preventing Medication Errors

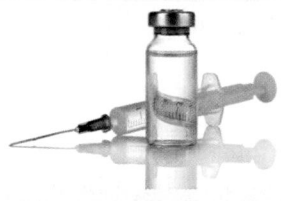

During your busy clinical day as a student nurse, the staff nurse assigned to your patient comes to you and says, "Would you like to give this injection? We have a 'now' order for octreotide acetate 200 mcg subcutaneously. I've already drawn it up; 200 mcg equals 2 mL. It needs to be given as soon as possible, so I drew it up to save time." She hands you a syringe that has 2 mL of a clear fluid in it, and the patient's medication administration record (MAR).

1. Should you give this medication "now," as ordered? Why or why not?

You decide to check the order that is handwritten on the MAR with the order written on the chart. The physician wrote, "Octreotide, 200 mcg now, SUBCUT, then 100 mcg every 8 hours as needed." Before you have a chance to find your instructor, the nurse returns and says, "Your instructor probably won't let you give the injection unless you can show the medication ampoules. Here are the ampoules I used to draw up the octreotide. Be quick— your patient needs it now!" You take the order, the MAR, the two ampoules, and the syringe to your instructor. Together, you read the order and then check the ampoules.

Each ampoule is marked "Sandostatin (octreotide acetate) 500 mcg/mL."

2. If the nurse drew up 2 mL from those two ampoules, how much octreotide acetate is in the syringe? How does that amount compare with the order?

The nurse is astonished when you point out that the ampoules read "500 mcg/mL." She goes into the automated medication dispenser and sees two identical boxes of Sandostatin® next to each other in the refrigerated section. One box is labelled "100 mcg/mL" and the other box is labelled "500 mcg/mL." She then realizes she chose an ampoule of the wrong strength of drug and drew up an incorrect dose.

3. What would have happened if you had given the injection?

4. What should be done at this point? What contributed to this potential ME, and how can it be prevented in the future?

Note: High-alert drugs include adrenal drugs (corticosteroids), analgesics (acetaminophen), anti-infectives and antibiotics, antihistamines, antineoplastics, asthma drugs, bronchodilators, heart drugs, electrolytes, vitamins, minerals, insulin, opioids, and sedatives.

For answers see http://evolve.elsevier.com/Canada/Lilley/pharmacology/.

KEY POINTS

❖ To prevent MEs from misinterpretation of the prescriber's orders, avoid abbreviations. MEs include giving the drug to the wrong patient, confusing sound-alike and look-alike drugs, administering the wrong drug or the wrong dose, giving the drug by the wrong route, or giving the drug at the wrong time.

❖ Measures to help prevent MEs include being prepared and knowledgeable and taking time always to triple-check for the right patient, drug, dosage, time, and route. It is also important for nurses always to be aware of the entire medication administration process and to take a system analysis approach to MEs and their prevention.

❖ Encourage patients to ask questions about their medications and to question any concern about the drug or any component of the medication administration process.

❖ Encourage patients to always carry drug allergy information on their persons and to keep a current list of medications in their wallets or purses and on their refrigerators. This list should include the drug's name, reason the drug is being used, usual dosage range and dosage prescribed, expected adverse effects and possible toxicity of the drug, and the prescriber's name and contact information.

❖ Report MEs. It is important to include in this documentation the assessment of the patient status before, during, and after the ME, as well as specific orders carried out in response to the error.

EXAMINATION REVIEW QUESTIONS

1. Which measures does the nurse keep in mind to reduce the risk of MEs?
   a. When questioning a drug order, keep in mind that the prescriber is correct.
   b. Be careful about questioning the drug order a board-certified physician has written for a patient.
   c. Always double-check the many drugs with sound-alike and look-alike names because of the high risk of error.
   d. If the drug route has not been specified, use the oral route.

2. During the medication administration process, it is important that the nurse remembers which guideline?
   a. When in doubt about a drug, ask a colleague about it before giving the drug.
   b. Ask what the patient knows about the drug before giving it.
   c. When giving a new drug, be sure to read about it after giving it.
   d. If a patient expresses a concern about a drug, stop, listen, and investigate the concerns.

3. If a student nurse realizes that a drug error has been made, the instructor should remind the student of what concept?
   a. The student bears no legal responsibility when giving medications.
   b. The major legal responsibility lies with the health care institution at which the student is placed for nursing practice experience.
   c. The major legal responsibility for drug errors lies with the faculty members.
   d. Once the student has committed a ME, the responsibility is to the patient and to being honest and accountable.

4. The nurse is giving medications to a newly admitted patient who is to receive nothing by mouth (NPO status) and finds an order written as follows: "Digoxin, 250 mcg stat." Which action is appropriate?
   a. Give the medication immediately (stat) by mouth because the patient has no intravenous (IV) access at this time.
   b. Clarify the order with the prescribing physician before giving the drug.
   c. Ask the charge nurse what route the physician meant to use.
   d. Start an IV line and then give the medication IV so that it will work faster, because the patient's status is NPO at this time.

5. The nurse is reviewing medication orders. Which digoxin dose is written correctly?
   a. digoxin .25 mg
   b. digoxin .250 mg
   c. digoxin 0.250 mg
   d. digoxin 0.25 mg

6. The nurse is administering medications. Examples of high-alert medications include (Select all that apply):
   a. Insulins
   b. Antibiotics
   c. Opiates
   d. Anticoagulants
   e. Potassium chloride for injection

7. Convert 250 micrograms to milligrams. Be sure to depict the number correctly according to the guidelines for decimals and zeroes.

CRITICAL THINKING ACTIVITIES

1. The health care provider has ordered a stat IV vancomycin infusion, but when the bag comes up from the pharmacy, the nurse notices that the dose is incorrect. It takes 2 hours for the pharmacy to send up an IV bag with the correct dose. While checking the medication, the nurse checks the medication rights and notes that it has been 2 hours since it was ordered stat. What are the priority actions of the nurse, if anything, before giving this medication?

2. Just after the nurse administers an oral antihypertensive drug, the patient asks, "Wasn't that supposed to be a half-tablet? I just took the whole tablet!" The nurse realizes that the patient was given twice the ordered amount; the order was for 25 mg, a half-tablet, and the entire 50-mg tablet was given. At this time, what would the nurse need to say to the patient? What are the nurse's priority actions?

3. The nurse is reviewing the orders on a newly admitted patient and reads this order: "Humalog insulin, 4 units daily." What problems, if any, would the nurse identify in this order?

For answers see http://evolve.elsevier.com/Canada/Lilley/pharmacology/.

CHAPTER 7

Patient Education and Drug Therapy

Objectives

After reading this chapter, the successful student will be able to do the following:

1. Discuss the importance of patient education in the safe and efficient administration of drugs (e.g., prescription drugs, over-the-counter drugs, natural health products).

2. Summarize the various teaching and learning principles appropriate to patient education and drug therapy across the lifespan as applicable to any health care setting.

3. Identify the impact of the various developmental phases (as described by Erikson) on patient education as it relates to drug therapy.

4. Develop a complete patient education plan as part of a comprehensive collaborative plan of care for drug therapy for the adult patient.

e-Learning Activities

Website
(http://evolve.elsevier.com/Canada/Lilley/pharmacology/)

evolve

- Answer Key—Textbook Case Studies
- Answer Key—Critical Thinking Activities
- Chapter Summaries—Printable
- Review Questions for Exam Preparation
- Unfolding Case Studies

Key Terms

Affective domain The most intangible domain of the learning process. It involves affective behaviour, which is conduct that expresses feelings, needs, beliefs, values, and opinions; the feeling domain. (p. 106)

Cognitive domain The domain involved in the learning and storage of basic knowledge. It is the thinking portion of the learning process and incorporates a person's previous experiences and perceptions; the learning or thinking domain. (p. 106)

Health literacy The degree to which individuals have the capacity to obtain and then process and understand basic health information and services needed to make appropriate health decisions (p. 106)

Learning The acquisition of knowledge or skill that involves a change in behaviour. (p. 106)

Psychomotor domain The domain involved in the learning of a new procedure or skill; often called the *doing domain*. (p. 106)

Teaching A system of directed and deliberate actions intended to induce learning. (p. 106)

OVERVIEW

Given the constant change in today's health care climate and increased consumer awareness, the role of the nurse as an educator continues to increase and remains a significant part of patient care, both in and out of the hospital environment. Patient education is essential in any health care setting and is a critical component of quality and safe health care. Patient education is a necessary nursing practice standard that meaningfully impacts a patient's health and quality of life. Without patient education, the highest quality and safest of care cannot be provided. Patient education is a process, much like the nursing process; it provides patients with a framework of knowledge that assists in the learning of healthy behaviours and assimilation of these behaviours into a lifestyle. Patient education is also crucial for assisting patients, family, significant others, and caregivers to adapt to illness, prevent illness, maintain wellness, and provide self-care. Being well informed provides patients with the opportunity to be more actively involved participants and advocates in their own health care needs. However, successful outcomes are often dictated by the willingness and capacity of patients to self-manage their health behaviours. The challenge is to develop strategies to engage patients in their own health care (Conn, 2015).

Patient education may be one of the more satisfying aspects of nursing care because it is essential to improved health outcomes. In fact, in the current era of increasing acuteness of patient conditions and the need to decrease length of stays in hospitals, patient education and family teaching become even more essential to effectively and efficiently meet outcome criteria. Patient education has also been identified as a valued and satisfying activity for the professional nurse as the nurse develops a therapeutic relationship and the trust of the patient, caregiver, and family. Nurses may often cite the lack of time and resources to adequately teach patients; however, while there may not always be optimum time for teaching, nurses need to consider how they can most effectively and efficiently teach in the time available.

Contributing to the effectiveness of patient education is an understanding of and attention to the three domains of learning: the cognitive, affective, and psychomotor domains. It is recommended that one or a combination of these domains be addressed in any patient educational session. The **cognitive domain** refers to the level at which basic knowledge is learned and stored. It is the thinking portion of the learning process and incorporates a person's previous experiences and perceptions. Previous experiences with health and wellness influence the learning of new materials, and prior knowledge and experience can serve as the foundation for adding new concepts. Thus, the learning process begins with identifying the experiences the person has had with the subject matter or content. However, it is important to remember that thinking involves more than the delivery of new information because a patient must build relationships between prior and new experiences to formulate new meanings. At a higher level in the thinking process, the new information is used to question something that is uncertain, recognize when to seek additional information, and make decisions during real-life situations.

The **affective domain** is the most intangible component of the learning process. Affective behaviour is conduct that expresses feelings, needs, beliefs, values, and opinions. It is well known that individuals view events from different perspectives and often choose to internalize feelings rather than express them. Nurses must be willing to approach patients in a nonjudgemental manner, listen to their concerns, recognize the nonverbal messages being communicated, and assess patient needs with an open mind. Being successful in gaining the trust and confidence of patients and family members may have a powerful effect on their attitudes and thus on the learning process.

The **psychomotor domain** involves the learning of a new procedure or skill and is often called the *doing domain*. Learning is generally accomplished by demonstration of the procedure or task using a step-by-step approach, with return demonstrations by the learner to verify that the procedure or skill has been mastered. Using a teaching approach that engages these domains—whether one, two, or a combination of all three—certainly adds to the quality and effectiveness of patient education sessions and subsequent learning.

The result of effective patient education is learning. **Learning** is defined as a change in behaviour, and **teaching** as a sharing of knowledge. Although you may never be certain that patients will take medications as prescribed, you may carefully assess, plan, implement, and evaluate the teaching you provide to help maximize outcome criteria. Just like the nursing process, the medication administration process and the teaching–learning process provide systematic frameworks for professional nursing practice. The remainder of this chapter provides a brief look at patient education as related to drug therapy.

ASSESSMENT OF LEARNING NEEDS RELATED TO DRUG THERAPY

The patient education process is similar to the nursing process. An important facet of the patient education process is a thorough assessment of learning needs. This assessment should be completed before patients begin any form of drug therapy. As related to patient education and drug therapy, a thorough assessment includes gathering subjective and objective data about the following:

- Adaptation to any illnesses
- Age
- Barriers to learning (Box 7-1)
- Cognitive abilities
- Coping mechanisms
- Cultural background (see Ethnocultural Implications: Patient Education)
- Developmental status for age group, with attention to cognitive and mental processing abilities
- Education level, including highest grade level completed and literacy level
- Emotional status
- Environment at home and at work
- Folk medicine, home remedies, or use of alternative/complementary therapies (e.g., physiotherapy, chiropractic therapy, osteopathic medicine, meditation, yoga, aromatherapy)
- Family relationships
- Financial status
- **Health literacy** (see Box 7-2)
- Psychosocial growth and developmental level according to Erikson's stages (see Box 7-3)

BOX 7-1   Strategies to Enhance Patient Education and Reduce Barriers to Learning

- Work with available educational resources in nursing and pharmacy to collect or order and distribute materials about drug therapy. Make sure that written materials are available to all individuals and are prepared at a reading level that is most representative of the geographical area, such as a Grade 8 reading level. Most acute care and other health care facilities have electronic resources, so that printing educational materials is easy.
- Be sure that written and verbal instructions are available in the language most commonly spoken. Identify resources within the facility and in the community that can provide assistance with translation, such as nurses or other health care providers who are proficient in languages other than one of the official languages. Have the information available so that education is carried out in a timely and effective manner.
- Perform a cultural assessment that includes questions about level of education, learning experiences, past and present successes of therapies and medication regimens, language(s) spoken, core beliefs, value system, meaning of health and illness, perceived cause of illness, family roles, social organization, and health practices or lack thereof.
- Make sure that written materials are available on the most commonly used medications and that all materials are updated annually to ensure that information is current.

- Have available information for patients on how they can prevent medication errors. The Institute for Safe Medication Practices Canada offers informative pamphlets on the patient's role in preventing medication errors as well as web-based resources such as alerts for consumers with the proper citation.
- Work collaboratively in the health care setting, inpatient and outpatient, to develop a listing of medications that may be considered error prone, such as cardiac drugs, chemotherapeutic drugs, low-molecular-weight heparin sodium, digoxin, metered-dose inhaled drugs, and acetaminophen. Lack of time for patient education is often a concern for nurses, but efforts should be undertaken to make materials available and review these with patients and those involved in their care. Use all available resources, such as videos, verbal instructions, pictures, and other health care providers.
- Educate the health care consumer about the accuracy or quality of online information and provide suggested reliable sites.
- For the adolescent, be sure to provide clear and simple directions for each medication, including clarification of information that may well be misinterpreted. For example, adolescent girls may have the false idea that oral contraceptives prevent them from contracting sexually transmitted diseases.

BOX 7-2   A Brief Look at Health Literacy

- In 2007, the Canadian Council on Learning estimated that 60% of adult Canadians have difficulty obtaining, understanding, and acting upon health information and services and consequently making appropriate decisions about their own health concerns. As related to patient education, assessing and addressing health literacy is only one aspect, though an important aspect, of health communication and the cognitive domain of learning.
- Studies have shown that poor health literacy is associated with issues of nonadherence to treatment regimens and disease complications as well as difficulty accessing health care, contributing to poor health as well as higher health care costs (Remshardt, 2011; Roter, Rude, & Comings, 1998).
- Poor health literacy has been associated with less education, lower socioeconomic status, decrease in

sensorial abilities, and multiple disease processes, so assessment of these factors is important to individualized patient education.
- Other areas to assess related to health literacy include reading level, ability to follow directions/instructions, as well as ability to manage everyday living activities such as self-care, grocery shopping, and meal preparation.
- Assessment of health literacy must be done with much sensitivity and relates not only to education but also to levels of stress or difficulty coping with a new diagnosis or process and new and complex information (i.e., patients with higher levels of education but who are stressed and unable to process information because of a disturbing diagnosis).

- Health beliefs, including beliefs about health, wellness, and illness
- Information the patient understands about past and present medical condition, medical therapy, and medications

- Language(s) spoken
- Level of knowledge about any medication(s) being taken
- Limitations (physical, psychological, cognitive, and motor)

BOX 7-3 Erikson's Stages of Development

Infancy (birth to 1 year of age): Trust versus mistrust. Infant learns to trust self, others, and the environment; learns to love and be loved.

Toddlerhood (1 to 3 years of age): Autonomy versus shame and doubt. Toddler learns independence; learns to master the physical environment and maintain self-esteem.

Preschool age (3 to 6 years of age): Initiative versus guilt. Preschooler learns basic problem solving; develops conscience and sexual identity; initiates activities as well as imitates.

School age (6 to 12 years of age): Industry versus inferiority. School-age child learns to do things well; develops a sense of self-worth.

Adolescence (12 to 18 years of age): Identity versus role confusion. Adolescent integrates many roles into self-identity through imitation of role models and peer pressure.

Young adulthood (18 to 45 years of age): Intimacy versus isolation. Young adult establishes deep and lasting relationships; learns to make commitment as spouse, parent, or partner.

Middle adulthood (45 to 65 years of age): Generativity versus stagnation. Adult learns commitment to community and world; is productive in career, family, and civic interests.

Older adulthood (over 65 years of age): Integrity versus despair. Older adult appreciates life role and status; deals with loss and prepares for death.

 # ETHNOCULTURAL IMPLICATIONS

Patient Education

Every health care encounter provides an opportunity to have a positive effect on patient health. Health care providers can maximize this potential by learning more about patients' cultures so they can respond in a respectful manner and be responsive to the preferences of each patient, with the goal of an individualized approach to nursing care. Culture is dynamic and multidimensional and may include gender, religion, sexual orientation, profession, values and beliefs, age, socioeconomic status, disability, ethnicity, and race. For example, with a Somali patient, aspects of nursing care need to be approached in a sensitive manner with strong consideration for the family, communication needs, and religion. The majority of Somalis are Sunni Muslims. Islamic religion is a significant part of Somali life. Islamic religious teachings provide meaning for living, dying, family life, child-rearing, and the maintenance of health. In Islam, prayer is performed five times a day; before prayer, the hands, face, and feet are washed. Islam forbids the eating of pork, drinking alcohol, or touching (or being near) dogs. Attitudes, social customs, and gender roles in Somalia are based primarily on Islamic tradition. Married Somali women cover their bodies and

veil their faces in a hijab. Elders are treated with respect. Health is considered a gift from Allah (God), so it is an expectation to maintain health. Taking preventative medications is not within the traditional Somali view. Illness prevention occurs because of the use of prayer and living a life according to Islam. Traditionally, men and women do not touch members of the opposite sex, except for close family members.

Somalis believe that spirits reside within each individual. When the spirits become angry, illnesses such as fever, headache, dizziness, and weakness can result. The cure involves a healing ceremony, including reading from the Koran, eating special foods, and burning incense. It is important to remember that the beliefs identified above cannot be generalized to all persons of Somali culture. To help meet the needs of Somali patients, it is important for the nurse to have a basic understanding, but it is more important to fully assess and include their needs and beliefs in their care.

Source: Based on Lewis, T. (2014). Somali cultural profile. Retrieved from http://ethnomed.org/culture/somali/somali-cultural-profile

- Medications currently taken (including OTC drugs, prescription drugs, and natural health products)
- Misinformation about drug therapy
- Mobility and motor skills
- Motivation
- Nutritional status
- Past and present health behaviours
- Past and present experience with drug regimens and other forms of therapy, including levels of adherence
- Race or ethnicity
- Religion or religious beliefs
- Self-care ability

- Sensory status
- Social support

During the assessment of learning needs, be astutely aware of the patient's verbal and nonverbal communication. Often a patient will not divulge true feelings to the nurse as the environment may not be conducive to a private conversation. Although it might be challenging to do so, the nurse should attempt to find a private area for the discussion. A seeming discrepancy is an indication that the patient's emotional or physical state may need to be further assessed in relation to readiness and motivation for learning for learning. Use of open-ended questions is encouraged, because they stimulate more discussion and greater clarification from the patient than closed-ended questions, which require only a "yes" or "no" answer. Ask questions about the following: (1) What do the patient and family know about the purpose, dose, and adverse effects of the medications? (2) Can the patient demonstrate how the treatments are done at home?, and (3) How confident are the patient and the family that the treatments can be carried out at home? Assess level of anxiety, because mild levels of anxiety have been identified as motivating, whereas moderate to severe levels may be obstacles. In addition, if there are physical needs that are not being met, such as relief from pain, vomiting, or other physical distress, these needs become obstacles to learning and must be managed appropriately before any patient teaching occurs.

NURSING DIAGNOSES RELATED TO LEARNING NEEDS AND DRUG THERAPY

Some of the most commonly used nursing diagnoses related to patient education and drug therapy are as follows:

- Deficient knowledge
- Readiness for enhanced knowledge
- Falls, risk for
- Ineffective self-health management
- Readiness for enhanced health management
- Impaired memory
- Injury, risk for
- Nonadherence
- Readiness for enhanced communication
- Readiness for enhanced power
- Readiness for enhanced decision making
- Sleep deprivation

As an example of how nursing diagnoses related to patient education are derived, the nursing diagnosis of *deficient knowledge* refers to a situation in which the patient, caregiver, or significant other has a limited knowledge base or skills with regard to the medication or medication regimen. A nursing diagnosis of *deficient knowledge* develops out of objective or subjective data showing that there is limited understanding, no understanding, or misunderstanding of the medication and its action, indications, adverse reactions, toxic effects, drug–drug or drug–food interactions, cautions, and contraindications. This diagnosis may also reflect decreased cognitive ability or impaired motor skill needed to perform self-medication. Deficient knowledge differs from nonadherence; nonadherence is when the patient does not take the medication as prescribed or at all—in other words, the patient does not adhere with the instructions given about the medication. Nonadherence is usually a patient's choice. A nursing diagnosis of *nonadherence* is made when data collected from the patient show that the condition or symptoms for which the patient is taking the medication have recurred or were never resolved because the patient did not take the medication per the prescriber's orders or did not take it at all. It is critical to assess factors to determine the cause of the nonadherance (e.g., lack of ability of the parent, family, or caregiver to administer the medication or other physical, emotional, or socioeconomic factors). These factors are associated with the nursing diagnosis of ineffective health maintenance and provide a patient-centred approach to the plan of care.

PLANNING RELATED TO LEARNING NEEDS AND DRUG THERAPY

The planning phase of the teaching and learning process occurs as soon as a learning need has been assessed and then identified in the patient, family, or caregiver. With mutual understanding, the nurse and patient identify goals and outcome criteria that are associated with the identified nursing diagnosis and are able to relate them to the specific medication the patient is taking. The following is an example of a measurable goal with an outcome criterion related to a nursing diagnosis of *readiness for enhanced knowledge* for a patient who is self-administering an oral antihyperglycemic drug and has many questions about the medication therapy. *Sample goal:* The patient safely self-administers the prescribed oral antihyperglycemic drug within a given time frame. *Sample outcome criterion:* The patient remains without signs or symptoms of overmedication while taking an oral antihyperglycemic drug, such as hypoglycemia with tachycardia, palpitations, diaphoresis, hunger, and fatigue. When drug therapy goals and outcome criteria are developed, appropriate time frames for meeting outcome criteria should also be identified (see Chapter 1 for more information on the nursing process). In addition, goals and outcome criteria need to be realistic, based on patient needs, stated in patient terms, and include behaviours that are measurable, such as list, identify, demonstrate, self-administer, state, describe, and discuss.

IMPLEMENTATION RELATED TO DRUG THERAPY

After the nurse has completed the assessment phase, identified nursing diagnoses, and created a plan of care, the implementation phase of the teaching–learning process begins. Nurses have a responsibility to address patients' needs but have an equal responsibility to teach. Providing "care" means ensuring that patients are fully educated about their condition and their proposed treatments so that they are able to make informed decisions about them. This phase includes conveying specific information about the medication to the patient, family, or caregiver. Teaching–learning sessions must

BOX 7-4 General Teaching and Learning Principles

- Make learning patient-centred and individualized to each patient's needs, including the patient's learning needs. This includes assessment of the patient's ethnocultural beliefs, educational level, previous experience with medications, level of growth and development (to best select a teaching–learning strategy), age, gender, family support system, resources, preferred learning style, and level of sophistication with health care and health care treatment.
- Assess the patient's motivation and readiness to learn.
- Assess the patient's ability to use and interpret label information on medication containers.
- It is estimated that 42% of Canadian adults between the ages of 16 to 65 have low literacy skills. Fifteen percent have serious problems reading printed materials and 27% have only simple reading skills. Less than 20% of individuals with the lowest literate skills are employed (Canadian Literacy and Learning Network, 2015). Sixty percent of immigrants have low literacy, compared with 37% of native-born Canadians (Life Literacy Canada, 2015). It is estimated that between 55 and 60% of adults and 88% of seniors over the age of 65 in Canada are not health literate (Public Health Agency of Canada, 2014). Indigenous people are also at risk for poor health literacy, many of whom have less than a Grade 9 education (Canadian Nurses Association, 2015). It is therefore important to ensure that that the educational strategies and materials are at a level the patient is able to understand, while taking care not to embarrass the patient.
- Patients who are illiterate still need to be instructed on safe medication administration; use pictures, demonstrations, and return demonstrations to emphasize instructions.
- Consider, assess, and appreciate language and ethnicity during patient teaching. Make every effort to educate non–English-speaking patients in their native languages. Ideally, the patient should be instructed by a health professional familiar with the patient's clinical situation who also speaks the patient's native language. At the least, provide the patient with detailed written instructions in the patient's native language.
- Assess the family support system for adequate patient teaching. Family living arrangements, financial status, resources, communication patterns, the roles of family members, and the power and authority of different family members should always be considered.
- Make the teaching–learning session simple, easy, fun, thorough, effective, and not monotonous. Make it applicable to daily life, and schedule it at a time when the patient is ready to learn. Avoid providing extraneous information that may be confusing or overwhelming to the patient.
- Remember that learning occurs best with repetition and periods of demonstration and with the use of audiovisuals and other educational aids.
- Patient teaching must focus on the various processes in the cognitive, affective, or psychomotor domains (see earlier discussion).
- Consult online resources for help in obtaining the most up-to-date and accurate patient teaching materials and information.
- Technology advances have increased the variety of methods available for teaching. For example, recorded information by telephone, telephone help-lines, videos, podcasts, websites, text messaging, webinars, and social networking are some of the options for creative approaches to teaching. In addition, there are various language translator applications such as Google Translate. Smart phone and tablet applications are also essential tools to aid in patient education.

incorporate clear, simple, concise written instructions (Box 7-4); oral instructions; and written pamphlets, pictures, videos, or any other learning aids that will help ensure patient learning. The nurse may have to conduct several brief teaching–learning sessions with multiple strategies, depending on the needs of the patient. Several changes related to the growth and aging of patients (although they may also apply to other age groups experiencing chronic diseases) may affect teaching–learning. Age-associated changes are most pronounced in people of advanced age—85 years or older. Table 7-1 lists educational strategies for accommodating these changes in a plan of care. The nurse may also need to identify aids to help the patient in the safe administration of medications at home, such as the use of medication day and time calendars, pill reminder stickers, daily medication containers with alarms, weekly pill containers with separate compartments for different dosing times for each day of the week, or a method of documenting doses taken to avoid overdosage or omission of doses. Many pharmacies now package a week's supply of pills, with a blister pack for each time of day. Medical technology companies are developing smart technology systems to assist patients to take and keep track of medications. For example, an ingestible sensor that when swallowed is activated by stomach fluids, initiating a heartbeatlike signal picked up by a patch worn on the chest. The patch records data from the sensor such as that the patient has ingested the medication and additional information such as heart rate. There are also patient-tracking apps that remind patients to take their medications. Certainly, there is a need for a large portfolio of technologies, from simple to complex, in order to meet the needs of all patients.

Special issues arise when the patient speaks limited or no English. Communicate with the patient in the patient's native language, if at all possible. If the nurse is not able to speak the patient's native language, including sign language, a translator needs to be made available to prevent communication problems, minimize errors, and

TABLE 7-1	
Strategies to Educate Older Adults With Age-Related Changes	
Changes Related to Aging	**Educational Strategy**

IMPAIRED MEMORY

Slowed cognitive functioning	Slow the pace of the presentation and attend to verbal and nonverbal patient cues to verify understanding.
Decreased short-term memory	Provide smaller amounts of information at one time. Repeat information frequently. Provide written instructions for home use.
Decreased ability to think abstractly	Use examples to illustrate information. Use a variety of methods, such as audiovisuals, props, videos, large-print materials, materials with vivid colours, return demonstrations, and practice sessions.
Decreased ability to concentrate. Increased reaction time (slower to respond)	Decrease external stimuli as much as possible. Always allow sufficient time and be patient. Allow more time for feedback.

ALTERED SENSORY PERCEPTION

Hearing

Diminished hearing	Perform a baseline hearing assessment. Use tone- and volume-controlled teaching aids; use bright, large-print material to reinforce learning.
Decreased ability to distinguish sounds (e.g., words beginning with *S, Z, T, D, F,* and *G*)	Face the patient. Speak distinctly and slowly, and articulate carefully.
Decreased conduction of sound	Sit on the side of the learner's "best" ear, but always make sure the patient can see your face as you speak.
Loss of ability to hear high-frequency sounds	Do not shout; speak in a normal voice but lower voice pitch.
Partial to complete loss of hearing	Face the patient so that lip reading is possible. Use visual aids to reinforce verbal instruction. Reinforce teaching with easy-to-read materials. Provide teaching in a room with no distractions and extraneous noise. If the patient uses sign language to communicate, find a sign language interpreter. If the patient uses a hearing aid(s), make sure the aid is/are in place and that batteries are functioning. Use community resources for the hearing impaired.

Vision

Decreased visual acuity	Ensure that the patient's glasses are clean and in place and that the prescription is current.
Decreased ability to read fine detail	Use large-print, clear, brightly coloured material.
Decreased ability to discriminate among blue, violet, and green: tendency for all colours to fade, with red fading the least	Use high-contrast materials, such as black on white. Avoid the use of blue, violet, and green in type or graphics; use red instead.
Thickening and yellowing of the lenses of the eyes, with decreased accommodation	Use nonglare lighting and avoid contrasts of light (e.g., darkened room with single light). Use additional lighting and avoid harsh lights, direct sunlight, and glossy paper.
Decreased depth perception	Adjust teaching to allow for the use of touch to gauge depth.
Decreased peripheral vision	Keep all teaching materials within the patient's visual field.

Touch and Vibration

Decreased sense of touch	Allow more time for the teaching of psychomotor skills, the number of repetitions, and the number of return demonstrations.
Decreased sense of vibration	Teach patient to palpate more prominent pulse sites (e.g., carotid and radial arteries).

Modified from Mullen, E. (2013). Health literacy challenges in the adult population. *Nursing Forum, 48*(4), 248–255; Speros, C. I. (2009). More than words: Promoting health literacy in older adults. *The Online Journal of Issues in Nursing, 14*(3). doi: 10.3912/OJIN.Vol14No03Man05

help boost the patient's level of trust and understanding. In practice, this translator may be another nurse or health care provider; a nonprofessional member of the health care team; or a layperson, family member, adult friend, or religious leader or associate. However, it is best to avoid using family members as translators if possible because of issues with bias and misinterpretation, as well as potential confidentiality issues. It is important to remember that some of these individuals may not be competent in or comfortable with communicating technical clinical information, and other resources must be used if this is the case. Canada has experienced a rapid growth in minority populations and our health care system has seen a staggering increase in the percentage of non–English-speaking patients. Demographic changes will be significant, with the numbers of visible minority groups doubling by 2031. This growth in cultural diversity will continue to demand that nursing and related health care professions provide patient education materials in English and Southeast Asian and East Asian languages (as well as other prominent languages). Publications provided for non–English-speaking patients may enable the nurse to convey a sufficient amount of information in the patient's language to help effectively educate the patient and also allow the nurse to share materials with family members and caregivers for their use. Companies now also publish a variety of patient education materials for the discharge process in both English and other languages.

Non–English-speaking patients tend to notice and appreciate their health care providers' efforts to speak their language and will often help teach them new words or phrases, if there is enthusiasm and interest. This experience may lead to significantly greater rapport, put patients at ease, and show respect for their culture or race/ethnicity. Obtaining and keeping available a foreign language dictionary for languages that are widely spoken in that geographical area may be helpful. Keeping notes about newly learned words, phrases, or sentences may be helpful, too. Even if the professional does not use the correct verb tenses, communication with the patient may often be sufficient to meet the immediate need. As one begins to learn a foreign language, a major challenge may be to speak with a patient over the telephone. The important goal is to try to increase one's *listening* speed to match the *speaking* speed of the patient. With effort, this can be accomplished. If one can grasp even a few words of what the patient is saying, one may be able, with continued conversation with the patient, to determine and respond to the patient's needs. However, be aware that patients who are native English speakers may also have challenges learning about their medications and treatment regimens because of learning deficits or difficulties, hearing and speech deficits, lack of education, or minimal previous exposure to treatment regimens and medication use.

The teaching of manual skills for specific medication administration is also part of the teaching–learning session. Sufficient time must be allowed for the patient to become familiar with any equipment and to perform several return demonstrations to the nurse or another health care provider. Teaching and learning needs will vary from patient to patient. Make every effort to include family members, significant others, or caregivers in the teaching sessions for reinforcement purposes. Audiovisual aids may be incorporated and should be based on findings from the learning needs and nursing assessment. One online resource for information about medications is the Pharmasave medication library (http://www.pharmasave.com/default/0/medications.aspx), which

provides information for the public. Another good resource is the *Compendium of Pharmaceuticals and Specialties: The Canadian Drug Reference for Health Professionals*, which has an Information for the Patient component written in lay language that is easier for patients to understand yet provides helpful advice and how-to information for patients on many drugs. This section is available only in the e-CPS. This type of resource may be helpful to the patient when seeking information about a medication (e.g., purpose, adverse effects, method of administration, drug interactions) and helpful to the nurse in developing a patient teaching plan. Create a safe, nonthreatening, nondistracting environment for learning needs, and be open and receptive to the patient's questions. The following strategies may help ensure an effective teaching–learning session:

- Begin the teaching–learning process upon the patient's admission to the health care setting (see the Legal and Ethical Principles box).
- Individualize the teaching session to the patient.
- Provide positive rewards or reinforcement for accurate return demonstration of a procedure, technique, or skill during the teaching session (e.g., a sticker or badge for a child).
- Complete a medication calendar that includes the names of the drugs to be taken along with the dosage and frequency. Allow the patient to see what the medications look like for future reference.
- Use audiovisual aids.
- Involve family members or significant others in the teaching session, as deemed appropriate.
- Keep the teaching on a level that is most meaningful to the given patient; general research on reading skills has shown that written materials must be written at a Grade 8 reading level.

Box 7-4 lists some general teaching and learning principles to consider in providing patient education.

Upon completion of any teaching–learning process or patient education session, complete the documentation and include notes about the content provided, strategies used, and patient response to the teaching session and an overall evaluation of learning. Because of the significance of patient education related to drug therapy and the nursing process, this textbook integrates patient education into each chapter in the implementation phase of the nursing process. In addition, a Patient Teaching Tips section is included at the end of most chapters.

EVALUATION OF PATIENT LEARNING RELATED TO DRUG THERAPY

Evaluation of patient learning is a critical component of safe and effective drug administration. To verify the success—or lack of success—of patient education, ask specific questions related to patient outcomes and request that the patient repeat information or give a return demonstration of skills. The patient's behaviour, such as adherence to the schedule for medication

LEGAL & ETHICAL PRINCIPLES

Discharge Teaching

The safest practices for discharge teaching include the following:

- Always follow the health care facility's policy on discharge teaching, focusing on how much information to impart to the patient.
- Do not assume that any patient has received adequate teaching before interacting with you.
- Always begin discharge teaching as soon as possible when the patient is ready.
- Minimize any distractions during the teaching session.
- Evaluate any teaching of the patient and significant others by having the individuals repeat the instructions you have given them.
- Contact the institution's social service department or the discharge planner if there are any concerns regarding the learning capacity of the patient.
- Document what you taught, who was present with the patient during the teaching, what specific written instructions were given, what the responses of the patient and significant other or caregiver were, and what your nursing actions were, such as specific demonstrations or referrals to community resources.

- Document teaching and learning strategies, such as videotapes and pamphlets.
- Case managers need to make sure patients have a follow-up phone call and the name and number of someone to contact if they have questions, can't get their medication, or have symptoms.
- (http://www.ahcmedia.com/articles/135610-work-with-nursing-to-make-sure-patients-understand-the-discharge-plan)

Sources: Modified from the U.S. Pharmacopeia Safe Medication Use Expert Committee Meeting, Rockville, MD, May 2003. http://www.usp.org; https://www.cmpa-acpm.ca/serve/docs/ela/goodpracticesguide/pages/communication/Informed_Discharge/informed_discharge-e.html; Okoniewska, B., Santana, M. J., Groshaus, H., et al. (2015). Barriers to discharge in an acute care medical teaching unit: A qualitative analysis of health providers' perceptions. *Journal of Multidisciplinary Healthcare, 8*: 83–89. doi: 10.2147/JMDH.S72633; https://www.ismp-canada.org/download/MedRec/BPMDP_Patient_Interview_Guide.pdf; http://www.nursingcenter.com/CEArticle?an=00152193-201505000-00012.

CASE STUDY

Patient Education and Anticoagulant Therapy

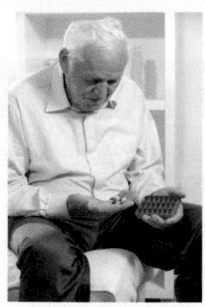

Martin, an 82-year-old retired civil servant, has developed atrial fibrillation. As part of his medical therapy, he is started on the oral anticoagulant warfarin sodium (Coumadin®). His wife reports that he has some trouble hearing yet refuses to consider getting hearing aids. In addition, this is his first illness and his wife states that he has "always hated taking medications. He's read about herbs and folk healing and would rather try natural therapy." The nurse is planning education about oral anticoagulant therapy, and Martin says that he'll

"give it a try" for now, but he "knows nothing about this drug."

1. What will the nurse assess, including possible barriers to learning, before teaching?
2. Formulate an education-related nursing diagnosis for this patient based on the information given above. In addition, provide a goal and one example of an outcome criterion for the nursing diagnosis.
3. What education strategies will the nurse plan to use, considering any age-related changes the patient may have?

For answers see http://evolve.elsevier.com/Canada/Lilley/pharmacology/.

administration with few or no complications, is one key to determining whether or not teaching was successful and learning occurred. If a patient's behaviour is characteristic of nonadherence or an inadequate level of learning, develop, implement, and evaluate a new plan of teaching.

SUMMARY

Patient education is a critical part of patient care, and patient education about medication administration, therapies, or regimens is no exception. From the time of

initial contact with the patient and throughout the time the nurse works with the patient, he or she is entitled to all information about medications prescribed as well as other aspects of patient care.

Evaluation of patient learning and adherence with the medication regimen remains a continuous process: be willing to listen to the patient about any aspects of his or her drug therapy. Professional nurses are teachers and serve as patient advocates and thus have a responsibility to facilitate learning for patients, families, significant others, and caregivers. Accurate assessment of learning needs and readiness to learn always requires a look at the whole patient, including cultural values, health practices, and literacy issues. Every effort needs to be made to see that the patient learns effectively to ensure successful outcomes with regard to drug therapy—and all parts of the patient's health care.

It is important to consult resources mentioned earlier, as well as the Institute for Safe Medication Practices Canada (ISMP) (at http://www.ismp-canada.org/). ISMP Canada provides nurses with a wealth of information related to patient education, safety, and prevention of medication errors. As a nonprofit organization, this institute works closely with nurses, prescribers, regulatory agencies, and professional organizations to provide education about medication errors and their prevention, and is a premier resource in all matters pertaining to safe medication practices in health care organizations.

Other resources available are medication checks. For example in Ontario, any Ontario resident with a chronic condition and taking three or more prescription medications, or anyone living with type 1 or type 2 diabetes, may qualify for a MedsCheck service. Such a service provides a 20- to 30-minute, one-to-one meeting with a community pharmacist to ensure that medications are being taken safely and appropriately. A similar program is available in New Brunswick, called PharmaCheck.

PATIENT TEACHING TIPS

❖ Teaching needs to focus on the cognitive, affective, or psychomotor domain or a combination of all three. The cognitive domain may involve recall for synthesis of facts, with the affective domain involving behaviours such as responding, valuing, and organizing. The psychomotor domain includes teaching someone how to perform a procedure.

❖ Realistic patient teaching goals and outcome criteria must be established with the involvement of the patient, caregiver, or significant other.

❖ Keep patient teaching on a level that is most meaningful to the individual. Most research indicates that reading materials need to be written at a Grade 8 reading level but adjusted accordingly to patient assessment.

❖ Follow teaching and learning principles when developing and implementing patient education.

❖ Be sure to control the environmental factors, such as lighting, noise, privacy, and odours. Provide dignified care while preparing the patient for teaching, and respect personal space. If there are distractions, such as television, radio, cellphone, or computer, work with the patient and family members to safely and appropriately quiet these items during teaching sessions.

❖ Make sure that all patient education materials are organized and at hand. If the patient wears glasses or hearing aids, be sure they are made available prior to education.

KEY POINTS

❖ The effectiveness of patient education relies on an understanding of and attention to the cognitive, affective, and psychomotor domains of learning. Once the assessment phase, identified nursing diagnoses, and plan of care are completed, the implementation phase of the teaching–learning process begins; re-evaluation of the teaching plan must occur frequently and as needed. The growth in cultural diversity, in particular the increase in the Asian and Southeast Asian population, demands that nursing and other health care providers make patient education materials available not only in English but also in other languages.

❖ Patients need to receive information through as many senses as possible, such as aurally and visually (as with pamphlets, videos, diagrams), to maximize learning.

Information should also be at the patient's reading level and in the language the patient speaks most fluently. For example, a person may be from Thailand, but speaks French and not English. Teaching, therefore, would be appropriate in French, not Thai. Information should also be suitable for the patient's level of cognitive development (see Erikson's stages in Box 7-3).

❖ Teaching and learning principles also must be integrated into patient education plans. Evaluation of patient learning is a critical component of safe and effective drug administration.

❖ To verify the success—or lack of success—of patient education, nurses need to be clear and specific in their questions related to patient outcomes and request that the patient repeat information or perform a return demonstration of skills, if appropriate.

EXAMINATION REVIEW QUESTIONS

1. Lucas, a 47-year-old patient with diabetes, is being discharged home on insulin injections twice a day. Which concepts should the nurse keep in mind when considering patient teaching?
a. Teaching needs to begin at the time of diagnosis or admission and is individualized to the patient's reading level.
b. The nurse can assume that because Lucas is in his forties he will be able to read any written or printed documents provided.
c. The majority of teaching can be done with pamphlets that Lucas can share with family members.
d. A thorough and comprehensive teaching plan designed for a Grade 11 reading level needs to be developed.

2. The nurse is developing a discharge plan regarding a patient's medication. Which statement about the discharge plan is true? The teaching will:
a. Be done right before the patient leaves the hospital.
b. Be developed only after the patient is comfortable or after pain medications are administered.
c. Include videos, demonstrations, and instructions written at least at a Grade 5 level.
d. Be individualized and based on the patient's level of cognitive development.

3. The nurse is responsible for preoperative teaching for a patient who is mildly anxious about receiving narcotics postoperatively. The nurse acknowledges that this level of anxiety may:
a. Impede learning because anxiety is always a barrier to learning.
b. Lead to major emotional unsteadiness.
c. Result in learning by increasing the patient's motivation to learn.
d. Reorganize the patient's thoughts and lead to inadequate potential for learning.

4. What action by the nurse is the best way to assess a patient's learning needs?
a. Quiz the patient daily on all medications.
b. Begin with validation of the patient's present level of knowledge.

c. Assess family members' knowledge of the medication even if they are not involved in the patient's care.
d. Ask the caregivers what the patient knows about the medications.

5. Which technique would be most appropriate for teaching a patient who does not understand English?
a. Obtain an interpreter who can speak in the patient's native tongue for teaching sessions.
b. Use detailed and lengthy explanations, speaking slowly and clearly.
c. Assume that the patient understands the information presented if the patient has no questions.
d. Provide only written instructions.

6. A nursing student is identifying situations that involve the psychomotor domain of learning as part of a class project. Which are examples of learning activities that involve the psychomotor domain? (Select all that apply.)
a. Teaching a patient how to self-administer eye drops
b. Having a patient list the adverse effects of an antihypertensive drug
c. Discussing what foods to avoid while taking antilipemic drugs
d. Teaching a patient how to measure the pulse before taking a β-blocker
e. Teaching a family member how to give an injection
f. Teaching a patient the rationale for checking a drug's blood level

7. The nurse is instructing an older adult patient on how to use his walker. Which education strategies are appropriate? (Select all that apply.)
a. Speak slowly and loudly.
b. Ensure a quiet environment for learning.
c. Repeat information frequently.
d. Allow for an increased number of return demonstrations.
e. Provide all the information in one teaching session.

Answers: 1. a, 2. d, 3. c, 4. b, 5. a, 6. a, d, e, 7. b, c, d

CRITICAL THINKING ACTIVITIES

1. Ed, a 65-year-old patient with diabetes mellitus, is to begin treatment with insulin injections. Using the guidelines and principles for patient education discussed in this chapter of your textbook, develop a 10-minute teaching plan for Ed on the basics of subcutaneous self-administration of insulin.

2. A nurse has been trying to communicate with a patient, Narinder, who does not speak English, but so far none of the communication techniques has been successful. What are the best strategies the nurse can use to develop a plan of care that addresses Narinder's need

for medication information on the cardiac drug digoxin and also focuses on the potential for toxicity? (Note: You may need to look up the drug in the textbook if you are not familiar with it.)

3. A patient has had hip replacement surgery and will be going home in a few days. The surgeon has requested that the nurses teach the patient and a family member how to give subcutaneous injections of the low-molecular-weight heparin that will be prescribed for him after his discharge. What is the priority regarding this patient's education? Explain your answer.

CHAPTER 8

Over-the-Counter Drugs and Natural Health Products

Objectives

After reading this chapter, the successful student will be able to do the following:

1. Discuss the differences between prescription drugs, over-the-counter (OTC) drugs, and natural health products.

2. Briefly discuss the differences between the federal legislation governing the promotion and sale of prescription drugs and the legislation governing OTC drugs and natural health products.

3. Describe the advantages and disadvantages of the use of OTC drugs and natural health products.

4. Discuss the role of nonprescription drugs, specifically natural health products and dietary supplements, in the integrative (often called *alternative* or *complementary*) approach to nursing and health care.

5. Discuss the potential dangers associated with the use of OTC drugs and natural health products.

6. Develop a collaborative plan of care for the patient who uses OTC drugs or natural health products.

e-Learning Activities

Website
(http://evolve.elsevier.com/Canada/
Lilley/pharmacology/)

evolve

- Answer Key—Textbook Case Studies
- Answer Key—Critical Thinking Activities
- Chapter Summaries—Printable
- Review Questions for Exam Preparation
- Unfolding Case Studies

Key Terms

Alternative medicine Herbal medicine, natural health approaches, chiropractic, acupuncture, massage, reflexology, and any other therapies that are not part of conventional medicine yet are popular with many patients. (p. 121)

Complementary medicine Alternative medicine used simultaneously with conventional medicine. (p. 121)

Conventional medicine The practice of medicine by medical doctors and the allied health professions to treat symptoms and diseases. Also referred to as *allopathic medicine* and *Western medicine*. (p. 121)

Dietary supplement A product that contains an ingredient intended to supplement the diet, including vitamins, minerals, herbs or other botanicals, amino acids, and substances such as enzymes, organ tissues, glandular preparations, metabolites, extracts, and concentrates. (p. 120)

Herbal medicine The practice of using herbs to heal. (p. 121)

Herbs Plant components including bark, roots, leaves, seeds, flowers, fruit of trees, and extracts of these plants and materials that are valued for their savoury, aromatic, or medicinal qualities. (p. 121)

Homeopathy A popular form of alternative medicine that uses microdoses of active ingredients, usually plants or minerals, to for the treatment of disease. (p. 121)

Iatrogenic effects Unintentional adverse effects caused by the actions of a prescriber or other health care provider or by a specific treatment. (p. 121)

Integrative medicine Simultaneous use of both conventional and alternative medicine. (p. 121)

Marihuana for Medical Purposes Regulations Guidelines that allow access to marihuana for medical purposes and define the circumstances and the manner in which such access is permitted. (p. 123)

Natural health products (NHPs) Umbrella term that includes vitamins and minerals, herbal remedies, homeopathic medicines, traditional medicines such as traditional Chinese medicines, probiotics, and other products such as amino acids and essential fatty acids. (p. 120)

Over-the-counter (OTC) drugs Medications that are legally available without a prescription. (p. 117)

Phytochemicals The pharmacological active ingredients in herbal remedies. (p. 123)

Phytomedicine The application of scientific research to the practice of herbal medicine. (p. 121)

OVER-THE-COUNTER DRUGS

Health care consumers are increasingly involved in the diagnosis and treatment of common ailments. This has led to a great increase in the use of nonprescription or over-the-counter (OTC) drugs. There are approximately 40 000 OTC medications currently available on the Canadian market (Ramsay, 2009). Over 80 therapeutic classes of OTC drugs exist, marketed to treat a variety of illnesses, including pain relievers, cold and allergy medications, laxatives, and weight control. Over the course of a year, 83% of adult Canadians take OTC medications, 59% take multivitamins or minerals, and 27% take herbal remedies (Ramsay, 2009). Clearly, OTC medications comprise a large percentage of all medications used in Canada. Health care consumers consider OTC drugs to be low risk and use them to prevent, cure, or treat more than 400 different ailments. In order to reduce health care costs, many medications that formerly required a prescription are now available OTC. It is estimated that 40 to 87% of people 65 years of age or older use one OTC product regularly, 26% of Canadians aged 65 years and older use OTC drugs daily, and 5.7% take five or more OTC or dietary supplements daily. It is also estimated that more than 50% of children under 12 years of age use one or more medicinal products, usually OTC drugs, in a given week (Goldman, 2011). Some of the most commonly used OTC products include acetaminophen (see Chapter 11), aspirin (see Chapter 27), ibuprofen (see Chapter 49), famotidine, omeprazole and antacids (see Chapter 39), loperamide (see Chapter 40), and cough and cold products (see Chapter 37).

For nurses to understand current OTC classification, it is helpful to have some knowledge of Health Canada's approval process for these medications. OTC drugs are regulated by the Food and Drug Regulations (see Chapter 3). The National Drug Scheduling Advisory Committee (NDSAC) of the National Association of Pharmacy Regulating Authorities (NAPRA) sets out the level of professional intervention and advice necessary for the safe and effective use of drugs by consumers. These drug schedules are based on cascading principles. Schedule I drugs are available only by prescription. Schedule II drugs are restricted-access drugs available only from a pharmacist and are retained in an area behind the counter where there is no opportunity for consumer self-selection. Examples include insulin and acetaminophen with codeine 8 mg. This strategy ensures that the consumer is not self-medicating inappropriately and that the use of these drugs is subject to counselling by the pharmacist. Schedule III drugs include pharmacy-only nonprescription drugs. The consumer has open access to Schedule III drugs, and a pharmacist is available to answer questions. Examples are antihistamines and ulcer medications. Schedule IV drugs are those that may be prescribed by a pharmacist according to specific guidelines. Unscheduled drugs are nonprescription drugs such as ibuprofen, acetaminophen, and nicotine gum that can be sold in any store by a nonpharmacist. OTC drugs may also be prescribed but legally do not require a prescription. Although OTC drugs are usually paid for by the consumer, sometimes they are covered by public or private drug plans.

In the 2006 report by the United States Institute of Medicine (IOM), eight major sources of medication errors related to labelling were identified. ISMP Canada (2013) acknowledged the emergence of similar concerns about the design and layout of information on nonprescription products, which are often self-selected by consumers and patients, without the assistance and intervention of health care providers. In Canada, an estimate of one in nine emergency room visits was related to adverse drug events, of which almost 70% were thought to be preventable. In response to the difficulties and safety risks assumed by consumers confronted with unclear prescription drug labelling, Health Canada in 2014 launched Regulations Amending the Food and Drug Regulations (Labelling, Packaging and Brand Names of Drugs for Human Use), a "plain language labelling initiative," requiring a new, stricter "drug facts" table for OTC products, in an easy-to-read format. The regulations includes information on the following: purpose and uses of the product, storage information, dosage instructions, inactive ingredients, specific warnings and adverse effects that could occur, when the product should not be used under any circumstances, and when it is appropriate to consult a doctor or pharmacist. This labelling also requires information to facilitate adverse event reporting and quality reporting, and evidence that drug names would not be confused with other products. In addition, manufacturers would be required to submit a mock-up drug label and packaging to regulators for review. Plans are to implement all changes in June 2015 for prescription drug products, with OTC medications following in 2017. See Figure 8-1 for an example of the proposed standardized labelling for an OTC drug.

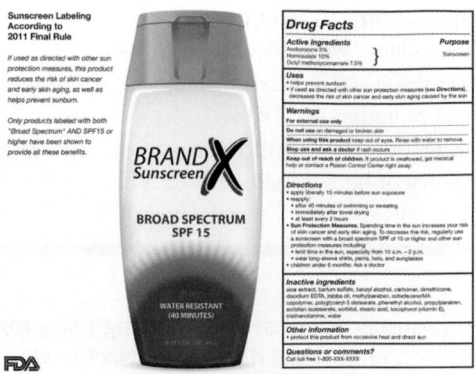

FIG. 8-1 Example of an over-the-counter (OTC) drug label incorporating plain language labelling. Source: U.S. Food and Drug Administration.

Drug ingredients can also be switched from prescription to nonprescription status. This used to involve a lengthy application process, taking 14 to 20 months from proposing a regulatory amendment to removing the ingredient from Schedule F. Schedule F of Health Canada's Food and Drug Regulations has been eliminated and replaced with the Prescription Drug List (see Chapter 3). Now, switches from prescription to nonprescription status are initiated by a request from a company in the form of a drug submission. After reviewing this data, Health Canada may determine that the ingredient should be available by prescription only, or that nonprescription sale is appropriate. Once the federal decision has been made, the provinces and territories can further restrict the conditions of sale of these products. The intent of the new process is to make nonprescription drugs available faster. The application must contain information and data about the safety, quality, and efficacy of the drug. The drug usually has been marketed in Canada and other countries long enough to demonstrate that it can be used safely by consumers on their own. Generally, to be switched from prescription to nonprescription status, a drug must meet the three criteria listed in Box 8-1. This information is obtained from clinical-trial results and postmarketing safety surveillance data, which are submitted to Health Canada by the manufacturer.

OTC status has many advantages over prescription status. Patients can conveniently and effectively self-treat many minor ailments. Some professionals argue that allowing patients to self-treat minor illnesses enables prescribers to spend more time caring for patients with serious health problems. Others argue that it delays patients from seeking medical care until they are quite ill. The financial effect of this status change is enormous: Expenditure on nonprescribed drugs was forecasted to have reached $12.1 billion in 2014 (Canadian Institutes of Health Research, 2014).

Reclassifying a prescription drug to an OTC drug may increase out-of-pocket costs for many patients because third-party health insurance plans usually do not cover OTC products. However, overall health care costs tend to

decrease when products are reclassified as OTC, due to a direct reduction in drug costs, elimination of physician office visits, and avoidance of pharmacy dispensing fees. Some examples of drugs that have recently been reclassified as OTC products appear in Box 8-2.

The importance of patient education cannot be overemphasized. Many patients are inexperienced in interpreting medication labels, which results in misuse of the products. This lack of experience and possibly lack of information or knowledge may lead to adverse events or drug interactions with prescription medications, other OTC medications, or NHPs. Small print on OTC package labels often complicates the situation, especially for older patients. In one study, parents gave children incorrect doses of OTC antipyretics over 50% of the time and another 15% administered subtherapeutic doses of acetaminophen or ibuprofen (Sullivan & Farrar, 2011). Use of OTC medications can be hazardous for patients with various chronic illnesses, including diabetes, liver, kidney disease (including acute kidney injury and chronic kidney disease), enlarged prostate, hypertension, cardiovascular disease, and glaucoma. Patients are encouraged to read labels carefully and consult a qualified health care provider when in doubt.

Another common problem associated with OTC drugs is that their use may postpone effective management of serious or life-threatening disorders. The OTC medication may relieve symptoms without necessarily addressing the cause of the disorder. This situation is often complicated when patients are afraid to visit a health care

---

BOX 8-1

Criteria for Over-the-Counter Status

I: Indications for Use

Consumer must be able to easily:
- Diagnose condition
- Monitor effectiveness
  Benefits of correct usage must outweigh risks.

II: Safety Profile

Drugs must have:
- Favourable adverse event profile
- Limited interaction with other drugs
- Low potential for misuse
- High therapeutic index*

III: Practicality for Over-the-Counter Use

Drugs must be:
- Easy to use
- Easy to monitor

---

*Ratio of toxic to therapeutic dosage.

BOX 8-2

Reclassified OTC Products

Analgesics

acetaminophen, codeine 8 mg, caffeine (Tylenol No. 1®)*
acetylsalicylic acid, codeine 8 mg, caffeine (222®, A. C. & C®)
ibuprofen (Advil®, Motrin®)
naproxen sodium (Aleve®, Anaprox®, Naprelan®, Naproxen®)

Histamine Blockers

H1 Receptors
cetirizine (Aller-Relief®, Reactine®)
chlorpheniramine maleate (Chlor-Tripolon®)
diphenhydramine hydrochloride (Benadryl®)
loratadine (Claritin®)

H2 Receptors
famotidine (Pepsid®)
ranitidine (Zantac®)

Smoking Deterrents

nicotine gum (Nicorette®)
nicotine transdermal patch (Nicoderm®, Habitrol®)

Topical Medications

clotrimazole (Canesten®)
miconazole nitrate (Micazole®, Monistat®)
minoxidil (Minox®, Rogaine®)

---

*Manitoba has recently classified Tylenol No. 1 ® as a schedule I drug

---

provider, are uninsured or underinsured, have impaired health literacy (see Chapter 7), lack access to a family physician or clinic, or perhaps wish to avoid visiting a health care provider and hope for a "quick fix" for themselves or their children.

OTC medications also have their own toxicity profiles. For example, cough and cold products usually include one or more of the following ingredients: nasal decongestants (for stuffy nose), expectorants (for loosening chest mucus), antihistamines (for sneezing and runny nose), and antitussives (for cough). In 2008, Health Canada issued recommendations that OTC cough and cold medicines (CCMs) not be used in children younger than 6 years of age. This followed numerous case reports of symptoms such as oversedation, seizures, tachycardia, and even death in toddlers medicated with such products. There is also evidence that such medications are simply not efficacious in small children. Numerous studies have shown a dramatic decrease in visits of young children to emergency departments since the recommendation (Hampton, Nguyen, Edwards, & Budnitz, 2013; Shehab, Schaefer, Kegler, & Budnitz, 2010). Health Canada continues to evaluate the safety and efficacy of cough and cold products for children but has issued no guidelines to date. Parents are advised to be mindful of how much medication they give to their children and to be careful not to give two products that contain the same active ingredient(s).

Two other examples of OTC drug dangers include products containing acetaminophen (e.g., Tylenol) and nonsteroidal anti-inflammatory drugs (NSAIDs) such as ibuprofen (e.g., Advil®, Motrin®), naproxen (e.g., Aleve®). Hepatic toxicity is associated with excessive doses of acetaminophen and is a leading cause of liver failure. Acetaminophen doses are not to exceed a total of 4 grams (4 000 mg) per day for patients with normal liver function (this dosage is currently being reviewed by Heath Canada; see Chapter 11 for more detail). The use of NSAIDs is associated with gastrointestinal ulceration, myocardial infarction, and stroke. Patients may sometimes choose excessive dosages of these and other OTC medications out of lack of knowledge or simply in hopes of easing their symptoms. Health Canada finalized regulations requiring specific labelling for acetaminophen (2009) and aspirin (2013) to enhance consumer awareness of these risks. The most current guidance document for NSAIDS is 2006. In addition, Johnson and Johnson, the manufacturers of Tylenol in Canada, developed a website with specific information for consumers on dosages, adverse effects, drug interactions and so on (http://www.tylenol.ca/adult-pain-relief).

Misuse can also be a potential hazard with the use of OTC drug products. Pseudoephedrine is found in a variety of cough and cold products (see Chapter 37); however, this drug is also used to manufacture the widely misused street drug methamphetamine. Because of the potential for misuse, products containing pseudoephedrine must be sold from behind the pharmacy counter. Many patients become addicted to OTC nasal sprays because they can cause rebound congestion and dependency. Dextromethorphan (used as a cough suppressant) is also commonly misused. It is known by the brand name Robitussin, and misusing it is called *Robotripping*.

Several other OTC products can cause specific problems. The use of sympathomimetics (e.g., epinephrine, pseudoepinephrine; see Chapter 19) can cause adverse effects in patients with type 1 diabetes (elevated plasma glucose levels), hypertension, or angina (e.g., dysrhythmias). Aspirin is not to be used in children as it can cause a rare condition called Reye's syndrome (see Chapter 27). Long-term use of antacids can result in constipation or impaction (see Chapter 39).

Normally, OTC medications should be used for only short-term treatment of common minor illnesses. An appropriate medical evaluation is recommended for all chronic health conditions, even if the final decision is to prescribe OTC medications. Patient assessment includes questions on OTC drug use, including on what conditions are being treated. Such questions may help uncover more serious ongoing medical problems. Inform patients that OTC drugs, including NHPs, are still medications.

Their use may have associated risks depending on the specific OTC drugs used, concurrent prescription medications, and the patient's overall health status and disease states.

Health care providers have an excellent opportunity to prevent common problems associated with the use of OTC drugs. Up to 60% of patients consult a health care provider when selecting an OTC product. Provide patients with information about choice of an appropriate product, correct dosing, common adverse effects, and drug interactions with other medications. For specific information on OTC drugs, see the appropriate drug chapters later in this text (see Table 8-1 for a cross-reference to these chapters).

NATURAL HEALTH PRODUCTS

History

In Canada, natural health products are subject to the Food and Drugs Act and Food and Drug Regulations. Internationally, the regulation of natural health products varies. There are many differences in how countries approach the regulation of health products. In Canada, as in European Union countries, natural health products are considered drugs, whereas in the United States, many natural health products are classified as "dietary supplements." Under the Natural Health Products Regulations, **natural health products (NHPs)** is the umbrella term that

includes vitamin and mineral supplements; herbal remedies; homeopathic preparations; traditional Chinese, Ayurvedic, and other traditional medicines; probiotics; and other products such as amino acids and essential fatty acids.

The language surrounding NHPs can be confusing. For example, in the United States, dietary supplements are considered to be food products. In Canada, they were considered NHPs and regulated as such. However, in 2013, Health Canada announced that it would transition products that more appropriately fit the definition of a food away from the Natural Health Products Regulations. Because of the differences in language and terminology, a brief discussion of the forms and history of various NHPs follows. Basic definitions are provided here to ensure complete understanding and to prevent confusion in how these terms are used.

Dietary supplement is a broad term for orally administered alternative medicines and includes the category of herbal supplements. Although there are differences in what is considered a dietary supplement, they are products intended to augment the diet and include ingredients such as vitamins, minerals, herbs or other botanicals, amino acids, dietary substances that supplement the diet by increasing the total dietary intake, concentrates, metabolites, constituents, or extracts (Health Canada, 2012). Dietary supplements are produced in many forms, such as tablets, capsules, softgels, gelcaps, liquids, and

TABLE 8-1

Common OTC Drugs Discussed in This Book

Type of OTC Drug	Examples	Where Discussed in This Book
Acid-controlling drugs (H2 blockers, proton pump inhibitors) and antacids	famotidine (Pepsid AC®), omeprazole® (heart burn control), ranitidine hydrochloride (Zantac®); aluminum- and magnesium-containing products (Maalox®, Mylanta®), calcium-containing products (Tums®)	Chapter 39: Acid-Controlling Drugs
Antifungal drugs (topical)	clotrimazole (Canesten®), miconazole nitrate (Micozole®, Monistat®)	Chapter 56: Dermatological Drugs
Antihistamines and decongestants	brompheniramine maleate (Dimetane®, Dimetapp®) cetirizine hydrochloride (Reactine®) chlorpheniramine maleate (Advil Cold and Sinus®, Chlor-Tripolon®, Triaminic®) diphenhydramine hydrochloride (Benadryl, Nadryl®) fexofenadine hydrochloride (Allerga®) guaifenesin (Balminil®) loratadine (Claritin®) desloratidine (Aerius®, Allernix), pseudoephedrine hydrochloride (Actifed®)	Chapter 37: Antihistamines, Decongestants, Antitussives, and Expectorants
Eye drops	Artificial tears (Murine®)	Chapter 57: Ophthalmic Drugs
Hair growth drugs (topical)	minoxidil (Rogaine®)	Chapter 56: Dermatological Drugs
Pain-relieving drugs (analgesics)	acetaminophen (Tylenol)	Chapter 11: Analgesic Drugs
Pain-relieving drugs (NSAIDs)	aspirin ibuprofen (Advil®, Motrin®) naproxen sodium (Aleve®, Naprelan®)	Chapter 49: Anti-Inflammatory and Antigout Drugs

powders. These supplements may also be found in nutritional, breakfast, snack, or health food bars; drinks; and shakes.

Herbs come from nature and include the leaves, bark, berries, roots, gums, seeds, stems, and flowers of plants. They have been used for thousands of years to help maintain good health. Herbs have been an integral part of society because of their culinary and medicinal properties. About 30% of all modern drugs are derived from plants (Table 8-2). In the early nineteenth century, scientific methods became more advanced, and the development and mass production of chemically synthesized drugs revolutionized health care in most parts of the world. During this time, the practice of botanical healing was dismissed as quackery. Nonetheless, **herbal medicine** (or the practice of **phytomedicine**) are now in great demand in the developing world for primary health care because they are inexpensive and have better cultural acceptability, are reasonably safe and effective, and have advantageous compatibility and minimal adverse effects (World Health Organization, 2015). However, use of traditional medicine is not limited to developing countries, and during the past two decades, public interest in natural therapies has increased greatly in industrialized countries, with expanding use of ethnobotanicals. Indeed, in the future, traditional herbal medicine research may play a critical role in global health. Herbs and plants can be processed and ingested in numerous ways and forms. This includes whole herbs, teas, essential oils, ointments, salves, syrup, tinctures, rubs, capsules, and tablets that contain a ground or powdered form of a raw herb or its dried extract. Plant and herb extracts vary in the solvent used for extraction, temperature, and extraction time and include alcoholic extracts (tinctures), vinegars (acetic acid extracts), hot water extracts (tisanes), long-term boiled extracts, usually roots or bark (decoctions), and cold infusion of plants (macerates). There is no standardization, and components of an herbal extract or a product are likely to vary significantly between batches and producers (Benzie & Wachtel-Galor, 2011). Herbs are generally to be taken intermittently, not in continuous daily dosing.

In the 1960s, concerns were expressed over the **iatrogenic effects** of **conventional medicine** (medicine taught in the West). These concerns, along with a desire for more self-reliance, led to a renewed interest in "natural health," and as a result, the use of NHPs, including the use of herbal products, increased. In 1974, the World Health Organization (WHO) encouraged developing countries to use traditional plant medicines. In 1978, the German equivalent of Health Canada published a series of herbal recommendations known as the *Commission E Monographs*. These monographs focus on herbs whose effectiveness for specific indications is supported by the research literature. Recognition of the rising use of herbal medicines and other nontraditional remedies, known as **alternative medicine**, led to the establishment of the Health of the Office of Alternative Medicine by the National Institutes of Health in 1992. This office was later renamed the National Center for Complementary and Alternative Medicine (NCCAM). **Complementary medicine** refers to the simultaneous use of both conventional and alternative medicine. This practice is also referred to as **integrative medicine.** NCCAM classifies complementary and alternative medicine into five categories: (1) alternative medical systems, (2) mind–body interventions, (3) biologically based therapies, (4) manipulative and body-based methods, and (5) energy therapies. A popular form of alternative medicine is **homeopathy**. Homeopathy is based on the belief that a disease can be treated by the administration of a microdose of a substance thought to cause the physical signs of that disease. Homeopathy is thought to stimulate the body's immune defences.

Many controversies remain about the safety and the control of NHPs, although they continue to be used in Canada and abroad. Their uses and touted advantages are widely publicized. As a result, these products are marketed and placed in grocery stores, pharmacies, health food stores, and fitness gyms and can even be ordered through television and radio ads and over the Internet. Adverse effects are considered minimal by the public as well as by the companies and businesses that sell these supplements. However, this belief has created a false sense of security because the public's view tends to be that if a product is "natural" then it is safe. The information listed in this book regarding NHPs does not imply author or publisher endorsement of such products.

Concerns over the accessibility and regulation of all NHPs led the Health Canada Directorate to establish the Advisory Panel on Natural Health in 1997. After consultations with interested stakeholders, the Minister of Health tabled *Natural Health Products: A New Vision*, which provided the framework for the development of the Office of Natural Health Products. This office would later be renamed the Natural and Non-prescription Health Products Directorate (NHPD). In 2004, the Natural Health Products Regulations came into effect. Manufacturers must obtain a product licence from Health Canada

TABLE	8-2

Conventional Medicines Derived From Plants

Medicine*	Plant
atropine	*Atropa belladonna*
capsaicin	*Capsicum frutescens*
cocaine	*Erythroxylon coca*
codeine	*Papaver somniferum*
digoxin	*Digitalis purpurea*
paclitaxel	*Taxis brevifolia*
quinine	*Cinchona officinalis*
scopolamine	*Datura fastuosa*
senna	*Cassia acutifolia*
vincristine	*Catharanthus roseus*

*Includes both OTC and prescription drugs.

to sell their products in Canada. If the product meets the NHPD criteria, then a Natural Product Number (NPN) will be issued. The Licensed Natural Health Products Database (LNHPD), managed by Health Canada, provides information on licensed NHPs. These include vitamin and mineral supplements, herb- and plant-based remedies, traditional medicines (e.g., traditional Chinese medicines or Ayurvedic [Indian] medicines), omega-3 and essential fatty acids, probiotics, homeopathic medicines, and numerous consumer products, such as certain toothpastes, antiperspirants, shampoos, facial products, and mouthwashes. This database can be accessed at http://www.hc-sc.gc.ca/dhp-mps/prodnatur/applications/licen-prod/lnhpd-bdpsnh-eng.php.

Homeopathic medicines (HMs) receive a Drug Identification Number (DIN)-HM, followed by a product number. Extensive product labelling must meet specific requirements regarded as essential to risk management. On the basis of information from the WHO, the European Scientific Cooperative on Phytotherapy, and the German Commission E, the NHPD developed the Compendium of Monographs. The regulations also impose standard labelling requirements to ensure that consumers can make informed choices about NHPs. Labels contain such details as the product name, the quantity of the product in the container, and the recommended conditions for use, which include recommended use or purpose and dose, warnings, cautionary statements, contraindications, and possible adverse reactions. With such regulations, Canada, similar to Germany, France, and the United Kingdom, enforces standards for the assessment of natural-product quality and safety.

Consumer Use of Natural Health Products

Consumer use of NHPs is growing. An estimated 73% of Canadians use some form of alternative medicine and regularly take NHPs such as vitamins and minerals, herbal products, and homeopathic medicines (Health Canada, 2015a), despite the fact that 12% who use them experience adverse reactions and only 41% who experience adverse effects report them. Canadians who take NHPs and prescription drugs are six times as likely to suffer unwanted adverse effects as those just using drugs (Necyk, Barnes, Tsuyuki, et al., 2013). Consumers select NHPs for the treatment and prevention of diseases and, proactively, to preserve health and wellness and boost the immune system (e.g., reduce cardiovascular risk factors, increase liver and immune system functions, increase feelings of wellness). In addition, herbs may be used as adjunct therapy to support conventional pharmaceutical therapies.

Some products may be used to treat minor conditions and illnesses (e.g., coughs, colds, stomach upset) in much the same manner as conventional Health-Canada–approved OTC nonprescription drugs are used. As the number of NHPs on the market increases, nurses will need to respond to patient educational needs about these products.

Safety

NHPs, particularly herbal medicines, are often perceived as natural and therefore healthier than conventional drugs; however, this is not always the case. There are examples of allergic reactions, toxic reactions, and adverse effects caused by herbs. Some herbs have been shown to have possible mutagenic effects and to interact with drugs (see Natural Health Products: Selected Natural Health Products and their Possible Drug Interactions). It is estimated that many patients using NHPs do not disclose this to their health care providers. Patients are reluctant to disclose use for fear of disapproval by their health care providers or that they will not give their full attention to the topic (Walji, Boon, Barnes, et al., 2010). In addition, there are concerns about the level of consumer knowledge of these products and their risks, even among regular users. This demonstrates the need for health care providers to develop a clinical knowledge base regarding these products and know where to find key information as the need arises. Because of underreporting, present knowledge may represent but a small fraction of potential safety concerns.

There are few published scientific data regarding the safety of NHPs. Two recent examples indicating some of the growing concerns with specific herbal remedies include Health Canada warnings about possible liver toxicity with the use of kava root and possible cardiovascular and stroke risks with the use of ephedra. Ephedra remains on the market and in 2012, after a 10-year ban, Health Canada has regulated kava root as a new drug. Also, a paper published in the *Journal of the American Association of Cardiology* suggests that many herbal products are best avoided in patients with cardiovascular diseases (Tachjian, Vigar, Jahanjir, et al., 2010). Herbal products can increase bleeding risk with warfarin sodium (see Chapter 26), potentiate digoxin toxicity (see Chapter 25), increase the effects of antihypertensive agents (see Chapter 23), and cause heart block or dysrhythmias (see Chapter 26).

In order to improve the NHP vigilance system, several initiatives have been put in place by Health Canada that are available to both consumers and health care providers. The Canada Vigilance Program is Health Canada's postmarket surveillance program that maintains an online database of suspected adverse reactions submitted by both consumers and health care providers. The database provides information only. Through the MedEffect program, consumers and health care providers can report adverse effects from NHPs via web, phone, fax, or mail. Also available is the Health Product Info Watch, published monthly, with health product advisories and summary safety information about marketed health products and information of new health product safety. Other authoritative references that can be utilized for herbal information include Pharmacist's Letter, Prescriber's Letter, and Natural Medicines (formerly Natural Medicines Comprehensive Database and Natural Standard), all available at http://www.naturalstandard.com/. Health care providers need to be on the alert for

NATURAL HEALTH PRODUCTS

Selected Natural Health Products and Their Possible Drug Interactions

Natural Health Product	Possible Drug Interaction
Chamomile	Increased risk for bleeding with anticoagulants
Cranberry	Decreased elimination of many drugs excreted by the kidneys
Echinacea	Possible interference with or counteraction to immunosuppressant drugs and antivirals
Evening primrose	Possible interaction with antipsychotic drugs
Garlic	Possible interference with hypoglycemic therapy and the anticoagulant warfarin sodium (Coumadin®)
Gingko biloba	May increase risk of bleeding with use of anticoagulants (warfarin sodium, heparin sodium) and antiplatelets (aspirin, clopidrogrel)
Ginger root	At high dosages, possible interference with cardiac, antidiabetic, or anticoagulant drugs
Grapefruit	Decreases metabolism of drugs used for erectile dysfunction
	Decreases metabolism of estrogens and some psychotherapeutic drugs (benzodiazepines, sertraline)
	Increases risk of toxicity of immunosuppressants, HMG-CoA reductase inhibitors, and of some psychotherapeutic drugs (pimozide, escitalopram)
	Increases intensity and duration of effects of caffeine
Hawthorn	May lead to toxic levels of cardiac glycosides (e.g., digitalis)
Kava	May increase the effect of barbiturates and alcohol
Saw palmetto	May change the effects of hormones in oral contraceptive drugs, patches, or hormonal replacement therapies
St. John's wort	May lead to serotonin syndrome if used with other serotonergic drugs (e.g., selective serotonin reuptake inhibitors [see Chapter 17])
	Strong CYP 3A4 inducer resulting in decreased concentrations of many drugs
Valerian	Increases central nervous system depression if used with sedatives

Modified from Bailey, D. G., Dresser, G., & Arnold, J. M. O. (2013). Grapefruit–medication interactions: Forbidden fruit or avoidable consequences? *Canadian Medical Association Journal, 185*(4). doi: 10.1503/cmaj.120951; Seden, K., Dickinson, L., Khoo, S., & Back, D. (2010). Grapefruit-drug interactions. *Drugs, 70*(18): 2373–2407.

announcements about the safe and effective use of NHPs as well as their reported adverse effects. The discriminating and proper use of some products may provide some therapeutic benefits, but the indiscriminate or excessive use of NHP supplements can be dangerous (see Ethnocultural Implications Box).

Level of Use

There are approximately 16 000 NHPs currently licensed for use in Canada, with many new products introduced annually. A great deal of public interest in the use of NHPs remains. Estimates of the prevalence of use differ greatly.

The many different herbs in these preparations contain a wide variety of active phytochemicals (plant compounds). Herbal medicine is based on the premise that plants contain natural substances that can promote health and alleviate illness. Some of the more common ailments and conditions treated with herbs are anxiety, arthritis, colds, constipation, cough, depression, fever, headache, infection, insomnia, intestinal disorders, premenstrual syndrome, menopausal symptoms, stress, ulcers, and weakness.

NHPs constitute the largest growth area in retail pharmacy and their use is increasing, exceeding the growth in the use of conventional drugs. Some of the most commonly used natural health herbal remedies are aloe, black cohosh, chamomile, echinacea, feverfew, garlic, ginger, ginkgo biloba, ginseng, goldenseal, hawthorn, St. John's wort, saw palmetto, and valerian.

Medical Use of Marihuana

Marihuana is an herb with a long history of use for its therapeutic and medicinal qualities. In Canada, marihuana remains an illegal and controlled substance. However, in 2003, Health Canada implemented the Marihuana Medical Access Regulations (MMAR) to allow access to and possession of marihuana for individuals suffering from specific grave and debilitating illnesses, while protecting public safety. These regulations were repealed in 2014 and the **Marihuana for Medical Purposes Regulations** (MMPR) became law. This transition from the MMAR to the MMPR program represents a substantial change in direction for the supply and acquisition of medical marihuana in Canada and allows for a wider variety of choice of strains of marihuana produced under controlled conditions. Access to marihuana for medical purposes has been transferred from Health Canada to the health care provider (e.g., physician or nurse practitioner) who provides medical documentation confirming a medical diagnosis and submits it directly to a licensed supplier of dry marihuana. The supplier then

BOX 8-3 Cannabis

Cannabis sativa, or cannabis from the hemp plant, is widely used for recreational purposes. After tobacco, it is the most frequently smoked substance worldwide. Cannabinoids are the psychoactive ingredients of marihuana, of which $1\text{-}\Delta^9\text{-}trans\text{-}tetrahydrocannabinol$ (THC), concentrated in the bud of the female plant, is the main psychoactive substance. When marihuana is smoked, the effect is almost immediate and lasts for one to three hours. THC is absorbed by most tissues and organs in the body; however, it is primarily found in fat tissues. The body attempts to eliminate the foreign chemical by chemically transforming THC into metabolites. The half-life of THC for an infrequent user is approximately 1.3 days and for frequent users 5 to 13 days (Sharma, Murthy, & Bharath, 2014). THC metabolites can be found in the urine, the preferred sample, for up to one week after smoking marihuana. Metabolites can also be detected retrospectively in hair. Once incorporated into the growing hair, the drug can be detected for 90 days after it has been eliminated from more conventional samples, such as blood and urine (Khajuria & Nayak, 2014). THC acts on cannabinoid receptors on brain cells and triggers a series of chemical reactions that ultimately lead to the "high" that users experience. Cannabinoid receptors are found in areas of the brain that influence pleasure, memory, thought, con-centration, sensory and time perception, and coordinated movement. There is evidence that THC acts on neurotransmitters and exerts either excitatory or inhibitory effects.

Cannabidiol (CBD) is the major nonpsychotropic cannabinoid found in marihuana. It has shown antiepileptic, anti-inflammatory, antiemetic, muscle relaxing, anxiolytic, neuroprotective, and antipsychotic activity; inhibits colon cancer cell proliferation; and reduces the psychoactive effects of THC (Romano et al., 2014). The mode of action of cannabidiol is not fully understood.

While there is sociopolitical concern around the medical use of marihuana, and the clinical therapeutic potential for marihuana has not yet been proven in controlled clinical trials beyond 6 weeks, there is anecdotal evidence that it may be beneficial in a variety of disorders. In Canada, marihuana is authorized based on promising clinical evidence for use as an adjunctive treatment for neuropathic pain in adults with multiple sclerosis and as adjunctive analgesic treatment in adult patients with advanced cancer, for acquired immunodeficiency syndrome (AIDS)–related anorexia associated with weight loss, as well as for severe nausea and vomiting associated with cancer chemotherapy.

ships the dried marihuana directly to the patient, who must be registered with the supplier. In 2015, the Supreme Court of Canada ruled against the federal government to expand the definition of medical marihuana beyond the "dried" form and allow the consumption of medical marihuana as well as use other extracts and derivatives (Do, 2015). See Box 8-3 for discussion of the use of marihuana (also known as *cannabis*) for medical purposes.

NURSING PROCESS

▨ Assessment

▪ Over-the-Counter Drugs

Nursing assessments are always important to perform, but they are especially important in situations in which the patient is self-medicating. Reading level, cognitive level, motor abilities, previous use of OTC drugs, successes versus failures with drug therapies and self-medication, and caregiver support are just a few of the variables to be assessed, as deemed appropriate. Other assessment data include questioning about allergies to any of the ingredients or additives (e.g., dyes, preservatives, or fillers) of the drug. Include a list of *all* medications and substances used by the patient in the medication history, including OTC drugs, prescription drugs, herbal products, vitamins, and minerals. Also note use of alcohol, tobacco, and caffeine. Assess past and present medical history so that possible drug interactions, contraindications, and cautions are identified. Screen patients carefully before recommending an OTC drug because patients often assume that if a drug is sold OTC it is completely safe to take and without negative consequences. This is not true—OTC drugs can be just as lethal or problematic as prescription drugs if they are not taken properly or are taken in high dosages and without regard to directions (see discussion earlier in the chapter).

Assessment of the patient's knowledge about the components of self-medication, including the positive and negative consequences of the use of a given OTC drug, must be included. Assessment of the patient's (or caregiver's or family member's) level of knowledge and experience with OTC self-medication is critical to the patient's safety, as is assessment of attitudes toward and beliefs about their use. This is especially true if a casual attitude is combined with a lack of knowledge, which could result in overuse, overdosage, and potential complications. See Chapter 7 for more information on patient education.

For the most part, laboratory tests are not ordered before the use of OTC drugs because they are self-administered and self-monitored. However, there are situations in which patients may be taking certain medications that react adversely with OTC drugs, and laboratory testing may be needed. Some patient groups are also at higher risk for adverse reactions to OTC drugs (as to most drugs in general), including: pediatric and older adult patients; patients with single and/or multiple acute and chronic illnesses; those who are frail or in poor

ETHNOCULTURAL IMPLICATIONS

Drug Responses and Ethnocultural Factors

Responses to drugs, including OTC drugs and NHPs, may be affected by beliefs, values, and genetics as well as by culture, race, and ethnicity. As one example of the impact of culture on drug response and use, if patients who are Japanese experience nausea, vomiting, or bowel changes as adverse effects of OTC drugs or NHPs, these often are not mentioned. The reason is that individuals in this culture find it unacceptable to report gastrointestinal symptoms and they may remain unreported to the point of causing risk to the patient.

NHPs, specifically herbal and alternative therapies, may also be used more extensively in some cultures than in others. Wide acceptance of herbal use without major concern for the effects on other therapies may be problematic because of the many interactions of conventional drugs with herbs and dietary supplements. For example, the Chinese herb ginseng may inhibit or accelerate the metabolism of a specific medication and significantly affect the drug's absorption or elimination.

One genetic factor that has an influence on drug response is acetylation polymorphism; that is, prescription drugs, OTC drugs, and NHPs may be metabolized in different ways that are genetically determined and vary with race or ethnicity. For example, populations of European or African descent contain approximately equal numbers of individuals showing rapid and slow acetylation (which affects drug metabolism), whereas Japanese and Inuit populations may contain more rapid acetylators. See Chapter 4 for a more in-depth discussion of these specific genetic attributes.

Source: Modified from Munoz, C., Hilgenberg, C: Ethnopharmacology, *Am J Nurs* 105(8):40–49, 2005.

health, debilitated and nutritionally deficient; and those with suppressed immune systems. OTC drugs must also be used with caution and may be contraindicated in patients with a history of kidney, liver, heart, or vascular dysfunction. More assessment information for OTC drugs and NHPs can be found in other chapters in this textbook, when relevant (see Table 8-1 on page 120). It is important to remember that consumer/patient safety and quality of care related to drug therapy of any kind begins with education. Thus, the best way for patients to help themselves is for them to learn how to assess each situation, weigh all the factors, and find out all they can about the OTC drug they wish to take *before* taking it.

◼ Natural Health Products

Many NHPs, including herbs, probiotics, and dietary supplements, are readily available in drug, health food, and grocery stores as well as in gardens, kitchens, and medicine cabinets. As noted earlier in the chapter, among the more commonly used herbals are aloe, echinacea, feverfew, garlic, ginger, ginkgo biloba, ginseng, goldenseal, hawthorn, St. John's wort, saw palmetto, and valerian. Although patients generally self-administer these products and do not perform an assessment, in various settings the health care provider may be able to assess the patient through a head-to-toe physical examination, medical and nursing history, and medication history. Share assessment data, factors, and variables to consider with the patient for the patient's safety. This sharing of assessment information allows the health care provider to be sure that the patient is taking the NHP in as safe a manner as possible.

Many NHPs may lead to a variety of adverse effects. For example, some may cause dermatitis when used topically, whereas some taken systemically may be associated with kidney disorders such as nephritis. Therefore, for example, patients with existing skin problems or kidney dysfunction must seek medical advice before using certain herbal products. It is also crucial to patient safety to consider any other contraindications, cautions, and potential drug–drug and drug–food interactions. See Natural Health Products on page 123 for more information on drug interactions.

◪ Nursing Diagnoses

Nursing diagnoses appropriate for the patient who is taking OTC drugs or NHPs include the following (without related causes because these are too numerous to include):

1. Impaired physical mobility
2. Impaired memory
3. Impaired urinary elimination
4. Acute pain or persistent pain
5. Fatigue
6. Activity intolerance
7. Insomnia
8. Ineffective health maintenance
9. Risk for injury
10. Readiness for enhanced self-care
11. Readiness for enhanced knowledge

◪ Planning

◼ Goals

1. Patient will be able to increase mobility as tolerated and without distress.
2. Patient will experience increased alertness and improved short-term and long-term memory with continued use of the NHP.

3. Patient will maintain normal elimination patterns during NHP use.
4. Patient will experience pain relief or relief of the symptoms of the disease process or injury.
5. Patient will experience increase in energy and function (or both).
6. Patient's tolerance for activity will remain within normal limits or improve during OTC drug or therapy.
7. Patient will experience limited sleep pattern disturbance while on OTC drug or NHP therapy.
8. Patient will seek healthy maintenance behaviours with questions about the OTC drug or NHP (or both), as well as its action, therapeutic effects versus adverse effects, toxicity, cautions, contraindications, drug–drug or drug–food interactions, and appropriate dosage formulation administration.
9. Patient will remain free from injury while taking the OTC drug or NHP (or both).

Expected Patient Outcomes

- Patient states that the actions of the OTC drug or NHP have been beneficial, with relief of symptoms and increased physical mobility.
- Patient experiences improving overall well-being and health status, with minimal adverse effects or complications.
- Patient reports any change in orientation to person, place, or time or in short-term or long-term memory immediately and seeks appropriate directions regarding discontinuing therapy.
- Patient describes nonpharmacological approaches to the treatment of acute and persistent pain, such as the use of hot or cold packs, physiotherapy, massage, relaxation therapy, biofeedback, imagery, and hypnosis.
- Patient identifies measures to increase urinary elimination and enhance urinary elimination patterns, such as increasing fluid intake to six to eight glasses of water per day, unless contraindicated, and taking time to void at regular intervals.
- Patient takes measures to minimize fatigue through the use of NHPs, sleeping 6 to 8 hours per night; increasing fluid intake; and maintaining an intake of recommended daily amounts of food, calories, and protein.
- Patient states that the actions of the OTC drug or NHP (or both) have been beneficial, with relief of symptoms and subsequent increased ability to participate in activities of daily living (ADLs) as well as increased participation in other physical activities.
- Patient states increased hours of sleep (i.e., 6 to 8 hours of sleep) and less difficulty with onset of sleep while using OTC drugs, herbal products, or dietary supplements.
- Patient experiences healthier behaviours as related to health maintenance, by being more knowledgeable about self-medication administration with OTC drugs or NHPs.
- Patient inquires of pharmacist or health care provider about the safe daily healthy maintenance behaviour of taking NHPs and deciphers information appropriately.
- Patient states the importance of taking drugs as directed and of immediately reporting any severe adverse effects or complications associated with the use of an OTC drug or NHP to the health care provider and pharmacist and contacting the poison control centre, if needed.
- Patient is able to self-administer OTC drugs or NHPs as directed and with proper administration technique (e.g., transdermal patch, suppository, liquid, quick-dissolve tablet) with minimal adverse effects and a decrease in risk for self-injury.

Implementation

With OTC drugs and NHPs, patient education is an important strategy to enhance patient safety. Patients need to receive as much information as possible about the safe use of these products and to be informed that, even though these are not prescription drugs, they are *not* completely safe and are not without toxicity. Include information about safe use, frequency of dosing and dose specifics of how to take the medication (e.g., with food or at bedtime), as well as strategies to prevent adverse effects, drug interactions, and toxicity in the patient instructions. Another consideration is the dosage form, because a variety of dosage forms are available, such as liquids, tablets, enteric-coated tablets, transdermal patches, gum, and quick-dissolve tablets or strips. Instructions must be provided and the need to recheck dosage emphasized. For transdermal patches (e.g., for smoking cessation), it is important to emphasize proper use and application. As previously mentioned, many consumers believe that no risks exist if a medication is available OTC or is a "natural" substance. See Box 8-1 for more information about the criteria for moving a drug from prescription to OTC status. The fact that a drug is a NHP does not mean that it can be safely administered to children, infants, pregnant or lactating women, or patients with certain health conditions that put them at risk.

Evaluation

Patients taking OTC drugs or NHPs need to carefully monitor themselves for unusual or adverse reactions and therapeutic responses to the medication to prevent overuse and overdosing. The range of therapeutic responses will vary, depending on the specific drug and the indication for which it is used. Therapeutic responses also vary depending on the drug's action—a few examples include decreased pain; decreased stiffness and swelling in joints; decreased fever; increased ease of carrying out ADLs; increased hair growth; increased ease in breathing; decreased constipation, diarrhea, bowel irritability, or gastrointestinal reflux or hyperacidity; resolution of allergic symptoms; decreased vaginal itching and discharge; increased healing; increased sleep; and decreased fatigue or improved energy.

For more specific nursing diagnoses, planning with goals and outcome criteria, implementation, and evaluation related to various OTC drugs and NHPs, see the appropriate chapters later in the textbook; Table 8-1 provides cross-references to these chapters.

 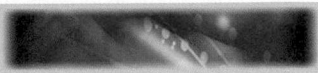

CASE STUDY

Over-the-Counter Drugs and Natural Health Products

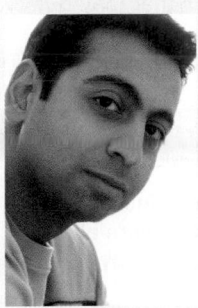

Jag, a 28-year-old graduate student, is at the student health clinic for a physical examination that is required before he goes on a research trip out of the country. As he completes the paperwork, he asks the nurse, "The form is asking about my medications. I don't have any prescribed medicines, but I take several herbal products and OTC medicines. Do you need to know about these?"

1. How should the nurse answer Jag?
   On the form, Jag lists the following items:
   1 low-dose (81 mg) aspirin daily to prevent blood clots
   Sleepwell® herbal product with valerian at night if needed
   Benadryl as needed for allergies, especially at night
   Stress Away® herbal product with ginseng as needed

   Generic ibuprofen, 3 or 4 tablets three times a day for muscle aches from working out
   Memory Boost herbal product with ginkgo biloba every morning

2. Examine the products on Jag's list, and state whether there are any concerns with interactions or adverse effects. It may be necessary to refer to descriptions of the individual herbal products (see the inside back cover for a complete listing of Natural Health Products boxes located throughout the textbook) or to the appropriate drug chapters for more information.

3. Upon further questioning, Jag remembers that he has had problems with "acid stomach" for about a year and takes Maximum Strength Pepcid® AC-OTC as needed to manage this problem. What concerns, if any, are there about this?

For answers see http://evolve.elsevier.com/Canada/Lilley/pharmacology/.

PATIENT TEACHING TIPS

❖ Provide verbal and written information about how to choose an appropriate OTC drug or NHP, as well as information about correct dosing, common adverse effects, and possible interactions with other medications.

❖ Many patients believe that no risks exist if a medication is herbal and "natural" or if it is sold OTC, so provide adequate education about the drug or product as well as all of the advantages and disadvantages of its use because this is crucial to patient safety.

❖ Provide instructions on how to read OTC and NHP labels. Encourage the reading of ingredients if using more than one product, as the ingredient or chemical may occur in both products. For example, a multivitamin supplement may contain ginseng, and taking additional ginseng supplements may lead to toxicity. Another example is with products containing acetaminophen (Tylenol). If the patient is taking acetaminophen and then also takes a cold/flu product, there may also be acetaminophen in that product, and consequently the risk of adverse effects and toxicity increases.

❖ Emphasize the importance of taking all OTC drugs, herbals, and dietary supplements with extreme caution and being aware of all the possible interactions and concerns associated with the use of these products.

❖ Instruct the patient that all health care providers (e.g., nurses, dentists, osteopathic and chiropractic physicians) need to be aware of the use of any OTC drugs and NHPs (and, of course, any prescription drug use).

❖ Encourage journalling of any improvement of symptoms noted with the use of a specific OTC drug or NHP.

❖ Encourage the use of appropriate and authoritative resources for patient information, such as a registered pharmacist, literature provided from the drug company or pharmacist, and web-based information from reliable sites at an appropriate reading level for the patient (e.g. www.Webmd.com).

❖ Instruct the patient that all medications, whether OTC drugs or NHPs should be kept out of the reach of children and pets.

❖ Provide thorough instructions regarding the various dosage forms of OTC drugs and NHPs

❖ Provide specific instructions, such as how to mix powders and how to properly use transdermal patches, inhalers, ointments, lotions, nose drops, ophthalmic drops, elixirs, suppositories, vaginal suppositories or creams, and all other dosage forms (see Chapter 10); also provide information about proper storage and cleansing of any equipment.

KEY POINTS

❖ Consumers use NHPs therapeutically for the treatment of diseases and pathological conditions, prophylactically for long-term prevention of disease, and proactively as agents for the maintenance of health and wellness.

❖ Health Canada has established the MedEffect program to track adverse events or problems related to drug therapy. The toll-free number is 1-866-678-6789 for marketed health products, including prescription and nonprescription medications and NHPs. Consumers and

health care providers may report adverse events anonymously and without consequence.

❖ NHPs are approved by Health Canada, with specific labelling requirements to provide adequate instructions for use and warnings.

❖ The fact that a drug is an NHP or an OTC medication is no guarantee that it can be safely administered to children, infants, pregnant or lactating women, or patients with certain health conditions that may put them at risk.

EXAMINATION REVIEW QUESTIONS

1. Which statement is true about current Canadian legislation regarding NHPs?
   a. Herbals were regulated in the early 1900s in reference to their efficacy and toxicity.
   b. The Natural Health Products Directorate (NHPD) regulates the safety, efficacy, and quality of NHPs.
   c. The Marihuana for Medical Purposes Regulations allow access to and possession of marihuana for individuals.
   d. The NHPD was specifically designed to encourage the freedom of choice and philosophical and ethnocultural diversity of NHPs.

2. What information about NHPs is important for the nurse to communicate to patients?
   a. Natural health and OTC products are not approved by Health Canada and are under strict regulation.
   b. These products are scrutinized for safety and tested repeatedly by Health Canada.
   c. No adverse effects are associated with these agents because they are "natural" and may be purchased without a prescription.
   d. Labelling is not 100% reliable for the provision of proper instructions or warnings, and the products should be taken with caution.

3. When taking a patient's drug history, the nurse asks about use of OTC drugs. The patient responds by saying, "Oh, I frequently take something for my headaches, but I didn't mention it because aspirin is nonprescription." What is the best response from the nurse?
   a. "That's true, OTC drugs are generally not harmful."
   b. "Aspirin is one of the safest drugs out there."
   c. "Although aspirin is over the counter, it is still important to know why you take it, how much you take, and how often."
   d. "We need you to be honest about the drugs you are taking. Are there any others that you haven't told us about?"

4. When making a home visit to a patient who was recently discharged from the hospital, the nurse notes that she has a small pack over her chest and that the pack has a strong odour. She also is drinking herbal tea. When asked about the pack and the tea, she says,

"Oh, my grandmother never used medicines from the doctor. She told me this plaster and tea were all I would need to fix things." Which response by the nurse is most appropriate?
   a. "You really should listen to what the doctor told you if you want to get better."
   b. "What's in the plaster and the tea? When do you usually use them?"
   c. "These herbal remedies rarely work, but if you want to use them, then it is your choice."
   d. "It's fine if you want to use this home remedy, as long as you use it with your prescription medicines."

5. A patient tells the nurse that he has been using an herbal supplement that contains kava for several years to help him to relax in the evening. However, the nurse notes that he has a yellow tinge to his skin and sclera and is concerned about liver toxicity. The nurse advises the patient to stop taking the kava and see his health care provider for an examination. What else, if anything, should the nurse do at this time?
   a. Report this incident to MedEffect.
   b. Notify the provincial or territorial pharmaceutical association.
   c. Contact the supplement manufacturer.
   d. No other action is needed.

6. The nurse is reviewing the drug history of a patient, and during the interview the patient asks, "Why are some drugs over the counter and others are not?" The nurse keeps in mind that criteria for OTC status include which of the following: (Select all that apply.)
   a. The condition must be diagnosed by a health care provider.
   b. The benefits of correct usage of the drug outweigh the risks.
   c. The drug has limited interaction with other drugs.
   d. The drug is easy to use.
   e. The drug company sells OTC drugs at lower prices.

7. A patient comes to the clinic reporting elbow pain after an injury. He states that he has been taking two pain pills, eight times a day, for the past few days. The medication bottle contains acetaminophen, 325-mg tablets. Calculate how much medication he has been taking per day. Is this a safe dose of this medication?

CRITICAL THINKING ACTIVITIES

1. The nurse is discussing OTC drugs and NHPs with neighbours. One neighbour comments, "Oh, the OTC drugs and NHPs are safe. As long as you use the recommended amounts, there won't be any bad side effects." What is the best response from the nurse?

2. The nurse is teaching a patient about pain control at home with OTC products. What teaching points are priorities during the discussion with the patient?

3. A patient tells the clinic nurse that he has been taking a "blood thinner" for several months and wants to ask about taking ginkgo biloba to prevent memory loss. He says his sister uses it and it "works wonders." He also says, "I think it would be safe because I can buy it at the grocery store. They wouldn't sell harmful drugs." What is the nurse's best response to this patient? (You may need to look up the drug warfarin and the herbal product elsewhere in the textbook.)

For answers see http://evolve.elsevier.com/Canada/Lilley/pharmacology/.

CHAPTER 9

Vitamins and Minerals

Objectives

After reading this chapter, the successful student will be able to do the following:

1. Discuss the importance of the various vitamins and minerals to the normal functioning of the human body.

2. Briefly describe the various acute and chronic disease states and conditions that may lead to various imbalances in vitamin and mineral imbalances.

3. Discuss the pathologies that result from vitamin and mineral imbalances.

4. Describe the treatment of these vitamin and mineral imbalances.

5. Identify mechanisms of action, indications, cautions, contraindications, drug interactions, dosages, recommended daily allowances, and routes of administration of each of the vitamins and minerals.

6. Develop a collaborative plan of care related to the use of vitamins and minerals that includes all phases of the nursing process.

e-Learning Activities

Website
(http://evolve.elsevier.com/Canada/
Lilley/pharmacology/)

evolve

- Answer Key—Textbook Case Studies
- Answer Key—Critical Thinking Activities
- Chapter Summaries—Printable
- Review Questions for Exam Preparation
- Unfolding Case Studies

Drug Profiles

- ascorbic acid (vitamin C), p. 145
- calcifediol (vitamin D), p. 137
- calcitriol (vitamin D), p. 137
- calcium, p. 132
- cyanocobalamin (vitamin B_{12}), p. 144
- dihydrotachysterol (vitamin D), p. 137
- ergocalciferol (vitamin D), p. 137
- magnesium, p. 148
- niacin (vitamin B_3), p. 142
- phosphorus, p. 149
- pyridoxine (vitamin B_6), p. 143
- riboflavin (vitamin B_2), p. 141
- thiamine (vitamin B_1), p. 140
- vitamin A, p. 134
- vitamin E, p. 138
- vitamin K_1, p. 139

Key Terms

Beriberi A disease of the peripheral nerves caused by a dietary deficiency of thiamine (vitamin B_1). Symptoms include fatigue, diarrhea, weight loss, edema, heart failure, and disturbed nerve function. (p. 140)

Coenzyme A nonprotein substance that combines with a protein molecule to form an active enzyme. (p. 131)

Enzymes Specialized proteins that catalyze chemical reactions. (p. 131)

Fat-soluble vitamins Vitamins that can be dissolved (i.e., are soluble) in fat. (p. 132)

Minerals Inorganic substances that are ingested and attach to enzymes or other organic molecules. (p. 131)

Pellagra A disease resulting from a deficiency of niacin or a metabolic defect that interferes with the conversion of tryptophan to niacin (vitamin B_3). (p. 140)

Rhodopsin   The purple pigment in the rods of the retina, formed by the protein opsin and a derivative of retinol (vitamin A). (p. 133)

Rickets   A condition caused by a deficiency of vitamin D. (p. 136)

Scurvy   A condition caused by a deficiency of ascorbic acid (vitamin C). (p. 144)

Tocopherols   Biologically active chemicals that make up vitamin E compounds. (p. 137)

Vitamins   Organic compounds essential in small quantities for normal physiological and metabolic functioning of the body. (p. 131)

Water-soluble vitamins   Vitamins that can be dissolved (i.e., are soluble) in water. (p. 132)

OVERVIEW

For the body to grow and maintain itself, it needs the essential building blocks provided by carbohydrates, fats, and proteins. Vitamins and minerals are needed to efficiently utilize these nutrients. **Vitamins** are organic molecules needed in small quantities for normal metabolism and other biochemical functions, such as growth or repair of tissue. Equally important are **minerals**, inorganic elements found naturally in the earth. **Enzymes** are proteins secreted by cells; they act as catalysts to induce chemical changes in other substances. A **coenzyme** is a substance that enhances or is necessary for the action of enzymes. Many enzymes are useless without the appropriate vitamins and minerals that cause them to function properly. Both vitamins and minerals act primarily as coenzymes, binding to enzymes (or other organic molecules) to activate anabolic (tissue-building) processes in the body. For example, coenzyme A is an important carrier molecule associated with the citric acid cycle, one of the body's major energy-producing metabolic reactions. However, it requires pantothenic acid (vitamin B_5) to complete its function in the citric acid cycle.

Vitamins and minerals are essential in our lives, whether or not we make conscious food choices. Under most circumstances, daily requirements of vitamins and minerals are met by ingestion of fluids and balanced meals. Ingesting food maintains adequate stores of essential vitamins and minerals, serves to preserve intestinal structure, provides chemicals for hormones and enzymes, and prevents harmful overgrowth of bacteria.

Various illnesses can cause acute or chronic deficiencies of vitamins, minerals, electrolytes, and fluids. These conditions require replacement or supplementation of these nutrients. Common examples include extensive burn injuries and acquired immune deficiency syndrome (AIDS). Excessive loss of vitamins and minerals may also be the result of poor dietary intake, an inability to swallow after cancer chemotherapy or radiation, or mental health disorders such as anorexia nervosa. Poor dietary absorption can also be caused by various gastrointestinal malabsorption syndromes such as celiac disease, Crohn's disease, or cystic fibrosis. In addition, drug and alcohol misuse are frequently associated with inadequate nutritional intake and absorption that warrants vitamin and mineral supplementation. Deficiencies in dietary protein, fat, and carbohydrates are also common. These nutrients are discussed in Chapter 42. Because of some of their distinct properties and functions in the body related to blood formation, iron and folic acid (vitamin B_9) are discussed separately in Chapter 55.

VITAMINS

The human body requires vitamins in specific minimum amounts on a daily basis, and these can be obtained from both plant and animal food sources. In some cases, the body synthesizes some of its own vitamin supply. Supplemental amounts of vitamin B complex and vitamin K are synthesized by normal bacterial flora in the gastrointestinal tract. Vitamin D can be synthesized by the skin when exposed to sunlight.

An inadequate diet will cause nutrition-related vitamin deficiencies. In 1942, the Nutrition Division of the federal government, in collaboration with the Canadian Council on Nutrition, published Canada's Official Food Rules. Based on six food groups, a list of recommended daily allowances (RDAs) of essential nutrients was identified. In 1944, the RDAs became Canada's Food Rules. There have since been six revisions of the RDAs, with the latest revision in 1992. A newer published standard is the list of dietary reference intakes (DRIs). Whereas the RDAs represented minimum nutrient requirements, the DRIs are designed to represent optimal nutrient requirements for good health. The estimated average requirement (EAR) and the tolerable upper intake level (UL) within the DRIs provide improved tools for use in dietary assessment and planning for individuals and for groups. In Canada, vitamins and minerals are considered natural health products (NHPs) and are governed under the Natural Health Products Regulations. Health Canada requires mandatory detailed nutritional information to be listed on any packaged food product. The values that appear on the labels are the percentage daily values and indicate what percentage of the DRI for a specific nutrient is met by a single serving of the food product. Information regarding DRIs and nutrition labelling is available from the following websites:

1. Health Canada Food and Nutrition: Dietary Reference Intakes   http://www.hc-sc.gc.ca/fn-an/nutrition/reference/index-eng.php

2. Health Canada: Dietary References Intakes Tables: recommended intakes for individuals available at http://www.hc-sc.gc.ca/fn-an/nutrition/reference/table/index-eng.php

Vitamins are classified as either fat soluble or water soluble. **Water-soluble vitamins** can be dissolved in water and are easily excreted in the urine. **Fat-soluble vitamins** are dissolvable in fat. Because water-soluble vitamins (the B-complex group and vitamin C) cannot be stored in the body over long periods, daily intake is required to prevent the development of deficiencies. Conversely, fat-soluble vitamins (vitamins A, D, E, and K) do not need to be taken daily unless one is deficient, because substantial amounts are stored in the liver and fatty tissues. Deficiencies of these vitamins occur only after prolonged deprivation from an adequate supply or from disorders that prevent their absorption. Table 9-1 lists the fat-soluble and water-soluble vitamins.

One controversial topic related to vitamins is that of nutrient "megadosing," as a strategy both for health promotion and maintenance and for treatment of various illnesses. Some cancer patients elect to use supplemental megadosing of specific nutrients in hopes of strengthening their body's response to more conventional cancer treatments. *Megadosing* refers to taking doses of a nutrient that are 10 or more times the recommended amount. A related term was coined in 1968 by the Nobel prize–winning chemist Linus Pauling. He defined *orthomolecular medicine* to be "the preventive or therapeutic use of high-dose vitamins to treat disease." The best-known claim of Dr. Pauling was that megadoses of vitamin C (at more than 100 times Canadian RDA) could prevent or cure the common cold and cancer. Many studies since have not substantiated this claim. However, there are some situations in which nutrient megadosing is known to be helpful, including the following:

- When concurrent long-term drug therapy depletes vitamin stores or otherwise interferes with the function of a vitamin. A common clinical example is the use of vitamin B_6 (pyridoxine) supplementation in patients receiving the drug isoniazid for the treatment of tuberculosis (see Chapter 46).
- In gastrointestinal malabsorption syndromes such as those seen in patients with severe colitis and cystic fibrosis (all major nutrient classes, including protein, fat, carbohydrates, vitamins, and minerals).
- For the treatment of pernicious anemia, which results from vitamin B_{12} (cyanocobalamin) deficiency. The gastrointestinal tract uses a complex mechanism to drive cyanocobalamin absorption. Specifically, a glycoprotein known as *intrinsic factor* is secreted by the parietal cells of the gastric glands (see Chapter 55). Intrinsic factor facilitates absorption of cyanocobalamin in the intestine. When this process is compromised (e.g., by disease), administration of megadoses of cyanocobalamin can bypass this absorption mechanism by allowing a small amount of the vitamin to diffuse on its own through the intestinal mucosa.
- When the vitamin acts as a drug when megadosed. The most common example is niacin (vitamin B_3, also called *nicotinic acid*). At doses of up to 20 mg daily, it functions as a vitamin, but at dosages 50 to 100 times higher, it reduces blood levels of both triglycerides and low-density lipoprotein (LDL) cholesterol (see Chapter 28).

In contrast with the aforementioned examples, there are some situations in which nutrient megadosing is known to be harmful. For example, any excess of one or more nutrients can result in deficiencies of other nutrients because of their chemical "competition" for sites of absorption in the intestinal mucosa. This is likely to be the case with megadosing of minerals, such as with calcium, copper, iron, and zinc, and is less likely to result from vitamin megadosing. Vitamin megadosing can lead to toxic accumulation known as *hypervitaminosis*, especially with the fat-soluble vitamins A, D, and K. Vitamin E appears safer, however, even at doses 10 to 20 times the recommended DRI. Hypervitaminosis is much less likely to occur with the water-soluble vitamins (B complex and C) because they are readily excreted through the urinary system. Nevertheless, it is known that megadosing with

TABLE 9-1

Fat- and Water-Soluble Vitamins

Fat Soluble		Water Soluble	
Designation	**Alternate Name**	**Designation Vitamin B Complex**	**Alternate Name**
vitamin A	retinol	vitamin B_1	thiamine
vitamin D	D_3, cholecalciferol	vitamin B_2	riboflavin
	D_2, ergocalciferol; dihydrotachysterol	vitamin B_3	niacin
vitamin E	tocopherols	vitamin B_5	pantothenic acid
vitamin K	K_1, phytonadione	vitamin B_6	pyridoxine
	K_2, menaquinone	vitamin B_9	folic acid
		vitamin B_{12}	cyanocobalamin
		vitamin B_7	biotin
		vitamin C	ascorbic acid

vitamin B$_6$ (pyridoxine) at 50 to 100 times the DRI can nonetheless cause nerve damage.

A person with an illness may be less tolerate of nutrient megadosing, although megadosing regimens are often prescribed to them. For example, megadosing may be more of a strain for a gastrointestinal tract that is already weakened by illness. Megadosing can interfere with chemotherapy drugs as well as with radiation treatments, because these therapies work to destroy cancer cells through oxidation processes. Nutritional supplementation with antioxidants may impede such treatment mechanisms. Patients need to tell their health care providers any unusual nutritional regimens that they plan to try, especially if they have a serious illness.

FAT-SOLUBLE VITAMINS

Fat-soluble vitamins are not readily excreted in the urine and are stored in the body. Thus, daily ingestion of these vitamins is not necessary to maintain good health and, in fact, is more likely to result in hypervitaminosis.

The fat-soluble vitamins are A, D, E, and K. As a group, they share the following characteristics:
- They are present in both plant and animal foods.
- They are stored primarily in the liver.
- They exhibit slow metabolism or breakdown.
- They are excreted via the feces.
- They can reach toxic levels (*hypervitaminosis*) if excessive amounts are consumed. Owing to their ability to accumulate in the body, fat-soluble vitamins have a higher potential for toxicity than water-soluble vitamins do. Iron-containing vitamins are the most toxic.

Table 9-2 lists the food sources for several nutrients.

VITAMIN A

Vitamin A (retinol) is derived from animal fats such as those found in dairy products, eggs, meat, liver, and fish liver oils. It is also derived from carotenes, which are found in plants (green and yellow vegetables, yellow fruits). Therefore, vitamin A is an exogenous substance for humans because it must be obtained from either plant or animal foods. There are more than 600 naturally occurring carotenoid compounds in plant-based foods. Of these, 40 to 50 occur commonly in the human diet. Beta carotene is the most prevalent of these, followed by alpha carotene and cryptoxanthin. These are known as *provitamin A carotenoids* because they are all metabolized to various forms of vitamin A in the body.

Mechanism of Action and Drug Effects

Vitamin A is essential for night vision and for normal vision because it is part of one of the major retinal pigments called **rhodopsin**. Beta carotene is metabolized in the body to retinal (retinaldehyde), and some of this retinal is reduced to the alcohol compound known as

TABLE 9-2

Food Sources of Selected Nutrients

Vitamins/Minerals	Food Sources
vitamin A	Liver; fish; dairy products; egg yolks; dark green, leafy, yellow–orange vegetables and fruits
vitamin D	Dairy products, fortified cereals and fortified orange juice, liver, fish liver oils, saltwater fish, butter, eggs
vitamin E	Fish, egg yolks, meats, vegetable oils, nuts, fruits, wheat germ, grains, fortified cereals
vitamin K	Cheese, spinach, broccoli, Brussels sprouts, kale, cabbage, turnip greens, soybean oils
vitamin B$_1$ (thiamine)	Yeast, liver, enriched whole-grain products, beans
vitamin B$_2$ (riboflavin)	Meats, liver, dairy products, eggs, legumes, nuts, enriched whole-grain products, green leafy vegetables, yeast
vitamin B$_3$ (niacin)	Liver, turkey, tuna, peanuts, beans, yeast, enriched whole-grain breads and cereals, wheat germ
vitamin B$_6$ (pyridoxine)	Organ meats, meats, poultry, fish, eggs, peanuts, whole-grain products, vegetables, nuts, wheat germ, bananas, fortified cereals
vitamin B$_{12}$ (cyanocobalamin)	Liver, kidney, shellfish, poultry, fish, eggs, milk, blue cheese, fortified cereals
vitamin C (ascorbic acid)	Broccoli, green peppers, spinach, Brussels sprouts, citrus fruits, tomatoes, potatoes, strawberries, cabbage, liver
Calcium	Dairy products, fortified cereals and calcium-fortified orange juice, sardines, salmon
Magnesium	Meats, seafood, milk, cheese, yogourt, green leafy vegetables, bran cereal, nuts
Phosphorus	Milk, yogurt, cheese, peas, meats, fish, eggs
Zinc	Red meats, liver, oysters, certain seafood, milk products, eggs, beans, nuts, whole grains, fortified cereals

retinol. Retinol is involved in the maintenance of the integrity of mucosal and epithelial surfaces as well as cholesterol and steroid synthesis. The remainder of the retinal may be oxidized to the carboxylic acid compound retinoic acid. Unlike retinal, retinoic acid has no direct role in vision, but it is essential for normal cell growth and differentiation and for the development of the physical shapes of the body's many parts—a process known as *morphogenesis*. It is also involved in the growth and development of bones and teeth and in other body processes, including reproduction, integrity of mucosal and epithelial surfaces, and cholesterol and steroid synthesis.

Indications

Supplements of vitamin A may be used to satisfy normal body requirements or an increased demand such as in infants and in pregnant and nursing women. A normal diet usually provides adequate amounts of vitamin A, but in cases of excessive need or inadequate dietary intake, vitamin A supplementation is indicated. Symptoms of vitamin A deficiency include night blindness, xerophthalmia, keratomalacia (softening of the cornea), hyperkeratosis of both the stratum corneum (outermost layer) of the skin and the sclera (outermost layer of eyeball), retarded infant growth, generalized weakness, and increased susceptibility of mucous membranes to infection. Vitamin A–related compounds, such as isotretinoin, are also used to treat various skin conditions, including acne, psoriasis, and keratosis follicularis.

Contraindications

Contraindications to vitamin A supplementation include known allergy to the individual vitamin product; known current state of hypervitaminosis; and excessive supplementation beyond recommended guidelines, especially in oral malabsorption syndromes. Vitamin A is considered highly teratogenic in pregnancy, particularly in the first 8 weeks, with daily intake more than 10 000 units (Rosenbloom, 2014).

Adverse Effects

There are minimal acute adverse effects associated with normal vitamin A ingestion. Only after long-term excessive ingestion of vitamin A do symptoms appear. Adverse effects are usually noticed in bones, mucous membranes, the liver, and the skin. Table 9-3 lists some of the symptoms of long-term excessive ingestion of vitamin A.

Toxicity and Management of Overdose

The major toxic effects of vitamin A result from ingestion of excessive amounts, which occurs most commonly in children. A few hours after administration of an excess dose of vitamin A, irritability, drowsiness, vertigo, delirium, coma, vomiting, or diarrhea may occur. In infants, excessive amounts of vitamin A can cause an increase in intracranial pressure, resulting in symptoms such as bulging fontanelles, headache, papilledema, exophthalmos (bulging eyeballs), and visual disturbances. Papilledema is the presence of edematous fluid, often including blood, in the optic disc. This is the portion of the eye in the back of the retina, where nerve fibres converge to form the optic nerve. Over several weeks, a generalized peeling of the skin and erythema (skin reddening) may occur. These symptoms seem to disappear a few days after discontinuation of the drug, which is the only treatment necessary in situations of overdose.

Interactions

Vitamin A is absorbed less when used together with lubricant laxatives and cholestyramine. In addition, the concurrent use of isotretinoin and vitamin A supplementation can result in additive effects and possible toxicity.

Dosages

For dosage information on vitamin A, refer to the table on p. 134.

TABLE 9-3

Vitamin A: Adverse Effects

Body System	Adverse Effects
Central nervous	Headache, increased intracranial pressure, lethargy, malaise
Gastrointestinal	Nausea, vomiting, anorexia, abdominal pain, jaundice
Integumentary	Dry skin, pruritus, increased pigmentation, night sweats
Metabolic	Hypomenorrhea, hypercalcemia
Musculoskeletal	Arthralgia, retarded growth

DRUG PROFILE

There are three forms of vitamin A: retinol, retinyl palmitate, and retinyl acetate. Medications containing vitamin A may require a prescription, but many over-the-counter products, such as vitamin A–containing multivitamins, are also available. All vitamin A products are safe to use during pregnancy.

▸▸*vitamin A*

Vitamin A, also known as *retinol*, *retinyl palmitate*, and *retinyl acetate*, is available in a variety of oral forms. Doses for vitamin A are expressed as *retinol activity equivalents (RAEs)*. One RAE is approximately equal to the following:

- 1 mcg of retinol (either dietary or supplemental)
- 2 mcg of supplemental β-carotene
- 12 mcg of dietary β-carotene
- 24 mcg of dietary carotenoids

PHARMACOKINETICS

Route	Onset of Action	Peak Plasma Concentration	Elimination Half-Life	Duration of Action
PO	N/A	4 hr	50–100 days	Unknown

DOSAGES   Selected Vitamins

Drug	Pharmacological Class	Usual Dosage Range	Indications/Uses
VITAMIN D–ACTIVE COMPOUNDS			
calcifediol	Fat-soluble	*Adults and children* PO: 50 mcg once daily	Hypocalcemia in patients receiving hemodialysis
calcitriol	Fat-soluble	*Adults and children* 6 yr and older PO/IV: 0.25–1 mcg/day	Hypoparathyroidism; hypocalcemia in patients receiving hemodialysis
cholecalciferol (vitamin D_3)	Fat-soluble	*Adults and children older than 9 yr* 600–800 units/day (max 4000 units/day) Children aged 0–4 yrs 400–600 units/day (max 1000–3000/day)	Vitamin D deficiency
VITAMIN B–ACTIVE COMPOUNDS			
vitamin B_1 (thiamine)	Water-soluble, B complex group	*Adults* 100 mg/day until normal dietary intake is established 5–30 mg/day × 30 days	Alcohol-induced deficiency Beriberi
vitamin B_2 (riboflavin)	Water-soluble, B complex group	*Adults* PO: 5–30 mg/day *Children* 3–10 mg/day	Deficiency
vitamin B_3 (niacin, niacinamide)	Water-soluble, B complex group	*Adults* PO: 1.5–6 g/day 300–500 mg/day Children IV: Up to 300 mg/day	Dyslipidemia Pellagra (deficiency) Deficiency
vitamin B_6	Water-soluble, B complex group	*Adults* PO/IV: 2.5–10 mg/day *Children* PO/IV: 5–25 mg/day × 3 wk, then give multivitamin product *Adults* PO/IV: 100–200 mg/day Children PO: 100–200 mg/kg/day	Deficiency Drug-induced neuritis (e.g., isoniazid for tuberculosis) Deficiency; anemia
vitamin B_{12} (cyanocobalamin)	Water-soluble, B complex group	*Adults and children* IM/Subcut: 100 mcg/mo PO: 50–100 mcg/day	Deficiency; anemia
VITAMINS A, C, E, AND K			
vitamin A	Fat-soluble	*Children 1–18 yr* PO: 30–3000 mcg RAE/day	Deficiency
vitamin C (ascorbic acid)	Water-soluble	*Adults* PO/IV/IM/SC: 100–250 mg daily–bid × 3 wk *Children* PO/IV: 100–300 mg/day	Deficiency (scurvy)
vitamin E	Fat-soluble	*Adults* PO: 60–75 units/day	Deficiency
vitamin K (phytonadione)	Fat-soluble	*Adults* IM/Subcut: 2.5–10 mg single dose Infants and Children IM/Subcut: 2.5–10 mg single dose; may repeat in 4–6 hr Infants IM/Subcut: 1 mg single dose	Deficiency; warfarin-induced hypoprothrombinemia Hemorrhagic disease of newborn

*Adequate dietary intake is always preferred over supplementation to prevent vitamin deficiencies.

VITAMIN D

Vitamin D, also called the *sunshine vitamin*, is responsible for the proper utilization of calcium and phosphorus in the body. The two most important members of the vitamin D family are vitamin D_2 (ergocalciferol) and vitamin D_3 (cholecalciferol). They have different sites of origin but similar functions in the body. Ergocalciferol is plant derived and is therefore obtained through dietary sources. The natural form of vitamin D produced in the skin by ultraviolet irradiation from the sun is chemically known as *7-dehydrocholesterol*. It is more commonly referred to as *cholecalciferol*. This endogenous synthesis of vitamin D_3 usually produces sufficient amounts to meet daily requirements. Vitamin D is obtained through both endogenous synthesis and consumption of vitamin D_2–containing foods such as fish oils, salmon, sardines, and herring; fortified milk, bread, and cereals; and animal livers, tuna fish, eggs, and butter. Normal serum levels are 50 nmol/L.

Mechanism of Action and Drug Effects

The basic function of vitamin D is to regulate the absorption and subsequent utilization of calcium and phosphorus. It is also necessary for the normal calcification of bone. Vitamin D in coordination with parathyroid hormone and calcitonin regulates serum calcium levels by increasing calcium absorption from the small intestine and extracting calcium from the bone. Ergocalciferol and cholecalciferol are inactive and require transformation into active metabolites for biological activity. Both vitamin D_2 and vitamin D_3 are biotransformed in the liver by the actions of the parathyroid hormone. The resulting compound, calcifediol, is then transported to the kidney, where it is converted to calcitriol, which is believed to be the most physiologically active form of vitamin D. Calcitriol promotes the intestinal absorption of calcium and phosphorus and the deposition of calcium and phosphorus into the structure of teeth and bones.

The drug effects of vitamin D are similar to those of vitamin A and essentially all vitamin and mineral compounds. It is used as a supplement to satisfy normal daily requirements or an increased demand, as in infants and in pregnant and nursing women.

Indications

Vitamin D can be used either to supplement dietary intake of vitamin D or to treat a deficiency of vitamin D. When used to supplement dietary intake, it is given prophylactically to prevent deficiency-related problems, and it is recommended for breastfed infants. Vitamin D may also be used to treat and correct the results of a long-term deficiency that leads to such conditions as infantile rickets, tetany (involuntary sustained muscular contractions), and osteomalacia (softening of bones). **Rickets** is specifically a vitamin D deficiency state. Symptoms include soft, pliable bones, which causes deformities such as bow legs and knock knees; nodular enlargement on the ends and sides of the bones; muscle pain; enlarged skull; chest deformities; spinal curvature; enlargement of the liver and spleen; profuse sweating; and general tenderness of the body when touched. Vitamin D can also help promote the absorption of phosphorus and calcium. For this reason, its use is important in preventing osteoporosis. Because of the role of vitamin D in the regulation of calcium and phosphorus, it may be used to correct deficiencies of these two elements. Other uses include dietary supplementation and treatment of osteodystrophy, hypocalcemia, hypoparathyroidism, pseudohypoparathyroidism, and hypophosphatemia. Many patients have vitamin D deficiency and it is common to see doses of 1 000 to 2 000 or more units daily prescribed.

There were some early indications that maintaining adequate levels of vitamin D may have a protective effect and lower the risk of developing multiple sclerosis. However, there have been no current, evidence-informed studies to support this theory.

Contraindications

Contraindications to vitamin D products include known allergy to the product, hypercalcemia, kidney dysfunction, kidney stones, and hyperphosphatemia.

Adverse Effects

Few acute adverse effects are associated with normal vitamin D ingestion. Only after long-term excessive ingestion of vitamin D do symptoms appear. Such effects are usually noticed in the gastrointestinal tract or the central nervous system (CNS) and are listed in Table 9-4.

Toxicity and Management of Overdose

The major toxic effects from ingesting excessive amounts of vitamin D occur most commonly in children. Discontinuation of vitamin D and reduced calcium intake reverse the toxic state. Toxicity occurs because vitamin D is fat-soluble and is stored in the body's fat supply. The amount of vitamin D considered to be toxic varies considerably among individuals. In adults, a dose of 50 000 IU per day of vitamin D can eventually increase blood levels to

TABLE 9-4	
Vitamin D: Adverse Effects	
Body System	**Adverse Effects**
Cardiovascular	Hypertension, dysrhythmias
Central nervous	Fatigue, weakness, drowsiness, headache
Gastrointestinal	Nausea, vomiting, anorexia, cramps, metallic taste, dry mouth, constipation
Genitourinary	Polyuria, albuminuria, increased blood urea nitrogen level
Musculoskeletal	Decreased bone growth, bone pain, muscle pain

more than 374 nmol/L; at these concentrations, abnormal levels of calcium and phosphorus can also build up in the blood. However, 10 000 to 14 000 units daily have not produced toxic effects.

The toxic effects of vitamin D are those associated with hypertension, such as weakness, fatigue, headache, anorexia, dry mouth, metallic taste, nausea, vomiting, ataxia, and bone pain. If not recognized and treated, these symptoms can progress to impairment of kidney function and osteoporosis.

Interactions

Reduced absorption of vitamin D occurs with the concurrent use of lubricant laxatives and cholestyramine.

Dosages

For dosage information on vitamin D, refer to the table on p. 135.

VITAMIN E

Four biologically active chemicals called **tocopherols** (alpha [α], beta [β], gamma [γ], and delta [δ]) make up the vitamin E compounds. Alpha-tocopherol is the most biologically active, natural form of vitamin E and can come from plant and animal sources.

Mechanism of Action and Drug Effects

Vitamin E is a powerful biological antioxidant and an essential component of the diet. Its exact nutritional function has not been fully demonstrated. The only recognized significant deficiency syndrome for vitamin E occurs in premature infants. In this situation, vitamin E deficiency may result in irritability, edema, thrombosis, and hemolytic anemia.

The drug effects of vitamin E are not as well defined as those of the other fat-soluble vitamins. It is believed to protect polyunsaturated fatty acids, a component of cellular membranes. It has also been shown to hinder the deterioration of substances such as vitamin A and ascorbic acid (vitamin C), two substances that are highly oxygen sensitive and readily oxidized; thus, it acts as an antioxidant.

Indications

Vitamin E is most commonly used as a dietary supplement to augment current daily intake or to treat a deficiency. Premature infants are at greatest risk of complications from vitamin E deficiency. Vitamin E has received much attention for its function as an antioxidant. Free radical damage contributes to the early stages of atherosclerosis and may also contribute to cancer, heart disease, and numerous other chronic diseases. Early studies such as the Nurses' Health Study showed promise for vitamin E's role as a scavenger for the damaging free radicals, with beneficial effects for patients with cancer, heart disease, Alzheimer's disease, premenstrual syndrome, and sexual dysfunction. Results from the Heart Outcomes Prevention Evaluation (HOPE) trial also showed no benefit of 4 years of vitamin E

 DRUG PROFILES

▸▸ vitamin D

There are four forms of vitamin D: calcifediol, calcitriol, dihydrotachysterol, and ergocalciferol. Vitamin D is available in over-the-counter preparations—such as multivitamin products—or by prescription. They are considered safe to use during pregnancy as long as the patient is not dosed at higher levels than recommended.

▸▸ calcitriol

Calcitriol (Rocaltrol®), a steroid hormone, is the 1,25-dihydroxylated form of cholecalciferol (vitamin D₃). It is a vitamin-D analogue used for the management of hypocalcemia in patients with chronic kidney failure, on dialysis, as well as for the management of secondary hyperparathyroidism in patients not yet on dialysis. Calcitriol is also used in the treatment of hypoparathyroidism and pseudohypoparathyroidism, vitamin D–dependent rickets, hypophosphatemia, and hypocalcemia in premature infants. Calcitriol is available for oral use.

▸▸ dihydrotachysterol

Dihydrotachysterol is a vitamin-D analogue that is administered orally, once daily, for the treatment of any of the previously mentioned conditions. It is available orally in combination with calcium carbonate.

▸▸ ergocalciferol

Ergocalciferol (Osto-D₂®) is vitamin D₂. It is indicated for use in patients with gastrointestinal, liver, or biliary disease associated with malabsorption of vitamin-D analogues. It is available orally.

PHARMACOKINETICS (ERGOCALCIFEROL, VITAMIN D₂)

Route	Onset of Action	Peak Plasma Concentration	Elimination Half-Life	Duration of Action
PO	30 days	Unknown	19 days	Months to years

PHARMACOKINETICS

Route	Onset of Action	Peak Plasma Concentration	Elimination Half-Life	Duration of Action
PO	Less than 3 hr	3–6 hr	3–6 hr	3–5 days

supplementation among the 9 500 men and women already diagnosed with heart disease or at high risk for it. In fact, when the HOPE trial was extended for an additional 4 years, researchers found a higher risk of heart failure in those subjects. The Heart and Stroke Foundation (2015) recommends a healthy diet that includes vitamin E (e.g., pecans, walnuts, almonds). As well, vitamin E supplement use has no immediate or long-term effects on cancer risk (Chan, 2015).

Free radicals can also damage collagen and cause skin dryness, fine lines, and wrinkles. Vitamin E is available in many skin creams and ointments; it is thought to provide protection against ultraviolent radiation.

Contraindications

Contraindications for vitamin E include known allergy to a specific vitamin E product. There are currently no approved injectable forms of this vitamin.

Adverse Effects

Few acute adverse effects are associated with normal vitamin E ingestion, because it is relatively nontoxic. Adverse effects are usually noticed in the GI tract or CNS and are listed in Table 9-5.

Dosages

For the dosage information on vitamin E, refer to the table on p. 135.

VITAMIN K

Vitamin K is the last of the four fat-soluble vitamins (A, D, E, and K). There are three types of vitamin K: phytonadione (vitamin K_1), menaquinone (vitamin K_2), and menadione (vitamin K_3). The body does not store large amounts of vitamin K; however, vitamin K_2 is synthesized by the intestinal flora, which provides an endogenous supply. Vitamin K is essential for the synthesis of blood coagulation factors, which takes place in the liver. Vitamin K–dependent blood coagulation factors are factors II, VII, IX, and X. Other names for these clotting factors are as follows: factor II (prothrombin), factor VII (proconvertin), factor IX (Christmas factor), and factor X (Stuart-Prower factor). Minimum daily requirements have been estimated at 1 to 5 mcg/kg for infants and 0.03 mcg/kg for adults. There is no commercially available oral formulation of vitamin K1; however, the injectable formulation has been used orally. It is usually administered by intramuscular or subcutaneous route, but the intravenous route can be used cautiously.

Vitamin K also plays a role in converting osteocalcin, a non-collagen protein found in the bone, into its active form. Osteocalcin, once activated, serves to anchor calcium into place within the bone.

Mechanism of Action and Drug Effects

Vitamin K activity is essential for effective blood clotting because, as noted earlier, it facilitates the liver biosynthesis of factors II, VII, IX, and X. Vitamin K deficiency results in coagulation disorders caused by hypoprothrombinemia. Coagulation defects affecting these clotting factors can be corrected with administration of vitamin K. Vitamin K deficiency is rare because intestinal flora is normally able to synthesize sufficient amounts. If a deficiency develops, it can be corrected with vitamin K supplementation.

Indications

Vitamin K is indicated for dietary supplementation and for treatment of deficiency states. Although rare, deficiency states can develop with inadequate dietary intake or inhibition of the intestinal flora resulting from the administration of broad-spectrum antibiotics. Deficiency states can also be seen in newborns because of malabsorption attributable to inadequate amounts of bile. For this reason, infants born in hospitals are often given a prophylactic intramuscular dose of vitamin K on arrival to the nursery. Vitamin K may also be used to reverse excessive anti-coagulation if the patient has evidence of bleeding (as measured by the international normalized ratio [INR]).

Vitamin K deficiency can also result from the administration and pharmacological action of the oral

TABLE 9-5
Vitamin E: Adverse Effects

Body System	Adverse Effects
Central nervous	Fatigue, headache, blurred vision
Gastrointestinal	Nausea, diarrhea, flatulence
Genitourinary	Increased blood urea nitrogen
Musculoskeletal	Weakness

DRUG PROFILE

▶▶*vitamin E*

Vitamin E is available as an over-the-counter medication. It has four forms: alpha (α), beta (β), gamma (γ), and delta (δ) tocopherol. It is available in many multivitamin preparations and is also available by prescription.

Vitamin E products are usually contraindicated only in cases of known drug allergy. Vitamin E (Aquasol E®) activity is generally expressed in US Pharmacopeia (USP) or international units. It is available for oral and injection use.

anticoagulant warfarin sodium (see Chapter 27). Warfarin sodium's anticoagulant effects occur by inhibiting vitamin K–dependent clotting factors II, VII, IX, and X in the liver. Administration of vitamin K overrides the mechanism by which the anticoagulant inhibits production of vitamin K–dependent clotting factors. Thus vitamin K can be used to reverse the effects of warfarin sodium. It is important to note that when vitamin K is used in this manner, the patient becomes unresponsive to warfarin sodium for approximately 1 week after vitamin K administration. When vitamin K_1 is deficient, it can lead to impaired mineralization of the bone due to diminished functioning of osteocalcin. Osteoporosis increases one's risk of fracture. It has been shown that the greater the deficiency in vitamin K, the greater the severity of the fracture.

Contraindications

The only usual contraindication to treatment with vitamin K is known drug allergy.

Adverse Effects

Vitamin K is relatively nontoxic and thus causes minimal adverse effects. Severe reactions limited to hypersensitivity or anaphylaxis have occurred rarely, during or immediately after intravenous administration. Adverse effects are usually related to injection-site reactions and hypersensitivity. See Table 9-6 for a list of such major effects by body system.

Toxicity and Management of Overdose

Toxicity is limited primarily to use in the newborn. Hemolysis of red blood cells (RBCs) can occur, especially in infants with low levels of glucose-6-phosphate dehydrogenase (G6PD). In severe cases, replacement with blood products may be indicated.

Dosages

For dosage information on vitamin K, refer to the table on p. 135.

WATER-SOLUBLE VITAMINS

The water-soluble vitamins include the vitamin B complex and vitamin C (ascorbic acid). They are present in a variety of plant and animal food sources. The vitamin B complex is a group of 10 vitamins that are often found together in food, although they are chemically dissimilar and have different metabolic functions. Because the B vitamins were originally isolated from the same sources, they were grouped together as B-complex vitamins. Vitamin C (ascorbic acid), the other principal water-soluble vitamin, is concentrated in citrus fruits and is not classified as part of the B complex. The numeric subscripts associated with the various B vitamins reflect the order in which they were discovered. In clinical practice, some B vitamins are more often referred to by their common name, whereas others are more often referred to by their numeric designation.

For example, *vitamin B_{12}* is used more often in clinical practice than the corresponding common name, *cyanocobalamin*. However, *folic acid* is rarely referred to as *vitamin B_9*, although this would also be correct. The most commonly used B-complex vitamins, as well as vitamin C, are listed in Table 9-1 on p. 132. Folic acid (vitamin B_9) has a special role in hematopoiesis and therefore is described further in Chapter 55.

TABLE	9-6

Vitamin K: Adverse Effects

Body System	Adverse Effects
Central nervous	Headache, brain damage (large doses)
Gastrointestinal	Nausea, decreased liver enzyme levels
Hematological	Hemolytic anemia, hemoglobinuria, hyperbilirubinemia
Integumentary	Rash, urticaria

 DRUG PROFILE

The most commonly used form of vitamin K is phytonadione (vitamin K_1), which is available by prescription only in parenteral form. Menadione (vitamin K_3) is not available in Canada and is contraindicated in patients with a known hypersensitivity. Its use is also contraindicated in patients who are in the last few weeks of pregnancy and in patients with severe liver disease. Vitamin K must be used with caution in patients taking warfarin sodium.

▶▶ vitamin K_1

Vitamin K_1 (phytonadione) is available in injectable form and is usually administered by the intramuscular or subcutaneous route. Because of its potential to cause anaphylaxis (due to the formulation), for intravenous use it is usually diluted and given over 30 to 60 minutes. Vitamin K is given IV and not intramuscularly when used to reverse the effects of warfarin sodium.

PHARMACOKINETICS

Route	Onset of Action	Peak Plasma Concentration	Elimination Half-Life	Duration of Action
IV	1–2 hr	12–14 hr	1.2 hr	24 hr

Water-soluble vitamins are a chemically diverse group sharing only the characteristic of being dissolvable in water. Like fat-soluble vitamins, they act primarily as coenzymes or oxidation-reduction agents in important metabolic pathways. Unlike fat-soluble vitamins, water-soluble vitamins are not stored in the body in appreciable amounts. Their water-soluble properties promote urinary excretion and reduce their half-life in the body. Therefore, dietary intake must be adequate and regular or deficiency states will develop. The body excretes what it does not need, which makes toxic reactions to water-soluble vitamins rare.

VITAMIN B₁

A deficiency of vitamin B_1 (thiamine) results in the classic disease **beriberi** or Wernicke's encephalopathy (cerebral beriberi). Common findings in beriberi include brain lesions, polyneuropathy of peripheral nerves, serous effusions (abnormal collections of fluids in body tissues), and cardiac anatomical changes. Vitamin deficiency can result from poor diet, extended fever, hyperthyroidism, liver disease, alcoholism, malabsorption, and pregnancy and breastfeeding. Normal serum levels are 0.75–222 nmol/L.

Mechanism of Action and Drug Effects

Vitamin B_1 (thiamine) is an essential precursor for the formation of thiamine pyrophosphate. When thiamine combines with adenosine triphosphate (ATP), the result is thiamine pyrophosphate coenzyme. This is required for the citric acid cycle (Krebs cycle), a major part of carbohydrate metabolism, as well as several other metabolic pathways. In addition, thiamine plays a key role in the integrity of the peripheral nervous system, cardiovascular system, and gastrointestinal tract.

Indications

The essential role of thiamine in many metabolic pathways makes it useful in treating a variety of metabolic disorders. These include subacute necrotizing encephalomyelopathy, maple syrup urine disease, and lactic acidosis associated with pyruvate carboxylase enzyme deficiency and hyper-β-alaninemia. Some of the deficiency states treated by thiamine are beriberi, Wernicke's encephalopathy syndrome, peripheral neuritis associated with **pellagra** (niacin deficiency), and neuritis of pregnancy. Thiamine is used as a dietary supplement to prevent or treat deficiency in cases of malabsorption, such as that induced by alcoholism, cirrhosis, or gastrointestinal disease. Other situations in which thiamine may have therapeutic value are poor appetite, ulcerative colitis, chronic diarrhea, and cerebellar syndrome or ataxia (impaired muscular coordination). Although it has been suggested, studies do not support the use of oral vitamin B as an insect repellent.

Contraindications

The only usual contraindication to any of the B-complex vitamins is known allergy to a specific vitamin product.

Adverse Effects

Adverse effects are rare but include hypersensitivity reactions, nausea, restlessness, pulmonary edema, pruritus, urticaria, weakness, sweating, angioedema, cyanosis, and cardiovascular collapse. Administration by intramuscular injection can produce local tenderness, and intravenous injections can produce anaphylaxis.

Interactions

Thiamine is incompatible with alkaline- and sulfite-containing solutions.

Dosages

For the dosage information on vitamin B_1, refer to the table on p. 140.

VITAMIN B₂

A deficiency of vitamin B_2 (riboflavin) results in cutaneous, oral, and corneal changes that include cheilosis (chapped or fissured lips), seborrheic dermatitis, and keratitis.

Mechanism of Action and Drug Effects

Riboflavin serves several important functions in the body. Riboflavin is converted into two coenzymes (flavin mononucleotide and flavin adenine dinucleotide) that are essential for tissue respiration. Riboflavin also plays an important part in carbohydrate catabolism. Another B vitamin, vitamin B_6 (pyridoxine), requires riboflavin for activation. Riboflavin is also needed to convert tryptophan into niacin and to maintain erythrocyte integrity. Deficiency is rare and does not usually occur in healthy people.

 ## DRUG PROFILE

▸▸*thiamine*

Thiamine is contraindicated in individuals with a known hypersensitivity to it. It is available for both oral (in combination) and parenteral use. It is safe to use during pregnancy.

PHARMACOKINETICS

Route	Onset of Action	Peak Plasma Concentration	Elimination Half-Life	Duration of Action
PO	Unknown	1–2 hr	1.2 hr	24 hr

Indications

Riboflavin is used primarily as a dietary supplement and for treatment of deficiency states. Patients who may experience riboflavin deficiency include those with long-standing infections, liver disease, alcoholism, or malignancy and those taking probenecid. Riboflavin supplementation may also be beneficial in the treatment of microcytic anemia; acne; migraine headache; congenital methemoglobinemia (presence in the blood of an abnormal, nonfunctional hemoglobin pigment); muscle cramps; and Gopalan's syndrome, a symptom of suspected riboflavin (and possibly pantothenic acid [vitamin B_5]) deficiency that involves a sensation of tingling in the extremities (for this reason, it is also called *burning feet syndrome*).

Contraindications

The only usual contraindication to riboflavin is known allergy to a given vitamin product.

Adverse Effects

Riboflavin is a safe and effective vitamin; to date, no adverse effects or toxic effects have been reported. In large doses, riboflavin will discolour urine to yellow–orange.

Dosages

For dosage information on riboflavin, refer to the table on p. 141.

VITAMIN B_3

The body is able to produce a small amount of vitamin B_3 (niacin) from dietary tryptophan, an essential amino acid occurring in dietary proteins and some commercially available nutritional supplements. A dietary deficiency of niacin will produce the classic symptoms known as *pellagra*. Symptoms of pellagra include various psychotic disorders; neurasthenic syndrome; crusting, erythema, and desquamation of the skin; scaly dermatitis; inflammation of the oral, vaginal, and urethral mucosa, including glossitis (inflamed tongue); and diarrhea or bloody diarrhea.

Mechanism of Action and Drug Effects

The metabolic actions of niacin (vitamin B_3) are not because of niacin in the ingested form but rather its metabolic product, nicotinamide. Nicotinamide is required for numerous metabolic reactions, including those involved in carbohydrate, protein, purine, and lipid metabolism, as well as tissue respiration (Figure 9-1). A key example involves two compounds, nicotinamide adenine dinucleotide (NAD) and nicotinamide adenine dinucleotide phosphate (NADP), both of which are necessary for the carbohydrate pathway known as *glycogenolysis* (the breakdown of stored glycogen to usable glucose). The parent compound, niacin, also has a pharmacological role as an antilipemic drug (see Chapter 28). The doses of niacin required for its antilipemic effect are substantially higher than those required for the nutritional and metabolic effects.

Indications

Niacin is indicated for the prevention and treatment of pellagra, a condition caused by a deficiency of vitamin B_3 that is most commonly the result of malabsorption. It is also used for management for certain types of dyslipidemia (see Chapter 28). Niacin also has a beneficial effect in peripheral vascular disease.

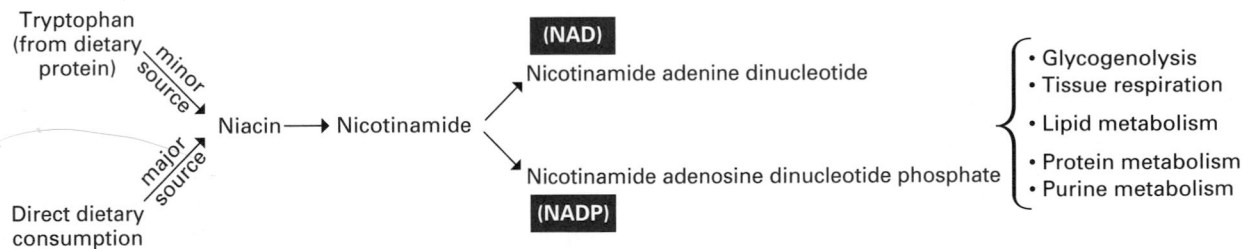

FIG. 9-1 Niacin, once in the body, is converted to nicotinamide adenine dinucleotide (NAD) and nicotinamide adenosine dinucleotide phosphate (NADP), which are coenzymes needed for many metabolic processes.

DRUG PROFILE

▸▸ *riboflavin*

Riboflavin (vitamin B_2) is needed for normal respiratory reactions. It is a safe, nontoxic water-soluble vitamin with almost no adverse effects. It is available for oral and parenteral use. It is safe to use during pregnancy.

PHARMACOKINETICS

Route	Onset of Action	Peak Plasma Concentration	Elimination Half-Life	Duration of Action
PO	Unknown	Unknown	66–84 min	24 hr

Contraindications

Niacin, unlike certain other B-complex vitamins, has additional contraindications besides drug allergy. These include liver disease, severe hypotension, arterial hemorrhage, and active peptic ulcer disease.

Adverse Effects

The most frequent adverse effects associated with the use of niacin are flushing, pruritus, and gastrointestinal distress. These usually subside with continued use and are most frequently seen when larger doses of niacin are used in the treatment of dyslipidemia. Table 9-7 lists adverse effects by body system.

Dosages

For dosage information on niacin, refer to the Drug Profile box below.

VITAMIN B$_6$

Vitamin B$_6$ (pyridoxine) is composed of three compounds: pyridoxine, pyridoxal, and pyridoxamine. Deficiency of vitamin B$_6$ can lead to a type of anemia known as *sideroblastic anemia*, neurological disturbances, seborrheic dermatitis, cheilosis, and xanthurenic aciduria (formation of xanthine crystals or "stones" in urine). It may also result in convulsions, especially in neonates and infants; hypochromic microcytic anemia; and glossitis (inflamed tongue) and stomatitis (inflamed oral mucosa). Pyridoxine deficiency also affects the peripheral nerves, skin, and mucous membranes. Inadequate intake or poor absorption of pyridoxine causes the development of these conditions. Vitamin B$_6$ deficiency may occur as a result of uremia, alcoholism, cirrhosis, hyperthyroidism, malabsorption syndromes, and heart failure. It may also be induced by various drugs, such as isoniazid and hydralazine.

Mechanism of Action and Drug Effects

Pyridoxine, pyridoxal, and pyridoxamine are all converted in erythrocytes to the active coenzyme forms of vitamin B$_6$, pyridoxal phosphate and pyridoxamine phosphate. These compounds are necessary for many metabolic functions, such as protein, carbohydrate, and lipid utilization in the body. They also play an important part in the conversion of amino acid tryptophan to niacin (vitamin B$_3$) and the neurotransmitter serotonin. They are essential in the synthesis of γ-aminobutyric acid (GABA), an inhibitory neurotransmitter in the central nervous system. They are important in the synthesis of heme and the maintenance of the hematopoietic system. In addition, these substances are necessary for the integrity of the peripheral nerves, skin, and mucous membranes.

Indications

Pyridoxine is used to prevent and treat vitamin B$_6$ deficiency. This includes deficiency that can result from therapy with certain medications, including isoniazid (for tuberculosis) and hydralazine (for hypertension). Although vitamin B$_6$ deficiency is rare, it can occur in conditions of inadequate intake or poor absorption of pyridoxine. Seizures that are unresponsive to usual therapy, morning sickness during pregnancy, and metabolic disorders may respond to pyridoxine therapy.

Contraindications

The only usual contraindication to pyridoxine use is known drug allergy.

Adverse Effects

Adverse effects with pyridoxine use are rare and usually do not occur at normal dosages; high dosages and long-term use may produce the adverse effects listed in

TABLE	9-7

Niacin: Adverse Effects

Body System	Adverse Effects
Cardiovascular	Postural hypotension, dysrhythmias
Central nervous	Headache, dizziness, anxiety
Gastrointestinal	Nausea, vomiting, diarrhea, peptic ulcer
Genitourinary	Hyperuricemia
Hepatic	Abnormal liver function tests, hepatitis
Integumentary	Flushing, dry skin, rash, pruritus, keratosis
Metabolic	Decreased glucose tolerance

 DRUG PROFILE

▶▶*niacin*

Niacin is used to treat pellagra, dyslipidemias, and peripheral vascular disease. Its use must be monitored closely in patients who have a history of coronary artery disease, gallbladder disease, jaundice, liver disease, or arterial bleeding. Niacin is available for oral use. It is safe to use during pregnancy.

PHARMACOKINETICS (NIACIN, VITAMIN B$_3$)

Route	Onset of Action	Peak Plasma Concentration	Elimination Half-Life	Duration of Action
PO	30–60 min	45 min	45 min	Variable

TABLE 9-8

Pyridoxine (Vitamin B$_6$): Adverse Effects

Body System	Adverse Effects
Central nervous	Paresthesias, flushing, warmth, headache, lethargy

Table 9-8. Toxic effects are a result of large dosages sustained for several months. Neurotoxicity is the most likely result, but this will subside upon discontinuation of the pyridoxine.

Interactions

Pyridoxine will reduce the activity of levodopa; therefore, vitamin formulations containing B$_6$ must be avoided in patients taking levodopa alone. However, the overwhelming majority of patients with Parkinson's disease take a combination of levodopa and carbidopa, and this interaction does not occur with combination therapy.

Dosages

For dosage information on vitamin B$_6$, refer to the table on p. 135.

VITAMIN B$_{12}$

Vitamin B$_{12}$ (cyanocobalamin) is a water-soluble B-complex vitamin that contains cobalt (hence, its name; *cyano-* means "blue"). It is synthesized by microorganisms and is present in the body as two different coenzymes: adenosylcobalamin and methylcobalamin. Cyanocobalamin is a required coenzyme for many metabolic pathways, including fat and carbohydrate metabolism and protein synthesis. It is also required for growth, cell replication, hematopoiesis, and nucleoprotein and myelin synthesis (Figure 9-2).

Vitamin B$_{12}$ deficiency results in gastrointestinal lesions, neurological changes that can result in degenerative central nervous system lesions, and megaloblastic anemia. The major cause of cyanocobalamin deficiency is malabsorption. Other possible but less likely causes are poor diet, chronic alcoholism, and chronic hemorrhage. Normal serum levels are 118–701 pmol/L.

Mechanism of Action and Drug Effects

Humans must have an exogenous source of cyanocobalamin because it is required for nucleoprotein and myelin synthesis, cell reproduction, normal growth, and the maintenance of normal erythropoiesis. The cells that have the greatest requirement for vitamin B$_{12}$ are those that divide rapidly, such as epithelial cells, bone marrow, and myeloid cells.

Reduced sulfhydryl (-5H) groups are required to metabolize fats and carbohydrates and synthesize protein. Cyanocobalamin is involved in maintaining 5H groups in the reduced form. Cyanocobalamin deficiency can lead to neurological damage that begins with an inability to produce myelin and is followed by gradual degeneration of the axon and nerve head.

Cyanocobalamin activity is identical to the activity of the antipernicious anemia factor present in liver extract, called *extrinsic factor* or *Castle factor*. The oral absorption of cyanocobalamin (extrinsic factor) requires the presence of intrinsic factor, which is a glycoprotein secreted by gastric parietal cells. A complex is formed between the two factors, which is then absorbed by the intestines. This mechanism is depicted in Figure 9-3.

Indications

Cyanocobalamin is used to treat deficiency states that develop because of an insufficient intake of the vitamin. It is also included in multivitamin formulations that are used as dietary supplements. Deficiency states are most

---

 ## DRUG PROFILE

▸▸ *pyridoxine*

Pyridoxine is a water-soluble B-complex vitamin composed of three components: pyridoxine, pyridoxal, and pyridoxamine. It has several vital roles in the body but is primarily responsible for the integrity of peripheral nerves, skin, mucous membranes, and the hematopoietic system. It is available only for oral use. It is safe to use in pregnancy.

PHARMACOKINETICS

Route	Onset of Action	Peak Plasma Concentration	Elimination Half-Life	Duration of Action
PO	Unknown	30–60 min	15–20 days	Unknown

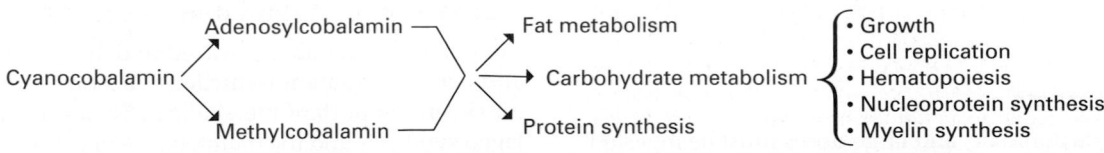

FIG. 9-2   Cyanocobalamin is a required coenzyme for many body processes.

DRUG PROFILE

▸▸*cyanocobalamin*

Cyanocobalamin is a water-soluble B-complex vitamin required for maintenance of body fat and carbohydrate metabolism and protein synthesis. It is also needed for growth, cell replication, blood cell production, and the integrity of normal nerve function. Cyanocobalamin is available both as an over-the-counter preparation and by prescription. Most of the over-the-counter, cyanocobalamin-containing products are multivitamin preparations, whereas many of the cyanocobalamin-containing products contain large doses for parenteral injection and are available by prescription only. Cyanocobalamin is safe for use during pregnancy.

PHARMACOKINETICS (CYANOCOBALAMIN, VITAMIN B$_{12}$)

Route	Onset of Action	Peak Plasma Concentration	Elimination Half-Life	Duration of Action
PO	Unknown	8–12 hr	6 days	Unknown

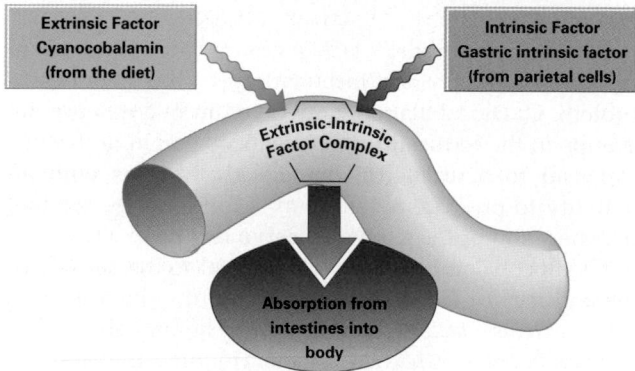

FIG. 9-3 Oral absorption of cyanocobalamin requires the presence of intrinsic factor, which is secreted by gastric parietal cells.

TABLE	9-9

Cyanocobalamin: Adverse Effects

Body System	Adverse Effects
Cardiovascular	Heart failure, peripheral, vascular thrombosis, pulmonary edema
Central nervous	Flushing, optic nerve atrophy
Gastrointestinal	Diarrhea
Integumentary	Pruritus, rash, pain at injection site
Metabolic	Hypokalemia

often the result of malabsorption or poor dietary intake, including consumption of a strict vegetarian diet, because the primary source of cyanocobalamin is foods of animal origin. The most common manifestation of untreated cyanocobalamin deficiency is pernicious anemia. The use of vitamin B$_{12}$ to treat pernicious anemia and other megaloblastic anemias results in the rapid conversion of megaloblastic bone marrow to normoblastic bone marrow. The preferred route of administration of vitamin B$_{12}$ in treating megaloblastic anemias is deep intramuscular injection. If not treated, deficiency states can lead to megaloblastic anemia and irreversible neurological damage. Cyanocobalamin is also useful in the treatment of pernicious anemia caused by an endogenous lack of intrinsic factor.

Contraindications

The only usual contraindication to cyanocobalamin (vitamin B$_{12}$) is known drug product allergies. This may include sensitivity to the chemical element cobalt, which is part of the structure of cyanocobalamin. Another contraindication is hereditary optic nerve atrophy (Leber's disease).

Adverse Effects

Vitamin B$_{12}$ is nontoxic, and large doses must be ingested to produce adverse effects, which include itching, transitory diarrhea, and fever. Other adverse effects are listed by body system in Table 9-9.

Interactions

Concurrent use with anticonvulsants, aminoglycoside antibiotics, or long-acting potassium preparations decreases the oral absorption of vitamin B$_{12}$.

Dosages

For dosage information on vitamin B$_{12}$, refer to the table on p. 135.

VITAMIN C

Vitamin C (ascorbic acid) can be used in many therapeutic situations. Prolonged ascorbic acid deficiency results in the nutritional disease **scurvy**, which is characterized by weakness, edema, gingivitis and bleeding gums, loss of teeth, anemia, subcutaneous hemorrhage, bone lesions, delayed healing of soft tissues and bones, and hardening of leg muscles. Scurvy has been recognized for several centuries, especially among sailors. In 1795, the British navy ordered ingestion of limes to prevent the disease.

Mechanism of Action and Drug Effects

Vitamin C is reversibly oxidized to dehydroascorbic acid and acts in oxidation-reduction reactions. It is required for several important metabolic activities, including collagen synthesis and the maintenance of connective tissue; tissue repair; maintenance of bone, teeth, and capillaries;

and folic acid metabolism (specifically, the conversion of folic acid into its active metabolite). It is also essential for erythropoiesis. Vitamin C enhances the absorption of iron and is required for the synthesis of lipids, proteins, and steroids. It has also been shown to aid in cellular respiration and resistance to infections.

Indications

Vitamin C is used to treat diseases associated with vitamin C deficiency and as a dietary supplement. It is most beneficial in patients who have larger daily requirements because of pregnancy, lactation, hyperthyroidism, fever, stress, infection, trauma, burns, smoking, exposure to cold temperatures, and the consumption of certain drugs (e.g., estrogens, oral contraceptives, barbiturates, tetracyclines, and salicylates). Because vitamin C is an acid, it can also be used as a urinary acidifier. The benefits of other uses of vitamin C are undocumented. For example, taking vitamin C to prevent or treat the common cold is common practice. However, most large, controlled studies have shown that ascorbic acid has little or no value as a prophylactic for the common cold.

Contraindications

The only usual contraindication for vitamin C use is known allergy to a specific vitamin product.

Adverse Effects

Vitamin C is usually nontoxic unless excessive dosages are consumed. Megadoses can produce nausea, vomiting, headache, and abdominal cramps and will acidify the urine, which can result in the formation of cystine, oxalate, and urate kidney stones. Furthermore, individuals who discontinue taking excessive daily doses of ascorbic acid can experience scurvylike symptoms.

Interactions

Ascorbic acid has the potential to interact with many classes of drugs. However, clinical experience concerning interactions is inconclusive. Coadministration with acid-labile drugs such as penicillin G or erythromycin must be avoided. Large doses of vitamin C can acidify the urine but may enhance the excretion of basic drugs and delay the excretion of acidic drugs.

Dosages

For dosage information on vitamin C, refer to the table on p. 135.

MINERALS

Minerals are essential nutrients that are classified as inorganic compounds. They act as building blocks for many body structures and thus are necessary for a variety of physiological functions. They are also needed for intracellular and extracellular body fluid electrolytes. Iron is essential for the production of hemoglobin, which is required for transport of oxygen throughout the body (see Chapter 55). Minerals are necessary for muscle contraction and nerve transmission and are required components of essential enzymes.

Mineral compounds are composed of metallic and nonmetallic elements that are chemically combined with ionic bonds. When these compounds are dissolved in water, they separate (dissociate) into positively charged metallic cations and electrolytes or negatively charged nonmetallic anions and electrolytes (Figure 9-4). Ingestion of minerals provides essential elements necessary for vital bodily functions. Elements that are required in larger amounts are called *macrominerals*; those required in smaller amounts are called *microminerals* or *trace elements*. Table 9-10 classifies these nutrient elements as either *macrominerals* or *microminerals* and as *metal* or *nonmetal*.

CALCIUM

Calcium is the most abundant mineral element in the human body, accounting for approximately 2% of the total body weight. The highest concentration of calcium is in bones and teeth. The efficient absorption of calcium requires adequate amounts of vitamin D.

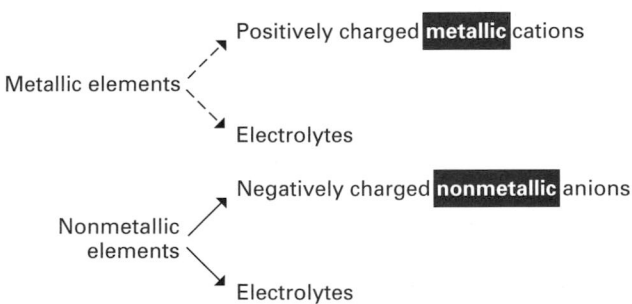

FIG. 9-4 When mineral compounds are dissolved in water, they separate into positively charged metallic cations and electrolytes or negatively charged nonmetallic anions and electrolytes.

 DRUG PROFILE

▶▶ *ascorbic acid*

Ascorbic acid is a water-soluble vitamin required for the prevention and treatment of scurvy. It is also required for erythropoiesis and the synthesis of lipids, protein, and steroids. It is available both in over-the-counter preparations such as multivitamin products and by prescription. Ascorbic acid is available in many oral dosage forms as well an injectable form. It is safe to use during pregnancy.

TABLE 9-10

Mineral Elements

Element	Symbol	Type	Ionic/Electrolyte Form
MACROMINERALS			
calcium*	Ca	Metal	Ca^{2+} calcium cation
chlorine	Cl	Nonmetal	Cl^- chloride anion
magnesium*	Mg	Metal	Mg^{2+} magnesium cation
phosphorus*	P	Nonmetal	PO_4^{3-} phosphate anion
potassium	K	Metal	K+ potassium cation
sodium	Na	Metal	Na^+ sodium cation
sulphur	S	Nonmetal	SO_4^{2-} sulphate anion
MICROMINERALS			
chromium	Cr	Metal	Cr^{3-} chromium cation
cobalt	Co	Metal	Co^{2+} cobalt cation
copper	Cu	Metal	Cu^{2+} copper cation
fluorine	F	Nonmetal	F^+ fluoride anion
iodine*	I	Nonmetal	I^+ iodide anion
iron*	Fe	Metal	Fe^{2+} ferrous cation
manganese	Mn	Metal	Mn^{2+} manganese cation
molybdenum	Mo	Metal	Mo^{6+} molybdenum cation
selenium*	Se	Metal	Se^{2-} selenium cation
zinc*	Zn	Metal	Zn^{2+} zinc cation

*Mineral elements that have a current recommended daily allowance (RDA).

Calcium deficiency results in hypocalcemia and can affect many bodily functions. Causes of calcium deficiency include inadequate calcium intake and insufficient vitamin D to facilitate absorption; hypoparathyroidism; and malabsorption syndrome, especially in older individuals. Calcium deficiency–related disorders include infantile rickets, adult osteomalacia, muscle cramps, osteoporosis (especially in postmenopausal females), hypoparathyroidism, and kidney dysfunction. Table 9-11 lists the possible causes of calcium deficiency and the resulting disorders. Normal serum levels are 2.05 to 2.55 mmol/L.

Mechanism of Action and Drug Effects

Calcium participates in a variety of essential physiological functions and is a building block for body structures.

TABLE 9-11

Calcium Deficiency: Causes and Disorders

Cause	Disorder
Inadequate intake	Infantile rickets
Insufficient vitamin D	Adult osteomalacia
Hypoparathyroidism	Muscle cramps
Malabsorption syndrome	Osteoporosis

Specifically, calcium is involved in the proper development and maintenance of teeth and skeletal bones. It is an important catalyst in many of the coagulation pathways in the blood. Calcium acts as a cofactor in clotting reactions involving the intrinsic and extrinsic pathways of thromboplastin. It is also a cofactor in the conversion of prothrombin to thrombin by thromboplastin and the conversion of fibrinogen to fibrin. Calcium is essential for the normal maintenance and function of the nervous, muscular, and skeletal systems and for cell membrane and capillary permeability. It is an important catalyst in many enzymatic reactions, including transmission of nerve impulses; contraction of cardiac, smooth, and skeletal muscles; renal function; respiration; and, as noted earlier, blood coagulation. Calcium also plays a regulatory role in the release and storage of neurotransmitters and hormones, in white blood cell (WBC) and hormone activity, in the uptake and binding of amino acids, and in intestinal absorption of cyanocobalamin (vitamin B_{12}) and gastrin secretion.

Indications

Calcium salts are used for the treatment or prevention of calcium depletion in patients for whom dietary measures are inadequate. Calcium requirements are also high for growing children and women who are pregnant or breastfeeding. Many conditions may be associated with calcium deficiency, including the following:
- Achlorhydria
- Alkalosis
- Chronic diarrhea
- Hyperphosphatemia
- Hypoparathyroidism
- Menopause
- Pancreatitis
- Pregnancy and lactation
- Premenstrual syndrome
- Kidney failure
- Sprue
- Steatorrhea
- Vitamin D deficiency

Calcium is also used to treat various manifestations of established deficiency states, including adult osteomalacia, hypoparathyroidism, infantile rickets or tetany, muscle cramps, and osteoporosis. In addition, calcium is used as a dietary supplement for women during pregnancy and lactation.

More than 12 different selected calcium salts are available for treatment or nutritional supplementation. Each calcium salt contains a different amount of elemental calcium per gram of calcium salt. Table 9-12 lists the available salts and their associated calcium contents.

Contraindications

Contraindications for administration of exogenous calcium include hypercalcemia, ventricular fibrillation, and known allergy to a specific calcium drug product.

Adverse Effects

Although adverse effects and toxicity are rare, hypercalcemia can occur. Symptoms include anorexia, nausea, vomiting, and constipation. In addition, when calcium salts are administered by intramuscular or subcutaneous injection, mild to severe local reactions, including burning, necrosis and sloughing of tissue, cellulitis, and soft tissue calcification, may occur. Venous irritation may occur with intravenous administration. Other adverse effects associated with both oral and parenteral use of calcium salts are listed in Table 9-13.

Toxicity and Management of Overdose

Long-term excessive calcium intake can result in severe hypercalcemia, which can cause heart irregularities, delirium, and coma. Management of acute hypercalcemia may require hemodialysis, whereas milder cases will respond to discontinuation of calcium intake.

Interactions

Calcium salts will chelate (bind) with tetracyclines and quinolones to produce an insoluble complex. If hypercalcemia is present in patients taking digoxin, serious cardiac dysrhythmias can occur. Calcium may interfere with the absorption of thyroid replacement medications; therefore, it is recommended to take the thyroid medication 2 hours before taking calcium.

Dosages

For dosage information on calcium and other selected minerals, refer to the table on p. 135.

TABLE 9-12	
Calcium Salts: Calcium Content	
Calcium Salt	**Calcium Content (Per Gram)**
phosphate tribasic	400 mg (20 mmol)
carbonate*	400 mg (20 mmol)
phosphate dibasic anhydrous	290 mg (14.5 mmol)
chloride	270 mg (13.5 mmol)
acetate	253 mg (12.7 mmol)
phosphate dibasic dihydrate	230 mg (11.5 mmol)
citrate*	210 mg (10.6 mmol)
glycerophosphate	191 mg (9.6 mmol)
lactate	130 mg (6.5 mmol)
gluconate*	90 mg (4.5 mmol)
gluceptate	82 mg (4.1 mmol)
glubionate	64 mg (3.2 mmol)

*Most commonly used forms for the prevention of osteoporosis.

TABLE 9-13	
Calcium Salts: Adverse Effects	
Body System	**Adverse Effects**
Cardiovascular	Hemorrhage, rebound hypertension
Gastrointestinal	Constipation, obstruction, nausea, vomiting, flatulence
Genitourinary	Kidney dysfunction, kidney stones, kidney failure
Metabolic	Hypercalcemia, metabolic alkalosis

 ## DRUG PROFILE

Calcium

Calcium salts are primarily used in the treatment or prevention of calcium depletion in patients in whom dietary measures are inadequate. Many calcium salts are available, all with a different content of elemental calcium per gram of salt. Calcium is available in both oral and parenteral (injectable) forms. Numerous calcium preparations are available that have different names and provide different dosages. Consult manufacturer instructions for recommended dosages. The pharmacokinetics of calcium is highly variable and depends on individual patient physiology and the characteristics of the specific drug product used. Medication errors and confusion are common with calcium products because the amount of salt is not the same as the amount of elemental calcium. For example, calcium carbonate 1 250 mg is equal to 500 mg of elemental calcium. Depending on the manufacturer, the drug may be profiled as 1 250 mg when the tablet is labelled as 500 mg. Additional confusion occurs with the injectable forms, calcium chloride and calcium gluconate. Calcium chloride provides about three times as much elemental calcium as calcium gluconate, but they are both ordered as 1 g or 1 ampule. Calcium chloride can cause severe problems if it infiltrates from the intravenous line. For that reason, it is recommended that it be diluted or given through a central line if it is given by intravenous push. Adding to the confusion is calcium acetate (acetic acid), which is used not for calcium replacement but to bind phosphate in patients with kidney disease. Calcium products are considered safe to use during pregnancy.

MAGNESIUM

Magnesium is one of the principal cations present in the intracellular fluid. It is an essential part of many enzyme systems associated with energy metabolism. Magnesium deficiency (hypomagnesemia) is usually caused by (1) malabsorption, especially in the presence of high calcium intake; (2) alcoholism; (3) long-term intravenous feeding; (4) diuretic use; and (5) metabolic disorders, including hyperthyroidism and diabetic ketoacidosis. Symptoms associated with hypomagnesemia include cardiovascular disturbances, neuromuscular impairment, and mental health disorders. Dietary intake from vegetables and other foods will usually prevent magnesium deficiency. However, magnesium is required in greater amounts in individuals with diets high in protein-rich foods, calcium, and phosphorus. Normal serum levels are 0.65 to 1.05 mmol/L.

Mechanism of Action and Drug Effects

The precise mechanism for the effects of magnesium has not been fully determined. Magnesium is a known cofactor for many enzyme systems. It is required for muscle contraction and nerve function. Magnesium produces an anticonvulsant effect by inhibiting neuromuscular transmission for selected convulsive states.

Indications

Magnesium is used for treatment of magnesium deficiency and as a nutritional supplement in total parenteral nutrition and multivitamin preparations. It is used as an anticonvulsant in magnesium deficiency–induced seizures; to manage complications of pregnancy, including pre-eclampsia and eclampsia; as a tocolytic drug for inhibition of uterine contractions in premature labour; for treatment of acute nephropathy in children; for management of various cardiac dysrhythmias; and for short-term treatment of constipation.

Contraindications

Contraindications to magnesium administration include known drug product allergy, heart block, kidney failure, adrenal gland failure (Addison's disease), and hepatitis.

Adverse Effects

Adverse effects of magnesium are due to hypermagnesemia, which results in tendon reflex loss, difficult bowel movements, central nervous system depression, respiratory distress and heart block, and hypothermia.

Toxicity and Management of Overdose

Toxic effects are extensions of symptoms caused by hypermagnesemia, a major cause of which is the long-term use of magnesium products (especially antacids in patients with kidney dysfunction). Severe hypermagnesemia is treated with intravenous calcium salt, administered intravenously, and possibly the diuretic furosemide.

Interactions

The use of magnesium with neuromuscular blocking agents and central nervous system depressants produces additive effects.

PHOSPHORUS

Phosphorus is widely distributed in foods, and thus a dietary deficiency is rare. Deficiency states are primarily due to malabsorption, extensive diarrhea or vomiting, hyperthyroidism, liver disease, and long-term use of aluminum or calcium antacids. Normal serum levels are 0.74 to 1.52 mmol/L.

Mechanism of Action and Drug Effects

Phosphorus in the form of the phosphate group or anion (PO_4^{3-}) is a required precursor for the synthesis of essential body chemicals and an important building block for body structures. Phosphorus is required as a structural unit for the synthesis of nucleic acid and the adenosine phosphate compounds (adenosine monophosphate [AMP], adenosine diphosphate [ADP], and adenosine triphosphate [ATP]) responsible for cellular energy transfer. It is also necessary for the development and maintenance of the skeletal system and teeth. Bones contain up to 85% of the phosphorus content of the body. In addition, phosphorus is required for the proper utilization of many B-complex vitamins, and it is an essential component of physiological buffering systems.

Indications

Phosphorus is used for treatment of deficiency states and as a dietary supplement in many multivitamin formulations.

Contraindications

Contraindications to phosphorus or phosphate administration include hyperphosphatemia and hypocalcemia.

 DRUG PROFILE

▶▶*magnesium*

Magnesium is a mineral that has a variety of dosage forms and uses. It is an essential part of many enzyme systems. When absent or diminished in the body, cardiovascular,

neuromuscular, and mental health disorders can occur. Magnesium sulphate is the most common form of magnesium used as a mineral replacement. It is available in injectable form. It is safe to use in pregnancy.

DRUG PROFILES

▸▸ phosphorus

Phosphorus is a mineral that is essential to our well-being. It is needed to make energy in the form of ADP and ATP for all bodily processes. Phosphorus is present in a large number of drug formulations and appears as a phosphate salt (PO_4). Phosphorus should be used with caution in patients with kidney impairment.

▸▸ zinc

The metallic element zinc is often taken orally in the form of the sulphate salt as a mineral supplement. Normally a dietary trace element, zinc plays a crucial role in the enzymatic metabolic reactions involving both proteins and carbohydrates. This makes it especially important for normal tissue growth and repair. It therefore also has a major role in wound repair.

DOSAGES   Selected Minerals

Drug	Pharmacological Class	Usual Dosage Range	Indications/Uses
calcium carbonate (Rolaids®, TUMS®)	Mineral salt	PO: 500 mg 2–4 times daily	Antacid, nutritional-calcium supplementation, hyperphosphatemia associated with chronic kidney failure

Adverse Effects

Adverse effects are usually associated with the use of phosphorus replacement products. These effects include diarrhea, nausea, vomiting, and other gastrointestinal disturbances. Other adverse effects include confusion, weakness, and breathing difficulties.

Toxicity and Management of Overdose

Toxic reactions to phosphorus are extremely rare and usually occur after ingestion of the pure element.

Interactions

Antacids can reduce the oral absorption of phosphorus.

NURSING PROCESS

Assessment

Before administering vitamins, assess the patient for nutritional disorders by reviewing the results of various laboratory tests such as hemoglobulin, hematocrit, WBC and RBC counts, serum albumin, and total protein levels. Assess the patient's dietary intake, dietary patterns, menu planning, grocery shopping/food practices and habits, and ethnocultural influences prior to giving any supplemental therapy. Assess contraindications, cautions, and drug interactions before giving any supplemental therapy. For vitamin A deficiencies, perform a baseline vision assessment, including night vision, and conduct a thorough examination of the skin and mucous membranes and document the findings. Assess for contraindications to vitamin A such as known allergy as well as a current state of excessive supplementation or hypervitaminosis. Additionally, assess for drug interactions with laxatives and cholestyramine leading to possible decreased absorption of the vitamin. Baseline assessment and documentation of level of consciousness, gastrointestinal functioning and concerns, vision, condition of the skin, and musculoskeletal status is also important due to the adverse effects and signs and symptoms of toxicity associated with overdosage of vitamin A (see the pharmacology discussion and Table 9-3).

For patients who are deficient in vitamin D, perform a baseline assessment of skeletal formation with attention to any deformities. Serum vitamin D (35 to 150 nmol/L) and calcium levels are usually ordered as baseline and then during therapy. It is also important to assess for known contraindications such as kidney dysfunction and hypercalcemia or hyperphosphatemia. Assess for drug interactions with laxatives and cholestyramine leading to possible decreased absorption of the vitamin.

Before vitamin E is administered, assess patients for hypoprothrombinemia because this condition may occur secondary to vitamin E deficiency. Document any baseline bleeding or hematological problems and conduct a thorough skin assessment with attention to skin integrity, presence of any edema, muscle weakness, easy bruising, or bleeding.

The last of the fat-soluble vitamins, vitamin K, is associated with clotting function; therefore, prior to its use, measure and document the patient's prothrombin time, INR, and platelet counts. Assess the skin for bruises, petechiae, and erythema. Examine the gums for gingival bleeding. Assess urine and stool for the presence of blood. Also assess vital signs with attention to blood pressure and pulse rate. If intravenous dosage forms are prescribed, baseline assessment must include vital signs because of the risk of anaphylactic reactions. This is particularly important for vitamin K_1 injection because of an associated higher risk of anaphylaxis. Assessment of liver function is also important. It is critical to patient safety to remember that fat-soluble vitamins are all stored in the body tissue when excessive quantities are consumed and may become toxic if taken in large doses. Assess and document baseline values of vitamin K; normal ranges are 0.29 to 2.64 nmol/L.

Vitamin B_1 (thiamine) hypersensitivity may cause skin rash and wheezing; therefore, document the presence of any allergic reactions to vitamin B compounds. Also document baseline assessment of vital signs. Because it is rare for a deficiency of only one B-complex vitamin to occur, rule out deficiencies of all the B vitamins before treatment begins. The normal Vitamin B_1 (thiamine) level is 0.75 nmol/L, and vitamin B_{12} (cyanocobalamin) levels range from 118 to 701 pmol/L. Urinary thiamine levels may also be ordered (in adults, urinary thiamine levels of less than 27 mcg/dL indicate deficiency). Vitamin B_1 deficiency may result in Wernicke's encephalopathy (see the pharmacology discussion); thus, there is a need for a thorough mental status assessment. Thoroughly assess the medication order for accuracy and for route of administration. Drug interactions include alkaline and sulfite-containing solutions, so be sure to assess for drugs being administered at the same time. Vitamin B_2 (riboflavin) has no major toxic effects or drug interactions, but assessing for known allergy to any vitamin product is important. Vitamin B_3 (niacin) has several important indications. Assess for contraindications such as liver disease, severe hypotension, and active peptic ulcer disease. With vitamin B_6 (pyridoxine), perform a thorough neurological assessment due to associated neurotoxicity with large dosages. Levodopa is a significant drug interaction to assess for with pyridoxine because the vitamin reduces the action of levodopa. Vitamin B_{12} (cyanocobalamin) requires thorough assessment of the medication order. Note the route of administration because the preferred route is deep IM injection. Drug interactions to assess for include anticonvulsants, aminoglycoside antibiotics, and long-acting potassium supplements because they decrease the oral absorption of vitamin B_{12}.

Vitamin C (ascorbic acid) is usually well tolerated; however, assess the patient for any history of nutritional deficits or problems with dietary intake as well as any allergies to a specific product. Assess for drug interactions that include acid-labile drugs such as penicillin G or erythromycin. Additionally, it is important to note that large doses of vitamin C may increase the excretion of many basic (opposite of acidic) drugs and delay the excretion of acidic drugs.

With the minerals calcium and magnesium, include in the baseline assessment allergies, nutritional status, use of medications, medical history, contraindications, cautions, and drug interactions. Laboratory studies that may be prescribed include serum calcium (2.05 to 2.55 mmol/L), magnesium (0.65 to 1.05 mmol/L), hemoglobin, hematocrit, and RBC and WBC counts. Calcium interacts with many medications, as described previously, so a thorough assessment of the patient's medication history is important to patient safety. The specific interaction of calcium is that of chelation or binding with the drug and, in this case, it is with levothyroxine, tetracycline and quinolone antibiotics. The chelation then forms an insoluble complex, rendering the antibiotic inactive. Another significant interaction occurs when a patient is hypercalcemic and takes digitalis, with the result of serious cardiac dysrhythmias. If there is a history of cardiac disease, a baseline electrocardiogram recording may be ordered prior to calcium therapy. Because of the various calcium preparations with different names and doses, always thoroughly assess the medication order and be certain that the right product is being given. Also note that the injectable forms of calcium (i.e., calcium chloride and calcium gluconate) may be easily confused, so be cautious. Assess patency of the intravenous site, if intravenous dosage forms are ordered, because infiltrates may lead to severe irritation of the vein and surrounding tissue.

Magnesium is also associated with several drug interactions. Review for potential interactions before drug therapy is initiated, such as with central nervous system depressants and neuromuscular blocking drugs. Assess the patient's kidney, heart, and liver functioning. It is important to document neurological functioning and grading of deep tendon reflexes prior to giving magnesium. Hyporeflexia may indicate toxicity. It is also important to assess the health care provider's order for completeness and reason for use to fully understand why the drug is being given (e.g., for replacement, antacid, or laxative purposes). In addition, thoroughly assess any order for the use of calcium, magnesium, or zinc within total parenteral nutrition infusions.

▨ Nursing Diagnoses

- Impaired physical mobility related to poorly developed muscles from vitamin D or vitamin E deficiency or from fatigue related to poor nutrition and vitamin B deficiency
- Impaired tissue integrity related to vitamin C deficiency and subsequent decreased healing
- Risk for injury related to possible night blindness or altered vision due to vitamin A deficiency

▨ Planning

▰ Goals

- Patient will regain or maintains normal or near-normal physical mobility and musculoskeletal functioning.
- Patient will maintain intact skin and tissue integrity.
- Patient will remain free from injury.

▰ Expected Patient Outcomes

- Patient increases mobility daily with performance of activities of daily living and usual exercise regimen or as prescribed.

- Patient states measures to increase energy, stamina, and strength, such as increase in dietary consumption of well-balanced diet and fluids with vitamin or mineral supplementation.
- Patient states measures to minimize injury and maximize intactness of skin and mucous membranes, such as performing frequent mouth care, keeping skin clean and dry and applying moisturizers as needed, as well as drinking at least 180 to 240 mL of water per day.
- Patient states measures to prevent injury such as minimizing obstacles in the home setting, removing area or throw rugs, and adding night lights.
- Patient states measures to replace vitamin A deficiencies through replacement therapy and dietary intake such as increased intake of liver, fish, dairy products, egg yolks, and yellow orange vegetables and fruits.

Implementation

Before administering vitamin A or any vitamin or supplement, document the patient's dietary intake for the preceding 24 hours. Document any signs and symptoms of hypervitaminosis and hypercarotenemia (excess vitamin A). Vitamin D is available in over-the-counter products (e.g., multivitamins) or by prescription (10 000 units), but attention to the product prescribed is important to patient safety. Combination intramuscular dosage forms are available for those with gastrointestinal, liver, biliary or malabsorptive syndromes. During therapy, advise the patient to report any palpitations or unresolved nausea, vomiting, constipation, or muscle pain. Instruct the patient to take vitamin B_1 (thiamine) as directed. Instruct the patient to take vitamin B_1 (thiamine) therapy as ordered. Vitamin B_2 (riboflavin) is not associated with any adverse or toxic effects but it is important to note that in large doses it may turn the urine yellowish-orange. Tell patients to take vitamin B_3 (niacin) with milk or food to decrease gastrointestinal upset. Niacin is often used for dyslipidemia (see Chapter 28) and in much larger doses. Vitamin B_6 (pyridoxine) is more commonly used to treat drug-induced B_6 deficiencies. Two examples of this are with the antituberculin drug isoniazid (INH) and antihypertensive drug hydralazine hydrochloride. Vitamin B_{12} (cyanocobalamin) is administered orally with meals to increase its absorption. Intranasal gel and sublingual tablets are other dosage forms available. If given for megaloblastic anemia, deep IM injection is the preferred route of administration. Give vitamin C (ascorbic acid) orally, and if oral effervescent forms are used, instruct the patient to dissolve it in at least 180 mL of water or juice. If vitamin C is administered for acidification of urine, it is important for the nurse to frequently assess urinary pH.

Various oral calcium products are available and, because of the differences in the amount of elemental calcium they provide (e.g., calcium carbonate 1 250 mg is equal to only 500 mg of elemental calcium), medication errors may occur and confusion may arise about the various dosages available OTC. A list of the various calcium salts available is found in Table 9-12. Instruct the patient to take oral dosage forms of calcium 1 to 3 hours after meals. Injectable dosage forms of calcium may also be confusing. Follow the medication order carefully and check policies and standards regarding infusions (see previous discussion in the pharmacology section and the Preventing Medication Errors box below). Because of problems with venous irritation, give intravenous calcium via an intravenous infusion pump and with proper dilution. Giving intravenous calcium too rapidly may precipitate severe hypercalcemia with subsequent heart irregularities, delirium, and coma. Administer intravenous calcium slowly, as ordered, and within the manufacturer guidelines (e.g., usually less than 1 mL/min). Patients need to remain recumbent for 15 minutes after the infusion to prevent further problems. Should extravasation of the intravenous calcium solution occur, the nurse should discontinue the infusion immediately and leave the IV catheter in place. The physician may then order an injection of 1% procaine or other antidotes or fluids to reduce vasospasm at the site and dilute the effects of the calcium on surrounding tissue. However, follow all facility policies and procedural guidelines and manufacturer insert information as appropriate. In addition, include the appearance of the intravenous site (e.g., erythema, swelling, and any drainage) in the documentation.

Administer magnesium according to manufacturer guidelines and as ordered. Always give intravenous magnesium sulphate cautiously; use an infusion pump, and follow manufacturer guidelines for dosage and dilution concentration. During intravenous magnesium infusion, monitor the patient's ECG and vital signs, and rate

PREVENTING MEDICATION ERRORS

All Calcium Forms Are Not the Same!

When calcium is given, it is essential to use the correct form. Calcium chloride has many uses, including treatment of cardiac arrest and hypocalcemic tetany. Both calcium carbonate (Rolaids®, TUMS®) and calcium citrate are used as antacids, and they are also used to treat or prevent calcium deficiency and treat hyperphosphatemia. However, calcium acetate is not used for calcium replacement. It is used only to control hyperphosphatemia in patients with end-stage kidney disease. Be cautious when giving calcium—the different forms are not interchangeable.

patellar (knee-jerk) reflexes. Impaired reflexes are used as an indication of drug-related central nervous system depressant effects. Central nervous system depression may quickly lead to respiratory or cardiac depression; thus, perform frequent monitoring. Document intravenous magnesium infusion and record each set of vital sign measurements with ratings of reflexes. If there is a decrease in the strength of reflexes or a decrease in respirations to less than 10 breaths per minute, contact the prescriber immediately, stop the infusion, and monitor the patient. Other signs that require immediate attention are confusion, irregular heart rhythm, cramping, unusual fatigue, lightheadedness, and dizziness. Calcium gluconate must be readily accessible for use as an antidote to magnesium toxicity. Administer oral dosage forms of magnesium as ordered and in the exact dosage prescribed. See the Patient Teaching Tips for more information related to the use of vitamins, minerals, and trace elements.

☑ Evaluation

In the patient's evaluation, always review whether goals and outcome criteria have been met. Monitor for therapeutic responses and adverse effects of each vitamin or mineral. Therapeutic responses to vitamin A therapy include restoration of normal vision and intact skin; adverse effects of vitamin A include lethargy, headache, nausea, and vomiting (see Table 9-3). Therapeutic responses to vitamin D include improved bone growth and formation and an intact skeleton, with decreased or no pain compared with baseline musculoskeletal deformity, weakness, and discomfort; adverse effects include hypertension, dysrhythmias, fatigue, weakness, headache, and decreased bone growth (see Table 9-4). Therapeutic responses to vitamin E include improved muscle strength, improved skin integrity, and α-tocopherol levels within normal limits; adverse effects are listed in Table 9-5. Therapeutic responses to vitamin K include return to normal clotting; adverse effects include headache, nausea, and hemolytic anemia (see Table 9-6). Therapeutic responses to vitamin B_1 (thiamine) include improved mental status and reduction in confusion. Therapeutic responses include improved skin integrity, normal vision, improved mental status, and normal RBC, hemoglobin, and hematocrit. Adverse effects from vitamin B (niacin) are rare, but they are associated with postural hypotension, dysrhythmias, headache, and nausea (see Table 9-7 for complete listing). Vitamin B_6 (pyridoxine) adverse effects include flushing, paresthesias, lethargy, and headache. Vitamin B_{12} (cyanocobalamin) has adverse effects of heart failure, flushing, diarrhea, itching, and hypokalemia. Therapeutic responses to vitamin C include improvements in capillary intactness, integrity of the skin and mucous membrane, healing, energy level, and mental health state. Therapeutic responses to calcium include improved deficiency states. Adverse effects are listed in Table 9-13. Therapeutic effects of magnesium include bolstering of many enzymatic functions in the body with other uses as an anticonvulsant, treatment of pre-eclampsia and eclampsia, and management of various dysrhythmias. Adverse effects include loss of deep tendon reflexes, central nervous system depression, constipation, respiratory distress, and heart block.

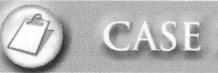

CASE STUDY

Vitamin Supplements

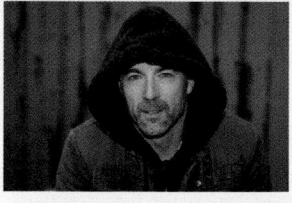

Brian, 49 years of age, was found unconscious in a vacant house and was brought to the emergency department. He had an elevated blood alcohol level and eventually manifested delirium tremens. Now, a week later, he is in stable condition on a medical–surgical unit. He is weak and malnourished, and he cannot remember how he got to the hospital. The nurse is reviewing his medication list and notes that several vitamin supplements are ordered.

1. Based on Brian's history, what vitamin deficiencies are possible?

2. Which vitamin supplement is especially used to treat complications associated with alcoholism? Explain your answer.

3. Brian is receiving large doses of several vitamins, and the nurse is concerned about vitamin toxicities. Which type of vitamin, water-soluble or fat-soluble, carries the risk of toxicities? Explain your answer.

4. Because of Brian's long-term malnourished state, the physician is concerned about the condition of his bones and starts Brian on phosphorus and calcium supplementation, along with vitamin D. Explain the rationale behind the addition of vitamin D.

For answers see http://evolve.elsevier.com/Canada/Lilley/pharmacology/.

PATIENT TEACHING TIPS

❖ Educate the patient about the best dietary sources of both water- and fat-soluble vitamins (vitamins A, B, C, D, E, and K), as well as about the best sources of elements and minerals. See Table 9-2 for the nutrient content of select food items.

❖ Monitor any patient taking vitamins or minerals closely for therapeutic and adverse effects. Encourage patients to monitor self-progress on how well they feel and to note any improvement in the related condition or health status. Encourage intake of fluids with all vitamin and mineral therapy.

❖ Inform patients who have had a gastrectomy or ileal resection and those with pernicious anemia of the necessity for vitamin B_{12} injections. In

the community, an oral supplementation may be used.

❖ Educate the patient taking up to 600 mg/day of vitamin C that there may be a slight increase in daily urination and that diarrhea is associated with intake of more than 1 g of vitamin C per day.

❖ Stress that patients taking calcium therapy and magnesium (see Table 9-10) must take the medication as prescribed and with adequate amounts of fluids.

❖ Educate the patient about calcium therapy and about food items and drugs that will chelate (or bind) with calcium. For example, calcium binds with tetracycline antibiotics and decreases or negates the effect of the antibiotic.

KEY POINTS

❖ Over-the-counter use of vitamins and minerals may lead to serious problems and adverse effects and requires careful consideration prior to self-medication. A health care provider may be consulted prior to use if there are any questions or concerns.

❖ Incorporate the nutritional status of the patient into the collaborative plan of care to provide comprehensive care during vitamin or mineral therapy.

❖ Provide information about dietary needs and the body's need for vitamins and minerals as part of the patient's health promotion.

❖ Focus patient education related to vitamin and mineral replacement on dietary sources of the specific nutrient, drug, and food interactions, and adverse effects. Instruct the patient on when it is necessary to contact the health care provider.

❖ Vitamins and minerals can be dangerous to the patient if given without concern or caution for the patient's overall condition and underlying disease processes.

❖ Never assume that because the drug is a vitamin or mineral it does not have adverse reactions or toxicity.

EXAMINATION REVIEW QUESTIONS

1. When giving calcium intravenously, the nurse needs to give it slowly, keeping in mind that rapid intravenous administration of calcium may cause which problem?
a. Ototoxicity
b. Kidney damage
c. Tetany
d. Cardiac dysrhythmias

2. The nurse will assess the results of which laboratory tests before administration of vitamin K?
a. Prothrombin time and INR
b. Red blood cell and white blood cell counts
c. Phosphorus and calcium levels
d. Total protein and albumin levels

3. A patient has gastrointestinal malabsorption due to severe intestinal damage from a gastrointestinal infection. The nurse will need to assess for signs of a deficiency of which vitamin?
a. Vitamin A (retinol)
b. Vitamin B_{12} (cyanocobalamin)
c. Vitamin B_6 (pyridoxine)
d. Vitamin E (tocopherols)

4. The nurse is providing wound care for a patient with a stage IV pressure ulcer and expects the patient will receive which supplement to assist with wound healing?
a. Vitamin K
b. Vitamin B_1
c. Zinc
d. Calcium

5. While caring for a newly admitted patient who has a long history of alcoholism, the nurse anticipates that part of the patient's medication regimen will include which vitamin?
a. Vitamin B_1 (thiamine)
b. Vitamin B_6 (pyridoxine)
c. Vitamin C (ascorbic acid)
d. Vitamin A (retinol)

6. When administering vitamin and mineral supplements, the nurse implements which appropriate interventions? (Select all that apply.)
a. Not administering oral calcium tablets along with oral tetracyclines
b. Administering intravenous calcium via a rapid intravenous push infusion
c. Monitoring the heart rhythm (ECG) of a patient receiving an intravenous magnesium infusion
d. Giving oral niacin with milk or food to decrease gastrointestinal upset
e. Monitoring for the formation of kidney stones in patients taking large doses of vitamin C

7. The order reads, "Give vitamin K 0.5 mg IM within 1 hour of birth." The medication is available in a vial that contains 1 mg/0.5 mL. How many millilitres will the nurse draw up for the injection?

CRITICAL THINKING ACTIVITIES

1. The nurse is about to administer calcium supplemental therapy to a patient with a history of cardiac disease. What is the most important assessment needed before the nurse gives the drug?

2. A patient with a stage III pressure ulcer is receiving daily doses of vitamin C and zinc. A new nurse asks the medication nurse, "Why is this patient receiving these two particular supplements?" What is the nurse's best answer?

3. A patient receiving a magnesium infusion has developed tendon reflex loss, CNS depression, and some respiratory distress. These problems are a result of what condition? What are the nurse's priority actions at this time?

For answers see http://evolve.elsevier.com/Lilley/pharmacology/.

CHAPTER 10

Principles of Drug Administration

PREPARING FOR DRUG ADMINISTRATION

When giving medications, remember safety measures and correct administration techniques to avoid errors and to ensure optimal drug actions. Keep in mind the following Rights for drug administration:

1. Right drug
2. Right dose
3. Right time
4. Right route
5. Right patient
6. Right reason

Refer to Chapter 1 for additional rights as per each province and territory's professional regulatory body. Other things to keep in mind when preparing to give medications are as follows:

- Remember to perform hand hygiene before preparing or giving medications (see Box 10-1).
- If unsure about a drug or dosage calculation, do not hesitate to double-check with a drug reference or pharmacist. **DO NOT** give a medication if you are unsure about it!
- Be punctual when giving drugs. Some medications must be given at regular intervals to maintain therapeutic blood levels.
- There are a variety of automated dispensing machines—decentralized medication distribution systems—that provide computer-controlled storage, dispensing, and tracking of medications. Figure 10-1 shows one example of a computer-controlled drug-dispensing system. To prevent errors, obtain the drugs for one patient at a time.
- Remember to check the drug at least three times before giving it. The first check is when the medications are removed from the automated dispensing machine, the medication drawer, or whatever system

is in place at a given institution. The nurse is responsible for checking medication labels against the transcribed medication order. In Figure 10-2, the nurse is checking the drug against the medication administration record (MAR) after removing the drug from the dispenser drawer. The second check is when preparing the medications for administration. The drug should be checked before opening the container, and again after opening it. It is recommended that some drugs (e.g., heparin sulphate and insulin) must be checked by two licensed nurses. Some agencies have specific policies related to the two-nurse, double-check practice for certain medications. Always follow agency policy. The final check occurs at the patient's bedside, just before medications are given. This check also provides the opportunity to teach the patient about the medications.

- Health care facilities have various means of checking the MAR when a new one is printed, so be sure that you are working from a MAR that has been checked or verified before giving the oral medication. If the patient's MAR has a new drug order on it, the best rule of practice is to double-check that order against the original medication order on the patient's chart.
- Check the expiration date of all medications. Medications used past the expiration date may be less potent or potentially harmful.
- Make sure that drugs that are given together are compatible. For example, bile acid sequestrants and antacids (see Chapters 28 and 39) must not be given with other drugs because they will interfere with drug absorption and action. Check with a pharmacist if unsure.
- Before administering any medication, check the patient's identification bracelet (Figure 10-3). Also assess the patient's drug allergies. Some hospitals use a bar code system, shown in Figure 10-4. Accreditation Canada standards require two patient identifiers (name and birthday, or name and account number, according to the facility policy). In some facilities, patient information is in a barcode system that is

---

NOTE: This chapter is designed to illustrate general aspects of drug administration. For detailed instructions, please refer to a nursing fundamentals or skills book.

BOX 10-1 Standard Precautions/Routine Practices

Always adhere to standard precautions/routine practices, including the following:

- Wear clean gloves when there is exposure or potential exposure to blood, body fluids, secretions, excretions, or any items that may contain these substances. Always wash hands immediately when there is direct contact with these substances or any item contaminated with blood, body fluids, secretions, or excretions. Follow agency policy about wearing gloves when giving injections and during medication preparation. Be sure to assess for latex allergies and use nonlatex gloves if indicated.
- Perform hand hygiene after removing gloves and between patient contacts. According to the World Health Organization and Centers for Disease Control and Prevention, the preferred method of hand decontamination is with an alcohol-based hand rub, but washing with an antimicrobial soap and water is an alternative to the alcohol rub. Use soap and water to wash hands when they are visibly dirty or visibly soiled with blood or other body fluids and after using the toilet.

- Perform hand hygiene in the following circumstances:
  - Before direct contact with patients
  - After contact with blood, body fluids, excretions, mucous membranes, wound dressings, or nonintact skin
  - After contact with a patient's skin (i.e., when taking a pulse or positioning a patient)
  - After removing gloves
- Wear a mask, eye protective gear, and face shield during any procedure or patient care activity with the potential for splashing or spraying of blood, body fluids, secretions, or excretions. Use of a gown may also be indicated for these situations.
- When administering medications, once the exposure or procedure is completed and exposure is no longer a danger, remove contaminated protective garments or gear and perform hand hygiene.
- Never remove, cap, recap, bend, or break any used needle or needle system. Be sure to discard any disposable syringes and needles in the appropriate puncture-resistant container.

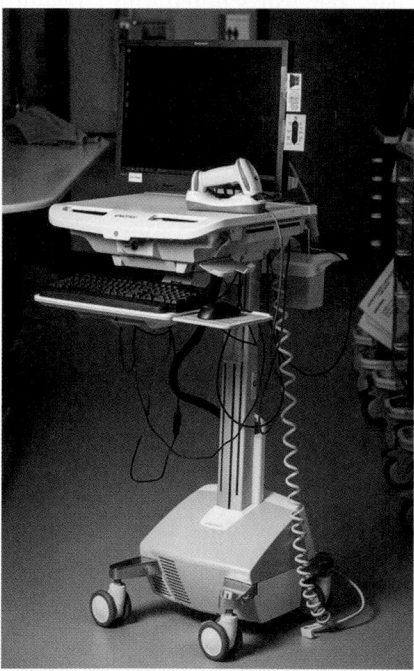

FIG. 10-1 Mobile computer-controlled medication workstation.

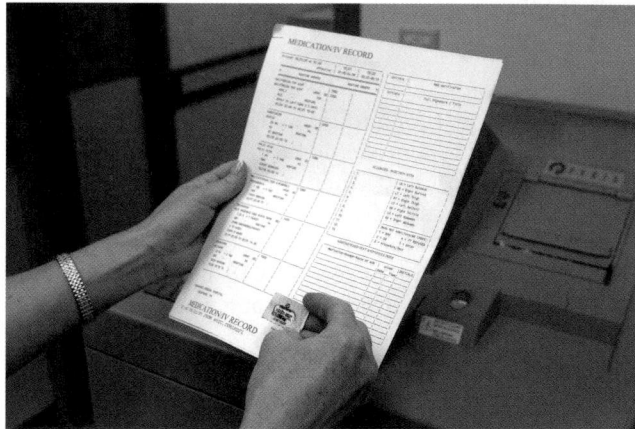

FIG. 10-2 Checking the medication against the order on the medication administration record (MAR).

scanned. Advanced bar code technology allows the nurse to scan her badge, the patient's hospital identification band, and the medication, to assure that the right patient is receiving the correct medication in the correct dose and by the correct route.

- Assess the patient's physical condition prior to administering a medication. This may be focused on a specific system or value (e.g., plasma glucose level prior to the administration of insulin, blood pressure and heart rate prior to the administration of an antihypertensive, or a pain assessment prior to administering an analgesic). The prescriber may provide certain parameters for when to administer or withhold a medication. This assessment provides a baseline for post-medication evaluation.
- In addition, assess the patient's drug allergies before giving any medication. Be aware of medications that may have adverse effects, such as mental status changes or bronchospasm.
- Be sure to take the time to explain to the patient and caregiver the purpose of each medication, its action, possible adverse effects, and any other pertinent

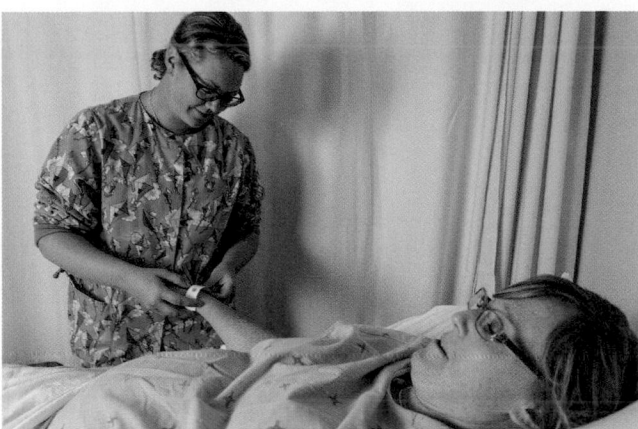

FIG. 10-3 Always check the patient's identification and allergies before giving medications.

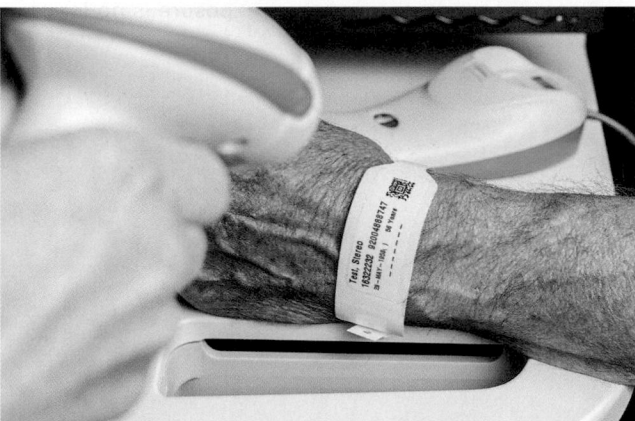

FIG. 10-4 Example of a hospital barcode.

TTH / PMH / OCI	Run from 06/03/17 07:31 to 06/03/18 07:30			

24 Hour Check Done
Date: _____
Time: _____
RN: _____

Location: TEST
Name: Test, Patient
Diagnosis:
Allergies: No Known Allergy
Physician: Doctor, John Q.
MRN #: 0012457   *Age:* 49
Visit #: 000012457

US/RN	START STOP	MEDICATION		07:31 – 19:30	19:31 – 07:30
		***** ROUTINE MEDS *****			
/	06/03/16 07/03/16	ENOXaparin Sodium Inj 80 MG/0.8 ML SYRINGE 80 MG = 0.8 ML SC every 12 hours	Q12H	10:00	22:00
/	06/03/16 07/03/16	Famotidine Inj 20 MG in Dextrose Inj 5% 50 ML Baxter Batch Infuse IV over 15–30 min	Q12H	10:00	22:00
/	06/03/16 07/03/16	Mycophenolate Susp 1000MG/5ML 1000 MG = 5 ML PO/NG 2 times a day	BID	10:00	22:00
		***** PREMEDS *****			
/	06/03/16 07/03/16	Acetaminophen Tab 325 MG 650 MG = 2 Tab orally as directed (For Tylenol) pre platelets infusion	UD		
		***** ANTIMICROBIAL PREMIXED INJECTABLES *****			
/	06/03/16 06/04/15	Ampicillin Inj 1 GM Sodium Chloride Inj 0.9% Infuse IV over 15 min	Q6H	12:00 18:00	00:00 06:00
		***** CHEMO & MISC. INJECTABLES *****			
/	06/03/16 06/03/18	Doxorubicin HCl Inj 100 MG For IV use **VESICANT** Total number of syringes: ____ Each syringe contains: ____MG per ____mL	Q24H	17:00	–
/	06/03/16 06/03/18	Granisetron HCl Inj 1 MG in Dextrose Inj 5% 25 ML Baxter Batch Infuse IV over 5 min	Q24H	15:00	–
		***** PRN ORDERS *****			
/	06/03/16 07/03/16	Docusate Sodium Cap 100 MG 100 MG = 1 Cap orally 2 times a day as needed (For Colace) Give with plenty of water	BIDPO		

FIG. 10-5 One example of a medication administration record (MAR).

information, especially drug–drug or drug–food interactions.

- Open the medication at the bedside into the patient's hand or into a medicine cup. Try not to touch the drugs with your hands. Leaving the drugs in their packaging until you get to the patient's room helps to avoid contamination and waste in case the patient refuses the drug.
- If the patient refuses a drug, the drug may be returned to the automated medication dispenser or to the pharmacy if the package is unopened. Check facility policy. Discard opened drugs per facility protocol. Scheduled drugs that are not given will need a witness if discarded. Note on the patient's record which drug was refused and the patient's reason for refusal.
- Discard any medications that fall to the floor or become contaminated by other means.
- Remain with the patient while the patient takes the drugs. Do not leave the drugs on the bedside table or the meal tray for the patient to take later.
- Chart the medication on the MAR as soon as it is given and before going to the next patient (Figure 10-5). Be sure to also document therapeutic responses, adverse effects (if any), and other concerns in the nurse's notes.

Some facilities use manual documentation, and others use electronic documentation.

- Return to evaluate the patient's response to the drug. Remember that the expected response time will vary according to the drug route. For example, responses to sublingual nitroglycerin or intravenous push medications need to be evaluated within minutes, but it may take an hour or more for a response to be noted after an oral medication is given.
- See Special Populations: Children: Pharmacokinetic Changes in Children in Chapter 4 for age-related considerations when administering medication to infants and children.

ENTERAL DRUGS

Administering Oral Drugs

Always begin by washing your hands, and maintain standard precautions/routine practices (see Box 10-1). When administering oral drugs, keep in mind the points outlined in the sections below.

Oral Medications

- Administration of some oral medications (and medications by other routes) requires special assessments. For example, it is recommended that the apical pulse be auscultated for 1 full minute before any digitalis preparation is given (Figure 10-6). Administration of other oral medications may require blood pressure

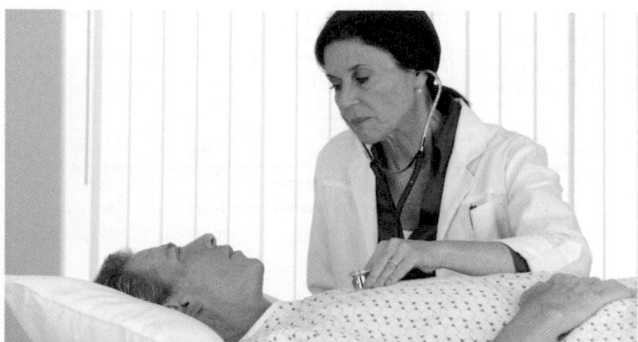

FIG. 10-6 Some medications require special assessment before administration, such as measuring the apical pulse rate.

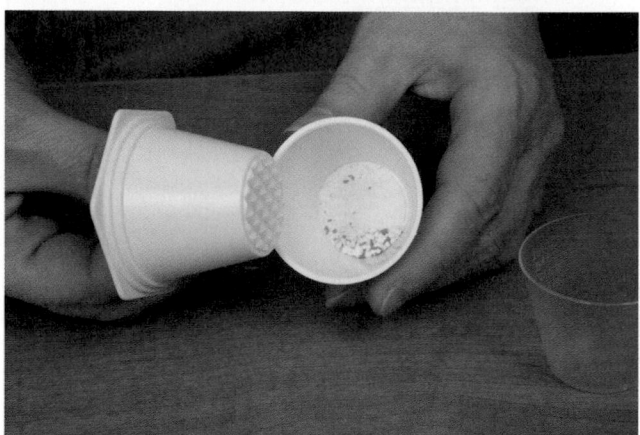

FIG. 10-7 Using a pill-crushing device to crush a tablet.

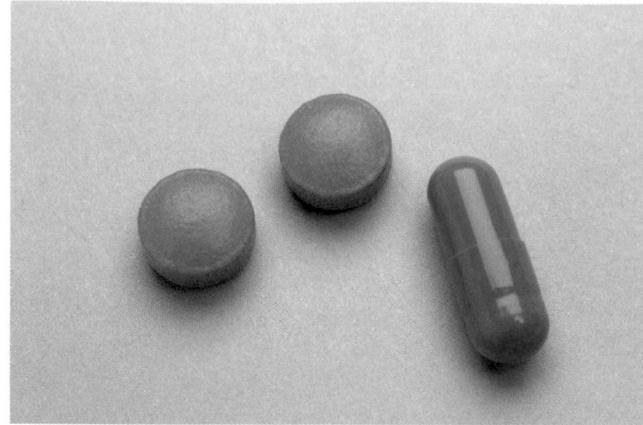

FIG. 10-8 Enteric-coated tablets and long-acting medications should not be crushed.

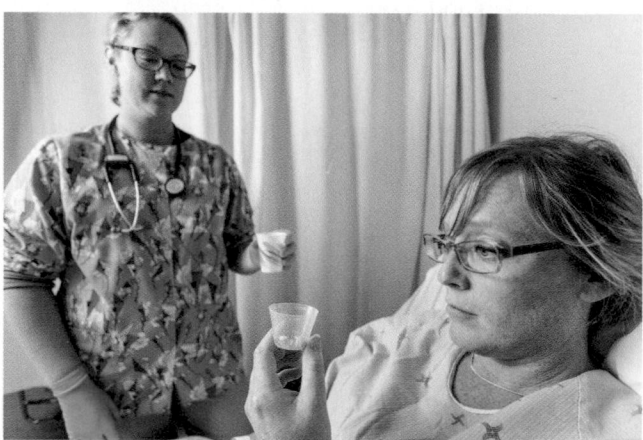

FIG. 10-9 Giving oral medications.

monitoring. Be sure to document all parameters on the MAR. In addition, do not forget to check the patient's identification and allergies before giving any oral medication (or medication by any other route).

- If the patient is experiencing difficulty swallowing (dysphagia), some types of tablets can be crushed with a pill-crushing device (Figure 10-7) for easier administration. Crush one type of pill at a time, because if you mix together all of the medications before crushing (instead of crushing them one at a time) and then spill some, there is no way to tell which drug has been wasted. Also, if all are mixed together, you cannot check the Five Rights three times before giving the drug. Mix the crushed medication in a small amount of soft food, such as applesauce or pudding. Be sure that the entire serving is consumed and the pill-crushing device is clean before and after you use it. See Chapter 2 for more information on medications that should not be crushed.
- **CAUTION**: Be sure to verify whether a medication can be crushed by consulting a drug reference book or a pharmacist. Some oral medications, such as capsules, enteric-coated tablets, and sustained-release or long-acting drugs, must *not* be crushed, broken, or chewed (Figure 10-8). These medications are formulated to protect the gastric lining from irritation or to protect the drug from destruction from gastric acids,

or are designed to break down gradually to slowly release the medication. If these drugs, designated with labels such as *sustained-release* or *extended-release*, are crushed or opened, then the intended action of the dosage form is destroyed. As a result, gastric irritation may occur, the drug may be inactivated by gastric acids, or the immediate availability of a drug that was supposed to be released slowly may cause toxic effects. Check with the health care provider or pharmacist to see if an alternate form of the drug is needed.

- Be sure to position the patient in a sitting or side-lying position to make it easier to swallow oral medications and to avoid the risk of aspiration (Figure 10-9). Always provide aspiration prevention measures as needed.
- Offer the patient a full glass of water; 120 to 180 mL of water or other fluid is recommended for the best dissolution and absorption of oral medications.
- Age-related and fluid-restricted considerations: Young patients and older adults may not be able to drink a full glass of water but need to take enough fluid to ensure that the medication reaches the stomach. If the patient prefers another fluid, be sure to check for interactions between the medication and the fluid of choice.

If fluid restriction is ordered, be sure to follow the guidelines.

- If the patient requests it, you may place the pill or capsule in his or her mouth with your gloved hand.
- Lozenges are not chewed unless this instruction is specifically given.
- Effervescent powders and tablets should be mixed with water and then given immediately after they are dissolved.
- Remain with the patient until all medication has been swallowed. If you are unsure whether a pill has been swallowed, ask the patient to open his or her mouth so that you can inspect to see if it is gone. Assist the patient to a comfortable position after the medication has been taken.
- Document the medication given on the MAR (see Figure 10-5) and monitor the patient for a therapeutic response as well as for adverse reactions.

Sublingual and Buccal Medications

The sublingual and buccal routes prevent destruction of the drugs in the gastrointestinal tract and allow for rapid absorption into the bloodstream through the oral mucous membranes. Be sure to provide instruction to the patient before giving these medications.

- Sublingual tablets are placed under the tongue (Figure 10-10). Buccal tablets are placed between the upper or lower molar teeth and the cheek.
- Be sure to wear gloves if you are placing the tablet into the patient's mouth. Adhere to standard precautions/routine practices (see Box 10-1).
- Instruct the patient to allow the drug to dissolve completely and not to swallow it.
- These drug forms are not taken with fluids. Instruct the patient not to drink anything until after the tablet has dissolved completely.
- Be sure to instruct the patient not to swallow the tablet; saliva should also not be swallowed until after the drug is dissolved.
- When using the buccal route, alternate sides with each dose to reduce possible oral mucosal irritation.

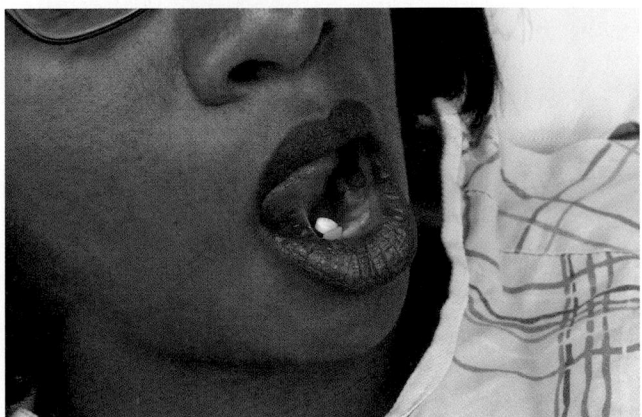

FIG. 10-10   Proper placement of a sublingual tablet.

- Document the medication given on the MAR (see Figure 10-5) and monitor the patient for a therapeutic response as well as for adverse reactions.

Liquid Medications

- Liquid medications may be packaged as a single-dose (unit-dose) package, be poured into a medicine cup from a multidose bottle, or be drawn up in an oral-dosing syringe (Figure 10-11).
- When pouring a liquid medication from a container, first shake the bottle gently to mix the contents if indicated. Remove the cap and place it upside down on a paper towel on the counter, upside down. Hold the bottle with the label against the palm of your hand to keep any spilled medication from altering the label. Place the medicine cup at eye level, and fill to the proper level on the scale (Figure 10-12). Pour the liquid so that the base of the meniscus is even with the appropriate line measure on the medicine cup.
- If you overfill the medicine cup, discard the excess in an environmentally appropriate way according to the agency policy. Do not pour it back into the multidose bottle. Before replacing the cap, wipe the rim of the bottle with a paper towel.

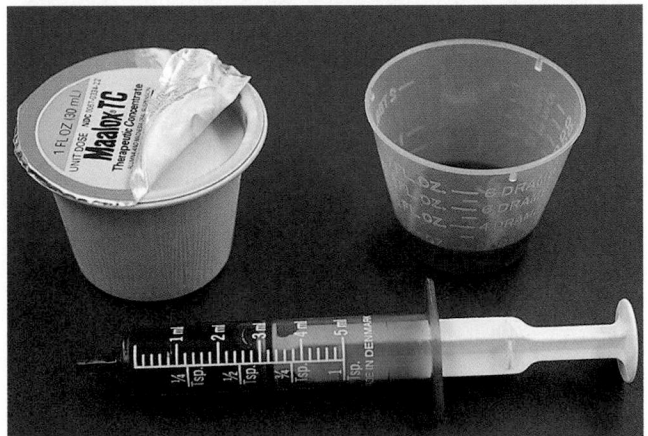

FIG. 10-11   **A,** Liquid medication in a unit-dose package. **B,** Liquid measured into a medicine cup from a multidose container. **C,** Liquid medicine in an oral-dosing syringe.

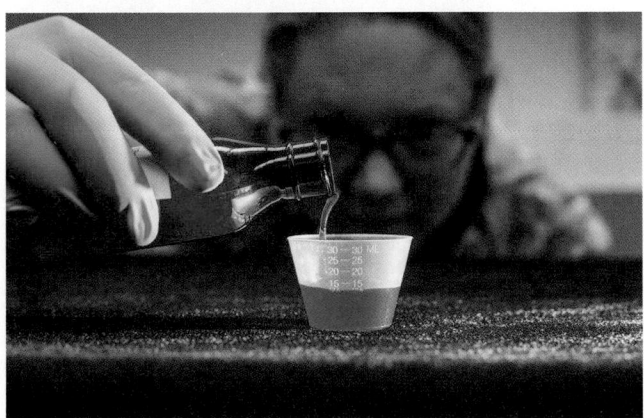

FIG. 10-12   Measuring liquid medication.

- Doses of medications that are less than 5 mL cannot be measured accurately in a calibrated medicine cup. For small volumes, use a calibrated syringe. Do not use a hypodermic syringe or a syringe with a needle or syringe cap. If hypodermic syringes are used, the drug may be inadvertently given parenterally, or the syringe cap or needle, if not removed from the syringe, may become dislodged and accidentally aspirated by the patient when the syringe plunger is pressed.
- Document the medication given on the MAR (see Figure 10-5), and monitor the patient for a therapeutic response as well as for adverse reactions.

Oral Medications for Infants and Children

- Liquids are usually ordered for infants and young children because they cannot swallow oral pills or capsules.
- A plastic, disposable oral-dosing syringe is recommended for measuring small doses of liquid medications. Use of an oral-dosing syringe prevents the inadvertent parenteral administration of a drug once it is drawn up into the syringe.
- Position the infant so that the head is slightly elevated to prevent aspiration. Not all infants will be cooperative, and many may need to be partially restrained (Figure 10-13).
- Place the plastic dropper or syringe inside the infant's mouth, beside the tongue, and administer the liquid in small amounts while allowing the infant to swallow each time.
- A clean, empty nipple may be used to administer the medication. Place the liquid inside the empty nipple and allow the infant to suck the nipple. Add a few millilitres of water to rinse any remaining medication into the infant's mouth, unless contraindicated.

- Take great care to prevent aspiration. A crying infant can easily aspirate medication. If the infant is crying, wait until the infant is calmer before trying again to give the medication.
- Do not add medication to a bottle of formula; the infant may refuse the feeding or may not drink all of it.
- Make sure that all of the oral medication has been taken, and then return the infant to a safe, comfortable position.
- A child will reject oral medications that taste bitter. The drug may be mixed with 5 mL (1 teaspoon) of a sweet-tasting food such as jelly, applesauce, ice cream, or sherbet. Using honey on infants is *not* recommended because of the risk of botulism. Do not mix the medication in an essential food item, such as formula, milk, or orange juice, because the child may reject that food later. After the medication is taken, offer the child diluted juice, a flavoured frozen popsicle, or water.

Administering Drugs Through a Nasogastric or Gastrostomy Tube

Always begin by performing hand hygiene, and maintain standard precautions/routine practices (see Box 10-1). Follow agency policy about wearing gloves during the procedure. When administering drugs via these routes, keep in mind the following points:

- Follow institution-specific protocols for medication administration through a nasogastric or gastrostomy tube. Institutions may require checking the placement of the nasogastric tube and assessing gastric residual volumes (how much of the previous feeding is in the stomach). Reinstill gastric residual per institutional policy, and then clamp the tube (Figure 10-14).

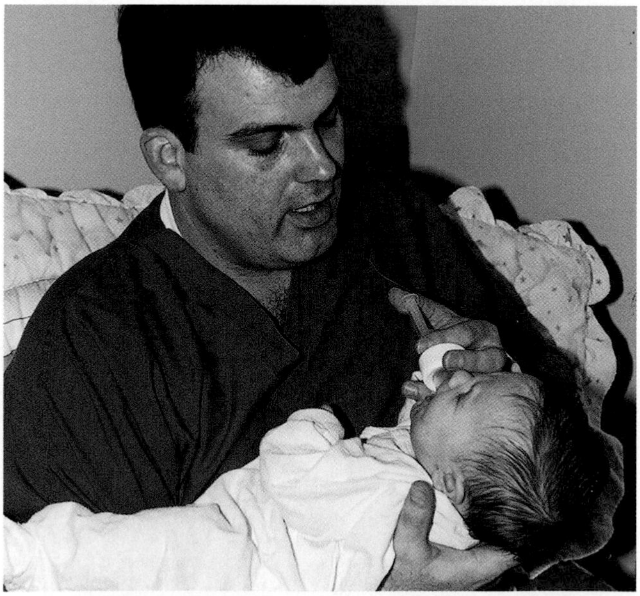

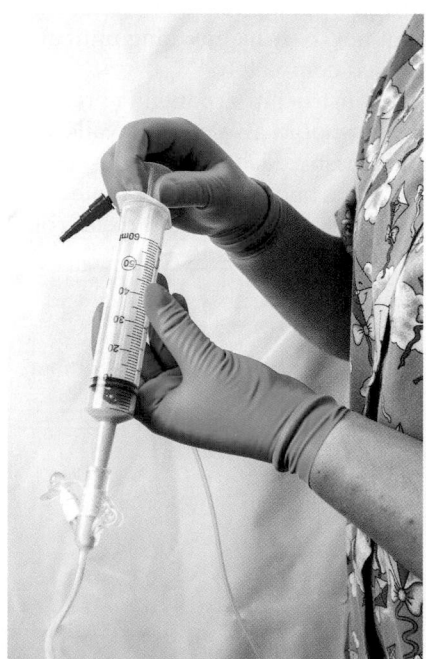

FIG. 10-13 Administering oral liquid medication to an infant.

FIG. 10-14 Check the gastric residual before administering medications.

- Before giving drugs via these routes, position the patient in a semi-Fowler's or high Fowler's position and leave the head of the bed elevated for at least 30 minutes afterward, to reduce the risk of aspiration (Figure 10-15).
- Assess whether fluid restriction or fluid overload is a concern. It will be necessary to give water along with the medications to flush the tubing.
- Check to see if the drug is recommended to be given on an empty or full stomach. In addition, some drugs are incompatible with enteral feedings. If the drug is to be taken on an empty stomach, or if incompatibility exists, the feeding may need to be stopped before and after giving the medication. Follow the guidelines for the specific drug if this is necessary. Examples of drugs that are not compatible with enteral feedings are phenytoin and carbidopa-levodopa. Whenever possible, give liquid forms of the drugs to prevent clogging of the tube.

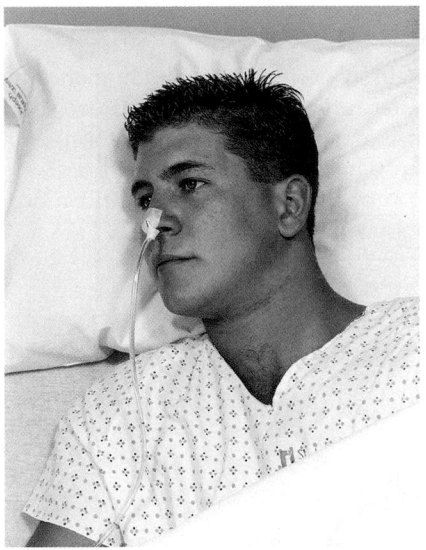

FIG. 10-15 Elevate the head of the bed before administering medications through a nasogastric tube.

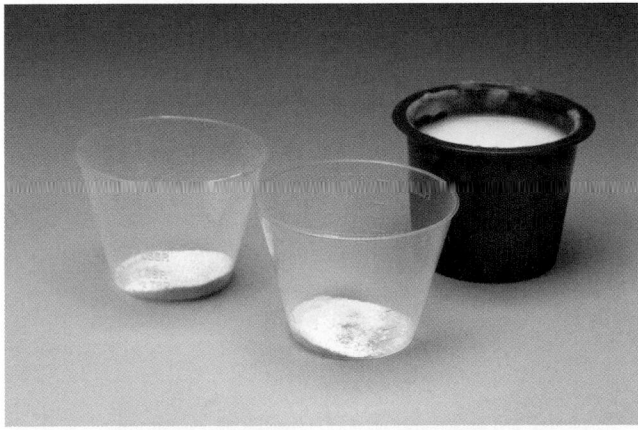

FIG. 10-16 Medications given through gastric tubes should be administered separately. Dilute crushed pills in 15 to 30 mL of water before administration.

- If tablets must be given, crush them individually into a fine powder. Administer the drugs separately (Figure 10-16). Keeping the drugs separate allows for accurate identification if a dose is spilled. Be sure to check whether the medication can be crushed; In general, do not administer sustained-release, chewable, long-acting, or enteric-coated tablets and capsules through an NG or gastrostomy tube. Check with a pharmacist if you are unsure.
- Dilute a crushed tablet or liquid medication in 15 to 30 mL of warm water. Some capsules may be opened and dissolved in 30 mL of warm water; check with a pharmacist.
- Remove the piston from an adaptable-tip syringe and attach it to the end of the tube. Unclamp the tube and pinch the tubing to close it again. Add 30 mL of warm water and release the pinched tubing. Allow the water to flow in by gravity to flush the tube, and then pinch the tubing closed again before all the water is gone to prevent excessive air from entering the stomach. If a stopcock valve device is present on the enteral tube, open and close the stopcock instead of pinching the tubing to clamp it.
- Pour the diluted medication into the syringe and release the tubing to allow it to flow in by gravity (Figure 10-17). Flush between each drug with 10 mL of warm water. Be careful not to spill the medication mixture. Adjust fluid amounts if fluid restrictions are ordered, but sufficient fluid must be used to dilute the medication and to flush the tubing.
- If water or medication does not flow freely, you may apply gentle pressure with the plunger of the syringe or the bulb of the syringe. Do not try to force the medicine through the tubing.

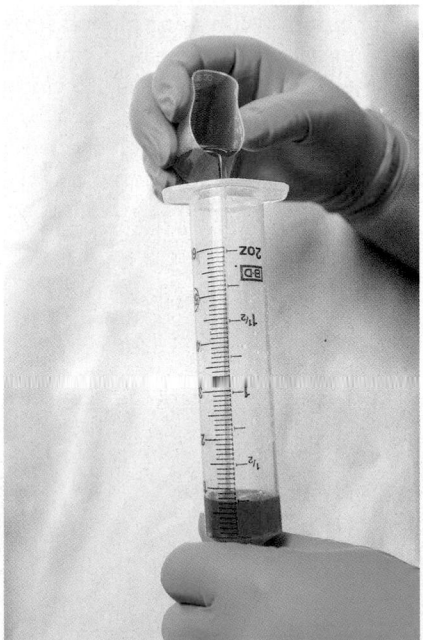

FIG. 10-17 Pour liquid medication into the syringe. Then unclamp the tubing and allow it to flow in by gravity.

- After the last drug dose, flush the tubing with 30 mL of warm water, and then clamp the tube. Resume the tube feeding when appropriate.
- Have the patient remain in a high Fowler's or slightly elevated right–side-lying position to reduce the risk of aspiration.
- Document the medications given on the MAR (see Figure 10-5), the amount of fluid given on the patient's intake and output record, and the patient's response in the patient's record.

Administering Rectal Drugs

Always begin by performing hand hygiene, and maintain standard precautions/routine practices (see Box 10-1). Gloves must be worn. When administering rectal drugs, keep in mind the following points:

- Assess the patient for the presence of active rectal bleeding or diarrhea, which generally are contraindications for the use of rectal suppositories.
- Suppositories should not be divided to provide a smaller dose. The active drug may not be evenly distributed within the suppository base.
- Position the patient on the left side, unless contraindicated. The uppermost leg needs to be flexed toward the waist (Sims' position). Provide privacy and drape.
- Do not insert the suppository into stool. Gently palpate the rectal wall for presence of feces. If possible, have the patient defecate. DO NOT palpate the patient's rectum if the patient has had rectal surgery.
- Remove the wrapping from the suppository and lubricate the rounded tip with water-soluble gel (Figure 10-18).
- Insert the tip of the suppository into the rectum while having the patient take a deep breath and exhale through the mouth. With your gloved finger, quickly and gently insert the suppository into the rectum, alongside the rectal wall, at least 2.5 cm beyond the internal sphincter (Figure 10-19).
- Have the patient remain lying on the left side for 15 to 20 minutes to allow absorption of the medication.

- Age-related considerations: With children, it may be necessary to gently but firmly hold the buttocks in place for 5 to 10 minutes until the urge to expel the suppository has passed. Older adults with loss of sphincter control may not be able to retain the suppository.
- If the patient prefers to self-administer the suppository, give specific instructions on its purpose and correct procedure. Be sure to tell the patient to remove the wrapper.
- Use the same procedure for medications administered by a retention enema, such as sodium polystyrene sulfonate (see Chapter 40). Drugs given by enemas are diluted in the smallest amount of solution possible. Retention enemas need to be held for 30 minutes to 1 hour before expulsion, if possible, for maximum absorption.
- Document the medication given on the MAR (see Figure 10-5), and monitor the patient for a therapeutic response as well as for adverse reactions.

Administering Vaginal Medications

Always begin by performing hand hygiene and maintain standard precautions/routine practices (see Box 10-1). Gloves must be worn. When administering vaginal preparations, keep in mind the following points:

- Vaginal suppositories are larger and more oval than rectal suppositories (Figure 10-20).

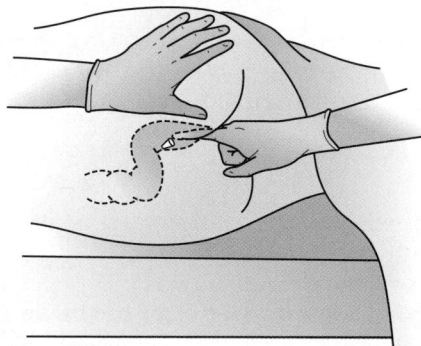

FIG. 10-19 Inserting a rectal suppository.

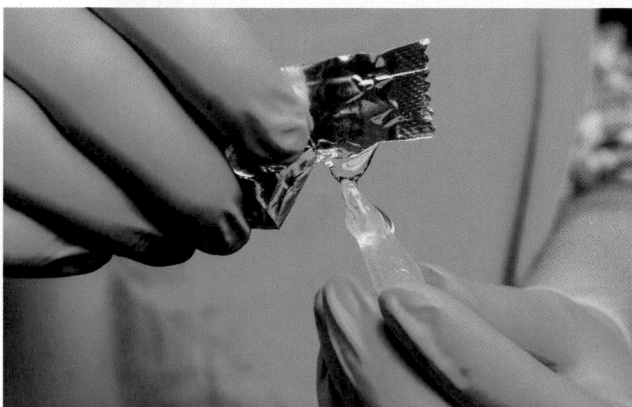

FIG. 10-18 Lubricate the suppository with a water-soluble lubricant.

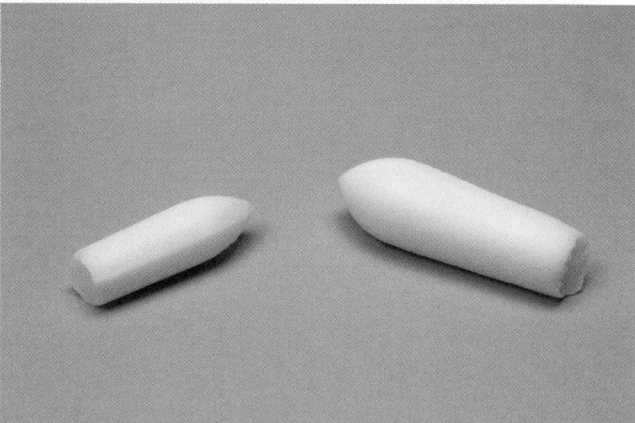

FIG. 10-20 Vaginal suppositories (right) are larger and more oval than rectal suppositories (left).

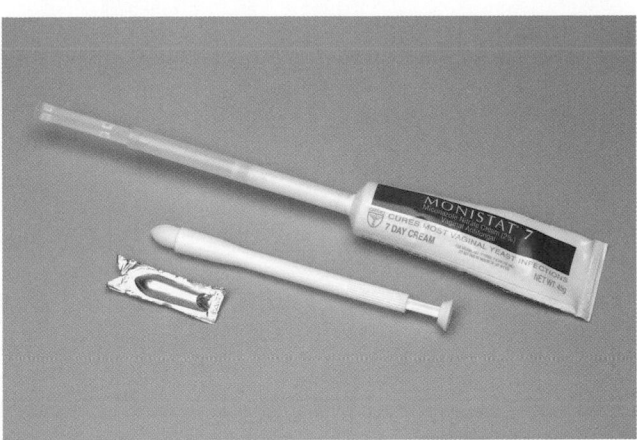

FIG. 10-21 Vaginal cream and suppository, with applicators.

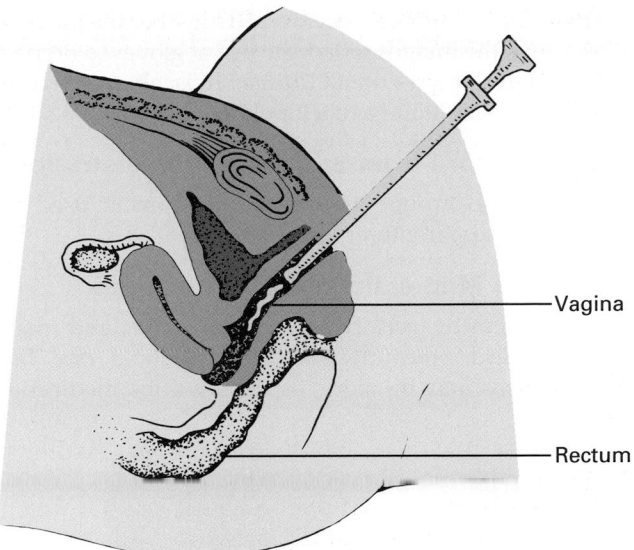

FIG. 10-22 Administering vaginal cream with an applicator.

- Figure 10-21 shows examples of a vaginal suppository in its applicator and vaginal cream in an applicator.
- Before giving these medications, explain the procedure to the patient, have her void to empty the bladder, and perform pericare.
- If possible, administer vaginal preparations at bedtime to allow the medications to remain in place for as long as possible.
- Some patients may prefer to self-administer vaginal medications. Provide specific instructions if necessary.
- Position the patient in the lithotomy position and elevate the hips with a pillow, if tolerated. Be sure to drape the patient to provide privacy.

Creams, Foams, Or Gels Applied With an Applicator

- Fit the applicator to the tube of the medication, and then gently squeeze the tube to fill the applicator with the correct amount of medication.
- Lubricate the tip of the applicator with a water-soluble lubricant.
- Use your nondominant hand to spread the labia and expose the vagina. Gently insert the applicator as far as possible into the vagina (Figure 10-22).
- Push the plunger to deposit the medication. Remove the applicator, and wrap it in a paper towel for cleaning.

Suppositories or Vaginal Tablets

- For suppositories or vaginal tablets, remove the wrapping and lubricate the suppository with a water-soluble lubricant. Be sure that the suppository is at room temperature.
- Using the applicator, insert the suppository or tablet into the vagina, and then push the plunger to deposit the suppository. Remove the applicator.
- If no applicator is available, use your dominant index finger to insert the suppository about 5 cm into the vagina (Figure 10-23).

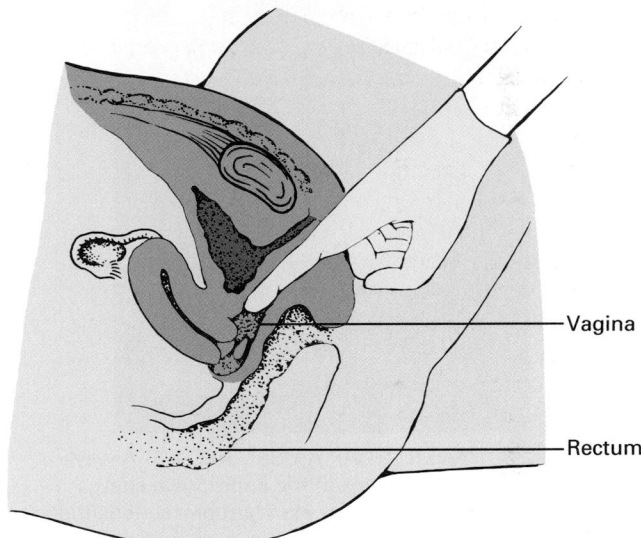

FIG. 10-23 Administering a vaginal suppository.

- Have the patient remain in the supine position with hips elevated for 5 to 10 minutes to allow the suppository to dissolve and the medication to absorb.
- If the patient desires, apply a perineal pad.
- If the applicator is to be reused, wash with soap and water and store in a clean container for the next use.
- Document the medication given on the MAR (see Figure 10-5) and monitor the patient for a therapeutic response as well as for adverse reactions.

PARENTERAL DRUGS

According to the World Health Organization (2010), gloves are not usually recommended for injections if the skin is intact. Gloves do not protect against a needle-stick injury. Practice may vary among institutions/agencies and educational settings about the use of gloves to prepare and administer parenteral drugs. For the purpose of this text, the images reflect the use of gloves to prepare and administer parenteral drugs. It is always recommended to follow the agency policy.

Preparing for Parenteral Drug Administration

Figures 10-24 through 10-34 show equipment used for administering parenteral drugs.

Removing Medications From Ampoules

Always begin by performing hand hygiene, and maintain standard precautions/routine practices (see Box 10-1). Gloves may be worn, especially if the medication

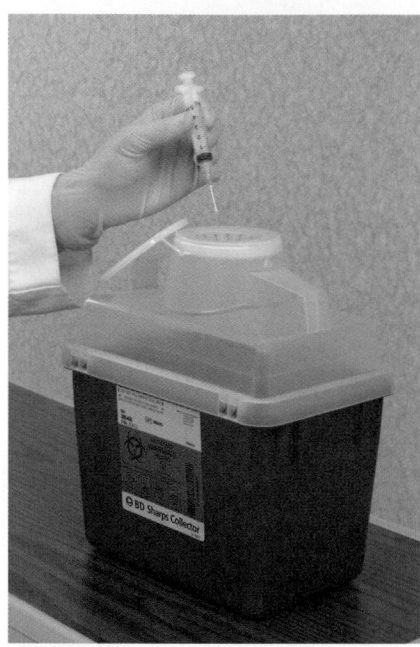

FIG. 10-24   NEVER RECAP A USED NEEDLE! Always dispose of uncapped needles in the appropriate sharps container. Refer to Box 10-1 for standard precautions/routine practices.

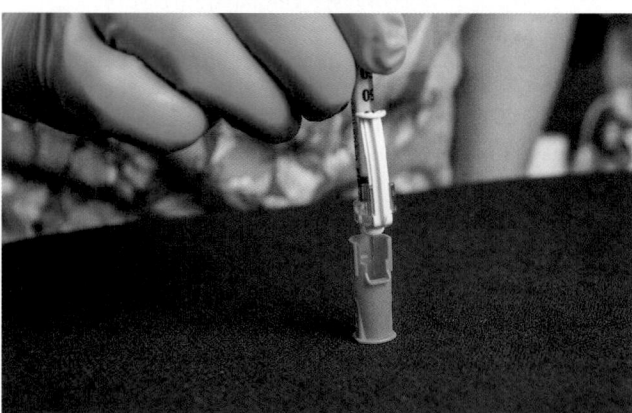

FIG. 10-25   An UNUSED needle may need to be recapped before the medication is given to the patient. The "scoop method" is one way to recap an unused needle safely. Be sure not to touch the needle to the countertop or to the outside of the needle cap.

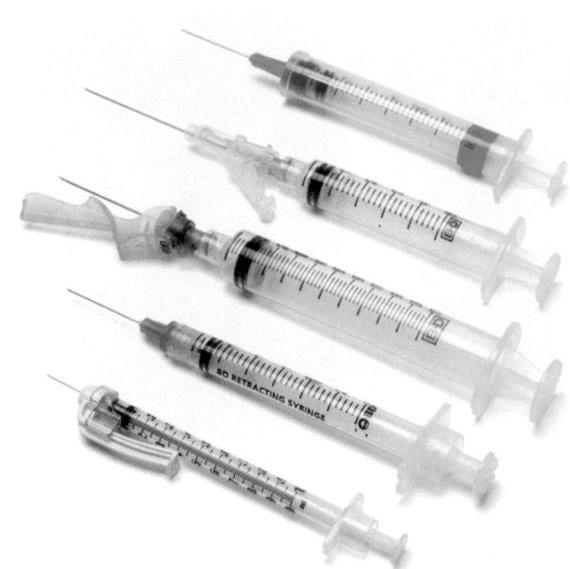

FIG. 10-26   Examples of several different types of needle-stick prevention syringes.

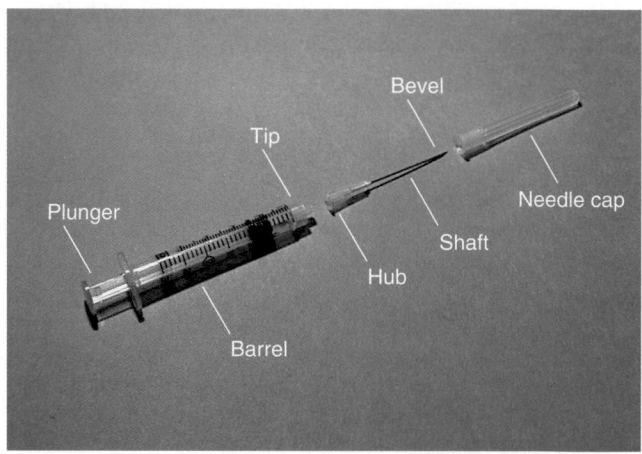

FIG. 10-27   The parts of a syringe and hypodermic needle.

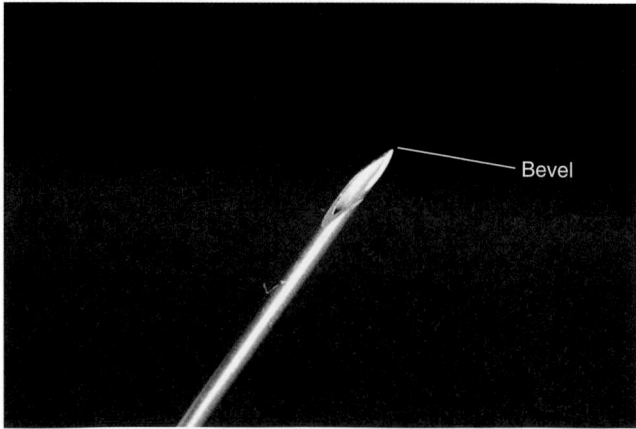

FIG. 10-28   Close-up view of the bevel of a needle.

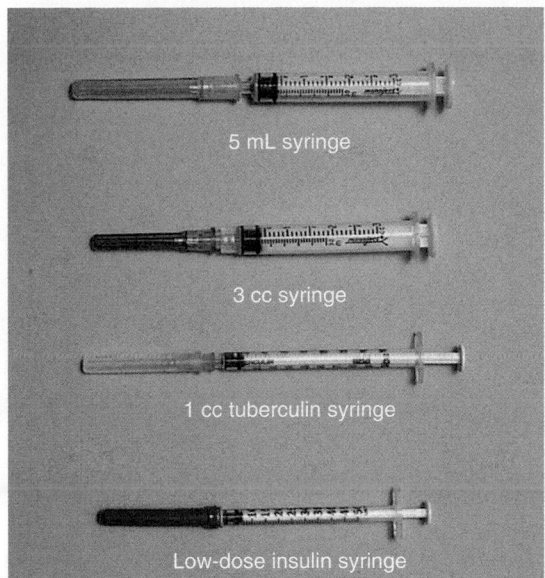

FIG. 10-29 Be sure to choose the correct size and type of syringe for the drug ordered.

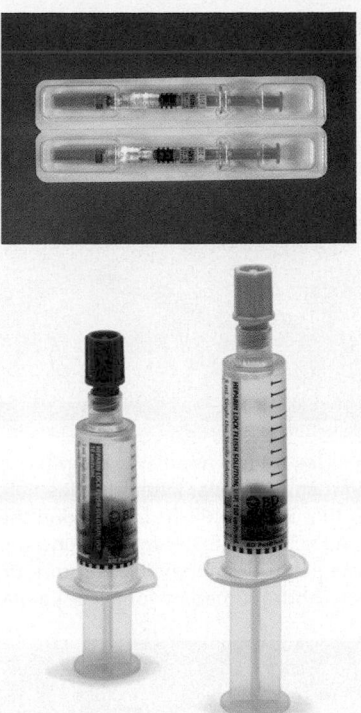

FIGS. 10-31 AND 10-32 Figure 10-31 is an example of prefilled low-molecular-weight heparin enoxaparin sodium. Figure 10-32 is an example of a saline lock prefilled syringe. After use, the syringe is disposed of in a sharps container.

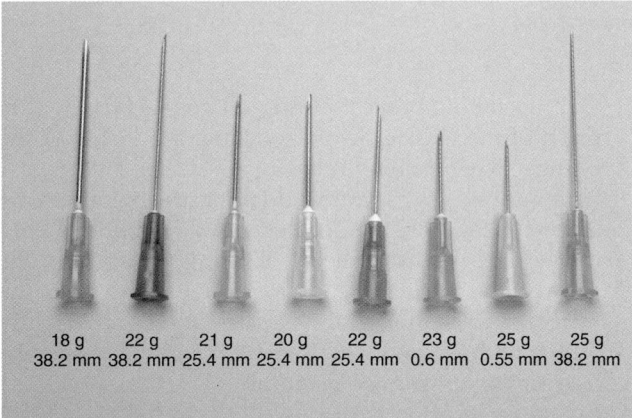

| 18 g | 22 g | 21 g | 20 g | 22 g | 23 g | 25 g | 25 g |
| 38.2 mm | 38.2 mm | 25.4 mm | 25.4 mm | 25.4 mm | 0.6 mm | 0.55 mm | 38.2 mm |

FIG. 10-30 Needles come in various gauges and lengths. The larger the gauge, the smaller the needle and often the shorter in length. Be sure to choose the correct needle—gauge and length—for the type of injection ordered.

is toxic. When performing these procedures, keep in mind the following points:

- Medication often rests in the top part of the ampoule. Tap the top of the ampoule lightly and quickly with your finger until all fluid moves to the bottom portion of the ampoule (Figure 10-35).
- When removing medication from an ampoule, use a sterile filter needle if available (see Figure 10-34). These needles are designed to filter out glass particles that may be present inside the ampoule after it is broken. The filter needle IS NOT intended for administration of the drug to the patient.
- Place a small gauze pad or dry alcohol swab around the neck of the ampoule to protect your hand. Snap the neck quickly and firmly and break the ampoule *away* from your body and away from any other open areas or individuals (Figure 10-36). There are many

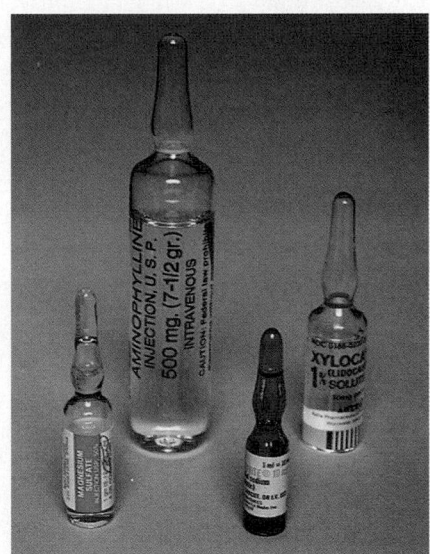

FIG. 10-33 Ampoules containing medications come in various sizes. The neck of the ampoule must be broken carefully before the medication is withdrawn.

varieties of ampoule breakers that are available to open ampoules and minimize the risk of potential injury from broken edges of glass. Many agencies also use a plastic sleeve that is placed over the neck of the ampoule. The ampoule is broken in the same manner as described above.

- To draw up the medication, either set the open ampoule on a flat surface or hold the ampoule upside

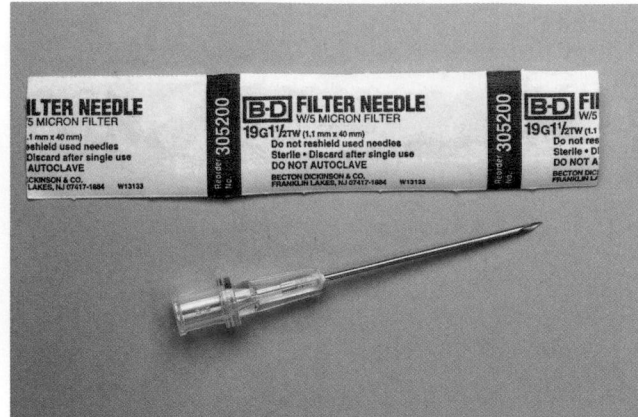

FIG. 10-34 Use a filter needle when withdrawing medication from an ampoule. Filter needles help remove tiny glass particles that may result from breaking the ampoule. DO NOT USE A FILTER NEEDLE for injecting medication into a patient! Some institutions may also require the use of a filter needle to withdraw medications from a vial.

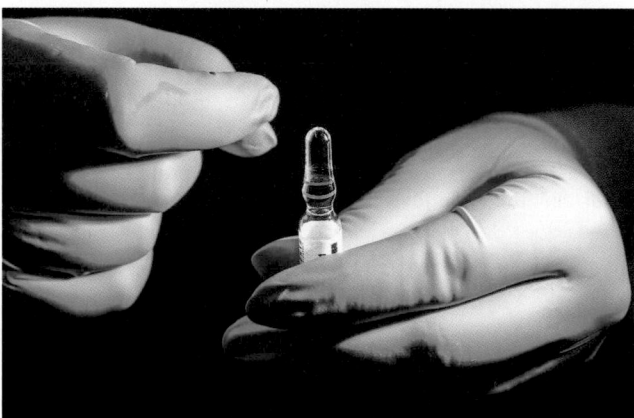

FIG. 10-35 Tapping the ampoule to move the fluid below the neck.

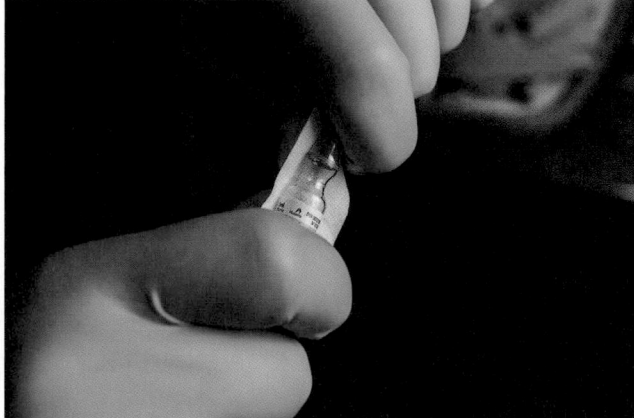

FIG. 10-36 Breaking an ampoule.

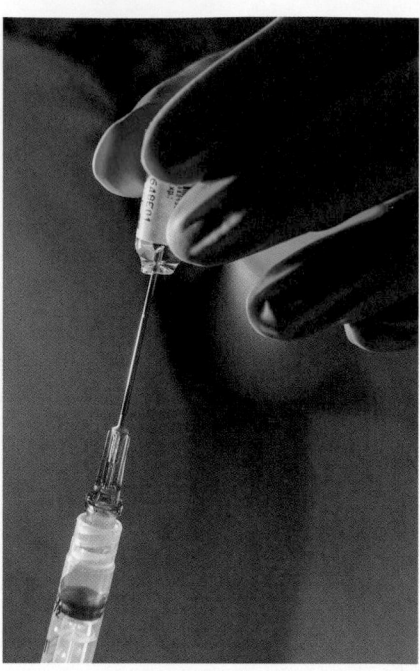

FIG. 10-37 Using a filter needle to draw medication from an ampoule.

vial; tip the ampoule to bring all of the fluid within reach of the needle. Avoid touching the inside of the plunger when pulling it back.

- If air bubbles are aspirated, do not expel them into the ampoule. Remove the needle from the ampoule, hold the syringe with the needle pointing up, and tap the side of the syringe with your finger to cause the bubbles to rise toward the needle. Draw back slightly on the plunger, and slowly push the plunger upward to eject the air. Do not eject fluid.
- Excess medication is disposed of into the sink. Hold the syringe vertically with needle tip up and slanted toward the sink. Slowly eject the excess fluid into the sink, and then recheck the fluid level by holding the syringe vertically.
- Remove the filter needle and replace with the appropriate needle for administration. NEVER use a filter needle to administer medications to a patient!
- Be sure to ensure the sterility of the injection needle throughout the process. Do not touch the open end of the needle hub, or the tip of the syringe, when attaching a needle to a syringe.
- Dispose of the glass ampule pieces and the used filter needle into the appropriate sharps container.

Removing Medications From Vials

Always begin by performing hand hygiene, and maintain standard precautions/routine practices (see Box 10-1). Gloves may be worn. When performing these procedures, keep in mind the following points:

- Vials can contain either a single dose or multiple doses of medications. Follow the institution's policy for using opened multidose vials, such as vials of insulin. Mark multidose vials with the date and time of

down. Insert the filter needle (attached to a syringe) into the centre of the ampoule opening. Do not allow the needle tip or shaft to touch the rim of the ampoule (Figure 10-37).

- Gently pull back on the plunger to draw up the medication. Keep the needle tip below the fluid within the

opening and the discard date (per institution policy). If you are unsure about the age of an opened vial of medication, discard it and obtain a new one.

- Check institutional policies regarding which type of needle to use to withdraw fluid from a vial.
- With the exception of insulin, which must be withdrawn using an insulin syringe, fluid may be withdrawn from a vial using a blunt fill needle or a filter needle. Using a blunt fill needle reduces the chance of injury.
- If the vial is unused, remove the cap from the top of the vial and clean well with an alcohol swab.
- If the vial has been previously opened and used, wipe the top of the vial vigorously with an alcohol swab.
- Air must first be injected into a vial before fluid can be withdrawn. The amount of air injected into a vial needs to equal the amount of fluid to be withdrawn.
- Determine the volume of fluid to be withdrawn from the vial. Pull back on the syringe's plunger to draw an amount of air into the syringe that is equivalent to the volume of medication to be removed from the vial (Figure 10-38). Insert the syringe into the vial, preferably using a needleless system.
- Some vials are not compatible with needleless systems and therefore require a needle for fluid withdrawals. Use a blunt fill needle if possible.
- Figure 10-39 shows a needleless vial adapter that may be used for safe and rapid transfer and reconstitution of drugs between vials and syringes. It can be used for a multidose vial. Adaptors are available in a variety of styles. Many have a blunt access device. Adaptors were created to reduce exposure to needle-stick injuries. To use the adaptor, remove the cover from the vial cap; on a firm surface, centre the needless adaptor directly over the top of the vial and press the adaptor firmly onto the vial until it is sealed. The adaptor can be cleansed with an alcohol wipe and the drug removed similarly to the steps described below.
- While holding onto the plunger, invert the vial and remove the desired amount of medication (Figure 10-40 and Figure 10-41).

- Gently but firmly tap the syringe to remove air bubbles. Excess fluid, if present, should be discarded into a sink.
- When an injection requires two medications from two different vials, begin by injecting air into the first vial (without touching the fluid in the first vial), and then inject air into the second vial. Immediately remove the desired dose from the second vial. Change needles (if possible), and then remove the exact prescribed dose of drug from the first vial. Take great care not to contaminate the drug in one vial with the drug from the other vial. Check with a pharmacist to make sure the two drugs are compatible for mixing in the same syringe.
- For injections, if a needle has been used to remove medication from a vial, always change the needle before administering the dose. Changing needles ensures that a clean and sharp needle is used for the injection. Medication that remains on the outside of the needle may cause irritation to the patient's tissues. In addition, the needle may become dull if used to puncture a rubber stopper. However, some syringes, such as insulin syringes, have needles that are fixed onto the syringe and cannot be removed.
- Ensure the sterility of the injection needle throughout the process. Do not touch the open end of the needle hub, or the tip of the syringe, when attaching a needle to a syringe.

Injections Overview

Current best practice for the administration of injections varies throughout health care agencies and practice environments (Crawford & Johnson, 2012). Aspiration for intramuscular injections is one controversial topic; the literature is unclear as to whether it is best practice to aspirate or not aspirate for blood before medication injections. Evidence recommends no aspiration is required for the intramuscular injections of vaccines and immunizations and subcutaneous injections of heparin sulphate and insulin (Centers for Disease Control and Prevention, 2015; Crawford & Johnson, 2012).

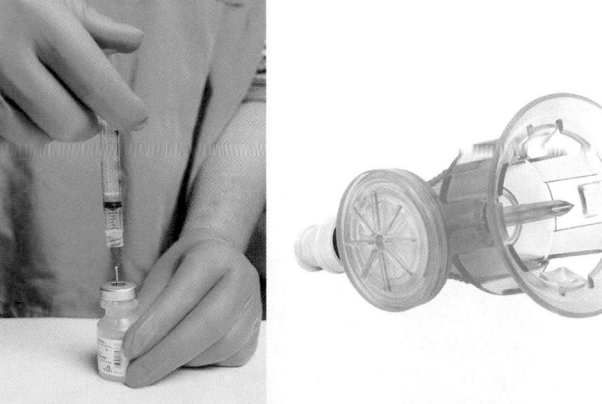
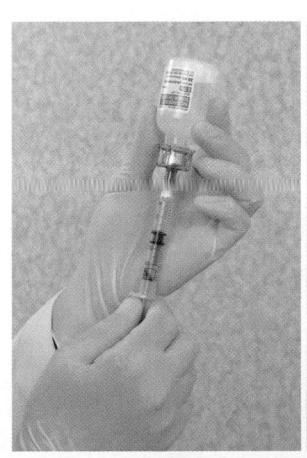
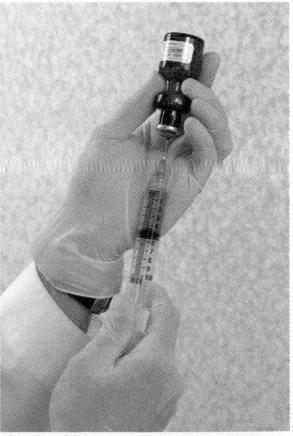

FIGS. 10-38 AND 10-39 Inject air into the vial before withdrawing medication (needlelss system shown). Needleless vial adaptor shows a needleless system of vial access.

FIGS. 10-40 AND 10-41 Using a needle and syringe to remove medication from a vial (needleless system shown on the right).

Needle Insertion Angles for Intramuscular, Subcutaneous, and Intradermal Injections

- For any injection, if syringes are prepared at a medication cart or in a medication room, each parenteral medication should be prepared separately and a label identifying the patient, the medication, the dose, and the route placed on the barrel of the syringe before the nurse leaves the preparation area.
- For intramuscular (IM) injections, insert the needle at a 90-degree angle (see Figure 10-42). Intramuscular injections deposit the drug deep into muscle tissue, where the drug is absorbed through blood vessels within the muscle. The rate of absorption of drug given by the intramuscular route is slower than that of drugs given by the intravenous route but faster than that of drugs given by the subcutaneous route. Intramuscular injections generally require a longer needle to reach the muscle tissue, but shorter needles may be needed for older patients, children, and adults who are malnourished. The site chosen will also determine the length of the needle needed. In general, aqueous drugs can be given with a 22- to 27-gauge needle; however, oil-based or more viscous (thick) drugs are given with an 18- to 25-gauge needle. Average needle lengths for children range from 16 mm to 25 mm, and needles for adults range from 25 mm to 38 mm. The nurse must choose the needle length based on the size of the muscle at the injection site, the age of the patient, and the type of drug used. For a normal, well-developed adult, 3 mL is the maximum amount used in a single injection. Follow agency policy. If more than 3 mL is needed for the ordered dose, then the drug will need to be given in two separate injections. However, if the patient is an older adult or thin, a smaller maximum volume, such as 2 mL, is recommended.
- For subcutaneous (subcut) injections, insert the needle at either a 45- or a 90-degree angle. Subcutaneous injections deposit the drug into the loose connective tissue under the dermis. This tissue is not as well supplied with blood vessels as is the muscle tissue; as a result, drugs are absorbed more slowly than drugs given intramuscularly. Doses are usually 0.5 to 1 mL. In general, use a 25-gauge, 12-mm to 16-mm needle (for insulin, a 6-mm or 8-mm needle is recommended). A 90-degree angle is used for a patient of average-size; a 45-degree angle may be used for patients who are thin, emaciated, or cachectic and for children. To ensure correct needle length, grasp the skin fold with the thumb and forefinger, and choose a needle that is approximately one half the length of the skin fold from top to bottom.
- Intradermal (ID) injections are given into the outer layers of the dermis in tiny amounts, usually 0.01 to 0.1 mL. These injections are used mostly for diagnostic purposes, such as when testing for allergies or tuberculosis and for local anaesthesia. Little of the drug is absorbed systemically. In general, choose a tuberculin or 1-mL syringe with a 26- or 27-gauge needle that is 10 mm to 16 mm long. The angle of injection is 5 to 15 degrees.
- For specific information about giving injections to children, see Box 10-2.

Air-Lock Technique

- Some facilities recommend administering intramuscular injections using the air-lock technique (Figure 10-43). Check institutional policy.
- After withdrawing the desired amount of drug into the syringe, withdraw an additional 0.2 mL of air. Be sure to inject using a 90-degree angle. The small air bubble that follows the medication during the injection may help prevent the medication from leaking through the needle track into the subcutaneous tissues.

Intradermal Injection

Always begin by performing hand hygiene, and maintain standard precautions/routine practices (see Box 10-1). When giving an intradermal injection, keep in mind the following points:

- Be sure to choose an appropriate site for the injection. Avoid areas of bruising, rashes, inflammation, edema, or skin discoloration.
- Help the patient to a comfortable position. Extend and support the elbow and forearm on a flat surface.
- In general, three to four finger-widths below the antecubital space and one hand-width above the wrist are the preferred locations on the forearm. Areas on the back that are also suitable for subcutaneous injections may be used if the forearm is not appropriate for the intradermal injection.

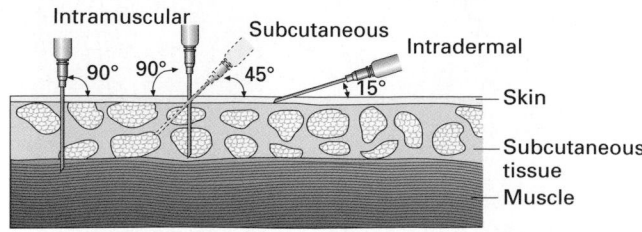

FIG. 10-42 Various needle angles.

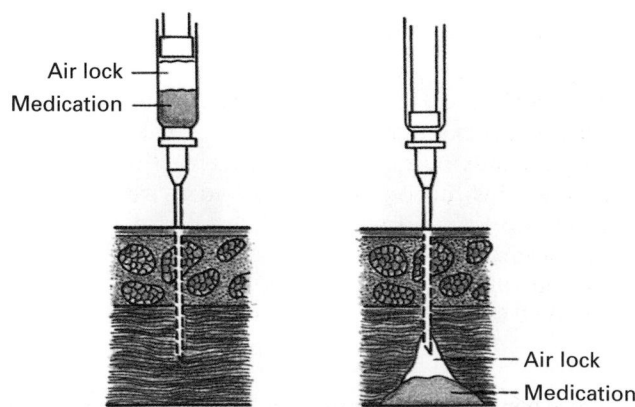

FIG. 10-43 Air-lock technique for intramuscular injections.

BOX 10-2   Pediatric Injections

For pediatric injections, site selection is crucial. Factors to consider are the age of the child, the size of the muscle at the injection site, the type of injection, the thickness of the solution, and the ease with which the child can be positioned properly. There is no universal agreement in the literature on the best intramuscular injection site for children. For infants, the preferred site is the vastus lateralis muscle. The ventrogluteal site may also be used in children of all ages. For immunizations in toddlers and older children, the deltoid muscle may be used *if* the muscle mass is well developed. Intramuscular injections for older infants and small children should not exceed 1 mL in a single injection. Refer to facility policy.

Children are often extremely fearful of needles and injections. Even a child who appears calm may become upset and lose control during an injection procedure. For safety reasons, it is important to have another person available for positioning and holding the child.

Distraction techniques are helpful. Say to the child, "If you feel this you can ask me to take it out, please." Be quick and efficient when giving the injection.

Have a small, colourful adhesive bandage on hand to apply after the injection. If the child is old enough, have the child hold the bandage and apply it after the injection. If possible, offer a reward sticker after the injection.

After the injection, allow the child to express feelings about the injection. For young children, encourage parents to offer comfort with holding and cuddling. Older children respond better if they receive praise.

EMLA (lidocaine/prilocaine) cream or a vapocoolant spray, if available, may be used before the injection to reduce the pain from the needle insertion. However, because these agents do not absorb down into the muscle, the child may still experience pain when the medication enters the muscle. Apply EMLA cream to the site at least 1 hour and up to 3 hours before the injection. Vapocoolant spray is applied to the site immediately before the injection. Another option is to apply a wrapped ice cube to the injection site for a minute before the injection. Infants also experience pain with the administration of injections. Breast feedings during the procedure or administering a glucose solution have both been effective strategies for pain management.

- Cleanse the site with an alcohol or antiseptic swab. Apply the swab at the centre of the site, and cleanse outward in a circular direction for about 5 cm; then let the skin dry. After cleansing the site, stretch the skin over the site with your nondominant hand.
- With the needle almost against the patient's skin, insert the needle, bevel up, at a 5- to 15-degree angle until resistance is felt, and then advance the needle through the epidermis, approximately 3 mm (Figures 10-44 and 10-45). The needle tip should still be visible under the skin.
- Do not aspirate. This area under the skin contains few blood vessels.
- Slowly inject the medication. It is normal to feel resistance, and a bleb that resembles a mosquito bite (about 6 mm in diameter) will form at the site if accurate technique is used.
- Withdraw the needle slowly while gently applying a gauze pad at the site, but do not massage the site.
- DO NOT RECAP the needle. Dispose of the syringe and needle in the appropriate container. Perform hand hygiene after administering the medication.
- Provide instructions to the patient as needed for a follow-up visit for reading the skin testing, if applicable.
- Document in the MAR the date of the skin testing and the date that results need to be read, if applicable.

Subcutaneous Injections

Always begin by performing hand hygiene, and maintain standard precautions/routine practices (see Box

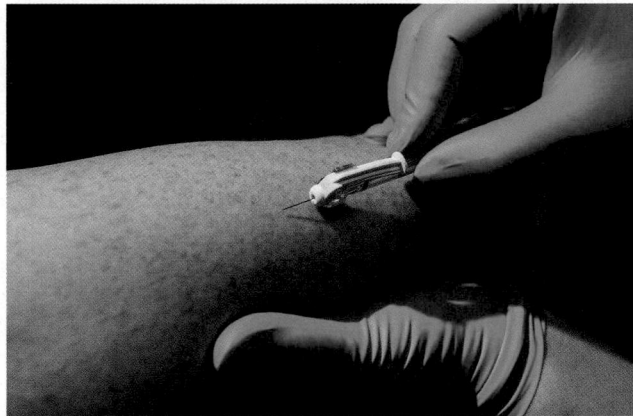
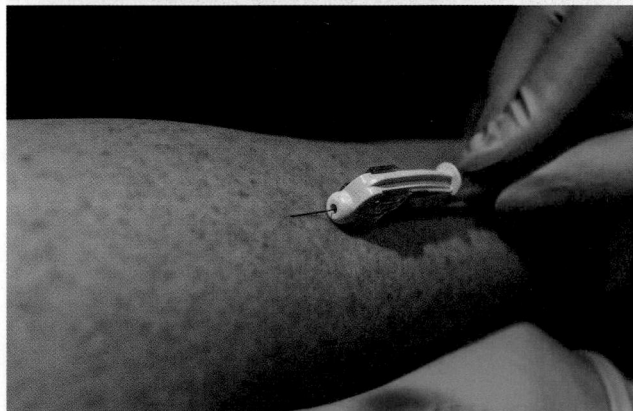

FIGS. 10-44 AND 10-45   Intradermal injection.

10-1). When giving a subcutaneous injection, keep in mind the following points:

- Be sure to choose an appropriate site for the injection. Avoid areas of bruising, rashes, inflammation, edema, or skin discolorations as well as scars, moles, or hair roots (Figure 10-46).
- Ensure that the needle size is correct. Grasp the skin fold between your thumb and forefinger and measure from top to bottom. The needle should be approximately one half of this length.
- Cleanse the site with an alcohol or antiseptic swab. Apply the swab at the centre of the site, and cleanse outward in a circular direction for about 5 cm (Figure 10-47); then let the skin dry.
- Tell the patient that he or she will feel a "stick" as you insert the needle.
- For a patient who is of average size, pinch the skin with your nondominant hand, and inject the needle quickly at a 45- or 90-degree angle (Figure 10-48).

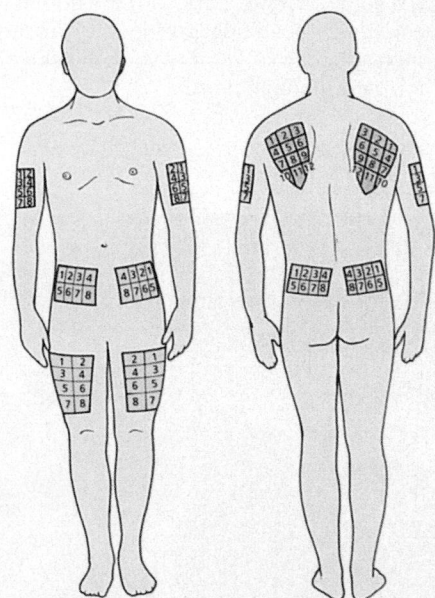

FIG. 10-46 Potential sites for subcutaneous injections.

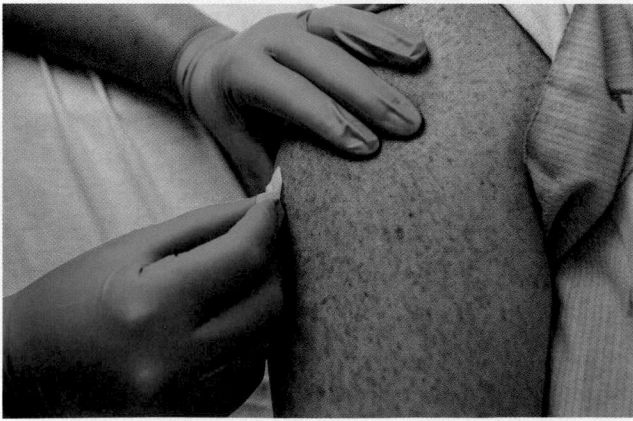

FIG. 10-47 Before giving an injection, cleanse the skin with an alcohol or antiseptic swab.

- For a patient who is obese, pinch the skin and inject the needle at a 90-degree angle. Be sure the needle is long enough to reach the base of the skin fold.
- Age-related considerations: For a child or a thin patient, pinch the skin gently and be sure to use a 45-degree angle when injecting the needle.
- Injections given in the abdomen must be given at least 5 cm away from the umbilicus because of the surrounding vascular structure (Figure 10-49). The injection site must also be 5 cm away from any incisions, stomas, or open wounds, if present.
- After the needle enters the skin, grasp the lower end of the syringe with your nondominant hand. Move your dominant hand to the end of the plunger—be careful not to move the syringe.
- Aspiration of medication to check for blood return is not necessary for subcutaneous injections or vaccinations (Public Health Agency of Canada, 2013). Heparin sulfate injections and insulin injections are absolutely NOT aspirated before injection.
- With your dominant hand, slowly inject the medication.
- Withdraw the needle quickly, and place a swab or sterile gauze pad over the site.

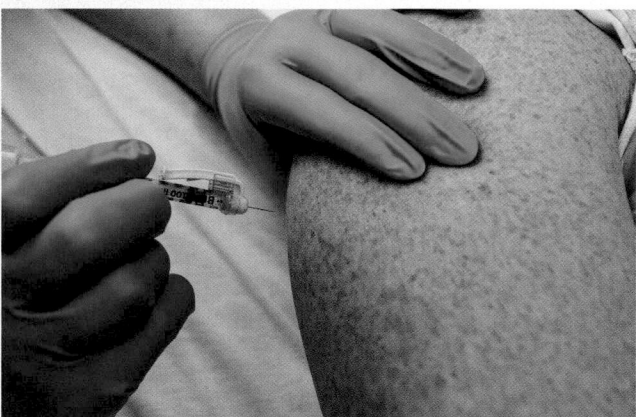

FIG. 10-48 Giving a subcutaneous injection at a 90-degree angle.

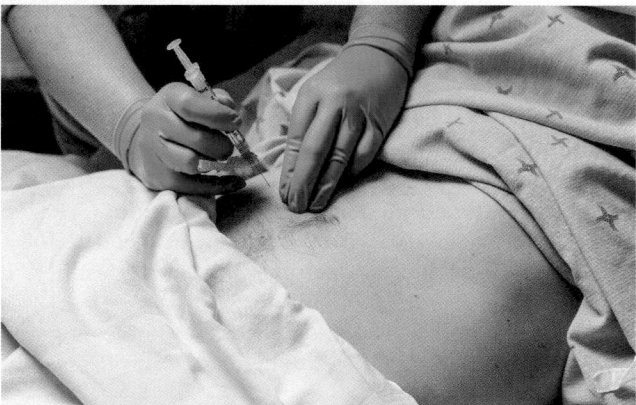

FIG. 10-49 When giving a subcutaneous injection in the abdomen, be sure to choose a site at least 5 cm away from the umbilicus.

- Apply gentle pressure but do not massage the site. If necessary, apply a bandage to the site.
- DO NOT RECAP the needle. Dispose of the syringe and needle in the appropriate container. Perform hand hygiene after administering the injection.
- Document the medication given on the MAR (see Figure 10-5), and monitor the patient for a therapeutic response as well as for adverse reactions.
- For heparin sulphate or other subcutaneous anticoagulant injections, follow the manufacturer's instructions for injection technique as needed. Many manufacturers recommend the area of the abdomen known as the "love handles" for injection of anticoagulants. DO NOT ASPIRATE before injecting, and DO NOT MASSAGE the site after injection. These actions may cause a hematoma at the injection site.
- Heparin doses are ordered in units, but it is important to note that units of heparin sulphate are not the same as units of insulin. Heparin sulphate is *never* measured with insulin syringes.
- Also available are prefilled syringes with air lock of low-molecular-weight heparin (e.g., enoxaparin sodium, dalteparin sodium). The air lock of 0.2 to 0.3 mL of air is left in the injector; when the drug is administered followed by the air, a lock is created where the needle is inserted to prevent the heparin from penetrating the skin. This reduces the possibility of developing a hematoma. In addition, all the drug is pushed by the air into the subcutaneous tissue and the precise dose of the drug is administered.

Insulin Syringes

- Always use an insulin syringe to measure and administer insulin. When giving small doses of insulin, use an insulin syringe that is calibrated for smaller doses. Figure 10-50 shows insulin syringes with two different calibrations. Notice that in the 100-unit syringe, each line represents 2 units; on the 50-unit syringe, each line represents 1 unit. NOTE: One unit of insulin is NOT equivalent to one millilitre of insulin.

- Figure 10-51 shows several examples of devices (syringe, insulin pen) that can be used to help patients self-administer insulin. These devices feature a multi-dose container of insulin and easy-to-read dials for choosing the correct dose. The needle is changed with each use. These devices are for single-patient use only, due to the risk of blood contamination of the medication reservoir.
- When two different types of insulin are drawn up into the same syringe, always draw up the clear (fast-acting) insulin into the syringe first. An easy way to remember which insulin is drawn up first is thinking "Fast/First."
- Disinfection of the site for insulin is usually not required; however, the use of alcohol or antiseptic swabs in the hospital or home care setting are often used.

Intramuscular Injections

Always begin by performing hand hygiene, and maintain standard precautions/routine practices (see Box 10-1). Gloves must be worn. When giving an intramuscular injection, keep in mind the following points:

- Choose the appropriate site for the injection by assessing not only the size and integrity of the muscle but also the amount and type of injection. Palpate potential sites for areas of hardness or tenderness, and note the presence of bruising or infection.
- The dorsogluteal injection site is no longer recommended for injections because of the close proximity to the sciatic nerve and major blood vessels. Injury to the sciatic nerve from an injection may cause partial paralysis of the leg. The dorsogluteal site is not to be used for intramuscular injections; instead, the ventrogluteal site is the preferred intramuscular injection site for adults and children.
- Assist the patient to the proper position, and ensure the patient's comfort.
- Locate the proper site for the injection and cleanse the site with an alcohol or antiseptic swab. Apply the

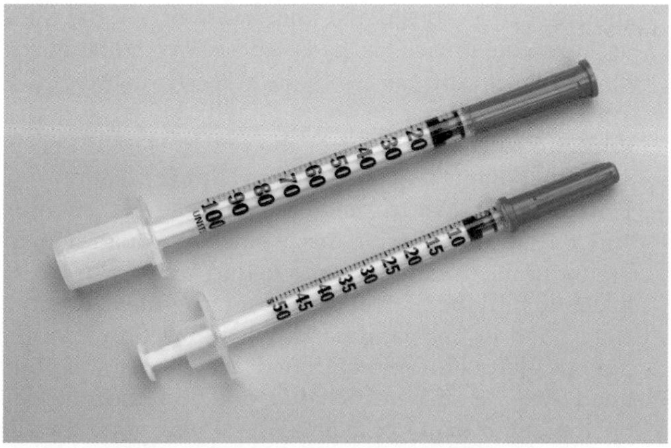

FIG. 10-50 Insulin syringes are available in 100-unit and 50-unit calibrations.

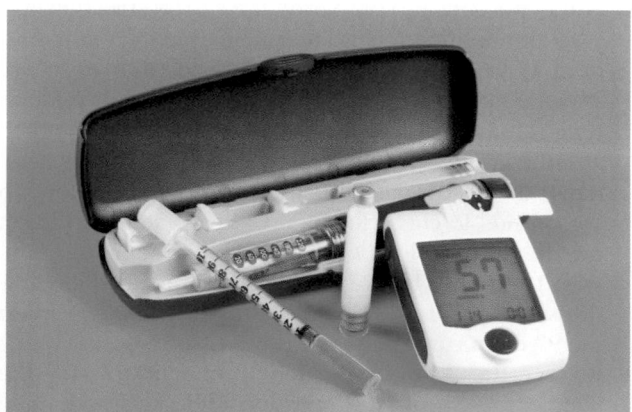

FIG. 10-51 A variety of devices are available for insulin injections.

swab at the centre of the site, and cleanse outward in a circular direction for about 5 cm (see Figure 10-47); then let the skin dry. Keep a sterile gauze pad nearby for use after the injection.

- With your nondominant hand, pull the skin taut. Follow the instructions for the Z-track method (see later), if appropriate.
- Grasp the syringe with your dominant hand between thumb and index finger, as if holding a dart, and hold the needle at a 90-degree angle to the skin. Tell the patient to expect a "stick" feeling as you insert the needle.
- Insert the needle quickly and firmly into the muscle. Grasp the lower end of the syringe with the nondominant hand while still holding the skin back, to stabilize the syringe. With the dominant hand, pull back on the plunger for 5 to 10 seconds to check for blood return.
- If no blood appears in the syringe, inject the medication slowly, at the rate of 1 mL every 10 seconds. After injecting the drug, wait 10 seconds, and then withdraw the needle smoothly while releasing the skin.
- Apply gentle pressure at the site and watch for bleeding. Apply a bandage if necessary.
- If blood does appear in the syringe, remove the needle, dispose of the medication and syringe, and prepare a new syringe with the medication.
- DO NOT RECAP the needle. Dispose of the syringe and needle in the appropriate container. Remove gloves and perform hand hygiene.
- Document the medication given on the MAR (see Figure 10-5), and monitor the patient for a therapeutic response as well as for adverse reactions.

Z-Track Method

- The Z-track method is used for injections of irritating substances such as iron dextran and hydroxyzine hydrochloride. The technique reduces pain, irritation, and staining at the injection site. Some facilities recommend this method for *all* intramuscular injections (Figures 10-52 and 10-53).
- After choosing and preparing the site for injection, use your nondominant hand to pull the skin laterally, and hold it in this position while giving the injection. When using this technique in the older adult population, it may not be necessary to pull the skin as much as in a younger adult because of loose skin turgor. Insert the needle at a 90-degree angle, aspirate for 5 to 10 seconds to check for blood return, and then inject the medication slowly. After injecting the medication, wait 10 seconds before withdrawing the needle. Withdraw the needle slowly and smoothly, and maintain the 90-degree angle.
- Release the skin immediately after withdrawing the needle to seal off the injection site. This technique forms a Z-shaped track in the tissue that prevents the medication from leaking through the more sensi-

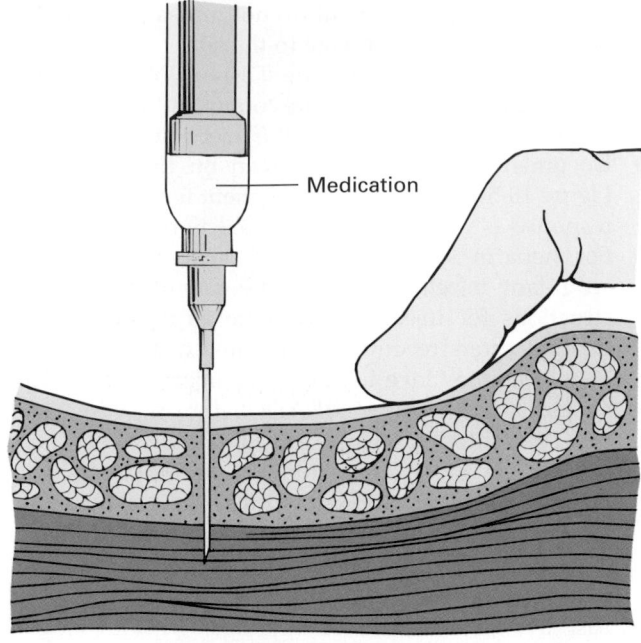

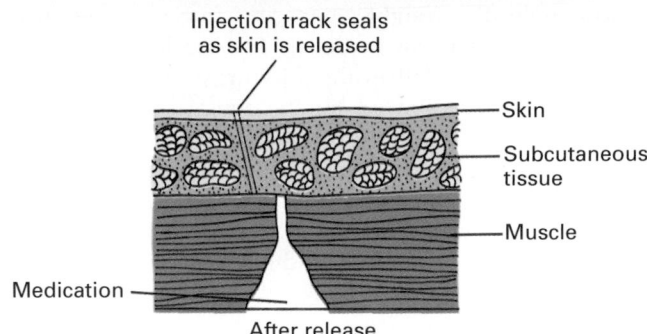

FIGS. 10-52 AND 10-53 The Z-track method for intramuscular injections.

tive subcutaneous tissue from the muscle site of injection. Apply gentle pressure to the site with a dry gauze pad.

Ventrogluteal Site

- The ventrogluteal site is the *preferred* site for adults and children. It is considered the safest of all the sites because the muscle is deep and away from major blood vessels and nerves (Figure 10-54).
- Position the patient on one side, with knees bent and upper leg slightly ahead of the bottom leg. If necessary, the patient may remain in a supine position.
- Palpate the greater trochanter at the head of the femur and the anterosuperior iliac spine. As illustrated in Figure 10-55, use the left hand to find landmarks when injecting into the patient's right ventrogluteal, and the right hand to find landmarks when injecting into the patient's left ventrogluteal site. Place the palm of your hand over the greater trochanter and your index finger on the anterosuperior iliac spine. Point your thumb toward the patient's groin and your fingers toward the patient's head. Spread the middle finger back along

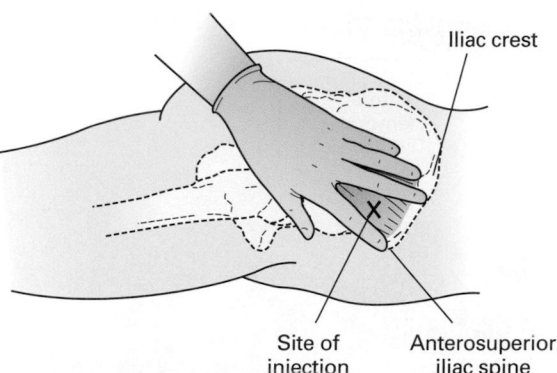

FIG. 10-54 Finding landmarks for a ventrogluteal injection.

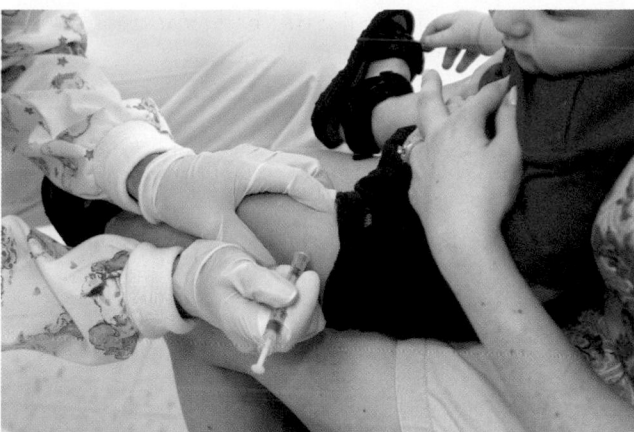

FIG. 10-57 Vastus lateralis intramuscular injection in an infant.

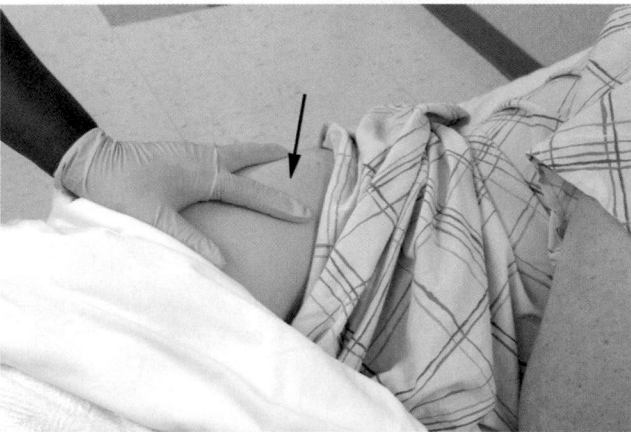

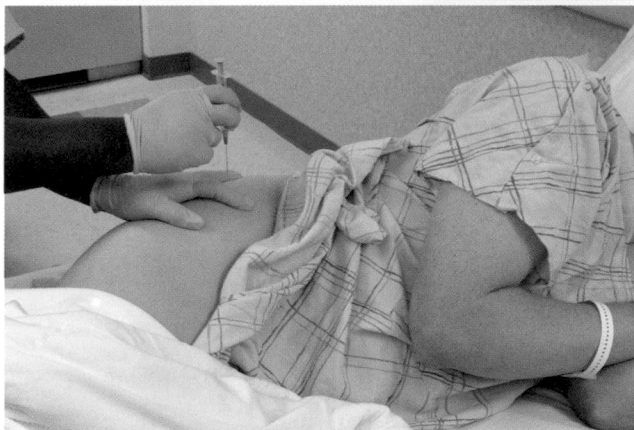

FIGS. 10-55 AND 10-56 Ventrogluteal intramuscular injection.

the iliac crest, toward the buttocks, as much as possible.
- The injection site is the centre of the triangle formed by your middle and index fingers (see arrow in Figure 10-55).
- Before giving the injection, you may need to switch hands so that you can use your dominant hand to give the injection (Figure 10-56).
- Follow the general instructions for giving an intramuscular injection.

Vastus Lateralis Site

- Generally, the vastus lateralis muscle is well developed and not located near major nerves or blood vessels. It is the preferred site of injection of drugs such as immunizations for infants (Figure 10-57). For specific information about giving injections to children, see Box 10-2.
- The patient may be sitting or lying supine; if supine, have the patient bend the knee of the leg in which the injection will be given.
- To find the correct site of injection, place one hand above the knee and one hand below the greater trochanter of the femur. Locate the midline of the anterior thigh and the midline of the lateral side of the thigh. The injection site is located within the rectangular area (Figures 10-58, 10-59, and 10-60).

Deltoid Site

- Even though the deltoid site (Figure 10-61) is easily accessible, it is *not* the first choice for intramuscular injections because the muscle may not be well developed in some adults, and the site carries a risk for injury because the axillary nerve lies beneath the deltoid muscle. In addition, the brachial artery and radial, brachial, and ulnar nerves are also located in the upper arm. Always check medication administration policies, because some facilities do not use the deltoid site for intramuscular injections. The deltoid site must only be used for giving immunizations to toddlers, older children, and adults (not infants) and only for small volumes of medication (0.5 to 1 mL).
- The patient may be sitting or lying down. Remove clothing to expose the upper arm and shoulder. Do not roll up tight-fitting sleeves. Have the patient relax the arm and slightly bend the elbow.
- Palpate the lower edge of the acromion process. This edge becomes the base of an imaginary triangle (Figure 10-62).
- Place three fingers below this edge of the acromion process. Find the point on the lateral arm in line with

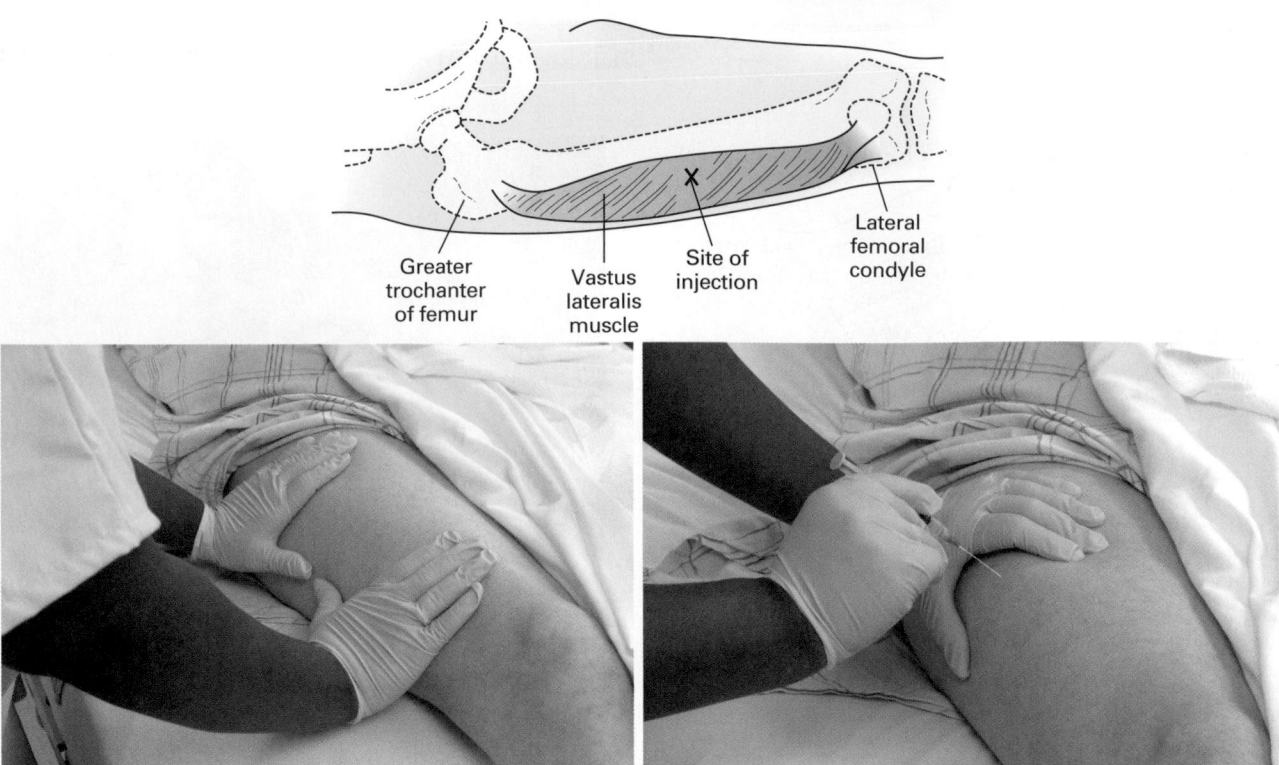

Greater trochanter of femur   Vastus lateralis muscle   Site of injection   Lateral femoral condyle

FIGS. 10-58, 10-59, AND 10-60 Vastus lateralis intramuscular injection.

Deltoid muscle

Site of injection

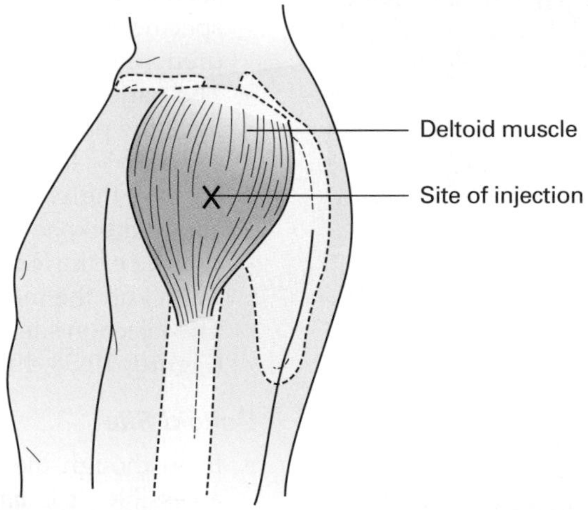

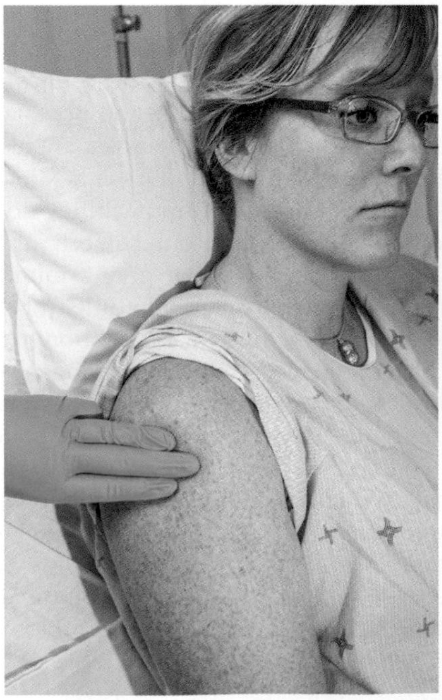

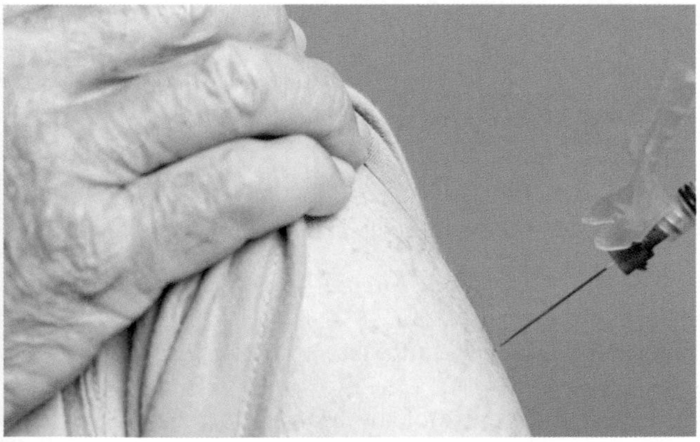

FIGS. 10-61, 10-62, AND 10-63 Deltoid intramuscular injection.

the axilla. The injection site will be in the centre of this triangle, three finger widths (2.5 to 5 cm) below the acromion process.

- Age-related considerations: In children and smaller adults, it may be necessary to bunch the underlying tissue together before giving the injection and use a shorter (16 mm) needle (Figure 10-63).
- To reduce patient anxiety, have the patient look away before you give the injection.

Preparing Intravenous Medications

Always begin by performing hand hygiene, and maintain standard precautions/routine practices (see Box 10-1). Gloves may be worn for these procedures. Check the agency policy. When administering intravenous drugs, keep in mind the following points:

- The intravenous route for medication administration provides for rapid onset and faster therapeutic drug levels in the blood than other routes. However, the intravenous route is also potentially more dangerous. Once an intravenous drug is given, it begins to act immediately and cannot be removed. The nurse must be aware of the drug's intended effects and possible adverse effects. In addition, hypersensitivity (allergic) reactions may occur quickly.
- Four provinces (Alberta, Manitoba, Ontario, and Saskatchewan) in Canada have passed laws or regulations pertaining to the use of safety-engineered devices (needleless systems for infusion lines); other provinces and territories are expected to follow.
- Before giving an intravenous medication, assess the patient's drug allergies, the intravenous line for patency, and the site for signs of phlebitis or infiltration.
- When more than one intravenous medication is to be given, check with the pharmacy for compatibility if medications are to be infused at the same time.
- Check the expiration date of both the medication and infusion bags.
- Age-related considerations: For children, infusion pumps *must* be used to prevent the risk of infusing the fluid and medication too fast.
- In many institutions, the pharmacy prepares the intravenous solutions and intravenous piggyback (IVPB) admixtures under a special laminar air-flow hood. Most IVPB medications come in vials that are added to the intravenous bag just before administration. When you dilute a drug for intravenous use, contact the pharmacist for instructions. Be sure to verify which type of fluid to use and the correct amount of solution for the dosage according to agency-specific guidelines or protocols for IV medication dilution and administration.
- Many IVPB medications are provided as part of an "add-a-vial" system that allows the intravenous medication vial to be attached to a small-volume minibag for administration. Figure 10-64 shows two examples

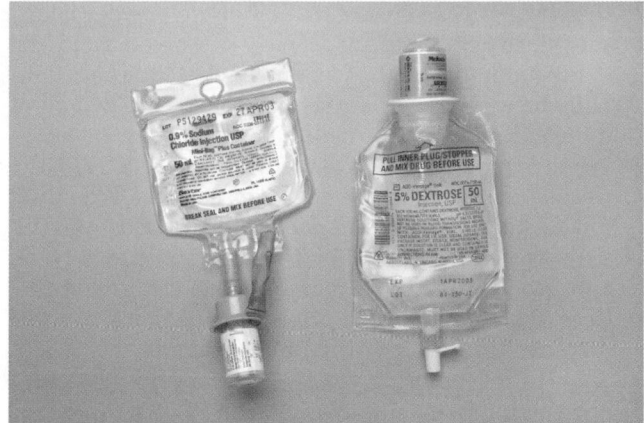

FIG. 10-64 Two types of intravenous piggyback (IVPB) medication delivery systems. These IVPB medications must be activated before administration to the patient.

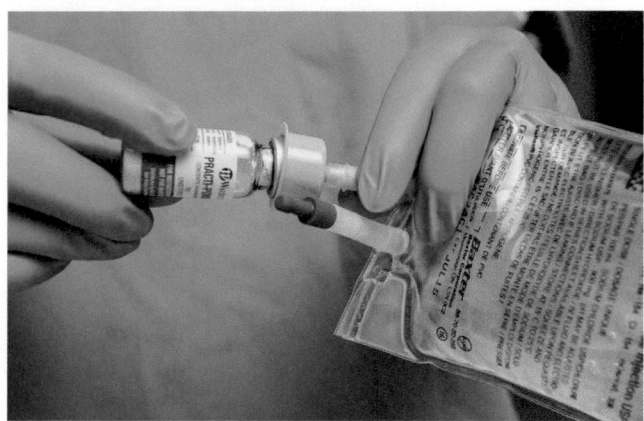

FIG. 10-65 Activating an IVPB infusion bag (step 1).

of IVPB medications attached to small-volume infusion bags.

- These IPVB medication setups allow for mixing of the drug and diluent immediately before the medication is given. Remember that if the seals are not broken and the medication is not mixed with the fluid in the infusion bag, then the medication stays in the vial! As a result, the patient does not receive the ordered drug dose; instead, the patient receives a small amount of plain intravenous fluid.
- It is important to choose the correct solution for diluting intravenous medications. For example, phenytoin must be infused with normal saline (NS), not dextrose solutions (see Chapter 15). Check with the pharmacist if necessary.
- One type of IVPB that needs to be activated before administration is illustrated in Figure 10-65. To activate this type of IVPB system, snap the connection area between the intravenous infusion bag and the vial (Figure 10-66). Gently squeeze the fluid from the infusion bag into the vial and allow the medication to dissolve (Figure 10-67). After a few minutes, rotate

the vial gently to ensure that all of the powder is dissolved. When the drug is fully dissolved, hold the IVPB apparatus by the vial and squeeze the bag; fluid will enter the bag from the vial. Make sure that all of the medication is returned to the IVPB bag.

- When hanging these IVPB medications, take care NOT to squeeze the bag. This may cause some of the fluid to leak back into the vial and alter the dose given.
- Always label the IVPB bag with the patient's name and room number, the name of the medication, the dose, the date and time mixed, your initials, and the date and time the medication was given.
- Some intravenous medications must be mixed using a needle and syringe. In many facilities, this procedure may be performed in the pharmacy. If you are mixing the IV medication, be sure to verify which type of fluid to use and the correct amount of solution for the

dosage according to agency-specific guidelines or protocols for IV medication dilution and administration. After checking the order and the compatibility of the drug and the intravenous fluid, wipe the port of the intravenous bag with an alcohol swab (Figure 10-68).

- Carefully insert the needle into the centre of the port and inject the medication (Figures 10-69 and 10-70). Note how the medication remains in the lower part of the intravenous infusion bag. Turn the bag gently,

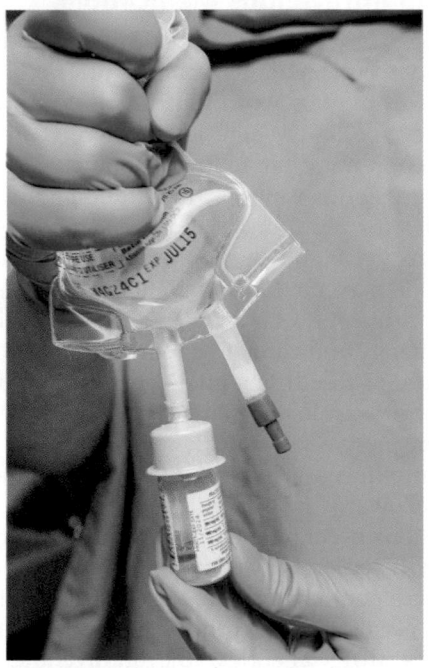

FIG. 10-67 Activating an IVPB infusion bag (step 3).

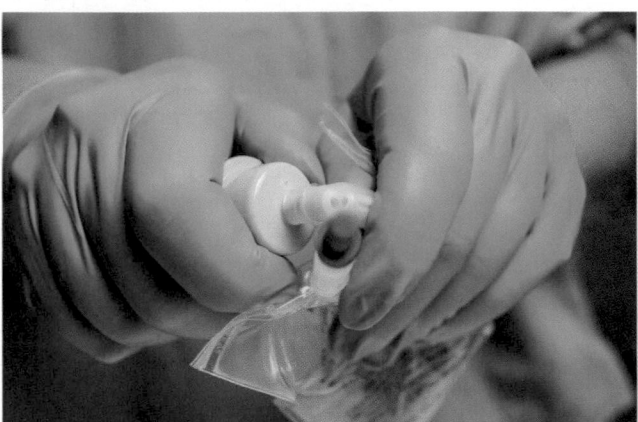

FIG. 10-66 Activating an IVPB infusion bag (step 2).

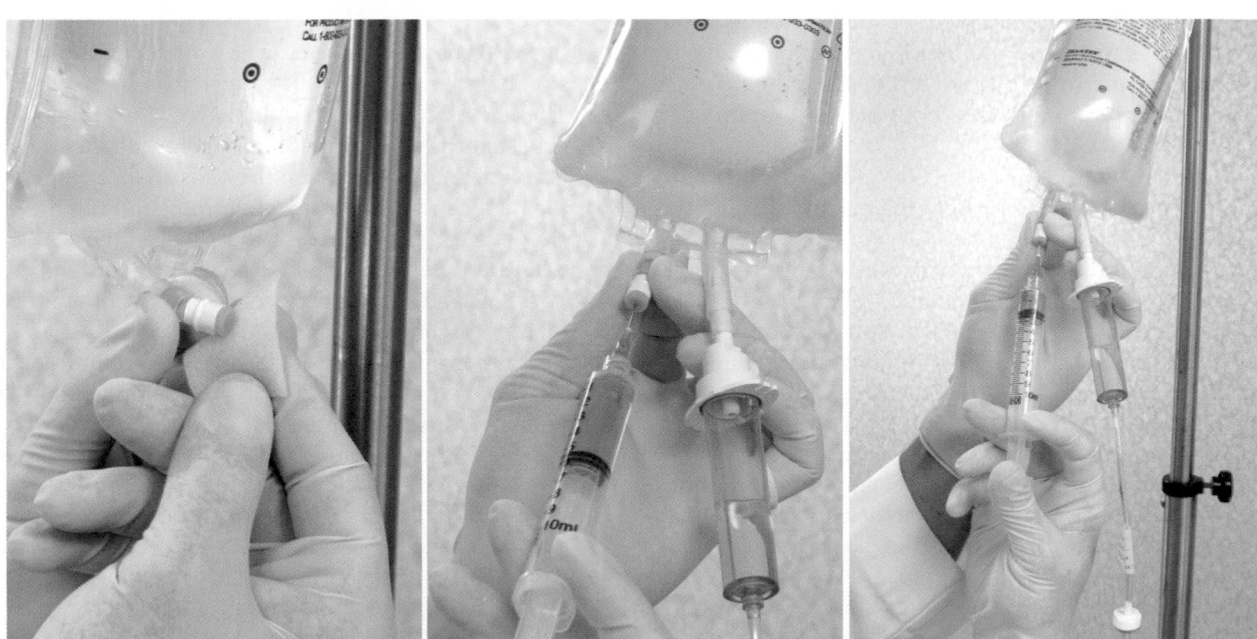

FIGS. 10-68, 10-69, AND 10-70 Adding a medication to a full intravenous infusion bag with a needle and syringe (prior to initiating the infusion).

end to end, to mix the fluid and added medication (Figure 10-71).

- Always add medication to a *new* bag of intravenous fluid, not to a bag that has partially infused. The concentration of the medication may be too strong if it is added to a partially full bag.
- Always label the intravenous infusion bag when a drug has been added (Figure 10-72). Label as per institution policy and include the patient's name and room number, the name of the medication, the date and time

mixed, your initials, and the date and time the infusion was started. In addition, label all intravenous infusion tubing per institution policy.

Infusions of Intravenous Piggyback Medications

Always begin by performing hand hygiene, and maintain standard precautions/routine practices (see Box 10-1). Gloves must be worn.

- Refrigerated medications may need to be left on the counter to warm to room temperature before administering. If you are infusing the IVPB medication for the first time, you will need to attach the medication bag to the appropriate tubing and "prime" the tubing by allowing just enough fluid through the tubing to flush out the air. Take care not to waste too much of the medication when flushing the tubing.
- If you are adding IVPB medication to an infusion that already has tubing, then use the technique of "backpriming" to flush the tubing (Figure 10-73). Backpriming allows for the administration of multiple intravenous medications without multiple disconnections, and thus reduces the risk of contamination of the intravenous tubing system.
- Backpriming allows the removal of the old medication fluid that has remained in the IVPB tubing from the previous dose of intravenous medication. After ensuring that the medication in the primary infusion (if any) is compatible with the medication in the IVPB bag, close the roller clamp on the primary infusion if the intravenous fluid is infusing by gravity flow (not necessary if an infusion pump is used). Remove the empty IVPB container from the intravenous pole, lower it to below the level of the primary infusion bag, and open

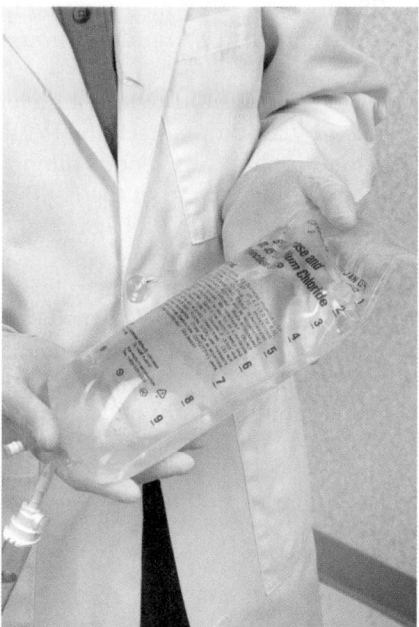

FIG. 10-71   Mix the medication thoroughly before infusing.

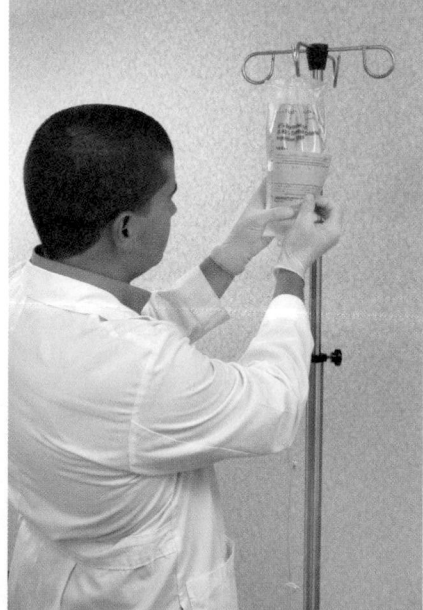

FIG. 10-72   Label the intravenous infusion bag when medication has been added.

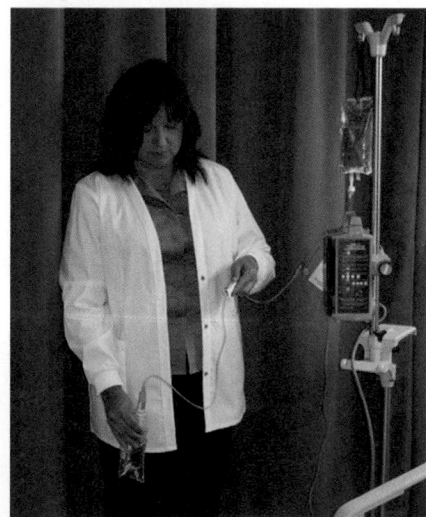

FIG. 10-73   Flush the intravenous piggyback (secondary) tubing by using the backpriming method. Fluid is drained through the tubing into the old intravenous piggyback bag, which is then discarded. The new dose of medication is then attached to the primed secondary tubing.

the clamp on the IVPB tubing. This will allow fluid to flow from the primary intravenous bag into the empty IVPB bag. Then, close the clamp on the IVPB tubing and squeeze the fluid that is in the drip chamber into the old IVPB bag to remove the old medication fluid. At this point, you may attach the new dose of intravenous medication to the IVPB tubing.

- Backpriming will not be possible if the primary intravenous infusion contains heparin sulphate, aminophylline, a vasopressor, or multivitamins. Check with a pharmacist if unsure about compatibility.

- Stopping intravenous infusions of medications such as vasopressors for an IVPB medication may affect a patient's blood pressure; stopping intravenous heparin may affect the patient's coagulation levels. Be sure to assess carefully before adding an IVPB medication to an existing infusion. A separate intravenous line may be necessary.

- Figure 10-74 shows an IVPB medication infusion (also known as the *secondary infusion*) with a primary gravity infusion. When the IVPB bag is hung higher than the primary intravenous infusion bag, the IVPB medication will infuse until empty, and then the primary infusion will take over again.

- When beginning the infusion, attach the IVPB tubing to the upper port on the primary intravenous tubing. A back-check valve above this port prevents the medication from infusing up into the primary intravenous infusion bag.

- Fully open the clamp of the IVPB tubing and regulate the infusion rate with the roller clamp of the primary infusion tubing. Be sure to note the drip factor of the tubing and calculate the drops per minute to count to set the correct infusion rate for the IVPB.

- Monitor the patient during the infusion. Observe for hypersensitivity and for adverse reactions. In addition, observe the intravenous infusion site for infiltration. Have the patient report if pain or burning occurs.

- Monitor the rate of infusion during the IVPB administration. Changes in arm position may alter the infusion rate.

- When the infusion is complete, clamp the IVPB tubing and check the primary intravenous infusion rate. If necessary, adjust the clamp to the correct infusion rate.

- Figure 10-75 shows an IVPB medication infusion with a primary infusion that is running through an electronic infusion pump.

- When giving IVPB drugs through an intravenous infusion controlled by a pump, attach the IVPB tubing to the port on the primary intravenous tubing above the pump. Open the roller clamp of the IVPB medication tubing. Make sure that the IVPB bag is higher than the primary intravenous infusion bag.

- Following the manufacturer's instructions, set the infusion pump to deliver the IVPB medication. Entering the volume of the IVPB bag and the desired time frame of the infusion (e.g., over a 60-minute period) will cause the pump to automatically calculate the IVPB rate. Start the IVPB infusion as instructed by the pump.

- Monitor the patient during the infusion, as described earlier.

- When the infusion is complete, the primary intravenous infusion will automatically resume.

- Document the medication given on the MAR (see Figure 10-5), and monitor the patient for a therapeutic response as well as for adverse reactions.

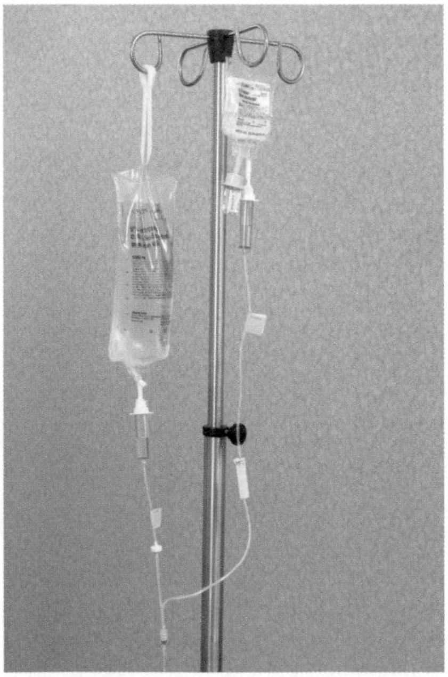

FIG. 10-74 Infusing an IVPB medication with a primary gravity intravenous infusion.

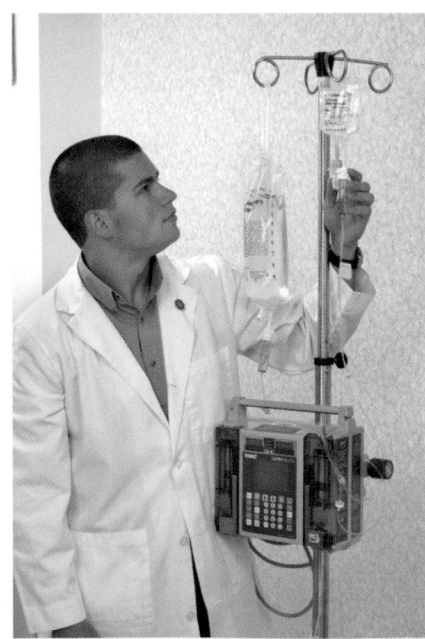

FIG. 10-75 Infusing an IVPB medication with the primary intravenous infusion on an electronic infusion pump.

- When giving intravenous medications through a saline (heparin) lock, follow the facility's guidelines for the flushing protocol before and after the medication is administered.
- In patient-controlled analgesia (PCA), a specialized pump is used to allow patients to self-administer pain medications, usually opiates (Figure 10-76). These pumps allow the patient to self-administer only as much medication as needed to control the pain, by pushing a button for intravenous bolus doses. Safety features of the pump prevent accidental overdoses. A patient receiving PCA pump infusions should be monitored closely for response to the drug, excessive sedation, hypotension, and changes in mental and respiratory status. Follow the facility's guidelines for setup and use.
- Figure 10-77 displays a smart pump, a type of intravenous infusion safety system designed to reduce intravenous medication errors. A smart pump contains built-in software that is programmed with facility-specific dosing profiles. The pump is able to "check" the dose-limits and other clinical guidelines, and when the pump is set up for patient use, it can warn the nurse if a potentially unsafe drug dose or therapy is entered.

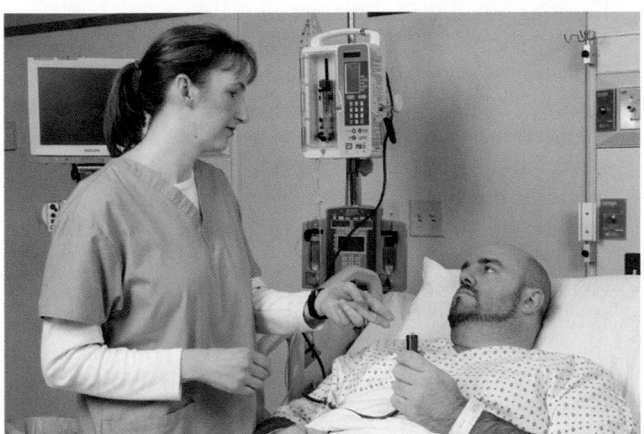

FIG. 10-76   Instructing the patient on the use of a patient-controlled analgesia (PCA) pump.

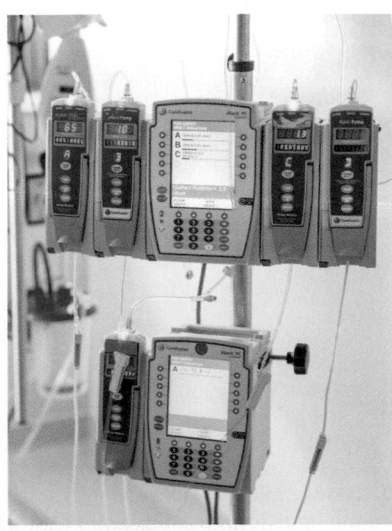

FIG. 10-77   A smart pump.

Intravenous Push Medications

Always begin by performing hand hygiene, and maintain standard precautions/routine practices (see Box 10-1). When administering intravenous push (or bolus) medications, keep in mind the following points:

- Registered nurses are usually the only nursing staff members allowed to give intravenous push medications. This may vary at different facilities.
- Intravenous push injections allow for rapid intravenous administration of a drug. The term *bolus* refers to a dose given all at once. Intravenous push injections may be given through an existing intravenous line, through an intravenous (saline or heparin) lock, or directly into a vein.
- Because the medication may have an immediate effect, monitor the patient closely for therapeutic effects as well as for adverse reactions.
- Follow the pharmacy/manufacturer's instructions carefully when preparing an intravenous push medication. Some drugs require careful dilution. Consult the pharmacist if unsure about the dilution procedure. Improper dilution may increase the risk of phlebitis and other complications. Always follow the agency guidelines/policies for dilution and administration of IV push medications.
- Some drugs are *never* given by intravenous push. Examples include dopamine, potassium chloride, and antibiotics such as vancomycin. Some medications administered by IV push require specific monitoring and are given only in specialty areas such as the emergency room and critical care unit. Follow agency protocols on the administration of drugs given by IV push.
- Small amounts of medication, less than 1 mL, need to be diluted in 5 to 10 mL of NS or another compatible fluid to ensure that the medication does not collect in a "dead space" of the tubing (such as the Y-site port). Check the facility's policy.
- Most drugs given by intravenous push injection are to be given over a period of 1 to 5 minutes to reduce local or systemic adverse effects. Always time the administration with your watch, because it is difficult to estimate the time accurately. Adenosine, however, must be given rapidly, within 2 to 3 seconds, for optimal action. ALWAYS check packaging information for guidelines, because many errors and adverse effects have been associated with too-rapid intravenous drug administration.

Intravenous Push Medications Through a Peripheral Intravenous Lock

- Obtain two syringes of 0.9% NS; both syringes should contain the required amount of fluid of solution according to agency policy. (Facilities may differ in protocol for intravenous lock flushes.) Many facilities provide prefilled syringes. Prepare medication for injection. If ordered, prepare a syringe with heparin sulphate flush solution.

- Follow the guidelines for a needleless system, if used.
- Cleanse the injection port of the intravenous lock with an alcohol or antiseptic swab for 15 seconds or according to agency protocol (Figure 10-78).
- Insert the syringe of NS into the injection port (Figure 10-79; a needleless system shown). Open the clamp of the intravenous lock tubing, if present.
- Gently aspirate and observe for blood return. Be sure to follow the agency policy regarding the need to aspirate for blood. Absence of blood return does not mean that the intravenous line is occluded; further assessment may be required.
- Flush gently with saline while assessing for resistance. A push-pause technique is recommended when instilling flush solution (e.g., give 2 mL to 3 mL of flush, pause, give another 3 ml of flush, pause, give another 2 mL to 3 mL of flush, and repeat until completed. The push-pause action creates turbulence within the needleless connector and catheter for more thorough

flushing. If you feel resistance, do not apply force. Stop and reassess the intravenous lock.

- Observe for signs of infiltration while injecting saline.
- Reclamp the tubing (if a clamp is present) and remove the NS syringe. Repeat cleansing of the port, and attach the medication syringe. Open the clamp again.
- Inject the medication over the prescribed length of time. Measure time with a watch or clock (Figure 10-80).
- When the medication is infused, clamp the intravenous lock tubing (if a clamp is present), and remove the syringe.
- Repeat cleansing of the port; attach a 2- 3-mL NS syringe and inject the contents into the intravenous lock slowly. If a heparin sodium flush is ordered, attach the syringe containing the heparin sulfate flush solution and inject slowly (per the institution's protocol).

Intravenous Push Medications Through an Existing Infusion

- Prepare the medication for injection. Follow the guidelines for a needleless system, if used.
- Check compatibility of the intravenous medication with the existing intravenous solution.
- Choose the injection port that is closest to the patient.
- Remove the cap, if present, and cleanse the injection port with an alcohol or antiseptic swab.
- Occlude the intravenous line by pinching the tubing just above the injection port (Figure 10-81). Attach the syringe to the injection port.
- Gently aspirate for blood return.
- While keeping the intravenous tubing clamped, slowly inject the medication according to administration guidelines. Be sure to time the injection with a watch or clock.
- After the injection, release the intravenous tubing, remove the syringe, and check the infusion rate of the intravenous fluid.

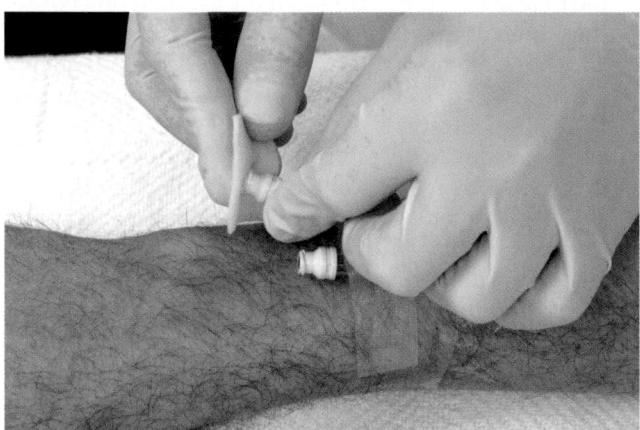

FIG. 10-78 Cleanse the port before attaching the syringe.

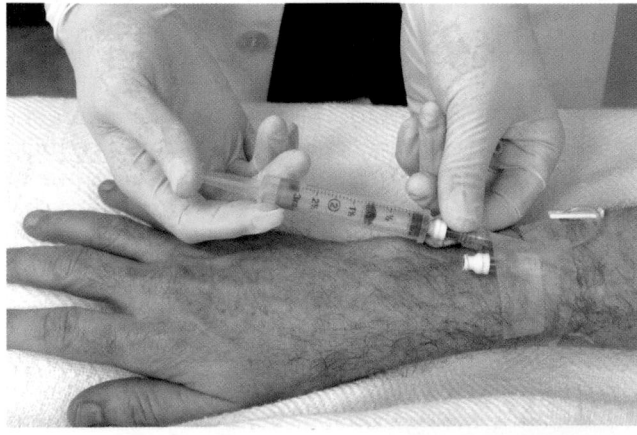

FIG. 10-79 Attaching the syringe to the intravenous lock.

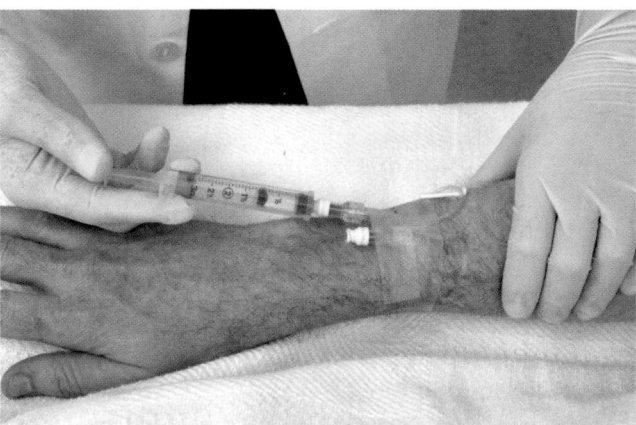

FIG. 10-80 Slowly inject the intravenous push medication through the intravenous lock; use a watch to time the injection.

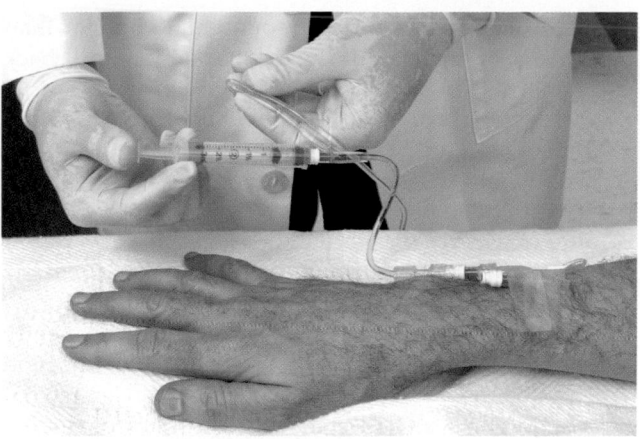

FIG. 10-81 When giving an intravenous push medication through an intravenous line, pinch the tubing just above the injection port.

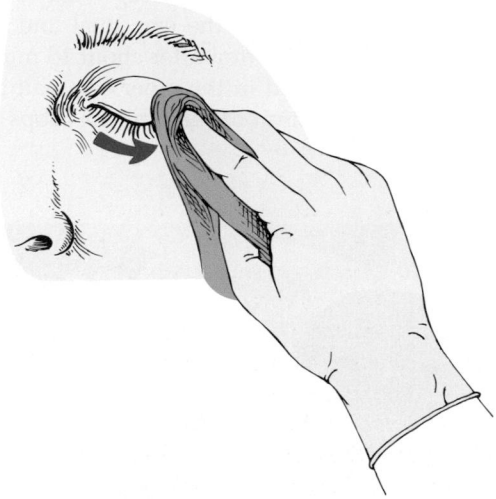

FIG. 10-82 Cleanse the eye, washing from the inner canthus to the outer canthus, before giving eye medications.

After Injecting an Intravenous Push Medication

- Monitor the patient closely for adverse effects. Monitor the intravenous infusion site for signs of phlebitis and infiltration.
- Document medication given on the MAR (see Figure 10-5), and monitor the patient for therapeutic response as well as adverse effects.

TOPICAL DRUGS

Administering Eye Medications

Always begin by performing hand hygiene, and maintain standard precautions/routine practices (see Box 10-1). Gloves may be worn. When administering eye preparations, keep in mind the following points:

- Assist the patient to a supine or sitting position. The patient's head should be tilted back slightly. Make sure the patient is not wearing contact lenses.
- Remove any secretions with a sterile gauze pad; be sure to wipe from the inner to the outer canthus (Figure 10-82).

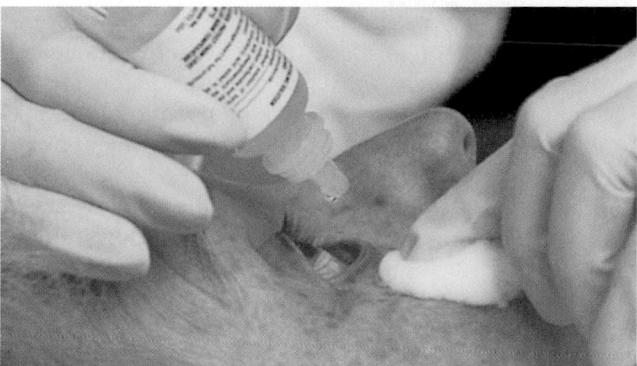

FIG. 10-83 Insert the eye drop into the lower conjunctival sac.

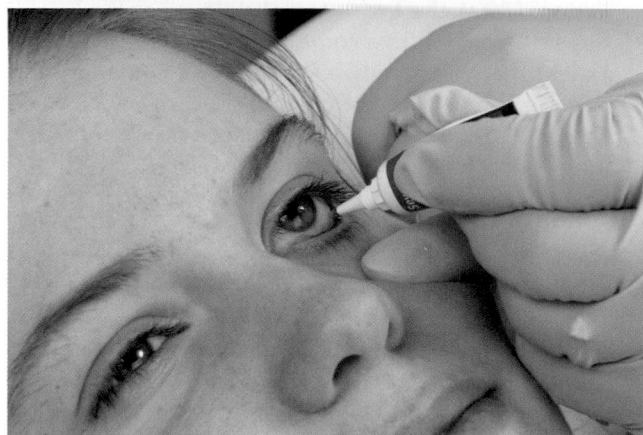

FIG. 10-84 Applying eye ointment.

- Instruct the patient to tilt the head slightly back. With your nondominant hand, gently pull the lower lid open to expose the conjunctival sac.

Eye Drops

- With your dominant hand resting on the patient's forehead, hold the eye medication dropper 1 to 2 cm above the conjunctival sac. Do not touch the tip of the dropper to the eye or with your fingers (Figure 10-83).
- Drop the prescribed number of drops into the conjunctival sac. Never apply eye drops to the cornea.
- If the drops land on the outer lid margins (if the patient moved or blinked), repeat the procedure.
- Age-related considerations: Infants often squeeze the eyes tightly shut to avoid eye drops. To give drops to an uncooperative infant, restrain the head gently and place the drops at the corner where the eyelids meet the nose. When the eye opens, the medication will flow into the eye.

Eye Ointment

Gently squeeze the tube of medication to apply an even strip of medication (about 1 to 2 cm) along the border of the conjunctival sac. Start at the inner canthus and move toward the outer canthus (Figure 10-84).

After Instilling Eye Medications

- Ask the patient to close the eye gently. Squeezing the eye shut may force the medication out of the conjunctival sac. A tissue may be used to blot liquid that runs out of the eye, but instruct the patient not to wipe the eye.
- You may apply gentle pressure to the patient's nasolacrimal duct for 30 to 60 seconds with a gloved finger wrapped in a tissue. This will help reduce systemic absorption of the drug through the nasolacrimal duct and may also help to reduce the taste of the medication in the oropharynx from the nasopharynx (Figure 10-85).
- If multiple eye drops are due at the same time, wait several minutes before administering the second medication. Check the instructions for the specific drug.
- Assist the patient to a comfortable position. Warn the patient that vision may be blurry for a few minutes.
- Document the medication given on the MAR (see Figure 10-5), and check the patient for a therapeutic response as well as for adverse reactions.

Administering Ear Drops

Always begin by performing hand hygiene, and maintain standard precautions/routine practices (see Box 10-1). Gloves may be worn. When administering ear medications, keep in mind the following points:

- After explaining the procedure to the patient, assist the patient to a side-lying position with the affected ear facing up. If drainage is noted in the outer ear canal, remove it carefully without pushing it back into the ear canal.
- Remove excessive amounts of cerumen before instilling medication.
- If refrigerated, warm the ear medication by taking it out of refrigeration for at least 30 minutes before administration. Instillation of cold ear drops can cause nausea, dizziness, and pain.
- Age-related considerations: For an adult or a child older than 3 years of age, pull the pinna up and back (Figure 10-86). For an infant or a child younger than 3 years of age, pull the pinna down and back (Figure 10-87).
- Administer the prescribed number of drops. Direct the drops along the sides of the ear canal rather than directly onto the eardrum.
- Instruct the patient to lie on one side for 5 to 10 minutes. Gently massaging the tragus of the ear with a finger will help distribute the medication down the ear canal.
- If ordered, a loose cotton pledget can be gently inserted into the ear canal to prevent the medication from flowing out. The cotton must remain somewhat loose to allow any discharge to drain out of the ear canal. To prevent the dry cotton from absorbing the ear drops that were instilled, moisten the cotton with a small amount of medication before inserting the pledget. Insertion of cotton too deeply may result in increased pressure within the ear canal and on the eardrum. Remove the cotton after about 15 minutes.
- If medication is needed in the other ear, wait 5 to 10 minutes after instillation of the first ear drops before administering.

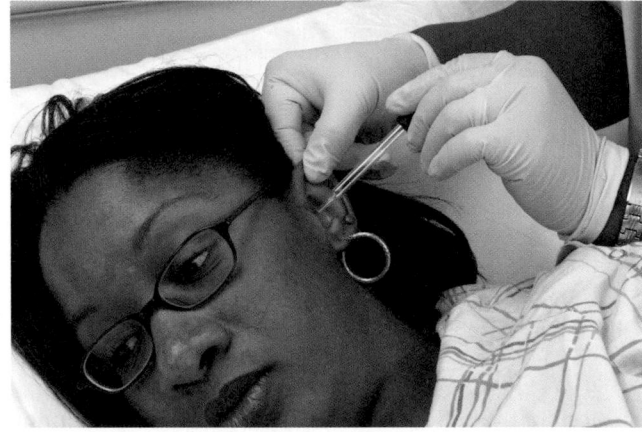

FIG. 10-86 With adults, pull the pinna up and back.

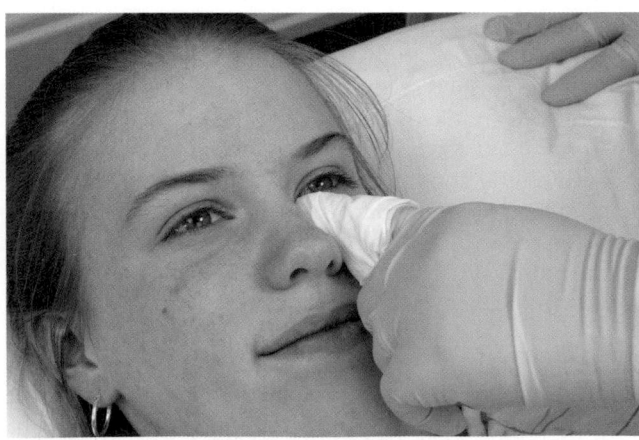

FIG. 10-85 Applying gentle pressure against the nasolacrimal duct after giving eye medications.

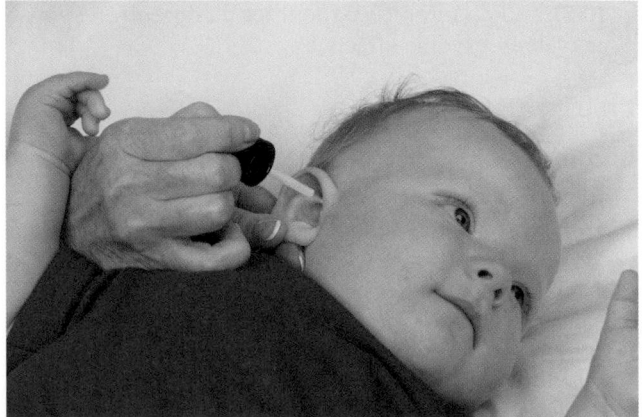

FIG. 10-87 With infants and children under 3 years of age, pull the pinna down and back.

- Document the medication given on the MAR (see Figure 10-5), and monitor the patient for a therapeutic response as well as for adverse reactions.

Administering Nasal Medications

Always begin by performing hand hygiene, and maintain standard precautions/routine practices (see Box 10-1). Patients may self-administer some of these drugs after proper instruction. Gloves must be worn. When administering nasal medications, keep in mind the following points:

- Before giving nasal medications, explain the procedure to the patient and tell the patient that temporary burning or stinging may occur. Instruct the patient that it is important to clear the nasal passages by blowing the nose, unless contraindicated (e.g., with increased intracranial pressure or nasal surgery), before administering the medication. Assess for deviated septum or a history of nasal fractures, because these may impede the patient's ability to inhale through the affected nostril.
- Figure 10-88 illustrates delivery forms for nasal medications: sprays, drops, and dose-measured sprays.
- Assist the patient to the supine position. Support the patient's head as needed.
- If specific areas are targeted for the medication, position the patient's head as follows:
- For the posterior pharynx, position the head backward.
- For the ethmoid or sphenoid sinuses, place the head gently over the top edge of the bed or place a pillow under the shoulders, and tilt the head back.
- For the frontal or maxillary sinuses, place the head back and turned toward the side that is to receive the medication.

Nasal Drops

- Hold the nose dropper approximately 1 cm above the nostril. Administer the prescribed number of drops toward the midline of the ethmoid bone (Figure 10-89).

- Repeat the procedure as ordered, instilling the indicated number of drops per nostril.
- Keep the patient in the supine position for 5 minutes.
- Age-related considerations: Infants are nose breathers, and the potential congestion caused by nasal medications may make it difficult for them to suck. If nose drops are ordered, administer them 20 to 30 minutes before a feeding.

Nasal Spray

- Have the patient sitting upright and occlude one nostril by pressing a finger against the outer naris. After gently shaking the nasal spray container, insert the tip into the nostril. Squeeze the spray bottle into the nostril while the patient inhales through the open nostril (Figure 10-90).
- Repeat the procedure as ordered, instilling the indicated number of sprays per nostril.
- Keep the patient in the supine position for 5 minutes.

After Administration of Nasal Medicines

- Offer the patient tissues for blotting any drainage, but instruct the patient to avoid blowing her nose for several minutes after instillation of the drops.

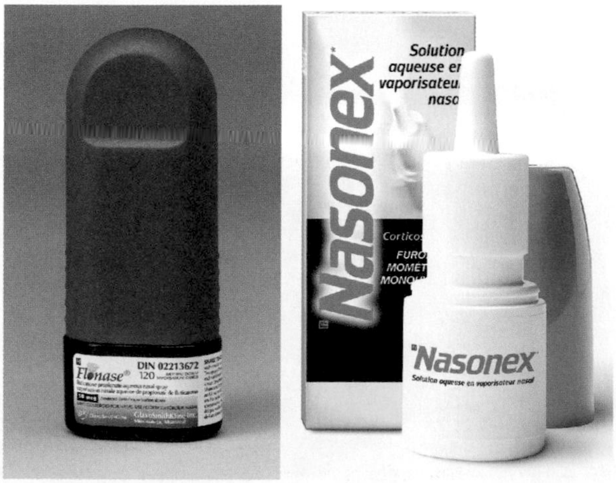

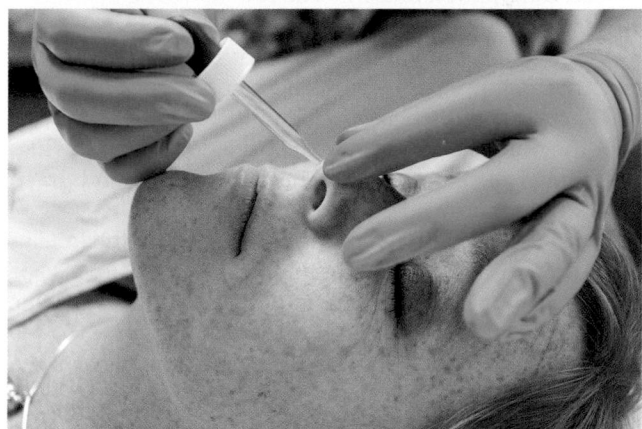

FIG. 10-89 Administering nose drops.

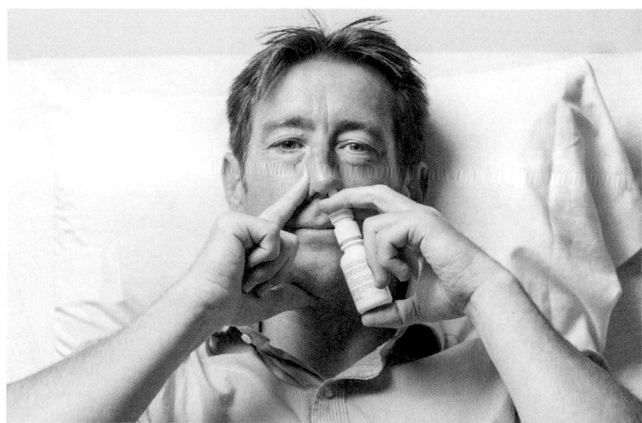

FIG. 10-90 Before self-administering the nasal spray, the patient should occlude the other nostril and spray the medication away from the septum.

FIG. 10-88 Nasal medications in various delivery forms.

- Assist the patient to a comfortable position.
- Document the medication administration on the MAR (see Figure 10-5), and document drainage, if any. Monitor the patient for a therapeutic response as well as for adverse reactions.

Administering Inhaled Drugs

Always begin by performing hand hygiene, and maintain standard precautions/routine practices (see Box 10-1). Gloves may be worn. Patients with asthma need to monitor their peak expiratory flow rates by using a peak flowmeter. A variety of inhalers are available (Figure 10-91). Be sure to check for specific instructions from the manufacturer as needed. Improper use will result in inadequate dosing and lack of therapeutic effect. When administering inhaled preparations, keep in mind the following points:

Metered-Dose Inhalers

- A spacer is always used with a pressured metered-dose inhaler (MDI) that delivers inhaled corticosteroids. Spacers can make it easier for medication to reach the lungs, and also mean that less medication gets deposited in the mouth and throat, where it can lead to irritation and mild infections.
- Shake the (MDI) gently before using.
- Remove the cap; hold the inhaler upright, and grasp with the thumb and first two fingers.
- Tilt the patient's head back slightly.
- If the MDI is used without a spacer, do the following: Remove the cap; hold the inhaler upright and grasp with the thumb and first two fingers.
1. Have the patient open his mouth; position the inhaler 3 to 5 cm away from the mouth (Figure 10-92). For self-administration, some patients may measure this distance as 1 to 2 finger-widths.
2. Have the patient exhale, then press down once on the inhaler to release the medication; have the patient breathe in slowly and deeply for 5 seconds.

3. Have the patient hold his or her breath for approximately 10 seconds, and then exhale slowly through pursed lips.
- Age-related consideration: Spacers can be used with children and adults who have difficulty coordinating inhalations with activation of metered-dose inhalers (see Chapter 38). If the inhaler is used with a spacer, do the following:
1. Attach the spacer to the mouthpiece of the inhaler after removing the inhaler cap.
2. Place the mouthpiece of the spacer in the patient's mouth.
3. Have the patient exhale.
4. Press down on the inhaler to release the medication, and have the patient inhale deeply and slowly through the spacer. The patient then breathes in and out slowly for 2 to 3 seconds, and then holds his breath for 10 seconds (Figure 10-93).
5. Clean the spacer. Take the spacer apart and gently move the parts back and forth in warm soapy water. Avoid the use of high-pressure or boiling hot water, rubbing alcohol, or disinfectant. Rinse the parts well in clean water. Do not dry the inside of

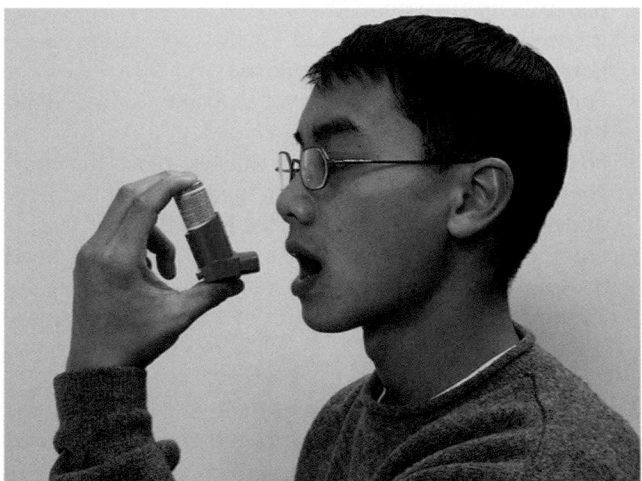

FIG. 10-92 Using an MDI without a spacer.

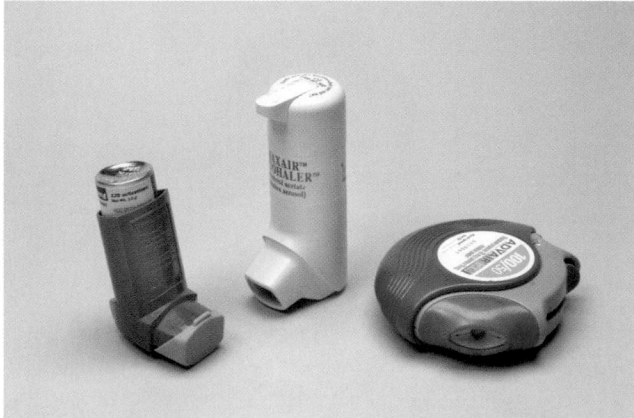

FIG. 10-91 **A,** Metered-dose inhaler (MDI). **B,** Automated MDI. **C,** "Disk-type" metered-dose inhaler for delivering powdered medication.

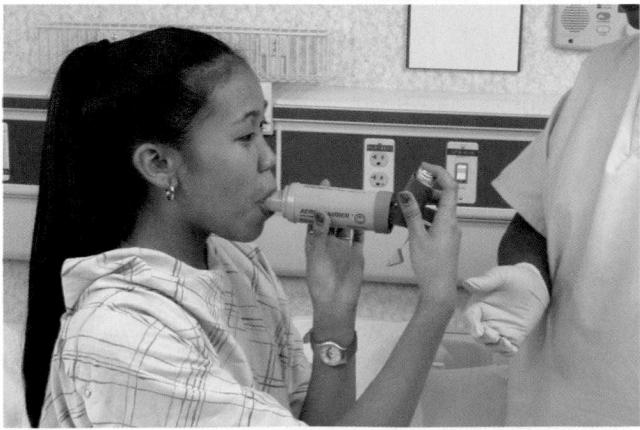

FIG. 10-93 Using a spacer device with an MDI.

the spacer with a towel as it will create static; rather, air dry.

- If a second puff of the same medication is ordered, wait 1 to 2 minutes between puffs.
- If a second type of inhaled medication is ordered, wait 2 to 5 minutes between medication inhalations or as prescribed.
- If both a bronchodilator and a corticosteroid inhaled medication are ordered, the bronchodilator should be administered first so that the air passages will be more open for the second medication.
- Instruct the patient to rinse his mouth with water after inhaling a steroid medication to prevent the development of an oral fungal infection.
- Document the medication given on the MAR (see Figure 10-5), and monitor the patient for a therapeutic response as well as for adverse reactions.
- It is important to teach the patient how to calculate the number of doses in the inhaler and to keep track of uses. Simply shaking the inhaler to "estimate" whether it is empty is not accurate and may result in its being used when it is empty. Many metered-dose inhalers now come with devices that help to count the remaining doses. If the inhaler does not have a dose-counting device, the patient should be taught to count the number of puffs needed per day (doses) and divide this amount into the actual number of actuations (puffs) in the inhaler to estimate the number of days the inhaler will last. Then, a calendar can be marked a few days before this date with a note that it is time to obtain a refill. In addition, the date can be marked on the inhaler with a permanent marker. For example, an inhaler with 200 puffs, ordered to be used 4 times a day (2 puffs per dose, 8 puffs per day), would last for 25 days (200 divided by 8). The patient may experience the sensation of a puff even when the canister is empty. This sensation occurs from the propellant but there is little or no drug in the puff, and it is, therefore, not effective. Dry powder inhalers have varied instructions, so follow the manufacturer's instructions closely. Instruct patients to cover the mouthpiece completely with their mouths. Capsules that are intended for use with these inhalers should NEVER be taken orally. Some dry powder inhalers also have convenient, built-in dose counters.

Small-Volume Nebulizers

- Check the doctor's order in regard to the use of compressed air or oxygen for the administration of the nebulizer treatment.
- In some facilities, the air compressor is located in the wall unit of the room. In other facilities and at home, a small, portable air compressor is used. Be sure to follow the manufacturer's instructions for use.
- In some facilities, nebulizer treatments may be performed by a respiratory therapist. However, closely monitor the patient before, during, and after the drug administration.

- Be sure to take the patient's baseline heart rate, especially if a β-adrenergic drug is used. Some drugs may increase the heart rate.
- After gathering the equipment, add the prescribed medication to the nebulizer cup (Figure 10-94). Some medications will require a diluent; others are premixed with a diluent. Be sure to verify before adding a diluent.
- Have the patient hold the mouthpiece between the lips (Figure 10-95).
- Age-related considerations: Use a face mask for a child or an adult who is too fatigued to hold the mouthpiece. Special adaptors are available if the patient has a tracheostomy.
- Before starting the nebulizer treatment, have the patient take a slow, deep breath, hold it briefly, then exhale slowly. Patients who are short of breath should

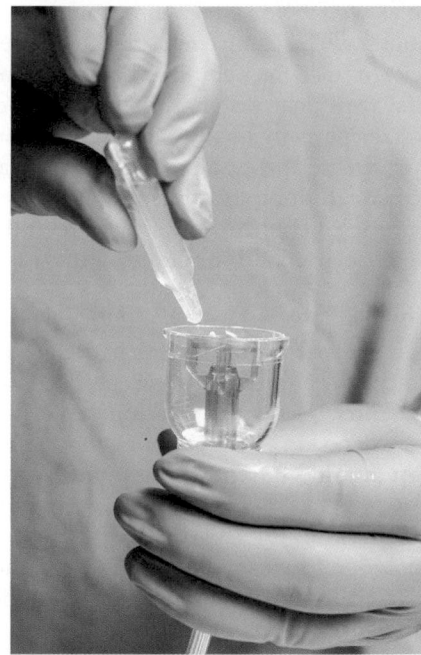

FIG. 10-94 Adding medication to the nebulizer cup.

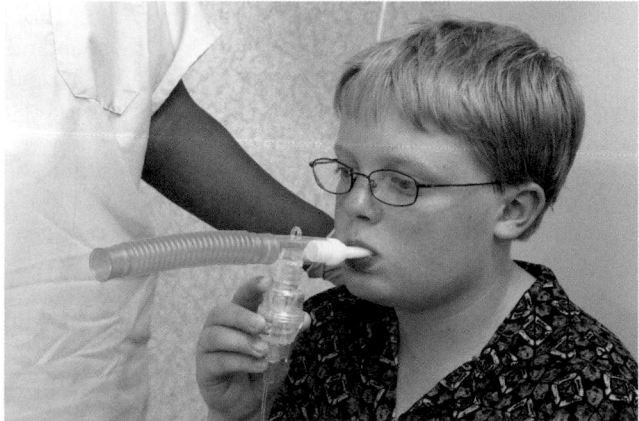

FIG. 10-95 Administering a small-volume nebulizer treatment.

be instructed to hold their breath every fourth or fifth breath.

- Turn on the small-volume nebulizer machine (or turn on the wall unit), and make sure that a sufficient mist is forming.
- Instruct the patient to repeat the breathing pattern mentioned previously during the treatment.
- Occasionally tap the nebulizer cup during the treatment and toward the end to move the fluid droplets back to the bottom of the cup.
- Monitor the patient's heart rate during and after the treatment.
- If inhaled steroids are given, instruct the patient to rinse his mouth afterward.
- After the procedure, clean and store the tubing per institution policy.
- Document the medication given on the MAR (see Figure 10-5), and monitor the patient for a therapeutic response as well as for adverse reactions.
- If the patient will be using a nebulizer at home, instruct the patient to rinse the nebulizer parts daily after each use with warm, clear water and allow to air dry. Soak the nebulizer parts in a solution of vinegar and water (four parts water and one part white vinegar) for 30 minutes; rinse thoroughly with clear, warm water; and air dry. Storing nebulizer parts that are still wet will encourage bacterial and mould growth.

Administering Medications to the Skin

Always begin by performing hand hygiene, and maintain standard precautions/routine practices (see Box 10-1). Gloves must be worn. Avoid touching the preparations to your own skin. When administering skin preparations, keep in mind the following points:

Lotions, Creams, Ointments, And Powders

- Apply powder to clean, dry skin. Have the patient turn her head to the other side during application to avoid inhalation of powder particles.
- Apply lotion to clean, dry skin. Remove residual from previous applications with soap and water.
- Before administering any dose of a topical skin medication, ensure that the site is clean and dry. Thoroughly remove previous applications using soap and water, if appropriate for the patient's condition, and dry the area thoroughly. Be sure to remove any debris, drainage, or pus if present.
- Age-related considerations: The skin of an older patient may be more fragile and easily bruised or damaged (e.g., skin tears and possible breakdown of skin from use of tape). Be sure to assess for appropriateness of the skin area before applying medication, and handle the skin gently when cleansing to prepare the site for medication and when applying medications.
- With lotion, cream, or gel, obtain the correct amount with your gloved hand (Figure 10-96). If the medication is in a jar, remove the dose with a sterile tongue depressor and apply to your gloved hand. Do not contaminate the medication in the jar.

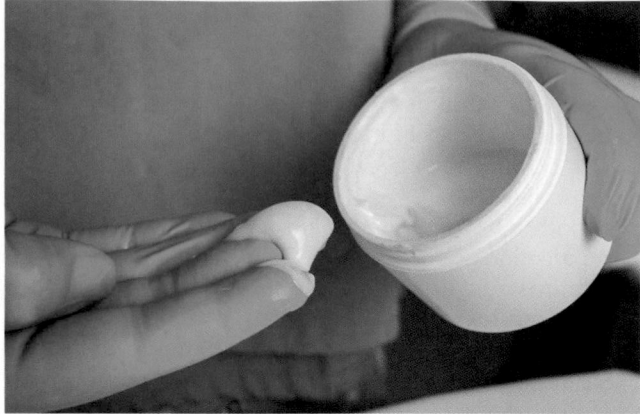

FIG. 10-96 Use gloves to apply topical skin preparations.

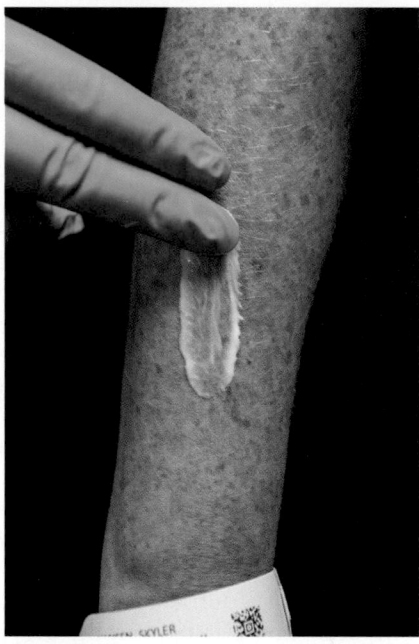

FIG. 10-97 Spread the lotion on the skin with long, smooth, gentle strokes.

- Some ointments and creams may soil the patient's clothes and linens. If these preparations are ordered, cover the affected site with gauze or a transparent dressing.
- Although nitroglycerin ointment is not used as frequently as the nitroglycerin transdermal patch, it is still available for use. Nitroglycerin ointment in a tube is measured carefully on clean, ruled application paper before it is applied to the skin. Do not massage nitroglycerin ointment into the skin. Apply the measured amount onto a clean, dry site and then secure the application paper with a transparent dressing or a strip of tape (Figure 10-97). Always remove the old medication before applying a new dose. Rotate application sites.

Transdermal Patches

- Be sure that the used patch is removed as ordered. Some patches may be removed before the next patch

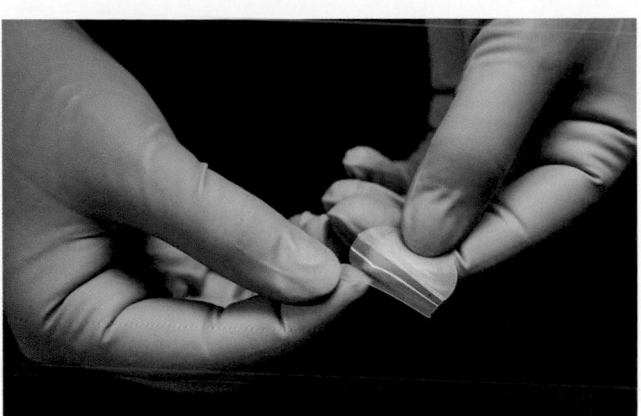

FIG. 10-98   Opening a transdermal patch medication.

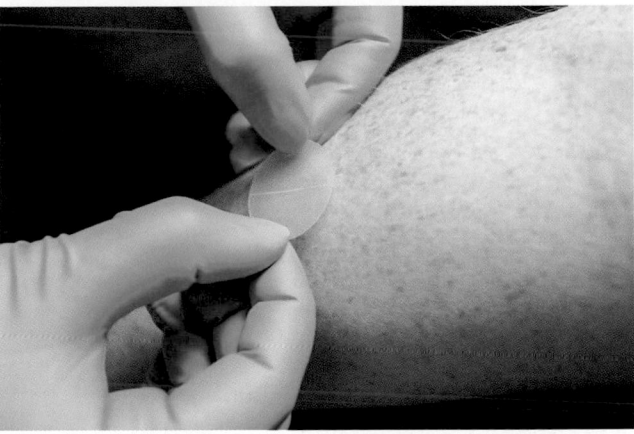

FIG. 10-99   Ensure that the edges of the transdermal patch are secure after applying.

is due—check the order. Clear patches may be difficult to find, and patches may be overlooked in obese patients with skin folds. Cleanse the site of the used patch thoroughly. Observe for signs of skin irritation at the old patch site. Rotate sites of application with each dose.

- Transdermal patches should be applied at the same time each day if ordered daily.
- The used patch can be pressed together and then wrapped in a glove as you remove the glove from your hand. Dispose in the proper container according to the facility's policy.
- Select a new site for application and ensure that it is clean and without powder or lotion. For best absorption and fewest adverse effects, the site needs to be hairless and free from scratches or irritation. If it is necessary to remove hair, clip the hair instead of shaving to reduce irritation to the skin. Application sites may vary. Follow the drug manufacturer's specific instructions as to where to apply the patch.
- Remove the backing from the new patch (Figure 10-98). Take care not to touch the medication side of the patch with your fingers.
- Place the patch on the skin site and press firmly (Figure 10-99). Press around the edges of the patch with one or two fingers to ensure that the patch is adequately secured to the skin. If an overlay is provided by the drug manufacturer, apply it over the patch.
- Instruct the patient not to cut transdermal patches. Cutting transdermal patches releases all of the medication at once and may result in a dangerous overdose.
- Instruct the patient to safely dispose of the old patch by folding the medicated side facing inward. Using this disposal method prevents contact with the drug-eluting portion of the patch.

After Administering Topical Skin Preparations

- Chart the medication given on the MAR (see Figure 10-5), and monitor the patient for a therapeutic response as well as for adverse reactions.
- Provide instruction on administration to the patient or caregiver.

ILLUSTRATION CREDITS

PART TWO

Drugs Affecting the Central Nervous System

STUDY SKILLS TIPS:
- VOCABULARY
- TEXT NOTATION
- LANGUAGE CONVENTIONS

VOCABULARY

For any subject matter, mastering the vocabulary is essential to mastering the content. However, in a complex, technical subject such as nursing pharmacology, if you do not master the vocabulary, understanding the content will be almost impossible. Each chapter in this text contains a list of key terms at the beginning, and as an independent learner, you should spend some time and energy on the vocabulary contained in the key terms. Do not expect to completely understand and master the words from the key terms alone; they are further defined and explained in the body of the chapter, and it is when you read the chapter that you should expect to fully master the vocabulary. However, the time you spend working on the key terms will pay off when you read the chapter.

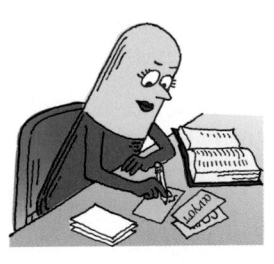

Consider the terms *agonist* and *antagonist* in the Chapter 11 key terms. These terms share a common word part, which means the words are related in meaning. This is an important first step in mastering them. What does *agonist* mean? What is the similarity between *agonist* and *antagonist*? What is the essential difference between the two? Remember, take an active role in your learning. Asking these questions as you start to work on Chapter 11 is a valuable technique for beginning to master the content. Do not simply memorize the terms. Learn what they mean and link relationships between words with common elements. As you practice this technique, it will

become easier to retain the meanings of terms. The Chapter 11 Key Terms also contain other words that should be viewed as a group that shares an important relationship. The first of these words is *pain*. The definition provided is clear and relatively easy to understand, but your focus should be not just on that single word because there are 13 other words that relate to pain: *acute, breakthrough, cancer, central, chronic, deep, neuropathic, phantom, referred, somatic, superficial, vascular,* and *visceral*. Each of these words defines and categorizes pain in a very specific way.

Consider using vocabulary cards. These are small pieces of paper or cards (ideally the size of your hand) that you can use to write on, both front and back. The front lists the vocabulary term, while the back lists the definition. At first, you will rely on the back to gain familiarity with the terminology; however, over time, you will be able to use the vocabulary card as a means to evaluate your knowledge of the terminology cards.

As you go about setting up vocabulary cards, look at the opening pages of Chapter 11. You will find considerable discussion of these terms, which is useful in helping you obtain the fullest understanding of the terms. Do not simply focus on the meaning of each term, but also ask what the similarities and differences are and how these words relate to one another.

TEXT NOTATION

The Study Skills Tips for Part 1 discussed a method for text underlining. Remember, text notation is an active process that facilitates your ability to comprehend material. If it is done carefully, this strategy is particularly useful for later review of text material. The object of text underlining is to pick out important terms, ideas, and information so you can come back to it later for quick review. The three key elements in successful text underlining are as follows:

1. Read the material once before attempting any underlining.
2. Be acutely aware of the author's language.
3. Be selective in underlining. The most common fault in underlining is to mark too much material.

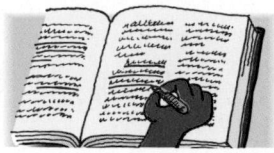

Following are three paragraphs from Chapter 11 that have been underlined. The underlining should be viewed as an example of what can be done. Each reader will mark the text somewhat differently, based on his or her background and experience. As you study this example, think not only about what has been underlined but also about why that material might have been chosen. Consider sample underline #1 and sample underline #2. Notice the difference in the words that are selected for underlining. Sample #1 underlined significantly more text material, whereas sample #2 underlined less. Now, compare both below and ask yourself, "What do I find more helpful?" "Why?"

(ORIGINAL TEXT WITHOUT HIGHLIGHTS)

Pain is most commonly defined as an unpleasant sensory and emotional experience associated with either actual or potential tissue damage. It is a personal and individual experience. Pain can be defined as whatever the patient says it is, and it exists whenever the patient says it does. Although the mechanisms of pain are becoming better understood, a patient's perception of pain is a complex process. Pain involves physical, psychological, and ethnocultural factors (see Ethnocultural Implications: The Patient Experiencing Pain: Considerations From a Holistic Perspective). Because pain intensity cannot be precisely quantified, health care providers must cultivate relationships of mutual trust with their patients to provide optimal care.

There is no single approach to effective pain management. Instead, it is tailored to each patient's needs. The cause of the pain, the existence of concurrent medical conditions, the characteristics of the pain, and the psychological and ethnocultural characteristics of the patient all need to be considered. It also requires ongoing reassessment of the pain and the effectiveness of treatment. The patient's emotional response to pain depends on the individual psychological experience of pain. Pain results from the stimulation of sensory nerve fibres known as **nociceptors**. These receptors transmit pain signals from various body regions to the spinal cord and brain, which leads to the sensation of pain, or **nociception** (Figure 11-1). Nociceptive pain is transitory in response and serves an important and protective role.

(SAMPLE UNDERLINE #1)

Pain is most commonly defined as an <u>unpleasant sensory and emotional experience associated with either actual or potential tissue damage.</u> <u>It is a personal and individual experience.</u> Pain can be defined as whatever the <u>patient says it is,</u> and it <u>exists</u> whenever the <u>patient says it does.</u> Although the mechanisms of pain are becoming better understood, <u>a patient's perception of pain is a complex process.</u> Pain involves <u>physical, psychological, and ethnocultural factors</u> (see Ethnocultural Implications: The Patient Experiencing Pain: Considerations From a Holistic Perspective). Because <u>pain intensity cannot be precisely quantified,</u> <u>health care providers must cultivate relationships of mutual trust with their patients to provide optimal care.</u>

There is <u>no single approach to effective pain management.</u> Instead, it is <u>tailored to each patient's needs.</u> The cause of the pain, the existence of concurrent medical conditions, the characteristics of the pain, and the psychological and ethnocultural characteristics of the patient all need to be considered. It also requires <u>ongoing reassessment of the pain and the effectiveness of treatment.</u> The patient's <u>emotional response to pain depends on the individual psychological experience of pain.</u> Pain results from the stimulation of sensory nerve fibres known as **nociceptors**. These receptors <u>transmit pain signals from various body regions to the spinal cord and brain, which leads to the sensation of pain, or **nociception**</u> (Figure 11-1). Nociceptive pain is transitory in response and serves an important and protective role.

(SAMPLE UNDERLINE #2)

Pain is most commonly defined as an <u>unpleasant sensory and emotional experience associated with either actual or potential tissue damage.</u> It is a personal and individual experience. Pain can be defined as whatever the patient says it is, and it exists whenever the patient says it does. Although the mechanisms of pain are becoming better understood, a patient's perception of pain is a complex process. Pain involves <u>physical, psychological, and ethnocultural factors</u> (see Ethnocultural Implications: The Patient Experiencing Pain: Considerations From a Holistic Perspective). Because <u>pain intensity cannot be precisely quantified,</u> health care providers must cultivate relationships of mutual trust with their patients to provide optimal care.

There is no single approach to effective pain management. Instead, it is <u>tailored to each patient's needs.</u> The cause of the pain, the existence of concurrent medical conditions, the characteristics of the pain, and the psychological and ethnocultural characteristics of the patient all need to be considered. It also requires ongoing reassessment of the pain and the effectiveness of treatment. The patient's emotional response to pain depends on the individual psychological experience of pain. Pain results from <u>the stimulation of sensory nerve fibres known as **nociceptors**.</u> These receptors transmit pain signals from various body regions to the spinal cord and brain, which leads to the sensation of pain, or **nociception** (Figure 11-1). Nociceptive pain is transitory in response and serves an important and protective role.

(ORIGINAL TEXT WITHOUT HIGHLIGHTS)

The physical impulses that signal pain activate various nerve pathways from the periphery to the spinal cord and to the brain. The level of stimulus needed to produce a painful sensation is referred to as the **pain threshold**. Because this is a measure of the physiological response of the nervous system, it is similar for most persons. However, variations in pain sensitivity may result from genetic factors.

(SAMPLE UNDERLINE #1)

The <u>physical impulses that signal pain activate various nerve pathways from the periphery to the spinal cord and to the brain.</u> The <u>level of stimulus needed to produce a painful sensation is referred to as the **pain threshold**.</u> Because this is a measure of the physiological response of the nervous system, it is similar for most persons. However, <u>variations in pain sensitivity may result from genetic factors.</u>

(SAMPLE UNDERLINE #2)

The physical impulses that signal pain activate various nerve pathways from the periphery to the spinal cord and to the brain. The level of <u>stimulus needed to produce a painful sensation is referred to as the **pain threshold**.</u> Because this is a measure of the physiological response of the nervous system, it is similar for most persons. However, variations in pain sensitivity may result from genetic factors.

LANGUAGE CONVENTIONS

Certain words and phrases are like signal lights at an intersection. They serve to tell the reader that something special, important, or noteworthy is happening. To the attentive, active reader, these conventions contribute significantly to understanding what the author is trying to convey. Whether you are highlighting, underlining, writing margin notes, or studying the material using the PURR model, it is important for you to become sensitive to these conventions.

In Chapter 11, the text following the topic heading Overview contains several examples. In the third paragraph, the first sentence contains the phrase *classified as*. Whenever an author says that something is being classified, it means that there are at least two (and perhaps several more) elements of the term or idea being classified. This means that you should immediately ask yourself questions about the reading, such as, "What is being classified? How many classifications are there for this?" These questions will help you focus on what to learn and keep your attention firmly fixed on the process of learning.

As you read this and other chapters, become aware of words and phrases like these that are intended to draw your attention to something the author wanted to emphasize. The more aware you are of language conventions, the easier it will be to become a selective reader. Selective readers do not try to remember everything they read—they select those concepts and terms that the writers tried to stress from the mass of information to read.

CHAPTER 11

Analgesic Drugs

Objectives

After reading this chapter, the successful student will be able to do the following:

1. Define acute pain and persistent (chronic or long-term) pain.

2. Contrast the signs, symptoms, and management of acute and persistent pain.

3. Discuss the pathophysiology and characteristics associated with cancer pain and other special pain situations.

4. Describe pharmacological and nonpharmacological approaches for the management and treatment of acute and persistent pain.

5. Discuss the use of nonopioids, nonsteroidal anti-inflammatory drugs (NSAIDs), and opioids (opioid agonists, opioids with mixed actions, opioid agonist–antagonists and antagonists), and miscellaneous drugs in the management of acute and persistent pain, cancer pain, and special pain situations.

6. Identify examples of drugs classified as nonopioids, nonsteroidal anti-inflammatory drugs, opioids (opioid agonists, opioids with mixed actions, opioid agonist–antagonists and antagonists), and miscellaneous drugs.

7. Briefly describe the mechanism of action, indications, dosages, routes of administration, adverse effects, toxicity, cautions, contraindications, and drug interactions of nonopioids, nonsteroidal anti-inflammatory drugs (see Chapter 49), opioids (opioid agonists, opioids with mixed actions, opioid agonist–antagonists and antagonists), and miscellaneous drugs.

8. Contrast the pharmacological and nonpharmacological management of acute and persistent pain associated with cancer and pain experienced in terminal conditions.

9. Briefly describe the specific standards of pain management as defined by the World Health Organization and the Canadian Pain Society.

10. Develop a collaborative plan of care based on the nursing process related to the use of nonopioid and opioid drug therapy and the nursing process for patients in pain.

11. Identify various resources, agencies, and professional groups that are involved in establishing standards for the management of all types of pain and for promotion of a holistic approach to the care of patients with acute or persistent pain and those in special pain situations.

e-Learning Activities

Website
(http://evolve.elsevier.com/Canada/
Lilley/pharmacology/)

evolve

- Answer Key—Textbook Case Studies
- Answer Key—Critical Thinking Activities
- Chapter Summaries—Printable
- Review Questions for Exam Preparation
- Unfolding Case Studies

Drug Profiles

▸▸ acetaminophen, p. 214
   codeine (codeine sulphate)*, p. 209
   fentanyl (fentanyl citrate), p. 209
   lidocaine, transdermal, p. 214
   meperidine (meperidine hydrochloride)*, p. 210
   methadone (methadone hydrochloride)*, p. 210
▸▸ morphine (morphine sulphate)*, p. 208
▸▸ naloxone (naloxone hydrochloride)*, p. 211
   naltrexone (naltrexone hydrochloride)*, p. 211
   oxycodone (oxycodone hydrochloride)*, p. 210
   tramadol (tramadol hydrochloride)*, p. 214

▸▸ Key drug

*Full generic name is given in parentheses. For the purposes of this text, the more common, shortened name is used.

Key Terms

Acute pain   Pain that is sudden in onset, usually subsides when treated, and typically occurs over less than a 6-week period. (p. 195)

Addiction   Strong psychological or physical dependence on a drug or other psychoactive substance, usually resulting from habitual use, that is beyond normal voluntary control. (p. 200)

Adjuvant analgesic drugs   Drugs that are added for combined therapy with a primary drug and may have additive or independent analgesic properties, or both. (p. 194)

Agonists   Substances that bind to a receptor and cause a response. (p. 201)

Agonist–antagonists   Substances that bind to a receptor and cause a partial response that is not as strong as that caused by agonists (also known as a *partial agonists*). (p. 202)

Analgesic ceiling effect   What occurs when a particular pain drug no longer effectively controls a patient's pain despite the administration of the highest safe dosages. (p. 202)

Analgesics   Medications that relieve pain (sometimes referred to as *painkillers*). (p. 194)

Antagonists   Drugs that bind to a receptor and prevent (block) a response, resulting in inhibitory or antagonistic drug effects; also called inhibitors. (p. 203)

Breakthrough pain   Pain that occurs between doses of pain medication. (p. 201)

Cancer pain   Pain resulting from any of a variety of causes related to cancer or the metastasis of cancer. (p. 196)

Central pain   Pain resulting from any disorder that causes central nervous system damage. (p. 198)

Gate control theory   A common and well-described theory of pain transmission and pain relief. It uses a gate model to explain how impulses from damaged tissues are sensed in the brain. (p. 198)

Narcotics   A legal term established under the *Narcotic Control Act* in 1961. It originally applied to drugs that produce insensibility or stupor, especially the opioids (e.g., morphine sulphate, heroin). Currently used to refer to any medically used controlled substances and in legal settings to refer to any illicit or "street" drug. (NOTE: This term is falling out of use in favour of *opioid* and will not be used further in this text.)

Neuropathic pain   Pain that results from a disturbance of function or pathologic change in a nerve. (p. 196)

Nociception   Processing of pain signals in the brain that gives rise to the feeling of pain. (p. 195)

Nociceptors   A subclass of sensory nerves (A and C fibres) that transmit pain signals to the central nervous system from other body parts. (p. 195)

Nociceptive pain   Pain that arises from mechanical, chemical, or thermal irritation of peripheral sensory nerves (e.g., after surgery or trauma or associated with degenerative processes). Two subtypes of nociceptive pain are visceral and somatic. (p. 195)

Nonopioid analgesics   Analgesics that are structurally and functionally different from opioids. (p. 207)

Nonsteroidal anti-inflammatory drugs (NSAIDs)   A large, chemically diverse group of drugs that are analgesics and possess anti-inflammatory and antipyretic properties but are not corticosteroids. (p. 218)

Opiate analgesics   Synthetic drugs that bind to opiate receptors to relieve pain. (p. 202)

Opioid naive   Describes patients who are receiving opioid analgesics for the first time or intermittently for a brief period of time and who therefore are not accustomed to their effects. (p. 206)

Opioid tolerant   The opposite of opioid naive; describes patients who have been receiving opioid analgesics (legally or otherwise) for a period of time (1 week or longer) and who are at greater risk of opioid withdrawal syndrome upon sudden discontinuation. (p. 200)

Opioid withdrawal   The signs and symptoms associated with abstinence from, withdrawal of or dose reduction an opioid analgesic when the body has become physically dependent on the substance. (p. 206)

Pain   An unpleasant sensory and emotional experience associated with actual or potential tissue damage. (p. 194)

Pain threshold   The level of stimulus that results in the sensation of pain. (p. 195)

Pain tolerance   The amount of pain a patient can endure without its interfering with normal function. (p. 195)

Partial agonist   A drug that binds to a receptor and causes a response that is less than that caused by a full agonist (same as *agonist–antagonist*). (p. 203)

Persistent pain   Recurring pain that is often difficult to treat. Includes any pain lasting longer than 3 to 6 months, pain lasting longer than 1 month after healing of an acute injury, or pain that accompanies a nonhealing tissue injury. (Also referred to as *chronic* or *long-term* pain). (p. 195)

Phantom pain   Pain experienced in an area of the body part that has been surgically or traumatically removed. (p. 196)

Physical dependence   A condition in which a patient takes a drug over a period of time and in which unpleasant physical symptoms (withdrawal symptoms) occur if the drug is stopped abruptly or smaller doses are given. The physical adaptation of the body to the presence of an opioid or other addictive substance. (p. 206)

Psychological dependence   A pattern of compulsive use of opioids or any other addictive substance characterized by a continuous craving for the substance and the need to use it for effects other than pain relief (also called *addiction*). (p. 200)

Referred pain   Pain occurring in an area away from the organ of origin. (p. 196)

Somatic pain   Pain that originates from skeletal muscles, ligaments, or joints.

Special pain situation   The general term for pain control situations that are complex and whose treatment typically involves multiple medications, various health care personnel, and nonpharmacological therapeutic modalities (e.g., massage, chiropractic care, surgery).

Superficial pain   Pain that originates from the skin or mucous membranes; opposite of *deep pain.*

Synergistic effects   Drug interactions in which the effect of a combination of two or more drugs with similar actions is greater than the sum of the individual effects of the same drugs given alone. For example, 1 + 1 is greater than 2. (p. 201)

Tolerance   The general term for a progressively decreased responsiveness to a drug as a result of which a larger dose of the drug is needed to achieve the effect originally obtained by a smaller dose. (p. 196)

Vascular pain   Pain that results from pathology of the vascular or perivascular tissues. (p. 196)

Visceral pain   Pain that originates from internal organs or smooth muscles.

World Health Organization (WHO)   An international body of health care providers, including clinicians and epidemiologists among many others, that studies and responds to health needs and trends worldwide. (p. 201)

OVERVIEW

The management of pain is an important aspect of nursing care in a variety of settings and across the lifespan. Pain is the more common reason that patients seek health care and is the underlying reason for 78% of emergency department visits annually in Canada. Surgical and diagnostic procedures often require pain management, as do several diseases including arthritis, diabetes, multiple sclerosis, cancer, and acquired immune deficiency syndrome (AIDS). Pain leads to much suffering and is a tremendous economic burden as a result of lost workplace productivity, workers' compensation payments, and other related health care costs.

To provide quality patient care, it is important to be well informed about both pharmacological and nonpharmacological methods of pain management. This chapter focuses on pharmacological methods of pain management. Some examples of nonpharmacological methods of pain management are listed in Box 11-1.

Medications that relieve pain are classified as **analgesics.** They are also commonly referred to as *painkillers.* There are various classes of analgesics, determined by their chemical structures and mechanisms of action. The focus of this chapter is primarily on the **opioid analgesics,** which are used to manage moderate to severe pain. Often drugs from other chemical categories are added to the opioid regimen as **adjuvant analgesic drugs** (or adjuvants), and these are described later. **Pain** is most commonly defined as an unpleasant sensory and emotional experience associated with either actual or potential tissue damage. It is a personal and individual experience. Pain can be defined as whatever the patient says it is, and it exists whenever the patient says it does. Although the mechanisms of pain are becoming better understood, a patient's perception of pain is a complex process. Pain involves physical, psychological, and ethnocultural factors (see Ethnocultural Implications: The Patient Experiencing Pain: Considerations From a Holistic Perspective). Because pain intensity cannot be precisely

BOX 11-1

Nonpharmacological Treatment Options for Pain

- Acupressure
- Acupuncture
- Art therapy
- Behavioural therapy
- Biofeedback
- Comfort measures
- Counselling
- Distraction
- Hot or cold packs
- Hypnosis
- Imagery
- Massage
- Meditation
- Music therapy
- Pet therapy
- Physical therapy
- Reduction of fear
- Relaxation
- Surgery
- Therapeutic baths
- Therapeutic communication
- Therapeutic touch
- Transcutaneous electrical nerve stimulation
- Yoga

quantified, health care providers must cultivate relationships of mutual trust with their patients to provide optimal care.

There is no single approach to effective pain management. Instead, it is tailored to each patient's needs. The cause of the pain, the existence of concurrent medical conditions, the characteristics of the pain, and the psychological and ethnocultural characteristics of the patient all need to be considered. It also requires ongoing

ETHNOCULTURAL IMPLICATIONS

The Patient Experiencing Pain: Considerations From a Holistic Perspective

- Pain is experienced by individuals, not by a particular culture. Health care providers often interpret pain behaviour through their own cultural lens and often make assumptions about patients by the behaviours they display.
- Know that there are environmental and ethnocultural variations in pain experience and expression and in health care–seeking treatment.
- Recognize the contributions and limitations of the social determinants of health to pain experience, pain expression, and treatment access.
- Know that pain behaviours and reports are best understood in the context of social interactions among the individual, family, employers, and health care providers and in the context of community, governmental, or legal procedures.
- Be aware of communication related to cultural and religious variation that health care providers should consider when assessing and managing pain.

- Recognize that social environmental factors, including the individual's beliefs about the origins and nature of pain and how one should access health care, can influence both experiential and expressive features of pain.
- Recognize the internal and exogenous barriers that impact access to the implementation of pain evaluation and treatment (e.g., individual motivation, beliefs, adverse effects, availability of opioids).
- Remain aware of all ethnocultural influences on health-related behaviours and on patients' attitudes toward medication therapy and thus, ultimately, on its effectiveness. A thorough assessment that includes questions about the patient's cultural background and practices is important to the effective and individualized delivery of nursing care.

reassessment of the pain and the effectiveness of treatment. The patient's emotional response to pain depends on the individual psychological experience of pain. Pain results from the stimulation of sensory nerve fibres known as **nociceptors**. These receptors transmit pain signals from various body regions to the spinal cord and brain, which leads to the sensation of pain, or **nociception** (Figure 11-1). Nociceptive pain is transitory in response and serves an important protective role.

The physical impulses that signal pain activate various nerve pathways from the periphery to the spinal cord and to the brain. The level of stimulus needed to produce a painful sensation is referred to as the **pain threshold**. Because this is a measure of the physiological response of the nervous system, it is similar for most persons. However, variations in pain sensitivity may result from genetic factors.

There are three main receptors believed to be involved in pain. The μ (mu) receptors in the dorsal horn of the spinal cord appear to play the most crucial role. Less important but still involved in pain sensations are the κ (kappa) and δ (delta) receptors. Pain receptors are located in both the central nervous system (CNS) and various body tissues. Pain perception—and, conversely, emotional well-being—is closely linked to the number of μ (mu) receptors. This number is controlled by a single gene, the μ (mu) opioid receptor gene. When the number of receptors is high, pain sensitivity is diminished. Conversely, when the receptors are reduced or missing altogether, relatively minor noxious stimuli may be perceived as painful.

The patient's emotional response to the pain is also moulded by the patient's age, gender, culture, previous pain experience, and anxiety level. Whereas pain thresh-

TABLE	11-1

Conditions That Alter Pain Tolerance

Pain Threshold	Conditions
Lowered	Anger, anxiety, depression, discomfort, fear, isolation, persistent pain, sleeplessness, tiredness
Raised	Diversion, empathy, rest, sympathy, medications (analgesics, antianxiety drugs, antidepressants)

old is the physiological element of pain, the psychological element of pain is called **pain tolerance**. This is the amount of pain a patient can endure without its interfering with normal function. Because it is a subjective response, pain tolerance can vary from patient to patient. Pain tolerance can be modulated by the patient's personality, attitude, environment, culture, and ethnic background. Pain tolerance can even vary within the same person depending on the circumstances involved. Table 11-1 lists the various conditions that can alter one's pain tolerance.

Pain can also be further classified in terms of its onset and duration as either acute or persistent. **Acute pain** is sudden and usually subsides when treated. One example of acute pain is postoperative pain. **Persistent pain** (also referred to as *chronic* or *long-term pain*) is recurring, lasting 3 to 6 months. It is often more difficult to treat, because changes occur in the nervous system that often require increasing drug dosages (see Evidence in Practice: Student Nurses' Misconceptions of Adults with Chronic Nonmalignant Pain Review). This situation is known by

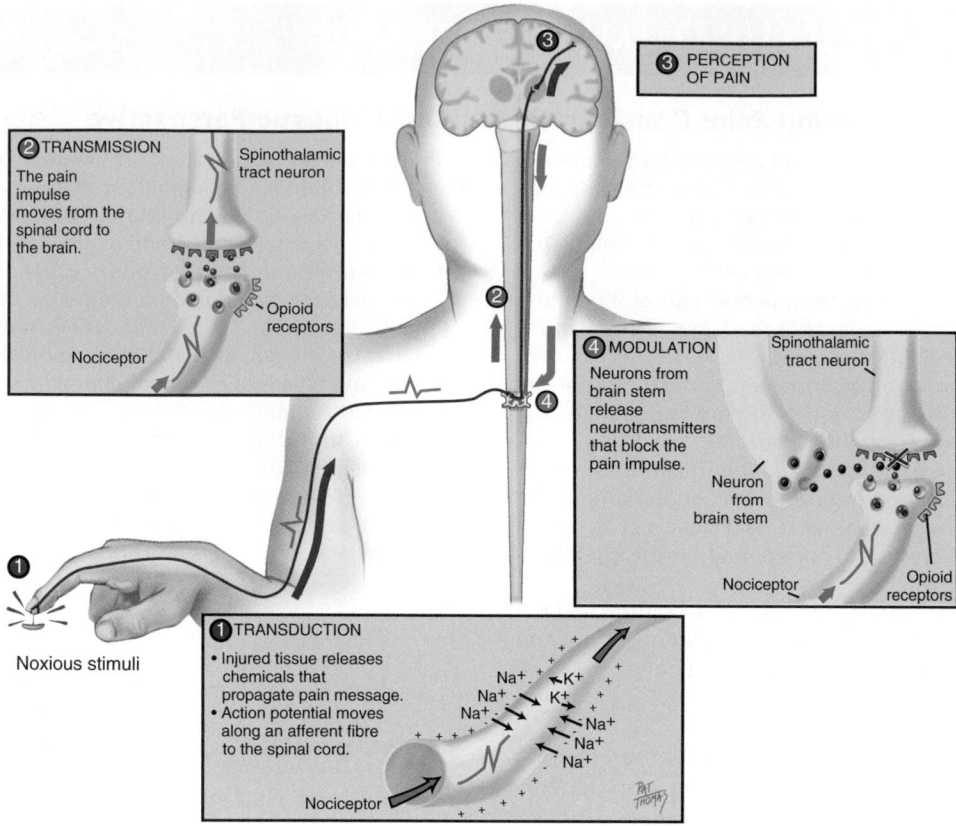

FIG. 11-1 Illustration of the four processes of nociception. (Source: Jarvis C., Browne, A. J., MacDonald-Jenkins, J., et al. (2014). *Physical examination and health assessment—Canadian 2nd Edition.* St Louis, MO: Saunders.)

TABLE	11-2

Acute Versus Persistent Pain

Type of Pain	Onset	Duration	Examples
Acute	Sudden (minutes to hours); usually sharp, localized; physiological response (SNS: tachycardia, sweating, pallor, increased blood pressure)	Limited (has an end)	Myocardial infarction, appendicitis, dental procedures, kidney stones, surgical procedures
Persistent	Slow (days to months); long duration; dull, long-lasting, aching	Long-lasting or recurring (endless)	Arthritis, cancer, lower back pain, peripheral neuropathy

SNS, sympathetic nervous system.

the general term **tolerance**. Tolerance is the state of progressively decreased responsiveness to a drug as a result of which a larger dose of the drug is needed to achieve the effect originally obtained by a smaller dose.(see Chapter 18). Acute and persistent pain differ in their onset and duration, their associated diseases or conditions, and the way they are treated. Table 11-2 lists the different characteristics of acute and persistent pain and various diseases and conditions associated with each.

Pain can be further classified according to the diseases or conditions that cause it. **Vascular pain** is believed to originate from the vascular or perivascular tissues and is thought to account for a large percentage of migraine headaches. **Referred pain** occurs when visceral nerve fibres synapse at a level in the spinal cord close to fibres that supply specific subcutaneous tissues in the body. An example is the pain associated with cholecystitis, which is often referred to the back and scapular areas. **Neuropathic pain** usually results from damage to peripheral or CNS nerve fibres by disease or injury but may also be idiopathic (unexplained). **Phantom pain** occurs in the area of a body part that has been removed—surgically or traumatically—and is often described as burning, itching, tingling, or stabbing. It can also occur in paralyzed limbs following spinal cord injury. **Cancer pain** can be acute or persistent or both. It most often results from pressure of the tumour mass against nerves, organs, or tissues. Other causes of cancer pain include hypoxia from blockage of

EVIDENCE IN PRACTICE

Student Nurses' Misconceptions of Adults With Chronic Nonmalignant Pain Review

The purpose of this study was to identify some of the misconceptions that student nurses have, across 3 years of undergraduate education, about adults who are experiencing chronic nonmalignant pain. Previously identified misconceptions about patients with chronic nonmalignant pain reported in an extensive literature search served as the basis of the study. The rationale for this study was to identify potential gaps in attitudes and knowledge of student nurses. The results were then used to discuss educational approaches focused on improving care of the patient experiencing chronic nonmalignant pain. The two major questions that this study sought to explore were as follows: (1) Do student nurses hold misconceptions about adults with chronic nonmalignant pain? and (2) if so, to what extent do they develop during their undergraduate education?

Type of Evidence

The researchers developed, tested, and validated a survey tool specifically for this cross-sectional study to evoke responses from students at three points during their undergraduate nursing education in New Zealand. The survey began with a vignette of a 22-year-old client who had been experiencing back pain for 6 months. The injury that caused the pain resulted when the woman suffered a fall while lifting a patient. It was thought that the vignette represented demographics that would be most familiar to the participants. Part of the vignette also purposely alluded to some of the basic details of misconceptions of pain (McCaffery and Pasero, 1999) but without giving many specific details. The patient in the vignette was also someone who was a healthy, fit young adult prior to the injury. There were two slight variations in the vignettes with the hopes of eliciting possible differences in responses toward patients, depending on whether a specific pathology had been identified. A series of eight items, the misconception items, were directly linked to each of the misconceptions identified by McCaffery, Ferrell, and Pasero (1990), and the responses were gathered using a seven-point Likert scale, seeking differing levels of agreement in relation to the items. A tool was designed and used with another group of students from a different discipline but within the same facility. This was done to get feedback from a group of students similar to the participants but prior to the final study. Some minor changes were made in the tool before moving forward with the study.

Results of Study

Some 435 students were approached to participate in the research study, and 430 completed and returned the surveys, for a total response rate of 99%. A convenience sampling was used because the students were easily accessible; they represented about 75% of students enrolled in the facility in semesters one, four, and six of the undergraduate nursing degree program in the city of Auckland and around 13% of those enrolled in New Zealand. These participants were distributed over a 3-year period of undergraduate studies during six semesters of full-time studies. The majority were female students, although there was no further specific demographic data collected about the participants. A cross-sectional design meant that data gathered came from each participant only once during the study. A research assistant—one who had not taught the students—met with the students and invited them to participate in the study. Sessions were held in the middle of the semester to increase the response rate as well as diminish anxiety during final exam time. More than 38% of the participants demonstrated a misconception about people with chronic pain and that they were tolerant to some degree of pain. More than 60% did not hold this misconception about tolerance to pain. More than one-half of the students' (59%) responses indicated that they held the misconception that psychological impairment is related to chronic pain. Approximately 79% of the students suggested that they believed stress was a contributory cause of chronic pain, whereas less than one-fourth indicated that they accurately understood that this was not the case. The misconception of compensation and exaggeration in chronic pain was held by 47.9% of the participants, and 51.7% did not hold this same misconception. About one-third of the students indicated that they held the misconception that patients with chronic pain were manipulative, and the majority indicated that they did not.

Approximately 64% of the participants held the misconception that depression plays a role in the chronic pain experience. Opioid addiction was a misconception held by about one-half of the participants, such that 54.8% believed that patients taking opioids were likely to be addicted. Some 58% of the students indicated that they held the misconception that patients with chronic pain were noncompliant and dependent, whereas 41.4% indicated that they did not hold this misconception. Another question that was posed to the students was the extent to which they had developed their misconceptions of patients with chronic pain during their undergraduate education. There were significantly positive trends across the semesters, suggesting that students held their misconceptions to a lesser degree as they progressed through their course of study. In summary, analysis of the results indicates that a substantial proportion of students who participated in the study hold misconceptions about patients with chronic pain to some extent.

The analysis of the misconception scores across the semesters indicates that the knowledge and attitudes of students toward adults experiencing chronic nonmalignant pain developed to some degree because their misconceptions were held to a lesser degree by the end of the program of study.

Link of Evidence to Nursing Practice

It is a known phenomenon that a gap exists between theory and practice across many areas of professional nursing practice. Therefore, it would be ideal for nursing educators and the nursing educational experience to

EVIDENCE IN PRACTICE—cont'd

equip students with the knowledge, skills, and attitudes to participate in the discussion, planning, and implementing of care for patients suffering from chronic nonmalignant pain. Nursing faculty and schools of nursing need to make available experiential learning situations that will enhance the blending of knowledge, skills, and attitudes into professional nursing practice so that these gaps in care are closed. The findings of this study show that students, like many practising nurses, hold misconceptions about adults with chronic nonmalignant pain, representing a lack of

knowledge and inappropriate attitudes. An integrated approach to teaching chronicity and disability needs to be included in the nursing curriculum; however, critical thinking, linking theory to practice, and developing compassion also need to be part of the educational process.

References: Shaw, S., & Lee, A. (2010). Student nurses' misconceptions of adults with chronic malignant pain. *Pain Management Nursing, 11*(1), 2–14.; McCaffrey, M., & Pasero, C. (1999): *Pain: Clinical manual* (2nd ed.) St. Louis, MO: Mosby.

TABLE 11-3

A and C Nerve Fibres

Type of Fibre	Myelin Sheath	Fibre Size	Conduction Speed	Type of Pain
A	Yes	Large	Fast	Sharp and well localized
C	No	Small	Slow	Dull and nonlocalized

blood supply to an organ; metastases; pathological fractures; muscle spasms; and adverse effects of radiation, surgery, and chemotherapy. **Central pain** occurs with tumours, trauma, inflammation, or disease (e.g., cancer, diabetes, stroke, multiple sclerosis) affecting CNS tissues.

The concept of pain has been influenced by the course of history, based on the current knowledge during the different periods. Most recent is the **gate control theory** proposed by Melzack and Wall in 1965. This theory elucidates the mechanism underlying the modulation of somatosensory afferents that act like a "gate" that is able to modulate pain signals transmitted from the periphery. Four distinct processes, all of which operate simultaneously, are required for nociceptive pain to occur and are widely believed to determine the perception of and response to acute pain.

The first process, *transduction*, corresponds to the transformation of mechanical, chemical, or thermal stimuli into electrochemical energy. At first, tissue injury prompts the release of numerous chemicals such as prostaglandins, bradykinin, serotonin, substance P, histamine, and potassium from injured cells. Some current pain medications work by altering the actions and levels of these substances (e.g., NSAIDs target prostaglandins; antidepressants target serotonin). The release of these pain-mediating chemicals initiates action potentials (electrical nerve impulses) at the distal end of sensory nerve fibres through pain receptors known as *nociceptors*. These nerve impulses are conducted along sensory nerve fibres and activate pain receptors in the dorsal horn of the spinal cord. This is where the so-called gates are located. These gates regulate the flow of sensory nerve impulses. If impulses are stopped by a gate at this junction, no impulses are transmitted to the higher centres of the brain. Conversely, if the gates permit a sufficient number

and intensity of action potentials to be conducted from the spinal cord to the cerebral cortex, the sensation of pain is then felt. This is known as *nociception*. Figure 11-2 depicts the gate control theory of pain transmission.

The second process, *transmission*, involves the propagation of pain impulses along pain fibres, as well as other sensory nerve fibres, to activate pain receptors in the spinal cord and brain. There are two types of nociceptor pain fibres: large-diameter, A-delta fibres and small-diameter, C fibres (Table 11-3). The A-delta fibres constitute the majority of myelinated fibres responsible for the first pain sensation. There are two types of A-delta fibres that exist, which are triggered by the specificity of their responses to different stimulation: the *mechanonociceptors* respond to intense and possibly harmful stimulation (flight or fight response); the polymodal A-delta fibres respond to mechanical, thermal, and chemical stimulation. The C fibres are unmyelinated and transmit poorly localized, dull, and aching pain.

The majority of nociceptive impulses travel through the anterolateral quadrant of the spinal cord. The spinothalamic tract is the most important pathway for transmission. The nociceptive fibres enter the spinal cord through an area known as the *dorsal (posterior) horn*. Here, neurotransmitters glutamate and substance P continue the pain impulse across the synaptic cleft between nociceptors and dorsal horn neurons. From the dorsal horn, numerous different ascending fibre tracts within the larger spinothalamic tract transmit pain into the thalamus, where the integration of nociceptive information takes place. From the thalamus, the pain impulses are relegated to the pain cortical structures.

It is at the dorsal horn that the so-called gates are located and control pain transmission. Closing of the gate seems to be affected by the activation of A fibres. This

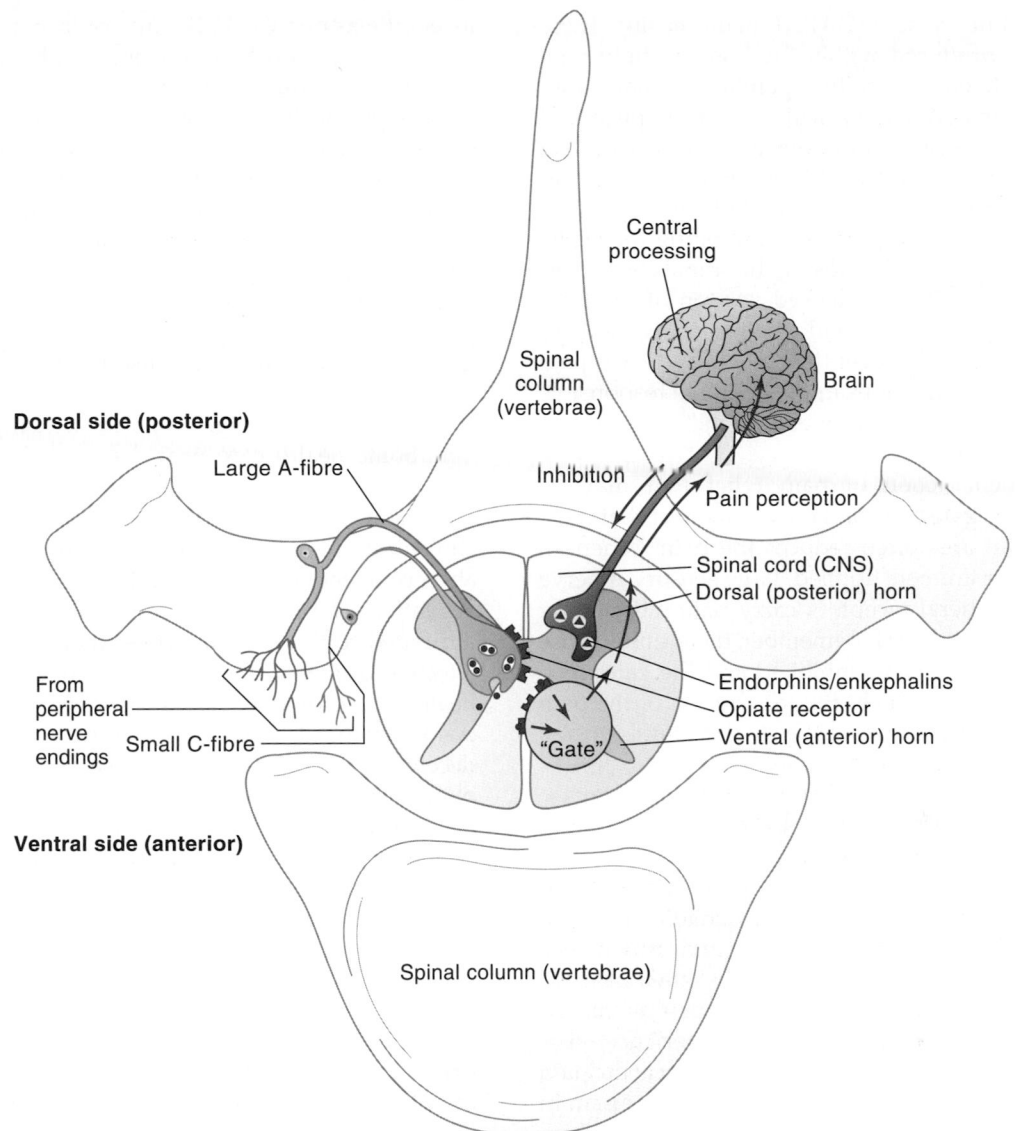

FIG. 11-2 Gate control theory of pain transmission. *CNS*, central nervous system.

causes the inhibition of impulse transmission to the brain and avoidance of pain sensation. Opening of the gate is affected by the stimulation of C fibres. This allows impulses to be transmitted to the brain and pain to be sensed. The gate is innervated by nerve fibres that originate in the brain and modulate the pain sensation by sending impulses to the gate in the spinal cord. These nerve fibres enable the brain to evaluate, identify, and localize the pain. Thus, the brain can control the gate, either by keeping the gate closed or allowing it to open so that the brain is stimulated and pain is sensed. The cells that control the gate have a threshold. Impulses that reach these cells must rise above this threshold before an impulse is permitted to travel up to the brain.

The third process, *perception*, is less an actual physiologic event than a subjective phenomenon of pain (how it feels) that encompasses complex behavioural, psychological, and emotional factors. An identical stimulus can evoke different types of pain from one individual to another. The μ (mu) receptors in the dorsal horn appear to play a crucial role. Pain perception and, conversely, emotional well-being, are closely linked to the number of μ receptors. Pain sensitivity is diminished when the receptors are present in relative abundance. When the receptors are reduced in number or missing altogether, relatively minor noxious stimuli may be perceived as painful.

Modulation is the fourth process. Modulation is a neural activity that controls pain transmission to neurons in both the peripheral and central nervous systems. The pathways involved are referred to as the *descending pain system* because the neurons originate in the brain stem and descend to the distal horn of the spinal cord. The descending nerve fibres release endogenous neurotransmitters known as *enkephalins* and *endorphins* (e.g., endogenous opioids, serotonin [5-HT], norepinephrine [NE], gamma aminobutyric acid [GABA], neurotensin). These substances are produced within the body to fight pain and are considered the body's painkillers. Both substances are capable of binding with opioid receptors and inhibiting the transmission of pain impulses by closing the spinal cord gates, in a manner similar to that of opioid analgesic drugs to produce analgesia. Both are capable of bonding with opioid receptors and inhibiting the transmission of pain impulses by closing the spinal cord gates. The term *endorphin* is a condensed version of the term *endogenous morphine*. These endogenous analgesic substances are released whenever the body experiences pain or prolonged exertion. For example, they are responsible for the phenomenon of "runner's high." Figure 11-1 depicts this entire process.

Another phenomenon of pain relief that may be explained by the gate control theory is the fact that massaging a painful area often reduces the pain. When an area is rubbed or liniment applied, large sensory A nerve fibres from peripheral receptors carry pain-modulating impulses to the spinal cord. Remember, the A fibres cause impulse transmission to be inhibited and the gate to be closed. This, in turn, reduces the recognition of the pain impulses arriving by means of the small fibres.

TREATMENT OF PAIN IN SPECIAL SITUATIONS

It is estimated that one of every five Canadians experiences persistent pain. Pain is poorly understood and often undertreated. In addition to enduring their baseline persistent pain, patients with illnesses such as cancer, AIDS, and sickle cell anemia may also experience crisis periods of acute pain. Effective management of acute pain is often different from management of persistent pain in terms of medications and dosage used. Routes of drug administration may include oral, intravenous (IV), intramuscular (IM), subcutaneous (subcut), transdermal, and rectal. One IV route commonly used in the hospital setting is patient-controlled analgesia (PCA). In this situation, patients are able to self-medicate by pressing a button on a PCA infusion pump. This has been shown to be effective and reduces the total opioid dose used. Morphine sulphate and fentanyl are commonly given by PCA.

Patients with complex pain syndromes often benefit from a holistic clinical or multimodal clinical approach that involves pharmacological or nonpharmacological treatment or a combination of both. The goals of pain management include reducing and controlling pain and improving body function and quality of life.

In situations such as pain associated with cancer, the main consideration in pain management is patient comfort and not trying to prevent **addiction** (or **psychological dependence**; see Chapter 18) to the pain medication. **Opioid tolerance** is a state of adaptation in which exposure to a drug causes changes in drug receptors that result in reduced drug effects over time. This can occur in as little as one week. Because of increasing pathology (e.g., tumour burden), patients with cancer usually require increasingly higher opioid doses and thus do become physically dependent on the drugs. Patients with cancer are likely to experience withdrawal symptoms (see Chapter 18) if opioid doses are abruptly reduced or discontinued; however, actual psychological dependence or addiction in such patients is unusual. For long-term pain control, oral, IV, subcut, transdermal, and sometimes even rectal dosing routes are favoured over multiple IM injections due to associated puncture trauma (bruising) and erratic drug absorption.

One controversial issue in pain management is the use of placebos, inert dosage forms that actually lack medication. Some health care providers feel that this practice may be helpful by taking advantage of the well-documented placebo effect. The placebo effect is a psychological therapeutic effect that occurs even in the absence of actual medication. It is believed to arise from activation of the patient's own endorphins. It is also attributed to the patient's belief that any "treatment" is effective, as well as the patient's high level of trust in the health care provider. Critics argue that the use of placebos is unethical, because it requires that the patient be deceived in the process. The use of placebos for pain management has fallen out of favour, and they are rarely used today (see Chapter 3 for further discussion).

The treatment of acute pain in patients who are addicted to opioids is of great concern to clinicians, who may be reluctant to prescribe opioid therapy. However, habitual opioid users are **opioid tolerant** and generally require high dosages. Longer-acting opioids such as methadone or extended-release oxycodone are usually better choices than shorter-acting immediate-release drug products for these patients. Genetic differences in cytochrome P450 enzymes (see Chapters 4 and 5) can cause different patients, with or without an addiction, to respond more or less effectively to a given drug. For this reason, patients must not automatically be viewed with suspicion if they report that a given drug does not work for them.

The label of *addict* can be used unfairly to justify refusal to prescribe pain medications, resulting in undertreatment of pain, even in patients who do not use street drugs. This is now regarded as an inappropriate and inhumane clinical practice. In these situations, control of the patient's pain takes ethical and clinical priority over concerns regarding drug addiction. Nonetheless, health care providers must contend with the reality of misuse of street or prescription drugs by patients (see Chapter 18). Such patients often request excessive numbers of prescriptions and may use multiple health care providers or pharmacies. At times, they may also forge prescriptions or use a telephone to call in prescriptions for opioid pain relievers such as those containing oxycodone, hydromorphone, fentanyl, morphine, and codeine. Community pharmacists work collaboratively to detect such abuses and notify law enforcement authorities.

Creating a phony prescription for a controlled substance is a felony. Nonetheless, Canada is the highest opioid-consuming country, per capita, in the world.

For patients receiving long-acting opioid analgesics, **breakthrough pain** often occurs between doses of pain medications. This is because the analgesic effects wear off as the drug is metabolized and eliminated from the body. Treatment with prn (as needed) doses of immediate-release dosage forms (e.g., oxycodone IR), given between scheduled doses of extended-release dosage forms (e.g., oxycodone ER), is often helpful in these cases. Chewing or crushing of any extended-release opioid drug can cause oversedation, respiratory depression, and even death due to rapid drug absorption. If the patient is requiring larger doses for breakthrough pain, the dose of the scheduled extended-release opioid may need to be increased, administered more frequently, or changed to a more potent opioid.

Drugs from other chemical categories are often added to the opioid regimen as adjuvant drugs. These assist the primary drugs in relieving pain. Such adjuvant drug therapy may include NSAIDs (see Chapter 49), antidepressants (see Chapter 17), antiepileptic drugs (see Chapter 15), and corticosteroids (see Chapter 50), all of which are discussed further in their corresponding chapters. This approach allows the use of smaller dosages of opioids and reduces some of the adverse effects that are seen with higher dosages of opioids, such as respiratory depression, constipation, and urinary retention. It permits drugs with different mechanisms of action to produce **synergistic effects.** Antiemetics (see Chapter 41) and laxatives (see Chapter 40) may also be needed to prevent or relieve associated constipation, nausea, and vomiting (Table 11-4).

One common use of adjuvant drugs is in the treatment of neuropathic pain. Opioids are not completely effective in such cases. Neuropathic pain usually results from some kind of nerve damage secondary to disease (e.g., diabetic neuropathy, postherpetic neuralgia secondary to shingles, trigeminal neuralgia, AIDS, or injury, including nerve damage secondary to surgical procedures [e.g., post-thoracotomy pain syndrome occurring after cardiothoracic surgery]). Common symptoms include hypersensitivity or hyperalgesia to mild stimuli such as light touch or a pinprick, or the bed sheets on a person's feet. This is also known as *allodynia*. It can also manifest as hyperalgesia to uncomfortable stimuli, such as pressure from an inflated blood pressure cuff on a patient's limb. It may be described as heat, cold, numbness and tingling, burning, or electrical sensations. Examples of adjuvants commonly used in these cases are the antidepressant amitriptyline hydrochloride and the anticonvulsants gabapentin and pregabalin.

The three-step analgesic ladder proposed by the **World Health Organization (WHO)** (Figure 11-3) is often applied as the pain management standard for cancer pain and to meet the therapeutic challenges presented by opioid tolerance. Examples of nonopioid analgesic drugs

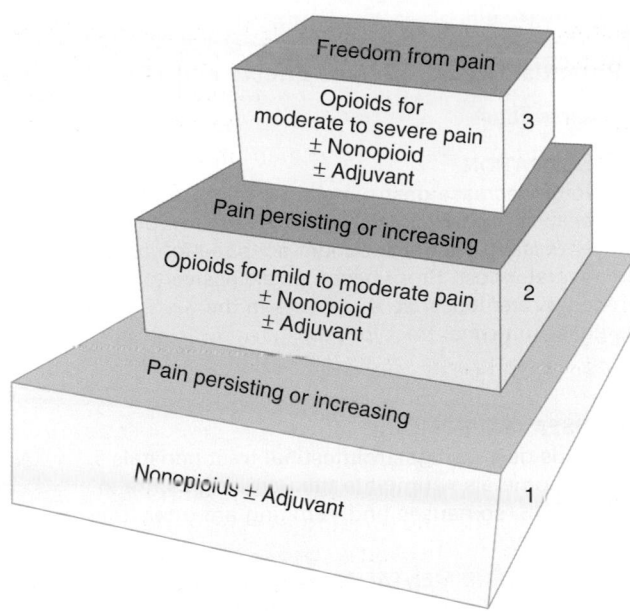

FIG. 11-3 Three-step analgesic ladder. (Source: World Health Organization. (2008). *WHO's pain ladder*. Retrieved from http://www.who.int/cancer/palliative/painladder/en/.)

include NSAIDs (see Chapter 49) as well as acetaminophen and tramadol hydrochloride (see Drug Profiles). Step 1 is the use of nonopioids (with or without adjuvant medications) once the pain has been identified and assessed. If pain persists or increases, treatment moves to step 2, which is defined as the use of opioids with or without nonopioids and with or without adjuvants. Should pain persist or increase, management then rises to step 3, which is the use of opioids indicated for moderate to severe pain, administered with or without nonopioids or adjuvant medications. The ultimate goal for patients, as confirmed by the WHO, is freedom from pain.

Not all patients will be treated effectively using the ladder method and some may need to seek an experienced pain management physician. In 2012, WHO developed evidence-informed guidelines on the *Pharmacological treatment of persisting pain in children with medical illnesses* and is developing guidelines on the *Pharmacological treatment of persisting pain in adults with medical illnesses* and the *Pharmacological treatment of acute pain*. (See http://www.who.int/medicines/areas/quality_safety/guide_on_pain/en/ for information.)

OPIOID DRUGS

Opioids are classified as both mild **agonists** (e.g., codeine, hydrocodone bitartrate) and strong agonists (e.g., morphine, hydromorphone hydrochloride, oxycodone, meperidine, fentanyl, methadone). Meperidine is not recommended for long-term use because of the accumulation of a neurotoxic metabolite, *normeperidine*. In fact, there is a move in hospitals to restrict the use of meperidine as a result of adverse events such as neurotoxicity from the normeperidine metabolite, delirium in older

TABLE 11-4	
Potential Opioid Adverse Effects and Their Management	
Adverse Effect	**Preventative Measures**

CONSTIPATION

Opioids decrease gastrointestinal tract peristalsis because of their central nervous system (CNS) depression, with subsequent constipation as an adverse effect. Stool becomes excessively dehydrated because it remains in the gastrointestinal tract longer.

Constipation may be managed with increased intake of fluids; stool softeners such as docusate sodium, or the use of stimulants such as bisacodyl or senna; and the use of agents such as lactulose, sorbitol, and polyethylene glycol (Clearlax®) solution. Less commonly used are bulk-forming laxatives such as psyllium, for which increased fluid intake is especially important to avoid fecal impactions or bowel obstructions. Ambulation is also a method of promoting bowel movement.

NAUSEA AND VOMITING

Opioids decrease gastrointestinal tract peristalsis, and some also stimulate the vomiting centre in the CNS, so nausea and vomiting are often experienced.

Nausea and vomiting may be managed with the use of antiemetics such as phenothiazines.

SEDATION AND MENTAL CLOUDING

Any change in mental status should always be evaluated to ensure that causes other than drug-related CNS depression are ruled out.

Persistent drug-related sedation may be managed with a decrease in the dose of opioid or change in drug used. The health care provider may also order various CNS stimulants (see Chapter 14).

RESPIRATORY DEPRESSION

Long-term opioid use is generally associated with tolerance to respiratory depression.

For severe respiratory depression, opioid antagonists (naloxone hydrochloride) may be used to improve respiratory status and, if they are titrated in small amounts, the respiratory depression may be reversed without analgesia reversal.

SUBACUTE OVERDOSE

Subacute overdose may be more common than acute respiratory depression and may progress slowly (over hours to days), with somnolence and respiratory depression. Before analgesic dosages are changed or reduced, advancing disease must be considered, especially in the dying patient.

Often, holding one or two doses of an opioid analgesic is enough to judge if the mental and respiratory depression is associated with the opioid. If there is improvement with this measure, the opioid dosage is often decreased by 25%.

OPIOID-INDUCED HYPERALGESIA (OIH)

Prolonged used of opioids such morphine sulphate can cause a paradoxical effect, where the patient develops a heightened sensitivity (hyperalgesia) to noxious stimuli. At times, this may even evolve to a painful response to non-noxious stimuli (allodynia).

Once OIH is diagnosed, the most straightforward intervention is to stop the opioid slowly to minimize adverse withdrawal. If the patient still requires some amount of analgesia, then titrating to reduce the dose has been found successful.

OTHER OPIOID ADVERSE EFFECTS

Dry mouth, urinary retention, pruritus, myoclonus, dysphoria, euphoria, sleep disturbances, sexual dysfunction, and inappropriate secretion of antidiuretic hormone may occur but are less common than the aforementioned adverse effects.

Ongoing assessment is needed for each adverse effect so that appropriate measures may be implemented (e.g., sucking of sugar-free hard candy or use of artificial saliva drops or gum for dry mouth; use of diphenhydramine hydrochloride for pruritus).

---

adult patients, and serotonin syndrome. Opiate **agonist–antagonists** such as pentazocine are associated with an **analgesic ceiling effect**. This means that the drug reaches a maximum analgesic effect, so that analgesia does not improve even with higher dosages (see Drug Profiles). Such drugs are useful only in patients who have not been previously exposed to opioids and can be used for non-escalating, moderate to severe pain. Finally, because of associated bruising and bleeding risks, as well as

injection discomfort, there is now a strong trend away from IM injections in favour of IV, subcut (e.g., via a subcutaneous butterfly), oral, and transdermal routes of drug administration.

The synthetic pain-relieving drugs currently known as **opioid analgesics** originated from the opium poppy plant. Natural opioids containing or derived from opium are known as **opiate analgesics**. The word *opium* is a Greek word that means "juice." More than 20 different

TABLE	11-5

Chemical Classification of Opioids

Chemical Category	Opioid Drugs
morphinelike drugs	morphine, heroin, hydromorphone, codeine, hydrocodone, oxycodone
meperidinelike drugs	meperidine, fentanyl, remifentanil, sufentanil, alfentanil
methadonelike drugs	methadone
Other	tramadol, tapentadol

TABLE	11-6

Opioid Receptors and Their Characteristics

Receptor Type	Prototypical Agonist	Effects
μ (mu)	morphine	Supraspinal analgesia, respiratory depression, euphoria, sedation*
κ (kappa)	butorphanol tartrate	Spinal analgesia, sedation, †miosis
δ (delta)	enkephalins	Analgesia

*Moderate level of sedation; †Twice as much sedation compared to μ (mu) receptors.

alkaloids are obtained from the unripe seed of the poppy plant. The properties of opium and its many alkaloids have been known for centuries. Opium-smoking immigrants brought opium to Canada, where unrestricted availability of opium prevailed until the early twentieth century.

Chemical Structure

Opioid analgesics are strong pain relievers. They can be classified according to their chemical structure or their action at specific receptors. Of the 20 different natural alkaloids available from the opium poppy plant, only three are clinically useful: morphine, codeine, and papaverine. Of these three, only morphine and codeine are pain relievers; papaverine is a smooth muscle relaxant. Relatively simple chemical modifications of these opium alkaloids have produced the three different chemical classes of opioids: morphinelike drugs, meperidinelike drugs, and methadonelike drugs (Table 11-5).

Mechanism of Action and Drug Effects

Opioid analgesics can also be characterized according to their mechanism of action. They are agonists or agonist–antagonists. An agonist binds to an opioid pain receptor in the brain and causes an analgesic response, the reduction of pain sensation. An agonist–antagonist, also called a **partial agonist**, binds to a pain receptor and causes a weaker pain response than a full agonist does. Different drugs in this class exert their agonist or antagonist effects by binding in different degrees to κ (kappa) and μ (mu) opioid receptors. Although not normally used as first-line analgesics, they are sometimes useful in pain management in patients who are addicted to opioids as well as obstetrical patients (because they avoid oversedation of the mother and fetus). **Antagonists** are nonanalgesics that bind to pain receptors but do not reduce pain signals. They function as competitive antagonists because they compete with and reverse the effects of agonist and agonist–antagonist drugs at the receptor sites.

The receptors to which opioids bind to relieve pain are listed in Table 11-6. The μ (mu), κ (kappa), and δ (delta) receptors are the most responsive to drug activity, with the μ (mu) being the most important. Many of the characteristics of a particular opioid, such as its ability to sedate, its potency, and its ability to cause hallucinations, can be attributed to relative affinity for these various receptors.

Understanding the relative potencies of various drugs becomes important in clinical settings. *Equianalgesia* refers to the ability to provide equivalent pain relief by calculating dosages of different drugs or routes of administration that provide comparable analgesia. Box 11-2 lists equianalgesic doses for several common opioids and shows how to calculate dosage conversions for patients. Because fentanyl is most commonly used transdermally, it is discussed separately in its drug profile.

Indications

The main use of opioids is to alleviate moderate to severe pain. The amount of pain control or unwanted adverse effects depends on the specific drug, the receptors to which it binds, and its chemical structure. Strong opioid analgesics such as fentanyl, sufentanil, and alfentanil are commonly used in combination with anaesthetics during surgery. These drugs are used not only to relieve pain but also to maintain a balanced state of anaesthesia. The practice of using combinations of drugs to produce anaesthesia is referred to as *balanced anaesthesia* (see Chapter 12). Use of fentanyl injection for management of postoperative and procedural pain has become popular because of its rapid onset and short duration. Transdermal fentanyl is available in a patch formulation for use in long-term pain management and is not be used for postoperative pain or any other short-term pain control (see Preventing Medication Errors: Fentanyl Transdermal Patches).

Strong opioids such as morphine, meperidine, hydromorphone, and oxycodone are often used to control postoperative and other types of pain. Because morphine and hydromorphone are available in injectable forms, they are often first-line analgesics in the immediate postoperative setting. There is a trend away from using meperidine due to its greater risk for toxicity (see Drug Profile). All available oxycodone dosage forms are orally administered. The brand name product OxyContin is a sustained-release form of oxycodone that contains more oxycodone

BOX 11-2 — Calculating Dosage Conversions Between Commonly Used Opioids

	Oral Dose (mg)	Parenteral Dose (mg)	Oral-to-Parenteral Dose Ratio	Dosing Interval (hr)
			Equianalgesic Doses	
morphine	30	10	3:1	12 (continuous release)
				4 (immediate release)
hydromorphone	7.5	1.5	5:1	4 (immediate release)
oxycodone	15	N/A	N/A	4 (immediate release)
hydrocodone bitartrate	30	N/A	N/A	N/A
fentanyl	See fentanyl drug profile			

Basic Conversion Equation

$$\frac{24 - hour\ amount\ of\ current\ drug}{x} = \frac{EA\ dose\ of\ current\ drug}{EA\ dose\ of\ desired\ drug}$$

Where x = amount of desired opioid in 24 hours and EA = equianalgesic dose obtained from the table above

For example: A patient with colon cancer is currently taking oral oxycodone 80 mg every 12 hours and needs to be converted to IV morphine due to a bowel obstruction. What is the equivalent IV morphine dose?

Step 1: **Determine the 24-hour amount of oxycodone taken by this patient:**

80 mg × 2 doses per 24 hours = 160 mg per 24 hours

Step 2: **Using the conversion table above, find the equianalgesic (EA) doses of oxycodone and parenteral morphine:**

15 mg oxycodone = 10 mg parenteral morphine

Step 3: **Use the above equation and solve for x by cross-multiplying:**

$$\frac{24 - hour\ amount\ of\ oxycodone\ (160\ mg)}{x}$$
$$= \frac{EA\ dose\ of\ current\ oxycodone\ (15\ mg)}{EA\ dose\ of\ parenteral\ morphine\ (10\ mg)}$$

Where x = amount of parenteral morphine in 24 hours (solve by cross-multiplying)

$$160\ mg \times 10\ mg = 15\ mg\ x \quad x = \frac{1\,600\ mg}{15\ mg}$$

X = 107 mg (approximately 100 mg of injectable morphine sulphate per 24 hours)

N/A, not applicable.

hydrochloride than the immediate-release formulation, with the intent to last up to 12 hours. The "Contin" in the product name stands for "continuous release," a synonym for long action in any drug product. If the tablet is chewed, crushed, or dissolved, however, the medication is released all at once. This may occur accidentally, or it may be done deliberately to achieve a euphoric high. Once crushed, the drug can also be snorted or injected. Because of this abuse and the increase in the number of addicted individuals, this formulation was removed from the Canadian market. It has been replaced with OxyNeo®, a formulation designed to reduce misuse; when the drug is crushed and combined with water, it becomes gel-like and difficult to inject. Similarly, the drug product MS Contin® is a long-acting or sustained-release form of morphine that is also designed to provide 8 to 12 hours of pain relief. The "MS" stands for the salt name, morphine sulphate. Morphine is generally available. There are immediate-release dosage forms of oxycodone and morphine in tablet, capsule, and liquid form. Meperidine is available only in immediate-release dosage forms, both oral and injectable. The analgesic effects of

immediate-release dosage forms of all three drugs typically last for about 4 hours.

Opioids also suppress the medullary cough centre, which results in cough suppression. The most commonly used opioid for this purpose is codeine (see Chapter 37). Hydrocodone is also used in many cough suppressants, either alone or in combination with other drugs. Sometimes opioid-related cough suppressants have a depressant effect on the CNS and cause sedation. To avoid this problem, dextromethorphan, a nonopioid cough suppressant, is often given instead (see Chapter 37).

Constipation from decreased gastrointestinal (GI) motility is often an unwanted adverse effect of opioids related to their anticholinergic effects. However, these effects are sometimes helpful in treating diarrhea. Some of the opioid-containing antidiarrheal preparations are opium/belladona tincture (paregoric) and diphenoxylate/atropine (Immodium®) tablets.

Contraindications

Contraindications to the use of opioid analgesics include known drug allergy and severe asthma. It is not

PREVENTING MEDICATION ERRORS

Fentanyl Transdermal Patches

When applying fentanyl (Duragesic Mat®) transdermal patches, the nurse needs to keep in mind several important points to avoid improper administration:

- These patches are recommended to be used only by patients who are considered opioid tolerant. To be considered opioid tolerant, a patient should have been taking, for a week or longer, morphine 60 mg daily, oral oxycodone 30 mg daily, or oral hydromorphone 8 mg daily (or an equianalgesic dose of another opioid). Applying fentanyl transdermal patches to non–opioid-tolerant patients may result in severe respiratory depression. Thorough assessment is important.
- Inform patients that heat, such as a sauna, hot tub, heating pad or heating pack, must never be applied over a fentanyl transdermal patch. The increased circulation that results from the application of heat may result in increased absorption of medication, causing an overdose.
- Teach patients to avoid the use of soap, alcohol, or other solvents on the skin surface where the patch is to be applied as these products may enhance the drug's ability to penetrate the skin. Recommend the use of plain water to wash the area. After applying or removing the patch, wash hands with water only.

- Teach patients that fentanyl patches should not be cut under any circumstances.
- Teach patients about the proper disposal of transdermal patches. Children have pulled used patches from the trash, which has resulted in deaths because of exposure to the drug. For disposal at home, the product insert recommends that the patch be folded so that the adhesive side of the system adheres to itself and then disposed of by flushing down the toilet. However, disposal practices may vary by area because of concerns for the water systems. Disposal policies in facilities also vary, but some require that used patches be placed in a sharps container rather than be flushed.
- Keep patches, as well as all medications, away from children and pets. Do not store medications in warm, moist places such as medicine cabinets in the bathroom.

The Institute for Safe Medication Practices has described examples of fatal patient incidents resulting from failure to follow the above points. It is essential for patients' safety to read the product labelling and follow instructions precisely. For more information, go to https://www.ismp-Canada.org.

---

uncommon for patients to state they are allergic to codeine, when, in the overwhelming majority of these patients, nausea was the "allergic" reaction. Many patients will claim to be allergic to morphine because it causes itching. Itching is a pharmacological effect due to histamine release and not an allergic reaction. Thus, it is important to determine the exact nature of a patient's stated allergy. Although not absolute contraindications, extreme caution is to be used in cases of respiratory insufficiency, especially when resuscitative equipment is not available; conditions involving elevated intracranial pressure (e.g., severe head trauma); morbid obesity or sleep apnea; myasthenia gravis; paralytic ileus (bowel paralysis); and pregnancy, especially with long-term use or high doses.

Adverse Effects

Many of the unwanted effects of opioid analgesics are related to their pharmacological effects in areas other than the CNS. Some of these unwanted effects can be explained by the drug's selectivity for the receptors listed in Table 11-6. The various body systems that the opioids affect and the corresponding adverse effects are summarized in Table 11-7.

Opioids that have an affinity for μ receptors, and that have rapid onset of action, produce marked euphoria. These are the opioids that are most likely to be misused and used recreationally by the lay public as well as by health care providers, who often have relatively easy

TABLE 11-7

Opioid-Induced Adverse Effects by Body System

Body System	Adverse Effect
Central nervous	Sedation, disorientation, euphoria, lightheadedness, dysphoria, lowered seizure threshold, tremors
Cardiovascular	Hypotension, palpitations, flushing
Respiratory	Respiratory depression and asthma exacerbation
Gastrointestinal	Nausea, vomiting, constipation, biliary tract spasm
Genitourinary	Urinary retention
Integumentary	Itching, rash, wheal formation

access. The person taking opioids to deliberately achieve an altered mental status will soon become psychologically dependent (addicted; see Chapter 18).

In addition, opioids cause histamine release. It is thought that this histamine release is responsible for many of the drugs' unwanted adverse effects, such as itching or pruritus, rash, and hemodynamic changes. Histamine release causes peripheral arteries and veins to dilate, which leads to flushing and orthostatic hypotension. The amount of histamine release that an opioid analgesic causes is related to its chemical class. The naturally occurring opiates (e.g., morphine) elicit the most histamine release; the synthetic opioids (e.g., meperidine) elicit the least histamine release. (See Table 11-5 for a list of the opioids and their respective chemical classes.)

The most serious adverse effect of opioid use is CNS depression, which may lead to respiratory depression. When death occurs from opioid overdose, it is almost always due to respiratory depression. When opioids are given, care must be taken to titrate the dose so that the patient's pain is controlled without affecting respiratory function. Individual responses to opioids vary, and patients may occasionally experience respiratory compromise despite careful dose titration. Respiratory depression can be prevented in part by using drugs with short duration of action and no active metabolites. Respiratory depression seems to be more common in patients with a pre-existing condition causing respiratory compromise, such as asthma or chronic obstructive pulmonary disease or sleep apnea. Respiratory depression is strongly related to the degree of sedation (see Toxicity and Management of Overdose, below).

GI tract adverse effects are common in patients receiving opioids due to stimulation of GI opioid receptors. Nausea, vomiting, and constipation are the most common adverse effects. Opioids can irritate the GI tract, stimulating the chemoreceptor trigger zone in the CNS, which, in turn, may cause nausea and vomiting. Opioids slow peristalsis and increase water absorption from intestinal contents. These two actions combine to produce constipation. This is more pronounced in hospitalized patients who are nonambulatory. Patients may require laxatives (see Chapter 40) to help maintain normal bowel movements.

Urinary retention, or the inability to void, is another unwanted adverse effect of opioid analgesics caused by increasing the sphincter tone of the bladder by sympathetic overstimulation, resulting in increased bladder outlet resistance. Opioids also decrease the sensation of bladder fullness by partially inhibiting the parasympathetic nerves that innervate the bladder. This is sometimes prevented by giving low dosages of an opioid agonist–antagonist, an opioid antagonist, or a cholinergic agonist (see Chapter 21) such as bethanechol.

Severe hypersensitivity or anaphylactic reaction to opioid analgesics is rare. Many patients will experience GI discomforts or histamine-mediated reactions to opioids and call these "allergic reactions." However, true anaphylaxis is rare, even with intravenously administered opioids. Some patients may report flushing, itching, or wheal formation at the injection site, but this is usually local and histamine mediated, and not a true allergy. Refer to Table 11-4 for additional information on opioid adverse effects and their management.

Toxicity and Management of Overdose

Naloxone and naltrexone are opioid antagonists that bind to and occupy all of these receptor sites (μ, κ, and δ). They are competitive antagonists with a strong affinity for these binding sites. Through such binding, they can reverse the adverse effects induced by the opioid drug,

TABLE 11-8		
Opioid Antagonists (Reversal Drugs)		
Generic Name	**Trade Name**	**Cautions**
naloxone hydrochloride (IV)	Naloxone hydrochloride injection	Raised or lowered blood pressure, dysrhythmias, pulmonary edema, withdrawal
naltrexone (PO)	ReVia	Nervousness, headache, nausea, vomiting, pulmonary edema, withdrawal

such as respiratory depression. These drugs are used in the management of opioid overdose and less commonly for opioid addiction. The commonly used opioid antagonists (reversal drugs) are listed in Table 11-8.

When treating an opioid overdose or toxicity, the symptoms of withdrawal need to be considered. However, regardless of potential withdrawal symptoms, when a patient experiences severe respiratory depression, naloxone must be given. Some degree of physical dependence is expected in opioid-tolerant patients. The extent of opioid tolerance is most visible when an opioid drug is discontinued abruptly or when an opioid antagonist is administered. This usually leads to symptoms of **opioid withdrawal**, also known as *abstinence syndrome* (see Chapter 18). This can occur after as little as two weeks of opioid therapy in patients who are **opioid naive**. Gradual dosage reduction after chronic opioid use, when possible, helps to minimize the risk and severity of withdrawal symptoms.

Respiratory depression is the most serious adverse effect associated with opioids. Stimulating the patient may be adequate to reverse mild hypoventilation. If this is unsuccessful, ventilatory assistance using a bag and mask or endotracheal intubation may be needed to support respiration. Administration of opioid antagonists (e.g., naloxone) may also be necessary to reverse severe respiratory depression. Careful titration of dose until the patient begins to breathe independently will prevent over-reversal. The effects of naloxone are short lived and usually last about one hour. With long-acting opioids, respiratory depressant effects may reappear, and naloxone may need to be redosed.

The onset of withdrawal symptoms is directly related to the half-life of the opioid analgesic being used. Withdrawal symptoms resulting from discontinuing or the reversal of therapy with short-acting opioids (codeine, hydrocodone bitartrate, morphine, and hydromorphone) will appear within 6 to 12 hours and peak at 24 to 72 hours. Withdrawal symptoms usually subside within 7 to 10 days but depend on a variety of factors (e.g., amount taken, length of time taking the drug, severity of dependence). Withdrawal symptoms associated with the long half-life drugs (methadone and transdermal fentanyl) may not appear for 24 hours or more after drug discontinuation and may be milder.

Interactions

Potential drug interactions with opioids are significant. Coadministration of opioids with alcohol, antihistamines, barbiturates, benzodiazepines, promethazine, and other CNS depressants can result in additive respiratory depressant effects. The combined use of opioids (such as meperidine) with monoamine oxidase inhibitors, such as selegiline, can result in respiratory depression, seizures, and hypotension.

Laboratory Test Interactions

Opioids can cause an abnormal increase in the serum levels of amylase, alanine aminotransferase, alkaline phosphatase, bilirubin, lipase, creatinine kinase, and lactate dehydrogenase (see Lab Values Related to Drug Therapy: Analgesics). Other abnormal results include a decrease in urinary 17-ketosteroid levels and an increase in urinary alkaloid and glucose concentrations.

Dosages

For the recommended initial dosages of selected analgesic drugs in opioid-naive patients, see the Dosages table on p. 212. Drug pharmacokinetics for selected drugs are provided in the Drug Profiles table.

NONOPIOID AND MISCELLANEOUS ANALGESICS

Acetaminophen (Tylenol) is the most widely used nonopioid analgesic. Over 4 billion doses of acetaminophen are sold each year in Canada, with approximately 15% of these sales for prescription products (Health Canada, 2015). Combination products (acetaminophen plus another medication) (see Table 11-9 for a common example of combination products including acetaminophen, codeine, and caffeine), including OTC cough and cold remedies and pain relievers containing opioids, make up more than half of all acetaminophen doses sold (Health Canada, 2015).

All of the drugs in the NSAID class (which includes aspirin, ibuprofen, naproxen, the cyclo-oxygenase-2 [COX-2] inhibitor, celecoxib [Celebrex®], and others) are nonopioid analgesics. These drugs are discussed in greater detail in Chapter 49. They are used for management of pain, especially pain associated with inflammatory conditions such as arthritis, because they have significant anti-inflammatory effects in addition to their analgesic effects.

Miscellaneous analgesics include tramadol and transdermal lidocaine and are discussed in depth in their respective drug profiles in this chapter. Capsaicin is a topical product made from several different types of peppers. It works by decreasing or interfering with substance P, a pain signal in the brain. Capsaicin is available over the counter. It can be used for muscle pain, joint pain, and nerve pain. Milnacipran is a selective serotonin and norepinephrine dual-uptake inhibitor. It is indicated for the treatment of fibromyalgia. It is thought that patients with fibromyalgia have reduced levels of norepinephrine in their brains, and milnacipran increases norepinephrine levels, which helps reduce pain associated with the disease. Milnacipran is in clinical trial in Canada as another alternative for pain and symptom relief in fibromyalgia for some patients. Longer-term and comparative studies are needed.

Mechanism of Action and Drug Effects

The mechanism of action of acetaminophen is similar to that of the salicylates. It blocks peripheral pain impulses by inhibition of prostaglandin synthesis. Acetaminophen also lowers febrile body temperature by acting on the hypothalamus, the structure in the brain that regulates body temperature. Heat is dissipated through resulting vasodilation and increased peripheral blood flow. In contrast to NSAIDs, acetaminophen lacks anti-inflammatory effects (although there is some controversy in this area). Although acetaminophen shares the analgesic and antipyretic effects of the salicylates and other NSAIDs, it does not have many of the unwanted effects of these drugs. For example, acetaminophen products are not usually associated with cardiovascular effects (e.g., edema) or platelet effects (e.g., bleeding), as aspirin and other NSAIDs are. They also do not cause the aspirin-related GI tract irritation or bleeding, nor any of the aspirin-related acid–base changes.

TABLE 11-9

Acetaminophen–Codeine Tablet Combinations

Combination	Amount of Acetaminophen*	Amount of Codeine	Amount of Caffeine
TYLENOL WITH CODEINE NO-1 TAB®	300 mg	8 mg	15 mg
TYLENOL WITH CODEINE NO-2 TAB®	300 mg	15 mg	15 mg
TYLENOL WITH CODEINE NO-3 TAB®	300 mg	30 mg	15 mg
TYLENOL WITH CODEINE NO-4 TAB®	300 mg	60 mg	None

*Depending on the pharmaceutical company, there are some variations in the amount of acetaminophen.

LAB VALUES RELATED TO DRUG THERAPY

Related to Drug Therapy for Analgesics

Laboratory Test	Normal Ranges	Rationale for Assessment
Alkaline phosphatase (ALP)	30–120 units/L	ALP is found in many tissues but in highest concentrations in the liver, biliary tract, and bone. Detection of this enzyme is important for determining liver and bone disorders. Enzyme levels of ALP are increased in both extrahepatic and intrahepatic obstructive biliary disease and cirrhosis or other liver abnormalities.
Alanine aminotransferase (ALT)	4–36 units/L Older adults may have slightly higher levels than adults	ALT is found mainly in the liver and lesser amounts in the kidneys, heart, and skeletal muscle. If there is injury or disease to the liver parenchyma (cells), it will cause a release of this liver cellular enzyme into the bloodstream and thus elevate serum ALT levels. Most ALT elevations are from liver disease. Therefore, if medications are then metabolized by the liver, this metabolic process will be altered and possibly lead to toxic levels of drugs.
Gamma-glutamyl transferase (GGT)	Male/female 45 years of age and older: 8–38 units/L	GGT is an enzyme that is present in liver tissue; when there is damage to the liver cells (hepatocytes) that manufacture bile, the enzyme will be released throughout the cell membranes and into the blood. The normal values for individuals of African ancestry are double those of individuals who are White.
Aspartate aminotransferase (AST)	0–35 units/L	AST is elevated with hepatocellular diseases. With disease or injury of liver cells, the cells lyse and the AST is released and picked up by the blood; the elevation of AST is directly related to the number of cells affected by disease or injury.
Lactic dehydrogenase (LDH)	100–190 units/L	LDH is found in cells of many body tissues including the heart, liver, red blood cells, kidneys, skeletal muscles, brain, and lungs. Because it is in so many tissues, the total LDH level is not a specific indicator of one disease. If there is disease or injury affecting cells containing LDH, the cells lyse and LDH is released from the cells into the bloodstream, thus increasing LDH levels. This enzyme is just part of the total picture of altered liver function which, if present, will then decrease the breakdown/metabolism of drugs and other chemical compounds, resulting in elevated blood levels of drugs.

Note: Usually levels that are 3 to 5 times the upper level of the normal range of the enzyme test are considered significant and are indicative of liver tissue damage. As well, elevation of a single test may not be clinically significant for liver damage.

DRUG PROFILES

Opioid Agonists

▶▶ morphine sulphate

Morphine sulphate, a naturally occurring alkaloid derived from the opium poppy, is the drug prototype for all opioid drugs. It is classified as a Schedule I controlled substance. Morphine is indicated for severe pain and has a high abuse potential. It is available in oral, injectable, and rectal dosage forms. Extended-release forms include MS Contin, M-Eslon®, Kadian®, and Avinza®. Morphine also has a potentially toxic metabolite known as morphine-6-glucuronide. Accumulation of this metabolite is more likely to occur in patients with kidney impairment. For this reason, other Schedule I opioids such as hydromorphone (Dilaudid®) and fentanyl (see fentanyl drug profile) may be safer analgesic choices for patients with kidney insufficiency. Drug profile information for hydromorphone is similar to that for morphine and meperidine. However, it is essential that all health care providers realize that hydromorphone is about eight times more potent than morphine. One milligram of IV, IM, or subcut hydromorphone hydrochloride is equivalent to 7 mg of IV, IM, or subcut morphine. This difference in potency often is not taken into account when prescribing, and deaths have been reported when larger doses of hydromorphone are given. Epidural dosage forms are injected onto the dura mater of the spinal cord. Epidural analgesics have the potential for causing increased intracranial pressure, especially with multiple injections, and increased CNS depression when given with other CNS depressant drugs. Other CNS depressant drugs are not to be given without orders from an anaesthesiologist.

DRUG PROFILES—cont'd

PHARMACOKINETICS

Route	Onset of Action	Peak Plasma Concentration	Elimination Half-Life	Duration of Action
IM	Rapid	30–60 min	1.7–4.5 hr	6–7 hr

codeine sulphate/phosphate

Codeine sulphate (oral) (codeine phosphate as injection) is a natural opiate alkaloid (Schedule I) obtained from opium. It is similar to morphine sulphate in terms of its pharmacokinetic and pharmacodynamic properties. In fact, about 10% of a codeine dose is metabolized to morphine in the body. However, codeine is less effective as an analgesic and is the only agonist to possess a ceiling effect (meaning increasing the dose will not increase the response). Therefore, it is more commonly used as an antitussive drug in an array of cough preparations (see Chapter 37). Codeine combined with acetaminophen (tablets or elixir) is classified as a Schedule I controlled substance and is commonly used for control of mild to moderate pain as well as cough. Codeine causes GI tract upset, and many patients will say they are allergic to codeine, when in fact it just upsets their stomach. Codeine is metabolized in the liver and converted to morphine through the enzyme CYP2D6. Some individuals have a genetic polymorphism to this enzyme, preventing them to metabolize it appropriately. There has been a growing concern for individuals who are so called "ultra-rapid metabolizers" as they convert codeine into morphine more rapidly, leading to dose-related opioid adverse effects. Current practice regarding codeine administration in pediatrics has been linked to serious morbidity and mortality. Two deaths and one resuscitation of North American children who were prescribed appropriate age–weight doses of codeine have occurred. These events prompted Health Canada to issue a recommendation that codeine and codeine-containing products are not to be used in children under the age of 12.

PHARMACOKINETICS

Route	Onset of Action	Peak Plasma Concentration	Elimination Half-Life	Duration of Action
PO	15–30 min	35–45 min	2.5–4 hr	4–6 hr

fentanyl

Fentanyl is a synthetic opioid (Schedule I) used to treat moderate to severe pain. Like other opioids, it also has a high misuse or abuse potential. It is available as a parenteral injection, transdermal patch, and sublingual tablet. The injectable form of fentanyl is used most commonly in perioperative settings and in critical care unit settings for sedation during mechanical ventilation. The parenteral form can be used subcutaneously or sublingually, depending on the patient's ability to manage sublingual administration. If administered sublingually, the drug must remain there for at least 5 minutes. Oral bioavailability of fentanyl is negligible and therefore this medication cannot be taken orally. Patients are generally unable to keep more than 1.5 mL to 2 mL under the tongue before it dribbles into the mouth, rendering it inactive. The oral (sublingual) and transdermal forms are used primarily for long-term control of both malignant and nonmalignant persistent pain. Fentanyl is a potent analgesic. Fentanyl at a dose of 0.1 mg given intravenously is roughly equivalent to 10 mg of morphine given intravenously.

The transdermal delivery system (patch) has been shown to be highly effective in the treatment of various persistent pain syndromes such as cancer-induced pain, especially in patients who cannot tolerate oral medications. This route is not to be used in opiate-naive patients or for acute pain relief. Fentanyl patches are difficult to titrate and are best used for nonescalating pain. To perform a conversion using the table in Box 11-2, first determine the daily (24-hour) opioid requirement of the patient. Second, if the opioid is not morphine, convert its dose to the equianalgesic dose of morphine using Box 11-2. Finally, calculate the equipotent transdermal fentanyl dosage. These tables are conservative in their dosages for achieving pain relief, and supplemental short-acting opioid analgesics should be added as needed.

Fentanyl patches take 6 to 12 hours to reach steady-state pain control after the first patch is applied, and supplemental short-acting therapy may be required. Most patients will experience adequate pain control for 72 hours with this method of fentanyl delivery. A new patch is to be applied every 72 hours. It is important to remove the old patch when applying a new one. It takes about 17 hours for the amount of fentanyl to reduce by 50% once the patch is removed.

Health Canada has issued many safety warnings about the use of fentanyl patches. Fentanyl patches are intended for management of persistent or cancer pain in opioid-tolerant patients whose pain is not adequately controlled by other types of medications. These patches are not recommended for acute pain situations such as postoperative pain. Deaths have occurred from drug-induced respiratory arrest when these conditions have not been met. Patients who are considered opioid tolerant are those who have been taking at least 60 mg of oral morphine daily or at least 30 mg of oral oxycodone daily or at least 8 mg of oral hydromorphone daily or an equianalgesic dose of another opioid. Other hazards associated with the use of fentanyl patches are cutting the patch and exposing the patch to heat (e.g., via a heating pad or sauna), both of which accelerate the diffusion of the drug into the patient's body. Fentanyl patches should not be cut for use. In the agency setting, fold used patches in half and place in the needle disposal container, or place in a tamperproof container and return to a community pharmacy, to prevent misuse.

PHARMACOKINETICS

Route	Onset of Action	Peak Plasma Concentration	Elimination Half-Life	Duration of Action
IV	Rapid	Minutes	1.5–6 hr	30–60 min
Transdermal	12–24 hr	48–72 hr	Delayed	1–2 hr
IM	7–15 min	20–30 min	1.5–6 hr	13–40 hr

Continued

DRUG PROFILES–cont'd

meperidine hydrochloride

Meperidine hydrochloride (Demerol®) is a synthetic opioid analgesic (Schedule I). Meperidine must be used with caution, if at all, in older adults and in patients who require long-term analgesia or who have kidney dysfunction. Meperidine has poor oral bioavailability, variable IM absorption and a short half-life of 3 to 4 hours. An active metabolite, normeperidine, can accumulate to toxic levels and predispose patients to normeperidine neurotoxicity, which does not respond to naloxone and makes meperidine overdose particularly dangerous. Recognition of the adverse consequences associated with meperidine use and its overall unfavourable risk–benefit profile in all patient populations has resulted in a progressive movement away from meperidine use, and it has been removed from stock in many agencies. It is not recommended for long-term pain treatment. However, it may still be used for acute pain during postoperative periods, as well as in emergency department settings for acute migraine headaches. Meperidine is available in tablet and injectable form. Although an oral tablet form is still available from one pharmaceutical company in Canada, the Institute for Safe Medication Practices (ISMP) Canada has recommended the removal of oral meperidine from hospital formularies, and is also establishing safe practices surrounding the prescribing of parenteral meperidine, including the use of other, safer alternatives for analgesia.

PHARMACOKINETICS

Route	Onset of Action	Peak Plasma Concentration	Elimination Half-Life	Duration of Action
IM	Rapid	30–60 min	3–4 hr	2–4 hr

methadone hydrochloride

Methadone hydrochloride (Metadol®) is a synthetic opioid analgesic (Schedule I). It is the opioid of choice for the detoxification treatment of persons addicted to opioids in methadone maintenance programs. Use of agonist–antagonist opioids (e.g., pentazocine) in patients addicted to heroin or those in methadone-maintenance programs can induce significant withdrawal symptoms. There has been renewed interest in the use of methadone for severe persistent (e.g., neuropathic) and cancer-related pain that requires daily, continuous, long-term opioid treatment, is opioid-responsive, and for which alternative options are inadequate. Methadone dosing for pain is different from methadone dosing for opioid dependence because of tolerance to the analgesic effects of opioids. The drug is readily absorbed through the GI tract with peak plasma concentrations at 4 hours for single dosing. Methadone is unique in that its half-life of 24 to 36 hours is longer than its duration of activity because it is bound to the tissues of the liver, kidneys, and brain. With repeated doses, the drug accumulates in these tissues and is slowly released, thus allowing for 24-hour dosing. Methadone is eliminated through the liver, which makes it a safer choice than some other opioids for patients with kidney impairment. There has been concern recently that the prolonged half-life of

the drug is a cause of unintentional overdoses and deaths. There is also concern that methadone may cause cardiac dysrhythmias. Methadone is available for oral use in liquid form. Methadone can only be prescribed by health care providers who have received an exemption pursuant to section 56 of the *Controlled Drugs and Substances Act* from the Minister of Health (Canada).

PHARMACOKINETICS

Route	Onset of Action	Peak Plasma Concentration	Elimination Half-Life	Duration of Action
PO	30–60 min	1.5–2 hr	25 hr	24–48 hr

oxycodone hydrochloride

Oxycodone hydrochloride is an analgesic drug that is structurally related to morphine and has comparable analgesic activity (Schedule I). It is also commonly combined in tablets with acetaminophen (Percocet®) and with aspirin (Ratio-Oxycodan®). Oxycodone is also available in immediate-release formulations (Oxy IR) and sustained-released formulations (OxyNeo). Oxycodone or naloxone (Targin®) is a new controlled-release combination offering a dual therapeutic effect. It is indicated for severe pain requiring daily, long-term opioid treatment, and the naloxone blocks and reduces the adverse effects of opioid analgesic-induced constipation. Naloxone blocks the pain-relieving effects of opioids in general, but this formulation of oral naloxone blocks only the bowel adverse effects and is not absorbed through the intestine to block the drug's pain-relieving properties in the body and brain. A somewhat weaker but commonly used opioid is hydrocodone bitartrate (Schedule I), which is available in a tablet and as a syrup. It is available in combination with phenyltoloxamine (Tussinex®) as a controlled-release resin. The addition of phenyltoloxamine potentiates the antitussive effect of hydrocodone bitartrate.

PHARMACOKINETICS (IMMEDIATE RELEASE)

Route	Onset of Action	Peak Plasma Concentration	Elimination Half-Life	Duration of Action
PO	10–15 min	1 hr	2–3 hr	3–6 hr

Opioid Agonist–Antagonists

Opioids with mixed actions are often called *agonist–antagonists* (Schedule I). They bind to the μ receptor and can therefore compete with other substances for these sites. They either exert no action (i.e., they are competitive antagonists) or have only limited action (i.e., they are partial agonists). They are similar to the opioid agonists in terms of their therapeutic indications; however, they have a lower risk of misuse and addiction. The antagonistic activity of this group can produce withdrawal symptoms in opioid-dependent patients. Their use is contraindicated in patients who have shown hypersensitivity reactions to the drugs.

These drugs have varying degrees of agonist and antagonist effects on the different opioid receptor subtypes. They are used in situations requiring short-term pain

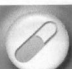

DRUG PROFILES—cont'd

control, such as after obstetrical procedures. They are sometimes chosen for patients who have a history of opioid addiction. These medications can both help prevent overmedication and reduce post-treatment addictive cravings in these patients. Combination products of buprenorphine hydrochloride and naloxone dehydrate offer physicians an in-office treatment of addiction (see Chapter 18). These drugs are normally not strong enough for management of longer-term persistent pain (e.g., cancer pain, persistent lower back pain). They are *not* to be given concurrently with full opioid agonists, because they may both reduce analgesic effects and cause withdrawal symptoms in opioid-tolerant patients. Adverse reactions are similar to opioids but with a lower incidence of respiratory depression. Four opioid agonist–antagonists are currently available: a buprenorphine transdermal patch (Butrans®), butorphanol tartrate, nalbuphine (Nubain®), and pentazocine (Talwin®). They are available in various dosage forms as indicated in the dosage table. Buprenorphine hydrochloride is also available in combination with the opioid antagonist naloxone (Suboxone) to enhance its opioid antagonistic effect, which is usually weaker than the agonistic effects of the drug.

Opioid Antagonists

Opioid antagonists produce their antagonistic activity by competing with opioids for CNS receptor sites.

▶▶ naloxone hydrochloride

Naloxone hydrochloride is a pure opioid antagonist. It has no agonist morphinelike properties and works as a blocking drug to the opioid drugs. Accordingly, the drug does not produce analgesia or respiratory depression. Naloxone is the drug of choice for the complete or partial reversal of opioid-induced respiratory depression. It is also indicated in cases of suspected acute opioid overdose. Failure of the drug to significantly reverse the effects of the presumed opioid overdose indicates that the condition may not be related to opioid overdose. The primary adverse effect is opioid withdrawal syndrome, which can occur with abrupt over-reversal in opioid-tolerant patients. Naloxone is available only in injectable dosage forms. Use of the drug is contraindicated in patients with a history of hypersensitivity to it.

PHARMACOKINETICS

Route	Onset of Action	Peak Plasma Concentration	Elimination Half-Life	Duration of Action
IV	<2 min	Rapid	C4 min	Variable depending on dose and route

naltrexone hydrochloride

Naltrexone hydrochloride (ReVia®) is an opioid antagonist used as an adjunct for the maintenance of an opioid-free state in former opioid addicts. It has been recognized as a safe and effective adjunct to psychosocial treatments of alcoholism. It is also indicated for reversal of postoperative opioid-induced respiratory depression. Nausea and tachycardia are the most common adverse effects and are related to reversal of the opioid effect. Use of naltrexone hydrochloride is contraindicated in cases of known drug allergy and in patients with hepatitis or liver dysfunction or failure.

PHARMACOKINETICS

Route	Onset of Action	Peak Plasma Concentration	Elimination Half-Life	Duration of Action
PO	Rapid	1 hr	3.9–12.9 hr	24–72 hr

Indications

Acetaminophen is indicated for the treatment of mild to moderate pain and fever. It is an appropriate substitute for aspirin because of its analgesic and antipyretic properties. Acetaminophen is a valuable alternative for those patients who cannot tolerate aspirin or for whom aspirin may be contraindicated. Acetaminophen is also the antipyretic (antifever) drug of choice in children and adolescents with flu syndromes because the use of aspirin in such populations is associated with a condition known as Reye's syndrome.

Contraindications

Contraindications to acetaminophen use include known drug allergy, severe liver disease, and the genetic disease known as *glucose-6-phosphate dehydrogenase (G6PD) enzyme deficiency*.

Adverse Effects

Acetaminophen is an effective and relatively safe drug. It is therefore available over the counter and in many combination prescription drugs. Acetaminophen is generally well tolerated. Possible adverse effects include rash, nausea, and vomiting. Much less common but more severe are the adverse effects of blood disorders or dyscrasias (e.g., anemias) and kidney function when acetaminophen is taken with light-to-moderate alcohol intake, and of most concern, hepatotoxicity.

Toxicity and Management of Overdose

Most people do not realize that acetaminophen, despite its over-the-counter status, is a potentially lethal drug when taken in overdose. Patients who are depressed (especially adolescents) may intentionally take an overdose of the drug without realizing the grave danger involved.

The ingestion of large amounts of acetaminophen, as in an acute overdose or even persistent unintentional misuse, can cause liver necrosis. This is the most serious acute toxic effect. Acute ingestion of acetaminophen doses of 150 mg/kg (approximately 7 to 10 grams) or more may result in liver toxicity. Acute hepatotoxicity

DOSAGES Selected Analgesic Drugs and Related Drugs

Drug	Pharmacological Class	Usual Dosage Range	Indications
OPIOIDS			
codeine sulphate (oral); codeine phosphate injection	Opioid; opiate; opium alkaloid	**Adults/Children (12 yr and older)** PO: 15–60 mg q4–6 hr IV: 30–60 mg q4–6 hr	Analgesia
		Adults/Children (12 yr and older) 15–60 mg tid–qid; maximum 120 mg/day 15–60 mg tid–qid; maximum 120 mg/day	Antitussive
fentanyl (Abstral®, Duragesic Mat, Fentanyl Citrate Injection®)	Opioid analgesic	All doses titrated to response, starting with lowest effective dose **Children (2–12 yr)** IV: 2–3 mcg/kg/dose **Adults** IV: 2–150 mcg/kg (range from minor to complicated procedures)	Procedural sedation or adjunct to general anaesthesia
		Adults Epidural: 100 mcg diluted in 8 mL 0.9% sodium chloride on demand; continuous infusion 1 mcg/kg/hr Duragesic (transdermal patch): 12–100 mcg/h q72 hr Sublingual tablets (Astral): Begin with lowest dosage 100 mcg and titrate as necessary	Relief of moderate to severe acute pain; relief of persistent pain, including cancer pain
meperidine hydrochloride (Demerol)	Opioid analgesic	**Children** IM/SC: 1.1–1.8 mg/kg q2–3 hr prn (max 100 mg/dose) IM/SC: 1.1–1.2 mg/kg 30–90 min before anaesthesia **Adults** PO (18 yr and older): 50–150 mg q3–4 hr prn IM/SC: 50–100 mg 30–90 min before anaesthesia; 50–150 mg q3 hr prn for pain	Meperidine hydrochloride use not recommended because of the unpredictable effects of neurometabolites at analgesic doses and risk for seizures; use for 2 days Obstetric analgesia; preoperative sedation
methadone hydrochloride (Astral®, Metadol®, Metadose®) (D)	Opioid analgesic	**Adults** PO for pain 2.5–10 mg q4 hr x 3–5 days; followed by fixed dose q8–12 hr depending on patient needs	Opioid analgesic, relief of persistent pain, opioid detoxification, opioid addiction maintenance
▶▶**morphine sulphate (M.O.S. Sulphate®, MS IR®, Statex®)** **morphine hydrochloride (Doloral syrup®)**	Opioid; opiate; opium alkaloid	**Children** PO: 0.1–0.5 mg/kg/dose q3–4 hr Subcut: 0.1–0.2 mg/kg q4 hr (maximum 15 mg/single dose) **Adults** PO: 10–30 mg q4 hr IV/IM/Subcut: 2.5–15 mg q2–4 hr	Opioid analgesia Opioid analgesia
morphine sulphate, continuous release (Kadian, M.O.S. Sulphate, MS Contin)	Opiate analgesic; opium alkaloid	**Adults only** PO: 10–100 mg q8 hr to 100 mg q12 hr daily	Relief of moderate to severe pain
oxycodone hydrochloride, immediate-release (Oxy-IR®)	Opioid, synthetic	**Children** PO: 1.25–2.5 mg q6 hr prn **Adults** PO: 5–20 mg q4–6 hr prn	Relief of moderate to severe pain
oxycodone hydrochloride, continuous-release (ACT Oxycodone SR®, OxyNeo)	Opioid, synthetic	**Adults only** PO: 10–20 mg q12 hr, titrated to relief	Relief of moderate to severe pain

DOSAGES   Selected Analgesic Drugs and Related Drugs—cont'd

Drug	Pharmacological Class	Usual Dosage Range	Indications
OPIOID ANTAGONISTS			
▸▸naloxone hydrochloride	Opioid antagonist	**Neonates** IM/IV/Subcut:0.1 mg/kg at 2–3-min intervals **Children** IV: 0.01 mg/kg IV followed by 0.1 mg/kg if needed; 0.005–0.01 mg/kg; repeat in 2–3-min intervals **Adults** IV: 0.4–2 mg; repeat in 2–3 min if needed; 0.1–0.2 mg; repeat in 2–3-min intervals	Opioid-induced depression Treatment of opioid overdose; postoperative anaesthesia reversal Treatment of opioid overdose; postoperative anaesthesia reversal
naltrexone hydrochloride (ReVia)	Opioid antagonist	**Adults** PO: 50 mg daily or 100 mg every other day PO: 50–100 mg q3 4 hr	Maintenance of opioid-free state
NONOPIOIDS			
▸▸acetaminophen (Tylenol®, others)	Nonopioid analgesic, antipyretic	**Children** PO/PR: Variable doses by age 40–480 mg q4–6 hr **Adults** PO/PR: 325–650 mg q4–6 hr; do not exceed 4 g/day In those with alcohol disorders, do not exceed 2 g/day	Relief of mild to moderate pain Relief of mild to moderate pain
tramadol hydrochloride immediate-release (Apo-Tramadol®) tramadol hydrochloride extended-release (Durela®, Ralivia®, Tridura®)	Nonopioid analgesic (with opioidlike activity)	**Adults 18 yr and older** PO: 50–100 q4–6 hr; not to exceed 400 mg/day PO: 100–300 mg q24 hr; not to exceed 300 mg/day	Relief of moderate to moderately severe pain

IM, intramuscular; IV, intravenous; PCA, patient-controlled analgesia; PO, oral; Subcut, subcutaneous; SL, sublingual

can usually be reversed with acetylcysteine, whereas long-term toxicity is more likely to be permanent.

The standard maximum daily dose of acetaminophen for healthy adults is 4 000 mg. At the time of writing this book, Health Canada is considering additional steps to minimize the risk of liver damage and improve acetaminophen safety, for example, reducing the maximum daily recommended dose for all oral and rectal forms of acetaminophen-containing products, decreasing the unit dose for some products, or both. As well, product labelling and packaging, such as requiring children's liquid products to be sold with an accurate dosing device in the package, are also being considered.

Limitation of acetaminophen dosages to 2 000 mg or less may be necessary for patients with risk factors such as advanced age or those with liver dysfunction. Excessive dosing may occur inadvertently with the use of combination products that include a fixed ratio of an opioid drug plus acetaminophen (e.g., hydrocodone plus acetaminophen). Health care providers must be mindful of recommended daily dose limits when prescribing these medications.

The long-term ingestion of large doses of acetaminophen is more likely to result in severe hepatotoxicity, which may be irreversible. Because the reported or estimated quantity of drug ingested is often inaccurate and not a reliable guide to the therapeutic management of the overdose, serum acetaminophen concentration should be determined no sooner than 4 hours after the ingestion. If a serum acetaminophen level cannot be determined, it should be assumed that the overdose is potentially toxic and treatment with acetylcysteine needs to be started. Acetylcysteine is the recommended antidote for acetaminophen toxicity and works by preventing the hepatotoxic metabolites of acetaminophen from forming. It is most effective when given within 10 hours of an overdose. Historically, the usual dosage regimen—140 mg/kg oral loading dose, followed by 70 mg/kg every 4 hours for 17 additional doses—is usually administered intravenously according to protocol.

The oral drug is notoriously bad tasting, with an odour of rotten eggs, and vomiting of an oral dose is common. It is recommended that the dose be repeated if vomiting occurs within 1 hour of dosing.

Interactions

A variety of substances may interact with acetaminophen. Alcohol is potentially the most dangerous. Persistent heavy alcohol abuse may increase the risk of liver toxicity from excessive acetaminophen use. For this reason, a maximum daily dose of 2 000 mg is generally recommended. Health care providers need to warn patients with regular intake of moderate to large amounts of alcohol not to exceed recommended doses of acetaminophen because of the risk of liver dysfunction and possible liver failure. Ideally, alcohol consumption is not to exceed the recommended guidelines of 15 drinks per week for men and 10 drinks per week for women. Other drugs that can potentially interact with acetaminophen include phenytoin, barbiturates, warfarin sodium, isoniazid, rifampin, β-blockers, and anticholinergic drugs, all of which are discussed in greater detail in later chapters. Drug pharmacokinetics for selected drugs are provided in the Drug Profiles table.

 # DRUG PROFILES

▸▸ *acetaminophen*

Acetaminophen (Tylenol) is an effective and relatively safe nonopioid analgesic used for mild to moderate pain relief. Acetaminophen is provided in oral and rectal dosage formulations. Acetaminophen is also a component of several prescription combination drug products, including oxycodone and acetaminophen (Endocet®, Percocet).

PHARMACOKINETICS

Route	Onset of Action	Peak Plasma Concentration	Elimination Half-Life	Duration of Action
PO	10–30 min	0.5–2 hr	1–4 hr	3–4 hr

tramadol hydrochloride

Tramadol hydrochloride (Ultram®) is categorized as a miscellaneous analgesic because of its unique properties. It is a centrally acting analgesic with a dual mechanism of action. It creates a weak bond to the μ (mu) opioid receptors and inhibits the reuptake of both norepinephrine and serotonin. Although it does have weak opioid receptor activity, tramadol is not currently classified as a controlled substance. Tramadol is indicated for the treatment of moderate to moderately severe pain. Tramadol is rapidly absorbed and its absorption is unaffected by food. It is metabolized in the liver to an active metabolite (O-dimethyl tramadol) and eliminated via renal excretion.

Tramadol has a relatively safe profile in comparison to other opiates; however, two potential significant adverse effects of this drug are seizures and serotonin syndrome. Seizures have been reported in patients taking tramadol and occur in patients taking both normal and excessive dosages. Patients who may be at risk are those receiving tricyclic antidepressants, selective serotonin reuptake inhibitors (SSRIs), monoamine oxidase inhibitors, neuroleptics, or other drugs that reduce the seizure threshold. There is also an increased risk of developing serotonin syndrome when tramadol is taken concurrently with SSRIs (see Chapter 17). Other adverse effects are similar to those of opioids and include drowsiness, dizziness, headache, nausea, constipation, and respiratory depression.

Use of tramadol is contraindicated in cases of known drug allergy, which may include allergy to opioids due to potential cross-reactivity. It is also contraindicated in cases of acute intoxication with alcohol, hypnotics, centrally acting analgesics, opioids, or psychotropic drugs. The drug is available only in oral dosage forms, including a combination with acetaminophen (Tramacet®), as well as extended-release formulation (Durela, Ravilia, Zytram XL®). A new drug, tapentadol hydrochloride (Nucynta®) is structurally related to tramadol, with a duel mechanism of action. It is a μ (mu) agonist and a norepinephrine reuptake inhibitor. It is currently recommended to be a scheduled opioid.

PHARMACOKINETICS

Route	Onset of Action	Peak Plasma Concentration	Elimination Half-Life	Duration of Action
PO	30 min	2 hr	5–8 hr	Unknown

lidocaine, transdermal

Transdermal lidocaine is a topical anaesthetic and cardiac antidysrhythmic (see Chapter 26 discussion) that is formulated into a patch (EMLA®), which is placed onto painful areas of the skin. It is indicated for the treatment of postherpetic neuralgia, a painful skin condition that remains after a skin outbreak of shingles. Shingles is caused by the herpes zoster virus, also known as the *varicella zoster virus*, which causes chickenpox in children. Lidocaine patches provide local pain relief, and up to three patches may be placed on a large painful area. However, the patches are not to be worn for longer than 12 hours a day to avoid potential systemic drug toxicity (e.g., cardiac dysrhythmias). Because they act topically, there are minimal systemic adverse effects. However, the skin at the site of treatment may develop redness or edema, and unusual skin sensations may occur. These reactions are usually mild and resolve within a few minutes to hours. Patches are applied only to intact skin with no blisters. They can be used either alone or as part of adjunctive treatment with systemic therapies such as antidepressants (see Chapter 17), opioids, or anticonvulsants (see Chapter 15). Used patches must be disposed of securely because they may be dangerous to children or pets. Specific pharmacokinetic data are not listed due to the continuous nature of dosing. Studies have demonstrated that a patch can provide varying degrees of pain relief for 4 to 12 hours.

NURSING PROCESS

Pain may be acute or persistent and occurs in patients in all settings and across the lifespan, thus leading to much distress. Patients experiencing pain pose many challenges to the nurse, prescribers, and other health care providers involved in their care. The challenge is that pain is a complex and multifaceted problem that requires astute assessment skills with appropriate interventions based on the individual, the specific type of pain, related diseases, or health status.

Medical associations, health care organizations, governing bodies, and professional nursing organizations have been involved in defining guidelines and outcomes of care related to assessment and management of pain. For example, the Canadian Guideline for Safe and Effective Use of Opioids (http://nationalpaincentre.mcmaster.ca/opioid/) is a national, evidence-informed guideline to help primary care providers and specialists safely and effectively use opioids to treat patients with persistent non-cancer pain. In addition, the WHO (www.who.int/en) has developed standards related specifically to cancer pain and are developing guidelines for management of acute pain and pain in children. Professional nursing organizations, such as the Registered Nurses' Association of Ontario, have also created standards of care related to pain assessment and management.

⬛ Assessment

Adequate analgesia requires a holistic, comprehensive, and individualized patient assessment with specific attention to the type, intensity, and characteristics of the pain and the levels of comfort. *Comfort*, in this situation, is defined as the extent of physical and psychological ease that an individual experiences. Perform a thorough health history, nursing assessment, and medication history as soon as possible or upon the first encounter with the patient, including questions about the following: (1) allergies to nonopioids, opioids, partial or mixed agonists, or opioid antagonists (see previous pharmacological discussion for examples of specific drugs); (2) potential drug–drug or drug–food interactions; (3) presence of diseases or CNS depression; (4) history of the use of alcohol, street drugs, or any illegal drug or substance and history of substance abuse, with information about the substance, dose, and frequency of use; (5) results of laboratory tests ordered, such as levels of serum ALT, ALP, GGT, 5'-nucleotidase, and bilirubin (indicative of liver function), or levels of blood urea nitrogen (BUN) and creatinine (reflective of kidney function); abnormal liver or kidney function that may require lower doses of analgesic to prevent toxicity or overdosage (see Lab Values Related to Drug Therapy: Analgesics on p. 208); (6) character and intensity of the pain, including onset, location,

and quality (e.g., stabbing/knifelike, throbbing, dull ache, sharp, diffuse, localized, referred); actual rating of the pain using a pain assessment scale (see later); and any precipitating, aggravating, or relieving factors; (7) duration of the pain (acute versus persistent); and (8) types of pharmacological, nonpharmacological, or adjunctive measures that have been implemented, with further explanation of the treatment's duration of use and overall effectiveness.

To be thorough and effective, include in the assessment the factors or variables that may impact an individual's pain experience, such as physical factors (e.g., age, gender, pain threshold, overall state of health, disease processes, pathologies) and emotional, spiritual, and cultural variables (e.g., reaction to pain; pain tolerance; fear; anxiety; stressors; sleep patterns; societal influences; family roles; phases of growth and development; religious, racial, or ethnic beliefs or practices). Age-appropriate assessment tools are recommended in assessing pain across the lifespan (see later discussion). For pediatric and older adult patients, nonverbal behaviour or cues and information from family members or caregivers may be helpful in identifying pain levels. In an older adult, physical or cognitive impairment may affect reporting of pain; however, this does not mean that the older adult patient is not experiencing pain—the patient's reporting may just be altered. Persistent pain and pain associated with cancer are both complex and multifactorial problems requiring a holistic approach with attention to other patient reports, such as a decrease in activities of daily living, insomnia, depression, social withdrawal, anxiety, personality changes, and quality of life issues.

Perform a system-focused nursing assessment with collection of both subjective and objective data as follows: neurological status (e.g., level of orientation and alertness, level of sedation, sensory and motor abilities, reflexes); respiratory status (e.g., respiratory rate, rhythm, and depth; breath sounds); GI status (e.g., presence of bowel sounds; bowel patterns; reports of constipation, diarrhea, nausea, vomiting, or abdominal discomfort); genitourinary (GU) status (e.g., urinary output, any burning or discomfort on urination, urinary retention); and cardiac status (e.g., pulse rate and rhythm, blood pressure, any problems with dizziness or syncope). Assess and document vital signs, including blood pressure, pulse rate, respirations, temperature, and level of pain (now considered the fifth vital sign). It is important to pull from one's knowledge base and remember that during the acute pain response, stimulation of the sympathetic nervous system may result in elevated values for vital signs, with an increase in blood pressure (120/80 mm Hg or higher), pulse rate (100 beats/min or higher), and respiratory rate and depth (20 breaths/min or higher and shallow breathing).

A variety of pain assessment tools are available that may be used to gather information about the fifth vital sign. One basic assessment tool is the Numeric Pain

Intensity Scale (0 to 10 pain rating scale); patients are asked to rate their pain intensity by picking the number that most closely represents their level of pain. The Verbal Rating Scale, another pain assessment tool, uses verbal descriptors for pain, including words such as *mild, moderate, severe, aching, agonizing,* or *discomfort.* The FACES Pain Rating Scale is helpful in assessing pain in patients of all ages and educational levels because it relies on a series of faces ranging from happy to sad to sad with tears. The patient is asked to identify the face that best represents the pain being experienced at that moment. When the patient is in acute pain, when pain intensity is a primary focus for assessment, or when the need is to determine the efficacy of pain management intervention, the simple, one-dimensional scales (e.g., the Numeric Pain Intensity Scale) work best. Older adult patients, especially those with cognitive impairment, may need more time to respond to the assessment tool and may also require large-print versions of written tools.

There are other assessment tools that are multi-dimensional scales and are more beneficial in assessing patients who experience persistent pain rather than acute pain. One example is the Brief Pain Inventory assessment tool, which includes a body map so that the patient can identify on the figure the exact area where pain is felt. This tool also helps in obtaining information about the impact of pain on functioning. Assess pain before, during, and after the pain intervention, as well as the level of pain during activity and at rest. The following sections provide assessment information for specific drug classes.

Nonopioids

For patients taking nonopioid analgesics, focus the assessment not only on general data as described earlier but also on the specific drug being given. For example, in those patients taking acetaminophen, begin the assessment determining whether the patient has allergies, is pregnant, or is breastfeeding. As mentioned in the pharmacology section, acetaminophen is contraindicated in those with severe liver disease and in patients with G6PD deficiency. Additionally, due to possible adverse effects of blood disorders (anemias), kidney or liver toxicity, cautious use is necessary. See pharmacology discussion for more information about acute overdose and persistent unintentional misuse. Also assess for any other medications the patient is taking, because of the risk of excessive doses when taking combination products containing acetaminophen. Inadvertent overdosing is a possible consequence of this situation. Other drug interactions and concerns are addressed in the pharmacology discussion.

Once therapy has been initiated, closely monitor for persistent acetaminophen poisoning, looking for symptoms such as rapid, weak pulse; dyspnea; and cold and clammy extremities. Long-term daily use of acetaminophen may lead to increased risk of permanent liver damage, and therefore frequently monitor the results of liver function studies. Adults who ingest higher-than-recommended dosages may be at higher risk of liver dysfunction as well as other adverse effects such as loss of appetite, jaundice, nausea, and vomiting. Children are also at high risk of liver dysfunction if the recommended dosage ranges are exceeded. With the use of NSAIDs (e.g., ibuprofen, aspirin, and COX-2 inhibitors), assess kidney and liver functioning and gather information about GI disorders such as ulcers (see Chapter 49 for more information on anti-inflammatory drugs). With aspirin, age is important; this drug is not to be given to children and adolescent patients because of the risk of Reye's syndrome. Aspirin may also lead to bleeding and ulcers, so ruling out conditions that represent contraindications and cautions to its use before therapy begins is important to patient safety. With tramadol, assessment of age is important because this drug is not recommended for use in individuals 75 years of age or older.

A miscellaneous nonopioid analgesic, lidocaine transdermal, is another option for managing different types of pain. For lidocaine transdermal patches, understand that this transdermal drug is indicated in those with postherpetic neuralgia, and thus assess the herpetic lesion(s) and surrounding skin. When these patches are used, they must be kept away from children and are not to be prescribed for young, small, or debilitated patients because they are at higher risk for toxicity. Liver function also needs to be assessed and monitored.

Opioids

When opioid analgesics or any other CNS depressants are prescribed, focus assessment on vital signs; allergies; respiratory disorders; respiratory function (rate, rhythm, depth, and breath sounds); presence of head injury (which will mask signs and symptoms of increasing intracranial pressure); neurologic status, with attention to level of consciousness or alertness and level of sedation; sensory and motor functioning; GI tract functioning (bowel sounds and bowel patterns); and GU functioning (intake and output). In addition, all opioids may cause spasms of the sphincter of Oddi. If kidney and liver function studies are ordered, monitor results because the risk of toxicity increases with diminished function of these organs.

An additional concern is any past or present history of neurological disorders such as Alzheimer's disease, dementia, multiple sclerosis, muscular dystrophy, myasthenia gravis, or cerebrovascular accident or stroke—the use of opioids may alter symptoms of the disease process, possibly masking symptoms or worsening the clinical presentation when no actual pathological changes have occurred. In these situations, use of another analgesic or pain protocol may be indicated. Attention to age is also important because both older adults and young patients are more sensitive to opioids, as to many other medications. In fact, older or younger age may be a contraindication to opioid use, depending on the specific drug. See

SPECIAL POPULATIONS: CHILDREN

Use of Opioids

- Assessment of children is challenging, and all types of behaviour that may indicate pain, such as muscular rigidity, restlessness, agitation, screaming, fear of moving, and withdrawn behaviour, must be carefully considered.
- Pain management is more difficult to determine in children; depending on age, children are less able or unable to express themselves. Frequently, the reason older children do not verbalize their pain is their fear of the treatment, such as injections. Compassionate and therapeutic communication skills, as well as the use of alternate routes of administration, as ordered, will help the nurse in these situations.
- The "ouch scale" is often used to determine the level of pain in children. This scale is used to obtain the child's rating of the intensity of pain from 0 to 5 by means of simple face diagrams, from a happy face for level 0 (no pain) to a sad, tearful face for level 5 pain. Parents and caregivers play an important role in pain management in the child and in noting any crying or distress.
- Pain assessment is important in children because they are often undermedicated. Always thoroughly assess a child's verbal and nonverbal behaviour, and never underestimate the child's reports. Remember that parents and caregivers can play an important role in this assessment.
- The child's baseline age, weight, and height are important to document because drug calculations are often based on these variables. With children, check and double-check *all* mathematical calculations for accuracy to avoid excessive dosages; this is especially true for opioids.
- Analgesics must be given before pain becomes severe, with oral dosage forms used first, if appropriate.

- If suppositories are used, be careful to administer the exact dose and not to split, halve, or divide an adult dose into a child's dose. This may result in the administration of an unknown amount of medication and possible overdose.
- When subcut, IM, and IV medications are used, the principle of nontraumatic care in the delivery of nursing care must be followed. One method to ensure nontraumatic care is the application of a mixture of local anaesthetics or other prescribed substances to the injection site before the injection is given. EMLA (lidocaine/prilocaine) is a topical cream that anaesthetizes the site of the injection; if ordered, apply 1 to 2-1/2 hours prior to the injection.
- Distraction and creative imagery may be used for younger children such as toddlers or preschool-aged children.
- Children should always be monitored closely for any unusual behaviour while they are receiving opioids.
- The following signs and symptoms should be reported to the physician immediately if they occur: CNS changes such as dizziness, lightheadedness, drowsiness, hallucinations, changes in level of consciousness, or sluggish pupil reaction. Do not administer further medication until receiving further orders from the physician.
- Always monitor and document vital signs before, during, and after the administration of opioid analgesics. An opioid medication is usually withheld if a patient's respiration rate is less than 10 breaths/min or if there are any changes in the level of consciousness. Always follow protocol, and never ignore a patient's status.
- Generally speaking, smaller doses of opioids (with close and frequent monitoring) are indicated for children. Giving oral medications with meals or snacks will help decrease GI tract distress.

---

the earlier pharmacology discussion regarding cautions, contraindications, and drug interactions. See Special Populations: Children and Special Populations: Older Adults for use of opioids in both of these age groups.

■ Opioid Agonist–Antagonists

In patients taking *opioid agonist–antagonists*, assess vital signs with attention to respiratory rate and breath sounds. Opioid agonist–antagonists still possess opioid agonist effects, and therefore the assessment information related to opioids is applicable to these drugs as well.

It is also important to remember during assessment that these drugs are still effective analgesics and will have CNS-depressant effects but are subject to the analgesic ceiling effect (see earlier definition). Given the action of these drugs, the assessment may help determine whether the patient is a misuser of opioids. This information is important because the simultaneous administra-

tion of agonist–antagonists with another opioid will lead to reversal of analgesia and possible opioid withdrawal. Age is another factor to assess because these drugs are not recommended for use in patients 18 years of age or younger. See previous discussion for a listing of contraindications, cautions, and drug interactions.

■ Opioid Antagonists

Remember that opioid antagonists are used mainly in reversing respiratory depression secondary to opioid overdosage. Naloxone may be used in patients of all ages, including neonates and children. Assess and document vital signs before, during, and after the use of the antagonist so that the therapeutic effects can be further assessed and documented and the need for further doses determined. In addition, remember that the antagonist drug may not work with just one dosing and that repeated doses are generally needed to reverse the effects of

SPECIAL POPULATIONS: THE OLDER ADULT

Opioid Use

- Record the patient's weight and height before the start of opioid treatment, if appropriate.
- Monitor the patient carefully for any changes in vital signs, level of consciousness, or central nervous system (CNS) depression, respiratory rate, as well as any changes indicative of respiratory function. Report and document these changes.
- Many institutionalized or hospitalized older adult patients can be stoic about pain; older adult patients may also have altered presentations of common illnesses so that the pain experience manifests in a different way, or may simply be unable to state how they feel in a clear manner. The older adult patient may also have complex pain needs such as both persistent and acute pain. Each patient, regardless of age, has the right to a thorough pain assessment and adequate and appropriate pain management. It is a myth that aging increases one's pain threshold. The challenge is that cognitive impairment and dementia are often major barriers to pain assessment. Nevertheless, many older adult patients are still reliable in their reporting of pain, even with moderate to severe cognitive impairment (see Evidence in Practice: Student Nurses' Misconceptions of Adults with Chronic Nonmalignant Pain Review on p. 197).
- Over time, older adults may lose reliability in recalling and accurately reporting persistent pain. Older adults, especially those 75 years of age or older, are at higher risk for too much or too little pain management, and it is important to remember that these drugs have a higher peak and longer duration of action in these patients than in their younger counterparts.
- Smaller dosages of opioids are generally indicated for older adults because of their increased sensitivity to the central nervous system depressant effects of the drugs and diminished kidney and liver function. Paradoxical (opposite) reactions and unexpected reactions may be more likely to occur in patients of this age group.
- In older adult male patients, benign prostatic hypertrophy or obstructive urinary diseases should be considered because of the urinary retention associated with the use of opioids. Urinary outflow can become further diminished in these patients and result in adverse reactions or complications. The physician may need to make dosage adjustments.
- Polypharmacy is often a problem in older adults; therefore, have a complete list of all medications the patient is currently taking, and assess for drug interactions and treatment (drug) duplication.
- Frequent assessments of older adult patients are needed. Pay attention to level of consciousness, alertness, and cognitive ability while ensuring that the environment is safe by keeping a call bell or light at the bedside. Using bed alarms is indicated where available.
- Decreased circulation causes variation in the absorption of IM or IV dosage forms and often results in the slower absorption of parenteral forms of opioids.
- Encourage older adults to ask for medications if needed. They often hesitate to ask for pain medication because they do not want to bother the nurse or give in to pain.
- Nonsteroidal anti-inflammatory drugs must be used with caution because of their potential for renal and GI toxicity. Acetaminophen is the drug of choice for relieving mild to moderate pain but with cautious dosing because of liver and kidney concerns. The oral route of administration is preferred for analgesia. The regimen should be as simple as possible to enhance adherence. Be sure to note, report, and document any unusual reactions to the opioid drugs. Hypotension and respiratory depression may occur more frequently in older adults taking opioids; thus, careful vital sign monitoring is needed.

the opioid. See the pharmacology section for information about contraindications, cautions, and drug interactions.

▨ Nursing Diagnoses

- Impaired gas exchange related to opioid-induced CNS effects and respiratory depression
- Acute pain related to specific disease processes or conditions and other pathologies leading to various levels and types of pain
- Persistent pain related to various disease processes, conditions, or syndromes causing pain
- Constipation related to the CNS-depressant effects on the GI system
- Deficient knowledge related to lack of familiarity with opioids, their use, and their adverse effects

▨ Planning

▧ Goals

- Patient will regain or maintain a respiratory rate between 10 and 20 breaths per minute without respiratory depression.
- Patient will state adequate acute pain relief associated with appropriate analgesic drug therapy regimen.
- Patient will experience relief from persistent pain associated with appropriate pharmacological therapy regimen.
- Patient will identify measures to help maintain normal bowel elimination patterns and avoid or minimize opioid-induced constipation.
- Patient will demonstrate adequate knowledge about the analgesic or other drug therapy and nondrug regimen.

■ Expected Patient Outcomes

- Patient states correct technique for coughing and deep breathing and adequate fluid intake while taking opioids or other analgesics for pain.
- Patient's respiratory rate is within normal depth, rate, and patterns with clearing breath sounds.
- Patient relates increased comfort levels as seen by decreased use of analgesics, increased activity and performance of activities of daily living, decreased reports of acute pain, as well as decreased levels of pain as rated on a scale of 1 to 10.
- Patient uses nonpharmacological measures such as relaxation therapy, distraction, and music therapy to help improve comfort and enhance any drug therapy regimens for persistent pain.
- Patient states various measures to help minimize or avoid the occurrence of constipation with forcing of fluids, increasing fibre in the diet, and improving mobility.
- Patient reports appropriate use of analgesics with minimal complications or adverse effects.
- Patient states rationale for the use, action, and therapeutic effects associated with analgesic drugs for management of acute or persistent pain.
- Patient states rationale for the use of nondrug approaches to pain management.
- Patient states importance of taking medication as prescribed.

■ Implementation

Once the cause of pain has been diagnosed or other assessment and data gathering have been completed, begin pain management immediately and aggressively according to the needs of each individual patient and situation. Pain management is varied and multifaceted and needs to incorporate pharmacological and nonpharmacological approaches (see Box 11-1 and Natural Health Products: Feverfew). Negotiate with patients by integrating religious ceremonies and traditional healing practices into pain care, rather than imposing Western cultural approaches. Pain management strategies must also include

consideration for the type of pain and pain rating as well as pain quality, duration, and precipitating factors, and interventions that help the pain. Some general principles of pain management are as follows:

1. Individualize a plan of care based on the patient as a holistic and cultural being (see Ethnocultural Implications: The Patient Experiencing Pain, p. 195).
2. Manage mild pain with the use of nonopioid drugs such as acetaminophen, tramadol hydrochloride, and NSAIDs (see Chapter 49).
3. Manage moderate to severe pain with a stepped approach, using opioids. Other analgesics or types of analgesics may be used in addition to other categories of medication (see pharmacology discussion).
4. Administer analgesics as ordered but before the pain gets out of control.
5. Always consider the use of nonpharmacological comfort measures (see Box 11-1) such as homeopathic and folk remedies, exercise, distraction, music or pet therapy, massage, and transcutaneous electrical stimulation. Although not always effective, these measures may prove beneficial for some patients. See Patient Teaching Tips for more information related to analgesics.

■ Nonopioids

Give nonopioid analgesics as ordered or as indicated for fever or pain. Acetaminophen should be taken as prescribed and within the recommended dosage range over a 24-hour period because of the risk of liver damage and acute toxicity. If a patient is taking other over-the-counter medications with acetaminophen, he or she needs to understand the importance of reading the labels (of other medications) carefully to identify the total amount of acetaminophen taken and any other drug–drug interactions. In educating the patient, emphasize the signs and symptoms of acetaminophen overdose: bleeding, loss of energy, fever, sore throat, and easy bruising (because of hepatotoxicity). These must be reported immediately by the patient, family member, or caregiver to the nurse or health care provider. Any worsening or change in the nature or characteristic of pain must also be reported.

NATURAL HEALTH PRODUCTS

FEVERFEW (*Chrysanthemum parthenium*)

Overview
A member of the marigold family known for its anti-inflammatory properties

Common Uses
Treatment of migraine headaches, menstrual cramps, inflammation, and fever

Adverse Effects
Nausea, vomiting, constipation, diarrhea, altered taste sensations, muscle stiffness, and joint pain

Potential Drug Interactions
Possible increase in bleeding with use of aspirin and other nonsteroidal anti-inflammatory drugs, dipyridamole, and warfarin sodium

Contraindications
Contraindicated in those with allergies to ragweed, chrysanthemums, and marigolds, as well as those about to undergo surgery

If taken by suppository, once the suppository is unwrapped, cold water may be run over it to moisten it for easier insertion. The suppository is inserted into the rectum using a gloved finger and water-soluble lubricating gel if necessary. Acetaminophen tablets may be crushed if needed. Adult patients who take more than 4 000 mg/day or greater are at risk for acute hepatotoxicity. Death may occur after ingestion of more than 15 g. Liver damage from acetaminophen may be minimized by timely dosing with acetylcysteine (see previous discussion). If acetylcysteine is indicated, warn the patient about the drug's foul taste and odour; many patients report that the drug smells and tastes like rotten eggs. Acetylcysteine is better tolerated if it is disguised by mixing with a drink such as cola or flavoured water to increase its palatability. Use of a straw may help minimize contact with mucous membranes of the mouth and is recommended. This antidote may be given through a nasogastric tube or intravenously, if necessary.

Tramadol may cause drowsiness, dizziness, headache, nausea, constipation, and respiratory depression. If dizziness, blurred vision, or drowsiness occurs, be sure to assist the patient with ambulation to minimize the risk of fall and injury. Educate the patient about injury prevention, including the need to dangle the feet over the edge of the bed before full ambulation, changing positions slowly, and asking for assistance when ambulating. In addition, while the patient is taking tramadol, as well as any other analgesics, and especially opioids, the patient needs to avoid any tasks that require mental clarity and alertness. Increasing fluids and fibre in the diet may help with constipation. Use of flat cola, ginger ale, or dry crackers may help to minimize nausea.

■ Opioids

When opioids (and other analgesics) are prescribed, administer the drug as ordered after checking for the "rights" of medication administration (see Chapter 1). After the health care provider's order has been double-checked, closely examine the medication profile and documentation to determine the last time the medication was given before administering another dose. Monitor the patient's vital signs at frequent intervals, with special attention to respiratory changes. A respiratory rate of 10 breaths/min (some protocols still adhere to the parameter of 12 breaths/min) may indicate respiratory depression and must be reported to the health care provider. The drug dosage, frequency, or route may need to be changed or an antidote (opioid antagonist) given if respiratory depression occurs. Naloxone must always be available, especially with the use of IV or other parenteral dosage forms of opioids, such as PCA (see Chapter 10 and the discussion to follow) or epidural infusions. Naloxone is indicated to reverse CNS depression, specifically respiratory depression, but remember that this antidote also reverses analgesia. Monitor the patient's urinary output as well; it should be at least 720 mL/24 hr. Monitor

bowel sounds during therapy; decreased peristalsis may indicate the need for a dietary change, such as increased fibre, or use of a stool softener or mild laxative (see Box 11-2). Assess the patient's pupillary reaction to light. Pinpoint pupils indicate a possible overdose.

Opioids or any analgesic must be given before the pain reaches its peak to help maximize the drug's effectiveness. Once the drug is administered, return at the appropriate time (taking into consideration the times of onset and peak effect of the drug and the route) to assess the effectiveness of the drug or other interventions as well as observe for the presence of adverse effects (see previous discussion of pain assessment tools). In regard to the route of administration, the recommendation is that oral dosage forms be used first, but only if ordered and if there is no nausea or vomiting. Taking the dose with food may help minimize GI upset. Should nausea or vomiting be problematic, an antiemetic may be ordered for administration before or with the dosing of medication. Crucial safety measures include keeping bed side rails up, turning bed alarms on (depending on facility policies and procedures), and making sure the call bell or alarm is within the patient's reach. These measures will help to prevent falls or injury related to opioid use. Opioids and similar drugs lead to CNS depression with possible confusion, altered sensorium or alertness, hypotension, and altered motor functioning. Because of these drug effects, all patients are at risk for falls or injury, and older adults are at higher risk (see Box 11-2 and Special Populations: Older Adults: Use of Opioids). See Table 11-10 below for more specific information concerning the handling of controlled substances and opioid counts.

When managing pain with morphine sulphate, meperidine hydrochloride, and similar opioid drugs, withhold the dose and contact the health care provider if there is any decline in the patient's condition or if vital signs are abnormal (see parameters mentioned earlier), and especially if the respiratory rate is less than 10 breaths/min. IM injections of analgesics are rarely used because of the availability of other effective and convenient dosage forms, such as PCA pumps, transdermal patches, constant subcut infusions, and epidural infusions. For transdermal patches (e.g., transdermal fentanyl), two systems are used. The older type of patch contains a reservoir system consisting of four layers, beginning with the adhesive layer and ending with the protective backing. Between these two layers are the permeable rate-controlling membrane and the reservoir layer, which holds the drug in a gel or liquid form. The newer type of patch has a matrix system consisting of two layers—one layer containing the active drug with the releasing and adhesive mechanisms, and the protective impermeable backing layer. The advantages of the matrix system over the reservoir system are that the patch is slimmer and smaller, it is more comfortable, it is worn for up to 7 days (the older reservoir system patch is worn for up to 3 to 4 days), and it appears to result in more constant serum

TABLE 11-10

Opioid Administration Guidelines

Opioid	Nursing Administration
buprenorphine and butorphanol tartrate	When giving IV, infuse over the recommended time (usually 3–5 min). Always assess respirations. Give IM as ordered.
codeine phosphate	Give PO doses with food to minimize gastrointestinal tract upset; ceiling effects occur with oral codeine phosphate, resulting in no increase in analgesia with increased dosage.
fentanyl	Administer parenteral doses as ordered and per manufacturer's guidelines in regard to mg/min to prevent CNS depression and possible cardiac or respiratory arrest. Transdermal patches come in a variety of dosages. Be sure to remove residual amounts of the old patch prior to application of a new patch. Dispose of patches properly to avoid inadvertent contact with children or pets. A fentanyl citrate sublingual effervescent tablet (Fentora®) is available for the management of breakthrough pain in patients with cancer that are 18 years of age and older who are already receiving and are tolerant to continuous opioid therapy for their persistent baseline cancer.
hydromorphone hydrochloride	May be given subcut, rectally, IV, IM, or PO.
meperidine hydrochloride	Given by a variety of routes: IV, IM, or PO; highly protein bound, so watch for interactions and toxicity. Monitor older adults for increased sensitivity.
morphine sulphate	Available in a variety of forms: subcut, IM, IV, PO, extended, and immediate release, and for epidural infusion. Always monitor respiratory rate.
nalbuphine hydrochloride	IV dosages of 10 mg given undiluted over 5 min
naloxone hydrochloride	Antagonist given for opioid overdose; 0.4 mg usually given IV over 15 sec or less. Reverses analgesia as well.
oxycodone hydrochloride	Often mixed with acetaminophen or aspirin; PO and suppository dosage forms. Available in both immediate and sustained-release tabs
pentazocine	PO, subcut, IV, and IM forms; mixed agonist–antagonist; IV dose of 5 mg to be given over 1 min

CNS, central nervous system; IM, intramuscular; IV, intravenous; PO, oral; subcut, subcutaneous.

drug levels. In addition, the matrix system is alcohol free; the alcohol in the reservoir system often irritates the patient's skin. It is important to know what type of delivery system is being used so that proper guidelines are followed to enhance the system's and drug's effectiveness.

Apply transdermal patches to only a clean, nonhairy area. When the patch is changed, place the new patch on a new site, but only after the old patch has been removed and the site cleansed of any residual medication. Rotation of sites helps decrease irritation and enhance drug effects. Transdermal patches require special discarding of old and used patches (see Preventing Medication Errors: Fentanyl Transdermal Patches on p. 205). Transdermal systems are beneficial for the delivery of many types of medications, especially analgesics, and have the benefits of allowing multiday therapy with a single application, avoiding first-pass metabolism, improving patient adherence, and minimizing frequent dosing. However, the patient should be watched carefully for the development of any type of contact dermatitis caused by the patch (contact the health care provider immediately if this occurs) and maintain a pain journal when at home. Journal entries are a valid source of information for the nurse, other health care providers, the patient, and family members to assess the patient's pain control and to monitor the effectiveness of not only transdermal analgesia but any medication regimen.

With the IV administration of opioid agonists, follow the manufacturer's guidelines and institutional policies regarding specific dilution amounts and solution as well as the time period for infusion. When PCA is used, the amounts and times of dosing should be noted in the appropriate records and tracked by appropriate personnel. The fact that a pump is being used, however, does not mean that it is 100% reliable or safe. Closely monitor and frequently check all equipment. Additionally, frequently monitor pain levels, response to medication, and vital signs with the use of other parenteral opioid administration. Always follow dosage ranges for all opioid agonists and agonist–antagonists, and pay special attention to the dosages of morphine and morphinelike drugs. For IV infusions, the nurse is responsible for monitoring the IV needle site and documenting any adverse effects or complications. Another point to remember when administering opioids, as well as other analgesics, is that each medication has a different onset of action, peak, and duration of action, with the IV route producing the most rapid onset (i.e., within minutes) (see Table 11-10).

To reverse an opioid overdose or opioid-induced respiratory depression, an opioid antagonist such as naloxone must be administered. If naloxone is used, 0.4 to 2 mg should be given intravenously in its undiluted form and should be administered over 15 seconds (or as ordered); if reconstitution is needed, 0.9% NaCl or 5%

dextrose injection should be used (see Table 11-8). However, the guidelines in the package insert should also be followed. Emergency resuscitative equipment should be nearby in the event of respiratory or cardiac arrest.

Opioid Agonist–Antagonists

When giving agonist–antagonists, remember that they react differently depending on whether they are given by themselves or with other drugs. When administered alone, they are effective analgesics because they bind with opiate receptors and produce an agonist effect (see discussion in pharmacology section). If given at the same time with other opioids, however, they lead to reversal of analgesia and acute withdrawal because of the blocking of opiate receptors. Be careful to check dosages and routes as well as perform the interventions mentioned for opioid agonist drugs, including closely assessing vital signs, especially respiratory rate. Emphasize with the patient the importance of reporting any dizziness, unresolved constipation, urinary retention, and sedation. See Table 11-7 for additional adverse effects of opioid agonists as they are similar to the opioid agonist–antagonist drugs. Other points to emphasize include that the drug also has the ability to reverse analgesia as well as precipitate withdrawal (if taken with other opioid agonists). A list of other opioid agonists must be shared with the patient as well.

Opioid Antagonists

Opioid antagonists must be given as ordered and be readily available, especially when the patient is receiving PCA with an opioid, is opioid naive, or is receiving continuous doses of opioids. Several doses of these drugs are often required to ensure adequate opioid agonist reversal (see earlier discussion). Encourage patients to report any nausea or tachycardia.

General Considerations

You are always responsible and accountable for maintaining a current, updated knowledge base on all forms of analgesics as well as protocols for pain management, with focus on the specific drug(s) as well as differences in the treatment of mild to moderate pain, severe pain, and pain in special situations (e.g., cancer pain). The WHO's three-step analgesic ladder provides a standard for pain management in patients with cancer and must be reviewed and considered, as needed. Dosing of medications for pain management is important to the treatment regimen. Once a thorough assessment has been performed, it is best to treat the patient's pain before it becomes severe, which is the rationale for considering pain the fifth vital sign. When pain is present for more than 12 hours a day, analgesic doses are individualized and best administered around the clock rather than on

an as-needed basis, while always staying within safe practice guidelines for each drug used. Around-the-clock (or scheduled) dosing maintains steady-state levels of the medication and prevents drug troughs and pain escalation. No given dosage of an analgesic will provide the same level of pain relief for every patient; thus there is a need for a process of titration, upward or downward, to be carried out based on the individual's needs. Aggressive titration may be necessary in difficult pain control cases and in cancer pain situations. Patients with severe pain, metastatic pain, or bone metastasis pain may need increasingly higher doses of analgesic. These special pain situations may require an opiate such as morphine that needs to be titrated, until the desired response is achieved or until adverse effects occur. A patient-rated pain level of less than 4 on a scale of 1 to 10 is considered an indication of effective pain relief.

If pain is not managed adequately by monotherapy, other drugs or adjuvants may need to be added to enhance analgesic efficacy. This includes the use of NSAIDs (for analgesic and anti-inflammatory effects), acetaminophen (for analgesic effects), corticosteroids (for mood elevation and anti-inflammatory, antiemetic, and appetite-stimulation effects), anticonvulsants (for treatment of neuropathic pain), tricyclic antidepressants (for treatment of neuropathic pain and opioid-potentiating effects), neuroleptics (for treatment of persistent pain syndromes), local anaesthetics (for treatment of neuropathic pain), hydroxyzine hydrochloride (for mild antianxiety properties as well as sedating effects and antihistamine and mild antiemetic actions), or psychostimulants (for reduction of opioid-induced sedation when opioid dosage adjustment is not effective). See Table 11-11 for a listing of drugs that should not be used in patients experiencing cancer pain.

Dosage forms are also important, especially with persistent pain and cancer pain. Oral administration is always preferred but is not always tolerated by the patient and may not even be a viable option for pain control. If oral dosing is not appropriate, less invasive routes of administration include rectal and transdermal routes. Rectal dosage forms are safe, inexpensive, effective, and helpful if the patient is experiencing nausea or vomiting or altered mental status; however, this route is not suitable for those with diarrhea, stomatitis, or low blood cell counts. Transdermal patches (e.g., the buprenorphine transdermal patch) may provide up to 7 days of pain control but are not for rapid dose titration and are used only when stable analgesia has been previously achieved. Long-acting forms of morphine and fentanyl may be delivered via transdermal patches when a longer duration of action is needed. Intermittent injections or continuous infusions via the IV or subcut routes are often used for opioid delivery and may be administered at home in special pain situations, such as in hospice care and in persistent cancer pain management. Subcut infusions are often used when there is no IV access. PCA

TABLE 11-11

Drugs Not Recommended for Treatment of Cancer Pain

Class	Drug	Reason for Not Recommending
Opioids with dosing around the clock	meperidine	Short (2–3 hr) duration of analgesia; administration may lead to CNS toxicity (tremor, confusion, or seizures)
Miscellaneous	cannabinoids	Adverse effects of dysphoria, drowsiness, hypotension, and bradycardia, which preclude their routine use as analgesics; may be indicated for use in treating severe chemotherapy-induced nausea and vomiting
Opioid agonist–antagonists	pentazocine butorphanol tartrate nalbuphine	May precipitate withdrawal in opioid-dependent patients; analgesic ceiling effect; possible production of unpleasant psychological adverse effects, including dysphoria, delusions, and hallucinations
	buprenorphine	Analgesic ceiling effect; can precipitate withdrawal if given with an opioid
Opioid antagonists	naloxone naltrexone	Reverses analgesia as well as CNS depressant effects, such as respiratory depression
Anxiolytics (as monotherapy) or sedative–hypnotics (as monotherapy)	Benzodiazepines (e.g., alprazolam)	Analgesic properties not associated with these drugs except in some situations of neuropathic pain; common risk of sedation, which may put some patients at higher risk for neurological complications
	Barbiturates	Analgesic properties not demonstrated; sedation is problematic and limits use

pumps may be used to help deliver opioids intravenously, subcutaneously, or even intraspinally and can be managed in home health care or hospice care for the patient at home. Use of the intrathecal or epidural route requires special skill and expertise, and delivery of pain medications using these routes is available only from certain home health care agencies for at-home care. The main reason for long-term intraspinal opioid administration is intractable pain. Transnasal dosage forms are approved only for butorphanol tartrate, an agonist–antagonist drug, and this dosage form is generally not used or recommended. Regardless of the specific drug or dosage form used, a fast-acting rescue drug needs to be ordered and available for patients with cancer pain or other special challenges in pain management. Regardless of the drug(s) used for the pain management regimen, always remember that individualization of treatment is one of the most important considerations for effective and quality pain control. Also consider implementing the following:

- At the initiation of pain therapy, conduct a review of all relevant histories, laboratory test values, nurse-related charting entries, and diagnostic study results in the patient's medical record.
- If there are underlying problems, consider them while never forgetting to treat with dignity and respect. Never let compounding variables or any other problems overshadow the fact that there is a patient who is in pain and deserving of safe, quality care.
- Develop goals for pain management in conjunction with the patient, family members, significant others, or caregiver. These goals include improving the level of comfort with increased levels of activities of daily living and ambulation.
- Collaborate with other members of the health care team to select a regimen that will be easy for the patient to follow while in the hospital and, if necessary, at home (e.g., for patients with cancer and other patients experiencing persistent pain).
- Be aware that most regimens for acute pain management include treatment with short-acting opioids plus the addition of other medications such as NSAIDs.
- Be familiar with equianalgesic doses of opioids because lack of knowledge of equivalencies may lead to inadequate analgesia or overdose.
- Use an analgesic appropriate for the situation (e.g., short-acting opioids for severe pain secondary to a myocardial infarction, surgery, or kidney stones). For cancer pain, the regimen usually begins with short-acting opioids with eventual conversion to controlled-release formulations.
- Use preventative measures to manage adverse effects. In addition, switch to another opioid as soon as possible if the patient finds that the medication is not controlling the pain adequately.
- Consider the option of analgesic adjuvants, especially in cases of persistent pain or cancer pain; these might include other prescribed drugs such as NSAIDs, acetaminophen, corticosteroids, anticonvulsants, tricyclic antidepressants, neuroleptics, local anaesthetics, hydroxyzine hydrochloride, or psychostimulants. Over-the-counter drugs and natural health products may also be helpful.
- Be alert to patients with special needs, such as patients with breakthrough pain. Generally, the drug used to manage such pain is a short-acting form of the longer-acting opioid being given (e.g., immediate-release morphine for breakthrough pain while sustained-release morphine is also used).
- Identify community resources that can assist the patient, family members, or significant others. These

CASE STUDY

Opioid Administration

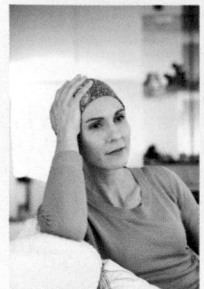

You are assigned to care for a patient, Daphna, who is in the terminal stage of breast cancer. As a community health care nurse, you have many responsibilities; however, you have not cared for many patients who are in the terminal stages of their illness. In fact, most of your patients are postoperative and have only required assessments, dressing changes, and wound care.

Daphna is 48 years of age and underwent bilateral mastectomy 4 years ago. She had lymph node involvement at the time of surgery and was recently diagnosed with metastasis to the bone. She has been taking sustained-release oxycodone (one 10-mg tab every 12 hours) at home but is not sleeping through the night and is now reporting increasing pain to the point that her quality of life has decreased significantly. She wants to stay at home during the terminal stage of her illness but needs to have adequate and safe pain control. Her husband of 18 years is supportive. They have no

children. They are both university graduates and have medical insurance.

1. Daphna's recent increase in pain has been attributed to bone metastasis in the area of the lumbar spine. At this time, the oxycodone is not beneficial, and you need to advocate for Daphna to receive adequate pain relief. When discussing her pain medications with her health care provider, what type of medication would you expect to be ordered to relieve the bone pain, and what is the rationale for this recommendation? Provide references from within this chapter for the selection of the specific opioid drug.

2. Daphna's husband confides in you that he is worried that she will become addicted to the new medication. He is not sure he agrees with round-the-clock dosing. How do you address his concerns?

3. What should Daphna's husband do if he feels that Daphna has had an overdose?

For answers see http://evolve.elsevier.com/Canada/Lilley/pharmacology/.

resources may include various websites for patient education such as http://www.canadianpainsociety.ca, http://www.chronicpaincanada.com, http://www.canadianpaincoalition.ca, and http://www.iasp-pain.org. Many other pain management sites may be found on the Internet by searching using the terms *pain*, *pain clinic*, or *pain education* and looking for patient-focused materials or sites.

- Conduct frequent online searches to remain current on the topic of pain management, pain education, drug and nondrug therapeutic regimens for pain and special pain situations.

- Because fall prevention is of utmost importance in patient care (after the ABCs [airway, breathing, circulation] of care are addressed), monitor the patient frequently after an analgesic is given. Frequent measurement of vital signs, inclusion of the patient in a frequent watch program, or use of bed alarms is encouraged.

☑ Evaluation

Positive therapeutic outcomes of acetaminophen use are decreased symptoms, fever, and pain. Monitor for adverse reactions of anemias and liver problems due to hepatotoxicity, and report patient reports of abdominal

pain or vomiting to the health care provider. During and after the administration of nonopiod analgesics such as tramadol, opioids, and mixed opioid agonists, monitor the patient for both therapeutic effects and adverse effects frequently and as needed. Therapeutic effects of analgesics include increased comfort periods as well as decreased reports of pain, with improvements in performance of activities of daily living, appetite, and sense of well-being. Monitoring for adverse effects varies with each drug (see earlier discussions), but adverse effects may consist of nausea, vomiting, constipation, dizziness, headache, blurred vision, decreased urinary output, drowsiness, lethargy, sedation, palpitations, bradycardia, bradypnea, dyspnea, and hypotension. Should vital signs change, the patient's condition decline, or pain continue, the physician should be contacted immediately and the patient closely monitored. Respiratory depression may be manifested by a respiratory rate of less than 10 breaths/min, dyspnea, diminished breath sounds, or shallow breathing. If the patient's vital signs change, the patient's condition declines, or pain continues, contact the prescriber immediately and continue to closely monitor. Include a review of the effectiveness of multimodal and nonpharmacological approaches to pain management in your evaluation.

PATIENT TEACHING TIPS

- Capsaicin is a topical product made from different types of peppers that may help with muscle pain and joint or nerve pain. It may cause local, topical reactions, so be sure to share information with the patient about its safe use.
- Opioids are not to be used with alcohol or with other CNS depressants, unless ordered, because of worsening of the depressant effects.
- A holistic approach to pain management may be appropriate, with the use of complementary modalities including the following: biofeedback, imagery, relaxation, deep breathing, humour, pet therapy, music therapy, massage, use of hot or cold compresses, and use of herbal products.
- Dizziness, difficulty breathing, low blood pressure, excessive sleepiness (sedation), confusion, or loss of memory must be promptly reported to the nurse or other health care provider.
- Opioids may result in constipation, so encouraging fluids (up to 3 L/day unless contraindicated), increased fibre consumption, and exercise as tolerated are recommended. Stool softeners may also be necessary.
- Report any nausea or vomiting. Antiemetic drugs may be prescribed.
- Any activities requiring mental clarity or alertness may need to be avoided if experiencing drowsiness or sedation. Ambulate with caution or assistance as needed.
- It is important for the patient to share any history of addiction with health care providers, but when such a patient experiences pain and is in need of opioid analgesia, understand that the patient has a right to comfort. Any further issues with addiction may be managed during and after the use of opioids. Keeping an open mind regarding the use of resources, counselling, and other treatment options is important in dealing with addictive behaviours.
- If pain is problematic and not managed by monotherapy, a combination of a variety of medications may be needed. Other drugs that may be used include antianxiety drugs, sedatives, hypnotics, or anticonvulsants.
- For the patient with cancer or special needs, the health care provider will monitor pain control and the need for other options for therapy or for dosing of drugs. For example, the use of transdermal patches, buccal tablets, and continuous infusions while the patient remains mobile or at home is often helpful in pain management. It is also important to understand that if morphine or morphinelike drugs are being used, the potential for addiction exists; however, in specific situations, the concern for quality of life and pain management is more important than the concern for addiction.
- Most hospitals have inpatient and outpatient resources such as pain clinics. Patients need to constantly be informed and aware of all treatment options and remain active participants in their care for as long as possible.
- Tolerance does occur with opioid use, so if the level of pain increases while the patient remains on the prescribed dosage, the prescriber or health care provider must be contacted. Dosages must not be changed, increased, or doubled unless prescribed.

KEY POINTS

- Pain is individual and involves senses and emotions that are unpleasant. It is influenced by age, ethnoculture, spirituality, and all other aspects of the person.
- Pain is associated with actual or potential tissue damage and may be exacerbated or alleviated depending on the treatment and type of pain.
- Types of analgesics include the following:
  - Nonopioids including acetaminophen and aspirin and other NSAIDs
  - Opioids, which are natural or synthetic drugs that either contain or are derived from morphine (opiates) or have opiatelike effects or activities (opioids), and opioid agonist–antagonist drugs
- Child dosages of morphine must be calculated cautiously with close attention to the dose and kilograms of body weight. Cautious titration of dosage upward is usually the standard. Older adult patients may react differently from what is expected to analgesics, especially opioids and opioid agonist–antagonists.
- Remember that older adult patients experience pain the same as the general population, but they may be reluctant to report pain and may metabolize opiates at a slower rate and thus are at increased risk for adverse effects such as sedation and respiratory depression. The best rule is to begin with low dosages, reevaluate often, and go slowly during upward titration.

EXAMINATION REVIEW QUESTIONS

1. For best results when treating severe pain associated with pathological spinal fractures related to metastatic bone cancer, the nurse should remember that the best type of dosage schedule is to administer the pain medication in which way?
   a. As needed
   b. Around the clock
   c. On schedule during waking hours only
   d. Around the clock, with additional doses as needed for breakthrough pain

2. A patient is receiving an opioid via a PCA pump as part of his postoperative pain management program. During rounds, the nurse finds him unresponsive, with respirations of 8 breaths/min and blood pressure of 102/58 mm Hg. After stopping the opioid infusion, what should the nurse do next?
   a. Notify the charge nurse
   b. Draw arterial blood gases
   c. Administer an opiate antagonist per standing orders
   d. Perform a thorough assessment, including mental status examination

3. A patient with bone pain caused by metastatic cancer will be receiving transdermal fentanyl patches. The patient asks the nurse what benefits these patches have. The nurse's best response includes which of these features?
   a. More constant drug levels for analgesia
   b. Less constipation and minimal dry mouth
   c. Less drowsiness than with oral opioids
   d. Lower dependency potential and no major adverse effects

4. IV morphine is prescribed for a patient who has had surgery. The nurse informs the patient that which common adverse effects can occur with this medication? (Select all that apply.)
   a. Diarrhea
   b. Constipation
   c. Pruritus
   d. Urinary frequency
   e. Nausea

5. Several patients have standard orders for acetaminophen as needed for pain. When the nurse reviews their histories and assessments, it is discovered that one of the patients has a contraindication to acetaminophen therapy. Which of the following patients should receive an alternate medication?
   a. A patient with a fever of 39.7°C
   b. A patient admitted with deep vein thrombosis
   c. A patient admitted with severe hepatitis
   d. A patient who had abdominal surgery 1 week earlier

6. The nurse is administering an IV dose of morphine to a 48-year-old postoperative patient. The dose ordered is 3 mg every 3 hours as needed for pain. The medication is supplied in vials of 4 mg/mL. How much will be drawn into the syringe for this dose?

7. An opioid analgesic is prescribed for a patient. The nurse checks the patient's medical history knowing this medication is contraindicated in which disorder?
   a. Renal insufficiency
   b. Severe asthma
   c. Liver disease
   d. Diabetes mellitus

Answers: 1. d, 2. c, 3. a, 4. b, c, e 5. c, 6. 0.75 mL, 7. b

CRITICAL THINKING ACTIVITIES

1. The nurse is about to administer 5 mg of morphine intravenously to a patient with severe postoperative pain, as ordered. What priority assessment data must be gathered before and after administering this drug? Explain your answer.

2. A patient reports that the drugs he is receiving for severe pain are not really helping. What is the nurse's priority action at this time?

3. A young woman is brought by ambulance to the emergency department because she was found unconscious next to an empty bottle of acetaminophen. While the medical team assesses her, the nurse goes to question the family about the situation. What is the most important piece of information to know about this possible overdose?

For answers see http://evolve.elsevier.com/Canada/Lilley/pharmacology/.

CHAPTER 12

General and Local Anaesthetics

Objectives

After reading this chapter, the successful student will be able to do the following:

1. Define anaesthesia.

2. Describe the basic differences between general and local anaesthesia.

3. List the most commonly used general and local anaesthetics and associated risks.

4. Discuss the differences between depolarizing neuromuscular blocking drugs and nondepolarizing blocking drugs and their impact on the patient.

5. Compare the mechanisms of action, indications, adverse effects, routes of administration, cautions, contraindications, and drug interactions of general anaesthesia and local anaesthesia, and of drugs used for procedural sedation.

6. Develop a collaborative plan of care for patients before anaesthesia (preanaesthesia), during anaesthesia, and after anaesthesia (postanaesthesia), related to general anaesthesia.

7. Develop a collaborative plan of care for patients undergoing local anaesthesia or procedural sedation.

e-Learning Activities

Website
(http://evolve.elsevier.com/Canada/Lilley/pharmacology/)

evolve

- Answer Key—Textbook Case Studies
- Answer Key—Critical Thinking Activities
- Chapter Summaries—Printable
- Review Questions for Exam Preparation
- Unfolding Case Studies

Drug Profiles

dexmedetomidine hydrochloride, p. 233
halothane, p. 233
isoflurane, p. 233
ketamine hydrochloride, p. 233
▸▸ **lidocaine (lidocaine hydrochloride*),** p. 237
nitrous oxide, p. 233
pancuronium (pancuronium bromide*), p. 240
▸▸ **propofol,** p. 233
sevoflurane, p. 233
▸▸ **succinylcholine,** p. 240
▸▸ **vecuronium bromide,** p. 240

▸▸ Key drug

*Full generic name is given in parentheses. For the purposes of this text, the more common, shortened name is used.

Key Terms

Adjunct anaesthetics Drugs used in combination with anaesthetic drugs to control the adverse effects of anaesthetics or to help maintain the anaesthetic state in the patient. (See *balanced anaesthesia*) (p. 229)

Anaesthesia The loss of the ability to feel pain resulting from the administration of an anaesthetic drug. (p. 228)

Anaesthetics Drugs that depress the central nervous system (CNS) or peripheral nerves to produce decreased sensation, loss of sensation, or muscle relaxation. (p. 228)

Balanced anaesthesia The practice of using combinations of different classes of drugs rather than a single drug to produce anaesthesia. (p. 229)

General anaesthesia A drug-induced state in which CNS nerve impulses are altered to reduce pain and other sensations throughout the entire body. It normally involves complete loss of consciousness and depression of normal respiratory drive. (p. 228)

Local anaesthesia A drug-induced state in which peripheral or spinal nerve impulses are altered to reduce or eliminate pain and other sensations in tissues innervated by these nerves. (p. 228)

Malignant hyperthermia A genetically linked, major adverse reaction to general anaesthesia characterized by a rapid rise in body temperature as well as tachycardia, tachypnea, and sweating. (p. 231)

Overton-Meyer theory A theory that describes the relationship between the lipid solubility of anaesthetic drugs and their potency. (p. 230)

Procedural sedation A milder form of general anaesthesia that causes partial or complete loss of consciousness but does not generally reduce normal respiratory drive (formerly referred to as *conscious sedation* or *moderate sedation*). (p. 231)

Spinal anaesthesia Local anaesthesia induced by injection of an anaesthetic drug near the spinal cord to anaesthetize nerves that are distal to the site of injection (also called *intraspinal anaesthesia*). (p. 232)

OVERVIEW

Anaesthetics are drugs that reduce or eliminate pain by depressing the central nervous system (CNS) or the peripheral nervous system (PNS). This state of reduced neurological function is called **anaesthesia**. Anaesthesia is further classified as general or local. **General anaesthesia** involves complete loss of consciousness, loss of body reflexes, elimination of pain and other sensations throughout the entire body, and skeletal and smooth muscle paralysis, including paralysis of respiratory muscles. **Local anaesthesia** does not involve paralysis of respiratory function but does involve elimination of pain sensation in the tissues innervated by anaesthetized nerves. Functions of the autonomic nervous system, which is a branch of the parasympathetic nervous system, may also be affected.

GENERAL ANAESTHETICS

General anaesthetics are drugs that induce general anaesthesia and are most commonly used to induce anaesthesia during surgical procedures. General anaesthetics are given only under controlled situations by anaesthesiologists. General anaesthesia is achieved by the use of one or more drugs. Often a synergistic combination of drugs is used, which allows lower doses of each drug and better control of the patient's anaesthetized state. Inhalational anaesthetics are volatile liquids or gases that are vaporized or mixed with oxygen to induce anaesthesia. For a historical perspective on general anaesthesia, see Box 12-1.

Parenteral anaesthetics (Table 12-1) are given intravenously and are used for induction or maintenance of general anaesthesia, for induction of amnesia, and as adjuncts to inhalation-type anaesthetics (Table 12-2). The specific goal varies with the drug. Common intravenous anaesthetic drugs include drugs classified solely as general anaesthetics, such as propofol.

BOX 12-1

General Anaesthesia: A Historical Perspective

Until recently, general anaesthesia was described as having several definitive stages. This was especially true with the use of many of the ether-based inhaled anaesthetic drugs. Features of these distinctive stages were easily observable to the trained eye. They included specific physical and physiological changes that progressed gradually and predictably with the depth of the patient's anaesthetized state. Gradual changes in pupil size, progression from thoracic to diaphragmatic breathing, vital sign changes, and several other changes all characterized the various stages. Newer inhalational and intravenous general anaesthetic drugs, however, often have a much more rapid onset of action and body distribution. As a result, the stages of anaesthesia once observed with older drugs are no longer sufficiently well defined to be observable. Thus, the concept of *stages of anaesthesia* is an outdated one in most modern surgical facilities. Registered nurses who pursue advanced training to become certified registered nurse anaesthetists often find this to be a rewarding and interesting area of nursing practice. In Canada, there is currently one program providing training for nurse practitioners in anaesthesia care (NP-A). The role of an anaesthesia assistant is also relatively new in Canada; however, training programs are not limited to registered nurses. Regulations about the role of anaesthesia assistants vary among provinces and territories. In addition, perianaesthesia nursing is a recognized specialty at a national level. Nurses who successfully write the certification exam are recognized for their knowledge and expertise by the Canadian Nurses Association.

TABLE 12-1

Parenteral General Anaesthetics

Generic Name	Trade Name
ketamine	Ketalar
propofol	Diprivan
thiopental	Pentothal®

TABLE 12-2

Inhaled General Anaesthetic Drugs

Generic Name	Trade Name
INHALED GAS	
nitrous oxide ("laughing gas")	
INHALED VOLATILE LIQUID	
desflurane	Suprame®
halothane	Halothane
isoflurane	Forane
sevoflurane	Sevorane AF®

Adjunct anaesthetics, or simply *adjuncts*, are also used. *Adjunct* is a general term for any drug that enhances clinical therapy when used simultaneously with another drug. Adjunct drugs can be thought of as "helper drugs" when their use complements the use of any other drug(s). They are used simultaneously with general anaesthetics for anaesthesia initiation (induction), sedation, reduction of anxiety, and amnesia. Adjuncts include neuromuscular blocking drugs (NMBDs; see Neuromuscular Blocking Drugs later in this chapter), sedative–hypnotics or anxiolytics (see Chapter 13) such as propofol (this chapter), benzodiazepines (e.g., diazepam, midazolam), barbiturates (e.g., thiopental, methohexital; see Chapter 13), opioid analgesics (e.g., morphine sulphate, fentanyl citrate, sufentanil citrate; see Chapter 11), anticholinergics (e.g., atropine sulphate; see Chapter 22), and antiemetics (e.g., ondansetron hydrochloride dihydrate; see Chapter 41). Note that propofol can be used as a general anaesthetic or sedative–hypnotic, depending on the dose. The simultaneous use of both general anaesthetics and adjuncts is called **balanced anaesthesia**. Common adjunct anaesthetic drugs are listed in Table 12-3.

TABLE 12-3

Adjunct Anaesthetic Drugs

Drug	Pharmacological Class	Usual Dosage Range	Indications/Uses

alfentanil hydrochloride (Alfenta®)	Opioid analgesic	Initial loading dose:
		  5–75 mcg/kg IV
		  (increments as needed)
		  0.5 to 1.5 mcg/kg/min
			Anaesthesia induction

fentanyl citrate (Fentanyl Citrate Injection®)		50–100 mcg/kg IV	
remifentanil hydrochloride		0.5–1 mcg/kg IV	
sufentanil citrate		doses up to 8 mcg/kg IV	
diazepam (Valium®)	Benzodiazepine	2–10 mg PO/IV/IM	Amnesia and anxiety reduction
midazolam		1–5 mg IV/IM	
atropine sulphate	Anticholinergic	0.02–0.6 mg/kg IM/Subcut	Drying up of excessive secretions
glycopyrrolate		0.004 mg/kg IM	
scopolamine		Children: 0.006 mg/kg IV/ IM/Subcut Adults: 0.3–0.6 mg IV/IM/ Subcut	
morphine sulphate	Opioid analgesic	5–20 mg IM/Subcut	Pain prevention and pain relief
hydroxyzine hydrochloride	Antihistamine	25–100 mg PO/IM	Sedation, prevention of nausea and vomiting, anxiety reduction
promethazine hydrochloride		25–50 mg IV/IM	
pentobarbital sodium	Sedative–hypnotic	150–200 mg IM	Amnesia and sedation
dexmedetomidine hydrochloride (Precedex)	α_2 agonist	0.2–1.1 mcg/hr (doses up to 1.4 mcg/kg/hr have been shown to be effective)	Sedation

IM, intramuscular; *IV*, intravenous; *PO*, oral; *Subcut*, subcutaneous.

Mechanism of Action and Drug Effects

Many theories have been proposed to explain the actual mechanism of action of general anaesthetics. The drugs vary widely in their chemical structures, and their mechanisms of action are not easily explained by a structure–receptor relationship. The concentrations of various anaesthetics required to produce a given state of anaesthesia also differ greatly. The **Overton-Meyer theory** has been used to explain some of the properties of anaesthetic drugs since the early days of anaesthesiology. In general terms, it proposes that, for all anaesthetics, potency varies directly with lipid solubility. In other words, across a continuum of drug potency, fat-soluble drugs are stronger anaesthetics than water-soluble drugs. Nerve cell membranes have a high lipid content, as does the blood–brain barrier (see Chapter 2). Lipid-soluble anaesthetic drugs can therefore easily cross the blood–brain barrier and concentrate in nerve cell membranes.

The overall effect of general anaesthetics is a progressive reduction of sensory and motor CNS functions. The degree and speed of this process varies with the anaesthetics and adjuncts used, along with their dosages and routes of administration. General anaesthesia initially produces a loss of the senses of sight, touch, taste, smell, and hearing, along with loss of consciousness. Cardiac and pulmonary functions are usually the last to be interrupted because they are controlled by the medulla of the brainstem. These are the classical "stages" of anaesthesia. Mechanical ventilatory support is absolutely necessary. In more extensive surgical procedures, especially those involving the heart, pharmacological cardiac support involving adrenergic drugs (see Chapter 19) and inotropic drugs (see Chapter 25) may also be required.

The reactions of various body systems to general anaesthetics are further described in Table 12-4.

Indications

General anaesthetics are used to produce unconsciousness and relaxation of skeletal and visceral smooth muscles for surgical procedures, as well as in electroconvulsive therapy for severe depression (see Chapter 17).

Contraindications

Contraindications to the use of anaesthetic drugs include known drug allergy. Depending on the drug type, contraindications may also include pregnancy, narrow-angle glaucoma, and known susceptibility to malignant hyperthermia (see Adverse Effects) from prior experience with anaesthetics.

Adverse Effects

Adverse effects of general anaesthetics are dose dependent and vary with the individual drug. The heart, peripheral circulation, liver, kidneys, and respiratory tract are the sites primarily affected. Pulmonary aspiration is a possible complication of general anaesthesia. Patient-related factors such as a full stomach and diabetes may place a patient at higher risk for aspiration; this is why adequate fasting is required prior to elective procedures requiring general anaesthesia). Myocardial depression is a common adverse effect. All of the halogenated anaesthetics are capable of causing hepatotoxicity.

With the development of newer drugs, many of the unwanted adverse effects characteristic of the older drugs (such as hepatotoxicity and myocardial depression) are now in the past. In addition, many bothersome adverse effects such as nausea, vomiting, and confusion are less common since balanced anaesthesia is widely used. This practice prevents many of the unwanted, dose-dependent adverse effects and toxicity associated with anaesthetic drugs while also achieving a more balanced general anaesthesia. Substance misuse (e.g., alcohol misuse; see Chapter 18) can predispose a patient to anaesthetic-induced complications (e.g., liver toxicity). A positive history of substance misuse may lead to dosage adjustments in one or more of the drugs used. A patient who misuses drugs and has a high tolerance for street drugs may also require higher doses of

TABLE 12-4

Effects of Inhaled and Intravenous General Anaesthetics

Organ/System	Reaction
Respiratory system	Depressed muscles and patterns of respiration; altered gas exchange and impaired oxygenation; depressed airway-protective mechanisms; airway irritation and possible laryngospasm
Cardiovascular system	Depressed myocardium; hypotension and tachycardia; bradycardia in response to vagal stimulation
Central nervous system	CNS depression; blurred vision; nystagmus; progression of CNS depression to decreased alertness and sensorium as well as decreased level of consciousness
Cerebrovascular system	Increased intracranial blood volume and increased intracranial pressure
Gastrointestinal system	Reduced liver blood flow and thus reduced liver clearance
Renal system	Decreased glomerular filtration
Skeletal muscles	Skeletal muscle relaxation
Cutaneous circulation	Vasodilation
Central nervous system (CNS)	CNS depression; blurred vision; nystagmus; progression of CNS depression to decreased alertness, sensorium, and level of consciousness

anaesthesia-related drugs (e.g., benzodiazepines, opioids) to achieve the desired sedative effects.

Malignant hyperthermia is an uncommon, but potentially fatal, genetically linked adverse metabolic reaction to general anaesthesia. It is classically associated with the use of volatile inhalational anaesthetics as well as the depolarizing neuromuscular blocking drug succinylcholine (see Neuromuscular Blocking Drugs later in this chapter). Signs include rapid rise in body temperature, tachycardia, tachypnea, and muscular rigidity. Patients known to be at greater risk for malignant hyperthermia include children, adolescents, and individuals with muscular or skeletal abnormalities such as hernias, strabismus, ptosis, scoliosis, and muscular dystrophy. Malignant hyperthermia is treated with cardiorespiratory supportive care as needed to stabilize heart and lung function, along with the skeletal muscle relaxant dantrolene sodium (see Chapter 13). All facilities that provide general anaesthesia must maintain a certain amount of dantrolene sodium on hand in case of malignant hyperthermia.

Toxicity and Management of Overdose

In large doses, anaesthetics are potentially life threatening, with cardiac and respiratory arrest as the ultimate causes of death. However, these drugs are almost exclusively administered in a controlled environment by personnel trained in advanced cardiac life support. These drugs are also quickly metabolized. In addition, the medullary centre, which governs the vital functions, is the last area of the brain to be affected by anaesthetics and the first to regain function. These factors combined make an anaesthetic overdose rare and easily reversible.

Interactions

Some of the common drugs that interact with general anaesthetics are antihypertensives and β-blockers, which have additive effects when given with general anaesthetics (increased hypotensive effects from antihypertensives; increased myocardial depression with β-blockers). Patients using long-term antihypertensives such as β-blockers are usually discontinued prior to the procedure requiring a general anaesthetic. No significant laboratory test interactions have been reported.

Dosages

For the recommended dosages of selected general anaesthetic drugs, see the Dosages table below.

DRUGS FOR PROCEDURAL SEDATION

Procedural sedation refers to anaesthesia that does not cause complete loss of consciousness and does not normally cause respiratory arrest. As more minor surgical procedures move from traditional operating room settings to outpatient surgery centres or office-based

DOSAGES	**Selected General Anaesthetic Drugs**		
Drug	Pharmacological Class	Usual Dosage Range	Indications
Halothane®	Inhalation general anaesthetic (halogenated hydrocarbon)	0.5–1.5% concentration	General anaesthesia
isoflurane (Forane®)	Inhalation general anaesthetic (enflurane isomer)	0.1–2% concentration with appropriate drugs	General anaesthesia
nitrous oxide ("laughing gas")	Inorganic inhalation general anaesthetic	20–40% with oxygen (e.g., 70% with 30% oxygen)	Analgesia Anaesthesia

 ## SPECIAL POPULATIONS: OLDER ADULTS

Anaesthesia

- Older adult patients are affected more adversely by anaesthesia than young or middle-aged adults. With aging comes organ system deterioration. Declining liver function results in decreased metabolism of drugs, and a decline in kidney functioning leads to decreased drug excretion. Either of these can lead to drug toxicity, unsafe levels, or overdose. If both of these organs are not functioning properly, the risk of drug toxicity or overdose is even greater. In addition, the older adult population is more sensitive to the effects of drugs affecting the central nervous system.
- Presence of cardiac and respiratory diseases places the older adult patient at higher risk for cardiac dysrhythmias, hypotension, respiratory depression, atelectasis, or pneumonia during the postanaesthesia and postoperative phases.
- The practice of polypharmacy is yet another concern in older adults in regard to administration of any type of anaesthetic. Because of the presence of various age-related diseases, older patients are generally taking more than one medication. The more drugs a patient is taking, the higher the risk of adverse reactions and drug–drug interactions, including interactions with anaesthetics.

SPECIAL POPULATIONS: CHILDREN

Anaesthesia

- Premature infants, neonates, and pediatric patients are more adversely affected by anaesthesia than young or middle-aged adult patients. The reason for this difference in response is the increased sensitivity of the pediatric patient to anaesthetics and related drugs because of immature functioning of the liver and kidneys, which leads to possible drug accumulation, toxicity, and subsequent complications. The central nervous system of pediatric patients is also more sensitive to the effects of anaesthetics. Because of these risks of toxicity and complications with all forms of anaesthesia, take every precaution to ensure that the patient remains safe and free from harm.
- Cardiac and respiratory systems are not fully developed in the neonate, premature infant, and newborn, which makes this age group more susceptible to problems with the metabolism and excretion of drugs. Some of the more common problems include central nervous system depression with subsequent respira-

tory and cardiac depression, development of atelectasis, pneumonia, and cardiac abnormalities.
- Neonates in particular (see age group definitions and further discussion in Chapter 4) are at higher risk of upper airway obstruction during general anaesthesia. During the anaesthetic process, the risk of laryngospasm related to the intubation process may be increased for neonates because of the specific physical characteristics of the larynx and respiratory structures in this age group. Their higher metabolic rate and small airway diameter also put neonates at greater risk of complications during general anaesthesia.
- Before any medications are given to the pediatric patient, perform a careful check and double-check of mathematical drug calculations. In addition to weight, take into consideration body surface area and laboratory test results that may indicate organ dysfunction when making the actual drug calculation.
- Resuscitative equipment should be readily available on any neonatal or pediatric nursing care unit.

practices, the use of procedural sedation will continue to increase. Procedural sedation allows patients to relax and have markedly reduced or no anxiety, yet still maintain their own open airway and respond to verbal commands. Standards must be followed when providing procedural sedation. Health care providers who administer procedural sedation are required to have advanced cardiac life support training; one professional must have no duties other than to monitor the patient, and someone with the ability to intubate the patient must be present in case the patient slips into a deeper state of sedation and is unable to maintain an open airway. The Canadian Anesthesiologists' Society has published guidelines on procedural sedation, which can be found at https://www.cas.ca.

The most commonly used drugs for procedural sedation include a benzodiazepine, usually midazolam (see Chapter 13), with an opioid, usually fentanyl citrate or morphine sulphate. Propofol is also a common drug used. Propofol is usually given by an anaesthesiologist. The doses of midazolam used in procedural sedation are 0.02 to 0.1 mg over a 2-minute period, not to exceed 2.5 mg. If needed, a repeat dose of 25% of the initial dose may be used. If midazolam is combined with an opioid such as fentanyl citrate or morphine sulphate, the dose should be reduced by 30 to 50%. The most common dose of fentanyl citrate is 1 to 2 mcg/kg, which may be repeated every 30 minutes. The dose of morphine sulfate for procedural sedation is 2 mg IV. When these drugs are combined with a benzodiazepine, lower doses should be used. The dose of propofol for procedural sedation is 0.5 to 1 mg/kg, followed by 0.5 mg/kg every 3 to 5 minutes. Mild amnesia is also a common effect, due to the midazolam. This is often desirable for helping

patients not to remember painful medical procedures. Procedural sedation is associated with a more rapid recovery time than general anaesthesia is; it is also associated with a better safety profile because of lower cardiopulmonary risks.

The oral route of drug administration is commonly used in pediatric patients. This often involves administering an oral syrup form of midazolam with or without concurrent use of injected medications such as opiates. This is especially helpful for pediatric patients who must undergo uncomfortable procedures—such as wound suturing—or diagnostic procedures requiring reduced movement, such as computed tomography and magnetic resonance imaging. See the Special Populations: Children box below for other considerations.

LOCAL ANAESTHETICS

Local anaesthetics are the second major class of anaesthetics. They reduce pain sensations at the level of peripheral nerves, although this can involve intraspinal anaesthesia (see later). They are also called *regional anaesthetics* because they render a specific portion of the body insensitive to pain without major reduction of CNS function and level of consciousness. They act by interfering with nerve transmission in specific areas of the body, blocking nerve conduction only in the area in which they are applied, without causing loss of consciousness. They are most commonly used in clinical settings in which loss of consciousness is undesirable or unnecessary. These include childbirth and other situations in which **spinal anaesthesia** is desired, dental procedures, suturing of skin lacerations, and diagnostic procedures (e.g., lumbar puncture, thoracentesis, biopsy).

DRUG PROFILES

The dose of any anaesthetic depends on the complexity of the surgical procedure to be performed and the physical characteristics of the patient. All general anaesthetics have a rapid onset of action along with rapid elimination upon discontinuation. Anaesthesia is maintained intraoperatively by continuous administration of the drug.

isoflurane

Isoflurane (Forane) is a fluorinated ether that is a chemical isomer of the older fluorinated ether enflurane. It has a more rapid onset of action, causes less cardiovascular depression, and has little or no toxicity. This is in contrast to enflurane, which can cause seizures, and halothane, which is associated with liver toxicity.

sevoflurane

Sevoflurane is a fluorinated ether and is now widely used. Its pharmacokinetics, with rapid onset and rapid elimination, make it especially useful in outpatient surgery settings. It is also nonirritating to the airway, which greatly facilitates induction of an unconscious state, especially in pediatric patients.

ketamine hydrochloride

Ketamine hydrochloride (Ketalar®) is a unique drug with multiple properties. Given intravenously, it can be used for both general anaesthesia and procedural sedation. It is commonly used in the emergency department for setting broken bones. It can also provide procedural sedation when given intravenously. It binds to receptors in both central and peripheral nervous systems, including opioid receptors. The most important receptors for the therapeutic activity of this drug, however, are the N-methyl-D-aspartate (NMDA) receptors located in the dorsal horn of the spinal cord. The drug is highly lipid soluble and penetrates the blood–brain barrier rapidly, which results in a rapid onset of action. It has a low incidence of reduction of cardiovascular, respiratory, and bowel function. Adverse effects can include disturbing psychomimetic effects, including hallucinations. However, these are less likely to occur when benzodiazepines (see Chapter 13) are coadministered with the drug. Interacting drugs include NMBDs (prolonged paralysis) and halothane (reduced cardiac output and blood pressure). The drug is contraindicated in cases of known drug allergy.

nitrous oxide

Nitrous oxide, also known as *laughing gas*, is the only inhaled gas currently used as a general anaesthetic. It is the weakest of the general anaesthetic drugs and is used primarily for dental procedures or as a useful supplement to other, more potent anaesthetics.

▸▸propofol

Propofol (Diprivan®) is a parenteral general anaesthetic used for the induction and maintenance of general anaesthesia and also for sedation for mechanical ventilation in the Critical Care Unit (CCU) and other critical care settings. Because it provides a rapid deep sedation, an anaesthesiologist or sedation team often administers it and monitors its use outside the operating room. It is thought to mediate gamma-aminobutyric acid (GABA) activity. Propofol has no analgesic properties. In lower doses, it can also be used as a sedative–hypnotic for procedural sedation. Propofol is typically well tolerated, producing few undesirable effects. However, it does lead to a dose-dependent reduction in arterial blood pressure and cardiac output; therefore, it must be used with caution in patients who are hemodynamically unstable. Propofol is a lipid-based emulsion, and prolonged use, or use in conjunction with total parenteral nutrition, requires serum lipids to be monitored.

dexmedetomidine

Dexmedetomidine (Precedex®) is an α_2-adrenergic receptor agonist (see Chapter 13). It produces dose-dependent sedation, decreased anxiety, and analgesia without respiratory depression. It is used for procedural sedation and for surgeries of short duration. It has a short half-life, and the patient awakens quickly upon withdrawal of the drug. Dexmedetomidine is also used in the critical care setting for sedation of mechanically ventilated patients. Lower doses may be needed with concurrent anaesthetics, sedatives, or opioids. Adverse effects include hypotension, bradycardia, transient hypertension, and nausea. Doses are listed in Table 12-3. Although the prescribing information states that dexmedetomidine is to be used for only 24 hours, multiple studies have shown it to be safe and effective at longer durations.

Most local anaesthetics belong to one of two major groups of organic compounds—esters or amides. They are classified as either *parenteral* (injectable) or *topical* anaesthetics. Parenteral anaesthetics are most commonly given intravenously but may also be administered by various spinal injection techniques (Box 12-2). Topical anaesthetics are applied directly to the skin and mucous membranes. They are available in the form of solutions, ointments, gels, creams, powders, suppositories, and ophthalmic drops. Their dosage strengths are listed in Table 12-5.

The injection of parenteral anaesthetic drugs into the area near the spinal cord is known as *spinal* or *intraspinal*

anaesthesia. This type of anaesthesia is generally used to block all peripheral nerves that branch out distal to the injection site. The result is elimination of pain and paralysis of the skeletal and smooth muscles of the corresponding innervated tissues. Some of the medications used for spinal anaesthesia include the opioids morphine sulphate, hydromorphone, and fentanyl citrate (see Chapter 11), and the local anaesthetics lidocaine and bupivacaine. Because spinal anaesthesia does not normally depress the CNS at a level that causes loss of consciousness, it can be thought of as a large-scale type of local rather than general anaesthesia. Common types of local anaesthesia are described in Box 12-2. The parenteral anaesthetic

SPECIAL POPULATIONS: CHILDREN

Procedural Anaesthesia*

- Procedural sedation (anaesthesia) is used to reduce anxiety, pain, and fear in the pediatric patient. The use of procedural anaesthesia in the pediatric patient allows a procedure to be performed restraint free in most situations while keeping the patient responsive.
- Pediatric dosing often conforms to the following guidelines:
  - Morphine sulphate—pediatric dosing may be at 0.05 to 0.1 mg/kg intravenously (IV) over a 2-minute period and is ideal for long procedures or cases in which pain is anticipated after the procedure.
  - Fentanyl citrate—pediatric dosing may be at 0.5 to 1 mcg/kg with increments over 3 minutes, to a maximum of 3 doses. Too rapid an IV injection may result in chest rigidity, which may need to be treated with muscle relaxants and possibly mechanical ventilation. Fentanyl citrate is used often for short procedures.
  - Hydromorphone hydrochloride—pediatric dosing is at 0.015 to 0.02 mg/kg.
- Discharge status of the pediatric patient depends on the types of drugs and drug combinations used.

Discharge after procedural sedation is based mainly on whether the following criteria are met:
- Patient is alert and oriented compared with the baseline neurological assessment.
- Protective swallowing and gag reflexes are intact.
- Vital signs are stable and consistent with baseline values for at least 30 minutes after the last dosing. Different health care facilities set different criteria that must be met and documented (blood pressure and pulse rate within normal limits or within 20 points of baseline, temperature lower than 38.3°C.
- Oxygen saturation is at least 95% on room air 30 minutes after the last dose.
- Pain rating is at baseline levels or less.
- Ambulation is at baseline level.
- An adult is present to take the child home and remain with him or her for at least two half-lives of the various drugs used for the anaesthesia.
- If a reversal drug was administered, there has been time for the drug to be excreted.

*Drugs given as anaesthesia for procedural sedation procedures are given only under controlled situations by anaesthesiologists.

BOX 12-2   Types of Local Anaesthesia

Central

Spinal or intraspinal anaesthesia: Anaesthetic drugs are injected into the area near the spinal cord within the vertebral column. Intraspinal anaesthesia is commonly accomplished by one of two injection techniques: intrathecal and epidural. Spinal anaesthesia is commonly used for surgery on the lower extremities, perineum (e.g., surgery on the genitalia or anus), or lower body wall (e.g., inguinal herniorrhaphy). Caesarean deliveries are routinely performed under spinal anaesthesia, as are total hip arthroplasty and total knee arthroplasty.

- **Intrathecal anaesthesia:** Anaesthetic drugs are injected into the subarachnoid space. Intrathecal anaesthesia is commonly used for patients undergoing major abdominal or orthopedic surgery or planned Caesarean sections for whom the risks of general anaesthesia are too high or who prefer this technique instead of complete loss of consciousness during their surgical procedure. More recently, intrathecal injection of anaesthetics through implantable drug pumps is being used on an outpatient basis in patients with severe persistent pain syndromes, such as those resulting from occupational injuries.
- **Epidural anaesthesia:** Anaesthetic drugs are injected via a small catheter into the epidural space without puncturing the dura. Epidural anaesthesia is commonly used to reduce maternal discomfort during labour and delivery, for planned Caesarean sections, orthopedic surgery, and to manage postoperative acute pain after major abdominal or pelvic surgery. This route is becoming more popular for the administration of opioids for pain management.

Peripheral

- **Infiltration:** Small amounts of anaesthetic solution are injected into the tissue that surrounds the operative site. This approach to anaesthesia is commonly used for such procedures as wound suturing and dental surgery. Often, drugs that cause constriction of local blood vessels (e.g., epinephrine, cocaine) are also administered to limit the site of action to the local area.
- **Nerve block:** Anaesthetic solution is injected at the site where a nerve innervates a specific area, such as a tissue. This allows large amounts of anaesthetic to be delivered to a specific area without affecting the whole body. This method is often reserved for more difficult-to-treat pain syndromes, such as cancer pain and chronic orthopedic pain.
- **Topical anaesthesia:** The anaesthetic drug is applied directly onto the surface of the skin, eye, or any other mucous membrane to relieve pain or prevent it from being sensed. It is commonly used for diagnostic eye examinations and skin suturing.

TABLE 12-5

Selected Topical Anaesthetics

Drug	Route	Dosage Strength
benzocaine (Cetacaine®, Lanacane®, Solarcaine®)	Topical, aerosol, and spray	18% gel
cocaine hydrochloride	Topical	4–10% solution
dibucaine hydrochloride (Nupercainal®)	Topical	0.5–1% ointment or cream
dyclonine hydrochloride (Sucrets®)	Topical	Lozenges
lidocaine (Bactine®, Betacaine®)	Topical	Jelly, ointment, cream, spray
prilocaine/lidocaine (EMLA)	Topical	2.5% prilocaine and 2.5% lidocaine cream, patch
tetracaine hydrochloride (Pontocaine®)	Injection, topical, and ophthalmic	0.5–2% solution, gel, ointment, or cream

TABLE 12-6

Selected Parenteral Local Anaesthetic Drugs*

Generic Name	Trade Name	Potency	Onset	Duration
lidocaine hydrochloride	Xylocaine	Moderate	Immediate	60–90 min
mepivacaine hydrochloride	Carbocaine®, Isocaine®	Moderate		120–150 min
tetracaine hydrochloride	Pontocaine	Highest	5–10 min	90–120 min

*Other common parenteral anaesthetic drugs include bupivacaine (Marcaine®, Sensorcaine®), chloroprocaine (Nesacaine®), and ropivacaine (Naropin®).

drugs and their pharmacokinetics are summarized in Table 12-6.

Local anaesthesia of specific peripheral nerves is accomplished either by nerve block anaesthesia or infiltration anaesthesia. Nerve block anaesthesia involves relatively deep injections of drugs into locations adjacent to major nerve trunks or ganglia. It focuses on a relatively large body region but not necessarily one as extensive as that affected by spinal anaesthesia. In contrast, infiltration anaesthesia involves multiple small injections (intradermal, subcutaneous, submucosal, or intramuscular) to produce a more limited or "local" anaesthetic field. Another subtype of local anaesthesia involves topical application of a drug (e.g., lidocaine) onto the surface of the skin, mucous membranes, or eye. A newer method of administering local anaesthetics is via a peripheral nerve catheter attached to a pump containing the local anaesthetic. These pumps are designed to infuse local anaesthetic around the nerves that innervate the surgical site for several days postoperatively. The catheter is implanted during surgery and is normally taken out by the patient at home once the anaesthetic has been infused. A common trade name is the ON-Q*® PainBuster pump.

Mechanism of Action and Drug Effects

Local anaesthetics act by rendering a specific portion of the body insensitive to pain by interfering with nerve transmission. Nerve conduction is blocked only in the area in which the anaesthetic is applied, and there is no loss of consciousness. Local anaesthetics block both the generation and conduction of impulses through all types of nerve fibres (sensory, motor, and autonomic) by blocking the movement of certain ions (sodium, potassium, and calcium) important to this process. They do this by making it more difficult for these ions to move in and out of the nerve fibre. For this reason, some of these drugs are also described as *membrane-stabilizing* because they alter the cell membrane of the nerve so that the free movement of ions is inhibited. The membrane-stabilizing effects occur first in the small fibres and then in the large fibres. In terms of paralysis, usually autonomic activity is affected first, and then pain and other sensory functions are lost; motor activity is the last to be lost. When the effects of the local anaesthetic wear off, recovery occurs in reverse order: motor activity returns first, then sensory functions, and finally autonomic activity.

Possible systemic effects of the administration of local anaesthetics include effects on circulatory and respiratory functions. The systemic adverse effects depend on where and how the drug is administered (e.g., injection at a certain level in the spinal cord or topical application of a drug that gains access to the circulatory system). Such adverse effects are unlikely unless large quantities of a drug are injected. Local anaesthetics also produce *sympathetic blockade*; that is, they block the action of the two neurotransmitters of the sympathetic nervous system, norepinephrine and epinephrine (see Chapter 19). The cardiac effects include a decrease in stroke volume, cardiac output, and peripheral resistance. The respiratory effects include reduced respiratory function and altered breathing patterns, but complete paralysis of respiratory function is unlikely.

Indications

Local anaesthetics are used for surgical, dental, or diagnostic procedures, as well as for the treatment of certain types of persistent pain. Spinal anaesthesia is used to control pain during surgical procedures and childbirth. Nerve block anaesthesia is used for surgical, dental, and diagnostic procedures and for the therapeutic management of persistent pain. Infiltration anaesthesia is used for relatively minor surgical and dental procedures.

Contraindications

Contraindications for local anaesthetics include known drug allergy. Only specially formulated dosage forms are intended for ophthalmic use (see Chapter 57).

Adverse Effects

The adverse effects of the local anaesthetics are limited and of little clinical importance in most circumstances. The undesirable effects usually occur with high plasma concentrations of the drug, which result from inadvertent intravascular injection, an excessive dose or rate of injection, slow metabolic breakdown, or injection into a highly vascular tissue. One notable complication of spinal anaesthesia is spinal headache. Spinal headache occurs in up to 70% of patients who either experience inadvertent dural puncture during epidural anaesthesia or undergo intrathecal anaesthesia. Spinal headache is most often self-limiting and is treated with bedrest and conventional analgesic medications. Oral forms of the CNS stimulant caffeine (see Chapter 14) are also sometimes used. Severe cases of spinal headache may be treated by the anaesthetist by injection of a small volume (approximately 15 mL) of venous sample of the patient's own blood into the patient's epidural space. The exact mechanism by which this blood patch provides relief is unknown, but it is effective in treating spinal headache in over 90% of cases.

True allergic reactions to local anaesthetics are rare. However, they can occur, ranging from skin lesions, urticaria, and edema, to anaphylactic shock. Such allergic reactions are generally limited to a particular chemical class of anaesthetics called the *ester type*. Box 12-3

categorizes the local anaesthetic drugs into the ester and amide chemical families. Different enzymes are responsible for the breakdown of these two groups of anaesthetics in the body. Anaesthetics belonging to the ester family are metabolized by cholinesterase in the plasma and liver. They are converted into a para-aminobenzoic acid (PABA) compound. This compound is responsible for the allergic reactions. In contrast, the amide type of anaesthetics is metabolized uneventfully to active and inactive metabolites in the liver by other enzymes. Often when an individual has an adverse reaction to one of the local anaesthetics, using a drug from the alternate chemical class avoids this problem.

Toxicity and Management of Overdose

Local anaesthetics have little opportunity to cause toxicity under most circumstances. However, systemic reactions are possible if sufficiently large quantities are absorbed into the systemic circulation. To prevent this from occurring, a vasoconstrictor such as epinephrine is often coadministered with the local anaesthetic to maintain localized drug activity (e.g., lidocaine with epinephrine or bupivacaine with epinephrine). This property of epinephrine also serves to reduce local blood loss during minor surgical procedures. If significant amounts of the locally administered anaesthetic are absorbed systemically, cardiovascular and respiratory function may be compromised. In extreme cases, such as inadvertent injection of a drug into a major blood vessel, symptomatic and supportive cardiovascular or respiratory therapy may be required until the drug is metabolized and eliminated.

Interactions

Few clinically significant drug interactions occur with local anaesthetics. When given with enflurane, halothane, or epinephrine, these drugs can lead to dysrhythmias.

NEUROMUSCULAR BLOCKING DRUGS

Historically, snakes and plants have played a role in the identification of substances that cause paralysis and in the discovery of related receptor proteins in animals and humans. The beginning steps involved study of the irreversible nerve transmission inhibition in muscles caused by toxins in the venom of the kraits snake and certain varieties of cobra.

Curare, a general term for various South American arrow poisons, has a long and intriguing history. It has been used for centuries by natives of the Amazon River region and other parts of South America to kill wild animals for food. Animals shot with arrows soaked in this plant substance normally die from paralysis of the respiratory muscles. Once the receptor sites of action of venoms and toxins were identified, pharmacological

---

BOX 12-3

Chemical Groups of Local Anaesthetics

Ester Type	Amide Type
benzocaine	bupivacaine hydrochloride
chloroprocaine	dibucaine hydrochloride
procaine	lidocaine
proparacaine	mepivacaine hydrochloride
propoxycaine	prilocaine hydrochloride
tetracaine	

DRUG PROFILES

Besides lidocaine, profiled here, local anaesthetics include bupivacaine hydrochloride, mepivacaine hydrochloride, prilocaine hydrochloride, and tetracaine hydrochloride. There are two major types of local anaesthetics as determined by their chemical structure: amides and esters. These designations refer to the type of linkage between the aromatic ring and the amino group of the chemical structures of the drug molecules. These structural components give these drugs their anaesthetic properties.

lidocaine hydrochloride

Lidocaine belongs to the amide class of local anaesthetics. Some patients may report that they have allergic or anaphylactic reactions to the "caines," as they may refer to lidocaine and the other amide drugs. In these situations, it may be wise to try a local anaesthetic of the ester type.

Lidocaine hydrochloride (Xylocaine®) is one of the most commonly used local anaesthetics. It is available in several strengths, both alone and in different concentrations with epinephrine, and is used for both infiltration and nerve block anaesthesia. Lidocaine hydrochloride is also available in topical forms, including the unique product EMLA®. This is a cream mixture of lidocaine hydrochloride and prilocaine hydrochloride that is applied to skin to ease the pain of needle punctures (e.g., starting an intravenous line). Parenteral lidocaine is also used to treat certain cardiac dysrhythmias (see Chapter 26). Contraindications include known drug allergy. There are no adequate, well-controlled studies in pregnant women on the effect of lidocaine hydrochloride on the developing fetus.

PREVENTING MEDICATION ERRORS

Neuromuscular Blocking Drugs

Neuromuscular blocking drugs are considered high-alert drugs, because improper use may lead to severe injury or death. The Institute for Safe Medication Practices Canada has reported several cases of patient death or injury as a result of medication errors involving neuromuscular blocking drugs. Because these drugs paralyze the respiratory muscles, incorrect administration without sufficient ventilator support has resulted in patient deaths. There have been medication errors due to "sound-alike" drug names as well (e.g., vancomycin and vecuronium). Most facilities have followed recommendations to restrict access to these drugs, provide warning labels and reminders, and increase staff awareness of the dangers of these drugs.

drugs were developed that mimic these substances. Curare can be considered the grandfather of modern NMBDs. Several curarelike drugs are now used in clinical practice. The first drug derived from curare to be used medicinally was d-tubocurarine, which was introduced into anaesthesia practice in 1940; it has now been replaced by newer drugs such as pancuronium. Pancuronium has a pharmacodynamic profile similar to that of curare but produces fewer adverse effects.

Neuromuscular blocking drugs (NMBDs) prevent nerve transmission in skeletal and smooth muscles, leading to paralysis. They are often used as adjuncts with general anaesthetics for surgical procedures. Neuromuscular blocking drugs also paralyze the skeletal muscles required for breathing: the intercostal muscles and the diaphragm. The patient is rendered unable to breathe independently, and mechanical ventilation is required to prevent brain damage or death by suffocation. Deaths have been reported when an NMBD is accidentally mistaken for a different drug and given to a patient who is not mechanically ventilated. Most hospitals have taken extra precautions to keep NMBDs separated from other drugs, or at least marked with warning stickers. It is essential that the nurse ensure that the patient is ventilated before giving an NMBD and double-check that an

NMBD is not inadvertently given. In the event of an error, the patient would experience a horrendous death, because the mind would be alert but the patient would not be able to speak or move (see Preventing Medication Errors: Neuromuscular Blocking Drugs).

Mechanism of Action and Drugs Effects

NMBDs are classified into two groups based on mechanism of action: depolarizing and nondepolarizing. Depolarizing NMBDs work similarly to the neurotransmitter acetylcholine (ACh). They bind in place of ACh to cholinergic receptors at the motor endplates of muscle nerves or neuromuscular junctions. Thus, they are competitive agonists (see Chapter 2). There are two phases of depolarizing block. During phase I (depolarizing phase), the muscles fasciculate (twitch). Eventually, after continued depolarization has occurred, muscles are no longer responsive to the ACh released; thus, muscle tone cannot be maintained and muscles become paralyzed. This is phase II, or the desensitizing phase. Depolarizing NMBDs include d-tubocurarine and succinylcholine (see later in this chapter). The duration of action of succinylcholine after a single dose to facilitate intubation is only about 5 to 9 minutes because of the rapid breakdown of the drug by cholinesterase, the enzyme responsible for metabolizing succinylcholine. Nondepolarizing NMBDs also bind to ACh receptors at the neuromuscular junction, but instead of mimicking ACh, they block its actions. Therefore, these drugs are competitive antagonists (see Chapter 2) of ACh. Consequently, the nerve cell membrane is not depolarized, the muscle fibres are not stimulated, and skeletal muscle contraction does not occur. Nondepolarizing NMBDs include vecuronium and pancuronium and are typically classified into three groups based on their duration of action: short-acting, intermediate-acting, and long-acting drugs (Table 12-7).

The typical time course of NMBD-induced paralysis during a surgical procedure is as follows. The first sensation typically experienced is muscle weakness. This is usually followed by a total flaccid paralysis. Small, rapidly moving muscles such as those of the fingers and eyes are typically the first to be paralyzed. The next are those of the limbs, neck, and trunk. Finally, the intercostal muscles and the diaphragm are paralyzed. The patient can no longer breathe independently. It must be noted that NMBDs, when used alone, do *not* cause sedation or relieve pain or anxiety. Therefore, the patient needs to also receive appropriate medications to manage pain or anxiety. Neuromuscular blocking drugs temporarily inactivate the body's natural drive to control respirations. Recovery of muscular activity after discontinuation of anaesthesia usually occurs in the reverse order to the initiation of paralysis, and thus the diaphragm is ordinarily the first muscle to regain function.

Indications

The main therapeutic use of NMBDs is for maintaining skeletal muscle paralysis to facilitate controlled ventilation during surgical procedures. Shorter-acting NMBDs

are often used to facilitate intubation with an endotracheal tube. This is commonly done for a variety of diagnostic procedures such as laryngoscopy, bronchoscopy, and esophagoscopy. When used for this purpose, NMBDs are frequently combined with anxiolytics or anaesthetics. Additional nonsurgical applications include reduction of laryngeal or general muscle spasms, reduction of spasticity from tetanus and neurological diseases such as multiple sclerosis, and prevention of bone fractures during electroconvulsive therapy (see Chapter 17). These drugs are also used for the diagnosis of myasthenia gravis, a disease characterized by chronic muscular weakness.

Contraindications

Contraindications to NMBDs include known drug allergy and also may include previous history of malignant hyperthermia, penetrating eye injuries, and narrow-angle glaucoma.

Adverse Effects

The key to limiting adverse effects with most NMBDs is to use only enough of the drug to block the neuromuscular receptors. If too much is used, the risk is increased that other ganglionic receptors will be affected. Blockade of these other ganglionic receptors leads to most of the undesirable effects of NMBDs. The effects of ganglionic blockade in various areas of the body are listed in Table 12-8.

The muscle paralysis induced by depolarizing NMBDs (e.g., succinylcholine) is sometimes preceded by muscle spasms, which may damage muscles. These muscle spasms are termed *muscle fasciculations* and are most pronounced in the muscle groups of the hands, feet, and face. Injury to muscle cells may cause postoperative muscle pain and release potassium into the circulation, resulting in hyperkalemia, which is usually self-limiting and reversible. Small doses of nondepolarizing NMBDs are sometimes administered with succinylcholine to minimize these muscle fasciculations. In spite of these disadvantages, succinylcholine is still popular due to its rapid onset of action, its depth of neuromuscular blockade, and its short duration of action. For these reasons, it is often preferred to nondepolarizing NMBDs for rapid-sequence induction of anaesthesia (e.g., for emergency intubation).

TABLE 12-7

Classification of Neuromuscular Blocking Drugs

DRUG
Intermediate-Acting
atracurium besylate
cisatracurium besylate
rocuronium bromide (Zemeron®)

Long-Acting
pancuronium bromide

TABLE 12-8

Effects of Ganglionic Blockade by Neuromuscular Blocking Drugs

Site	Part of Nervous System Blocked	Physiological Effect
Arterioles	Sympathetic	Vasodilation and hypotension
Veins	Sympathetic	Dilation
Heart	Parasympathetic	Tachycardia
Gastrointestinal	Parasympathetic	Reduced tone and tract motility; constipation
Urinary bladder	Parasympathetic	Urinary retention

The effects on the cardiovascular system vary depending on the NMBD used and the individual patient. Increases and decreases in blood pressure and heart rate have been seen. Some NMBDs cause a release of histamine, which can result in bronchospasm, hypotension, and excessive bronchial and salivary secretion. The gastrointestinal tract is seldom affected by NMBDs. When it is affected, decreased tone and motility typically result, which can lead to constipation or even ileus. Use of succinylcholine has been associated with hyperkalemia; dysrhythmias; fasciculations; muscle pain; myoglobinuria; increased intraocular, intragastric, and intracranial pressure; and malignant hyperthermia.

Toxicity and Management of Overdose

The primary concern when NMBDs are overdosed is prolonged paralysis requiring prolonged mechanical ventilation (see the Preventing Medication Errors: Neuromuscular Blocking Drugs box on p. 237). Cardiovascular collapse may be seen and is thought to be the result of histamine release. Multiple medical conditions can predispose an individual to toxicity. These conditions increase the sensitivity of the individual to NMBDs and prolong their effects and are listed in Box 12-4. Some conditions make it more difficult for NMBDs to work, and therefore higher doses of NMBDs are required in these cases. Although these conditions do not necessarily lead to toxicity or overdose, they are worthy of mention and are listed in Box 12-5.

Anticholinesterase drugs such as neostigmine methylsulphate, pyridostigmine bromide, and edrophonium chloride are antidotes and are used to reverse muscle paralysis. They work by preventing the enzyme cholinesterase from breaking down ACh. This causes ACh to build up at the motor endplate, and it eventually displaces the nondepolarizing NMBD molecule, returning the nerve to its original state. Dysmetabolic syndrome, known as *malignant hyperthermia* (see General Anaesthetics earlier in the chapter) can also occur with NMBDs, especially succinylcholine.

Interactions

Many drugs can interact with NMBDs, which may lead to either synergistic or opposing effects. Aminoglycoside antibiotics, when given with an NMBD, can have additive effects. Tetracycline antibiotics can also produce neuromuscular blockade, possibly by chelation of calcium, and calcium channel blockers have also been shown to enhance neuromuscular blockade. Other notable drugs that interact with NMBDs are listed in Box 12-6.

Dosages

For dosage information of selected NMBDs, refer to the Dosages table on p. 241.

PHARMACOKINETIC BRIDGE TO NURSING PRACTICE

With procedural sedation or anaesthesia, it is always important to understand the pharmacokinetic properties of the drug(s) used. For example, the intravenous form of midazolam has an onset of action of 1 to 5 minutes, a peak plasma effect time of 20 to 60 minutes, an elimination half-life of 1 to 4 hours (time it takes for 50% of the drug to be excreted), and a duration of action of 2 to 6

BOX 12-4

Conditions That Predispose Patients to Toxic Effects From Neuromuscular Blocking Drugs

Acidosis	Myasthenia gravis
Amyotrophic lateral sclerosis	Myasthenic syndrome
Hypermagnesemia	Neonatal status
Hypocalcemia	Neurofibromatosis
Hypokalemia	Paraplegia
Hypothermia	Poliomyelitis

BOX 12-5

Conditions That Oppose the Effects of Neuromuscular Blocking Drugs

Cirrhosis with ascites	Hyperkalemia
Clostridial infections	Peripheral nerve transection
Hemiplegia	Peripheral neuropathies
Hypercalcemia	Thermal burns

BOX 12-6

Drugs That Interact With Neuromuscular Blocking Drugs

Additive Effects	Opposing Effects
Aminoglycosides	carbamazepine
Calcium channel blockers	Corticosteroids
clindamycin	phenytoin
cyclophosphamide	
cyclosporine	
dantrolene	
furosemide	
Inhalation anaesthetics	
Local anaesthetics	
magnesium	
quinidine	

DRUG PROFILES

Neuromuscular blocking drugs are one of the most commonly used classes of drugs in the operating room. They are given primarily with general anaesthetics to facilitate endotracheal intubation and to relax skeletal muscles during surgery. In addition to their use in the operating room, they are given in the CCU to paralyze mechanically ventilated patients. There are two basic types of NMBDs: depolarizing and nondepolarizing drugs. Nondepolarizing drugs are generally classified by their duration of action. Table 12-8 lists examples of currently used nondepolarizing drugs.

DEPOLARIZING NEUROMUSCULAR BLOCKING DRUGS

succinylcholine

Succinylcholine (Quelicin®) is the only currently available drug in the depolarizing subclass of NMBDs. Succinylcholine has a structure similar to that of the parasympathetic neurotransmitter ACh. It stimulates the same neurons as ACh and produces the same physiological responses initially. Compared to ACh, however, succinylcholine is metabolized more slowly. Because of this slower metabolism, succinylcholine subjects the motor endplate to ongoing depolarizing stimulation. Repolarization cannot occur. As long as sufficient succinylcholine concentrations are present, the muscle loses its ability to contract, and flaccid muscle paralysis results. Because of its quick onset of action, succinylcholine is most commonly used to facilitate endotracheal intubation. It is seldom used over long periods because of its tendency to cause muscular fasciculations. It is contraindicated in patients with personal or familial history of malignant hyperthermia, skeletal muscle myopathies, and known hypersensitivity to the drug. For dosage information, refer to the Dosages table on p. 241.

PHARMACOKINETICS

Route	Onset of Action	Peak Plasma Concentration	Elimination Half-Life	Duration of Action
IV	Rapid, less than 1 min	Rapid	Less than 1 min	4–6 min

NONDEPOLARIZING NEUROMUSCULAR BLOCKING DRUGS

Nondepolarizing NMBDs are commonly used to facilitate endotracheal intubation, reduce muscle contraction, and facilitate a variety of diagnostic procedures. They are often combined with anxiolytics or anaesthetics. They may also be used to induce respiratory arrest in patients on mechanical ventilation. Nondepolarizing NMBDs are typically classified into three groups based on their duration of action: short-, intermediate-, and long-acting drugs (see Table 12-7).

pancuronium bromide

Pancuronium bromide is a long-acting nondepolarizing NMBD. It is used as an adjunct to general anaesthesia to facilitate endotracheal intubation and to provide skeletal muscle relaxation during surgery or mechanical ventilation. It is most commonly employed for long surgical procedures that require prolonged muscle paralysis. Use of pancuronium is contraindicated in cases of known drug allergy. It is available only in injectable form. For dosage information, refer to the Dosages table on p. 241.

PHARMACOKINETICS

Route	Onset of Action	Peak Plasma Concentration	Elimination Half-Life	Duration of Action
IV	3–5 min	5 min	100 min	45–60 min

vecuronium bromide

Vecuronium bromide is an intermediate-acting nondepolarizing NMBD. It is used as an adjunct to general anaesthesia to facilitate tracheal intubation and to provide skeletal muscle relaxation during surgery or mechanical ventilation, and it is one of the most commonly used NMBDs. Long-term use in the CCU setting has resulted in prolonged paralysis and subsequent difficulty weaning from mechanical ventilation. This is believed to be due to an active metabolite, 3-desacetyl vecuronium, which tends to accumulate with prolonged use. Use of vecuronium bromide is contraindicated in cases of known drug allergy. For dosage information, refer to the Dosages table on p. 241.

PHARMACOKINETICS

Route	Onset of Action	Peak Plasma Concentration	Elimination Half-Life	Duration of Action
IV	2.5–3 min	3–5 min	65–76 min	25–40 min

hours. Therefore, if midazepam is used for procedural sedation, you will begin to see the sedating properties within 1 to 5 minutes and peak effects on the patient between 20 and 60 minutes. Since the drug's action lasts for only 2 to 6 hours, midazolam is an attractive option for use in outpatient procedures because of fast onset and short duration of action. Therefore, as noted with this drug's pharmacokinetic properties, you may then be able to predict the drug's onset of action, peak effect, and duration of action.

NURSING PROCESS

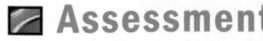

Assessment

It is important to note that anaesthetics are not typically given by the registered nurse unless the nurse is a licensed nurse anaesthetist. Exceptions to this statement are orders for topical forms, such as oral swish-and-

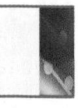

DOSAGES   Selected Neuromuscular Blocking Drugs

Drug	Pharmacological Class	Usual Dosage Range	Indications
pancuronium bromide	Nondepolarizing NMBD (long acting)	*Adults, children older than 1 month* IV: 0.046–0.1 mg/kg Neonates up to 1 month Because neonates are especially sensitive to nondepolarizing NMBDs, give a test dose of 0.02 mg/kg IV Adults IV: 0.04–0.1 mg Continuous infusion: 0.1 mg/kg/hr *Children* IV: 0.6 mg/kg *Adults* IV: 0.6–1.2 mg/kg Continuous infusion: 0.01–0.012 mg/kg/min; 0.1 mg/kg/hr *Children* IV: 1–2 mg/kg	Intubation Adjunct to balanced anaesthesia
▶▶succinylcholine chloride (Quelicin Chloride Injection®)	Depolarizing NMBD (short acting)	IM: 32.5–4 mg/kg *Adults* IV: 0.3–1.1 mg/kg over 10–30 sec IM: 2.5–4 mg/kg *Children* IV: 0.08–0.1 mg/kg	Intubation Mechanical ventilation
▶▶vecuronium bromide (Norcuron®)	Nondepolarizing NMBD (intermediate acting)	*Adults* IV: 0.08–0.1 mg/kg Continuous infusion: 0.16–1.8 mcg/kg/hr	Intubation Mechanical ventilation

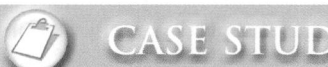

CASE STUDY

Procedural Sedation

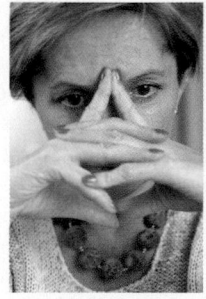

Helen is a 53-year-old woman who is scheduled to have a colonoscopy this morning, and she is extremely anxious. The anaesthesiologist has explained the procedural sedation that is planned, but the patient says after the anaesthesiologist leaves the room, "I'm so afraid of feeling it during the test. Why don't they just put me to sleep?"

1. How does procedural sedation differ from general anaesthesia?
2. What is the nurse's best answer to Helen's question?
3. What is important for the nurse to assess before this procedure is performed?
4. Explain the purpose of these two medications during procedural sedation. How are the dosages adjusted when these are given together?

For answers see http://evolve.elsevier.com/Canada/Lilley/pharmacology/.

swallow solutions that may be used during chemotherapy and lidocaine patches for pain relief. Associated with each drug used for general and local anaesthesia are some broad as well as specific assessment parameters. First, for any form of anaesthesia, and during any of the phases of anaesthesia, the major parameters to assess are airway, breathing, and circulation (ABCs). Include in your assessment questions regarding allergies and use of prescription as well as over-the-counter drugs, natural health products (NHPs), and social and illegal drugs.

Another important area to consider is the use of alcohol and nicotine. Excessive use of alcohol may alter the patient's response to general anaesthesia, especially if there is liver impairment. Also, if the patient has a history of alcohol misuse, withdrawal symptoms may occur during the recovery from anaesthesia or surgery. Perform a respiratory assessment (e.g., respiratory rate, rhythm, and depth; breath sounds; oxygen saturation level), especially if the patient has a history of smoking or is currently a smoker. The patient's history of smoking is important because nicotine has a paralyzing effect on the cilia within the respiratory system. Once they are malfunctioning, these cilia cannot perform their main function of keeping foreign bodies out of the lungs and allowing mucus and secretions to be coughed up with ease. Malfunctioning of the cilia can potentially lead to atelectasis or pneumonia.

Other objective data to be collected include weight and height because these parameters are often used in determining the dosing of anaesthesia. Other studies that may be ordered by the anaesthesiologist or surgeon include an electrocardiogram, a chest radiograph, and tests of kidney function (e.g., BUN level, creatinine level, urinalysis with specific gravity) and liver function (e.g., total protein and albumin levels; bilirubin level; ALP, AST, ALT levels). Additional laboratory tests may include Hgb, Hct, WBC with differential, and tests that indicate clotting abilities, such as PT-INR, aPTT, and platelet count. Also assess results of tests for serum electrolytes, specifically potassium, sodium, chloride, phosphorus, magnesium, and calcium because abnormalities may lead to further complications from the anaesthesia. You must assess the results of a pregnancy test in females of childbearing age, if ordered, because of the possibility of teratogenic effects (adverse effects on the fetus) related to the anaesthetic drug.

Neurological assessment is extremely important and includes performing and documenting thorough a baseline survey. Determine and document level of consciousness, alertness, and orientation to person, place, and time prior to the anaesthesia. Additional neurological assessment includes motor assessments, with left–right and upper extremity versus lower extremity comparisons of strength, reflexes, grasp, and ability to move on command. Sensory assessment focuses on the same anatomical areas, with comparisons of the response to various types of stimuli such as sharp, dull, soft, and cold versus warm. Swallowing ability and gag reflex are also important to assess and document for baseline status and comparisons. When these motor, sensory, and cognitive parameters are within normal limits, there is proof of an intact neurological system.

One significant reaction to assess for in patients receiving general anaesthesia is that of malignant hyperthermia. This is a rapid progression of hyperthermia that may be fatal if not promptly recognized and aggressively treated. The tendency is inherited, so questions about related signs and symptoms in the patient's and family's medical histories are important to document and report. A familial history of malignant hyperthermia would put the patient at risk. Signs and symptoms of malignant hyperthermia include a rapid rise in body temperature, tachycardia, tachypnea, muscle rigidity, cyanosis, irregular heartbeat, mottling of the skin, diaphoresis (profuse sweating), and an unstable blood pressure. If there is no documented problem with general anaesthesia or if the patient is undergoing general anaesthesia for the first time, perform an astute and careful examination of all medical and medication histories. With any type of

anaesthesia, it is often slight changes in vital signs, other vital parameters, and laboratory test results that may provide nurses and other health care providers with a possible clue to the patient's reaction to anaesthesia. Note that malignant hyperthermia occurs during the anaesthesia process and in the surgical suite; nevertheless, close observation after anaesthesia is still important and much needed. Intravenously administered anaesthetic drugs are usually combined with adjunct drugs (given at the same time) such as sedative–hypnotics, antianxiety drugs, opioid and nonopioid analgesics, antiemetics, and anticholinergics. These drugs are used to decrease some of the undesirable aftereffects of inhaled anaesthetics. If they are used, perform a complete assessment for each of the drugs, including obtaining a medical history and medication profile. Liver and kidney function studies are important in these patients as well, so that any risks of toxicity and complications can be anticipated.

For patients about to undergo anaesthesia with neuromuscular blocking drugs (NMBDs), perform a complete head-to-toe assessment with a thorough medical and medication history. Which specific drug is being used and whether it is depolarizing or nondepolarizing will guide your assessment because of the action of NMBDs on the patient's neuromuscular functioning (see previous discussion in this chapter). Assess all cautions, contraindications, and drug interactions. Another concern with the use of these drugs is that they are associated with an increase in intraocular pressure and intracranial pressure. Therefore, these anaesthetic drugs should not be used, or should be used with extreme caution (close monitoring of these pressures), in patients with glaucoma or closed head injuries.

Paralysis of respiratory muscles allows patient relaxation to the point where the patient will not fight against the breaths delivered by the ventilator. Complete a thorough respiratory assessment in patients receiving NMBDs because of the effect of these drugs on the respiratory system. In particular, these drugs have a paralyzing effect on the muscles used for breathing and—for this reason—are used to facilitate intubation for mechanical ventilation. Also indicated with the use of NMBDs is careful assessment of serum electrolyte levels, specifically potassium and magnesium levels. Imbalances in these electrolytes may lead to increased action of the NMBD with exacerbation of the drug's actions and toxic effects. Allergic reactions to these drugs are most commonly characterized by rash, fever, respiratory distress, and pruritus. Drug interactions with natural health products are outlined in the Natural Health Products box below. For more specific information on the differences between depolarizing and nondepolarizing NMBDs, see the pharmacology section of this chapter.

With the use of procedural sedation, as with any anaesthesia technique, assessment for allergies, cautions, contraindications, and drug interactions is important.

NATURAL HEALTH PRODUCTS

Potential Effects of Popular Natural Health Products When Combined With Anaesthetics

Feverfew: Migraine headaches, insomnia, anxiety, joint stiffness, risk of increased bleeding times with increased risk of bleeding

Garlic: Changes in blood pressure, risk of increased bleeding

Ginger: Sedating effects; risk of bleeding, especially if taken with either aspirin or ginkgo biloba

Ginseng: Irritability and insomnia, risk of cardiac adverse effects

Kava: Sedating effects, potential liver toxicity, risk of additive effects with medications

St. John's wort: Sedation, blood pressure changes, risk of interaction with other medications that prolong the effects of anaesthesia

---

Because procedural sedation is commonly used across the lifespan, closely assess organ function and note diseases or conditions that could lead to excessive levels of the drug in the body, such as liver or kidney impairment. See Chapters 11 and 13 for more information about the assessment associated with the use of opioids and sedative–hypnotics/CNS depressants.

Use of spinal anaesthesia requires thorough assessment with an emphasis on the ABCs, respiratory function, and vital signs, specifically blood pressure. Baseline respirations with attention to rate, rhythm, depth, and breath sounds are important to note, as are oxygen saturation levels obtained via pulse oximetry. Because of possible problems with vasodilatation from the spinal anaesthetic, document baseline blood pressure levels and pulse rate. Assess platelet count as a hematoma may be an adverse effect, especially for patients with thrombocytopenia. Record history of previous reactions to this form of anaesthesia, allergies, and a listing of all medications, and report any abnormal reactions to the anaesthesiologist and surgeon. Neurological assessment with notation of sensory and motor intactness in the lower extremities, as well as documentation of any abnormalities, is important. The use of epidural anaesthesia requires special attention to overall hemostasis through monitoring of vital signs and oxygen saturation levels. Assess baseline sensory and motor function in the extremities, and document an intact neurological system (see Implementation for more detailed discussion). Spinal headaches may occur with either spinal anaesthesia or epidural injections, and thus baseline assessment for the presence of headaches is important. Many institutions have care-flow assessment monitoring sheets specifically for assessing the patient with an epidural.

Topical local anaesthetics such as lidocaine, used for either infiltration or nerve block anaesthesia, may be administered with or without a vasoconstrictor (e.g., epinephrine). Vasoconstrictors are used to help confine the local anaesthetic to the injected area, prevent systemic absorption of the anaesthetic, and reduce bleeding. If there is systemic absorption of the vasoconstrictor into the bloodstream, the patient's blood pressure could elevate to life-threatening levels, especially in patients who are at high risk (e.g., those with underlying arterial

disease). Therefore, review the patient's medical history to assess for any pre-existing illnesses, such as vascular disease, aneurysms, or hypertension because these may be contraindications to the use of the vasoconstrictor with the anaesthetic. In addition, with these local anaesthetics, assess for allergies to the drug as well as baseline vital signs. Also assess for possible drug interactions, and note prescription medications, natural health products, and over-the-counter medications. In summary, with any type of anaesthesia, it is important to assess the patient's level of homeostasis prior to actual administration of the drug. This assessment may include taking vital signs as well as checking the ABCs. Other parameters of interest may be oxygen saturation levels measured by pulse oximetry, cardiovascular and respiratory function, and neurological function.

Nursing Diagnoses

1. Impaired gas exchange related to the general anaesthetic's CNS-depressant effects with altered respiratory rate and effort (decreased rate, decreased depth)
2. Decreased cardiac output related to systemic effects of anaesthesia
3. Acute pain related to the adverse effect of spinal headache from epidural anaesthesia
4. Deficient knowledge related to lack of information about anaesthesia
5. Risk for injury related to the impact of any form of anaesthesia on the CNS (e.g., CNS depression and decreased sensorium)

Planning

Goals

- Patient will state the adverse effects of general or local anaesthesia, including decreased sensorium.
- Patient will state potential complications of anaesthesia involving the cardiac system.
- Patient will experience minimal to no respiratory complications related to anaesthesia.
- Patient will adhere to postanaesthesia care to help decrease the chance of complications.

- Patient will follow instructions regarding his or her care during the postoperative period.
- Patient will communicate (as needed) anxiety regarding preanaesthesia and postanaesthesia care.
- Patient will communicate anxiety, fears, and concerns regarding anaesthesia.
- Patient will understand the purpose, adverse effects, and complications of anaesthesia.

■ Expected Patient Outcomes

1. Patient states measures to increase respiratory expansion, through coughing, deep breathing, turning, and ambulating (when allowed).
2. Patient remains well hydrated, with increase in fluids and remains ambulating to help increase circulation and minimize complications, unless contraindicated.
3. Patient states measures to help minimize or prevent acute pain from possible complication of spinal headache, with bedrest, hydration, and following postanaesthesia and postepidural orders for up to 24 to 48 hours after procedure.
4. Patient experiences maximal effects of anaesthesia as noted by following preanaesthesia orders, such as remaining NPO (nothing by mouth) and taking medications only as prescribed, and also experiences minimal adverse effects due to adequate knowledge about the postanaesthesia period and ways to minimize problems (see all measures listed in Expected Patient Outcomes 1 to 3 and 5).
5. Patient remains free of injury or falls by asking for assistance while ambulating or having assistance if at home and recovering, as well as by taking medications only as prescribed, sitting up for brief periods prior to ambulating, staying well hydrated, and resuming adequate nutritional intake during the postanaesthesia period.

■ Implementation

Regardless of the type of anaesthesia used, one of the most important nursing considerations during the preanaesthesia, intra-anaesthesia, and postanaesthesia periods is close and frequent observation of all body systems. Begin with a focus on the ABCs of nursing care, vital signs, and oxygen saturation levels measured by pulse oximetry as well as by the clinical presentation of the patient. Remember that the way a patient looks is very important at any point in time! Document the observations from these interventions, and repeat the interventions as needed, depending on the patient's status and in keeping with the standard of care for the type of anaesthesia. Monitor vital signs frequently and as needed, and based on the patient's condition, including assessing the fifth vital sign of pain (see discussion later in this section and in Chapter 11).

For patients undergoing general anaesthesia, assessing the patient's temperature is especially important because of the risk of malignant hyperthermia, and close monitoring is required if malignant hyperthermia occurred during the anaesthesia process. A sudden elevation in the patient's body temperature (e.g., higher than 40°C) not only requires critical care during and immediately after anaesthesia but also calls for close monitoring even during regular postoperative care (see earlier discussion).

When intravenous, inhaled, or other forms of anaesthesia are used, resuscitative equipment and medications, including opioid antidotes, should be readily available in the surgical and postsurgical areas in case of cardiorespiratory distress or arrest. The anaesthesiologist keeps control of the anaesthetic drug and is well prepared for any emergency—as is the entire group of individuals in the surgical suite and postanaesthesia recovery area. Continual monitoring of the status of breath sounds is an important intervention because hypoventilation may be a complication of general and other forms of anaesthesia. Oxygen is administered after a patient has received general or other forms of anaesthesia to compensate for the respiratory depression that may have occurred during the anaesthesia and surgical process. Because oxygen is a drug, a doctor's order is needed for its administration.

Continuous monitoring of oxygen saturation levels is therefore an important intervention. In addition, hypotension and orthostatic hypotension are possible problems after anaesthesia, so postural blood pressure measurements (supine and standing), in addition to regular blood pressure monitoring, may be needed. Additional nursing interventions include monitoring of neurological parameters such as reflexes, response to commands, level of consciousness or sedation, and pupil reaction to light. Monitor for changes in sensation and movement in the extremities, distal pulses, temperature, and colour when nerve blocks and spinal anaesthesia are used because it is important to confirm that areas distal to the anaesthetic site have remained intact.

Should the patient require pain management once the anaesthesia has been terminated, remember that the anaesthetic and any adjunct drugs used continue to have an effect on the patient until the period of the drugs' action has passed. Therefore, administer sedative–hypnotics, opioids, nonopioids, and other CNS depressants for pain relief cautiously and *only* with close monitoring of vital signs. If the patient has received some of these medications during postanaesthesia, document dosages of drugs used, and then pass them on during a report when the patient is transferred to another unit. Additional orders are usually provided by the physician, surgeon, or anaesthesiologist regarding doses of analgesics to administer once the patient has been transferred or discharged to home. If such orders have not been provided, however, and the patient is experiencing pain, contact the appropriate prescriber. The concern here is that the patient may receive either too much or not enough analgesic.

Patients who receive NMBDs as part of an induction process for mechanical ventilation need to be monitored closely during and after initiation of mechanical ventilation. Patients receiving NMBDs and who are awake may need to receive other medications for sedation or pain. These patients are in CCUs, and many protocols are provided regarding interventions after the intubation. These protocols include measurement of vital signs and determination of neurological status, including sensation and hand grasp strength. When mechanical ventilation is used, educate patients and family members about the purpose of the drug-induced paralysis during mechanical ventilation (e.g., to prevent the patient from fighting against the ventilation provided by the machine or resisting the effects of the mechanical ventilatory assistance, which could lead to hypoventilation). Inform the family, and remember that, during the care of these patients, they can still hear the spoken word. Knowing what to expect is key to helping decrease fears and anxiety—for both the patient and those visiting the patient.

Patients undergoing procedural sedation as the method of anaesthesia should receive patient education before the procedure. As noted earlier in the chapter, recovery from this type of anaesthesia is more rapid, and the safety profile is better, than with general anaesthesia, with its inherent cardiorespiratory risks. As with general anaesthesia, however, monitor the ABCs of care, vital signs, pulse oximetry oxygen saturation levels, and level of consciousness or sedation. See Box 12-7 for more information on procedural sedation.

With spinal anaesthesia, nursing interventions need to include constant monitoring for a return of sensation and motor activity below the anaesthetic insertion site. Because of the risk that the anaesthetic drug may move upward in the spinal cord and breathing may be affected, continually monitor respiratory and breathing status. Remember, though, that this complication is usually iden-

---

BOX 12-7   Procedural Sedation: What to Expect and Questions to Ask

1. What questions should the patient or caregiver ask about the technique of procedural sedation?
- Who will be providing this type of anaesthesia?
- Who will be monitoring me or my loved one?
- Will there be constant monitoring of blood pressure, pulse rate, respiratory rate, and temperature?
- Will there be emergency equipment in the room, in case of need?
- Are the personnel qualified to administer these drugs? To administer advanced cardiac life support, if needed?
- What do I need to know about care at home? Will I need help? Can I drive after having the procedure?

2. What are the adverse effects of procedural sedation?
- Brief periods of amnesia (loss of memory)
- Headache
- Hangover
- Nausea and vomiting

3. What should be expected immediately following the procedure?
- Frequent monitoring
- Written postoperative instructions and care
- If the patient is of driving age, no driving for at least 24 hours after undergoing procedural sedation
- A follow-up contact by phone to check on the patient

4. Who can administer the procedural sedation?
- Procedural sedation is safe when administered by qualified health care providers. Certified registered nurse anaesthetists, anaesthesiologists, other physicians, dentists, and oral surgeons are qualified to administer procedural sedation.

5. Which procedures generally require procedural sedation?
- Breast biopsy
- Vasectomy
- Minor foot surgery
- Minor bone fracture repair
- Plastic or reconstructive surgery
- Dental prosthetic or reconstructive surgery
- Endoscopy (such as diagnostic studies and treatment of stomach, colon, and bladder cancer)

6. What are the overall benefits of this type of anaesthesia?
- It is a safe and effective option for patients undergoing minor surgeries or diagnostic procedures.
- It allows patients to recover quickly and resume normal activities in a relatively short period of time.

7. Are there any concerns about daily medications or natural health products for patients undergoing procedural sedation?
- As with any form of anaesthesia, it is important for patient safety that the patient be open and honest with the anaesthesiologist or other attending professional about all medications and natural health products taken.
- Be sure to follow instructions closely in regard to the intake of all medications including natural health products, food, or liquids before anaesthesia, as such substances may react negatively with the drugs being administered.
- Inquire about any brochures or written pamphlets that provide further information on medications, including natural health products, and procedural sedation.

tified and treated by the anaesthesiologist, and patients will not return to their rooms on a nursing unit until all respiratory risks are identified and managed appropriately. Another major area of concern with spinal anaesthesia is the risk for a sudden decrease in blood pressure. This drop in blood pressure is secondary to vasodilation caused by the anaesthetic block to the sympathetic vasomotor nerves. Vital signs and oxygen saturation levels should return to normal before the patient is transferred out of postanaesthesia care; however, continue to monitor these vital signs frequently after transfer.

Another adverse reaction to intraspinal anaesthesia is the occurrence of spinal headaches. These may occur with both intrathecal and epidural injections but are actually more frequent with the latter. Because intrathecal spinal needle designs have been technologically improved, the occurrence of spinal headaches has become rare. Larger-bore needles are used to deliver epidural anaesthetics, however, and these are more likely to give rise to spinal headache.

A spinal headache can occur as a result of penetration into and through the dura mater of the spinal cord (the covering that encloses the spinal cord and cerebrospinal fluid); a leakage of cerebrospinal fluid occurs from the insertion site. Because this is a pressurized system that extends from the intracranial cavity down to the sacrum, any fluctuation in pressure can result in headache. If enough spinal fluid leaks out, a spinal headache results. Patients say that these headaches are worse than any other type! They are more severe when the patient is in an upright position and improve upon lying down. They may occur up to five days after the procedure and may be prevented with bedrest after the epidural procedure. Adequate hydration using intravenous fluids is often tried, to help increase cerebrospinal fluid pressure. Other recommendations include drinking beverages that are high in caffeine and strict bedrest for 24 to 48 hours. If the headaches are intolerable, however, the anaesthesiologist may create a blood patch to help close up or seal the leak. This procedure requires insertion of a needle into the same space or right next to the area that was injected with the anaesthesia. A small amount of blood is then taken from the patient and injected into the epidural space. The blood clots and forms a seal over the hole that caused the leak, and the headache is relieved.

The use of epidural anaesthesia (also called *regional anaesthesia* in some textbooks) does not pose the same risk of respiratory complications as general anaesthesia; however, monitoring is still needed to confirm overall homeostasis. You must measure vital signs and pulse oximetry to determine oxygen saturation levels. In addition, patients undergoing this form of anaesthesia require monitoring for the return of motor function and tactile sensation. Check the patient frequently for the return of sensation bilaterally along the dermatome (area of the skin innervated by a specific segment of the spinal cord); such monitoring is important to ensure patient safety as well as to maximize comfort. Assess touch sensation through hand pressure or a gentle pinch of the skin. You need to know the level at which the epidural anaesthesia was given to monitor properly for return of sensation. This monitoring process generally occurs in a postanaesthesia care unit, and the patient is not returned to a regular nursing unit until all sensation or voluntary movement of the lower extremities is regained.

Solutions of topical or local anaesthetics (e.g., lidocaine with or without epinephrine) that are not clear and appear cloudy or discoloured are not to be used. Some anaesthesiologists mix the solution with sodium bicarbonate to minimize local pain during infiltration, but this also causes a more rapid onset of action and a longer duration of sensory analgesia. If an anaesthetic ointment or cream is used, the nurse thoroughly cleanses and dries the area to be anaesthetized before applying the drug. If a topical or local anaesthetic is being used in the nose or throat, remember that it may cause paralysis or numbness of the structures of the upper respiratory tract, which can lead to aspiration. If the patient receives a solution form of anaesthetic, exact amounts of the drug are used, at exact dosing times or intervals. Local anaesthetics are not to be swallowed unless the physician has so instructed. Should this occur, closely observe the patient, check for the gag reflex, and expect to withhold food or drink until the patient's sensation and gag reflex have returned.

Once the patient has recovered from the anaesthesia and procedure and is ready for discharge, complete your patient teaching. Focus the patient education on the patient's needs and how these needs can be met at home. Home health care or rehabilitation services may be indicated, and arrangements should be made before the patient is discharged. If additional resources are needed at home (e.g., for a patient who lives alone), these arrangements should be completed in a timely fashion. Some examples of procedures for which help might be needed are wound care, dressing changes, surgical site care, drawing of blood for laboratory studies, and administration of various medications through the intravenous, intramuscular, or subcutaneous route. Some patients may also need assistance with taking oral medications at home. Pain management requires thorough and individualized patient teaching and also includes any necessary education for patients who will require home health care. Refer to Chapter 11 for more information on analgesics.

Provide simple instructions, using age-appropriate teaching strategies. Sharing of information about community resources is also important, especially for patients who need transportation, assistance with meals, housekeeping during recovery, or the services of additional health care providers (e.g., physiotherapists, occupational therapists) in the home setting. Some of these community resources may include agencies supported by municipal, provincial, or territorial social service programs; Meals on Wheels; older adult support groups; and church-sponsored groups, to name just a few. Many of these resources are free or have income-based fees.

Additional suggestions regarding patient education are provided in the Patient Teaching Tips.

Evaluation

The therapeutic effects of any general or local anaesthetic include loss of consciousness (during general anaesthesia) or loss of sensation to a particular area (during local anaesthesia—e.g., loss of sensation to the eye during corneal transplantation). Constantly monitor patients who have undergone general anaesthesia for the occurrence of adverse effects of the anaesthesia. These may include myocardial depression, convulsions, respiratory depression, allergic rhinitis, and decreased kidney or liver function. Constantly monitor patients who have received a local anaesthetic for the occurrence of adverse effects, including bradycardia, myocardial depression, hypotension, and dysrhythmias. In addi-

tion, as mentioned earlier in the chapter, significant overdoses of local anaesthetic drugs or direct injection into a blood vessel may result in cardiovascular collapse or cardiac or respiratory depression. For those receiving spinal anaesthesia, therapeutic effects include loss of sensation below the area of administration, while adverse effects include hypotension, hypoventilation, urinary retention, the possibility of a prolonged period of decreased sensation or motor ability, and infection at the site. With epidural anaesthesia, therapeutic effects are similar to those seen with intrathecal anaesthesia; however, adverse effects include possible spinal headache (often severe) or loss of motor function or sensation below the area of administration. Procedural sedation provides the therapeutic effect of a decreased sensorium but without the complications of general anaesthesia; however, there are CNS depressant effects associated with the drugs used.

PATIENT TEACHING TIPS

❖ Whenever general anaesthesia is used, emphasize the prescriber's recommendations and orders about whether any medications should be discontinued or tapered before anaesthetic administration.

❖ Make sure information about the anaesthetic, route of administration, adverse effects, and special precautions is included in preprocedure and surgical education.

❖ Openly discuss with the patient all fears and anxieties about anaesthesia and related procedures or surgery.

❖ Share with the patient and family instructions about the postanaesthesia process and the need for close monitoring of vital signs, breath sounds, and neurological intactness. Patients should expect frequent turning, coughing, and deep breathing to prevent atelectasis or pneumonia.

❖ Encourage patients to ambulate with assistance as needed and as ordered. Mobility helps increase circulation and improve ventilation to the alveoli of the lungs; consequently, circulation to the legs will be improved (which helps prevent stasis of blood and possible blood clot formation in the leg veins). Assistance is needed to prevent falls or injury until recovery from the anaesthetic.

❖ Encourage the patient to request pain medication, if needed, before pain becomes moderate to severe. Inform the patient that, even though anaesthesia has been administered, there may still be discomfort or

pain from the procedure or surgery. The anaesthesia will wear off, and adequate analgesia will be needed. Ask the patient to rate the pain on a scale of 0 to 10, with 0 being no pain and 10 being the worst possible pain. See Chapter 11 for more information on pain assessment and its management.

❖ Explain the rationale for any other treatments or procedures related to the anaesthesia (e.g., epidural catheter placement; delivery of oxygen; administration of a gas; use of various tubes, catheters, or intravenous lines). Adequate patient education will help ease fears and anxieties and help prevent adverse effects or complications.

❖ For a patient with diminished sensorium, the bed side rails should be up and a call button should be available at the bedside. These precautions are crucial to patient safety. Note that bed alarms may be used instead of side rails. Everyone involved in the postanaesthesia and postsurgical care (e.g., family members) should be educated about these safety measures.

❖ With local anaesthesia, the patient should understand the purpose and action of the local anaesthetic, as well as adverse effects.

❖ Inform a patient receiving spinal anaesthesia about the need for frequent assessments, measurement of vital signs, and system assessments during and after the procedure.

KEY POINTS

❖ Anaesthesia is the loss of the ability to feel pain resulting from the administration of an anaesthetic drug. General anaesthesia is a drug-induced state in which the nerve impulses of the CNS are altered to reduce pain and other sensations throughout the

entire body and normally involves complete loss of consciousness and depression of respiratory drive.

❖ General anaesthetics are drugs that induce general anaesthesia, including the administration of specific parenteral anaesthetics. Inhalational anaesthetic drugs

Continued

KEY POINTS—cont'd

are also general anaesthetics and include volatile liquids or gases.

❖ Local anaesthetics are used to induce a state in which peripheral or spinal nerve impulses are altered to reduce or eliminate pain and other sensations. Spinal anaesthesia, or regional anaesthesia, is a form of local anaesthesia.

❖ Procedural sedation is a form of general anaesthesia resulting in partial or complete loss of consciousness but without reducing normal respiratory drive.

❖ Adjunct anaesthetics are drugs that assist with the induction of general anaesthesia and include neuromuscular blocking drugs (NMBDs), sedative–hypnotics or anxiolytics, and antiemetics.

❖ Nondepolarizing NMBDs are used as an adjunct to general anaesthesia to provide skeletal muscle relaxation during surgery or mechanical ventilation.

❖ Nursing assessment is important to patient safety during and after all forms of anaesthesia. With general anaesthesia, however, one major problem is malignant hyperthermia, which may be fatal if not promptly recognized and aggressively treated. Signs and symptoms include rapid rise in body temperature, increased pulse rate (tachycardia), increased respiratory rate (tachypnea), muscle rigidity, and unstable blood pressure.

EXAMINATION REVIEW QUESTIONS

1. The prescriber has requested "lidocaine *with* epinephrine." The nurse recognizes that the most accurate rationale for adding epinephrine is that it:
   a. Helps calm the patient before the procedure
   b. Minimizes the risk of an allergic reaction
   c. Enhances the effect of the local lidocaine
   d. Reduces bleeding in the surgical area

2. The surgical nurse is reviewing operative cases scheduled for the day. Which of these patients is more prone to complications from general anaesthesia?
   a. A 79-year-old woman who is about to have her gallbladder removed
   b. A 49-year-old male athlete who quit heavy smoking 12 years ago
   c. A 30-year-old woman who is in perfect health but has never had anaesthesia
   d. A 50-year-old woman scheduled for outpatient laser surgery for vision correction

3. Which nursing diagnosis is possible for a patient who is now recovering after having been under general anaesthesia for 3 to 4 hours during surgery?
   a. Impaired urinary elimination related to the use of vasopressors as anaesthetics
   b. Increased cardiac output related to the effects of general anaesthesia
   c. Risk for falls related to decreased sensorium for 2 to 4 days postoperatively
   d. Impaired gas exchange due to the CNS depressant effect of general anaesthesia

4. A patient is recovering from general anaesthesia. What is the nurse's main concern during the immediate postoperative period?
   a. Airway
   b. Pupillary reflexes
   c. Return of sensations
   d. Level of consciousness

5. A patient is about to undergo cardioversion, and the nurse is reviewing the procedure and explaining procedural sedation. The patient says, "I am afraid of feeling it when they shock me." What is the nurse's best response?
   a. "You won't receive enough of a shock to feel anything."
   b. "You will feel the shock but you won't remember any of the pain."
   c. "The medications you receive will reduce any pain and help you not to remember the procedure."
   d. "They will give you enough pain medication to prevent you from feeling it."

6. The nurse is administering an NMBD to a patient during a surgical procedure. Number the following phases of muscle paralysis in the order in which the patient will experience them. (Number 1 is the first step.)
   a. Paralysis of intercostal muscles and diaphragm
   b. Muscle weakness
   c. Paralysis of muscles of the limbs, neck, and trunk
   d. Paralysis of small, rapidly moving muscles (e.g., fingers, eye)

7. During a patient's recovery from a lengthy surgery, the nurse monitors for signs of malignant hyperthermia. In addition to a rapid rise in body temperature, which assessment findings would indicate the possible presence of this condition? (Select all that apply.)
   a. Respiratory depression
   b. Tachypnea
   c. Tachycardia
   d. Seizure activity
   e. Muscle rigidity

Answers: 1. d, 2. a, 3. d, 4. a, 5. c, 6. a=4, b=1, c=3, d=2, 7. b, c, e

CRITICAL THINKING ACTIVITIES

1. The nurse is monitoring a patient in the postanaesthesia care unit. The patient had a colectomy with formation of a colostomy because of colon cancer. During this time, what is the priority focus of the nurse's assessment of the patient?

2. The nurse on the orthopedic surgery unit is monitoring the vital signs of a patient who had hip replacement surgery 2 hours earlier. At this time, the certified nursing assistant reports that the patient's temperature has changed from 37.2°C to 40.4°C. Another nurse comments that the patient must be developing an infection from the hip replacement. What is the nurse's priority action at this time?

3. The nurse is assessing a patient who is receiving mechanical ventilation because of respiratory problems. The patient's wife is visiting and asks the nurse, "Is he awake? Can he hear me?" What would be the nurse's best answer?

For answers see http://evolve.elsevier.com/Canada/Lilley/pharmacology/.

Central Nervous System Depressants and Muscle Relaxants

Objectives

After reading this chapter, the successful student will be able to do the following:

1. Briefly describe the functions of the central nervous system.

2. Contrast the effects of central nervous system depressant drugs and central nervous system stimulant drugs (see Chapter 14) pertaining to their basic actions.

3. Define the terms *hypnotic, rapid eye movement, rapid eye movement sleep interference, rapid eye movement rebound, sedative, sedative–hypnotic, sleep,* and *therapeutic index.*

4. Briefly discuss the problem of sleep disorders.

5. Identify the specific drugs within each of the following categories of central nervous system depressant drugs: benzodiazepines, nonbenzodiazepines, muscle relaxants, and miscellaneous drugs.

6. Contrast the mechanisms of action, indications, adverse effects, toxic effects, cautions, contraindications, dosage forms, routes of administration, and drug interactions of the following medications: benzodiazepines, nonbenzodiazepines, muscle relaxants, and miscellaneous drugs.

7. Discuss the nursing process as it relates to the nursing care of a patient receiving any central nervous system depressants or muscle relaxants.

8. Develop a collaborative plan of care related to the use of pharmacological and nonpharmacological approaches to the treatment of sleep disorders.

e-Learning Activities

Website
(http://evolve.elsevier.com/Canada/ Lilley/pharmacology/)

evolve

- Answer Key—Textbook Case Studies
- Answer Key—Critical Thinking Activities
- Chapter Summaries—Printable
- Review Questions for Exam Preparation
- Unfolding Case Studies

Drug Profiles

▸▸ baclofen, p. 259
▸▸ cyclobenzaprine (cyclobenzaprine hydrochloride)*, p. 259
midazolam, p. 255
dantrolene (dantrolene sodium)*, p. 259
pentobarbital (pentobarbital sodium)*, p. 258
phenobarbital (phenobarbital sodium)*, p. 258
ramelteon, p. 255
▸▸ temazepam, p. 255
▸▸ zolpidem tartrate, p. 255
▸▸ zopiclone, p. 255

▸▸ Key drug

*Full generic name is given in parentheses. For the purposes of this text, the more common, shortened name is used.

Key Terms

Barbiturates A class of drugs that are chemical derivatives of barbituric acid. They are used to induce sedation. (p. 256)

Benzodiazepines A chemical category of drugs most frequently prescribed as anxiolytic drugs and less frequently as sedative–hypnotic agents. (p. 252)

Gamma-aminobutyric acid (GABA) The primary inhibitory neurotransmitter found in the brain. A key compound affected by sedative, anxiolytic, psychotropic, and muscle-relaxing medications. (p. 253)

Hypnotics Drugs that, when given at low to moderate doses, calm or soothe the central nervous system (CNS) without inducing sleep but when given at high doses cause sleep. (p. 251)

Non–rapid eye movement (NREM) sleep The largest portion of the sleep cycle. It has four stages and precedes REM sleep. Most of a normal sleep cycle consists of non-REM sleep. (p. 251)

Rapid eye movement (REM) sleep One of the stages of the sleep cycle. Some of the characteristics of REM sleep are rapid movement of the eyes, vivid dreams, and irregular breathing. (p. 251)

REM interference A drug-induced reduction of REM sleep time. (p. 251)

REM rebound Excessive REM sleep following discontinuation of a sleep-altering drug. (p. 251)

Sedatives Drugs that have an inhibitory effect on the CNS to the degree that they reduce nervousness, excitability, and irritability without causing sleep. (p. 251)

Sedative–hypnotics Drugs that can act in the body either as sedatives or hypnotics. (p. 251)

Sleep A transient, reversible, and periodic state of rest in which there is a decrease in physical activity and consciousness. (p. 251)

Sleep architecture The structure of the various elements involved in the sleep cycle, including normal and abnormal patterns of sleep. (p. 251)

Therapeutic index The ratio between the toxic and therapeutic concentrations of a drug. If the index is low, the difference between the therapeutic and toxic drug concentrations is small, and use of the drug is more hazardous. (p. 256)

OVERVIEW

Sedatives and hypnotics are drugs that have a calming effect or that depress the central nervous system (CNS). A drug is classified as either a sedative or a hypnotic drug, depending on the degree to which it inhibits the transmission of nerve impulses to the CNS. **Sedatives** reduce nervousness, excitability, and irritability without causing sleep, but a sedative can become a hypnotic if it is given in large enough doses. **Hypnotics** cause sleep and have a much more potent effect on the CNS than do sedatives. Many drugs can act as either a sedative or a hypnotic, depending on dose and patient responsiveness, and for this reason are called sedative–hypnotics. **Sedative–hypnotics** can be classified chemically into three main groups: barbiturates, benzodiazepines, and nonbenzodiazepine sedatives.

PHYSIOLOGY OF SLEEP

Sleep is defined as a transient, reversible, and periodic state of rest in which there is a decrease in physical activity and consciousness. Normal sleep is cyclic and repetitive, and a person's responses to stimuli are markedly reduced during sleep. During waking hours, the body is bombarded with stimuli that provoke the senses of sight, hearing, touch, smell, and taste. These stimuli elicit voluntary and involuntary movements or functions. During sleep, a person is no longer aware of the sensory stimuli within the immediate environment.

Sleep research involves study of the patterns of sleep, or what is sometimes referred to as **sleep architecture**. The architecture of sleep consists of two basic stages that occur cyclically: **rapid eye movement (REM) sleep** and **non–rapid eye movement (NREM) sleep**. The normal cyclic progression of the stages of sleep is summarized in Table 13-1. Various sedative–hypnotic drugs affect different stages of the normal sleep pattern. Prolonged sedative–hypnotic use may reduce the cumulative amount of REM sleep; this is known as **REM interference**. This interference can result in daytime fatigue, since REM sleep provides a certain component of the "restfulness" of sleep. Upon discontinuance of a sedative–hypnotic drug, **REM rebound** can occur, during which the patient has an abnormally large amount of REM sleep, often leading to frequent and vivid dreams. Misuse of sedative–hypnotic drugs is common and is discussed in Chapter 18. In Ethnocultural Implications, sleep aids used by different ethnocultural groups are listed.

Melatonin is a natural health product (NHP) and a commonly used sleep aid. Melatonin, chemically N-acetyl-5-methoxytryptamine, is a hormone secreted by the pineal gland in the human brain. It helps regulate other hormones and maintains the body's circadian rhythm. The pineal gland is inactive during the day, and during darkness (at around 2100 hours) the pineal gland secretes melatonin, which promotes drowsiness. Nocturnal melatonin levels and the quality of sleep both decline at puberty, while in older adults, periods of sleep tend to become shorter and the quality of sleep becomes poorer. Melatonin is often taken for insomnia, sleep difficulties associated with menopause, and jet lag, and it may promote sleep in children with attention deficit hyperactivity disorder or autism spectrum disorder. Adverse effects may include daytime fatigue, drowsiness, headaches, and dizziness. It should not be used in any patients who are using anticoagulants, immunosuppressants, antihyperglycemics, or birth control medications. It is contraindicated in patients under the age of 20 and patients with depression, hypertension, impaired liver function, or seizure disorder.

TABLE 13-1

Stages of Sleep

Stage	Characteristics	Average Percentage of Time in Each Stage (for Young Adults)
NON-REM SLEEP		
1	Dozing or feelings of drifting off to sleep; person can be easily awakened; those with insomnia have longer stage 1 periods than normal	2–5%
2	Relaxed, but person can easily be awakened; person has occasional REMs and also slight eye movements	50%
3	Deep sleep; difficult to wake person; respiratory rates, pulse, and blood pressure may decrease	5%
4	Difficult to wake person; person may be groggy if awakened; dreaming occurs, especially about daily events; sleepwalking or bedwetting may occur	10–15%
REM SLEEP		
	REMs occur; vivid dreams occur; breathing may be irregular	25–33%

Modified from George, N. M., & Davis, J. E. (2013). Assessing sleep in adolescents through a better understanding of sleep physiology. *American Journal of Nursing, 113*(6), 26–32. doi:10.1097/01.NAJ.0000430921.99915.24; McKenry, L., Tessier, E., & Hogan, M. (2006). *Mosby's pharmacology in nursing* (22nd ed.). St. Louis, MO: Mosby.

 ETHNOCULTURAL IMPLICATIONS

Understanding Your Patients' Sleep Needs

- Question patients of ethnocultures you are unfamiliar with about usual sleep patterns and habits and what the patient practises to promote sleep.
- Collect a thorough health, medication, and diet history to identify food and natural health practices used to manage common everyday problems such as insomnia.
- People from Africa and Asia as well as Indigenous peoples have a high incidence of lactose intolerance, so use of warm milk at bedtime to help with sleep may lead to gastrointestinal (GI) distress, abdominal cramping, and bloating. Lactose-free milk may be used.
- Some Canadians of Asian descent may practice meditation, herbalism, nutritional interventions, and acupuncture to aid sleep.
- Some Chinese patients have been found to require lower doses of benzodiazepines (e.g., diazepam [Valium®]).

- Some Hispanic people believe that maintaining a balance in diet and physical activity prevents evil or poor health. Nondrug therapies or home remedies of vegetables and herbs may be used for sleep.
- Some people may tend to be less accepting of therapeutic touch, whether because of their culture or religion or for some other reason. Nurses should be sensitive to this and find alternatives to massage.
- There are numerous sleep traditions that Muslim people may follow in accordance with the practice of the Prophet. For example, some Muslims must not be involved in any activity after the darkness prayer (1.5 to 2 hours after sunset) and before Fajr prayer (1 hour before sunrise).

BENZODIAZEPINES AND MISCELLANEOUS HYPNOTIC DRUGS

Historically, **benzodiazepines** were the most commonly prescribed sedative–hypnotic drugs and continue to be prescribed; nonbenzodiazepine drugs are also frequently prescribed. Other drugs commonly used for sleep include the antihistamine diphenhydramine hydrochloride (see Chapter 37), and the antidepressants trazodone hydrochloride and amitriptyline hydrochloride (see Chapter 17). The benzodiazepines show favourable adverse effect profiles, efficacy, and safety when used therapeutically in the short-term. Benzodi-

azepines are classified as either sedative–hypnotics or anxiolytics, depending on their primary usage. Anxiolytic drugs are used to reduce the intensity of feelings of anxiety. However, any of these drugs can function along a continuum as a sedative or hypnotic or anxiolytic, depending on the dosage and patient sensitivity. See Chapter 17 for a further discussion of the anxiolytic use of benzodiazepines. There are five benzodiazepines commonly used as sedative–hypnotic drugs. In addition, there are several miscellaneous drugs that are used as hypnotics. They function much like benzodiazepines but are chemically distinct from them. All are listed in Table 13-2.

TABLE 13-2

Sedative–Hypnotic Benzodiazepines and Miscellaneous Drugs

Generic Name	Trade Name
LONG ACTING	
clonazepam	Rivotril®, Clonapam®
diazepam	Diastat®, Diazemuls®, Valium
flurazepam hydrochloride	Dalmane®, Som-Pam®
INTERMEDIATE ACTING	
alprazolam	Xanax
bromazepam	Lectopam®
lorazepam	Ativan®
oxazepam	Oxpam
temazepam	Restoril
SHORT ACTING	
midazolam hydrochloride (IM/IV only)	
triazolam	
zolpidem tartrate*	Sublinox
zopiclone*	Imovane

*These drugs share many characteristics with the benzodiazepines but is classified as a miscellaneous hypnotic drug.

Mechanism of Action and Drug Effects

The sedative and hypnotic action of benzodiazepines is related to their ability to depress activity in the CNS. The specific areas affected include the hypothalamic, thalamic, and limbic systems of the brain. Although the mechanism of action is not certain, research suggests that there are specific receptors in the brain for benzodiazepines. These receptors are thought to be either **gamma-aminobutyric acid (GABA)** receptors or other adjacent receptors. GABA is the primary inhibitory neurotransmitter in the CNS of the brain, and it serves to modulate CNS activity by inhibiting overstimulation. Like GABA itself, benzodiazepines' activity appears to be related to their ability to inhibit stimulation of the brain. They have many favourable characteristics compared with the older drug class *barbiturates* (see the next section of this chapter). They do not suppress REM sleep to the same extent, nor do they induce liver microsomal enzyme activity as the barbiturates do. They are safe to administer to patients who are taking medications metabolized by this enzyme system.

Indications

Nonebnzodiazepines are used for the short-term treatment and symptomatic relief of insomnia. Benzodiazepines have a variety of therapeutic applications. They are commonly used for sedation, relief of agitation or anxiety, treatment of anxiety-related depression, sleep induction, skeletal muscle relaxation, sedation, and treatment of acute seizure disorders. Benzodiazepines are often combined with anaesthetics, analgesics, and neuromuscular blocking drugs in balanced anaesthesia and also procedural sedation (see Chapter 12) for their amnesic properties to reduce memory of painful procedures. Finally, benzodiazepine receptors in the CNS are in the same area as those that play a role in alcohol addiction. Therefore, some benzodiazepines (e.g., diazepam, chlordiazepoxide) are used in the treatment and prevention of the symptoms of alcohol withdrawal (see Chapter 18). When benzodiazepines are used to treat insomnia, it is recommended that they be used short term, if clinically feasible, to avoid dependency.

Contraindications

Contraindications to the use of benzodiazepines include known drug allergy, narrow-angle glaucoma, and pregnancy.

Adverse Effects

Adverse effects associated with the use of benzodiazepines usually involve the CNS and include confusion, ataxia, amnesia, and drowsiness. These effects are more pronounced in the older adult population, who are most commonly prescribed with this class of drugs. Other commonly reported undesirable effects are headache, paradoxical excitement or nervousness, dizziness or vertigo, and lethargy. Benzodiazepines can create a significant fall hazard in older adults, and the lowest effective dose must be used in this patient population. Although these drugs have comparatively less intense effects on the normal sleep cycle, a "hangover" effect is sometimes reported (e.g., daytime sleepiness). Withdrawal symptoms such as rebound insomnia (i.e., greater insomnia than pretreatment) may occur with abrupt discontinuation. Long-term use of benzodiazepines is associated with tolerance. Physical dependence can occur after a few weeks or months of use.

Toxicity and Management of Overdose

An overdose of benzodiazepines may result in one or all of the following symptoms: somnolence, confusion, coma, or diminished reflexes. Overdose of benzodiazepines alone rarely results in hypotension and respiratory depression. These symptoms are more commonly seen when benzodiazepines are taken with other CNS depressants, such as alcohol or barbiturates. The same holds true for their lethal effects. In the absence of the concurrent ingestion of alcohol or other CNS depressants, benzodiazepine overdose rarely results in death.

Treatment of benzodiazepine intoxication is generally symptomatic and supportive. Flumazenil, a benzodiazepine antidote, can be used to acutely reverse the sedative effects of benzodiazepines. Flumazenil antagonizes the action of benzodiazepines on the CNS by directly competing with them for binding at the receptors. Flumazenil is used in cases of oral overdose or excessive intravenous sedation. The dosage regimen to be followed for the reversal of procedural sedation or general anaesthesia induced by benzodiazepines and the management of suspected benzodiazepine overdose are summarized in Table 13-3.

TABLE 13-3

Flumazenil Treatment Regimen

Indication	Recommended Regimen	Duration
Reversal of procedural sedation or general anaesthesia	0.2 mg IV, given over 15 sec; if consciousness does not occur in 60 sec, give 0.1 mg; may be repeated at 60-sec intervals (maximum total dose, 1 mg; usual dose is 0.3–0.6 mg)	1–4 hr
Management of suspected benzodiazepine overdose	0.3 mg IV, given over 30 sec; wait 30 sec, then give 0.3 mg over 30 sec if consciousness does not occur; further doses of 0.3 mg can be given over 30 sec at intervals of 60 sec to a cumulative maximum total dose of 2 mg	1–4 hr

TABLE 13-4

Benzodiazepines: Drug Interactions

Drug	Mechanism	Result
Azole antifungals, verapamil, diltiazem, protease inhibitors, macrolide antibiotics, grapefruit juice	Decreased benzodiazepine metabolism	Prolonged benzodiazepine action
CNS depressants	Additive effects	Increased CNS depression
olanzapine	Unknown	Increased benzodiazepine effects
rifampin	Increased metabolism	Decreased benzodiazepine effects

 # NATURAL HEALTH PRODUCTS

KAVA (*Piper methysticum*)

Overview
Kava consists of the dried rhizomes of *Piper methysticum*. The drug contains kava pyrones (kawain). Extended continuous intake can cause a temporary yellow discoloration of the skin, hair, and nails.

Common Uses
Relief of anxiety, stress, restlessness; promotion of sleep

Adverse Effects
Skin discoloration, possible accommodative disturbances and papillary enlargement, and scaly skin (with long-term use). In 2002, Health Canada banned the selling of kava supplements because of the risk of severe liver damage and toxicity; however, individuals can import kava for personal use.

POTENTIAL DRUG INTERACTIONS

Alcohol, barbiturates, psychoactive drugs

Contraindications
Contraindicated in patients with Parkinson's disease, liver disease, depression, or alcoholism; in those operating heavy machinery; and in pregnant and breastfeeding women

VALERIAN (*Valeriana officinalis*)

Overview
Valerian root, consisting of fresh underground plant parts, contains essential oil with monoterpenes and sesquiterpenes (valerianic acids).

Common Uses
Relief of anxiety, restlessness, sleep disorders

Adverse Effects
Central nervous system depression, hepatotoxicity, nausea, vomiting, anorexia, headache, restlessness, insomnia

Potential Drug Interactions
Central nervous system depressants, monoamine oxidase inhibitors, phenytoin, warfarin sodium; may have enhanced relative and adverse effects when taken with other drugs (including other natural health products) that have known sedative properties (including alcohol)

Contraindications
Contraindicated in patients with heart disease, liver disease, or those operating heavy machinery

Interactions

Potential drug interactions with the benzodiazepines are significant because of their intensity, particularly when they involve other CNS depressants (e.g., alcohol, opioids, muscle relaxants). These drugs result in further CNS-depressant effects (including decreased blood pressure, reduced respiratory rate, sedation, confusion, and diminished reflexes). These and other major drug interactions are listed in Table 13-4. Natural health product interactions include those with kava and valerian, which may also lead to further CNS depression (see Natural Health Products: Kava and Valerian). Food–drug interactions with grapefruit and grapefruit juice, which alter drug metabolism via inhibition of the cytochrome P450 system, can result in prolonged effect, increased effect, and toxicity.

Dosages

For dosage information, see the table on p. 256.

DRUG PROFILES

The benzodiazepines and miscellaneous sedative–hypnotic drugs are prescription-only drugs and are designated as Schedule IV controlled substances. Uses for benzodiazepines can vary, including treatment of insomnia, moderate sedation (see Chapter 12), muscle relaxation, anticonvulsant therapy (see Chapter 15), and anxiety relief (see Chapter 17). The miscellaneous drugs are normally used only for their hypnotic purposes to treat insomnia. Dosage information appears in the Dosages table on page 256.

BENZODIAZEPINES

diazepam

Diazepam (Valium) was the first clinically available benzodiazepine drug. It has varied uses, including for treatment of anxiety, procedural sedation (and as an anaesthesia adjunct), anticonvulsant therapy, and skeletal muscle relaxation following orthopedic injury or surgery.

PHARMACOKINETICS

Route	Onset of Action	Peak Plasma Concentration	Elimination Half-Life	Duration of Action
IV	Immediate	8 min	20–50 hr	15–60 min
PO	30 min	1–2 hr	20–60 hr	12–24 hr

midazolam

Midazolam is most commonly used preoperatively and for procedural sedation (see Chapter 12). It is useful for this indication due to its ability to cause amnesia and anxiolysis (reduced anxiety) as well as sedation. This helps patients to feel less anxious about, and avoid remembering, uncomfortable medical procedures. Refer to Chapter 12 for dosage information.

PHARMACOKINETICS

Route	Onset of Action	Peak Plasma Concentration	Elimination Half-Life	Duration of Action
IV	1–5 min	20–60 min	1–4 hr	2–6 hr

▶▶temazepam

Temazepam (Restoril®), an intermediate-acting benzodiazepine, is actually one of the metabolites of diazepam and normally induces sleep within 20 to 40 minutes. Temazepam has a long onset of action, so it is recommended that patients take it about 1 hour prior to going to bed. Although it is still an effective hypnotic, it has been replaced by newer drugs.

PHARMACOKINETICS

Route	Onset of Action	Peak Plasma Concentration	Elimination Half-Life	Duration of Action
PO	30–60 min	2–3 hr	9.5–12 hr	7–8 hr

NONBENZODIAZEPINES

▶▶zolpidem tartrate

Zolpidem tartrate (Sublinox®), available as a sublingual, orally disintegrating tablet, is also a short-acting nonbenzodiazepine hypnotic. Its relatively short half-life and its lack of active metabolites contribute to a lower incidence of daytime sleepiness compared with benzodiazepine hypnotics.

PHARMACOKINETICS

Route	Onset of Action	Peak Plasma Concentration	Elimination Half-Life	Duration of Action
PO	30 min	1.6 hr	1.4–4.5 hr	6–8 hr

▶▶zopiclone

Zopiclone (Imovane®, Rhovane®) is a short-acting benzodiazepinelike drug. It is indicated for the short-term treatment of insomnia and should be limited to 7 to 10 days of treatment.

PHARMACOKINETICS

Route	Onset of Action	Peak Plasma Concentration	Elimination Half-Life	Duration of Action
PO	30 min	90 min	5 hr	6–8 hr

ramelteon

Ramelteon is included here because Canadians see televised advertisements about this drug, although it is currently not available in Canada. This drug is structurally similar to the hormone melatonin, which is believed to regulate circadian rhythms (day–night sleep cycles) in the body. Over-the-counter natural health products containing melatonin have been available for several years. This hypnotic has a new mechanism of action. Ramelteon works as an agonist at melatonin receptors in the CNS. Technically, it is not a CNS depressant, but it is included here because of its use as a hypnotic. It is also not classified as a controlled substance because of its lack of observed dependency risk. It has a shorter duration of action than other hypnotics and is therefore indicated primarily for patients who have difficulty with sleep *onset* rather than sleep maintenance. Its use is contraindicated in cases of severe liver dysfunction. It is best avoided in patients receiving fluvoxamine (see Chapter 17), fluconazole, or ketoconazole (see Chapter 48), all of which can impede its metabolism. Rifampin (see Chapter 46) can reduce the efficacy of ramelteon by speeding its metabolism via the induction of hepatic enzymes.

PHARMACOKINETICS

Route	Onset of Action	Peak Plasma Concentration	Elimination Half-Life	Duration of Action
PO	30–60 min	45 min	1–2.5 hr	6–8 hr

DOSAGES	Benzodiazepines: Selected Hypnotic Drugs		
Drug	**Onset and Duration**	**Usual Dosage Range**	**Indications/Uses**
diazepam (Valium)	Long acting	**Adults** PO: 2–10 mg 3–4 times daily IV: 2–10 mg IV (supplied 5 mg/mL) IM: infrequent use	Muscle relaxation, preprocedure sedation, status epilepticus, acute anxiety or agitation
lorazepam (Ativan)	Intermediate acting	**Adults** PO: 1-4 mg daily IV/IM: 0.05 mg/kg	PO: Generalized anxiety disorder IV: Status epilepticus IM: Excessive anxiety prior to surgery
▶▶temazepam (Restoril)	Intermediate acting	**Adults** PO: 15–30 mg at bedtime	Sleep induction
▶▶zolpidem tartrate (Sublinox)		**Adults** Sublingual: 5–10 mg at bedtime	Sleep induction
▶▶zopiclone (Imovane, Rhovane)	Short acting	**Adults** PO: 3.75–7.5 mg at bedtime	Sleep induction

BARBITURATES

Barbiturates were first introduced into clinical use in 1903 and were the standard drugs for treating insomnia and producing sedation. Chemically, they are derivatives of barbituric acid. There are few in clinical use today due to the favourable safety profile and proven efficacy of the benzodiazepines. Barbiturates can produce many unwanted adverse effects. They are physiologically habit forming and have a low **therapeutic index** (i.e., there is only a narrow dosage range within which the drug is effective, and above that range it is rapidly toxic).

Mechanism of Action and Drug Effects

Barbiturates are CNS depressants that act primarily on the brain stem in an area called the *reticular formation*. Their sedative and hypnotic effects are dose related, and they act by reducing the nerve impulses travelling to the area of the brain called the *cerebral cortex*. Their ability to inhibit nerve impulse transmission is due in part to their ability to potentiate the action of the inhibitory neurotransmitter GABA, which is found in high concentrations in the CNS. Barbiturates also raise the seizure threshold and can be used to treat seizures (see Chapter 15).

Indications

All barbiturates have the same sedative–hypnotic effects but differ in their potency, time to onset of action, and duration of action. They can be used as hypnotics, sedatives, and anticonvulsants, as well as for anaesthesia during surgical procedures.

Contraindications

Contraindications to barbiturate use include known drug allergy, pregnancy, significant respiratory difficulties, and severe kidney or liver disease. These drugs must be used with caution in older adults due to the drugs' sedative properties and increased fall risk.

Adverse Effects

Adverse effects of barbiturates relate to the CNS and include drowsiness, lethargy, dizziness, hangover (prolongation of drowsiness, lethargy, and dizziness), and paradoxical restlessness or excitement. Their long-term effects on normal sleep architecture can be detrimental. Common adverse effects of barbiturates are listed in Table 13-5.

Toxicity and Management of Overdose

An overdose of barbiturates produces CNS depression, ranging from sleep to profound coma and death. Respiratory depression progresses to Cheyne-Stokes respirations, hypoventilation, and cyanosis. Patients often have cold, clammy skin or are hypothermic, and later they can exhibit fever, areflexia, tachycardia, and hypotension. Because phenobarbital is also used to treat status epilepticus (prolonged uncontrolled seizures), in extreme cases, patients may be intentionally overdosed to cause therapeutic phenobarbital or pentobarbital coma. Because of the inhibitory effects on nerve transmission in the brain (possibly GABA mediated), uncontrollable seizures can

TABLE 13-5

Barbiturates: Adverse Effects

Body System	Adverse Effects
Cardiovascular	Vasodilation and hypotension, especially if given too rapidly
Gastrointestinal	Nausea, vomiting, diarrhea, constipation
Hematological	Agranulocytosis, thrombocytopenia
Nervous	Drowsiness, lethargy, vertigo
Respiratory	Respiratory depression, cough
Other	Hypersensitivity reactions: urticaria, angioedema, rash, fever, Stevens-Johnson syndrome

be stopped until sufficient serum levels of anticonvulsant drugs are achieved.

Treatment of an overdose is mainly symptomatic and supportive. The mainstays of therapy are maintenance of an adequate airway, assisted ventilation, and oxygen administration if needed, along with fluid and pressor support as indicated. Barbiturates are highly metabolized by the liver, where they also induce enzyme activity. In an overdose, however, the amount of barbiturate may overwhelm the liver's ability to metabolize it. This is a situation in which administration of activated charcoal may be helpful. Activated charcoal adsorbs (binds to) drug molecules in the stomach. It also has the effect of drawing the drug from the circulation into the GI tract for elimination. Multiple-dose (every 4 hours) nasogastric administration of activated charcoal is a common regimen. Phenobarbital is relatively acidic and can be eliminated more quickly by the kidneys when the urine is alkalized (pH is raised). This keeps the drug in the urine and prevents it from being resorbed back into the circulation. Alkalization, along with forced diuresis using diuretics (e.g., furosemide [see Chapter 29]), can hasten elimination of the barbiturate.

Interactions

Barbiturates as a class are notorious enzyme inducers. They stimulate the action of enzymes in the liver that are responsible for the metabolism or breakdown of many drugs. By stimulating the action of these enzymes, they cause many drugs to be metabolized more quickly, which usually shortens their duration of action. Other drugs that are enzyme inducers are warfarin sodium, rifampin, and phenytoin.

Additive CNS depression occurs with the coadministration of barbiturates with alcohol, antihistamines, benzodiazepines, opioids, and tranquilizers. Most of the drug–drug interactions are secondary to the effects of barbiturates on the hepatic enzyme system. Barbiturates increase the activity of hepatic microsomal or cytochrome P450 enzymes (see Chapter 2). This process is called *enzyme induction*. Induction of this enzyme system results in increased drug metabolism and breakdown. However, if two drugs are competing for the same enzyme system, the result can be inhibited drug metabolism and possibly increased toxicity for the wide variety of drugs that are metabolized by these enzymes. Drugs most likely to

have marked interactions with the barbiturates include monoamine oxidase inhibitors (MAOIs), tricyclic antidepressants (see Chapter 17), anticoagulants (see Chapter 27), glucocorticoids (see Chapter 49), and oral contraceptives (see Chapter 35) with barbiturates. Coadministration of MAOIs and barbiturates can result in prolonged barbiturate effects. Coadministration of anticoagulants with barbiturates can result in decreased anticoagulation response and possible clot formation. Coadministration of barbiturates with oral contraceptives can result in accelerated metabolism of the contraceptive drug and possible unintended pregnancy. Women taking both types of medication concurrently need to be advised to consider an additional method of contraception as a backup.

Dosages

Barbiturates can act as either sedatives or hypnotics, depending on the dosage. For information on selected barbiturates and their recommended sedative and hypnotic dosages, see the table on page 257.

MUSCLE RELAXANTS

A variety of conditions such as trauma, inflammation, anxiety, and pain can be associated with acute muscle spasms. Although there is no perfect therapy available for relief of skeletal muscle spasticity, muscle relaxant drugs are capable of providing some relief. Muscle relaxants are a group of compounds that act predominantly within the CNS to relieve pain associated with skeletal muscle spasms. Most muscle relaxants are known as *centrally acting* skeletal muscle relaxants because their site of action is the CNS. These compounds are similar in structure and action to other CNS depressants such as diazepam. It is believed that the muscle relaxant effects are related to this CNS depressant activity. Only one of these compounds, dantrolene, acts directly on skeletal muscle. It belongs to a group of relaxants known as *direct acting* skeletal muscle relaxants and closely resembles GABA. Muscle relaxants are most effective when used in conjunction with rest and physiotherapy. When taken with alcohol, other CNS depressants, or opioid analgesics, enhanced CNS depressant effects are seen. In such cases, close monitoring and dosage reduction of one or both drugs need to be considered.

DOSAGES	**Selected Barbiturates**		
Drug	**Onset and Duration**	**Usual Dosage Range**	**Indications/Uses**
phenobarbital	Long acting	**Pediatric** PO: 2 mg/kg in 3 divided doses IM/IV: 1–3 mg/kg 1–2 hr before surgery	 Sedative Preoperative sedative
		Adults PO: 15–30 mg bid or tid IM/IV: 130–200 mg 1–2 hr before surgery	 Sedative Preoperative sedative

DRUG PROFILES

Like benzodiazepines, barbiturates can also have varied uses, including preoperative sedation, anaesthesia adjunct, and anticonvulsant therapy. All barbiturates are controlled substances. Dosage information appears in the Dosages table for barbiturates.

phenobarbital

Phenobarbital is the most commonly prescribed barbiturate, either alone or in combination with other drugs. It is considered the prototypical barbiturate and is classified as a long-acting drug. Phenobarbital is used for the prevention of generalized tonic–clonic seizures and fever-induced convulsions. In addition, it has been useful in the treatment of hyperbilirubinemia in neonates. It is only rarely used today as a sedative and is no longer recommended as a hypnotic drug. It is available in oral and injectable forms.

PHARMACOKINETICS

Route	Onset	Peak	Half-Life	Duration
IV	5 min	30 min	50–120 hr	6–12 hr
PO	30 min	1–6 hr	50–120 hr	6–12 hr

OVER-THE-COUNTER HYPNOTICS

Nonprescription sleep aids often contain antihistamines (see Chapter 37), which have a CNS depressant effect. The most common antihistamines contained in over-the-counter sleep aids are doxylamine succinate (Unisom-2®) and diphenhydramine hydrochloride (Sleep-Eze®, Unisom®). Analgesics (e.g., acetaminophen [see Chapter 11]) are sometimes added to offer some pain relief if pain is a component of the sleep disturbance (e.g., acetaminophen/diphenhydramine hydrochloride [Extra Strength Tylenol® Nighttime]). As with other CNS depressants, concurrent use of alcohol can cause respiratory depression or arrest.

Mechanism of Action and Drug Effects

The majority of muscle relaxants work within the CNS. Their beneficial effects are believed to come from their sedative effects, rather than from direct muscle relaxation. Dantrolene acts directly on the excitation–contraction coupling of muscle fibres and not at the level of the CNS. It directly affects skeletal muscles by decreasing the response of the muscle to stimuli. It appears to exert its action by decreasing the amount of calcium released from storage sites in the sarcoplasmic reticulum of muscle fibres. All other muscle relaxants have no direct effects on muscles, nerve conduction, or muscle–nerve junctions and have a depressant effect on the CNS. Their effects are the result of CNS depression in the brain, primarily at the level of the brain stem, thalamus, and basal ganglia, as well as at the spinal cord.

The effects of muscle relaxants are relaxation of striated muscles, mild weakness of skeletal muscles, decreased force of muscle contraction, and muscle stiffness. Other effects include generalized CNS depression manifested as sedation, somnolence, ataxia, and respiratory and cardiovascular depression. Baclofen is one of the more effective drugs in this class and is a derivative of GABA. It is believed to work by depressing nerve transmission in the spinal cord. The other drugs in this class are not derivatives of GABA but act by enhancing GABA's central inhibitory effects at the level of the spinal cord.

Indications

Muscle relaxants are used primarily for the relief of painful musculoskeletal conditions, such as muscle spasms, often following injuries such as low back strain. They are most effective when used in conjunction with physiotherapy. They may also be used in the management of spasticity associated with severe chronic disorders, such as multiple sclerosis and other types of cerebral lesions, cerebral palsy, and rheumatic disorders. Some relaxants are used to reduce choreiform movement in patients with Huntington's disease, to reduce rigidity in patients with parkinsonian syndromes, or to relieve the pain associated with trigeminal neuralgia. Intravenous dantrolene is used for the management of the hypermetabolic muscle spasms that accompany the crisis condition of malignant hyperthermia (see Chapter 12). Baclofen has been shown to be effective in relieving hiccups.

Contraindications

The only usual contraindication to the use of muscle relaxants is known drug allergy, but contraindications for some of these drugs may include severe renal impairment.

Adverse Effects

The primary adverse effects of muscle relaxants are an extension of their effects on the CNS and skeletal muscles. Euphoria, lightheadedness, dizziness, drowsiness, fatigue, confusion, and muscle weakness are often experienced early in treatment. These adverse effects are generally short-lived, as patients grow tolerant of them over time. Less common adverse effects seen with muscle relaxants include diarrhea, GI upset, headache, slurred speech, muscle stiffness, constipation, sexual difficulties in males, hypotension, tachycardia, and weight gain.

Toxicity and Management of Overdose

The toxicities and consequences of an overdose of muscle relaxants primarily involve the CNS. There is no specific antidote (or reversal drug) for muscle relaxant overdoses. They are best treated with conservative supportive measures. More aggressive therapies are generally needed when muscle relaxants are taken along with other

CNS-depressant drugs as an overdose. Gastric lavage and close observation of the patient are recommended. An adequate airway must be maintained, and means of artificial respiration should be readily available. Electrocardiographic monitoring needs to be instituted and large quantities of intravenous fluids are administered to avoid crystalluria.

Interactions

When muscle relaxants are administered along with other depressant drugs, such as alcohol and benzodi-

azepines, caution needs to be used to avoid overdose. The combination of propoxyphene and orphenadrine has resulted in additive CNS effects. Mental confusion, anxiety, tremors, and additive hypoglycemic activity have been reported with this combination as well. A dosage reduction or discontinuance of one or both drugs is recommended.

Dosages

For dosage information for commonly used muscle relaxants, refer to the table below.

DOSAGES	Selected Muscle Relaxants		
Drug	**Pharmacological Class**	**Usual Dosage Range**	**Indications**
▶▶baclofen (Lioresal)	Central acting	*Adults* PO: 5 mg tid daily ×3 days, then 10 mg daily tid ×3 days, then 15 mg daily tid ×3 days, then 20 mg tid daily ×3 days, then titrated to response to max of 80 mg daily	Spasticity
▶▶cyclobenzaprine hydrochloride (Novo-Cycloprine, Riva-Cycloprine)	Central acting	Adults PO: 10 mg tid	Spasticity
dantrolene sodium (Dantrene)	Direct-acting	*Children* PO: 0.5 mg/kg/bid up to 3 mg/kg/day given in divided doses bid–qid *Adults* PO: 25 mg/day; may increase to 25–100 mg bid–qid *Children/Adults* IV: 1 mg/kg; may repeat to total dose of 10 mg/kg	Chronic spasticity and malignant hyperthermia Malignant hyperthermia
tizanidine hydrochloride	Direct-acting	*Adults* PO: 2 mg increased by 2–4 mg to optimum effect up to 36 mg/day divided tid	Spasticity

DRUG PROFILES

With the exception of dantrolene (Dantrium®), which acts directly on skeletal muscle tissues, muscle relaxants are classified as centrally acting relaxants because of their site of action in the CNS. These include baclofen (Lioresal®), chlorzoxazone (Acetazone Forte C8®), cyclobenzaprine, methocarbamol (Robaxacet®, Robaxacin®), orphenadrine citrate (Norflex®), and tizanidine hydrochloride. Muscle relaxants are not controlled substances. Use of all muscle relaxants is contraindicated in patients who have shown a hypersensitivity reaction to them or have compromised pulmonary function, active liver disease, or impaired myocardial function. Dosage information appears in the Dosages table for muscle relaxants.

▶▶baclofen

Baclofen (Lioresal) is available in both oral and injectable dosage forms. The injectable form is for use with an implantable baclofen pump device. This method is sometimes used to treat chronic spastic muscular conditions. With this route, a test dose needs to be administered initially to test for a positive response. The injection is diluted

before infusion. Both oral and injectable doses are titrated to desired response.

PHARMACOKINETICS

Route	Onset of Action	Peak Plasma Concentration	Elimination Half-Life	Duration of Action
PO	0.5–1 hr	2–3 hr	2.5–4 hr	8 hr or longer

▶▶cyclobenzaprine hydrochloride

Cyclobenzaprine hydrochloride is available in a 10-mg dose. Cyclobenzaprine is a centrally acting muscle relaxant that is structurally and pharmacologically related to the tricyclic antidepressants. It is the most commonly used drug in this class to reduce spasms following musculoskeletal injuries. It is very common for patients to exhibit marked sedation from its use.

PHARMACOKINETICS

Route	Onset of Action	Peak Plasma Concentration	Elimination Half-Life	Duration of Action
PO	1 hr	3–8 hr	8–37 hr	12–24 hr

NURSING PROCESS

Assessment

Before administering any CNS-depressant drug, such as a benzodiazepine, nonbenzodiazepine, miscellaneous drug, muscle relaxant, or barbiturate, perform an assessment focusing on some of the more common parameters and data, including the following: (1) reports of any insomnia with attention to onset, duration, frequency, and pharmacological as well as nonpharmacological measures used (see Box 13-1); (2) any concerns of the patient or family about sleep disorders, sleep patterns, difficulty in sleeping, or frequent awakenings; (3) the time it typically takes to fall asleep and energy level upon awakening; (4) vital signs with attention to blood pressure (both supine and standing measurements); pulse rate and rhythm; respiratory rate, rhythm, and depth; body temperature; and presence of pain; (5) thorough physical assessment or examination for baseline comparisons; (6) neurological findings with a focus on any changes in mental status, memory, cognitive abilities, alertness, level of orientation (to person, place, and time), level of sedation, mood changes, depression or other mental disorder, sensation, anxiety, or panic attacks; and (7) miscellaneous information about medical history; allergies; use of alcohol; smoking history; caffeine intake; past and current medication profile, with notation of use of any prescription drugs, over-the-counter drugs, and natural health products; alternative or folk practices; and any changes in health status, weight, nutrition, exercise, life stressors (including loss and grief), or lifestyle.

For patients taking benzodiazepines and benzodiazepinelike drugs, assessment needs to also include the identification of disorders or conditions that represent cautions or contraindications to the use of these drugs, as well as drugs the patient is taking that might interact with benzodiazepines or benzodiazepinelike drugs (see pharmacology discussion). Closely monitor those who are anemic, are suicidal, or have a history of misusing drugs, alcohol or other substances. Other significant cautions pertain to use of these drugs in older adults and very young children because of their increased sensitivity to these drugs, as well as in women who are pregnant or are lactating. Older adults and very young children may require lower dosages due to potential ataxia and

---

BOX 13-1   Sleep Diaries and Nonpharmacological Treatment of Sleep Disorders

Information for a Sleep Diary

- What time do you usually go to bed and wake up?
- How long and how well do you sleep?
- When were you awake during the night, and for how long?
- How easy was it to go to sleep?
- How easy was it to wake up in the morning?
- How much caffeine do you consume?
- What time did you last eat or drink (if after dinner)?
- Did you have a bedtime snack?
- What emotions or stressors do you have?
- What medications do you take daily?
- Do you smoke? If so, how many cigarettes do you smoke a day, and how long have you been smoking?
- Do you consume alcohol? If so, how often do you have a drink and how long have you been drinking that amount?
- Do you take any over-the-counter drugs? If so, what drugs do you take and for what reason? How often do you take these drugs and in what dosages? How long have you been taking them?
- Do you take any natural health products? If so, which ones? What do you take them for and how long have you been taking them?

Nonpharmacological Sleep Interventions

- Establish a set sleep pattern with a time to go to bed at night and a regular time to get up in the morning, and stick to it. This will help to reset your internal clock.
- Sleep only as much as you need to feel refreshed and renewed. Too much sleep may lead to fragmented sleep patterns and shallow sleep.
- Keep the temperature in the bedroom moderate, if possible.
- Avoid caffeine-containing beverages and food within 6 hours of bedtime.
- Decrease exposure to loud noises while you sleep.
- Avoid daytime napping.
- Avoid exercise late in the evening (i.e., not past 1900 hours).
- Avoid alcohol in the evening. Rather than putting you to sleep, it actually causes fragmented sleep.
- Avoid tobacco at bedtime because it disturbs sleep.
- Try to relax before bedtime with soft music, yoga, relaxation therapy, deep breathing, or light reading on a topic that is not intense or anxiety provoking.
- Drink a warm, noncaffeinated beverage, such as warm milk or chamomile tea, 30 minutes to 1 hour before bedtime.
- If you are still awake 20 minutes after going to bed, get up and engage in a relaxing activity (as noted previously) and go back to bed once you feel drowsy. Repeat as necessary.

excessive sedation. In addition, before initiating drug therapy with benzodiazepines or other sedative–hypnotic drugs, including barbiturates, the prescriber may order blood studies, such as a complete blood count (CBC). Kidney function studies (blood urea nitrogen [BUN] or creatinine levels) or liver function studies (alkaline phosphatase isoenzyme level) may be ordered to rule out organ impairment and prevent potential toxicity or complications resulting from decreased excretion or metabolism. Potential drug interactions are presented in Table 13-4. Pay particular attention to the concurrent use of other CNS depressants (e.g., opioids), because this may lead to severe decreases in blood pressure, respiratory rate, reflexes, and level of consciousness.

With the nonbenzodiazepines such as zaleplon, zopiclone, and zolpidem tartrate, include a head-to-toe physical assessment and a thorough medication history with measurement of vital signs and other parameters (see above discussion). Assess and document for allergies to these drugs and to aspirin. If the patient is allergic to aspirin, there is an associated risk of allergies to nonbenzodiazepines. Other considerations include the need for assessment of any confusion and lightheadedness, especially in older adults, because of their increased sensitivity. Do not use zaleplon and zopiclone in those younger than 18 years of age, and use extreme caution if there is a history of compromised respiratory status or drug, alcohol, or other substance abuse. Drug interactions include other CNS depressants.

For muscle relaxants, always note drug allergies before use, and perform a complete head-to-toe assessment with focus on the neurological system. In older adults, there is increased risk of CNS toxicity with possible hallucinations, confusion, and excessive sedation. Assessment includes taking a thorough health and medication history and examining the complete patient profile with results of associated laboratory studies. See pharmacology discussion about cautions, contraindications, and drug interactions.

The miscellaneous drug ramelteon is a newer medication that is used for insomnia but is not associated with CNS depression, does not carry the potential for abuse or dependence, and does not lead to withdrawal symptoms when treatment stops. Therefore, this drug can be used for patients who are likely to misuse CNS depressants. Include inquiry into sleep patterns and habits in your assessment. Because this drug is not to be used in patients with liver impairment, liver function studies are needed prior to beginning the medication. Perform respiratory assessment and assessment of other vital signs as well. If the patient has a history of respiratory disorders such as chronic obstructive pulmonary disease or sleep apnea, or if the patient is a child, this medication would not be indicated.

Barbiturates are discussed further in Chapter 15 along with other antiepileptic drugs. However, a brief description is needed to emphasize the importance of conducting a thorough patient assessment as well as evaluating

for cautions, contraindications, and drug interactions. Barbiturates are not to be used by pregnant or lactating women. These drugs cross the placenta and breast–blood barriers, posing a risk of respiratory depression in the fetus and neonate. Withdrawal symptoms may appear in neonates born to women who have taken barbiturates during their last trimester of pregnancy. Barbiturates may also produce paradoxical excitement in children and confusion and mental depression in older adults, so baseline neurological assessment is needed. Assessment of kidney and liver function is also important in those with compromised organ function and in older adults to help avoid toxicity.

Nursing Diagnoses

- Impaired gas exchange related to the respiratory depression associated with CNS depressants
- Deficient knowledge related to inadequate information about the various CNS drugs and their first-time use
- Disturbed sleep pattern related to the drug's interference with REM sleep
- Risk for injury and falls as related to the adverse effect of decreased sensorium
- Risk for injury related to possible drug overdose or adverse reactions related to drug–drug interactions (e.g., combined use of the drug with alcohol, tranquilizers, or analgesics) and decreased level of alertness and an unsteady gait
- Risk for injury and addiction related to physical or psychological dependency on CNS drugs

Planning

Goals

- Patient will maintain normal gas exchange and be free of respiratory depression.
- Patient will demonstrate adequate knowledge about the drugs, how they work, and their adverse effects and interactions.
- Patient will remain free of further disturbed sleep patterns.
- Patient will remain free of self-injury and falls due to safety measures for decreased sensorium.
- Patient will remain free of injury due to adequate information about drug interactions that lead to further CNS depression.
- Patient will remain free of injury to self with no drug dependence.

Expected Patient Outcomes

- Patient states measures to maintain normal gas exchange such as coughing, deep breathing, taking only the prescribed amount of medication, and reporting any difficulty breathing to prescriber.

- Patient demonstrates adequate knowledge about the medication(s) used, including their sedating or hypnotic properties, CNS-depressant effects, and adverse effects of altered respirations, decreased depth and rate of respirations, altered cough, confusion, drowsiness, and interactions with other CNS depressants.
- Patient states risk for REM interference from sedative–hypnotic drugs with associated sleep interference with most of these drugs, as well as known hangover effects.
- Patient states importance of trying nonpharmacological measures for enhancing sleep as appropriate prior to drug therapy, such as massage, relaxation therapy, music, or biofeedback.
- Patient demonstrates understanding of safety measures to decrease risk of injury or falls while taking sedatives or hypnotics, such as taking medication only as prescribed, removing all throw rugs from walking areas (especially at night), moving and changing positions slowly, ambulating with caution, and reporting any excessive drowsiness or sedation to prescriber.
- Patient states common drug interactions associated with, and to avoid with, sedatives or hypnotics (i.e., other CNS depressants, opioids, natural health products [e.g., kava, valerian], alcohol, and sedating products found over the counter [e.g., diphenhydramine hydrochloride]).
- Patient remains free of risk of drug dependence issues through appropriate use of sedatives or hypnotics, taking medication only as prescribed, reporting any problems with increased resistance to the drug's effects, as well as excessive sedation and the feeling that more medication is needed to get the same drug effect.
- Patient tries nonpharmacological measures to promote sleep, as needed.

Implementation

Patients taking benzodiazepines and other CNS depressants experience sedation and possible ataxia; thus patient safety measures are needed. Hospital or facility policies mandate the type of safety precautions to be taken, such as the use of side rails or bed alarms. Ambulation needs to occur safely and with assistance when patients are sedated or are experiencing the adverse effects of these drugs. In addition, dependence may be a problem with benzodiazepines. While taking these drugs, patients need to avoid driving or participating in any activities that require mental alertness. It is recommended that these drugs be taken on an empty stomach for faster onset of action; however, this often results in GI upset. So, practically speaking, they need to be taken with food—a light snack or meal. Orally administered benzodiazepines have an onset of action of 30 minutes to 6 hours depending on the drug (see the Pharmacokinetics tables in the Drug Profiles section), and the appropriate timing and intervals of dosing will be determined by

these characteristics. For example, if a patient takes a benzodiazepine or other CNS drug to induce sleep and the drug's onset of action is 30 to 60 minutes, then the drug needs to be dosed 60 minutes prior to bedtime. In addition, it is crucial to patient adherence and safety to understand that the patient may develop drug tolerance to many of these drugs, and so may require larger dosages to produce the same therapeutic effect at some point. Interrupting therapy helps to decrease drug tolerance.

Among the benzodiazepines, REM interference is less problematic with flurazepam, primarily because it produces fewer active metabolites. Educate patients about the REM interference and rebound insomnia that may occur with just a 3- to 4-week regimen of drug therapy. To minimize REM interference, benzodiazepines and other drugs are used only when nonpharmacological methods fail and must be used with caution and for short periods of time in all patients with sleep disorders. Gradual weaning-off periods are recommended with benzodiazepines and all CNS depressants. Hangover effects are also associated with many of the CNS depressants but occur less frequently with benzodiazepines and nonbenzodiazepines than with barbiturates.

It is recommended that nonbenzodiazepines be taken for the prescribed time. Zolpidem tartrate sublingual, orally disintegrating tablets have optimal absorption if taken at bedtime on an empty stomach with no crushing or chewing, and they are not to be taken with water. Place the tablet under the tongue, where it will disintegrate. This drug may infrequently lead to temporary memory loss. To help avoid this adverse effect, it is important to encourage the patient to not take a dose of the drug without a full night's sleep (i.e., at least 7 to 8 hours) the previous night. As with any CNS-depressant drug, the patient should avoid tasks requiring mental alertness until response to the drug is known. Tolerance and dependence are possible with prolonged use, and this drug is to be gradually weaned before discontinuation.

Muscle relaxants have different indications from those of barbiturates and benzodiazepines and are not used to treat insomnia. They are generally indicated for some forms of spasticity (e.g., from upper motor neuron syndromes or muscular pain or spasms from peripheral musculoskeletal conditions). However, they may lead to adverse effects and toxicities, so frequently monitor airway, breathing, and circulation. Early identification of toxicity is critical to provide prompt treatment and prevent respiratory and other CNS-depressant effects. Closely monitor all vital parameters, level of consciousness, and presence of sedation when these muscle relaxants are used. Encourage cautious ambulation. Recommend that the patient change positions purposefully and slowly to prevent syncope or dizziness. The greatest risk for hypotension associated with these drugs is usually within 1 hour of dosing, so the patient must be more cautious about activity during this time.

Barbiturates are to be used with close monitoring and extreme caution. Observe and document the patient's level of consciousness or sedation; orientation to person, place, and time; respiratory rate; oxygen saturation; and other vital signs. Advise the patient to take oral doses with food or a light snack and not to alter dosage forms. Use a bed alarm system or side rails and provide assistance with ambulation, as needed or indicated, to help prevent injury. Barbiturates also produce a hangover effect; this residual drowsiness occurs upon awakening and results in impaired reaction times. Intermediate- and long-acting hypnotics are often the culprits of this adverse effect. Abrupt withdrawal of barbiturates after prolonged therapy may produce adverse effects ranging from nightmares, hallucinations, and delirium to seizures. In addition, while the patient is taking barbiturates, monitor red blood cell (RBC) count and hemoglobin and hematocrit levels because of the possible adverse effect of anemia. Long-term use of barbiturates also requires monitoring of therapeutic blood levels of the drug. For example, the therapeutic level of phenobarbital must range between 10 and 40 mcg/mL. Patients with serum levels above 40 mcg/mL may experience toxicity, manifested by cold and clammy skin, a respiratory rate of less than 10 breaths per minute, and other signs of severe CNS depression.

Intravenous use of barbiturates, as with some benzodiazepines (e.g., diazepam), requires dilution of the drug with normal saline or other recommended solutions. Recommendations regarding diluents and rates of intravenous administration must be strictly followed for safe use. Most of the drugs are not to be given any faster than 1 mg/kg per minute, and a maximum amount per minute may be specified. Consult authoritative drug sources (e.g., the agency parenteral administration policy, a current drug handbook or reference, or the manufacturer's insert) for the recommended rate of infusion before giving any of these drugs. Too rapid an infusion of a barbiturate may produce profound hypotension and marked respiratory depression. If intravenous infiltration is present, the site may become swollen, erythematous, and tender. Tissue necrosis may occur with this infiltration, depending on the irritating qualities of the particular drug. There are antidote protocols for some of the intravenous barbiturates. For example, with phenobarbital intravenous infiltration, the solution must be discontinued, a 0.5% procaine solution injected into the affected area and moist heat applied, as per institutional policy or procedure. Always check protocol for management of infiltration of an intravenous drug before intervening because, in certain situations, the intravenous catheter may be left in place until antidotes are administered. Another area of concern with intravenous drugs is incompatibilities with other intravenously administered medications, and barbiturates have several. Some intravenous drugs that are incompatible with barbiturates include amphotericin B, hydrocortisone, and hydromorphone. Give these particular drugs only after the intravenous line has been adequately flushed with normal saline. With intramuscular injection, give the solution deep into a large muscle mass to prevent tissue sloughing; however, avoid this route and use only when absolutely necessary.

In summary, before giving any CNS depressant, it is always important to try nonpharmacological measures to induce sleep. However, if medication therapy is indicated, preventing respiratory depression and other problems associated with CNS depression is of prime importance, as is maintaining patient safety and preventing injury. Documentation must be timely, clear, and concise and reflect follow-up of the patient's response to the drug. After each dose is given, it is also important to document the dose, route, time of administration, and safety measures taken.

Evaluation

Some of the criteria by which to confirm a patient's therapeutic response to a CNS depressant include the following: an increased ability to sleep at night, fewer awakenings, shorter sleep induction time, few adverse effects such as hangover effects, and an improved sense of well-being because of improved sleep. Therapeutic effects related to muscle relaxants include decreased spasticity, reduction of choreiform movements in patients with Huntington's disease, decreased rigidity in parkinsonian syndromes, and relief of pain from trigeminal neuralgia. Constantly watch for and document the occurrence of any of the adverse effects of benzodiazepines, barbiturates, and muscle relaxants. See the previous discussion on adverse effects for each type of drug. Evaluation for CNS-depressant toxic effects includes monitoring for severe CNS depression of all body systems, especially respiratory and circulatory collapse, with decrease in respiratory rate or depth (or both), and decrease in blood pressure.

CASE STUDY

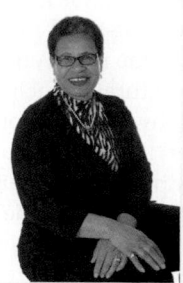

Drugs for Sleep

Pamela, a 68-year-old retired administrative assistant, comes to the office stating that she feels "so tired" during the day. She has had trouble sleeping off and on for years, and a few weeks ago she received a prescription for the benzodiazepine alprazolam (Xanax®) to take "as needed for nerves." Upon closer questioning, the nurse discovers that Pamela has been using alprazolam almost every night for 3 weeks to help her get to sleep. She says, "I just could not fall asleep before! I am sleeping very well, but I'm so tired during the day. I don't understand how I can get such good sleep and still feel tired!"

1. Can you explain the reason for her tiredness?
2. Pamela's nurse practitioner prescribes a period of decreasing doses of the alprazolam each evening, then every other evening, until the medication is stopped. Explain the rationale behind the tapering dosage schedule.
3. Pamela receives a prescription for zolpiderm tartrate (Sublinox). How is this drug different from alprazolam?
4. What nonpharmacological measures can Pamela try to improve her sleep?

For answers see http://evolve.elsevier.com/Canada/Lilley/pharmacology/.

PATIENT TEACHING TIPS

❖ Encourage the patient to keep a journal where they record sleep habits and their response to both drug and nondrug therapy (Box 13-1).

❖ To enhance sleep, implement nonpharmacological measures first. This is important because the use of CNS depressants for treatment of sleep deficit or insomnia often leads to interference with the REM stage of sleep, hangover effects, and tolerance, as well as other adverse effects.

❖ Always check with the prescriber or pharmacist before taking any over-the-counter medications because of the many drug interactions with CNS depressants.

❖ Instruct the patient to keep these drugs and all medications out of the reach of children.

❖ Emphasize that medications are to be taken only as prescribed. The patient is usually told that if one dose does not work, not to double up on the dosage unless otherwise prescribed or directed.

❖ Educate the patient about any time constraints while taking these medications, related to driving, operation of heavy machinery or equipment, and participation in activities requiring mental alertness.

❖ Instruct the patient not to abruptly discontinue or withdraw these medications, if possible, to avoid rebound insomnia.

❖ Sedative–hypnotic drugs (for sleep promotion) are not intended for long-term use because of their adverse effects, interference with REM sleep, and addictive properties.

❖ Advise the patient that hangover effects may occur with most of these drugs and that this is more problematic in older adults or patients with altered kidney and liver function.

❖ Provide the patient with thorough instructions about safety with these drugs, such as avoiding smoking in bed or when lounging.

❖ Teach the patient about significant drug–drug and drug–food interactions with all these medications.

❖ Educate patients about the effect of grapefruit and grapefruit juice on benzodiazepines. The grapefruit results in decreased drug metabolism via inhibition of the cytochrome P450 system and may lead to a prolonged effect and possible toxicity (of the benzodiazepine).

KEY POINTS

❖ Nonpharmacological measures to improve sleep should be tried before resorting to treatment with medications.

❖ Recognize and understand the classification and pharmacokinetic properties of barbiturates. The short-acting barbiturate is pentobarbital sodium but there are no short-acting or intermediate-acting barbiturates available in Canada. The long-acting barbiturate is phenobarbital.

❖ The pharmacokinetics of each group of barbiturates lends specific characteristics to the drugs in that group.

The nurse needs to understand how these drugs are absorbed orally and used parenterally, as well as their onset, peak, and duration of action. In addition, the nurse must understand the life-threatening potential of these drugs because too rapid an infusion may precipitate respiratory or cardiac arrest.

❖ Benzodiazepines are commonly used for sedation, relief of anxiety, skeletal muscle relaxation, and treatment of acute seizure disorders.

❖ Most sedative–hypnotic drugs suppress REM sleep and should be used only for the recommended period of

KEY POINTS—cont'd

time. This time frame varies, depending on the specific drug used.

❖ Long-acting benzodiazepines include clonazepam, diazepam, and flurazepam. Intermediate-acting benzodiazepines include alprazolam, lorazepam, and temazepam. Short-acting benzodiazepines include midazolam and triazolam.

❖ Zolpidem and zopiclone are nonbenzodiazepine hypnotics.

EXAMINATION REVIEW QUESTIONS

1. A patient has been admitted to the emergency department because of an overdose of an oral benzodiazepine. He is extremely drowsy but still responsive. The nurse will prepare for which immediate intervention?
   a. Hemodialysis to remove the medication
   b. Administration of flumazenil
   c. Administration of naloxone
   d. Intubation and mechanical ventilation

2. An older adult had been given a barbiturate for sleep induction, but the night nurse noted that the patient was awake most of the night, watching television and reading in bed. The nurse documents that the patient has had which type of reaction to the medication?
   a. Allergic
   b. Teratogenic
   c. Paradoxical
   d. Idiopathic

3. The nurse is preparing to administer a medication for sleep. Which intervention applies to the administration of a nonbenzodiazepine, such as zolpidem tartrate (Sublinox)?
   a. These drugs need to be taken about 1 hour before bedtime.
   b. Because of their rapid onset, these drugs need to be taken just before bedtime.
   c. The patient needs to be cautioned about the high incidence of morning drowsiness that may occur after taking these drugs.
   d. These drugs are less likely to interact with alcohol.

4. The nurse will monitor the patient who is taking a muscle relaxant for which adverse effect?
   a. CNS depression
   b. Hypertension

   c. Peripheral edema
   d. Blurred vision

5. A hospitalized patient is reporting having difficulty sleeping. Which action will the nurse take first to address this problem?
   a. Administer a sedative–hypnotic drug if ordered.
   b. Offer tea made with the herbal preparation valerian.
   c. Encourage the patient to exercise by walking up and down the halls a few times if tolerated.
   d. Provide an environment that is restful, and reduce loud noises.

6. Which considerations are important for the nurse to remember when administering a benzodiazepine as a sedative–hypnotic drug? (Select all that apply.)
   a. These drugs are intended for long-term management of insomnia.
   b. The drugs can be administered safely with other CNS depressants for insomnia.
   c. The dose needs to be given about 1 hour before the patient's bedtime.
   d. The drug is used as a first choice for treatment of sleeplessness.
   e. The patient needs to be evaluated for the drowsiness that may occur the morning after a benzodiazepine is taken.

7. A child is to receive phenobarbital 2 mg/kg IV on call as a preoperative sedative. The child weighs 29 kilograms (64 pounds). How many milligrams will the child receive for this dose?

Answers: 1. b, 2. c, 3. b, 4. a, 5. d, 6. c, e, 7. 58.2 mg

CRITICAL THINKING ACTIVITIES

1. A patient has a prescription for zopiclone (Imovane) because he has had trouble sleeping. The nurse is reviewing the use of this medication, and the patient says, "I've been drinking a glass of wine before bedtime to help me sleep. Can I still do that? This medication is not like Valium, right?" What is the nurse's best response?

2. During rounds on the night shift, the nurse finds a patient lying in bed, wide awake, at 0400 hours. The patient reports, "I can't sleep. I need my sleeping pill.

Can I have it now?" The patient's medication administration record has a prn (as needed) order for temazepam (Restoril). What is the nurse's priority action at this time?

3. The nurse is talking to a patient about what adverse effects to expect when taking a muscle relaxant for injuries the patient received in an automobile accident. What is the priority adverse effect the nurse needs to discuss with the patient? Explain your answer.

For answers see http://evolve.elsevier.com/Canada/Lilley/pharmacology/.

CHAPTER 14

Central Nervous System Stimulants and Related Drugs

Objectives

After reading this chapter, the successful student will be able to do the following:

1. Briefly review the anatomy, physiology, and functions of the central nervous system (CNS) with attention to the effects of stimulant on its function.

2. Understand the key terms as they relate to the central nervous system and stimulant drugs.

3. Identify the CNS stimulant drugs.

4. Discuss the mechanisms of action, indications, dosages, routes of administration, contraindications, cautions, drug interactions, adverse effects, and any related toxicities of the various CNS stimulants and related drugs.

5. Develop a collaborative plan of care based on the nursing process for patients using CNS stimulant and related drugs.

e-Learning Activities

Website
(http://evolve.elsevier.com/Canada/Lilley/pharmacology/)

evolve

- Answer Key—Textbook Case Studies
- Answer Key—Critical Thinking Activities
- Chapter Summaries—Printable
- Review Questions for Exam Preparation
- Unfolding Case Studies

Drug Profiles

▸▸ amphetamines, p. 273
    atomoxetine (atomoxetine hydrochloride)*, p. 273
▸▸ caffeine, p. 277
▸▸ methylphenidate (methylphenidate hydrochloride)*, p. 273
    modafinil, p. 273
    orlistat, p. 276
▸▸ sumatriptan, p. 276

▸▸ Key drug

*Full generic name is given in parentheses. For the purposes of this text, the more common, shortened name is used.

Key Terms

Amphetamines A class of stimulant drugs that includes amphetamine sulfate and all of its drug derivatives. (p. 270)

Analeptics CNS stimulants that have generalized effects on the brain stem and spinal cord, which produce an increase in responsiveness to external stimuli and stimulate respiration. (p. 275)

Anorexiants Drugs used to control or suppress appetite. (p. 271)

Attention deficit hyperactivity disorder (ADHD) A syndrome characterized by difficulty in maintaining concentration on a given task or hyperactive behaviour; may affect children, adolescents, and adults. The term *attention deficit disorder (ADD)* has been absorbed under this broader term. (p. 268)

Cataplexy A condition characterized by abrupt attacks of muscular weakness and hypotonia triggered by an emotional stimulus, such as joy, laughter, anger, fear, or surprise. It is often associated with narcolepsy. (p. 268)

Central nervous system (CNS) stimulants Drugs that stimulate specific areas of the brain or spinal cord. (p. 267)

Ergot alkaloids Drugs that narrow or constrict blood vessels in the brain and provide relief of pain for certain migraine headaches. (p. 272)

Migraine A common type of recurring painful headache characterized by a pulsatile or throbbing quality, incapacitating pain, and photophobia. (p. 269)

Narcolepsy A syndrome characterized by sudden sleep attacks, cataplexy, sleep paralysis, and visual or auditory hallucinations at the onset of sleep. (p. 268)

Serotonin receptor agonists A class of CNS stimulants used to treat migraines; work by stimulating 5-hydroxytryptamine 1 receptors in the brain and are sometimes referred to as *selective serotonin receptor agonists* or *triptans*. (p. 272)

Sympathomimetic drugs CNS stimulants such as noradrenergic drugs (and, to a lesser degree, dopaminergic drugs) whose actions resemble or mimic those of the sympathetic nervous system. (p. 267)

OVERVIEW

The central nervous system (CNS) is a complex system in the human body. Many therapeutic drugs either work in the CNS or cause adverse effects in the CNS. Activity of the CNS is regulated by a checks-and-balances system that consists of excitatory and inhibitory neurotransmitters and their corresponding receptors in the brain and spinal cord tissues. CNS stimulation results from either excessive stimulation of the excitatory neurons or blockade of the inhibitory neurons.

Central nervous system (CNS) stimulants are a broad class of drugs that stimulate specific areas of the brain or spinal cord. Most CNS stimulants act by stimulating the excitatory neurons in the brain. These neurons contain receptors for excitatory neurotransmitters, including dopamine (dopaminergic drugs), norepinephrine (adrenergic drugs), and serotonin (serotonergic drugs). Dopamine is a metabolic precursor of norepinephrine, which is also a neurotransmitter in the sympathetic nervous system. The actions of adrenergic drugs often resemble or mimic the actions of the sympathetic nervous system. For this reason, adrenergic drugs (and, to a lesser degree, dopaminergic drugs as well) are also called **sympathomimetic drugs**. Other sympathomimetic drugs are discussed further in Chapter 19.

CNS stimulant drugs are classified in three ways. The first is on the basis of chemical structural similarities. Major chemical classes of CNS stimulants include amphetamines, serotonin agonists, sympathomimetics, and xanthines (Table 14-1). Second, these drugs can be classified according to their site of therapeutic action in the CNS (Table 14-2). Finally, they can be categorized according to five major therapeutic usage categories for CNS stimulant drugs (Table 14-3). These include anti—attention deficit, antinarcoleptic, anorexiant, antimigraine, and analeptic drugs. There is some therapeutic overlap among these drug categories.

TABLE 14-1

Structurally Related CNS Stimulants

Chemical Category	CNS Stimulant
Amphetamines and related stimulants	amphetamine aspartate monohydrate, dextroamphetamine sulfate, lisdexanfetamine dimesylate, methylphenidate
Serotonin agonists	almotriptan malate, eletriptan hydrobromide, frovatriptan succinate, naratriptan hydrochloride, rizatriptan benzoate, sumatriptan succinate, zolmitriptan
Sympathomimetics	Not available in Canada
Xanthines	caffeine, theophylline, aminophylline
Miscellaneous	modafinil, sodium oxybate (CNS depressant), orlistat (lipase inhibitor)

TABLE 14-2

CNS Stimulants: Site of Action

CNS Stimulant	Site of Action
Serotonin agonists	Cerebrovascular system, $5\text{-HT}_{1D/1B}$ receptors
Amphetamines, phenidates, modafinil	Cerebral cortex
Anorexiants	Hypothalamic and limbic regions
Analeptics	Medulla and brain stem

TABLE 14-3

CNS Stimulants and Related Drugs: Therapeutic Categories

Category	Drugs
Anti-ADHD	amphetamine aspartate monohydrate, dextroamphetamine sulfate, methamphetamine hydrochloride, methylphenidate, atomoxetine (norepinephrine reuptake inhibitor)
Antinarcoleptic	dextroamphetamine (adjunct), methamphetamine hydrochloride, methylphenidate, sodium oxybate (CNS depressant used for cataplexy)
Anorexiant	methamphetamine hydrochloride, orlistat (lipase inhibitor)
Antimigraine (serotonin agonists)	almotriptan malate, eletriptan hydrobromide, frovatriptan succinate, naratriptan hydrochloride, rizatriptan benzoate, sumatriptan succinate, zolmitriptan
Analeptic	caffeine, aminophylline, theophylline, modafinil (antinarcoleptic)

ADHD, attention deficit hyperactivity disorder; *CNS*, central nervous system.

ATTENTION DEFICIT HYPERACTIVITY DISORDER

Attention deficit hyperactivity disorder (ADHD), formerly known as *attention deficit disorder (ADD)*, is the most commonly diagnosed neurodevelopmental disorder in children, affecting 3 to 10% of school-aged children. Boys are estimated to be affected from two to nine times as often as girls, although the disorder may be underdiagnosed in girls. Primary symptoms of ADHD centre on a developmentally inappropriate inability to maintain attention span along with the presence of hyperactivity and impulsivity. The disorder may involve predominantly attention deficit, predominantly hyperactivity or impulsivity, or a combination of both. It often begins before 7 years of age, sometimes earlier than 3 years. Previously, a diagnosis of ADHD required at least some symptoms of ADHD to have been present by age 7 years. This age criterion has been raised to the age of 12 years or earlier. Symptoms must be present for at least 6 months and occur in at least two different settings (e.g., home and school). For diagnosis in adults 17 years or older, five symptoms of either inattention or either hyperactivity or impulsivity are required. According to the *Diagnostic and Statistical Manual of Mental Disorders-5 (DSM-5)*, an individual with ADHD can have mild, moderate, or severe ADHD based on the number of symptoms an individual has and how difficult those symptoms make daily life. Many children outgrow ADHD, but adult ADHD is also common. New to the DSM-5 is that an individual can be diagnosed with ADHD and autism spectrum disorder. Drug therapy for both childhood and adult ADHD is essentially the same. There is some social controversy regarding the possible overdiagnosis of, and overmedication for, this disorder. Studies in twins indicate a degree of genetic predisposition and familial heritability. The disorder is commonly associated with other forms of mental health disorders, including depression, bipolar disorder, anxiety, and learning difficulties. Sleep and alertness difficulties have also been identified in children and adults with ADHD. It is unclear if ADHD stimulants directly affect sleep onset or if insomnia is a result of reduced blood concentrations of the drug at night, or if insomnia is a symptom of mental health comorbidities.

NARCOLEPSY

Narcolepsy is a common, disabling, incurable sleep disorder in which patients experience excessive daytime sleepiness (EDS) and may unexpectedly fall asleep in the middle of normal daily activities. As a consequence of sleepiness, patients may report inattention, poor memory, blurry vision, diplopia, and automatic behaviours such as driving without awareness. Another major symptom of the disease is dysfunctional rapid eye movement (REM) sleep. REM sleep manifestations that intrude into wakefulness include **cataplexy** (sudden loss of muscle tone triggered by strong emotions; commonly the knees buckle and the individual falls to the floor while still awake), sleep paralysis, *hypnagogic/hypnopompic hallucinations* (sensory events that occur at the transition from wakefulness to sleep), and sleep-onset REM periods. Men and women are equally affected. The prevalence of narcolepsy in Canada is approximately 1 in 2 000 individuals. Symptoms often begin during adolescence. Some genetic markers have been identified. Approximately one half of patients with narcolepsy experience migraine headaches as well.

OBESITY

Currently, there are approximately 7 million obese adults and 600 000 obese school-aged children in Canada. Prevalence estimates based on waist circumference indicate that 37% of adults and 13% of youth are abdominally obese (Janssen, 2013). The prevalence of obesity is expected to continue to rise at a predicted rate of 4 to 5% per year. Obesity was formerly defined as being 20% or more above one's ideal body weight, based on population statistics for height, body frame, and gender. More recent data are based on a measurement known as the body mass index (BMI), defined as weight in kilograms divided by height in metres squared (i.e., BMI = weight [kg] ÷ [height (m)]^2). *Overweight* is now defined as a BMI of 25 to 29.9, whereas *obesity* is now defined as a BMI of 30 or higher. Waist circumference is also a gauge of health risk associated with excess fat or central obesity around the waist. It provides an independent estimate of health risk beyond the BMI. A waist circumference of 102 cm or more in men or 88 cm or more in women is associated with increased health risks. Waist circumferences for each gender for Ethnicity-specific populations are associated with increased risks as follows: for people of European, Sub-Saharan African, Eastern Mediterranean and Middle Eastern (Arab) descent, greater than 94 cm for men and 80 cm for women respectively; for people of South Asian, Chinese, Japanese, South and Central American descent, greater than 90 cm for men and 80 cm for women, respectively. Moreover, the incidence of obesity in young people aged 6 to 19 years has more than doubled since 1980. Almost one in three children and adolescents is overweight (19.8%) or obese (11.8%). Most adolescents do not outgrow this problem and, in fact, many continue to gain excess weight. The pathophysiology of obesity is not fully understood, but calorie excess, disordered metabolism, inadequate sleep, and other factors are hypothesized. Obesity increases the risk for hypertension; dyslipidemia; coronary artery disease; stroke; type 2 diabetes mellitus; gallbladder disease; gout; osteoarthritis; sleep apnea; nonalcoholic fatty liver disease; and certain types of cancer, including breast and colon cancer. An estimated 80% of diabetes risk in Canada can be attributed to excess weight. The burden of obesity is estimated at $4.6 billion. Yet, many people who attempt weight loss do so for cosmetic reasons rather than health reasons. Obese people are often stigmatized, at times even by the health care providers treating them.

MIGRAINE

A **migraine** is a common type of recurring headache, usually lasting from 4 to 72 hours. Typical features include a pulsatile quality with pain that worsens with each pulse. The pain is most commonly unilateral but may occur on both sides of the head. Associated symptoms include nausea, vomiting, photophobia (avoidance of light), and phonophobia (avoidance of sounds). In addition, some migraines are accompanied by an aura, which is a predictive set of altered visual or other senses (formerly termed *classic migraine*). However, the majority of migraines are without an aura (formerly termed *common migraine*). Migraines affect about 8% of Canadians over the age of 12, with a reported incidence in females three times that in males. Migraines are most commonly experienced by both men and women between the ages of 25 and 39, although approximately 8% of children and adolescents suffer from migraines. Migraine headaches have been classified by the World Health Organization (WHO) as one of the 19 most disabling diseases worldwide. Migraines commonly begin after 10 years of age and peak between the mid-twenties and

early forties. They often fade after 50 years of age. Familial inheritance of migraine is well recognized, and environmental factors, stress, and psychological factors also play a role in the development of migraines. There are several conditions that coexist commonly with migraine headaches, including depression and anxiety, with risk increasing in those with daily headaches. Individuals who experienced adverse childhood events such as abuse and unfavourable family conditions, and whose symptoms are complicated by anxiety and depression, are more likely to experience disabling pain and be more challenging to treat.

Historically, there have been several theories regarding the cause of migraines, including the "vascular hypothesis" and the "neurovascular hypothesis"—most recent evidence points to decreased serotonin levels. Thus, the majority of current investigations involve drugs that can increase serotonin levels.

It is believed that repeated migraine attacks cause neuroplastic changes in the brain's structure and function over time, resulting in chronic daily headaches rather than episodic ones. These chronic migraines alter brain metabolism, cause atrophy of grey matter, and result in generalized hyperexcitability of the central nervous system, and central sensitization. Sensitization tends to progress from isolated trigeminal nerve throbbing pain to more centralized allodynia (i.e., resulting from a stimulus that does not normally cause pain). More severe allodynia may not respond to serotonin receptor agonists.

ANALEPTIC-RESPONSIVE RESPIRATORY DEPRESSION SYNDROMES

Neonatal apnea, or periodic cessation of breathing in newborn babies, is a common condition seen in neonatal intensive care units. It occurs in about 25% of premature infants whose pulmonary and CNS structures, including the medullary centres that control breathing, have not completed their gestational development because of preterm birth. Infants undergoing prolonged mechanical ventilation, especially at high pressures, often develop a chronic lung disease known as *bronchopulmonary dysplasia*, for which caffeine can be helpful. Postanaesthetic respiratory depression occurs when a patient's spontaneous respiratory drive does not resume adequately and in a timely manner after general anaesthesia. Respiratory depression may also be secondary to abuse of some drugs. Hypercapnia, or elevated blood levels of carbon dioxide, is often associated with later stages of chronic obstructive pulmonary disease (COPD). Analeptic drugs such as theophylline, aminophylline, and caffeine may be used to treat one or more of these conditions. Analeptic drugs are now used much less frequently than they were in the earlier days of general anaesthesia. This is because of advances in intensive respiratory care, including mechanical ventilation and improved anaesthetic techniques, as well as the availability of newer medications with less toxicity.

DRUGS FOR ATTENTION DEFICIT HYPERACTIVITY DISORDER AND NARCOLEPSY

CNS stimulants are the first-line drugs of choice for both ADHD and narcolepsy. They are potent drugs with a strong potential for tolerance and psychological dependence (addiction; see Chapter 18). They are classified as Schedule III drugs under the *Controlled Drugs and Substances Act*. Although there has been some public controversy regarding their use in ADHD, these drugs have led to a 65 to 75% improvement in symptoms in treated patients, compared with a placebo. In general, CNS stimulants elevate mood, produce a sense of increased energy and alertness, decrease appetite, and enhance task performance impaired by fatigue or boredom. Two of the oldest known stimulants are cocaine and amphetamine, which are prototypical drugs for this class. Caffeine, contained in coffee and tea, is another plant-derived CNS stimulant.

Amphetamine sulfate was first synthesized in the late 1800s. It was subsequently used to treat narcolepsy and then to prolong the alertness of soldiers during World War II. Later derivatives of this drug, which are still used clinically, include its d-isomer dextroamphetamine sulfate, methamphetamine hydrochloride, and mixed amphetamine salts—salts of both amphetamine and dextroamphetamine. They are often collectively referred to simply as *amphetamines*. Methylphenidate, a synthetic amphetamine derivative, was first introduced for the treatment of hyperactivity in children in 1958. Its d-isomer is the drug dexmethylphenidate. The phenidates are also Schedule III drugs. All of these amphetamine-related drugs are used to treat ADHD or narcolepsy. The sole nonamphetamine stimulant is modafinil.

Atomoxetine is a nonstimulant drug that is also used to treat ADHD. Atomoxetine is a norepinephrine reuptake inhibitor. Because it is not an amphetamine, it is associated with a low incidence of insomnia and has low misuse potential. Another advantage is that phone-in refills are allowed for this drug (as opposed to Schedule III drugs, which require a written prescription). One of the newest drugs in the ADHD arsenal is lisdexamfetamine dimesylate (Vyvanse®), recommended for use in children aged 6 to 12 years at a dosage of 30 mg once daily in the morning. It is a prodrug for dextroamphetamine, meaning it is converted in the body to dextroamphetamine.

Mechanism of Action and Drug Effects

Amphetamines stimulate areas of the brain associated with mental alertness, such as the cerebral cortex and the thalamus. Pharmacological actions of CNS stimulants are similar to the actions of the sympathetic nervous system, in that the CNS and respiratory systems are the primary body systems affected. CNS effects include mood elevation or euphoria, increased mental alertness and capacity for work, decreased fatigue and drowsiness, and prolonged wakefulness. The respiratory effects most commonly seen are relaxation of bronchial smooth muscle, increased respiration, and dilation of pulmonary arteries. Stringent controls have greatly reduced their medical use in Canada, as CNS stimulants are potent drugs with a strong potential for tolerance and psychological dependence. They are therefore classified as Schedule III drugs under the *Controlled Drugs and Substances Act* (see Legal & Ethical Principles on the proper handling of prescription drugs).

The amphetamines and phenidates increase the effects of norepinephrine and dopamine in CNS synapses by increasing their release and blocking their reuptake. As a result, both neurotransmitters are in contact with their receptors for longer, which lengthens their duration of action. The sole nonamphetamine stimulant available in Canada is modafinil (Alertec®). Modafinil is also

---

 LEGAL & ETHICAL PRINCIPLES

Handling of Prescription Drugs

It is important for nurses to understand the federal laws that apply to the handling of all prescription drugs by the registered nurse. (Note: This is a summary and does not reflect the laws in their entirety. Currently, nurse practitioners can prescribe in Canada. As well, in some provinces and territories, nurses can also dispense [see Chapter 3].)

The registered nurse is prohibited from doing the following:

- Compounding or dispensing the designated drugs for legal distribution and administration
- Distributing the drugs to any individuals who are not licensed or authorized by federal or provincial or

territorial law to receive the drugs (e.g., those individuals outside the health care provider–patient relationship); the penalties for such actions are generally severe.

- Making, selling, keeping, or concealing any counterfeit drug equipment
- Possessing any type of stimulant or depressant drug unless authorized to do so by a legal prescription (as a patient); any unauthorized possession is illegal

It is important to adhere to these legal guidelines in the practice of drug administration to avoid legal penalties, including possible loss of licensure or other severe penalties.

classified as an analeptic. It promotes wakefulness like the amphetamines and phenidates. It lacks sympathomimetic properties, however, and appears to work primarily by reducing gamma-aminobutyric acid (GABA)–mediated neurotransmission in the brain. (GABA is the principle inhibitory neurotransmitter in the brain.) The nonstimulant drug atomoxetine is also being used to treat ADHD. It works in the CNS by selective inhibition of norepinephrine reuptake.

Indications

Various amphetamine derivatives, including methylphenidate, are currently used to treat both ADHD and narcolepsy. The newer nonstimulant drug atomoxetine is also now used to treat ADHD. Amphetamine sulfate was also used to treat obesity in the early to mid-twentieth century. In Canada, amphetamines are not currently approved for this indication due to safety concerns. The nonamphetamine stimulant modafinil is indicated for narcolepsy. Specialists sometimes recommend periodic "drug holidays" (e.g., 1 day per week) without medication to diminish the addictive tendencies of the stimulant drugs. School-aged children often do not take these drugs on weekends or during school vacations.

Contraindications

Contraindications to the use of amphetamine and non-amphetamine stimulants include known drug allergy or cardiac structural abnormalities. These drugs can also exacerbate the following conditions: marked anxiety or agitation, Tourette's syndrome and other tic disorders (hyperstimulation), hypertension, and glaucoma (can increase intraocular pressure; see Chapter 57). The drugs must not be used in patients who have received therapy with any monoamine oxidase inhibitor (MAOI) in the preceding 14 days (see Chapter 16). Contraindications specific to atomoxetine include drug allergy, glaucoma, and recent MAOI use.

Adverse Effects

Both amphetamine and nonamphetamine stimulants have a wide range of adverse effects that most often arise when these drugs are administered at high doses. These drugs tend to "speed up" body systems. For example, effects on the cardiovascular system include increased heart rate and blood pressure. Other adverse effects include angina, anxiety, insomnia, headache, tremor, blurred vision, increased metabolic rate, gastrointestinal distress, dry mouth, and worsening of or new onset of psychiatric disorders, including mania, psychoses, or aggression. Common adverse effects associated with atomoxetine include headache, abdominal pain, vomiting, anorexia, and cough.

In 2015, Health Canada issued a safety communication with strong warnings on the risk of suicidal thoughts and behaviours related to all drugs used in the treatment of ADHD. Health Canada opinion is that the benefits of these drugs in the effective management of ADHD continue to outweigh their risks. The product monographs will now contain information about the possible occurrence of psychiatric adverse effects with ADHD drugs in a warning section. The need for focus on monitoring moods, behaviours, thoughts and feelings in adults and children taking these medications is highlighted, as is the significance of taking psychiatric disorders into account when prescribing these drugs.

Interactions

Drug interactions associated with these drugs vary greatly from class to class. Refer to Table 14-4 for a summary of some of the more common interactions for all drug classes in this chapter.

Dosages

For dosage information, refer to the table on p. 274.

ANOREXIANTS

By definition, an anorexiant is any substance that suppresses appetite. **Anorexiants** are CNS stimulant drugs used to promote weight loss in obesity; however, their effectiveness has not been proven. Stringent regulations have greatly reduced their medical use in Canada and none are currently approved for treating obesity. Orlistat (Xenical) is a related nonstimulant drug used to treat obesity. It works locally in the small and large intestines where it inhibits absorption of caloric intake from fatty foods.

Mechanism of Action and Drug Effects

Orlistat differs from other antiobesity drugs in that it is not a CNS stimulant. It works by irreversibly inhibiting the enzyme lipase. This results in reduced absorption of dietary fat from the intestinal tract and increased fat elimination in the feces.

Indications

Orlistat is to be used in conjunction with a mildly hypocaloric diet; it is indicated for obesity management, including weight loss, weight maintenance and reduction of the risk of weight regain after prior weight loss. Orlistat is for obese patients with a BMI of 30 or higher, or patients with a BMI of 27 or higher who are also hypertensive or have high cholesterol or type 2 diabetes.

Contraindications

Orlistat is contraindicated in patients with known drug allergy, chronic malabsorption syndrome (e.g. Crohn's disease, colitis, short bowel syndrome) or cholestasis.

Adverse Effects

The most common adverse effects of orlistat include headache, upper respiratory tract infection (mechanism

TABLE 14-4			
CNS Stimulants: Common Drug Interactions			
Drug	**Interacting Drugs**	**Mechanism**	**Result**
AMPHETAMINE AND NONAMPHETAMINE STIMULANTS			
Amphetamines (various salts), methylphenidate	CNS stimulants	Additive toxicities	Cardiovascular adverse effects, nervousness, insomnia
	MAOIs	Increased release of catecholamines	Headaches, dysrhythmias, severe hypertension
Atomoxetine	Sympathomimetic drugs	Enhanced SNS effects	Cardiovascular adverse effects (dysrhythmias, tachycardia, hypertension)
	CYP2D6 inhibitors (MAOIs, paroxetine)	Reduced metabolism of atomoxetine	Enhanced atomoxetine toxicity
ANOREXIANTS AND ANALEPTICS			
phentermine	CNS stimulants	Additive toxicities	Nervousness, insomnia, seizures
	MAOIs	Increased release of catecholamines	Headaches, dysrhythmias, severe hypertension
	Serotonergic drugs	Additive toxicity	Cardiovascular adverse effects, nervousness, insomnia, convulsions
SEROTONIN AGONISTS			
sumatriptan and others	Ergot alkaloids, SSRIs, MAOIs	Additive toxicity	Cardiovascular adverse effects, nervousness, insomnia, convulsions
ERGOT ALKALOIDS			
dihydroergotamine mesylate (DHT®)	Protease inhibitors, azole antifungals, macrolide antibiotics	Increased ergot levels	Acute ergot toxicity, nausea, vomiting, hypotension or hypertension, seizures, coma, death; use with ergot alkaloids is contraindicated

CNS, central nervous system; *CYP2D6,* cytochrome P450 enzyme 2D6; *MAOIs,* monoamine oxidase inhibitor; *SNS,* sympathetic nervous system; *SSRIs,* selective serotonin reuptake inhibitors.

uncertain), and gastrointestinal distress, including fecal incontinence.

Interactions

Drug interactions for orlistat are listed in Table 14-4.

Dosages

For dosage information, refer to the table on p. 274.

ANTIMIGRAINE DRUGS

Serotonin receptor agonists, first introduced in the 1990s, have revolutionized the treatment of migraine headache. They work by stimulating serotonin receptors in the brain. They include sumatriptan succinate (Imitrex), almotriptan malate (Axert®), eletriptan hydrobromide (Relpax®), naratriptan hydrochloride (Amerge®), rizatriptan benzoate (Maxalt®), zolmitriptan (Zomig®), and frovatriptan succinate (Frova®). Collectively, these drugs are referred to as *triptans.* They are to be used cautiously in patients with severe cardiovascular disease (especially angina pectoris). Historically, **ergot alkaloids** were the mainstay of migraine headaches treatment, but these have been replaced by the triptans for first-line therapy. The ergot alkaloids are obtained from a fungus and cause vasoconstriction of dilated blood vessels in the brain and the carotid arteries. They are contraindicated in patients with peripheral vascular disease, coronary artery disease, sepsis, impaired renal or hepatic function, or severe hypertension.

Mechanism of Action and Drug Effects

The chemical name for serotonin is 5-hydroxytryptamine, or 5-HT. Physiologists have further identified two 5-HT receptor subtypes on which these drugs have their greatest effect: 5-HT_{1B} and 5-HT_{1D}. Triptans stimulate these receptors in cerebral arteries, causing vasoconstriction and normally reducing or eliminating headache symptoms. They also reduce the production of inflammatory neuropeptides. This is known as *abortive* drug therapy because it treats a headache that has already started. Ergot alkaloids also narrow or constrict blood vessels in the brain. Although the cause of migraines is not fully understood, they are thought to be related to abnormal dilation of the blood vessels within the brain.

Indications

The triptan antimigraine drugs, also referred to as *selective serotonin receptor agonists (SSRAs),* are indicated for abortive therapy of an acute migraine headache. Although

DRUG PROFILES

Amphetamines and Related Stimulants

The principal drugs used to treat ADHD and narcolepsy are the amphetamines and nonamphetamine stimulants. Atomoxetine, a nonstimulant drug, is also used for ADHD.

▶▶ amphetamines

The various amphetamine salts are the prototypical CNS stimulants used to treat ADHD and narcolepsy. Amphetamine is available in prescription form only for oral use, as dextroamphetamine sulfate (Dexedrine®) and amphetamine aspartate monohydrate (Adderall®).

PHARMACOKINETICS

Route	Onset of Action	Peak Plasma Concentration	Elimination Half-Life	Duration of Action
PO	30–60 min	90–120 min	7–14 hr	10 hr

▶▶ methylphenidate hydrochloride

Methylphenidate hydrochloride (Ritalin®) was the first prescription drug indicated for ADHD and continues to be the most widely prescribed drug for its treatment. It is also used to treat narcolepsy. Extended-release (XR) dosage forms include Ritalin SR®, Concerta®, and Biphetin® and are often preferred over the immediate-release (IR) stimulants. Short-acting stimulants peak after several hours and must be taken two to three times a day, compared with the longer-acting or extended-release stimulants which last for 8 to 12 hours and are usually taken once a day. Children with ADHD taking XR stimulant medication are less likely to visit an emergency room and also less likely to be hospitalized (and are hospitalized for a shorter period of time) than those initially prescribed IR stimulants. This may be due to improved adherence and the resulting effectiveness or as a result of the prolonged therapeutic effect of the XR medications, leading to fewer inattentive or impulsive behaviours in the evening. However, the XR drugs may not be covered by public or private drug plans.

There is some controversy regarding drug therapy for ADHD. Some parents may be understandably apprehensive regarding this type of drug therapy. However, with proper diagnosis of the disorder, proper dosing of the drug, and regular medical monitoring, many children can achieve significant improvement in school performance and social skills. Psychosocial problems within a child's family need to be ruled out or addressed if they are contributing to the child's problems, regardless of whether the medication is prescribed.

PHARMACOKINETICS (IMMEDIATE RELEASE)

Route	Onset of Action	Peak Plasma Concentration	Elimination Half-Life	Duration of Action
PO	30–60 min	6–8 hr	1—3 hr	4–6 hr

atomoxetine hydrochloride

Atomoxetine hydrochloride (Strattera®) is approved for treating ADHD in children older than 6 years of age and in adults. This medication is not a controlled substance because it lacks addictive properties, unlike amphetamines and phenidates. For this reason, it has rapidly gained popularity as a therapeutic option for treating ADHD. However, Health Canada and the drug manufacturer did issue a warning describing cases of suicidal thinking and behaviour in a small number of adolescent patients receiving this medication, similar to its previous warnings regarding adolescent use of antidepressant medications (Chapter 17). With each prescription or refill of Strattera, pharmacists are to provide the medicine guide to patients, families, or caregivers. Health care providers are advised to work with parents in providing prudent monitoring of any young patients taking this medication and to promptly re-evaluate patients showing any behavioural symptoms of concern.

PHARMACOKINETICS

Route	Onset of Action	Peak Plasma Concentration	Elimination Half-Life	Duration of Action
PO	60 min	1–2 hr	5–24 hr	24–120 hr

modafinil

Modafinil (Alertec) is indicated for improvement of wakefulness in patients with excessive daytime sleepiness associated with narcolepsy and also with shift work sleep disorder. It has less misuse potential than amphetamines and methylphenidate and is available by prescription.

PHARMACOKINETICS

Route	Onset of Action	Peak Plasma Concentration	Elimination Half-Life	Duration of Action
PO	1–2 months for therapeutic effect	2–4 hr	8–15 hr	Unknown

they may be taken during aura symptoms in patients who have auras with their headaches, these drugs are not indicated for preventive migraine therapy. Preventive therapy is indicated if migraine attacks occur one or more days per week. A variety of drugs are used for preventive therapy; most of them are discussed in more detail in other chapters. First-line drugs for preventive therapy include propranolol (see Chapter 20), amitriptyline (see Chapter 17), valproic acid, and topiramate (see Chapter 15). Second-line therapies include the ergot alkaloid dihydroergotamine mesylate (DHE®); nonsteroidal anti-inflammatory drugs, including naproxen (see Chapter 49); calcium channel blockers; and angiotensin receptor blockers (see Chapter 23). In many cases, preventive drug therapy is sufficient to prevent a full-blown migraine. However, when prevention fails, treatment is needed,

DOSAGES Selected CNS Stimulants and Related Drugs

Drug	Pharmacological Class	Usual Dosage Range	Indications/Uses
▸▸amphetamine aspartate monohydrate (mixed salts) (Adderall XR®)	CNS stimulant	*Children 6–12 yr* PO: 5–10 mg once daily in morning, increased weekly until desired effect to a daily max of 30 mg *Adolescents 13–17 yr, Adults* PO: 10 mg once daily in morning, increased weekly to a daily max of 20 mg (not to exceed 30 mg/day)	ADHD, narcolepsy
atomoxetine hydrochloride (Strattera)	Selective norepinephrine reuptake inhibitor	*Children 6 yr and older, adolescents (less than 70 kg)* PO: 0.5–1.4 mg/kg/day divided once or twice daily *Children/Adolescents/Adults (70 kg or more)* PO: 40–100 mg/day divided once or twice daily	ADHD
methylphenidate hydrochloride, extended-release (Concerta)	CNS stimulant	*Children 6–12/adolescents 13–18* PO: 18–54 mg/day, single dose *Adults over 18* PO: 18–72 mg/day, single dose	ADHD
▸▸methylphenidate hydrochloride (Ritalin, Ritalin SR)	CNS stimulant	*Children/adolescents, 6 yr and older* PO: 5–10 mg tid, max 60 mg *Adults* PO: 20–60 mg/day divided bid–tid	ADHD ADHD
modafinil (Alertec)	CNS stimulant	*Adult over 18* PO: 200mg qAM; if second dose is needed, give at noon	Narcolepsy
orlistat (Xenical®)	Lipase inhibitor	*Adults* PO: 120 mg tid with each meal	Obesity
▸▸sumatriptan (Imitrex®, Imitrex DF®)	Serotonin receptor agonist	*Adults* PO: 50 mg, repeat after 2 hr to max 200 mg/day Subcut: 6 mg, repeat in 1 hr; max 12 mg/day) Nasal spray: 5–20 mg, repeat after 2 hr; max 40 mg/day	Acute migraine with or without aura

ADHD, attention deficit hyperactivity disorder; *CNS*, central nervous system.

and the triptans are the most commonly prescribed drug class. Another frequently used product for abortive therapy is Fiorinal®, a combination of either acetaminophen or aspirin, plus the barbiturate butalbital, plus the analeptic caffeine. In addition to potentiating the effects of the analgesics, caffeine can also enhance intestinal absorption of the ergot alkaloids and has a vasoconstricting effect, which can reduce cerebral blood flow to ease headache pain. Caffeine also has a diuretic effect, which may ultimately also reduce cerebral blood flow, owing to reduced vascular volume secondary to enhanced urinary output.

Contraindications

Contraindications to triptans include known drug allergy and the presence of serious cardiovascular disease, because of the vasoconstrictive potential of these medications. Contraindications to the use of ergot alkaloids include uncontrolled hypertension; cerebral, cardiac, or peripheral vascular disease; dysrhythmias; glaucoma; and coronary or ischemic heart disease.

Adverse Effects

Triptans have potential vasoconstrictor effects, including effects on coronary circulation. Injectable dosage forms may cause local irritation at the site of injection. Other adverse effects include tingling, flushing (skin warmth and redness), or a congested feeling in the head or chest. Ergot alkaloids are associated with the adverse effects of nausea, vomiting, cold or clammy hands and feet, muscle pain, dizziness, numbness, a vague feeling of anxiety, a bitter or foul taste in the mouth or throat, and irritation of the nose (with the nasal spray dosage form). Overuse of abortive therapy may result in rebound headaches.

Interactions

Drug interactions for antimigraine drugs are presented in Table 14-4.

Dosages

For dosage information, refer to the table on p. 274.

EVIDENCE IN PRACTICE

Ibuprofen May Help Relieve Acute Migraine Headaches

Review

Migraine headache is a common, disabling condition that has a major impact on individuals, health care services, and society. Many migraine sufferers do not seek proper medical attention and often rely on the use of over-the-counter (OTC) medications. The goal of this review of literature is to assess the effectiveness and tolerability of ibuprofen on migraine headaches in adults. Additionally, this review is to assess ibuprofen when given as monotherapy or together with an antiemetic, as compared to placebo treatment or other drug treatment for the relief of acute migraines in adults.

Type of Evidence

The investigators searched the databases of Cochrane CENTRAL, MEDLINE, and EMBASE, as well as the Oxford Pain Relief Database. These sources were used to identify studies published through April 2010 about ibuprofen and migraines. Criteria used to determine inclusion included randomized, double-blind trials of self-given ibuprofen versus active comparators to treat a migraine episode with outcome data for at least 10 participants per treatment group. Once data were collected, two independent investigators performed a methodological trial from which nine studies comparing ibuprofen and placebo or other active drugs were identified. Over 4 300 participants were studied for a total of over 5 220 migraine attacks. Of these studies, none were representative of the protocol of using ibuprofen and an antiemetic. Single doses of medications were used to treat all the attacks. Relative risk and number needed to treat (NNT) or harm versus placebo or other active drug were calculated from the participants.

Results of Study

When comparing ibuprofen 400 mg with use of the placebo, the NNTs were 7.2 for 2 hours pain-free (26% versus 12%), 3.2 for 2 hours of headache relief (57% versus 25%), and 4.0 for 24-hour sustained headache relief (45% versus 19%). Ibuprofen 200 mg versus the placebo showed that the NNTs were 9.7 for 2 hours pain-free (20% versus 10%) and 6.3 for 2 hours of headache relief (52% versus 37%). The ibuprofen dose of 400 mg offered significantly better 2-hour headache relief than the 200-mg dose, and the soluble dosage forms of ibuprofen offered better 1-hour relief but not the 2-hour headache relief, as compared to standard tablet dosage forms. Another set of symptoms that was looked at included nausea, vomiting, photophobia, phonophobia, and functional disability. These symptoms were reduced within 2 hours with the ibuprofen versus placebo. Additionally, fewer participants used rescue medication. Side effects were mostly mild and temporary and occurred similarly in participants across treatment groups. The major limitation of this review includes weaknesses inherent in the reviewed studies, as well as the fact that a small number of events were used to calculate some of the results.

Link of Evidence to Nursing Practice

About 8% of the Canadian population over the age of 12 experience migraines with significant impacts on quality of life. Migraine management remains a huge challenge for health care providers and has a subsequent negative impact on health care costs. As migraines have been classified as one of the 19 most disabling diseases worldwide, adequate management or treatment is crucial to patient quality of life and to helping trim the costs of health care. Ibuprofen has been identified as an effective treatment for acute migraine headaches, leading to pain relief in about 50% of sufferers but only complete relief from pain (and other symptoms) in a minority of participants. This review is just one example of the need for more effective studies with larger sample sizes. Additionally, there is a need for further studies on migraines, looking at a variety of outcomes for pain relief, types of management, and multi-symptom management. Dosage formulations and their advantages and effectiveness also need to be studied. Nurse researchers need to continue to take the lead in identifying patient problems as well as help to identify a variety of medical, holistic, and alternative approaches to their short- and long-term treatment.

Reference: Rabbie, R., Derry, S., Moore, R. A., et al. (2010). Ibuprofen with or without an antiemetic for acute migraine headaches in adults. *Cochrane Database of Systematic Reviews, 2010*(10). doi:10.1002/14651858.CD008039.pub2

ANALEPTICS

Analeptics include the methylxanthines aminophylline, theophylline, and caffeine. The drugs are mentioned here, although they are in use to treat neonatal and postoperative respiratory depression. Postoperative respiratory depression is a less common problem today due to the design of newer anaesthetic drugs with shorter durations of action.

Mechanism of Action and Drug Effects

Analeptics work by stimulating areas of the CNS that control respiration, mainly the medulla and spinal cord. Methylxanthine analeptics (caffeine, aminophylline, and theophylline) also inhibit the enzyme phosphodiesterase. This enzyme breaks down a substance called cyclic adenosine monophosphate (cAMP). When analeptics block this enzyme, cAMP accumulates. This results in relaxation of smooth muscle in the respiratory tract, dilation of pulmonary arterioles, and stimulation of the CNS in general. Aminophylline is a prodrug (a drug that is formulated for greater solubility to facilitate administration but must be metabolized to an active form); it is hydrolyzed to theophylline in the body. Theophylline, in turn, is metabolized to caffeine. Caffeine is inherently a

DRUG PROFILES

Anorexiants

Amphetamine salts are no longer used for treatment of obesity because of their high misuse potential. The non-stimulant drug orlistat, a lipase inhibitor, is available by prescription.

orlistat

Orlistat (Xenical) works by binding to gastric and pancreatic enzymes called *lipases*. Blocking these enzymes reduces fat absorption by approximately 30%. Restricting dietary intake of fat to less than 30% of total calories can help reduce some of the gastrointestinal adverse effects, which include oily spotting, flatulence, and fecal incontinence in 20 to 40% of patients. Decreases in serum concentrations of vitamins A, D, and E and β-carotene are seen as a result of the blocking of fat absorption. Supplementation with fat-soluble vitamins corrects this deficiency.

PHARMACOKINETICS

Route	Onset of Action	Peak Plasma Concentration	Elimination Half-Life	Duration of Action
PO	3 mo for therapeutic effect	6–8 hr	1–2 hr	Unknown

DRUG PROFILES

Serotonin Receptor Agonists

Serotonin receptor agonists are used to treat migraine headache. They can produce relief from moderate to severe migraines within 2 hours in 70 to 80% of patients. They work by stimulating 5-HT$_1$ receptors in the brain. They are available in a variety of formulations, including oral tablets, sublingual tablets, subcutaneous self-injections, and nasal sprays. A common effect of migraines is nausea and vomiting. Orally administered medications are therefore not tolerated by some patients. Non-oral (including sublingual) forms are advantageous for this reason. They also often have a more rapid onset of action, producing relief in some patients in 10 to 15 minutes, compared with 1 to 2 hours for tablets taken orally. For dosage information, refer to the table on p. 274.

▶▶sumatriptan

Sumatriptan (Imitrex) was the original prototype drug for this class. There are now seven triptans. Slight pharmacokinetic differences exist between some of these products, but their effects are comparable overall.

PHARMACOKINETICS

Route	Onset of Action	Peak Plasma Concentration	Elimination Half-Life	Duration of Action
PO	0.5–1 hr	2.5 hr	2.5 hr	4 hr

ERGOT ALKALOIDS

Ergot alkaloids, such as ergotamine, are still used in the treatment and prevention of migraines but are rapidly being replaced by the triptans. Dihydroergotamine mesylate (DHE) is available in injectable form and as a nasal spray (Migranal®).

stronger CNS stimulant, hence its popularity in coffee, tea, and soft drinks. It also helps to potentiate the effects of analgesics used for migraine therapy and has a diuretic effect. The stimulant effects of caffeine are attributed to its antagonism (blocking) of adenosine receptors in the brain. Adenosine is associated with sleep promotion.

Indications

Analeptics are used primarily to stimulate respirations.

Contraindications

Contraindications to the use of analeptics include drug allergy, peptic ulcer disease (especially for caffeine), and serious cardiovascular conditions. Concurrent use of other phosphodiesterase-inhibiting drugs such as sildenafil and similar drugs is also not recommended.

Adverse Effects

At higher dosages, analeptics stimulate the vagal, vasomotor, and respiratory centres of the medulla in the brain stem, as well as skeletal muscles. Vagal effects include stimulation of gastric secretions, diarrhea, and reflex tachycardia. Vasomotor effects are flushing (warmth, redness) and sweating of the skin. Respiratory effects include elevated respiratory rate (which is normally desired). Skeletal muscle effects are muscular tension and tremors. Neurological effects include reduced deep tendon reflexes.

Interactions

Drug interactions for the analeptics are presented in Table 14-4.

Dosages

For dosage information, refer to the table on p. 274.

DRUG PROFILES

Analeptic drugs include the methylxanthines aminophylline, theophylline, and caffeine. The profiles for aminophylline and theophylline can be found in Chapter 38. The antinarcoleptic drug modafinil is discussed in the Narcolepsy section of this chapter.

▶▶ *caffeine*

Caffeine is a CNS stimulant that can be found in over-thecounter drugs and combination prescription drugs. It is also contained in many beverages and foods. A few of the many foods and drugs that contain caffeine are listed in Table 14-5. Caffeine is contraindicated in patients with a known hypersensitivity to it and should be used with

caution in patients who have recently suffered a myocardial infarction or who have a history of peptic ulcers or cardiac dysrhythmias. In Canada, pure caffeine is regulated as a food additive. It may only be added to carbonated soft drinks and it must be declared in the ingredients list on the product label. Caffeine may not be added to any other food. It is available in oral forms.

PHARMACOKINETCS

Route	Onset of Action	Peak Plasma Concentration	Elimination Half-Life	Duration of Action
PO	15–45 min	1 hr	3–4 hr	6 hr

TABLE 14-5

Caffeine-Containing Foods and Drugs

Medication or Beverage	Amount of Caffeine
SELECTED NONPRESCRIPTION MEDICATIONS	
Analgesics	
acetaminophen compound caplets or tablets with 8 mg codeine (Atasol®, Extrol-8®)	15–30 mg/caplet or tab
acetylsalicylic acid 325 mg with caffeine 32 mg (Anacin); acetylsalicylic acid 500 mg with caffeine 32 mg (Anacin Extra-Strength®)	32 mg/tab
acetylsalicylic acid compound tablets with 8 mg codeine (A.C. & C. Tablets)	15–30 mg/tab
acetaminophen 500 mg with caffeine 65 mg (Excedrin Extra-Strength®)	65 mg/tab
PRESCRIPTION MEDICATIONS (FOR MIGRAINE)	
acetylsalicylic acid 330 mg, butalbital 50 mg, caffeine 40 mg, codeine phosphate 30 mg (Fiorinal C1/2®)	40 mg/tab

Beverages	Amount of Caffeine
Cocoa	5–40 mg/237 mL (1 cup)
Coffee (brewed)	135 mg/237 mL (1 cup)
Coffee (decaffeinated)	3 mg/237 mL (1 cup)
Coffee (instant)	76–106 mg/237 mL (1 cup)
Cola beverage (regular)	36–46 mg/355 mL (1 can)
Cola beverage (diet)	39–50 mg/355 mL (1 can)
Tea (brewed, average blend)	43 mg/237 mL (1 cup)
Supplemented water (Red Bull®, Amp Energy®, Rockstar®, Monster Energy®)	80–100 mg /250 mL (1 can)

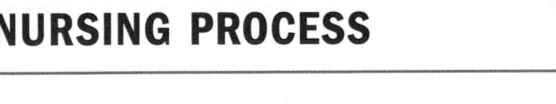

NURSING PROCESS

✐ Assessment

CNS stimulants are used for a variety of conditions and disorders. They have addictive potential, and so the following assessment data need to be collected before CNS stimulant use, regardless of indication: (1) a thorough medical history with attention to pre-existing diseases or conditions, especially those of the cardiovascular, cerebrovascular, neurological, renal, and hepatic systems; (2)

past and current history of addictive or substance misuse behaviours; (3) complete medication profile with a listing of prescription, over-the-counter, and natural health products and any use of alcohol, nicotine, or social or illegal drugs; and (4) a complete nutritional and dietary history. Assess all of these areas because of the mechanism of action of CNS stimulants, which increases pulse rate and blood pressure and can lead to seizures, intracerebral bleeding, and toxicity (due to decreased drug metabolism and excretion). Stimulation of the respiratory system is actually desirable, and this action is beneficial in those patients suffering from CNS depression, such as postoperatively. Improvement of attention span is beneficial for those in need of the medication, but the

NATURAL HEALTH PRODUCTS

SELECTED HERBAL COMPOUNDS USED FOR NERVOUS SYSTEM STIMULATION

Common Name(s)	Uses	Possible Drug Interactions (Avoid Concurrent Use)
Ginkgo biloba, ginkgo	To enhance mental alertness; to improve memory or reduce dementia	Warfarin sodium, aspirin
Ginseng	To enhance impaired mental function and concentration	Drugs for diabetes that lower blood sugar (e.g., insulin, oral hypoglycemic drugs), monoamine oxidase inhibitors
Guarana	To stimulate nervous system, suppress appetite	Adenosine, quinolones, oral contraceptives, β-blockers, iron, lithium carbonate, phenylephrine maleate (e.g., nasal spray), cimetidine, theophylline, tobacco

possibility of adverse effects requires a thorough assessment to obtain baseline information. The anorexiant action may cause complications if the drugs are used or ordered inappropriately. When these drugs are taken for appetite suppression, assess and document baseline height, weight, and dietary intake. Measure vital signs with specific attention to blood pressure and pulse rate whenever these drugs are used.

To add to the thoroughness of the assessment, include in your nursing history the following information: inquiry about lifestyle, exercise, nutritional habits and patterns, (e.g., a reduction in fat-soluble vitamins, history of any type of eating disorder), educational level, previous teaching and learning successes and failures, available support structures (e.g., family and friends), self-esteem, stress levels, mental status and mental health problems (drugs may exacerbate psychosis), presence of diabetes (patients with diabetes need closer monitoring and tighter glucose control when taking stimulant medications due to increased glycogenolysis), and information related to contraindications, cautions, and drug interactions (see Table 14-4).

With drugs used for the management of ADHD, cautiously and continuously assess the patient. For pediatric patients, gather the following information during assessment: baseline weight, height, growth and development patterns, and vital signs. Complete blood counts may be ordered. Thoroughly document any changes in emotional status as well. Adults also require thorough assessment of baseline weight, height, and vital signs. Assess and document usual sleep habits and patterns so that sleep disturbances may be anticipated and managed appropriately. Atypical behaviour, loss of attention span, and history of social problems or problems in school are also important to assess and document before and during therapy for baseline comparison. For children with ADHD, parental support is important to the success of treatment; therefore, a home assessment may be needed. Attention to and documentation of daily dietary intake before drug therapy is initiated is important because of the risk of drug-related weight loss. It is also important

that the pediatric patient not experience too rapid or too much weight loss; a thorough nutritional and dietary assessment is needed. Cardiac assessment is important because of CNS stimulation. Blood pressure, pulse rate, heart sounds, and any history of chest pain or palpitations must be noted. Other data to gather during assessment include possible contraindications, cautions, and drug interactions (see previous discussion). Document findings and note the patient's use of any prescription drugs, over-the-counter drugs (e.g., nasal decongestants, which are also stimulants), and natural health products, specifically ginseng and caffeine (see Natural Health Products: Selected Herbal Compounds Used for Nervous System Stimulation above).

The serotonin receptor agonists commonly used in the treatment of migraines are not without adverse reactions, contraindications, cautions, and drug interactions (see previous discussion). Include in the assessment a thorough cardiac history as well as measurement of blood pressure, pulse rate, and rhythm. If a patient has a history of hypertension, there is risk of further increases in blood pressure to dangerous levels with use of these drugs; hence the need for careful assessment and documentation. In fact, generally these drugs are not prescribed for patients with migraines who also have coronary artery disease unless a thorough heart evaluation has been performed. Conduct a careful assessment to identify other drugs the patient is taking that might lead to significant drug interactions, such as ergot alkaloids, selective serotonin receptor inhibitors, and MAOIs. If serotonin agonists are taken within 2 weeks of the use of these drugs, there is high risk for an additive toxicity. Such toxicity would be manifested by nervousness, insomnia, cardiovascular complications, and convulsions (serotonin syndrome).

Ergot alkaloids also have cautions, contraindications, and drug interactions (see previous discussion), which you need to assess for and document. Obtain a history of the migraines and their pattern, exacerbating factors, measures that provide relief, and previous treatments.

Analeptics are used as central respiratory stimulants. The same concerns regarding contraindications, cautions, and drug interactions exist for this drug as for all CNS stimulants, and even closer attention must be paid to vital signs, especially heart rate, rhythm, and blood pressure. Any elevations in blood pressure and pulse rate may put the patient at a higher risk of complications. Perform a thorough neurological assessment with specific attention to any possibility of seizures. Assess baseline deep tendon reflexes, and document for comparative purposes.

Nursing Diagnoses

- Decreased cardiac output related to the adverse effects of CNS stimulants (e.g., palpitations and tachycardia)
- Imbalanced nutrition, less than body requirements, related to adverse effects of CNS stimulants (e.g., amphetamines and anorexiants)
- Chronic pain related to the experience of or a history of migraine headaches
- Disturbed sleep patterns related to the action and adverse effects of CNS stimulants

Planning

Goals

- Patient will remain free of cardiac symptoms and adverse effects.
- Patient's nutritional status will remain intact and without excess weight loss.
- Patient will regain adequate comfort level with adequate and efficient management of migraines.
- Patient will experience minimal disturbed sleep patterns.

Expected Patient Outcomes

- Patient vital signs, especially blood pressure (120/80) and pulse rate (60 to 100) remain within normal limits and without major fluctuations or changes.
- Patient states symptoms (e.g., palpitations, chest pain) that need to be reported to the prescriber immediately.
- Patient maintains appropriate weight without too rapid losses during drug therapy regimen.
- Patient regains or maintains near-normal body weight and BMI during therapy.
- Patient continues to undergo close-to-normal growth and development while taking medications.
- Patient reports a decrease in headaches and improved well-being and participation in activities of daily living while taking medications as prescribed.
- Patient reports minimal adverse effects from antimigraine medications.

- Patient states improved quality of life with efficient and adequate self-administration of medication.
- Patient experiences more restful sleep while experiencing efficient drug therapy.
- Patient uses nonpharmacological measures to enhance sleep, such as massage, biofeedback, music therapy, relaxation breathing, and keeping the room quiet and at a comfortable temperature.

Implementation

With drugs used for the treatment of attention deficit hyperactivity disorder, some pediatric patients may respond better to certain dosage forms, such as immediate release. However, dosing needs to be individualized and based on the patient's needs at different times during the school day (e.g., a noon dose to help with music lessons later in the afternoon). Well-planned scheduling of these medications and close communication among the school, teachers, school nurse, and the family and patient is very important to successful treatment. It is also important to time the dosing of medications—as ordered—for periods in which symptom control is most needed but without causing alterations in sleep patterns. In general, once-a-day dosing is used with extended-release or long-acting preparations. Adequate and proper dosing will be manifested by good control of inattentive or impulsive behaviour during school time. If extended-release dosage forms lead to acceptable outcomes for the pediatric patient, taking medications at school may not be necessary. Often, a stigma is associated with taking medications at school. The need to do so may be avoided with the use of long-acting preparations or other scheduling. To help decrease the occurrence of insomnia, it is recommended that the last daily dose be taken 4 to 6 hours before bedtime, as ordered. During therapy, monitor the patient for continued physical growth, with specific attention to weight and height. The prescriber may order medication-free times on weekends, holidays, or vacations; that is, the drug may be discontinued periodically so that the need for the medication can be reassessed and sensitivity increased.

Because anorexiants are generally used for a short period, emphasize to the patient and all members of the patient's support system that a suitable diet, appropriate independent or supervised exercise program, and behavioural modifications are necessary to support a favourable outcome and to help the patient cease overeating and experience healthy weight loss. With a drug regimen, medications are usually taken first thing in the morning, as ordered, to minimize interference with sleep. Therefore, it is recommended that these drugs not be taken within 4 to 6 hours of sleep. If the patient has been taking anorexiants for a prolonged period, an interval period of weaning upon discontinuation is needed to avoid withdrawal symptoms and any chance of a rebound increase in appetite. Weight must be assessed weekly or as ordered. Encourage the patient to keep a journal with a record of food intake as well as responses to the drug regimen, any adverse effects, socialization, exercise, and mood. Dry mouth may be managed with frequent mouth care and the use of sugar-free gum or hard candy. Sucking ice chips, as well as keeping a bottle of fresh water on hand at all times, may also be helpful. If headaches occur, acetaminophen will most likely be suggested. Caffeine in any form needs to be avoided, including coffee, tea, sodas, and chocolate. Other products that may contain caffeine include some over-the-counter analgesics; over-the-counter compounds to treat menstrual symptoms; over-the-counter products for cough, cold, flu, or congestion; and prescription drugs such as analgesics with ergotamine and caffeine, and butalbital with aspirin and caffeine. Supplementation with fat-soluble vitamins may be indicated with use of these drugs. It is also important to watch for tolerance to the anorexiant during the course of treatment. Other nursing considerations include emphasis on a holistic approach to the treatment of obesity, including the possible use of hypnosis, biofeedback, and guided imagery, as ordered. Encourage patients to keep follow-up visits with all those involved in their care.

SSRAs are available in a variety of dosage forms. Rizatriptan is available in a disintegrating tablet or a wafer that dissolves on the tongue. The latter dosage form leads to more rapid absorption. Use of the nasal spray or self-injectable forms of the serotonin agonists is especially desirable in patients experiencing the nausea and vomiting that may occur with migraine headaches. Self-injectable forms and nasal sprays also have the benefit of an onset of action of 10 to 15 minutes, compared with 1 to 2 hours with tablet forms. Administration of a test dose of the injectable and all other dosage forms is usually recommended. If the injectable form is prescribed, provide instructions and demonstrations of the technique. Refer to Patient Teaching Tips for more information.

Ergot alkaloids should be taken exactly as prescribed; for example, tablets need to be taken with 180 to 240 mL (6 to 8 ounces) of water or other fluid and work best when taken at the first sign of the migraine; these steps allow for more successful treatment. With ergotamine tartrate and related drugs, the maximum dose is usually 6 tablets for a single headache and 10 tablets in any 7-day period. Dependence may occur with the ergots, and if they are withdrawn suddenly, rebound headaches may occur. Encourage the patient to report to the prescriber any headaches that are uncharacteristic or unusual, as well as any persistent headache, worsening of headaches, or severe nausea, vomiting, dizziness, or restlessness. Any of the following also need to be reported immediately to the prescriber: slow, fast, or irregular heartbeat; tingling, pain, or coldness in the fingers or toes; loss of feeling in the fingers or toes; muscle pain or weakness; chest pain; severe stomach or abdominal pain; lower back pain; or little or no urine. Emphasize that the patient must seek immediate medical attention if there is any chest pain, change in vision, confusion, or slurred speech. As mentioned previously, these medications are not to be taken with triptans.

Evaluation

Therapeutic responses to drugs for attention deficit hyperactivity disorder include decreased hyperactivity, increased attention span and concentration, improved behaviour and, for adults, increased effectiveness at work. Adverse effects range from loss of appetite to increased irritability, insomnia, palpitations, nausea, and headaches. Therapeutic effects of anorexiants include appetite control and weight loss for the treatment of obesity. Adverse effects of these drugs include dry mouth, headache, insomnia, constipation, cardiac irregularities, hypertension, changes in mental status or sensorium, changes in mood or affect, alteration of sleep patterns, and seizures (all due to excessive CNS stimulation). Evaluating for any increased irritability and withdrawal symptoms (e.g. nausea and vomiting) is also important. If the anorexiant affects fat metabolism, then there may be adverse effects such as flatulence with an oily discharge, spotting, and fecal urgency. The patient also needs to be closely evaluated for decreased levels of fat-soluble vitamins (A, D, E, and K), because their levels may be affected by the decrease in absorption of fats. For drugs used to treat narcolepsy, therapeutic responses include a decrease in sleepiness. Adverse effects for which to monitor include headache, nausea, nervousness, and anxiety.

Therapeutic responses to the serotonin agonists include the aborting of migraine headache with improved daily functioning and performance because of the reduction in headaches. Adverse effects for which to monitor include pain at the injection site (if a self-injectable form is used, such pain should be temporary), flushing, chest tightness or pressure, weakness, sedation, dizziness, sweating, increase in blood pressure and pulse rate, and bad taste with the nasal spray formulation (which may precipitate nausea).

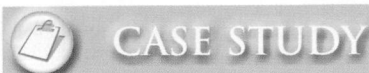

CASE STUDY

Methylphenidate for Attention Deficit Hyperactivity Disorder

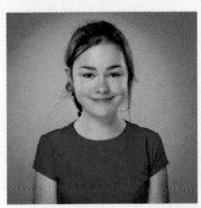

Nina, a 13-year-old girl, has been diagnosed with attention deficit hyperactivity disorder. She is in Grade 7 at a local middle school and plays the clarinet in the school's after-school band. Her parents have noticed that she has had trouble focusing on assignments and music practice for the last year and have discussed her problems with Nina's pediatrician. The physician has prescribed methylphenidate (Ritalin), 5 mg, twice a day for 2 weeks, then increasing the dose to 10 mg twice a day if no improvement is noted.

1. What are the therapeutic effects of methylphenidate?

2. After 3 weeks, Nina's mother calls the physician's office to say that Nina has been doing better at school, as reported by her morning teacher, but the band teacher has reported that Nina gets restless during after-school rehearsals. Nina's mother also reports that Nina seems unable to get to sleep at night and has been staying up too late. What should the nurse suggest?

3. At the 2-month checkup, the physician suggests that Nina's mother hold the medication on weekends, giving the drug only during the weekdays while Nina is at school. In addition, careful height and weight measurements are taken. What is the reason for this "drug holiday," as described by the physician? What is the purpose of the height and weight measurements?

4. When it is time for a refill, Nina's mother calls the pharmacy. The pharmacist tells her, "I can't refill this medication by phone. You will need to bring in a new prescription." What is the reason for this?

For answers see http://evolve.elsevier.com/Canada/Lilley/pharmacology/.

PATIENT TEACHING TIPS

General Information

❖ Medications need to be taken exactly as prescribed without skipping, omitting, or adding doses.

❖ Alcohol, nicotine, over-the-counter cold products, cough syrups that contain alcohol, and caffeine-containing food items or beverages must be avoided when taking CNS stimulants.

❖ Keep a journal of daily activities, response to drug therapy and any adverse effects.

❖ Avoid any abrupt or sudden withdrawal of medications.

Drugs Used to Treat Attention Deficit Hyperactivity Disorder

❖ For maximal drug effects, medications are to be taken on an empty stomach 30 to 45 minutes before eating.

❖ Keeping all follow-up appointments is important to monitoring drug therapy.

❖ If the prescriber decides to discontinue the medication, a weaning process with careful supervision is recommended.

❖ Extended-release or long-acting preparations are to be taken in their original dosage form and only as directed. They are not to be crushed, chewed, broken, or altered in any way.

❖ Dosage amounts are not to be increased or decreased by the patient or family, because this may lead to drug-related complications. If there is any concern about the drug and its dosage amount or adverse effects, encourage parents or caregivers to contact the prescriber.

Anorexiants

❖ The patient must follow all prescriber instructions regarding medications, diet, and exercise.

❖ Some of these medications may impair alertness and the ability to think, so patients need to remain cautious if engaging in activities in which their performance may be adversely affected by these impairments.

❖ An unpleasant taste from the medication and dry mouth may be minimized by use of mouth rinses, ice chips, sugar-free chewing gum, and hard candies.

Antimigraine Drugs

❖ Encourage patients who experience migraines to avoid foods or beverages that are known triggers to such headaches.

❖ Other triggers for some individuals may include food additives, preservatives (including monosodium glutamate, nitrates, and nitrites), artificial sweeteners (especially aspartame when consumed for extended periods of time), and chocolate.

❖ Before using a nasal spray dosage form of an antimigraine drug, instruct the patient to first gently blow the nose to clear the nasal passages. With the head upright, the patient then closes one nostril and inserts the nozzle into the open nostril. While a breath is taken through the nose, the spray is released. The nozzle is removed, and then the patient gently breathes in through the nose and out through the mouth for 10 to 20 seconds. Some bad taste may be experienced.

❖ Until a migraine is resolved, the patient may find comfort by avoiding doing things that require alertness and rapid skilled movements. It may be helpful to keep the room darkened and noise to a minimum. If the headache is not resolved or vomiting occurs, the patient may need further medical attention to help avoid additional problems, such as dehydration.

❖ Encourage the patient to keep a journal about the experience of all headaches, including precipitators,

Continued

PATIENT TEACHING TIPS—cont'd

relievers and the rating of each headache on a scale of 0 to 10, (where 0 is no pain and 10 is the worst pain ever). The patient should also record other symptoms (e.g., photophobia, nausea, and vomiting) as well as their frequency and duration.

❖ When taking SSRAs, the patient must understand the importance of contacting the physician immediately if there are any problems with palpitations, chest pain, or pain or weakness in the extremities.

❖ Injectable forms of sumatriptan succinate are to be given subcutaneously and as ordered. Have the patient practice administering injections (without the medication) at the prescriber's office so that proper technique is learned and a moderate comfort level is achieved.

❖ Autoinjectors with prefilled syringes may be used. The syringe needs to be discarded in an appropriate container or receptacle after use and kept out of the reach of children.

❖ Administer no more than two injections of sumatriptan succinate during a 24-hour period; at least 1 hour should be allowed between injections.

❖ When using injectable sumatriptan succinate, contact the prescriber or emergency services immediately if there is swelling around the eyes,

pain or tightness in the chest or throat, wheezing, or heart throbbing.

❖ Treatment for migraine headaches may relieve the pain and symptoms of a migraine attack as well as prevent further migraine attacks. Some abortive therapies, such as sumatriptan succinate, may offer rapid relief if drugs are given as ordered and before the headache worsens. Drugs may be given orally, sublingually, or by subcutaneous injection in the thigh. When a triptan does not work, an ergot alkaloid (e.g., dihydroergotamine mesylate or ergotamine tartrate) may be ordered but is not to be used concurrently. Other drugs that may also be used to try to prevent migraine headaches include antidepressants, antiseizure medications, and β-blockers.

❖ Serotonin agonists are to be taken as prescribed on a prn (as needed) basis at the onset of the migraine but within the frequency and dosage amount prescribed.

❖ Medications or foods and beverages identified as triggers to a migraine may vary from person to person. Encourage the patient to track food and beverage intake as well as sleep habits and other practices or factors that may be identified as precipitators of migraines.

KEY POINTS

❖ CNS stimulants are drugs that stimulate the brain or spinal cord.

❖ The actions of these stimulants mimic those of the neurotransmitters of the sympathetic nervous system (e.g., norepinephrine, dopamine, and serotonin).

❖ Sympathomimetic drugs mimic the sympathetic division of the autonomic nervous system.

❖ Included in the family of CNS stimulants are amphetamines, analeptics, and anorexiants with therapeutic uses for attention deficit hyperactivity disorder, narcolepsy, and appetite control.

❖ Adverse effects associated with CNS stimulants include changes in mental status or sensorium, changes in mood or affect, tachycardia, loss of appetite, nausea, altered sleep patterns (e.g., insomnia), physical dependency, irritability, and seizures.

❖ Serotonin agonists may be administered as a subcutaneous injection, as a nasal spray, and as oral tablets. Any chest pain or tightness, tremors, vomiting,

or worsening symptoms need to be reported to the prescriber immediately.

❖ Anorexiants control or suppress appetite. They are used to stimulate the CNS and they result in the suppression of appetite control centres in the brain.

❖ Contraindications to the use of anorexiants, as well as other CNS stimulants, include hypersensitivity, seizure activity, convulsive disorders, and liver dysfunction.

❖ The SSRAs are a newer class of CNS stimulants and are used to treat migraine headaches. They are not to be given to patients with coronary heart disease.

❖ Amphetamines elevate mood or produce euphoria, increase mental alertness and capacity for work, decrease fatigue and drowsiness, and prolong wakefulness.

❖ Journals are helpful in evaluating the effects of all drugs used to treat attention deficit hyperactivity disorder, obesity, migraines, and narcolepsy.

EXAMINATION REVIEW QUESTIONS

1. A patient with narcolepsy will begin treatment with a CNS stimulant. The nurse expects to see which adverse effect?
   a. Bradycardia
   b. Nervousness
   c. Mental clouding
   d. Drowsiness at night

2. A patient at a weight management clinic who was given a prescription for orlistat (Xenical) calls the clinic hotline because of a "terrible adverse effect." The nurse suspects the patient is referring to which problem?
   a. Nausea
   b. Sexual dysfunction
   c. Urinary incontinence
   d. Fecal incontinence

EXAMINATION REVIEW QUESTIONS—cont'd

3. The nurse is developing a plan of care for a patient receiving an anorexiant. Which nursing diagnosis is the most appropriate?
a. Deficient fluid volume
b. Sleep deprivation
c. Impaired memory
d. Imbalanced nutrition, more than body requirements

4. A patient has a new prescription for sumatriptan succinate (Imitrex). The nurse providing patient teaching on self-administration will include which information?
a. Correct technique for intramuscular injections
b. Take the medication before the headache worsens
c. Allow at least 30 minutes between injections
d. Take no more than 4 doses in a 24-hour period

5. The nurse is reviewing the history of a patient who will be starting the triptan sumatriptan succinate (Imitrex) as part of treatment for migraine headaches. Which condition, if present, may be a contraindication to triptan therapy?
a. Cardiovascular disease
b. Chronic bronchitis
c. History of renal calculi
d. Diabetes mellitus type 2

6. The nurse is reviewing medication therapy with the parents of an adolescent with ADHD. Which statement(s) is/are correct? (Select all that apply.)
a. "Be sure to have your child blow his nose before administering the nasal spray."
b. "This medication is used only when symptoms of ADHD are severe."
c. "The last dose should be taken 4 to 6 hours before bedtime to avoid interference with sleep."
d. "Be sure to contact the physician right away if you notice expression of suicidal thoughts."
e. "We will need to check your child's height and weight periodically to monitor physical growth."
f. "If adverse effects become severe, stop the medication for 3 to 4 days."

7. The medication order reads: "Atomoxetine (Strattera) 1.2 mg/kg/day in 2 divided doses." The child weighs 30 kg. How much will be given with each dose?

Answers: 1. b, 2. d, 3. d, 4. b, 5. a, 6. c, d, e, 7. 18 mg per dose

CRITICAL THINKING ACTIVITIES

1. The parents of a 10-year-old boy are concerned about the effects of the medication their son is taking for ADHD. They ask, "What should we be looking for when he starts this medicine?" What is the nurse's best response?

2. A patient calls the headache clinic because she is unhappy about her medication. She says, "I've been taking zolmitriptan (Zomig) to prevent headaches, but I am still having them." What is the nurse's priority action?

3. A patient who is obese is discussing options for appetite suppressant therapy and says, "I want to lose weight, but I can't help myself—I'm hungry all the time! The doctor wants me to take a pill to stop my appetite, but I'm afraid there will be bad effects." What is the priority action by the nurse at this time?

For answers see http://evolve.elsevier.com/Canada/Lilley/pharmacology/.

CHAPTER 15

Antiepileptic Drugs

Objectives

After reading this chapter, the successful student will be able to do the following:

1. Briefly describe the pathophysiology of epilepsy.

2. Discuss the rationale for the use of the various classes of antiepileptic drugs in the management of the different forms of epilepsy.

3. Identify the various drugs in each of the following drug classes: iminostilbenes, benzodiazepines, barbiturates, hydantoins, and miscellaneous drugs.

4. Identify the mechanisms of action, indications, cautions, contraindications, dosages, routes of administration, adverse effects, toxic effects, therapeutic blood levels, and drug interactions for each antiepileptic drug.

5. Develop a collaborative plan of care, including patient education, based on the nursing process for patients receiving antiepileptic drugs.

e-Learning Activities

Website
(http://evolve.elsevier.com/Canada/Lilley/pharmacology/)

evolve

- Answer Key—Textbook Case Studies
- Answer Key—Critical Thinking Activities
- Chapter Summaries—Printable
- Review Questions for Exam Preparation
- Unfolding Case Studies

Drug Profiles

▸▸ carbamazepine, p. 292
▸▸ gabapentin, p. 293
ethosuximide, p. 293
lamotrigine, p.293
levetiracetam, p. 294
oxcarbazepine, p. 292
perampanel, p. 293
▸▸ phenobarbital (phenobarbital sodium)*, p. 291
▸▸ phenytoin (phenytoin sodium)*, p. 291
pregabalin, p. 293
topiramate, p. 294
▸▸ valproic acid, p. 294

▸▸ Key drug

*Full generic name is given in parentheses. For the purposes of this text, the more common, shortened name is used.

Key Terms

Anticonvulsants Substances or procedures that prevent or reduce the severity of epileptic or other convulsive seizures. (p. 286)

Antiepileptic drugs Prescription drugs that prevent or reduce the severity of epilepsy and different types of epileptic seizures, not just convulsive seizures. (p. 286)

Autoinduction A metabolic process in which a drug stimulates the production of enzymes that enhance its own

metabolism over time, which leads to a reduction in therapeutic drug concentrations. (p. 292)

Convulsion A type of seizure involving excessive stimulation of neurons in the brain and characterized by the spasmodic contraction of voluntary muscles. (See also *seizure*.) (p. 285)

Electroencephalogram (EEG) A recording of the electrical activity that arises from spontaneous currents in nerve cells in the brain, derived from electrodes placed on the outer skull. (p. 285)

Epilepsy A general term for any of a group of neurological disorders characterized by recurrent episodes of convulsive seizures, sensory disturbances, abnormal behaviour, loss of consciousness, or any combination of these. (p. 285)

Generalized onset seizures Seizures originating simultaneously in both cerebral hemispheres. (p. 285)

Gingival hyperplasia Overgrowth of gum tissue; often an adverse effect of phenytoin. (p. 292)

Partial onset seizures Seizures originating in a more localized region of the brain. Also called *focal* seizures. (p. 286)

Primary epilepsy Epilepsy in which there is no identifiable cause. Also known as *idiopathic* seizures. (p. 285)

Seizure Excessive stimulation of neurons in the brain, leading to a sudden burst of abnormal neuron activity that results in temporary changes in brain function, primarily affecting sensory and motor activity. (p. 285)

Status epilepticus A medical emergency of prolonged seizure activity, that lasts for 5 minutes or longer, of continuous clinical or electrographic seizure activity or recurrent seizure activity without recovery (returning to baseline) between seizures. (p. 286)

Tonic–clonic seizures Seizures involving initial muscular contraction throughout the body (tonic phase), progressing to alternating contraction and relaxation (clonic phase). (p. 285)

EPILEPSY

Epilepsy is a syndrome of central nervous system (CNS) dysfunction that can cause symptoms ranging from momentary sensory disturbances to convulsive seizures. It is the most common chronic neurological illness, affecting 0.6% of the Canadian population and 50 million people worldwide, approximately 60% of whom experience partial seizures. It results from excessive electrical activity from neurons (nerve cells) located in the superficial area of the brain known as the *cerebral cortex* or *grey matter*. The terms *seizure, convulsion,* and *epilepsy* are often used interchangeably, but they do not have the same meaning. A **seizure** is the excessive stimulation of the neurons in the brain, leading to a brief episode of abnormal neuron activity that results in temporary changes in brain function, primarily affecting sensory and motor activity. A seizure may lead to a convulsion. A **convulsion** is a more severe seizure characterized by involuntary spasmodic contractions of any or all voluntary muscles throughout the body, including skeletal, facial, and ocular muscles. Commonly reported symptoms include abnormal motor function, loss of consciousness, altered sensory awareness, and psychic changes. In contrast, **epilepsy** is a chronic, recurrent pattern of seizures. Excessive electrical discharges can often be detected by an **electroencephalogram (EEG)**, which is obtained to help diagnose epilepsy. Fluctuations in the brain's electrical potential are seen in the form of waves. These waves correlate well with different neurological conditions and are used as diagnostic indicators. In the case of epilepsy, they are used to identify specific seizure subtypes.

Up to 50% of the cases of epilepsy have normal EEGs; therefore, a careful history is very important for accurate diagnosis. Other applicable diagnostic tests include skull radiography, computed tomography, and magnetic resonance imaging. These procedures help to rule out structural causes of epilepsy, such as brain tumours. In particularly severe cases, patients may be observed in a hospital setting or sleep study laboratory. This allows for continuous EEG and video monitoring to identify detailed patterns of seizure activity and to allow tailoring of an effective treatment.

Epilepsy occurs most commonly in children and older adults. Epilepsy without an identifiable cause is known as **primary epilepsy** or idiopathic epilepsy. Primary epilepsy accounts for roughly 50% of cases. Evidence indicates genetic predispositions, but these have yet to be clearly defined. Studies in the field of pharmacogenomics (see Chapter 5) are beginning to clarify genetic factors that can help optimize antiepileptic drug therapy. In other cases, epilepsy has a distinct cause, such as trauma, infection, cerebrovascular disorder, or other illness. This type is known as secondary or symptomatic epilepsy. The chief causes of secondary epilepsy in children and infants are developmental defects, metabolic disease, and injury at birth. Febrile seizures occur in children 6 months to 5 years of age, and by definition are caused by fever. Children usually outgrow the tendency to have such seizures, and thus they do not constitute a chronic illness. Antipyretic drugs (e.g., acetaminophen [see Chapter 11]) are normally adequate for acute treatment.

In adults, acquired brain disorder is the major cause of secondary epilepsy. Examples include head injury, disease or infection of the brain and spinal cord, stroke, metabolic disorders, adverse drug reactions (e.g., meperidine hydrochloride [see Chapter 11], theophylline [see Chapter 38]), primary or metastatic brain tumour, or other nonspecific neurological diseases. Older adults have the highest incidence of new-onset epilepsy. Fortunately, seizures in older adults are often well controlled with drug therapy.

Generalized onset seizures are characterized by neuronal activity that originates simultaneously in the grey matter of both hemispheres. There are several subtypes of generalized seizures. **Tonic–clonic seizures** begin with muscular contraction throughout the body (tonic phase) and progress to alternating contraction and relaxation (clonic phase). Tonic seizures involve spasms of the upper trunk with flexion of the arms. Clonic seizures are the same as tonic–clonic seizures but without the tonic phase. Atonic seizures, also known as *drop attacks*, involve

TABLE 15-1

Antiepileptic Drugs Used to Treat Status Epilepticus

Drug	IV Dose	Onset	Duration	Half-Life	Adverse Effects
diazepam*	5–10 mg (repeat in 2–4 hr if necessary)	3–10 min	Minutes	35 hr	Apnea, hypotension, somnolence
fosphenytoin	15–20 phenytoin equivalents/kg	15–30 min	12–24 hr	10–60 hr	Comparable to those for phenytoin (see below)
lorazepam	0.05 mg/kg up to a maximum of 4 mg	1–20 min	Hours	12–15 hr	Apnea, hypotension, somnolence
phenobarbital	**Adults:** 20 mg/kg **Children:** 20 mg/kg	5 min	6–12 hr	50–120 hr	Apnea, hypotension, somnolence
phenytoin	**Adults:** 150–200 mg **Children:** 250 mg/m^2	1–2 hr	12–24 hr	7–42 hr	Cardiac dysrhythmias, hypotension

*Rectal products are also available for emergency use for both adults and children of all ages.

sudden global muscle weakness and syncope. Myoclonic seizures are characterized by brief muscular jerks, but which are not as extreme as in other subtypes. Finally, absence seizures involve a brief loss of awareness that commonly occurs with repetitive spasmodic eye blinking for up to 30 seconds. This type occurs primarily in childhood and rarely after 14 years of age.

Partial onset seizures originate in a localized or focal region (e.g., one lobe) of the brain. There are three types of partial onset seizures. Simple partial onset seizure is characterized by brief loss of awareness (e.g., blank stare) but without loss of consciousness or spasmodic eye blinking as in absence seizures. In complex partial onset seizure, the level of consciousness is reduced but is not completely lost. Partial onset seizures can progress to generalized tonic–clonic seizures in up to 40% of patients. This third type is known as a secondary generalized tonic–clonic seizure. The latter two types are also associated with postictal confusion, a term for the confused mental state that follows seizure activity. Unclassified seizures are those that do not clearly fit into any of the other categories.

Seizure episodes can sometimes start off as partial and then become generalized. If the partial component is not noticed, the patient may be misdiagnosed and receive suboptimal drug therapy. Another important seizure condition is **status epilepticus.** In status epilepticus, multiple seizures occur that last for 5 minutes or longer of continuous clinical or electrographic (or both) seizure activity or recurrent seizure activity without recovery (returning to baseline) between seizures (Brophy, Bell, Classen, et al., 2012).

Status epilepticus may be precipitated by an exacerbation of a pre-existing seizure disorder, the initial manifestation of a seizure disorder, or an insult other than a seizure disorder. In patients with known epilepsy, the most common cause is a change in medication. Numerous physiological changes occur with a generalized convulsive status epilepticus, such as tachycardia, cardiac arrhythmias, and hyperglycemia, occur from the release of catecholamines. This is followed by hypotension, elevated body temperature from the robust muscle activity,

followed by metabolic acidosis, hypoxia, brain damage, and possibly death. Thus, status epilepticus is considered a true medical emergency and must be treated promptly and aggressively. Initially, ABCs must be maintained, followed by intravenous administration of drugs (see Table 15-1 for drugs used to treat status epilepticus). Management protocols will vary among institutions, and a gold standard is lacking (Friedman, Canadian Paediatric Society, & Acute Care Committee, 2014). Management is often labelled as *first-*, *second-*, and *third-line* drugs; however, the Neurocritical Care guidelines (2012) recommend the terms *emergent*, *urgent*, and *refractory* to reflect timing urgency and the sequencing of drug administration. For example, lorazepam IV or diazepam rectally are initial emergent drugs, while emergent control drugs include phenytoin, fosphenytoin, and phenobarbital. Once status epilepticus is controlled, long-term drug therapy is started with other drugs for the prevention of future seizures.

In addition, febrile seizures can also sometimes progress to status epilepticus. In addition to the website of the International League Against Epilepsy, other helpful websites include http://www.ninds.nih.gov/disorders/epilepsy/epilepsy.htm and www.epilepsy.ca.

ANTIEPILEPTIC DRUGS

Antiepileptic drugs are also called *anticonvulsants*. *Antiepileptic drugs* is a more appropriate term because many of these medications are indicated for the management of all types of epilepsy, and not necessarily just convulsions. **Anticonvulsants**, on the other hand, are medications that are used to prevent the convulsive seizures typically associated with epilepsy.

The goal of antiepileptic drug therapy is to control or prevent seizures while maintaining a reasonable quality of life. Approximately 70% of patients can expect to become seizure free while taking only one drug (monotherapy). The remaining 30% of cases are more complicated and often require multiple medications. Single-drug therapy must fail before multidrug therapy is attempted.

Patients are normally started on a single antiepileptic drug, and the dosage is slowly increased until the seizures are controlled or until clinical toxicity occurs. If the first antiepileptic drug is not effective, the drug is tapered slowly while a second drug is introduced. Antiepileptic drugs are never to be stopped abruptly unless a severe adverse effect occurs.

Antiepileptic drugs have many adverse effects, and it is often difficult to achieve seizure control while avoiding adverse effects. In many cases, the therapeutic goal is not to eliminate seizure activity but rather to maximally reduce the incidence of seizures while minimizing drug-induced toxicity. Many patients must take these drugs for their entire lives. Treatment may eventually be stopped in some, but others will experience repeated seizures if constant levels of antiepileptic drugs are not maintained in the blood. Abrupt discontinuation of these drugs can result in withdrawal seizures. In both children and adults, there is only a 40% chance of recurrence after the first partial or generalized seizure. Therefore, antiepileptic drug therapy is *not* recommended after a single isolated seizure event.

There are numerous antiepileptic drugs available. To optimize drug selection, neurologists must consider the known efficacy of the drug for a certain type of seizure, adverse effects and drug interaction profile, cost, ease of use, and availability of pediatric dosage forms. Many antiepileptic drugs are also used to treat other types of illnesses, including mental health disorders such as depression and bipolar disorder (see Chapter 17), migraine headaches (see Chapter 14), and neuropathic pain syndromes (see Chapter 11).

Therapeutic drug monitoring (see Chapter 2) of serum drug concentrations provides a useful guideline in assessing the effectiveness of and adherence to therapy. For example, if the serum level is low, it may mean the patient is not taking the medication as prescribed. This gives the nurse an opportunity to ask about why the patient may not be taking the medication. If the level is above normal, the nurse needs to contact the prescriber before giving the next dose.

Maintaining serum drug levels within therapeutic ranges helps not only to control seizures but also to reduce adverse effects. Drugs that are routinely monitored in this way have a narrow therapeutic index (see Chapter 2). There are established normal therapeutic ranges for many antiepileptic drugs, but these are only guidelines. The serum concentrations of phenytoin, phenobarbital, carbamazepine, and primidone correlate better with seizure control and toxicity than those of valproic acid, ethosuximide, and clonazepam. Each patient must be monitored and dosed individually. It may be possible to achieve maintenance at levels below or above the usual therapeutic range. The goal is to slowly titrate to the lowest effective serum drug level that controls the seizure disorder. This reduces the risk for adverse drug effects and drug interactions. Successful control of a seizure disorder hinges on selection of the appropriate

TABLE 15-2

Currently Available Antiepileptic Drugs

Generic Name	Trade Name	Route
TRADITIONAL ANTIEPILEPTIC DRUGS		
Barbiturates		
phenobarbital	Generic	PO
	Generic	IV
primidone	Generic	PO
Hydantoins		
phenytoin	Dilantin, Tremytoine INJ®	PO IV
fosphenytoin	Cerebyx	IV, IM
Iminostilbenes		
carbamazepine	Tegretol, Mazepine	PO
oxcarbazepine	Trileptal	PO
MISCELLANEOUS ANTIEPILEPTIC DRUGS		
gabapentin	Neurontin	PO
lacosamide	Vimpat®	PO, IV
lamotrigine	Lamictal	PO
levetiracetam	Keppra	PO
pregabalin	Lyrica	PO
topiramate	Topamax	PO
valproic acid (divalproex sodium)	Depakene, Diprovalex, Epival ECT	PO

drug class and drug dosage, avoidance of drug toxicity, and patient adherence with the treatment regimen.

The antiepileptic drugs traditionally used to manage seizure disorders include barbiturates, hydantoins, and iminostilbenes, plus valproic acid. Second- and third-generation antiepileptics are also available (Table 15-2). The latter drugs may have fewer adverse effects and drug interactions than the more traditional drugs. This may benefit older adults, who are more likely to be taking multiple medications, and, therefore, are more prone to drug interactions. However, there is current debate in the neurological literature as to whether patients actually benefit more from newer than from older drugs. It is now believed that the majority of pediatric and adult patients with epilepsy who have been seizure free for 1 to 2 years while taking antiepileptic drugs can eventually stop taking them with medical supervision.

Mechanism of Action and Drug Effects

As with many classes of drugs, the exact mechanism of action of the antiepileptic drugs is not known with certainty. However, evidence indicates that they alter the movement of sodium, potassium, calcium, and magnesium ions. The changes in the movement of these ions result in more stabilized and less responsive cell membranes.

The major pharmacological effects of antiepileptic drugs are threefold. First, they increase the threshold of activity in the area of the brain called the *motor cortex*. In other words, they make it more difficult for a nerve to be excited, or they reduce the nerve's response to incoming electrical or chemical stimulation. Second, they act to limit the spread of a seizure discharge from its origin. They do this by suppressing the transmission of impulses from one nerve to the next. Third, they can decrease the speed of nerve impulse conduction within a given neuron. Less well understood are mechanisms that involve drug effects outside the neuron. For example, some drugs may indirectly affect seizure foci (locations) in the brain by altering the blood supply to these areas. However, the overall effect is that antiepileptic drugs stabilize neurons and keep them from becoming hyperexcited and generating excessive nerve impulses to adjacent neurons. Some drugs work by enhancing the effects of the inhibitory neurotransmitter gamma-aminobutyric acid (GABA). GABA plays a role in regulating neuron excitability in the brain. Low levels of GABA are associated with seizures. Many antiepileptic drugs increase GABA levels to the normal range, and thus reduce the potential for seizures. Regardless of the mechanism, the overall effect is that antiepileptics stabilize neurons and keep them from becoming hyperexcited and generating excessive nerve impulses to adjacent neurons.

Indications

Antiepileptic drugs are used to prevent or control seizure activity. As evidenced by the wide range of seizure disorders discussed earlier in this chapter, epilepsy is a diverse disorder. As a result, specific indications vary among drugs. The most recent indications are noted, drug by drug, in Table 15-3, the Dosages table on p. 295, and in specific drug profiles. It is important to have an accurate diagnosis of the seizure type because some drugs may not be ideal for specific seizures. For example, it is known that carbamazepine may worsen myoclonic

or absence seizures. Other evidence supports the following generalizations: Phenobarbital, phenytoin, primidone, carbamazepine, and valproic acid are equally effective for partial onset seizures. Lamotrigine, topiramate, gabapentin, and levetiracetam are all effective as adjunct therapy for refractory (not responsive to other therapy) partial-onset seizures. Specific antiepileptic drugs and the seizure disorders they are used to treat are listed in Table 15-3.

Patients who undergo brain surgery or who have suffered severe head injuries may receive prophylactic antiepileptic drug therapy. These patients are at high risk for acquiring a seizure disorder, and often severe complications will arise if seizures are not controlled.

Contraindications

The only usual contraindication to antiepileptics is known drug allergy. Pregnancy is also a common contraindication; however, the prescriber must consider the risks to mother and infant of untreated maternal epilepsy and the increased risks for seizure activity. Many women take antiepileptics throughout their pregnancy. The newer generation antiepileptic drugs appear to be safer in pregnancy than the traditional drugs.

Adverse Effects

Antiepileptics have numerous adverse effects that often limit their usefulness. Many patients cannot tolerate the adverse effects, and therapy must be withdrawn. Skin rashes and immune reactions (e.g., Stevens-Johnson's syndrome) are extremely common in patients taking antiepileptic drugs. Birth defects in the infants of mothers who have epilepsy are higher than normal, regardless of whether the mother was receiving drug therapy. Women with epilepsy need to be monitored closely during pregnancy by both an obstetrician and a neurologist. Each antiepileptic drug is associated with

TABLE 15-3

Common Seizure Indications for Antiepileptic Drugs

	Partial	Secondary General	Generalized Tonic–Clonic	Absence	Myoclonic
FIRST-LINE DRUGS	carbamazepine phenobarbital primidone phenytoin fosphenytoin	carbamazepine phenobarbital primidone phenytoin fosphenytoin	carbamazepine phenobarbital primidone phenytoin fosphenytoin valproic acid	valproic acid	valproic acid
ADJUNCT DRUGS	clonazepam clorazepate oxcarbazepine gabapentin perampanel pregabalin lamotrigine levetiracetam topiramate	clonazepam oxcarbazepine gabapentin lamotrigine levetiracetam topiramate	clonazepam lamotrigine topiramate zonisamide	acetazolamide ethosuximide	clonazepam

its own diverse set of adverse effects. The various antiepileptic drugs and their most common adverse effects are listed in Table 15-4.

Interactions

Drug interactions that can occur with antiepileptic drugs are numerous and are summarized in Table 15-5. Many of the antiepileptic drugs can interact with each other, requiring close monitoring of the patient. Since many of these drugs induce hepatic metabolism, the effects of other drugs may be reduced, including oral contraceptives. There is a prime opportunity to counsel the patient about the need for alternative birth control methods due to reduced efficacy. Carbamazepine is not to be given with grapefruit because this leads to increased toxicity of the antiepileptic drug.

TABLE 15-4
Adverse Effects of Selected Antiepileptic Drugs

Drug or Drug Class	Adverse Effects
FIRST-LINE DRUGS	
Barbiturates: phenobarbital, primidone	Dizziness, drowsiness, lethargy, paradoxical restlessness
Hydantoins: phenytoin, fosphenytoin	Nystagmus, ataxia, drowsiness, rash, gingival hyperplasia, thrombocytopenia, agranulocytosis, hepatitis
Iminostilbenes: carbamazepine, oxcarbazepine	Nausea, headache, dizziness, unusual eye movements, visual change, behavioural changes, rash, abdominal pain, abnormal gait
valproic acid and derivatives, including valproate sodium and divalproex sodium	Dizziness, drowsiness, gastrointestinal upset, weight gain, hepatotoxicity, pancreatitis
ADJUNCT DRUGS	
gabapentin	Dizziness, drowsiness, nausea, visual and speech changes, edema
perampanel	Dizziness, drowsiness
pregabalin	Dizziness, drowsiness, peripheral edema, blurred vision
lamotrigine	Drowsiness, ataxia, headache, benign skin rashes, nausea, blurred or double vision
levetiracetam	Dizziness, drowsiness, hyperactivity, behaviour changes such as anxiety, hostility, agitation, or suicidal ideation, incoordination
Succinimides: ethosuximide	Nausea, abdominal pain, dizziness, drowsiness
topiramate	Dizziness, drowsiness, GI upset, ataxia

TABLE 15-5
Significant Drug Interactions of Antiepileptic Drugs

AED Drug or Drug Class	Interacting Drug	Mechanism	Results
BARBITURATES			
	β-blockers, corticosteroids (e.g., prednisone), oral contraceptives, dihydropyridine, calcium channel blockers, metronidazole, quinidine, theophylline	Altered CYP450 enzyme metabolism	Reduced effects of listed drugs
	ethanol (alcohol)	Enhanced CNS depression	Can be fatal
HYDANTOINS phenytoin	amiodarone, benzodiazepines, azole antifungals, isoniazid, proton pump inhibitors, sulfonamide antibiotics, SSRIs	Altered CYP450 enzyme metabolism	Reduced hydantoin clearance and increased effects
	carbamazepine	Altered CYP450 enzyme metabolism	Increased hydantoin clearance and reduced effects
	cyclosporine, loop diuretics, meperidine, methadone, rifampin, quinidine, quetiapine, theophylline	Increased metabolism	Reduced effects of listed drugs
	warfarin sodium	Displacement of warfarin from plasma protein binding sites	Increased free warfarin levels and bleeding risk

Continued

TABLE 15-5

Significant Drug Interactions of Antiepileptic Drugs—cont'd

AED Drug or Drug Class	Interacting Drug	Mechanism	Results
IMINOSTILBENES			
carbamazepine	Azole antifungals, diltiazem, isoniazid, macrolides, protease inhibitor antiretrovirals, SSRIs, valproic acid, verapamil	Altered CYP450 enzyme metabolism	Increased carbamazepine levels and toxicity risk
	Barbiturates, hydantoins, rifampin, succinimides, theophylline	Altered CYP450 enzyme metabolism	Reduced carbamazepine levels and efficacy
	acetaminophen	Altered CYP450 enzyme metabolism	Increased hepatic metabolism of acetaminophen and toxicity risk, and reduced efficacy
	Antipsychotics, antidepressants, benzodiazepines, cyclosporine, oral contraceptives	Altered CYP450 enzyme metabolism	Reduced efficacy; patient response must be monitored
	Monoamine oxidase inhibitors (MAOIs)	Altered CYP450 metabolism	Increased MAOI toxicity risk
oxcarbazepine	Barbiturates, hydantoins	Altered CYP450 enzyme metabolism	Increased barbiturate and hydantoin levels and reduced oxcarbazepine levels
	valproic acid, verapamil	Altered CYP450 enzyme metabolism	Reduced oxcarbazepine levels
	lamotrigine	Altered CYP450 enzyme metabolism	Reduced lamotrigine levels
	Oral contraceptives	Altered CYP450 enzyme metabolism	Reduced oral contraceptive levels and increased likelihood of pregnancy
VALPROIC ACID AND DERIVATIVES			
valproic acid and divalproex sodium	aspirin	Displacement of valproic acid from plasma protein binding sites	Increased free valproic acid levels and toxicity risk
	carbamazepine, oxcarbazepine, lamotrigine	Altered CYP450 enzyme metabolism	Reduced valproic acid efficacy; increased lamotrigine levels; increased or decreased carbamazepine levels
	lorazepam	Altered hepatic metabolism	Increased lorazepam toxicity risk
	rifampin	Altered CYP450 enzyme metabolism	Reduced valproic acid efficacy
	Tricyclic antidepressants	Altered CYP450 enzyme metabolism	Increased tricyclic antidepressant toxicity risk
SUCCINIMIDES			
ethosuximide	Hydantoins, barbiturates, valproic acid	Altered CYP450 enzyme metabolism	Increased or reduced involved drug clearance
MISCELLANEOUS AEDS			
gabapentin	Alcohol	Additive CNS depression	Increased CNS depression
perampanel	Carbamazepine, phenytoin, oxcarbazepine	Altered CYP450 enzyme metabolism	Reduced perampanel levels by up to 67%
pregabalin	None listed		
lamotrigine	Hydantoins, oral contraceptives, oxcarbazepine, rifampin	Altered CYP450 enzyme metabolism	Reduced lamotrigine levels and efficacy; may need dosage increase
lamotrigine	CNS depressants	Additive effects	Increased CNS depression
lamotrigine	valproic acid	Altered CYP450 enzyme metabolism	Increased lamotrigine levels and toxicity risk; may need dosage reduction
levetiracetam	None listed		
topiramate	carbamazepine, hydantoins, valproic acid, oral contraceptives	Altered CYP450 enzyme metabolism	Reduced object drug activity

Dosages

For certain antiepileptic drugs, the therapeutic range is narrow. Drugs that have a narrow difference between safe and toxic levels are called *narrow therapeutic index (NTI) drugs*. Table 15-6 lists the various drugs for which monitoring of therapeutic plasma levels is required as well as their corresponding therapeutic levels. For dosage information, refer to the table on p. 295.

TABLE 15-6	
Therapeutic Plasma Levels of Antiepileptic Drugs with a Narrow Therapeutic Range	
Antiepileptic Drug	**Therapeutic Plasma Level (mcg/L)**
carbamazepine	4–12
phenobarbital	15–40
phenytoin	10–20
primidone	5–12
valproic acid	40–100

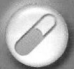

DRUG PROFILES

In most children and adults, epilepsy can be controlled with a first-line antiepileptic drug such as carbamazepine (Tegretol®), phenobarbital, phenytoin (Dilantin®), or valproic acid (Depakene®, Diprovalex®). For patients who do not respond to these first-line antiepileptic drugs, there are a number of second-line or adjunct antiepileptic drugs that are used occasionally, such as ethosuximide (Zarontin®); primidone; the benzodiazepines diazepam (Valium®), clonazepam (Clonapam®, Rivrotril®), and clorazepate dipotassium (see Chapter 17); and the diuretic acetazolamide (see Chapter 29).

After valproic acid was introduced in 1978, no major new drugs for the treatment of epilepsy were introduced in Canada until the 1990s. Gabapentin (Neurontin®) and lamotrigine were approved during this decade. These two drugs are used primarily as add-on drugs in adults who have partial seizures alone or with secondary generalized seizures. Antiepileptic drugs most recently approved include levetiracetam (Keppra®), topiramate (Topamax®), and pregabalin (Lyrica®). These drugs fall under the miscellaneous category of antiepileptics and have greatly expanded the options currently available to patients with seizure disorders. Common adverse effects and drug interactions are listed in the individual drug profiles or in Tables 15-3 and 15-4. For dosage information, see the table on p. 291.

BARBITURATES

▶▶*phenobarbital sodium and primidone*

Historically, two of the most commonly used antiepileptic drugs were the barbiturates phenobarbital and primidone. Primidone is metabolized in the liver to phenobarbital and phenylethylmalonamide, both of which have anticonvulsant properties. Use of primidone can provide anticonvulsant activity with a lower serum level of phenobarbital than that attained with phenobarbital alone. This combination can reduce the likelihood of sedation and fatigue associated with phenobarbital. Phenobarbital is a Schedule IV controlled substance, whereas primidone is not controlled. Phenobarbital has been used since 1912, principally for controlling tonic–clonic and partial seizures. Phenobarbital is used for the management of status epilepticus and is an effective prophylactic drug for the control of febrile seizures. Although phenobarbital is still used to treat seizure emergencies, the use of oral phenobarbital for seizure prevention is much less common. In developing countries, oral phenobarbital is often the drug of choice for routine seizure prophylaxis because of its low cost. The most common adverse effect of phenobarbital is sedation, although tolerance to this effect usually develops with continued therapy. Therapeutic effects are generally seen at serum drug levels of 15 to 40 mcg/mL (in children, 15 to 30 mcg/mL). A major advantage of this drug is its long half-life, which allows once-a-day dosing. This can be a substantial advantage for patients who have a difficult time remembering to take their medication or for those who have erratic schedules. Even if a patient takes a dose 12 or even 24 hours late, therapeutic blood levels may still be maintained. Contraindications include known drug allergy, porphyria (a disorder of the synthesis of heme, a component of hemoglobin), liver or kidney impairment, and respiratory illness. Adverse effects include cardiovascular, CNS, gastrointestinal (GI), and dermatological reactions (see Table 15-4). Phenobarbital interacts with many drugs because it is a major inducer of hepatic microsomal enzymes, including the cytochrome P450 system enzymes (see Chapter 2), which causes more rapid clearance of some drugs (see Table 15-5). Phenobarbital is available in oral and injectable forms, whereas primidone is available only for oral use.

PHARMACOKINETICS (PHENOBARBITAL SODIUM)

Route	Onset of Action	Peak Plasma Concentration	Elimination Half-Life	Duration of Action
PO	20–60 min	8–12 hr	50–120 hr	6–12 hr
IV	5 min	30 min	50–120 hr	6–12 hr

PHARMACOKINETICS (PRIMIDONE)

Route	Onset of Action	Peak Plasma Concentration	Elimination Half-Life	Duration of Action
PO	Unknown	3–4 hr	10–12 hr*	Unknown

*Longer for active metabolites, including phenobarbital.

HYDANTOINS

▶▶*phenytoin sodium and fosphenytoin*

Phenytoin sodium (Dilantin) has been used as a first-line drug for seizures for many years and is the prototypical drug. It is indicated for the management of tonic–clonic and partial seizures. Contraindications include known drug allergy and heart conditions that involve bradycardia or blockage of electrocardiac function. Adverse effects and drug interactions both are numerous and are listed in

Continued

DRUG PROFILES—cont'd

Tables 15-4 and 15-5, respectively. The most common adverse effects are lethargy, abnormal movements, mental confusion, and cognitive changes. **Gingival hyperplasia** is a well-known adverse effect of long-term oral phenytoin therapy. Scrupulous dental care can help prevent gingival hypertrophy. Long-term phenytoin therapy can cause gingival hyperplasia, acne, hirsutism, and hypertrophy of subcutaneous facial tissue, resulting in an appearance known as *Dilantin facies*. Another long-term consequence of phenytoin therapy is osteoporosis. Vitamin D therapy may help to prevent this condition, particularly in women. Therapeutic drug levels are usually 10 to 20 mcg/mL. At toxic levels, phenytoin can cause nystagmus, ataxia, dysarthria, and encephalopathy. Phenytoin can interact with other medications, for two main reasons. First, it is highly bound to plasma proteins and competes with other highly protein-bound medications for binding sites. Second, it induces liver microsomal enzymes, mainly the cytochrome P450 enzymes (see Chapter 2). This increases the metabolism of other drugs that are metabolized by these enzymes and reduces their blood levels.

Exaggerated phenytoin effects can be seen in patients with extremely low serum albumin concentrations. This most commonly occurs in patients who are malnourished or have chronic kidney failure. In these patients, it may be necessary to maintain phenytoin levels well below 80 μmol/L. With lower levels of albumin in a patient's body, more of the free, unbound, pharmacologically active phenytoin molecules will be present in the blood.

Phenytoin has many advantages for long-term therapy. It is usually well tolerated, highly effective, and relatively inexpensive. It can also be given intravenously if needed. Most often, however, phenytoin is taken orally. The long half-life allows twice- or even once-daily drug therapy. If a patient has to remember to take medication only once or twice a day, adherence will be increased and thus the likelihood of therapeutic drug levels being reached is increased, leading to better seizure control.

Parenteral phenytoin is adjusted chemically to a pH of 12 for reasons of drug stability. It is extremely irritating to veins when injected and must be given slow intravenous (IV) push (not exceeding 50 mg/min in adults), directly into a large vein through a large-gauge needle (20-gauge or higher) venous catheter. Phenytoin is only to be diluted in normal saline (NS) for IV infusion, and a filter must be used. Follow each dose with an injection of saline flush to avoid local venous irritation. Soft-tissue irritation and inflammation can occur at the site of injection with or without extravasation. This can vary from slight tenderness to extensive necrosis and sloughing, and, in rare instances, can require amputation. Avoid improper administration, including subcutaneous or perivascular injection, to help prevent the possibility of such occurrences.

Fosphenytoin (Cerebyx®) is an injectable prodrug of phenytoin that was developed in an attempt to overcome some of the chemical disadvantages of phenytoin injectable. Fosphenytoin is a water-soluble phenytoin derivative that can be given intramuscularly or intravenously—by IV push or continuous infusion—without causing the burning on injection associated with phenytoin. Fosphenytoin is dosed in phenytoin equivalents (PE), as indicated in Table 15-7. Fosphenytoin is given at a rate of 150 mg/min or less to avoid hypotension or cardiorespiratory depression. If dysrhythmias or hypotension occur, discontinue the infusion. Implement fall prevention measures after infusion of either phenytoin or fosphenytoin because of possible ataxia and dizziness. Take vital signs up to 2 hours after infusion. Check available references or consult with a pharmacist before administering because there are numerous IV incompatibilities with both drugs.

PHARMACOKINETICS (PHENYTOIN SODIUM)

Route	Onset of Action	Peak Plasma Concentration	Elimination Half-Life	Duration of Action
PO	Unknown	12 hr	7–42 hr	12–36 hr
IV	1–2 hr	2–3 hr	7–42 hr	12–24 hr

IMINOSTILBENES

▶▶ *carbamazepine*

Carbamazepine (Mazepine®, Tegretol) is the second-most commonly prescribed antiepileptic drug in Canada, after phenytoin. It was marketed in the late 1960s for the treatment of epilepsy after its efficacy and safety were proven for the treatment of trigeminal neuralgia (a painful facial nerve condition). It is chemically related to the tricyclic antidepressants (see Chapter 17) and is considered a first-line treatment for partial seizures and generalized tonic–clonic seizures. It may actually worsen myoclonic or absence seizures. Therefore its use is contraindicated in both of these conditions as well as in cases of known drug allergy and bone marrow depression. Carbamazepine is associated with **autoinduction** of hepatic enzymes. Autoinduction is a process in which, over time, a drug stimulates the production of enzymes that enhance its own metabolism, which leads to lower-than-expected drug concentrations. With carbamazepine this process usually occurs within the first 2 months after the start of therapy. Carbamazepine has numerous adverse reactions and drug interactions; examples are given in Tables 15-4 and 15-5. It is available for oral use only.

PHARMACOKINETICS

Route	Onset of Action	Peak Plasma Concentration	Elimination Half-Life	Duration of Action
PO	Slow	4–8 hr	25–65 hr	12–24 hr

oxcarbazepine

Oxcarbazepine (Trileptal®) is a chemical analogue of carbamazepine. Its precise mechanism of action has not been identified, although it is known to block voltage-sensitive sodium channels, which aids in stabilizing excited neuronal membranes. It is indicated for partial seizures and secondarily generalized seizures. Contraindications include known drug allergy. Common adverse reactions include headache, dizziness, and nausea (see

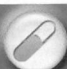

DRUG PROFILES—cont'd

also Table 15-4). Unlike carbamazepine, this drug is not a hepatic enzyme inducer. As a result, it is associated with far fewer common drug interactions than is carbamazepine (see Table 15-5). Oxcarbazepine is available for oral use only.

PHARMACOKINETICS

Route	Onset of Action	Peak Plasma Concentration	Elimination Half-Life	Duration of Action
PO	2–4 hr	2–3 days	2–9 hr	Unknown

SUCCINIMIDE

ethosuximide

Ethosuximide (Zarontin) is used in the treatment of uncomplicated absence seizures. It is not effective for secondary generalized tonic–clonic seizures. The only listed contraindication for either use is known allergy to succinimides. Adverse effects include GI and CNS effects (see Table 15-4). Drug interactions most commonly involve hepatic enzyme–inducing drugs (see Table 15-5). Succinimides are available for oral use only.

PHARMACOKINETICS

Route	Onset of Action	Peak Plasma Concentration	Elimination Half-Life	Duration of Action
PO	Unknown	4 hr	60 hr	Unknown

MISCELLANEOUS DRUGS

▶▶ gabapentin

Gabapentin (Neurontin) is a chemical analogue of GABA, a neurotransmitter that inhibits brain activity. The exact mechanism of action of gabapentin is unknown. Many believe that it works by increasing the synthesis and accumulation of GABA between neurons; hence, the drug name. It is indicated as an adjunct drug for the treatment of partial seizures and for prophylaxis of partial seizures. Evidence also shows gabapentin to be effective as single-drug therapy for new-onset epilepsy. It is most commonly used to treat neuropathic pain (see Chapter 11). Contraindications include known drug allergy. Adverse effects include CNS and GI symptoms (see Table 15-4). Drug interactions are listed in Table 15-5. Gabapentin is available for oral use only.

PHARMACOKINETICS

Route	Onset of Action	Peak Plasma Concentration	Elimination Half-Life	Duration of Action
PO	Unknown	Unknown	5–7 hr	Unknown

perampanel

Perampanel (Fycompa®) is a selective, noncompetitive antagonist of the ionotropic α-amino-3-hydroxy-5-methyl-4-isoxazolepropionic acid (AMPA) glutamate receptor on postsynaptic neurons, although its precise mechanism is still unknown. Glutamate is the excitatory neurotransmitter in the brain; elevated levels of glutamate have been suspected to trigger seizure activity. Perampanel reduces the neuronal hyperexcitation associated with seizures by targeting glutamate activity. As it binds to the postsynaptic AMPA receptors, perampanel does not directly block glutamate from binding but inhibits activation of the receptor. The drug is indicated as adjunct therapy for partial seizures. Adverse drug reactions are primarily CNS related (see Table 15-4). No clinically significant drug interactions are listed to date; however, as with all antiepileptic drugs, the potential for additive CNS depression exists when other sedating drugs are used. It is contraindicated in individuals with severe liver or kidney disease. Perampanel is available for oral use only.

PHARMACOKINETICS

Route	Onset of Action	Peak Plasma Concentration	Elimination Half-Life	Duration of Action
PO	Unknown	1 hr	105 hr	Unknown

pregabalin

Pregabalin (Lyrica), like gabapentin, is structurally related to the inhibitory neurotransmitter GABA. However, it does not bind to GABA receptors but rather to the α_2-delta receptor sites, which affect calcium channels in CNS tissues. Its mechanism of action is still not fully understood. The drug is indicated as adjunct therapy for partial seizures, although it is most commonly used for neuropathic pain (see Chapter 11) and postherpetic neuralgia (see Chapter 45). Contraindications include known drug allergy. Adverse drug reactions are primarily CNS related (see Table 15-5). No clinically significant drug interactions are listed to date; however, as with all antiepileptic drugs, the potential for additive CNS depression exists when other sedating drugs are used. Pregabalin is available for oral use only.

PHARMACOKINETICS

Route	Onset of Action	Peak Plasma Concentration	Elimination Half-Life	Duration of Action
PO	Unknown	1.5 hr	6 hr	Unknown

lamotrigine

Lamotrigine (Lamictal®) is indicated for simple or complex partial seizures, for generalized seizures related to Lennox-Gastaut syndrome (an atypical form of absence epilepsy that may persist into adulthood), and, most recently, for primary generalized tonic–clonic seizures. It is also used for the treatment of bipolar disorder. It has no known contraindications other than drug allergy. Common adverse effects include relatively minor CNS and GI symptoms (see Table 15-4). One potentially serious adverse effect is a rash that can progress to the major dermatological reaction known as Stevens-Johnson syndrome. This condition involves inflammation and sloughing of skin, potentially over the entire body, in a manner that resembles a third-degree burn. It is often reversible but can also be fatal. To avoid this condition, doses are slowly titrated over several weeks. Drug interactions chiefly involve other antiepileptic drugs as well as other CNS depressants and

Continued

DRUG PROFILES—cont'd

oral contraceptives (see Table 15-5). Lamotrigine is available for oral use only.

PHARMACOKINETICS

Route	Onset of Action	Peak Plasma Concentration	Elimination Half-Life	Duration of Action
PO	Unknown	1.4–2.3 hr	24 hr	Unknown

levetiracetam

Levetiracetam (Keppra) is indicated as adjunct therapy for partial seizures with and without secondary generalization. It is contraindicated in cases of known drug allergy. Its mechanism of action is unknown. It is generally well tolerated, with the most common adverse effects being CNS related (see Table 15-4). No drug interactions are currently listed; however, like all antiepileptic drugs, the potential for excessive CNS depression exists when it is used in combination with other sedating drugs. Levetiracetam is available in both oral and injectable forms.

PHARMACOKINETICS

Route	Onset of Action	Peak Plasma Concentration	Elimination Half-Life	Duration of Action
PO	Rapid	1 hr	6–8 hr	Unknown

topiramate

Topiramate (Topamax) is a structurally unique drug that's chemically related to fructose. It is indicated as adjunct therapy for partial and secondarily generalized seizures, for generalized tonic–clonic seizures, and for drop attacks in Lennox-Gastaut syndrome. Contraindications include known drug allergy. Its exact mechanism of action is unknown. Common adverse effects are primarily CNS related (see Table 15-4). Angle-closure glaucoma can also occur, and the patient must immediately report any visual changes. Common drug interactions involve chiefly other antiepileptic drugs and oral contraceptives (see Table

15-5). Topiramate is available for oral use only. There is an increased risk of cleft palate in children born to mothers who were taking topiramate during pregnancy.

PHARMACOKINETICS

Route	Onset of Action	Peak Plasma Concentration	Elimination Half-Life	Duration of Action
PO	Unknown	2–4 hr	21 hr	Unknown

▸▸ valproic acid

Valproic acid (Epival®) is used primarily in the treatment of generalized seizures (absence, myoclonic, and tonic–clonic). It is also used for bipolar disorder (see Chapter 17) and has been shown to be effective in controlling partial seizures. Contraindications include known drug allergy, liver impairment, and urea cycle disorders (genetic disorders of urea metabolism). Common adverse effects include drowsiness; nausea, vomiting, and other GI disturbances; tremor; weight gain; and transient hair loss (see Table 15-4). The most serious adverse effects are hepatotoxicity and pancreatitis. Valproic acid can interact with many medications (see Table 15-5). The main reasons for these interactions are protein binding and liver metabolism. It is highly bound to plasma proteins and competes with other highly protein-bound medications for binding sites. It also is metabolized by hepatic microsomal enzymes and competes for metabolism with other drugs. In contrast to phenobarbital and phenytoin, it is not a hepatic enzyme inducer. It is available in both oral and injectable forms. Valproic acid is chemically the simplest dosage form and is available as an oral syrup and tablet.

PHARMACOKINETICS

Route	Onset of Action	Peak Plasma Concentration	Elimination Half-Life	Duration of Action
PO, IV	15–30 min	1–4 hr	6–16 hr	4–6 hr

TABLE 15-7

Phenytoin Sodium Versus Fosphenytoin Sodium

	Phenytoin Sodium (Dilantin) IV	Fosphenytoin Sodium (Cerebyx) IM/IV
pH	12	8.6–9
Maximum infusion rate	50 mg/min	150 mg PE*/min
Admixtures	0.9% saline	0.9% saline or 5% dextrose

IM, intramuscular; *IV*, intravenous; *PE*, phenytoin sodium equivalents.
*150 mg fosphenytoin sodium = 100 mg phenytoin sodium.

NURSING PROCESS

✐ Assessment

With the use of any of the antiepileptic drugs, perform a thorough physical assessment and obtain a comprehensive health and medication history, so that any possible allergies, drug interactions, adverse reactions, cautions, and contraindications can be indicated. Include an assessment for Steven-Johnson's syndrome, a serious immune reaction, that occurs about 1 to 3 weeks after a drug is started. It produces mucosal lesions, usually multiple blisters and is often preceded fever, sore throat, chills, and malaise. Thoroughly review the patient's medical history, and note any type of seizure disorder; precipitating events; and the duration, frequency, and intensity of

DOSAGES Selected Antiepileptic Drugs

Drug	Pharmacological Class	Usual Dosage Range	Indications
▸▸carbamazepine (Mazepine, Tegetrol)	Iminostilbene	*Children (6–12 yr)* PO: 100–1000 mg/day (to best response) *Adults/Children over 12 yr* PO: 800–1200 mg/day	Partial, secondary generalized, generalized tonic–clonic seizures
ethosuximide (Zarontin)	Succinimide	*Children* PO: 3–6 yr, 250 mg/day then adjust; older than 6 yr, 500 mg/day then adjust *Adults* PO: 500 mg/day then adjust	Absence seizures
▸▸fosphenytoin (Cerebyx)	Hydantoin	*Children* IV: 15–20 PE*/kg loading dose; may begin maintenance dosing 8–12 hr later using child phenytoin dosing guidelines (see below) *Adults* IV: 15–20 PE*/kg loading dose; maintenance dose 4–6 PE/kg/day	Control of generalized convulsive status epilepticus
▸▸gabapentin (Neurontin)	GABA analogue	*Children* PO: not recommended *Adults* PO: over 18 yr, 900–1800 mg/day	Adjunctive therapy for partial seizures
lamotrigine (Lamictal)	Miscellaneous	*Children* PO: 2–12 yr, 1–5 mg/kg/day depending on other AEDs used *Adults* PO: 100–200 mg/day	Partial, secondary generalized, generalized tonic–clonic seizures; seizures associated with Lennox-Gastaut syndrome
levetiracetam (Keppra)	Miscellaneous	*Adults* PO: 500 mg bid–3000 mg/day	Partial, secondary generalized seizures
oxcarbazepine (Trileptal)	Iminostilbene	*Children (6–16 yr)* PO: 8–10 mg/kg/day divided bid; max 600 mg/day *Adults* 300–600 mg bid	Adjunctive therapy, monotherapy of partial seizures
▸▸phenobarbital (oral, injectable)	Barbiturate	*Children* PO: 15–50 mg bid or tid/day IV: 20 mg/kg over 20 min *Adults* PO: 50–100 mg bid or tid/day IV: 20 mg/kg at 50–75 mg/min	Partial, secondary generalized, generalized tonic–clonic seizures, prophylaxis for febrile seizures Status epilepticus Partial, secondary generalized, generalized tonic–clonic seizures Status epilepticus
▸▸phenytoin (Dilantin)	Hydantoin	*Children under 18 yr* PO: 4–8 mg/kg/day individualized IV: 250 mg/m² *Adults* PO: 300–600 mg/day IV: 15–18 mg/kg	Partial, secondary generalized, generalized tonic–clonic seizures Status epilepticus Partial, generalized tonic–clonic, psychomotor seizures Status epilepticus
perampanel (Fycompa)	Miscellaneous	Adults over 18 years PO: 2–12 mg/day, at bedtime	Partial seizures
pregabalin (Lyrica)	Miscellaneous	*Adults* PO: 150–600 mg/day divided	Off label for partial seizures

Continued

DOSAGES   Selected Antiepileptic Drugs—cont'd

Drug	Pharmacological Class	Usual Dosage Range	Indications
primidone	Barbiturate	*Children younger than 8 yr* PO: 125 mg bid/day divided *Children older than 8 yr/Adults* PO: 350 mg qid/day divided	Partial, secondary generalized, generalized tonic–clonic seizures
topiramate (Topamax)	Miscellaneous	*Children, 2–16 yr* PO: 5–9 mg/kg/day divided bid *Adults (over 17 yr)* PO: 200–400 mg/day divided bid *Children over 6 yr/Adults* PO: 100–400 mg/day divided bid	Adjunct therapy Adjunct therapy Monotherapy partial, secondary generalized, generalized tonic–clonic seizures
▸▸valproic acid (Depakene, Epival ECT®)	Miscellaneous	*Children/Adults* PO: 15–60 mg/kg/day divided bid	Generalized tonic–clonic, absence, myoclonic seizures

ECT, enteric coated; *IM,* intramuscular; *IV,* intravenous; *PO,* oral.
*PE = phenytoin equivalent: 1.5 mg fosphenytoin to be given for each milligram of phenytoin desired. One PE = 1.5 mg fosphenytoin = 1 mg phenytoin.

the seizure activity. Also assess for the occurrence of any other problems or signs and symptoms occurring before, during, or after the seizure. Question the patient about the occurrence of panic attacks because of the possible association between high levels of anxiety or stress and the precipitation of seizures in those at risk. Assess the patient for signs and symptoms of autonomic nervous system responses associated with anxiety or stress such as cold, clammy hands, excessive sweating (diaphoresis), agitation, and trembling of the extremities. Additional assessment about other problems or symptoms is important because some antiepileptic medications may be indicated for other medical diagnoses, such as prevention of migraines or treatment of postherpetic neuralgia and neuropathic pain. A complete neurological assessment with documentation of baseline CNS functioning is also important before administering antiepileptic drugs. This may include testing and grading the response of deep tendon reflexes; bilateral and upper and lower extremity sensory and motor testing; and questioning about the presence of any headaches, photosensitivity, auras, or visual changes.

Before giving these drugs, review the laboratory test results, which may include the results of red blood cell and white blood cell counts, clotting studies, and kidney or liver function studies. Knowing baseline levels of these laboratory values is important to help identify any initial abnormalities as well as to provide a comparison value when assessing for possible adverse effects, cautions, contraindications, and interactions. Assess urinary output (at least 30 mL/hr) and urine specific gravity. Conditions other than epilepsy or seizure disorders may also cause loss of or alterations in consciousness and are worthy of consideration during assessment. These conditions include syncope, breath-holding practices, transient ischemic attacks, drug use, metabolic disorders, infections, head trauma, tumours, and psychogenic problems.

Therefore, an attempt will most likely be made to rule out or eliminate many of these disorders or conditions during the diagnosing of epilepsy, and therein lies the importance of analyzing all available points of data. An EEG may also be ordered to provide more information related to the diagnosis of epilepsy. Another diagnostic procedure, magnetic resonance imaging, may be performed for neuroimaging and further data gathering.

The use of a succinimide, such as ethosuximide, requires assessment for the specific indication for this medication, that is, generalized absence seizures. In addition to performing a baseline neurological assessment, ask the patient about any problems with nausea, abdominal pain, or dizziness. Always assess for any allergies to this drug.

The miscellaneous drug topiramate is a more recently approved antiepileptic drug and has significant contraindications, cautions, and drug interactions (previously discussed in the pharmacology section in this chapter and summarized in Tables 15-4 and 15-5). Assess vital signs and mental status with attention to the patient's sensorium; level of alertness or consciousness; and any mental depression before, during, and after drug therapy and seizure activity. Document any of the following baseline problems if administering tiagabine or topiramate: dizziness, drowsiness, GI upset, ataxia, or agitation.

If barbiturates have been ordered, carefully assess not only the patient's neurological system but also vital signs because of the CNS depression associated with this class of drugs. Obtain and document all of the aforementioned general assessment data when barbiturates are prescribed. In addition, for safety purposes, identify patients at high risk for excessive. If the patient is in an acute care facility, assess the room and environment to ensure that safety measures are in place (e.g., side rails up or use of a bed alarm system in use, depending on facility policy).

Also ensure that noise level is controlled and seizure precautions are available (oxygen, suctioning equipment, and airway devices nearby; padded side rails being used; and IV access per facility policy). Note the patient's age because extremely young patients and older adults react with more sensitivity to these drugs with paradoxical reactions, irritability, and hyperactivity (as compared to CNS depressant effects). Cautions, contraindications, and drug interactions were previously discussed, earlier in the chapter.

With hydantoins like phenytoin, the previously mentioned assessment data are also appropriate. Perform a skin assessment and document intactness and the presence or absence of any rashes because of the possibility of a measleslike rash. In addition, baseline dental hygiene habits and an oral assessment, including the status of the patient's gums and teeth, are important because of the adverse effects of gingival hyperplasia. Assessment of baseline neurological functioning is crucial with the use of these CNS-altering medications and needs to include the following: (1) a focus on vision with attention to any abnormalities, especially those related to eye movement; (2) baseline neuromuscular stability with attention to coordinated movements, gait, and reflexes; and (3) assessment of speech for clarity and ability to form and express words appropriately. In addition, when phenytoins are taken, baseline liver function studies and complete blood counts (CBCs) are needed. Attention must also be given to specific drug-related cautions, contraindications, and drug interactions.

Before administering carbamazepine, an iminostilbene, a CBC is often ordered. Document these laboratory findings for baseline comparisons because of the possible adverse effect of drug-related anemias (e.g., aplastic anemia). Measure baseline vision and any abnormalities because of the potential visual changes. Significant contraindications include conditions involving bone marrow suppression because it is an adverse effect (though rare).

Gabapentin requires a thorough neurological assessment with attention to baseline energy levels, visual intactness, sensory and motor functioning, and any changes in speech. It is also important to understand the rationale for gabapentin's use so that appropriate education and instructions can be shared with the patient and family. For example, gabapentin may be used for seizure therapy, but it is also used to treat postherpetic neuralgia and neuropathic pain and to prevent migraines. Thus, an individualized plan of care with proper education needs to be developed from the appropriate assessment data. Pregabalin is similar to gabapentin and requires the same assessment.

Valproic acid requires a careful assessment as well. Gather and document information about the patient's medical history, medication profile, and neurological system, with information about seizure activity (see previous discussion). Assessment for drug allergies, cautions, contraindications, and drug interactions has been previously discussed. Other assessment areas include baseline weight, liver function studies, and notation of a history of pancreatitis.

Lamotrigine use requires a thorough neurological assessment and documentation of baseline energy levels, vision acuity, and history of headaches for comparative purposes due to the common adverse effects of headaches, vision changes, and drowsiness. Several newer miscellaneous antiepileptic drugs are available, such as levetiracetam, topiramate, and pregabalin. These miscellaneous drugs require the same thorough, general assessment as other antiepileptic drugs do. A few additional points must be kept in mind. For example, in patients taking levetiracetam, you must document the presence of any neuropsychiatric symptoms because of the potential for drug-related agitation, depression, anxiety, and other mood or behavioural changes. Although these adverse effects are rare, the assessment data must still be thorough. One interesting fact, as noted in the pharmacology section, is the lack of drug interactions with levetiracetam; however, because all antiepileptic drugs depress the CNS in some manner, assessment for the use of other CNS depressant drugs is important to note. In addition, assess liver and kidney functioning before therapy is initiated. Topiramate is used not only for management of seizures but also for other indications such as cluster headaches and neuropathic pain. Therefore, include a thorough review of the medical and medication history in the assessment to understand the reason for the drug's use. Document energy levels as well.

Nursing Diagnoses

- Deficient knowledge related to lack of familiarity and minimal experience with and lack of information concerning the use of antiepileptic drugs
- Nonadherence with the therapeutic regimen related to patient's misuse of drugs or lack of understanding about the seizure disorder and its treatment
- Chronic low self-esteem related to diagnosis of a lifelong disease and the adverse effects associated with antiepileptic drugs
- Risk for injury related to decreased sensorium and CNS depression associated with the actions and adverse effects of antiepileptic drugs

Planning

Goals

- Patient will demonstrate adequate knowledge about diagnosis and associated drug therapy.
- Patient will remain compliant with the therapy regimen, avoid adverse effects as much as possible, and experience minimal problems with either overtreatment or undertreatment.
- Patient will maintain positive self-esteem and body image.

CASE STUDY

Medications for Seizures

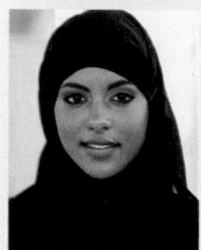

Nahla, a 21-year-old patient, has been brought to the emergency department in status epilepticus. Measures are taken to ensure her safety and prevent injury, and an intravenous (IV) line is started. The emergency department physician has ordered diazepam (Valium) 8 mg IV push, STAT.

1. The diazepam is supplied in a vial of 5 mg/mL. How much medication will the nurse draw up into the syringe?

The IV diazepam is given at a rate of 2 mg/min. Soon after the IV diazepam is given, Nahla's seizures stop, and she regains consciousness. She is admitted to a medical–surgical unit, and her mother goes to the room with her. The admitting orders call for an initial IV dose of phenytoin, followed by oral doses twice a day.

2. Why was the loading dose given intravenously?

After 2 days of observation, Nahla is ready for discharge to her mother's home. Her phenytoin level is 16 mcg/mL. She is extremely concerned about how the phenytoin will affect her.

3. Evaluate the phenytoin level of 16 mcg/mL.

4. What teaching should the patient receive regarding self-care and the adverse effects of phenytoin?

5. After 4 months, the patient's mother calls to report that Nahla has seemed "very sad lately" and has not wanted to join her friends for evenings out. "Nahla just goes to work, then comes home and stays in her room." What is the priority in this situation?

For answers, see http://evolve.elsevier.com/Canada/Lilley/pharmacology/.

• Patient will remain free from injury during drug therapy.

Expected Patient Outcomes

• Patient states the therapeutic drug effects (e.g., minimal to no seizure activity) as well as adverse effects of antiepileptic drugs and measures to decrease drug-related sedation, confusion, ataxia, and drowsiness.

• Patient or family states the importance of taking the medication exactly as prescribed, such as at the same time every day, to help maximize therapeutic effectiveness and minimize adverse effects.

• Patient states the dangers associated with sudden withdrawal of the medication, such as rebound seizure activity.

• Patient communicates openly and frequently about diagnosis-related and drug-related changes in self-esteem as well as increase in feelings of anxiety, stress, or altered body image.

• Patient experiences a safe and protective environment while at home and work while implementing safety measures to minimize injury to self, such as changing positions slowly and purposely and keeping throw rugs off the floor.

• Patient reports any symptoms of excessive sedation, confusion, lethargy, and dizziness to prescriber.

Implementation

For patients taking antiepileptic drugs, interventions are aimed at monitoring the patient while providing safety measures (see previous discussion) and securing the airway, breathing, and circulation. Airway maintenance is of critical importance for patients with epilepsy because the tongue relaxes during seizure activity, falling backward, and subsequently blocking the airway. Maintain the patient's airway in the same way as during cardiopulmonary resuscitation, using the chin lift or jaw thrust method. Provide rescue breathing, if the patient is not breathing, at a rate of 1 breath every 5 seconds. If the patient is breathing, keep the airway open through proper positioning (as just described). In addition to performing these critical components of care, maintain seizure precautions according to hospital policy. This may include making sure the patient is gently kept in bed or kept from falling, putting the side rails up, or placing the patient in a side-lying position if needed. Avoid use of a tongue blade or other instrument to pry open the patient's mouth or clenched teeth, and ensure quick access to oxygen and suctioning equipment at all times. See Special Populations: Antiepileptic Drugs.

With antiepileptic drug administration, adhere closely to the drug dose and frequency of dosing, as ordered. Close monitoring of dosing is important to attain therapeutic blood levels. For example, if an antiepileptic drug is ordered to be administered every 6 hours, it is crucial to dose the drug so that it is given around the clock to maintain blood levels. Administering the antiepileptic drug at the same time every day is also important to maintain blood levels. Educate patients on the importance of adhering to the medication regimen due to the impact one dose may have on maintaining steady states and therapeutic blood levels (see Chapter 2). If one or more doses of the antiepileptic drug is missed, the prescriber needs to be contacted immediately due to the increased risk of seizure activity. See Patient Teaching Tips for more information.

SPECIAL POPULATIONS: CHILDREN

Antiepileptic Drugs

- If a skin rash develops in a child or infant taking phenytoin, discontinue the drug immediately and notify the prescriber.
- Chewable dosage forms of antiepileptic drugs are not recommended for once-a-day administration. Intramuscular injections of barbiturates or phenytoin must never be used.
- Encourage family members, parents, significant others, or caregivers to keep a journal with a record of the signs and symptoms before, during, and after a seizure, and before, during, and after treatment with an antiepileptic drug.
- Encourage the child to wear a medical alert bracelet or necklace at all times with information about the diagnosis, drug therapy, and any drug allergies.
- Shake suspension dosage forms thoroughly before use. A graduated device or oral syringe may be used for more accurate dosing of this liquid.
- Pediatric patients are more sensitive to barbiturates and may respond to lower-than-expected dosages.

They may also experience more profound central nervous system depressive effects related to the antiepileptic drug or show depression, confusion, or excitement (a paradoxical reaction).

- Any excessive sedation, confusion, lethargy, hypotension, bradypnea, tachycardia, or decreased movement in pediatric patients taking any antiepileptic drug must be reported to the prescriber immediately.
- Carbamazepine may be given with meals to reduce risk of GI distress. All suspension forms are to be shaken and mixed thoroughly before use.
- Oral forms of valproic acid are not to be given with milk because this may cause the drug to dissolve early and irritate the mucosa. Carbonated beverages must also be avoided.

_____

GI, gastrointestinal.

With oral dosing, it is recommended that these drugs be taken with at least 180 to 240 mL of fluid—preferably water—and with food (a meal or snack) to help decrease the risk of GI upset, a frequently encountered adverse effect. Juices, milk, and carbonated beverages are best avoided because of possible interactions with the drug. Oral suspensions are to be shaken and the solution mixed thoroughly. Capsules are *not* to be crushed, opened, or chewed—especially if extended- or long-release forms. Chewing or altering these long-release formulations would allow for the entire dosage to be released at once versus over a period of time. Extended-release dosage forms are usually ordered once a day, so checking and double-checking the dosage and frequency is critical to patient safety. These actions will help to prevent the patient from experiencing either too high or too low drug serum levels.

If there are any questions regarding the type of capsule, pill, or tablet or questions about other dosage forms and recommended administration guidelines, use appropriate authoritative sources to find the answers. These sources include a licensed pharmacist, manufacturer package insert, or a current (within last 3 years) nursing drug handbook or pharmacology book. If there are any questions about the medication order or the medication prescribed, contact the prescriber immediately for clarification. Topiramate and valproic acid tablets and delayed- or extended-release dosage forms are not to be altered in any way and must be given as prescribed.

The following interventions are specific to drugs or drug classes:

- Carbamazepine: This drug is *not* to be given with grapefruit or grapefruit juice because it leads to increased toxicity of the antiepileptic drug. Grapefruit is a potent inhibitor of the intestinal cytochrome P450 CYP3A4 system, which is responsible for the first-pass effect of many medications. This interaction can lead to increases in bioavailability and result in elevated serum drug levels. If the drug is to be replaced with another antiepileptic drug, a plan must be in place to decrease the dosages of the older drug before beginning low doses (at first) of the newer drug. Serum therapeutic levels are given in Table 15-6.
- Hydantoins: As a point of reference, 150 mg of fosphenytoin is the equivalent of 100 mg of phenytoin, and the dose, concentration solution, and infusion rate of fosphenytoin is expressed as a phenytoin equivalent (PE). With parenteral forms, the only dilutional fluid to use with these drugs is normal saline (NS). A filter must also be used. Rates of infusion must follow manufacturer's guidelines and are usually 150 mg PE/min or less to avoid hypotension and cardiorespiratory depression. If dysrhythmias or hypotension occur, discontinue the infusion immediately, monitor patient vital signs, and contact the prescriber immediately. Implement safety measures, such as assisting the patient with ambulation and having the patient move slowly and purposefully, when this drug (or any other antiepileptic drug) is given because of the adverse effects of ataxia and dizziness.
- IV dose administration requires even more cautious use because of the rapid onset of action. CNS depression is always a concern; thus, there is a need to frequently monitor the patient's vital signs. If existing intravenous lines contain D5W or other solutions, the line must be flushed with normal saline before and

after dosing to avoid precipitate formation. If infiltration of the IV site leads to subcutaneous tissue access, ischemia and sloughing may occur because of the high alkalinity of the drug. Review hospital or facility policy as well as manufacturer's guidelines regarding use of possible antidotes. If infiltration occurs, discontinue infusion of the solution immediately, but leave the IV catheter and needle in place until all orders from the prescriber have been received. This practice allows any antidote medication to be administered through the IV catheter, if ordered.

- Gingival hyperplasia is an adverse effect and requires that the patient receive daily oral care as well as frequent dental visits. Complete blood counts are often monitored very closely within the first year of therapy (e.g., measured monthly for 1 year, then every 3 months). Sustained or extended release should never be opened, punctured, chewed, or broken in pieces. Other regular forms of the drug may be crushed, as needed.

- Barbiturates (e.g., phenobarbital): Abrupt withdrawal of these drugs or any antiepileptic drug must be avoided due to possible rebound seizure activity. Most of the oral dosage forms of this class of drugs are to be taken with water. Elixir dosage forms may be safely mixed with fruit juice, milk, or water. If IV infusions are indicated, calculate the dose carefully and use an IV infusion pump to administer the drug. Too-rapid infusion of IV dosage forms may lead to cardiovascular collapse and respiratory depression. In addition, frequently monitor vital signs and IV infusion rates and document in the patient's chart. If any signs or symptoms of cardiovascular or respiratory depression are noted, withhold the drug and contact the prescriber immediately, while providing supportive care through maintenance of the airway, breathing, and circulation.

- Gabapentin: This is one of the antiepileptic drugs that can be taken without regard to meals. If discontinuation of the drug is indicated, taper the dosage, as ordered, over at least 1 week to avoid rebound seizures.

- Lamotrigine: The dosing regimen for this drug must be followed, as ordered. Checking for possible drug interactions is important for patient safety. If the patient shares any suicidal thoughts or actions, contact the prescriber immediately.

- Levetiracetam: The most common adverse effect for this drug is sleepiness. Contact the prescriber if any extreme adverse effects or any problems with moving, walking, or changes in mood or behaviour occur. Any

suicidal thoughts or psychotic symptoms must also be reported immediately. With the beginning of antiepileptic therapy, due to the sedation and CNS depression, encourage the patient not to drive, operate heavy machinery, or make major decisions.

- Oxcarbazepine: This drug is to be taken as prescribed and is usually given in two divided doses. Always check for any potential drug interactions before administering (see previous discussion). The drug must be taken with food or snacks. Rash, abnormal walking or moving, or abdominal pain must also be reported, if present.

- Pregabalin: The daily dosage of this drug is usually given in two or three divided doses. Sudden or abrupt withdrawal is to be avoided. Monitor the patient for any excessive dizziness, ocular or visual changes, or edema. If these are present, report this information immediately.

- Valproic acid: Oral dosage forms of this drug are not to be taken with carbonated beverages. It is recommended that this drug be taken with at least 180–240 mL of water, food, or a snack to minimize GI upset.

Evaluation

The occurrence of a therapeutic response to antiepileptic drugs does not mean that the patient has been cured of the seizures but that seizure activity is decreased or absent. Thoroughly document any response to the medication in the nurses' notes. Because these classes of medications have other indications, such as management of chronic pain, neuropathic pain, fibromyalgia, migraines, and aggressive behaviours in children, the existing problem or disorder should show improvement with minimal adverse effects. In addition, when monitoring and evaluating the effects of antiepileptic drugs, constantly assess the patient for changes in mental status and level of consciousness, affect, eye problems, or visual disorders. Monitoring CBC is also important because of the occurrence of blood dyscrasias. Measurements of serum levels of the specific antiepileptic drug are ordered at baseline or at the start of therapy and frequently thereafter to determine if subsequent serum levels are subtherapeutic, therapeutic, or toxic. Subtherapeutic levels indicate that the dosage may need to be increased (by the prescriber), and toxic levels require withholding or decreasing the dose—but only if prescribed! Serum therapeutic levels are found in Table 15-6.

PATIENT TEACHING TIPS

❖ Educate the patient about the sedating effects of drug therapy so that appropriate steps can be taken to ensure patient safety until a steady state is achieved (usually after four or five drug half-lives). The patient is not to drive, operate heavy machinery, or make major decisions until a steady state is achieved.

❖ The patient needs to understand the importance of reporting any suicidal thoughts or ideas immediately. Alcohol, caffeine intake, and smoking are common and modifiable risk factors that may influence the risk of seizures or epilepsy and are to be avoided.

❖ Antiepileptic drugs must never be abruptly discontinued as it may precipitate rebound seizure activity.

❖ Advise female patients contemplating pregnancy to seek education and medical advice from the prescriber due to the teratogenic effects of some of the medications.

❖ Educate the patient about drug interactions between antiepileptic drugs and β-blockers, corticosteroids, calcium channel blockers, ethanol (alcohol), and other CNS depressants.

❖ The adverse effects most commonly associated with these drugs are drowsiness, GI upset, and CNS-depressing effects. Remind the patient that these adverse effects often decrease after the drug has been taken for several weeks. Taking the antiepileptic drug with food or 180 to 240 mL of fluids will help to minimize GI upset, unless otherwise noted.

❖ Inform the patient that a recurrence of seizure activity is usually due to a lack of adherence with the drug regimen. If a dose or doses of medication are missed, the prescriber needs to be contacted for further instructions. Adherence to the medication regimen is critical to the prevention of seizure activity.

❖ Emphasize to the patient that treatment of epilepsy is lifelong and that adherence with the treatment regimen is important for effective therapy. Share information with the patient and family about community and other appropriate resources (e.g., national and local support groups).

❖ Discuss with the patient important ways to improve safety in day-to-day activities while taking antiepileptic drugs. *In the kitchen:* Use an electric stove with no open flame, wear oven mitts, and cook only on rear burners. Cook in the microwave—it is the safest option.

Have a plumber install a heat-control device on faucets to avoid burns. Cover floors in carpet to help cushion falls, and use plastic dishes and containers instead of glass when possible. *In the bathroom:* Use heat-control devices on faucets. Cover floors in carpet instead of using tile. Do not put a lock on the bathroom door so that help can be obtained if needed. Bathe with only a few inches of water in the tub, and if seizure activity has not been fully controlled, bathe while someone else is present in the home. *During activities:* Always have someone along when engaging in sports, and make sure the person is knowledgeable about the management of airway and seizures. Bike riding with a helmet, swimming, and water sports are okay if an accompanying adult is present who knows how to manage seizure activity and its consequences.

❖ Each province and territory has different driving regulations for individuals with epilepsy, and provides specific requirements and guidelines. In all of these jurisdictions, the individual driver is required by law to report to the authorities any health problems, such as epilepsy, that could interfere with driving. In general, a person is legally able to drive when seizures appear to be controlled by medication, the person has been free from seizures for 6 months, and medications do not cause drowsiness or poor coordination. Other restrictions may apply. Contact each provincial or territorial's Ministry of Transportation for current and relevant information.

❖ Many people with epilepsy work at steady jobs and have successful careers. Some are unable to work, but epilepsy should not prevent people from getting a job. The Canadian Human Rights Act prohibits discrimination against persons with disabilities, while the Equality Rights section of the Canadian Charter of Rights and Freedoms guarantees people with disabilities equal benefit and protection before and under the law.

❖ Encourage the patient to wear a MedicAlert bracelet or necklace and to carry a medical alert card at all times.

❖ Keeping a daily diary or journal is important and is a helpful tool for the patient, prescriber, or caregivers. Entries need to include the date and time of any seizure as well as any details such as omitted drug doses, illnesses, and so on.

KEY POINTS

❖ Epilepsy is a disorder of the brain manifested as a chronic, recurrent pattern of seizures. A seizure is abnormal electrical activity in the brain.

❖ Seizures are classified as follows: partial-onset seizures or those originating in a more localized region of the brain; status epilepticus, a life-threatening emergency characterized by generalized tonic–clonic convulsions that occur repeatedly in succession; and tonic–clonic seizures, involving initial muscular contraction throughout the body (tonic) and progressing to alternating contraction and relaxation (clonic phase).

❖ It is important to distinguish between the different types of seizure and assess and document all symptoms, events, and problems that occur before, during, and after any seizure activity. This information may aid in the diagnosis of the type of seizure the patient is experiencing.

❖ Nonadherence with the drug regimen is the most important factor leading to treatment failure.

❖ Monitor therapeutic blood levels at all times. Avoid abrupt withdrawal of the antiepileptic drug to prevent rebound seizure activity.

❖ IV infusions of antiepileptic drugs are dangerous and must be managed cautiously, with adherence to hospital or facility policy and manufacturer's guidelines. Avoid rapid infusions because of the risk for cardiac or respiratory arrest.

❖ Older adult patients may experience paradoxical reactions to antiepileptic drugs, resulting in hyperactivity and irritability versus sedation.

EXAMINATION REVIEW QUESTIONS

1. The nurse is preparing to give medications. Which of the following is the most appropriate nursing action for intravenous (IV) phenytoin (Dilantin)?
   a. Give IV doses via rapid IV push.
   b. Administer in normal saline solutions.
   c. Administer in dextrose solutions.
   d. Ensure continuous infusion of drug.

2. The nurse is reviewing the drugs currently taken by a patient who will be starting drug therapy with carbamazepine (Tegretol). Which drug may raise a concern for interactions?
   a. digoxin (Lanoxin®)
   b. acetaminophen (Tylenol®)
   c. diazepam (Valium)
   d. warfarin sodium (Coumadin®)

3. Which response would the nurse expect to find in a patient with a phenytoin (Dilantin) level of 35 mcg/L?
   a. Ataxia
   b. Hypertension
   c. Seizures
   d. No unusual response; this level is therapeutic

4. A patient is taking pregabalin (Lyrica) but does not have a history of seizures. The nurse recognizes that this drug is also indicated for which of the following?
   a. Postherpetic neuralgia
   b. Viral infections
   c. Parkinson's disease
   d. Depression

5. The nurse is assessing a newly admitted patient who has a history of seizures. During the assessment, the patient has a generalized seizure that does not stop for several minutes. The nurse expects that which drug will be ordered for this condition?
   a. valproic acid (Depakote®)
   b. gabapentin (Neurontin)
   c. carbamazepine (Tegretol)
   d. diazepam (Valium)

6. The nurse is administering an antiepileptic drug and will follow which guidelines? (Select all that apply.)
   a. Monitor the patient for drowsiness.
   b. Stop medications if seizure activity disappears.
   c. Give the medication at the same time every day.
   d. Give the medication on an empty stomach.
   e. Notify the prescriber if the patient is unable to take the medication.

7. The nurse is preparing to administer valproic acid to a child. The order reads: "Give valproic acid, 15 mg/kg/day PO in three divided doses." The child weighs 15 kg. How many milligrams will the child receive with each dose?

CRITICAL THINKING ACTIVITIES

1. The nurse is about to administer the morning dose of phenobarbital to Paul, a patient with a history of seizures. Before the dose is given, the laboratory calls to report that Paul's phenobarbital blood level is 8 mcg/mL. What is the priority action at this time?

2. The laboratory results indicate that Paul's valproic acid level is at toxic levels, but Paul insists that he has not taken extra doses of medication. "I take it the same way at the same time every morning," he states emphatically. Upon further questioning, the patient mentions that he also takes aspirin two or three times a day for muscle aches. "Could that have any effect on my drug level?" he asks. What is the nurse's best response?

3. A patient is starting an antiepileptic drug and has many questions about it. The patient states, "I can't wait to be able to drive to work." What is the priority issue for the nurse to consider when replying?

For answers see http://evolve.elsevier.com/Canada/Lilley/pharmacology/.

CHAPTER 16

Antiparkinsonian Drugs

Objectives

After reading this chapter, the successful student will be able to do the following:

1. Briefly discuss the impact of acetylcholine and dopamine on the brain.

2. Describe the pathophysiology of Parkinson's disease (PD).

3. Identify the different classes of medications used to manage PD and list the drugs in each class.

4. Discuss the mechanisms of action, dosages, indications, routes of administration, contraindications, cautions, drug interactions, adverse effects, and toxic effects of antiparkinsonian drugs.

5. Develop a collaborative plan of care that includes all phases of the nursing process for patients taking antiparkinsonian drugs.

e-Learning Activities

Website
(http://evolve.elsevier.com/Canada/Lilley/pharmacology/)

evolve

- Answer Key—Textbook Case Studies
- Answer Key—Critical Thinking Activities
- Chapter Summaries—Printable
- Review Questions for Exam Preparation
- Unfolding Case Studies

Drug Profiles

amantadine (amantadine hydrochloride)*, p. 313
▸▸ benztropine (benztropine mesylate)*, p. 315
bromocriptine (bromocriptine mesylate)*, p. 310
entacapone, p. 314
▸▸ levodopa–carbidopa, p. 311
▸▸ ropinirole (ropinirole hydrochloride)*, p. 310
▸▸ selegiline (selegiline hydrochloride)*, p. 313
rasagiline (rasagiline mesylate)*, p. 313

▸▸ Key drug

*Full generic name is given in parentheses. For the purposes of this text, the more common, shortened name is used.

Key Terms

Adjunctive drugs Drugs added as a second drug for combined therapy with a primary drug and may have additive or independent properties. (p. 311)

Akinesia Classically defined as "without movement"; absence or poverty of movement that results in a mask-like facial expression and impaired postural reflexes. (p. 306)

Bradykinesia Slowness of movement; a classic symptom of Parkinson's disease. (p. 306)

Chorea A condition characterized by involuntary, purposeless, rapid motions, such as flexing and extending the fingers, raising and lowering the shoulders, or grimacing. (p. 306)

Dyskinesia Abnormal, often distressing involuntary movements; involves inability to control movements, which often occurs as an adverse effect of levodopa therapy. (p. 306)

Dystonia Impaired or distorted voluntary movement, often involving the head, neck, or feet. (p. 306)

Exogenous Any substance produced outside of the body that may be taken into the body (e.g., a medication, food, or environmental toxin). (p. 309)

On–off phenomenon Common in patients taking medication for Parkinson's disease; phenomenon in which the person experiences periods of greater symptomatic control ("on" time) alternating with periods of lesser symptomatic control ("off" time). (p. 306)

Parkinson's disease (PD) A slowly progressive, degenerative neurological disorder characterized by resting tremor, pill-rolling of the fingers, masklike faces, shuffling gait, forward flexion of the trunk, loss of postural reflexes, and muscle rigidity and weakness. (p. 305)

Postural instability A decrease or change in motor and muscle movements that leads to unsteadiness and hesitation in movement and gait when the individual starts or stops walking, or causes leaning to one side when sitting; occurs in Parkinson's disease. (p. 306)

Presynaptic In reference to drugs, those that exert their antiparkinsonian effects before the nerve synapse. (p. 312)

Rigidity Resistance of the muscles to passive movement; leads to the "cogwheel" rigidity seen in Parkinson's disease. (p. 306)

TRAP An acronym for symptoms of Parkinson's disease; stands for **T**remor, **R**igidity, **A**kinesia, **P**ostural instability. (p. 306)

Tremors In Parkinson's disease, shakiness of the extremities, seen mostly at rest. (p. 306)

Wearing-off phenomenon A gradual worsening of parkinsonian symptoms as a patient's medications begin to lose their effectiveness, despite maximal dosing with a variety of medications. (p. 306)

PARKINSON'S DISEASE

Parkinson's disease (PD) is a chronic, progressive, neurodegenerative disorder affecting the dopamine-producing neurons in the brain. It is the second-most common neurodegenerative disorder after Alzheimer's disease. PD was initially recognized in 1817, at which time it was called *shaking palsy*. James Parkinson later described in more detail the symptoms of both the early and advanced stages of the disease. The underlying pathological defect was not discovered until the 1960s, when it was recognized that PD involves a dopamine deficit. This deficit occurs in the area of the cerebral cortex called the substantia nigra, which is contained within another brain structure known as the basal ganglia. Also relevant is the adjacent structure called the globus pallidus. All three structures make up the extrapyramidal system, which is involved in the coordination of movement and the regulation of motor function, including posture, muscle tone, and smooth-muscle activity. In addition, the thalamus serves as a relay station for brain impulses, whereas the cerebellum regulates muscle coordination (Figure 16-1).

Dopamine is an inhibitory neurotransmitter and *acetylcholine* is an excitatory neurotransmitter in this area of the brain. A correct balance between these two neurotransmitters is needed for the proper regulation of posture, muscle tone, and voluntary movement. PD results from an imbalance in these two neurotransmitters in the basal ganglia. This imbalance is caused by failure of the nerve terminals in the substantia nigra to produce dopamine. Dopamine acts in the basal ganglia to control movements. Destruction of the substantia nigra by PD leads to dopamine depletion. This often results in excessive, unopposed acetylcholine (cholinergic) activity due to the lack of a normal dopaminergic balancing effect. Figure 16-2 illustrates the difference in neurotransmitter concentrations in persons with normal balance and in those with PD.

Some experts theorize that PD is the result of a previous head injury or of excess iron in the substantia nigra,

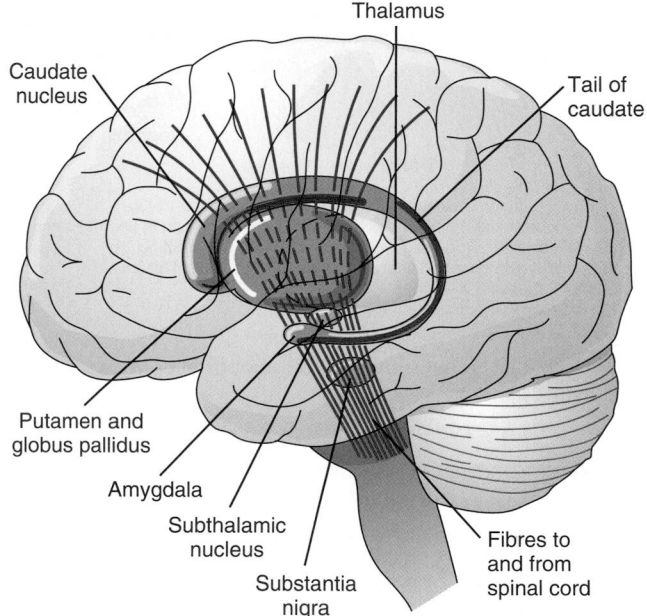

FIG. 16-1 Basal ganglia and related structures of the brain. (From Copstead-Kirkhorn, L. C., & Banasik, J. L. (2010). *Pathophysiology* (4th ed.). St. Louis, MO: Elsevier Saunders.)

which undergoes oxidation and causes the generation of toxic free radicals. Another theory postulates that because dopamine levels naturally decrease with age, PD represents a premature aging of the nigrostriatal cells of the substantia nigra, resulting from environmental or intrinsic biochemical factors, or both. Evidence from animal studies suggests that environmental toxins, such as pesticides and metals, may also contribute to the development of PD.

PD affects over 100 000 Canadians and 4.1 million people worldwide. Approximately 6 600 new cases are diagnosed each year in Canada. The average age of diagnosis is 60 years, although 85% of cases are diagnosed in those 65 years of age and older. The number of patients with PD is expected to rise dramatically due to the aging

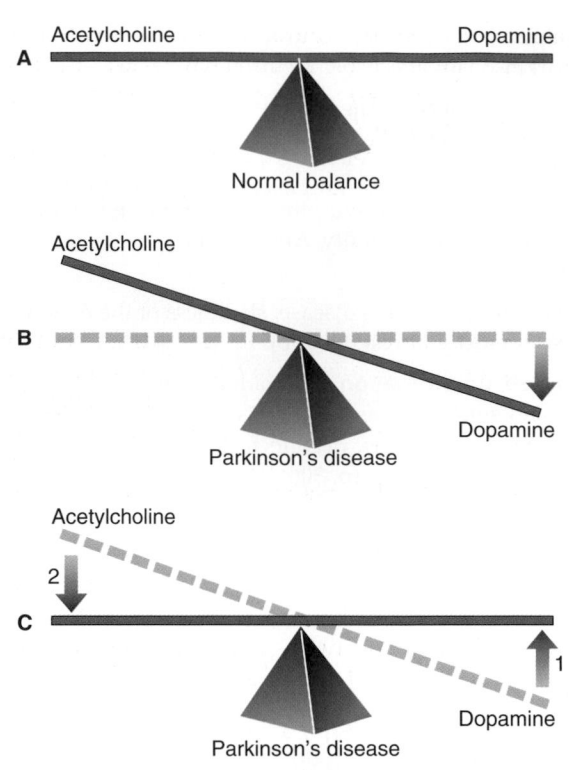

A, Normal balance of acetylcholine and dopamine in the CNS.
B, In Parkinson's disease, a decrease in dopamine results in an imbalance.
C, Drug therapy in Parkinson's disease is aimed at correcting the imbalance between acetylcholine and dopamine. This can be accomplished by either
   1. increasing the supply of dopamine or
   2. blocking or lowering acetylcholine levels.

FIG. 16-2 The neurotransmitter abnormality of Parkinson's disease.

TABLE	16-1

Classic Parkinsonian Symptoms

Symptom	Description
Akinesia	Absence of psychomotor activity, resulting in masklike facial expression
Bradykinesia	Slowness of movement
Rigidity	Cogwheel rigidity, resistance to passive movement
Tremor	Pill-rolling—tremor of the thumb against the forefinger, seen mostly at rest, is less severe during voluntary activity; usually begins on one side and progresses to the other; is a presenting sign in 70% of cases; also seen as tremor of the hand and extremities
Postural instability	Unsteadiness (associated with bradykinesia and rigidity) that leads to danger of falling; leaning to one side, even when sitting

of the baby boomer population, with a 2 to 4% risk among individuals over the age of 60 (Parkinson's Disease Foundation, 2016). Between 2011 and 2031, the prevalence of Canadians diagnosed with PD is expected to increase to more than 163 700 (Public Health Agency of Canada 2014), while the estimated number of patients with PD will increase to 8.7 million in 2030. Young-onset PD can occur in individuals under the age of 40, especially after acute encephalitis or carbon monoxide or metallic poisoning. However, the disease etiology is usually idiopathic. Overall, there is a 2% lifetime chance of developing the disease. Men are affected more often than women, in a ratio of 3:2. Evidence now suggests a possible genetic link, with up to 20% of patients having a family history of the disease.

There are no readily available laboratory tests that can detect or confirm PD. The diagnosis is usually made on the basis of the classic symptoms and physical findings. The classic symptoms of PD include **bradykinesia, postural instability, rigidity,** and **tremors** (**TRAP** [tremor, rigidity, akinesia, postural instability] with **akinesia** really manifesting as bradykinesia; refer to Table 16-1). Computed tomography (CT), magnetic resonance imaging (MRI), cerebrospinal fluid analysis, and electroencephalography (EEG) are usually normal and of little diagnostic value. Positron emission tomography (PET)

may offer some additional information. CT, MRI, and PET may be useful tools for ruling out other possible diseases as causes of the symptoms, as well as for follow-up imaging after drug and surgical treatments.

PD is a progressive condition. As the disease advances, there is substantial degeneration of surviving dopaminergic terminals that can take up pharmacologically administered levodopa and convert it into dopamine. Various types of motor complications may occur: (1) end-of-dose wearing off (diminishing dopamine effect towards end of dose associated with increasing loss of neuronal storage capability); (2) delayed on or no on response (due to delayed gastric emptying); (3) start hesitation "freezing"; and (4) peak-dose dyskinesia. Swings in the response to levodopa—called the **on–off phenomenon**—can occur. Plasma levels may fluctuate erratically because of the 90-minute half-life of levodopa and the frequently unpredictable intestinal absorption of this medication. The result is worsening of the symptoms when too little dopamine is present, or dyskinesias when too much is present. In contrast, the **wearing-off phenomenon** occurs when antiparkinsonian medications begin to lose their effectiveness, despite maximal dosing, as the disease progresses. **Dyskinesia** is the difficulty in performing voluntary movements that is commonly seen in PD. The two types of dyskinesias most frequently associated with antiparkinsonian therapy are **chorea** and **dystonia.** *Chorea* is irregular, spasmodic, involuntary movements of the limbs or facial muscles. *Dystonia* is a movement disorder that commonly involves the head, neck, and tongue and is a symptom common to patients with PD. These motor complications make PD a prominent cause of disability. Dementia may also be a result of the disease and is referred to as *Parkinson's disease–associated dementia.*

Symptoms of PD do not appear until approximately 80% of the dopamine store in the substantia nigra has been depleted. This means that by the time the disease is diagnosed, only approximately 20% of the patient's original dopaminergic terminals are functioning normally.

TREATMENT OF PARKINSON'S DISEASE

The first step in the treatment of PD is a full explanation of the disease to the patient, family members, and significant others. Physiotherapy, speech-language therapy, and occupational therapy are almost always needed in the later stages of the disease.

Treatment of the disease is primarily drug therapy, which relieves symptoms. Physical activity is also a priority for patients with PD. Many experts believe that physical activity is as important as any drug therapy, and together they greatly improve mobility. For severe cases, the surgical technique of deep brain stimulation may be used. This involves electrical stimulation of dopamine-deficient brain tissues in a way that helps to reduce

Parkinson-associated dyskinesias. Surgical treatments are for more severe cases, and patients must still respond well to drug therapy. Stem cell research is ongoing, using embryonic stem cells, induced pluripotent stem cells, and adult stem cells to find ways to regenerate, repair, or replace dopamine-producing cells to restore functioning.

DRUG THERAPY

Because PD is thought to be due to an imbalance of dopamine and acetylcholine, drug therapy is aimed at increasing the levels of dopamine or antagonizing the effects of acetylcholine. Current drug therapy is used not to slow the progression of the disease, but of symptoms. Drugs available for the treatment of PD are listed in Table 16-2.

Antiparkinsonian drug therapy is based upon the fact that nerve terminals can take up substances, store them, and release them for use when needed. As long as there are functioning nerve terminals that can take

TABLE 16-2

Review of Pharmacological Therapy for Parkinson's Disease

Generic Name	Trade Name	Route	Indications
INDIRECT-ACTING DOPAMINE RECEPTOR AGONISTS (MAO-B INHIBITORS)			
selegiline		PO	Used in conjunction with levodopa–carbidopa in early stages
rasagiline mesylate	Azilect	PO	of disease; helpful with symptom fluctuations
DOPAMINE MODULATOR			
amantadine hydrochloride		PO	Used in early stages; can be effective in moderate or advanced stages; reduces tremor or muscle rigidity
COMT INHIBITORS			
entacapone	Comtan	PO	Usually added to levodopa–carbidopa to treat symptom fluctuations; delays "off" periods; has levodopa dose-sparing effect
DIRECT-ACTING DOPAMINE RECEPTOR AGONISTS			
Ergot			
bromocriptine		PO	Usually used as drug of choice for young patients; first- or second-line therapy of choice for older adults; can be used as
Nonergot			adjunct to levodopa for "off" periods; can be used to reduce
pramipexole dihydrochloride monohydrate	Mirapex	PO	dyskinesia associated with later stages
ropinirole hydrochloride	Requip	PO	
DOPAMINE REPLACEMENT DRUGS			
levodopa–carbidopa	Duodopa®, Sinemet	PO	Usually started as soon as patient becomes functionally impaired; drug of choice for most older adult patients
ANTICHOLINERGIC DRUGS*			
benztropine mesylate		PO	Combination of levodopa and benztropine that diminishes the
ethopropazine hydrochloride	Parsitan®	PO	incidence of the levodopa-induced peripheral adverse effects
procyclidine hydrochloride		PO	of nausea, vomiting, and possibly cardiac arrhythmias; used
trihexyphenidyl hydrochloride		PO	as secondary drug for tremors and muscle rigidity
ANTIHISTAMINES†			
diphenhydramine hydrochloride	Benadryl	PO, IV	Used as secondary drug for tremors and muscle rigidity

PO, oral; *IV*, intravenous.
*See Chapter 22.
†See Chapter 37.

up dopamine, the symptoms of PD can be at least partially controlled. Since PD is essentially a deficiency of dopamine in certain areas of the brain, it seems logical that drug therapies focus primarily on restoring and enhancing dopaminergic activity in these neurons. A variety of both direct-acting and indirect-acting drugs are available for this purpose. The indirect-acting drugs are often administered first in the disease process.

DIRECT-ACTING DOPAMINE RECEPTOR AGONISTS

Direct-acting dopamine receptor agonists are drugs used to treat PD, often as first-line agents used upon diagnosis. These drugs include two subclasses: 1) nondopamine dopamine receptor agonists and 2) dopamine replacement drugs. Nondopamine dopamine receptor agonists are further subdivided into the ergot derivative bromocriptine and the nonergot drugs pramipexole dihydrochloride monohydrate (Mirapex®) and ropinirole (Requip®).

NONDOPAMINE DOPAMINE RECEPTOR AGONISTS

Mechanism of Action and Drug Effects

All of the nondopamine dopamine receptor agonists work by direct stimulation of presynaptic or postsynaptic dopamine receptors in the brain. They may be used in early or late stages of the disease. These drugs are preferred in younger patients.

Chemically, bromocriptine is an ergot alkaloid similar to ergotamine (see Chapter 14). (*Ergot* is the name of a pathological fungal growth on plants.) Bromocriptine works by activating presynaptic dopamine receptors to stimulate the production of more dopamine. Its chief site of activity is the D_2 subclass of dopamine receptors. Pramipexole dihydrochloride monohydrate and ropinirole are two newer, nonergot nondopamine dopamine receptor agonists. Both are effective in early and late stages of PD.

Indications

Both ergot and nonergot nondopamine dopamine receptor agonists are used to treat various stages of PD, either alone or in combination with other drugs. There is less risk of motor complications with ergot/nonergot nondopamine receptor agonists monotherapy. This approach is preferred in younger patients. Bromocriptine also inhibits the production of the hormone prolactin, which stimulates normal lactation. For this reason, it is used to treat women with excessive or undesired breast milk production (galactorrhea) and for the treatment of prolactin-secreting tumours.

Contraindications

Known allergy is a contraindication to dopaminergic drug therapy. These drugs are not to be used concurrently with adrenergic drugs (see Chapter 19) due to the cardiovascular risks of excessive catecholamine activity.

Adverse Effects

Many potential adverse effects are associated with dopaminergic drugs. These effects are listed in Table 16-3.

TABLE 16-3

Adverse Effects of Selected Antiparkinsonian Drugs

Drug or Drug Class	Adverse Effects
MAO-B inhibitor: selegiline	Dizziness, insomnia, hallucinations, ataxia, agitation, depression, paresthesia, somnolence, headache, dyskinesia, nausea, diarrhea, hypotension or hypertension, chest pain, weight loss, dermatological reactions, rhinitis, pharyngitis
Dopamine modulator: amantadine	Dizziness, insomnia, agitation, anxiety, headache, hallucinations, nausea, orthostatic hypotension, peripheral edema, dry mouth
COMT inhibitor: entacapone	GI upset, dyskinesia, urine discoloration, orthostatic hypotension, syncope, dizziness, fatigue, hallucinations, anxiety, somnolence, rash, dyspnea, worsening of dyskinesia
Anticholinergic agent: benztropine	Tachycardia; confusion; memory impairment; rash; hyperthermia; constipation; dry throat, nose, or mouth; nausea; vomiting; urinary retention; blurred vision; fever
Ergot derivative: bromocriptine mesylate	Ataxia, dizziness, headache, depression, drowsiness, GI upset, visual changes
Nonergot derivatives: pramipexole dihydrochloride monohydrate, ropinirole hydrochloride	Edema, fatigue, syncope, dizziness, drowsiness, GI upset
Dopamine replacement drug: levodopa–carbidopa combination	Palpitations, hypotension, urinary retention, depression, dyskinesia

COMT, catechol ortho-methyltransferase; *GI,* gastrointestinal; *MAO-B,* monoamine oxidase type B.

TABLE 16-4

Selected Drug Interactions of Antiparkinsonian Drugs

Drug or Drug Class	Interacting Drug	Mechanism	Result
MAO-B inhibitor: selegiline hydrochloride	meperidine hydrochloride and other opioids, tramadol hydrochloride, cyclobenzaprine hydrochloride, dextromethorphan hydrobromide, other MAOIs, serotonergic antidepressants, oxcarbazepine	Additive CNS stimulation	Serotonin syndrome
	carbamazepine, oral contraceptives	Reduced selegiline hydrochloride clearance	Potential selegiline hydrochloride toxicity
	buspirone hydrochloride	Uncertain	Hypertension
Dopamine modulator: amantadine	Anticholinergics	Additive effects	Increased anticholinergic adverse effects
COMT inhibitor: entacapone	MAOIs, catecholamines	Reduced catecholamine metabolism	Tachycardia, cardiac dysrhythmias, hypertension
Ergot derivative: bromocriptine	erythromycin	Cytochrome P450 interactions	Increased bromocriptine effects with risk of toxicity
	Sympathomimetics	Additive effects	Hypertension, cardiac dysrhythmias
	Antihypertensives	Additive effects	Hypotension
Nonergot: ropinirole	warfarin sodium, ciprofloxacin	Cytochrome P450 interactions	Reduced ropinirole clearance with risk of toxicity
	Antipsychotics	Antidopaminergic activity	Reduced efficacy of ropinirole
Dopamine replacement: levodopa, carbidopa	Nonselective MAOIs	Additive toxicity	Hypertensive reactions
	Benzodiazepines, antipsychotics	Reduced levodopa effects	Reduced therapeutic effects

CNS, central nervous system; *COMT,* catechol ortho-methyltransferase; *MAO-B,* monoamine oxidase type B; *MAOI,* monoamine oxidase inhibitor.

Interactions

Interactions vary among drugs and are listed in Table 16-4.

Dosages

For dosage information, refer to the table on p. 312.

DOPAMINE REPLACEMENT THERAPY

The drug levodopa has been the traditional cornerstone of therapy for PD. It is a biological precursor of dopamine, required by the brain for dopamine synthesis. However, levodopa cannot be used by itself in the brain and must be combined with another substance, carbidopa. The combination product levodopa–carbidopa provides **exogenous** sources of dopamine that directly replace dopamine in the substantia nigra. These drugs are thus classified as *dopamine replacement* drugs and are drugs of choice in the later stages of PD.

Mechanism of Action and Drug Effects

Dopamine replacement drugs stimulate presynaptic dopamine receptors to increase brain levels of dopamine. Dopamine must be administered orally as levodopa, because exogenously administered dopamine cannot pass through the blood–brain barrier. Levodopa is the biological precursor of dopamine and can penetrate into the central nervous system (CNS).

Levodopa is given in combination with carbidopa. Large oral doses of levodopa are required to obtain adequate dopamine replacement because much of the levodopa administered is broken down outside the CNS by the enzyme dopa decarboxylase. Large doses result in high peripheral levels of dopamine and lead to many unwanted adverse effects (see Table 16-3), including confusion, involuntary movements, gastrointestinal (GI) distress, hypotension, and even cardiac dysrhythmias. These problems may be avoided when levodopa is given with carbidopa. Carbidopa is a peripheral decarboxylase inhibitor with little or no pharmacological activity when given alone. When given in combination with levodopa, carbidopa inhibits the breakdown of levodopa in the periphery and thus allows smaller doses of levodopa to be used. Lesser amounts of levodopa result in fewer unwanted adverse effects.

Indications

Dopamine replacement drugs are used to directly restore dopaminergic activity in PD. Dopamine is also given by

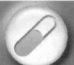

DRUG PROFILES

The traditional role of the nondopamine dopamine receptor agonists bromocriptine, pramipexole dihydrochloride monohydrate, and ropinirole has been as adjuncts to levodopa for management of motor fluctuations; however, they are now often used as first-line therapy. These drugs differ from levodopa in that they do not replace dopamine itself but act by stimulating dopaminergic receptors in the brain. They have been used as initial monotherapy and as combination therapy with low-dose levodopa in an attempt to either delay levodopa therapy or reduce the dosage of levodopa and its associated motor complications (see drug profile for levodopa).

bromocriptine mesylate

Bromocriptine mesylate stimulates only the D_2 receptors and antagonizes the D_1 receptors. Eventually, levodopa–carbidopa is needed to control the patient's symptoms. Using amantadine or a nondopamine agonist until it fails may postpone the need for levodopa therapy for up to 3 years. Bromocriptine may also be given with levodopa–carbidopa so that lower dosages of the levodopa are needed. This often results in prolonging the "on" periods and minimizing the "off" periods of the symptoms. Bromocriptine is indicated for PD as well as for hyperprolactinemia. Bromocriptine is contraindicated in cases of known drug allergy to any ergot alkaloids. It is also contraindicated in patients with severe ischemic disease of any kind (e.g., peripheral vascular disease) due to the ability of bromocriptine to stimulate dopamine receptors in the peripheral tissues outside of the brain. This stimulation can result in vasoconstriction, which can worsen peripheral vascular disease. Adverse reactions are listed in Table 16-3. Drug interactions occur with erythromycin (see Chapter 43) and adrenergic drugs (see Chapter 19).

Drug interactions are listed in Table 16-4. Bromocriptine is available only for oral use.

PHARMACOKINETICS

Route	Onset of Action	Peak Plasma Concentration	Elimination Half-Life	Duration of Action
PO	0.5–1.5 hr	1–3 hr	3–5 hr	4–8 hr

ropinirole hydrochloride

Ropinirole hydrochloride (Requip) is a nonergot nondopamine dopamine receptor agonist. A similar drug is pramipexole dihydrochloride monohydrate (Mirapex). These nonergot drugs have a better adverse effects profile (e.g., fewer dyskinesias) than bromocriptine. Ropinirole is more specific than bromocriptine for the D_2 subfamily of dopamine receptors (D_2, D_3, D_4). This in turn results in more specific antiparkinsonian effects with fewer of the adverse effects associated with more generalized dopaminergic stimulation. Ropinirole can be effective in both early- and late-stage PD and appears to delay the need for levodopa therapy. Ropinirole is indicated for both monotherapy and adjunctive therapy with levodopa. The drug is contraindicated in patients with known drug allergy. Adverse effects are listed in Table 16-3. Drug interactions occur with any drug metabolized by cytochrome P450 enzyme 1A2 (e.g., warfarin sodium, ciprofloxacin; refer to Table 16-4). Ropinirole is available only for oral use.

PHARMACOKINETICS

Route	Onset of Action	Peak Plasma Concentration	Elimination Half-Life	Duration of Action
PO	30 min	1–2 hr	3–5 hr	6–10 hr

injection in critical care settings (see Chapter 19) as a pressor drug to raise blood pressure and enhance kidney perfusion.

Contraindications

Levodopa and carbidopa are both contraindicated in cases of primary angle-closure glaucoma because they can raise intraocular pressure. However, they may be used cautiously in patients with open-angle glaucoma (see Chapter 57). Neither drug is to be used in patients with any undiagnosed skin condition because both drugs can activate malignant melanoma.

Adverse Effects

Adverse effects of dopamine replacement drugs include cardiac dysrhythmias, hypotension, chorea, muscle cramps, and GI distress (see Table 16-3).

Interactions

A possible drug interaction can occur with pyridoxine (vitamin B_6). Other interactions are listed in Table 16-4.

Dosages

For the recommended dosages of dopaminergic drugs, refer to the table on p. 312.

INDIRECT-ACTING DOPAMINERGIC DRUGS

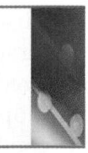

MONOAMINE OXIDASE INHIBITORS

The enzyme monoamine oxidase (MAO) causes the breakdown of the catecholamines dopamine, norepinephrine, and epinephrine in the body. There are two subclasses of MAO in the body: MAO-A and MAO-B. As early as 1965, nonselective monoamine oxidase inhibitors (MAOIs), which inhibit both MAO-A and MAO-B, were being used to improve the therapeutic effect of levodopa by preventing its metabolic breakdown. They were also among the

DRUG PROFILES

levodopa–carbidopa

Levodopa–carbidopa (Sinemet®), available orally, is one of the most commonly used drugs for PD. Carbidopa alone is not used as therapy, but rather as an adjunct to treat nausea associated with Sinemet. A variety of studies have shown that the controlled-release product Sinemet CR® (or generic) increases "on" time and decreases "off" time. As with all controlled-release products, Sinemet CR must not be crushed or chewed. Drug interactions occur with tricyclic antidepressants and other drugs (see Table 16-4). A possible drug interaction may occur with pyridoxine hydrochloride (vitamin B$_6$). Pyridoxine hydrochloride reduces the effectiveness of levodopa–carbidopa; however, the dose can usually be adjusted to overcome this interaction. See the nursing implementation section for discussion of the possible interaction of levodopa–carbidopa with dietary protein. Levodopa–carbidopa is best taken on an empty stomach; however, to minimize GI adverse effects, it can be taken with food.

Levodopa–carbidopa dosage is individualized, and drug administration is continuously matched to the needs and tolerance of the patient. Because the therapeutic range of Sinemet is narrow compared to that of levodopa alone, due to its greater milligram potency, titration and adjustment of dosage should be made incrementally. Recommended dosage ranges should usually not be exceeded. The goal of treatment is maximal benefit without dyskinesias, which are a sign of toxicity. Dosage is usually started at one tablet of Sinemet 100/25 three times a day (providing 75 mg of levodopa), increased by one tablet every 3 days until the optimal dosage has been achieved without dyskinesias. During titration, dosing is usually four times a day.

PHARMACOKINETICS

Route	Onset of Action	Peak Plasma Concentration	Elimination Half-Life	Duration of Action
PO	2–3 wk for therapeutic effect	0.5–2 hr	1.5 hr	5 hr

first medications used to treat depression, but their use for this purpose has been widely replaced by newer drug categories (see Chapter 17). A major adverse effect of the nonselective MAOIs is that they interact with tyramine-containing foods and beverages (e.g., cheese, red wine, beer, yogourt) because of their inhibitory activity against MAO-A. This has been called the *cheese effect*, and it can result in severe hypertension. Selegiline, a selective MAO-B inhibitor, is much less likely to elicit the classic cheese effect. It is approved for use in conjunction with levodopa therapy in the treatment of PD. There was earlier speculation that selegiline, as well as possibly vitamins E and C, might have antiparkinsonian effects due to neuroprotective activity at the neuronal (nerve cell) level. The results of some animal studies suggested this as a possibility; however, no studies to date have conclusively demonstrated this to be true. Nonetheless, this theoretical neuroprotective effect is still debated in the literature.

Rasagiline is the newest antiparkinsonian drug. Like selegiline, rasagiline is a selective MAO-B inhibitor. It is approved to be given once a day as monotherapy in the early stages of the disease and as adjunctive therapy, in combination with other drugs, in advanced cases. Drug interactions and adverse effects are similar to those of selegiline.

Mechanism of Action and Drug Effects

The MAO enzymes are widely distributed throughout the body, with the highest concentrations found in the liver, kidney, stomach, intestinal wall, and brain. Most MAO-B occurs in the CNS, primarily in the brain. The primary role of MAO enzymes is the breakdown of catecholamines such as dopamine, norepinephrine, and epinephrine, as well as serotonin. Giving an MAO-B inhibitor such as selegiline or rasagiline causes an increase in the levels of dopaminergic stimulation in the CNS. This helps to counter the dopaminergic deficiency seen in PD. Administration of selegiline can also allow the dose of levodopa (discussed previously in this chapter) to be reduced. Improvement in functional ability and decrease in severity of symptoms can occur; however, only approximately 50 to 60% of patients show a positive response.

Indications

Selegiline and rasagiline are currently approved for use in combination with levodopa–carbidopa. They are **adjunctive drugs** used when a patient's response to levodopa is fluctuating. As adjunctive drugs, selegiline and rasagiline can prolong the effects of levodopa and reduce fluctuations in motor control. These benefits decline within 12 to 24 months. Both drugs may also delay the need for taking levodopa when used as monotherapy in the early stages of the disease. As PD progresses, it becomes more difficult to manage it with levodopa. Ultimately, levodopa no longer controls the disease, and the patient becomes seriously debilitated. This generally occurs between 5 and 10 years after the start of levodopa therapy.

Contraindications

Selegiline and rasagiline are contraindicated in cases of known drug allergy. Concurrent use of the opioid drug meperidine hydrochloride (see Chapter 11) is contraindicated due to well-documented drug interactions between MAOIs and meperidine hydrochloride.

Adverse Effects

The most common adverse effects associated with selegiline and rasagiline use are mild and are listed in Table 16-3. At recommended dosages of 10 mg/day, the drugs maintain their selective MAO-B inhibition. However, at dosages that exceed 10 mg/day, selegiline becomes a nonselective MAOI, which contributes to the development of the cheese effect described earlier.

Interactions

Selegiline interacts with meperidine hydrochloride and has been associated with delirium, muscle rigidity, hyperpyrexia (high fever), and hyperirritability. Other reported reactions are listed in Table 16-4. Selegiline may be taken safely concurrently with catechol ortho-methyltransferase (COMT) inhibitors (see later drug section). Patients taking higher doses of selegiline need to avoid tyramine-containing foods (see Box 16-1 for a list of tyramine-containing foods).

Dosage

For the recommended dosage of selegiline see the table below.

DOPAMINE MODULATOR

Only one drug is currently known to function as a dopamine modulator. Amantadine was first recognized as an antiviral drug and was used for treating influenza virus infections. It is still used for this purpose (see Chapter 45) as well as for management of PD.

Mechanism of Action and Drug Effects

Amantadine appears to work by causing the release of dopamine and other catecholamines from their storage sites, or vesicles, in the **presynaptic** fibres of nerve cells within the basal ganglia that have not yet been destroyed by the disease process. Amantadine also blocks the reuptake of dopamine into the nerve fibres. This results

---

BOX 16-1

Foods Containing Tyramine

Food Containing Tyramine	Examples
Aged cheeses	Cheddar, stilton, blue, camembert, gorgonzola
Alcoholic beverages	Draft beer, vermouth
Meat, poultry, fish	Dry sausages, salami, smoked or pickled fish, caviar, soups or casseroles containing meat extracts (e.g., bouillon, beef broth), soy products, sauerkraut

---

DOSAGES	**Selegiline and Selected Dopaminergic Drugs**		
Drug	**Pharmacological Class**	**Usual Dosage Range**	**Indications**
amantadine hydrochloride	Dopamine modulator	*Adults* PO: 100–300 mg/day divided q12h	Parkinson's disease
benztropine	Anticholinergic	PO: 0.5–6 mg/day	
bromocriptine	Direct-acting dopamine agonist; ergot derivative	*Adults* PO: 2.5–40 mg/day divided	Parkinson's disease
entacapone (Comptan®, Stalevo®)	COMT inhibitor	*Adults* PO: 200 mg with each dosage of levodopa	Parkinson's disease
levodopa–benserazide hydrochloride (Prolopa®)	Combination direct-acting dopamine agonist/ replacement and decarboxylase inhibitor	*Adults* PO: 100–125, 400–800 mg/day based on levodopa divided into 4–6 doses	Parkinson's disease
▶levodopa–carbidopa (Sinemet, Sinemet CR, Parcopa®)	Antiparkinsonian agent	*Adults* PO: 100/10, 100/25, 250/25; titrated to optimum dosage (1500 mg levodopa max/day; 70–100 mg carbidopa max/day) CR: 200–50, 1–2 tab bid; up to 8 tabs/day; 100–25: 1–4 tab bid	Parkinson's disease
▶ropinirole (ReQuip)	Direct-acting dopamine agonist	*Adults* PO: 0.25 mg tid slowly titrating to max dose of 24 mg/day	Parkinson's disease
▶selegiline (Anipril®)	Selective MAO-B inhibitor	*Adults* PO: 5 mg bid with breakfast and lunch	Parkinson's disease

COMT, catechol ortho-methyltransferase; *CR,* controlled release; *MAO-B,* monoamine oxidase type B; *PO,* oral.

DRUG PROFILES

▸▸*selegiline hydrochloride and rasagiline mesylate*

Selegiline hydrochloride is a selective MAO-B inhibitor indicated for PD. It is used as an adjunct drug along with levodopa to reduce the dosage of levodopa needed for symptom control. Adverse effects that are increased with doses greater than 10 mg—when it loses its selectivity for MAO-B—are listed in Table 16-3. Drug interactions are listed in Table 16-4. Rasagiline mesylate (Azilect®) is a

newer selective MAO-B inhibitor comparable to selegiline. Its advantage is that it is approved as monotherapy for PD, whereas selegiline is normally used adjunctively with the dopamine replacement drug levodopa.

PHARMACOKINETICS

Route	Onset of Action	Peak Plasma Concentration	Elimination Half-Life	Duration of Action
PO	1 hr	0.5–2 hr	2 hr	1–3 days

DRUG PROFILE

amantadine hydrochloride

Amantadine—an antiviral drug—is indicated for treatment of moderate PD, for which it helps to control symptoms of tremor, including motor rigidity, by virtue of both its dopaminergic and anticholinergic effects. Interacting drugs include anticholinergics (due to additive effects; see Table 16-4). Amantadine is available only for oral use.

PHARMACOKINETICS

Route	Onset of Action	Peak Plasma Concentration	Elimination Half-Life	Duration of Action
PO	48 hr	2–4 hr	11–15 hr	6–12 wk

in higher levels of dopamine in the synapses between nerves and improved dopamine neurotransmission between neurons. Because amantadine does not directly stimulate dopaminergic receptors, it is considered indirect acting. Amantadine also has some anticholinergic properties (see Chapter 22). This may help further control dyskinesias.

Indications

Amantadine is generally indicated in the early stages of PD, while there are still some intact neurons in the basal ganglia. However, it can be used in the moderate to advanced stages. It is usually effective for only 6 to 12 months, after which it often fails to relieve hypokinesia and rigidity. Once it becomes ineffective, a dopamine agonist such as bromocriptine is usually tried (see later drug section). It is often used to treat dyskinesia associated with levodopa–carbidopa.

Contraindications

Amantadine is contraindicated in cases of known drug allergy.

Adverse Drug Effects

Common adverse effects associated with amantadine are relatively mild and include dizziness, insomnia, and nausea.

Drug Interactions

When given with anticholinergic drugs, amantadine causes increased anticholinergic adverse effects.

Dosage

For dosage information, refer to the table on p. 312.

CATECHOL ORTHO-METHYLTRANSFERASE INHIBITORS

The third category of indirect-acting dopaminergic drugs is COMT inhibitors. The sole drug in this category is entacapone (Comtan).

Mechanism of Action and Drug Effects

Entacapone, like amantadine, works presynaptically. This drug blocks COMT, the enzyme that catalyzes the breakdown of the body's catecholamines. Entacapone cannot cross the blood–brain barrier and therefore can act only peripherally. The positive effect of this drug is that it prolongs the duration of action of levodopa. This is especially true when levodopa is given with carbidopa (see section on dopamine replacement drugs earlier in the chapter). This results in reduction of the wearing-off phenomenon.

Indications

COMT inhibitors are indicated for the treatment of PD.

Contraindications

Entacapone is contraindicated in cases of known drug allergy.

Adverse Effects

Commonly reported adverse effects with entacapone include GI upset and urine discoloration. In addition, it also can worsen dyskinesia that may already be present (see Table 16-3).

Interactions

Entacapone is to be taken with nonselective MAOIs because of cardiovascular risk due to reduced catecholamine metabolism. However, the selective MAO-B inhibitor selegiline may be safely taken concurrently with COMT inhibitors.

Dosages

For dosage information, see the table on p. 312.

ANTICHOLINERGIC THERAPY

Anticholinergic drugs—drugs that block the effects of acetylcholine—are sometimes useful in treating the muscle tremors and muscle rigidity associated with PD. These two symptoms are caused by excessive cholinergic activity, which occurs because of a lack of normal dopamine balance. Anticholinergics do little, however, to relieve the bradykinesia associated with PD. The rationale for the use of anticholinergics is to reduce excessive cholinergic activity in the brain. The first drugs in this category to be used were the belladonna alkaloids—atropine and scopolamine. However, the anticholinergic adverse effects of dry mouth, urinary retention, and blurred vision can be excessive; therefore, new synthetic anticholinergics and antihistamines with better adverse effect profiles (e.g., benztropine, trihexyphenidyl) were developed.

Mechanism of Action and Drug Effects

Anticholinergic drugs block the effects of the neurotransmitter acetylcholine at cholinergic receptors in the brain as well as in the rest of the body. They are discussed in greater detail in Chapter 22. Anticholinergics are used as adjunct drug therapy in PD due to their antitremor

properties. The purpose of their use is to reduce excessive cholinergic activity in the brain. Accumulation of acetylcholine in PD causes an overstimulation of the cholinergic excitatory pathways, which results in tremors and muscle rigidity. Rigidity tends to be prominent in the flexor muscles of the trunk and limbs, which results in the stooped posture characteristic of PD. It is often associated with pain. *Lead-pipe rigidity* refers to a constant resistance to motion throughout the range of motion; it is the result of an increase in muscle tone. Cogwheel rigidity is a combination of lead-pipe rigidity and tremors. It occurs as jerky resistance that starts and stops as the limb is moved through its range of motion (the muscles contract and relax). Muscle tremors are usually worse when the patient is at rest and consist of a pill-rolling movement and bobbing of the head. Anticholinergic drugs help to alleviate these bothersome and often disabling symptoms. However, anticholinergics do little to relieve the bradykinesia that is also associated with PD.

Acetylcholine is responsible for causing increased **s**alivation, **l**acrimation (tearing of the eyes), **u**rination, **d**iarrhea, increased **g**astrointestinal motility, and possible **e**mesis (vomiting). The acronym SLUDGE is often used to describe these cholinergic effects. Anticholinergics have the opposite effects—they can cause dry mouth or decreased salivation, urinary retention, decreased GI motility (constipation), dilated pupils (mydriasis), and smooth-muscle relaxation. Anticholinergic drugs readily cross the blood–brain barrier and therefore can get to the site of PD pathology in the brain, the substantia nigra.

Historically, the anticholinergic drugs atropine sulphate and scopolamine hydrobromide were used. However, the anticholinergic adverse effects of dry mouth, urinary retention, and blurred vision associated with these original anticholinergics can be excessive. Therefore, synthetic anticholinergics were developed that have better adverse effect profiles. The anticholinergics most commonly used include benztropine and trihexyphenidyl hydrochloride. Antihistamines (see Chapter 37) also have significant anticholinergic properties; they can also be used to manage cholinergic symptoms in PD. The

 DRUG PROFILE

Inhibition of the enzyme in the body known as COMT is a strategy for prolonging the duration of action of levodopa. Entacapone (Comtan) is a reversible inhibitor of COMT.

entacapone

Entacapone (Comtan) is a COMT inhibitor indicated for the adjunctive treatment of PD. It is taken with levodopa and is effective from the first dose; a patient can feel the benefit of entacapone within a few days. Entacapone benefits patients who are experiencing wearing-off effects. When used with levodopa, it can also reduce on–off effects; the levodopa dosage can often be reduced. Entacapone is

contraindicated in patients who have shown a hypersensitivity reaction to it and should be used with caution in patients with pre-existing liver disease. Entacapone is available only for oral use. It is also available in combination tablets that contain various doses of entacapone, carbidopa, and levodopa (Stalevo).

PHARMACOKINETICS

Route	Onset of Action	Peak Plasma Concentration	Elimination Half-Life	Duration of Action
PO	1 hr	0.5–1.5 hr	1.5–3.5 hr	6 hr

DRUG PROFILES

▶▶*benztropine mesylate*

Benztropine mesylate is an anticholinergic drug used for PD and also for extrapyramidal symptoms from antipsychotic drugs (see Chapter 17). Benztropine is to be used with caution in hot weather or during exercise because it may cause hyperthermia. Other adverse effects include tachycardia, confusion, disorientation, toxic psychosis, urinary retention, dry throat, constipation, nausea, and vomiting. Anticholinergic syndrome can occur when this drug is given with other drugs such as amantadine or tricyclic antidepressants that are associated with a high incidence of anticholinergic effects. Alcohol is to be avoided as it can increase drowsiness and dizziness. Benztropine is available as tablets and in injectable form. The normal dosage is 0.5 to 6 mg/day in one or two divided doses.

PHARMACOKINETICS

Route	Onset of Action	Peak Plasma Concentration	Elimination Half-Life	Duration of Action
PO	1 hr	2–4 hr	4–8 hr	6–10 hr

most common choice of antihistamine is diphenhydramine hydrochloride (Benadryl®). Anticholinergics must be used cautiously in older adults because of significant potential adverse effects such as confusion, urinary retention, visual blurring, palpitations, and increased intraocular pressure.

NURSING PROCESS

 ## Assessment

After patients are diagnosed with PD, they soon experience the impact of the disease with every movement and activity of daily living. Not only will their lives never be the same, they soon learn that their quality of life depends on drug therapy and nondrug measures. Before medications for PD are given, assess and document vital signs (e.g., blood pressure, pulse, respirations, temperature, pain) and ABCs (airway, breathing, and circulation). In addition, obtain a complete nursing history with a thorough physical assessment, including compilation of a comprehensive medication profile. Because it may take several weeks to see a therapeutic response to medication regimens, a keen assessment and careful patient monitoring are critical to quality nursing care. Also assess the symptoms of PD (e.g., akinesia, tremors, pill-rolling, shuffling gait, masklike facies, twisting motions, drooling) during drug therapy. The on–off phenomenon may cause symptoms to appear or improve suddenly. A thorough assessment includes a health history, a review of systems, and determination of sensory and motor abilities. Also gather the following information: report(s) upon admission or the symptom(s) or event that led the patient to obtain medical treatment; past and current medical history with a focus on the presence or absence of head injury, seizures, diabetes, hypertension, heart disease, or cancer; family history of any neuromuscular or neurological disorders, heart disease, diabetes, cancer, seizures, cerebrovascular accident (stroke), or PD.

Additionally, complete a thorough systems assessment, including the gathering of subjective and objective information in the following areas as related to the possible impact of PD:

- *Central nervous system*—Inquire about any headaches, fatigue, weakness, paralysis, dizziness, or syncope. Note any changes in walking or mobility, increases in rigidity or muscle movements, or changes in the ability to carry out activities of daily living. Also important are any changes in sensation in the extremities, changes in vision or hearing, loss of or changes in coordination, changes in gait and balance, or changes in energy level. Also include questions about any changes in baseline levels of alertness; changes in memory (short term or long term); blackouts or seizures; numbness, tingling, or abnormal sensations in the extremities; changes in mood; changes in muscle movement or strength (e.g., paralysis) or motor control; and any muscle rigidity or tremors. Assess response to stimuli, and assess pupils with attention to size, shape, response to light, and symmetry (in reactions). Assess deep tendon reflexes with attention to strength bilaterally. Observe and document the patient's ability to walk and the person's gait and extremity strength. Also assess and document the ability carry out activities of daily living, including self-care.
- *Gastrointestinal and genitourinary (GU) systems*—Perform a general survey of the abdominal area with inspection, auscultation of bowel sounds, and palpation for any distention or tenderness. Determine daily baseline urinary and bowel patterns with attention to any changes in or loss of control of bladder or bowel functioning, as well as the patient's ability to engage in toileting activities. Inquire about the need for assistance with these daily functions. Ask the patient about any difficulty in swallowing (dysphagia) and any problems in self-feeding or preparing meals. Also ask if the patient has any difficulties swallowing medications. If such difficulties are identified, assess further for any subsequent nutrition imbalance.
- *Skin and oral mucous membranes*—Assess the skin colour, texture, turgor, and fragility, and note any

breaks in the skin, bruises, lesions, masses, or swelling. Also document colour and moisture of the oral cavity and mucous membranes.

- *Respiratory system*—Focus attention on respiratory rate, rhythm, depth, effort, and breath sounds.
- *Psychological and emotional status*—Assess the patient for any recent or past changes in mood, affect, or personality. Also note any other disease-related concerns such as depression, emotional ups and downs, increase in irritability, social withdrawal, or changes in sexual functioning or intimacy.
- *Functional abilities*—Inquire about any changes in everyday function in the patient's personal and professional life. Note any changes in daily task performance at work or any sick leave or sick days taken, as well as the patient's ability to exercise, drive, or shop for groceries and other necessities.

With indirect-acting dopamine receptor agonists—such as amantadine—and direct-acting dopamine receptor agonists—such as levodopa–carbidopa and ropinirole—include in your assessment vital signs with supine and standing blood pressures (because of drug-related orthostatic hypotension), height, weight, medication and medical history, and nursing history. Include family, significant others, and caregivers in the assessment and data collection process. Note contraindications, cautions, and drug interactions prior to administering these drugs (see previous pharmacology discussion). Assess motor skills, including abilities and deficiencies, and for the presence of akinesia, bradykinesia, postural instability, rigidity, tremors, staggering gait, or drooling (see Key Terms and Table 16-1).

Assessment of urinary patterns is also important because of the possibility of drug-induced urinary retention. If blood urea nitrogen (BUN) and creatinine measurements are ordered, the results need to be routinely examined because these values are indicators of kidney function. Alkaline phosphatase levels are indicators of liver function and also need to be assessed, if ordered. It is important to determine these laboratory values in patients with decreased kidney or liver function so that dosages of antiparkinsonian drugs may be altered by the health care provider.

Related to lifespan considerations, it is important to understand the gynecological history of the patient and to know if the patient is pregnant or lactating. Some of the dopamine replacement drugs cross into the placenta and into breast milk and have unknown actions in fetuses. Interactions related to these drugs are presented in Table 16-4. Refer to Table 16-3 for a listing of selected antiparkinsonian drugs and their related classifications and subclassifications.

When anticholinergic drugs are prescribed, assess the patient carefully to determine gross level of organ functioning—especially in those systems most affected by PD, including the GI, GU, visual, cardiac, and neurological systems. Assess mental status, and pay close attention to any present or past changes as well as to any presence of confusion, disorientation, or psychoticlike behaviour. It is important to consider this aspect in older adults because of decline in liver function and a subsequent higher risk for adverse effects and possible toxicity (with antiparkinsonian drugs and drugs in general) and an overall increased sensitivity to the effects of drugs (see Chapter 4). Cautions, contraindications, and drug interactions have been previously discussed.

For the indirect-acting dopamine receptor agonist drugs (a subclass of presynaptic dopamine release enhancers) that are also antiviral (e.g., amantadine), the previously discussed baseline and general assessment information is also applicable. The patient's knowledge of the drug's use for PD (versus its use as an antiviral) and awareness that its onset of action will be delayed for several days or longer needs to be confirmed. Continuous assessment of the patient's status and improvement in disease-related symptoms is important because a decline in this drug's effectiveness (specifically a failure in the ability to control hypokinesia and rigidity) may occur within 6 to 12 months after initiation of therapy. If amantadine (also a prolactin inhibitor) is prescribed, the nurse must understand that this drug is also used for suppression of lactation and must assess for the appropriateness of its use. Patients taking these drugs also require additional CNS assessment because of the possible adverse effects of dizziness, headache, insomnia, and anxiety. Also, if the patient is taking this medication long term, assessment for orthostatic hypotension and dizziness is crucial to patient safety.

The antiparkinsonian drugs classified as indirect-acting dopamine receptor agonists (a subclass of MAO-B inhibitors), such as selegiline, require assessment of many of the same parameters discussed earlier. In addition, however, cardiac status is important to assess and document because of the possible adverse effects of hypotension or hypertension and chest pain. Assessment of dosing is also important because, as with other antiparkinsonian drugs, a low dose is used initially, with gradual increases over an approximately 3- to 4-week period. The lowest possible dose is recommended for initiation of therapy so that there is plenty of room for further increases in dosing as the disease progresses. These drugs also require careful neurological assessment due to the adverse effects of depression, hallucinations, ataxia, and agitation (see Table 16-3).

For the indirect-acting dopamine receptor agonist COMT inhibitors (e.g., entacapone), assessment of baseline vital signs is also required, with a focus on standing and supine blood pressure because of the adverse effects of orthostatic hypotension and syncope. These adverse effects occur with more frequency with the COMT inhibitors than with the other antiparkinsonian drugs, and thus increased caution and concern are needed. Assessment of dosing time is also important because if these drugs are not given 1 hour before or 2 hours after levodopa, the bioavailability of the drug may be adversely affected. Assess serum transaminase levels before and

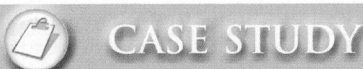

CASE STUDY

Drugs for Parkinson's Disease

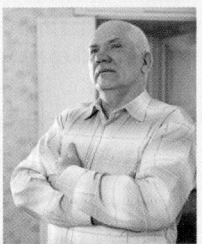

Boris, a 62-year-old retired contractor, is undergoing surgery to repair an umbilical hernia. He has had Parkinson's disease for 5 years and is currently taking levodopa–carbidopa (Sinemet CR) and selegiline. Other than the Parkinson's disease, he has no health problems. He has enjoyed fairly good control up until this week but is now experiencing more "bad times," as he calls them.

1. Patients who are taking long-term levodopa treatment often experience an "on–off" phenomenon in symptoms. Explain the physiology behind this phenomenon.

2. Explain the reason for giving selegiline along with the levodopa–carbidopa.

3. Are there any concerns regarding drug interactions? Explain your answer.

4. What is the purpose of the entacapone?

5. Before administering the entacapone, the nurse reviews Boris's history for any potential contraindications. What condition(s) would be a potential contraindication to entacapone?

_____

For answers, see http://evolve.elsevier.com/Canada/Lilley/pharmacology/.

during drug therapy. If the patient's alanine aminotransferase level is elevated to the upper range of normal or higher, the health care provider will most likely discontinue the drug because of the increased risk of liver failure.

Nursing Diagnoses

- Impaired urinary retention related to the pathophysiological effects of the disease process on the bladder with incomplete emptying
- Constipation related to decreased GI peristalsis associated with the disease process
- Imbalanced nutrition, less than body requirements, related to the disease process as well as adverse effects of drug therapy
- Impaired physical mobility related to the disease process and adverse effects of the various antiparkinsonian medications
- Disturbed body image related to changes in appearance and mobility due to the disease process
- Deficient knowledge related to lack of exposure to and experience with a complex and long-term treatment regimen
- Risk for injury related to the physical limitations and changes in mobility, gait, balance, and coordination produced by the disease process

Planning

Goals

- Patient will regain as normal as possible bladder elimination patterns.
- Patient will maintain as normal as possible bowel elimination patterns.
- Patient will maintain adequate and balanced nutritional status.

- Patient will be able to maintain safe mobility and activities of daily living.
- Patient will maintain a positive self-image and body image.
- Patient will demonstrate adequate knowledge and comprehension about the illness, medication therapy, and drug-related adverse and toxic effects.
- Patient will remain free from injury and self-harm.

Outcome Criteria

- Patient discusses ways to minimize problems associated with drug-induced alterations in bladder elimination patterns (retention), such as consuming plenty of fluids, taking medications as prescribed, attempting to empty the bladder at regular intervals, and reporting any unresolved urinary problems.
- Patient implements various measures to decrease constipation, such as increasing bulk and fibre in the diet with fruits and vegetables, consuming plenty of fluids, and remaining as active as possible.
- Patient states the importance of maintaining proper nutrition, including the use of nutritional supplements and vitamins and gives examples of daily menus designed to increase dietary protein and intake from the major food groups (divided into six small, frequent meals).
- Patient participates in ambulation and daily care with the use of assistive devices, as appropriate.
- Patient removes any barriers to safe mobility in the home environment and uses handrails throughout the home.
- Patient maintains mobility and activity participation through involvement in physiotherapy and occupational therapy interventions, as well as through the use of active and passive range of motion exercises.

- Patient openly verbalizes fears, anxieties, and changes in self-image with family, members of the health care team, support staff, and support groups.
- Patient, family, significant others, and caregivers openly discuss the effects of the disease process on relationships, daily activities, and future plans, as well as the impact of any drug-related adverse effects (e.g., dizziness, nausea, vomiting, GI upset, palpitations) and the lifelong need for daily medication and monitoring.
- Patient states purposes of medication therapy, such as decrease in symptoms of PD, improved comfort, enhanced participation in activities of daily living, and increased nutritional status.
- Patient states information required to contact the health care provider and states symptoms that should reported, such as dry mouth, unresolved nausea or vomiting, fainting, or loss of appetite.
- Patient and family, significant others, and caregivers describe ways of preventing injury, such as using assistive devices, removing throw rugs, using night lights, and installing handrails throughout the home.

Implementation

Nursing interventions associated with antiparkinsonian drugs vary somewhat depending on the drug class, but close monitoring and comprehensive patient education are required for all of these drugs. With the onset of drug therapy, educate patients, family, and caregivers to keep a daily drug calendar or journal, with entries including the drugs prescribed, dosage, frequency and timing, therapeutic changes, and adverse effects. During the start of dopaminergic drug therapy, the patient will most likely need assistance when walking because of dizziness and possible syncope. Doses are given several hours before bedtime to decrease the incidence of insomnia, a known adverse effect of dopaminergic drugs. Oral doses are given with food to help minimize GI upset. Interaction of vitamin B_6 (pyridoxine hydrochloride) with levodopa was once a major concern because this vitamin was found to block the uptake of plain levodopa. However, the majority of patients taking a levodopa–carbidopa combination drug have no problems with vitamin B_6. If it is a problem, the health care provider needs to be consulted for further instructions. In addition, amino acids from dietary protein may interfere with the uptake of levodopa in the brain. While taking levodopa–carbidopa, the patient may continue to eat high-protein foods (e.g., meat, fish, poultry, and dairy products) but use portion control (limiting meat portions to about the size of a deck of cards) and take the drug dose a half hour before a protein-containing meal. Timing is the most important factor, not the quantity of protein consumed over the course of the day. A nutritional consult may be beneficial to assist the patient in menu planning. A registered dietitian or nutritionist may also be helpful in teaching the patient about how to divide daily intake of protein among small, frequent meals so that minimal amounts of protein are ingested throughout the day and are consumed at the proper time. Consumption of well-balanced meals is important, as is increasing fluid intake. Patients should aim to drink at least 3 000 mL/day unless contraindicated. Drinking water is important even if the patient is not thirsty or in need of hydration, to prevent and manage the adverse effect of constipation. Encourage the intake of foods that are natural laxatives, such as prunes, vegetables, and other foods high in fibre. If the adverse effect of dry mouth is problematic, taking fluids and sucking on hard candies or lozenges may be helpful. Regular dental hygiene should be encouraged. If nausea or vomiting occurs or problems with edema are persistent (the patient gains 1 kg or more in 24 hours or 2.3 kg or more in 1 week), the health care provider should be contacted immediately.

With anticholinergic drugs, patients must take the medication as prescribed, after meals or at bedtime and not at the same time as other medications. Patients also need to know that it may take a few days to several weeks for the drugs to show their therapeutic effectiveness (e.g., improvement in tremors). Because of the risk of GI upset (i.e., nausea, vomiting), it is recommended that these drugs be taken with a light, bland snack, such as crackers or plain bread. These medications are generally taken at night because of their sedating properties. Measures to help prevent and treat dry mouth are encouraged, such as increasing fluid intake and sucking on sugar-free hard candies. See Chapter 22 for further information about the use of these drugs, related interventions, and adverse effects to report. Bromocriptine is to be taken as prescribed and not abruptly stopped. Because this drug may cause GI upset, it is best taken with a snack. Any severe dizziness, GI upset, ataxia, extreme drowsiness, or visual changes must be reported immediately.

MAO-B inhibitors, such as selegiline, must be given exactly as ordered. Selegiline is often given in upwardly titrated dosages, while levodopa–carbidopa dose amounts are decreased. Orthostatic hypotension may be a transient problem, so the patient must move and change positions slowly and purposefully. If dizziness is severe or if the patient experiences hallucinations, the health care provider should be contacted for further instructions.

The newer COMT inhibitors have been shown to have greater efficacy in patients with advanced forms of PD. After treatment using the various dosage forms of levodopa–carbidopa, a COMT inhibitor may be added to the therapeutic regimen. Onset of therapeutic effects is rapid. These drugs must be administered as prescribed and may be taken without regard to meals or food. These and other antiparkinsonian drugs must never be discontinued abruptly and require a gradual weaning period to avoid worsening of PD or other dangerous effects. Emphasize to patients and caregivers that all appointments with health care providers must be kept and all laboratory testing performed as ordered. Patients must also understand the importance of changing positions slowly and with purpose to avoid syncope due to drug-related orthostatic hypotension. Inform patients that entacapone may turn their urine brownish orange but that this is not harmful. As with all medications, patients must keep with them at all times a written list of prescription drugs, over-the-counter (OTC) drugs, vitamins, minerals, and natural health products they are taking. This list of medications needs updating frequently and should be taken each time patients visit the health care provider or are hospitalized. Having this list allows continuity of information with health care providers and helps to prevent errors or omission of medications.

It is most important in the care of patients with PD to be aware of all other forms of therapies that may be beneficial, such as support groups, water aerobics, and occupational therapy and physiotherapy. Some community resources that are available include community recreation facilities, transportation services, and Meals on Wheels. Educational materials and emotional support resources must be made available and shared with family members, caregivers, and significant others because of the long-term and progressive nature of the disease. Contacting research institutes about new treatment protocols may be a viable option for patients and family members during the course of the disease. See Patient Teaching Tips for more specific information.

Evaluation

Monitoring patients' responses to any of the antiparkinsonian drugs is crucial to documenting treatment success or failure. Therapeutic responses to antiparkinsonian drugs include an improved sense of well-being, improved mental status, increased appetite, ability to perform activities of daily living, improved concentration and ability to think clearly, and a decrease in intensity of symptoms of PD (e.g., less tremor, a less shuffling gait, decreased muscle rigidity, fewer involuntary movements). In addition to monitoring for therapeutic responses, also monitor for adverse effects such as dizziness, hallucinations, nausea, insomnia (associated with indirect-acting dopamine receptor agonists such as selegiline, amantadine, and entacapone), ataxia, depression (associated with direct-acting dopamine receptor agonists such as bromocriptine and dopamine replacement drugs such as levodopa–carbidopa), palpitations, hypotension, and urinary retention. Patients need to understand the importance of immediately reporting to their health care provider any of the following signs and symptoms that indicate possible overdose: excessive twitching, drooling, or eye spasms. Therapeutic effects of COMT inhibitors (e.g., entacapone) may be noticed within a few days, whereas therapeutic effects of other antiparkinsonian drugs may take weeks to manifest. Adverse effects for which to monitor with COMT inhibitors include those mentioned previously, but fewer dyskinesias are seen than with dopamine agonists. See Special Populations: Older Adults for points related to PD in older adults.

SPECIAL POPULATIONS: OLDER ADULTS

Antiparkinsonian Drugs

- Levodopa–carbidopa must be used cautiously and with close monitoring in older adults, especially those with a history of heart, kidney, liver, endocrine, pulmonary, ulcer, or mental health disorders.
- Levodopa–carbidopa is often started at a low dose because of the increased sensitivity of older patients to these medications and the need to save larger dosages for a later time during treatment.
- Overheating is a problem in patients taking anticholinergics, so older adults taking these medications must avoid excessive exercise during warm weather and excessive heat exposure.
- One of the main challenges with the long-term use of levodopa–carbidopa is that its duration of effectiveness decreases over time; this is even more problematic for older adult patients. COMT inhibitors hold much promise for older adult patients who are experiencing the wearing-off phenomenon; they help turn the "off" times into "on" times so that the drug begins to work throughout the day.

PATIENT TEACHING TIPS

- ❖ Patients should be aware that all medications must be taken exactly as ordered. Around-the-clock dosing is usually prescribed to achieve steady blood levels, especially with dopamine agonists.
- ❖ Some patients will be allowed a certain amount of freedom in the dosing of their medications, depending on their individual needs. For example, when a patient is travelling or attending an important function, an extra dose of medication may be indicated to help with movement disorders.
- ❖ Patients should avoid alcohol, OTC drugs, and natural health products unless approved by the health care provider.
- ❖ Emphasize to patients the importance of taking medication as prescribed and not stopping the medication. It is important for patients,

Continued

PATIENT TEACHING TIPS—cont'd

family, and caregivers to understand that medications must be taken at the dosage and time prescribed. Inability to adhere or remain adherent to protocols may lead to exacerbation of symptoms and development of complications. Missing a dose by even 30 minutes may lead to an "off" period that lasts hours. Parkinson Society Canada has a "get it on time" campaign designed to improve the quality of life of individuals with Parkinson's disease. This is an educational program helping health care providers, patients, families, and caregivers to understand the disease and the adverse effects that occur if medications are not administered on time.

❖ If a patient misses a dose of medication, the health care provider must be contacted for further instructions. Some health care providers inform patients initially that if they miss a dose to take it as soon as they remember, and, if it is close to the next dose time, to skip the missed dose and take the next dose.

❖ If experiencing orthostatic hypotension, patients need to understand the rationale for changing positions slowly and the need to increase intake of fluids and wear compression stockings, unless contraindicated. Patients with a history of heart failure must be monitored for signs and symptoms of fluid overload.

❖ Patients should be aware that sustained-release drug forms are not to be crushed, chewed, or altered in any way. The drug is to be taken in its whole form.

❖ With anticholinergics, warn patients about the adverse effect of dry mouth. Using artificial saliva drops or gum, engaging in frequent mouth care, drinking fluids, and sucking on sugarless gum or hard candy may be helpful.

❖ Inform patients taking entacapone that urine colour may darken and that this adverse effect is harmless.

❖ Encourage patients to report any change in vision (e.g., blurring), decline in mental alertness, confusion, or lethargy while taking any of the antiparkinsonian drugs. Any difficulty with urination, irregular pulse rate, or severe uncontrolled movements of the arms or legs must also be reported.

❖ Educate patients and their families that some antiparkinsonian drugs are often titrated to the patient's

response and that it may take 3 to 4 weeks for a therapeutic response to become evident.

❖ The nonergot drug ropinirole may result in drowsiness, fatigue, and syncope. Emphasize to patients the importance of safety and instruct them on how to handle these adverse effects.

❖ Encourage patients to increase intake of fluids and dietary fibre to help prevent constipation associated with the disease process. Constipation is also an adverse effect of drug therapy.

❖ Inform patients that the COMT inhibitor entacapone needs to be taken with a meal or snack to minimize GI upset. Patients using this medication should also report to their health care providers any signs and symptoms of possible liver dysfunction such as jaundice or back or abdominal pain.

❖ Patients must immediately report to their health care providers any abnormal contractions of the head, neck, or trunk, as well as any syncope, falls, itching, or jaundice.

❖ Educate patients about the goal of therapy, especially if entacapone is being used to help manage the wearing-off phenomenon. This phenomenon is a waning of the effects of a dose of levodopa before the scheduled time of the next dose, resulting in diminished motor ability and performance and the experience of more disease symptoms. If a COMT inhibitor is added to levodopa–carbidopa, the wearing-off phenomenon is minimized, and the therapeutic effects of the regimen are maximized. The patient can then expect that the "off" time will be minimized and that the drugs will work throughout the day, which is the goal in the treatment of PD.

❖ Suggest resources such as Parkinson Society Canada (http://www.parkinson.ca/). This organization provides educational materials and support services for patients, families, and caregivers.

❖ Recommend involvement with an interdisciplinary team as required in the management of PD (including, for example, movement disorder neurologist, geriatrician, nurse with experience in PD care, physiotherapist, occupational therapist, speech-language pathologist, registered dietitian, social worker, and spiritual care professional).

KEY POINTS

❖ The neurotransmitter abnormalities caused by PD include chronic, progressive degeneration of dopamine-producing neurons in the brain. Patients with this disease also have elevated acetylcholine levels and lowered dopamine levels.

❖ Signs and symptoms of this disease include bradykinesia (slow movements), muscle rigidity (cogwheel rigidity), tremors (e.g., pill-rolling), postural instability, and dystonias (abnormal muscle tone in any tissue).

❖ Dyskinesias occur as adverse effects of some of the antiparkinsonian drugs. Dyskinesias include

motor difficulties while performing voluntary movements.

❖ Drugs used in the treatment of PD include amantadine, benztropine, bromocriptine, levodopa–carbidopa, entacapone, ropinirole, and selegiline.

❖ Patient considerations include providing individual and family support along with options for care of the family member with PD. The disease is long term and lifelong, as well as debilitating. A holistic approach in which all aspects of the patient and family are considered and respected is the key to quality nursing care.

EXAMINATION REVIEW QUESTIONS

1. Which condition will alert the nurse to a potential caution or contraindication in regard to the use of a dopaminergic drug for treatment of mild PD?
a. Diarrhea
b. Tremors
c. Angle-closure glaucoma
d. Unstable gait

2. A patient is taking entacapone as part of the therapy for PD. Which intervention by the nurse is appropriate at this time?
a. Notify the patient that this drug causes discoloration of the urine.
b. Limit the patient's intake of tyramine-containing foods.
c. Monitor results of kidney studies because this drug can seriously affect kidney function.
d. Force fluids to prevent dehydration.

3. During patient teaching for antiparkinsonian drugs, the nurse will include which statement?
a. "The drug will be stopped when tremors and weakness are relieved."
b. "If a dose is missed, take two doses to avoid significant decreases in blood levels."
c. "Be sure to notify your physician if your urine turns brownish-orange."
d. "Take care to change positions slowly to prevent falling due to a drop in blood pressure."

4. A patient will be taking selegiline, 10 mg daily, in addition to dopamine replacement therapy for PD. The nurse will implement which precautions regarding selegiline?
a. Teach the patient to avoid foods containing tyramine.
b. Monitor for dizziness.

c. Inform the patient that this drug may cause urine discoloration.
d. Monitor for tachycardia and palpitations.

5. A patient with PD will start taking entacapone along with the levodopa–carbidopa he has been taking for a few years. The nurse recognizes that the advantage of taking entacapone is that
a. The entacapone can reduce on-off effects.
b. The levodopa may be stopped in a few days.
c. There is less GI upset with entacapone.
d. It does not cause the cheese effect.

6. The nurse is assessing a patient who has begun therapy with amantadine for PD. The nurse will look for which possible adverse effects? (Select all that apply.)
a. Nausea
b. Palpitations
c. Dizziness
d. Insomnia
e. Edema

7. The order reads: bromocriptine 10 mg per day PO. The medication is available in 2.5-mg tablets. How many tablets will the nurse give per dose?

Answers: 1. c, 2. a, 3. d, 4. b, 5. a, 6. a, c, d, 7. 4 tablets

CRITICAL THINKING ACTIVITIES

1. A patient has been taking levodopa for a few years and is now experiencing an increase in symptoms of PD. His physician gave him a new prescription for entacapone, and the patient is excited, stating, "My doctor said that I should see improvement in a few days." When the nurse reviews the patient's health history, the nurse notes a previous medical condition that may be of concern. What condition would this be, and what is the nurse's priority action?

2. A patient with PD will be starting therapy with amantadine. He asks the nurse, "How long will I have to take this medicine?" What would be the nurse's best response?

3. The nurse is assessing a patient who is visiting the clinic for a 2-month follow-up appointment after starting selegiline, 10 mg daily. The patient is pleased with the improvement in his PD symptoms but states, "My wife looked up this drug and told me that I can't eat cheese or drink wine anymore. I hate that, and I really don't want to take this medicine." What is the nurse's priority action at this time?

For answers, see http://evolve.elsevier.com/Canada/Lilley/pharmacology/.

CHAPTER 17

Psychotherapeutic Drugs

Objectives

After reading this chapter, the successful student will be able to do the following:

1. Briefly discuss the etiology and pathophysiology of the various mental health disorders.

2. Identify the psychotherapeutic drug classes, such as anxiolytic drugs, antidepressants, mood-stabilizing drugs, and antipsychotics.

3. Discuss the mechanisms of action, indications, therapeutic effects, adverse effects, toxic effects, drug interactions, contraindications, and cautions associated with psychotherapeutic drugs.

4. Develop a collaborative plan of care that includes all phases of the nursing process for patients taking psychotherapeutic drugs.

5. Develop patient education guidelines for patients taking psychotherapeutic drugs.

e-Learning Activities

Website
(http://evolve.elsevier.com/Canada/Lilley/pharmacology/)

evolve

- Answer Key—Textbook Case Studies
- Answer Key—Critical Thinking Activities
- Chapter Summaries—Printable
- Review Questions for Exam Preparation
- Unfolding Case Studies

Drug Profiles

- ▶▶ alprazolam, p. 329
- ▶▶ amitriptyline (amitriptyline hydrochloride)*, p. 335
- ▶▶ bupropion (bupropion hydrochloride)*, p. 338
  buspirone (buspirone hydrochloride)*, p. 329
- ▶▶ clozapine, p. 344
- ▶▶ diazepam, p. 329
  duloxetine (duloxetine hydrochloride)*, p. 339
- ▶▶ fluoxetine (fluoxetine hydrochloride)*, p. 338
  haloperidol, p. 343
- ▶▶ lithium (lithium carbonate)*, p. 331
- ▶▶ lorazepam, p. 329
- ▶▶ mirtazapine, p. 339
- ▶▶ risperidone, p. 344
  trazodone (trazodone hydrochloride)*, p. 338

▶▶ Key drug

*Full generic name is given in parentheses. For the purposes of this text, the more common, shortened name is used.

Key Terms

Affective disorders Emotional disorders that are characterized by changes in mood. (p. 325)

Agoraphobia An anxiety disorder that involves an intense fear of being in unfamiliar situations or places that may be difficult to leave or in which help may not be available in the event of having an unexpected panic attack or pani-clike symptoms. (p. 325)

Akathisia A movement disorder in which there is an inability to sit still; motor restlessness; can occur as an adverse effect of psychotropic medications. (p. 341)

Anxiety The unpleasant state of mind in which real or imagined dangers are anticipated or exaggerated. (p. 324)

Biogenic amine hypothesis (BAH) A theory suggesting that depression and mania are caused by alterations in the concentrations of dopamine, norepinephrine, serotonin, and histamine. (p. 328)

Bipolar disorder (BPD)   A major psychological disorder characterized by episodes of mania or hypomania, cycling with depression. (p. 325)

Cardiometabolic syndrome   A cluster of risk factors (increased glucose level, increased blood pressure, abnormal cholesterol levels, excess body fat around the waist) occurring together that increases the risk of heart disease, stroke, and type 2 diabetes. (p. 341)

Depression   An abnormal emotional state characterized by exaggerated feelings of sadness, melancholy, dejection, worthlessness, emptiness, and hopelessness that impact the patient's life and may be out of proportion to reality. Signs include withdrawal from social contact, loss of appetite, and insomnia. (p. 325)

Dopamine hypothesis   A theory suggesting that dopamine dysregulation in certain parts of the brain is one of the primary contributing factors to the development of psychotic disorders (psychoses). (p. 325)

Dysregulation hypothesis   A theory that views depression and affective disorders as caused not simply by decreased or increased catecholamine and serotonin activity but by failure of the brain to regulate the levels of these neurotransmitters. (p. 328)

Dystonia   A syndrome of abnormal muscle contraction that produces repetitive involuntary twisting movements and abnormal posturing of the neck, face, trunk, and extremities; often an adverse reaction to psychotropic medications. (p. 341)

Extrapyramidal symptoms   Signs and symptoms that result from pathological changes to the pyramidal portions of the brain. Such symptoms include various motion disorders similar to those seen in Parkinson's disease and are an adverse effect associated with the use of various antipsychotic drugs. (p. 341)

Gamma-aminobutyric acid (GABA)   An amino acid in the brain that functions to inhibit nerve transmission in the central nervous system. (p. 324)

Hypomania   A less severe and less potentially hazardous form of mania. (p. 325)

Mania   An acute illness characterized by an expansive emotional state, extreme excitement, elation, hyperactivity, agitation, talkativeness, flight of ideas, reduced attention span, increased psychomotor activity, impulsivity, insomnia, anorexia, and sometimes violent, destructive, and self-destructive behaviour. (p. 325)

Neuroleptic malignant syndrome   An uncommon but serious adverse effect associated with the use of antipsychotic drugs and characterized by symptoms such as fever, cardiovascular instability, and myoglobinemia (presence in the blood of muscle breakdown proteins). (p. 341)

Neurotransmitters   Endogenous chemicals in the body that serve to conduct nerve impulses between nerve cells (neurons). (p. 323)

Permissive hypothesis   A theory postulating that reduced concentrations of serotonin (5-hydroxytriptamine) is the predisposing factor in individuals with affective disorders. (p. 328)

Psychosis   (plural: psychoses) A type of serious mental health disorder that can take several different forms and is associated with being out of touch with reality; that is, the individual is unable to distinguish imaginary from real circumstances and events. (p. 325)

Psychotherapeutics   Drugs used in the treatment of emotional and mental health disorders. (p. 324)

Psychotropic   Capable of affecting mental processes; usually said of a medication. (p. 325)

Serotonin syndrome   A rare collection of symptoms resulting from elevated levels of the neurotransmitter serotonin; may occur with the use of any psychotropic drug that enhances brain serotonin activity (e.g., antidepressants, buspirone, tramadol; see Box 17-1). (p. 337)

Stigma   Widespread negative perceptions of and prejudice toward a specific group of people, such as those with mental health disorders. (p. 324)

Tardive dyskinesia   A serious adverse drug reaction characterized by abnormal and distressing involuntary body movements and muscle tension that is associated with antipsychotic medications. (p. 341)

OVERVIEW

Many people periodically experience the normal emotions of anxiety, depression, and grief. Often, such emotions are simply situational. They arise because of a specific event and subside with time. Treatment, if any, is often limited to psychotherapy and possibly short-term drug therapy. However, longer-term pharmacotherapy in conjunction with psychotherapy is usually recommended when a person's emotions or behaviours compromise quality of life, ability to carry out normal activities of daily living (ADLs), social functioning (interactions and relationships with others), or functioning in productive occupations (e.g., employment, school) over a prolonged period (at least several months).

The exact causes of mental health disorders are not fully understood. There are numerous theories that attempt to explain the etiology and pathophysiology of mental dysfunction. In the biochemical imbalance theory, mental health disorders are thought to arise as the result of abnormal levels of endogenous chemicals in the brain, referred to as **neurotransmitters**. The conduction of messages between neurons (nerve cells) by neurotransmitters is called *neurotransmission*. Neurotransmission occurs in both the central nervous system (CNS) and the peripheral nervous system. The proposed mechanisms of both the pathology of and drug therapy for mental health disorders centre around neurotransmission within the brain. There is evidence indicating that brain levels of catecholamines (especially dopamine and norepinephrine; see Chapter 19) and indolamines (serotonin and histamine) play an important role in maintaining mental health. Other biochemicals necessary for the maintenance of normal mental function are the inhibitory neurotransmitter **gamma-aminobutyric acid (GABA)**, the cholinergic neurotransmitter acetylcholine (see Chapter 21), and some inorganic ions such as sodium, potassium, calcium, and magnesium. Drugs used to treat mental health disorders including anxiety, affective disorders, and psychoses work by blocking or stimulating the release of these endogenous neurotransmitters.

The symptoms of the different mental health disorders often overlap, which can make them difficult to accurately diagnose. Complicating this issue further is the subjectivity of patients' experience of their symptoms. A widely used reference is the *Diagnostic and Statistical Manual of Mental Disorders*, 5th edition, *(DSM-5)*, published by the American Psychiatric Association and updated in 2013. It provides demographic information and diagnostic criteria for recognized mental health disorders. The *DSM-5* differs from previous editions as it uses a developmental approach and supports the examination of disorders across the lifespan, including in children and older adults. Often, a patient has a range of ongoing symptoms that meet the criteria for several mental health disorders. Such patients may be said to have a spectrum disorder; one example is autism spectrum disorder. As well, adults with chronic depression may also have a comorbid personality disorder, a comorbid anxiety disorder, or a substance use disorder. The challenge of comorbid substance use is especially troublesome and complex. Comorbidity between substance use disorders and other mental health disorder requires a comprehensive approach that identifies and evaluates both. Accordingly, any patient requesting assistance for substance use or another mental health disorder should be assessed for both and treated accordingly.

Patients with mental health disorders may also be more susceptible to various physical health problems than the general population. In particular, these patients are at greater risk for physical illnesses associated with cardiometabolic syndrome. Economic, educational, and psychosocial issues may preclude a person with mental health disorder from seeking mental health care. Thus, many patients self-medicate with alcohol, tobacco, and illegal drugs or unauthorized prescription drugs. This compounds the problem of their baseline mental health disorder.

Despite the development of newer, more effective treatments for mental health disorders, a longstanding societal **stigma** continues to be an obstacle for diagnosed patients. In 2009, The Mental Health Commission of Canada launched "Opening Minds," the largest-ever national effort to reduce the stigma of mental health disorders in Canada. More recently, Bell Canada's "Let's Talk" popular awareness campaign was launched, and in 2011 and subsequent years, a designated day was dedicated to opening discussions about mental health disorders. The goal of this campaign is to end the impact of and the stigma around mental health issues across Canada. In addition, as mental health is the leading cause of 15% of workplace disability in Canada (Mood Disorders Society of Canada, 2011), Bell Canada is working with corporate Canada and the health care community to develop and adopt mental health best practices in the workplace (Bell Canada, 2015).

The treatment of mental health disorders is called **psychotherapeutics.** Ideal mental health care involves many components, including a carefully detailed patient interview (to help ensure accurate and complete diagnosis) and carefully chosen and regularly monitored drug therapy. Nonpharmacological treatments include psychotherapy, support groups, social and family support systems, and spiritual support systems. Many patients benefit from a combination of cognitive behavioural therapy and drug therapy. Other practices that promote mental health include physical exercise, good nutrition, and relaxation exercises, such as meditation and visualization. For individuals who experience refractory depression, a variety of options are available, such as electroconvulsive therapy (ECT), vagal nerve stimulation, transcranial magnetic therapy, electrical brain stimulation, or deep brain stimulation.

OVERVIEW OF MENTAL HEALTH DISORDERS

This chapter focuses on three common types of mental health disorders: anxiety disorders, affective disorders, and psychotic disorders. Anxiolytics, antidepressants, mood stabilizers, and antipsychotics are the main classes of psychotropic medications used to treat these mental conditions.

Anxiety occurs as "multiple, excessive, age-inappropriate worries about a variety of issues that occur for an extended period of time" (McBride, 2015, p. 29). There are often associated symptoms, including feeling on edge or restless, being easily fatigued, muscle tension, difficulty sleeping, and problems with concentration. Anxiety may be based on anticipated or past experiences. It may also stem from exaggerated responses to imaginary negative situations or to common, everyday experiences. According to the *DSM-5*, persistent anxiety is divided clinically into several distinct disorders, including the following:

- Separation anxiety disorder
- Selective mutism

- Specific phobia
- Social anxiety disorder (social phobia)
- Panic disorder (e.g., depressive disorder with panic attacks, post-traumatic stress disorder [PTSD] with panic attacks)
- Panic attack (specifier)
- Agoraphobia
- Generalized anxiety disorder
- Substance- or medication-induced anxiety disorder
- Anxiety disorder due to another medical condition
- Other specified anxiety disorder
- Unspecified anxiety disorder

Anxiety is a normal reaction to stress. Generalized anxiety disorder affects 3% of the general population; lifetime prevalence is 5%. Panic disorder has an incidence rate and lifetime prevalence of 1.6% and 3.7%, respectively, while **agoraphobia** (the fear of being in unfamiliar situations or places) has an incidence of 0.7% and a lifetime prevalence of 1.5% (Langlois, Samokhvalov, Rehm, et al., 2012). Anxiety may occur as a result of medical illnesses (e.g., cardiovascular or pulmonary disease, hypothyroidism, hyperthyroidism, pheochromocytoma, Cushing's syndrome, or hypoglycemia).

Affective disorders, also called *mood disorders*, are characterized by changes in mood and range from **mania** to **depression.** Bipolar disorder has a lifetime prevalence of 2.4% and a 12-month prevalence of 1% of the Canadian population (Langlois et al., 2012). A manic episode is characterized by an abnormally elevated, expansive, or irritable mood for at least 1 week, plus the presence of at least three of the following additional symptoms: grandiosity (exaggerated belief in one's importance), decreased need for sleep, pressured (intense) speech, flight of ideas (thoughts rapidly skip to distantly related ideas in no logical progression), distractibility, increased involvement in goal-directed activities; or involvement in pleasurable activities that have a high potential for painful consequences. The manic episode must be severe enough to cause impairments in social or occupational functioning or to require hospitalization (Brenner & Shyn, 2015). Some patients may exhibit both mania and depression, experiencing periodic swings in emotions between these two extremes. This is referred to as **bipolar disorder (BPD)**. An episode of **hypomania** is similar to one of mania, but less intense; it lasts for at least 4 days and has an impact on the individual's functioning. Some patients may exhibit rapid cycling (patients who experience at least four depressive/hypomanic episodes per year.) These patents have a poorer prognosis and require frequent hospitalizations and complex management.

The burden of depression and other mental health disorders is on the rise globally. Even when they are successfully treated and remission is achieved, depressive disorders still inflict significant burden. Remission is rarely accompanied by a total disappearance of all symptoms. Residual symptoms, especially cognitive impairment or social dysfunction, can continue to reduce performance and cause considerable distress. The ever-present risk of relapse and recurrence also weighs heavily, generally reducing quality of life. The World Health Organization estimates that depressive disorders will be the leading cause of disease burden worldwide by 2030 (Lépine & Briley, 2011). Depression is currently reported to have lifetime prevalence in Canadian adults over 18 of about 12% (Langlois et al., 2012). Depressive disorders are characterized by the presence of sad, empty, or irritable mood, accompanied by somatic and cognitive changes that significantly affect the individual's capacity to function (American Psychological Association [APA], 2013). A major depressive episode is characterized by a depressed mood and a loss of interest or pleasure in daily activities for longer than 2 weeks. At least five of the following symptoms must be present almost daily: depressed mood or irritability, feelings of worthlessness/guilt, loss of interest in normally pleasurable activities (anhedonia), fatigue or reduced energy level, reduced motivation and ability to meet routine responsibilities, drastic increase or decrease in appetite, lack of concentration, insomnia or hypersomnia, and recurrent thoughts of death or suicide (APA, 2013). In addition to being associated with reductions in quality of life and occupational and social functioning, depression is also accompanied by the occurrence of major sleep disturbances in up to 80% of patients. Despite recent advances in pharmacotherapy for depression, it remains undertreated and underdiagnosed.

Psychosis is a symptom or feature of severe mental health disorders that often impairs mental function to the point of causing significant disability in performing ADLs. A hallmark of psychosis is a loss of contact with reality. The primary psychotic disorders are schizophrenia and depressive and drug-induced psychoses. Schizophrenia may trigger hallucinations, paranoia, and delusions (false beliefs), and it is estimated to affect 1% of the population. The **dopamine hypothesis** of psychotic illness grows out of the observation that patients who experience psychosis often have excessive dopaminergic activity in the brain. Drug therapy is therefore aimed at reducing this activity. Note that this is in direct contrast to the treatment of Parkinson's disease (see Chapter 16), in which the therapeutic goal is to enhance brain dopaminergic activity.

Psychotropic drugs are among the most commonly prescribed drugs in Canada. Because of the inherent variability in description of symptoms and diagnoses, the effects of these drugs are less easily quantified than those of many other types of medications. Drug response may vary considerably between patients and the dosage of psychotropic drugs as these drugs are highly dependent on clinical response. Drug selection is often a trial-and-error process, which can be long and frustrating for both health care providers and patients.

It is hoped that the emerging field of pharmacogenomics (see Chapter 5 and the Ethnocultural Implications box below) will eventually allow more proactive and improved customization of psychotropic drug therapy.

Also, as more is learned about a drug after initial marketing, it is common for the approved indications for a given drug to expand over time. For example, a drug initially approved to treat depression may later be approved to treat social anxiety disorder or additional conditions. Most antidepressants are effective anxioloytic drugs and are often first-line treatment for anxiety disorders.

A common problem with psychotropic drug therapy, as with other types of drug therapy, is nonadherence to the prescribed regimen. Many people do not want to accept a diagnosis of a mental health disorder because of the associated stigma. As a result, they may remain in denial about the reality of their mental health disorder, including the need to take psychotropic medications. They may also have legitimate fears about adverse effects, as well as fear of the unknown regarding their illness. For example, the weight gain associated with antipsychotics can be a reason for patient nonadherance. Finally, they may dread the prospect of having to remain on medication to control their symptoms. Such patients can often be helped by support groups and other social supports. As they adjust to their diagnoses, it is hoped that they will gain insight into the benefits of treatment to strengthen their own roles in maintaining their mental health.

ANXIETY DISORDERS

Anxiolytic Drugs

Primary anxiolytic drugs include the benzodiazepine drug class and the miscellaneous drug buspirone (Table 17-1). Although antidepressants are usually first-line drug therapy for the treatment of anxiety disorders, the benzodiazepines are the focus of this section. In addition, other drugs that are effective as anxiolytics include selective serotonin reuptake inhibitors (SSRIs), tricyclic anti-

depressants (TCAs), and monoamine oxidase inhibitors (MAOIs), all discussed in the section on antidepressants), antipsychotics (see later section on antipsychotic drugs), propanolol and the antihistamine hydroxyzine hydrochloride (see Chapter 37).

Mechanism of Action and Drug Effects

All anxiolytic drugs reduce anxiety by reducing overactivity in the CNS. Benzodiazepines exert their anxiolytic effects by depressing activity in the brainstem and the limbic system. Benzodiazepines are believed to increase the action of GABA, which is an inhibitory neurotransmitter (i.e., inhibits reuptake of neurotransmitters such as serotonin, norepinephrine, and dopamine) in the brain that blocks nerve transmission in the CNS.

The drug buspirone is a miscellaneous anxiolytic in its own class and is described in further detail in its drug profile.

Indications

Benzodiazepines are the classic anxiolytic drug class; however, they are also associated with physical tolerance/dependence and misuse potential. Withdrawal and adverse effects do not offer any advantage over other classes such as SSRIs. They are sometimes used for other indications, such as ethanol withdrawal (see Chapter 18), insomnia and muscle spasms (see Chapter 13), seizure disorders (see Chapter 15), and as adjuncts in anaesthesia (see Chapter 12). They are also used as adjunct therapy for depression because depressive and anxious symptoms often occur together. Benzodiazepines are effective for the short-term treatment of anxiety, as they stop symptoms of anxiety quickly. They do not prevent anxiety, nor are they effective for treating depressive symptoms. Therefore, they are not effective for use in patients with anxiety and co-morbid depression.

Contraindications

Contraindications to benzodiazepines include known drug allergy; narrow-angle glaucoma, due to their ability to cause mydriasis; and pregnancy, due to their sedative properties and risk for teratogenic effects.

Adverse Effects

The most common undesirable adverse effect of benzodiazepines is an overexpression of their therapeutic effects, in particular CNS depression. Benzodiazepines can also cause hypotension. Of particular note are paradoxical (opposite of what would normally be expected) reactions to the benzodiazepines, including hyperactivity and aggressive behaviour. Such reactions are relatively uncommon. They are more likely to occur in children, in adolescents, and in older adults with dementia. Rebound disinhibition can occur in older adult patients upon tapering of doses or discontinuation of the benzodiazepines. In rebound disinhibition, an older adult patient experiences marked sedation for 1 to 2 hours, followed by marked agitation and confusion for several hours afterward. All benzodiazepines are potentially habit

TABLE 17-1

Currently Available Anxiolytic Drugs

Generic Name	Trade Name	Route
BENZODIAZEPINES		
Alprazolam	Xanax	PO
clorazepate dipotassium		PO
chlordiazepoxide hydrochloride	Librax®	PO
Clonazepam	Clonapam®	PO
Diazepam	Valium	PO, IM, IV
Lorazepam	Ativan	PO, IM, IV, sublingual
Oxazepam	Oxpam®	PO
MISCELLANEOUS		
buspirone hydrochloride		PO
hydroxyzine hydrochloride	Atarax®	PO, IM

PO, oral; *IM*, intramuscular; *IV*, intravenous.

TABLE 17-2

Adverse Effects of Selected Anxiolytic Drugs*

Drug or Drug Class	Adverse Effects
Benzodiazepines	Amnesia, anorexia, sedation, lethargy, fatigue, confusion, drowsiness, dizziness, ataxia, headache, visual changes, hypotension, weight gain or loss, nausea, weakness
MISCELLANEOUS buspirone hydrochloride	Paradoxical anxiety, dizziness, blurred vision, headache, nausea

*See also drug profiles for drug-specific information.

forming and addictive. They have a rapid onset and duration of action and, therefore, can provide significant symptom relief; however, they must be used judiciously and at the lowest effective doses for the shortest period of time needed for symptom control.

Refer to Table 17-2 for more information on adverse effects. Older adult patients tend to be particularly sensitive to the CNS sedating effects of benzodiazepines, which can increase their risk for falls; thus, lower doses are usually needed. Benzodiazepines taken by older adult patients may also have longer elimination half-lives due to decreased hepatic metabolism. In general, dosages of benzodiazepines for older adult patients should be approximately one third to one half of the recommended dose for younger adults. In addition, it is possible to administer dosages of benzodiazepines every other day to reduce toxic effects.

Toxicity and Management of Overdose

Overdose of anxiolytics is usually not severe but may be associated with excessive sedation, hypotension, and seizures. There is no specific antidote, but in extreme cases, a cholinergic drug (see Chapter 21) may be used to treat anticholinergic adverse effects associated with anxiolytics. When benzodiazepines are taken alone, an overdose is generally not life threatening. When they are combined with alcohol or other CNS depressants, the outcome is much more severe. An overdose of benzodiazepines may result in any of the following symptoms: somnolence, confusion, coma, and respiratory depression. When overdose is suspected, gastric lavage may be instituted as soon as possible and 50 to 100 g of activated charcoal may be introduced to and left in the stomach. Flumazenil is a benzodiazepine receptor blocker (antagonist) that is used as adjunctive therapy to reverse the effects of benzodiazepines. It is usually given to reverse benzodiazepine effects after procedures involving procedural sedation (see Chapter 12). The treatment regimen for the acute reversal of benzodiazepine effects is summarized in Chapter 13. Flumazenil may cause acute withdrawal syndrome, including seizures in patients taking benzodiazepines long term or those with a history of substance misuse.

Interactions

Several notable drug interactions occur with the use of benzodiazepines. Alcohol and other CNS depressants, when coadministered with benzodiazepines, can result in additive CNS depression, respiratory depression and subsequent death. This serious consequence is more likely to occur in patients with kidney or liver compromise (e.g., older adults). Other drug interactions are listed in Table 17-3.

Dosages

Recommended dosages of selected antianxiety drugs are given in the table on p. 330.

AFFECTIVE DISORDERS

Several classes of drugs are used in the treatment of affective (emotional) disorders. The two main drug categories are mood-stabilizing drugs and antidepressant drugs.

MOOD-STABILIZING DRUGS

Mood stabilizers are drugs used to treat bipolar disorder (cycles of mania, hypomania, and depression). Clinical evidence indicates that the catecholamines (dopamine and norepinephrine) play an important pathophysiological role in the development of mania. Serotonin also appears to be involved. Lithium has been in use for many years and is still used to effectively alleviate the symptoms of acute mania. Lithium is available in two salt forms: lithium carbonate and lithium citrate. Lithium is also effective for the maintenance treatment of bipolar disorder as well as bipolar depression and mixed episodes. Lithium is thought to potentiate serotonergic neurotransmission. A variety of medications may be used in conjunction with lithium to regulate mood or achieve stability; they include benzodiazepines (described earlier), antipsychotic drugs (see later in the chapter), antiepileptic drugs (see Chapter 15), and dopamine receptor agonists (see Chapter 16). The antiepileptics valproic acid, lamotrigine, oxcarbazepine, and topiramate may be used when patients do not tolerate lithium. Lithium has a narrow therapeutic range and requires blood level monitoring. These drugs are often effective in treating mania, hypomania, and, to a lesser degree, depressive symptoms. Other evidence has shown that the atypical antipsychotic drugs risperidone, olanzapine, quetiapine, lurasidone hydrochloride, and ziprasidone hydrochloride monohydrate (see later) can also be effective in the acute treatment of mania and hypomania and also maintenance treatment of bipolar disorder. Available mood-stabilizing drugs are listed in Table 17-4.

ANTIDEPRESSANT DRUGS

Antidepressants are the pharmacological treatment of choice for major depressive disorders. In 2012, 42.6 million prescriptions for antidepressants were filled in Canada. The highest use for men is between the ages of

TABLE 17-3

Drug Interactions of Selected Anxiolytic Drugs*

Drug Class	Interacting Drug(s)	Mechanism	Result
BENZODIAZEPINES	CNS depressants (e.g., alcohol, opioids)	Additive effects	Enhanced CNS depression (e.g., sedation, confusion, ataxia)
	Oral contraceptives, azole antifungals, SSRIs, verapamil hydrochloride, diltiazem hydrochloride, opioids, valproic acid	Impaired liver elimination of benzodiazepine	Enhanced benzodiazepine effects (e.g., CNS depression)
	rifampin	Enhanced benzodiazepine clearance	Reduced therapeutic effects
	theophylline	Antagonistic effects	Reduced sedative effects
	phenytoin	Reduced clearance	Potential for digoxin toxicity and phenytoin toxicity
MISCELLANEOUS buspirone hydrochloride	CYP3A4 inhibitors, azole antifungals, verapamil hydrochloride, diltiazem hydrochloride	Impaired liver metabolism of buspirone hydrochloride	Enhanced buspirone hydrochloride effects
	rifampin	Enhanced buspirone hydrochloride clearance	Reduced therapeutic effects
	MAOIs	Unknown	Increased blood pressure

*See also drug profiles for drug-specific information.
CNS, central nervous system; *MAOIs*, monoamine oxidase inhibitors.

25 to 44 and for women between the ages of 25 to 79 (Rotermann, Sanmartin, Hennessy, et al., 2014). Not only are antidepressants effective in treating depression, they are also useful for treating other disorders, such as anxiety disorders, dysthymia (chronic low-grade depression), schizophrenia (as an adjunctive drug), eating disorders, and personality disorders. Some of the antidepressants are also used in the treatment of various medical conditions, including migraine headaches, chronic pain syndromes, sleep disorders, premenstrual syndrome, and hot flashes associated with menopause. Available antidepressants are listed in Table 17-4.

Many of the drugs currently used to treat affective disorders increase the levels of neurotransmitter concentrations in the CNS; these neurotransmitters include serotonin (also known as 5-hydroxytryptamine, or 5-HT), dopamine, and norepinephrine. This treatment is based on the belief that alterations in the levels of these neurotransmitters are responsible for causing depression. A widely held hypothesis advanced to explain depression in these terms is the **biogenic amine hypothesis (BAH)**. It postulates that depression results from a deficiency of neuronal and synaptic catecholamines (primarily norepinephrine), and mania results from an excess of amines at the adrenergic receptor sites in the brain. This hypothesis is illustrated in Figure 17-1.

Another hypothesis to explain the cause of depression is the **permissive hypothesis,** which led to the creation of the SSRI drug class. The permissive theory postulates that reduced concentrations of serotonin are the predis-

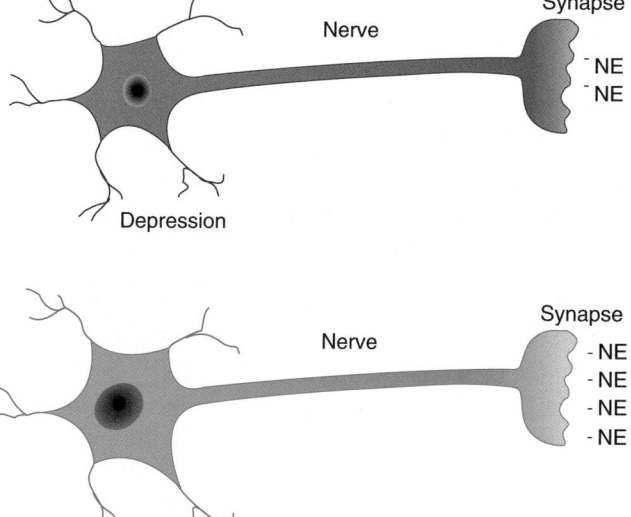

FIG. 17-1 Biogenic amine hypothesis (BAH). *NE,* norepinephrine.

posing factor in patients with affective disorders. Depression results from decreases in both the serotonin and catecholamine levels, whereas mania results from increased dopamine and norepinephrine levels but decreased serotonin levels. The permissive hypothesis is illustrated in Figure 17-2. The **dysregulation hypothesis** is essentially a reformulation of the BAH. This theory views depression and other affective disorders not simply

DRUG PROFILES

BENZODIAZEPINES

Benzodiazepines are widely used anxiolytic drugs. They are targeted substances and classified as Schedule IV controlled substances. For dosage and indication information, refer to the table on p. 336.

▶ *alprazolam*

Alprazolam (Xanax®) is most commonly used as an anxiolytic. It is also indicated for the specific anxiety disorder known as *panic disorder*. Adverse effects include confusion, ataxia, headache, and others listed in Table 17-2. Interacting drugs include alcohol, antacids, oral contraceptives, and others listed in Table 17-3. It has moderate withdrawal effects. Alprazolam is available only for oral use, in tablet form.

PHARMACOKINETICS

Route	Onset of Action	Peak Plasma Concentration	Elimination Half-Life	Duration of Action
PO	30–60 min	1–2 hr	10–15 hr	6 hr

▶ *diazepam*

Diazepam (Valium®), the longest-acting benzodiazepine, used to be the most commonly prescribed benzodiazepine; however, for treatment of anxiety, it has generally been replaced by the shorter-acting benzodiazepines alprazolam and lorazepam. Diazepam is indicated for relief of anxiety, management of alcohol withdrawal, reversal of status epilepticus or preoperative sedation, and, less frequently, as an adjunct for the relief of skeletal muscle spasms. Diazepam has active metabolites that can accumulate in patients with liver dysfunction because it is metabolized primarily in the liver. This accumulation can result in additive, cumulative effects that may be manifested as prolonged sedation, respiratory depression, or coma. For this reason, it is probably best avoided in patients with major liver compromise. Adverse drug effects include headache, confusion, slurred speech, and others listed in Table 17-2. Diazepam interacts with alcohol, oral contraceptives, and others, as shown in Table 17-3. Diazepam is available in oral and injectable dosage forms. It is generally not administered by intramuscular (IM) injection due to its poor and inconsistent absorption rate.

PHARMACOKINETICS

Route	Onset of Action	Peak Plasma Concentration	Elimination Half-Life	Duration of Action
PO	30–60 min	1–2 hr	20–80 hr	12–24 hr

▶ *lorazepam*

Lorazepam (Ativan®) is an intermediate-acting benzodiazepine. Lorazepam is available in oral and injectable forms. It may be given intravenously or intramuscularly.

It has excellent absorption and bioavailability when given intramuscularly, but it is irritating to the muscle and must be diluted. The conversion between injectable and oral dosage forms is 1:1. Lorazepam can be given by intravenous push, which is useful in the treatment of an acutely agitated patient. It is often administered as a continuous infusion to agitated patients who are undergoing mechanical ventilation. It is also used to treat or prevent alcohol withdrawal (see Chapter 18). Lorazepam has fewer active metabolites and less drug interactions.

PHARMACOKINETICS

Route	Onset of Action	Peak Plasma Concentration	Elimination Half-Life	Duration of Action
PO	30–60 min	2 hr	11–16 hr	8 hr

MISCELLANEOUS DRUG

buspirone hydrochloride

Buspirone hydrochloride is an anxiolytic drug that is different both chemically and pharmacologically from the benzodiazepines. Its precise mechanism of action is unknown, but it appears to have agonist activity at both serotonin and dopamine receptors. It is indicated for treatment of anxiety and is always administered on a scheduled (not "as-needed") basis, as opposed to the benzodiazepines that may be administered as needed or on a schedule. The only reported contraindication is drug allergy. Buspirone lacks the sedative properties and dependency potential of the benzodiazepines. Adverse effects include paradoxical anxiety, dizziness, blurred vision, headache, and nausea. Potential drug interactions include a risk for serotonin syndrome (see section on antidepressants). Patients receiving buspirone and antidepressants together need to be monitored carefully. It is recommended that MAOIs not be used concurrently with buspirone due to the risk of hypertension. A washout period of at least 14 days after discontinuation of MAOI therapy must be allowed before buspirone is started. Other drugs that interact with buspirone include *inhibitors* of the cytochrome P450 enzyme system (see Chapter 2)—specifically with CYP3A4 (e.g., ketoconazole [see Chapter 48], clarithromycin [see Chapter 43])—which can reduce buspirone clearance; and *inducers* of these same enzymes, which can enhance buspirone clearance and decrease its therapeutic effect. In either case, the buspirone dosage may need to be adjusted. Other interactions are listed in Table 17-3. Buspirone is available only for oral use.

PHARMACOKINETICS

Route	Onset of Action	Peak Plasma Concentration	Elimination Half-Life	Duration of Action
PO	2–3 wk	40–60 min	2–3 hr	Unknown

DOSAGES Selected Anxiolytic Drugs

Drug	Pharmacological Class	Usual Dosage Range	Indications
alprazolam (Xanax)	Benzodiazepine	**Adults** PO: 0.25–1 mg bid/tid; do not exceed 3 mg/day	Generalized anxiety disorder
		Older adults PO: 0.125 mg bid/tid	Generalized anxiety disorder
▸diazepam (Valium)	Benzodiazepine	**Adults** PO: 2–10 mg bid/qid/day	Anxiety
		Children PO: 1–2.5 mg tid/qid/day	
▸lorazepam (Ativan)	Benzodiazepine	**Adults** PO: 0.5–6 mg/day prn in 2–3 divided doses	Generalized anxiety disorder

TABLE 17-4

Currently Available Mood Stabilizers and Antidepressants

Generic Name	Trade Name	Route
MOOD STABILIZERS		
lithium carbonate*	Carbolith®, Lithane®	PO
lithium citrate		PO
Antiepileptics (valproic acid, lamotrigine, topiramate. oxcarbazepine)	Depakene®, Epival®, Lamictal®, Topamax®, Trileptal®	PO
ANTIDEPRESSANTS		
First Generation		
Tricyclics		
amitriptyline hydrochloride	Elavil, Levate	PO
clomipramine hydrochloride	Anafranil®,	PO
desipramine hydrochloride		PO
doxepin hydrochloride	Silenor®, Sinequan®	PO
imipramine hydrochloride		PO
nortriptyline hydrochloride	Aventyl®	PO
trimipramine maleate		PO
Tetracyclics		
maprotiline hydrochloride (first generation)		PO
mirtazapine (second generation)	Remeron®, Remeron RD®	PO
MAOIs		
phenelzine sulfate	Nardil®	PO
tranylcypromine sulfate	Parnate®	PO
Second Generation		
SSRIs		
citalopram hydrobromide	Celexa®	PO
escitalopram oxalate	Cipralex®, Cipralex Meltz®	PO
fluoxetine hydrochloride	Prozac®	PO
fluvoxamine maleate	Luvox®	PO
paroxetine hydrochloride	Paxil®, Paxil CR®	PO
sertraline hydrochloride	Zoloft®	PO
SNRIs		
duloxetine hydrochloride	Cymbalta®	PO
venlafaxine hydrochloride	Effexor XR®	PO
Miscellaneous		
bupropion hydrochloride	Wellbutrin®	PO
trazodone hydrochloride	Oleptro®	PO

*Also classified as an antipsychotic.
PO, oral; *MAOIs*, monoamine oxidase inhibitors; *SNRIs*, serotonin-norepinephrine reuptake inhibitors; *SSRIs*, selective serotonin reuptake inhibitors.

DRUG PROFILES

lithium

The mood-stabilizing effect of lithium is not fully understood. Lithium ions are thought to alter sodium ion transport in nerve cells, which results in a shift in catecholamine metabolism. The levels of lithium required to produce a therapeutic effect are close to the toxic levels (i.e., it has a narrow therapeutic index). For the management of acute mania, a lithium serum level of 1 to 1.5 mmol/L is usually required. Desirable long-term maintenance levels range between 0.6 and 1.2 mmol/L. Blood levels are best measured 8 to 12 hours after the last dose (roughly the midpoint of the drug half-life) because the half-life is usually between 18 and 24 hours. Both sodium and lithium are monovalent positive ions, and one can affect the other. Therefore, the patient's serum sodium levels require monitoring. Keeping sodium levels in the normal range (135 to 145 mmol/L) helps to maintain therapeutic lithium levels. Patients should be advised not to drastically change their sodium intake while taking lithium and to avoid overhydration as well as dehydration.

Lithium is indicated for the treatment of manic episodes in bipolar disorder as well as for maintenance therapy to prevent such episodes. Contraindications to lithium therapy are relative and include dehydration, known sodium imbalance, and major kidney or cardiovascular disease because all of these conditions increase the risk of lithium toxicity. Kidney dysfunction of any degree can increase lithium levels. Older adult patients are particularly prone to this effect because kidney function normally declines with advancing age. Adverse effects tend to correlate with serum levels. Mild to moderate toxic reactions can occur at lithium levels from 1.5 to 2 mmol/L, and moderate to severe reactions occur at levels above 2 mmol/L. Toxicity manifestations include gastrointestinal (GI) discomfort, tremor, confusion, somnolence, seizures, and possibly death. The most serious adverse effect is cardiac dysrhythmia. Other effects include drowsiness, slurred speech, epilepsy-type seizures, choreoathetotic movements (involuntary wavelike movements of the extremities), ataxia (generalized disturbance of muscular coordination), and hypotension. Long-term treatment may cause hypothyroidism. Potentially interacting drugs include the thiazide diuretics (see Chapter 29), angiotensin-converting enzyme inhibitors (see Chapter 23), and nonsteroidal anti-inflammatory drugs (see Chapter 49), all of which can increase lithium toxicity. Lithium is available only for oral use.

PHARMACOKINETICS

Route	Onset of Action	Peak Plasma Concentration	Elimination Half-Life	Duration of Action
PO	7–14 days to therapeutic effect	0.5–2 hr	18–24 hr	2–24 hr

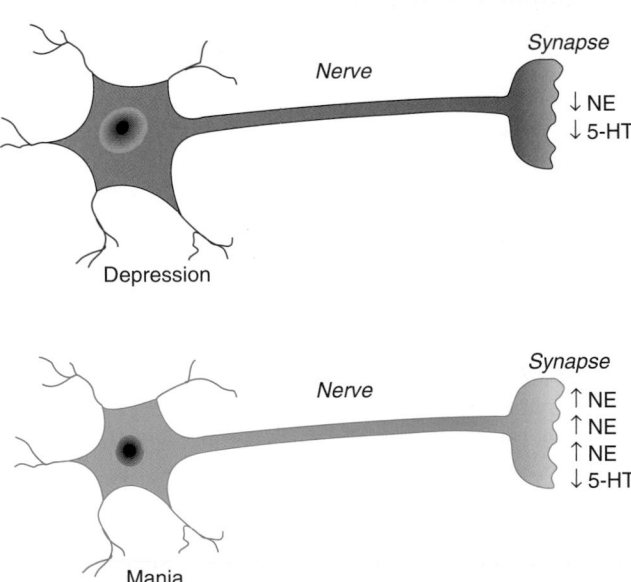

FIG. 17-2 Permissive hypothesis. *NE*, norepinephrine; *5-HT*, serotonin.

in terms of decreased or increased catecholamine activity but as a failure of the regulation of these systems.

Early and aggressive antidepressant treatment increases the chances for full remission. The first 6 to 8 weeks of therapy constitute the acute phase. The primary goals during this time are to obtain a response to drug therapy and improve the patient's symptoms. It is currently recommended that antidepressant drug therapy be maintained at the effective dose for an additional 8 to 14 months after remission of depressive symptoms. In choosing an antidepressant, the patient's previous psychotropic drug response history (if any) needs to be considered. Family history of depression with known drug responses is also helpful. Therapeutic response is measured primarily by subjective patient feedback. In addition, there are measurement tools available that attempt to quantify the patient's response to drug therapy, such as the Hamilton Rating Scale for Depression and the Symptom Checklist-90 anxiety factor scale.

Anxiety and depression commonly occur together and reinforce each other. Similarly, there is much crossover in terms of symptom control between antidepressant and anxiolytic drugs. There is a wide variation in response to antidepressant drug therapy, which can be attributed to genetic polymorphism (see Chapter 5). An early response (within 2 weeks) to antidepressant therapy is thought to reflect the true effect of antidepressant therapy and is also a predictor of a stable response (Fabbri, Marsano, Balestri, et al., 2013). Efficacy may take 3 to 6 weeks in many patients. Adverse effects may occur earlier than efficacy.

A nonresponse to antidepressant drug therapy is defined as failure to respond to at least 6 weeks of therapy with adequate drug dosages (Al-Harbi, 2012). The 20 to

30% of patients who do not respond to the usual dosage of an antidepressant will respond to higher doses. Therefore, dose optimization, which involves careful upward titration of the dose for several weeks, is recommended before concluding that a given drug is ineffective. Often, a switch to a different pharmacological class of antidepressant is necessary; 40 to 60% of patients will respond to the second drug class tried. Benzodiazepine and antipsychotic drugs may also be used, either alone or as adjunct therapy. Evidence suggests that psychotherapy given with antidepressant medication is more effective than medication alone, although access to psychotherapy may be an issue.

The most severe cases of refractory depression may warrant ECT. ECT is a safe and effective treatment carried out in a postanaesthesia care unit setting under short-acting brief anaesthesia and a muscle relaxant. There is some controversy over the positioning of electrodes; they can be positioned in the bifrontotemporal, right unilateral, and bifrontal positions. The electrical stimulus must be sufficient to stimulate seizure activity in the brain and lasts around 25 to 150 seconds. The number of treatments required for an effective course of ECT varies substantially between individuals. A typical course requires 6 to 12 treatments over a 2- to 4-week period, while patients with mania or schizophrenia may require a somewhat higher number of treatments. A typical adverse effect is memory impairment, both retrograde (patient forgets events prior to the seizure) and anterograde (patient forgets events after the seizure), which usually subsides within 1 to 6 months (Enns & Reiss, 2015).

Another newer alternative treatment to ECT is magnetic seizure therapy (MST). Rather than using electrical currents to create seizures throughout the entire brain as with ECT, MST uses repetitive magnetic stimulation to produce targeted seizures in the prefrontal cortex, avoiding adverse effects on cognition. Another treatment that has gained attention is the use of ketamine (see Chapter 12) intravenously to relieve depression symptoms (Melville, 2012).

Treatment failure in cases of depression may be due to a misdiagnosis or failure to treat a concurrent mental health disorder (e.g., anxiety disorder, substance misuse) or comorbid nonpsychiatric illness (e.g., hypothyroidism). It may also be due to nonadherence to drug therapy. Careful choice of drug therapy to minimize adverse effects may improve patient adherence with treatment and therapeutic outcomes. Another reason for treatment failure may be the discouragement associated with depression itself. This alone may cause patients to give up prematurely on their drug therapy, especially because antidepressants often take several weeks to reach their full effect. Effective psychotherapy and support groups can help encourage patients to be consistent with prescribed psychotropic drug therapy through patient education.

In 2004, Health Canada issued special warnings regarding the use of all classes of antidepressants in both adult and pediatric patient populations (in the United States, these are known as black box warnings; Health Canada uses a "box warning" on product monographs). Clinical trials and postmarketing reports indicated an increased risk for suicide and agitation-type emotional and behavioural changes in patients receiving these medications. As a result, current recommendations for all patients receiving antidepressants include regular monitoring for signs of worsening depressive symptoms, especially when the medication is first started or the dosage is changed. Patients need immediate evaluation if they report, or others observe, signs of worsening depression or other emotional instability. Most patients do not experience severe adverse effects from these medications, and many patients obtain significant relief.

TRICYCLIC ANTIDEPRESSANTS

Tricyclic antidepressants (TCAs) were the original first-generation antidepressants. Their use has largely been replaced with the SSRIs and serotonin-norepinephrine reuptake inhibitors (SNRIs). TCAs are considered second-line drug therapy in patients for whom SSRIs are ineffective or as adjunct therapy with newer drugs. TCAs are so named because of their characteristic three-ring chemical structure.

Mechanism of Action and Drug Effects

TCAs are believed to work by correcting imbalance in the neurotransmitter concentrations of serotonin and norepinephrine at the nerve endings in the CNS (the BAH). This is accomplished by blocking the presynaptic reuptake of the neurotransmitters, which makes them available for transmission of nerve impulses to adjacent neurons in the brain. Some also believe that these drugs may help regulate malfunctioning neurons (the dysregulation hypothesis).

Indications

Currently, TCAs are most commonly used to treat neuropathic pain syndromes and insomnia. With the advent of the newer-generation antidepressant classes, their use as antidepressants is rare. Some TCAs have additional specific indications. For example, imipramine hydrochloride is used as an adjunct in the treatment of childhood enuresis (bedwetting), and clomipramine hydrochloride is useful in the treatment of obsessive-compulsive disorder. Because TCAs tend to increase appetite, leading to weight gain, they are sometimes used to treat anorexia nervosa.

Contraindications

Contraindications for TCAs include known drug allergy, use of MAOIs within the previous 14 days, and pregnancy. TCAs are also not recommended in patients with any acute or chronic cardiac problems or a history of seizures because both conditions are associated with a greater likelihood of death upon TCA overdose.

Adverse Effects

Undesirable effects of TCAs are a result of their effects on various receptors, especially the muscarinic receptors (a type of cholinergic receptor) and, to a lesser degree, adrenergic, histaminergic, dopaminergic, and serotonergic receptors. Blockade of cholinergic receptors results in undesirable anticholinergic adverse effects, the most common being constipation and urinary retention. Nortriptyline hydrochloride and desipramine hydrochloride have less anticholinergic activity, and they are preferred for use in older adults. Adrenergic and dopaminergic receptor blockade can lead to disturbances in cardiac conduction and hypotension. Histaminergic blockade can cause sedation, and serotonergic blockade can alter the seizure threshold and cause sexual dysfunction (see Table 17-5).

Toxicity and Management of Overdose

TCA overdoses are notoriously lethal. It is estimated that 70 to 80% of patients who die of TCA overdose do so before reaching the hospital, especially if the drugs are taken with alcohol. The primary organ systems affected are the CNS and the cardiovascular system. Death usually results from either seizures or dysrhythmias. Historically, it was taught that patients should not receive more than a 1-month supply of antidepressants because of the risk of suicide attempts. Many people choose to receive a 3-month supply to avoid paying more dispensing fees each time they fill a prescription.

There is no specific antidote for TCA poisoning. Management efforts are aimed at reducing drug absorption by administering multiple doses of activated charcoal. Administration of sodium bicarbonate speeds up elimination of the TCA by alkalinizing the urine. CNS damage may be minimized by the administration of diazepam, and cardiovascular events may be minimized by giving antidysrhythmics. Other care includes basic life support in an intensive care setting to maintain vital organ functions. These interventions must continue until enough of the TCA is eliminated to permit restoration of normal organ function.

Interactions

Increased anticholinergic effects are seen when TCAs are taken with anticholinergics and phenothiazines. When MAOIs are taken with TCAs, the result may be increased therapeutic and toxic effects, including hyperpyretic

---

TABLE 17-5

Adverse Effects of Selected Mood Stabilizers and Antidepressants*

Drug or Drug Class	Adverse Effects
MOOD STABILIZERS	
lithium salts	GI discomfort, tremor, confusion, sedation, seizures, cardiac dysrhythmia, drowsiness, slurred speech, slowed motor abilities, weight gain, ataxia, hypotension
Antiepileptic drugs	Dizziness, drowsiness, GI upset, weight gain, hepatotoxicity, pancreatitis, unusual eye movements, visual changes, behavioural changes, ataxia
ANTIDEPRESSANTS	
First Generation	
Tricyclics	Anorexia, dry mouth, blurred vision, constipation, gynecomastia, sexual dysfunction, altered blood glucose level, urinary retention, agitation, anxiety, ataxia, cognitive impairment, sedation, headache, insomnia, skin rash, photosensitivity, weight gain, orthostatic hypotension, blood dyscrasias
MAOIs	Dizziness, dyskinesias, nausea, syncope, hypotension
Second Generation	
Tetracyclics	
mirtazapine, maprotiline hydrochloride	Drowsiness, abnormal dreams, dry mouth, constipation, increased appetite, asthenia (muscle weakness)
SSRIs	Anxiety, dizziness, drowsiness, headache, mild GI disturbance, sexual dysfunction, asthenia, tremor
SNRIs	Dizziness, drowsiness, headache, GI upset, anorexia, hepatotoxicity
Miscellaneous	
trazodone hydrochloride, bupropion hydrochloride	Dizziness, headache, sedation, nausea, blurred vision, tachycardia

*See also drug profiles for drug-specific information.
GI, gastrointestinal; *MAOIs*, monoamine oxidase inhibitors; *SNRIs*, serotonin-norepinephrine reuptake inhibitors; *SSRIs*, selective serotonin reuptake inhibitors.

crisis (excessive fever). Other drug interactions are listed in Table 17-6.

Dosages

Recommended dosages of selected TCA drugs are given in the table on p. 336.

MONOAMINE OXIDASE INHIBITORS

Monoamine oxidase inhibitors (MAOIs), along with TCAs, represent the first generation of antidepressant drug therapy; they are now rarely used as antidepressants but are used to treat Parkinson's disease, atypical depression, or mood disorder with phobic trait. A serious

---

TABLE   17-6

Drug Interactions of Selected Mood-Stabilizing and Antidepressant Drugs*

Drug Class	Interacting Drug(s)	Mechanism	Result
MOOD STABILIZERS			
lithium salts	Thiazide diuretics, angiotensin converting enzyme inhibitors, verapamil, diltiazem, NSAIDs	Decreased lithium excretion	Increased lithium toxicity
Antiepileptic drugs	See Table 15-5.		
ANTIDEPRESSANTS			
First Generation			
Tricyclics (TCAs)	carbamazepine, rifamycins	Enhanced TCA clearance	Reduced therapeutic effects
	carbamazepine	Reduced carbamazepine clearance	Potential for carbamazepine toxicity
	MAOIs	Enhance serotonergic effects	Potential for serotonin syndrome
	valproic acid	Reduced TCA clearance	Potential for TCA toxicity
	Anticholinergics	Additive anticholinergic effects	Potential for paralytic ileus
	Sympathomimetics	Enhanced sympathomimetic effects	Potential for cardiac dysrhythmias
Second Generation			
Tetracyclics			
mirtazapine, maprotiline hydrochloride	Alcohol, CYP inhibitors	Additive effects	Increased toxicity
SSRIs	MAOIs, linezolid, lithium, metoclopramide hydrochloride, buspirone hydrochloride, sympathomimetics, tramadol hydrochloride	Additive effects	Potential for serotonin syndrome
	Benzodiazepines	Reduced metabolism	Potential benzodiazepine toxicity
	warfarin sodium, phenytoin	Protein binding displacement	Potential for warfarin sodium or phenytoin toxicity
	propafenone hydrochloride	Increased propafenone levels	Potential for propafenone hydrochloride toxicity
SNRIs			
Duloxetine	SSRIs, triptans	Additive effects	Risk of serotonin syndrome
	NSAIDs, warfarin sodium	Additive effects	Risk of bleeding
	Alcohol	Additive liver toxicity	Increased risk of hepatotoxicity
MISCELLANEOUS			
trazodone, bupropion	Azole antifungals, phenothiazines, protease inhibitors	Impaired hepatic metabolism	Increased effects
	carbamazepine	Increased metabolism	Decreased therapeutic effects
	Alcohol, CNS depressants	Additive effects	Increased CNS depression

*See also drug profiles for drug-specific information.
CNS, central nervous system; *NSAIDs*, nonsteroidal anti-inflammatory drugs; *MAOIs*, monoamine oxidase inhibitors; *SNRIs*, serotonin-norepinephrine reuptake inhibitors; *SSRIs*, selective serotonin reuptake inhibitors; *TCAs*, tricyclic antidepressants.

DRUG PROFILES

TCAs are effective drugs in the treatment of various affective disorders, but they are associated with serious adverse effects. Therefore, patients taking them need to be monitored closely. For this reason, all antidepressants are available only with a prescription. Some natural health products used to treat depression, such as St. John's wort (see the Natural Health Products: St. John's wort box on p. 335), are available over the counter but should not be taken with prescription antidepressants due to the risk of serotonin syndrome.

▶▶ amitriptyline hydrochloride

Amitriptyline hydrochloride (Elavil®, Levate®) is the oldest and most widely used of all the TCAs. Its original

indication was depression, but it is now more commonly used to treat insomnia and neuropathic pain. Contraindications include known drug allergy, pregnancy, and recent myocardial infarction. It has potent anticholinergic properties, which can lead to many adverse effects such as dry mouth, constipation, blurred vision, urinary retention, and dysrhythmias (see Table 17-5). Drug interactions are listed in Table 17-6. Amitriptyline is available only for oral use.

PHARMACOKINETICS

Route	Onset of Action	Peak Plasma Concentration	Elimination Half-Life	Duration of Action
PO	7–21 days	2–12 hr	10–50 hr	6–12 hr

NATURAL HEALTH PRODUCTS

ST. JOHN'S WORT (Hypericum perforatum)

Overview
St. John's wort preparations consist of the dried, above-ground parts of the plant species *Hypericum perforatum* gathered during flowering season. St. John's wort is available over the counter in numerous oral dosage forms. It is sometimes referred to as the "herbal Prozac."

Common Uses
Depression, anxiety, sleep disorders, nervousness

Adverse Effects
GI upset, allergic reactions, fatigue, dizziness, confusion, dry mouth, possible phototoxicity (especially in fair-skinned individuals)

Potential Drug Interactions
MAOIs, SSRIs, TCAs, cyclosporine, sympathomimetic amines, piroxicam, tetracycline, tyramine-containing foods, opioids, digoxin, estrogens, theophylline, warfarin

Contraindications
St. John's wort is contraindicated in patients with bipolar disorder, schizophrenia, Alzheimer's disease, and other forms of dementia.

---

disadvantage to MAOI use is their potential to cause a hypertensive crisis when taken with stimulant medications or with a substance containing tyramine, which is found in many common foods and beverages (Table 17-7).

Currently, three MAOI antidepressants are available. Phenelzine sulfate and tranylcypromine sulfate are nonselective inhibitors of both monoamine oxidase (MAO) type A and MAO type B. Selegiline hydrochloride is a selective MAO-B inhibitor, also used to treat Parkinson's disease (see Chapter 16). Because these drugs inhibit the MAO enzyme system in the CNS, amines such as dopamine, serotonin, and norepinephrine are not broken down, and therefore higher levels of these substances occur. This higher level, in turn, alleviates the symptoms of depression.

Most adverse effects of MAOIs stem from their interactions with food and other medications. A variety of over-the-counter (OTC) drugs (especially for coughs and colds) also can interact with MAOIs to cause adverse cardiovascular effects. For example, MAOIs may increase the CNS depressant effects of diphenhydramine hydro-

chloride and cetirizine hydrochloride. Patients taking MAOIs need to read labels or consult the pharmacist when using any such products. Dosage information for selected MAOIs is given in the table on p. 336.

Sympathomimetic drugs can also interact with MAOIs, and together these drugs can cause a hypertensive crisis. MAOIs can markedly potentiate the effects of meperidine hydrochloride, and therefore their concurrent use is contraindicated. In addition, concurrent use of MAOIs with SSRIs carries the risk for serotonin syndrome. A washout period of 2 to 5 weeks between drugs is recommended.

Toxicity and Management of Overdose

Clinical symptoms of MAOI overdose generally do not appear until about 12 hours after ingestion. The primary signs and symptoms are cardiovascular and neurological in nature. The most serious cardiovascular effects are tachycardia and circulatory collapse, and the neurological symptoms of major concern are seizures and coma. Hyperthermia and miosis are also generally present in overdose. Treatment is aimed at eliminating the ingested toxin and protecting the organs at greatest risk for

DOSAGES Selected Mood-Stabilizing and Antidepressant Drugs

Drug	Pharmacological Class	Usual Dosage Range*	Current Health Canada–Approved Indications/Uses
Mood Stabilizers			
▶▶**lithium carbonate**	Inorganic salt	600–1800 mg/day divided bid–tid	Acute mania, prevention of mania
Antidepressants			
First Generation			
▶▶**amitriptyline hydrochloride** (Elavil, Levate)	Tricyclic	PO: 10–300 mg/day	Depression (more commonly used for insomnia and neuropathic pain)
Second Generation			
▶▶**bupropion hydrochloride** (Wellbutrin®, Zyban®)	Miscellaneous	PO, SR: 100–300 mg/day, divided bid	Depression (Wellbutrin), smoking cessation (Zyban)
duloxetine hydrochloride (Cymbalta®)	SNRI	PO: 30–60 mg/day	Depression, generalized anxiety disorder, neuropathic pain associated with diabetic peripheral neuropathy
▶▶**fluoxetine hydrochloride** (Prozac®)	SSRI	PO: 20–60 mg/day, in the morning	Depression, obsessive-compulsive disorder, bulimia nervosa, panic disorder, premenstrual dysphoric disorder
▶▶**mirtazapine (Remeron®)**	Tetracyclic	PO: 15–45 mg at bedtime	Depression, bipolar disorder
trazodone hydrochloride (Trazorel®)	Triazolopyridine	PO: 150–600 mg/day, divided bid–tid	Depression (more commonly used for insomnia)

*All dosages reflect usual adult dosage ranges. Pediatric dosages may be more variable and are best prescribed by a pediatrician.
PO, oral; *SNRI*, serotonin norepinephrine reuptake inhibitor; *SSRI*, selective serotonin reuptake inhibitor.

TABLE 17-7

Food and Drink to Avoid When Taking Monoamine Oxidase Inhibitors

Food/Drink	Examples
HIGH TYRAMINE CONTENT—NOT PERMITTED	
Aged mature cheeses	Cheddar, blue, Swiss
Smoked or pickled meats	Herring, sausage, corned beef, smoked fish or poultry, salami, pepperoni
Aged or fermented meats	Chicken or beef liver paté, game fish or poultry
Yeast extracts	Brewer's yeast
Red wines	Chianti, burgundy, sherry, vermouth
Italian broad beans	Fava beans
MODERATE TYRAMINE CONTENT—LIMITED AMOUNTS ALLOWED	
Meat extracts	Bouillon, consommé
Pasteurized, light and pale beer	
Ripe avocado	
LOW TYRAMINE CONTENT—PERMISSIBLE	
Distilled spirits	Vodka, gin, rye, Scotch (in moderation)
Non-aged cheeses	Processed cheese, mozzarella, cottage cheese, cream cheese
Chocolate and caffeinated beverages	
Fruit	Figs, bananas, raisins, grapes, pineapple, oranges
Soy sauce	
Yogourt, sour cream	

damage—the brain and heart. Recommended treatments are urine acidification to a pH of 5 and hemodialysis. Treatment of hypertensive crisis resulting from consumption of tyramine-containing foods or beverages may require intravenous administration of hypotensive drugs, along with careful monitoring in an intensive care setting.

SECOND GENERATION ANTIDEPRESSANTS

The period from the 1980s to the present was one of much development in psychotropic pharmacotherapy. Several new antidepressants were introduced, including trazodone (Oleptro®, Trazorel) and bupropion

(Wellbutrin); both are still commonly used. The SSRIs were also introduced. These include fluoxetine (Prozac), sertraline hydrochloride (Zoloft®), paroxetine hydrochloride (Paxil®), fluvoxamine maleate (Luvox®), citalopram hydrobromide (Celexa®), and escitalopram oxalate (Cipralex®). The SNRIs venlafaxine hydrochloride (Effexor®) and the mirtazapine (Remeron) which has norepinephrine and specific serotonergic activity, came later, followed by two new SNRIs, duloxetine hydrochloride (Cymbalta) and desvenlafaxine succinate (Pristiq®). Desvenlafaxine succinate is the major active metabolite of venlafaxine. Currently available second-generation drugs are listed in Table 17-4. Second-generation antidepressants are generally considered superior to TCAs and MAOIs in terms of their adverse effect profiles. It takes approximately the same amount of time to reach maximum clinical effectiveness with these drugs as it does with the TCAs and MAOIs—typically 4 to 6 weeks.

Mechanism of Action and Drug Effects

The inhibition of serotonin reuptake is the primary mechanism of action of the SSRIs, although these drugs may also have weak effects on norepinephrine and dopamine reuptake (see individual drug profiles). SNRIs inhibit the reuptake of both serotonin and norepinephrine with the exception of bupropion which is a weak norepinephrine-dopamine reuptake inhibitor. Patients should be educated about the time it takes for before full therapeutic effects of antidepressant drugs are realized—commonly several weeks.

Indications

Although depression is their primary indication, SSRIs and SNRIs have shown benefit in treating a variety of other mental and physical disorders. Examples include bipolar disorder, obesity, eating disorders, obsessive-compulsive disorder, panic attacks or disorders, social anxiety disorder, post-traumatic stress disorder, premenstrual dysphoric disorder, the neurologic disorder myoclonus, and various substance misuse problems such as alcoholism. Bupropion (Zyban) is also used for smoking cessation.

Contraindications

Contraindications include known drug allergy and use of MAOIs in the previous 14 days. In addition, a significant history of heart disease or seizure may be a contraindication due to the relatively uncommon, but reported, cardiac effects and alterations in seizure threshold (see later discussion). Bupropion is also contraindicated in cases of eating disorders as well as in seizure disorders because it can lower the seizure threshold.

Adverse Effects

Second-generation antidepressants offer advantages over TCAs and MAOIs due to their improved adverse effect profiles. However, up to two thirds of all depressed patients may still discontinue therapy due to drugs'

adverse effects. Some of the most common adverse effects are insomnia (partly due to reduced rapid eye movement sleep), weight gain, and sexual dysfunction. Sexual dysfunction caused by SSRIs is primarily related to inability to achieve orgasm.

One potentially hazardous adverse effect of any drug or combination of drugs that have serotonergic activity is **serotonin syndrome**. Serotonin syndrome results from excessive effects of serotonin on the CNS; the agonist effects on 5-HT 2A receptors contributes most substantially to serotonin syndrome (Cooper & Senjnowski, 2013). As mentioned, it usually results from taking medications, such as SSRIs, that elevate levels of serotonin either therapeutically or with intentional overdoses. However, it may also result from unintended drug interactions that elevate the effects of the serotonergic medication. The symptoms of this condition are listed in Box 17-1. Fortunately, it is usually self-limiting on discontinuation of the causative drugs. (Refer to Table 17-5.)

Interactions

Second-generation antidepressants are highly bound to albumin. When given with other drugs that are also highly bound to protein (e.g., warfarin sodium, phenytoin), they compete for binding sites on the surface of albumin. This results in a more free, unbound drug and therefore a more pronounced drug effect.

Some of these drugs may also inhibit cytochrome P450 enzymes, although there is debate about this in the literature. The cytochrome P450 system is an enzyme system in the liver that is responsible for the metabolism of several drugs (see Chapter 2). Inhibition of this enzyme system results in higher levels of drugs, with the potential for toxicity.

BOX 17-1

Common Symptoms of Serotonin Syndrome

Common symptoms include:
- Delirium
- Agitation
- Tachycardia
- Sweating
- Myoclonus (muscle spasms)
- Hyperreflexia
- Shivering
- Coarse tremors
- Extensor plantar muscle (sole of foot) responses

In more severe cases, the following may occur:
- Hyperthermia
- Seizures
- Rhabdomyolysis
- Chronic kidney disease
- Cardiac dysrhythmias
- Disseminated intravascular coagulation

To prevent potentially fatal pharmacodynamic interactions (e.g., serotonin syndrome) that can occur between these drugs and the MAOIs, a 2- to 5-week washout period is recommended between use of these two classes of medications. Other drug interactions are listed in Table 17-6.

Dosages

Recommended dosages of selected newer-generation antidepressants are given in the table on p. 336.

PSYCHOTIC DISORDERS

ANTIPSYCHOTIC DRUGS

Antipsychotic drugs are used to treat serious mental health disorders such as psychoses, schizophrenia, and autism. Antipsychotics are also used to treat extreme

---

 DRUG PROFILES

Second-generation drugs have proved to be effective antidepressants. They also have generally better adverse effect profiles than first-generation antidepressants. They are now considered first-line drugs in the treatment of patients with depression, including patients with concurrent symptoms of anxiety and patients with depression with suicidal ideation.

trazodone hydrochloride

Trazadone hydrochloride (Trazorel, Oleptro) belongs to the triazolopyridine drug class. It was the first of the second-generation antidepressants that could selectively inhibit serotonin reuptake but minimally affect norepinephrine reuptake. Trazodone has minimal adverse effects on the cardiovascular system, which is an advantage over the TCAs. It is indicated for the treatment of depression, and it is also commonly used as a nonaddictive drug treatment for insomnia. Contraindications include known drug allergy. Adverse effects include strong sedative qualities; these can be severe and can impair cognitive function in older adults. However, the sedating effect of trazodone is often advantageous in helping depressed patients—who commonly have comorbid anxiety or insomnia—to obtain effective sleep. Trazodone has also been associated, in rare cases, with transient nonsexual *priapism*. This is a dangerously sustained penile erection that is reportedly the result of α-adrenergic blockade. Trazodone interacts with azole antifungals (see Chapter 47), phenothiazines (see later in the chapter), and protease inhibitors (see Chapter 45), all of which can increase the risk of trazodone toxicity; carbamazepine (see Chapter 15), which can reduce trazodone levels at the same time as carbamazepine levels are increased; and CNS depressants (e.g., alcohol), whose effects can be potentiated by trazodone. It is also recommended that trazodone be started gradually after a patient has recently stopped MAOI therapy. Trazodone is available only for oral use.

PHARMACOKINETICS

Route	Onset of Action	Peak Plasma Concentration	Elimination Half-Life	Duration of Action
PO	1–2 wk	2–4 wk	6–9 hr	Several weeks

▶▶fluoxetine hydrochloride

Fluoxetine hydrochloride (Prozac) was the first SSRI marketed for the treatment of depression and is considered the prototypical SSRI. Since that time, it has become one of the most commonly prescribed of all drugs. Although it was initially indicated for the treatment of depression, the indications for fluoxetine have since expanded to include bulimia nervosa and obsessive-compulsive disorder. Contraindications include known drug allergy and concurrent MAOI therapy. Adverse effects include anxiety, dizziness, drowsiness, insomnia, and others listed in Table 17-5. Interacting drugs include benzodiazepines (reduced benzodiazepine clearance; see Chapter 13), buspirone (reduced buspirone effects; see earlier in the chapter), antipsychotics (elevated antipsychotic levels), and propafenone hydrochloride (see Chapter 25). Other drug interactions are listed in Table 17-6. Fluoxetine is available only for oral use.

PHARMACOKINETICS

Route	Onset of Action	Peak Plasma Concentration	Elimination Half-Life	Duration of Action
PO	1–4 wk	6–8 hr	1–3 days*	2–4 wk

*Active metabolite has a half-life of 7 to 10 days.

▶▶bupropion hydrochloride

Bupropion hydrochloride is a unique antidepressant in terms of both its structure and mechanism of action. It has relatively weak, but measurable, effects on brain serotonin activity but little to no activity on monoamine oxidase. It is a norepinephrine dopamine reuptake inhibitor. Its strongest therapeutic action appears to be primarily on the dopaminergic and noradrenergic pathways.

Bupropion was originally indicated for treatment of depression but is now also indicated as an aid in smoking cessation. It is sometimes added as an adjunct antidepressant for patients experiencing sexual adverse effects secondary to SSRI therapy. Although the mechanism is unclear, the drug is often effective in this situation. A sustained-release form of bupropion, Zyban, was approved for smoking cessation treatment. Sustained-release bupropion was an innovative new treatment because it was the first nicotine-free prescription medicine used to treat nicotine dependence. Its exact mechanism of action in treating nicotine dependence is unknown, but it is believed to be related to the drug's ability to modulate dopamine and norepinephrine levels in the brain. Both of these neurotransmitters are thought to play an important role in maintaining nicotine addiction. However, the newer smoking

DRUG PROFILES—cont'd

cessation drug varenicline tartrate (Champix®; see Chapter 18) is becoming popular for this purpose.

Bupropion is contraindicated in patients who have a known drug allergy, those with a seizure disorder (bupropion can lower the seizure threshold), those who currently have or previously have had anorexia nervosa or bulimia nervosa, and those currently taking an MAOI. Common adverse effects include dizziness, confusion, tachycardia, agitation, tremor, and dry mouth. Drugs that interact with bupropion include the azole antifungals (see Chapter 47) as well as other drugs metabolized by the cytochrome P450 enzyme system (see Chapter 2) and CNS depressants. Other drug interactions are listed in Table 17-6. Bupropion is available only for oral use.

PHARMACOKINETICS

Route	Onset of Action	Peak Plasma Concentration	Elimination Half-Life	Duration of Action
PO	Up to 4 wk	3 hr	10–14 hr	Weeks to months

▶▶ mirtazapine

Mirtazapine (Remeron) is unique in that it promotes the presynaptic release of both serotonin and norepinephrine in the brain. This is due to its antagonist activity in the presynaptic α_2-adrenergic receptors. It does not inhibit the reuptake of either of these neurotransmitters. It is strongly associated with sedation in more than 50% of patients because of its histamine 1 (H_1) receptor activity and therefore is usually dosed once daily at bedtime. Furthermore, although clearance of the drug may be somewhat reduced in older adults, no dosage adjustment is currently recommended. Mirtazapine is indicated for the treatment of depression, including that associated with bipolar disorder. It is also sometimes helpful (mechanism unknown) in reducing sexual adverse effects experienced by male patients receiving SSRI therapy. Mirtazapine is known to be an appetite stimulant and thus can be helpful in

underweight depressed patients or harmful in those who are already overweight. Mirtazapine is contraindicated in cases of drug allergy and concurrent use of MAOIs. Adverse effects include drowsiness, abnormal dreams, dry mouth, constipation, increased appetite, and asthenia. Drug interactions include additive CNS depressant effects with alcohol and CYP (liver enzymes) inhibitors (see Chapter 2). Mirtazapine is available only for oral use.

PHARMACOKINETICS

Route	Onset of Action	Peak Plasma Concentration	Elimination Half-Life	Duration of Action
PO	1–3 wk	2 hr	20–40 hr	Unknown

duloxetine hydrochloride

Duloxetine hydrochloride (Cymbalta), like venlafaxine hydrochloride, is a delayed-release serotonin-norepinephrine reuptake inhibitor (SNRI). These two drugs along with trazodone are the three top-selling antidepressants in Canada. Duloxetine hydrochloride is considered an analgesic/antidepressant/anxiolytic and is indicated for depression and generalized anxiety disorder. It is also indicated for pain resulting from diabetic peripheral neuropathy, fibromyalgia, chronic low back pain, and osteoarthritis of the knee. It is contraindicated in cases of known drug allergy and concurrent MAOI use, and it can worsen uncontrolled angle-closure glaucoma. Adverse effects include dizziness, drowsiness, headache, GI upset, anorexia, and hepatotoxicity. Drugs with which duloxetine hydrochloride interacts include SSRIs and triptans (increased risk of serotonin syndrome) and alcohol (increased risk of liver injury). Duloxetine hydrochloride is available only for oral use.

PHARMACOKINETICS

Route	Onset of Action	Peak Plasma Concentration	Elimination Half-Life	Duration of Action
PO	2–6 weeks	6 hr	12 hr	Unknown

mania (as an adjunct to lithium), bipolar disorder, depression that is resistant to other therapy, certain movement disorders (e.g., Tourette's syndrome), and certain other medical conditions (e.g., nausea, intractable hiccups). Antipsychotic use in children is increasing, such as for disruptive behavioural disorders in children and adolescents (Loy, Merry, Hetrick, & Stasiak, 2012).

Antipsychotic drugs represent a significant advance in the treatment of mental health disorders, highlighted by the fact that early treatment of mental health disorders (before the 1950s) consisted of such extreme measures as isolation, physical restraint, shock therapy, and even lobotomy.

Phenothiazines are the largest chemical class of antipsychotic drugs, constituting about two thirds of all antipsychotics. They were also the original drugs in this category. As with many other drugs, phenothiazines were

discovered by chance, in this case during research for new antihistamines. Chlorpromazine, isolated in 1951, was the first phenothiazine to be discovered in this way. The currently available antipsychotics are listed in Table 17-8.

Overall, there are few differences among conventional, or first-generation, antipsychotics in their mechanisms of action. Therefore, selection of an antipsychotic is based primarily on the patient's tolerance and the need to minimize adverse effects. Of the currently available antipsychotic drugs, no single drug stands out for all patients as either more or less effective in the treatment of psychotic symptoms. Antipsychotic drug therapy does not normally provide a cure for psychoses but is a way of chemically controlling the symptoms of the illness.

More recently, a new generation of antipsychotic medications has evolved. These are referred to as *atypical*

TABLE 17-8

Currently Available Antipsychotic Drugs

Generic Name	Trade Name	Route
CONVENTIONAL		
Phenothiazines		
chlorpromazine hydrochloride		PO, IM, IV
fluphenazine		PO, IM, SUBCUT
perphenazine		PO
prochlorperazine		PO, PR, IM, IV
trifluoperazine hydrochloride		PO
Thioxanthene		
thiothixene	Navane®	PO
Phenylbutylpiperidines		
haloperidol		PO, IM
pimozide	Orap®	PO
ATYPICAL		
Dibenzodiazepines		
clozapine	Clozaril®	PO
loxapine succinate	Xylane	PO
loxapine hydrochloride	Loxapac®	IM
olanzapine	Zyprexa®	PO, IM
quetiapine fumurate	Seroquel®	PO
asenapine maleate	Saphris®	Sublingual
Benzisoxazoles		
lurasidone hydrochloride	Latuda®	PO
paliperidone	Invega®	PO, IM
risperidone	Risperdal®	PO, IM
ziprasidone hydrochloride monohydrate	Zeldox®	PO, IM
Quinolinone		
aripiprazole	Abilify®	PO, IM

IM, intramuscular; *IV*, intravenous; *PO*, oral; *PR*, per rectum; *SUBCUT*, subcutaneous.

antipsychotics, as opposed to the conventional drugs, which can also be thought of as older-generation antipsychotics. Atypical antipsychotics differ from conventional drugs in that they tend to have better adverse effect profiles. The atypical antipsychotics still have adverse effects, but they are usually not as severe as those of conventional antipsychotic drugs.

Mechanism of Action and Drug Effects

All antipsychotics block dopamine receptors in the brain, which decreases dopamine concentration in the CNS. Specifically, the conventional phenothiazines block the dopamine receptors postsynaptically in certain areas of the CNS, such as the limbic system and the basal ganglia. These are the areas associated with emotions, cognitive function, and motor function. This receptor blocking produces a tranquilizing effect in patients who are psychotic. Both the therapeutic and toxic effects of these drugs are the direct result of the dopamine blockade in these areas. The atypical antipsychotic drugs block specific dopamine receptors called *dopamine 2 (D_2) receptors*, as well as specific serotonin receptors in the brain known as *2 (5-HT_2) receptors*. These more refined mechanisms of action of the

atypicals are responsible for their improved efficacy and safety profiles, compared with older drugs (see Adverse Effects).

All antipsychotics show efficacy in improving the positive symptoms of schizophrenia, and these beneficial effects may even increase over time. Positive symptoms include auditory and visual hallucinations, delusions, and conceptual disorganization. The first-line treatment option for hallucinations in schizophrenia is antipsychotic medication (which blocks the dopamine D_2 receptors), producing a rapid decrease in severity. Unfortunately, conventional drugs are less effective in managing negative symptoms. Negative symptoms are apathy, social withdrawal, blunted affect, poverty of speech, and catatonia. It is these negative symptoms that account for most of the social and occupational dysfunction caused by schizophrenia. Fortunately, atypical antipsychotics have improved efficacy in treating both positive and negative symptoms.

Indications

Antipsychotic drugs are indicated for psychosis associated with mental health disorders, most commonly schizophrenia. As more has been learned about these drugs, especially the atypical antipsychotic drugs, their indications have expanded to include anxiety and mood disorders. Certain antipsychotics (e.g., prochlorperazine maleate) are used as antiemetics (see Chapter 41). They block serotonin receptors and dopamine receptors in the chemoreceptor trigger zone in the brain and inhibit neurotransmission in the vagus nerve in the GI tract. Additional blocking of dopamine receptors in the brainstem reticular system also allows atypical drugs to have anxiolytic, or antianxiety, effects.

Contraindications

Contraindications to the use of antipsychotic drugs include known drug allergy, comatose state, significant CNS depression, brain damage, liver or kidney disease, blood dyscrasias, or uncontrolled epilepsy.

Adverse Effects

Common adverse effects caused by blockade of the α-adrenergic, dopamine, endocrine, histamine, and muscarinic (cholinergic) receptors are listed in Table 17-9. Possible severe hematological effects include agranulocytosis (low numbers of white blood cells [WBCs] in the blood) and hemolytic anemia. Integumentary effects may include exfoliative dermatitis. CNS effects include drowsiness, neuroleptic malignant syndrome, extrapyramidal symptoms, and tardive dyskinesia. **Neuroleptic malignant syndrome** is a relatively rare but potentially life-threatening adverse effect that is triggered by a reaction associated with antipsychotic medications or other medications that cause reduced dopamine activity (either through blockage of D_2 receptors or decreased availability of dopamine) in the CNS. Due to blockade of dopamine neurotransmission in the nigrostriatum, muscular rigidity can result. Dopamine blockade in the hypothalamus can produce altered thermoregulation (high fever), vital sign instability, and autonomic instability (irregular pulse or blood pressure, tachycardia, diaphoresis, and cardiac dysrhythmias; Agar, 2010). Additional signs may include elevated creatine phosphokinase, myoglobinuria (rhabdomyolysis), and acute kidney injury. Treatment involves prompt withdrawal of the causative medication and supportive treatment.

Extrapyramidal symptoms are involuntary motor symptoms similar to those associated with Parkinson's disease (see Chapter 16). This drug-induced state is known as *pseudoparkinsonism* and is characterized by symptoms such as **akathisia** (distressing motor restlessness) and acute **dystonia** (painful muscle spasms). Two anticholinergic medications, benztropine mesylate (Kynesia®) and trihexyphenidyl hydrochloride, are commonly used to treat these symptoms (see Chapter 15).

Tardive means "late-appearing"; **tardive dyskinesia** is characterized by involuntary contractions of oral and facial muscles (e.g., involuntary tongue-thrusting) and choreoathetosis (wavelike movements of the extremities) and usually appears only after continuous long-term antipsychotic therapy. Theoretically, these effects are possible with atypical antipsychotics as well, however, evidence suggests that the incidence with these drugs is lower.

Cardiovascular effects, caused by α-receptor blockade, include orthostatic hypotension. In addition, electrocardiogram (ECG) changes, notably prolonged QT interval, are associated with all classes of antipsychotic drugs. Baseline and periodic ECGs, as well as measurement of serum potassium and magnesium levels, can help to determine if a patient is at risk for such effects or to diagnose newly acquired cardiac dysrhythmias. Conventional drugs such as phenothiazines and haloperidol can also augment prolactin release, which can result in swelling of the breasts and milk secretion in women. Gynecomastia (breast tissue enlargement) can also be a distressing adverse effect in male patients (Table 17-10).

Adverse effects on the endocrine system associated with antipsychotics include insulin resistance, weight gain, and changes in serum lipid levels. Antipsychotics are associated with development of **cardiometabolic syndrome** (see Box 17-2), which can cause serious long-term health problems.

In 2011, Health Canada required manufacturers to update product labelling to include stronger wording regarding the use of antipsychotics in pregnant women. The new labelling includes more consistent information about the potential risk for abnormal muscle movements (extrapyramidal symptoms) and withdrawal symptoms

TABLE 17-9

Antipsychotics: Receptor-Related Adverse Effects

Receptor	Adverse Effect	Drug Category
α-Adrenergic	Orthostatic hypotension, lightheadedness, reflex tachycardia	Conventional drugs
Dopamine	Extrapyramidal movement disorders, dystonia, parkinsonism, akathisia, tardive dyskinesia	Atypical drugs
Histamine	Sedation, drowsiness, hypotension, weight gain	Conventional drugs
Muscarinic (cholinergic)	Blurred vision, worsening of angle-closure glaucoma, dry mouth, tachycardia, constipation, urinary retention, decreased sweating	Conventional drugs

TABLE 17-10

Adverse Effects of Selected Psychotropic Drugs*

Drug or Drug Class	Adverse Effects
Conventional (e.g., haloperidol)	Akathisia, extrapyramidal symptoms, hypertension, neuroleptic malignant syndrome, confusion, headache, mild GI disturbance, dry mouth, amenorrhea, gynecomastia, visual disturbances, hyperpyrexia, edema, tardive dyskinesia, skin rash, photosensitivity, weight gain, urinary retention
Atypical (e.g., clozapine, risperidone)	Tachycardia, akathisia, agitation, asthenia, ataxia, seizures, dyskinesia, dizziness, drowsiness, headache, insomnia, dry mouth, dyspepsia, anxiety, increased appetite, weight gain

*See also drug profiles for drug-specific information.
GI, gastrointestinal.

BOX 17-2 — Antipsychotic Use and Cardiometabolic Syndrome

Cardiometabolic syndrome involves the presence of at least three abnormal values out of the five following criteria: visceral obesity measured by waist circumference, blood pressure, fasting plasma glucose [FPG], high-density lipoprotein cholesterol level (HDL-C), and triglycerides (TGs; Leiter et al., 2011). Although not well understood, psychotropic drugs (especially atypical antipsychotics) are associated with increased weight gain and metabolic adverse effects. Several neurotransmitter systems have been implicated, such as histamine receptor blockade. Genetic predisposition may also play a role. Patients with schizophrenia who are treated with antipsychotic medications develop features of cardiometabolic syndrome at a rate that is approximately one and a half to two times higher than in the general population (Riordan, Antonini, & Murphy, 2011). All ages of patients are susceptible to the metabolic adverse effects of antipsychotics; however, children and adolescents are most vulnerable (Riordan et al., 2011). Complicating the risk for developing cardiometabolic syndrome are lifestyle factors (sedentary lifestyle, food insecurity, high rates of smoking, and substance misuse) combined with stress and the negative symptoms of schizophrenia. Those on more than one drug may be at elevated risk for developing higher rates of cardiometabolic syndrome than those on monotherapy (Yogaratnam, Biswas, Vadivel, et al., 2013).

The mean age of death for individuals with schizophrenia is 61 years of age; life expectancy is reduced by 20%, with the majority of mortality due to physical illness (Yogaratnam et al., 2013). Indeed, cardiovascular disease is the most common cause of mortality in patients with schizophrenia; incidence of diabetes is two to four times higher in patients with schizophrenia than in the general population (Riordan, Antonini, & Murphy, 2011).

All patients receiving treatment with antipsychotic medications require ongoing metabolic and lifestyle monitoring.

Sources: Leiter, L. A., Fitchett, D. H., Gilbert, R. E., et al. (2011). Cardiometabolic risk in Canada: A detailed analysis and position paper by the cardiometabolic risk working group. *Canadian Journal of Cardiology, 27*(2), e1–e33. doi:10.1016/j.cjca.2010.12.054

Riordan, H. J., Antonini, P., & Murphy, M. F. (2011). Atypical antipsychotics and metabolic syndrome in patients with schizophrenia: Risk factors, monitoring, and healthcare implications. *American Health and Drug Benefits, 4*(5), 292–302.

Yogaratnam J., Biswas, N., Vadivel, R., et al. (2013). Metabolic complications of schizophrenia and antipsychotic medications— An updated review. *East Asian Archives of Psychiatry, 23*(1), 21–28.

---

in newborns whose mothers were treated with these drugs during the third trimester of pregnancy.

Interactions

Major drug interactions are listed in Table 17-11. Antihypertensives may have additive hypotensive effects and CNS depressants may have additive CNS depressant effects when taken with antipsychotics. Grapefruit juice can enhance the effects of clozapine (by reducing its metabolism via the cytochrome P450 enzyme system). Because grapefruit juice affects many enzymes in the liver P450 system, it is wise for patients taking multiple medications to avoid this food.

Dosages

Recommended dosages of selected antipsychotic drugs are given in the table on p. 345.

NURSING PROCESS

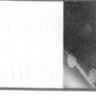 **Assessment**

Before administering any of the psychotherapeutic drugs, perform a complete head-to-toe physical assessment and

TABLE 17-11

Drug Interactions of Selected Antipsychotics*

Drug Class	Interacting Drug(s)	Mechanism	Result
Conventional and Atypical	Alcohol, other CNS depressants	Additive drug effects	Enhanced CNS depression; dystonia with alcohol
	Antihypertensives	Enhanced antihypertensive effects	Potential for hypotension
Conventional: Phenothiazines	Anticholinergics	Additive and antagonistic drug effects	Reduced phenothiazine efficacy; enhanced anticholinergic effects
	β-blockers	Additive drug effects	Potential toxicity of either drug
	Oploids	Addltlve drug effects	Excessive sedation, hypotenslon
	Levodopa–carbidopa	Uncertain	Diminished antiparkinsonian effects
	phenytoin	Uncertain	Can increase or reduce phenytoin levels
Atypicals*	Thiazide diuretics	Reduced diuretic clearance	Potential for hypotension
	CYP3A4 inhibitors (e.g., ketoconazole)	Reduced antipsychotic clearance	Potential for antipsychotic toxicity
	carbamazepine	Enhanced antipsychotic clearance	Reduced therapeutic effects

*See also drug profiles for drug-specific information.
CNS, central nervous system; *CYP3A4,* cytochrome P450 enzyme 3A4.

 # DRUG PROFILES

Conventional antipsychotic drugs are still available on the Canadian market (see Table 17-8). However, much of their use in common clinical practice has been replaced by the atypical antipsychotic drugs, which generally have better adverse effect profiles. All antipsychotics are prescription-only medications that are indicated for the treatment of various psychotic disorders. No single drug stands out as more or less effective in the treatment of the symptoms of psychosis. Some of the factors to be considered before selecting an antipsychotic are the patient's history of response to a drug and the possible adverse effect profile. Starting at a low dose with titration to the lowest effective dose helps achieve a balance between symptom relief and adverse effects. For dosage information on profiled drugs, see the table on p. 336.

BUTYROPHENONE

haloperidol

Haloperidol is structurally different from the thioxanthenes and the phenothiazines but has similar antipsychotic properties. It is indicated primarily for the long-term treatment of psychosis. However, it has been largely replaced by the atypical antipsychotics because of its adverse effects (see later). Haloperidol blocks D₂ receptors found in the chemoreceptor trigger zone and consequently may be used for the management of nausea in palliative patients. Haloperidol is contraindicated in patients who have shown a hypersensitivity reaction to it, those in a comatose state, those taking large amounts of CNS depressants, and those with Parkinson's disease (due to its antidopaminergic effects). It is a high-potency neuroleptic drug that has a favourable cardiovascular, anticholinergic, and sedative adverse effect profile, but it can cause extrapyramidal symptoms as well as tardive dyskinesia. Haloperidol is available in two salt forms: base (for oral use) and decanoate injection (for IM use only). Haloperidol decanoate has an extremely long duration of action, which has historically made it useful in treating patients with schizophrenia who were nonadherent to their drug regimen. Other adverse effects are listed in Table 17-10. Drugs with which haloperidol interacts are listed in Table 17-11.

PHARMACOKINETICS

Route	Onset of Action	Peak Plasma Concentration	Elimination Half-Life	Duration of Action
PO	2 hr	2–6 hr	13–35 hr	8–12 hr
IM (decanoate)	3–9 days	Unknown	13–35 hr	Decanoate: 1 mo

ATYPICAL ANTIPSYCHOTICS

Between 1975 and 1990, no new antipsychotic drug was approved in Canada. In 1991, clozapine (Clozaril®), the first of the atypical antipsychotics, was approved. Clozapine was followed by risperidone (Risperdal®), olanzapine (Zyprexa®), quetiapine (Seroquel®), ziprasidone (Zeldox®), aripiprazole (Abilify®), paliperidone (Invega®), asenapine maleate (Saphris®), and lurasidone hydrochloride (Latuda®).

Atypical antipsychotics have several advantageous properties, including reduced effect on prolactin levels compared with conventional drugs and improvement in the negative symptoms associated with schizophrenia. They also seem to show a lower risk for neuromuscular malignant syndrome and tardive dyskinesia. All 10 of the currently available atypical drugs have several

Continued

DRUG PROFILES—cont'd

pharmacological properties in common. Antagonist activity at the dopamine D_2 receptor is believed to be the mechanism of their antimanic activity. Serotonergic (serotonin agonist) activity at various serotonin (5-HT) receptor subtypes and α_2-adrenergic (agonist) activity are both associated with antidepressant activity. α_1-adrenergic receptor antagonist activity is associated with orthostatic hypotension, and histamine H_1 receptor antagonist activity is associated with both sedative and appetite-stimulating effects. This last effect accounts for the common adverse effect of weight gain that is associated to various degrees with atypical antipsychotic drugs. This effect can cause or worsen obesity and can result in type 2 diabetes (see Research Box). Clozapine and olanzapine are associated with the most weight gain, risperidone and quetiapine with less, and ziprasidone is considered weight neutral. Other atypical antipsychotics fall between the aforementioned drugs.

Sedative effects may diminish over time and can actually be helpful to patients with insomnia. Although these drugs all have similar pharmacological properties, they vary in their degree of affinity for the various types of receptors. These subtle pharmacological differences, along with often unknown and unpredictable physiological patient differences, help to explain why some patients respond better (or do not respond) to one medication than another. In 2005, Health Canada issued a public health advisory concerning the use of atypical antipsychotic drugs in older adults for off-label, nonapproved uses. These medications are currently approved to treat schizophrenia and mania. In practice, however, they are also used to control behavioural symptoms of agitation in older adults with dementia, including dementia related to Alzheimer's disease. Data showed that older adults given atypical antipsychotics for this reason were up to 1.7 times more likely to die during treatment than if they had not had the treatment. Health Canada recommends that health care providers re-evaluate the treatment plans of patients treated with these drugs and recommend nondrug approaches to manage behaviour symptoms.

Dosage information for atypical antipsychotics is given in the table on p. 326.

clozapine

Clozapine (Clozaril) was the first of the atypical antipsychotics. Compared to conventional antipsychotic drugs, it more selectively blocks the dopaminergic receptors in the mesolimbic region of the brain. Conventional antipsychotic drugs block dopamine receptors in an area of the brain called the neostriatum, but blockade in this area is believed to cause extrapyramidal adverse effects. Because clozapine has weak dopamine-blocking abilities in the neostriatum, it causes minor or no extrapyramidal symptoms. Clozapine is therefore often the drug of choice for treatment of psychotic disorders in patients who also have Parkinson's disease because it will not worsen motor symptoms.

Clozapine has been extremely useful for the treatment of patients for whom therapy with other antipsychotic drugs have not been effective, especially those with schizophrenia. In particular, it is indicated for patients with schizophrenia who have shown high risk for suicidal behaviour and are resistant to other antipsychotics. Adverse effects include the potential for drug-induced agranulocytosis, a dangerous lack of WBC production. The occurrence of agranulocytosis is highest between 6 weeks and 18 weeks after starting clozapine treatment. For this reason, patients beginning clozapine therapy require weekly monitoring of WBC count for the first 6 months of therapy. The drug needs to be withheld if the count falls below 3.5×10^9/L and until it rises above this value. It is also recommended that WBC counts be evaluated weekly for 4 weeks after discontinuation of the drug. Clozaril is available only through the Clozapine Risk Management Program, with which both the patient and health care provider must be registered. Other adverse effects are listed in Table 17-10.

Clozapine is contraindicated in patients with known drug allergy; in those with myeloproliferative disorders, severe granulocytopenia, CNS depression, or narrow-angle glaucoma; and in patients who are comatose. Interacting drugs include alcohol and other CNS depressants (increased CNS depression), levodopa (diminished therapeutic effects), antihypertensives (risk of hypotension), and others listed in Table 17-11. Clozapine is available only for oral use.

Other atypical antipsychotics have features comparable to those of clozapine but do not require extensive WBC monitoring. Risperidone is described in the following profile as an example of these drugs. Orally disintegrating tablets are available for risperidone, and asenapine is available as a sublingual tablet. These dosage forms may improve adherence. The dosage is the same as for regular tablets (refer to the table on p. 345).

PHARMACOKINETICS

Route	Onset of Action	Peak Plasma Concentration	Elimination Half-Life	Duration of Action
PO	1–6 hr	Weeks	6 hr	4–12 hr

▶▶ risperidone

Risperidone (Risperdal) is an atypical antipsychotic that was introduced a few years after clozapine. It is even more active than clozapine at the serotonin (5-HT_{2A} and 5-HT_{2C}) receptors. It also has high affinity for α_1- and α_2-adrenergic receptors and histamine H_1 receptors. It has lower affinity for the serotonin 5-HT_{1A}, 5-HT_{1C}, and 5-HT_{1D} receptors and the dopamine D_1 receptor. This drug is indicated for refractory schizophrenia, including negative symptoms, and causes minimal extrapyramidal symptoms at therapeutic dosages of 1 to 6 mg/day. Risperidone is contraindicated in cases of known drug allergy. Adverse effects include elevated serum prolactin levels, abnormal dreams, insomnia, dizziness, headache, and others listed in Table 17-10. It is available in both oral and long-acting injectable forms.

In 2015, the drug manufacturer and Health Canada issued a limitation to the use of risperidone to severe dementia of the Alzheimer type for psychosis and

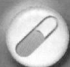 DRUG PROFILES—cont'd

aggression. Tablets, oral solutions, and oral disintegrating tablets are affected. There is a higher risk of cerebrovascular adverse events in patients with the mixed or vascular dementia, compared to those with dementia of the Alzheimer type.

Drugs interacting with risperidone include CNS depressants, antihypertensives, and others listed in Table 17-11. Risperidone is available for oral and injectable use. The long-acting injectable form is called Risperdal Consta®, and one IM injection lasts approximately 2 weeks. This form is at least one option for helping patients maintain adherence with the prescribed drug regimen. Patients must continue to take oral risperidone for 3 weeks after the first injection of the Consta dosage form to ensure adequate blood levels from the injection. Paliperidone palmitae is a long-acting injection (Invega Sustenna®) that lasts 1 month.

PHARMACOKINETICS

Route	Onset of Action	Peak Plasma Concentration	Elimination Half-Life	Duration of Action
PO	1–2 wk	1–2 hr	20–30 hr	7 days
IM	3 wk	Unknown	20–30 hr	2 wk

DOSAGES   Selected Antipsychotic Drugs

Drug	Pharmacological Class	Usual Dosage Range*	Indications/Uses
First Generation (Conventional)			
haloperidol	Butyrophenone, phenylbutylpiperidine	**Adults** PO: 0.5–5 mg bid–tid IM: 2.5–5 mg prn **Children** PO: 0.25–0.5 bid–tid	Acute psychosis of schizophrenia and mania, Tourette's syndrome, severe aggression or agitation
Second Generation (Atypical)			
clozapine (Clozaril)	Dibenzodiazepine	PO: 12.5 mg bid, titrate up to maximum of 300–900 mg/day, divided	Treatment-resistant schizophrenia
▸risperidone (Risperdal)	Benzisoxazole	PO: 4–6 mg/day in either one or two doses IM depot form (Risperdal Consta): 25–50 mg every 2 wk	Schizophrenia, mania, aggression or psychosis associated with dementia

IM, intramuscular; *PO*, oral
*All dosages reflect usual adult dosage ranges. Pediatric doses may be more variable and should be specified by a pediatric health care provider.

mental status examination. Document your findings. This data will serve as a comparative baseline for the patient during and after initiation of therapy.

Thoroughly assess the patient's neurological functioning, including level of consciousness, mental alertness, and level of motor and cognitive functioning. The Mini-Mental Status Examination (MMSE) is one tool that may be used to assess cognitive status and help identify impairments often found in mental health disorders. The MMSE is simple to use, is cost-effective, and can be completed in about 20 minutes. The MMSE is available in most nursing assessments, nursing fundamentals, or psychiatric or mental health nursing textbooks. Points are scored in the areas of level of orientation, attention and calculation ability, recall, and language skills. Other mental health assessment tools include the Beck Depression Inventory, the Burns Anxiety Inventory, the six-item Blessed Orientation-Memory-Concentration Test, clock-drawing tasks, the Functional Activities Questionnaire (for those with dementia), the Alzheimer's Disease Assessment Scale, the Mattis Dementia Rating Scale, the Severe Impairment Battery, and the Hamilton Rating Scale for Depression. In addition to performing assessments such as these, note baseline levels of motor responses and reflexes as well as the presence of any tremors or personality changes. Assess for the presence of cold, clammy hands; sweating; and pallor—these particular findings may be indicative of altered autonomic nervous response.

Constantly assess the patient for any suicidal ideations or tendencies, with attention to not only overt cues and behaviours but also to covert thoughts and ideation. This is important because of the potential for suicide with the use of psychotherapeutic drugs, with or without the concurrent use of other medications or alcohol. Suicide assessment tools are available and may help you identify an individual's risk for suicidal behaviours. One such tool, the Suicide Assessment Scale, has been found to be valid, reliable, and easy to use. The following are some questions that may be helpful: "What brings you to the doctor's office today?" "How has life been treating you?" "What are some of your worries or concerns?" "How would you describe your mood?" "Tell me about your thoughts." People at the highest risk for committing suicide in the near future have a specific suicide plan, the means to carry out the plan, a time frame for doing it, and an intention to do it. An immediate response is required—call 911, call a crisis centre, or take the person to an emergency room. Asking the direct question, "Are you thinking about wanting to die?" or "Are you thinking about committing suicide?" to someone who may be considering suicide is also recommended. IS PATH WARM is a 10–warning sign mnemonic for assessing suicide risk, developed by the American Association for Suicidology (2015), including: **I**deation; **S**ubstance use; **P**urposelessness; **A**nxiety; **T**rapped; **H**opelessness; **W**ithdrawal; **A**nger; **R**ecklessness; **M**ood changes.

Remember that many of the patients who require psychotherapeutic drugs are depressed and, as such, suffer from insomnia and possibly from self-neglect. Deterioration in health status and weight loss or gain may also occur. Therefore, it is important to assess sleep habits and nutritional intake and to perform a head-to-toe physical examination for baseline and comparative purposes. Note any drug allergies as well as any contraindications, cautions, and potential drug interactions (see pharmacology discussion and Tables 17-3, 17-6, and 17-11). Assess and document blood pressure and pulse rate before, during, and after drug therapy. Postural blood pressures (i.e., blood pressure taken supine and then standing) are particularly important to note because of the possible drug-related adverse effects of orthostatic hypotension and dizziness. The more potent older drugs (e.g., MAOIs or TCAs) may lead to a significant drop in blood pressure and possible syncope, warranting even more skillful assessment and close monitoring (of blood pressure readings).

Review the results of any laboratory studies performed before and during the drug therapy. This is particularly important for patients who are receiving long-term drug therapy to prevent or identify any early complications or other possible adverse effects or toxicity. Laboratory studies may include, but are not limited to, tests to confirm serum therapeutic levels of the specific drug, and, if appropriate, a complete blood cell count, erythrocyte sedimentation rate, serum electrolyte and glucose levels, blood urea nitrogen, liver function studies, kidney function tests, serum levels of vitamin B_{12}, lipid and triglyceride levels, and thyroid studies. If the patient is experiencing dementia, other types of testing may be needed, such as genetic studies, computed tomography, or magnetic resonance imaging.

With psychotherapeutic drug therapy, assess the patient's mouth and oral cavity to make sure the patient has swallowed the entire oral dosage. This helps prevent hoarding or "cheeking" of medications, a form of nonadherence that may lead to drug toxicity or overdose. If the assessment shows that this is a potential risk, using liquid or rapid dissolving tablets dosage forms, when available, may minimize such problems. Other areas to assess include the patient's appetite, sleeping patterns, addictive behaviours, elimination difficulties, and allergic reactions. Note any new symptoms or problems.

■ Benzodiazepines

Anxiety disorders are treated with the benzodiazepine drugs. Anxiolytic drugs, specifically the benzodiazepines, are associated with many contraindications, cautions, and drug interactions (see pharmacology discussion). When these drugs are used, the health care provider may order laboratory studies, such as complete blood counts, serum electrolyte levels, and liver and kidney function studies (see earlier discussion). Blood pressure readings are also important to assess because of drug-related orthostatic hypotension. The baseline neurological examination needs to include assessment of alertness, orientation, and sensory and motor functioning, as well as any reports of ataxia, headache, or other neurological abnormalities. To complete a thorough medication profile, create a list of all medications taken, including any other psychotherapeutic drugs, all prescription drugs, OTC drugs, and natural health products. Diazepam, although one of the more commonly prescribed benzodiazepines, is generally used for seizure disorders and preoperative sedation and requires assessment related to these uses (see Chapters 12 and 15). Specific concerns for children and older adult patients are presented in the Special Populations: Children box and the Special Populations: Older Adults box on p. 347. Closely observe and assess older adult patients for oversedation or profound CNS depression during drug therapy. Falls and resulting fractures are a common risk factor in older adults taking benzodiazepines. Older adults are often more sensitive to drugs and therefore more likely to experience adverse effects; their safety needs to be a constant concern.

Since eye problems may occur with the use of benzodiazepines, baseline visual testing using a Snellen chart or an eye examination conducted by the appropriate health care provider (i.e., an ophthalmologist or optometrist) is recommended. Allergic reactions to some of these medications (e.g., clonazepam) are characterized by a red raised rash. In addition, patients who are obese may experience toxicity in a shorter period of time. This susceptibility occurs because several anxiolytic drugs are lipid soluble and have greater affinity for fatty tissues; therefore, their half-life is increased in patients who are obese. Give lorazepam cautiously (under close supervision) if a patient is suicidal because its use may be associated with suicide attempts. Administer alprazolam only after careful assessment of mental status, mood, sensorium, and sleep patterns.

Buspirone is another anxiolytic drug that is not a benzodiazepine. It is used because it has fewer adverse effects, such as decreased sedation and lack of dependency potential. However, it is associated with many drug

SPECIAL POPULATIONS: CHILDREN

Psychotherapeutic Drugs

- Children are more likely to experience adverse effects from psychotropic drugs, especially extrapyramidal effects.
- The incidence of Reye's syndrome and other adverse effects is greater in children taking psychotropic drugs who have had chicken pox, CNS infections, measles, acute illnesses, or dehydration.
- Lithium may lead to decreased bone density or bone formation in children; therefore, children receiving it need to be closely monitored for signs and symptoms of lithium toxicity and bone disorders. The safety and efficacy of lithium dosing for those younger than 6 years of age is not established.

- TCAs generally are not prescribed for patients younger than 12 years of age. However, some antidepressants are used in children with enuresis, attention deficit hyperactivity disorder, or major depressive disorders and may be associated with adverse effects such as electrocardiographic changes, nervousness, sleep disorders, fatigue, elevated blood pressure, and GI upset.
- Children are generally more sensitive to the effects of most drugs, and psychotherapeutic drugs are no exception. Be aware of the risk of toxicity, which can be fatal. If confusion, lethargy, visual disturbances, insomnia, tremors, palpitations, constipation, or eye pain occur, contact the prescribing health care provider immediately.

 SPECIAL POPULATIONS: OLDER ADULTS

Psychotherapeutic Drugs

- Older adults show higher serum levels of psychotherapeutic drugs because they have age-related changes in drug distribution and metabolism, less serum albumin, decreased lean body mass, less water in tissues, and increased body fat. They also have decreased kidney function. Because of these changes, older adults generally require lower doses of antipsychotic and antidepressant drugs than younger adults, and they are at greater risk for toxicity.
- Orthostatic hypotension, anticholinergic adverse effects, sedation, and extrapyramidal symptoms are more common in older adults taking psychotherapeutic drugs.
- Careful evaluation and documentation of baseline parameters, including neurological findings, are

important to the safe use of psychotherapeutic drugs.
- Increased anxiety is often associated with the use of TCAs.
- Patients with a history of heart disease may be at greater risk for experiencing dysrhythmias, tachycardia, stroke, myocardial infarction, or heart failure.
- Lithium toxicity is more common older adults, and lower doses are often necessary to achieve therapeutic levels. Close monitoring is important to its safe use in this age group. CNS toxicity, lithium-induced goitre, and hypothyroidism are more common in older adult patients.

interactions, cautions, and contraindications (see pharmacology discussion). It is also important to complete a general assessment of the neurological system and a mental health assessment.

■ Mood-Stabilizing Drugs

As previously discussed in the pharmacology section, affective disorders are treated with mood-stabilizing drugs, antipsychotics, and antidepressant drugs. Before antimanic drugs such as lithium are administered, perform a thorough neurological examination. Also assess vital signs, especially blood pressure, hydration status, dietary intake, skin tone, and presence of edema. It is also important to assess baseline levels of consciousness and alertness, gait and mobility levels, and overall motor functioning. Poor coordination, tremors, and weakness may be symptoms of toxic blood levels of antimanic

drugs. Laboratory studies often ordered before and during drug therapy include serum sodium, albumin, and uric acid levels. Serum levels of sodium are important to know because lithium toxicity is potentiated by the presence of hyponatremia and hypovolemia. During the initial phase of therapy, serum lithium levels must be assessed every 3 to 4 days (therapeutic levels are 0.6 mEq/L to 1.2 mEq/L; toxic levels are above 1.5 mEq/L). A urinalysis with specific gravity may also be ordered to assess volume status.

■ Antidepressants

Assess for the many cautions, contraindications, and drug interactions before giving antidepressants (see pharmacology discussion). An assessment of suicide risk based on the identification and appraisal of warning signs that are present is important for all patients with a history of prior suicide attempt or suicidal ideation. Suicide must always be considered a potential risk when any psychotherapeutic medication, whether an antidepressant or other CNS-altering drug, is taken alone or in combination with other drugs or alcohol. Patients may hoard drugs for the purpose of suicide.

Second-generation antidepressants are associated with fewer and less severe adverse effects compared to the older TCAs and MAOI antidepressants. These second-generation drugs include SSRIs (fluoxetine [Prozac]) and SNRIs (duloxetine hydrochloride [Cymbalta]). However, with SSRIs, it is still important to assess and document neuromuscular and GI systems. Cautious use in older adults is recommended due to their increased risk for toxicity. Additionally, there is concern for the occurrence of serotonin syndrome (see Box 17-1), which includes symptoms such as agitation, tachycardia, sweating, and muscle tremors. Contraindications include the use of these drugs with some antipsychotic drugs and within 14 days of use of MAOIs. Assess for significant drug interactions, such as warfarin sodium and phenytoin, due to their increased protein binding. Do not give SNRIs, such as duloxetine hydrochloride (Cymbalta), to patients with closed-angle glaucoma or those taking MAOIs. Liver function studies may be ordered prior to use of this drug because of the risk of liver toxicity. The miscellaneous antidepressant bupropion may be preferred over some of the other antidepressants because of fewer anticholinergic, antiadrenergic, and cardiotoxic effects (see pharmacology discussion). Assess the patient's baseline neurological, mental, and cardiac status before the drug is used. Because of delayed therapeutic effects, closely assess the patient for any suicidal tendencies or ideas. Assess the availability of family support systems as well as the need for any supportive resources.

TCAs, as an older class of antidepressants, are effective drugs but are associated with serious adverse effects. However, some patients do tolerate them. When patients are taking TCAs, monitor closely for potential adverse effects. Use with the natural health product St. John's wort is not recommended. Amitriptyline is not to be used in patients with recent myocardial infarction and is associated with potent anticholinergic properties leading to dry mouth, constipation, blurred vision, urinary retention, and alterations in cardiac rhythm.

MAOIs are particularly dangerous and can cause death if taken in an overdose. It is important to closely monitor patients receiving MAOIs who have a history of suicide attempts or suicidal ideation. Patients should be monitored closely by a health care provider (e.g., psychiatrist, physician, or nurse practitioner) to ensure their safety and prevent harm to themselves or others. MAOIs are also known for their significant drug interactions (see Table 17-4), such as with meperidine hydrochloride, other opioids, other MAOIs, SSRIs, oral contraceptives, and buspirone. MAOIs, if taken with foods high in tyramine (see Table 17-7), are associated with a hypertensive crisis; therefore, closely monitor blood pressure

readings, including postural blood pressure measurements. Orthostatic hypotension, an adverse effect of MAOIs, may lead to a high risk of dizziness, fainting, and possible falls or injury. If the patient is hospitalized, monitor supine and standing or sitting blood pressures at least every 8 hours or more frequently, if needed. Allow 1 to 2 minutes to elapse after taking the supine blood pressure before measuring standing or sitting pressures and pulse rate. Laboratory tests that are often ordered for patients taking these drugs include complete blood counts and renal and liver function studies. In addition, it is crucial to understand that older adult patients should be given these drugs only if it is deemed absolutely necessary by a health care provider, and only with careful monitoring. The extrapyramidal adverse effects (e.g., tremors) are often worse in older adults and may result in an inability to perform ADLs. This extrapyramidal reaction may lead to progressive deterioration of motor activities; thus, a thorough motor and neurological assessment is needed.

■ Antipsychotics

To be safe and effective, the use of antipsychotics requires careful and skillful assessment of cardiovascular, cerebrovascular, neurological, GI, genitourinary, kidney, liver, and hematological functioning before and during drug therapy. The presence of significant disease in one or several organ systems may lead to a more adverse response to a drug and may be dose limiting. Weight gain may occur, and if the patient is experiencing deleterious health effects because of weight gain, a drug may be ordered. Numerous adverse effects may be associated with many of these drugs (see earlier discussion); therefore, perform and document a thorough nursing history and mental status examination prior to the initiation of drug therapy. Identify possible drug interactions with any prescription drugs, OTC medications, or natural health products the patient is taking, as well as any conditions that represent cautions or contraindications to use of the antipsychotic drug (see pharmacology discussion).

Haloperidol is similar to other high-potency antipsychotics because its sedating effects are low but the incidence of extrapyramidal symptoms (see earlier discussion and Chapter 16) is high.

Atypical antipsychotics such as clozapine and risperidone have many contraindications, cautions, and drug interactions (see earlier discussion). Monitor liver and kidney function studies, complete blood count, and urinalysis before and during therapy. Clozapine is associated with neutropenia and monitoring of WBCs is required. Make sure to document blood pressure readings with close attention to postural readings because of the potential for the adverse effect of orthostatic hypotension. A drop of 20 mmHg or more in the systolic blood pressure requires immediate attention and implementation of safety precautions. In addition, for older adults, health care providers may order reduced dosages to help prevent toxicity. Atypical antipsychotics are also associated with a high degree of sedation and must be used only when absolutely necessary and with extreme caution (close monitoring) in older adults and other patients who are at risk for falls or harm or who have limited motor and sensory capabilities. Carefully monitor heart sounds and assess for any abnormal heart rhythms in patients taking these drugs.

Nursing Diagnoses

- Imbalanced nutrition, less than body requirements, related to consequences of the mental health disorder or the use of psychotherapeutic drugs
- Urinary retention related to the adverse effects of psychotherapeutic drugs
- Constipation related to the adverse effects of psychotherapeutic drugs
- Sexual dysfunction related to the adverse effects of psychotherapeutic drugs
- Sleep deprivation related to the mental health disorder or related drug therapy
- Deficient knowledge related to lack of information about specific psychotherapeutic drugs and their adverse effects
- Impaired social interaction related to various inadequacies felt by the patient due to illness or isolation from others
- Situational low self-esteem related to the mental health disorder and from the adverse effects of psychotherapeutic drugs, including sexual dysfunction
- Risk for injury to self related to the mental health disorder or possible adverse effects of psychotherapeutic drugs

Planning

Goals

- Patient will exhibit improved nutritional status, without weight loss.
- Patient will remain free from any alterations in urinary elimination patterns.
- Patient will regain or maintain normal bowel elimination patterns.
- Patient will remain free from or experience minimal alterations in sexual function.
- Patient will implement measures to minimize sleep deprivation.
- Patient will be adherent to medication therapy, take medication(s) as ordered, and remain free from complications associated with drug therapy.
- Patient will regain or maintain social interaction and open communication with family, friends, significant others, and members of the health care team.
- Patient will exhibit more positive self-image, healthier thought processes, and interactive processes.
- Patient will maintain safety with drug therapeutic regimen and without injury to self.

Expected Patient Outcomes

- Patient shows healthy nutritional habits with appropriate weight gain and maintains a diet that includes foods from each section of *Canada's Food Guide*. (Culturally-sensitive food guides are available on the Health Canada website for First Nations, Inuit, and Métis individuals [2011], as are suggestions of culturally-specific foods that can make the Food Guide more accessible to Canada's diverse population.
- Patient reports any problems with urinary hesitancy, urgency, or retention, or other discomfort over the lower abdominal area.
- Patient states measures to increase bowel elimination, such as increasing dietary fibre with fruits and vegetables while also increasing fluid intake.
- Patient reports any problems with bowel elimination, such as constipation or passing of hard stool.
- Patient openly communicates with partner and health care providers about difficulty with sexual functioning as related to drug therapy.
- Patient openly identifies and discusses options for improving sexual functioning to assist with any altered patterns of sexual behaviour.
- Patient reports measures to increase healthier sleeping habits, including journalling and maintaining optimal sleep hygiene through retiring at a regular time nightly, decreasing room noise and light, listening to calming music, using aromatherapy, and avoiding caffeine in the late afternoon or evening (see Chapter 13 for sleep hygiene nursing interventions).
- Patient states reasoning for adherence to medication regimen, acknowledges the need to take the medication exactly as prescribed, and shows understanding of related drug safety measures.
- Patient has assistance at home in the daily monitoring of self-administration of medication(s).
- Patient states common adverse effects of psychotherapeutic drug therapy, such as confusion, sedation, constipation, nausea, dizziness, unsteady gait, dry mouth, changes in sexual performance, weight gain or loss, and loss or increase in appetite.
- Patient states adverse effects that necessitate reporting to the health care provider, such as unresolved constipation, urinary retention, increasing levels of sedation, and dizziness or fainting upon standing or changing of positions.
- Patient demonstrates improved or no further deterioration in social integration, with healthier

patterns of communication and participation in activities.

- Patient interacts openly and frequently with family, friends, significant others, and members of the health care team without suspicion or paranoia.
- Patient participates daily or more frequently in social interactions and activities and plans to engage in more social activities, as appropriate.
- Patient demonstrates improved self-concept and self-esteem in daily interactions with family, friends, and significant others, while experiencing fewer episodes of self-destructive and negative behaviours.
- Patient feels more positive about self, demonstrated by increased participation in ADLs, social activities, and family functions.
- Patient demonstrates safety with ADLs, including self-care measures, by moving slowly, changing positions slowly, and reporting excess dizziness or fainting episodes.

Implementation

Regardless of the psychotherapeutic drug prescribed, several general nursing actions are important for safe administration. Once the patient's reading level and the most effective means of teaching and learning are identified, provide the patient with simple explanations about the drug, its action, and the length of time before therapeutic effects can be expected. Always use a psychosocial and holistic approach when caring for any patient with any illness. Monitor vital signs and document findings, especially during the initiation of therapy. The administration of psychotherapeutic medications to older adults and to patients with a history of hypertension and heart disease should be done with great care. All of the psychotherapeutic drugs are to be taken exactly as prescribed, at the same time every day, and without failure. If omission occurs, contact the health care provider immediately. Abrupt withdrawal may have negative effects on the patient's physical and mental status. Solicit help from family members or others providing support in the care of the patient so that there are options for assistance with drug administration. Adherence to the medication regimen is crucial to effective symptom management; identify and utilize all support systems and resources to accomplish this.

Benzodiazepines

Specific nursing interventions related to the use of anxiolytic drugs include frequent monitoring of vital signs with special attention to blood pressure and postural blood pressures. Encourage the use of elastic compression stockings and recommend that the patient change positions slowly to minimize dizziness and falls from orthostatic hypotension. Create a therapeutic environment for open communication—especially of all disturbing thoughts, including those of suicide. Check the patient's oral cavity for hoarding or cheeking of drugs. If medications are crushed, make sure they are not extended-release formulations. As well, some medications (e.g., olanzapine oral disintegrating tablet) melt instantly on the tongue, so caution needs to be used when opening so as not to touch the tablet. Use intravenous routes of administration only as prescribed and give over the recommended time, with the proper diluents and at a rate indicated by the manufacturer and health care provider. Always administer IM dosage forms in a large muscle mass and only as ordered or indicated (see Chapter 10 for more information on parenteral administration). See Patient Teaching Tips for more information.

Mood-Stabilizing Drugs

Safe use of the mood-stabilizing drug lithium depends on adequate hydration and electrolyte status because lithium may become toxic with dehydration and hyponatremia. See Patient Teaching Tips for more information.

Antidepressants

With second-generation antidepressants, emphasize that it may take up to 4 to 6 weeks before therapeutic effects are evident. This 4- to 6-week time frame also applies to TCAs and MAOIs. Make sure the patient understands the need for patience and continues to take the medication as prescribed, even if the patient feels the condition is not improving. Carefully monitor the patient, be readily available, and provide supportive care during this time. The period just before therapeutic effects are seen, when the patient has increased energy, may be the time the patient is at highest risk for self-harm or suicide. Advise the patient to take the drug(s) with food and at least 120 to 180 mL of fluid. Assist with ambulation and other activities if the patient is weak or dizzy (from orthostatic hypotension) or if the patient is an older adult. Counsel the patient about potential sexual dysfunction (if appropriate) if this is an adverse effect of the drug. If sexual dysfunction occurs, provide information to the patient about various options (e.g., waiting to see if the adverse effect resolves, reducing the current dosage of the drug as ordered, taking a "drug holiday" if ordered by the health care provider). A drug holiday, if indicated, generally occurs in a hospital setting, and the drug is removed only under close monitoring. See Patient Teaching Tips for more specific information regarding SSRIs and SNRIs.

With the use of TCAs and MAOIs, educate the patient on adverse effects and drug or food interactions. Emphasize the importance of keeping a list of all medications with the patient at all times. This can be on a smartphone or tablet. Pharmacies can also provide a list of medications for the patient to keep. Advise the patient to change positions purposefully and slowly. All health care providers need to be informed that the patient is taking these

CASE STUDY

Antidepressants

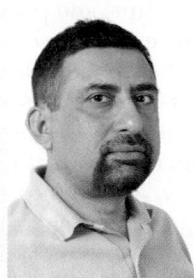

A 49-year-old patient, Alim, comes to the clinic with a history of depression. He tells you that he was treated for it by a doctor in another country, but he "ran out of pills" a week ago and did not know how to get a refill. He could not remember the name of the medication but said it was for "depression." He has also been having trouble sleeping. After a psychiatric evaluation, he is given a 2-week prescription for fluoxetine (Prozac).

1. A few days later, Alim's wife calls to describe "a terrible reaction" that he is having. She says that he is shaking and shivering, has a fever, and is somewhat confused and upset. She thinks he has a bad infection. What do you think has happened, and why?
2. What could have been done to prevent this problem?
3. After 2 weeks, Alim is given a prescription for trazodone (Trazorel) and is instructed to return to the office in 2 weeks. What advantage does this medication have for this patient?

For answers, see http://evolve.elsevier.com/Canada/Lilley/pharmacology/.

ETHNOCULTURAL IMPLICATIONS

Psychotherapeutic Drugs

Many racial and ethnic groups respond to drugs differently. For example, Asian people have lower drug metabolism activity than White people, related to lower levels of various enzymes. Asian people often require lower dosages of benzodiazepines and TCAs because they have lower levels of the enzymes metabolizing these drugs (e.g., CY02D6) and are therefore more sensitive to the drugs.

Diazepam follows a different metabolic pathway in Chinese and Japanese populations. These two groups are found to be poor metabolizers of this drug and its metabolite. Approximately 20% of Chinese and Japanese individuals metabolize diazepam poorly, which results in rapid drug accumulation. To prevent possible toxicity, lower dosages are generally required. Nurses need to be aware of this cultural variable and assess these patients for sedation, overdosage, and other adverse reactions.

Researchers have also identified genetic variations that may explain individual differences in response to antidepressants. The serotonin transporter gene (5-HTT) may influence antidepressant response to SSRIs. This is an area of ongoing research.

drugs and that if the drugs are to be discontinued, the patient must be weaned off them. With TCAs, advise the patient to report any of the following to the health care provider if they occur: blurred vision, excessive drowsiness, sleepiness, urinary retention, constipation, or cognitive impairment. It is also important to inform patients that tolerance to sedation will occur with some second-generation antidepressants.

Antipsychotics

Antipsychotic drugs must be taken exactly as prescribed to be effective. Different levels of paranoia or delusions may lead the patient to mistrust the nurse and other members of the health care team, so maintain a sufficient level of trust through consistency, empathy, and the establishment of a strong therapeutic relationship to help ensure adherence. Adherence is always a crucial issue for patients with psychotic illnesses because they are at higher risk for not taking medications, often because they begin to feel better and do not keep follow-up appointments. Nonadherence to the medical and treatment regimen is of major concern because the serum levels of drugs such as haloperidol must be within a therapeutic range for the patient to feel better, be functional, and not relapse. If serum levels of haloperidol are less than 4 ng/mL, the patient may show symptoms of the mental health disorder, whereas levels greater than 22 ng/mL may result in toxicity. Therefore, selection of an antipsychotic drug and its dosage, route of administration, risk for toxicity, and suicidal potential, as well as therapeutic communication and patient education, are all important factors for successful therapy. If an antipsychotic medication is determined to no longer be effective or necessary and the patient has been in therapy for a period of 3 to 6 months or longer, it may be advantageous to slowly taper the dose until the antipsychotic medication is discontinued or until the lowest effective dose is determined. While there is no best practice for tapering antipsychotics, it is recommended to do so slowly to avoid symptoms of withdrawal or rebound effects. Because most antipsychotic drugs are quite potent, be sure that oral dosage forms have actually been swallowed and not intentionally hidden in the side of the mouth (see previous discussion on cheeking of medications). Oral forms of antipsychotics are generally well absorbed and will cause less GI upset if taken with food or a full glass of water. Sucking on hard candy or gum may help to relieve dry mouth. With any of the dosage forms, perspiration may be increased; therefore, encourage the patient to avoid being exposed to heat or humidity or engaging in excessive activity. Excessive sweating can lead to dehydration and subsequent drug toxicity.

Haloperidol may not necessarily be the best drug to use because of the risk for undermedication or overmedication and troubling adverse effects (see Table 17-10). Therefore, other antipsychotics (e.g., clozapine and risperidone) may be preferred, as previously discussed. Clozapine and risperidone are therapeutically effective and carry a minimal risk of tardive dyskinesia and extrapyramidal symptoms. In addition, they usually lead to improvement in cognitive behaviour. Clozapine is to be taken as ordered and is usually given in divided doses; proper dosing is important for therapeutic effectiveness. If any changes in blood counts (e.g., leukopenia) are noted or if abnormal cardiac functioning (e.g., tachycardia) is identified, contact the health care provider immediately. In such a case, the medication may need to be discontinued, but only as ordered, and the patient should be monitored closely. Titration of doses of clozapine, either upward or downward, needs to be done carefully, with close monitoring of the patient for any exacerbation of the mental health disorder or suicidal tendencies.

Risperidone is to be given as ordered and administered by injection into a deep muscle mass. Always check hospital or facility policy or drug insert guidelines regarding the administration of this drug. IM injection dosage forms may be ordered along with oral doses of risperidone or possibly another antipsychotic drug for several weeks, with maintenance doses of an IM injection given every 2 to 4 weeks, as ordered. Always alternate IM injection sites to maintain tissue integrity and muscle mass, and be sure that the site is not red, swollen, or irritated. Document and report any changes. Oral solution, tablets, and orally disintegrating tabs are other available dosage forms. Do not give oral solutions with cola or tea. Disintegrating tabs need to be dissolved under the tongue before swallowing with or without liquid. Always follow the health care provider's orders for administering this and all other drugs. The daily amount is usually given in two divided doses, with dosage decreased in older adults and in those with impaired kidney or liver function. Make sure you report any excess sedation, anxiety, extrapyramidal symptoms, tardive dyskinesia, seizures, or strokelike symptoms immediately. Measuring vital signs and monitoring for any orthostatic hypotension are also important during treatment.

Once therapy with any of the antipsychotic drugs has been initiated, it is important for the nurse and other health care providers involved in the patient's care to monitor drug therapy closely during follow-up visits, including serum drug levels. If the patient is suspected of being nonadherent and serum drug levels are subtherapeutic, the patient needs to be re-evaluated by the prescribing health care provider for a possible change of drug or dosage form. The parenteral dosage form is available in a depot (longer-releasing) dosage preparation that releases the drug over 2 to 4 weeks, leading to increased adherence and often a better therapeutic outcome.

Patient education (see Patient Teaching Tips) and patient adherence with the drug regimen are keys to successful treatment, regardless of the mental health disorder. Often, it is the mental health disorder itself that causes patient nonadherence. Keeping communication open with the patient and family or caregivers is important to developing trust and a sense of empathy. Although patient education may have been thorough, emphasize that the patient may call the health care provider, clinic, or a hotline 24 hours a day. Keep phone numbers continuously updated. Make available ongoing professional counselling with a mental health care provider (psychiatrist, nurse practitioner, or other licensed mental health professional), as needed, so that the patient's progress is consistently monitored. Group therapy and support groups are also available for the patient and significant others.

Evaluation

Both the therapeutic effects of psychotropic medications and the patient's progress within the treatment regimen must be monitored at all times during and even after therapy. Mental alertness, cognition, mood, ability to carry out ADLs, appetite, and sleep patterns are all areas that need to be closely monitored and documented. Encourage the patient to continue with other forms of therapy, in addition to drug therapy, with the goal of acquiring more effective coping skills. Other forms of treatment may include intense psychotherapy, relaxation therapy, stress reduction, and lifestyle changes. It is important to mention that blood levels of psychotropic drugs will need to be measured during follow-up visits to ensure that therapeutic levels are maintained. Such monitoring of serum drug levels helps identify both subtherapeutic and toxic levels.

The therapeutic effects of anxiolytic drugs are evidenced by improved mental alertness, cognition, and mood; fewer anxiety and panic attacks; improved sleep patterns and appetite; more interest in self and others; less tension and irritability; and fewer feelings of fear, impending doom, and stress. Watch for the adverse effects of hypotension, lethargy, fatigue, drowsiness, and confusion in patients taking anxiolytic drugs. In general, adverse reactions to antidepressants include drowsiness, dry mouth, constipation, dizziness, orthostatic hypotension, sedation, blood dyscrasias, sexual dysfunction, and dyskinesias. Overdose is evidenced by seizures or dysrhythmias.

Therapeutic effects of the mood stabilizer lithium are decreased mania and stabilization of the patient's mood. Lithium is usually better tolerated by the patient during manic phases than depressive phases. Adverse reactions to lithium include dysrhythmias, hypotension, sedation, slurred speech, slowed motor abilities, weight gain, and GI discomfort.

When used as antidepressants, SSRIs and SNRIs may take up to 6 weeks to reach full therapeutic effect. A therapeutic response to these drugs includes improved depression or mental status, improved ability to carry out ADLs, decreased insomnia, and improved mood, with minimal adverse effects of weight gain, headache, GI discomfort, insomnia, dizziness, drowsiness, and sexual dysfunction. Monitor the patient for symptoms of serotonin syndrome such as agitation, tachycardia, hyperreflexia, and tremors.

The therapeutic effects of the antipsychotic drugs include improvement in mood and affect, as well as alleviation of or decrease in psychotic symptoms (hallucinations, paranoia, delusions, garbled speech) once the patient has been taking the medication for several weeks. Careful monitoring of the patient's potential to injure self or others during the delay between the start of therapy and symptomatic improvement is crucial. Evaluation for adverse effects includes monitoring blood counts (clozapine) as well as noting any tic-like trembling movements of the hands, face, neck, and head; hypotension; and dry mouth (haloperidol).

PATIENT TEACHING TIPS

❖ Anxiolytic Drugs
- Encourage patients to avoid operating heavy machinery and driving until the adverse effects of sedation or drowsiness have resolved.
- Educate patients about the development of tolerance to the sedating properties of benzodiazepines with chronic use (see Chapter 13).
- Instruct patients not to take OTC drugs or natural health products without seeking advice from the health care provider.
- Remind patients to keep these and all psychotherapeutic drugs out of the reach of children.
- Inform patients that they must avoid alcohol and other CNS depressants.
- Advise patients to carry a medical alert or other identification bracelet/necklace with their diagnoses and a list of their drugs and allergies at all times. The drug list needs to be updated at least every 3 months.
- Emphasize to patients that medications must always be taken exactly as ordered and that sudden withdrawal should be avoided. If withdrawal of a drug is necessary, tapering or weaning of doses is needed. Benzodiazepines are usually recommended for short-term use.

❖ Mood-Stabilizing Drugs
- Instruct patients that lithium must be taken at the same time each day and give specific instructions on how to handle missed doses. Make sure the patient understands the importance of adequate hydration.
- Inform patients that the adverse effects of lithium are usually transient; however, excessive tremors, seizures, confusion, ataxia, and excessive sedation must be reported to the health care provider immediately.

❖ Monoamine Oxidase Inhibitors and Tricyclic Antidepressants
- Advise patients taking MAOIs to contact the prescriber immediately if any of the following signs and symptoms of overdosage or toxicity occur: tachycardia, hyperthermia, or seizures.
- If a patient is taking an MAOI, caution about avoiding OTC cold and flu products. Foods or beverages high in tyramine must also be avoided (see Table 17-7).

- When a patient is taking a TCA, any blurred vision, agitation, urinary retention, or ataxia needs to be reported to the prescriber immediately.
- Encourage patients to wear a medical alert necklace or bracelet indicating diagnoses and a list of current drugs.

❖ Selective Serotonin Reuptake Inhibitors and Serotonin-Norepinephrine Reuptake Inhibitors
- Inform patients that consumption of fibre supplements must occur at least 2 hours before or after the dosing of medication to avoid interference with drug absorption; however, dietary fibre intake is appropriate.
- Encourage patients to openly discuss any concerns about the medication and adverse effects, such as GI upset, sexual dysfunction, or tremors.
- Provide a listing of drug–drug interactions, such as the strong interaction between SSRIs and MAOIs, St. John's wort (a natural health product), and tryptophan (a serotonin precursor found in foods). Such interactions may pose a risk for the occurrence of serotonin syndrome (see earlier discussion). Cold products and OTC medications must be approved by the health care provider.
- Stress to patients that SSRIs must be taken carefully and as prescribed. Any increase in suicidal thoughts or extreme changes in mood need to be reported immediately to the health care provider.
- Emphasize the importance of regularly attending follow-up visits and contacting health care providers if there are any concerns. Many patients use antidepressants inconsistently or stop taking them prematurely. Inform the patient that discontinuation of SSRIs and SNRIs requires a tapering period of up to 1 to 2 months, as ordered. Discontinuation syndrome may occur with or without a tapering period; this includes symptoms of dizziness, diarrhea, movement disorders, insomnia, irritability, visual disturbance, lethargy, anorexia, and lowered mood.
- Tell patients that if there is ever any doubt as to whether too much of an antidepressant has been taken, they should contact the health care provider or seek emergency medical treatment immediately.

Continued

PATIENT TEACHING TIPS—cont'd

❖ Antipsychotics
- Advise patients to avoid hot baths, saunas, and hot climates with the use of antipsychotics because of the risk of further drop in blood pressure, especially upon standing (orthostatic hypotension). Injury may occur because of dizziness or fainting.
- Warn patients that haloperidol and other antipsychotics must never be stopped abruptly because of the high risk of inducing a withdrawal psychosis.

- Inform patients that drug interactions with clozapine include alcohol, CNS depressants, levodopa, and antihypertensives.
- Counsel patients taking clozapine that any sore throat, malaise, fever, or bleeding must be reported to a health care provider immediately because of possible drop in WBC counts.
- Educate patients with schizophrenia that they may require antipsychotics for their lifetime.

KEY POINTS

❖ Psychosis is a symptom of a mental health disorder that impairs mental function.
❖ A person experiencing psychosis cannot participate in everyday life and shows the hallmark sign of loss of contact with reality.
❖ Affective disorders are emotional disorders characterized by changes in mood. They range from mania (abnormally elevated emotions) to depression (abnormally reduced emotions) and include anxiety, a normal emotion that may be a healthy reaction but becomes pathological when it is life altering.

❖ Situational anxiety arises in response to specific life events, and nursing assessment is key to identifying patients who are at risk.
❖ SSRIs and SNRIs are often prescribed because of their superiority to older antidepressants.
❖ Nursing considerations related to psychotherapeutic drugs include the need for skillful patient assessment with an emphasis on past and present medical history, a physical examination, and a thorough medication history and profile.

EXAMINATION REVIEW QUESTIONS

1. The nurse is caring for a patient experiencing ethanol withdrawal. The nurse expects to administer which medication or medication class as treatment for this condition?
a. lithium (Carbolith®)
b. Benzodiazepines
c. buspirone
d. Antidepressants

2. The nurse is teaching a patient receiving an MAOI. What food product should the nurse teach the patient to avoid?
a. Orange juice
b. Milk
c. Shrimp
d. Swiss cheese

3. The nurse calls a patient to schedule a follow-up visit after the patient has been treated for depression for 4 weeks. What concern will the nurse assess for during the conversation with the patient?
a. Weakness
b. Hallucinations
c. Suicidal ideation
d. Difficulty with urination

4. The nurse is caring for a patient who has been taking clozapine (Clozaril®) for 2 months. Which laboratory test(s) should be performed regularly while the patient is on this medication?
a. Platelet count
b. WBC count

c. Liver function studies
d. Kidney function studies

5. The nurse is giving medications to a patient. Which drug or drug class, when administered with lithium, increases the risk for lithium toxicity?
a. Thiazides
b. levofloxacin
c. calcium citrate
d. β-blockers

6. The nurse is teaching a patient about treatment with an SSRI antidepressant. Which teaching considerations are appropriate? (Select all that apply.)
a. The patient should be told which foods contain tyramine and instructed to avoid these foods.
b. The patient should be instructed to use caution when standing up from a sitting position.
c. The patient should not take any products that contain the natural health product St. John's wort.
d. This medication should not be stopped abruptly.
e. Drug levels may become toxic if dehydration occurs.
f. The patient should be told to check with the health care provider before taking any OTC medications.

7. A patient with a feeding tube will be receiving risperidone (Risperdal®) 8 mg in 2 divided doses via the feeding tube. The medication is available in a 1 mg/mL solution. How many millilitres will the nurse administer for each dose?

CRITICAL THINKING ACTIVITIES

1. A 22-year-old patient who has been taking lithium for 3 months has had severe vomiting and diarrhea from a gastrointestinal flu. What is the nurse's priority assessment at this time?

2. A 68-year-old patient has been taking an SSRI antidepressant for 5 weeks. His wife calls and expresses concern because he has started to give away some of his keepsakes. What is the nurse's priority action?

3. A patient has been admitted to the hospital because of a suspected overdose of a TCA. What two problems are the nurse's priorities during this time?

For answers, see http://evolve.elsevier.com/Canada/Lilley/pharmacology/.

CHAPTER 18

Substance Misuse

Objectives

After reading this chapter, the successful student will be able to do the following:

1. Discuss substance misuse and the significance of the problem in Canada.

2. Identify the drugs or chemicals that are most frequently misused.

3. Contrast the signs and symptoms of the most commonly misused drugs or chemicals.

4. Compare the treatments for drug withdrawal for the most commonly misused opioids; central nervous system depressants; amphetamines and other CNS stimulants; nicotine; and alcohol.

5. Describe alcohol misuse syndrome with a focus on signs and symptoms, mild to severe alcohol withdrawal symptoms, and associated treatment.

6. Describe other drug misuse syndromes, including their signs and symptoms, withdrawal symptoms, and treatment regimens.

7. Identify various assessment tools used in the nursing assessment of substance misuse.

8. Develop a collaborative plan of care, encompassing all phases of the nursing process, for a patient undergoing treatment for substance misuse and dependency.

e-Learning Activities

Website
(http://evolve.elsevier.com/Canada/
Lilley/pharmacology/)

evolve

- Answer Key—Textbook Case Studies
- Answer Key—Critical Thinking Activities
- Chapter Summaries—Printable
- Review Questions for Exam Preparation
- Unfolding Case Studies

Key Terms

Addiction Strong psychological or physical dependence on a drug or other psychoactive substance. (p. 357)

Amphetamine A drug that stimulates the central nervous system. (p. 359)

Detoxification A process of eliminating a toxic substance from the body; a medically supervised program for alcohol or opioid addiction. (p. 359)

Habituation Development of tolerance to a substance following prolonged medical use but without psychological or physical dependence (addiction). (p. 357)

Illicit drug use The use of a drug or substance in a way that it is not intended to be used or that is not legally approved for human administration. (p. 359)

Intoxication Stimulation, excitement, or stupefaction produced by a chemical substance. (p. 357)

Korsakoff's psychosis A syndrome of amnesia with confabulation (making up of stories) associated with chronic alcohol misuse; it often occurs together with Wernicke's encephalopathy. (p. 364)

Narcolepsy A sleep disorder characterized by sleeping during the day, disrupted night-time sleep, cataplexy, sleep paralysis, and hallucinations. (p. 361)

Opioid analgesics Synthetic pain-relieving substances that were originally derived from the opium poppy. Naturally occurring opium derivatives are called *opiates*. (p. 358)

Physical dependence A condition characterized by physiological reliance on a substance, usually indicated by tolerance to the effects of the substance and development of withdrawal symptoms when use of the substance is terminated. (p. 357)

Psychoactive properties Drug properties that affect mood, behaviour, cognitive processes, and mental status. (p. 360)

Psychological dependence A condition characterized by strong desires to obtain and use a substance. (p. 357)

Raves All-night parties that typically involve dancing, drinking, and the use of illicit drugs. (p. 360)

Roofies Pills that are classified as benzodiazepines; gained popularity as a recreational drug; chemically known as *flunitrazepam*. (p. 362)

Substance misuse The use of a mood- or behaviour-altering substance in a maladaptive manner that often compromises health, safety, and social and occupational functioning and causes legal problems. (p. 357)

Wernicke's encephalopathy A neurological disorder characterized by apathy, drowsiness, ataxia, nystagmus, and ophthalmoplegia; caused by thiamine (vitamin B_1) deficiency secondary to chronic alcohol misuse. (p. 364)

Withdrawal A substance-specific mental health disorder that occurs as a group of symptoms, varying in severity, following the cessation or reduction in use of a psychoactive substance that has been taken regularly. (p. 357)

OVERVIEW

Substance misuse affects individuals of all ages, genders, and ethnic and socioeconomic backgrounds. **Physical dependence** and **psychological dependence** on a substance are complex chronic disorders with remissions and relapses, such as with any other chronic illness. Relapses are common and are often reflective of other social issues that are yet to be addressed (e.g., housing, social support). Recognizing physical or psychological dependence and understanding the various treatment guidelines are important skills for health care providers caring for patients with these conditions. *Habituation* refers to situations in which a patient becomes accustomed to a certain drug (develops tolerance) and may have mild psychological dependence on it but does not show compulsive dose escalation, drug-seeking behaviour, or major withdrawal symptoms on drug discontinuation. This might occur, for example, in a postsurgical patient who receives opioid pain therapy regularly for only a few weeks.

According to the 2012 *Canadian Community Health Survey*, approximately 21.6% of Canadians, about 6 million over the age of 15, meet the criteria for a substance use disorder over their lifetimes (Pearson, Janz, & Ali, 2015). Alcohol was the most commonly misused substance, at 18.1%. Marihuana was identified as the most commonly misused illicit drug (6.8%), followed by psychotherapeutic drugs, pain relievers, tranquilizers, stimulants, and sedatives used for nonmedical purposes. Youth aged 15 to 24 had the highest rate of substance misuse disorder (11.9%), while the lowest rate, 1.9%, was among those aged 45 and older.

Substance misuse is strongly associated with many types of mental health disorders. Treatment of both disorders is often difficult, in part because of the much greater risk of drug interactions with the misused substances. Assessment, intervention, use of certain medications, specific **addiction** treatment strategies, and recovery monitoring are essential to the care of this patient population.

The focus of this chapter is on the three major classes of commonly misused substances (opioids, stimulants, and depressants) and two commonly misused individual drugs (alcohol and nicotine). A description of the category or the individual drug, possible effects, signs and symptoms of **intoxication** and **withdrawal**, peak period and duration of withdrawal symptoms, and drugs used to treat withdrawal are discussed. The list of substances of misuse in Box 18-1 is not all-inclusive, but it contains some of the substances most commonly misused at this time. Not all of these substances are discussed in this chapter. Refer to the Centre for Addiction and Mental Health's website (http://www.camh.ca) for more information.

Specific drugs used to treat withdrawal symptoms are discussed in the sections covering the drug whose

BOX 18-1

Commonly Misused Substances

Major Categories

Opioids
Stimulants
Depressants

Individual Drugs

Alcohol
Anabolic steroids (see Chapter 36)
Cocaine
Fentanyl
Heroine
Dextromethorphan hydrobromide
Lysergic acid diethylamide (LSD)
Marihuana
Methamphetamine
Methylenedioxymethamphetamine (MDMA, ecstasy, E)
Nicotine
Phencyclidine (PCP)

withdrawal symptoms they are intended to treat. Pharmacological therapies are indicated for patients with addictive disorders to prevent life-threatening withdrawal complications, such as seizures and delirium tremens, and to increase adherence to psychosocial forms of addiction treatment.

OPIOIDS

Opioid analgesics are synthetic versions of pain-relieving substances that were originally derived from the opium poppy plant (see Chapter 11). More than 20 different alkaloids are obtained from the unripe seed of the opium poppy plant, only a few of which are clinically useful, including morphine and codeine. The other opioid analgesics currently used in medical practice are synthetic or semisynthetic derivatives of these two drugs.

Diacetylmorphine (better known as *heroin*) and opium are also opioids; they are classified as Schedule I drugs and are not available in Canada for therapeutic use. Heroin was banned in Canada in 1908 because of its high potential for misuse and the increasing number of heroin addicts. In Europe, heroin is available for medical treatment of pain, and governmental programs also exist to provide heroin to addicts with the goal of reducing crime.

Heroin is one of the most commonly misused opioids. Some others in the opioid category are codeine phosphate, hydrocodone, hydromorphone, meperidine hydrochloride, morphine, fentanyl, and oxycodone. For example, residual fentanyl remaining in used patches can be extracted and used in a number of ways, including chewing or smoking. Currently, heroin remains one of the top 10 most misused drugs in Canada and often is used in combination with the stimulant drug cocaine (discussed later in Stimulants). It can be mixed with marihuana and smoked. When heroin is injected (also called *mainlining* or *skin-popping*), sniffed (known as *snorting*), or smoked, it binds with opiate receptors found in many regions of the brain. The result is intense euphoria, often referred to as a *rush*. This rush lasts only briefly and is followed by a relaxed, contented state that persists for a couple of hours. In large doses, heroin, like other opioids, can reduce or stop respiration.

Mechanism of Action and Drug Effects

Opioids work by blocking receptors in the central nervous system (CNS). When these receptors are blocked, the perception of pain is blocked. There are three main receptor types to which opioids bind. These receptors and their physiological effects when stimulated are discussed in Chapter 11. The unique mixture of receptor affinities that a specific opioid possesses determines its therapeutic and toxic effects. One of the reasons that opioids are misused is their ability to produce euphoria.

The drug effects of opioids are primarily centred in the CNS. However, these drugs also act outside the CNS, and many of their unwanted effects stem from these actions. In addition to analgesia, opioids produce drowsiness, euphoria, tranquility, and other alterations of mood. The mechanism by which opioids produce the latter effects is not entirely clear. The effects of opioids can be collectively referred to as *narcosis* or *stupor*, which involves reduced sensory response, especially to painful stimuli. For this reason, opioid analgesics, along with other classes of drugs that produce similar effects, are also referred to as *narcotics* (see Chapter 3), especially by law enforcement authorities.

Indications

The intended drug effects of opioids are to relieve pain, reduce cough, relieve diarrhea, and induce anaesthesia. Many have a high potential for problematic use and are therefore classified as Schedule I controlled substances. Relaxation and euphoria are the most common drug effects that lead to misuse and psychological dependence. Sustained-release oxycodone is one example of an opioid analgesic that is controversial because it is often overprescribed and grossly misused. Numerous deaths have been reported when the sustained-release form of oxycodone hydrochloride was crushed and the entire 12-hour supply was released at one time. OxyContin was removed from the Canadian market and replaced with OxyNeo®, a form that is more difficult to crush. With the unavailability of OxyContin, however, the illicit use of fentanyl has risen. Fentanyl, which can be over 40 times more potent than heroin, has accounted for hundreds of deaths in Canada alone over recent years. Often, the user has no knowledge of the fentanyl being mixed into fake OxyContin pills and heroin. The exempted codeine preparation Tylenol 1 is widely available in Canada without a prescription and is also subject to misuse.

Certain opioid drugs are used to treat opioid dependence. Historically, methadone has been used for this purpose. Its long half-life of 12 to 24 hours allows patients to be dosed once daily at federally approved methadone maintenance clinics and at pharmacies (witnessed ingestion). Methadone is a long-acting opioid agonist that reduces the craving for opioids, suppresses euphoria, and prevents withdrawal symptoms. In theory, the goal of such programs is to reduce the patient's dosage gradually, so that eventually the patient can live permanently drug free. Unfortunately, relapse rates are often high in these programs. However, patients who remain on long-term opioid maintenance therapy in a medical setting still benefit by avoiding the hazards associated with obtaining and using illegal "street" drugs.

Contraindications

Contraindications to the therapeutic use of opioid medications include known drug allergy, pregnancy (high dosage or prolonged use is contraindicated), respiratory depression or severe asthma when resuscitative equipment is not available, and paralytic ileus.

Adverse Effects

Adverse effects of opioids can be separated into two groups: CNS and non-CNS. The primary adverse effects of opioids are related to their actions in the CNS, and the major ones include drowsiness, diuresis, miosis, convulsions, nausea, vomiting, and respiratory depression. Many of the non-CNS adverse effects are secondary to the release of histamine caused by opioids. Histamine release can cause vasodilation leading to hypotension, spasms of the colon leading to constipation, increased spasms of the ureter resulting in decreased urinary retention, and dilation of cutaneous blood vessels leading to flushing of the skin of the face, neck, and upper thorax. The release of histamine is also thought to cause sweating, urticaria, and pruritus.

Management of Withdrawal, Toxicity and Overdose

Box 18-2 lists the signs and symptoms of opioid drug withdrawal. The box also indicates the time when these symptoms are most likely to occur and their duration. Many patients require a formal **detoxification** program while withdrawal symptoms are occurring. See Chapter 11 for a detailed discussion of physical dependence and the management of acute intoxication, toxicity, and overdose. Withdrawal symptoms include nausea, dysphoria, muscle aches, lacrimation, rhinorrhea, pupillary dilation, piloerection (hair standing on end), sweating, diarrhea, yawning, fever, and insomnia. Medications listed in Box 18-3 are intended to help decrease the desire for the misused opioid and reduce the severity of these withdrawal symptoms. The most serious adverse effect and the most common cause of death with opioids is respiratory depression.

Certain medications are used to prevent relapse drug use once an initial remission is achieved. They are useful only when concurrent counselling is provided, offering additional insurance against return to **illicit drug use.** For opioid misuse or dependence, naltrexone hydrochloride, an opioid antagonist, is administered. Naltrexone, which is also available as an injection called methylnatroxone bromide (Relistor®), works by blocking the opioid receptors so that use of opioid drugs does not produce euphoria. When euphoria is eliminated, the reinforcing effect of the drug is lost. The patient needs to be free from opioids for at least 1 week before beginning this medication because naltrexone can produce withdrawal symptoms if given too soon. Naltrexone is also approved for use by patients who are alcohol-dependent to reduce cravings for alcohol and the likelihood of a full relapse if a slip occurs. Another opioid antagonist, naloxone hydrochloride, is used for opioid overdose and respiratory depression. It can be used alone or more commonly combined with buprenorphine hydrochloride (Suboxone®) or hydromorphone hydrochloride (Targin®; see Chapter 11). Health Canada is reviewing the prescription-only status of naloxone (Branswell, 2015). Currently, some provinces and cities (e.g., Edmonton, Toronto) have initiated harm reduction programs in which they provide "rescue" kits containing naloxone and syringes to opioid users or their families and friends.

STIMULANTS

The misuse of stimulants is related to their ability to cause elevation of mood, reduction of fatigue, a sense of increased alertness, and invigorating aggressiveness. **Amphetamine** is a stimulant drug that is commonly misused. Chemically, three classes of amphetamine exist: salts of racemic amphetamine, dextroamphetamine, and methamphetamine. These classes vary with respect to their potency and peripheral effects. Another stimulant drug of misuse is cocaine, which also produces strong CNS stimulation. Cocaine was originally classified as a narcotic. It is considered a controlled substance by the

TABLE 18-1	
Various Forms of Amphetamine and Cocaine With Street Names*	
Chemical Name	**Street Names**
dimethoxymethylamphetamine	DOM, STP
methamphetamine (crystallized form)	Ice, crystal, glass, jibb, Tina
methamphetamine (powdered form)	Speed, meth, crank
methylenedioxyamphetamine	MDA
methylenedioxymethamphetamine	MDMA, ecstasy, E, Molly, love drug
methylenedioxypyrovalerone	Ivory wave, purple wave, cloud nine, rave, vanilla sky, bliss, plant food
cocaine (powdered form)	Coke, dust, snow, flake, blow, girl, icing
cocaine (crystallized form)	Crack, crack cocaine, freebase rocks, rock, candy

*Street names for drugs are extensive and change along with societal trends.

correctional system and has been treated as a controlled substance in terms of secured storage in health care facilities. However, unlike the opioid analgesics, cocaine does not normally induce a state of narcosis or stupor and is therefore more correctly categorized as a stimulant drug. It is a Schedule I drug under the *Controlled Drugs and Substances Act* of Canada. Other commonly misused substances in the category of stimulants include methylphenidate hydrochloride and dextroamphetamine sulphate. Multiple slight chemical derivations of amphetamine exist. These "designer drugs" have **psychoactive properties** (affecting mood, behaviour, cognitive processes, and mental status) along with their stimulant properties that further enhance their misuse potential. Table 18-1 lists commonly misused forms of amphetamine and cocaine with some of their street names.

Methamphetamine is a chemical class of amphetamine, but it has a much stronger effect on the CNS than the other two classes of amphetamine. Methamphetamine is generally used in pill form orally or in powder form by snorting or injecting. Methamphetamine has 15 to 20 times the potency of amphetamine sulphate, the original drug in this class. Crystallized methamphetamine, known as *ice, crystal*, or *crystal meth*, is a smokable and more powerful form of the drug. Methamphetamine users who inject the drug and share needles are at risk HIV infection and AIDS, as well as hepatitis B and C. Marihuana and alcohol are commonly listed as additional drugs of misuse in those admitted for treatment of methamphetamine misuse. Most recorded methamphetamine-related deaths involved the use of methamphetamine in combination with at least one other drug, such as alcohol, heroin, or cocaine. The over-the-counter (OTC) decongestant pseudoephedrine is commonly used to synthesize methamphetamine in secret drug laboratories, often in private homes. This practice has led to a dramatic increase in the misuse of this drug. Canada's Precursor Control Regulations include requirements to control precursors and other substances used in the production of methamphetamine, including ephedrine, pseudoephedrine, and red phosphorus. In 2006, the National Drug Scheduling Advisory Committee recommended restricted retail sales of all nonprescription drug products containing pseudoephedrine. Specific restrictions include allowing sales only from *behind* the pharmacy counter (Schedule II) and that combination formulations be sold only in pharmacies (Schedule III).

Another synthetic amphetamine derivative is methylenedioxymethamphetamine (MDMA, ecstasy, or E), which is also usually prepared in home laboratories. This drug tends to have more calming effects than other amphetamine drugs. It is usually taken in pill form but can also be snorted or injected. Users often feel a strong sense of social bonding with and acceptance of other people, hence the nickname "love drug." The drug can also be energizing, which makes it popular at **raves** (all-night dance parties). Originally synthesized by Merck Pharmaceuticals in 1914, it was studied by the U.S. Army as a "brainwashing" drug in the 1950s. In 2005, methamphetamine was reclassified from a Schedule III drug to a Schedule I drug of the *Controlled Drugs and Substances Act* on the basis of harms caused by methamphetamine production, trafficking, and misuse.

The newest synthetic stimulant to appear in Canada is bath salts, named because of the similarity to bath salt packaging that is used for distribution. Bath salts is composed of the primary chemical cathinone, 3,4-methylenedioxypyrovalerone (MDPV). Bath salts can be orally ingested, sniffed, snorted, smoked, or injected. The desired effects of euphoria, increased energy, expanded consciousness, and increased libido begin rapidly and typically last for 3 to 4 hours. Physiological symptoms include tachycardia, hypertension, pupil dilation, diaphoresis, tremor, and anxiety. Individuals ingesting this drug may also experience paranoia, restlessness, bizarre behaviour, and persecutory hallucinations. It is because of these latter effects that individuals co-ingest "downers" such as marihuana.

Cocaine is a white powder that is derived from leaves of the South American coca plant. Cocaine is either snorted or injected intravenously. It tends to give a temporary illusion of limitless power and energy but afterward leaves the user feeling depressed, edgy, and craving more. Cocaine and crack (a crystallized form of cocaine that is generally smoked) are highly addictive.

Psychological and physical dependence can erode physical and mental health and can become so strong that these drugs dominate all aspects of an addict's life.

Mechanism of Action and Drug Effects

Stimulants work by releasing biogenic amines from their storage sites in the nerve terminals. The primary biogenic amine released is norepinephrine. Its release results in stimulation of the CNS, as well as cardiovascular stimulation, leading to increased blood pressure and heart rate and possible cardiac dysrhythmias. The effect on smooth muscle is seen primarily in the urinary bladder and results in contraction of the sphincter. This is helpful in treating enuresis but results in painful and difficult micturition otherwise.

Stimulants, particularly amphetamines, are potent CNS stimulants. This CNS stimulation commonly results in wakefulness, alertness, and a decreased sense of fatigue; elevation of mood, with increased initiative, self-confidence, and ability to concentrate; often elation and euphoria; and an increase in motor and speech activity.

Indications

Stimulants have many therapeutic uses. Currently, their most common use is in the treatment of attention deficit hyperactivity disorder (see Chapter 14). Stimulants may be used to prevent or reverse fatigue and sleep, such as when they are used to treat **narcolepsy** (episodes of acute sleepiness). Another therapeutic effect of amphetamines is their ability to stimulate the respiratory centre. Stimulants are also used to reduce food intake and treat obesity; however, this therapeutic effect is limited because of rapid development of tolerance.

Contraindications

Contraindications to the therapeutic use of stimulant medications include drug allergy, diabetes, cardiovascular disorders, states of agitation, hypertension, known history of problematic drug use, and Tourette's syndrome.

Adverse Effects

Adverse effects of stimulants are commonly an extension of their therapeutic effects. The CNS-related adverse effects are restlessness, syncope (fainting), dizziness, tremor, hyperactive reflexes, talkativeness, tenseness, irritability, weakness, insomnia, fever, and sometimes euphoria. Confusion, aggression, increased libido, anxiety, delirium, paranoid hallucinations, panic states, and suicidal or homicidal tendencies can also occur, especially in patients who are mentally ill. Fatigue and depression usually follow CNS stimulation. Cardiovascular effects are common and include headache, chilliness, pallor or flushing, palpitations, tachycardia, cardiac dysrhythmias, anginal pain, hypertension or hypotension, and cardiac arrest. Excessive sweating can also occur. Gastrointestinal (GI) effects include dry mouth, metallic taste, anorexia, nausea, vomiting, diarrhea, and abdominal cramps. A sometimes fatal hyperthermia can also occur, driven partly by excessive drug-induced muscular contractions.

Management of Withdrawal, Toxicity, and Overdose

Box 18-4 lists the signs and symptoms of withdrawal from stimulants and also indicates the peak period when these symptoms are most likely to occur and their duration. Death due to poisoning or toxic levels is usually a result of convulsions, coma, or cerebral hemorrhage and may occur during periods of either intoxication or withdrawal. Treatment of overdose is supportive and generally requires sedation of the patient.

DEPRESSANTS

Depressants are drugs that relieve anxiety, irritability, and tension when used as intended. They are also used to treat seizure disorders and induce anaesthesia. The two main pharmacological classes of depressants are benzodiazepines and barbiturates. Both of these drug classes are discussed further in Chapter 13.

Benzodiazepines are relatively safe although highly addictive with prolonged use. They offer many advantages over older drugs used to relieve anxiety and insomnia. However, they are often intentionally and unintentionally misused. Ingestion of benzodiazepines together with alcohol can be lethal. Another depressant that is neither a benzodiazepine nor a barbiturate is marihuana. Derived from the cannabis plant, marihuana (*pot*, *grass*, or *weed*) is the most commonly misused illicit drug worldwide. Canada has one of the highest rates of marihuana use in the world (Centre for Addiction and Mental

---

BOX 18-4

Signs and Symptoms of Stimulant Withdrawal

Peak Period

1–3 days

Duration

5–7 days

Signs

Social withdrawal, psychomotor retardation, hypersomnia, hyperphagia

Symptoms

Depression, suicidal thoughts and behaviour, paranoid delusions

Treatment

No specific pharmacological treatments to reduce cravings or reverse acute toxicity and no known antidotes

Health, 2014). Marihuana is generally smoked as a cigarette (*joint*), rolled in a cigar wrapper (*blunt*), through a pipe, or in a water-chamber (*bong*) and can be mixed in food or tea.

A benzodiazepine that has gained popularity as a recreational drug is flunitrazepam (Rohypnol®). Flunitrazepam is not legally available for prescription in Canada, but it is legally sold in over 60 countries for the treatment of insomnia. This drug is often known as **roofies** and creates a sleepy, relaxed, drunken feeling that lasts 2 to 8 hours. Roofies are commonly used in combination with alcohol and other drugs. They are sometimes taken to enhance a heroin high or to mellow or ease the experience of coming down from a cocaine or crack high. Used with alcohol, roofies produce disinhibition and amnesia.

Roofies have gained a reputation as the "date rape" drug. Individuals have reported being sexually assaulted after being involuntarily sedated with roofies, which were often slipped into their drinks by their attackers. The drug has no taste or odour, so the victims do not realize what is happening. About 10 minutes after ingesting the drug, victims may feel dizzy and disoriented, simultaneously too hot and too cold, and nauseated. They may experience difficulty speaking and moving and then pass out. Individuals will have no memories of what happened while under the influence of the drug. Another popular date rape drug used in similar fashion is gamma-hydroxybutyric acid (GHB). GHB works by mimicking the natural inhibitory brain neurotransmitter gamma-aminobutyric acid (GABA). It is also known as *liquid ecstasy*. These drugs are also used simply for their depressant and hallucinogenic effects.

Mechanism of Action and Drug Effects

Benzodiazepines and barbiturates work by increasing the action of GABA. GABA is an amino acid in the brain that inhibits nerve transmission in the CNS. The alteration of GABA in the CNS results in relief of anxiety, sedation, and muscle relaxation. The effects of depressants are primarily limited to the CNS. They can also cause amnesia and unconsciousness. They have moderate effects outside the CNS, causing slight blood pressure decreases.

The active ingredients of the marihuana plant are cannabinoids, the most active of which is Δ-9-transtetrahydrocannabinol (THC). THC exerts its effects on the body by chemically binding to and stimulating two cannabinoid receptors in the CNS (CB1 and CB2). Smoking the drug leads to acute sensorial changes that start within 3 minutes, peak in 20 to 30 minutes, and last for 2 to 3 hours. Effects last longer when the drug is taken via the oral route. Specific effects include mild euphoria, memory lapses, dry mouth, enhanced appetite, motor awkwardness, and distorted sense of time and space. THC also stimulates sympathetic receptors and inhibits parasympathetic receptors in heart tissue, which leads to tachycardia. Other effects include hallucinations, anxiety, paranoia, and unsteady gait.

Indications

There are many therapeutic uses of depressants. Benzodiazepines are used primarily to relieve anxiety, induce sleep, sedate, and prevent seizures. Barbiturates are used as sedatives and anticonvulsants and to induce anaesthesia. Medical uses for marihuana include treatment of persistent pain, reduction of nausea and vomiting associated with cancer treatment, and appetite stimulation in those with wasting syndromes, such as in patients with cancer or AIDS. However, it is often not popular with those who claim it is not as effective as inhaled marihuana. Under the Marihuana for Medical Purposes Regulations, authorized individuals have access to dried marihuana for medical use and, as of 2015, edible products as well as other derivatives. For example, patients approved for medical marihuana are now able to brew marihuana leaves in tea or bake cannabis into brownies or cookies for consumption.

Contraindications

Contraindications to the therapeutic use of depressant medications include known drug allergy, dyspnea or airway obstruction, angle-closure glaucoma, and porphyria (a metabolic disorder).

Adverse Effects

The most common undesirable effect of benzodiazepines and barbiturates is an overexpression of their therapeutic effects. The CNS is the primary area of the body adversely affected by these drugs. Drowsiness, sedation, loss of coordination, dizziness, blurred vision, headaches, and paradoxical reactions (insomnia, increased excitability, hallucinations) are the primary CNS adverse effects. Occasional GI effects include nausea, vomiting, constipation, dry mouth, and abdominal cramping. Other possible adverse effects are pruritus and skin rash.

Several essential neurodevelopment phases occur during adolescence before the brain matures. Initially, the brain prunes inefficient neurons and insulating axons, which ensure optimal functioning; however, these changes also make the brain susceptible to the effects of marihuana use. The area of the brain where the majority of fine-tuning takes place is the frontal lobe, where executive functions develop (e.g., decision making, judgement, planning, and problem solving). This underdeveloped area is most susceptible to the effects of marihuana. Consequently, long-term use of marihuana during adolescence can lead to issues with cognitive and psychomotor functioning, dependence, and mental health disorders such as schizophrenia, mood and anxiety disorders, eating disorders, and childhood behavioural disorders (e.g., attention deficit hyperactivity disorder; Centre for Addiction and Mental Health, 2014). Marihuana use is also associated with chronic respiratory symptoms (similar to those of tobacco misuse). A chronic, depressive "amotivational" syndrome has also been observed, especially among younger users. This is a complex issue and other recent studies have produced results that

BOX 18-5

Signs, Symptoms, and Treatment of Depressant Withdrawal

Peak Period

2–4 days for short-acting drugs
4–7 days for long-acting drugs

Duration

4–7 days for short-acting drugs
7–12 days for long-acting drugs

Signs

Increased psychomotor activity; agitation; muscular weakness; hyperthermia; diaphoresis; delirium; convulsions; elevated blood pressure, pulse rate, and temperature; tremors of eyelids, tongue, and hands

Symptoms

Anxiety; depression; euphoria; incoherent thoughts; hostility; grandiosity; disorientation; tactile, auditory and visual hallucinations; suicidal thoughts

Treatment of Benzodiazepine Withdrawal

A 7- to 10-day taper (10- to 14-day taper with long-acting benzodiazepines). Treat with diazepam (Valium®) 10 to 20 mg orally qid on day 1, and then taper until the dosage is 5 to 10 mg orally on the last day. Avoid giving the drug as needed (prn). Adjustments in dosage according to the patient's clinical state may be indicated.

Treatment of Barbiturate Withdrawal

A 7- to 10-day taper or 10- to 14-day taper. Calculate barbiturate equivalence, and give 50% of the original dosage (if actual dosage is known before detoxification); taper. Avoid giving the drug prn.

contradict the above long-term effects (Bechtold, Simpson, White, et al., 2015).

Toxicity and Management of Overdose

Box 18-5 lists the signs and symptoms of withdrawal from depressants and also indicates the peak periods when these symptoms are most likely to occur and their duration. Fatal poisoning is unusual with benzodiazepines when they are taken alone. When they are ingested with alcohol or barbiturates, however, the combination can be lethal. Death is typically due to respiratory arrest. Abrupt withdrawal of benzodiazepines when they have been taken for prolonged periods has resulted in autonomic withdrawal symptoms, seizures, delirium, rebound anxiety, myoclonus (involuntary muscle contractions), myalgia, and sleep disturbances.

Flumazenil is a benzodiazepine reversal drug. It antagonizes the action of benzodiazepines on the CNS by directly competing for binding at the benzodiazepine receptors in the CNS, thereby reversing sedation. The dosage regimen to be followed for the reversal of procedural sedation or general anaesthesia induced by a benzodiazepine and the management of suspected benzodiazepine overdoses are summarized in Chapter 13 (Table 13-3).

Barbiturates and benzodiazepines are commonly implicated in suicides, especially in combination with alcohol. Depressants are not regularly prescribed over a long period. Relatively safe hypnotic drugs such as the benzodiazepines are preferred whenever possible, especially in patients who are emotionally unstable. Combinations of sedative–hypnotic compounds or hypnotics in combination with alcohol need to be avoided. Long-term use of hypnotic drugs leads to ineffective control of insomnia, decreased rapid eye movement sleep, dependence, and drug withdrawal symptoms. Effects of marihuana use are usually self-limiting and resolve within a few hours.

ALCOHOL

Alcohol has been used since the beginning of human civilization. Individuals of Arab descent introduced the technique of distillation to Europe in the Middle Ages. Alcohol has been called the "elixir of life" and has been promoted as a remedy for practically all diseases, which led to the term *whisky*, which is Gaelic for "water of life." Over time, it has been determined that the therapeutic value of ethanol is extremely limited, and long-term ingestion of excessive amounts is a major social and medical problem.

Mechanism of Action and Drug Effects

Alcohol, which is more accurately known as *ethanol* and abbreviated as ETOH, is a CNS depressant. It results in CNS depression by dissolving in lipid membranes in the CNS. The latest hypothesis is that ethanol causes a local disordering in the lipid matrix of the brain. This action has been termed *membrane fluidization*. Some also believe that ethanol may augment GABA-mediated synaptic inhibition and fluxes of chloride. As GABA is an inhibitory neurotransmitter in the brain, its enhancement causes CNS depression. The CNS is continuously depressed in the presence of ethanol. Effects of ethanol on circulation are relatively minor. In moderate doses, ethanol causes vasodilation, especially of the cutaneous vessels but also gastric vessels, and it produces warm, flushed skin, creating a feeling of warmth. Increased sweating may also occur. Heat is therefore lost more rapidly, and internal body temperature consequently falls. Although the short-term ingestion of ethanol, even in intoxicating doses, produces little lasting change in liver function, long-term ingestion is one of the primary causes of liver failure. Ethanol exerts a diuretic effect by inhibiting antidiuretic hormone secretion resulting in a decrease in renal tubular reabsorption of water.

Indications

Few legitimate uses of ethanol and alcoholic beverages exist. Ethanol is an excellent solvent for many drugs and is commonly employed as a vehicle for medicinal mixtures. When applied topically to the skin, ethanol acts as a coolant. Ethanol may also be used in liniments (oily medications used on the skin). Applied topically, ethanol is a popular skin disinfectant. More commonly, however, the type of alcohol used on the skin is isopropyl alcohol, which is similar in structure to ethanol but is more toxic and not drinkable.

Systemic uses of ethanol are primarily limited to the treatment of methyl alcohol and ethylene glycol intoxication (e.g., from drinking automotive antifreeze solution).

Adverse Effects

Long-term excessive ingestion of ethanol is associated with serious neurological and mental health disorders. These neurological disorders can result in seizures. Nutritional and vitamin deficiencies, especially of the B vitamins, can occur and can lead to **Wernicke's encephalopathy**, **Korsakoff's psychosis**, polyneuritis, and nicotinic acid deficiency encephalopathy.

Moderate amounts of ethanol may stimulate or depress respirations. Large amounts produce dangerous or lethal depression of respiration. Although circulatory effects of ethanol are relatively minor, acute severe alcoholic intoxication may cause cardiovascular depression. Long-term excessive use of ethanol has irreversible effects on the heart, such as cardiomyopathy.

When consumed on a regular basis in large quantities, ethanol produces a constellation of dose-related negative effects, such as alcoholic hepatitis or liver cirrhosis. Teratogenic effects are caused by the direct inhibitory action of ethanol on embryonic cellular proliferation early in gestation. This alcohol exposure can cause a wide spectrum of cognitive, behavioural, functional, and neurological deficits. *Fetal alcohol spectrum disorder* (FASD) is the nondiagnostic umbrella term for the wide range of effects of exposure to alcohol in utero. A diagnosis of FASD is complex and requires a comprehensive, multidisciplinary assessment. Fetal alcohol syndrome is the most severe form, characterized by craniofacial abnormalities, CNS dysfunction, and both prenatal and postnatal growth restriction in the infant. The current version of the *Diagnostic and Statistical Manual of Mental Disorders (DSM-5)* includes proposed criteria for neurodevelopmental disorder associated with prenatal alcohol exposure (ND-PAE). Pregnant women need to be educated about the effects of the consumption of alcohol during pregnancy, and appropriate treatment and counselling need to be arranged for pregnant women addicted to alcohol or any other drug of misuse.

Interactions

Alcohol can intensify the sedative effects of any medications that work in the CNS (e.g., sedative–hypnotics, benzodiazepines, antidepressants, antipsychotics, opioids). It can interact with the antibiotic metronidazole, causing a disulfiram reaction. (See below for details.) Alcohol can also cause severe hepatotoxicity when taken with acetaminophen. Acute ingestion of alcohol can increase the bioavailability of the anticoagulant warfarin sodium, which increases the chances of bleeding. Chronic ingestion can cause warfarin sodium to be less effective, leading to increased risks of clots.

Toxicity and Management of Overdose

Box 18-6 lists the common signs and symptoms of ethanol withdrawal. Withdrawal can begin 6 to 12 hours after the last drink. Signs and symptoms may vary depending on the individual's usage pattern, the preferred type of ethanol, and the presence of concurrent disorders. Symptoms usually peak at 2 to 3 days, although they can last up to 7 days. A subacute withdrawal syndrome may last for weeks, characterized by insomnia, irritability, and craving. Older adults tend to have more severe withdrawal. Treatment of ethanol toxicity is supportive and strives to stabilize the patient and maintain the airway. Ethanol withdrawal can be life threatening. Alcohol withdrawal protocols involving symptom-triggered administration of benzodiazepines have been established to reduce the duration of treatment and the cumulative benzodiazepine dose. The Clinical Institute Withdrawal Assessment for Alcohol, Revised (CIWA-Ar) is a validated assessment tool to guide benzodiazepine dosing in alcohol withdrawal. It is used extensively as part of symptom-triggered dosing regimens for benzodiazepines. This type of regimen promotes real-time coordination of the benzodiazepine dose to the severity of symptoms.

One pharmacological option for the treatment of alcoholism is disulfiram. (Disulfiram [Antabuse®] is no longer manufactured by a pharmaceutical company in Canada; it is available only from pharmacies that compound it.) Disulfiram works by altering the metabolism of alcohol. It is not a cure for alcoholism but helps patients who have a sincere desire to stop drinking. The rationale for its use is that patients know that if they are to avoid acetaldehyde syndrome (refer to Table 18-2), they cannot drink for at least 3 or 4 days after taking disulfiram. The adverse effects are uncomfortable and potentially dangerous for someone with any other major illnesses. For this reason, disulfiram is usually reserved as the treatment of last resort for patients who misuse alcohol, for whom other treatment options (e.g., Alcoholics Anonymous, psychotherapy) have failed but who still hope to avoid continued alcohol misuse. When ethanol is ingested by an individual previously treated with disulfiram, the blood acetaldehyde concentration rises 5 to 10 times higher than that in an untreated individual. Within 5 to 10 minutes of alcohol ingestion, the individual's face feels hot, and soon afterward it is flushed and scarlet. After this, throbbing in the head and neck, nausea, copious vomiting, diaphoresis, dyspnea, hyperventilation, vertigo, blurred vision, and confusion occur. As little as 7 mL of alcohol will cause mild

BOX 18-6 — Signs, Symptoms, and Treatment of Ethanol Withdrawal

Mild Withdrawal

Signs and Symptoms
Systolic blood pressure higher than 150 mm Hg, diastolic blood pressure higher than 90 mm Hg, pulse rate greater than 110 beats per min, temperature above 37.7°C, tremors, insomnia, agitation

Moderate Withdrawal

Signs and Symptoms
Systolic blood pressure 150 to 200 mm Hg, diastolic blood pressure 90 to 140 mm Hg, pulse 110 to 140 beats per min, temperature 37.7 to 38.3°C, tremors, insomnia, agitation

Severe Withdrawal (Delirium Tremens)

Signs and Symptoms
Systolic blood pressure higher than 200 mm Hg, diastolic blood pressure higher than 140 mm Hg, pulse rate higher than 140 beats per min, temperature above 38.3°C, tremors, insomnia, agitation

Treatment

Treatments include counselling and education, inpatient detoxification programs, and the 12-step program (Alcoholics Anonymous). Benzodiazepines are the drug treatment of choice for ethanol withdrawal. The dosages are variable and differ from institution to institution. Lower dosages are used for mild symptoms, and higher dosages are needed for severe withdrawal. The oral route is preferred; however, it is often necessary to use the intravenous route for patients experiencing severe withdrawal, who often require monitoring in an intensive care unit for cardiac and respiratory function, fluid and nutrition replacement, vital signs, and mental status. Restraints are indicated for a patient who is confused or agitated to protect the patient from self and to protect others (delirium tremens can be a terrifying and life-threatening state). Thiamine administration, hydration, and magnesium replacement may be indicated, depending on the severity of the withdrawal state.

TABLE 18-2

Disulfiram Adverse Effects: Acetaldehyde Syndrome

Body System Affected	Body System Result
Cardiovascular	Vasodilation over the entire body, hypotension, orthostatic syncope, chest pain
Central nervous	Intense throbbing of the head and neck, leading to a pulsating headache, sweating, marked uneasiness, weakness, vertigo, blurred vision, confusion
Gastrointestinal	Nausea, copious vomiting, thirst
Respiratory	Difficulty breathing

symptoms in a sensitive person. The effects last from 30 minutes to several hours. Once the symptoms wear off, the patient is exhausted and may sleep for several hours. Most of the signs and symptoms observed after the ingestion of disulfiram plus alcohol are attributable to the resulting increase in the concentration of acetaldehyde in the body. Acetaldehyde is a product of alcohol metabolism that is more toxic than alcohol itself. There have been a few published reports of localized disulfiram–alcohol skin reactions when alcohol preparations—even beer-containing shampoo—were placed on the skin. The usual dosage of disulfiram is 250 mg per day, or 125 mg per day in patients who experience adverse effects such as sedation, sexual dysfunction, and elevated liver enzyme levels.

A less noxious drug therapy option is the use of naltrexone (refer to the section on opioids earlier in the chapter). The newest drug treatment indicated for alcoholism is acamprosate calcium. It is used to prevent relapse in patients who are abstinent when starting the drug and who have additional psychosocial support. Its mechanism of action is not completely understood, but it may modulate glutamate and GABA receptors in the brain. Acamprosate calcium appears to restore the balance between these neurotransmitters, which are altered as a result of long-term alcohol intake. The usual dosage is two 333-mg tablets taken three times daily for 1 year. Diazepam is used for the treatment of seizures, the most common complication of alcohol withdrawal, and delirium tremens. Delirium tremens usually begins 5 to 7 days after the last drink and can last for several days. It is the most severe form of ethanol withdrawal and is characterized by disorientation, visual hallucinations, paranoid delusions, and sympathetic overdrive (fever, sweating, tachycardia, vomiting), which can progress to dysrhythmias and cardiovascular collapse.

NICOTINE

Nicotine was first isolated from the leaves of tobacco in 1828. The medical significance of nicotine stems from its toxicity, presence in tobacco, and propensity for eliciting dependence in its users. The long-term effects of nicotine and the untoward effects of the long-term use of tobacco are considerable. Although many people smoke because they believe cigarettes calm their nerves, smoking releases epinephrine, a hormone that creates physiological stress rather than relaxation in the smoker. The apparent calming effects may be related to the increased deep breathing associated with smoking. The use of tobacco is addictive. Most users develop tolerance for nicotine and need greater amounts to produce the desired effect. Tobacco smokers become physically and psychologically dependent and will suffer withdrawal symptoms. Smoking is particularly dangerous in adolescents because their bodies are still developing and changing. The chemicals, including 200 known poisons, present in cigarette smoke can adversely affect adolescents' maturation. One third of young people who are "just experimenting" end up becoming addicted by the time they are 20 years of age.

Mechanism of Action and Drug Effects

Nicotine works by directly stimulating the autonomic ganglia of the nicotinic receptors (see Chapter 21). Its site of action is the ganglion rather than the preganglionic or postganglionic nerve fibre. The organs throughout the body that are innervated by nerves stimulated by nicotine contain nicotinic receptors. These receptors are so named because they were originally tested with nicotine to measure their responses. Nicotine can have multiple unpredictable and dramatic effects on the body because nicotinic receptors are found in several systems, including the adrenal glands, skeletal muscles, and the CNS.

The major action of nicotine is transient stimulation, followed by more persistent depression of all autonomic ganglia. Small doses of nicotine stimulate the ganglion cells directly and facilitate the transmission of impulses. When larger doses of the drug are applied, the initial stimulation is followed quickly by a blockade of transmission.

Nicotine markedly stimulates the CNS, including respiratory stimulation. This stimulation of the CNS is followed by depression. Nicotine can have dramatic effects on the cardiovascular system as well, resulting in increases in heart rate and blood pressure. The GI system is generally stimulated by nicotine, which produces increased tone and activity in the bowel. This often leads to nausea and vomiting and occasionally to diarrhea.

Indications

The nicotine found in nature (i.e., tobacco plants) has no therapeutic uses. It is medically significant because of its addictive and toxic properties. Once nicotine is formulated into products to reduce cravings and promote smoking cessation, then it can be considered a therapeutic drug. It is available as treatment to stop smoking as chewing gum, transdermal patches, and nasal spray.

Adverse Effects

Nicotine primarily affects the CNS. Large doses can produce tremors and even convulsions. Respiratory stimulation also commonly occurs. The initial stimulation of the CNS induced by nicotine is quickly followed by depression. Death can even result from respiratory failure, which is thought to occur due to both central paralysis and peripheral blockade of respiratory muscles.

The cardiovascular effects of nicotine are increased heart rate and blood pressure. The effects of nicotine on the GI system are largely due to parasympathetic stimulation, which results in increased tone and motor activity of the bowel. Nicotine induces vomiting by both central and peripheral actions. Centrally, nicotine's emetic effects result from stimulation of the chemoreceptor trigger zone in the brain.

Management of Withdrawal, Toxicity, and Overdose

Acute nicotine toxicity generally occurs in children who accidentally ingest cigarettes. Treatment is supportive and may include activated charcoal. Smoking cessation is the primary cause for nicotine withdrawal, although discontinuation of any tobacco product can lead to this syndrome. An important and often overlooked problem in hospitalized patients is nicotine withdrawal, which manifests largely as cigarette craving. Irritability, restlessness, and a decrease in heart rate and blood pressure occur. Cardiac symptoms resolve over 3 to 4 weeks, but cigarette craving may persist for months or even years.

The nicotine transdermal system (patch), nicotine polacrilex (gum), and inhalers can be used to provide nicotine without the carcinogens found in tobacco and are now available over the counter. The patch uses a stepwise reduction in subcutaneous delivery to gradually decrease the nicotine dose, and patient treatment adherence seems to be higher than with the gum. Acute relief from withdrawal symptoms is most easily achieved with the use of the gum because rapid chewing releases an immediate dose of nicotine. The dose is approximately one half of the dose the average smoker receives in one cigarette, however, and the onset of action is 30 minutes, versus 10 minutes or less from smoking. These pharmacological changes in delivery minimize the immediate reinforcement and self-reward effects that are prominent with the rapid nicotine delivery of cigarette smoking.

A sustained-release form of the antidepressant bupropion hydrochloride (Zyban®; see Chapter 17) is approved as first-line therapy to aid in smoking cessation treatment. Extended-release bupropion hydrochloride is an innovative treatment because it is the first nicotine-free prescription medicine to treat nicotine dependence. Table 18-3 lists the currently available drugs for nicotine withdrawal therapy.

Varenicline tartrate (Champix®) both activates and antagonizes the α-4-β-2 nicotinic receptors in the brain. This effect provides some stimulation to nicotine receptors, while also reducing the pleasurable effects of nicotine from smoking. This drug has demonstrated greater efficacy than bupropion. The recommended 12-week treatment regimen begins with 0.5 mg orally twice daily, titrating up to 1 mg twice daily by day 8. An optional second 12-week regimen may be prescribed to help the patient maintain tobacco abstinence. The most common adverse effects are nausea, vomiting, headache, flatulence, insomnia, and taste disturbances. Drowsiness has also been reported, so it is important to advise patients about driving and engaging in other potentially

TABLE 18-3		
Nicotine Cessation Therapies		
Drug	**Dosage**	**Recommended Duration of Use**
TRANSDERMAL NICOTINE SYSTEMS		
Habitrol®, Nicoderm®	7 mg/24 hr	2–4 wk
	14 mg/24 hr	2–4 wk
	21 mg/24 hr	4–8 wk
ProStep Patch®	11 mg/24 hr	2–4 wk
	22 mg/24 hr	4–8 wk
Nicorette® inhaler	10 mg/inhalation	6–12 wk
nicotine gum (Resin®)	When the patient has a strong urge to smoke, a stick of gum is chewed; use gradually reduced over a 2–3 mo period	
ANTIDEPRESSANT		
bupropion hydrochloride (Zyban®)	15-mg sustained-release tabs	15 mg on days 1–3; then 150 mg bid for 7–12 wk
PARTIAL NICOTINE AGONIST		
Varenicline tartrate (Champix)	0.5- or 1-mg tabs	12-wk regimen, beginning with 0.5 mg orally bid, titrated to 1 mg daily by day 8

hazardous activities until patients can determine how the drug may affect them. Although many highly addicted smokers are reporting significant success with varenicline tartrate, there are other warnings regarding its use. Specifically, case reports of psychiatric symptoms while using the drug have emerged, including agitation, depression, and suicidality, as well as worsening of preexisting psychiatric illness. Appropriate patient education and follow-up regarding these adverse effects should be undertaken. Varenicline tartrate should not be used during pregnancy.

One of the newer trends to stop smoking is electronic cigarettes (vapour- or e-cigarettes). Typically, an e-cigarette consists of a cartridge that contains nicotine, water, and a flavouring in a base of propylene glycol and glycerine; an atomizer with a heating element that turns the liquid into a vapour; and a battery for a light that glows similarly to a lit cigarette. Not all e-cigarettes contain nicotine. E-cigarettes are not approved by Health Canada for sale or use.

NURSING PROCESS

Assessment

The purpose of a substance misuse assessment is to determine whether substance misuse exists, to evaluate the relationship between the misuse and other health concerns, and to begin the implementation of an effective health promotion and health restoration plan. Because of the prevalence of substance misuse and the role played by the professional nurse in a variety of settings, the nurse may be the first person to identify risky behaviour in a patient. Indications of misuse problems in patients may also become evident during hospitalization for an injury, illness, or surgery. However, even when substance misuse is not suspected, include questions about the use of alcohol, nicotine, opioids, and so on in the general nursing assessment and medication history (see Pharmacology section). Question all patients about the use and misuse of substances because addiction is found across the lifespan, in all cultures and in all types of individuals and may therefore be encountered in all clinical specialties. It is important to recognize that patients may underestimate or deny the use of and amount of substances taken. As well, misuse of substances including prescription medications may need to be assessed in family members because adolescents and other individuals in the home may be diverting parents' or other adults' prescription drugs.

The nurse's responsibilities relative to drug misuse and the nursing process must begin with the cultivation of excellent interpersonal communication skills and a nonjudgemental attitude. It is important to acknowledge and address your own individual beliefs about drug and alcohol use as well as any personal history of coping with addiction or dealing with addicted family members. This process will allow you to anticipate potential responses and behaviours toward this patient population and seek out resolution about these feelings. Acknowledging feelings and beliefs about this group of patients within a balanced perspective and ethical framework will allow you to resolve any personal animosity, judgemental attitudes, rejection, or enabling behaviours. Once detrimental behaviours and possible barriers to responsible and nonjudgemental care have been dealt with, focus on the patient and avoid being drawn into a misuser's manipulative behaviours and other negative conduct.

A thorough patient assessment and history must include specific questions about the substance(s) being used, the duration of misuse, related physical and mental health concerns, and withdrawal potential. In patients with suspected or confirmed substance misuse, honesty—on the part of the patient as well as the family or significant other—may be problematic when answering questions about drug use. Therefore, establishing an environment conducive to communication is necessary and may be possible through use of open-ended questions during assessment. Additionally, be sure to maintain a nonjudgemental approach during the assessment as well as other phases of the nursing process. A medication history needs to include information about all drugs being used, including prescription drugs, OTC drugs, natural health products, and illicit or street drugs. Include the names of the drugs, doses, frequency and duration of use. Be attentive to any clues a patient, family, or significant other may reveal, including behavioural and mood changes. A patient's reported use of multiple prescribed drugs as well as contact with multiple prescribers raises concern as a possible sign of drug misuse. In addition, laboratory findings are important to assess, including results of kidney and liver function studies and any drug screening studies. Assess and monitor results of HIV and hepatitis laboratory tests, if ordered. Monitor and document baseline vital signs.

A number of assessment tools with established validity and reliability are available to nurses and health care providers for use with patients suspected of drug or substance misuse. The goal of adequate screening for alcohol and other drug misuse or addiction is to identify patients who have or are at risk for developing alcohol- or drug-related problems and to further engage them in discussion. This may help in further diagnosing and more accurately treating the patient's misuse problem. Laboratory tests are available to detect alcohol and other drugs in the blood or urine. These are used to identify recent drug misuse rather than long-term use or dependence. However, there are other tests that are best used when assessing someone for confirmation of a diagnosis (Box 18-7).

The CAGE Questionnaire is available as a screening tool for alcohol use in adults and is used by many HCPs in the field of alcohol addiction. Even though it is simple and brief (consisting of only four questions), it has a noted accuracy rate of 93%. The CAGE Questionnaire has also been adapted to include drug use in adults (CAGE-AID). The CAGE or CAGE-AID should be preceded by the following two questions: (1) Do you drink alcohol? and (2) Have you ever experimented with drugs? If the patient has experimented with drugs, ask the CAGE-AID questions (modified by the italicized text). If the patient only drinks alcohol, ask the CAGE questions. See Box 18-8 for the CAGE and CAGE-AID questions. Each affirmative response earns one point. One point indicates a possible problem, while two points indicate a probable problem.

Other available screening tools include the Substance Abuse Subtle Screening Inventory (SASSI), the Michigan Alcoholism Screening Test—Geriatric Version (MAST-G) for use in geriatric patients, and the Problem Oriented Screening Instrument for Teenagers (POSIT). If the findings of an assessment questionnaire are positive, the next step is to explore the history of the patient's alcohol or drug use (or both) and problems. Further observation is needed to identify any physical, psychological, and social

---

BOX 18-7

Diagnosis of Substance Use Disorder

The *Diagnostic and Statistical Manual of Mental Disorders (DSM-5*; American Psychiatric Association, 2013) combines the *DSM-IV* categories of substance abuse and substance dependence into a single disorder measured on a continuum from mild to severe. Each specific substance is identified as a separate use disorder; however, the criteria for diagnosis remain the same for each substance. The occurrence of two or three symptoms indicates a mild substance use disorder, four or five symptoms indicate a moderate substance use disorder, and six or more symptoms indicate a severe substance use disorder:

1. Taking the substance in larger amounts or for longer than you meant to
2. Wanting to cut down or stop using the substance but not managing to
3. Spending a lot of time getting, using, or recovering from use of the substance
4. Cravings and urges to use the substance
5. Not managing to do what you should at work, home, or school because of substance use
6. Continuing to use, even when it causes problems in relationships
7. Giving up important social, vocational, or recreational activities because of substance use
8. Using substances again and again, even when it puts you in danger
9. Continuing to use, even when you know you have a physical or psychological problem that could have been caused or made worse by the substance
10. Needing more of the substance to get the effect you want (tolerance)
11. Development of withdrawal symptoms, which can be relieved by taking more of the substance

---

BOX 18-8

CAGE and CAGE-AID Questions

In the past, have you ever:
1. Felt that you wanted or needed to **C**ut down on your drinking or *drug use*?
2. Been **A**nnoyed or **A**ngered by others complaining about your drinking or *drug use*?
3. Felt **G**uilty about the consequences of your drinking or *drug use*?
4. Had a drink or *taken a drug* in the morning (**E**ye-opener) to decrease hangover or withdrawal symptoms?

signs of dependence and dysfunction. Maintaining communication with family members may also provide useful information. If misuse is identified by a history-taking process, physical assessment, drug history profile, screening tests, or patient's confession, then confidentiality, privacy, and nonjudgemental behaviour are keys to ethical nursing practice. Refer to local laws for the reporting of the substance(s) and adhere to the Canadian Nurses Association *Code of Ethics for Registered Nurses* in making a report (see Chapter 3).

Assessment of opioid misuse includes, in addition to the assessment data mentioned earlier, determination of the route being used for drug delivery (e.g., oral versus intravenous use). The use of intravenous drugs may give rise to other concerns such as HIV and AIDS or hepatitis. Respiratory assessment with attention to rate and rhythm are important because of the risk for respiratory depression with opioid overdose. Other, more specific signs and symptoms were described earlier in the chapter.

Assessment of CNS stimulant misuse requires careful questioning about and observation for adverse effects, toxicity, and withdrawal signs and symptoms. Some of the more commonly misused CNS stimulants are dextroamphetamine, methamphetamine (crystallized and powdered forms), and cocaine (see Table 18-1). Signs and symptoms of CNS stimulant misuse were previously discussed, such as changes in blood pressure and increased heart rate. However, the following information needs to be assessed and documented: (1) frequent vital signs; (2) thorough head-to-toe physical examination; (3) assessment of neurological functioning with attention to mydriasis (pupil dilation), hyperactive reflexes, headache, increased motor or speech activity, agitation, syncope, tremors, altered level of consciousness, and seizure activity; and (4) cardiac assessment with attention to increased heart rate (tachycardia), irregular heart rhythm (dysrhythmia), and hypertension or hypotension. Document and immediately report any abnormal assessment findings or the presence of an elevated temperature (hyperthermia, which may be fatal), reports of vomiting or headache, or flushing of the face.

The most dangerous substances in terms of withdrawal are CNS depressants such as alcohol, barbiturates, benzodiazepines, and synthetic cannabinoids (*K2*, *zinger*, or *spice* is a mixture of herbs, spices or shredded plant material that is typically sprayed with a synthetic compound chemically similar to THC, the psychoactive ingredient in marihuana). Misuse of CNS depressants is manifested by a decrease in vital signs and mental functioning (see previous discussion); therefore, frequent monitoring of vital signs and neurological status is needed for safe and prudent care. As with any drug, obtain a comprehensive, thorough nursing history and medication profile. Additional signs and symptoms of misuse are tremors and agitation, with possible progression to hallucinations and sometimes death with continued misuse. Because of the risk of respiratory and circulatory depression, always perform an assessment of the patient's CABs (circulation, airway, and breathing). Early withdrawal (see Box 18-5) may be manifested by increased blood pressure and pulse rate and altered mental status. See Pharmacology section for more specific information. Marihuana, as a depressant, may cause dizziness, disorientation, euphoria, and difficulty with speech and motor activities. Long-term use of marihuana may lead to chronic, depressive, amotivational behaviour. Be sure you always assess for any different or unusual behaviours. Assessment of marihuana use includes appraisal of cognitive and motor function and assessment for the ability to carry out minor tasks.

The signs and symptoms of ethanol (alcohol) withdrawal and toxicity are presented in Box 18-6. Include gathering data about possible drug interactions, especially the use of other CNS depressants such as opioids, sedatives, and hypnotics in the assessment. It is important to monitor blood alcohol levels because they are directly related to the health issues and signs and symptoms that appear.

Misuse of nicotine (a CNS stimulant) is associated with adverse effects such as increase in heart rate and blood pressure. It can also result in vomiting and increased bowel tone and motor activity. If the patient has a history of malnutrition, chronic lung disease, stroke, cancer, cardiac disease, or kidney or liver dysfunction, relevant laboratory tests are generally ordered, and their results need to be examined by the nurse and all those involved in the patient's care. Assessment needs to include vital signs, breath sounds, oxygen saturation levels, and monitoring for changes in neurological functioning (e.g., level of consciousness, sensory and motor problems). Remember that smoking cessation and signs and symptoms of nicotine withdrawal may happen abruptly in hospitalized patients. Signs and symptoms of a craving for nicotine include irritability, restlessness, and decrease in pulse rate and blood pressure, the observation of which will help in early identification of serious problems (see Special Populations: Older Adults and Special Populations: Adolescents).

Nursing Diagnoses

- Ineffective health management of self, related to perceived barriers of care due to substance misuse
- Deficient knowledge related to lack of information about addictive behaviours and drugs being misused
- Chronic low self-esteem related to the influence of substance misuse
- Risk for injury and falls related to substance misuse or abrupt withdrawal

Planning

Goals

- Patient will demonstrate patterns of more effective health maintenance.

SPECIAL POPULATIONS: OLDER ADULTS

Alcohol and Substance Misuse

Alcohol and substance misuse among older adults is a hidden national epidemic. A substantial number of older adults are drinking at higher-than-recommended levels; thus, alcohol misuse is becoming a growing problem in this population and one that is often ignored or missed by many HCPs.

Alcohol misuse and alcoholism cut across gender, race, and nationality. In people 15 years of age or older, 75% of individuals identified as current drinkers. Alcohol remains the main substance of misuse among older adults. Approximately 58% of women and 75% of men over 65 years of age use alcohol. Problematic alcohol use occurs in approximately 6 to 10% of people over 65 years of age. Obviously, alcohol misuse is of major concern for the older population and necessitates thorough assessment for drug and chemical misuse in this group.

Misuse of other substances by older adults is also an overlooked and often ignored problem. Older drug misusers are often poor, frail, and hidden from health care and service providers. The stigma associated with these problems keeps them, as well as family members, from coming forward to report problems. Although the overall rate of substance misuse is lower in older adults than in younger people, substance misuse in older adults is a significant and growing problem. It is complicated by the fact that many in this age group also use prescription and OTC

medications. OTC drugs may cause adverse effects even when taken alone, and serious consequences may result when they are taken with alcohol. Significant problems are seen when the combination of alcohol with a drug results in intensification of the drug's action (e.g., heightened hypotensive effects when an antihypertensive drug is taken with alcohol); this can lead to increased adverse effects with significant negative consequences (such as dizziness and possible syncope due to a greater-than-intended drop in blood pressure, which can result in falls and injury). Some of the signals indicating an alcohol- or alcohol and medication–related problem in an older adult include trouble with memory after having a drink or taking a medication; loss of coordination, unsteadiness in walking or frequent falls; changes in sleeping habits; unexplained bruises; and irritability, sadness, depression, and being unsure of oneself.

HCP, health care providers; *OTC*, over-the-counter.

Source: Public Health Agency of Canada. (2010). *The Chief Public Health Officer's report on the state of public health in Canada. Chapter 3: The health and well-being of Canadian seniors.* Retrieved from http://www.phac-aspc.gc.ca/cphorsphc-respcacsp/2010/fr-rc/cphorsphc-respcacsp-06-eng.php.

- Patient will openly discuss the substance misuse and the benefits of a treatment regimen.
- Patient will gain improved self-esteem during treatment for substance misuse.
- Patient will remain free from injury during treatment for substance misuse and addiction.

Expected Patient Outcomes

- Patient openly discusses perceived barriers to effective health maintenance.
- Patient exhibits healthy participation and cooperation with the therapeutic regimen for substance misuse disorders.
- Patient demonstrates a knowledge base about behaviours related to substance misuse and addiction through discussion of expectations of recovery, benefits and short- and long-term effects of treatment, as well as signs and symptoms of withdrawal regimen.
- Patient verbalizes feelings of improved self-esteem and discusses healthy adaptation and coping skills in an open and secure treatment environment.
- Patient undergoes safe withdrawal from the misused substance with stabilization of the aggravated and dysfunctional physical and emotional state without injury to self or others.

Implementation

The nurse plays a vital role in the care of patients manifesting misuse behaviours, intoxication, and withdrawal. It is also the nurse who, through the nursing process, helps to meet the patient's basic needs after developing a therapeutic relationship and teaches the patient, family, or significant others about addiction and its effect on the entire family. Nursing strategies for meeting actual or potential health problems are implemented for nursing diagnoses generated from assessment data. Nurses working with patients who misuse substances need a sound knowledge base as well as special understanding and empathy. Participation in training, seminars, and education about the process of substance misuse and related lifestyles is encouraged, to assist in understanding patients and developing comprehensive plans of care. Nursing interventions involve maximizing all of the therapeutic plans and minimizing those factors that contribute to maladaptive or dysfunctional behaviours. Once therapeutic rapport has been established and a patient–nurse–health care provider contract has been agreed upon, maximizing recovery is the plan. Interventions are based on the patient's specific physical and emotional problems and carried out accordingly and in order of priority of basic needs. For example, if a patient is experiencing hallucinations from either use of a substance or

SPECIAL POPULATIONS: ADOLESCENTS

Misuse of Alcohol, Misuse of Over-the-Counter and Prescription Drugs, and Huffing Practices in Adolescents

Although statistics vary by province, as many as 85% of Canadian adolescents have consumed alcohol while 50% have consumed illegal drugs (Health Canada, 2013). Rates of illicit drug use and risky drinking are higher in youth under the age of 25 than in other age groups. Surveys on student drug use have been conducted intermittently over the years in 9 of Canada's 10 provinces, as well as nationally. These include the British Columbia Adolescent Health Survey; the Alberta Youth Experience Survey; the Manitoba Student Alcohol and Drug Use Survey; the Ontario Student Drug Use and Health Survey; the Québec Health Survey of High School Students; the Student Drug Use Survey in the Atlantic Provinces; the Canadian Student Tobacco, Alcohol and Drugs Survey; and the Health Behaviour of School-Aged Children study. The Ontario Student Drug Use and Health Survey is used as an example in this chapter.

Adolescent patients are exposed to real drug hazards connected with some everyday products within the home. According to the 2013 Ontario Student Drug Use and Health Survey, a survey of Ontario students in Grades 7 to 12, the use of OTC and prescription drugs is rising, while alcohol consumption and smoking are at an all-time low. One percent of respondents reported using stimulant drugs that are normally used to treat attention deficit hyperactivity disorder. This is consistent with the British Columbia 2013 survey. The misuse of OTC cold products, specifically dextromethorphan-containing products, is a significant issue and appears to be on the rise. Dextromethorphan is the most commonly used and most effective nonprescription cough suppressant and is an ingredient in several OTC products, including Robitussin DM® cough syrup and liquid gel capsules. Some adolescents have discovered that taking dextromethorphan in large amounts leads to a "high" that is accompanied by hallucinations. The hallucinations have been documented to be similar to those associated with the street drug phencyclidine (PCP) and the anaesthetic ketamine (see Chapter 12). In 2013, almost 10% of Ontario students in Grades 7 to 12 reported use of cough or cold medication at least once in the past year to "get high." This statistic reflects an increasing trend from previous surveys. Two percent of students reported use of cough and cold medications six or more times in the past year. Dextromethorphan is available in over 140 preparations of the OTC drugs sold in the Canada, and for teens experimenting with drugs, it is cheap, easily obtained, and legal. Many of these OTC drugs also contain acetaminophen, which creates a potential consequence of acetaminophen toxicity.

Another, potentially new concoction is called *sizzurp*, made of pop, dissolved Jolly Rancher candy, and prescription cough syrup containing the antihistamine promethazine hydrochloride and the opioid codeine phosphate. While this prescription drug is only available in the United States, numerous products may be substituted in Canada.

One in five students admitted to abusing prescription drugs and 75% of these admitted to stealing them, often from the home medicine cabinet. One in eight reported using a prescription opioid pain medication recreationally in the last year.

Additionally, it has been found that teens who misuse dextromethorphan and prescription medications may also misuse other drugs. Another problem is that of huffing or the misuse of inhalants, including the following substances: (1) volatile solvents—nail polish and paint thinner, (2) aerosols—deodorants and cooking sprays, (3) gases butane cigarette lighter fluid and nitrous oxide (laughing gas), and (4) nitrites—cyclohexyl nitrite (found in room deodorizers) and amyl nitrite and butyl nitrite (sold on the street in small, sealed containers). Students may also inhale "computer duster," pressurized gases (e.g., etrafluoroethane or difluoroethane) used to clean electronic equipment. When inhaled, chemicals are quickly absorbed into the bloodstream via the lungs and then into organs with a large blood distribution, such as the brain and liver. The solvents lead to effects similar to those of alcohol intoxication. Long-term use can lead to kidney, liver, or brain damage. The hazardous short- or long-term effects that may occur with the additive effects of drugs include nausea, hot flashes, reduced mental status, dizziness, seizures, loss of coordination and balance, brain damage, and death.

The 2013 survey of Ontario students reported that 3.4% had sniffed glue or solvents at least once in the past year, which is a significant decrease from the previous report. The at-risk groups for inhalant misuse are students who have dropped out of school, people who have been physically or sexually abused or neglected, people who have been incarcerated or who are homeless, and members of Indigenous communities. Inhalant use often results in a euphoric feeling, but brain damage and even death can occur with just one huff. There is still a tremendous need for continued prevention and treatment efforts related to inhalant use. Education needs to begin early on in elementary school, so that children learn of the dangers of inhalant use and its potential damaging effects on the brain. Education and awareness are important to prevent misuse and abuse behaviours, and a child is never too young to learn about these types of dysfunctional and life-threatening behaviours. Parents, other family members and relatives, and caregivers need to be actively involved in any educational sessions about drugs that are misused and related signs and symptoms.

OTC, over-the-counter.

Source: Baydala, L. (2010 [Reaffirmed 2014]). Inhalant abuse. *Paediatrics and Child Health, 15*(7), 443–448; Boak, A., Hamilton, H. A., Adlaf, E. M., et al. (2013). *Drug use among Ontario students, 1977–2013: OSDUHS highlights (CAMH Research Document Series No. 37).* Toronto, ON: Centre for Addiction and Mental Health.

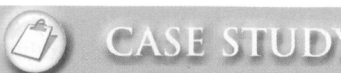

CASE STUDY

Substance Misuse and Adolescents

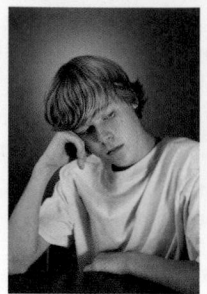

You are having a discussion with a neighbour, Jared, who has a 14-year-old son, Cayden. Jared expresses concern about Cayden and substance misuse problems he has heard about.

1. Jared describes one of Cayden's friends, who was once a bright and motivated student but has become sullen and withdrawn, lacking the motivation he once had. In addition, he has a chronic cough but denies that he smokes cigarettes. This behaviour change may indicate misuse of what substance? Are there any long-term effects?

2. Jared mentions "huffing," which Cayden told him has happened at several parties this year. Jared says, "Huffing is not harmful, right?" What will you tell him? A few weeks later, Jared calls you because Cayden is extremely drowsy and unable to speak. Jared notes that his bottle of alprazolam (Xanax®) is almost empty and worries that his son has taken an overdose.

3. What will you do first? What treatment would you expect his son to receive?

For answers, see http://evolve.elsevier.com/Canada/Lilley/pharmacology/.

from the withdrawal, the priority will be to manage the ABCs of care (airway, breathing, and circulation) and monitor vital signs and neurological and mental status, while providing a calm, quiet, nonjudgemental, and non-threatening environment. Seizures may occur, so safety precautions are needed, including the use of protective measures such as padding of side rails and implementation of other seizure precautions (consult facility policies and procedures). For more information see Special Populations: Older Adults and Special Populations: Adolescents).

Substance withdrawal is treated with a multimodal approach that includes pharmacological and nonpharmacological interventions. Remain nonjudgemental while assisting in a patient's recovery and rehabilitation. Also, remain current in your knowledge about the different substances being misused as well as the various treatment and rehabilitation protocols in use. In all interventions, ensuring patient safety is of utmost importance. The patient's movement through the plan of care for withdrawal, recovery, and rehabilitation must be individualized and take place in a safe, secure, and non-threatening environment. Patient education remains an essential part of patient care to help the patient, family, or significant others understand the need for long-term lifestyle changes. Whether it is disulfiram treatment for alcohol misuse or bupropion hydrochloride therapy for nicotine withdrawal, patients need careful instructions and information about their treatment regimen. In addition, patients need to be encouraged to be actively engaged in their treatment regimen, including planning, delivery, and ongoing decision making.

Substance misuse has a major impact on family members and significant others. Families will also be in need of treatment and therapeutic support. It is the caring, empathic, supportive, and educative responses by the nurse that will convey acceptance to the patient and family and help in the overall process of recovery and rehabilitation. A nonjudgemental attitude, caring,

BOX 18-9

Organizations and Agencies Concerned With Substance Misuse

Alcoholics Anonymous
Canadian Assembly of Narcotics Anonymous
Canadian Centre for Substance Abuse
Centre for Addiction and Mental Health
Drug Education and Awareness for Life
National Kids Help Phone
Health Canada Drug Strategy and Controlled Substances Program
Kaiser Foundation
Partnership for a Drug-Free Canada
Royal Canadian Mounted Police Drug Awareness
Think About It (formerly Safegrad)
Teen Challenge Canada
TeenNet CyberIsle

empathy, and quality care must always be at the centre of patient rights, as should be the Canadian Nurses Association's *Code of Ethics for Registered Nurses* (see Chapter 3), regardless of the admitting diagnosis or the type of substance being misused. Lifelong treatment is often indicated; the need for support during the long-term process of recovery must be emphasized and support recommended from within the family unit and extending outward to the community. (See Box 18-9 for a listing of various organizations and resources). Methods to encourage recovery and minimize relapse need to be individualized for each patient and draw on all available resources, whether private or public. Communication techniques must be reinforcing and firm, yet sensitive to the patient's values and beliefs. Family members must be an integral part of all treatment and must participate in all educational sessions.

▨ Evaluation

Patient safety is of utmost importance at all times during patient care but especially when the patient is experiencing the signs and symptoms of withdrawal. Patients may go from mild withdrawal to severe withdrawal and enter into life-threatening situations within a period of a day or two, and therefore complete evaluation of the patient and environment must be ongoing. Evaluation of the recovery and rehabilitation process is important as well, with monitoring of the therapeutic effects of the treatment regimen as well as for any ill effects from the physiological or psychological withdrawal from the substance. Also part of this evaluation process is review of the availability of needed resources during and after hospitalization, including family support. In addition, report any abnormality in vital signs, laboratory test results, mental status, or other parameters immediately. An ongoing evaluation needs to also examine the availability of emotional, social, cultural, spiritual, and financial support, and the nursing care plan should be revised as needed.

PATIENT TEACHING TIPS

❖ Ensure that relevant, nondiscriminatory, current, and accurate information—at various reading levels—is available to the patient, family, or significant others in regard to the specific misuse disorder, signs and symptoms, withdrawal, and treatment regimens. Making an informed decision about the treatment plan is best for everyone involved in the process of recovery and rehabilitation.

❖ Educate the patient, family, or significant others about available support groups and community resources.

❖ Be sure that the patient understands the importance of having a current list of all medications readily available at all times, including treatment regimens for the misuse disorder. Include information about the drug, its action, why it is used and how, adverse effects, cautions, drug–drug and drug–food interactions, cautions, contraindications, dosing, and consequences of missed doses.

❖ Patients must be educated about their rights to ethical and empathic treatment, regardless of the reason for treatment. Two online resources available are: http://www.ccsa.ca/ and http://www.camh.ca/. These sites provide downloadable information, resources, and treatment options for drug and chemical misuse.

KEY POINTS

❖ Physical dependence is a condition characterized by physiological reliance on a substance, usually indicated by tolerance to the effects of the substance and development of withdrawal symptoms when use of the substance is terminated.

❖ Psychological dependence is a condition characterized by strong desires to obtain and use a substance.

❖ *Habituation* refers to situations in which a patient becomes accustomed to a certain drug (develops tolerance) and may have mild psychological dependence on it but does not show compulsive dose escalation, drug-seeking behaviour, or major withdrawal symptoms upon drug discontinuation.

❖ Acamprosate calcium is used to maintain abstinence from alcohol in patients who are abstinent when starting the drug and who have additional psychosocial support. Its mechanism of action is not completely understood.

❖ A new medication for smoking cessation is varenicline tartrate, which has shown better efficacy than bupropion hydrochloride.

❖ Drug withdrawal symptoms vary with the class of drug and may even be the opposite of the drug's action.

❖ Signs and symptoms of opioid withdrawal include mydriasis (pupil dilatation), rhinorrhea, diaphoresis, piloerection (goose bumps), lacrimation, diarrhea, insomnia, and elevated blood pressure and pulse rate. Signs and symptoms of CNS stimulant withdrawal include social isolation or withdrawal, psychomotor retardation, and hypersomnia. Signs and symptoms of CNS depressant withdrawal include increased psychomotor activity; agitation; muscular weakness; hyperthermia; diaphoresis; delirium; convulsions; elevated blood pressure, pulse rate, and temperature; and eyelid tremors. Ethanol withdrawal produces varying degrees of signs and symptoms, depending on the specific blood alcohol level. Delirium tremens is characterized by hypertensive crisis, tachycardia, and hyperthermia; it may be life threatening.

❖ Evaluation of the recovery and rehabilitation process is important, including monitoring of the therapeutic effects of the treatment regimen and monitoring for any physiological or psychological ill effects from the withdrawal of the misused substance.

EXAMINATION REVIEW QUESTIONS

1. A patient is experiencing withdrawal from opioids. The nurse expects to see which assessment finding most commonly associated with acute opioid withdrawal?
a. Elevated blood pressure
b. Decreased pulse
c. Lethargy
d. Constipation

2. During treatment for withdrawal from opioids, the nurse expects which medication to be ordered?
a. amphetamine (Dexedrine®)
b. clonidine (Catapres)
c. diazepam (Valium)
d. disulfiram (Antabuse)

3. The nurse is presenting a seminar on substance misuse. Which drug is the most commonly used illicit drug in Canada?
a. Crack cocaine
b. Heroin
c. Marihuana
d. Methamphetamine

4. A patient who is taking disulfiram as part of an alcohol treatment program accidentally takes a dose of cough syrup that contains a small percentage of alcohol. The nurse expects to see which symptom as a result of acetaldehyde syndrome?
a. Lethargy
b. Copious vomiting
c. Hypertension
d. No ill effect because of the small amount of alcohol in the cough syrup

5. The nurse is assessing a patient for possible substance misuse. Which assessment finding indicates possible use of amphetamines?
a. Lethargy and fatigue
b. Cardiovascular depression
c. Talkativeness and euphoria
d. Difficulty swallowing and constipation

6. A patient experiencing ethanol withdrawal is beginning to show severe manifestations of delirium tremens. The nurse will plan to implement which interventions for this patient? (Select all that apply.)
a. Doses of an oral benzodiazepine
b. Doses of an intravenous benzodiazepine
c. Restraints if the patient becomes confused, agitated, or a threat to himself or others
d. Thiamine supplementation
e. Oral disulfiram (Antabuse) treatment
f. Monitoring in the intensive care unit

7. A patient has been admitted to the emergency department after a suspected overdose of benzodiazepines mixed with alcohol. The patient is lethargic and cannot speak. The nurse expects which immediate measures to be implemented? (Select all that apply.)
a. Prepare to administer naloxone (Suboxone)
b. Prepare to administer flumazenil
c. Monitor the patient for convulsions
d. Prepare for potential respiratory arrest
e. Apply restraints

Answers: 1. a, **2.** b, **3.** c, **4.** b, **5.** c, **6.** b, c, d, f, **7.** b, c, d

CRITICAL THINKING ACTIVITIES

1. A friend has revealed to the nurse that she has used crack cocaine often in the past few months and states that even though she enjoys the sensations, she can "stop at any time." What is the nurse's priority action in this situation?

2. A patient is admitted to the hospital for major abdominal surgery, and the physician has ordered a transdermal nicotine patch to be used while the patient is hospitalized because the patient was a heavy smoker. While the patch is applied, the patient

asks, "Why in the world would you want to give me nicotine when I'm trying to stop smoking?" What is the nurse's priority when answering the patient's question?

3. A patient has been admitted to the labour and delivery unit. She has a history of heavy use of alcohol and appears to be intoxicated. What are the potential effects of alcohol use on a fetus, and what would be priority concerns during the first few months of the newborn's life?

For answers, see http://evolve.elsevier.com/Canada/Lilley/pharmacology/.

PART THREE

Drugs Affecting the Autonomic Nervous System

STUDY SKILLS TIPS:

- PURR APPLICATION
- STUDY GROUPS

PURR APPLICATION

Planning for the Part

The basic explanation provided for the PURR (**p**repare, **u**nderstand, **r**ehearse, **r**eview) model in the Study Skills Tips for Part 1 demonstrates the application process as it relates to individual chapters. There is another application for the PURR model that can be very useful. This application encourages you to take a broader view of your readings. In the case of this text, did you notice how chapters are grouped together? Consider why they may be grouped this way.

Chapters are grouped into multiple chapter blocks called *parts*. Part organization is not a random process applied by the author to complicate the material. It is a carefully considered process of putting content together in a fashion that is both logical and meaningful for your learning. Since the authors have spent considerable time trying to link chapters together in the most logical pattern, it is to your benefit as a student to learn to take advantage of the work already done for you.

Part Title

Begin the process of part planning by looking at the Part 3 title, "Drugs Affecting the Autonomic Nervous System." Then look at the part's structure. There are four chapters contained in Part 3. What is common among these four chapters that allows them to be grouped together? They must all be concerned with the autonomic nervous system. Even before you have read any of the chapters, you can begin to look for the links that will establish relationships—not only the links among the

ideas in individual chapters, but also the broader links that connect the four chapters in this part with each other as well as with the ideas that have come in earlier parts and will follow in later parts.

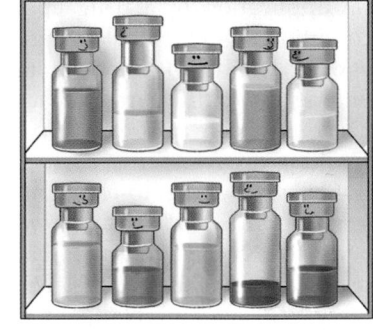

Here is a clear example of the way in which parts relate to one another. Look back at Part 2, "Drugs Affecting the Central Nervous System." Clearly, that part deals with some aspect of the nervous system, as this part does. Now, challenge yourself. What is the relationship between Part 2 and Part 3? Determining this relationship is a learning objective you should establish for yourself. You must be able to define and explain *central nervous system* and *autonomic nervous system*. However, merely defining these terms limits the learning you can achieve. Ask yourself some additional questions that will help you establish a connection between these parts. What are the differences in the functioning of the central and the autonomic nervous systems? Are there pharmacological drugs that have applications in both the central and autonomic nervous systems? Continue stressing the links that must exist throughout all the parts and chapters you are studying. The normal study pattern that most students apply is one that focuses on the individual chapters, but it is essential to remain aware of the broader scopes of chapters and parts.

Part Chapters

After considering the part title and looking for relationships between the new part and the previous parts, the next step in applying the *prepare* step of PURR is to spend a few minutes studying the chapter titles and looking for the relationships that must exist. Part 3 has four chapters, and there is a clear pattern in these chapters. Chapters 19 and 20 both contain the term *adrenergic*. Clearly, these two chapters deal with the same broad topic. However, Chapter 19 covers adrenergic drugs and Chapter 20 covers adrenergic-blocking drugs. Remember to take an active role in your reading; apply questioning strategies at this point. What does *adrenergic* mean? What is an *adrenergic drug*? These two questions are essential in mastering the content of Chapter 19 and are questions you should ask yourself almost without thinking.

The next step, though easily overlooked, is one that can greatly enhance your understanding when you start to read the material. Notice that Chapter 19 deals with drugs and Chapter 20 deals with blocking drugs. There must be a difference between a *drug* and a *blocking drug*. Hone your focus with a few questions that will keep you aware that the content in Chapter 19 has a direct relationship to the content in Chapter 20. Consider the following questioning strategies: "What is the difference between a drug and a blocking drug?"; "When is the pharmacological application of a drug appropriate?"; "Under what conditions should a blocking drug be chosen?" Then, ask a question to help maintain focus on the concept linking the entire part: "What aspects of the autonomic nervous system are related to the adrenergic drugs and blocking drugs?"

Once you begin to focus on the relationship of chapters within a part, certain connections and details will begin to become apparent. Chapters 21 and 22 also cover drugs and blocking drugs. These two chapters develop these concepts in relation to cholinergics rather than adrenergics. However, the same questions you used as a focus for Chapters 19 and 20 can be recycled in setting up the study of Chapters 20 and 21. Simply replace the term *adrenergic* with *cholinergic* and you are ready to begin reading these two chapters with clear personal learning objectives.

Active Questioning

Active questioning is a crucial concept to master when working through the process of planning your learning for an entire part, rather than for individual chapters. The idea is to view the part as a whole, as opposed to seeing only the content of individual chapters. The preceding discussion has provided a number of sample questions to help you begin the questioning process. The suggested questions should not be seen as an exhaustive list but rather as examples to help you develop a questioning process.

Keep in mind that you may or may not ask questions that are useful and appropriate when you are using only chapter titles as stimuli for questions. Some of the questions you devise will prove to be very useful when reading the chapter, while some of the initial questions you generate may have little or no application as you read and understand the content of an individual chapter. Do not worry about the quality of your questions when preparing at the part level. Questions can (and sometimes should) be revised or discarded when the details of the chapter become clearer. What is important is that you begin the part with some questions to help you focus your reading and learning. Also, you will find that the more you apply active questioning as a part of your learning strategy, the better your questions will become.

STUDY GROUPS

A significant part of the PURR approach to learning is active questioning and rehearsing. When we engage others in this process, we have access to their thoughts and understanding. We then must also think through our own ideas and make them clear to others. The best way to learn is to teach others. It is worth noting that members of a study group should individually make every effort to utilize the PURR method to learn the required content prior to working in a group setting, which fosters a learning environment that is collaborative and efficient.

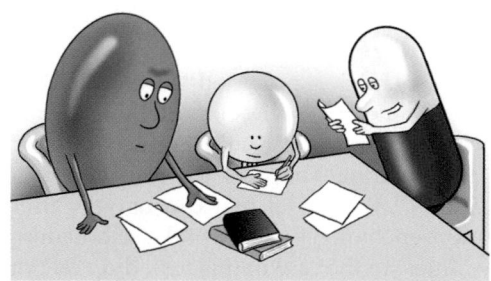

Study groups are particularly helpful when trying to anticipate test questions. With several minds working, you increase the odds of being correct. In nursing, your textbook learning is of no value until you are able to apply the knowledge and skills covered. Study groups provide a discussion venue to stimulate thinking about the nursing process. Study group members can share lecture notes, which is of value if you need to be absent or if you have an instructor who talks too quickly for you to take thorough notes. Relating with a study group keeps you alert while you are studying. It is unlikely that you will fall asleep or daydream when you are in the middle of a discussion. There are many advantages to working with a study group; however, you must be careful when selecting people to be in your group. Consider these four guidelines when establishing your study group:

1. Choose classmates who have **similar abilities and motivation** to yours. Socializing can take up valuable study time. Noncommitted and underprepared classmates can present additional barriers and challenges.

2. Look for students who share a **consistent and convenient time to meet.**

3. Select classmates who have learning styles **different** from yours. They might understand the reading material or lecture material better than you. They may be able to draw diagrams that will help your learning.

4. Find students who have **good communication skills—** that is, people who know how to listen, ask good questions, and explain concepts.

Study groups are not for everyone; however, they may be helpful to you if you are having difficulty staying focused during your personal study time.

Adrenergic Drugs

Objectives

After reading this chapter, the successful student will be able to do the following:

1. Briefly describe the functions of the sympathetic nervous system and the specific effects of adrenergic stimulation.

2. List the various drugs classified as adrenergic agonists or sympathomimetics.

3. Discuss the mechanisms of action, therapeutic effects, indications, adverse and toxic effects, cautions, contraindications, interactions, and available antidotes to overdosage of the adrenergic agonists or sympathomimetics.

4. Develop a collaborative plan of care that includes all phases of the nursing process for patients taking adrenergic agonists.

e-Learning Activities

Website
(http://evolve.elsevier.com/Canada/Lilley/pharmacology/)

evolve

- Answer Key—Textbook Case Studies
- Answer Key—Critical Thinking Activities
- Chapter Summaries—Printable
- Review Questions for Exam Preparation
- Unfolding Case Studies

Drug Profiles

▸▸ dobutamine (dobutamine hydrochloride)*, p. 385
▸▸ dopamine (dopamine hydrochloride)*, p. 385
▸▸ epinephrine (epinephrine hydrochloride)*, p. 385
   midodrine, p. 385
▸▸ norepinephrine (norepinephrine bitartrate)*, p. 386
   phenylephrine hydrochloride, p. 386

▸▸ Key drug

*Full generic name is given in parentheses. For the purposes of this text, the more common, shortened name is used.

Key Terms

Adrenergic agonists Drugs that stimulate and mimic the actions of the sympathetic nervous system; also called *sympathomimetics*. (p. 379)

Adrenergic receptors Receptor sites for the sympathetic neurotransmitters norepinephrine and epinephrine. (p. 380)

α-Adrenergic receptors A class of adrenergic receptors that is further subdivided into α_1- and α_2-receptors; α_1- and α_2-receptors exist postsynaptically, and α_2-receptors also

exist presynaptically. Both types are differentiated by their anatomical location in the tissues, muscles, and organs regulated by specific autonomic nerve fibres. (p. 380)

Autonomic functions Bodily functions that are involuntary and result from the physiological activity of the autonomic nervous system. The functions often occur in pairs of opposing actions between the sympathetic and parasympathetic divisions of the autonomic nervous system. (p. 379)

Autonomic nervous system   A branch of the peripheral nervous system that controls autonomic bodily functions; it consists of the sympathetic and parasympathetic nervous systems. (p. 379)

β-adrenergic receptors   A class of adrenergic receptors that is further subdivided into β_1- and β_2-receptors; located on postsynaptic cells that are stimulated by specific autonomic nerve fibres; β_1-adrenergic receptors are located primarily in the heart, whereas β_2-adrenergic receptors are located in the smooth muscle fibres of the bronchioles, arterioles, and visceral organs. (p. 380)

Catecholamines   Substances that can produce a sympathomimetic response; either endogenous catecholamines (such as epinephrine, norepinephrine, and dopamine) or synthetic catecholamine drugs (such as dobutamine). (p. 379)

Dopaminergic receptor   A third type of adrenergic receptor (in addition to α-adrenergic and β-adrenergic receptors); located in various tissues and organs and activated by the binding of the neurotransmitter dopamine, which can be either endogenous or a synthetic drug form. (p. 380)

Mydriasis   Pupillary dilation, whether natural (physiological) or drug induced. (p. 383)

Ophthalmics   Drugs that are used in the eye. (p. 383)

Positive chronotropic effect   An increase in heart rate. (p. 383)

Positive dromotropic effect   An increase in the conduction of cardiac electrical impulses through the atrioventricular node, which results in the transfer of nerve action potentials from the atria to the ventricles; ultimately leads to a systolic heartbeat (ventricular contractions). (p. 383)

Positive inotropic effect   An increase in the force of contraction of the heart muscle (myocardium). (p. 383)

Sympathomimetics   Drugs used therapeutically that mimic the catecholamines epinephrine, norepinephrine, and dopamine; also called *adrenergic agonists*. (p. 379)

Synaptic cleft   The space between either two adjacent nerve cell membranes or a nerve cell membrane and an effector organ cell membrane (also called a *synapse*). This space is bordered by the presynaptic cleft, from which neurotransmitters are generally released, and the postsynaptic cleft, on which neurotransmitters generally act. (p. 380)

OVERVIEW

The body's nervous system is divided into two major branches: the central nervous system (CNS) and the peripheral nervous system (PNS; Figure 19-1). The CNS contains the brain and the spinal cord. The PNS is further subdivided into the somatic and autonomic nervous systems. The autonomic nervous system (ANS) is yet further subdivided into the parasympathetic (cholinergic) and the sympathetic (adrenergic) nervous systems. Understanding the ANS and its subclasses is critical in the study of pharmacology, as numerous drugs act in these systems. This chapter will focus on the adrenergic nervous system and related compounds.

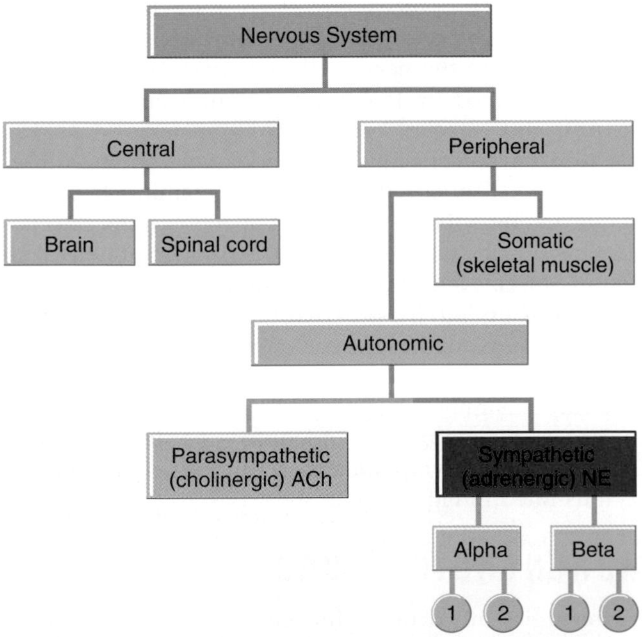

Adrenergic compounds include several exogenous (synthetic) and endogenous (naturally produced in the body) substances. They have a wide variety of therapeutic uses, depending on their site of action and their effect on different types of adrenergic receptors. Adrenergics stimulate the sympathetic nervous system (SNS) and are also called *adrenergic agonists*. They are also known as *sympathomimetics* because they mimic the effects of the SNS neurotransmitters norepinephrine, epinephrine, and dopamine. These three neurotransmitters are chemically classified as *catecholamines*. In considering the adrenergic class of medications, it is helpful to understand how the SNS operates in relation to the rest of the nervous system.

SYMPATHETIC NERVOUS SYSTEM

Figure 19-1 depicts the divisions of the nervous system and shows the relationship of the SNS to the entire nervous system. The SNS is the counterpart to the parasympathetic nervous system—together they make up the **autonomic nervous system.** They provide a check-and-balance system for maintaining the normal homeostasis of the **autonomic functions** of the human body.

There are receptor sites for the catecholamines norepinephrine and epinephrine throughout the body. These

FIG. 19-1   The sympathetic nervous system in relation to the entire nervous system. *ACh*, acetylcholine; *NE*, norepinephrine.

are referred to as **adrenergic receptors.** It is these receptor sites where adrenergic drugs bind and produce their effects. Many physiological responses are produced when they are stimulated or blocked. Adrenergic receptors are further divided into **α-adrenergic receptors** and **β-adrenergic receptors,** depending on the specific physiological responses caused by their stimulation. Both types of adrenergic receptors have subtypes (designated 1 and 2), which provide a further means of checks and balances that control stimulation and blockade, vasoconstriction and vasodilation of blood vessels, and the increased and decreased production of various substances. The α_1- and α_2-adrenergic receptors are differentiated by their location relative to nerves. The α_1-adrenergic receptors are located on postsynaptic effector cells (the tissue, muscle, or organ that the nerve stimulates). The α_2-adrenergic receptors are located on the presynaptic nerve terminals. They control the release of neurotransmitters. The predominant α-adrenergic agonist response is vasoconstriction and CNS stimulation.

The β-adrenergic receptors are all located on postsynaptic effector cells. The β_1-adrenergic receptors are located primarily in the heart (a useful mnemonic to help remember this: β_1—the *body* has *1* heart); the β_2-adrenergic receptors are located in the smooth muscle fibres of the bronchioles (a complementary mnemonic: β_2—the *body* has *2* lungs), arterioles, and visceral organs. A β-adrenergic agonist response results in bronchial, gastrointestinal (GI), and uterine smooth muscle relaxation; glycogenolysis; and heart stimulation. Table 19-1 provides a more detailed listing of the adrenergic receptors and the responses elicited when they are stimulated by a neurotransmitter or a drug that acts like a neurotransmitter (Figure 19-2).

Another type of adrenergic receptor is the **dopaminergic receptor.** When stimulated by dopamine, these receptors cause the vessels of the renal, mesenteric, coronary, and cerebral arteries to dilate, which increases blood flow to these tissues. Dopamine is the only substance that can stimulate these receptors. Catecholamine neurotransmitters are produced by the SNS and are stored in vesicles located at the ends of nerves. When a nerve is stimulated, the vesicles move to the walls of the nerve endings and release their contents into the space between the nerve ending and the effector organ, known as the *synaptic cleft* or *synapse.* The released contents of the vesicle (catecholamines) then have the opportunity to bind to the receptor sites located along the effector organ (see Figure 19-2). Once the neurotransmitter binds to the receptors, the effector organ responds. The sympathetic branch of the ANS is often described as having a "fight-or-flight" function because it allows the body to respond in a self-protective manner to dangerous situations. Depending on the function of the particular organ, this response involves muscle contraction (e.g., skeletal muscles) or relaxation (e.g., smooth muscles in the GI system and airway), an increased heart rate, the increased production of one or more substances (e.g., stress hormones), or blood vessel

TABLE 19-1

Adrenergic Receptor Responses to Stimulation

Location	Receptor	Response
CARDIOVASCULAR		
Blood vessels	α_1	Vasoconstriction
	β_2	Vasodilation
Heart muscle	β_1	Increased contractility
Atrioventricular node	β_1	Increased heart rate
Sinoatrial node	β_1	Increased heart rate
ENDOCRINE		
Kidney	β_2	Increased renin secretion
Liver	β_2	Glycogenolysis
GASTROINTESTINAL		
Muscle	α_1, β_2	Decreased motility (relaxation of gastrointestinal smooth muscle)
GENITOURINARY		
Bladder sphincter	α_1	Constriction
Penis	α_1	Ejaculation
Uterus	α_1	Contraction
	β_2	Relaxation
RESPIRATORY		
Bronchial muscles	β_2	Dilation (relaxation of bronchial smooth muscles)
Pupillary muscles of iris	α_1	Mydriasis (dilated pupils)

constriction. This process is halted by the action of specific enzymes and by reuptake of the neurotransmitter molecules back into the nerve cell (neuron). Catecholamines are metabolized by two enzymes, monoamine oxidase (MAO) and catechol ortho-methyltransferase (COMT). Each enzyme breaks down catecholamines but in a different area. MAO breaks down the catecholamines inside the nerve ending, whereas COMT breaks down the catecholamines outside the nerve ending, at the synaptic cleft (see Figure 19-2). Neurotransmitter molecules may also be taken back up into the presynaptic nerve fibre by various protein pumps within the cell membrane. This phenomenon is known as *active transport.* This reuptake restores the catecholamine to the vesicle and provides another means of maintaining an adequate supply of the substance for future sympathetic nerve impulses. This process is illustrated in Figure 19-2.

ADRENERGIC DRUGS

Adrenergics are drugs with effects that are similar to or mimic the effects of the SNS neurotransmitters norepinephrine, epinephrine, and dopamine (collectively referred to as *catecholamines*). Catecholamines produce a

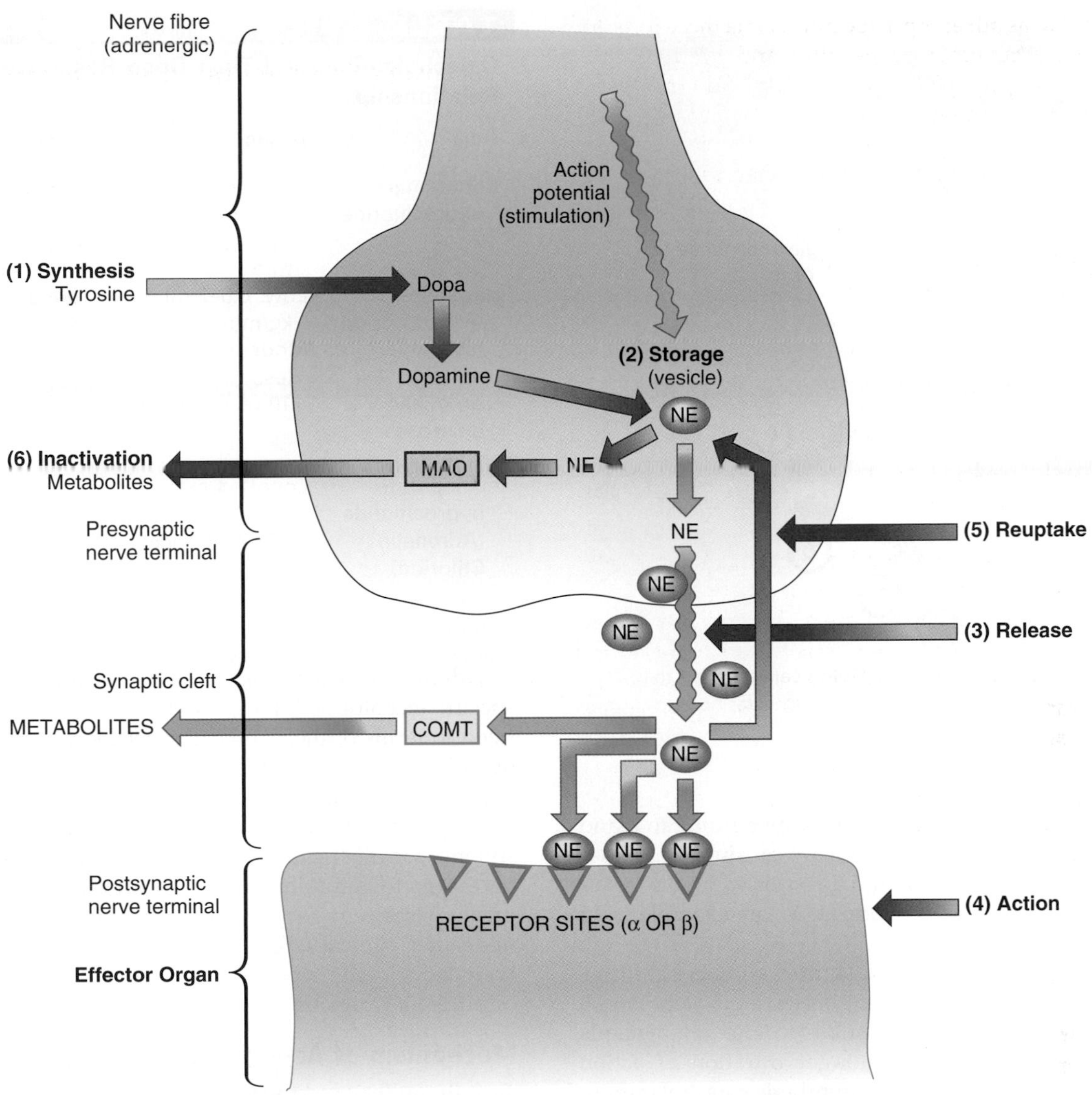

Nerve fibre
(adrenergic)

Action
potential
(stimulation)

(1) Synthesis
Tyrosine → Dopa

Dopamine

(2) Storage
(vesicle)
NE

(6) Inactivation
Metabolites ← MAO ← NE

NE

Presynaptic
nerve terminal

NE ← **(5) Reuptake**

NE

NE ← **(3) Release**

NE

Synaptic cleft

METABOLITES ← COMT ←

NE

Postsynaptic
nerve terminal

NE NE NE

RECEPTOR SITES (α OR β) ← **(4) Action**

Effector Organ

FIG. 19-2 Mechanism by which stimulation of a nerve fibre results in a physiological process; adrenergic drugs mimic this same process. *COMT*, catechol ortho-methytransferase; *MAO*, monoamine oxidase; *NE*, norepinephrine.

sympathomimetic response. They are either endogenous substances such as epinephrine, norepinephrine, and dopamine or synthetic substances such as dobutamine and phenylephrine hydrochloride. The three endogenous catecholamines are also available in synthetic drug form.

Catecholamine drugs that are used therapeutically produce the same result as endogenous catecholamines. When any of the adrenergic drugs is given, it bathes the area between the nerve and the effector cell (i.e., the synaptic cleft). Once there, the drug has the opportunity to induce a response. This can be accomplished in one of three ways: by direct stimulation, by indirect stimulation, or by a combination of the two (mixed-acting).

A direct-acting sympathomimetic binds directly to the receptor and causes a physiological response (Figure 19-3). Epinephrine is an example of such a drug. An indirect-acting sympathomimetic causes the release of

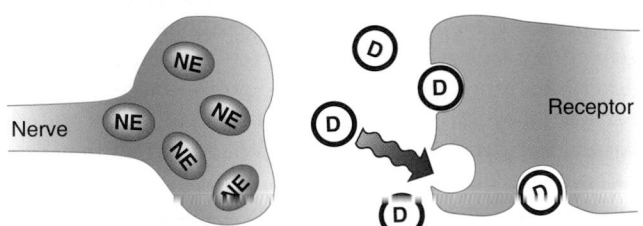

FIG. 19-3 Mechanism of physiological response to direct-acting sympathomimetics. *D*, drug; *NE*, norepinephrine.

catecholamine from the storage sites (vesicles) in the nerve endings; it then binds to the receptors and causes a physiological response (Figure 19-4). Amphetamines and other related anorexiants (see Chapter 14) are examples of such drugs. A mixed-acting sympathomimetic

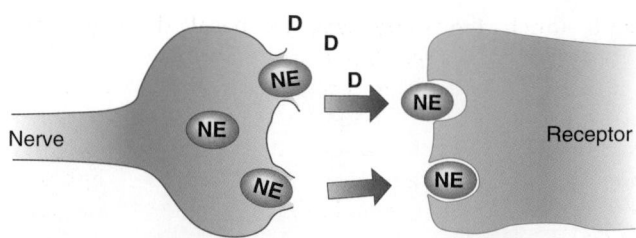

FIG. 19-4 Mechanism of physiological response to indirect-acting sympathomimetics. *D*, drug; *NE*, norepinephrine.

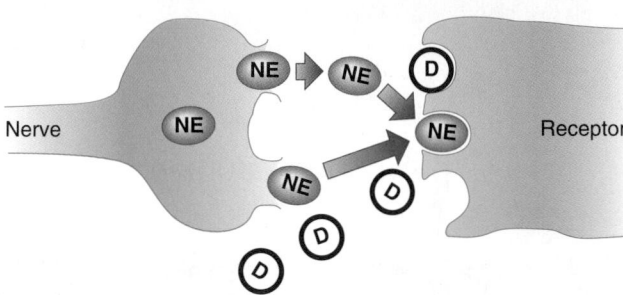

FIG. 19-5 Mechanism of physiological response to mixed-acting sympathomimetics. *D*, drug; *NE*, norepinephrine.

TABLE 19-2

Catecholamines and Their Dose–Response Relationship

Drug	Dosage	Receptor
dobutamine hydrochloride	Maintenance: 2–15 mcg/kg/min	β_1 more than β_2
	High: 40 mcg/kg/min	β_2 more than α_1
dopamine hydrochloride (available only in premixed 5% dextrose solution)	Low: 0.5–2 mcg/kg/min	Dopaminergic β_1
	Moderate: 2–4 or less than 10 mcg/kg/min	
epinephrine hydrochloride (Adrenalin Chloride)	Low: 1–4 mcg/min	β_1 more than β_2 and α_1
	High: 4–40 mcg/min	α_1 more than or equal to β_1

both directly stimulates the receptor by binding to it and indirectly stimulates the receptor by causing the release of the neurotransmitter stored in vesicles at the nerve endings (Figure 19-5). Ephedrine is an example of a mixed-acting adrenergic drug.

There are also noncatecholamine adrenergic drugs such as phenylephrine hydrochloride and salbutamol. These are structurally dissimilar to the endogenous catecholamines and have a longer duration of action than either the endogenous or synthetic catecholamines. The noncatecholamine drugs show similar patterns of activity.

Adrenergic agents can also be classified as either selective or nonselective in their actions. For example, phenylephrine is considered a selective agonist, meaning it only affects one receptor subtype (α-1). Epinephrine and norepinephrine are considered nonselective agonists because they have action at both α- and β-receptors. Adrenergic drugs can act at different types of adrenergic receptors depending on the amount of drug administered. For example, dopamine may produce dopaminergic, β_1, or α_1 effects, depending on the dose given. See Table 19-2 for other examples of catecholamines and the dose-specific selectivity.

Although adrenergics work primarily at postganglionic receptors (the receptors that immediately innervate the effector organ, gland, or muscle) peripherally, they may also work more centrally in the nervous system at the preganglionic sympathetic nerve trunks. Their ability to do so depends on the potency of the specific drug and the dose used.

Adrenergic drugs are classified technically by their specific receptor activities, but they may also be categorized in terms of their clinical effects. For example, phenylephrine hydrochloride is both an α_1-agonist and a vasopressive drug (pressor), whereas salbutamol is both a β_2-agonist and a bronchodilator. Both classifications are suitable for most clinical purposes. Clinically, it may be necessary to carefully choose an adrenergic drug with greater selectivity for a particular receptor type to avoid undesired clinical effects. In such a situation, detailed knowledge of the type and degree of receptor selectivity of different drugs becomes important.

Mechanism of Action and Drug Effects

To fully understand the mechanism of action of adrenergics, one must have a working knowledge of normal adrenergic transmission. This transmission takes place at the junction between the nerve (postganglionic sympathetic neuron) and the receptor site of the innervated organ or tissue (effector). The process of SNS stimulation is illustrated in Figure 19-2 and was discussed earlier in this chapter. When adrenergic drugs stimulate α_1-adrenergic receptor sites located on smooth muscles, vasoconstriction usually occurs. Binding to these α_1-adrenergic receptors can also cause the relaxation of gastrointestinal smooth muscle, contraction of the uterus and bladder sphincter, male ejaculation, and contraction of the ciliary muscles of the eye, which causes the pupils to dilate (see Table 19-1). Stimulation of α_2-adrenergic receptors, by contrast, actually tends to reverse sympathetic activity, but this action is not of great significance either physiologically or pharmacologically.

There are β_1-adrenergic receptors on the myocardium and in the conduction system of the heart, including the sinoatrial node and the atrioventricular node. When these β_1-adrenergic receptors are stimulated by an adrenergic drug, three effects result: (1) an increased force of contraction (**positive inotropic effect**), (2) an increase in heart rate (**positive chronotropic effect**), and (3) an increase in the conduction of cardiac electrical nerve impulses through the atrioventricular node (**positive dromotropic effect**). In addition, stimulation of β_1-receptors in the kidney causes an increase in renin secretion. Activation of β_2-adrenergic receptors produces relaxation of the bronchi (bronchodilation) and uterus and also causes increased glycogenolysis (glucose release) from the liver (see Table 19-1).

Indications

Adrenergics, or sympathomimetics, are used in the treatment of a wide variety of illnesses and conditions. Their selectivity for either α or β adrenergic receptors and their affinity for certain tissues or organs determine the settings in which they are most commonly used. Some adrenergics are used as adjuncts to dietary changes in the short-term treatment of obesity. These drugs are discussed in greater detail in Chapter 14.

Respiratory Indications

Bronchodilators are adrenergic drugs that have an affinity for the adrenergic receptors located in the respiratory system. Bronchodilators tend to preferentially stimulate the β_2-adrenergic receptors rather than the α-adrenergic receptors and cause bronchodilation. Of the two subtypes of β-adrenergic receptors, these drugs are attracted more to the β_2-adrenergic receptors, located on the bronchial, uterine, and vascular smooth muscles, and less so to the β_1-adrenergic receptors, located on the heart. The β_2-agonists are helpful in treating conditions such as asthma, bronchitis, and anaphylaxis. Common bronchodilators that are classified as predominantly β_2-selective adrenergic drugs include formoterol fumarate dihydrate, salbutamol, salmeterol xinafoate, and terbutaline sulphate. These drugs are discussed in more detail in Chapter 38. At low doses, epinephrine can selectively stimulate β_2-receptors, producing muscle relaxation and a decrease in peripheral resistance. However, once epinephrine concentrations that bind to the α_1-receptor are reached, vasoconstriction will occur.

Indications for Topical Nasal Decongestants

The intranasal application of certain adrenergics can cause the constriction of dilated arterioles and a reduction in nasal blood flow, which then decreases congestion. These adrenergic drugs work by stimulating α_1-adrenergic receptors and have little or no effect on β-adrenergic receptors. The nasal decongestants include oxymetazoline hydrochloride, xylometazoline hydrochloride, and phenylephrine hydrochloride. They are discussed in more detail in Chapter 38.

Ophthalmic Indications

Some adrenergics are applied to the surface of the eye. These drugs are called **ophthalmics**. Ophthalmics work much the same way as nasal decongestants except that they affect the vasculature of the eye. They stimulate α-adrenergic receptors located on small arterioles in the eye and temporarily relieve conjunctival congestion by causing arteriolar vasoconstriction. The ophthalmic adrenergics include epinephrine, naphazoline hydrochloride, phenylephrine hydrochloride, and tetrahydrozoline.

Adrenergics can also be used to reduce intraocular pressure, which makes them useful in the treatment of open-angle glaucoma. They can also dilate the pupils (**mydriasis**); both of these properties make them useful for diagnostic eye examinations. Adrenergics produce these effects by stimulating α- or β_2-adrenergic receptors, or both. The adrenergic used for this purpose is dipivefrin hydrochloride. Ophthalmic adrenergic drugs are discussed in more detail in Chapter 57.

Cardiovascular Indications

The final group of adrenergic agents is used to support the cardiovascular system during heart failure or shock. These drugs are referred to as *vasoactive sympathomimetics*, *vasoconstrictive drugs* (also known as *vasopressive drugs*, *pressor drugs*, or *pressors*), *inotropes*, or *cardioselective sympathomimetics*. They have a variety of effects on the various α- and β-adrenergic receptors, and the effects can be related to the specific dose of the adrenergic drug. Common vasoactive adrenergic drugs include dobutamine, dopamine, epinephrine, midodrine hydrochloride, norepinephrine, and phenylephrine hydrochloride.

Contraindications

The only usual contraindications to the use of adrenergic drugs are known drug allergy and severe hypertension.

It is important to note that a common medication error is confusion between norepinephrine bitartrate and the brand name for phenylephrine hydrochloride, Neo-Synephrine®. These drugs are often both ordered for a patient at the same time, and, because the names sound alike, the wrong drug may be given. To avoid this confusion, pharmacies list these drugs by their trade names as well: norepinephrine bitartrate is called Levophed® and phenylephrine hydrochloride is called Neo-Synephrine.

Adverse Effects

Unwanted CNS effects of the adrenergic drugs include headache, restlessness, tremors, nervousness, dizziness, insomnia, and euphoria. Possible cardiovascular adverse effects include chest pain, vasoconstriction, hypertension, tachycardia (positive chronotropy), fluctuations in blood pressure, and palpitations or dysrhythmias. Effects on other body systems include anorexia, dry mouth, nausea, vomiting, and, rarely, taste changes. Adrenergics administered as ophthalmics or by nebulizer can have systemic effects. Other significant effects include sweating, nausea, vomiting,

SPECIAL POPULATIONS: OLDER ADULTS

Use of β-Adrenergic Agonists

- Several physiological changes occur in the cardiovascular system of older adults, including a decline in the efficiency and contractile ability of the heart muscle, a decrease in cardiac output, and diminished stroke volume. In most cases, older adults adjust to these changes without too much difficulty; however, if unusual demands are placed on the aging heart, problems and complications may arise. Examples of unusual demands include strenuous activities, excess stress, heat, and medication use. For instance, stress, heat, and use of β-adrenergic agonists may lead to significant increases in blood pressure and pulse rate. Older adults may then react negatively, with a diminished ability to compensate adequately for these changes.
- Baroreceptors do not work as effectively in older adults. Reduced baroreceptor activity may lead to orthostatic hypotension, even without the impact of certain medications and their associated mechanism of action or adverse effects.

- Because of the possible presence of concurrent medical conditions (e.g., hypertension, peripheral vascular disease, and cardiovascular disease or cerebrovascular disease), monitor older adults carefully before, during, and after administration of adrenergic drugs.
- Advise older adult patients that any occurrence of chest pain, palpitations, headache, or seizures must be reported immediately to the health care provider (HCP), or emergency care should be accessed.
- Caution patients about the use of over-the-counter (OTC) drugs, natural health products, and other medications. This caution is due to possible drug–drug interactions as well as older adults' increased sensitivity to many drugs and other chemicals.
- Older adults may have decreased motor function and cognitive decline. Therefore, use additional equipment and certain facilitating aids (e.g., walkers, reachers, computer adaptations), and provide detailed instructions to help ensure proper dosing of medications.

and muscle cramps. See Special Populations: Older Adults—Use of β-Adrenergic Agonists box above for additional information.

Toxicity and Management of Overdose

The toxic effects of adrenergic drugs are an extension of their common adverse effects (e.g., seizures from excessive CNS stimulation, hypotension or hypertension, dysrhythmias, palpitation, nervousness, dizziness, fatigue, malaise, insomnia, headache, tremor, dry mouth, and nausea). The two most life-threatening toxic effects involve the CNS and cardiovascular system. The first is seizures, which in the acute setting can be effectively managed with diazepam. The second, intracranial bleeding, occurs as the result of an extreme elevation in blood pressure. Such elevated blood pressure increases the risk of hemorrhage not only in the brain but elsewhere in the body as well. The most effective treatment in this situation is to lower the blood pressure using a rapid-acting sympatholytic (e.g., esmolol; see Chapter 20). This can directly reverse the adrenergic-induced state.

The majority of adrenergic compounds have extremely short half-lives, and thus their effects are transient. Therefore, when these drugs are taken in an overdose or toxicity develops, stopping the drug causes the toxic symptoms to subside in a relatively short period of time. The recommended treatment for overdose is often managing the symptoms and supporting the patient. If death occurs, it is usually the result of either respiratory failure or cardiac arrest. The treatment of overdose is therefore aimed at supporting the respiratory and cardiac systems.

Interactions

Numerous drug interactions can occur with adrenergic drugs. Although many of the interactions result in a diminished adrenergic effect because of direct antagonism at and competition for receptor sites, as in the concurrent use of adrenergic antagonists (e.g., for hypertension) and adrenergics, some reactions can be life threatening. The following are some of the more serious drug–drug interactions involving adrenergic drugs. Administration of adrenergics with anaesthetic drugs or digoxin (see Chapter 12) can increase the risk of cardiac dysrhythmias. Tricyclic antidepressants (see Chapter 17), when given with adrenergics, can cause increased vasopressor effects and acute hypertensive crisis. Administration of adrenergic drugs with MOAIs may cause a possibly life-threatening hypertensive crisis (see Chapter 17). Antihistamines (see Chapter 37) and thyroid preparations (see Chapter 32) can also increase the effects of adrenergic drugs.

Laboratory Test Interactions

The α-adrenergic drugs can cause an increase in the serum levels of endogenous corticotropin (i.e., adrenocorticotropic hormone), corticosteroids, and glucose. Therefore, the results of laboratory tests for these substances need to be interpreted with caution in patients receiving any of these medications.

Dosages

For dosage information on various adrenergic drugs, see the table on p. 386.

DRUG PROFILES

The four frequently used classes of adrenergic drugs are the bronchodilators (Chapter 38), ophthalmic drugs (Chapter 57), nasal decongestants (Chapter 37), and vasoactive drugs, which are emphasized in this Drug Profile and in Chapter 25. The receptor selectivity for the α_1-, β_1-, and β_2-receptor subtypes is relative, as opposed to absolute. Thus, there may be some overlap of drug effects between the different adrenergic classes of drugs, especially at higher dosages. In contrast, dopamine receptors are more specific for dopamine itself or for specific dopaminergic drugs.

VASOACTIVE ADRENERGICS

Adrenergics used to support the cardiovascular system (e.g., a failing heart or shock) or to treat orthostatic hypotension are referred to as *vasoactive adrenergics*. The vasoactive adrenergics are potent, quick-acting, injectable drugs. Although dosage recommendations are provided in the table on p. 386, all of these drugs are titrated to the desired physiological response. For this reason, dosages for children are not given in the table. All of the vasoactive adrenergics (with the exception of midodrine) are rapid in onset, and their effects quickly cease when administration is stopped. Therefore, careful titration and monitoring of vital signs and electrocardiogram (ECG) are required.

dobutamine hydrochloride

Dobutamine hydrochloride is a β_1-selective vasoactive adrenergic drug that is structurally similar to the naturally occurring catecholamine dopamine. Through stimulation of the β_1-receptors on heart muscle (myocardium), it increases cardiac output by increasing contractility (positive inotropy), which increases the stroke volume, especially in patients with heart failure. Dobutamine is available only as an intravenous drug and is given by continuous infusion (see Dosages table on p. 386).

PHARMACOKINETICS

Route	Onset of Action	Peak Plasma Concentration	Elimination Half-Life	Duration of Action
IV	Less than 2 min	Less than 10 min	2–5 min	Less than 10 min

dopamine hydrochloride

Dopamine hydrochloride is a naturally occurring catecholamine neurotransmitter. It has potent dopaminergic as well as β_1- and α_1-adrenergic receptor activity, depending on the dosage. When used at low doses, dopamine can dilate blood vessels in the brain, heart, kidneys, and mesentery, which increases blood flow to these areas (dopaminergic receptor activity). For example, dopamine is used to maintain blood pressure in organs to be used for transplantation. At higher infusion rates, dopamine can improve heart contractility and output (β_1-adrenergic receptor activity). At highest doses, dopamine causes vasoconstriction (α_1-adrenergic receptor activity). Use of dopamine is contraindicated in patients who have a

catecholamine-secreting tumour of the adrenal gland known as a *pheochromocytoma*. The drug is available only as a 5% dextrose solution and is given by continuous infusion. (see Dosages table on p. 386).

PHARMACOKINETICS

Route	Onset of Action	Peak Plasma Concentration	Elimination Half-Life	Duration of Action
IV	2–5 min	Rapid	Less than 2 min	10 min

epinephrine hydrochloride

Epinephrine hydrochloride (Adrenalin®) is also an endogenous vasoactive catecholamine. It acts directly on both the α- and β-adrenergic receptors of tissues innervated by the SNS. It is considered the prototypical nonselective adrenergic agonist. Epinephrine is administered in emergency situations and is one of the primary vasoactive drugs used in many advanced cardiac life support protocols. The physiological response it elicits is dose related. At low dosages, it stimulates primarily β_1-adrenergic receptors, increasing the force of contraction and heart rate. It is also used to treat acute asthma (see Chapter 38) and anaphylactic shock because it has significant bronchodilatory effects via the β_2-adrenergic receptors in the lungs. In patients with anaphylaxis, epinephrine has potent, life-saving α_1-adrenergic vasoconstrictor effects. As a result of the vasoconstriction, mucosal edema is reduced, which prevents and relieves upper airway obstruction and increases blood pressure. Consequently, shock is prevented and relieved. The β_1-adrenergic effects lead to an increased rate and force of cardiac contractions. β_2 effects result in increased bronchodilation and decreased release of histamine, as well as other mediators of inflammation from mast cells and basophils. At high dosages (e.g., when given intravenously), epinephrine stimulates primarily α-adrenergic receptors, causing vasoconstriction, which elevates the blood pressure (see Dosages table on p. 386).

PHARMACOKINETICS

Route	Onset of Action	Peak Plasma Concentration	Elimination Half-Life	Duration of Action
Subcut	5–10 min	20 min	Variable	Unknown
IV	Less than 2 min	Rapid	Less than 5 min	5–30 min

midodrine hydrochloride

Midodrine hydrochloride is a prodrug (pharmacologically inactive form of the drug) that is converted metabolically in the liver to its active form, desglymidodrine. This active metabolite is responsible for the primary pharmacological action of midodrine hydrochloride, which is α_1-adrenergic receptor stimulation. This α_1 stimulation increases the vascular tone of both arterioles and veins, resulting in peripheral vasoconstriction and increased systemic vascular resistance. Midodrine hydrochloride is primarily indicated for the treatment of symptomatic orthostatic

Continued

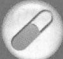 **DRUG PROFILES—cont'd**

hypotension. Midodrine hydrochloride is available as 2.5- and 5-mg tablets (see the Dosages table below). Midodrine hydrochloride is usually given two to three times per day. The last dose of the day should not be given after 1800 hours to prevent supine hypertension.

PHARMACOKINETICS

Route	Onset of Action	Peak Plasma Concentration	Elimination Half-Life	Duration of Action
PO	45–90 min	1 hr	More than 3–4 hr	6–8 hr

norepinephrine bitartrate

Norepinephrine bitartrate (Levophed) acts predominantly by directly stimulating α-adrenergic receptors, which leads to vasoconstriction. It also has some direct-stimulating β-adrenergic effects on the heart (β₁-adrenergic receptors) but none on the lung (β₂-adrenergic receptors). Norepinephrine is directly metabolized to dopamine and is used primarily in the treatment of hypotension and shock. It is given only by continuous infusion (see Dosages table).

PHARMACOKINETICS

Route	Onset of Action	Peak Plasma Concentration	Elimination Half-Life	Duration of Action
IV	Rapid	1–2 min	Less than 5 min	1–2 min

▶▶phenylephrine hydrochloride

Phenylephrine hydrochloride (Neo-Synephrine) works almost exclusively on the α-adrenergic receptors. It is used primarily for short-term treatment to raise blood pressure in patients in shock, to control specific dysrhythmias (supraventricular tachycardias), and to produce vasoconstriction in regional anaesthesia. It is also administered topically as an ophthalmic drug (see Chapter 57) and in some nasal decongestants (see Chapter 37; see Dosages table).

PHARMACOKINETICS

Route	Onset of Action	Peak Plasma Concentration	Elimination Half-Life	Duration of Action
IV	Rapid	Rapid	Less than 5 min	15–20 min

DOSAGES Selected Vasoactive Adrenergics

Drug	Pharmacological Class	Usual Dosage Range	Indications
▶▶dobutamine hydrochloride	β₁-adrenergic and dopaminergic	*Adults* IV infusion: 2.5–40 mcg/kg/min	Cardiac decompensation
▶▶dopamine hydrochloride (premixed ready-to-use solution)	β₁-adrenergic	*Adults* IV infusion: 2–50 mcg/kg/min	Shock syndrome, chronic cardiac decompensation
▶▶epinephrine hydrochloride (Adrenalin Chloride®)	α- and β-adrenergic	*Adults* IV: 1–4 mcg/min (β dose); more than 20 mcg/min dose titrated to effect (α dose)	β dose used to treat bradycardias, severe left ventricular dysfunction or anaphylaxis; α dose used to treat profound hypotension or pulseless cardiac arrest
midodrine hydrochloride	α₁-adrenergic	*Adults* PO: 10 mg tid, max 40 mg/day	Orthostatic hypotension
▶▶norepinephrine bitartrate (Levophed)	α- and β-adrenergic	*Adults* IV infusion: 2–30 mcg/min	Hypotensive states
phenylephrine hydrochloride (Neo-Synephrine)	α-adrenergic	*Adults* IV infusion: 10 mg/250 or 500 mL IV solution, start at 100–180 mcg/min and titrate down to 40–60 mcg/min IM/Subcut: 2–5 mg IV: 0.1–0.5 mg	Hypotension or shock

IM, intramuscular; *IV,* intravenous; *PO,* oral; *Subcut,* subcutaneous.

NURSING PROCESS

Assessment

Adrenergic agonist drugs have a variety of effects depending on the receptors they stimulate. Stimulation of the α-adrenergic receptors results in vasoconstriction. Stimulation of β_1-adrenergic receptors produces heart stimulation, and stimulation of the β_2-adrenergic receptors results in bronchodilation. Because of these properties, the use of adrenergic agonists requires careful patient assessment and monitoring to maximize therapeutic effects and minimize possible adverse effects. Focus assessment on a comprehensive health history, including past and present medical history. Include specific system-based questions, and identify cautions, contraindications, and drug interactions. Include the following health history questions in your assessment: (1) Medication history and allergies: What prescription medications do you regularly use (including self-administration of OTC drugs and natural health products)? Do you have allergies to any medication, foods, topical products, or environmental products? (2) Respiratory: Do you have a history of asthma and if so, how frequent and severe are the acute episodes? What factors exacerbate or help to alleviate asthma? Do you experience any other asthma-related symptoms such as dyspnea or chest pain? What treatments have you used for asthma and what have been their successes or failures? (3) Kidneys and liver: Do you have a history of kidney problems? Has anyone ever reported that your kidney or liver function studies are abnormal? Do you have a history of chronic kidney infections or any jaundice? (With altered kidney or liver function, there is the risk for altered excretion and metabolism of drugs, thus leading to possible toxicity.)

Performing a thorough head-to-toe physical assessment is also a significant part of data collection with adrenergic drugs. Thorough assessment of the cardiac system is important because the adrenergic agonist drugs may exacerbate pre-existing cardiac disorders. Baseline vital signs need to be thoroughly assessed with the use of adrenergic drugs; assess and document breath sounds, heart sounds, peripheral pulses, skin colour, and capillary refill. In addition to measurement of postural blood pressures and pulse rates, inquire about other relevant symptoms such as dizziness, lightheadedness, and syncope. Assessment of the patient's symptoms and the patient's perception of either disease progression or a decrease in symptoms is important for effective and successful treatment.

With other adrenergic drugs, such as those used for bronchodilating effects, perform a thorough respiratory assessment and document the patient's respiratory rate, rhythm, and depth, as well as the presence of normal or adventitious (abnormal) breath sounds. Ask about any reports of difficulty breathing or intolerance of activity or exercise. Assess and document pulse oximetry readings for oxygen saturation levels. Include in the assessment measurement of respiratory peak flow using a flow metre, as well as measurement of the anterior–posterior diameter of the chest wall. A decrease in peak flow readings may indicate bronchospasms, whereas an increased anterior–posterior chest wall diameter is seen in chronic lung disorders, such as chronic obstructive pulmonary disease. Health care providers may also order additional respiratory function studies such as measurement of arterial blood gas levels. Older adults and young patients may react with increased sensitivity to adrenergic drugs. In addition, some of these drugs are used only for acute episodes of asthma, whereas other drugs are used long term as preventative drugs. For example, the drugs salmeterol xinafoate (see Chapter 30) and formoterol fumarate are *not* used to treat acute asthmatic episodes, whereas salbutamol is indicated for treatment of acute episodes.

Epinephrine and similar drugs are used for their cardiac, bronchial, antiallergic, ocular, and vasopressor effects. Focus assessment on vital signs, breath sounds, arterial blood gas levels, and ECG findings, if ordered. Assess and document liver and kidney function test results. In addition, assess each system related to the specific action of the drug.

Overall, adrenergic drugs work in similar ways, but individual drugs may have some differences in actions, indications, and overall considerations. If the general class of drugs and the way in which they work is known, then the relative assessment parameters, cautions, contraindications, drug interactions, and lifespan considerations are easy to determine. If the drug is a pure adrenergic agonist, the net effect is stimulation of α-adrenergic receptors with vasoconstriction of blood vessels and subsequent elevation of blood pressure and heart rate; expect specific effects from the drug and anticipate certain adverse effects. The drug may be used for the therapeutic effect of increased blood pressure, but an unwanted adverse effect could be a hypertensive crisis. If the drug is a β-adrenergic agonist, it will stimulate both β_1- and β_2-receptors, which will lead to heart stimulation and bronchodilation. This β_1 action can also result in too much stimulation, with severe tachycardia and possibly chest pain if coronary artery disease is present. Thus, by knowing the actions of a given drug, it is possible to draw conclusions about, anticipate, and be alert to the drug's therapeutic actions, adverse effects, cautions, contraindications, drug interactions, and toxicity.

Nursing Diagnoses

- Impaired gas exchange related to asthma-induced bronchospasms
- Decreased cardiac output related to cardiovascular adverse effects of adrenergic agonist drugs
- Ineffective peripheral tissue perfusion related to intense vasoconstrictive reactions of medications

- Acute pain related to adverse effects of tachycardia and palpitations
- Disturbed sleep pattern related to CNS stimulation caused by adrenergic drugs
- Deficient knowledge of the therapeutic regimen, adverse effects, drug interactions, and precautions related to the use of adrenergic drugs
- Nonadherence with drug therapy related to lack of information about the importance of taking the medication as ordered
- Risk for injury related to possible adverse effects (nervousness, vertigo, hypertension, or tremors) or to potential drug interactions

▨ Planning

■ Goals

- Patient will experience normal patterns of gas exchange and maintain an open airway.
- Patient will maintain normal cardiac output status.
- Patient will display adequate peripheral vascular or tissue perfusion.
- Patient will experience relief of pain and increased levels of comfort.
- Patient will experience improved sleep patterns.
- Patient will demonstrate adequate knowledge about the use of specific medication.
- Patient will remain adherent to the drug therapy regimen and without drug-related complications.
- Patient will remain free from injury related to drug therapy.

■ Outcome Criteria

- Patient shows improvement in gas exchange and respiratory status with normal respiratory rate (12 to 20 breaths per minute), regular rhythm and depth, clearing breath sounds, and a normal pulse oximetry reading above 95%.
- Patient's blood pressure and pulse rate remain within normal limits (BP 120/80; pulse 60 to 100 beats per minute; mean arterial pressure (MAP) greater than 65).
- Patient's capillary refill is less than 3 seconds in fingers and toes.
- Patient's circulation in extremities remains intact.
- Patient's capillary refill is intact, with skin colour being pink and extremities warm to the touch.
- Patient's pedal pulse is intact and strong to palpation.
- Patient remains comfortable during drug therapy and takes medications exactly as prescribed.
- Patient remains free of increased heart rate and irregular heart rhythm.
- Patient uses relaxation therapy or massage and maintains healthy sleep patterns in a quiet, temperate room environment.
- Patient demonstrates proper use of drug therapy regimen and avoids overuse of medication, decreasing adverse effects.
- Patient states rationale for use of medications as well as timing, dosing, and scheduling of drug therapy.
- Patient states most common adverse effects of drug therapy.
- Patient states which adverse effects to report if they occur, such as chest pain, irregular heart rhythm,

◎ CASE STUDY

Dopamine Infusion

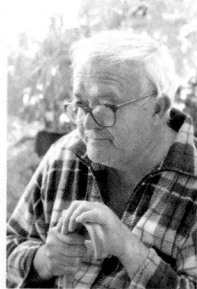

Janos, an 82-year-old retired real estate agent, is receiving dopamine at a dose of 5 mcg/kg/min via infusion pump for heart failure. He is being monitored by a cardiac monitor. He has a history of hypothyroidism and takes a daily dose of thyroid replacement hormone. Yesterday, Janos's vital signs were as follows:
Blood pressure: 150/88 mm Hg
Pulse rate: 92 beats/min
Respiration rate: 16 breaths/min

His heart rhythm showed sinus rhythm with rare ectopic beats. While at rest, he had no shortness of breath but did experience some dyspnea when getting up to the bedside commode. He has edema in his lower legs rated as 2+ edema.

1. Explain how this dose of dopamine works to help treat Janos's heart failure.

2. What would you expect to happen if the dose were set to 1 mcg/kg/min? 20 mcg/kg/min?

This morning, you make rounds and find that Janos's vital signs are as follows:
Blood pressure: 170/94 mm Hg
Pulse rate: 120 beats/min
Respiration rate: 22 breaths/min

The heart monitor shows sinus tachycardia with two to three ectopic beats per minute. Janos is reporting palpitations and some shortness of breath at rest but says, "I've felt this before when I've had bad spells with my heart. I'm sure it will pass."

3. Do you think there is a concern at this time? Explain your reasoning and what should be done.

4. The physician decides to titrate the dopamine infusion to 3 mcg/kg/min, which you do immediately. How quickly should you see a response from the patient to this decrease in dosage?

For answers, see http://evolve.elsevier.com/Canada/Lilley/pharmacology/.

dizziness, increased occurrence of palpitations, and overall feeling of discomfort, anxiety, or restlessness.

- Patient reports taking medication exactly as prescribed for maintenance or acute use and without adverse or toxic reactions.
- Patient remains free from self-injury as related to safe and as-prescribed self-administration of drug therapy.

Implementation

Many of the drugs discussed in this chapter are often only administered in specialty care areas, such as critical care units or the emergency department. Always refer to agency-specific protocols for administration of adrenergic drugs. There are several nursing interventions that may maximize the therapeutic effects of adrenergic drugs and minimize their adverse effects. These interventions include checking the package inserts concerning dilutional solutions to ensure compatibility with parenteral dosage forms. For example, subcutaneous administration of the adrenergic agonist epinephrine for patients with asthma requires careful calculations and accurate dosing to ensure safety. A tuberculin syringe used with subcutaneous epinephrine may be used to help with accurate dosing for both adults and children.

Use of epinephrine and some of the other pure α-adrenergics may not be indicated for shock-related symptoms because these drugs lead to vasoconstriction of the renal vessels and potential kidney damage or shutdown. Therefore, when a patient is in shock and requires medications, norepinephrine is generally the drug of choice. Norepinephrine is used because in specific dosage ranges, it helps treat a shock-related syndrome through its ability to produce vasoconstriction of peripheral blood vessels and increase blood pressure without vasoconstriction of the renal vasculature. This lack of renal vasculature vasoconstriction helps improve perfusion through the kidneys and thus salvages the kidneys (while increasing blood pressure). With administration of norepinephrine and similar drugs, check the intravenous site frequently (e.g., every hour, as needed) to be sure that the site remains intact and that the drug is being infused at the proper rate. Phentolamine mesylate is often used for the treatment of infiltration (see Chapter 20). Also, with intravenous infusions, use only clear solutions and a proper dilutional solution, always administer the drug with an intravenous infusion pump, and closely monitor the cardiac system (through attention to vital signs, heart sounds, or ECG monitoring). For example, patients receiving drugs such as dopamine and dobutamine by intravenous infusion would be on a cardiac monitor and require frequent nursing assessments. Give all of these drugs per the manufacturer's directions and at suggested infusion rates to avoid precipitating dangerously high blood pressure and pulse rate and subsequent complications. (See Legal & Ethical Principles regarding issues

that can arise with incorrect intravenous infusions causing infiltration.)

When adrenergics are administered via an inhaler or nebulizer, provide the patient with complete, thorough, and age-appropriate instructions about the correct use, storage, and care of equipment. Instruct the patient on how to use a spacer correctly, as use of this device with the inhaler is often ordered. A spacer provides more effective delivery of inhaled doses of drugs (see Patient Teaching Tips as well as Chapter 7). When the adrenergics are dosed for bronchodilating effects, often two adrenergics are prescribed. This is because different medications are associated with different pharmacokinetics and actions. One inhaler may be for use in acute situations, and the other may be for long-term and preventative use. With this type of treatment regimen, the patient needs to receive thorough, simple, and complete instructions and explanations about the method of delivery and about the drugs used. This will help to minimize risk of overdosage and reduce potential severe adverse effects such as hypertension, severe tachycardia, tremors, and CNS overstimulation.

Emphasize in patient teaching that adrenergic medications are to be used only as prescribed in regard to amount, timing, and spacing of doses. Because of their synergistic effects, when adrenergic medications are used in combination with other types of bronchodilators (especially in patients with asthma), the patient must be clear about what to do before, during, and after the dose is delivered. If the patient is taking an inhaled dosage form, an oral or parenteral form of a drug of the same class or a similar drug may also be prescribed. The reason for the use of more than one drug of the same drug class, and the use of more than one route of administration, is to achieve combined therapeutic effects. In educating the patient, pay extremely close attention to these regimes in order to prevent exacerbation of adverse effects, minimize drug interactions, and prevent severe vascular and cardiovascular adverse effects. Advise the patient to immediately report any chest pain, palpitations, blurred vision, headache, or seizures.

Patients with chronic lung disease who are receiving adrenergic drugs also need to avoid anything that may exacerbate their respiratory condition (e.g., certain foods or allergens, cigarette smoking) and implement measures that may help diminish their risk of respiratory infection. These measures may include avoiding those who are ill with colds and flu, avoiding crowded areas, remaining well nourished and rested, and maintaining fluid intake of up to 3 000 mL per day to ensure adequate hydration (unless contraindicated). Keeping a journal of symptoms and noting any improvement or worsening in the treated condition while taking the medications may be helpful.

Salmeterol xinafoate is not to be used for relief of acute symptoms, and education about its dosing is important. The dosage of salmeterol xinafoate is usually 1 puff twice daily at 12 hour intervals. Always recheck orders and

LEGAL & ETHICAL PRINCIPLES

Infiltrating Intravenous Infusions

Nurses often encounter an infiltrating infusion in the routine care of many of their patients. Every action taken is in ensuring that the nurse has acted as any prudent nurse would, and this prudence is essential to maintain the standard of care for the patient. The assessment and action taken by the nurse can be important for the patient, as in the case of *Macon-Bibb County Hospital Authority v. Ross* (1985).

Situation

At approximately 1452 hours, Ms. Ross arrived at the emergency department with dyspnea, bradycardia, and a blood pressure of 250/150 mm Hg. She became unresponsive, and at 1455 hours went into respiratory arrest. She was intubated by a respiratory therapist. At approximately 1458 hours, she received intravenous sodium nitroprusside in an intravenous site in her right wrist. Sodium nitroprusside was used to decrease her severely elevated blood pressure. By 1513 hours, Ms. Ross's blood pressure was 120/90 and the sodium nitroprusside was discontinued as prescribed. Actual events are documented as follows: At 1528 hours, the patient had no blood pressure at all and the physician had prescribed intravenous administration of dopamine to elevate her blood pressure; dopamine was actually administered at 1531 hours to increase her then nonexistent blood pressure. She was then transferred to the cardiac care unit at approximately 1630 hours, after the blood pressure stabilized. At midnight, a nurse noted that the intravenous catheter site had a "bruise bluish in colour." The next notation was at 1100 hours the following day. The patient's right arm was noted

to be swollen and sore, with a large blistered area around the intravenous catheter site. The same description was noted again at 1600 hours. There was no evidence that a physician was consulted or informed until 1850 hours. At this time, the blistered area was shown to a physician, but it was not until later in the evening that another physician cleansed the blistered area and treated it as a burn. The patient's lower right arm was permanently scarred and it was undisputed that the injury was a result of the infiltration of the dopamine.

It was noted that although an infiltration may result from an improper technique, it may also be related to the size of the needle, the status of the patient's veins, or specific intolerance to an intravenous catheter. However, according to the expert nurse's testimony, supported by evidence-informed references, dopamine should be infused into a "large vein," such as in the antecubital fossa, to minimize the risk of extravasation (leakage of fluid). In addition, dopamine needs to be monitored continuously and the infusion very closely regulated. The antidote to counter the effects of dopamine extravasation is phentolamine mesylate (Regitine®), and damage may be decreased or reversed if this is given within a specified time period. It is essential that nurses are educated about the intravenous administration of dopamine in order to minimize the consequences of extravasation, as in this case.

Data adapted from Macon-Bibb County Hospital Authority v. Ross, 335 SE2d 633 GA (176 Ga. App. 221 1985). Retrieved from http://www.leagle.com/decision/1985397176GaApp221_1302.xml/MACON-BIBB%20COUNTY%20HOSP.%20AUTH.%20v.%20ROSS

directions. If another type of inhalant is used, such as a corticosteroid, instruct the patient to use the bronchodilator first, with a 5-minute waiting period prior to taking the second drug. All equipment should be rinsed after use. Educate patients about the importance of rinsing the mouth thoroughly after the use of any inhalant form of medication. Oral rinsing and mouth care after use of inhaled drugs is needed to prevent irritation and infection. See Chapter 38 for further discussion of salmeterol xinafoate. If ophthalmic forms of adrenergic drugs are used, make sure that the medication has not expired and is also a clear solution. Do not allow the eyedropper to touch the eye when the drug is applied, to help prevent contamination of the remaining solution. With ophthalmic administration, drops and ointments should be applied into the conjunctival sac—not directly onto the cornea.

Oral midodrine hydrochloride is to be taken exactly as prescribed. This medication is usually ordered to be given with fluids before the patient gets out of bed in the morning. Doses of the drug are also often front-loaded in the dosing schedule so that most of the doses occur in the morning, when patients with orthostatic intolerance are

usually more symptomatic. Patients need to avoid taking this medication after 1800 hours if possible, to prevent insomnia and possible supine hypertension.

Evaluation

Therapeutic effects of adrenergic drugs are summarized as follows. For vasoactive drugs, therapeutic effects include improved cardiac output (with increased urinary output), return to normal vital signs (e.g., blood pressure of 120/80 mm Hg or higher, or gradual increases in blood pressure as indicated, and pulse rate greater than 60 but less than 100 beats per minute), improved skin colour (from pallor to pink) and temperature (from cool to warm) in the extremities, improved peripheral pulses, and increased level of consciousness. Therapeutic effects of drugs given for bronchial indications include a return to a normal respiratory rate (more than 12 but less than 20 breaths per minute), improved breath sounds throughout the lung field with fewer adventitious sounds than prior to intervention, increased air exchange in all areas of the lungs, decreased to no coughing, less dyspnea, improved partial pressure of oxygen and pulse oximeter readings, and tolerance of slowly increasing levels of activity. Therapeutic effects of midodrine hydrochloride include improved levels of functioning and improved performance of activities of daily living, fewer episodes of postural intolerance (dizziness, lightheadedness, and syncopal episodes), and increased energy.

To evaluate for the occurrence of adverse effects with adrenergic drugs, monitor for stimulation of the systems that are affected, such as the cardiac system and the CNS. Adverse effects such as dysrhythmias, hypertension, and tachycardia may occur. Be sure to monitor for chest pain.

PATIENT TEACHING TIPS

❖ Patients should be informed that medications must always be taken as prescribed. Excessive dosing may cause CNS and cardiovascular stimulation, with tremors, nervousness, insomnia, tachycardia, and palpitations.

❖ Instructions to patients for the use of inhaled forms of medication, including nebulizers, inhalers, and metered-dose inhalers (see Chapter 10), must be clear and concise.

❖ Instruct patients to report any dyspnea, distress, chest pain, heart palpitations, or worsening of respiratory symptoms.

❖ OTC medications and natural health products are to be avoided without consulting an HCP.

❖ Midodrine hydrochloride requires careful dosing, as ordered. Encourage patients taking this medication to keep a journal to record adverse effects, improvements in symptoms, and any worsening of symptoms.

KEY POINTS

❖ Catecholamines are substances that produce a sympathomimetic response. The naturally occurring or endogenous catecholamines include epinephrine, norepinephrine, and dopamine. An example of an exogenous catecholamine is dobutamine.

❖ Patients with a chronic respiratory disease, such as chronic obstructive pulmonary disease or chronic asthma, must avoid contact with individuals who may have infections, to help minimize situations that would exacerbate the original problem. Respiratory irritants must be avoided.

❖ Midodrine hydrochloride use requires careful blood pressure monitoring, so patient education about supine blood pressures and regular documentation of measured blood pressure values are crucial to the effective use of the drug.

❖ Inhaled forms of β_2-agonists are used for their bronchodilating action and must be taken only as prescribed, with caution to avoid overuse of the drug. Overdosage of these drugs may lead to severe cardiovascular, CNS, and cerebrovascular adverse effects and stimulation.

EXAMINATION REVIEW QUESTIONS

1. The nurse caring for a patient who is receiving β_1-agonist drug therapy needs to be aware that these drugs cause which effect?
   a. Increased heart contractility
   b. Decreased heart rate
   c. Bronchoconstriction
   d. Increased GI tract motility

2. During a teaching session for a patient receiving inhaled salmeterol xinafoate, the nurse emphasizes that the drug is indicated for which condition?
   a. Rescue treatment of acute bronchospasm
   b. Prevention of bronchospasm
   c. Reduction of airway inflammation
   d. Long-term treatment of sinus congestion

3. For a patient receiving a vasoactive drug such as intravenous dopamine, which action by the nurse is most appropriate?
   a. Monitor the gravity drip infusion closely and adjust as needed.
   b. Assess the patient's heart function by checking the radial pulse.
   c. Assess the intravenous site hourly for possible infiltration.
   d. Administer the drug by intravenous boluses, according to the patient's blood pressure.

4. A patient is receiving dobutamine for shock and is reporting feeling more "skipping beats" than yesterday. What will the nurse do next?
   a. Monitor for other signs of a therapeutic response to the drug.
   b. Titrate the drug to a higher dose to reduce the palpitations.
   c. Discontinue the dobutamine immediately.
   d. Assess the patient's vital signs and cardiac rhythm.

5. When a drug is characterized as having a negative chronotropic effect, the nurse knows to expect which effect?
   a. Reduced blood pressure
   b. Decreased heart rate
   c. Decreased ectopic beats
   d. Increased force of heart contractions

Continued

EXAMINATION REVIEW QUESTIONS—cont'd

6. The nurse is monitoring a patient who is receiving an infusion of a β-adrenergic agonist. Which adverse effects may occur with this infusion? (Select all that apply.)
a. Mild tremors
b. Bradycardia
c. Tachycardia
d. Palpitations
e. Drowsiness
f. Nervousness

7. An order reads, "Dopamine 3 mcg/kg/min IV." The solution available is 400 mg in 250 mL D₅W, and the patient weighs 176 pounds. The nurse will set the intravenous infusion pump to run at how many mL/hour?

Answers: 1. a, 2. b, 3. c, 4. d, 5. b, 6. a, c, d, f, 7. 9 mL/h

CRITICAL THINKING ACTIVITIES

1. While making initial morning rounds, the nurse checks the insertion site of a patient's dopamine infusion and finds the area swollen and cool to the touch. What is the nurse's priority action? Describe what the nurse will do following the initial action.

2. A patient with chronic obstructive pulmonary disease is experiencing an episode of bronchospasm and wants to use his salmeterol xinafoate inhaler. What is the priority action in this situation?

3. A patient is experiencing a severe anaphylactic reaction after a dose of an antibiotic, and the emergency team is present. The nurse is expecting to give what drug first? Explain your answer.

For answers, see http://evolve.elsevier.com/Canada/Lilley/pharmacology/.

CHAPTER 20

Adrenergic-Blocking Drugs

Objectives

After reading this chapter, the successful student will be able to do the following:

1. Briefly review the functions of the sympathetic nervous system and the specific effects of adrenergic-blocking drugs.

2. List the various drugs categorized as adrenergic antagonists (blockers) or sympatholytics.

3. Discuss the mechanisms of action, therapeutic effects, indications, adverse and toxic effects, cautions, contraindications, drug interactions, dosages, routes of administration, and any antidotal management for the α-antagonists (blockers), nonselective β-blockers, and the β$_1$- and β$_2$-blockers.

4. Develop a collaborative plan of care that includes all phases of the nursing process for patients taking adrenergic antagonists.

e-Learning Activities

Website
(http://evolve.elsevier.com/Canada/Lilley/pharmacology/)

evolve

- Answer Key—Textbook Case Studies
- Answer Key—Critical Thinking Activities
- Chapter Summaries—Printable
- Review Questions for Exam Preparation
- Unfolding Case Studies

Drug Profiles

▸▸ atenolol, p. 399
   carvedilol, p. 399
▸▸ esmolol (esmolol hydrochloride)*, p. 400
   labetalol (labetalol hydrochloride)*, p. 400
▸▸ metoprolol (metoprolol tartrate)*, p. 400
▸▸ phentolamine (phentolamine mesylate)*, p. 397
▸▸ propranolol (propranolol hydrochloride)*, p. 400
   sotalol (sotalol hydrochloride)*, p. 400
   tamsulosin hydrochloride, p. 397

▸▸ Key drug

*Full generic name is given in parentheses. For the purposes of this text, the more common, shortened name is used.

Key Terms

Acrocyanosis Decreased amount of oxygen delivered to the extremities, causing the feet or hands to turn blue. (p. 394)

Adrenergic receptors Specific receptor sites located throughout the body for the endogenous sympathetic neurotransmitters norepinephrine and epinephrine. (p. 394)

Agonists Drugs with a specific receptor affinity that produce a "mimic" response. (p. 394)

Angina Paroxysmal (sudden) chest pain caused by myocardial ischemia. (p. 398)

Antagonists Drugs that bind to specific receptors and inhibit or block the response of the receptors. (p. 394)

Dysrhythmias Irregular heart rhythms; almost always called *arrhythmias* in clinical practice. (p. 398)

Extravasation The leaking of fluid from a blood vessel into the surrounding tissues, as in the case of an infiltrated intravenous infusion. (p. 395)

First-dose phenomenon Severe and sudden drop in blood pressure after the administration of the first dose of an α-adrenergic blocker. (p. 395)

Intrinsic sympathomimetic activity The paradoxical action of some β-blocking drugs (e.g., acebutolol) that mimics the activity of the sympathetic nervous system. (p. 396)

Lipophilicity The chemical attraction of a substance (e.g., drug molecule) to lipid or fat molecules. (p. 398)

Orthostatic hypotension A sudden drop in blood pressure when a person stands up; also referred to as *postural hypotension* or *orthostasis*. (p. 395)

Pheochromocytoma A vascular adrenal gland tumour that is usually benign but secretes epinephrine and norepinephrine and thus often causes central nervous system stimulation and substantial blood pressure elevation. (p. 394)

Raynaud's disease A narrowing of small arteries that limits the amount of blood circulation to the extremities, causing numbness of the nose, fingers, toes, and ears in response to cold temperatures or stress. (p. 394)

Sympatholytics Drugs that inhibit the postganglionic functioning of the sympathetic nervous system. (p. 394)

OVERVIEW

The autonomic nervous system consists of the parasympathetic and sympathetic nervous systems. The class of drugs discussed in this chapter works primarily on the sympathetic nervous system (SNS). As discussed in Chapter 19, the adrenergic agonist drugs stimulate the SNS. These drugs are called **agonists** because they bind to receptors and cause a response. Adrenergic blockers have the opposite effect and are therefore referred to as **antagonists**. They bind to adrenergic receptors, but in doing so inhibit or block stimulation by the SNS. They are also referred to as *sympatholytics* because they lyse, or inhibit, SNS stimulation.

Throughout the body, there are receptor sites for the endogenous sympathetic neurotransmitters norepinephrine and epinephrine (see Table 19-1). Such receptors are known as *adrenergic receptors,* and two basic types are found—α and β. There are subtypes of both the α- and β-adrenergic receptors, designated 1 and 2. The $α_1$- and $α_2$-adrenergic receptors are differentiated by their location on nerves. The $α_1$-adrenergic receptors are located on the tissue, muscle, or organ that the nerve is stimulating (postsynaptic effector cells). The $α_2$-adrenergic receptors are located on the actual nerves that stimulate the presynaptic effector cells. The $α_2$-receptors are inhibitory in nature. Thus, it is actually the stimulation of $α_2$-receptors that causes inhibitory effects of the SNS. $α_2$ active drugs (e.g., clonidine) are discussed in Chapter 23. The $β_1$-adrenergic receptors are located primarily on the heart; the $β_2$-adrenergic receptors are located primarily on the smooth muscles of the bronchioles and blood vessels. It is at these various receptors that adrenergic blockers act. They are classified by the type of adrenergic receptor they block—α or β—or, in a few cases, both. Hence, they are called α-*blockers,* β-*blockers,* or α–β-blockers.

α-BLOCKERS

The α-adrenergic–blocking drugs, or α-blockers, interrupt stimulation of the SNS at the $α_1$-adrenergic receptors. More specifically, α-blockers work either by direct competition with norepinephrine or by a noncompetitive process. Figure 20-1 illustrates these two mechanisms. α- blockers have a greater affinity for the α-adrenergic receptor than norepinephrine does, and therefore can chemically displace norepinephrine molecules from the receptor. Selective adrenergic blockade at these receptors leads to effects such as vasodilation, reduced blood pressure (by decreasing total systemic vascular resistance and venous return), miosis (constriction of the pupil), and reduced smooth muscle tone in organs such as the bladder and prostate. Currently available α-blockers are listed in Table 20-1.

Mechanism of Action and Drug Effects

The α-blockers such as alfuzosin, doxazosin, prazosin, and terazosin cause both arterial and venous dilation, which reduces systemic vascular resistance and blood pressure. These drugs are used to treat hypertension (see Chapter 23). There are also α-adrenergic receptors in the prostate and bladder. By blocking or inhibiting $α_1$-receptors, these drugs reduce smooth muscle contraction of the bladder neck and the prostatic portion of the urethra. For this reason, α-blockers are given to patients with benign prostatic hyperplasia (BPH) to decrease resistance to urinary outflow. This reduces urinary obstruction and relieves some of the effects of BPH. Tamsulosin and alfuzosin are used exclusively for treating BPH, whereas terazosin and doxazosin can be used for both hypertension and BPH.

Other α-blockers can inhibit responses to adrenergic stimulation. These drugs noncompetitively block α-adrenergic receptors on smooth muscle and various exocrine glands. Because of this action, they are useful in controlling or preventing hypertension in patients who have a **pheochromocytoma,** a tumour that forms on the adrenal gland on top of the kidney and secretes norepinephrine, causing SNS stimulation. The α-blockers are also useful in the treatment of patients with increased endogenous α-adrenergic agonist activity, which results in vasoconstriction. Three conditions in which this occurs are **Raynaud's disease, acrocyanosis,** and frostbite. Phentolamine in particular can reverse potent vasoconstriction and restore blood flow to ischemic tissue.

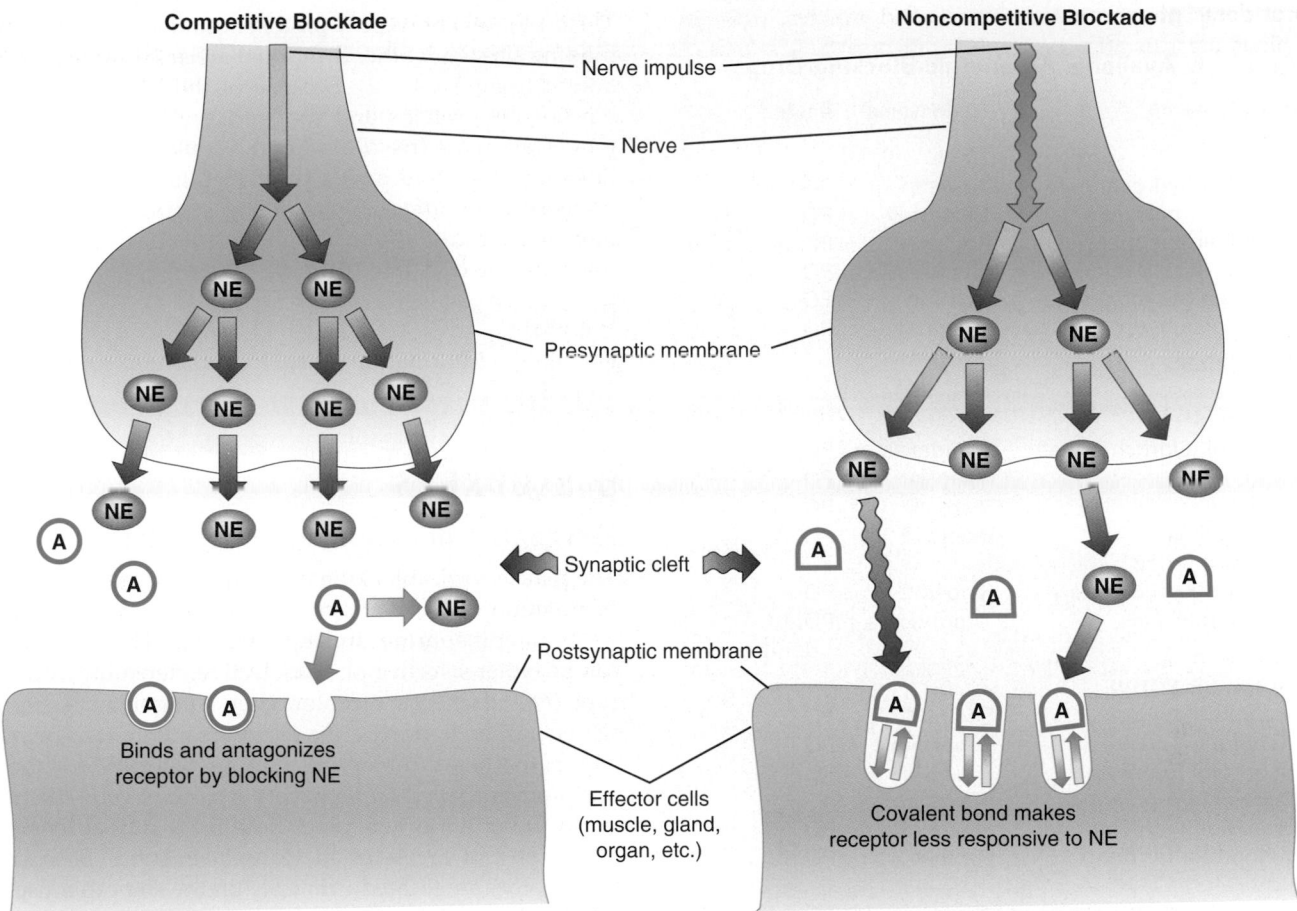

FIG. 20-1 α-Blocker mechanisms for α-adrenergic competitive and noncompetitive blockade. *A*, antagonist; *NE*, norepinephrine.

Still other α-blockers are effective at counteracting the effects of injected epinephrine and norepinephrine. They do this by causing systemic vasodilation and reducing systemic resistance by blocking catecholamine-stimulated vasoconstriction. Because of their potent vasodilating properties and their fast onset of action, they are used to prevent skin necrosis and sloughing after the **extravasation** (infiltration) of vasopressors such as norepinephrine or epinephrine. When these drugs extravasate (leak out of the blood vessel into the surrounding tissue), they cause vasoconstriction and ultimately tissue death, or necrosis. If the vasoconstriction is not reversed quickly, an entire limb can be lost.

Contraindications

Contraindications to the use of α-blocking drugs include known drug allergy and peripheral vascular disease, and may also include liver or kidney disease, coronary artery disease, peptic ulcer, and sepsis.

Adverse Effects

The primary adverse effects of α-blockers are those related to their effects on the vasculature. **First-dose phenomenon,** which is a severe and sudden drop in blood pressure after the administration of the first dose of an α-adrenergic blocker, can cause patients to fall or faint. All patients must be warned about this adverse effect before they take their first dose of an α- blocker. **Orthostatic hypotension** can occur with any dose of an α-blocker, and patients must be warned to rise and transfer slowly from a supine position. The primary adverse effects of the α-blockers are listed by body system in Table 20-2.

Toxicity and Management of Overdose

In an acute oral overdose, consultation with a Poison Control Centre is recommended. The patient's stomach should be emptied, usually by gastric lavage. After this, activated charcoal is administered to bind to the drug and remove it from the stomach and the circulation. With overdoses of both oral and injectable forms, symptomatic and supportive measures are to be instituted as needed. Blood pressure support with the administration of fluids, volume expanders, and vasopressor drugs, and the administration of anticonvulsants such as diazepam for the control of seizures, are examples of such measures.

Interactions

The most severe drug interactions with α-blockers are those that potentiate the effects of the α-blockers.

TABLE 20-1

Currently Available Adrenergic-Blocking Drugs

Generic Name	Trade Name	Route
α_1-BLOCKERS		
alfuzosin hydrochloride	Xatral®	PO
doxazosin mesylate	Cardura®	PO
phentolamine mesylate	Rogitine®	IM, IV
prazosin hydrochloride	Minipress®	PO
terazosin hydrochloride	Hytrin®	PO
tamsulosin hydrochloride	Flomax®	PO
β-BLOCKERS		
Nonselective		
carvedilol*		PO
labetalol hydrochloride*	Trandate®	PO, IV
nadolol	Nadol®	PO
pindolol	Visken®	PO
propranolol hydrochloride*	Inderal®	PO, IV
sotalol hydrochloride	Rylosol®	PO
timolol maleate	Timoptic®	PO, IV, ophthalmic
CARDIOSELECTIVE		
acebutolol hydrochloride	Sectral®	PO
atenolol	Tenormin®	PO
bisoprolol fumarate		PO
esmolol hydrochloride	Brevibloc®	IV
nebivolol hydrochloride	Bystolic®	PO
metoprolol tartrate	Lopressor®	PO, IV

IM, Intramuscular; *IV*, intravenous; *PO*, oral.
*Has antagonist activity at α_1-, β_1-, and β_2-receptors.

TABLE 20-2

α-Blockers: Adverse Effects

Body System	Adverse Effects
Cardiovascular	Palpitations, orthostatic hypotension, tachycardia, edema, chest pain
Central nervous	Dizziness, headache, anxiety, depression, weakness, numbness, fatigue
Gastrointestinal	Nausea, vomiting, diarrhea, constipation, abdominal pain
Other	Incontinence, dry mouth, pharyngitis

The α-blockers are highly protein bound and compete for binding sites with other drugs that are also highly protein bound (see Chapter 2). Because of the limited sites for binding on proteins and the increased competition for these sites, more free α-blocker molecules circulate in the bloodstream. More active drug results in a more pronounced drug effect. Some of the common drugs that interact with α-blockers and the results of these interactions are listed in Table 20-3.

Dosages

For dosage information on α-blockers, refer to the table on p. 397.

β-BLOCKERS

Mechanism of Action and Drug Effects

The β-adrenergic–blocking drugs (β-blockers) block SNS stimulation of the β-adrenergic receptors by competing with norepinephrine and epinephrine. The β-blockers can be either selective or nonselective, depending on the type of β-adrenergic receptors they antagonize. As mentioned earlier, β_1-adrenergic receptors are located primarily in the heart. β-blockers that are selective for these receptors are called *cardioselective β-blockers*, or *β_1-blocking drugs*. Other β-blockers block both β_1- and β_2-adrenergic receptors and are referred to as *nonselective β-blockers*. β_2-receptors are located primarily on the smooth muscles of the bronchioles and blood vessels. In addition, β-blockers can be further categorized according to whether they do or do not have **intrinsic sympathomimetic activity**. Drugs with intrinsic sympathomimetic activity (acebutolol, pindolol) not only block β-adrenergic receptors but also partially stimulate them. This was initially believed to be an advantageous characteristic, but clinical experience has not borne this out. Two β-blockers, carvedilol and labetalol, also have an α-receptor blocking activity, especially at higher doses. Table 20-1 lists currently available β-blockers.

Cardioselective β_1-blockers block the β_1-receptors on the surface of the heart. This reduces myocardial stimulation, which in turn reduces heart rate, slows conduction through the atrioventricular (AV) node, prolongs sinoatrial (SA) node recovery, and decreases myocardial

TABLE 20-3

α-Blockers: Common Drug Interactions

Drug	Interacting Drug	Mechanism	Result
phentolamine	β-blockers, alcohol, erectile dysfunction drugs	} Additive effects	} Profound hypotension
	epinephrine	Antagonism	Reduced phentolamine effects
tamsulosin	warfarin	Competition for plasma protein-binding sites	Risk of bleeding
	antihypertensives, erectile dysfunction drugs, alcohol	} Additive effects	} Risk of hypotension

DRUG PROFILES

The α-blockers are commonly used to treat hypertension or BPH. They include phentolamine, terazosin, alfuzosin, tamsulosin, and prazosin. Prazosin is discussed in Chapter 23.

▶▶phentolamine mesylate

Phentolamine mesylate (Rogitine®) is an α-blocker that reduces systemic vascular resistance and is sometimes used to treat hypertension. It is used to treat the high blood pressure caused by pheochromocytoma and also in the diagnosis of this catecholamine-secreting tumour. To help establish a diagnosis of pheochromocytoma, a single intravenous dose of phentolamine is given to the hypertensive patient. If blood pressure falls rapidly, it is highly likely that the patient has a pheochromocytoma. Phentolamine is available only as an intravenous preparation. It is most commonly used to treat the extravasation of vasoconstricting intravenous drugs such as norepinephrine, epinephrine, and dopamine, which when given intravenously can leak out of the vein, especially if the intravenous tube is not correctly positioned. If such a drug is allowed to extravasate into the surrounding tissue, the result is intense vasoconstriction, decreased blood flow, necrosis, and potential loss of the limb. Phentolamine 5 to 15 mg in 10 mL of normal saline solution is administered into the interstitial catheter prior to removal to direct phentolamine into the area of extravasation as soon as possible. This action causes α-adrenergic receptor blockade and vasodilation, which in turn increases blood flow to the ischemic tissue and prevents permanent damage. The use of the drug may be effective up to 12 hours post extravasation of the vasoconstrictor. Its use is contraindicated in patients who have shown a hypersensitivity to it, those who have experienced a myocardial infarction, and those with coronary artery disease. Adverse effects include tachycardia, dizziness, gastrointestinal upset, and others listed in Table 20-2. Drugs with which phentolamine interacts include alcohol (a disulfiramlike reaction; see Chapter 18)

and erectile dysfunction medications such as sildenafil citrate (causing additive hypotensive effects; see Chapter 36). Epinephrine and ephedrine can counteract the desired effects of phentolamine. Phentolamine is also available for intraoral submucosal injection (Oraverse®) for reversal of soft tissue anaesthesia. The recommended dosages are given in the table below.

PHARMACOKINETICS

Route	Onset of Action	Peak Plasma Concentration	Elimination Half-Life	Duration of Action
IV	2 min	20 min	19 min	30–45 min

tamsulosin hydrochloride

Tamsulosin hydrochloride (Flomax®) is an α-blocker used primarily to treat BPH and is exclusively indicated for male patients. A similar drug with the same indication is alfuzosin. These drugs block α-adrenergic receptors on smooth muscle within the prostate and bladder. This results in relaxation of the smooth muscle fibres and improved urinary flow. Terazosin and doxazosin mesylate are used to treat BPH as well as hypertension. Contraindications to tamsulosin hydrochloride include known drug allergy and concurrent use of erectile dysfunction drugs such as sildenafil citrate. Adverse effects include headache, abnormal ejaculation, rhinitis, and others listed in Table 20-2. Interacting drugs include other α-blockers, calcium channel blockers, and erectile dysfunction drugs (which cause additive hypotensive effects); drugs that induce or inhibit liver enzymes may reduce or enhance the effects of tamsulosin hydrochloride, respectively. It is available only for oral use.

PHARMACOKINETICS

Route	Onset of Action	Peak Plasma Concentration	Elimination Half-Life	Duration of Action
PO	Unknown	4–7 hr	15 hr	Unknown

DOSAGES   Selected α-Adrenergic–Blocking Drugs

Drug	Pharmacological Class	Usual Dosage Range	Indications
▶▶phentolamine mesylate (Rogitine)	α-blocker	*Adults* IV: 1–5 mg bolus; 0.1–2 mg/min infusion *Adults* 5–10 mg diluted in 10 mL NS injected into extravasation site within 12 hr *Children* 0.1–0.2 mg/kg into extravasation site	Hypertensive episodes with pheochromocytoma α-adrenergic drug extravasation
tamsulosin hydrochloride (Flomax)	α₁-blocker	*Adults* PO: 0.4 mg once daily	Benign prostatic hypertrophy

IV, intravenous; *NS*, normal saline; *PO*, oral.

oxygen demand by decreasing myocardial contractile force (contractility). Nonselective β-blockers not only have these cardiac effects, but they block β$_2$-receptors on the smooth muscle of the bronchioles and blood vessels as well.

Smooth muscle surrounds the airways, or bronchioles, in the lungs. When the β$_2$-receptors in the bronchioles are blocked, the result is smooth muscle contraction and narrowing of the airways. This may lead to shortness of breath. In addition, the smooth muscle that surrounds blood vessels can cause dilation or constriction, depending on whether the β$_1$- or β$_2$-receptors are stimulated. When β$_2$ stimulation is blocked, the muscles are then stimulated by unopposed sympathetic activity at the β$_1$-receptors, which causes them to contract. This contraction causes increased systemic vascular resistance. Furthermore, catecholamines promote glycogenolysis, the production of glucose from glycogen, and mobilize glucose in response to hypoglycemia. Nonselective β-blockers impair this process and impede the secretion of insulin from the pancreas, which causes elevation of blood glucose levels.

Finally, β-blockers can cause the release of free fatty acids from adipose tissue. This may result in moderately elevated blood levels of triglycerides and reduced levels of high-density lipoprotein (HDL).

Indications

Indications for β-blockers include **angina**, myocardial infarction, cardiac dysrhythmias, hypertension, and heart failure. β-blockers possess anti-ischemic as well as antiatherogenic and antidysrhythmic properties.

β-blockers work by decreasing the demand for myocardial energy and oxygen consumption, which helps to shift the supply-and-demand ratio to the supply side and allows more oxygen to reach the heart muscle. This in turn helps relieve pain in the heart muscle caused by the lack of oxygen.

β-blockers are also considered to be cardioprotective because they inhibit stimulation by the circulating catecholamines. Myocardial infarction causes catecholamines to be released. Unopposed stimulation by catecholamines would further increase the heart rate and the contractile force, thereby increasing myocardial oxygen demand. When a β-blocker occupies myocardial β$_1$-receptors, circulating catecholamines molecules are prevented from binding to the receptors. Thus, β-blockers protect the heart from being stimulated by catecholamines. Because of this characteristic, β-blockers are commonly given to patients after they have experienced a myocardial infarction.

β-blockers also have a profound effect on the conduction system of the heart. The AV node normally receives impulse stimulation from the SA node and slows it down so that the ventricles have time to fill before they are stimulated to contract. Conduction in the SA node, which spontaneously depolarizes at the most frequent rate, is slowed by β-blockers, which results in a decreased heart rate. β-blockers also slow conduction through the AV node. These effects on the conduction system of the heart make the drugs useful in the treatment of various types of irregular heartbeat rhythms called **dysrhythmias** (see Chapter 26).

β-blockers are useful in treating hypertension because of their ability to reduce SNS stimulation of the heart, including reducing heart rate and the force of myocardial contraction (systole). Traditionally, β-blockers were thought to worsen heart failure. However, recent studies have shown the benefit of using β-blockers. Certain β-blockers such as carvedilol and metoprolol have produced the best results to date. The form of heart failure that includes a component of diastolic dysfunction responds favourably to β-blockers.

Because of their **lipophilicity** (attraction to lipid or fat), some β-blockers (e.g., propranolol) can easily gain entry into the central nervous system and are used for the prophylaxis of migraine headaches rather than for acute attacks. In addition, the topical application of timolol maleate to the eye has been effective in treating ocular disorders such as glaucoma (see Chapter 57).

Contraindications

Contraindications of β-blockers include known drug allergies and may include acute decompensated heart failure (i.e., an acute exacerbation), cardiogenic shock, heart block or bradycardia, pregnancy, severe pulmonary disease, and Raynaud's disease.

Adverse Effects

The adverse effects of β-blockers are primarily extensions of their pharmacological activity. Most effects are mild and diminish with time. Some of the most serious undesirable effects can be caused by acute withdrawal of the drug. For example, sudden withdrawal may exacerbate underlying angina and precipitate a myocardial infarction or cause rebound hypertension.

β$_2$-receptors normally induce glucose production by stimulating both hepatic glycogen breakdown (glycogenolysis) and pancreatic release of glucagon and delivering that glucose to the system. When this process is blocked, low blood sugar may occur. Therefore, blockage of β$_2$-receptors can cause hypoglycemia. β-blockers also delay recovery from hypoglycemia in patients with type 1 diabetes (but rarely in those with type 2). In addition, the nonselective β-blockers can interfere with the normal responses to hypoglycemia, such as tremor, tachycardia, and nervousness, in essence masking the signs and symptoms of hypoglycemia. Conversely, nonselective β-blockers such as metoprolol and atenolol are thought to contribute to the development of hyperglycemia by impairing the release of insulin from the pancreatic β-cell (Fonseca, 2010). It is theorized that the lipoprotein effects of β-blockers may be from unopposed α-adrenergic stimulation, which leads to reduced peripheral lipoprotein lipase activity and thus reduced catabolism of very low-density lipoproteins and triglycerides. Cardioselective β-blockers such as carvedilol, labetalol, and nebivolol have a more favourable effect on glucose and cholesterol control. Lower doses have little to no effect on lipoprotein parameters (Fonseca, 2010).

Adverse effects induced by β-blockers are listed by body system in Table 20-4.

Toxicity and Management of Overdose

For overdoses of both oral and injectable dosage forms, treatment consists primarily of symptomatic and supportive care. Consultation with a Poison Control Centre is recommended. For oral overdose, the stomach should be emptied immediately by induction of emesis or by gastric lavage. Atropine sulphate may be given for the management of bradycardia. If bradycardia persists, norepinephrine or dopamine may be administered. If the bradycardia still persists, placement of a transvenous heart pacemaker may be considered. For the treatment of severe hypotension, vasopressors are titrated until the desired blood pressure and heart rate are achieved. Intravenously administered diazepam may be useful for the treatment of seizures. Most β-blockers are dialyzable; therefore, hemodialysis may be useful in enhancing elimination in the event of a severe overdose.

Interactions

Most of the drug interactions with β blockers result from either the additive effects of coadministered medications with similar mechanisms of action or the antagonistic effects of various drugs. Nonselective β-blockers may mask the tachycardia from hypoglycemia caused by insulin and sulfonylureas, and the hypoglycemic effect of insulin and sulfonylureas may be enhanced (see Chapter 33). Some of the common drugs that interact with β-blockers and the resulting effects are given in Table 20-5.

Dosages

For dosage information on selected β-blockers, refer to the table on p. 401.

TABLE	20-4

β-Blockers: Common Adverse Effects

Body System	Adverse Effects
Cardiovascular	Atrioventricular block, bradycardia, heart failure
Central nervous	Dizziness, fatigue, depression, drowsiness, unusual dreams
Gastrointestinal	Nausea, vomiting, constipation, diarrhea
Hematologic	Agranulocytosis, thrombocytopenia
Metabolic	Hyperglycemia or hypoglycemia, dyslipidemia
Other	Erectile dysfunction, alopecia, bronchospasm, wheezing, dry mouth

TABLE	20-5

β-Blockers: Drug Interactions

Drug	Mechanism	Result
Antacids (aluminum hydroxide type)	Decrease absorption	Decreased β-blocker activity
Antimuscarinics, anticholinergics	Antagonism	Reduced β-blocker effects
Diuretics, cardiovascular drugs, alcohol	Additive	Additive hypotensive effects
Neuromuscular blocking drugs	Additive	Prolonged neuromuscular blockade
Oral antihyperglycemic drugs	Mask effects of hypoglycemia	Delayed recovery from hypoglycemia

 DRUG PROFILES

The numerous β-blockers that are currently available are listed in Table 20-1. Several β-blockers are profiled in the following sections. Contraindications, adverse reactions, and drug interactions are comparable for these drugs and are listed previously (see Table 20-4 and Table 20-5).

▶▶atenolol

Atenolol (Tenormin®) is a cardioselective β-blocker that is commonly used to prevent future myocardial infarctions in patients who have previously had one. It is also used in the treatment of hypertension and angina and in the management of thyrotoxicosis to help block the symptoms of excessive thyroid activity. Atenolol is available for oral use. Recommended dosages are given in the table on p. 401.

PHARMACOKINETICS

Route	Onset of Action	Peak Plasma Concentration	Elimination Half-Life	Duration of Action
PO	1 hr	2–4 hr	6–7 hr	24 hr

carvedilol

Carvedilol has many effects, including acting as a nonselective β-blocker, an α_1-blocker, a calcium channel blocker (at high dosages), and possibly an antioxidant. Its action on β-receptors is 10 times stronger than that on α_1-receptors. It is used primarily in the treatment of heart failure but it is also beneficial in the treatment of hypertension and angina. It has been shown to slow the

Continued

DRUG PROFILES—cont'd

progression of heart failure and to decrease the frequency of hospitalization in patients with mild to moderate (class II or III) heart failure. Carvedilol is most commonly added to digoxin, furosemide, and angiotensin-converting enzyme inhibitors when used to treat heart failure. Carvedilol is available for oral use. Recommended dosages are given in the Dosages table on p. 401.

PHARMACOKINETICS

Route	Onset of Action	Peak Plasma Concentration	Elimination Half-Life	Duration of Action
PO	20–120 min	1–4 hr	6–8 hr	8–24 hr

esmolol hydrochloride

Esmolol hydrochloride (Brevibloc®) is a strong, short-acting β_1-blocker. It is primarily used in acute situations to provide rapid temporary control of the ventricular rate in patients with supraventricular tachydysrhythmias. Because of its very short half-life, it is given only as an intravenous infusion and is titrated to achieve the serum levels that control the patient's symptoms. Recommended dosages are given in the table on p. 401.

PHARMACOKINETICS

Route	Onset of Action	Peak Plasma Concentration	Elimination Half-Life	Duration of Action
IV	Immediate	6 min	9 min	15–20 min

labetalol hydrochloride

Labetalol hydrochloride (Trandate®) is unusual in that it can block both α- and β-receptors. It is used in the treatment of severe hypertension and in hypertensive emergencies to quickly lower blood pressure before permanent damage occurs. Labetalol is available for oral and parenteral use. Recommended dosages are given in the table on p. 401.

PHARMACOKINETICS

Route	Onset of Action	Peak Plasma Concentration	Elimination Half-Life	Duration of Action
IV	2–5 min	5–15 min	2.5–8 hr	2–4 hr
PO	20–120 min	1–4 hr	2.5–8 hr	8–24 hr

▸▸metoprolol tartrate

Metoprolol tartrate (Lopressor®) is a β_1-blocker that has become a favourite of cardiologists for use in patients after myocardial infarction. Recent studies of metoprolol have shown increased survival in patients given the drug after they have experienced a myocardial infarction. Metoprolol is available for oral and parenteral use. Recommended dosages are given in the table on p. 401.

PHARMACOKINETICS

Route	Onset of Action	Peak Plasma Concentration	Elimination Half-Life	Duration of Action
IV	1 min	20 min	3–8 hr	5–8 hr
PO	1 hr	2–4 hr	3–8 hr	10–20 hr

▸propranolol hydrochloride

Propranolol hydrochloride (Inderal®) is the prototypical nonselective β_1- and β_2-receptor–blocking drug. It was one of the first β-blockers to be used. Lengthy experience with the use of propranolol has revealed its many uses. In addition to the indications mentioned for metoprolol, propranolol has also been used in the treatment of the tachydysrhythmias associated with cardiac glycoside intoxication and for the treatment of hypertrophic subaortic stenosis, pheochromocytoma, thyrotoxicosis, migraine headache, essential tremor, and many other conditions. The same contraindications that apply to the cardioselective β-blockers discussed earlier apply to propranolol as well. Its use is contraindicated in patients with bronchial asthma. Propranolol is available for oral and parenteral use. Recommended dosages are given in the table on p. 401.

PHARMACOKINETICS

Route	Onset of Action	Peak Plasma Concentration	Elimination Half-Life	Duration of Action
IV	2 min	1–4 hr	3–5 hr	3–6 hr
PO	1–2 hr	1–4 hr	3–5 hr	6–12 hr

sotalol hydrochloride

Sotalol hydrochloride (Rylosol®) is a nonselective β-blocker that has potent antidysrhythmic properties. It is commonly used for the management of difficult-to-treat dysrhythmias. Often, these dysrhythmias are life-threatening ventricular dysrhythmias such as sustained ventricular tachycardia. Sotalol has properties characteristic of both a class II and a class III antidysrhythmic drug (see Chapter 26). Because it is a nonselective β-blocker, it causes some of the unwanted adverse effects typical of these drugs (e.g., hypotension) and dysrhythmias. It is used in select patients due to its potentially serious adverse effects. Sotalol is available only for oral use. Recommended dosages are given in the table on p. 401.

PHARMACOKINETICS

Route	Onset of Action	Peak Plasma Concentration	Elimination Half-Life	Duration of Action
PO	1–2 hr	2.5–4 hr	12 hr	8–16 hr

DOSAGES   Selected β-Adrenergic–Blocking Drugs

Drug	Pharmacological Class	Usual Dosage Range	Indications
▸▸atenolol (Tenormin)	β_1-blocker	*Adults* PO: 50–200 mg/day once daily or divided bid	Hypertension, angina pectoris
carvedilol	α- and β-blocker	*Adults* PO: 3.125 mg bid; may double dose every 2 wk to highest tolerated dose, max 50 mg/day	Heart failure
▸▸esmolol hydrochloride (Brevibloc)	β_1-blocker	*Adults* IV: Loading dose, 0.5 mg/kg/min over 1 min, followed by 4 min maintenance of 0.05 mg/kg/min and evaluate	Supraventricular tachydysrhythmias
labetalol hydrochloride (Trandate)	α_1- and β-blocker	*Adults* PO: 200–1200 mg/day divided bid IV: 20 mg over 2 min with additional doses of 40 mg at 10-min intervals until desired effect to max 300 mg; maintenance infusion of 2 mg/min initially and titrated to response	Hypertension Severe hypertension
▸▸metoprolol tartrate (Lopressor)	β_1-blocker	*Adults* PO: 100–400 mg/day divided bid SR tabs: 100–200 mg/day a.m. IV/PO: 3 bolus injections of 5 mg at 2-min intervals followed in 15 min by 50 mg PO q6h for 48 hr; thereafter 100 mg PO bid	Hypertension angina pectoris, late myocardial infarction Early myocardial infarction
▸▸propranolol hydrochloride (Inderal LA)	β-blocker	*Adults* PO: 80–320 mg/day divided tid–qid PO: 10–30 mg tid–qid before meals and at bedtime PO: 80–160 mg/day divided	Angina pectoris, hypertension Dysrhythmias Migraine prophylaxis
sotalol hydrochloride (Rylosol)	β-blocker (potassium blockage)	*Adults* PO: 160–320 mg/day divided	Life-threatening ventricular dysrhythmias

IV intravenous; *PO* oral; *SR* sustained release.

NURSING PROCESS

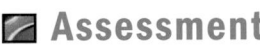

Assessment

Adrenergic-blocking drugs, or sympatholytics, produce a variety of effects on the patient, depending on the type of receptor(s) blocked. Because of the impact of these drugs on the cardiac and respiratory systems, their use requires careful assessment to minimize adverse effects and maximize therapeutic effects. Understanding the basic anatomy and physiology of adrenergic receptors and their subsequent actions if stimulated or blocked is critical to carrying out assessment and other aspects of the nursing process and drug therapy. If an adrenergic-blocking drug is nonselective, it blocks both α- and β- (β_1- and β_2-) receptors. α-receptor blocking affects blood vessels, whereas β_1-receptor blocking affects heart rate and β_2-blocking affects bronchial smooth muscle. Therefore, a nonselective adrenergic blocker will have the following actions: (1) α-blocking leading to blockade of the sympathetic stimulation of blood vessels, resulting in vasodilation and a subsequent decrease in blood pressure; (2) β_1-blocking leading to blockade of the sympathetic effects on heart rate, contractility, and conduction with resulting bradycardia, negative inotropic effects (i.e., decrease in contractility), and a decrease in conduction; and (3) β_2-blocking leading to blockade of the sympathetic effects on bronchial smooth muscle with the net effect of bronchoconstriction. However, if the drug is only an α-, β_1-, or β_2-adrenergic blocker, the resulting effect will be related to the specific receptor being blocked (or combination of receptors, depending on the drug). An understanding of these basic physiological concepts is necessary to critical thinking and decision making in the administration of these drugs.

Begin a thorough assessment by gathering information about the patient's allergies and past and present medical conditions. Conducting a system overview and taking a thorough medication history is also part of this process. It is essential to perform a cardiac assessment, including blood pressure and heart rate, prior to the administration of adrenergic-blocking drugs. Specifically, an apical pulse rate must be taken for 1 minute prior to the administration of a β-blocker. Ask the following questions and document the findings: Do you have any allergies to medications or foods? Do you have any history of chronic obstructive pulmonary disease, asthma, other respiratory diseases, hypertension or hypotension, heart disease, bradycardia, heart failure, or cardiac dysrhythmias? This information is crucial because the action and adverse effects of α- and β-blockers may cause additional health risks to individuals with these problems. For example, α-blockers may precipitate hypotension; thus patients with baseline low blood pressure readings need more frequent blood pressure monitoring, or they may not tolerate the drug at all. β-blocking drugs may precipitate bradycardia, hypotension, heart block, heart failure, bronchoconstriction, or increased airway resistance. Therefore, any pre-existing condition that might be worsened by the concurrent use of any of these medications may then represent a contraindication or caution. More specifically, with $β_1$-blocking drugs, patients with pre-existing bradycardia, decreased heart contractility, heart failure, or decreased conduction with heart block cannot take these drugs without exacerbation of these conditions. As another example, patients with a history of asthma, emphysema, bronchitis, or any condition causing increased airway resistance or bronchoconstriction cannot take $β_2$-blocking drugs without experiencing further bronchoconstriction and negative effects on their underlying disease condition. Given the actions and adverse effects of the drug, it is also important to assess intake and output, daily weights, breath sounds, and blood glucose levels, especially if the patient has diabetes. For a complete listing of drug interactions, see Tables 20-3 and 20-5.

Nursing Diagnoses

- Ineffective airway clearance related to the adverse effect of bronchoconstriction caused by β-adrenergic drugs as well as any underlying restrictive airway conditions
- Ineffective peripheral tissue perfusion related to the adverse effects of hypertension and the adverse effects of the adrenergic-blocking drugs (hypotension)
- Imbalanced nutrition, less than body requirements, due to nausea and vomiting related to the adverse effects of the adrenergic blockers
- Deficient knowledge related to lack of information about the therapeutic regimen, drug adverse effects, drug interactions, and precautions to be taken during drug treatment
- Risk for injury related to possible adverse effects of the adrenergic-blocking drugs (e.g., orthostatic hypotension, dizziness, syncope, numbness and tingling of the fingers and toes)

Planning

Goals

- Patient will maintain or regain effective airway clearance and airway exchange.
- Patient will maintain or regain adequate peripheral tissue perfusion.
- Patient will experience improved nutritional status.
- Patient will demonstrate adequate knowledge about use of specific medications, their adverse effects, and the appropriate dosing routine to be followed at home.
- Patient will remain free from injury related to adverse effects of drug therapy.

Outcome Criteria

- Patient states that respirations are performed with ease and in a regular rhythm, without any bronchospasm, wheezing, or difficulty.
- Patient states that blood pressure readings are within normal ranges.
- Patient experiences minimal adverse effects of drug therapy, specifically minimal hypotension.
- Patient states adequate dietary intake of the following: grains, vegetables, fruits, dairy, and protein-rich foods.
- Patient states the rationale for both pharmacological and nonpharmacological treatment of hypertension or other indications for drug therapy.
- Patient states the importance of adhering to the medication therapy regimen and taking medication as prescribed.
- Patient reports effective blood pressure lowering or other desired therapeutic effects of treatment with an adrenergic blocker without risks and complications such as syncope, dizziness, and hypotension.
- Patient demonstrates the correct method of self-measurement of blood pressure using a digital cuff device.
- Patient states the potentially occurring conditions that necessitate informing the health care provider (HCP), such as palpitations, chest pain, insomnia, and excessive agitation.
- Patient remains free from injury due to taking medication as prescribed and preventing or managing adverse reactions.
- Patient keeps all follow-up appointments with the HCP to maintain safe therapy.
- Patient follows instructions to avoid sudden withdrawal of hypertensive drugs to prevent rebound hypertensive crises and experiences minimal complications.

Implementation

Several nursing interventions can maximize the therapeutic effects of adrenergic-blocking drugs and minimize their adverse effects. To help minimize dry mouth, encourage intake of water within any restrictions and

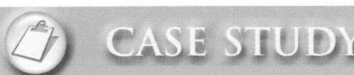

CASE STUDY

β-Blockers

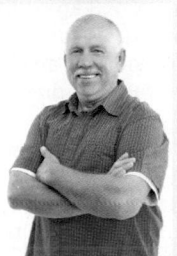

Frank, a 58-year-old high school music teacher, has been hospitalized after experiencing a myocardial infarction. He is married with two adult children. His physician told him that his myocardial infarction was "mild" but that Frank must make some lifestyle changes, including exercise and dietary changes. Frank has a history of asthma; he stopped smoking cigarettes 5 years ago and has had no recent problems. His history also includes gallbladder removal at 50 years of age. Frank's pulse rate has ranged from 78 to 112 beats/min; his blood pressure has been within normal range, 118/74 to 122/80 mm Hg. He is preparing for discharge and has the following prescriptions:

Aspirin, enteric-coated, 81 mg daily, PO

Propranolol 60 mg three times a day, clopidrogrel 75 mg daily, ramipril 5 mg BID, atorvastatin 80 mg daily, nitro-spray BID, PO

1. Explain the purpose of the propranolol order for Frank.

After Frank has been home for a week, the home health nurse calls him to check on how he is doing. Frank tells the nurse that he was "about to call the doctor" because he has been feeling more and more short of breath, even though he has been resting at home.

2. What could be causing this problem? What do you expect will happen as a result?

Two months later, Frank is in the office for a follow-up visit. He seems upset, even though his blood pressure is within normal range, his cardiac function is stable, and he has had no further breathing problems. He tells the nurse, "I don't care what the doctor tells me, I'm going to stop that new pill. I'm having a terrible problem and I know it's because of that medicine."

3. What do you suspect is causing Frank to be so upset, and what will be done about it? Will the β-blocker be discontinued today? Explain your answer.

For answers, see http://evolve.elsevier.com/Canada/Lilley/pharmacology/.

---

frequent rinsing or spraying of the mouth with over-the-counter dental products indicated for dry mouth. Sugarless gum or candy may also be helpful for dry mouth. When adrenergic-blocking medications are given intravenously, this usually takes place in specialty care areas and according to agency protocols. Heart monitoring is usually recommended. Encourage patients taking α-blockers to change positions slowly and with purpose to prevent or minimize orthostatic hypotension with subsequent dizziness or syncope. α-blockers and their indications in treatment of hypertensive disease or hypertensive crises are discussed further in Chapter 23. Use of the newer α-blocker tamsulosin hydrochloride in patients with BPH is quite common, and patients taking this drug need to inform all HCPs—including dentists—that this is part of their medical regimen, especially before any type of surgery. In addition, anything leading to vasodilation needs to be avoided to prevent orthostatic hypotension with resultant dizziness, lightheadedness, and syncope. This includes alcohol intake, excessive exercise, exposure to hot climates, and use of saunas, hot tubs, and hot showers or baths. When either an α-blocker or β-blocker is used, count the apical pulse rate for 1 full minute. Measure and document both supine and standing blood pressures. Contact the HCP immediately if the patient has any problems with dizziness, fainting, or lightheadedness; if the systolic blood pressure is lower than 100 mm Hg; or if the pulse rate is lower than 60 beats per minute. Daily weight measurement is important to monitor the progress of therapy and monitor for the adverse effect of edema. A good rule of thumb is to follow up if the patient shows an increase of 1 kg or more over a 24-hour period or 2.3 kg or more within 1 week. Keeping a daily journal documenting weights, blood pressure readings, pulse rates, adverse effects, and overall feelings of wellness or lack thereof will be important to the monitoring of the therapeutic regimen. Other symptoms to report to HCPs include muscle weakness, shortness of breath, and collection of fluid in the lower extremities as manifested by weight gain or difficulty in putting on shoes or socks. Patients taking any of the adrenergic-blocking medications must be weaned off the drug slowly because an abrupt discontinuation could lead to rebound hypertension or chest pain. The HCP will designate a period of time for weaning, generally over a period of 1 to 2 weeks. Understanding basic anatomy and physiology and how receptors work will help guide nursing actions related to these drugs. See Patient Teaching Tips for more specific information.

Evaluation

Therapeutic effects for which to monitor in patients receiving adrenergic-blocking drugs include, but are not limited to, a decrease in blood pressure, pulse rate, and palpitations (in patients with related problems before drug therapy); alleviation of the symptoms of the disorder for which the drug was indicated; a return to normal blood pressure and pulse with lowering of the blood pressure toward 120/80 mm Hg and the pulse toward 60 beats per minute in patients with diagnosed hypertension; and a decrease in chest pain in patients with angina. Also monitor patients for adverse effects associated with these medications, including bradycardia, depression, fatigue, and hypotension. See Tables 20-2 and 20-4 for other potential adverse effects.

PATIENT TEACHING TIPS

❖ Provide patients with written and verbal information about drug indications, actions, adverse effects, cautions, contraindications, and interactions with other drugs. This information needs to be age-appropriate and tailored to the specific learning needs of the patient.

❖ Emphasize the need to wear a medical alert bracelet or necklace identifying the specific medical diagnosis and provide a list of all medications. The patient needs to understand the importance of carrying this information (in handwritten or electronic form), having it available at all times, and updating it regularly and whenever there are major changes in the diagnosis and treatment regimen. Recommend to patients that they maintain a record of blood pressure readings by date and time. This information may then be shared with other HCPs.

❖ Caution patients to take medications exactly as prescribed and to never abruptly discontinue them due to the risk of rebound hypertension. If there is concern about omitted or skipped doses, patients need to contact their HCPs immediately.

❖ Caffeine and other central nervous system stimulants must be avoided while taking adrenergic-blocking drugs to prevent further irritability of the cardiac and central nervous systems and subsequent negative effects on health status.

❖ Encourage patients to contact their HCP upon the occurrence of palpitations, chest pain, confusion, weight gain (1 kg or more in 24 hours or 2.3 kg or more in 1 week), dyspnea, nausea, or vomiting. Other problems to report include swelling in the feet and ankles, shortness of breath, excessive fatigue, dizziness, and syncope.

❖ The α-blocker tamsulosin hydrochloride must be taken as directed and with caution in patients with blood pressure problems (e.g., hypotension). The drug must also be used with caution by older adults and while driving or engaging in other activities requiring alertness because the adverse effects of this drug include blurred vision, dizziness, and drowsiness.

❖ Caution patients to change positions slowly to avoid dizziness and syncope. Excessive exercise, exposure to hot climates, use of a sauna or tanning bed, and alcohol consumption exacerbate vasodilation from the adrenergic-blocking drugs and lead to a greater drop in blood pressure with additional risk of dizziness and syncope.

❖ Constipation may develop as an adverse effect. Increasing intake of fluids and fibre, as well as increasing exercise, may help to prevent constipation.

KEY POINTS

❖ Adrenergic-blocking drugs block the stimulation of the α-, β_1-, or β_2-adrenergic receptors, with the net result of blocking the effects of either norepinephrine or epinephrine on the receptor. This blocking action leads to a variety of physiological responses, depending on which receptors are blocked. Knowing how these receptors work allows the nurse to understand and predict the expected therapeutic effects of the drugs as well as the expected adverse effects.

❖ With α-blockers, the predominant response is vasodilation. This is due to the blocking of the α-adrenergic effect of vasoconstriction, which results in blood vessel relaxation.

❖ Vasodilation of blood vessels with the α-blockers results in a drop in blood pressure and a reduction in urinary obstruction, which may lead to increased urinary flow rates. Monitor for these effects in patients taking α-blockers.

❖ β-blockers inhibit the stimulation of β-adrenergic receptors by blocking the effects of the SNS neurotransmitters norepinephrine, epinephrine, and dopamine. Stimulation of β_1-receptors leads to an *increase* in heart rate, conduction, and contractility. Stimulation of β_2-receptors leads to an increase in bronchial smooth muscle relaxation or bronchodilation.

Blocking of β_1-receptors leads to a *decrease* in heart rate, conduction, and contractility. Blocking of β_2-receptors leads to a *decrease* in bronchial smooth muscle relaxation or bronchoconstriction.

❖ β-blockers are classified as either selective or nonselective. Selective β-blockers are also called cardioselective β-blockers and block only the β-adrenergic receptors in the heart that are located on the postsynaptic effector cells (i.e., the cells that nerves stimulate). The beneficial effects of the cardioselective β-blockers include decreased heart rate, reduced cardiac conduction, and decreased myocardial contractility with no bronchoconstriction. These drugs are a good choice for patients with hypertension who also experience bronchospasm associated with asthma or another pulmonary disease.

❖ Nursing considerations for patients taking α- and β-blockers include teaching patients that they must weigh themselves daily, avoid sudden changes in position, and increase their intake of fluids and fibre. Weight gain, dizziness, fainting, or a decrease in apical heart rate below 60 beats per minute or a blood pressure of less than 100 mm Hg systolic or less than 60 mm Hg diastolic need to be reported immediately.

EXAMINATION REVIEW QUESTIONS

1. When a patient has experienced extravasation of a systemic infusion of dopamine, the nurse will inject the α-blocker phentolamine (Rogitine) into the area of extravasation and expect which effect?
   a. Vasoconstriction
   b. Vasodilation
   c. Analgesia
   d. Hypotension

2. When administering β-blockers, the nurse will follow which guideline for administration and monitoring?
   a. The drug may be discontinued at any time.
   b. Orthostatic hypotension rarely occurs with this drug.
   c. Tapering off the medication is necessary to prevent rebound hypertension.
   d. The patient needs to stop taking the medication at once upon a 1.5- to 2-kg weight gain in a week.

3. The nurse providing teaching for a patient who has a new prescription for β₁-blockers will anticipate that these drugs may result in which effect?
   a. Tachycardia
   b. Tachypnea
   c. Bradycardia
   d. Bradypnea

4. A patient who has recently had a myocardial infarction has started therapy with a β-blocker. The nurse explains that the main purpose of the β-blocker for this patient is to:
   a. Cause vasodilation of the coronary arteries
   b. Prevent hypertension
   c. Increase conduction through the SA node
   d. Protect the heart from circulating catecholamines

5. Before initiating therapy with a nonselective β-blocker, the nurse will assess the patient for a history of which condition?
   a. Hypertension
   b. Liver disease
   c. Pancreatitis
   d. Asthma

6. A patient is taking an α-blocker as treatment for benign prostatic hyperplasia. The nurse will monitor for which potential drug effects? (Select all that apply.)
   a. Orthostatic hypotension
   b. Increased blood pressure
   c. Increased urine flow
   d. Headaches
   e. Bradycardia

7. A child in the pediatric intensive care unit has been receiving a dopamine infusion. This morning while on rounds, the nurse noted that the intravenous infusion has infiltrated. After stopping the infusion, the nurse prepares to administer phentolamine (Regitine). The ordered dose is 0.2 mg/kg, to be injected into the area of extravasation. The child weighs 39 lb. How many milligrams will the nurse administer? (Round to tenths.)

Answers: 1. b, 2. c, 3. c, 4. d, 5. d, 6. a, c, d, 7. 3.5 mg

CRITICAL THINKING ACTIVITIES

1. A 46-year-old woman has been prescribed labetalol (Trandate) for the control of tachycardia and hypertension. What is the nurse's priority in answering if the patient states, "Well, if it doesn't work after a month or two, I'll just quit taking it!"?

2. You are reviewing orders and find one for propranolol. When going to the automated drug-dispensing machine to retrieve the drug, the nurse finds propranolol (Inderal LA) in the drawer. Should you give the drug? What is your priority action at this time?

3. A 73-year-old man is given a new prescription for tamsulosin hydrochloride (Flomax) for treatment of BPH. He lives at home with his wife and uses a cane to help him walk because of the effects of a stroke he had 5 years ago. During the patient education session, the nurse should emphasize which issue of highest priority?

For answers, see http://evolve.elsevier.com/Canada/Lilley/pharmacology/.

CHAPTER 21

Cholinergic Drugs

Objectives

After reading this chapter, the successful student will be able to do the following:

1. Briefly review the functions of the autonomic nervous system and the impact of the parasympathetic division.

2. List the various drugs classified as cholinergic agonists (also called parasympathomimetics).

3. Discuss the mechanisms of action, therapeutic effects, indications, adverse and toxic effects, drug interactions, cautions, contraindications, dosages, routes of administration, and any antidotal management for the various cholinergic agonists (or parasympathomimetics).

4. Develop a collaborative plan of care that includes all phases of the nursing process for patients taking cholinergic agonists.

e-Learning Activities

Website
(http://evolve.elsevier.com/Canada/Lilley/pharmacology/)

evolve

- Answer Key—Textbook Case Studies
- Answer Key—Critical Thinking Activities
- Chapter Summaries—Printable
- Review Questions for Exam Preparation
- Unfolding Case Studies

Drug Profiles

▸▸ bethanechol (bethanechol chloride)*, p. 410
▸▸ donepezil (donepezil hydrochloride)*, p. 410
   memantine (memantine hydrochloride)*, p. 411
▸▸ physostigmine (physostigmine salicylate)*, p. 411

▸▸ Key drug

*Full generic name is given in parentheses. For the purposes of this text, the more common, shortened name is used.

Key Terms

Acetylcholine (ACh)   The neurotransmitter responsible for transmission of nerve impulses to effector cells in the parasympathetic nervous system. (p. 407)

Acetylcholinesterase (AChE)   The enzyme responsible for the breakdown of acetylcholine (also referred to simply as *cholinesterase*). (p. 408)

Alzheimer's disease   A disease of the brain characterized by progressive mental deterioration manifested by confu-

sion, disorientation, and loss of memory, ability to calculate, and visual–spatial orientation. (p. 409)

Atony   A lack of normal muscle tone. (p. 408)

Cholinergic crisis   Severe muscle weakness and respiratory paralysis due to excessive acetylcholine; often seen in patients with myasthenia gravis as an adverse effect of drugs used to treat the disorder. (p. 410)

Cholinergic receptor   A nerve receptor that is stimulated by acetylcholine. (p. 407)

Miosis   Contraction of the pupil. (p. 408)

Muscarinic receptors   Cholinergic receptors located postsynaptically in the effector organs, such as smooth muscle, heart muscle, and glands supplied by parasympathetic fibres. (p. 407)

Nicotinic receptors   Cholinergic receptors located in the ganglia (where presynaptic and postsynaptic nerve fibres meet) of both the parasympathetic nervous system and the sympathetic nervous system, so named because they can be stimulated by the alkaloid nicotine. (p. 407)

Parasympathomimetics   Drugs that mimic the parasympathetic nervous system; also referred to as *cholinergic agonist drugs*. (p. 412)

OVERVIEW

Cholinergics, cholinergic agonists, and *parasympathomimetics* are terms referring to the class of drugs that stimulate the parasympathetic nervous system.

PARASYMPATHETIC NERVOUS SYSTEM

The parasympathetic nervous system is the branch of the autonomic nervous system with nerve functions generally opposite to those of the sympathetic nervous system (Figure 19-1 and Figure 21-1). The parasympathetic nervous system controls homeostasis and the body at rest. It restores the body to a state of calm (e.g., slows heart rate, relaxes smooth muscle, constricts bronchioles, constricts pupils**). Acetylcholine (ACh)** is the neurotransmitter responsible for the transmission of nerve impulses to effector cells in the parasympathetic nervous system. A **cholinergic receptor** is a receptor that binds the ACh and mediates its actions. There are two types of cholinergic receptors, as determined by their location and their action. **Nicotinic receptors** are located in the ganglia of both the parasympathetic and sympathetic nervous systems. They are called *nicotinic* because they can be stimulated by nicotine. The other type of cholinergic receptor is the muscarinic receptor. **Muscarinic receptors** are located postsynaptically in the effector organs (i.e., smooth muscle, heart muscle, and glands) supplied by the parasympathetic fibres. They are called *muscarinic* because they are stimulated by the alkaloid muscarine, a substance isolated from mushrooms. Figure 21-2 shows how the nicotinic and muscarinic receptors are arranged in the parasympathetic nervous system.

CHOLINERGIC DRUGS

Cholinergic drugs mimic the effects of ACh. These drugs can stimulate cholinergic receptors directly or indirectly. *Direct-acting* cholinergic agonists bind directly to cholinergic receptors and activate them. *Indirect-acting* cholinergic agonists stimulate the postsynaptic release of ACh at the receptor site; this then allows the ACh to bind to and stimulate the receptor. Indirect-acting cholinergic

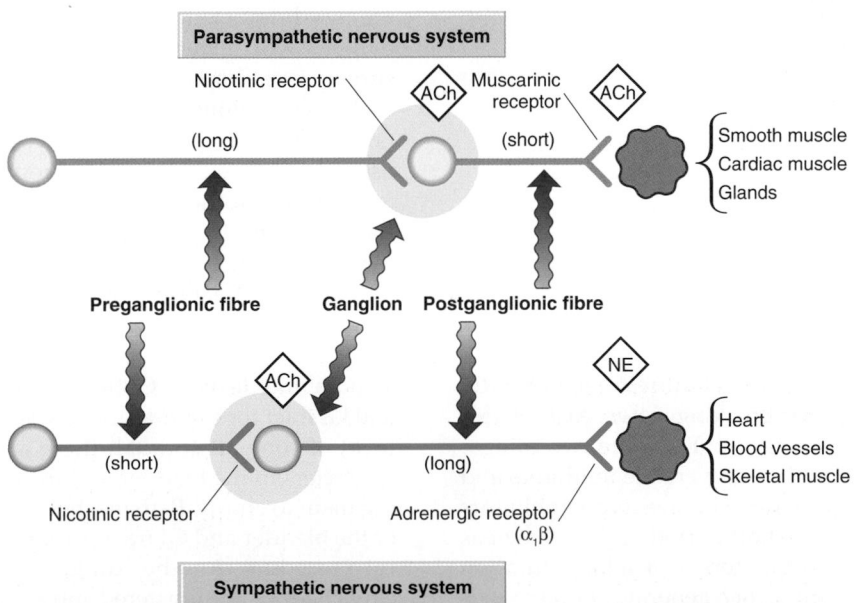

FIG. 21-1   The parasympathetic and sympathetic nervous systems and their relationships to one another. *ACh,* acetylcholine; *NE,* norepinephrine.

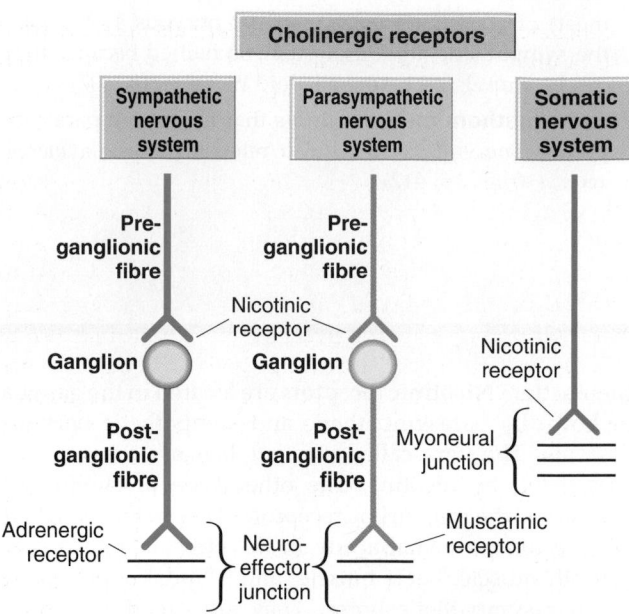

FIG. 21-2 The sympathetic, parasympathetic, and somatic nervous systems. Note the location of the nicotinic and muscarinic receptors within the parasympathetic nervous system.

BOX 21-1

Cholinergic Drugs

Direct-Acting Drugs

bethanechol chloride (Duvoid)
carbachol (Miostat Ophthalmic)
pilocarpine hydrochloride (Akarpine®, Salagen®, Diocarpine® [see Chapter 57], others)
succinylcholine chloride (Quelicin®; see Chapter 12)

Indirect-Acting Drugs

donepezil hydrochloride (Aricept)
edrophonium chloride (Tensilon®)
galantamine hydrobromide (Reminyl®)
neostigmine methylsulfate (Prostigmin®)
pyridostigmine bromide (Mestinon®)
rivastigmine hydrogen tartrate (Exelon)

drugs (also known as cholinesterase inhibitors) work by inhibiting the action of **acetylcholinesterase (AChE)**, the enzyme responsible for breaking down ACh. AChE is also referred to as *cholinesterase*. There are two categories of cholinesterase inhibitors: reversible inhibitors and irreversible inhibitors. *Reversible* cholinesterase inhibitors bind to cholinesterase for a short period of time, whereas *irreversible* cholinesterase inhibitors have a long duration of activity, and the body must then generate new enzymes to override the effects of the irreversible drugs. Box 21-1 lists the direct- and indirect-acting cholinergics.

Mechanism of Action and Drug Effects

When ACh binds directly to its receptor, stimulation occurs. Once binding takes place on the membranes of an effector cell of the target tissue or organ, the permeability of the cell changes, and calcium and sodium are permitted to flow into the cell. This then depolarizes the cell membrane and stimulates the effector organ.

The effects of direct- and indirect-acting cholinergics are seen when the parasympathetic nervous system is stimulated. There are many mnemonics to aid in remembering these effects. One is to think of the parasympathetic nervous system as the "rest-and-digest" system, in contrast to the "fight-or-flight" sympathetic nervous system.

Cholinergic drugs are used primarily for their effects on the gastrointestinal (GI) tract, bladder, and eye. These drugs stimulate the intestines and bladder, which results in increased gastric secretions, GI motility, and urinary frequency. They also stimulate constriction of the pupil, termed *miosis*; this helps to decrease intraocular pressure. In addition, cholinergic drugs cause increased salivation and sweating. Cardiovascular effects include decreased heart rate and vasodilation. Pulmonary effects include constriction of the bronchi of the lungs and narrowing of the airways.

At recommended doses, cholinergic drugs primarily affect the muscarinic receptors, but at high doses the nicotinic receptors can also be stimulated. The desired effects come from muscarinic receptor stimulation; many of the undesirable adverse effects are due to nicotinic receptor stimulation. The various effects of the cholinergic drugs are listed in Table 21-1, according to the receptors stimulated.

Indications
Direct-Acting Drugs

Direct-acting drugs, such as carbachol and pilocarpine, are used topically to reduce intraocular pressure in patients with glaucoma or in those undergoing ocular surgery (see Chapter 57). These drugs are poorly absorbed orally, which limits their use to primarily topical application. However, pilocarpine hydrochloride tablets are used to treat excessively dry mouth (xerostomia) resulting from a disorder known as *Sjögren's syndrome* and for salivary gland hypofunction caused by radiotherapy for cancer of the head and neck.

The direct-acting cholinergic drug bethanechol (Urecholine®) is administered orally. Bethanechol affects the detrusor muscle of the urinary bladder and also the smooth muscle of the GI tract. It causes increased bladder and GI tract tone and motility, which increases the movement of contents through these areas. It also causes the sphincters in the bladder and the GI tract to relax, allowing them to empty. Bethanechol is also used to treat **atony** of the bladder and GI tract. Atony can occur after a surgical procedure. Another direct-acting cholinergic is succinylcholine, administered intravenously, which is used as a neuromuscular blocker in general anaesthesia (see Chapter 12).

TABLE 21-1

Cholinergic Drugs: Drug Effects

Body Tissue	Response to Stimulation	
	Muscarinic	**Nicotinic**
PULMONARY		
Bronchi (lungs)	Increased secretion, constriction	None
CARDIOVASCULAR		
Blood vessels	Dilation	Constriction
Heart rate	Slowed	Increased
Blood pressure	Decreased	Increased
OCULAR		
Eye	Miosis (pupil constriction), decreased accommodation	Miosis (pupil constriction), decreased accommodation
GASTROINTESTINAL		
Tone	Increased	Increased
Motility	Increased	Increased
Sphincter	Relaxed	None
GENITOURINARY		
Tone	Increased	Increased
Motility	Increased	Increased
Sphincter	Relaxed	Relaxed
GLANDULAR SECRETIONS		
	Increased intestinal, lacrimal, salivary, and sweat gland secretion	No response
SKELETAL MUSCLE		
	No response	Increased contraction

Indirect-Acting Drugs

Indirect-acting drugs work by increasing ACh concentrations at the receptor sites, which leads to stimulation of the effector cells. Indirect-acting drugs cause skeletal muscle contraction and are used for the diagnosis and treatment of myasthenia gravis. Myasthenia gravis is a rare autoimmune neuromuscular disease characterized by varying degrees of weakness of the skeletal muscles of the body. It is caused by a defect in the function of ACh at the neuromuscular junctions. Indirect-acting drugs' ability to inhibit AChE also makes them useful for the reversal of neuromuscular blockade produced either by neuromuscular blocking drugs (NMBDs) or by anticholinergic poisoning. For this reason, the indirect-acting drug physostigmine is considered the antidote for anticholinergic poisoning and poisoning by irreversible cholinesterase inhibitors such as organophosphates and carbonates, common classes of insecticides. Physostigmine is a restricted drug in Canada and only available through the Special Access Programme.

Indirect-acting cholinergic drugs are also used to treat **Alzheimer's disease,** a neurological disorder in which patients have decreased levels of ACh. In the treatment of Alzheimer's disease, cholinergic drugs increase concentrations of ACh in the brain by inhibiting cholinesterase. These drugs do not stop or reverse the progression of Alzheimer's disease; however, the increase in ACh helps to enhance or maintain memory and learning capabilities. There are three cholinesterase inhibitors used to treat Alzheimer's disease: donepezil (Aricept®), galantamine (Reminyl®), and rivastigmine hydrogen tartrate (Exelon®). All are indirect-acting cholinergic drugs. It has been reported that as few as 15 to 30% of patients treated actually see benefit. However, indirect-acting drugs may cause small improvements in cognitive, functional, and global effects in those with mild to moderate disease, while marginal effects are seen in patients with severe disease, who are on long-term treatment, and who are of advanced age (Buckley & Salpeter, 2015). The efficacy of cholinesterase inhibitors appears to taper off over time, with minimal benefit seen after 1 year.

The most commonly used of these medications is donepezil. Patient response to these drugs is highly variable. For this reason, a failure to respond to maximally titrated doses of one of these drugs should not necessarily rule out an attempt at therapy with another drug in this same class. In the absence of any recently approved new therapies, the focus of manufacturers of the cholinesterase inhibitors has been on altering the formulations and dosage of current medications. One example is the rivastigmine patch ($18mg/10 \text{ cm}^2/24$ hr and $27 \text{ mg}/15 \text{ cm}^2/24$ hr) for use across all stages. Memantine (Ebixa®) is also used to treat Alzheimer's disease, but it is not a cholinesterase inhibitor. Memantine monotherapy produces small benefits in cognitive function in moderate to severe dementia, without significant adverse effects. For dosage information for all of these drugs, refer to the table on p. 411.

Contraindications

Contraindications to the use of cholinergic drugs include known drug allergy, GI or genitourinary (GU) tract obstruction, bradycardia, defects in cardiac impulse conduction, hyperthyroidism, epilepsy, hypotension, or chronic obstructive pulmonary disease. Parkinsonism (see Chapter 16) is listed as a precaution to these drugs; however, rivastigmine hydrogen tartrate (Exelon) is used in patients with Parkinson's disease who also have dementia.

Adverse Effects

The primary adverse effects of cholinergic drugs are the consequence of overstimulation of the parasympathetic nervous system. They are extensions of the cholinergic reactions that affect many body functions. The major effects are listed by body system in Table 21-2. The effects on the cardiovascular system are complex and may include syncope, hypotension with reflex tachycardia, hypertension, or bradycardia, depending on whether the muscarinic or nicotinic receptors are stimulated.

Toxicity and Management of Overdose

There is little systemic absorption of topically administered cholinergic drugs and therefore little systemic toxicity. When administered locally in the eye, they can cause temporary ocular changes such as transient blurring and dimming of vision. Systemic toxicity with topically applied cholinergics is seen most commonly when longer-acting drugs are given repeatedly over a long period. This can result in overstimulation of the

TABLE 21-2

Cholinergic Drugs: Adverse Effects

Body System	Adverse Effects
Cardiovascular	Bradycardia or tachycardia, hypotension or hypertension, conduction abnormalities (atrioventricular block and cardiac arrest), syncope
Central nervous	Headache, dizziness, convulsions, ataxia
Gastrointestinal	Abdominal cramps, increased secretions, nausea, vomiting, diarrhea, weight loss
Respiratory	Increased bronchial secretions, bronchospasms
Other	Lacrimation, sweating, salivation, miosis

parasympathetic nervous system and all the attendant responses. Treatment is generally symptomatic and supportive, and the administration of a reversal drug (e.g., atropine sulphate) is rarely required.

The likelihood of toxicity is greater for cholinergics that are given orally or intravenously. The most severe consequence of an overdose of a cholinergic drug is a **cholinergic crisis**. Symptoms include circulatory collapse, hypotension, bloody diarrhea, shock, and cardiac arrest. Early signs include abdominal cramps, salivation, flushing of the skin, nausea, and vomiting. Transient syncope, transient complete heart block, dyspnea, and orthostatic hypotension may also occur. These symptoms can be reversed promptly by the administration of atropine sulphate, a cholinergic antagonist. Severe cardiovascular reactions or bronchoconstriction may be alleviated by epinephrine, an adrenergic agonist. One way of remembering the effects of cholinergic poisoning is to use the acronym SLUDGE, which stands for **s**alivation, **l**acrimation, **u**rinary **i**ncontinence, **d**iarrhea, **g**astrointestinal cramps, and **e**mesis.

Interactions

Anticholinergics (such as atropine sulphate), antihistamines, and sympathomimetics may antagonize cholinergic drugs and lead to a reduced response to them. Other cholinergic drugs may have additive effects.

Dosages

For recommended dosages of the cholinergic drugs, refer to the table on p. 411.

 DRUG PROFILES

▶▶ bethanechol chloride

Bethanechol chloride (Duvoid®) is a direct-acting cholinergic agonist. It is used in the treatment of acute postoperative and postpartum nonobstructive urinary retention and for the management of urinary retention associated with neurogenic atony of the bladder. It has also been used to prevent and treat bladder dysfunction induced by phenothiazine and tricyclic antidepressants (TCAs) (see Chapter 17). In addition, it is used in the treatment of postoperative GI atony and gastric retention, chronic refractory heartburn, and in diagnostic testing for infantile cystic fibrosis. Bethanechol is available orally. Contraindications include known drug allergy, hyperthyroidism, peptic ulcer, active bronchial asthma, heart disease or coronary artery disease, epilepsy, and Parkinson's disease. The drug is to be avoided in patients in whom the strength or integrity of the GI tract or bladder wall is questionable or who have conditions in which increased muscular activity could prove harmful, such as known or suspected mechanical obstruction.

Adverse effects include syncope, hypotension with reflex tachycardia, headache, seizures, GI upset, and asthmatic attacks. Drugs that interact with bethanechol include AChE inhibitors (i.e., indirect-acting cholinergics), which

can enhance the adverse effects of bethanechol. For recommended dosages refer to the table on page 411.

PHARMACOKINETICS

Route	Onset of Action	Peak Plasma Concentration	Elimination Half-Life	Duration of Action
PO	30–90 min	Less than 30 min	Unknown	1–6 hr

▶▶ donepezil hydrochloride

Donepezil hydrochloride (Aricept) is a cholinesterase inhibitor drug that works centrally in the brain to increase levels of ACh by inhibiting AChE. It is used in the treatment of mild to moderate Alzheimer's disease. Similar cholinesterase inhibitors include galantamine hydrobromide and rivastigmine hydrogen tartrate. Rivastigmine hydrogen tartrate is also approved for treating dementia associated with Parkinson's disease. Contraindications for donepezil include known drug allergy. Adverse effects are normally mild and resolve on their own. These effects can often be avoided by careful dose titration. They include GI upset (including ulcer risk due to increased gastric secretions), drowsiness, dizziness, insomnia, and muscle cramps. The

DRUG PROFILES—cont'd

effects on the cardiovascular system are complex and may include bradycardia, syncope, hypotension with reflex tachycardia, or hypertension. Interacting drugs include anticholinergics (which counteract donepezil effects) and nonsteroidal anti-inflammatory drugs (see Chapter 49). Donepezil is available only for oral use as both a tablet and a rapid-acting, orally disintegrating tablet. Recommended dosages are given in the table on this page.

PHARMACOKINETICS

Route	Onset of Action	Peak Plasma Concentration	Elimination Half-Life	Duration of Action
PO	3 wk	3–4 hr	70 hr	2 wk

▸▸ memantine hydrochloride

Memantine hydrochloride (Ebixa) is not a cholinergic drug but is included here in the discussion of drugs for Alzheimer's disease. It is classified as an N-methyl-D-aspartate (NMDA) receptor antagonist owing to its inhibitory activity at the NMDA receptors in the central nervous system. NMDA receptors are glutamate-activated ion channel receptors found throughout the nervous system. The NMDA receptor is significant for its role in controlling synaptic plasticity and memory function (Yu & Popescu, 2013). Stimulation of these receptors is believed to be part of the Alzheimer's disease process. Memantine blocks this stimulation and thereby helps to reduce or arrest the patient's symptoms of cognitive degeneration. As with all other currently available medications for this debilitating illness, the effects of this drug are likely to be temporary but may still afford some improvement in quality of life and general functioning for some patients. Its only current contraindication is known drug allergy. Reported adverse effects are relatively uncommon but include hypotension, headache, GI upset, musculoskeletal pain, dyspnea, ataxia, and fatigue. No clearly defined drug interactions are listed. Memantine is available only for oral use. For the recommended dosage, refer to the table on this page.

PHARMACOKINETICS

Route	Onset of Action	Peak Plasma Concentration	Elimination Half-Life	Duration of Action
PO	Unknown	5 hr	70 hr	Unknown

▸▸ pyridostigmine bromide

Pyridostigmine bromide (Mestinon®, Mestinon SR®) is a synthetic quaternary ammonium compound and is structurally similar to other drugs in this class, including edrophonium chloride and neostigmine. All are indirect-acting cholinergic drugs that work to increase ACh by inhibiting AChE. Pyridostigmine bromide has been shown to improve muscle strength and is used to relieve the symptoms of myasthenia gravis; it is the most commonly used drug for the symptomatic treatment of this disease. Edrophonium chloride (Tensilon®) is an indirect-acting cholinergic drug that is commonly used to diagnose myasthenia gravis. It can also be used to differentiate between myasthenia gravis and cholinergic crisis. Edrophonium prevents the breakdown of ACh, which then helps stimulate the muscles. Cholinergic crisis causes the muscles to stop responding to ACh, resulting in flaccid paralysis and respiratory failure. The flaccid paralysis from cholinergic crisis can be distinguished from myasthenia gravis by the use of edrophonium, which worsens the paralysis caused by cholinergic crisis, but strengthens the muscle in the case of myasthenia gravis.

Neostigmine and pyridostigmine bromide are also useful for reversing the effects of nondepolarizing neuromuscular blocking drugs (see Chapter 12) after surgery. They are also used in the treatment of severe overdoses of TCAs because of the significant anticholinergic effects associated with the TCAs. Neostigmine and pyridostigmine are also used as an antidote after toxic exposure to nondrug anticholinergic agents, including those used in chemical warfare. Contraindications to these drugs include known drug allergy, prior severe cholinergic reactions, asthma, gangrene, hyperthyroidism, cardiovascular disease, and mechanical obstruction of the GI or GU tracts. Interacting drugs include the anticholinergic drugs, which counteract the therapeutic effects of indirect-acting cholinergic drugs. Pyridostigmine bromide is available in oral form. Recommended dosages are given in the Dosages table below.

PHARMACOKINETICS

Route	Onset of Action	Peak Plasma Concentration	Elimination Half-Life	Duration of Action
PO	15–45 min	1–2 hr	3–4 hr	Up to 6 hr

DOSAGES   Selected Cholinergic Agonist Drugs

Drug	Pharmacological Class	Usual Dosage Range	Indications/Uses
▸▸ bethanechol chloride (Duvoid)	Muscarinic (direct-acting)	*Adults* PO: 10–50 mg tid–qid (usually start with 5–10 mg, repeating hourly until urination, max 50 mg/cycle)	Postoperative and postpartum functional urinary retention; neurogenic atony
▸▸ donepezil hydrochloride (Aricept)	Anticholinesterase inhibitor (indirect-acting)	*Adults* PO: 5–10 mg/day as a single dose	Alzheimer's disease
pyridostigmine bromide (Mestinon)	Anticholinesterase (indirect-acting)	*Adults* PO: 180–540 mg/day divided bid	Myasthenia gravis; antidote for neuromuscular blocker toxicity

PO, oral.

NURSING PROCESS

▨ Assessment

Cholinergic drugs, or **parasympathomimetics**, produce a variety of effects stemming from their ability to stimulate the parasympathetic nervous system and mimic the action of ACh. These effects include a decrease in heart rate, an increase in GI and GU tone through increased contractility of the smooth muscle of the bowel and bladder, an increase in the contractility and tone of bronchial smooth muscle, increased respiratory secretions, and miosis or papillary constriction. Therefore, if the patient has any pre-existing conditions, such as heart block, or the patient is taking other drugs that mimic the actions of the parasympathetic nervous system, adverse effects or toxicity may increase. Before cholinergic drugs are given, perform a thorough head-to-toe physical assessment and obtain a nursing history and medication history (including prescription drugs, over-the-counter drugs [OTC], and natural health products). Document drug allergies and past and present medical conditions as well. Identify cautions, contraindications, and drug interactions. Assess and document vital signs, with special attention to baseline blood pressure readings because of the potential for orthostatic hypotension.

Before a drug for Alzheimer's disease such as donepezil or memantine is used, assess the patient for allergies, cautions, contraindications, and drug interactions. Perform a close assessment and documentation of the patient's neurological status, with attention to short- and long-term memory; level of alertness; motor, cognitive, and sensory functioning; any suicidal tendencies or ideations; musculoskeletal intactness; and GI, GU, and cardiovascular functioning. Assess urinary patterns so that any problems with urinary retention may be identified.

Report any abnormalities or patient-reported discomfort to the prescriber immediately. Presence or absence of family support systems is important to note because of the chronic nature of this illness. Once the patient has begun taking medication, it is critical for the nurse to continue to assess the patient's response to the drug. Note any changes in symptoms within the first 6 weeks of therapy. Journalling by the patient or a family or caregiver may be helpful to the health care provider (HCP) when assessing for any positive changes, adverse effects, or lack of improvement. Ginkgo may be used by some patients for additional cognitive benefits when added to conventional treatment with cholinesterase inhibitors, despite controversy over its efficacy in the prevention and treatment of dementia (Canevelli et al., 2014; see Natural Health Products: Ginkgo).

▨ Nursing Diagnoses

- Decreased cardiac output related to the adverse cardiovascular effects of hypotension and bradycardia
- Deficient knowledge of the therapeutic regimen, adverse effects, drug interactions, and precautions for cholinergic drugs related to lack of experience with drug therapies
- Risk for injury related to the possible adverse effects of cholinergic drugs, such as bradycardia and hypotension, with subsequent risk for falls or syncope

▨ Planning

▰ Goals

- Patient will maintain normal cardiac output and status due to taking medication exactly as prescribed.
- Patient will demonstrate adequate knowledge about the safe use of prescribed medication, its adverse effects, and appropriate dosing at home.

 NATURAL HEALTH PRODUCTS

GINKGO (*Ginkgo biloba*)

Overview
The dried leaf of the Ginkgo tree contains flavonoids, terpenoids, and organic acids that help ginkgo preparations exert their positive effects as an antioxidant and inhibitor of platelet aggregation.

Common Uses
To prevent memory loss, peripheral arterial occlusive disease, vertigo, tinnitus

Adverse Effects
Stomach or intestinal upset, headache, bleeding, allergic skin reaction

Potential Drug Interactions
Aspirin, nonsteroidal anti-inflammatory drugs, warfarin, heparin, anticonvulsants, ticlopidine, clopidogrel, dipyridamole, tricyclic antidepressants

Contraindications
None

- Patient will remain free from injury resulting from the adverse effects of the medication.

■ Outcome Criteria

- Patient, caregiver, or family member states the symptoms to report to an HCP immediately, such as dizziness, syncope, excess fatigue, and lightheadedness with heart rate changes.
- Patient has blood pressure and pulse rate monitored and recorded daily.
- Patient's blood pressure and pulse rate stay within normal ranges or without significant drops while on medication.
- Patient, caregiver, or family member states the importance of scheduling and keeping follow-up appointments with HCPs related to the management of the disorder for which medication has been prescribed and the monitoring for therapeutic or adverse effects.
- Patient, caregiver, or family member demonstrates understanding that medications are not curative but are for symptomatic control.
- Patient, caregiver, or family member demonstrates understanding that it may take several weeks for medications (e.g., medications for Alzheimer's disease) to have therapeutic effects.
- Patient, caregiver, or family member demonstrates an understanding about the need to implement safety measures to avoid falls, such as taking time to move slowly from lying or sitting to standing, making purposeful movements, and using compression stockings.

⬛ Implementation

Several nursing interventions may help to maximize the therapeutic effects of cholinergic drugs and minimize their adverse effects. If the patient has undergone surgery and cholinergic drugs are indicated, encourage ambulation and increased intake of fluids and fibre, unless contraindicated. Early ambulation helps to increase GI peristalsis and possibly prevent the need for drugs such as bethanechol, which is used to treat decreased or absent peristalsis related to surgery or anaesthesia. However, do not administer these drugs if a mechanical obstruction is suspected. Use of these drugs in such a situation may possibly result in bowel perforation. It is always preferable to use nonpharmacological measures rather than pharmacological regimens to treat the anticipated postoperative problems of decreased peristalsis or urinary retention. For drugs used to treat myasthenia gravis, give the oral medication approximately 30 minutes before meals to allow for onset of action and therapeutic effects (e.g., decreased dysphagia [difficulty swallowing]). Atropine sulphate is the antidote to cholinergic overdose; therefore, this medication needs to be readily available and given per the HCP's order.

None of the drugs used for Alzheimer's disease provides a cure, but these drugs do improve function and cognition to some degree. It is crucial to discuss, with empathy and compassion, the fact that the disease has no cure. The diagnosis of Alzheimer's disease or other causes of dementia is shocking, at best. Those involved in the care of the patient need to be honest in sharing

---

📋 CASE STUDY

Donepezil (Aricept) for Alzheimer's Disease

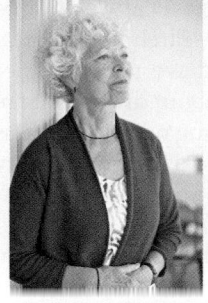

Elsa is a 72-year-old woman married to Fred, age 73 years. Fred has noticed that Elsa is becoming more forgetful, but he did not worry about it until she got lost while driving home from the grocery store. Fred makes an appointment for Elsa to see their health care provider, Dr. Sapienza. After the examination, Dr. Sapienza tells Fred, in private, that she thinks that Elsa is in the early stages of Alzheimer's disease but will order some tests to rule out other problems. Fred then accompanies Dr. Sapienza while she tells Elsa of the tentative diagnosis. Understandably, Elsa is upset to hear this news.

1. In her discussion with Elsa and Fred, Dr. Sapienza mentioned a drug called donepezil (Aricept) that can be used in the early stages of Alzheimer's disease. It may be started after a few diagnostic tests are performed. After Dr. Sapienza leaves the room, Elsa asks the nurse, "What will this drug do for me? Will it stop the Alzheimer's disease?" How will the nurse reply?

Several diagnostic tests are performed, including a complete blood count, serum electrolyte levels, vitamin B_{12} levels, liver and thyroid function tests, and a magnetic resonance imaging scan to rule out other neurological disease. Results of all tests are within normal limits. Dr. Sapienza decides to prescribe donepezil, 5 mg daily, for Elsa.

2. After a week, Fred calls the nurse to ask about giving Elsa an OTC antihistamine for her allergies. "She always needs an allergy pill this time of year." He also says that she needs to take a pain pill for her mild arthritis but is not sure whether to use acetaminophen or ibuprofen. What will the nurse tell Fred?

3. After 6 weeks, Fred brings Elsa back to the doctor's office for a follow-up appointment. Fred privately tells Dr. Sapienza that he is "upset" because he has noticed little improvement. Elsa tells Dr. Sapienza that she feels "fine" and has not noticed any problems. What do you think will be Dr. Sapienza's next order at this time? Is Elsa's response to the donepezil typical? Explain your answer.

For answers, see http://evolve.elsevier.com/Canada/Lilley/pharmacology/.

information with the patient, family, significant others, and caregivers about the fact that any of these drugs are given only for symptomatic improvement and not for a cure. Always follow ethical standards of practice when working with patients, and adhere to the Canadian Nurses Association's *Code of Ethics for Registered Nurses*. This code outlines behaviours required to maintain a high level of professionalism as well as specific actions that demonstrate respect for patients' rights in any patient care situation. However, any sharing of information with the patient, family, significant others, and caregivers must be done with the approval of the HCP, with good intent, in adherence with any research protocol, and with the goal of being a patient advocate.

When beginning any of these medications, the patient will most likely require continued assistance with activities of daily living and ambulation (because the medication may increase dizziness and cause gait imbalances at the initiation of treatment). The patient, family members, and caregivers also need to understand the importance of taking the medication exactly as ordered. Correct dosages and exact scheduling of medications are critical for the patient and family or caregiver to understand in order to achieve the drug's maximum therapeutic effects. In addition, instruct the patient and anyone involved in the patient's daily care about how the medication should be taken (e.g., taking the drug with food to decrease GI upset). Blister packaging of medications may assist patients and caregivers to enhance patients' adherence to their medication schedule. This is especially important for those who are older, have cognitive impairment, or are taking a large number of medications. The patient must be weaned off all drugs over a period of time designated by the HCP because of the potential for a rapid decline in cognitive functioning. Educate the patient and family or caregiver about the use of the drug, its adverse effects, possible interactions, and potential for harm, and emphasize the importance of *not* withdrawing the medication abruptly. Provide additional resources as needed.

Most of the cholinergic agonists have dose-limiting adverse effects that include severe GI disturbances such as nausea and vomiting. Blood pressure readings and pulse rates need to be taken and recorded before, during, and after initiation of therapy. Maintenance of a journal that records daily doses of drugs, ability of the patient to participate in activities of daily living, motor ability, gait, mental status, cognition, and any adverse effects will provide valuable information to any HCP or caregiver involved in the patient's day-to-day care.

Dosages of these medications may be changed by the HCP after about 6 weeks if no therapeutic response occurs. Monitor blood pressure, pulse rate, and electrocardiogram results throughout therapy. Instruct the patient, family, or caregiver to report any heart problems such as decrease in pulse rate (less than 60 beats per minute) or drop in blood pressure. A cholinergic crisis, resulting from overdosage of medication, may be manifested by abdominal cramps, flushing of the skin, and nausea and vomiting (early signs and symptoms) progressing to circulatory collapse, hypotension, and cardiac arrest. Dissolving forms of the medication donepezil are to be placed on the tongue and allowed to dissolve before the patient drinks fluids or swallows.

In summary, because most of the cholinergic drugs are used to treat patients diagnosed with Alzheimer's disease, monitor the patient's family and other support personnel closely, and be sure that their questions are answered fully and their needs met. Often family members, significant others, and caregivers have many questions as well as short- and long-term concerns. Preplanning education addressing these concerns is an important part of a holistic approach to patient care and to the meeting of patient needs. Often the best place to begin in terms of education is to prepare answers to the following questions that are often posed: What should we expect for our loved one? What will happen to the person emotionally and physically? What treatments are available and what drugs are deemed safe? What are the common adverse effects of drug therapy, and how can they be minimized? What are appropriate diet, fluid intake, and exercise for our loved one (See Evidence in Practice box: Exercise and Improved Cognition)? Are there natural health products or OTC drugs that would help with the disease, or should they be avoided? What will we need to do for long-term care or other living situations for our loved one? What are the expected costs of our loved one's care now and in the future? What are the costs of drug therapy? What might other costs be? What kind of help can we all receive emotionally? What about emotional support for our loved one? How can this disease affect intimate relationships? What about durable power of attorney and living wills? Other types of wills? Are these needed right away if we do not have these legal documents already? How do we all go on with our lives when our loved one is changing so drastically? Will life ever be normal again? What about research and clinical trials for treatment regimens? Should we pursue other treatments or do nothing new? What about drugs that are not Health Canada–approved? How long will this process take? What can we expect over time? Alzheimer Society Canada (http://www.alzheimer.ca) provides information, resources, support, counselling, and education that can address many of the above questions. An additional resource is The Canadian Geriatrics Society (http://www.canadiangeriatrics.ca), which promotes excellence in the medical care of older Canadians.

Evaluation

Monitor patients for the following therapeutic effects: (1) in patients with myasthenia gravis, a decrease in the signs and symptoms of the disease; (2) in patients experiencing a decrease in GI peristalsis postoperatively, an increase in bowel sounds, the passage of flatus, and the occurrence of bowel movements (all indicating an increase in peristalsis); and (3) in patients who have a hypotonic bladder with urinary retention, micturition (voiding) within approximately 60 minutes of the administration of bethanechol. Also monitor for adverse effects of these medications, including increased respiratory secretions, bronchospasm, nausea, vomiting, diarrhea, hypotension, bradycardia, and conduction abnormalities. For other adverse effects, refer to Table 21-2.

Therapeutic effects of the drugs used to manage Alzheimer's disease–related dementia or cognitive impairment include an improvement of the symptoms of the disease, but in most cases it takes up to 6 weeks for these effects to become apparent. Varying degrees of improvement in mood and a decrease in confusion usually occur. Adverse effects include nausea, vomiting, dizziness, and others (see individual drug profiles for specific information).

EVIDENCE IN PRACTICE

Exercise and Improved Cognition

Review

As the average age of the population in Canada and elsewhere continues to increase, the number of people worldwide living with Alzheimer's disease is expected to rise from the current 44.4 million to more than 135.5 million by 2050. It has been estimated that if the onset of dementia could be delayed by about 12 months, there would be approximately 9.2 million fewer cases worldwide. Several clinical trials have examined the ability of pharmacological therapies such as cholinesterase inhibitors (e.g., donepezil), and vitamin E to prevent progression to dementia in those at risk for Alzheimer's disease, but outcomes have been largely negative. Many studies have suggested that physical activity may reduce the risk for cognitive decline. This study is one of the first to demonstrate that exercise improves memory recall and brain function (measured by functional magnetic resonance imaging [fMRI]) in older adults experiencing mild cognitive impairment.

Type of Evidence

This study was a randomized, controlled trial consisting of two physically inactive groups of individuals (average age of 78); the study group of 17 participants had mild cognitive impairment while the control group of 18 participants had healthy brain function. Both groups were of similar age, gender, education, and genetic risk and had similar medication use. Both groups participated in a 12-week exercise program consisting of walking on a treadmill at moderate intensity under the supervision of a personal trainer.

Before and after the exercise program, both groups completed memory tests. The first was an fMRI famous name discrimination task. This memory test requires the participants to identify famous names as their brain activity is measured. The second was a neuropsychological battery. This test involves having participants recall words read to them from a list over five consecutive attempts, and once more after being distracted with a different list.

Results of Study

The participants with mild cognitive impairment and the control group significantly improved their memory scores from baseline on the list-learning memory retrieval test of the Rey Auditory Verbal Learning Test. The participants in both groups significantly increased their cardiorespiratory fitness by 10%.

Link of Evidence to Nursing Practice

An important achievement of this study is its demonstration of the potential benefit of the simple, nonpharmacological intervention of exercise, which is almost universally available, in the prevention of cognitive decline. For these participants as well as many other patients with physical or mental disease, the benefits of exercise go beyond improvement in cognition and include a positive impact on mood, quality of life, and cardiovascular function, as well as a decrease in falls and disability. Although advances are being made in health and technology and people are living longer, there is a need to find alternative therapies, as well as therapies that are nonpharmacological and simple, to implement to prevent and treat diseases such as Alzheimer's disease and other catastrophic brain disorders. Nurses can educate patients and family members on the importance of habitual exercise as well as encourage the provision of consistent medical care, a suitable environment, adequate nutritional intake, and social interaction to help prevent mental and physical deterioration associated with certain disease states. These simple measures are easy to implement and may contribute significantly to the improvement of the individual's well-being in later life.

Source: Smith, J. C., Nielson, K. A., Antuono, P., et al. (2013). Semantic memory functional MRI and cognitive function after exercise intervention in mild cognitive impairment. *Journal of Alzheimer's Disease, 37*(1), 197–215. doi:10.3233/JAD-130467

PATIENT TEACHING TIPS

❖ Instruct patients and caregivers that medications must be taken exactly as ordered and with meals to minimize GI upset. Medications are never to be increased except on the advice of the HCP. Give specific instructions on what to do if a medication dose has been omitted.

❖ Establish that intervals between doses of medication need to be timed consistently to optimize therapeutic effects and minimize adverse effects and toxicity.

❖ Encourage patients, family, significant others, or caregivers to call the HCP if there is any increased muscle weakness, abdominal cramps, diarrhea, dizziness, ataxia, or difficulty breathing.

❖ Share information about community resources with patients, caregivers, family, and significant others. Such resources may include, but are not be limited to, Meals on Wheels; local, provincial or territorial, and national chapters of the Alzheimer Society; adult day programs or alternate care resources; special prescription services; and respite care or home health care services.

❖ Signs and symptoms of improvement of myasthenia gravis include a decrease in or absence of ptosis (eyelid drooping) and diplopia (double vision), a decrease in difficulty chewing and swallowing, and an improvement in muscle weakness. If a medication is being taken for myasthenia gravis, the patient needs to take it 30 minutes before meals so that the drug begins to act before the patient chews and swallows. This will help strengthen the muscles required for eating.

❖ Patients should be informed that sustained-released or extended-release dosage forms must be taken in their entirety and should not be crushed, chewed, or broken in any way.

❖ Patients need to have a medical alert bracelet or necklace or carry a medical alert card at all times—these should include all medical diagnoses and provide access to a list of medications and allergies and outline any special requirements in regard to emergency treatment.

KEY POINTS

❖ *Cholinergics, cholinergic agonists,* and *parasympathomimetics* are all appropriate terms for the class of drugs that stimulate the parasympathetic nervous system, which is the branch of the autonomic nervous system that opposes the sympathetic nervous system.

❖ The primary neurotransmitter of the parasympathetic nervous system is acetylcholine, and there are two types of cholinergic receptors: nicotinic and muscarinic.

❖ Nursing considerations for the administration of cholinergic drugs include giving the drug as directed

and monitoring the patient carefully for the occurrence of bradycardia, hypotension, headache, dizziness, respiratory depression, and bronchospasms. If these occur in a patient taking cholinergics, the HCP must be contacted immediately.

❖ It may take about 6 weeks for a therapeutic response to occur with some of the medications used with Alzheimer's disease.

❖ Patients taking cholinergics need to change positions slowly to avoid dizziness and fainting that may result from the adverse effect of orthostatic hypotension.

EXAMINATION REVIEW QUESTIONS

1. The nurse is reviewing the use of bethanechol (Duvoid) in a patient who is experiencing postoperative urinary retention. Which statement best describes the mechanism of action of bethanechol?
   a. It causes decreased bladder tone and motility.
   b. It causes increased bladder tone and motility.
   c. It increases the sensation of a full bladder.
   d. It causes the sphincters in the bladder to become tighter.

2. The family of a patient who has recently been diagnosed with Alzheimer's disease asks about the new drug prescribed to treat this disease. The patient's wife says, "I'm so excited that there are drugs that can cure this disease! I can't wait for him to start treatment." Which reply from the nurse is appropriate?
   a. "The sooner he starts on the medicine, the sooner it can have this effect."
   b. "These effects won't be seen for a few months."
   c. "These drugs do not cure Alzheimer's disease. Let's talk about what the HCP said to expect with this drug therapy."
   d. "His response to this drug therapy will depend on how far along he is in the disease process."

3. The nurse is giving a dose of bethanechol (Urecholine) to a postoperative patient. The nurse is aware that contraindications to bethanechol include:
   a. Bladder atony
   b. Peptic ulcer
   c. Urinary retention
   d. Hypothyroidism

4. A patient took an accidental overdose of a cholinergic drug while at home. He comes to the emergency department with severe abdominal cramping and bloody diarrhea. The nurse expects that which drug will be used to treat this patient?
   a. atropine sulphate
   b. physostigmine
   c. bethanechol (Duvoid)
   d. phentolamine (Rogitine®)

EXAMINATION REVIEW QUESTIONS—cont'd

5. The nurse is reviewing the orders for a newly admitted patient and sees an order for edrophonium chloride (Tensilon). The nurse expects that this drug is ordered for which reason?
 a. To reduce symptoms and delay the onset of Alzheimer's disease
 b. To treat the symptoms of myasthenia gravis
 c. To aid in the diagnosis of myasthenia gravis
 d. To reverse the effects of nondepolarizing neuromuscular blocking drugs after surgery

6. When giving intravenous cholinergic drugs, the nurse must watch for symptoms of a cholinergic crisis, such as: (Select all that apply.)
 a. Peripheral tingling
 b. Hypotension
 c. Dry mouth
 d. Syncope
 e. Dyspnea
 f. Tinnitus

7. A patient who has had an accidental overdose of tricyclic antidepressants is to receive physostigmine, 1.5 mg IM stat. The medication is available in a vial that contains 2 mL, with a concentration of 1 mg/mL. How much medication will the nurse draw up into the syringe for this dose?

Answers: 1. b, 2. c, 3. b, 4. a, 5. c, 6. b, d, e, 7. 1.5 mL

CRITICAL THINKING ACTIVITIES

1. An older adult neighbour wants to take ginkgo (*Ginkgo biloba*) because he is worried about "losing his mind." He asks you if this drug would help him. He has lived alone since being widowed last year and does not have any family members in the area. What is your best answer for this neighbour? Review the Natural Health Products: Ginkgo box in this chapter as well as other sources, if desired.

2. A patient who has been newly diagnosed with myasthenia gravis received a dose of pyridostigmine bromide (Mestinon) in the morning, just before breakfast. She says, "Oh, I know this won't cure me, but I'm so glad that this drug makes me feel better. Will it last all day?" What is the priority when the nurse is teaching this patient about pyridostigmine bromide?

3. A patient is admitted to the emergency department after an industrial accident in which he was exposed to a large amount of organophosphate insecticide. The patient is having difficulty breathing. What is the nurse's priority of action at this time, and what antidote will be prepared?

For answers, see http://evolve.elsevier.com/Canada/Lilley/pharmacology/.

CHAPTER 22

Cholinergic-Blocking Drugs

Objectives

After reading this chapter, the successful student will be able to do the following:

1. Briefly review the functions of the sympathetic nervous system and the specific effects of blocking cholinergic receptors (also referred to as parasympatholytic effects).

2. List the drugs classified as cholinergic antagonists or parasympatholytics.

3. Discuss the mechanisms of action, therapeutic effects, indications, adverse and toxic effects, drug interactions, cautions, contraindications, dosages, routes of administration, and any antidotal management for the cholinergic antagonists.

4. Develop a collaborative plan of care that includes all phases of the nursing process for patients taking cholinergic antagonists.

e-Learning Activities

Website
(http://evolve.elsevier.com/Canada/Lilley/pharmacology/)

evolve

- Answer Key—Textbook Case Studies
- Answer Key—Critical Thinking Activities
- Chapter Summaries—Printable
- Review Questions for Exam Preparation
- Unfolding Case Studies

Drug Profiles

▸▸ atropine (atropine sulphate)*, p. 422
▸▸ dicyclomine (dicyclomine hydrochloride)*, p. 423
   glycopyrrolate, p. 423
   oxybutynin chloride, p. 423
   scopolamine (scopolamine hydrobromide)*, p. 423
▸▸ tolterodine (tolterodine L-tartrate)*, p. 424

▸▸ Key drug

*Full generic name is given in parentheses. For the purposes of this text, the more common, shortened name is used.

Key Terms

Cholinergic-blocking drugs Drugs that block the action of acetylcholine and substances similar to acetylcholine at receptor sites in the brain. (p. 419)

Mydriasis Dilation of the pupil of the eye caused by contraction of the dilator muscle of the iris. (p. 420)

Parasympatholytics Drugs that reduce the activity of the parasympathetic nervous system; also called *anticholinergics*. (p. 419)

OVERVIEW

The parasympathetic nervous system is the branch of the autonomic nervous system with nerve functions generally opposite those of the sympathetic nervous system (refer to Chapters 19 and 20 for a discussion of the sympathetic nervous system and Chapter 21 for further discussion of the parasympathetic nervous system). For example, the parasympathetic nervous system slows the heart rate, increases intestinal and gland activity, and relaxes sphincter muscles in the gastrointestinal (GI) tract. Acetylcholine is the neurotransmitter responsible for the transmission of nerve impulses to effector cells in the parasympathetic nervous system. A cholinergic receptor is one that binds acetylcholine and mediates its actions. This chapter focuses on cholinergic-blocking drugs, which inhibit the effects of the parasympathetic nervous system.

CHOLINERGIC-BLOCKING DRUGS

Cholinergic blockers, anticholinergics, **parasympatholytics,** and *antimuscarinic drugs* are all terms that refer to the class of drugs that block or inhibit the actions of acetylcholine in the parasympathetic nervous system. These drugs were first discussed in Chapter 16 in relation to treatment of Parkinson's disease.

Cholinergic blockers have many therapeutic uses and are one of the oldest groups of therapeutic drugs. Originally, they were derived from various plant sources, but today they are only part of a larger group of cholinergic blockers that also include synthetic and semisynthetic drugs. Box 22-1 lists the currently available cholinergic blockers.

Mechanism of Action and Drug Effects

Cholinergic-blocking drugs block the action of the neurotransmitter acetylcholine at the muscarinic receptors in the parasympathetic nervous system. Acetylcholine that is released from a stimulated nerve fibre is then unable to bind to the receptor site and fails to produce a cholinergic effect. That is why the cholinergic blockers are also referred to as *anticholinergics*. Blocking the parasympathetic nerves allows the sympathetic (adrenergic) nervous system to dominate. Because of this, cholinergic blockers have many of the same effects as the adrenergics (see Chapter 19). Figure 22-1 illustrates the site of action of the cholinergic blockers in the parasympathetic nervous system.

Cholinergic blockers are largely *competitive antagonists*, as they compete with acetylcholine for binding at the muscarinic receptors of the parasympathetic nervous system. Once they have bound to the receptor, they inhibit cholinergic nerve transmission. This generally occurs at the neuroeffector junction, or the point where the nerve ending reaches the effector organs such as smooth muscle, heart muscle, and glands. Cholinergic blockers have little effect at the nicotinic receptors, although at high doses they can have partial blocking effects there.

BOX 22-1

Cholinergic Blockers Grouped According to Chemical Class

Natural Plant Alkaloids

atropine sulphate
belladonna (Belladonna tincture®)
scopolamine hydrobromide

Synthetic and Semisynthetic Drugs

benztropine mesylate (Kynesia®; see Chapter 16)
clidinium bromide
dicyclomine hydrochloride (Bentylol®, Protylol®)
fesoterodine fumurate (Toviaz®)
glycopyrrolate
homatropine hydrochloride (Isopto Homatropine®; see Chapter 57)
ipratropium bromide (Atrovent®, Ipravent®; see Chapter 38)
oxybutynin chloride (Ditropan®)
solifenacin succinate (Vesicare®)
tolterodine tartrate (Detrol®)
trihexyphenidyl hydrochloride (generic; see Chapter 16)
trospium chloride (Allergan®)

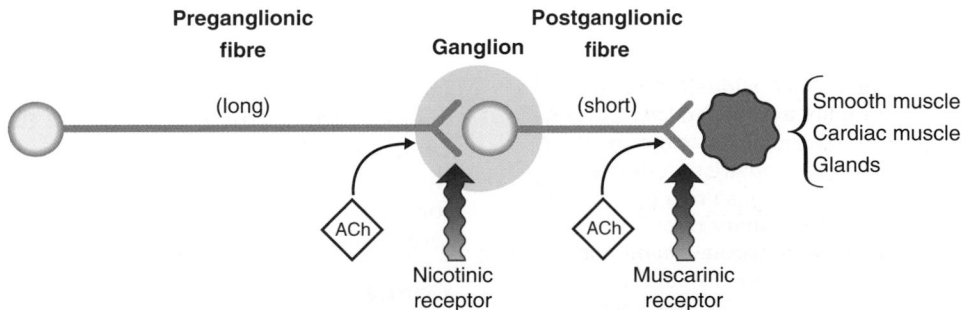

FIG. 22-1   Site of action of cholinergic blockers within the parasympathetic nervous system. *ACh,* acetylcholine.

The major sites of action of the cholinergic-blocking drugs are the heart, respiratory tract, GI tract, urinary bladder, eye, and exocrine glands (e.g., sweat gland, salivary gland). Anticholinergics have the opposite effects of the cholinergics (see Chapter 21) at these sites of action. Anticholinergic effects on the cardiovascular system are seen as an increase in heart rate. Respiratory system effects are dry mucous membranes and bronchial dilation. In the GI tract, cholinergic blockers cause a decrease in GI motility, GI secretions, and salivation. In the genitourinary (GU) system, anticholinergics lead to decreased bladder contraction, which can result in urinary retention. In the skin, anticholinergics reduce sweating. Finally, they increase intraocular pressure and cause the pupils to dilate. This occurs because the ciliary muscles and the sphincter muscle of the iris are innervated by cholinergic nerve fibres. Cholinergic blockers keep the sphincter muscle of the iris from contracting. The result is dilation of the pupil (**mydriasis**) and paralysis of the ocular lens (cycloplegia). This can be detrimental to patients with glaucoma because it results in increased intraocular pressure (see Chapter 57). These and other effects are listed by body system in Table 22-1. Many of the cholinergic-blocking drugs are available in a variety of forms, including intravenous, intramuscular, oral, and subcutaneous preparations.

Indications

In the central nervous system (CNS), cholinergic blockers (e.g., benztropine) have the therapeutic effect of decreasing muscle rigidity and diminishing tremors. This is beneficial in the treatment of both Parkinson's disease (see Chapter 16) and drug-induced extrapyramidal reactions such as those associated with antipsychotic drugs (see Chapter 17). These conditions involve dysfunction of the extrapyramidal parts of the brain and include motor dysfunctions such as chorea, dystonia, and dyskinesia.

Cardiovascular effects of anticholinergics are related to their cholinergic-blocking effects on the heart's conduction system. At low dosages, the anticholinergics may slow the heart rate through their effects on the cardiac centre in the medulla. At high dosages, cholinergic blockers block the inhibitory vagal (i.e., parasympathetic or cholinergic) effects on the pacemaker cells of the sinoatrial and atrioventricular nodes, which leads to acceleration of the heart rate because of unopposed sympathetic activity. Atropine is used primarily in the management of cardiovascular disorders, such as in the diagnosis of sinus node dysfunction, the treatment of patients with symptomatic second-degree atrioventricular block, and the provision of advanced life support in the treatment of sinus bradycardia that is accompanied by hemodynamic compromise. It also has ophthalmic uses such as relaxing the ciliary muscle of the eye, causing the pupil to dilate to facilitate an eye examination (see Chapter 57).

When the cholinergic stimulation of the parasympathetic nervous system is blocked by cholinergic blockers, the sympathetic nervous system's effects go unopposed. In the respiratory tract, this results in decreased secretions from the nose, mouth, pharynx, and bronchi. It also causes relaxation of the smooth muscles in the bronchi and bronchioles, which results in decreased airway resistance and bronchodilation. Because of this, the cholinergic blockers have proved beneficial in treating exercise-induced bronchospasms, asthma, and chronic obstructive pulmonary disease. They are also used preoperatively to reduce salivary secretions, which aids in intubation and other procedures (e.g., endoscopy) involving the oral cavity.

Gastric secretions and the smooth muscles responsible for producing gastric motility are all controlled by the parasympathetic nervous system, which is primarily under the control of muscarinic receptors. Cholinergic blockers antagonize these receptors, causing decreased secretions, relaxation of smooth muscle, and reduced GI motility and peristalsis. For these reasons, cholinergic blockers are commonly used in the treatment of irritable bowel disease and GI hypersecretory states.

Anticholinergics are useful in the treatment of GU tract disorders such as reflex neurogenic bladder and incontinence. They relax the detrusor muscles of the bladder and increase constriction of the internal sphincter. The ability of cholinergic blockers to decrease glandular secretions also makes them potentially useful drugs for reducing gastric and pancreatic secretions in patients with acute pancreatitis.

Contraindications

Contraindications to the use of anticholinergic drugs include known drug allergy, angle-closure glaucoma,

TABLE 22-1	
Cholinergic Blockers: Drug Effects	
Body System	**Cholinergic-Blocking Effects**
Cardiovascular	Small doses: decrease heart rate Large doses: increase heart rate
Central nervous	Small doses: decrease muscle rigidity and tremors Large doses: cause drowsiness, disorientation, hallucinations
Eye	Dilate pupils (mydriasis), decrease accommodation by paralyzing ciliary muscles (cycloplegia)
Gastrointestinal	Relax smooth muscle tone of GI tract, decrease intestinal and gastric secretions, decrease motility and peristalsis
Genitourinary	Relax detrusor muscle of bladder, increase constriction of internal sphincter; these two effects may result in urinary retention
Glandular	Decrease bronchial secretions, salivation, and sweating
Respiratory	Decrease bronchial secretions, dilate bronchial airways

acute asthma or other respiratory distress, myasthenia gravis, acute cardiovascular instability (some exceptions were listed previously), GI or GU tract obstruction (e.g., benign prostatic hyperplasia), GI (e.g., ulcerative colitis, paralytic ileus) or GU (e.g., urinary retention) illness, and cognitive impairment.

Adverse Effects

Anticholinergic drugs cause widely varied adverse effects. The adverse effects of cholinergic blockers are listed by body system in Table 22-2. Certain patient populations are more susceptible to the effects of anticholinergics. These populations include infants, children with Down syndrome, individuals with spastic paralysis or brain damage, and older adults. Older adults are extremely sensitive to the CNS effects of anticholinergics, and it is not uncommon them to develop cognitive impairments and delirium, as well as an increased risk for falls, due to anticholinergic effects. The risk of adverse effects increases with the use of medications with strong anticholinergic properties, higher doses of medications with anticholinergic properties, and the greater total number of medications with anticholinergic properties. Moreover, older adult patients, as a result of normal age-related physiological changes (e.g., decreased kidney function) and pre-existing clinical conditions (e.g., dementia), are much more sensitive to the adverse effects of medications with anticholinergic properties (see Evidence in Practice box).

Toxicity and Management of Overdose

The dosage of cholinergic blockers is particularly important, because there is a small difference between therapeutic and toxic dosages. Drugs with this characteristic are commonly referred to as having a *low therapeutic index* (see Chapter 2). The treatment of cholinergic-blocker overdose consists of symptomatic and supportive therapy. Consultation with a provincial or territorial Poison Control Centre is recommended. The patient should be hospitalized, with continuous monitoring, including continuous electrocardiographic monitoring. The stomach should be emptied by whichever means is most appropriate, usually through lavage. Activated charcoal has proven to be effective in removing from the GI tract any drug that has not yet been absorbed. For charcoal to be "activated," common charcoal is heated in the presence of a gas that causes the charcoal to develop porous spaces that, when ingested, trap chemicals. Fluid therapy and other standard measures used for the treatment of shock are instituted as needed. Delirium, hallucinations, coma, and cardiac dysrhythmias respond favourably to treatment with the cholinergic drug physostigmine (see Chapter 21). Its routine use as an antidote for cholinergic-blocker overdose is controversial because it has the potential to produce severe adverse effects (e.g., seizures, cardiac asystole), so it is usually reserved for the treatment of patients who show extreme delirium or agitation. It is available in Canada only through the Special Access Programme.

TABLE 22-2	
Cholinergic Blockers: Adverse Effects	
Body System	**Cholinergic-Blocking Effects**
Cardiovascular	Increased heart rate, dysrhythmias (tachycardia, palpitations)
Central nervous	Excitation, restlessness, irritability, disorientation, hallucinations, delirium, ataxia, drowsiness, sedation, confusion
Eye	Dilated pupils (causing blurred vision), increased intraocular pressure
Gastrointestinal	Decreased salivation, dry mouth (xerostomia), gastric secretions, and motility (causing constipation)
Genitourinary	Urinary retention
Glandular	Decreased sweating
Respiratory	Decreased bronchial secretions

 EVIDENCE IN PRACTICE

Cumulative Use of Strong Anticholinergics and Incident Dementia: A Prospective Cohort Study

Review

Anticholinergics block the action of acetylcholine activity and function to balance the neurotransmitters dopamine and acetylcholine. Anticholinergics affect the area of the brain that facilitates memory and learning. These drugs are used to treat a variety of disorders, including incontinence, GI cramps, and urinary muscular spasms. Medications with strong anticholinergic effects (e.g., antihistamines, with the adverse effect of drowsiness) may cause acute cognitive impairment and increase the risk for dementia.

Type of Evidence

The researchers tracked 3 434 men and women 65 years or older with no dementia at study entry. This prospective population-based cohort study used participants from Adult Changes in Thought (ACT), a long-term study conducted by the University of Washington and Group Health, based in Seattle. Recruitment occurred from 1994 through 1996 and from 2000 through 2003. Participants who died were replaced. All participants were followed every 2 years. Group Health's pharmacy records were used to

Continued

EVIDENCE IN PRACTICE—cont'd

identify both prescription and over-the-counter medications that each participant took in the 10 years before starting the study. Participants' health was tracked for an average of 7 years.

Results of Study

The most common anticholinergic classes used over the 7 years were tricyclic antidepressants, first-generation antihistamines, and bladder antimuscarinics. Over the mean follow-up of 7.3 years, 797 participants (23.2%) developed dementia. The majority of these, or 637 (79.9%), developed Alzheimer's disease. Dementia risk increased as the cumulative dose increased. Taking an anticholinergic drug for 3 years or more was associated with a 54% higher dementia risk than taking the same dose for 3 months or less.

Link of Evidence to Nursing Practice

It is important to note that this study found that high cumulative anticholinergic use is correlated with an increased risk for dementia. Although further research is necessary, increased attention to this potential medication-related risk is important. Adverse effects are associated with anticholinergic use over time. Assessment of high-risk prescription and over-the-counter anticholinergics by health care providers (HCPs), particularly those in use by older adults, is recommended. While avoiding all anticholinergics is not always clinically possible, increasing awareness of the most problematic medications is important. Medications with anticholinergic properties should be avoided in older adult patients whenever possible. If clinically necessary, anticholinergics should be used at the lowest dose and for the shortest duration possible.

Source: Gray, S. L., Anderson, M. L., Dublin, S., et al. (2015). Cumulative use of strong anticholinergics and incident dementia: A prospective cohort study. *Journal of the American Medical Association Internal Medicine*, 175(3), 401–407. doi:10.1001/jamainternmed.2014.7663

Interactions

The drug interactions most commonly reported for the anticholinergics are additive anticholinergic effects when taken with other drugs that possess anticholinergic adverse effects, such as amantadine hydrochloride (see Chapter 16), antihistamines (see Chapter 37), and tricyclic antidepressants (see Chapter 17). Reduced antipsychotic effects of phenothiazines (see Chapter 17) are seen when they are taken with anticholinergic drugs, and increased effects of digoxin (see Chapter 25) are seen when it is combined with anticholinergics.

Dosages

For dosage information on selected cholinergic blockers, refer to the table on p. 424.

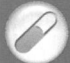

DRUG PROFILES

Among the oldest and best-known, naturally occurring cholinergic blockers are the belladonna alkaloids. Of these, atropine is the prototypical drug. It has been in use for hundreds of years and continues to be widely administered because of its effectiveness. Besides atropine, scopolamine is the other major, naturally occurring drug, derived from a variety of plants within the potato family.

Cholinergic blockers are used in the treatment of a variety of illnesses and conditions, ranging from irritable bowel syndrome to the symptoms of the common cold, and are also administered preoperatively to dry up secretions. Cholinergic blockers minimize gurgling and crackling sounds and can be used prophylactically in patients who are unconscious and dying; however, there is controversy about their usefulness. These drugs are the synthetic counterparts of the plant-derived belladonna alkaloids and are more specific in binding predominantly with muscarinic receptors. Synthetic cholinergic blockers are also associated with fewer adverse effects than plant-derived ones. Adverse effects and drug interactions are comparable for the different anticholinergic drugs and are detailed in Table 22-2 and previous text, respectively, unless otherwise noted.

▶ *atropine sulphate*

Atropine sulphate is a naturally occurring antimuscarinic. It is used for its cholinergic-blocking effects on the heart and its effects on the smooth muscles of the bronchi and intestines. Atropine is effective in the treatment of many of the conditions that are previously listed in the Indications section. Because atropine causes increased heart rate, it is used to treat bradycardia and ventricular asystole. Atropine is also used as an antidote for anticholinesterase inhibitor toxicity or poisoning. It is also used preoperatively to reduce salivation and GI secretions, as is glycopyrrolate. Atropine use is contraindicated in patients with angle-closure glaucoma, adhesions between the iris and lens, certain types of asthma (that are not cholinergic associated), advanced liver or kidney disease, hiatal hernia associated with reflux esophagitis, intestinal atony, obstructive GI or GU conditions, and severe ulcerative colitis. It is available as a parenteral injection in

DRUG PROFILES–cont'd

several concentrations, as well as in ophthalmic forms (Chapter 57). It is also combined with the opiate diphenoxylate hydrochloride to make Lomotil® tablets, a common antidiarrheal preparation. Adverse effects may include bloating, constipation, loss of appetite, and severe stomach pain with nausea and vomiting. Overdose of atropine (usually from taking excessive Lomotil) is associated with flushing, dry skin and mucous membranes, mydriasis, altered mental status, and fever. Other serious effects include sinus tachycardia, urinary retention, hypertension, hallucinations, respiratory depression, and cardiovascular collapse. See previous discussion on toxicity management. Recommended dosages are given in the table on p. 424.

PHARMACOKINETICS

Route	Onset of Action	Peak Plasma Concentration	Elimination Half-Life	Duration of Action
IV	Immediate	2–4 min	2.5 hr	4–6 hr

▸▸ dicyclomine hydrochloride

Dicyclomine hydrochloride (Bentylol, Protylol) is a synthetic antispasmodic cholinergic blocker used primarily in the treatment of functional disturbances of GI motility such as irritable bowel syndrome and spastic constipation. It is available in injectable and oral form. Recommended dosages are given in the table on this page.

It has also been used for the treatment of colic and enterocolitis in infants. It is contraindicated in patients who have a known hypersensitivity to anticholinergics and in those with angle-closure glaucoma, GI tract obstruction, myasthenia gravis, paralytic ileus, GI atony, or toxic megacolon. It is available in parenteral oral form. Recommended dosages are given in the table on p. 424.

PHARMACOKINETICS

Route	Onset of Action	Peak Plasma Concentration	Elimination Half-Life	Duration of Action
PO	1–2 hr	60–90 min	9–10 hr	3–4 hr

glycopyrrolate

Glycopyrrolate is a synthetic antimuscarinic drug that blocks receptor sites in the autonomic nervous system, controlling the production of secretions and the concentration of free acids in the stomach. It may be used as a preoperative medication to reduce salivation and excessive secretions in the respiratory and GI tracts. It is contraindicated in patients who are hypersensitive to it and in those with angle-closure glaucoma, myasthenia gravis, GI or GU obstruction, tachycardia, liver disease, myocardial ischemia, ulcerative colitis, or toxic megacolon. Glycopyrrolate is available parenterally. Recommended dosages are given in the table on p. 424.

PHARMACOKINETICS

Route	Onset of Action	Peak Plasma Concentration	Elimination Half-Life	Duration of Action
IV	1 min	10–15 min	Variable	4 hr

oxybutynin chloride

Oxybutynin chloride (Ditropan®) is a synthetic antimuscarinic drug used for the treatment of overactive bladder. It is also used as an antispasmodic for neurogenic bladder associated with spinal cord injuries and congenital conditions such as spina bifida. Contraindications include drug allergy, urinary or gastric retention, and uncontrolled angle-closure glaucoma. Oxybutynin chloride is available for oral use. A transdermal patch (Oxytrol®) and a gel (Gelnique®) are also available and approved for treatment of overactive bladder. Recommended dosages are given in the table on p. 424.

PHARMACOKINETICS

Route	Onset of Action	Peak Plasma Concentration	Elimination Half-Life	Duration of Action
PO	Unknown	1 hr	2–3 hr	Unknown

scopolamine hydrobromide

Scopolamine hydrobromide is a naturally occurring cholinergic blocker and one of the principal belladonna alkaloids. It is the most potent antimuscarinic for the prevention of motion sickness. It works by correcting the imbalance between acetylcholine and norepinephrine in the medulla, particularly in the vomiting centre. Ipratropium bromide, a derivative of scopolamine, has potent therapeutic effects on the lungs and is discussed in Chapter 38. For the prevention of motion sickness, scopolamine is available in a transdermal delivery system, a patch that can be applied just behind the ear 12 hours before travel (see Chapter 41). It is considered a natural health product by Health Canada. Transdermal scopolamine may cause drowsiness, dry mouth, and blurred vision.

Although not Health Canada approved, scopolamine (either by patch or by subcutaneous injection) has been used in palliative and end-of-life care. Loss of the ability to swallow may result from weakness and decreased neurological function. Consequently, the gag reflex and reflexive clearing of the oropharynx decline, resulting in the accumulation of secretions. This buildup of saliva and oropharyngeal secretions may lead to gurgling, crackling, or rattling sounds as air moves across pooled secretions, collectively known by the unfortunate term "death rattle." During the last stages of life, these secretions can be distressing to families. Blockade of the parasympathetic nervous system results in decreased production of secretions in the salivary, bronchial, and GI tracts; however, it is not effective on secretions that are already present. Scopolamine crosses the blood–brain barrier, and may result in more CNS effects such as sedation, disorientation, hallucinations, and delirium, particularly in older adults.

Using scopolamine with CNS depressants or alcohol may increase sedation. Scopolamine is also available in parenteral formulations for injection by various routes: intravenous, intramuscular, and subcutaneous. The contraindications that apply to atropine apply to scopolamine as well. Recommended dosages are given in the table on p. 424.

Continued

DRUG PROFILES–cont'd

PHARMACOKINETICS

Route	Onset of Action	Peak Plasma Concentration	Elimination Half-Life	Duration of Action
IV	30–60 min	30–45 min	Variable	4 hr
Transdermal	4–12 hr	6 hr	Variable	72 hr

▸▸*tolterodine tartrate*

Tolterodine tartrate (Detrol, Detrol LA) is muscarinic receptor blocker used for the treatment of urinary frequency, urgency, and urge incontinence caused by bladder (detrusor) overactivity. Another drug that is commonly used to treat these conditions is oxybutynin chloride (profiled previously), which is also one of the most commonly prescribed. Other older-generation drugs include hyoscine butylbromide and the tricyclic antidepressant imipramine hydrochloride. These drugs are less commonly used today because of their antimuscarinic adverse effects, particularly dry mouth. Newer drugs for this purpose include solifenacin succcinate (Vesicare), darifenacin hydrobromide (Enablex®), trospium chloride (Sanctura®), and fesoterodine fumarate (Toviaz). The newer drugs are associated with a much lower incidence of dry mouth, in part because of their pharmacological specificity for the bladder as opposed to the salivary glands.

Tolterodine is to be avoided in patients with angle-closure glaucoma or urinary retention. In patients with markedly decreased liver function or who are poor metabolizers of drugs that inhibit cytochrome P450 enzyme 3A4 (e.g., erythromycin or ketoconazole), the dose is reduced to 1 mg twice a day rather than the recommended dose of 2 mg twice a day. Tolterodine is available only for oral use. Recommended dosages are given in the table below.

PHARMACOKINETICS

Route	Onset of Action	Peak Plasma Concentration	Elimination Half-Life	Duration of Action
PO	1 hr	1–2 hr	2–4 hr	5 hr

DOSAGES   Selected Cholinergic-Blocking (Anticholinergic) Drugs

Drug	Pharmacological Class	Usual Dosage Range	Indications
▸▸atropine sulphate	Anticholinergic	*Infants and Children* IM/Subcut: 0.01–0.02 mg/kg/dose; max 0.5 mg	Treatment of bradycardia
		IV: 0.02–0.05 mg/kg every 15–20 minutes until effect	Anticholinesterase effect for organophosphate or carbamate poisoning (e.g., insecticides)
		Adults IM: 0.5 mg q3–5 minutes (max 3 mg)	Treatment of bradycardia, cardiopulmonary resuscitation
		IV: 1–2 mg/dose; repeat every 5–60 min until disappearance of muscarinic symptoms	Anticholinesterase effect for organophosphate or carbamate poisoning (e.g., insecticides)
▸▸dicyclomine hydrochloride (Bentylol)		*Children* PO: 5–10 mg tid–qid *Adults* PO: 10–20 mg tid–qid	Treatment of irritable bowel syndrome
glycopyrrolate		*Children and Adults* IM/IV: 0.005 mg/kg 30–60 min preoperative	Preoperative control of secretions
		Children and Adults 0.2 mg for each 1 mg of neostigmine or 5 mg of pyridostigmine	Reversal of neuromuscular blockade
oxybutynin chloride (Ditropan XL, Oxytrol [transdermal patch]), Gelnique [topical gel])		*Children over 5 yr* PO: 5 mg bid–tid *Adult and child older than 5 yr* PO: 5 mg bid–tid *Adults only* PO ER tab: 5–30 mg/day as single or divided doses Transdermal patch: 1 patch (3.9 mg/day) applied twice weekly (every 3–4 days) (for overactive bladder) Topical gel: 1 sachet (1 g)/day	Antispasmodic for neurogenic bladder (e.g., following spinal cord injury), overactive bladder

DOSAGES	Selected Cholinergic-Blocking (Anticholinergic) Drugs—cont'd		
Drug	**Pharmacological Class**	**Usual Dosage Range**	**Indications**
scopolamine hydrobromide (generic, transdermal patch)		*Children* IM/IV/Subcut: 0.006 mg/kg/dose *Adults* IM/IV/Subcut: 0.3–0.8 mg Transdermal patch: 1.5 mg patch behind ear q3days (delivers approx 1 mg scopolamine over 3 days); apply at least 12 hr before transportation	Preoperative control of secretions Preoperative control of secretions Motion sickness
▸▸tolterodine tartrate (Detrol, Detrol LA)		*Adults* PO: 1–2 mg bid PO ER cap: 2–4 mg daily	Treatment of overactive bladder

ER, extended release; *IM*, intramuscular; *IV*, intravenous; *PO*, oral; *Subcut*, subcutaneous.

NURSING PROCESS

☑ Assessment

The drugs known as *parasympatholytics, cholinergic blockers, cholinergic antagonists,* or *anticholinergics* produce a number of physiological effects that result from the blocking of cholinergic receptors. These effects include smooth muscle relaxation, decreased glandular secretion, and mydriasis (pupil dilation). Knowing the way these drugs work and the related physiology will assist you in the safe assessment and nursing care of patients taking these drugs. A thorough medical history; a complete medication history with a listing of prescription drugs, over-the-counter (OTC) drugs, and natural health products; as well as a thorough head-to-toe assessment will help to identify the presence of any contraindications, cautions, or potential drug interactions associated with the cholinergic-blocking drugs (see earlier discussion). The assessment data will help in documenting baseline findings and provide information for evaluating drug effectiveness. Lifespan considerations for young patients and older adults include the need for close assessment and monitoring because of the increased susceptibility of these groups to the adverse effects of restlessness, irritability, disorientation, constipation, urinary retention, blurred vision (from pupil dilation), and tachycardia; thus, older adults require more careful assessment and monitoring. See Special Populations: Older Adults for information about the care of older adults with an overactive bladder. It is of upmost importance to assess adult patients for the use of medications that have cholinergic-blocking properties. Using anticholinergic rating scales to assess the magnitude of anticholinergic burden can help HCPs to achieve this goal and ultimately enhance safety in older adult patients. A variety of anticholinergic risk rating scales are available. One tool is the Anticholinergic Risk Scale, a ranked categorical list of commonly prescribed medications with anticholinergic potential (Salahudeen, Duffull, & Nishtala, 2015). Medications are classified on a scale of 0 to 3 points, based on their probability of causing anticholinergic effects, such as dry mouth, dry eyes, constipation, and dizziness and confusion, which may result in falls.

In assessment associated with atropine and other cholinergic blockers, check for allergies, glaucoma, certain eye conditions (e.g., adhesions in the iris and lens of the eye), gastroesophageal reflux disease, poor intestinal motility, obstructions of the GI and GU systems, and severe ulcerative colitis. These conditions and others may be exacerbated by the cholinergic blockers (see earlier discussion in this chapter and in Chapters 19 to 21) and would be considered contraindications. Address the associated cautions, contraindications, and drug interactions with dicyclomine, glycopyrrolate, and oxybutynin chloride. Also, note any disorders of the bladder or GI tract. Apply the transdermal dosage form of scopolamine only after the order has been reviewed and the skin assessed.

☑ Nursing Diagnoses

- Constipation related to adverse effects of cholinergic-blocking drugs
- Deficient knowledge related to the lack of information about the therapeutic regimen, adverse effects, drug interactions, and precautions for the use of cholinergic-blocking drugs
- Risk for injury related to decreased sweating and loss of normal heat-regulating mechanisms due to the impact of the drug on temperature-regulating mechanisms

☑ Planning

■ Goals

- Patient will experience minimal adverse effects such as constipation.

SPECIAL POPULATIONS: OLDER ADULTS

Overactive Bladder

Overactive bladder is estimated to affect approximately 18.5% of Canadians (21.2% of women and 14.8% of men) over the age of 35, and its incidence increases with age (Cameron Institute, 2014). Some questions to pose to adults and older adults about this condition include the following:

- Do you suddenly experience a strong urge to urinate?
- Do you urinate more than eight times in a 24-hour period?
- Do you have to get up more than two times during the night to urinate?
- Do you have "wetting" accidents?
- Are these "wetting" accidents related to the uncontrollable urge to urinate?

NOTE: If a patient answers yes to some of these questions, the patient needs to be encouraged to contact the primary HCP. Referral to a urologist may or may not be necessary.

Various treatments are available in Canada, including the use of solifenacin succinate (Vesicare), which is to be taken once daily and treats all of the major symptoms of overactive bladder, including urgency, frequency, and urge-related incontinence. Solifenacin succinate was found to reduce the number of incontinence episodes over 12 weeks, in studies of the drug involving more than 3 000 patients with overactive bladder symptoms. With 5- to 10-mg dosing of the drug, there was alleviation of all of the major symptoms. Use of this drug is contraindicated in patients with glaucoma, certain GI or GU tract problems, severe constipation, or urinary retention. Adverse effects include dry mouth, constipation, and blurred vision. If a patient experiences severe abdominal pain or is constipated for 3 or more days, the patient should contact an HCP immediately.

Sources: Cameron Institute (2014). *Incontinence: A Canadian perspective.* Retrieved from http://www.canadiancontinence.ca/pdfs/en-incontinence-a-canadian-perspective-2014.pdf; HealthlinkBC (2013). *Overactive bladder.* Retrieved from http://www.healthlinkbc.ca/healthtopics/; Astellas. (2013) *VESIcare (solifenacin succinate).* Retrieved from http://www.vesicare.com/.

- Patient will demonstrate adequate knowledge about the use of the specific medications, adverse effects, and appropriate dosing at home.
- Patient will remain free from injury resulting from the adverse effect of inability to regulate sweating.

■ Outcome Criteria

- Patient states various measures to regain normal bowel patterns and avoids constipation by consuming additional fluids and increasing fibre in daily dietary intake.
  - Patient increases fluids up to 2 000 mL (preferably of water) per day.
  - Patient eats foods high in fibre, such as generous amounts of vegetables, fruits, and legumes, to help take in approximately 40 g per day.
  - Patient uses a natural fibre supplement, if not contraindicated, such as a psyllium-based fibre product.
- Patient states the rationale for the use of cholinergic blockers, such as in preoperative preparation, for decreasing adverse effects associated with drugs used for Alzheimer's disease, and in irritable bowel syndrome.
  - Patient states the more common adverse effects associated with cholinergic blockers, such as dry mouth, constipation, and urinary retention.
  - Patient states those adverse effects that need to be reported immediately to an HCP if they occur, such as unresolved constipation, pain over the bladder region and inability to urinate, or chest pain.

- Patient states measures to help decrease the impact of reduced ability to sweat, such as avoiding the following: hot climates, vigorous exercising (especially in heated or hot environments), saunas, and hot tubs.
  - Patients who are older identify their increased risk of being overwhelmed by the decreased ability to sweat and the need for adherence to the above stipulations.

■ Implementation

A preventive focus for nursing care is important to the effective use of cholinergic-blocking drugs. Some conditions may be amenable to lifestyle modification rather than pharmacotherapy, and minimal doses may be used to achieve desired effects. There are several nursing interventions that may maximize the therapeutic effects of these drugs and minimize the adverse effects. Some important nursing interventions include giving the drug at the same time each day and according to the HCP's order and giving the medication with adequate fluid intake (1 400 to 2 000 mL of water daily).

Because drugs such as atropine and glycopyrrolate are compatible with some of the commonly used opioids (e.g., meperidine hydrochloride, morphine sulphate), they may be used in combination with these drugs and mixed in the same syringe for parenteral dosing. Checking for the compatibility of drugs combined in the same syringe is important with any medication. Always double-check compatibility for patient safety. If a cholinergic-blocking drug is given via the ophthalmic route, always check the concentration of the drug and, once it is given, apply light pressure with a tissue to the inner canthus of the eye for approximately 30 to 60 seconds. This helps to minimize the possibility of systemic absorption of the drug.

Atropine may be combined with other cholinergic-blocking drugs for treatment of lower urinary tract discomfort or to help decrease GI and GU hypermotility, but give the drug via the correct route and with proper dosing as prescribed. The anticholinergic adverse effect of dry mouth may be managed with frequent mouth care, oral rinses, increase in fluids, and use of sugar-free gum or hard candy. Oxybutynin chloride needs to be taken as directed either 1 hour before or 2 hours after meals, if tolerated. Tolterodine must be taken as directed and with food. Transdermal forms of these medications (e.g., scopolamine, oxybutynin) are to be applied to the skin only after the previous dosage form has been removed and the area gently cleansed of residual medication. Transdermal patches may be applied to any dry, nonhairy, nonirritated area. Rotation of transdermal sites is recommended to decrease skin irritation. Also associated with the cholinergic-blocking drugs are the adverse effects of constipation and inability to sweat or perspire. Because these may be significant to patients, include education on how to minimize these adverse effects. See the Patient

Teaching Tips below for more information on these specific drugs.

Evaluation

Monitoring of goals and outcome criteria is a starting point for effective evaluation of therapy with cholinergic-blocking drugs. In particular, their therapeutic effects include the following: (1) in patients with Parkinson's disease, improved ability to carry out activities of daily living and fewer problems with tremors, salivation, and drooling; (2) decreased GI symptoms, such as hyperacidity, abdominal pain, heartburn, nausea, and vomiting, with improved comfort; (3) decreased GU hypermotility, with increased comfort and improved patterns of voiding with an increase in time between voidings; (4) fewer bronchospasms with induction of anaesthesia and fewer problems with thickened, viscous secretions in patients before, during, and after surgery. Monitor patients for the occurrence of adverse effects such as constipation, tachycardia, palpitations, confusion, sedation, drowsiness, hallucinations, urinary retention, and decreased sweating leading to hot and dry skin. Toxic effects of cholinergic-blocking drugs include delirium, hallucinations, and cardiac dysrhythmias.

CASE STUDY

Transdermal Scopolamine

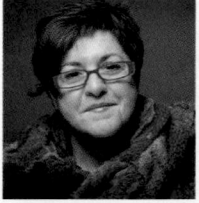

Julie, a 53-year-old elementary schoolteacher, is going on a cruise to Alaska with her husband, Terry, for their 30th anniversary. She is extremely excited about the trip but is also worried because she gets "so seasick" whenever she is on a boat. She calls her doctor's office for a prescription for a medicine for motion sickness. Her HCP prescribes transdermal scopolamine.

1. Before Julie picks up the prescription, the nurse assesses for contraindications to scopolamine. What are the contraindications to the use of the scopolamine patch?

The nurse provides patient education, and Jan indicates that she understands how to use the patch. On the first day of the cruise, she applies the patch 12 hours before she and her husband board the ship.

2. That evening, Julie and Terry go to dinner. Julie is feeling somewhat drowsy and thirsty. The waiter asks

if they would like to have champagne as part of the first-night-of-the-cruise celebration. How should Julie respond?

3. The next morning, while out on the deck, Terry and Julie are taking pictures of the bright, snow-covered shoreline views. Terry looks at Julie and exclaims, "Look at your eyes! Is that a side effect of that patch?" What has Terry noticed about Julie's blue eyes? What would you suggest for Julie because of what Terry has noticed?

4. Later that day, Julie tells Terry, "I'm feeling great! I don't think I need this patch. I'm going to take it off, but I'll save it for later in case I get nauseated." Is this a good idea? Explain your answer.

For answers, see http://evolve.elsevier.com/Canada/Lilley/pharmacology/.

PATIENT TEACHING TIPS

❖ Patients should be informed that medications need to be taken exactly as prescribed. Overdosage of cholinergic-blocking drugs may cause life-threatening problems, especially in the cardiovascular and central nervous systems.

❖ Cholinergic blockers may lead to dry mouth. Regular and thorough oral hygiene is required of patients taking these drugs, including brushing teeth twice daily and using dental floss. Dry mouth may be minimized by increasing fluid intake, if not contraindicated, using

Continued

PATIENT TEACHING TIPS—cont'd

- artificial saliva drops, chewing sugar-free gum, or sucking on sugar-free hard candy, as needed. Encourage regularly scheduled dental visits because of the risk of dental caries and gum disease with dry mouth. The use of Waterpik® devices may stimulate gums and help prevent gum disease.
- Patients should exercise with caution and avoid excessive sweating because of drug-induced altered sweating. This may cause hyperthermia in older adults or those with already altered sweating mechanisms.
- If there is sedation or blurred vision, patients need to avoid driving or engaging in activities that require quick decision making, alertness, or clear vision, such as operating heavy machinery, taking tests, and making important decisions. The adverse effects of sedation will decrease over time.
- Encourage patients to wear dark or tinted glasses or sunglasses because of the increased sensitivity to light associated with these medications.
- Patients must understand the importance of always consulting an HCP before taking any other medications, including prescription drugs, OTC medications, or natural health products.

- Older adult patients have existing age-related changes in body temperature–regulating mechanisms. With these medications, especially at high dosages, there is an increased risk of heat stroke or hyperthermia because of the drug's interference with the body's heat-regulating mechanisms. To prevent hyperthermia, older adults need to stay in shaded areas or inside an air-conditioned or cooled environment when external temperatures are warm; remain well-hydrated with cool fluids; wear protective clothing and hats; avoid saunas, hot tubs, excessive heat, and strenuous exercise in warm environments; keep portable fans on hand; and maintain adequate ventilation in heated environments.
- For patients taking cholinergic blockers, all HCPs need to be informed about the treatment regimen, and must be given a list of the patient's drugs. The primary HCP needs to be contacted if there is any unresolved constipation, palpitations, alterations in gait, excessive dizziness, or inability to void.
- Patients may manage constipation with increased dietary intake of fluids and fibre or through the use of OTC fibre-containing supplements, such as psyllium products.

KEY POINTS

- *Cholinergic blockers*, *parasympatholytics*, *anticholinergics*, and *antimuscarinics* are all terms that refer to the drugs that block or inhibit the actions of acetylcholine in the parasympathetic nervous system.
- The use of cholinergic blockers allows the sympathetic nervous system to dominate. These drugs are classified chemically as natural, semisynthetic, and synthetic cholinergic blockers. They may be competitive antagonists (blockers) and compete with acetylcholine

at the muscarinic receptors. In high dosages, they result in partial blocking actions at the nicotinic receptors. Anticholinergics bind to and block acetylcholine at muscarinic receptors located on the cells stimulated by the parasympathetic nervous system.
- The nurse should assess for possible contraindications such as benign prostatic hypertrophy, glaucoma, tachycardia, myocardial infarction, heart failure, and hiatal hernia.

EXAMINATION REVIEW QUESTIONS

1. The nurse is providing education about cholinergic-blocking drug therapy to an older adult patient. Which is an important point to emphasize for this patient?
   a. Avoid exposure to high temperatures.
   b. Limit liquid intake to avoid fluid overload.
   c. Begin an exercise program to avoid adverse effects.
   d. Stop the medication if excessive mouth dryness occurs.
2. The nurse is giving a cholinergic-blocking drug. The nurse will assess the patient for which contraindication to these drugs?
   a. Chronic bronchitis
   b. Peptic ulcer disease
   c. Irritable bowel syndrome
   d. Benign prostatic hypertrophy

3. When assessing for the adverse effects of cholinergic-blocking drug therapy, the nurse would expect to find that the patient reports which drug effect?
   a. Diaphoresis
   b. Dry mouth
   c. Diarrhea
   d. Urinary frequency
4. The nurse administering a cholinergic-blocking drug to a patient experiencing drug-induced extrapyramidal effects would assess for which therapeutic effect?
   a. Decreased muscle rigidity and tremors
   b. Increased heart rate
   c. Decreased bronchial secretions
   d. Decreased GI motility and peristalsis

EXAMINATION REVIEW QUESTIONS—cont'd

5. During the assessment of a patient about to receive a cholinergic-blocking drug, the nurse will determine whether the patient is taking any drugs that may potentially interact with the anticholinergic, including:
   a. Opioids, such as morphine sulphate
   b. Antibiotics, such as penicillin
   c. Tricyclic antidepressants, such as amitriptyline
   d. Anticonvulsants, such as phenobarbital

6. A patient has been given a prescription for transdermal scopolamine patches for motion sickness to use during a cruise vacation. The nurse will include which instructions? (Select all that apply.)
   a. "Apply the patch as soon as you board the ship."
   b. "Apply the patch 12 hours before boarding the ship."
   c. "The patch needs to be placed on a nonhairy area on your upper chest or upper arm."
   d. "The patch needs to be placed on a nonhairy area just behind your ear."
   e. "Change the patch every 3 days."
   f. "Rotate the application sites."

7. The preoperative order for an adult patient reads: "Give scopolamine hydrobromide, 0.7 mg IM on call for surgery." The medication is available in vials of 0.4 mg/mL. How many millilitres will the nurse administer for this dose? (Round to tenths.)

Answers: 1. a, 2. d, 3. b, 4. a, 5. c, 6. b, d, e, f, 7. 1.8 mL.

CRITICAL THINKING ACTIVITIES

1. The nurse is preparing to administer atropine and an opioid, ordered as standard preoperative medications, to a 75-year-old woman who will be undergoing minor surgery. When checking her medical history, the nurse notes that she has a history of smoking and has angle-closure glaucoma. What is your priority action at this time in regard to administration of the preoperative medications? Explain your answer.

2. In preparing a patient for emergency surgery, the order was to give 0.5 mg of atropine sulphate to the patient intravenously. The vial concentration is 1 mg/mL. In the haste of this emergency situation, 5 mL of the atropine solution is given. How much atropine did the patient receive? What is the nurse's priority action?

3. A patient who has a history of heart failure starts taking oxybutynin (Ditropan) for urge incontinence. One week later, she calls the office and tells the nurse, "I get so thirsty on this drug. I've been drinking lots of water, but it seems that I can't drink enough water to keep from getting thirsty!" What is the nurse's best response to this patient?

For answers, see http://evolve.elsevier.com/Canada/Lilley/pharmacology/.

Drugs Affecting the Cardiovascular and Renal Systems

STUDY SKILLS TIPS:
- LINKING LEARNING
- TEXT NOTATION

LINKING LEARNING

The Part Three Study Skills Tips stressed the importance of planning for the part as a whole. With that in mind, what is the focus of Part Four? The part title is "Drugs Affecting the Cardiovascular and Renal Systems." What do you think is the first question you should ask about this part? You might begin by asking, "What are cardiovascular and renal systems?" This is an obvious question and might seem so basic that it need not be asked, but the next eight chapters will all develop around concepts related to this part title. Asking the obvious question is sometimes the best way to get started.

Chapter Structure

Just as there is a structure to each part in the text, there is also a structure in the chapters. This structure is a repeating model created to organize the material and present it in the clearest way possible.

Chapter Objectives

Each chapter begins with a set of objectives. It is tempting to ignore these objectives and get right on with the task of reading the chapter, but it is helpful to spend a little time reading them and thinking about what they reveal about the content of the chapter.

Example Based on Chapter 25 Objectives

Objective 1. Differentiate between the terms *inotropic*, *chronotropic*, and *dromotropic*.

What can you learn from this objective? First, there is the vocabulary. This objective makes it clear that you have some terms to learn, and it may be helpful to have

some blank note cards available to start creating vocabulary cards for this chapter. Write each of the terms on a separate card and complete the card as the terms are introduced and explained in the chapter.

The next point that stands out is that the three terms contain a common element, *tropic*. This should bring active questioning into play. What does the suffix *tropic* mean? Asking this question now helps to note that these three terms do have some common meaning.

Objective 2: Briefly discuss the pathophysiology of heart failure.

From this statement comes the potential for a new question relating to the first objective. What do *inotropic*, *chronotropic*, and *dromotropic* have to do with the heart? Just as it is essential to see the relationship between parts and chapters, it is also essential to see relationships within the chapters. These two objectives should cause you to consider those relationships and make your own learning much more active.

Chapter Headings

The next aspect of chapter structure to consider in this exploration is the chapter headings. Chapter 25 has the major sections Overview, Drug Therapy, Angiotensin-Converting Enzyme Inhibitors, Angiotensin II Receptor Blockers, β-Blockers, Aldosterone Antagonists, Miscellaneous Heart Failure Drugs, Omega-3 Polyunsaturated Fatty Acids, Phosphodiesterase Inhibitors, Cardiac Glycosides, and Nursing Process. Now, ask yourself, "What is the importance of this heading structure?" It tells you that the authors will focus on the pharmacological aspects first and then explain how these relate to nursing.

The section Cardiac Glycosides is divided into smaller subsections in this chapter. Spend several minutes considering the organization of these subsections. The first subtopic to tackle is Mechanism of Action and Drug Effects. What is the mechanism of action of cardiac glycosides? How do they act? What effect do they have on the heart? It does not matter that you cannot answer these questions at this point. What is important is that you ask them as a means of fostering an active and participatory learning attitude when you begin to read the chapter. Think, question, anticipate, and then read. This sequence will enhance your learning.

Continue this process of looking at the subtopics and thinking ahead to what will be explained in the chapter. These subsections are the same in every chapter, and this thinking process should quickly become automatic.

Key Terms

This aspect of chapter structure was already stressed in previous Study Skills Tips, and it is essential to learning. The list of key terms is a miniature dictionary for each chapter—words that were not introduced earlier in the text and that are central to the content of this chapter are presented here. The listing is in alphabetical order, which means that the key terms will not necessarily appear in the same order as in the body of the chapter.

As you read the key terms, be aware of the nature of the definition. A key term definition is specific and brief. It is a useful place to begin to learn the new terms in the chapter, but the definition presented may not be enough to give you a full understanding. You will find that this will come after reading the chapter and encountering the term within the context of sentences and paragraphs of text that explain not only the term but also how it applies in the described situations.

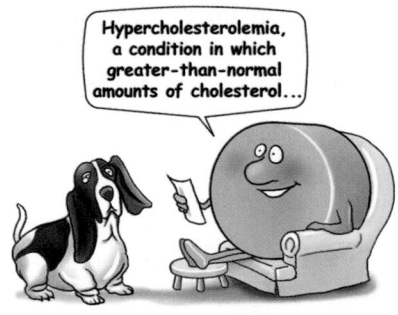

> Hypercholesterolemia, a condition in which greater-than-normal amounts of cholesterol...

Key Terms and Text Relationship

The term *inotropic drugs* is defined in the Chapter 25 key terms list. As you read the definition, you understand that inotropic has to do with force or energy of muscle contractions. The key term states that inotropic drugs affect myocardial contractility. Some of this information is clear, and some of it is still somewhat hazy. It should become clearer when connected with the chapter text. The first paragraph of the drug therapy section introduces inotropic drugs: "Drugs that increase the force of myocardial contraction are called positive **inotropic drugs,** and they have a role in the treatment of a failing heart muscle."

After reading this sentence, you should have a much clearer understanding of what is meant by *inotropic agents*, in addition to your knowledge that positive inotropic drugs exist. You see the core definition as presented in the key terms list and you read to determine how that core definition is expanded and exemplified in the body of the text. It would be useful to make note of expanded definitions on the vocabulary note cards previously mentioned.

When preparing vocabulary cards, it is not a good idea to simply copy the definition from the key terms list and assume that this definition will serve your purpose. Wait to fill out the card until after you encounter the term in the body of the chapter, and then pick and choose the information from the key terms list and the text that will provide you with the clearest summary of the term. Also, when writing information on vocabulary cards, it is always useful to include the chapter number and page numbers so that you can locate the source of your definition quickly later.

Chapter structures can provide you with a clear picture of what you are expected to learn and the organizational pattern in which the material will be presented. Being aware of these structures and making use of them in this way will improve your concentration, understanding, and memory when you begin to read the chapter. Time spent considering chapter structure is not wasted and does not significantly increase time spent studying the chapter. In fact, the time you spend working with the objectives, headings, and key terms will generally save time later when you are doing intensive reading and study.

TEXT NOTATION

Highlighting or underlining text materials can be helpful when rehearsing and reviewing materials after reading. The problem is that it is often difficult to limit the quantity of material that you mark. Although a good general guideline is to try to limit yourself to marking no more than 20 to 25% of the total text, this guideline applies to large blocks of material (Remember Part 2). However, some paragraphs contain essential information and must be marked extensively, whereas other paragraphs may need only one or two sentences marked. In this Study Skills Tips section, the object is to look at how the author's structure and language can help you select what should be marked.

Text Notation Application

Reproduced below are the first two paragraphs from Chapter 30, with model underlining completed, followed by a discussion of the reasons for these particular choices. You should not view the underlining shown here as a "perfect" model. The decision as to what to mark is an individual choice based on a number of factors, including prior experience with the subject matter and awareness of personal learning objectives and needs. This example is intended to provide you with a basic model to adapt to your own learning style and needs.

Chapter 30, 1st Paragraphs Under "Overview" and "Physiology of Fluid Balance"

"<u>Fluid and electrolyte management</u> is one of <u>the corner-stones of patient care</u>. Most disease processes, tissue injuries, and surgical procedures greatly influence the physiological status of fluids and electrolytes in the body. <u>Understanding fluid and electrolyte management requires knowledge of the extent and composition of the various body fluid compartments.</u>"

"Approximately 60% of the adult human body is water. This is referred to as *total body water* (TBW), and it is distributed among the three main compartments in the following proportions: **intracellular fluid (ICF)**, <u>67%;</u> **interstitial fluid (ISF)**, <u>25%</u>; and plasma volume (PV), <u>8%</u>. This distribution is illustrated in Figure 30-1. The actual volume of fluid that would normally be distributed in each compartment in an average 70-kg man with a TBW content of 60% is shown in Table 30-1."

Discussion. The first thing you should notice is that the underlining here exceeds the 20 to 25% guideline. These are the first paragraphs in the chapter. First paragraphs are usually introductions to the topic and may vary a great deal in the quantity of important information therein. This selection seemed to contain a number of key points that must be considered. Because the content seems important, more is underlined.

The first sentence was chosen because of the word "cornerstones." This word suggests that fluid management is extremely important in <u>patient</u> care—the reader must be sure to keep that focus throughout the chapter. Paying careful attention to the author's word choices plays a major role in selecting materials for text notation.

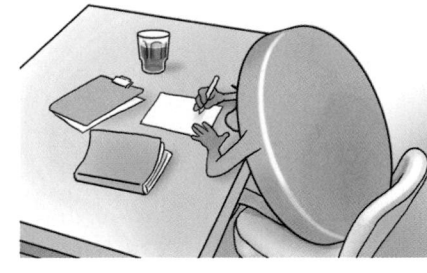

Paying attention to language led to the third sentence, which includes, "Understanding ... requires knowledge of ..." These words should immediately capture your attention. There is something that must be understood before anything else that follows will make complete sense. The phrase should also serve as a cue to generate a question for reading: "What knowledge is required in order to gain understanding of fluid and electrolyte management?" This question is answered directly by the sentence. Language clues suggest that you will probably want to underline or highlight some information. The

question helps you select what should be marked. Everything you do at this point serves as a guide to help you establish clear learning objectives and makes the process of selecting the best information for marking easier.

The next segment was chosen because it stands out from the body of the paragraph. *"Total body water"* is italicized. This is a print convention used as a means of putting emphasis on something that the author believes to be of special importance. The decision to underline words and phrases that are already emphasized is a personal one. You may feel that since the author has already marked it, you don't need to add your own marks. Some students find that their own marking, even of italicized or bolded print material, serves as an extra reminder of the importance of the information. Remember, text notation is highly personal. Whether you choose to add your own marking or not, there is one aspect of this phrase that is essential. *Total body water* is part of the vocabulary of fluids and electrolytes. That means it is time to add to your vocabulary cards.

This term served as a lead-in to the next key point marked. The next statement is "it [total body water] is distributed among the three main compartments ... " Whenever you see a phrase with a number and a word such as *main*, you should be aware that this is potentially important material. This phrase should generate a new question that will aid in your selection of material to mark: "What are the three main compartments?" You see immediately that the rest of this sentence answers that question and therefore identifies what needs to be marked. This marking also identifies three additional vocabulary items to be added to your cards for this chapter. As you set up your cards, be careful—one fluid is "intra-," and the second is "inter-." It would be easy to confuse the two, but they have different meanings. If you are not sure what the difference is between *intra-* and *inter-*, consult a dictionary source. (Make sure you consult a reliable and credible source. Consider that while it is easy to utilize the most convenient source, the information it provides may not be accurate.)

Chapter 30, Paragraph Two of "Physiology of Fluid Balance"

" . . . <u>The TBW</u> can be <u>described as being inside or outside of the blood vessels (vasculature)</u>. If this point of reference is used, then the <u>term</u> **intravascular fluid (IVF)** <u>describes fluid inside the blood vessels</u>, and the term **extravascular fluid (EVF)** <u>refers to the fluid outside the blood vessels</u>. Examples of EVF include lymph and cerebrospinal fluid. As these concepts are learned, it is important to remember the difference between the prefixes *intra-* (inside), *inter-* (between), and *extra-* (outside). The term **plasma** is used to describe the <u>fluid that flows through the blood vessels (IVF)</u> . . . ISF is the fluid that is in the <u>spaces between cells, tissues, and organs</u>. Both <u>plasma and ISF make up extracellular volume</u>. When discussing blood vessels, the term *extravascular volume* is used; extravascular volume is made up of plasma and ISF. When discussing cells, the term *extracellular volume* is used; extracellular volume is composed of ISF and ICF. These terms are often confused and misused."

Discussion. The language conventions and the print conventions **bold** and *italic* are the same as those used to help in the previous paragraph. This paragraph also makes a point about the possibility of confusing or misusing the terms introduced. Being told that there is confusing material suggests that it is crucial that you be able to identify, define, and explain each of the terms used, and that it will take some careful thinking to do so. While not referred to in this paragraph, there are many tables in this text. Tables are often used to simplify complex material and to clarify the relationships between the items presented.

CHAPTER 23

Antihypertensive Drugs

Objectives

After reading this chapter, the successful student will be able to do the following:

1. Briefly discuss the normal anatomy and physiology of the autonomic nervous system, including the events that take place within the sympathetic and parasympathetic divisions as related to long-term and short-term control of blood pressure.

2. Define *hypertension.*

3. Compare primary (essential) and secondary hypertension and their related manifestations.

4. Describe the protocol for treating hypertension as detailed in the Canadian Hypertension Education Program Guidelines, including the rationale for its use.

5. List the criterion pressure values (in millimetres of mercury) for the hypertension categories of normal pressure, prehypertension, hypertension stage 1, and hypertension stage 2.

6. Using the most recent guidelines, compare the various drugs used in the pharmacological management of hypertension in regard to mechanisms of action, specific indications, adverse effects, toxic effects, cautions, drug interactions, contraindications, dosages, and routes of administration.

7. Discuss the rationale for the nonpharmacological management of hypertension.

8. Develop a collaborative plan of care that includes all phases of the nursing process for patients receiving antihypertensive drugs.

e-Learning Activities

Website
(http://evolve.elsevier.com/Canada/Lilley/pharmacology/)

evolve

- Answer Key—Textbook Case Studies
- Answer Key—Critical Thinking Activities
- Chapter Summaries—Printable
- Review Questions for Exam Preparation
- Unfolding Case Studies

Drug Profiles

  aliskiren (aliskiren fumarate)* , p. 450
  bosentan (bosentan monohydrate)*, p. 451
▸▸ captopril, p. 446
▸▸ clonidine (clonidine hydrochloride)*, p. 444
  doxazosin mesylate, p. 444
  enalapril (enalapril sodium)*, p. 446
  eplerenone, p. 451
▸▸ hydralazine (hydralazine hydrochloride)*, p. 450
▸▸ losartan (losartan potassium)*, p. 448
  nebivolol hydrochloride, p. 444
  sodium nitroprusside, p. 450
  treprostinil (treprostinil sodium)*, p. 451

▸▸ Key drug

*Full generic name is given in parentheses. For the purposes of this text, the more common, shortened name is used.

Key Terms

α₁-blockers Drugs that primarily cause arterial and venous dilation through their action on peripheral sympathetic neurons. (p. 439)

Antihypertensive drugs Medications used to treat hypertension. (p. 438)

Cardiac output The amount of blood ejected from the left ventricle, measured in litres per minute. (p. 436)

Centrally acting adrenergic drugs Drugs that modify the function of the sympathetic nervous system in the brain by stimulating α₂-receptors. α₂-receptors are inhibitory in nature and thus have a reverse sympathetic effect and cause a decrease in blood pressure. (p. 439)

Essential hypertension Elevated systemic arterial pressure for which no cause can be found; also called *primary* or *idiopathic hypertension*. (p. 437)

Hypertension A common, often asymptomatic disorder in which blood pressure persistently exceeds 140 mm Hg or diastolic pressure exceeds 90 mm Hg. (p. 436)

Malignant hypertension Extremely high blood pressure, usually above 180/120. (p. 437)

Orthostatic hypotension A common adverse effect of adrenergic-blocking drugs involving a sudden drop in blood pressure when patients change position, especially when rising from a seated or horizontal position. (p. 441)

Prodrug A drug that is inactive in its given form and which must be metabolized to its active form in the body, generally by the liver, to be effective. (p. 444)

Secondary hypertension High blood pressure caused by another disease, such as kidney, pulmonary, endocrine, or vascular disease. (p. 437)

OVERVIEW

Hypertension, defined as a persistent systolic pressure of greater than 140 mm Hg or a diastolic pressure greater than 90 mm Hg, affects an estimated 7.5 million Canadians (Hypertension Canada, 2015c). Globally, the prevalence of hypertension is highest in Africa and other low- and middle-income nations, and it affects approximately 1 billion people worldwide, designating it the most common disease state (World Health Organization, 2013). Indigenous Canadians, Canadians of South Asian or Black ethnicities, and individuals of low socioeconomic status are at greater risk for developing hypertension (Heart and Stroke Foundation, 2015; see Ethnocultural Implications box). As the population ages, the incidence of hypertension will continue to increase (Heart and Stroke Foundation, 2015).

Hypertension is a major risk factor for coronary artery disease, cardiovascular disease, and death resulting from cardiovascular causes. It is the most important risk factor for stroke and heart failure, and it is also a major risk factor for kidney failure and peripheral vascular disease. There is indisputable evidence in regard to the relationship between blood pressure and risk of cardiovascular disease; the higher the blood pressure, the greater the chance of developing cardiovascular disease. For people 40 to 70 years of age, the risk of developing cardiovascular disease doubles with each 20 mm Hg increase in

systolic blood pressure or 10 mm Hg increase in diastolic pressure.

To gain insight into the treatment of hypertension, requires a basic understanding of blood pressure. Blood pressure is determined by the product of **cardiac output** (4 to 8 L/min) and systemic vascular resistance (SVR). The mean arterial pressure (MAP) is a product of CO and SVR. The MAP is calculated as 1/3 DBP and 2/3 DBP. The MAP may be a better indicator of tissue perfusion as two thirds of the cardiac cycle are spent in diastole; a MAP of 60 is believed to be necessary to maintain adequate tissue perfusion. Cardiac output is the amount of blood ejected from the left ventricle and is measured in litres per minute. SVR, or afterload, is the resistance to blood flow that is determined by the diameter of the blood vessel and the vascular musculature. It is calculated by dividing blood pressure by cardiac output. Numerous factors interact to regulate these two major variables and keep blood pressure within normal limits. These are illustrated in Figure 23-1 and are the same factors that can cause hypertension and are the targets of action of many of the antihypertensive drugs.

The diagnosis and management of hypertension have varied considerably over the years, resulting in a great deal of misunderstanding in how to treat this disorder. Since 2000, the Canadian Hypertension Education

ETHNOCULTURAL IMPLICATIONS

Antihypertensive Drug Therapy

The following are some important generalizations about demographics and the drugs used to treat hypertension:

- β-blockers and angiotensin-converting enzyme inhibitors have been found to be more effective in lowering blood pressure in White people than in Black people.
- Calcium channel blockers and diuretics have been shown to be more effective in patients who are Black than in patients who are White.
- Captopril used as monotherapy to treat hypertension has been found to elicit a lesser response in patients who are Black because they are considered to have lower renin levels than in the general treatment population.
- Losartan sodium, used as monotherapy for hypertension, has been found to be less effective in patients who are Black than in other racial groups because of their lower renin levels.

These findings are important to remember in the care of patients, whether they are in an inpatient setting, are being seen by a health care provider (HCP), or are being screened by a nurse in the community. The significance of these ethnocultural factors is that they allow a better understanding of the dynamics of pharmacological treatment in patients with hypertension of different ethnic groups and also underscore the importance of a thorough nursing assessment that includes attention to ethnocultural influences. Such ethnocultural factors also allow an appreciation of individual responses to drug therapy and aid in selecting first-line drugs and achieving more successful treatment of the disease.

Based on: Bope, E. T. & Kellerman, R. D. (2014). *Conn's current therapy 2014.* St. Louis, MO: Elsevier.

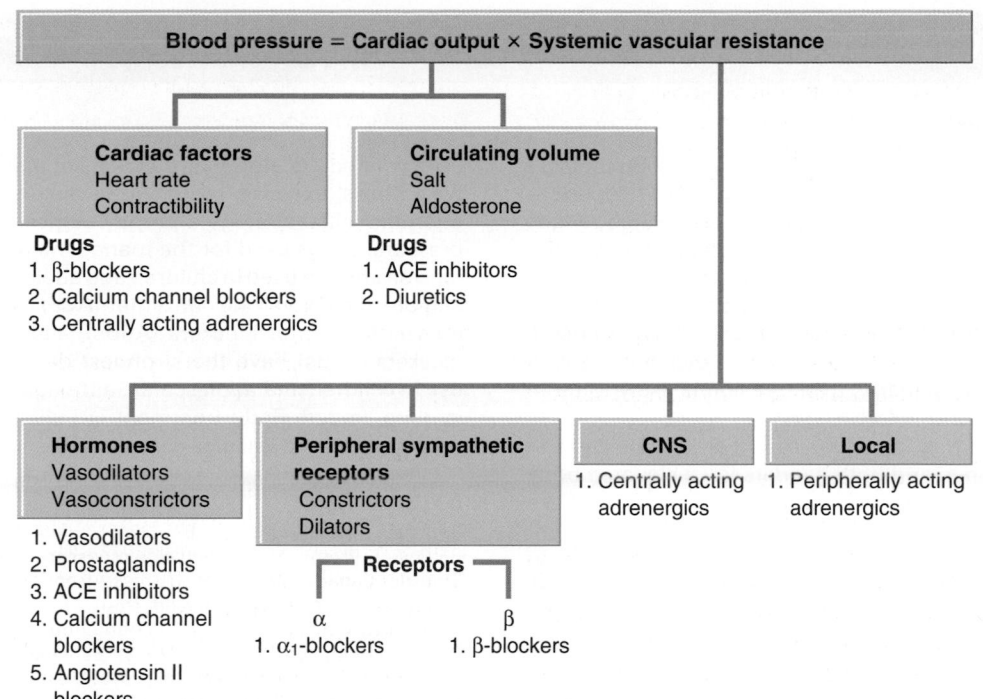

Blood pressure = Cardiac output × Systemic vascular resistance

Cardiac factors
Heart rate
Contractibility

Drugs
1. β-blockers
2. Calcium channel blockers
3. Centrally acting adrenergics

Circulating volume
Salt
Aldosterone

Drugs
1. ACE inhibitors
2. Diuretics

Hormones
Vasodilators
Vasoconstrictors

1. Vasodilators
2. Prostaglandins
3. ACE inhibitors
4. Calcium channel blockers
5. Angiotensin II blockers

Peripheral sympathetic receptors
Constrictors
Dilators

Receptors
α   β
1. α₁-blockers   1. β-blockers

CNS
1. Centrally acting adrenergics

Local
1. Peripherally acting adrenergics

FIG. 23-1 Normal regulation of blood pressure and corresponding mechanisms. *ACE*, angiotensin-converting enzyme; *CNS*, central nervous system.

Program (CHEP) and the Heart and Stroke Foundation of Canada have produced and updated yearly evidence-informed recommendations for the detection, assessment, and treatment of hypertension, assembled by the 43 members of the CHEP evidence-based recommendations task force. Each year, the recommendations focus on a change from previous guidelines or an important initiative (See https://www.hypertension.ca/en/chep for CHEP guidelines). CHEP's intent is to educate HCPs and the general public about the consequences of hypertension and the importance of adequate prevention and treatment in order to reduce the burden of cardiovascular disease. Nurses have a key role to play in the primary prevention, detection, and treatment of hypertension.

To identify those with hypertension, all adults require ongoing regular assessment of blood pressure. More recent CHEP guidelines include the classification of high-normal blood pressure. Those individuals who have high-normal blood pressure (130–139/85–89 mm Hg) are considered at higher risk of developing hypertension. It is estimated that of those who have high-normal blood pressure and are overweight, 40% will develop hypertension within 2 years, while an additional 20% will develop hypertension within 4 years. Previous guidelines had recommended a stepped-care pharmacological approach to treating hypertension; many HCPs believe that this approach no longer adequately reflects the current range of pharmacological alternatives available. Individualized therapy was proposed as a more appropriate treatment strategy. The individualized approach continues to be emphasized. Many patients will require two or more medications, even as initial therapy, depending on their

individual cardiovascular risk factors such as obesity, diabetes, and family history.

The classification scheme used to categorize individual cases of hypertension has been simplified based on blood pressure measurements. See www.hypertension.ca for the CHEP algorithm for the assessment of patients with hypertension.

Hypertension can also be defined by its cause. When the specific cause of hypertension is unknown, it may be called *essential hypertension* (or *idiopathic* or *primary hypertension*). About 90 to 95% of cases of hypertension are of this type. **Secondary hypertension** accounts for the other 5 to 10%. Secondary hypertension is most commonly the result of another disease such as a pheochromocytoma (adrenal tumour), pre-eclampsia of pregnancy (a pregnancy complication involving acute hypertension, among other symptoms), renal artery disease, sleep apnea, thyroid disease, or parathyroid disease. It may also result from the use of certain medications such as atypical antipsychotics (see Chapter 17). If the cause of secondary hypertension can be eliminated, blood pressure usually returns to normal. If untreated, hypertension can cause damage to end organs such as the heart, brain, kidneys, and eyes. **Malignant hypertension** is extremely high blood pressure, with levels usually above 180/120, and is considered and treated as a medical emergency. It develops rapidly and usually results in organ damage.

Hypertension in children is increasing in prevalence and may persist into adulthood with the associated long-term health risks that are common with a diagnosis of hypertension (see Special Populations: Children).

SPECIAL POPULATIONS: CHILDREN

Hypertension

It is estimated that 4% of children and adolescents in Canada have prehypertension (high-normal) or hypertension (Statistics Canada, 2013), although calculated ranges vary between 1 and 5%. Because hypertension is considered a "silent killer," as it is usually is asymptomatic, it is reasonable to assume that many children and adolescents remain undiagnosed. A secondary cause of hypertension is likely to be found in patients who have not reached adolescence; after puberty, hypertension is likely to be of primary (essential) etiology.

The strongest risk factor for essential hypertension in children of all ages and both genders is an elevated body mass index (BMI). Children who are overweight or obese have a twofold to threefold increased risk of hypertension. Insulin resistance and an adverse lipid profile often accompany adiposity (visceral obesity) and it is suggested that this trio of manifestations progress more rapidly in children and adolescents who are prehypertensive or hypertensive, compared with children who are normotensive.

As with adults, nonpharmacological management (e.g., weight loss, exercise, reduction of dietary salt and fat) is often the initial strategy and may suffice to reduce blood pressure. Drugs used for the management of adult hypertension are also used in children and adolescents; however, angiotensin-converting enzyme (ACE) inhibitors, angiotensin II receptor blockers (ARBs), and calcium channel blockers (CCBs) have the strongest data to support their use in children and adolescents, although data availability is quite limited. Early treatment is indicated to decrease the risk of cardiovascular complications in adulthood.

Sources: Rodriguez-Cruz, E. (2015). *Pediatric hypertension.* Retrieved from http://emedicine.medscape.com/article/889877; Statistics Canada. (2013). *Blood pressure of Canadian children and youth, 2009 to 2011.* Retrieved from http://www.statcan.gc.ca/pub/82-625-x/2012001/article/11713-eng.htm; Thompson, M., Dana, T., Bougatsos, C., et al. (2013). Screening for hypertension in children and adolescents to prevent cardiovascular disease. *Pediatrics, 131*(3), 490–525. doi:10.1542/peds.2012-3523

The objective of antihypertensive therapy is the reduction of cardiovascular and renal morbidity and mortality. According to the 2015 CHEP guidelines, the goal is to achieve a pressure of less than 140/90, which is associated with a decrease in cardiovascular disease complications. In patients with hypertension and concurrent diabetes or concurrent nondiabetic chronic kidney disease, the goal is less than 130/80 mm Hg and 140/90 mm Hg, respectively.

Fortunately, many significant advances have been made in both the methods of treating hypertension and in the understanding of the disease process. Large numbers of clinical trials have shown that adequately treating hypertension can prevent or delay cardiovascular disease. Over the past 40 years, the development of new antihypertensive medications has had an enormous impact on the quality of life of people with hypertension. Drug therapy for hypertension first became available in the early 1950s, with the introduction of ganglionic blocking drugs. However, unpleasant adverse effects and inconsistent therapeutic effects were common problems with these **antihypertensive drugs.** In 1953, the vasodilator hydralazine was introduced, and in 1958 the thiazide diuretics became available.

Since that time, several additional drug categories have been developed, including loop diuretics (also called potassium-depleting diuretics), potassium-sparing diuretics, β-blockers (β-receptor antagonists), angiotensin-converting enzyme (ACE) inhibitors, α_1-antagonists, α_2-agonists, angiotensin II receptor blockers (ARBs), calcium channel blockers (CCBs), vasodilators, and the newest class, the direct renin inhibitors. Although some of the medications mentioned in this chapter represent older classes of drugs, all are current therapeutic options listed in the CHEP treatment guidelines for hypertension.

ANTIHYPERTENSIVE DRUGS

Drug therapy for hypertension needs to be individualized. Important considerations in planning drug therapy are whether the patient has multiple medical problems and what impact drug therapy will have on the patient's quality of life. For example, sexual dysfunction in males is a common adverse effect of almost any antihypertensive drug and is the most common reason for nonadherence to drug therapy. Demographic factors, ethnocultural implications, the ease of medication administration (e.g., a once-a-day dosing schedule or transdermal administration), and cost are other important considerations.

There are seven main categories of pharmacological drugs used to treat hypertension: diuretics, adrenergic drugs, ACE inhibitors, ARBs, CCBs, vasodilators, and direct renin inhibitors. All of these antihypertensive drugs (with the exception of diuretics) have some vasodilatory action. Drugs in any of these classes may be used alone or in combination. The various categories and subcategories of antihypertensive drugs are listed in Box 23-1. The diuretics are discussed in detail in Chapter 29.

REVIEW OF AUTONOMIC NEUROTRANSMISSION

There are two divisions of the autonomic nervous system (ANS): the parasympathetic (PSNS) and

DIURETICS

The diuretics are a highly effective class of antihypertensive drugs. They are first-line antihypertensives in the CHEP guidelines for the treatment of hypertension. They may be used as monotherapy or in combination with drugs of other antihypertensive classes. Their primary therapeutic effect is decreasing volumes of plasma and extracellular fluid, which results in decreased preload. This leads to a decrease in cardiac output and total peripheral resistance, all of which decrease the workload of the heart. This large group of antihypertensives is discussed in detail in Chapter 29. The thiazide diuretics (e.g., hydrochlorothiazide and chlorthalidone) are the most commonly used diuretics for hypertension.

ADRENERGIC DRUGS

Adrenergic drugs are a large group of antihypertensive drugs, as shown in Box 23-1. The α-blockers and combined α- and β-blockers were described in detail in Chapter 20. The adrenergic drugs discussed here exert their antihypertensive action at different sites.

Mechanism of Action and Drug Effects

Five specific drug subcategories are included in the adrenergic antihypertensive drugs, as indicated in Box 23-1. Each of these subcategories of drugs can be described as having central action (in the brain) or peripheral action (at the heart and blood vessels). These drugs include the adrenergic neuron blockers (central and peripheral), the α_2-receptor agonists (central), the α_1-receptor blockers (peripheral), the β-receptor blockers (peripheral), and the combination α_1- and β-receptor blockers (peripheral).

The centrally acting α_2-adrenergic receptor agonists clonidine and methyldopa act by modifying the function of the SNS. Stimulation of the SNS leads to an increased heart rate and force of contraction, the constriction of blood vessels, and the release of renin from the kidneys; the result is hypertension. The **centrally acting adrenergic drugs** act by stimulating the α_2-adrenergic receptors in the brain. The α_2-adrenergic receptors are unique in that receptor stimulation actually reduces sympathetic outflow, in this case from the central nervous system (CNS). This reduction results in a lack of norepinephrine production, which reduces blood pressure. Stimulation of the α_2-adrenergic receptors also affects the kidneys, reducing the activity of renin. Renin is the hormone and enzyme that converts the protein precursor angiotensinogen to the protein angiotensin I, the precursor of angiotensin II, a potent vasoconstrictor that raises blood pressure.

In the periphery, the α_1-**blockers** doxazosin mesylate, prazosin hydrochloride, and terazosin hydrochloride also modify the function of the SNS. They do so by blocking the α_1-adrenergic receptors. When α_1-adrenergic receptors are stimulated by circulating norepinephrine, they produce increased blood pressure. When these

sympathetic (SNS) nervous systems. Stimulation of the ANS is controlled by the neurotransmitters acetylcholine and norepinephrine. Receptors for both divisions of the ANS are located throughout the body in a variety of tissues. ANS physiology can be reviewed in greater detail in the introductory sections of Chapters 19 to 22. Receptors in the SNS are called *adrenergic* or *noradrenergic* receptors (i.e., α- or β-receptors). Receptors located between the postganglionic fibre and the effector cells (i.e., postganglionic receptors) are called the *muscarinic* or *cholinergic* receptors in the PSNS. Physiological activity at muscarinic receptors is stimulated by acetylcholine and cholinergic agonist drugs (see Chapter 21) and is inhibited by cholinergic antagonists (anticholinergic drugs; see Chapter 22). Similarly, physiological activity at adrenergic receptors is stimulated by norepinephrine, epinephrine, and adrenergic agonist drugs (see Chapter 19) and inhibited by antiadrenergic drugs (adrenergic blockers, i.e., α- or β-receptor blockers; see Chapter 20). Nicotinic receptors are found on the postganglionic cell bodies in all autonomic ganglia and cause depolarization by opening both sodium and potassium channels. Figure 23-2 shows how these various receptors are arranged in both the PSNS and SNS and indicates their corresponding neurotransmitters.

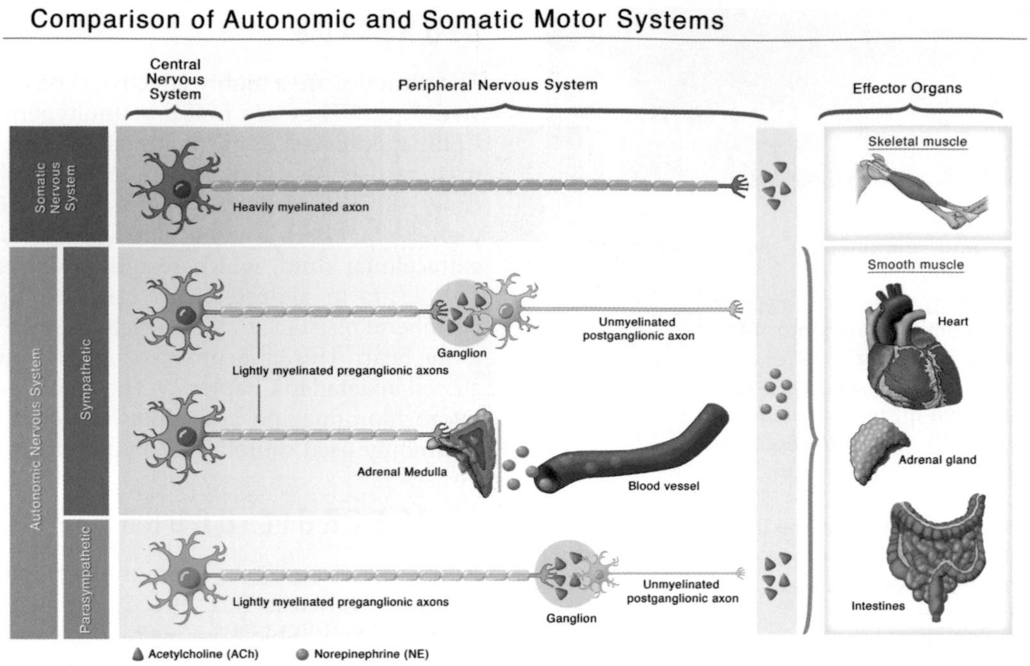

Comparison of Autonomic and Somatic Motor Systems

FIG. 23-2 Location of the acetylcholine and norepinephrine receptors within the parasympathetic and sympathetic nervous systems.

receptors are blocked, blood pressure is decreased. The drug effects of the α_1-blockers are primarily related to their ability to dilate arteries and veins, which reduces peripheral vascular resistance and subsequently decreases blood pressure. This reduction produces a marked decrease in the systemic and pulmonary venous pressures and an increase in cardiac output. The α_1-blockers also increase urinary flow rates and decrease outflow obstruction by preventing smooth muscle contractions in the bladder neck and urethra. This can be beneficial in cases of benign prostate hyperplasia (BPH).

The β-blockers also act in the periphery and include propranolol hydrochloride, metoprolol tartrate, and atenolol, as well as several other drugs. These drugs are discussed in more detail in Chapters 24 and 26 because they are also used for angina and conduction problems. Their effects are related to their reduction of the heart rate through β_1-receptor blockade. Furthermore, β-blockers also cause a reduction in the secretion of the hormone renin (see section on ACE inhibitors), which in turn reduces both angiotension II-mediated vasoconstriction and aldosterone-mediated volume expansion. Long-term use of β-blockers also reduces peripheral vascular resistance.

The dual-action α_1- and β-receptor blocker labetalol hydrochloride (Trandate®) acts in the periphery at the heart and blood vessels. They have the dual antihypertensive effects of reduction in heart rate (β_1-receptor blockade) and vasodilation (α_1-receptor blockade). Figure 23-3 illustrates the site and mechanism of action for the various antihypertensive drugs.

Indications

All of the drugs mentioned in this section are used primarily for the treatment of hypertension, either alone or in combination with other antihypertensive drugs. Various forms of glaucoma may also respond to treatment with some of these drugs. Clonidine is also used for menopausal flushing and has several off-label uses (that is, uses not approved by Health Canada but still common), including prophylaxis for migraine headaches and managing withdrawal symptoms in opioid, nicotine, or alcohol withdrawal (see Chapter 18). The α_1-blockers doxazosin mesylate, prazosin hydrochloride, and terazosin hydrochloride have been used to relieve the symptoms associated with BPH (see Chapter 20). They have also proven to be effective in the management of severe heart failure when used with cardiac glycosides (see Chapter 25) and diuretics (see Chapter 29).

Contraindications

Contraindications to the use of the adrenergic antihypertensive drugs include known drug allergy and may also include acute heart failure, concurrent use of monoamine oxidase inhibitors (see Chapter 17), severe depression, peptic ulcer, and severe liver or kidney disease. Asthma may also be a contraindication to the use of any noncardioselective β-blocker. The use of vasodilating drugs may also be contraindicated in cases of heart failure that is secondary to diastolic dysfunction.

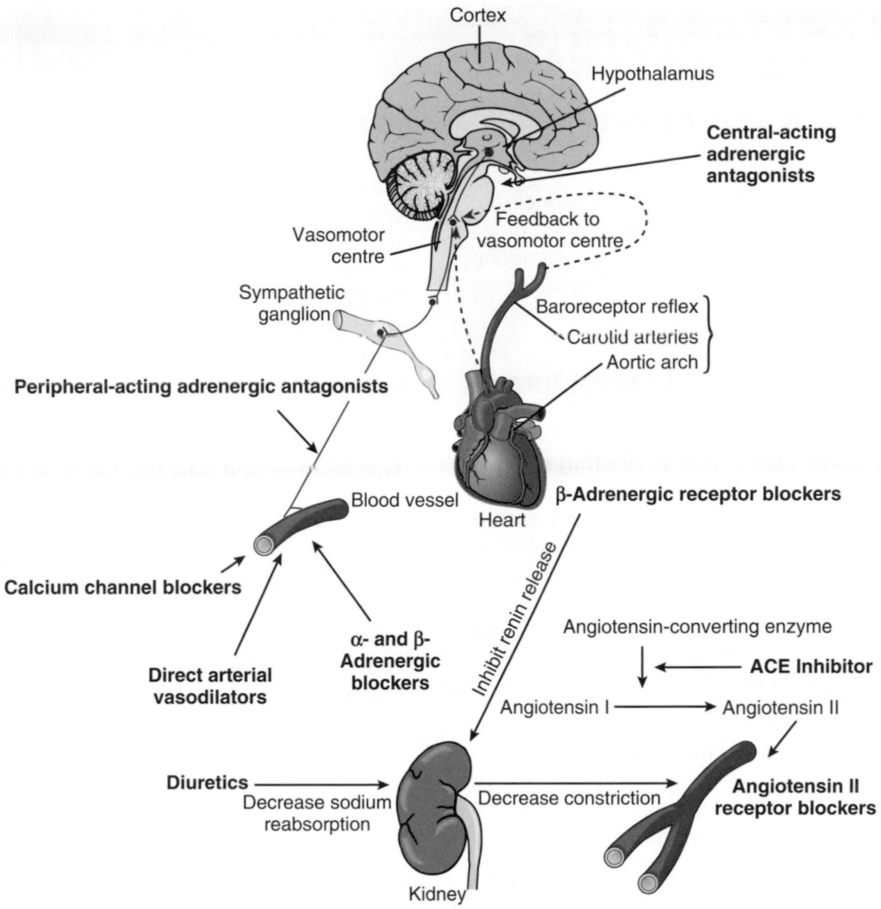

FIG. 23-3 Site and mechanism of action for the antihypertensive drugs. (Source: Lewis, S. M., Dirksen, S. R., Heitkemper, M. M., et al. (2014). *Medical-surgical nursing in Canada: Assessment and management of clinical problems* (3rd Canadian ed., M. A. Barry, S. Goldsworthy, & D. Goodridge, Canadian Eds.). Toronto, ON: Mosby. (Figure 35–7, p. 882.)

Adverse Effects

The most common adverse effects of adrenergic drugs are bradycardia with reflex tachycardia, orthostatic and postexercise hypotension, dry mouth, drowsiness, dizziness, depression, edema, constipation, and sexual dysfunction (e.g., erectile dysfunction; see Chapter 36 for drugs related to sexual dysfunction). Other effects include headaches, sleep disturbances, nausea, rash, and palpitations. There is a high incidence of **orthostatic hypotension** (defined as a sudden drop in systolic BP of greater than or equal to 20 mmHg or a drop in diastolic BP grater than or equal to 10 mmHg when assuming a standing position) in patients taking α-blockers. When the patient changes positions, a situation known as *first-dose syncope*, in which the hypotensive effect is severe enough to cause the patient to lose consciousness with even the first dose of medication, can occur. Educate patients taking these medications to change positions slowly.

In addition, the abrupt discontinuation of the centrally acting α2-receptor agonists can result in rebound hypertension, characterized by a sudden and high elevation of blood pressure. This may also be true for other antihypertensive drug classes, especially β-blockers. Nonselective blocking drugs are also commonly associated with bronchoconstriction (due to unrestrained parasympathetic tone) as well as metabolic inhibition of glycogenolysis in the liver, which can lead to hypoglycemia. However, hyperglycemic episodes are also among the adverse effects reported for this drug class.

Any change in the dosing regimen for cardiovascular medications should be undertaken gradually and with appropriate patient monitoring and follow-up. Although the same is also true for most other classes of medications, abrupt dosage changes of cardiovascular medications, either up or down, can be especially hazardous for the patient. Some of these drugs can also cause disruptions in blood counts as well as in serum electrolyte levels and kidney function. Periodic monitoring of white blood cell count, serum potassium and sodium levels (see also Evidence in Practice), and urinary protein levels is recommended.

EVIDENCE IN PRACTICE

Reduced Dietary Sodium in Hypertension Management

Background

This Canadian survey investigated Canadians' concerns, actions, and reported barriers related to limiting sodium intake, as well as support for a 2010 government-led policy geared toward lowering Canadians' sodium intakes.

Type of Evidence

The researchers from the University of Toronto and University of Guelph conducted an online survey of Canadians about their knowledge, attitudes, and behaviours related to sodium, as well as barriers to limiting sodium consumption. A representative sample of the Canadian population in terms of age, sex, province, and education was used in the survey. In addition, taking into consideration the proposed federal Bill C-460, intended to legislate a formal set of recommendations, the researchers also sought to determine the level of support Canadians had for a number of sodium reduction initiatives.

Results of Study

There is strong public support for sodium reduction strategies, with 76% of Canadians supporting mandatory warning labels on high-sodium products and 68% believing that regulations about maximum allowable levels of sodium in foods in grocery stores, restaurants, and public facilities such as hospitals, schools, and government buildings. Eighty percent would like the food industry to lower the amount of sodium in food. However, little support for taxing foods high in sodium or for subsidization of foods lower in sodium was reported. Of interest, 67% of respondents were concerned about their sodium intake (particularly those with high blood pressure and older adults). Fifty percent were actively lowering their sodium intake but thought that not adding salt at the table was adequate. In contrast, others were not limiting their salt intake because they had good health and normal blood pressure.

Link of Evidence to Nursing Practice

Approximately 2 million Canadians have hypertension as a consequence of excess dietary intake of sodium, which is a key risk contributing to the disease burden in (Hypertension Canada, 2016). Hypertension is the leading risk factor for mortality in Canada and worldwide. Recommendations for salt intake vary depending on the source, with a range of 2 000 to 3 200 mg of sodium per day. According to Health Canada (2012), the average Canadian has a daily sodium intake of over 3 400 mg (equivalent to 1.5 teaspoons), and more than 90% of Canadian children aged 4 to 8 years of age exceed dietary sodium guidelines. The majority of this sodium intake (77%) is found primarily in processed, packaged, and restaurant foods. Foods that make up 19% of the sodium in individuals' diets are pizzas, hamburgers, hotdogs, and sandwiches, with soups accounting for 7%, and pasta, 6%. Estimates are that one quarter of Canadian adults (approximately 7.5 million)

have hypertension, with more than 9 in 10 Canadians expected to develop high blood pressure if they have an average lifespan of about 80 years. While Health Canada's new *Eating Well with Canada's Food Guide* publication recommends that Canadians reduce their sodium intake, the World Health Organization (WHO; WHO, 2014) advocates a regulated approach. The WHO suggests that governmental policies restricting the amount of sodium added to food by food industries is more effective than simply recommending a reduction in sodium intake. Nurses can play a significant role in educating their patients about hypertension and how to reduce sodium intake. Reducing dietary sodium intake within the context of a healthy diet can substantially reduce the incidence of hypertension among Canadians with normal blood pressure. Therefore, a population health approach to reducing dietary sodium is an appropriate strategy.

The CHEP recommendations for lifestyle modifications to prevent and treat hypertension include the following:

- Recommended dietary sodium intake was updated in 2014 and raised to less than 87 mmol, or 5 g per day (equal to 2 000 mg of sodium per day). Previously, the recommendation was 1 500 mg per day. NOTE: The terminology of sodium and salt content is confusing. Conversion: 2 300 mg sodium is approximately one teaspoon of salt (sodium chloride), 100 mmol of sodium or salt, or 5.8 g (5 800 mg) of salt (NaCl).
- Perform 30 to 60 minutes of aerobic exercise 4 to 7 days per week.
- Maintain a healthy body weight (body mass index 18.5 kg/m² to 24.9 kg/m²) and waist circumference (smaller than 102 cm for men and smaller than 88 cm for women).
- Limit alcohol consumption to no more than 15 drinks per week in men or 10 drinks per week in women.
- Follow a diet that is reduced in saturated fat and cholesterol and that emphasizes fruits, vegetables, and low-fat dairy products, dietary and soluble fibre, whole grains, and protein from plant sources.
- Consider stress management in selected individuals with hypertension.

Based on: Arcand, J., Mendoza, J., Qi, Y., et al. (2013). Results of a national survey examining Canadians' concern, actions, barriers, and support for dietary sodium reduction interventions. *Canadian Journal of Cardiology, 29*(5), 628–631. doi:10.1016/j.cjca.2013.01.018; Health Canada. (2012). *Sodium in Canada.* Retrieved from http://www.hc-sc.gc.ca/fn-an/nutrition/sodium/index-eng.php; Heart and Stroke Foundation. (2014). *Dietary sodium, heart disease, and stroke.* Retrieved from http://www.heartandstroke.com/site/c.ikIQLcMWJtE/b.5263133/k.696/Dietary_sodium_heart_disease_and_stroke.htm; Hypertension Canada. (2014). *The case for sodium reduction in Canada: Fact sheet.* Retrieved from http://www.hypertensiontalk.com/wp-content/uploads/2014/03/FactSheet-Sodium-HTalk.pdf; World Health Organization. (2014). *Fact sheet: Salt reduction.* Retrieved from http://www.who.int/mediacentre/factsheets/fs393/en/.

TABLE 23-1

Adrenergic Drugs: Drug Interactions

Drug	Interacts With	Mechanism	Result
clonidine	TCAs, MAOIs, appetite suppressants, amphetamines	Opposing actions	Decreased hypotensive effects
	Diuretics, nitrates, other antihypertensive drugs	Additive	Increased hypotensive effects
	β-blockers	Additive	May potentiate bradycardia and increase the rebound hypertension in clonidine withdrawal
doxazosin mesylate	CNS depressants, alcohol	Additive	Increased CNS depression
	β-blockers and other hypotensive drugs	Additive	Increased hypotension
	verapamil hydrochloride	Increased serum prazosin levels	Increased hypotension

CNS, central nervous system; *MAOIs*, monoamine oxidase inhibitors; *TCAs*, tricyclic antidepressants.

TABLE 23-2

ACE Inhibitors: Distinguishing Characteristics

Drug (Trade Name)	Combination With Hydrochlorothiazide	Dose Schedule
benazepril hydrochloride (Fortekor®, Lotensin®)	None	Once a day
captopril (Capoten®)	None	Multiple
cilazapril (Inhibace®)	Inhibace Plus®	Once a day
enalapril sodium (Vasotec®)	Vaseretic®	Multiple
fosinopril sodium	None	Once a day
lisinopril (Prinivil®, Zestril®)	Zestoretic®	Once a day
perindopril erbumine (Coversyl®)	None	Once a day
quinapril hydrochloride (Accupril®)	Accuretic®	Once a day
ramipril (Altace®)	Altace HCT®	Once to twice daily
trandolapril (Mavik®)	None	Once a day

ACE, Angiotensin-converting enzyme; *HCT*, hydrochlorothiazide.

Interactions

Adrenergic drugs can cause additive CNS depression when taken with alcohol, benzodiazepines, and opioids. Other drug interactions that can occur with selected adrenergic drugs are summarized in Table 23-1. This list is merely representative and is not exhaustive. Always keep a drug information handbook available to check when a specific drug interaction is suspected. Pharmacists are also excellent resources.

Dosages

For dosage information on selected adrenergic antihypertensive drugs, refer to the table on p. 444.

ANGIOTENSIN-CONVERTING ENZYME INHIBITORS

The ACE inhibitors are members of a large group of antihypertensive drugs. There are a number of ACE inhibitors available for clinical use in addition to various combination drug products in which a thiazide diuretic or a CCB is combined with an ACE inhibitor. Combination products tend to improve adherence since the patient is taking fewer drugs. ACE inhibitors are safe and efficacious and are often used as one of the first-line drugs in the treatment of both heart failure and hypertension. It is also used as first-line in patients with concurrent diabetes for kidney protection. The available ACE inhibitors, drug combinations, and dosing schedules are summarized in Table 23-2. The drugs that make up the class of ACE inhibitors are quite similar to one another and differ in only a few of their chemical properties; however, there are some differences among them in their clinical properties.

Captopril has the shortest half-life and therefore must be dosed more frequently than any of the other ACE inhibitors. This may be an important drawback for patients with a history of nonadherence to their medication regimen. On the other hand, it may be best to start with a drug that has a short half-life in a patient who is critically ill, so that if problems arise they will be short-lived. Both captopril and enalapril can be dosed multiple times a day.

DRUG PROFILES

α_2-Adrenergic Receptor Stimulators (Agonists)

Of the two α_2-receptor agonists—clonidine and methyldopa—clonidine is by far the most commonly used and the prototype drug for this class. Methyldopa is commonly used to treat hypertension in pregnancy. However, these drugs are not typically prescribed as first-line antihypertensive drugs because their use is associated with a high incidence of adverse effects such as orthostatic hypotension, fatigue, and dizziness. They may be used as adjunct drugs in the treatment of hypertension after other drugs have failed or may be used in conjunction with other antihypertensives such as diuretics.

▶▶ *clonidine hydrochloride*

Clonidine hydrochloride (Catapres®, Dixarit®) is used primarily for its ability to decrease blood pressure. It is also useful in the management of opioid withdrawal. Clonidine has a better safety profile than the other centrally acting adrenergics. It must not be discontinued abruptly, as this will lead to severe rebound hypertension. Its use is contraindicated in patients who have shown hypersensitivity reactions to it. It is available for oral use only. For recommended dosages refer to the table below.

PHARMACOKINETICS

Route	Onset of Action	Peak Plasma Concentration	Elimination Half-Life	Duration of Action
PO	30–60 min	3–5 hr	6–20 hr	8 hr

α_1-Blockers

The α_1-blockers include doxazosin mesylate (Cardura®), prazosin hydrochloride (Minipress®), tamsulosin hydrochloride (Flomax CR®), and terazosin hydrochloride (Hytrin®). Their use is contraindicated in patients who have shown a hypersensitivity to them. They are not recommended for use during pregnancy. They are available only as oral preparations. Tamsulosin hydrochloride is not used to manage blood pressure but is indicated solely for symptomatic management of BPH. This use is described further in Chapters 19 and 35.

doxazosin mesylate

Doxazosin mesylate (Cardura) is a commonly used α_1-blocker. It reduces peripheral vascular resistance and blood pressure by dilating both arterial and venous blood vessels. It has been shown to be beneficial in the treatment of hypertension and the relief of the symptoms of obstructive BPH. It is available for oral use. For recommended dosages refer to the table on this page.

PHARMACOKINETICS

Route	Onset of Action	Peak Plasma Concentration	Elimination Half-Life	Duration of Action
PO	1–2 hr	2–3 hr	15–22 hr	Less than 24 hr

Dual-Action α_1- and β-Receptor Blockers
β-RECEPTOR BLOCKER

nebivolol hydrochloride

Nebivolol hydrochloride (Bystolic®) is the newest β-blocker, released in 2013. It is a β_1-selective blocker approved for use in hypertension. Nebivolol hydrochloride is similar to other β_1-selective blockers; however, in addition to blocking β_1-receptors, it also produces an endothelium-derived, nitric oxide–dependent vasodilation, which results in a decrease in SVR. It is promoted as causing less sexual dysfunction. Like other β-blockers, it should not be stopped abruptly but must be tapered over 1 to 2 weeks. Dosing starts at 5 mg/day and may be increased at 2-week intervals to a maximum of 20 mg/day.

DOSAGES	Selected Antihypertensive Drugs: Adrenergic Agonists and Antagonists		
Drug	**Pharmacological Class**	**Usual Dosage Range**	**Indications**
▶▶ clonidine hydrochloride (Catapres, Dixarit)	Centrally acting α_2-receptor agonist	*Adults* PO: Initial dose 0.2–0.6 mg/day divided bid	Hypertension (may have other off-label uses including treatment of psychiatric, opioid withdrawal, menopausal hot flashes cardiovascular, and gastrointestinal problems)
doxazosin mesylate (Cardura)	Peripherally acting α_1-receptor antagonist	*Adults* PO: Initial dose 0.1 mg/day; titrate up to maximum of 16 mg/day	Hypertension

PO, oral.

Captopril and lisinopril are the only two ACE inhibitors that are not prodrugs. A **prodrug** is a drug that is inactive in its administered form and must be metabolized to its active form by the liver and or gastrointestinal (GI) tract to be effective. This characteristic of captopril and lisinopril is an important advantage in treating a patient with liver dysfunction; all of the other ACE inhibitors are prodrugs, and their transformation to active form is dependent upon liver function to reveal the active drug.

Enalaprilat is the only ACE inhibitor available in a parenteral preparation. All of the newer ACE inhibitors, such as benazepril hydrochloride, fosinopril sodium, lisinopril, quinapril hydrochloride, and ramipril have long half-lives and long durations of action, which allows once-a-day dosing. A once-a-day medication regimen promotes better patient adherence.

When used in pregnancy during the second and third trimesters, ACE inhibitors may cause significant fetal morbidity or mortality, so they should be discontinued as soon as possible if pregnancy is detected. ACE inhibitors are to be used by pregnant women only if there are no safer alternatives.

Mechanism of Action and Drug Effects

The development of ACE inhibitors was spurred by the discovery of an animal substance found to have beneficial effects in humans. This particular substance was the venom of a South American viper, which was found to inhibit kininase activity. Kininase is an enzyme that normally breaks down bradykinin, a potent vasodilator in the human body.

As their name implies, these drugs inhibit angiotensin-converting enzyme, which is responsible for converting angiotensin I (formed through the action of renin) to angiotensin II. Angiotensin II is a potent vasoconstrictor and induces aldosterone secretion by the adrenal glands. Aldosterone stimulates sodium and water resorption, which can raise blood pressure. Together, these processes are referred to as the renin–angiotensin–aldosterone system. By inhibiting this process, blood pressure is lowered.

The primary effects of the ACE inhibitors are cardiovascular and renal. Their cardiovascular effects are due to their ability to reduce blood pressure by decreasing SVR. They do this by preventing the breakdown of the vasodilating substance bradykinin and substance P (another potent vasodilator), thus preventing the formation of angiotensin II. These combined effects decrease afterload, or the resistance against which the left ventricle must pump to eject its volume of blood during contraction. ACE inhibitors are beneficial in the treatment of heart failure because they prevent sodium and water resorption by inhibiting aldosterone secretion. This causes diuresis, which decreases blood volume and return to the heart. This in turn decreases preload, or the left ventricular end-diastolic volume, and the work required of the heart.

Indications

The therapeutic effects of the ACE inhibitors are related to their potent cardiovascular effects. They are excellent antihypertensives and adjunctive drugs for the treatment of heart failure. They may be used alone or in combination with other drugs such as diuretics in the treatment of hypertension or heart failure.

The beneficial hemodynamic effects of the ACE inhibitors have been studied extensively. Because of their ability to decrease SVR (a measure of afterload) and preload, ACE inhibitors can stop the progression of left ventricular hypertrophy, which is sometimes seen after a myocardial infarction. This pathologic process is known as *ventricular remodelling*. The ability of ACE inhibitors to prevent this process is termed a *cardioprotective effect*. ACE inhibitors have been shown to decrease morbidity and mortality rates in patients with heart failure. They are considered the drugs of choice for hypertensive patients with heart failure. ACE inhibitors also have been shown to have a protective effect on the kidneys because they reduce glomerular filtration pressure. This is one reason why they are among the cardiovascular drugs of choice for patients diagnosed with diabetes. Numerous studies have shown that the ACE inhibitors reduce proteinuria, and they are considered by many to be standard therapy for patients with diabetes to prevent the progression of diabetic nephropathy. The various therapeutic effects of the ACE inhibitors are listed in Table 23-3, which lists the biochemicals on which ACE inhibitors act and the resulting beneficial hemodynamic effects.

Contraindications

Contraindications to the use of ACE inhibitors include known drug allergy, especially a previous reaction of angioedema (e.g., laryngeal swelling) to an ACE inhibitor. Patients with a baseline potassium of 5 mmol/L or higher may not be suitable candidates for ACE inhibitor therapy because these drugs can promote hyperkalemia (see later discussion). Kidney function decline is a precaution. Although kidney protective, starting an ACEI in a patient with significant kidney decline would be further detrimental to kidney function. All ACE inhibitors are contraindicated in women who are lactating, in children, and in patients with bilateral renal artery stenosis.

TABLE 23-3			
ACE Inhibitors: Therapeutic Effects			
Body SUBSTANCE	**Effect in Body**	**ACE Inhibitor Action**	**Resulting Hemodynamic Effect**
aldosterone	Causes sodium and water retention	Prevents its secretion	Diuresis = ↓ plasma volume = ↓ filling pressures or ↓ preload
angiotensin II	Potent vasoconstrictor	Prevents its formation	↓ SVR = ↓ afterload
bradykinin	Potent vasodilator	Prevents its breakdown	↓SVR = ↓ afterload

ACE, angiotensin-converting enzyme; ↓, decreased; *SVR*, systemic vascular resistance.

Adverse Effects

Major CNS effects of ACE inhibitors include fatigue, dizziness, mood changes, and headaches. A characteristic dry, nonproductive cough may occur that is reversible with discontinuation of the therapy (the ACE inhibitor is usually switched to an ARB). A first-dose hypotensive effect can cause a significant decline in blood pressure. Other adverse effects include loss of taste, hyperkalemia, rash, anemia, neutropenia, thrombocytosis, and agranulocytosis. In patients with severe heart failure whose kidney function may depend on the activity of the renin–angiotensin–aldosterone system, treatment with ACE inhibitors may cause acute kidney failure. ACE inhibitors promote potassium resorption in the kidney, although they promote sodium excretion because of their reduction of aldosterone secretion. For this reason, serum potassium levels must be monitored regularly. This is particularly true when there is concurrent therapy with potassium-sparing diuretics, although many patients tolerate both types of drug therapy with no major problems. One rare, but potentially fatal, adverse effect is angioedema, a strong vascular reaction involving inflammation of submucosal tissues, which can progress to anaphylaxis.

Toxicity and Management of Overdose

The most pronounced symptom of an overdose of an ACE inhibitor is hypotension. Treatment is symptomatic and supportive and includes the administration of intravenous fluids to expand blood volume. Hemodialysis is effective for the removal of captopril and lisinopril.

Interactions

Nonsteroidal anti-inflammatory drugs (NSAIDS), such as ibuprofen, can reduce the antihypertensive effect of ACE inhibitors (see Chapter 49). The use of NSAIDs and ACE inhibitors may also predispose patients to the development of acute kidney injury. Concurrent use of ACE inhibitors and other antihypertensives or diuretics can have hypotensive effects. Giving lithium carbonate and ACE inhibitors together can result in lithium toxicity. Potassium supplements and potassium-sparing diuretics, when administered with ACE inhibitors, may result in hyperkalemia. The monitoring of serum potassium levels becomes important in these cases. False-positive results on tests for acetone in the urine may occur in patients taking captopril.

Dosages

For dosage information on selected ACE inhibitors, refer to the table on p. 447.

ANGIOTENSIN II RECEPTOR BLOCKERS

Angiotensin II receptor blockers (ARBs) are similar to ACE inhibitors. The class includes losartan (Cozaar®),

DRUG PROFILES

ACE Inhibitors

▸▸*captopril*

Captopril (Capoten) was the first available ACE inhibitor and is considered the prototypical drug for the class. Several large multicentre studies have shown its clinical efficacy in minimizing or preventing the left ventricular dilation and dysfunction (also called *ventricular remodelling*) that can arise in the acute period after a myocardial infarction, and thereby improve the patient's chances of survival. It can also reduce the risk of heart failure in these patients. It has the shortest half-life of all of the currently available ACE inhibitors, and it must be given three or four times a day. For recommended dosages refer to the table below.

PHARMACOKINETICS

Route	Onset of Action	Peak Plasma Concentration	Elimination Half-Life	Duration of Action
PO	15 min	1–2 hr	2 hr	2–6 hr

enalapril sodium

Enalapril sodium (Vasotec) is the only ACE inhibitor currently marketed that is available in both oral and parenteral preparations. The parenteral formulation (enalaprilat) is an active drug. It offers the hemodynamic benefit of inhibiting ACE activity in an acutely ill patient who cannot tolerate oral medications. The other benefit to intravenous enalapril is that it does not require cardiac monitoring as the intravenous β-blockers and CCBs do. Although its half-life is slightly longer than that of captopril, it may still have to be given twice a day. The oral form of enalapril differs from captopril in that it is a prodrug, and the patient must have a functioning liver for the drug to be converted into its active form. As with captopril, it has been shown in many large studies to improve a patient's chances of survival after a myocardial infarction and to reduce the incidence of heart failure. For recommended dosages refer to the table below.

PHARMACOKINETICS

Route	Onset of Action	Peak Plasma Concentration	Elimination Half-Life	Duration of Action
PO	1 hr	4–6 hr	2 hr	12–24 hr
IV	15 min	1–4 hr	2 hr	4–6 hr

DOSAGES   Selected Antihypertensive Drugs: Ace Inhibitors and Angiotensin II Receptor Blockers

Drug	Pharmacological Class	Usual Dosage Range	Indications
▸▸captopril (Capoten)	ACE inhibitor	*Adults* PO: 25–150 mg bid–tid	Hypertension, heart failure
enalapril sodium (Vasotec)	ACE inhibitor	*Children (less than 16 years)* PO: 0.08 mg/kg (up to 5 mg) once daily *Adults* PO: 10–40 mg/day as a single dose or in 2 divided doses PO: .25–40 mg/day as a single or divided dose IV: 1.25 mg q6h over a 5-min period	Hypertension Hypertension Heart failure Hypertension
▸▸losartan potassium (Cozaar)	Angiotensin II receptor blocker	*Adults* PO: 50–100 mg once daily	Hypertension

ACE, angiotensin converting enzyme; IV, intravenous, PO, oral.

eprosartan mesylate (Teveten®), valsartan (Diovan®), irbesartan, candesartan cilexetil (Atacand®), telmisartan (Micardis®), and azilsartan medoxomil potassium (Edarbi®).

Mechanism of Action and Drug Effects

The ARBs block the binding of angiotensin II to type 1 angiotensin II receptors. These type 1 receptors are thought to mediate the effects of important effectors in controlling blood pressure and volume in the cardiovascular system. The type 1 receptor is activated by angiotensin II with resulting effects that include vasoconstriction and aldosterone synthesis and secretion. The ACE inhibitors such as enalapril block conversion of angiotensin I to angiotensin II, but angiotensin II may be formed by other enzymes that are not blocked by ACE inhibitors. For comparison, recall that ACE inhibitors block the breakdown of bradykinins and substance P, which accumulate and may cause adverse effects such as cough but might also contribute to the drugs' antihypertensive and heart and nephroprotective effects. Bradykinins are potent vasodilators and help to reduce blood pressure by dilating arteries and decreasing SVR.

In contrast to ACE inhibitors, ARBs affect primarily vascular smooth muscle and the adrenal gland. By selectively blocking the binding of angiotensin II to the type 1 angiotensin II receptors in these tissues, ARBs block vasoconstriction and the secretion of aldosterone. Angiotensin II receptors have been found in other tissues throughout the body, but the effects of ARB blocking of these receptors is unknown.

Clinically, ACE inhibitors and ARBs appear to be equally effective for the treatment of hypertension. Both are well tolerated, but ARBs do not cause cough. There is evidence that ARBs are better tolerated and have lower mortality after myocardial infarction than ACE inhibitors. It is not yet clear whether ARBs are as effective as ACE inhibitors in treating heart failure or in protecting the kidneys, as in diabetes. Both types of drugs are contraindicated for use in the second or third trimester of pregnancy. Whether one or more of these drugs, particularly the newer drugs, could prove to have unique adverse effects with long-term use is unknown at this time.

Indications

The therapeutic effects of ARBs are related to their potent vasodilating properties. They are excellent antihypertensives and adjunctive drugs for the treatment of heart failure. They may be used alone or in combination with other drugs such as diuretics in the treatment of hypertension or heart failure. The beneficial hemodynamic effect of ARBs is their ability to decrease SVR (a measure of afterload). Their use is rapidly growing, and many more studies are verifying their beneficial effects. Currently, these drugs are used primarily in patients who have been intolerant of ACE inhibitors.

Contraindications

Contraindications to the use of ARBs are known drug allergy, pregnancy, and lactation. They need to be used cautiously in older adults and in patients with kidney dysfunction because of increased sensitivity to their effects and risk for more adverse effects in these patients. As with other antihypertensives, blood pressure and apical pulse rate need to be assessed before and during drug therapy.

Adverse Effects

The most common adverse effects of ARBs are upper respiratory infections and headache. Occasionally, dizziness, inability to sleep, diarrhea, dyspnea, heartburn, nasal congestion, back pain, and fatigue can occur. Rarely, anxiety, muscle pain, sinusitis, cough, and insomnia can also occur. Hyperkalemia is much less likely to occur with ARBs than with the ACE inhibitors.

Toxicity and Management of Overdose

Overdose may manifest as hypotension and tachycardia; bradycardia occurs less often. Treatment is symptomatic and supportive and includes the administration of intravenous fluids to expand blood volume.

Interactions

The drugs that interact with ARBs, the mechanisms responsible, and the results of the interaction are summarized in Table 23-4. In addition, as is the case with ACE inhibitors, ARBs can promote hyperkalemia, especially when taken concurrently with potassium supplements (although this occurs much less frequently than with ACE inhibitors). Patients' individual chemistry varies widely, however, so monitoring of serum potassium level is necessary for all patients. Potassium supplements may still be indicated for those patients with a tendency toward hypokalemia (whether acute or chronic).

Dosages

For dosage information on the ARBs, refer to the table on p. 447.

CALCIUM CHANNEL BLOCKERS

CCBs are also discussed in detail in the chapters on antidysrhythmic drugs (see Chapter 26) and antianginal drugs (see Chapter 24). As a class of medications, they are used for several indications and have many beneficial effects and relatively few adverse effects. CCBs are used primarily for the treatment of hypertension and angina. Their effectiveness in treating hypertension is related to their ability to cause smooth muscle relaxation by blocking the binding of calcium to its receptors. Because of their effectiveness and safety, they are also a first-line drug for the treatment of hypertension. Amlodipine mesylate (Norvasc®) is the CCB most commonly used for hypertension. CCBs are effective antidysrhythmics (see Chapter 26). One specific CCB, nimodipine, can prevent the cerebral artery spasms that can occur after a subarachnoid hemorrhage. CCBs are sometimes used in the treatment of Raynaud's disease and migraine headache. Finally, they are also used in combination with other drugs—for example, amlodipine mesylate/atorvastatin calcium (Caduet®), an antihypertensive and cholesterol-lowering drug (see Chapter 28) and amlodipine mesylate/temisartan (Twynsta®), an antihypertensive and angiotension II AT_1 receptor blocker.

VASODILATORS

Vasodilators act directly on arterial and venous smooth muscle to cause relaxation. They do not work through adrenergic receptors. Vasodilator drugs include minoxidil (Loniten®), hydralazine (Apresoline®), diazoxide (Proglycem®), and sodium nitroprusside (Nipride®).

TABLE	23-4

Angiotensin II Receptor Blockers: Drug Interactions

Drug	Mechanism	Result
NSAIDs	Decreased antihypertensive	Decreased effect of ARB and potential to kidney failure
lithium	Inhibits lithium carbonate elimination	Increased lithium concentrations
phenobarbital	Increases metabolism	Decreased ARB effectiveness
potassium supplements and potassium-sparing diuretics	Additive potassium-increasing effects	Possible hyperkalemia

ARB, angiotensin II receptor blocker.

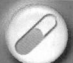 **DRUG PROFILES**

▸▸ *losartan potassium*

Losartan potassium (Cozaar) is beneficial for patients with hypertension and heart failure. Studies indicate that ARBs are better tolerated and produce a marginally lower mortality rate after myocardial infarction than treatment with ACE inhibitors.

The use of losartan is contraindicated in patients who are hypersensitive to any component of this product. It is to be used with caution in patients with kidney or liver dysfunction and in patients with renal artery stenosis. Breastfeeding women must not take losartan because it can cause serious adverse effects on the nursing infant. For recommended dosages, refer to the table on p. 447.

PHARMACOKINETICS

Route	Onset of Action	Peak Plasma Concentration	Elimination Half-Life	Duration of Action
PO	1 hr	6 hr	6–9 hr	24 hr

Mechanism of Action and Drug Effects

Direct-acting vasodilators are useful as antihypertensive drugs because of their ability to cause peripheral vasodilation. This results in a reduction in SVR. In general, the most notable effect of the vasodilators is their hypotensive effect. However, minoxidil (Rogaine®, its topical form) has received attention because of its effectiveness in restoring hair growth. This application is further described in Chapter 56. Diazoxide, hydralazine, and minoxidil work primarily through arteriolar vasodilation, whereas sodium nitroprusside has both arteriolar and venous effects.

Indications

All of the vasodilators can be used to treat hypertension, either alone or in combination with other antihypertensives. Sodium nitroprusside and intravenous diazoxide are reserved for the management of hypertensive emergencies, in which blood pressure is severely elevated.

Contraindications

Contraindications include known drug allergy and may also include hypotension, cerebral edema, head injury, acute myocardial infarction, and coronary artery disease. They may also be contraindicated in cases of heart failure secondary to diastolic dysfunction.

Adverse Effects

Adverse effects of hydralazine include dizziness, headache, anxiety, tachycardia, edema, dyspnea, nausea, vomiting, diarrhea, hepatitis, systemic lupus erythematosus (SLE), vitamin B_6 deficiency, and rash. Minoxidil adverse effects include T-wave electrocardiographic changes, pericardial effusion or tamponade, angina, breast tenderness, rash, and thrombocytopenia. Adverse effects of sodium nitroprusside include bradycardia, decreased platelet aggregation, rash, hypothyroidism, hypotension, methemoglobinemia, and, rarely, cyanide toxicity. Cyanide ions are a byproduct of sodium nitroprusside metabolism. Cyanide and thiocyanate toxicity are seen clinically when sodium nitroprusside is used at high dosages for long periods of time or in patients with renal insufficiency. When sodium nitroprusside is combined with sodium thiosulphate, the potential for cyanide toxicity is greatly reduced.

Toxicity and Management of Overdose

Hydralazine toxicity or overdose produces hypotension, tachycardia, headache, and generalized skin flushing. Treatment is supportive and symptomatic and includes the administration of intravenous fluids, digitalization if needed, and the administration of β-blockers for the control of tachycardia.

Minoxidil overdose or toxicity can precipitate excessive hypotension. Treatment is supportive and symptomatic and includes the administration of intravenous fluids. Norepinephrine and epinephrine should not be used to reverse the hypotension because of the possibility of excessive cardiac stimulation.

The main symptom of sodium nitroprusside overdose or toxicity is severe hypotension. This drug is normally administered only to patients receiving intensive care. Under these conditions, the infusion rate is usually carefully titrated, yielding immediately visible results on a cardiovascular monitor that provides constant measurements of blood pressure from centrally placed venous or arterial catheters. For this reason, excessive hypotension is usually avoidable. When it does occur, discontinuation of the infusion has an immediate effect because the drug is metabolized rapidly (with a half-life of 10 minutes). Treatment for the hypotension is supportive and symptomatic; if necessary, pressor drugs can be infused to quickly raise blood pressure. The chemical structure of sodium nitroprusside contains cyanide groups, which are released upon its metabolism in the body and can result in cyanide or thiocyanate toxicity. This usually occurs clinically when the drug is used at high dosages for prolonged periods or in patients with kidney failure. If cyanide or thiocyanate toxicity occurs, treatment can be administered using a standard cyanide antidote kit that includes sodium nitrite and sodium thiosulfate for injection and amyl nitrite for inhalation.

Interactions

The incidence of drug interactions is low for the direct-acting vasodilators as a class. Hydralazine can produce additive hypotensive effects when given with adrenergic or other antihypertensive drugs.

Dosages

For dosage information for selected vasodilator drugs, refer to the table on p. 450.

NURSING PROCESS

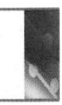

Over the last several decades, the diagnosis and treatment of hypertension has changed greatly from a stepped approach to a medical regimen that is now based on guidelines from CHEP. These guidelines apply to adults 18 years of age and older and describe evaluation, classification, diagnosis, risk factors, identifiable causes, and blood pressure measurement techniques. A new recommendation is the assessment of global cardiovascular risk using a multifactorial risk assessment model. The CHEP guidelines identify a high-normal blood pressure, often referred to as *prehypertension*, defined as a systolic blood pressure of 120 to 139 mm Hg or diastolic blood pressure of 80 to 89 mm Hg, or both. The CHEP guidelines were developed and implemented to encourage the management, both pharmacological and nonpharmacological, of hypertension early in the disease process instead of later

DRUG PROFILES

▸▸ hydralazine hydrochloride

Hydralazine hydrochloride (Apresoline) is less commonly used now than when it first became available, but it is still effective for selected patients. It can be taken orally for routine cases of essential hypertension. It is also available in injectable form for hypertensive emergencies and is useful for patients who cannot tolerate oral therapy in the hospital. Some hospitals may not require cardiac monitoring when it is given intravenously. Contraindications include drug allergy, coronary artery disease, and mitral valve dysfunction, such as that related to childhood rheumatic fever.

PHARMACOKINETICS

Route	Onset of Action	Peak Plasma Concentration	Elimination Half-Life	Duration of Action
IV	5–20 min	30–45 min	2–8 hr	1–4 hr
PO	20–30 min	1–2 hr	2–8 hr	8 hr

sodium nitroprusside

Sodium nitroprusside (Nipride), like diazoxide, is normally used in the critical care setting for severe hypertensive emergencies and is titrated to effect by intravenous infusion. Its use is contraindicated in patients with a known hypersensitivity to the drug, severe heart failure, and known inadequate cerebral perfusion (especially during neurosurgical procedures). For recommended dosages refer to the table below.

PHARMACOKINETICS

Route	Onset of Action	Peak Plasma Concentration	Elimination Half-Life	Duration of Action
IV	Less than 2 min	2–5 min	2 min	1–10 min

DOSAGES	**Selected Antihypertensive Drugs: Vasodilators**		
Drug	**Pharmacological Class**	**Usual Dosage Range**	**Indications**
▸▸hydralazine hydrochloride (Apresoline)	Direct-acting peripheral vasodilator	*Adults* PO: 10 mg qid for 2–4 days, followed by 25 mg qid for balance of week; second and subsequent weeks 50 mg qid, then adjust to lowest effective dose for maintenance IV: 5–40 mg prn	Hypertension
sodium nitroprusside (Nipride)		*Children/Adults* IV: 0.5–8 mcg/kg/min	

PO, oral; *IV*, intravenous.

DRUG PROFILES

Direct Renin Inhibitors

Direct renin inhibitors are the most recent classification of drugs to be used in the treatment of primary hypertension. The sole drug in this class is aliskiren.

▸▸ aliskiren fumarate

Aliskiren fumarate (Rasilez®) is the only drug in the class of low-molecular-weight direct renin inhibitors. This drug is indicated for the treatment of mild to moderate hypertension. Its use is currently recommended as monotherapy or in combination with other antihypertensive drugs such as thiazide diuretics, ACE inhibitors, or dihydropyridine CCBs because of its synergistic effects.

Aliskiren has a unique mechanism of action: it binds directly to the renin enzyme and blocks the conversion of angiotensinogen to angiotensin I and angiotensin II. This action results in the reduction of plasma renin activity and angiotensin I, angiotensin II, and aldosterone. Use of other antihypertensive drugs that work on the renin–angiotensin–aldosterone system, such as the ACE inhibitors and ARBs, results in a compensatory rise in the plasma renin levels because of their suppression of the negative feedback loop. Because of aliskiren's extended half-life, this compensatory rise in plasma renin does not occur. Antihypertensive effect occurs within 2 weeks after initiating therapy with 150 mg per day, and a maximum effect is reached after 4 weeks.

Its use is contraindicated in those who are hypersensitive to it. Aliskiren is generally well tolerated. The most common adverse effects include headache, dizziness, fatigue, and dose-related GI effects such as diarrhea. The concomitant use of aliskiren with cyclosporine is not recommended. Aliskiren is available for oral use. It is also available in combination with hydrochlorothiazide (Rasilez HCT®). The common adult dosage for this drug is 150 to 300 mg PO, once daily. It is also not recommended for use during pregnancy.

PHARMACOKINETICS

Route	Onset of Action	Peak Plasma Concentration	Elimination Half-Life	Duration of Action
PO	30 min	1–3 hr	31–41 hr	7 days

DRUG PROFILES

Miscellaneous Antihypertensive Drugs

Four newer medications exemplify some of the antihypertensives most recently made available in Canada. These include eplerenone, bosentan monohydrate, treprostinil sodium, and epoprostenol sodium. All of these drugs are currently indicated for adult use only.

eplerenone

Eplerenone (Inspra®) is currently the only drug in a new class of antihypertensive drugs called *selective aldosterone blockers*. It reduces blood pressure by blocking the actions of the hormone aldosterone at its corresponding receptors in the kidney, heart, blood vessels, and brain. Eplerenone is indicated for both routine treatment of hypertension and postmyocardial infarction heart failure. Its use is contraindicated in patients with known drug allergy, elevated serum potassium levels (higher than 5.5 mmol/L), or severe kidney impairment and in those using a medication that inhibits the action of cytochrome P450 enzyme 3A4. Many commonly used medications inhibit the action of this enzyme, including several antibiotic, antifungal, and antiviral drugs. Recommended dosages are given in the table on this page.

bosentan monohydrate

Bosentan monohydrate (Tracleer®) works by blocking the receptors of the hormone endothelin. Normally this hormone acts to stimulate the narrowing of blood vessels by binding to endothelin receptors (ET_A and ET_B) in the endothelial (innermost) lining of blood vessels and in vascular smooth muscle. Bosentan reduces blood pressure by blocking this action. However, currently its use is specifically indicated only for the treatment of pulmonary artery hypertension in patients with moderate to severe heart failure. Its use is contraindicated in patients with known drug allergy, with significant liver impairment, who are pregnant, and who are receiving concurrent drug therapy with cyclosporine or glyburide.

Ambrisentan (Volibris®) is a new drug similar to bosentan. Other drugs used to treat pulmonary hypertension include epoprostenol, and treprostinil. The erectile dysfunction drugs sildenafil citrate and tadalafil are also used (see Chapter 36); Both sildenafil citrate and tadalafil have different trade names when used for pulmonary hypertension—sildenafil citrate (commonly known as Viagra®) also has the trade name Revatio®, and tadalafil (commonly known as Cialis®) is Adcirca® when used for pulmonary hypertension.

treprostinil sodium

Treprostinil sodium (Remodulin®) and epoprostenol are analogues of prostacyclin, a metabolite of arachidonic acid, a naturally occurring prostaglandin that lowers blood pressure through a combined mechanism of action by dilating both pulmonary and systemic blood vessels and by inhibiting platelet aggregation. Like bosentan, treprostinil is indicated specifically for long-term management of pulmonary artery hypertension in patients with moderate to severe heart failure. Its only current contraindication is known drug allergy. Both drugs are unique in that they are diluted to the nanogram level for administration. For recommended dosages of treprostinil, refer to the table below.

DOSAGES	**Miscellaneous Antihypertensive Drugs**		
Drug	**Pharmacological Class**	**Usual Dosage Range**	**Indications**
bosentan monohydrate (Tracleer)	Endothelin-receptor antagonist	*Adults* PO: Initial dose of 62.5 mg bid × 4 wk, then increase as tolerated to maintenance dose of 125 mg bid	Pulmonary artery hypertension in patients with moderate to severe heart failure
eplerenone (Inspra)	Aldosterone receptor antagonist	*Adults* PO: Initial dose of 50 mg once/day × 4 wk, then increase as tolerated to max dose of 50 mg bid	Hypertension and postmyocardial infarction status (to improve postmyocardial infarction survival in patients with stable heart failure)
treprostinil sodium (Remodulin)	Vasodilator and platelet aggregation inhibitor	*Adults* Continuous subcutaneous infusion: 0.625–1.25 ng/kg/min	Pulmonary artery hypertension in patients with severe heart failure

PO, oral.

when multiple-organ damage may be present. Recommendations for management of high-normal blood pressure are annual follow-up and lifestyle management. The nursing process discussion that follows provides both general and specific information related to the pharmacological and nonpharmacological treatment of all stages of hypertension.

Assessment

Before any antihypertensive drug is given to a patient, obtain a thorough health history and perform a head-to-toe physical examination. Measure and document blood pressure (including consideration for an orthostatic blood pressure), pulse rate, respirations, and pulse oximetry readings. *Orthostatic hypotension* is defined as a decrease in systolic blood pressure of 20 mm Hg or in diastolic blood pressure of 10 mm Hg within 3 minutes of standing compared with blood pressure from the sitting or supine position. Monitor laboratory tests, including: (1) serum sodium, potassium, chloride, magnesium, and calcium levels; (2) serum levels of troponin, which is usually elevated within 4 to 6 hours after onset of a myocardial infarction and may be a reliable indicator up to 14 days after a heart attack; (3) kidney function studies, including blood urea nitrogen, serum and urinary creatinine levels; and (4) liver function studies, including serum alanine aminotransferase (ALT) and aspartate aminotransferase (AST).

Laboratory tests will most likely be complemented by more sophisticated scans and imaging studies. Noninvasive ophthalmoscopic examination of the eye structures (e.g., optic nerve, optic disc, vessels) by a professional trained to do eye examinations (e.g., nurse practitioner, ophthalmologist, optometrist) allows easy visualization of the structures impacted by hypertension. If hypertensive retinopathy is present, the examination will reveal narrowing of blood vessels in the eye, oozing of fluid from these blood vessels, spots on the retina, swelling of the macula and optic nerve, or bleeding in the back of the eye. These problems may be prevented by controlling blood pressure or treating hypertension with appropriate follow-up once it is diagnosed.

Assess also for conditions, factors, risk factors, or variables that may contribute to a patient's hypertension, such as:
- Addison's disease
- Coarctation of the aorta
- Coronary heart disease
- Culture, race, or ethnicity
- Cushing's disease
- Family history of hypertension
- Nicotine use
- Obesity
- Peripheral vascular disease
- Pheochromocytoma
- Pre-eclampsia of pregnancy

- Renal artery stenosis
- Kidney or liver dysfunction
- Stressful lifestyle

Many of these factors demand cautious use of antihypertensive drugs. Other cautions and contraindications relate to the use of these drugs in older adults and those with chronic illnesses. These individuals are at increased risk for further compromise of their physical condition due to uncontrolled or untreated hypertension or the adverse effects of antihypertensives (e.g., fluid loss, dehydration, electrolyte imbalances, hypotension). For a complete listing of adverse effects and drug interactions associated with antihypertensive drugs, see the pharmacology section in this chapter.

Use of α-adrenergic agonists demands close assessment of the patient's blood pressure, pulse rate, and weight before and during treatment because of their strong vasodilating properties and subsequent hypotensive adverse effects. These drugs may also be associated with fluid retention and edema, so assess heart and breath sounds, intake and output, as well as dependent edema. The α-adrenergic antagonists need to be used cautiously because of potential for hypotension-induced dizziness and syncope. The use of either of these groups of drugs requires close assessment of all parameters, especially in older adults or other patients with pre-existing dizziness or syncope (or an otherwise debilitated state). With doxazosin mesylate, first-dose orthostatic hypotension may occur within 2 to 6 hours; therefore, carefully assess blood pressures (supine and standing) and measure corresponding pulse rates before the first dose and 2 to 6 hours afterward, as well as with any subsequent increase in the dosage. When any antihypertensive drug is used, measure blood pressures and pulse rates (supine and standing), and assess for cautions, contraindications, and drug interactions. With centrally acting α-blockers, also assess white blood cell counts, serum potassium and sodium levels, and level of protein in the urine (to identify proteinuria).

Review the β-blockers and their mechanisms of action before administering these drugs to a patient because of the risk of complications in certain patient populations. If a drug is a nonselective β-blocker, it blocks both β_1- and β_2-receptors and will have both heart and respiratory effects, whereas if a drug is a β_1-blocking drug, the cardiac system will be affected (pulse rate and blood pressure will decrease), but there will be no β_2 effects. This limits any concern regarding respiratory problems. Therefore, if a patient needs a β-blocker but has restrictive airway problems, a β_1-blocker is recommended (to avoid bronchoconstriction). However, if there is no history of respiratory illnesses or concerns, the nonselective β-blockers may be effective as antihypertensives. In addition, for patients with heart failure, understand that β-blockers also have a negative inotropic effect on the heart (decrease contractility); their use would lead to worsening of heart failure, which calls for a completely different type of antihypertensive.

With the use of β-blockers, assess blood pressure and apical pulse rate immediately before each dose. If the systolic blood pressure is less than 90 mm Hg or the pulse rate is less than 60 beats/min, notify the HCP because of the risk of adverse effects (e.g., hypotension, bradycardia). In such cases, the drug would usually be withheld, as ordered or per protocol. These blood pressure and pulse rate parameters are also applicable to the use of other antihypertensives. Also assess breath sounds and heart sounds before and during drug therapy.

With the use of ACE inhibitors, assess blood pressure, apical pulse rate, and respiratory status (because of the adverse effect of a dry, hacking, chronic cough). Take blood pressure readings immediately before initial and subsequent doses of the drug so that extreme fluctuations may be identified early. Also assess serum potassium, sodium, chloride, and creatinine levels as ordered. Tests of baseline heart functioning will most likely be ordered prior to initiation of therapy. Because of potential adverse effects of neutropenia and other blood disorders, assess complete blood count before and during therapy, as ordered. ARBs are to be used cautiously in older adults and in patients with kidney dysfunction because of their increased sensitivity to the drug's effects and increased risk for more adverse effects. If the serum creatinine increases more than 30% over baseline, the ACEI should be stopped.

Perform a baseline neurological assessment with the use of vasodilators, with attention to level of consciousness and cognitive ability. Use these drugs with extreme caution with older adults because they are more sensitive to the drugs' blood pressure–lowering effects and may experience more problems with hypotension, dizziness, and syncope.

In summary, many assessment parameters are similar for the various groups of antihypertensives. The difference in the level of assessment depends on the drug's impact on blood pressure as well as the individual's response to the medication and any pre-existing illnesses or conditions. Other factors to be assessed in any patient receiving these drugs, as well as most other drugs, include the patient's cultural background, racial or ethnic group, reading level, learning needs, developmental and cognitive status, financial status, mental health status, support systems, and overall physical health status. Encourage patients to learn how to assess and monitor themselves and their individual responses to drug therapy.

Nursing Diagnoses

- Ineffective peripheral tissue perfusion related to the impact of the hypertensive disease process or possible severe hypotensive adverse effects associated with antihypertensive drug therapy
- Sexual dysfunction related to adverse effects of some antihypertensive drugs
- Constipation related to the adverse effects of antihypertensive drugs
- Nonadherence with drug therapy related to lack of familiarity with or acceptance of the disease process
- Risk for injury (e.g., possible falls) related to possible antihypertensive drug–induced orthostatic hypotension with dizziness and syncope

Planning

Focus nursing goals for antihypertensive therapy on educating patients, family members, and caregivers about the crucial importance of adequate management to prevent end-organ damage. Goals must include making sure patients understand the nature of the disease, its symptoms, and treatment, as well as the importance of adhering to the treatment regimen. Patients must also come to terms with their diagnoses, the fact that there is no cure for the hypertension, and that treatment will be lifelong. Emphasize the influence of chronic illness on daily life and the importance of nonpharmacological therapy, stress reduction, and follow-up care. Plan for ongoing assessment of blood pressure, weight, diet, exercise, smoking habits, alcohol intake, adherence with therapy, and sexual function in patients receiving therapy for hypertension.

Goals

- Patient will regain control of hypertension with return of adequate tissue perfusion.
- Patient will experience minimal changes in sexual functioning while managing adverse drug effects.
- Patient will experience minimal changes in bowel elimination patterns.
- Patient will remain adherent with antihypertensive drug therapy.
- Patient will remain free from injury during drug therapy.

Outcome Criteria

- Patient states the importance of taking antihypertensive drug therapy as prescribed to maintain normal to near-normal blood pressure control.
  - Patient regains control of hypertension with a return of blood pressure to a level below the ranges set by CHEP, that is, below a systolic blood pressure of 120 to 139 mm Hg or a diastolic blood pressure of 80 to 89 mm Hg.
  - Patient states the importance of keeping follow-up appointments with HCPs as well as monitoring blood pressure.
- Patient openly discusses any difficulty in sexual functioning during antihypertensive therapy.
  - Patient implements suggestions or interventions as shared by the HCP to assist in decreasing any problems with sexual function.

- Patient states the importance of avoiding abrupt discontinuation of drug therapy with antihypertensives while experiencing changes in sexual functioning to avoid rebound hypertension and risk for complications.
- Patient manages constipation with healthy lifestyle and dietary changes.
  - Patient improves constipation by increasing fluid intake (unless contraindicated), increasing dietary fibre through consuming more fruits and vegetables or by taking HCP-suggested psyllium-based product for improving constipation.
- Patient demonstrates an understanding of the importance of taking antihypertensive medication(s) exactly as prescribed.
  - Patient reports to HCP any adverse effects such as dizziness, syncope, excessive fatigue, constipation, or changes in sexual functioning while continuing medication regimen unless prescribed by HCP.
  - Patient's blood pressure begins to return to a range as defined by the HCP and CHEP.
- Patient follows instructions to maintain safety and minimize dizziness and syncope while on medication regimen.
  - Patient changes position slowly, carefully, and purposefully.
- Patient keeps daily journal with entries about diet, exercise, adverse effects, blood pressure readings, and daily weights.

Implementation

Nursing interventions may help patients achieve stable blood pressure while minimizing adverse effects. Many patients have problems adhering to treatment because the disease is silent or without symptoms. Because of this, some patients are unaware of their blood pressure or think that if they do not feel ill there is nothing wrong with them, which poses many problems for treatment. Also, the antihypertensives are associated with multiple adverse effects that may impact patients' self-concept and sexual integrity. These adverse effects may lead patients to abruptly stop taking the medication. Inform patients that any abrupt withdrawal is a serious concern because of the risk of developing rebound hypertension, which is a sudden and extremely high elevation of blood pressure. This places the patient at risk for a stroke or other cerebral or cardiac adverse events. It is important to understand that with *all* antihypertensives there is a risk of rebound hypertension (with abrupt withdrawal), and prevention of this through patient education is critical to patient safety. Other interventions related to each major group of drugs are discussed in the following paragraphs. See the Patient Teaching Tips for more information.

Because of the potential for drug-related orthostatic hypotensive effects, patients taking α-adrenergic agonists will need to monitor their blood pressure and pulse rate at home or have these parameters measured by a family member who has received instructions or by other qualified medical personnel. The blood pressure machines found in pharmacies and grocery stores do not provide as accurate readings as measurement in the aforementioned ways. The α-adrenergic agonists are associated with first-dose syncope, so to avoid injury, advise patients to remain supine for the first dose of the drug. These drugs will often be prescribed to be given at bedtime to allow the patient to sleep through the drug's first-dose syncope. It may take 4 to 6 weeks for the drug to achieve its full therapeutic effects. Educate the patient about this delayed onset of action and bedtime dosing to avoid injury. The patient needs continual monitoring for dizziness, syncope, edema, and other adverse effects (e.g., shortness of breath, exacerbation of pre-existing heart disorders). Diuretics may be ordered as adjunctive therapy to minimize the adverse effects of edema, but they may lead to more dizziness and electrolyte imbalances. Centrally acting α-blockers require the same type of nursing interventions as other α-blockers; however, as their name indicates, the mechanism of action of these drugs is central, so adverse effects are often more pronounced (e.g., hypotension, sedation, bradycardia, edema). See the Patient Teaching Tips for more information.

The β-blockers are either nonselective (block both β_1- and β_2-receptors; e.g., propranolol hydrochloride) or cardioselective (block mainly β_1-receptors; e.g., atenolol). With any β-blocker, careful adherence to the drug regimen is crucial to patient safety. Patients taking β-blockers may experience an exacerbation of respiratory diseases such as asthma, bronchospasm, and chronic obstructive pulmonary disease (because of increased bronchoconstriction due to β_2-blocking), or an exacerbation of heart failure (because of the drug's negative inotropic effects, i.e., decreased contractility due to β_1-blocking). Provide clear and concise instructions about reporting adverse effects and instructions for taking blood pressure and pulse rates. If a β_1-blocker causes shortness of breath, it is most likely because of edema or exacerbation of heart failure. Any dizziness, orthostatic hypotension, edema, constipation, or sexual dysfunction needs to be reported to the HCP immediately. See the Patient Teaching Tips for more information.

ACE inhibitors must also be taken exactly as prescribed. If angioedema occurs, contact the HCP immediately. If the drug must be discontinued, weaning is recommended (as with all antihypertensives) to avoid rebound hypertension. Monitor serum sodium and potassium levels during therapy. Serum potassium levels increase as an adverse effect of these drugs, resulting in hyperkalemia and possible complications. Impaired taste may occur as an adverse effect and last up to 2 to 3 months after the drug has been discontinued. It is also important to educate the patient that it takes several weeks to see full therapeutic effects and that potassium supplements are not needed with the ACE inhibitors because of the adverse effect of hyperkalemia.

ARBs must also be taken exactly as prescribed. They are often tolerated best with meals, as with many antihypertensives. The dosage must not be changed nor the medication discontinued except on the order of the HCP. With ARBs, if the patient has hypovolemia or liver dysfunction, the dosage may need to be reduced. A diuretic such as hydrochlorothiazide may be ordered in combination with an ARB for patients who have hypertension with left ventricular hypertrophy. Most importantly, with ARBs, report any unusual dyspnea, dizziness, or excessive fatigue to the HCP immediately.

Nursing considerations for vasodilators are similar to those for other antihypertensives; however, the impact of the vasodilators on blood pressure may be more drastic, depending on the specific drug and dosage. Hydralazine given by injection may result in reduced blood pressure within 10 to 80 minutes after administration and requires close monitoring of the patient. With hydralazine, systemic lupus erythematosus (SLE) may be an adverse effect if the patient is taking more than 200 mg orally per day. If signs and symptoms of SLE occur, such as photosensitivity, characteristic skin rashes, CNS changes, or various blood dyscrasias (hemolytic anemia, leukopenia, thrombocytopenia), discontinue the drug, contact the HCP immediately, and continue to closely monitor the patient. Electrocardiographic changes, cardiovascular inadequacies, and hypotension may have pronounced effects on the patient's heart status, so *never* give the drug without adequate monitoring and frequent assessment. Always dilute sodium nitroprusside per manufacturer guidelines. Because this drug is a potent vasodilator, it may lead to extreme decreases in the patient's blood pressure. Close monitoring is therefore important for preventing further complications. Severe drops in blood pressure may lead to irreversible ischemic injuries and even death, so close monitoring is needed during drug administration. Remember that sodium nitroprusside should never be infused at the maximum dose rate for more than 10 minutes. If this drug does not control a patient's blood pressure after 10 minutes, it will most likely be discontinued by the HCP.

Cyanide ions are a by-product of sodium nitroprusside metabolism. Cyanide and thiocyanate toxicity are seen clinically when sodium nitroprusside is used at high dosages for long periods of time or in patients with kidney insufficiency. When sodium nitroprusside is combined with sodium thiosulfate, the potential for cyanide toxicity is greatly reduced. To help prevent complications of cyanide and thiocyanate toxicity, (1) dilute the medication properly and avoid use of any solution that has turned blue, green, or red; (2) infuse only with use of a volumetric infusion pump, not through ordinary intravenous sets; (3) continuously monitor blood pressure during the infusion (often by invasive measures); and (4) when more than 500 mcg/kg of sodium nitroprusside is administered at a rate faster than 2 mcg/kg/min, be aware that this may result in production of cyanide at a more rapid rate than can be eliminated by the patient unaided (see Lab Values Related to Drug Therapy for more information.)

 ## LAB VALUES RELATED TO DRUG THERAPY

Related to Drug Therapy for Sodium Nitroprusside

Laboratory Test	Normal Ranges	Rationale for Assessment
Serum methemoglobin and serum cyanide	Normally there are no detectable amounts with appropriate drug levels of sodium nitroprusside	Use of sodium nitroprusside may be associated with sequestration of hemoglobin as methemoglobin. The appearance of this clinically significant adverse effect of methemoglobinemia is rare (less than 10% of cases). Serum laboratory testing is used to measure the amount of methemoglobin. One significant clinical sign of this adverse effect is impaired oxygen delivery despite adequate cardiac output. When the sequestration is diagnosed, the treatment of choice is 1 to 2 mg/kg of methylene blue given intravenously over several minutes to allow binding of the metabolic by-product of cyanide to methemoglobin as cyanmethemoglobin, but this must be given as ordered and with extreme caution.
		In addition, sodium nitroprusside may lead to toxic reactions, even with doses that are within recommended dosage ranges. Toxic reactions are evident by extreme hypotension, cyanide toxicity, or thiocyanate toxicity. Cyanide toxicity is manifested by severe hypotension. Cyanide assays are performed to detect if cyanide levels are in body fluids, but the results of this test are difficult to interpret and so it is not the most reliable method of monitoring. Other laboratory tests that may be helpful in diagnosing cyanide toxicity are alterations of acid–base balance and venous oxygen concentrations. Actual cyanide levels in the blood may lag behind peak cyanide levels by an hour or more.

CCBs and related nursing interventions are discussed only briefly here because these drugs are covered in other chapters. Drugs like enalapril are to be taken exactly as prescribed with the warning to the patient not to puncture, open, or crush the extended-release or sustained-release tablets and capsules. Be aware that CCBs are negative inotropic drugs (decrease cardiac contractility) because this action may induce more signs of heart failure if CCBs are given with drugs that are used to increase heart contractility, such as digoxin. Monitoring of blood pressure and pulse rate before and during therapy will aid in prevention or early detection of any problems related to the negative inotropic effects (decreased contractility), negative chronotropic effects (decreased heart rate), and negative dromotropic effects (decreased conduction).

Remember always to base nursing interventions on a thorough assessment and plan of care that includes consideration of the patient's cultural and ethnic group. This is particularly important with antihypertensives because research studies have documented differences in responses to antihypertensives among different racial and ethnic groups. Some ethnic groups respond less favourably to certain drugs than to others. As for patients with any disease, patients with hypertension must be treated with respect and with an appreciation for a holistic approach to health care in which all physical, psychosocial, and spiritual needs are taken into consideration. Remember also that patient education is of critical importance and plays an important role in ensuring adherence to the drug regimen and in decreasing the incidence of problems related to these medications.

Evaluation

Because patients with hypertension are at high risk for cardiovascular injury, it is critical for them to adhere to both their pharmacological and nonpharmacological treatment regimens. Monitoring patients for the adverse effects (e.g., orthostatic hypotension, dizziness, fatigue) and toxic effects of the various types of antihypertensive drugs helps the nurse to identify potentially life-threatening complications. The most important aspect of the evaluation process is collecting data and monitoring patients for evidence of controlled blood pressure. Blood pressure must be maintained at values lower than 140/90 mm Hg or below the levels set by the CHEP guidelines for high-normal hypertension (prehypertension), namely, below a systolic blood pressure of 120 to 139 mm Hg or a diastolic blood pressure of 80 to 89 mm Hg. If compelling indications are present, such as diabetes mellitus or kidney disease, the blood pressure goal is often 130/80. Blood pressure needs to be monitored at periodic intervals. Patient education about self-monitoring is important to the safe use of antihypertensives. Updated information on hypertension and its diagnosis, treatment, and evaluation is available on Hypertension Canada's website at https://www.hypertension.ca.

In addition to measuring blood pressure, the HCP will examine the fundus of the patient's eye. Because of the changes in the vasculature of the eye caused by high blood pressure, changes in the fundus have been found to be a more reliable indicator of the long-term effectiveness of treatment than blood pressure readings. Continually monitor the patient for the development of

CASE STUDY

Hypertension

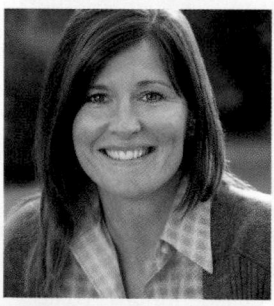

Gloria, a 45-year-old lawyer, has been diagnosed with hypertension. Both her mother and sister have hypertension, and both were also in their 40s when it was diagnosed. Gloria's most current blood pressure reading is 150/96 mm Hg, and for this reason the nurse practitioner has recommended drug therapy with captopril, light exercise in the form of walking, and relaxation therapy. After 1 month of therapy, Gloria's blood pressure is 145/86 mm Hg. Stress reduction has been the biggest obstacle in her treatment because of her work at a prominent law firm. She has found that her blood pressure is consistently elevated (160/100 mm Hg) whenever she measures it at work. At this follow-up visit, she is also given a prescription for a diuretic to help with her blood pressure control.

1. What type of diuretic was probably prescribed for Gloria at this time? Explain your answer.
2. What possible adverse effects does Gloria need to be aware of while taking captopril?
3. Gloria tells you that she uses an over-the-counter (OTC) pain reliever for occasional headaches. What potential interaction is of concern?
4. Gloria states that she and her husband are planning to start a family in 1 year. What will you, as her nurse, tell her about pregnancy and therapy with these drugs?
5. What lifestyle changes would you, as her nurse, recommend that she make, and, even more important, what information would you give her to help her change her lifestyle and more effectively reduce the stress in her life?

For answers, see http://evolve.elsevier.com/Canada/Lilley/pharmacology/.

end-organ damage and for the presence of the specific problems that the medication can cause. Counsel and carefully monitor male patients receiving antihypertensives for any sexual dysfunction. This is important because the patient may experience sexual dysfunction and, if he is not expecting it, may not report the problem and decide to stop taking the medication abruptly. Once an antihypertensive drug is stopped abruptly, the patient is the placed at high risk for rebound hypertension and possible stroke or other complications. Communication is critical in these situations. Follow-up visits to the HCP are important for monitoring these and other adverse effects and for confirming patient adherence to the drug regimen.

Therapeutic effects of antihypertensives in general include a return to a normal baseline level of blood pressure with improved energy levels and decreased signs and symptoms of hypertension, such as reduced edema, improved breath sounds, no abnormal heart sounds, capillary refill in less than 5 seconds, and reduced shortness of breath. Monitor for the adverse effects discussed in the pharmacology section of the chapter as well as those described for each group of drugs earlier in the Nursing Process section.

PATIENT TEACHING TIPS

Antihypertensives in General

- Patients should be informed that medications are to be taken exactly as ordered; doubling up or omitting doses is to be avoided.
- Stress to patients that successful therapy requires adherence to the medication regimen as well as to any dietary restrictions (e.g., decreasing consumption of fatty foods or high-cholesterol foods as well as dietary salt).
- Patients needs to monitor stress levels and use techniques such as biofeedback, imagery, relaxation techniques, or massage, as needed. Exercise, if approved by the HCP, may also help in the management of hypertension and serve to relieve stress; supervised, prescribed exercise is usually ordered.
- Educate patients about the importance of safety and the need to avoid smoking and excessive alcohol intake as well as excessive exercise, hot climates, saunas, hot tubs, and hot environments. Heat may precipitate vasodilation and lead to worsening of hypotension with the risk of syncope and injury to self.
- Frequent laboratory tests may be needed for the duration of therapy; emphasize to patients the importance of keeping follow-up appointments.
- All medications must be kept out of the reach of children because of the potential for extreme toxicity.
- Encourage patients to wear a medical alert bracelet or necklace and carry medical information, either in written or electronic form, specifying their diagnoses, noting allergies, and listing all medications taken (including prescribed drugs, OTC medications, and natural health products). The same information should be kept in a visible location in the patient's car and in the patient's home on the refrigerator for the use of emergency medical personnel.
- Emphasize to patients the importance of recording blood pressure readings (including orthostatic blood pressure readings) and daily weights in a journal or on an electronic device. Daily weights are to be done each morning, before breakfast, at the same time, and with the same amount of clothing. The patient must report to the HCP an increase in weight by 1 kg or more over a 24-hour period or 2.3 kg or more in 1 week.

- Assess patients' proficiency and comfort taking their own blood pressures and pulse rates. Monitor to ensure the use of proper techniques.
- Encourage patients to inform all HCPs about their antihypertensive regimens.
- Careful, purposeful, and cautious changing of positions is encouraged because of the possible adverse effect of orthostatic hypotension and associated risk for dizziness, lightheadedness, and possible fainting and falls.
- Instruct patients to always keep an adequate supply of hypertensive medications on hand, especially while travelling.
- Scheduling of periodic eye examinations is recommended every 6 months due to the need to evaluate treatment effectiveness because of the impact of hypertension on the vasculature of the eyes.
- With successful therapy, patients' hypertension will improve; however, patients must understand that they should never abruptly stop taking antihypertensive medications because they are feeling better. Lifelong therapy is usually required.
- Saliva substitutes, use of sugar-free hard candy or gum, and frequent fluid intake (unless contraindicated) may help with dry mouth. Increasing fluids and dietary fibre may help with constipation. Instruct patients to contact an HCP if constipation remains a problem.
- Sexual dysfunction may occur with antihypertensives, so encourage patients to be open in reporting and discussing any problems or concerns. Inform patients that if this adverse effect occurs, options are available to help alleviate the problem, such as combination therapy that allows lower dosages of drugs to be used, or the use of other types of antihypertensives. Always reinforce the fact that these medications are never to be abruptly stopped because of the risk of severe rebound hypertension.
- Inform patients that antihypertensives may lead to depression and to report any changes in mood to the HCP.

α-Adrenergic Agonists

- First-dose syncope is associated with α-adrenergic agonists, so patients need to avoid conditions, situations, and drugs that would exacerbate this.

Continued

PATIENT TEACHING TIPS—cont'd

❖ Caution patients to be careful at first with driving and other activities requiring alertness. Patients may have to postpone driving and other activities until drug-related drowsiness subsides.

❖ Instruct patients to report any dizziness, palpitations, and orthostatic hypotension to an HCP immediately.

❖ Because centrally acting α-blockers may also affect patients' sexual functioning (e.g., causing erectile dysfunction or reduced libido), inform patients of these adverse effects and advise them to contact an HCP if these effects are problematic. Other treatment options may be indicated.

β-Blockers

❖ Encourage patients to move and change positions slowly to avoid possible dizziness, syncope, and falls. Instruct patients to report a pulse rate of less than 60 beats per minute, dizziness, or a systolic blood pressure of 90 mm Hg or lower to the HCP.

❖ Prolonged sitting or standing and excessive physical exercise may also lead to exacerbation of hypotensive effects, so counsel the patient to avoid these activities or counteract them, such as by pumping the feet up and down while sitting.

❖ Heat may also exacerbate hypotensive effects of β-blockers. Educate patients to avoid saunas, hot tubs, and excessive heat, or syncope (fainting) may result.

KEY POINTS

❖ All antihypertensives in some way affect cardiac output. Cardiac output is the amount of blood ejected from the left ventricle and is measured in litres per minute.

❖ The major groups of antihypertensives are the diuretics (see Chapter 29), α-blockers, centrally active α-blockers, β-blockers, ACE inhibitors, vasodilators, CCBs, and ARBs. Direct renin inhibitors form a new class of antihypertensive drugs.

❖ ACE inhibitors work by blocking a critical enzyme system responsible for the production of angiotensin II (a potent vasoconstrictor). They prevent (1) vasoconstriction caused by angiotensin II, (2) aldosterone secretion and therefore sodium and water resorption, and (3) the breakdown of bradykinin (a potent vasodilator) by angiotensin II.

❖ Angiotensin receptor blockers work by blocking the binding of angiotensin at the receptors; the result is a decrease in blood pressure.

❖ CCBs may be used to treat angina, dysrhythmias, and hypertension and help to reduce blood pressure by causing relaxation of smooth muscles and dilation of blood vessels. If calcium is not present, the smooth muscle of the blood vessels cannot contract.

❖ A thorough nursing assessment includes determining whether a patient has any underlying causes of hypertension, such as kidney or liver dysfunction, a stressful lifestyle, Cushing's disease, Addison's disease, renal artery stenosis, peripheral vascular disease, or a pheochromocytoma.

❖ Always assess for the presence of contraindications, cautions, and potential drug interactions before administering any of the antihypertensive drugs. Contraindications include a history of myocardial infarction or chronic kidney disease. Cautious use is recommended in patients with kidney insufficiency or glaucoma. Drugs that interact with antihypertensive drugs include other antihypertensive drugs, anaesthetics, and diuretics.

❖ Hypertension is managed by both pharmacological and nonpharmacological measures. Patients with hypertension need to consume a diet low in fat, make any other necessary modifications in their diet (such as a decrease in sodium intake and an increase in fibre intake), engage in regular supervised exercise, and reduce the amount of stress in their lives.

EXAMINATION REVIEW QUESTIONS

1. A nurse is administering antihypertensive drugs to older adult patients. The nurse knows which adverse effect is of most concern for these patients?
  a. Dry mouth
  b. Hypotension
  c. Restlessness
  d. Constipation

2. When giving antihypertensive drugs, the nurse will consider giving the first dose at bedtime for which class of drugs?
  a. α-blockers such as prazosin (Minipress)
  b. Diuretics such as furosemide (Lasix®)
  c. ACE inhibitors such as captopril (Capoten)
  d. Vasodilators such as hydralazine (Apresoline)

EXAMINATION REVIEW QUESTIONS—cont'd

3. A 56-year-old man started antihypertensive drug therapy 3 months ago and is in the office for a follow-up visit. While the nurse is taking his blood pressure, he informs the nurse that he is having some problems with sexual intercourse. What would be the most appropriate response by the nurse?
a. "Not to worry. Tolerance will develop."
b. "Your health care provider can work with you on changing the dosage or drugs."
c. "Sexual dysfunction happens with this therapy, and you will learn to accept it."
d. "This is an unusual occurrence, but it is important to stay on your medications."

4. When a patient is being taught about the potential adverse effects of an ACE inhibitor, which of these effects should the nurse mention as possibly occurring when this drug is taken to treat hypertension?
a. Diarrhea
b. Nausea
c. Dry, nonproductive cough
d. Sedation

5. A patient has a new prescription for an ACE inhibitor. During a review of the patient's list of current medications, which would cause concern about a possible interaction with this new prescription? (Select all that apply.)
a. A benzodiazepine taken as needed for allergies
b. A potassium supplement taken daily
c. An oral anticoagulant taken daily
d. An opioid used for occasional severe pain
e. A nonsteroidal anti-inflammatory drug taken as needed for headaches

6. The order reads: Give hydralazine (Apresoline) 0.75 mg/kg/day. The child weighs 16 pounds. How much hydralazine will be given? Round to hundredths.

Answers: 1. b, **2.** a, **3.** b, **4.** c, **5.** b, e, **6.** 5.45 mg/kg/day

CRITICAL THINKING ACTIVITIES

1. A 53-year-old woman with a history of hypothyroidism and asthma has been diagnosed with primary hypertension. The nurse is reviewing the new orders and notes an order for labetalol (Trandate) as part of the treatment for hypertension. Considering the patient's history, what is the priority action at this time?

2. A 79-year-old woman has been admitted to the emergency department after experiencing severe headaches and "feeling faint." Upon admission, her blood pressure is measured as 286/190 mm Hg. A sodium nitroprusside infusion is started, and the nurse is monitoring the patient closely. After 8 minutes of infusion, the nurse notes that the patient's blood pressure suddenly drops to 100/60. What is the nurse's priority action?

3. During a follow-up appointment, a 58-year-old man is pleased to hear that his blood pressure is 118/64 mm Hg. He says, "I've been hoping to hear this good news! Now I can stop taking these pills, right?" What is the nurse's best answer?

For answers, see http://evolve.elsevier.com/Canada/Lilley/pharmacology/.

CHAPTER 24

Antianginal Drugs

Objectives

After reading this chapter, the successful student will be able to do the following:

1. Briefly describe the pathophysiology of myocardial ischemia and the subsequent occurrence of angina.

2. Describe the various factors that may precipitate angina as well as measures that decrease its occurrence.

3. Contrast the major classes of antianginal drugs (nitrates, calcium channel blockers, and β-blockers) according to their mechanisms of action, dosage forms, routes of administration, cautions, contraindications, drug interactions, adverse effects, patient tolerance, and toxicity.

4. Develop a collaborative plan of care incorporating all phases of the nursing process related to the administration of antianginal drugs.

e-Learning Activities

Website
(http://evolve.elsevier.com/Canada/Lilley/pharmacology/)

evolve

- Answer Key—Textbook Case Studies
- Answer Key—Critical Thinking Activities
- Chapter Summaries—Printable
- Review Questions for Exam Preparation
- Unfolding Case Studies

Drug Profiles

amlodipine (amlodipine besylate)*, p. 468
➤➤ atenolol, p. 467
➤➤ diltiazem (diltiazem hydrochloride)*, p. 468
➤➤ isosorbide (isosorbide dinitrate)*, p. 464
➤➤ isosorbide mononitrate, p. 465
➤➤ metoprolol (metoprolol tartrate)*, p. 467
➤➤ nitroglycerin, p. 464

➤➤ Key drug

*Full generic name is given in parentheses. For the purposes of this text, the more common, shortened name is used.

Key Terms

Acute coronary syndrome (ACS) A spectrum of clinical presentations compatible with acute myocardial ischemia, ranging from those for ST-segment elevation myocardial infarction (STEMI) to presentations found in non–ST-segment elevation myocardial infarction (NSTEMI) or in unstable angina. (p. 461)

Angina pectoris Chest pain that occurs when the heart's supply of blood carrying oxygen is insufficient to meet the demands of the heart. (p. 461)

Atherosclerosis A common form of arteriosclerosis involving deposits of fatty, cholesterol-containing material (plaques) within arterial walls. (p. 461)

Chronic stable angina Chest pain that is primarily caused by atherosclerosis, which results in long-term but relatively stable levels of obstruction in one or more coronary arteries. (p. 461)

Coronary arteries Arteries that deliver oxygen-carrying blood to the heart muscle. (p. 461)

Coronary artery disease (CAD) Any one of the abnormal conditions that can affect the arteries of the heart and produce pathological effects, especially a reduced supply of oxygen and nutrients to the myocardium. (p. 461)

Ischemia Poor blood supply to an organ. (p. 461)

Ischemic heart disease Poor blood supply to the heart via the coronary arteries. (p. 461)

Myocardial infarction (MI) Necrosis of the myocardium following interruption of blood supply; almost always caused by atherosclerosis of the coronary arteries. Commonly called a *heart attack*. (p. 461)

Reflex tachycardia A rapid heartbeat caused by a variety of autonomic nervous system effects, such as blood pressure changes, fever, or emotional stress. (p. 463)

Unstable angina Clinical presentation of acute coronary syndrome with cardiac ischemia, without persistent ST-segment elevation on electrocardiogram and no detectable release of the enzymes and biomarkers of myocardial necrosis. (p. 461)

Vasospastic angina Ischemia-induced myocardial chest pain caused by spasms of the coronary arteries; also referred to as *Prinzmetal's* or *variant angina*. (p. 461)

OVERVIEW

The heart is an efficient organ that pumps blood to all the tissues and organs of the body. It is demanding in an aerobic sense because it requires a large supply of oxygen to meet the extraordinary demands placed on it. The heart's much-needed oxygen supply is delivered to the myocardium through the **coronary arteries**. When the heart's supply of blood carrying oxygen and energy-rich nutrients is insufficient to meet the demands of the heart, the heart muscle (or myocardium) aches. This is called **angina pectoris**, or chest pain. Poor blood supply to an organ is referred to as **ischemia**. When the heart is involved, the condition is called **ischemic heart disease**.

Ischemic heart disease is currently the second most prevalent cause of death in Canada. The primary cause is a disease of the coronary arteries known as **atherosclerosis** (fatty plaque deposits in the arterial walls). When atherosclerotic plaques project from the walls into the lumens of the coronary vessels, they become narrow. The supply of oxygen and energy-rich nutrients needed for the heart to meet its demand is then decreased. This disorder is called **coronary artery disease (CAD)**. An acute result of CAD and of ischemic heart disease is **myocardial infarction (MI)**, or heart attack. An MI occurs when blood flow through the coronary arteries to the myocardium is completely blocked so that part of the myocardium (heart muscle) cannot receive any oxygen or blood-borne nutrients. It is almost always associated with rupture of an atherosclerotic plaque and partial or complete thrombosis of the infarct-related artery. If this process is not reversed immediately, that area of the heart will die and become necrotic (dead or nonfunctioning). Damage to a large enough area of the myocardium can be disabling or fatal.

The rate at which the heart pumps and the strength of each heartbeat (contractility) influence oxygen demands on the heart. There are numerous influences that can increase heart rate and contractility and thus increase oxygen demand. These include caffeine, exercise, and stress, among others, and result in stimulation of the sympathetic nervous system, which leads to increased heart rate and contractility. In a patient with CAD who has an already overburdened heart, this stimulation can worsen the balance between myocardial oxygen supply and demand and result in angina. Some of the drugs used to treat angina are aimed at correcting the imbalance between myocardial oxygen supply and demand by decreasing heart rate and contractility.

The pain of angina is a result of the following process. Under ischemic conditions, when the myocardium is deprived of oxygen, the heart shifts to anaerobic metabolism to meet its energy needs. One of the by-products of anaerobic metabolism is lactic acid. Accumulation of lactic acid and other mediators, such as bradykinin and adenosine, stimulate the pain receptors surrounding the heart, which produces the heart pain known as *angina*. This is the same pathophysiological mechanism responsible for causing the soreness in skeletal muscles after vigorous exercise. The Canadian Cardiovascular Society classifies exertion-induced angina to allow for the gauging of symptom severity according to the amount of physical activity (grade I to grade IV) that patients can tolerate before pain occurs (Christensen, 2014). There are three classic types of chest pain, or angina pectoris. **Chronic stable angina**, also referred to as *classic angina* and *effort angina*, occurs as a result of atherosclerosis. Chronic stable angina can be triggered by either exertion or other stress (e.g., cold, emotions). The nicotine in tobacco, as well as alcohol, caffeine, and other substances that stimulate the sympathetic nervous system, can also exacerbate angina. The pain of chronic stable angina is commonly intense but subsides within 15 minutes of either rest or appropriate antianginal drug therapy. **Unstable angina** is the most dangerous, as it is the clinical presentation of **acute coronary syndrome (ACS)** with cardiac ischemia without persistent ST-segment elevation on electrocardiogram (ECG) and no detectable release of the enzymes and biomarkers of myocardial necrosis. It often ends in an MI (ST elevation or STEMI) in subsequent years. For this reason, unstable angina is also called *preinfarction angina*. Unstable angina does not follow any predictable pattern and can occur without exertion. Pain increases in severity, as does the frequency of attacks. Unstable angina usually is diagnosed when it meets one or more of the following criteria: (1) angina at rest; (2) recent onset (less than 2 months) of severe angina; and (3) recent (less than 2 months) increase in severity of angina (increased intensity as well as duration, frequency, or both). **Vasospastic angina** results from spasm of the layer of smooth muscle that surrounds the atherosclerotic coronary arteries. In contrast to chronic stable angina, this type of pain often occurs at rest and without any precipitating cause. It does seem to follow a regular pattern, however, usually occurring at the same time of day. This type of angina is also called *Prinzmetal's angina* or *variant angina*. Dysrhythmias and ECG changes often accompany these different types of anginal attacks.

ANTIANGINAL DRUGS

The three main classes of drugs used to treat angina pectoris are the nitrates and nitrites, the β- blockers, and the calcium channel blockers (CCBs). Their various therapeutic effects are summarized and compared in Table 24-1. There are three main therapeutic objectives of antianginal drug therapy: (1) minimize the frequency of attacks and decrease the duration and intensity of the angina pain; (2) improve the patient's functional capacity with as few adverse effects as possible; and (3) prevent or delay the worst possible outcome—MI. The overall goals of antianginal drug therapy are to increase blood flow to the ischemic myocardium, decrease myocardial oxygen demand, or both. Figure 24-1 illustrates how drug therapy works to alleviate angina. Existing evidence suggests that drug therapy may be at least as effective as angioplasty in treating this condition.

NITRATES

Nitrates have long been the mainstay of both the prophylaxis and treatment for angina and other heart problems. Today, there are several chemical derivatives of the early precursors, all of which are organic nitrate esters. They are available in a wide variety of preparations, including sublingual, chewable, and oral tablets; capsules; ointments; patches; a translingual spray; and intravenous solutions. The following nitrates are the rapid- and long-acting nitrates available for clinical use:

- nitroglycerin (both rapid and long acting)
- isosorbide (both rapid and long acting)
- isosorbide-5-mononitrate (long acting)

Mechanism of Action and Drug Effects

The nitrates dilate all blood vessels. They predominantly affect venous vascular beds; however, they also have a dose-dependent arterial vasodilator effect. These

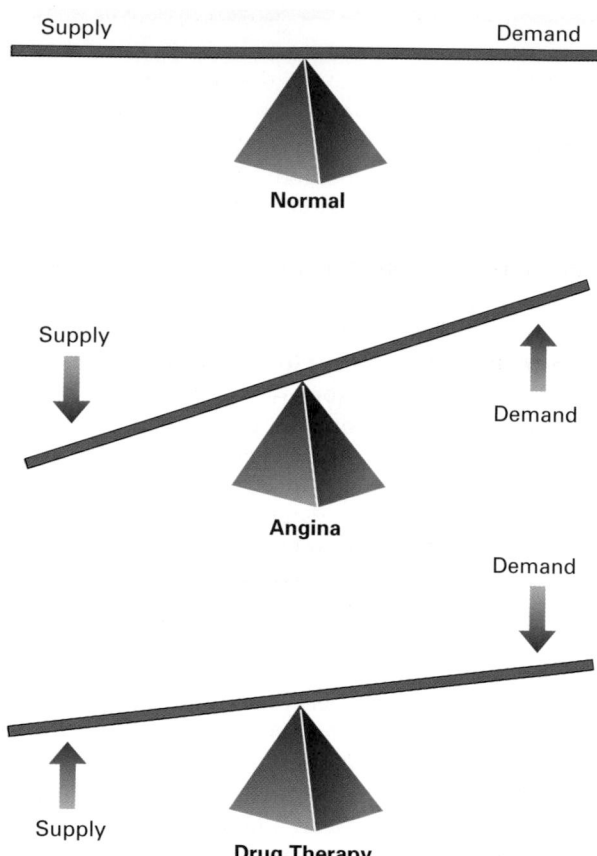

FIG. 24-1 Benefit of drug therapy for angina through increasing oxygen supply and decreasing oxygen demands.

TABLE	24-1

Antianginal Drugs: Therapeutic Effects

Therapeutic Effect	Nitrates	β-Blockers*	Amlodipine Besylate	Verapamil	Diltiazem
SUPPLY					
Blood flow	↑↑	↑	↑↑↑	↑↑↑	↑↑↑
Duration of diastole	0	↑↑↑	0/↑	↑↑↑	↑↑
DEMAND					
Preload†	↓↓	↑	↓/0	0	0/↓
Afterload	↓	0/↓	↓↓↓	↓↓	↓↓
Contractility	0	↓↓↓↓	↓	↓↓↓	↓↓
Heart rate	0/↑	↓↓↓	0/↓	↓↓	↓↓

*In particular, those that are cardioselective and do not have intrinsic sympathomimetic activity.

↓, Decrease; ↑, increase; 0, little or no effect.

†*Preload* is pressure in the heart caused by blood volume. The nitrates effectively move part of this blood out of the heart and into blood vessels, thereby decreasing preload or filling pressure.

vasodilatory effects are the result of relaxation of the vascular smooth muscle cells that are part of the wall structure of veins and arteries. Particularly notable, however, is the potent dilating effect of nitrates on the coronary arteries, both large and small. This effect causes redistribution of blood and therefore oxygen to previously ischemic myocardial tissue and a reduction of anginal symptoms. By causing venous dilation, the nitrates reduce venous return and, in turn, reduce the left ventricular end-diastolic volume (or preload). The reduced afterload (pressure that the left ventricle needs to overcome) that nitrates produce is due to its dose-dependent relaxation of arteries in addition to its decreased left ventricular tension; this effect is less than the dilation effects. The drug effects of the nitrate drugs listed above and others are summarized in Table 24-1.

Coronary arteries that have been narrowed by atherosclerosis can still be dilated as long as there remains smooth muscle surrounding the coronary artery and the atherosclerotic plaque does not completely obstruct the arterial lumen. Exercise-induced spasms in atherosclerotic coronary arteries can also be reversed or prevented by the administration of nitrates, which encourages healthy physical activity.

Indications

Nitrates are used to treat stable, unstable, and vasospastic angina. Long-acting dosage forms are used more for prevention of anginal episodes. Rapid-acting dosage forms, most often sublingual nitroglycerin tablets or spray, or an intravenous drip in the hospital setting, are used to treat acute anginal attacks.

Contraindications

Contraindications to the use of nitrates include known drug allergy as well as severe anemia, closed-angle glaucoma, hypotension, and severe head injury—the vasodilation effects of nitrates can worsen these conditions. In anemia, a drug-induced hypotensive episode can further compromise already reduced tissue oxygenation. Nitrates are also contraindicated with the use of the erectile dysfunction drugs sildenafil citrate (Revatio®, Viagra®), tadalafil (Adcirca®, Cialis®), and vardenafil hydrochloride (Levitra®, Staxyn®; see Chapter 36).

Adverse Effects

Nitrates are well tolerated, and most adverse effects are usually transient and involve the cardiovascular system. The most common undesirable effect is headaches, which generally diminish in intensity and frequency soon after the start of therapy. Other cardiovascular effects include tachycardia and orthostatic hypotension. If nitrate-induced vasodilation occurs too rapidly, the cardiovascular system overcompensates and increases the heart rate, a condition referred to as **reflex tachycardia**. This may occur when significant vasodilation involves the systemic veins. In this situation, there is a large shift in blood volume toward the systemic venous circulation and

away from the heart. Pressor sensors (baroreceptors) in the carotid sinus and aortic arch falsely sense that there has been a dramatic loss of blood volume. At this point, the heart begins beating more rapidly to move the apparently smaller volume of blood more quickly throughout the body, especially toward the vital organs (including the heart itself). However, the same baroreceptors soon sense that there has not been a loss of blood volume but that the volume of blood missing in the heart is now in the periphery (e.g., in the venous system), and the heart rate slows back to normal.

Topical nitrate dosage forms can produce various types of contact dermatitis (skin inflammations), but these are actually reactions to the dosage delivery system and not to the nitroglycerin contained within it, thus not a true drug allergy. It is important for the nurse to document the type of allergic reaction, so that clinicians do not avoid this important drug class if the reaction is only a contact dermatitis.

Tolerance to the antianginal effects of nitrates can occur surprisingly quickly in some patients, especially in those taking long-acting formulations or taking nitrates around the clock. In addition, cross-tolerance can arise when a patient receives more than one nitrate dosage form. To prevent this, a regular nitrate-free period (usually for 12 hours [e.g., on at 0800 hours and off at 2000 hours]) is arranged to allow certain enzymatic pathways to replenish themselves. A common regimen with transdermal patches is to remove them at night for 8 hours and apply a new patch in the morning. This has been shown to prevent tolerance to the beneficial effects of nitrates. However, some studies have questioned the advisability of this practice.

Interactions

Nitrate antianginal drugs can produce additive hypotensive effects when taken in combination with alcohol, β-blockers, CCBs, phenothiazines, and erectile dysfunction drugs such as sildenafil citrate, tadalafil, and vardenafil hydrochloride. Numerous deaths have been reported due to interactions with erectile dysfunction drugs.

Dosages

The organic nitrates are available in an array of forms and dosages. For more dosage information, refer to the table on p. 464.

β-BLOCKERS

The β-adrenergic blockers, more commonly referred to as β-blockers, have become the mainstay in the treatment of several cardiovascular diseases. These include angina, MI, hypertension (Chapter 23), and dysrhythmias (see Chapter 26). Most available β-blockers demonstrate antianginal efficacy, although not all have been approved for this use. Those β-blockers approved as antianginal drugs are atenolol, metoprolol, nadolol, and propranolol hydrochloride (see also Chapter 20).

DRUG PROFILES

▶▶isosorbide dinitrate

Isosorbide dinitrate (ISDN®) is an organic nitrate. It exerts the same effects as the other nitrates. When isosorbide is metabolized in the liver, it is broken down into two active metabolites, both of which have the same therapeutic actions as isosorbide. Isosorbide is available as rapid-acting sublingual tablets and long-acting oral dosage forms.

PHARMACOKINETICS

Route	Onset of Action	Peak Plasma Concentration	Elimination Half-Life	Duration of Action
PO	30 min	Unknown	3–5 hr	4–6 hr

▶▶isosorbide-5-mononitrate

Isosorbide-5-mononitrate (Imdur®) is one of the two active metabolites of isosorbide, but it has no active metabolites itself. Because of these qualities, it produces a more consistent, steady therapeutic response, with less variation in response within the same patient and between patients. It is available in extended-release oral dosage form.

PHARMACOKINETICS

Route	Onset of Action	Peak Plasma Concentration	Elimination Half-Life	Duration of Action
PO (extended-release)	Gradual release over 10 hr	4 hr	5 hr	5–12 hr

▶▶nitroglycerin

Nitroglycerin is the prototypical nitrate and is made by many pharmaceutical companies; therefore, it has many different trade names (e.g., Minitran®, Nitro-Dur®, Nitrol®, Trinipatch®). It has traditionally been the most important drug used in the symptomatic treatment of ischemic heart conditions such as angina. When given orally, nitroglycerin is metabolized in the liver before it can become active in the body. During this process, a large amount of the nitroglycerin is removed from the circulation (a large first-pass effect [see Chapter 2]). For this reason, nitroglycerin is administered by many other routes to bypass the first-pass effect. Sublingual tablets or pump sprays are used for the treatment of chest pain or angina of acute onset. They are also used for the prevention of angina when patients find themselves in situations likely to provoke an attack. Use of the sublingual route is advantageous for relieving acute conditions because the area under the tongue and inside the cheek is highly vascular; the nitroglycerin is absorbed quickly and directly into the bloodstream, with its therapeutic effects occurring rapidly. Sublingual nitroglycerin tablets must be stored in their original container because exposure to air and moisture can inactivate the drug.

Nitroglycerin is also available as a metered-dose pump that is sprayed under the tongue. It is available in an intravenous form that is used perioperatively for blood pressure control in hypertensive patients; for the treatment of ischemic pain, heart failure, and pulmonary edema associated with acute MI; and in hypertensive emergency situations. Oral and topical dosage formulations are used for the long-term prophylactic management of angina pectoris. The topical formulations offer the same advantages as the sublingual formulation in that they also bypass the liver and the first-pass effect. This formulation also allows for the continuous slow delivery of the drug, so that a steady dose of nitroglycerin is supplied to the patient.

PHARMACOKINETICS

Route	Onset of Action	Peak Plasma Concentration	Elimination Half-Life	Duration of Action
Sublingual	2–3 min	Unknown	1–4 min	0.5–1 hr

DOSAGES	**Selected Antianginal Nitrate Coronary Vasodilators**	
Drug	**Usual Dosage Range**	**Indications**
▶▶isosorbide dinitrate (ISDN)	*Adults* PO: 5–30 mg qid	Angina
▶▶isosorbide-5-mononitrate (Imdur)	*Adults* PO (ER): 30–120 mg/day	
▶▶nitroglycerin (Minitran, Nitro-Dur, Nitrol, Nitrostat, Trinipatch)	*Adults* IV (continuous infusion): 5–20 mcg q3–5 min Ointment, 2%: 2.5–5 cm (up to 10–12.5 cm) ribbon q3–8h Spray: 0.4–0.8 mg (1–2 sprays) onto or under the tongue, repeated twice, prn SL: 0.3–0.6 mg q5 min, 3 times Patch: 0.2–0.8 mg applied once daily	Angina

IV, intravenous; *PO*, oral; *SL*, sublingual; *ER*, extended-release; *prn*, as needed.

Mechanism of Action and Drug Effects

The primary effects of β-blockers are related to the cardiovascular system. As discussed in Chapters 19 and 20, the predominant β-adrenergic receptors in the heart are the $β_1$-adrenergic receptors. $β_1$-receptors are located in the heart's conduction system and throughout the myocardium. The $β_1$-receptors are normally stimulated by the binding of the neurotransmitters epinephrine and norepinephrine. These catecholamines are released in greater quantities during times of exercise or other stress to stimulate the heart muscle to contract more strongly. At the normal heart rate of 60 to 100 beats per minute, the heart spends 60 to 70% of its time in diastole. As the heart rate increases during stress or exercise, the heart spends more time in systole and less time in diastole.

In an ischemic heart, the increased oxygen demand from increasing contractility (systole) also leads to increasing degrees of ischemia and chest pain. The physiological act of systole requires energy in the form of adenosine triphosphate (ATP) and oxygen. Therefore, any decrease in the energy demands on the heart is beneficial for alleviating conditions such as angina. When β-receptors are blocked by β-blockers, the rate at which the pacemaker (sinoatrial [SA] node) fires decreases, and the time it takes for the node to recover increases.

β-blockers also slow conduction through the atrioventricular (AV) node and reduce myocardial contractility (negative inotropic effect). Both of these effects serve to slow the heart rate (negative chronotropic effect). These effects reduce myocardial oxygen demand, which aids in the treatment of angina by reducing the workload of the heart. Slowing the heart rate is also beneficial in patients with ischemic heart disease because the coronary arteries have more diastolic time to fill with oxygen- and nutrient-rich blood and deliver these substances to the myocardial tissues.

β-blockers also have many therapeutic effects after an MI. Following an MI, there is a high level of circulating catecholamines (norepinephrine and epinephrine). These catecholamines will produce harmful consequences if their actions go unopposed. They cause the heart rate to increase, which leads to a further imbalance in the supply-and-demand ratio, and they irritate the conduction system of the heart, which can result in potentially fatal dysrhythmias. β-blockers block all of these harmful effects, and their use has been shown to improve the chances for survival after an MI. Unless strongly contraindicated, they are given to all patients in the acute stages after an MI.

β-blockers also suppress the activity of the hormone renin, which is the first step in the renin–aldosterone–angiotensin system. Renin is a potent vasoconstrictor released by the kidneys when they are not being adequately perfused. When β-blockers inhibit the release of renin, blood vessels to and in the kidney dilate, causing reduced blood pressure (see Chapter 23).

Indications

β-blockers are most effective in the treatment of exertional angina. This is because the usual physiological effects of an increase in heart rate and systolic blood pressure that occurs during exercise or stress is blunted by β-blockers, thereby decreasing the myocardial oxygen demand. For individuals (often older adults) with significant angina, "exercise" may simply be carrying out activities of daily living such as bathing, dressing, cooking, or housekeeping. Performing such activities with significant angina can become a major stressor for these patients. β-blockers are also approved for the treatment of MI, hypertension (see Chapter 23), cardiac dysrhythmias (see Chapter 26), and essential tremor. Some uses that are common but are not Health Canada–approved are treatment of migraine headaches and, in low dosages, even treatment of the tachycardia associated with stage fright.

Contraindications

There are a number of contraindications to the use of β-blockers, including acute stage of decompensated heart failure and serious conduction disturbances because of the effects of β-blockade on heart rate and myocardial contractility. These drugs should be used with caution in patients with bronchial asthma because any level of blockade of $β_2$-receptors can promote bronchoconstriction. These contraindications are relative rather than absolute and depend on patient-specific risks and expected benefits of this drug therapy. Other relative contraindications include diabetes mellitus (because of masking of hypoglycemia-induced tachycardia) and peripheral vascular disease (the drug may further compromise cerebral or peripheral blood flow).

Adverse Effects

The adverse effects of β-blockers result from their ability to block β-adrenergic receptors ($β_1$- and $β_2$-receptors) in various areas of the body. Blocking of $β_1$-receptors can lead to a decrease in heart rate, cardiac output, and cardiac contractility. Blocking of $β_2$-receptors can result in bronchoconstriction and increased airway resistance in patients with asthma or chronic obstructive pulmonary disease. β-blockers may lead to cardiac rhythm problems, decreased SA and AV nodal conduction, decrease in systolic and diastolic blood pressures, peripheral receptor blockade, and decreased renin release from the kidneys. β-blockers can mask the tachycardia associated with hypoglycemia, and patients with diabetes may not be able to tell when their blood sugar falls too low. Fatigue, insomnia, and weakness may occur because of negative effects on the heart and the central nervous system. β-blockers can also cause both hypoglycemia and hyperglycemia, which is of particular concern in patients with diabetes. Other common β-blocker–related adverse effects are listed in Table 24-2.

Interactions

There are many important drug interactions that involve β-blockers. The more common and important of these interactions are listed in Table 24-3.

Dosages

For information on the dosages of selected β-blockers, refer to the table on p. 467.

CALCIUM CHANNEL BLOCKERS

There are three chemical classes of CCBs: phenylalkylamines, benzothiazepines, and dihydropyridines, commonly represented by verapamil hydrochloride, diltiazem, and amlodipine, respectively (Table 24-4).

Although they all block calcium channels, their chemical structures and, thus, mechanisms of action differ slightly. Many CCBs are available. Those used for the treatment of chronic stable angina are diltiazem, amlodipine, nifedipine, and verapamil hydrochloride.

Mechanism of Action and Drug Effects

Calcium plays an important role in the excitation–contraction coupling process that occurs in the heart and vascular smooth muscle cells, as well as in skeletal muscle. Preventing calcium from entering into this process thus prevents muscle contraction and promotes relaxation. Relaxation of the smooth muscles that surround the coronary arteries causes them to dilate. This dilation increases blood flow to the ischemic heart, which in turn increases the oxygen supply and helps shift the supply-and-demand ratio back to normal. Dilation also occurs in the arteries throughout the body, which results in a decrease in the force (systemic vascular resistance) against which the heart has to exert when delivering blood to the body (afterload). Decreasing the afterload reduces the workload of the heart and therefore reduces myocardial oxygen demand. This is the primary beneficial antianginal effect of the dihydropyridine CCBs, such as amlodipine and nifedipine. These drugs have a less negative inotropic effect than verapamil hydrochloride and diltiazem do.

Another cardiovascular effect of the CCBs is depression of the automaticity of and conduction through the sinoatrial (SA) and atrioventricular (AV) nodes. For this reason, they are useful in treating cardiac dysrhythmias

TABLE 24-2

β-Blockers: Adverse Effects

Body System	Adverse Effects
Cardiovascular	Bradycardia, hypotension, atrioventricular block
Central nervous	Dizziness, fatigue, depression, lethargy
Metabolic	Hyperglycemia and hypoglycemia, hyperlipidemia
Other	Wheezing, dyspnea, erectile dysfunction

TABLE 24-3

β-Blockers: Common Drug Interactions

Interacting Drug	Mechanism	Result
Diuretics and antihypertensives	Additive effects	Hypotension
Calcium channel blockers (diltiazem hydrochloride, verapamil hydrochloride)	Additive atrioventricular node suppression	Hypotension, bradycardia, heart block
Insulin and oral antihyperglycemic drugs	Masking of hypoglycemic effects	Unrecognized hypoglycemia

TABLE 24-4

Classification of Calcium Channel Blockers

Generic Name	Trade Name	Available Routes
BENZOTHIAZEPINES		
diltiazem hydrochloride	Cardizem®, Tiazac®, others	PO/IV
DIHYDROPYRIDINES		
amlodipine besylate	Caduet®, Norvasc®, Twynsta®, others	PO
felodipine	Plendil®, Renedil®	PO
nifedipine	Adalat XL®	PO
nimodipine	Nimotop®	PO
PHENYLALKYLAMINES		
verapamil hydrochloride	Isoptin SR®, Tarka®, Verelan®	PO/IV

IV, intravenous; *PO,* oral, *SR,* sustained release.

DRUG PROFILES

β-blockers are a mainstay in the treatment of a wide range of cardiovascular diseases, primarily hypertension, angina, and the acute stages and postmanagement of MI. The three most commonly used β-blockers are carvedilol, metoprolol, and atenolol. Carvedilol is not indicated for angina, but is instead indicated for heart failure, essential hypertension, and left ventricular dysfunction. The newest β-blocker, nebivolol hydrochloride (Bystolic®), is used to treat hypertension. As indicated, atenolol, metoprolol, nadolol, and propranolol hydrochloride all are indicated for angina. The drug profile for carvedilol appears in Chapter 20 on p. 399.

▶▶ atenolol

Atenolol (Tenorim®) is a cardioselective β₁-adrenergic receptor blocker and is indicated for the prophylactic treatment of angina pectoris. Use of atenolol after an MI has been shown to decrease mortality. It is available in oral form.

PHARMACOKINETICS

Route	Onset of Action	Peak Plasma Concentration	Elimination Half-Life	Duration of Action
PO	1 hr	2–4 hr	6–7 hr	24 hr

▶▶ metoprolol tartrate

Metoprolol tartrate (Betaloc®, Lopresor®, Lopresor SR®) is also a cardioselective β₁-adrenergic receptor blocker that is used for the prophylactic treatment of angina and has many of the same characteristics as atenolol. It has shown similar efficacy in reducing mortality in patients after MI and in treating angina. It is available in both oral (immediate-release and long-acting) and parenteral forms. Intravenous metoprolol is commonly administered to hospitalized patients after an MI and is used for treatment of hypertension in patients unable to take oral medicine.

PHARMACOKINETICS

Route	Onset of Action	Peak Plasma Concentration	Elimination Half-Life	Duration of Action
PO	1 hr	2–4 hr	3–8 hr	10–20 hr

DOSAGES   Selected β₁-Adrenergic Drugs

Drug	Pharmacological Class	Usual Dosage Range	Indications
▶▶ atenolol (Tenorim)	β₁-blocker	*Adults* PO: 50–200 mg/day as a single dose	Angina
▶▶ metoprolol tartrate (Lopresor, Lopresor SR)	β₁-blocker	*Adults* PO: 100–400 mg/day divided bid SR: 100–200 mg taken in the morning	Angina

PO, oral; *SR*, sustained release.

(Chapter 23). Finally, the CCBs reduce myocardial contractility and peripheral and coronary artery tone. Verapamil and diltiazem also decrease heart rate. Their strongest antianginal properties are secondary to their effects on myocardial contractility and the smooth muscle tone of peripheral and coronary arteries.

Indications

The therapeutic benefits of the CCBs are numerous. Because of their acceptable adverse effect and safety profiles, they are considered first-line drugs for the treatment of angina, hypertension, and supraventricular tachycardia. They are often effective for the treatment of coronary artery spasms (vasospastic or Prinzmetal's angina). However, they may not be as effective as the β-blockers in blunting exercise-induced elevations in heart rate and blood pressure. CCBs are also used for the short-term management of atrial fibrillation and flutter (see Chapter 26), migraine headaches (see Chapter 14), and Raynaud's disease (a type of peripheral vascular disease). The dihydropyridine nimodipine is indicated solely as an adjunct for cerebral artery spasms associated with aneurysm rupture.

Contraindications

Contraindications include known drug allergy, acute MI, second- or third-degree AV block (unless the patient has a pacemaker), and hypotension.

Adverse Effects

The adverse effects of the CCBs are limited and primarily relate to overexpression of their therapeutic effects. The most common adverse effects are listed in Table 24-5.

Interactions

Important drug interactions are listed in Table 24-6. A particular food interaction of note is grapefruit juice, which can increase the bioavailability of CCBs, especially nifedipine. Nifedipine is metabolized by the cytochrome P450 enzyme system, and compounds found in grapefruit juice inhibit the P450 system; hence, the intake of grapefruit juice increases plasma levels of nifedipine and augments its pharmacodynamic effects.

TABLE 24-5

Calcium Channel Blockers: Adverse Effects

Body System	Adverse Effects
Cardiovascular	Hypotension, palpitations, tachycardia or bradycardia
Gastrointestinal	Constipation, nausea
Other	Dermatitis, dyspnea, rash, flushing, peripheral edema

Dosages

For dosage information on selected CCBs, refer to the table on p. 469.

SUMMARY OF ANTIANGINAL PHARMACOLOGY

In patients with CAD, the clinical symptoms result from a lack of or inadequate delivery of blood carrying oxygen and nutrients to the heart, which results in ischemic heart disease. Antianginal drugs such as nitrates, β-blockers, and CCBs are used to reduce ischemia by increasing the delivery of oxygen- and nutrient-rich blood to cardiac tissues or by reducing oxygen consumption by the coronary vessels. Either of these mechanisms can reduce ischemia and lead to a decrease in anginal pain. Nitrates and nitrites work primarily by decreasing venous return

TABLE 24-6

Calcium Channel Blockers: Common Drug Interactions

Drug	Mechanism	Result
β-blockers	Additive effects	Bradycardia and atrioventricular block
digoxin	Interference with elimination	Possible increased digoxin levels
amiodarone hydrochloride	Decreased metabolism	Bradycardia and decreased cardiac output
Azole antifungals, clarithromycin, erythromycin, HIV drugs	Decreased metabolism	Elevated levels and effects of CCBs
Statins	Inhibited statin metabolism	Increased risk of statin toxicity
cyclosporine	Decreased metabolism of either drug	Possible toxicity of either drug

CCBs, calcium channel blockers; *HIV*, human immunodeficiency virus.

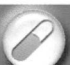 ## DRUG PROFILES

▶▶ diltiazem hydrochloride

Diltiazem hydrochloride (Cardizem, Tiazac) is the only benzothiazepine CCB. It has a particular affinity for the cardiac conduction system and is effective for the treatment of angina pectoris resulting from coronary insufficiency and hypertension. It is one of the few CCBs that is available in parenteral form, in which it is used for the treatment of atrial fibrillation and flutter along with paroxysmal supraventricular tachycardia (see Chapter 26). Verapamil hydrochloride is another CCB with similar indications. Several sustained-delivery formulations of diltiazem are available, which can be confused with each other. For example, there is Apo-diltiaz®, an immediate-release tablet; Apo-diltiaz SR®, sustained-release capsules that are taken twice a day; and Apo-diltiaz CD®, a controlled-delivery capsule taken once a day. In addition to other brands of these dosage forms, the drug is also available in several strengths of immediate-release tablets as well as in intravenous form.

PHARMACOKINETICS

Route	Onset of Action	Peak Plasma Concentration	Elimination Half-Life	Duration of Action
PO	0.5–1 hr	2–3 hr	3.5–9 hr	4–12 hr

amlodipine besylate

Amlodipine besylate (Caduet, Norvasc, Twynsta, others) is currently the most popular CCB of the dihydropyridine subclass. It is indicated for both angina and hypertension and is available only for oral use.

PHARMACOKINETICS

Route	Onset of Action	Peak Plasma Concentration	Elimination Half-Life	Duration of Action
PO	30–50 min	6–12 hr	30–50 hr	24 hr

DOSAGES   Selected Calcium Channel–Blocking Drugs

Drug	Pharmacological Class	Usual Dosage Range	Indications
amlodipine besylate (Caduet, Norvasc Twynsta, others)	CCB	*Adults* PO: 5–10 mg/day	Angina
▸▸**diltiazem hydrochloride** (Apo-Diltiaz TZ, Cardizem CD, Tiazac, Taztia XC)	CCB	*Adults* PO: Initial dose 30 mg qid before meals and at bedtime; range of 240–360 mg divided in 3–4 doses Sustained-released capsule: 120–360 mg, divided bid Controlled-delivery capsule: 120–360 mg once daily	Angina

PO, oral; *CCB*, calcium channel blocker.

to the heart (preload) and decreasing systemic vascular resistance (afterload). The CCBs decrease calcium influx into the smooth muscle, causing vascular relaxation. This either reverses or prevents the spasms of coronary vessels that cause the anginal pain associated with Prinzmetal's or chronic angina. The β-blockers slow the heart rate and decrease contractility, thereby decreasing oxygen demands. Although these groups of drugs have similar clinical effects, the nursing process required for each is somewhat specific in terms of the characteristics and effects of the drugs and the indications for and contraindications to their use.

PHARMACOKINETIC BRIDGE TO NURSING PRACTICE

Not only are the pharmacokinetic properties of nitrates interesting, but knowledge of these specific properties is critical to safe and accurate nursing care. Moreover, patients' understanding of nitrate pharmacokinetics is also important because the level of a patient's knowledge may strongly influence adherence to the drug regimen and the effectiveness of treatment for angina. The pharmacokinetics differ for the various dosage forms of nitroglycerin and include the following:

- Intravenous infusion: Onset of action 1 to 2 minutes (fastest of all dosage forms), peak action not applicable, duration of action 3 to 5 minutes
- Sublingual tablet: Onset of action 2 to 3 minutes, peak action unknown, duration of action 30 to 60 minutes
- Topical ointment: Onset of action 15 to 60 minutes, peak action within 0.5 to 2 hours, duration of action 3 to 8 hours
- Transdermal patch: Onset of action 30 to 60 minutes, peak action 1 to 3 hours, duration of action 8 to 12 hours.
- Translingual spray: Onset of action 2 minutes, peak action 4 to 10 minutes, duration of action 30 to 60 minutes

If the goal of treatment is to abort or treat a sudden attack of angina, then *rapid* onset of action is needed, so the clinical decision (by the health care provider) would be to order either an intravenous infusion, or a sublingual tablet (or translingual spray, which has a similar onset

time). These dosage forms have pharmacokinetics that allow quick entry of the drug to the bloodstream and lead to more rapid vasodilation. This provides more oxygenated blood to the myocardium and aborts acute attacks. If symptoms persist, more drastic medical management would be indicated. The quick-onset nitroglycerin dosage forms may also be used by the patient 5 to 10 minutes before engaging in activities known to provoke angina, such as increased physical activity, sexual intercourse, or other forms of physical exertion. If the purpose of treatment is maintenance therapy, the nitrate form must have other pharmacokinetic properties, such as a longer duration of action to provide protection against angina; a longer onset of action is acceptable because stopping an attack is not needed in this situation. Use of ointments, transdermal patches, or extended-release preparations would be appropriate in such cases. If an acute episode of angina occurs while the patient is taking maintenance therapy, a dosage form with a rapid onset of action is indicated (as ordered). It is easy to see that thorough knowledge about a drug and its pharmacokinetics allows for safe and sound decisions about drug therapy for patients with angina.

NURSING PROCESS

▨ Assessment

Before antianginal drugs are administered, obtain a thorough nursing history and medication history (including a listing of all prescription drugs, over-the-counter products, and natural health products being taken) and document the findings. Also measure weight, height, and vital signs, with attention to supine, sitting, and standing blood pressures. Report a systolic blood pressure reading of less than 100 mm Hg (or as specified) to the health care provider before administering a dose of any of these drugs. With the use of any drugs affecting blood pressure or pulse rate, such as antianginals, take the apical pulse rate for 1 full minute. If the pulse rate is 60 beats per minute or lower, or 100 beats per minute or greater, contact the health care provider for further instructions.

In addition to rate, assess the quality and rhythm of the heartbeat and document prior to the administration of antianginal drugs. If the patient is experiencing any chest pain, include in your assessment a description of onset, character (e.g., sharp, dull, piercing, squeezing, radiating), intensity, location, duration, precipitating factors (e.g., physical exertion, exercise, eating, stress, sexual intercourse), alleviating factors, and any presence of nausea or vomiting. The health care provider may order an ECG, in which case the nurse must review the results of this as well. Thoroughly assess for any contraindications, cautions, and drug interactions prior to giving these drugs. Significant interactions include alcohol, β-blockers, CCBs, phenothiazines, and erectile dysfunction drugs such as sildenafil citrate, tadalafil, and vardenafil hydrochloride. Taking these drugs with nitrates will result in worsening of hypotensive responses, paradoxical bradycardia, and a resultant increase in angina with subsequent significant risk of heart or cerebrovascular complications due to decreased perfusion. Older adult patients often have difficulty with blood pressure control because of the occurrence of normal, age-related orthostatic hypotension, and the use of antianginals may lead to worsening of hypotensive responses. If patients are taking nitrates on a long-term basis, it is important to assess continued therapeutic responses because of the development of tolerance to the drug's effects. During assessment and initiation of drug therapy, it is crucial to patient safety to notify the health care provider of any increased angina because another antianginal or vasodilating drug may be needed.

Concerns arise with the use of nonselective β-blockers and β$_2$-blockers (as vasodilators) in patients with bronchospastic disease because of the drug-related effects of bronchoconstriction and increased airway resistance, which results in wheezing and dyspnea as adverse effects. Therefore, if asthma or other respiratory problems are present, β-blockers would not be indicated because bronchoconstriction could be exacerbated. In addition, there are also concerns about the use of β-blockers in patients with peripheral vascular disease, hypotension, hyperglycemia or hypoglycemia (see pharmacology discussion), and bradycardia. Nonselective β-blockers may also exacerbate pre-existing heart failure. Assessment for edema is important in patients with cardiac risk factors and a weight gain of 1 kg or more over 24 hours or 2.3 kg or more in 1 week. Weight gain of this nature must be reported to the health care provider immediately. Assess for significant drug interactions, including the concurrent use of other antihypertensives, CCBs, and oral antihyperglycemic drugs (see Table 24-3 for more information).

In patients taking CCBs, assess for possible drug–food interactions, including grapefruit. Grapefruit juice reduces the metabolism of nifedipine, leading to possible toxicity; grapefruit must be avoided. Another area to be thoroughly assessed is that of the dosage form of nifedipine, which is available in extended- and immediate-release forms. Therefore, follow the orders for administration of nifedipine carefully, and closely monitor the patient (e.g., vital signs). Diltiazem (Cardizem) is available in several sustained-delivery forms; closely assess orders to avoid medication errors. Cautious use is important in patients with a history of hypotension, palpitations, tachycardia or bradycardia, constipation, dyspnea, and edema. Significant drug interactions are included in Table 24-6.

Nursing Diagnoses

- Decreased cardiac output related to the pathology of CAD
- Deficient knowledge related to first-time use of antianginal drugs and a new diagnosis of CAD
- Risk for injury to self, related to the possible adverse drug effect of hypotension with subsequent dizziness, syncope, and falls

Planning

Goals

- Patient will exhibit therapeutic effects of antianginal drug therapy, such as improved cardiac output, with fewer episodes of chest pain.
- Patient will demonstrate increased knowledge about disease process and drug therapy.
- Patient will remain free from injury while receiving antianginal drug therapy.

Outcome Criteria

- On follow-up with the health care provider, patient states that there are more frequent periods of comfort while carrying out activities of daily living, engaging in supervised exercise, and participating in moderate activity, without recurring angina and without major adverse effects.
  - Patient experiences fewer to no episodes of chest pain (angina).
- Patient states rationale for antianginal drug therapy and the importance of taking medication exactly as prescribed.
  - Patient states adverse effects of antianginal drug therapy, such as orthostatic hypotension, dizziness, and severe headaches, as well as measures to decrease their occurrence.
  - Patient states the appropriate time frame of when to seek out emergency care (i.e., if finding no relief 5 minutes after 1 dose of sublingual nitrates) and call 911.
- Patient states measures to decrease risk for injury, such as changing positions slowly, keeping legs moving when in a still position, increasing fluid intake with medication regimen, and removing rugs or carpets that can cause slips, trips, or falls.

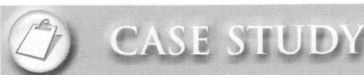

CASE STUDY

Nitroglycerin for Angina

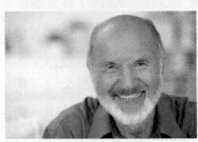

Sherman, a 68-year-old accountant, has been diagnosed with CAD after experiencing chest pain at times when he jogs. After undergoing a thorough physical examination, including cardiac catheterization, he is given a prescription for extended-release nitroglycerin capsules, 6.5 mg, three times a day. He also has a prescription for 0.4-mg sublingual nitroglycerin tablets to take as needed for chest pain.

1. What type of angina is Sherman experiencing, and what are the therapeutic goals of the drug therapy he has received?

Sherman asks you, "Why do I have two prescriptions for the same drug? It doesn't make sense to me!"

2. What is the best answer to his question?

3. Two days after he begins the nitroglycerin, Sherman calls the office and says, "I'm having awful headaches. What is wrong?" What is the best explanation, and what can he do about the headaches?

After 1 month, Sherman is switched from the extended-release capsules to a transdermal nitroglycerin patch. He says that he is glad he does not have to remember to "take those pills" three times a day. However, 2 months later, he calls and says, "I don't think this patch is working. I'm having more episodes of chest pain now when I jog."

4. What could be the explanation for this, and what can be done?

For answers, see http://evolve.elsevier.com/Canada/Lilley/pharmacology/.

Implementation

Always review and record patients' vital signs and descriptions of chest pain for the duration of therapy. Take into account the following considerations associated with the use of the various dosage forms and routes of administration:

1. For any dosage form: Administer the drug while the patient is seated to avoid falls or injury from drug-induced hypotension. This hypotension may last for up to 30 minutes after dosing of the drug. When administering nitrates, monitor the patient's chest pain, and have the patient rate the pain on a scale of 1 to 10, before, during, and after therapy. Monitor the patient's response to drug therapy by measuring blood pressure and pulse rate, as well as assessing for the presence of headache, dizziness, or lightheadedness. When the patient is in a supine position, an appropriate dose of a nitrate should produce a clinical response of a fall in blood pressure of about 10 mm Hg or a rise in heart rate of 10 beats per minute. However, the following parameters are alerts that the patient may have a problem and the health care provider should be contacted: a systolic blood pressure of 100 mm Hg or lower (or as specified), a pulse rate of 60 beats per minute or lower, or a pulse rate greater than 100 beats per minute.

2. For oral dosage forms: Counsel the patient that these are to be taken as ordered before meals and with 180 mL of water. Extended-release preparations must not be crushed, chewed, or altered in any way. Acetaminophen may be given if there is a drug-related headache, if not contraindicated.

3. For sublingual forms: Advise the patient to place the tablet under the tongue as directed and *not* to swallow until the drug is completely dissolved. Metered-dose pump sprays are applied onto or under the tongue (see Dosages table). Instruct the patient to keep nitrates in their original packaging or container (e.g., sublingual tablets come in a small, amber-coloured glass container with a metal lid). Exposure to light, plastic, cotton filler, and moisture must be avoided.

4. For ointment: Use the proper dosing paper supplied by the drug company to apply a thin layer on clean, dry, hairless skin of the upper arms or upper body. Avoid areas below the knees and elbows. Do not apply the ointment with the fingers unless using a glove, to avoid contact with the skin and subsequent absorption. A tongue depressor may also be used, but in most situations the ointment may be squeezed directly from the tube onto the proper dosing paper. Once the ointment is in place, do *not* rub it into the skin; cover the area with an occlusive dressing (e.g., plastic wrap). Rotate application sites and remove all residue from the previous dose of ointment gently with soap and water and pat the area dry.

5. For transdermal forms: Apply patches to a clean, residue-free, hairless area, and rotate sites. If cardioversion or use of an automated electrical defibrillator is required, remove the transdermal patch to avoid burning of the skin and damage to the defibrillator paddles. Before a new patch is applied, locate and remove the old patch and clean the skin of any residual drug. Carefully dispose of used, unneeded, or defective transdermal patches, from any medication, as indicated by hospital policy or per discharge instructions. It is important to follow any packaging insert instructions or facility policy because transdermal patches delivering potent medications need to be folded in half with the sticky sides together and placed in a garbage can that is out of reach of people and pets

(see Chapter 2). For more information, visit http://healthycanadians.gc.ca/drugs-products-medicaments-produits/drugs-medicaments/disposal-defaire-eng.php.

6. For intravenous forms: Intravenous dosing is for use in emergency situations only and in settings with close automatic monitoring of blood pressure and pulse as well as constant ECG monitoring. Intravenous administration of nitrates may lead to sudden and severe hypotension, cardiovascular collapse, and shock. Always check for incompatibilities and the proper diluent. Only give intravenous solutions through an infusion pump and as ordered. Intravenous dosage forms are available as ready-to-use injectable doses and are administered using specific nonpolyvinylchloride (non-PVC) plastic intravenous bags and tubing. Non-PVC infusion kits are used to avoid absorption or uptake of the nitrate by intravenous tubing and bags. This method prevents decomposition of the nitrate with breakdown into cyanide when the drug is exposed to light. Intravenous forms of nitroglycerin are stable for about 96 hours after preparation. If parenteral solutions are not clear and are discoloured, discard the solution.

With isosorbide, tablets are best taken on an empty stomach; however, if the patient reports headache or gastrointestinal upset, the medicine should be taken with meals. Oral tablets of isosorbide can be crushed; however, the sublingual and extended-release forms are *not* to be crushed or chewed. As with sublingual nitroglycerin, instruct patients not to swallow the medication until it is completely dissolved. If dizziness or lightheadedness occurs, assist the patient and encourage slow changing of positions. Closely monitor blood pressure, including orthostatic blood pressures. Document the occurrence of anginal episodes, their character, precipitating factors, severity, and frequency.

β-blockers need to be given as ordered and may be taken with or without food. Abrupt withdrawal must be avoided. Weights must be measured every day at the same time and with the patient wearing the same amount of clothing. If there is a weight gain of 1 kg or more in 24 hours or 2.3 kg or more in 1 week, contact the health care provider immediately. When these drugs are used, take measures to reduce the incidence of orthostatic hypotension, such as advising the patient to dangle the legs on the side of the bed before standing and to move slowly and purposefully. Instruct the patient to contact the health care provider immediately if any excessive or intolerable dizziness, fatigue, wheezing, or dyspnea occurs (see Chapter 20 for further discussion).

CCBs are to be taken as ordered and without sudden withdrawal. Abrupt withdrawal can precipitate rebound hypertension and worsening of tissue ischemia. Weight needs to be measured daily (see later discussion). Constantly monitor the patient for edema and shortness of breath. Instruct the patient to move and change positions slowly and cautiously to prevent syncope. Constipation may be prevented by increasing intake of fluids and fibre in the diet. If the patient experiences palpitations, pronounced dizziness, nausea, or dyspnea, contact the health care provider immediately. Intravenous administration of any CCB requires the use of an infusion pump and careful monitoring (see Chapter 26).

Patients taking any of the vasodilators must avoid alcohol, saunas, hot tubs, hot showers, and hot weather or environments. These conditions will exacerbate vasodilation and increase the occurrence of orthostatic hypotension, increasing the risk for dizziness, syncope, and falls. Caution patients that with certain sustained-release forms of medication, the wax matrix may appear in the stool; advise them that this occurs after the drug has been absorbed and that, even though the matrix is visible, it is of no concern. Instruct patients on how to self-monitor blood pressure and pulse rate, as well as how to document these findings in a journal or electronic device so that the information can be shared with health care providers. The journal or electronic device can also keep a record of daily weights, response to the medication regimen, and any adverse effects. See the Patient Teaching Tips for more information.

☑ Evaluation

Carefully monitor patients taking antianginals for the occurrence of an allergic reaction, which may be manifested by dyspnea, swelling of the face, or hives. Include in your evaluation a review for accomplishments of goals and outcome criteria, such as appropriate decrease in blood pressure, increase in cardiac output and tissue perfusion, decrease in angina, gradual increase in activity level, and improvement in performance of activities of daily living without exacerbation of anginal episodes. In addition, monitor the patient for adverse reactions such as headache, lightheadedness, dizziness, and decreased blood pressure, which may indicate the need to decrease the dosage. If the patient is receiving intravenous nitroglycerin, evaluate for excessive drops in blood pressure, worsening of angina, and significant changes in pulse rate (to less than 60 beats per minute or more than 100 beats per minute), and contact the health care provider immediately if any of these conditions occurs.

PATIENT TEACHING TIPS

❖ Nitroglycerin
- Emphasize to patients the importance of keeping a daily journal (in handwritten or electronic form), documenting number of anginal episodes and noting their intensity, frequency, duration, and character, as well as precipitating and relieving factors. Any evidence of possible tolerance to the medication is important to note and report to the health care provider.
- Capsules or extended release dosage forms are never to be chewed, crushed, or altered in any way.
- Instruct patients taking pump (spray) dosage forms not to shake the canister before lingual spraying and to avoid inhaling or swallowing until the drug is dispersed. Each metered dose contains 0.4 mg nitroglycerin. With the onset of an acute attack of angina pectoris, 1 or 2 metered doses (0.4 or 0.8 mg of nitroglycerin), as determined by experience, may be administered onto or under the tongue, without inhaling. The optimal dose may be repeated twice, at 5- to 10-minute intervals. With sublingual tablets, the medication must be taken at the first sign of chest pain and not delayed until the pain is severe. The patient needs to sit or lie down and take one sublingual tablet. According to current guidelines, if the chest pain or discomfort is not relieved in 5 minutes, after *one* dose, the patient (or a family member) must call 911 immediately. The patient can take one more tablet while awaiting emergency care and a third tablet 5 minutes later, but no more than three tablets total. These guidelines reflect the fact that angina pain that does not respond to nitroglycerin may indicate an MI. The sublingual dose is to be placed under the tongue and patients must avoid swallowing until the tablet is dissolved. Instruct patients not to eat or drink until the drug has completely dissolved.
- Educate patients about the best place to store their medication, such as keeping it away from moisture, light, heat, and cotton filler material. The sublingual dosage form of nitroglycerin needs to be kept in its original, amber-coloured glass container with metal lid, to avoid loss of potency from exposure to heat, light, moisture, and cotton filler.
- Patients should know that the potency of the sublingual nitroglycerin can be noted if there is burning or stinging once the medication is placed under the tongue; if the medication does not burn, then the drug has lost its potency, and a new prescription must be obtained.
- It is important to emphasize to patients that the sublingual nitroglycerin is potent for only 3 to 6 months. Remind them to always have a fresh supply of the drug on hand, to plan ahead if travelling, and (no matter what the dosage form) to sit or lie down when taking the medication to avoid falls secondary to a drop in blood pressure.
- With patients taking any form of nitrates, educate about adverse effects such as flushing of the face, dizziness, fainting, brief throbbing headaches, increase in heart rate, and lightheadedness. Headaches associated with nitrates last approximately 20 minutes (with sublingual forms) and may be easily managed with acetaminophen. If headaches are bothersome when taking an oral dosage form, the drug may be taken with meals, and the patient must contact the health care provider if adverse effects continue. Blurred vision, dry mouth, or severe headaches may indicate drug overdose and require immediate medical attention. While taking an antianginal, patients must avoid alcohol, hot environmental temperatures, saunas, hot tubs, and excessive exertion; these conditions increase vasodilation with subsequent worsening of hypotension, which can possibly lead to syncope (fainting) or other cardiac events.
- In many situations, the health care provider specifies that nitroglycerin be taken *before* stressful activities or events that may exacerbate angina, such as emotional situations, consumption of large meals, smoking, or sudden increase in activity (e.g., sexual intercourse). The patient needs to closely follow the HCP's directions regarding prophylactic dosing.
- With ointment forms, remind patients to use the appropriate dosage paper for application of ointment and not to use the fingers to apply the medicine. The medication can be pressed evenly and directly from the tube onto the printed dosing line on the paper. Instruct the patient to squeeze a thin line of ointment onto the paper and follow instructions regarding its application, such as measuring and applying 1.3 centimetres of ointment. An occlusive dressing must be used, such as applying a piece of plastic wrap taped around the edges to adhere the dose to the skin. Only clean, nonirritated, and nonhairy areas free of residual medication are to be used for these ointments. The use of ointments has been largely replaced by the more effective use of transdermal patches.
- With transdermal nitrate use, patients must apply the patch at the same time each day, be sure to have only one patch in place at a time, and cleanse all residue off the skin before applying a new patch. Advise patients to avoid skin folds, hairy areas, and any area distal to the knees or elbows as application sites. A transdermal patch must never be applied on irritated or open skin, and if the patch becomes loose, the patient needs to remove it, gently wash off the residue with lukewarm water and soap, *pat* the area dry, and place another patch in another area. Encourage rotation of sites to prevent irritation (with ointments as well). The health care provider may order the removal of the patch for an 8-hour period on specific days to help decrease or prevent drug tolerance, which may develop over time. Provide all instructions both verbally and in written format.

❖ Isosorbide Dinitrate or Isosorbide-5-Mononitrate
- Educate patients about the basic differences in oral nitrates (e.g., the mononitrate form is well absorbed after oral dosing; the dinitrate form is poorly

Continued

PATIENT TEACHING TIPS—cont'd

absorbed, but its metabolite, isosorbide mononitrate, is active and well absorbed). It is important that patients know that these drugs are *not interchangeable.*

- Instruct patients to take the medication exactly as ordered, with emphasis on the need to lie down when doses are taken to avoid injury from sudden drop in blood pressure, which may lead to dizziness, lightheadedness, and fainting.
- Isosorbide is generally given three times a day with a 12-hour drug-free interval, such as dosing at 0700 hours, 1300 hours, and 1900 hours. The 12-hour drug-free interval helps prevent the development of tolerance.

- Oral dosage forms are not to be altered in any way and must be taken with at least 180 to 240 mL of water.
- Patient must be cautious while taking these drugs and should be encouraged to rise slowly and move the legs around before standing up from a lying or sitting position to help prevent dizziness, syncope, and falls. The importance of avoiding of alcohol, heat, and saunas must be emphasized because these factors exacerbate the hypotensive effects of the drug and may result in injury.
- Advise patients that these and other antianginals are not to be stopped abruptly.

KEY POINTS

❖ Angina pectoris (chest pain) occurs because of a mismatch between oxygen supply and oxygen demand, with either too high a demand for oxygen or too little oxygen delivery.

❖ The heart is an aerobic (oxygen-requiring) muscle; when it does not receive enough oxygen, pain (angina) occurs. When the coronary arteries that deliver oxygen to the heart muscle become blocked, a heart attack or MI occurs.

❖ CAD is an abnormal condition of the arteries that deliver oxygen to the heart muscle. These arteries may become narrowed, which results in reduced flow of oxygen and nutrients to the myocardium.

❖ Nitrates, CCBs, and β-blockers may be used to treat the symptoms of angina.

❖ Nitroglycerin is the prototypical nitrate. Nitrates dilate constricted coronary arteries, helping to increase the supply of oxygen and nutrients to the heart muscle. Nitrates also dilate all other blood vessels. The venous dilation results in a decrease of blood return to the heart (decreased preload), whereas the arterial dilation results in a decrease of peripheral resistance (decreased afterload—that is, the pressure or force against which the left ventricle must pump). Isosorbide dinitrates were the first group of oral drugs

used to treat angina; isosorbide-5-mononitrates are new and improved nitrates used for angina therapy; β-blockers are also used to relieve angina, which they do by decreasing the heart rate, reducing the workload on the heart, and decreasing oxygen demands.

❖ Dosage forms for nitrates include conventional tablets, sublingual spray, controlled-release and sustained-release capsules, transdermal patches, topical ointments, and intravenous injections.

❖ Quick-onset nitrates are used to treat acute anginal attacks, while longer-onset nitrates are used for prophylaxis. Instruct patients to always keep a fresh supply of sublingual nitroglycerin on their persons and in their homes because the drug is stable for only 3 to 6 months.

❖ CCBs and β-blockers may be associated with the adverse effects of postural hypotension, dizziness, headache, and edema.

❖ The nonselective β-blockers may exacerbate heart failure, problems related to respiratory bronchospasm, and hypoglycemia.

❖ Check the patient's pulse rate before drug administration, and if it is 60 beats per minute or lower, contact the health care provider for further instructions.

EXAMINATION REVIEW QUESTIONS

1. A patient has a new prescription for transdermal nitroglycerin patches. The nurse teaches the patient that these patches are most appropriately used for which purpose?
   a. To relieve exertional angina
   b. To prevent palpitations
   c. To prevent the occurrence of angina
   d. To stop an episode of angina

2. A nurse with adequate knowledge about the administration of intravenous nitroglycerin will recognize which statement as correct?
   a. The intravenous form is given by intravenous push injection.
   b. Because the intravenous forms are short-lived, the dosing must be every 2 hours.
   c. Intravenous nitroglycerin must be protected from exposure to light through use of special tubing.
   d. Intravenous nitroglycerin can be given via gravity drip infusions.

EXAMINATION REVIEW QUESTIONS—cont'd

3. Which statement by the patient reflects the need for additional patient education about the calcium channel blocker diltiazem (Cardizem)?
   a. "I can take this drug to stop an attack of angina."
   b. "I understand that food and antacids can change how well I can absorb this drug when I take it as a pill."
   c. "When the long-acting forms are taken, the drug cannot be crushed."
   d. "This drug may cause my blood pressure to drop, so I should be careful when getting up."

4. While assessing a patient with angina who is to start β-blocker therapy, the nurse is aware that the presence of which condition may be a problem if these drugs are used?
   a. Hypertension
   b. Essential tremors
   c. Exertional angina
   d. Asthma

5. A 68-year-old man has been taking the nitrate isosorbide dinitrate (ISDN) for 2 years for angina. He has recently been experiencing erectile dysfunction and wants a prescription for sildenafil citrate (Viagra). Which response would the nurse most likely hear from the health care provider?

   a. "He will have to be switched to isosorbide-5-mononitrate if he wants to take sildenafil citrate."
   b. "Taking sildenafil citrate with the nitrate may result in a contraindication and cause severe hypotension."
   c. "I'll write a prescription, but if he uses it, he needs to stop taking the isosorbide for one dose."
   d. "These drugs are compatible with each other, so I'll write a prescription."

6. The nurse is reviewing drug interactions with a male patient who has a prescription for isosorbide (ISDN) as treatment for angina symptoms. Which substances listed below could potentially result in a drug interaction? (Select all that apply.)
   a. A glass of wine
   b. Thyroid replacement hormone
   c. tadalafil (Cialis), an erectile dysfunction drug
   d. metformin hydrochloride (Glucophage®), an antihyperglycemic drug
   e. carvedilol, a β-blocker

7. The order reads, "Give metoprolol (Lopresor) 300 mg/day PO in 2 divided doses." The tablets are available in 50-mg strength. How many tablets will the patient receive per dose?

Answers: 1. c, 2. c, 3. a, 4. d, 5. b, 6. a, c, e, 7. 3 tablets per dose (150 mg per dose)

CRITICAL THINKING ACTIVITIES

1. Your neighbour Angela has been shovelling snow all morning. As you shovel the snow in your yard, you see her suddenly sit down in her driveway. When you go over to check on her, she says that she has nitroglycerin tablets in her jacket pocket but she has forgotten how to take them. What is your priority action at this time?

2. Your patient has been switched from oral nitroglycerin capsules to a transdermal form. What are the priorities

for patient teaching regarding transdermal nitroglycerin therapy?

3. Johan has chronic stable angina, and has recently been prescribed sublingual nitroglycerin tablets for the relief of his anginal attacks. What teaching instructions does Johan require in order to take the nitroglycerin appropriately?

For answers, see http://evolve.elsevier.com/Canada/Lilley/pharmacology/.

CHAPTER 25

Heart Failure Drugs

Objectives

After reading this chapter, the successful student will be able to do the following:

1. Differentiate between the terms *inotropic*, *chronotropic*, and *dromotropic*.

2. Briefly discuss the pathophysiology of heart failure.

3. Identify the approach to treatment of heart failure.

4. Compare the mechanisms of action, pharmacokinetics, indications, dosages, contraindications, dosage forms, routes of administration, cautions, adverse effects, and toxicity of the drugs used in the treatment of heart failure.

5. Briefly discuss rapid versus slow digitalization as well as the use of the antidote digoxin immune Fab.

6. Identify significant drug–drug, drug–laboratory test, and drug–food interactions associated with digoxin and other heart failure drugs.

7. Develop a collaborative plan of care that includes all phases of the nursing process for patients undergoing treatment for heart failure.

e-Learning Activities

Website
(http://evolve.elsevier.com/Canada/
Lilley/pharmacology/)

evolve

- Answer Key—Textbook Case Studies
- Answer Key—Critical Thinking Activities
- Chapter Summaries—Printable
- Review Questions for Exam Preparation
- Unfolding Case Studies

Drug Profiles

▸▸ digoxin, p. 486
     digoxin immune Fab, p. 486
▸▸ dobutamine, p. 480
     hydralazine and isosorbide dinitrate, p. 480
▸▸ lisinopril, p. 479
▸▸ milrinone (milrinone lactate)*, p. 482
▸▸ valsartan, p. 480

▸▸ Key drug

*Full generic name is given in parentheses. For the purposes of this text, the more common, shortened name is used.

Key Terms

Atrial fibrillation A common cardiac dysrhythmia involving atrial contractions that are so rapid that they prevent full repolarization of myocardial fibres between heartbeats. (p. 481)

Automaticity A property of specialized excitable tissue in the heart that allows self-activation through the spontaneous development of an action potential, such as in the pacemaker cells of the heart. (p. 480)

Chronotropic drugs Drugs that influence the rate of the heartbeat. (p. 478)

Dromotropic drugs Drugs that influence the conduction of electrical impulses within tissues. (p. 479)

Ejection fraction The proportion of blood that is ejected during each ventricular contraction compared with the total ventricular filling volume. (p. 477)

Heart failure An abnormal condition in which the heart cannot pump enough blood to keep up with the body's demand. It is often the result of myocardial infarction, ischemic heart disease, or cardiomyopathy. (p. 477)

Inotropic drugs   Drugs that affect the force or energy of muscular contractions, particularly contraction of the heart muscle. (p. 478)

Left ventricular end-diastolic volume (LVEDV)   The total amount of blood in the ventricle immediately before it contracts, or the preload. (p. 477)

Refractory period   The period during which a *pulse generator* (i.e., the sinoatrial node of the heart) is unresponsive to an electrical input signal, and during which it is impossible for the myocardium to respond; during this period, the cardiac cell is readjusting its sodium and potassium levels and cannot be depolarized again. (p. 484)

OVERVIEW

Heart failure is a not a specific disease per se but rather a clinical syndrome caused by numerous different cardiac disorders. Approximately 600 000 people in Canada live with heart failure and 50 000 new patients are diagnosed each year (Heart and Stroke Foundation, 2016). It is one of the most common causes for hospitalization in Canada. This is especially true for the patient population over the age of 65. Heart failure also causes more than 5 000 deaths annually in Canada. The findings of one of the largest and most frequently cited studies involving patients with heart failure, the Framingham study, show that the 5-year survival rate in patients with heart failure is approximately 50%. The best way to prevent heart failure is to control risk factors associated with heart failure, including hypertension, coronary artery disease, obesity, and diabetes.

Heart failure is a pathological condition in which the heart is unable to pump blood in sufficient amounts from the ventricles (i.e., insufficient cardiac output) to meet the body's metabolic needs or can do so only at elevated filling pressures. The signs and symptoms typically associated with this insufficiency make up the syndrome of heart failure. Initially, the patient is asymptomatic. As the disease progresses, so do the symptoms. Failure of the ventricle(s) to eject blood efficiently results in fluid volume overload, chamber dilation, and elevated intracardiac pressure. This syndrome can affect the left ventricle, the right ventricle, or both ventricles simultaneously. Left ventricular or "left-sided" heart failure often leads to pulmonary edema, coughing, shortness of breath, and dyspnea (remember: left equals lung). Right ventricular heart failure typically involves systemic venous congestion, pedal edema, jugular venous distension, ascites, and hepatic congestion. Both syndromes occur due to increased hydrostatic pressure from the ventricles into the pulmonary or systemic circulation. Left-sided failure can be further divided into systolic and diastolic failure. Systolic dysfunction or failure is characterized by a decrease in myocardial contractility and a resulting reduction in the left ventricular ejection fraction (e.g., the left ventricle cannot pump with sufficient force to push blood into the circulation). Diastolic dysfunction or failure refers to cardiac dysfunction in which left ventricular filling is abnormal and is accompanied by elevated filling pressures during diastole. The ventricle is unable to relax as the muscle becomes stiff.

More specifically, heart failure occurs due to a reduced ratio of **ejection fraction** to **left ventricular end-diastolic volume (LVEDV)**. The ejection fraction is the amount of blood ejected with each contraction, whereas the left ventricular end-diastolic volume is the total amount of blood in the ventricle just before contraction. The ejection fraction is an index of left ventricular function, and the normal value is approximately 65% (0.65) of the total volume in the ventricle.

When a person has heart failure, the heart cannot meet the increased demands, and the blood supply to certain organs is reduced. The organs that are most dependent on blood supply—the brain and heart—are the last to be deprived of blood. The kidney is relatively less dependent on blood supply, and its blood supply is shunted away from it. Therefore, the filtration of fluids and removal of waste products is impaired. This can lead to acute kidney injury or chronic kidney failure. Reduced blood supply also contributes to conditions such as pulmonary edema (resulting in shortness of breath) and peripheral edema.

The physical defects producing heart failure are of two types: (1) a heart defect (myocardial deficiency such as myocardial infarction or valve insufficiency), which leads to inadequate cardiac contractility and ventricular filling, and (2) a defect outside the heart (e.g., systemic defects such as coronary artery disease, pulmonary hypertension, or diabetes), which results in an overload on an otherwise normal heart. Either or both of these defects may be present in a given patient. Common causes of myocardial deficiency and systemic defects are listed in Box 25-1.

The emphasis of this chapter is on systolic dysfunction or inadequate ventricular contractions (systole) during the pumping of the heart. Less common, but still important, is diastolic dysfunction or inadequate ventricular filling during ventricular relaxation (diastole). This condition is most commonly associated with left ventricular hypertrophy secondary to chronic hypertension. However, it may also result from cardiomyopathy (e.g., virus induced), pericardial disease, or diabetes.

Heart failure is stratified into classes, using The New York Heart Association's functional classification. Class I describes a patient who is not limited in normal physical activity by symptoms. Class II is said to occur when ordinary physical activity results in fatigue, dyspnea, or other symptoms. Class III is characterized by a marked limitation in normal physical activity. Class IV is defined by symptoms at rest or with any physical activity at all.

BOX 25-1

Myocardial Deficiency and Increased Workload: Common Causes

Myocardial Deficiency

Inadequate Contractility
Coronary artery disease
Myocardial infarction
Cardiomyopathy
Valvular insufficiency

Inadequate Filling
Atrial fibrillation
Infection
Tamponade
Ischemia

Increased Workload

Pressure Overload
Pulmonary hypertension
Systemic hypertension
Outflow obstruction

Volume Overload
Hypervolemia
Congenital abnormalities
Anemia
Thyroid disease
Infection
Diabetes

The American Heart Association (AHA) and American Colleges of Cardiology (ACC) (2013) developed a new classification designed to complement the NYHA classification. The evolution and progression of heart failure is now emphasized via the following stages: (1) Stage A includes patients who are at high risk for developing HF but have no structural disorder of the heart; (2) Stage B includes patients with structural disorders of the heart who have never had symptoms of HF; (3) Stage C includes patients with past or current symptoms of HF associated with underlying structural heart disease; and (4) Stage D includes patients with end-stage disease who require specialized treatment strategies, such as mechanical circulatory support, continuous IV inotrope infusions, cardiac transplantation, or hospice care. Drug therapy is individualized based on a patient's class or stage of heart failure.

DRUG THERAPY

Drugs that increase the force of myocardial contraction are called positive **inotropic drugs,** and they have a role in the treatment of failing heart muscle. Negative inotropic drugs reduce the force of contraction. Drugs that increase the rate at which the heart beats are called positive **chronotropic drugs.** Negative chronotropic drugs do the opposite. Drugs may also affect how quickly electrical impulses travel through the conduction system of the heart (the sinoatrial [SA] node, atrioventricular [AV] node, bundle of His, and Purkinje fibres) (Figure 25-1). Drugs that accelerate conduction are referred to as

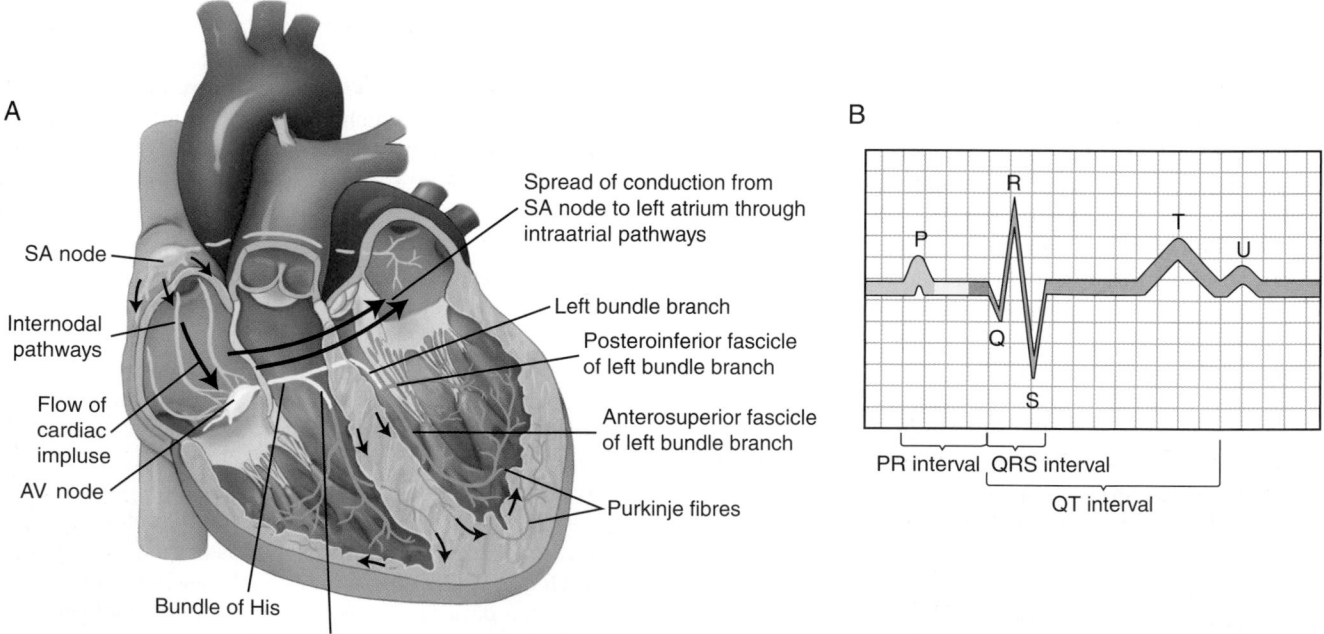

A

SA node
Internodal pathways
Flow of cardiac impulse
AV node
Bundle of His
Right bundle branch

Spread of conduction from SA node to left atrium through intraatrial pathways
Left bundle branch
Posteroinferior fascicle of left bundle branch
Anterosuperior fascicle of left bundle branch
Purkinje fibres

B

P   R   T   U   Q   S

PR interval   QRS interval
QT interval

FIG. 25-1   Conduction system of the heart. *AV,* atrioventricular; *SA,* sinoatrial. (Source: Lewis, S. M., Dirksen, S. R., Heitkemper, M. M., et al. (2014). *Medical-surgical nursing in Canada: Assessment and management of clinical problems* (3rd Canadian ed., M. A. Barry, S. Goldsworthy & D. Goodridge, Canadian Eds.). Toronto, ON: Mosby. Figure 34-4, p. 845.)

positive **dromotropic drugs.** This chapter focuses on the positive inotropic drugs, phosphodiesterase inhibitors (PDIs), and cardiac glycosides. Although several other drugs are used in the treatment of heart failure, they are discussed in detail in other chapters; for example, angiotensin-converting enzyme (ACE) inhibitors and angiotensin II receptor blockers (ARBs) are covered in Chapter 23; β-blockers are discussed in Chapters 20, 23, and 24; the vasodilator nitroglycerin used in acute heart failure is discussed in Chapter 24, and the mainstays of early treatment—diuretics—are discussed in Chapter 29. These drugs are mentioned in this chapter as well, but for specifics, refer to the indicated chapters.

The treatment of heart failure has changed dramatically over the past decade. The positive inotrope digoxin was once the drug of choice in heart failure treatment, but because of adverse effects and drug interactions, it has been replaced by other drugs. Its usefulness is still debated in the literature; however, it remains an important drug in the symptom management of severe end-stage heart failure and may reduce hospitalizations but not mortality. Inotropes do not improve patient outcomes. According to the 2012 Canadian Cardiovascular Society Heart Failure Management Guidelines Update: Focus on Acute and Chronic Heart Failure (McKelvie, Moe, Ezekowitz, et al., 2013), the proper approach to the treatment of chronic heart failure revolves around reducing the effects of the renin–angiotensin–aldosterone system and the sympathetic nervous system. Therefore, the drugs of choice at the start of therapy are the ACE inhibitors (lisinopril, enalapril, captopril, and others) or the ARBs (valsartan, candesartan, losartan, and others) and certain β-blockers (metoprolol or bisoprolol fumarate, cardioselective β-blockers; carvedilol, a nonspecific β-blocker). Loop diuretics (furosemide) are used to reduce the symptoms of heart failure secondary to fluid overload, and the aldosterone inhibitors (spironolactone, eplerenone) are added as the heart failure progresses. Only after these drugs are used is digoxin added. Dobutamine, a positive inotropic drug, has also been used to treat heart failure. A combination of hydralazine and isosorbide dinitrate is recommended specifically for use in patients who are Black.

ANGIOTENSIN-CONVERTING ENZYME INHIBITORS

ACE inhibitors comprise a class of drugs that, as their name implies, inhibit angiotensin-converting enzyme, which is responsible for converting angiotensin I (formed through the action of renin) to angiotensin II. Angiotensin II is a potent vasoconstrictor and induces aldosterone secretion by the adrenal glands. Aldosterone stimulates sodium and water resorption, which can raise blood pressure. Together, these processes are referred to as the renin–angiotensin–aldosterone system. ACE inhibitors are beneficial in the treatment of heart failure because they prevent sodium and water resorption by inhibiting aldosterone secretion. This action causes diuresis, which decreases blood volume and blood return to the heart. This result in turn decreases preload, or the left ventricular end-diastolic volume, and the work required of the heart. According to the 2012 Canadian Cardiovascular Society Heart Failure Management Guidelines Update: Focus on Acute and Chronic Heart Failure (McKelvie, Moe, Ezekowitz et al., 2013), an ACE inhibitor should not be started in the acute setting (e.g., within the first 8 to 12 hours) unless elevated blood pressure is present and should be initiated after the acute event (e.g., 24 hours). It is to be continued particularly if the patient is already being treated with chronic ACE inhibitor therapy. The ACE inhibitors (as well as ARBs) are also effective in slowing the progression of ventricular remodeling and hypertrophy.

Numerous ACE inhibitors are available, including lisinopril, enalapril maleate, fosinopril sodium, quinapril hydrochloride, captopril, ramipril, trandolapril, and perindopril erbumine. These drugs are all similar, and lisinopril will be used as the example for this class of drugs used to treat heart failure.

 DRUG PROFILE

▸▸ *lisinopril*

Lisinopril (Prinivil®, Zestril®) is a commonly used ACE inhibitor and is available in a generic form. It is used for hypertension, heart failure, and acute myocardial infarction. Like all ACE inhibitors, it can cause injury or fetal death when used in pregnancy. Hyperkalemia may occur with any ACE inhibitor, and potassium supplementation or potassium-sparing diuretics need to be used with caution. Like all ACE inhibitors, lisinopril can cause a dry cough, which will not harm patients but can be annoying. The cough is a result of bradykinins, insoluble by-products of the ACE inhibitors, building up in the blood and lodging in the lungs' bronchial tubes. The coughing spells represent the body's attempt to expel the kinins from the lungs. The cough usually resolves in a month, but patients may be switched to an angiotensin II receptor antagonist. Lisinopril (and all ACE inhibitors) may also be associated with a decrease in kidney function. For drug interactions, see Chapter 23.

PHARMACOKINETICS

Route	Onset of Action	Peak Plasma Concentration	Elimination Half-Life	Duration of Action
PO	1 hr	6 hr	11–12 hr	24 hr

ANGIOTENSIN II RECEPTOR BLOCKERS

The therapeutic effects of ARBs in heart failure are related to their potent vasodilating properties. They may be used alone or in combination with other drugs such as diuretics in the treatment of hypertension or heart failure. The beneficial hemodynamic effect of ARBs is their ability to decrease systemic vascular resistance (a measure of afterload). Seven ARBs are currently available: valsartan, candesartan cilexetil, eprosartan mesylate, irbesartan, telmisartan, olmesartan medoximil, and losartan potassium. All of the ARBs are similar in action. Valsartan will be used as the example for this class of drugs used to treat heart failure.

β-BLOCKERS

β-blockers (also discussed in Chapters 20, 23, and 24) work by reducing or blocking sympathetic nervous system stimulation to the heart and the heart's conduction system. By doing this, β-blockers prevent catecholamine-mediated actions on the heart. This is known as a cardioprotective quality of β-blockers. The resulting cardiovascular effects include reduced heart rate, delayed AV node conduction, reduced myocardial contractility, and decreased myocardial **automaticity.** Three β-blockers have been shown to reduce mortality: bisoprolol, extended-release metoprolol, and carvedilol. Metoprolol tartrate is the β-blocker most commonly used to treat heart failure. It is available as an immediate-release and an extended-release product, as well as an intravenous formulation.

Carvedilol has many effects, including acting as a nonselective β-blocker, an α_1-blocker, and possibly a calcium channel blocker and antioxidant. It is used primarily in the treatment of heart failure but is also beneficial for hypertension and angina. It has been shown to slow the progression of heart failure and to decrease the frequency of hospitalization in patients with mild to moderate (class II or III) heart failure. Carvedilol is most commonly added to digoxin, furosemide, and ACE inhibitors when used to treat heart failure. It is available only for oral use.

ALDOSTERONE ANTAGONISTS

Aldosterone antagonists spironolactone and eplerenone are useful in severe stages of heart failure. Activation of the renin–angiotensin–aldosterone system causes increased levels of aldosterone, which causes retention of sodium and water, leading to edema that can worsen heart failure. Spironolactone (Aldactone®) is a potassium-sparing diuretic and is discussed in detail in Chapter 29. It also acts as an aldosterone antagonist, which has been shown to reduce the symptoms of heart failure. Eplerenone (Inspra®) is a selective aldosterone blocker, blocking aldosterone at its receptors in the kidney, heart, blood vessels, and brain. It is discussed in detail in Chapter 23.

DRUG PROFILE

▶▶*valsartan*

Valsartan (Diovan®) is a commonly used ARB. Like all ARBs, it can cause fetal and neonatal morbidity and death when used during pregnancy. Valsartan shares many of the same adverse effects as lisinopril, profiled earlier. The ARBs are not as likely to cause the cough associated with ACE inhibitors, nor are they as likely to cause hyperkalemia. For drug interactions, see Chapter 23.

PHARMACOKINETICS

Route	Onset of Action	Peak Plasma Concentration	Elimination Half-Life	Duration of Action
PO	2 hr	Unknown	6 hr	12 hr

MISCELLANEOUS HEART FAILURE DRUGS

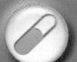

DRUG PROFILES

hydralazine/isosorbide dinitrate

Hydralazine and isosorbide dinitrate are approved specifically for individuals who are Black. A combination of the two drugs is available in the United States but not in Canada. The individual drugs are discussed in detail in Chapter 23 (hydralazine) and Chapter 24 (isosorbide). Peak plasma levels of hydralazine and isosorbide dinitrate are achieved in 1 hour.

▶▶*dobutamine hydrochloride*

Dobutamine hydrochloride is a β_1-selective vasoactive adrenergic drug that is structurally similar to the naturally occurring catecholamine dopamine. Through stimulation of the β_1-receptors on heart muscle (myocardium), it increases cardiac output by increasing contractility (positive inotropy), which increases the stroke volume, especially in patients with heart failure. Dobutamine hydrochloride is available only as an intravenous drug and is given by continuous infusion. See Chapter 18 for further discussion of this drug. The 2012 Canadian Cardiovascular Society Heart Failure Management Guidelines (McKelvie et al., 2013) recommend that dobutamine hydrochloride be used only for patients who are hemodynamically unstable.

OMEGA-3 POLYUNSATURATED FATTY ACIDS

The natural health product omega-3 polyunsaturated fatty acids (PUFA) is included in this chapter because it is recommended by the 2012 Canadian Cardiovascular Society Heart Failure Management Guidelines Update: Focus on Acute and Chronic Heart Failure (McKelvie et al., 2013), as adjunctive therapy for patients with chronic heart failure. Studies found that mortality is reduced by 21% in patients post–myocardial infarction who are taking 1 g of omega-3 PUFA (850 to 882 mg of eicosapentaenoic acid [EPA] and docosahexaenoic acid [DHA] as ethyl esters in the ratio of 1:1.2) daily.

PHOSPHODIESTERASE INHIBITORS

PDIs are a group of inotropic drugs that work by inhibiting the action of an enzyme called phosphodiesterase. These drugs were discovered in the search for positive inotropic drugs with a wider therapeutic window than that of digoxin. Currently, only one drug in this category is available: milrinone.

Mechanism of Action and Drug Effects

The mechanism of action of PDIs differs from other inotropic drugs such as digoxin and the catecholamines. PDIs share a similar pharmacological action with methylxanthines such as theophylline (see Chapter 38). Both types of drug inhibit the action of phosphodiesterase, which results in an increase in intracellular cyclic adenosine monophosphate (cAMP). However, milrinone is more specific for phosphodiesterase type III, which is commonly found in the heart and vascular smooth muscles.

The beneficial effects of milrinone are from the intracellular increase in cAMP, which results in two beneficial effects in a patient with heart failure: a positive inotropic response and vasodilation. For this reason, this class of drugs may also be referred to as *inodilators* (inotropics and dilators). Milrinone has a 10 to 100 times greater affinity for smooth muscle fibres surrounding pulmonary and systemic blood vessels than it does for cardiac muscle. This suggests that the primary beneficial effects of inodilators come from their vasodilating effects, which cause a reduction in the force against which the heart must pump to eject its volume of blood.

Finally, inhibition of phosphodiesterase results in the availability of more calcium for myocardial muscle contraction. This increased availability of calcium leads to an increase in the force of contraction (i.e., positive inotropic action). The increased calcium present in heart muscle is taken back up into its storage sites in the sarcoplasmic reticulum at a much faster rate than normal. As a result, the heart muscle relaxes more than normal and is also more compliant. In summary, PDIs have positive inotropic and vasodilatory effects. They may also increase heart rate in some instances and therefore may have positive chronotropic effects as well.

Indications

PDIs are primarily used in the intensive care unit setting for the short-term management of acute heart failure. The 2012 Canadian Cardiovascular Society Heart Failure Management Guidelines (McKelvie et al., 2013) do not recommend long-term infusion of PDIs. The guidelines place a high focus on the relief of dyspnea symptoms.

Contraindications

Contraindications to the use of PDIs include known drug allergy and may include the presence of severe aortic or pulmonary valvular disease and heart failure resulting from diastolic dysfunction.

Adverse Effects

The primary adverse effect seen with milrinone therapy is dysrhythmia. Milrinone-induced dysrhythmias are mainly ventricular. Ventricular dysrhythmias occur in approximately 12% of patients treated with this drug. Some other adverse effects associated with milrinone therapy are hypotension, angina (chest pain), hypokalemia, tremor, and thrombocytopenia.

Toxicity and Management of Overdose

No specific antidote exists for an overdose of milrinone. Hypotension secondary to vasodilation is the primary effect seen with excessive dosages. The recommendation is to reduce the dosage or temporarily discontinue the drug if excessive hypotension occurs. This is to be done until the patient's condition has stabilized. Initiation of general measures for circulatory support is also recommended.

Interactions

Concurrent administration of diuretics may cause significant hypovolemia and reduced cardiac filling pressure. Appropriately monitor the patient in an intensive care setting to detect and respond to these problems. Additive inotropic effects may be seen with coadministration of digoxin. Furosemide must not be injected into intravenous lines with milrinone because it will precipitate immediately.

Dosages

For dosage information, refer to the table on p. 482.

CARDIAC GLYCOSIDES

Cardiac glycosides comprise one of the oldest groups of cardiac drugs. Not only do they have beneficial effects on the failing heart, but they also help control the ventricular response to **atrial fibrillation**. They were originally obtained from either the *Digitalis purpurea* or the *Digitalis lanata* plant, both commonly known as *foxglove*. For this reason, cardiac glycosides are often referred to as *digitalis glycosides*. Cardiac glycosides were the mainstay of therapy for heart failure for more than 200 years; however, they are no longer used as first-line drugs. ACE inhibitors and diuretics are recommended as the key drugs to offer

DRUG PROFILE

▶▶*milrinone lactate*

Milrinone lactate is the only currently available PDI after the discontinuation of the production of inamrinone. Milrinone is also referred to as an *inodilator* because it exerts both a positive inotropic effect and a vasodilatory effect. Milrinone is contraindicated in cases of known drug allergy. Adverse effects include cardiac dysrhythmias, headache, hypokalemia, tremor, thrombocytopenia, and elevated liver enzyme levels. Interacting drugs include diuretics (causing additive hypotensive effects) and digoxin (causing additive inotropic effects). Milrinone is available only in injectable form. Recommended dosages are given in the table below.

PHARMACOKINETICS

Route	Onset of Action	Peak Plasma Concentration	Elimination Half-Life	Duration of Action
IV	5–15 min	1 hr	2.3 hr	1 to several hr

DOSAGES   Selected Drugs for Heart Failure

Drug	Pharmacological Class	Usual Dosage Range	Indications
▶▶digoxin (Lanoxin®)	Digitalis cardiac glycoside	*Children* Digitalizing dose: IV: 8–50 mcg/kg, divided into 3–4 doses, depending on age, from premature infant to child older than 10 yr PO: 10–60 mcg/kg, divided into 3–4 doses, depending on age, from premature infant to child older than 10 yr Usual maintenance dose: 20–35% of digitalizing dose *Adults* PO/IV: Usual digitalizing dose: 0.5–0.75 mg followed by 0.125–0.375 mg divided into 3–4 doses; usual oral maintenance dose: 0.125–0.5 mg/day	Heart failure, supraventricular dysrhythmias
▶▶milrinone lactate	Phosphodiesterase inhibitor	*Adults* IV loading dose: 50 mcg/kg IV continuous infusion dose: 0.375–0.75 mcg/kg/min	Heart failure

IV, intravenous; *PO*, oral.

---

therapeutic benefit; nevertheless, digoxin may still offer benefit in some patients (see Evidence in Practice: Digoxin Use in Heart Failure). According to The 2012 Canadian Cardiovascular Society Heart Failure Management Guidelines (McKelvie et al., 2013), digoxin is recommended for patients with normal sinus rhythm who continue to have moderate to severe symptoms, despite optimized heart failure therapy to relieve symptoms and reduce hospitalizations. Digoxin is the only cardiac glycoside currently available. Although digoxin is a powerful positive inotropic drug, it has not been shown to reduce mortality.

See Special Populations: Children for information on the use of cardiac glycosides in children with heart failure.

While the emphasis in this chapter regarding heart failure is on systolic dysfunction or inadequate ventricular contractions (systole) during the pumping of the heart, it is also important to note the less common condition of diastolic dysfunction, or inadequate ventricular filling, during ventricular relaxation (diastole). This condition is most commonly associated with left ventricular hypertrophy secondary to chronic hypertension. However, it may also result from cardiomyopathy (e.g., virus induced), pericardial disease, and diabetes. Unlike with systolic heart failure, inotropic drugs (including digoxin) and vasodilators (see Chapter 23) may not be the drugs of choice for diastolic failure. Diuretic drugs (see Chapter 29), on the other hand, are often used as part of therapy for both conditions.

Mechanism of Action and Drug Effects

The beneficial effect of digoxin is thought to be an increase in myocardial contractility, or a *positive inotropic effect*. This effect occurs secondarily to the inhibition of the sodium–potassium adenosine triphosphatase pump. When the action of this enzyme complex is inhibited, cellular sodium and calcium concentrations increase. The overall result is enhanced myocardial contractility. Digoxin also augments cholinergic stimulation via the vagus nerve of the parasympathetic nervous system. This effect is more commonly referred to as *vagal tone* and results in increased diastolic filling between heartbeats secondary to reduced heart rate. Vagal tone is also believed to sensitize cardiac baroreceptors, which reduces sympathetic stimulation from the central nervous system (CNS). All of these processes further enhance cardiac efficiency and output.

Digoxin changes the electrical conduction properties of the heart, and this change markedly affects the conduction system and cardiac automaticity. Digoxin decreases

EVIDENCE IN PRACTICE

Digoxin Use in Heart Failure

Background

Heart failure is a major public health problem in Canada and other developed countries. Digoxin was long established as a positive inotrope in heart failure and for its negative chronotropic activity in atrial fibrillation; however, the use of digoxin has declined recently, possibly over concerns about safety after the publication of observational studies reporting increased mortality with its use. The Digitalis Investigation Group (DIG) trial, conducted in 2006, was a multicentre randomized, double-blind, placebo-controlled trial conducted in Canada and the United States that evaluated the effects of digoxin on all-cause mortality and on hospitalization for heart failure in patients with heart failure. The DIG trial study was the largest randomized controlled trial of digoxin in heart failure and showed neutral effects on overall mortality and a reduction in admissions to hospital compared with placebo, as well as a decrease in mortality among those with low serum digoxin concentrations.

Type of Evidence

In order to clarify the concerns over the impact of digoxin on death and clinical outcomes, the authors conducted a systematic review and meta-analysis of observational and controlled trial data. A total of 52 studies published between 1960 and 2014 were reviewed, comprising a total of 621 845 patients.

The researchers assessed the safety and efficacy of digoxin by comprehensively meta-analyzing all available observational and experimental studies. The hypothesis was that study design would have a significant impact on the observed mortality associated with digoxin (Ziff, Lane, & Samra, 2015).

Results of Study

Overall, the researchers established that in studies with sound methodology and low risk of bias, there was a neutral association of digoxin with cardiovascular death. However, for all study types, digoxin led to a small but significant reduction in all-cause hospital admission.

Link of Evidence to Nursing Practice

Heart failure is the most common cause of cardiovascular hospital admission. Digoxin has been available for over 200 years and is widely used. The implementation of evidence-informed therapy for heart failure management is clinically efficacious. However, there is still uncertainty surrounding the appropriateness of its role and its value in treating patients with heart failure. The 2012 Canadian Cardiovascular Society Heart Failure Management Guidelines Update: Focus on Acute and Chronic Heart Failure (2013) strongly recommend the use of digoxin in patients in normal sinus rhythm who continue to have moderate to severe symptoms of chronic heart failure, despite optimized heart failure therapy to relieve symptoms and reduce hospitalizations. This recommendation is made with the understanding that the use of digoxin remains controversial in the literature. Nurses should be informed of current evidence to support management of heart failure but also be familiar with potential pitfalls.

Sources: Ahmed, A., Rich, M. W., Love, T. E., et al. (2006). Digoxin and reduction in mortality and hospitalization in heart failure: A comprehensive *post hoc* analysis of the DIG trial. *European Heart Journal, 27*(2), 178–186 doi:10.1093/eurheartj/ehi687; McKelvie, R. S., Moe, G. W., Ezekowitz, J. A., et al. (2013). The 2012 Canadian Cardiovascular Society Heart Failure Management Guidelines Update: Focus on acute and chronic heart failure. *Canadian Journal of Cardiology, 29*(2), 168–181. doi:10.1016/j.cjca.2012.10.007; Ziff, O. J., Lane, D. A., Samra, M., et al. (2015). Safety and efficacy of digoxin: Systematic review and meta-analysis of observational and controlled trial data. *The BMJ, 351*, h4451. doi:10.1136/bmj.h4451

SPECIAL POPULATIONS: CHILDREN

Heart Failure

- The causes, symptoms, treatments, and prognoses of heart failure in children vary depending on age. In infants, the cause of heart failure is generally congenital heart defects or other structural problems. In older children, the structure of the heart may be normal but the heart muscle may be weakened. Symptoms of heart failure differ depending on age and become worse with age because the heart must keep up with increased oxygen demands and energy demands with increased growth.
- Symptoms in infants and young children may include poor growth, difficulty in feeding (reflux, vomiting, feeding refusal), diaphoresis, pallor, and tachypnea; in older children, they include fatigue, inability to tolerate exercise and other activities, the need to rest often, dyspnea with minimal exertion, abdominal pain, orthopnea, nausea, and vomiting.
- Treatment is generally age- and cause-specific. For septal defects, surgery or medication may be indicated. For more complex problems, surgery may be needed within the first few weeks of life.

- Drug therapy may include furosemide (a loop diuretic) and a thiazide diuretic if required, ACE inhibitors, β-blockers, and sometimes digoxin to improve heart pumping efficiency.
- Correct calculation of dosages for any of the medications used is important for safe and cautious nursing care. A one-decimal-point placement error will result in a 10-fold dosage error, which could be fatal.
- Digoxin toxicity is manifested in children by nausea, vomiting, bradycardia, anorexia, and dysrhythmias.
- The health care provider needs to be notified immediately if any of the following develop or worsen: fatigue, sudden weight gain (1 kg or more in 24 hours), palpitations, tachycardia or bradycardia, or respiratory distress.

Source: Kantor, P. F., Lougheed, J., Dancea, A., et al. (2013). Presentation, diagnosis, and medical management of heart failure in children: Canadian Cardiovascular Society Guidelines. *Canadian Journal of Cardiology, 29*(12), 1535–1552. doi:10.1016/j.cjca.2013.08.008

the velocity (rate) of electrical conduction and prolongs the **refractory period** in the conduction system. The particular site in the conduction system where this occurs is the area between the atria and the ventricles (SA node to AV node). The cardiac cells remain in a state of depolarization for a longer period and are unable to start another electrical impulse, which also reduces heart rate and improves cardiac efficiency.

The following is a summary of the inotropic, chronotropic, dromotropic, and other effects produced by digoxin:

- A positive inotropic effect—an increase in the force and velocity of myocardial contraction without a corresponding increase in oxygen consumption
- A negative chronotropic effect—reduced heart rate
- A negative dromotropic effect—decreased automaticity at the SA node, decreased AV nodal conduction, reduced conductivity at the bundle of His, and prolongation of the atrial and ventricular refractory periods
- An increase in stroke volume
- A reduction in heart size during diastole
- A decrease in venous blood pressure and vein engorgement
- An increase in coronary circulation
- Promotion of tissue perfusion and diuresis as a result of improved blood circulation
- Decrease in exertional and paroxysmal nocturnal dyspnea, cough, and cyanosis
- Improved symptom control, quality of life, and exercise tolerance, but no apparent reduction in mortality

Indications

Digoxin is primarily used in the treatment of systolic heart failure and atrial fibrillation. However, the latest heart failure treatment guidelines recommend that it be used as an adjunct to drugs of other classes, including β-blockers, diuretics, ACE inhibitors, and ARBs.

Contraindications

Contraindications to the use of digoxin include known drug allergy and may include second- or third-degree heart block, atrial fibrillation, ventricular tachycardia or fibrillation, heart failure resulting from diastolic dysfunction, and subaortic stenosis (obstruction in the left ventricle below the aortic valve) and should be used with caution in those with reduced kidney function. However, digoxin may be used to treat some of these conditions, if recommended by a cardiologist, depending on the given clinical situation.

Adverse Effects

The common undesirable effects associated with digoxin use are cardiovascular, CNS, ocular, and gastrointestinal (GI) effects. These are outlined in Table 25-1.

Toxicity and Management of Overdose

Digoxin has a low therapeutic index (see Chapter 2). Digoxin levels are monitored when the patient first starts taking the drug. However, monitoring of digoxin

TABLE 25-1

Digoxin: Common Adverse Effects

Body System	Adverse Effect
Cardiovascular	Bradycardia, tachycardia, hypotension
Central nervous	Headache*, fatigue, confusion*, convulsions
Eye	Coloured vision (i.e., green, yellow, or purple)*, halo vision*
Gastrointestinal	Anorexia*, nausea*, vomiting*, diarrhea

*These are symptoms of toxicity.

levels after the drug reaches a steady state is usually necessary only if there is suspicion of toxicity, nonadherence, or deteriorating kidney function. Normal therapeutic levels for digoxin are 0.8 to 2 ng/mL although lower target levels (0.5–0.9 ng/mL) are recommended by the 2013 ACCF/AHA guidelines for the management of heart failure. Low potassium or magnesium levels may increase the potential for digoxin toxicity. Therefore, frequent monitoring of serum electrolytes is also important. A decrease in kidney function is also a common cause of digoxin toxicity because digoxin is excreted almost exclusively via the kidneys. Signs and symptoms of digoxin toxicity include bradycardia, headache, dizziness, confusion, nausea, and visual disturbances (blurred vision or yellow vision). With toxicity, electrocardiogram (ECG) findings may include heart block, atrial tachycardia with block, or ventricular dysrhythmias. Predisposing factors to digoxin toxicity are listed in Table 25-2.

Treatment strategies for digoxin toxicity depend on the severity of the symptoms. These strategies can range from simply withholding the next dose to instituting more aggressive therapies. The steps usually taken in the management of digoxin toxicity are listed in Table 25-3.

When significant toxicity develops as a result of digoxin therapy, the administration of digoxin immune Fab may be indicated. Digoxin immune Fab is an antibody that recognizes digoxin as an antigen and forms an antigen–antibody complex with the drug, thus inactivating the free digoxin. Digoxin immune Fab therapy is not indicated for every patient who is showing signs of digoxin toxicity. The following are the clinical situations in which its use may be indicated:

- Hyperkalemia (a serum potassium level higher than 5 nmoL/L) in a patient with digoxin toxicity
- Life-threatening cardiac dysrhythmias, sustained ventricular tachycardia or fibrillation, and severe sinus bradycardia or heart block unresponsive to atropine treatment or cardiac pacing
- Life-threatening digoxin overdose—more than 10 mg of digoxin in adults; more than 4 mg of digoxin in children

TABLE 25-2

Conditions Predisposing to Digitalis Toxicity

Condition/Disease	Significance
Use of cardiac pacemaker	A patient with this device may exhibit digoxin toxicity at lower dosages than usual.
Hypokalemia	The patient's risk of serious dysrhythmias is increased, and the patient is more susceptible to digoxin toxicity.
Hypercalcemia	The patient is at higher risk of experiencing sinus bradycardia, dysrhythmias, and heart block.
Atrioventricular block	Heart block may worsen with increasing levels of digoxin.
Dysrhythmias	Dysrhythmias may occur that did not exist before digoxin use and thus could be related to digoxin toxicity.
Hypothyroidism, respiratory, or kidney disease	Patients with these disorders require lower dosages because they cause delayed kidney drug excretion.
Advanced age	Because of decreased kidney function and the resultant diminished drug excretion, along with decreased body mass in this patient population, a lower dosage than usual is needed to prevent toxicity. The practice of polypharmacy may also lead to toxicity.
Ventricular fibrillation	Ventricular rate may actually increase with digoxin use.

Interactions

A wide variety of significant drug interactions are possible with digoxin. Common examples are provided in Table 25-4. The most important drug–drug interactions occurring with digoxin are interactions with amiodarone hydrochloride, quinidine sulfate, and verapamil hydrochloride. These three drugs can increase digoxin levels by 50%. When large amounts of bran are ingested, the absorption of oral digoxin may be decreased. Certain natural health products may interact with digoxin. For example, ginseng may increase digoxin levels, hawthorn may potentiate the effects of digoxin, licorice may increase the risk of cardiac toxicity due to potassium loss, and St. John's wort may reduce digoxin levels. Drugs that lower serum potassium or magnesium levels can predispose patients to digoxin toxicity.

Dosages

For dosage information, refer to the table on p. 482. Also refer to the Preventing Medication Errors: The Importance of Decimal Points.

TABLE 25-3

Digoxin Toxicity: Step-by-Step Management

Step	Instructions
1	Discontinue (hold) administration of the drug, take vital signs, assess for toxicity, and contact the health care provider.
2	Begin continuous electrocardiographic monitoring for cardiac dysrhythmias; administer any appropriate antidysrhythmic drugs, as ordered.
3	Determine serum digoxin and electrolyte levels.
4	Administer potassium supplements for hypokalemia if indicated, as ordered.
5	Institute supportive therapy for GI symptoms (nausea, vomiting, or diarrhea).
6	Administer digoxin antidote (i.e., digoxin immune Fab) if indicated, as ordered.

GI, gastrointestinal.

TABLE 25-4

Cardiac Glycosides: Drug Interactions

Interacting Drug	Mechanisms	Result
Antidysrhythmics calcium (parenteral) cholestyramine colestipol sucralfate	Increase cardiac irritability Decrease oral absorption	Increased digoxin toxicity Reduced therapeutic effect
β-blockers Calcium channel blockers	Block β_1-receptors in heart Block calcium channels in myocardium	Enhanced bradycardic effect of digoxin Enhanced bradycardic and negative inotropic effects of digoxin
quinidine, verapamil, amiodarone, dronedarone ciclosporin Azole antifungals	Decrease clearance	Digoxin levels increased by 50%; digoxin dose should be reduced by 50%

PREVENTING MEDICATION ERRORS

The Importance of Decimal Points

Incorrect decimal placement can be lethal when calculating digoxin dosages. According to the Institute for Safe Medication Practices Canada (ISMP Canada), trailing zeros are *not* be used after decimal points. This is extremely important in the case of digoxin, since when a 1 mg dose is ordered and written as "1.0 mg," the order could be misread as "10 mg," and the patient would receive 10 times the ordered dose.

ISMP Canada also recommends that leading zeroes be used if a dose is less than a whole number. For example, ".25 mg" can look like "25 mg," resulting in a dose that is 100 times the ordered dose. Rather, the order should be written as "0.25 mg" to avoid errors.

Of course, such an error hopefully would be caught when the nurse realizes how many 250-mcg digoxin tablets it would take to give a 25-mg dose, or how many millilitres would be needed for an intravenous dose. However, such errors have occurred. Consider what would happen if a digoxin overdose led to digoxin toxicity and the serious effect this would have on the patient.

For more information, visit www.ismp-canada.org/download/caccn/CACCN-Fall05.pdf

DRUG PROFILES

▶▶ *digoxin*

Digoxin (Lanoxin) is indicated for the treatment of both heart failure and atrial fibrillation and flutter. Digoxin use is contraindicated in patients who have shown a hypersensitivity to it and in those with ventricular tachycardia or fibrillation. Normal therapeutic drug levels of digoxin should be between 0.5 and 1 ng/mL levels higher than 2.4 ng/mL often precipitates manifestations of toxicity. However, levels higher than 0.8–1.5 ng/mL is the traget for the treatment of atrial fibrillation. Because of digoxin's long duration of action and half-life, a loading, or *digitalizing*, dose is often given to bring serum levels of the drug up to a desirable therapeutic level more quickly. For recommended digitalizing doses and the daily oral and intravenous adult and pediatric dosages, refer to the table on p. 482.

PHARMACOKINETICS

Route	Onset of Action	Peak Plasma Concentration	Elimination Half-Life	Duration of Action
PO	1–2 hr	2–8 hr	35–48 hr	3–4 days
IV	5–30 min	1–4 hr	35–48 hr	3–4 days

digoxin immune Fab

Digoxin immune Fab (Digifab®) is the antidote for severe digoxin overdose and is indicated for the reversal of such life-threatening cardiotoxic effects as severe bradycardia, advanced heart block, ventricular tachycardia or fibrillation, and severe hyperkalemia. It has a unique mechanism of action. Use of digoxin immune Fab is contraindicated in patients who have known hypersensitivity to it. It is available only in parenteral form. It is dosed on the basis of the patient's serum digoxin level in conjunction with the patient's weight. The recommended dosages vary according to the amount of digoxin ingested. One vial binds 0.5 mg of digoxin. For recommended dosages, the nurse should consult the manufacturer's latest dosage recommendations. It is important to remember that after digoxin immune Fab is given, all subsequent measures of serum digoxin levels will be elevated for days to weeks. Therefore, after its administration, the clinical signs and symptoms of digoxin toxicity, rather than the serum digoxin levels, should be the primary focus in monitoring for the effectiveness of reversal therapy. Digoxin immune Fab is made from immunoglobulin fragments from sheep immunized with a digoxin derivative. Because papain is used to cleave the antibody into the Fab fragments, individuals who are allergic to papaya, papain, or sheep protein need to be monitored for anaphylactic shock.

PHARMACOKINETICS

Route	Onset of Action	Peak Plasma Concentration	Elimination Half-Life	Duration of Action
IV	Immediate	Immediate	14–20 hr	Days to weeks

NURSING PROCESS

 Assessment

Before a drug used to treat heart failure is administered, perform a thorough assessment, including the patient's medical history, drug allergies, and family medical history, with emphasis on any history of cardiac, hypertensive, or kidney diseases. The nurse's review may yield findings that either dictate cautious use of the drug or represent contraindications to its use. Assess the following clinical parameters and other data:

- Blood pressure
- Pulse rate—both apical and radial, measured for 1 full minute
- Peripheral pulse location and grading of strength
- Capillary refill
- Presence or absence of edema
- Heart sounds

- Breath sounds
- Weight
- Intake and output amounts
- Serum laboratory values such as potassium, sodium, magnesium, and calcium levels
- Electrocardiogram
- Results of kidney function tests, including urea nitrogen and creatinine levels
- Results of liver function tests, such as levels of aspartate aminotransferase, alanine aminotransferase, creatine phosphokinase, lactate dehydrogenase, and alkaline phosphatase
- Medication history and profile, including all prescription drugs, over-the-counter drugs, and natural health products (e.g., Siberian ginseng may increase digoxin drug levels; consumption of large amounts of bran with digoxin will decrease the drug's absorption)
- Dietary habits and all meals and snacks consumed over the previous 24 hours
- Smoking history
- Alcohol intake

ACE inhibitors, such as lisinopril, require thorough assessment of cautions, contraindications, and drug interactions (see Chapter 23). Hyperkalemia is an adverse effect; therefore, perform an assessment of serum potassium before giving these drugs and use caution when administering potassium supplementation or potassium-sparing diuretics. Assess respiratory history, specifically any previous problems of cough. ACE inhibitors may cause a dry cough, which is not harmful but may be annoying. Patients may be switched to an ARB, such as valsartan (see Chapter 23), if the cough becomes problematic for them.

As mentioned earlier, metoprolol tartrate is the β-blocker most commonly used to treat heart failure. Carvedilol also has many therapeutic effects, as does bisoprolol (see Chapter 20), and is commonly added to existing regimens of furosemide (loop diuretic) and ACE inhibitors in the management of heart failure. Related assessment information for α- and β-blocking drugs may be found in Chapter 20. Dobutamine hydrochloride, a β₁-selective adrenergic, is also used to treat heart failure and is discussed further in Chapter 19. The status of the patient's veins is important to assess when this drug is indicated because it is given only intravenously.

Aldosterone antagonists, such as spironolactone and eplerenone, require close assessment of heart and breath sounds as well as assessment for the occurrence of edema, which is a known adverse effect (see Chapter 23 for more information). Hydralazine (discussed further in Chapter 23) combined with isosorbide dinitrate is used mainly in patients who are Black.

With any medication regimen, it is always important to assess support systems at home because safe and effective therapy depends on close observation, monitoring of appropriate parameters (e.g., daily weight), attention to patient concerns, and evaluation of how the patient is feeling and functioning. With milrinone, a PDI, closely monitor cardiac status, which is crucial to patient safety. Patients who are administered this drug are usually in a critical care setting and require frequent assessment of heart sounds, vital signs, and any evidence of ventricular dysrhythmias on ECG readings. Assess also for any history of angina, hypotension, and hypokalemia, which may all be exacerbated with this drug. Significant drug interactions for which to assess include parenteral furosemide, which will precipitate immediately if milrinone is present in intravenous lines.

Before giving digoxin, closely monitor serum electrolytes. Calcium levels should be checked as calcium is required for cardiac contractility. Specifically, assess potassium levels because low levels or hypokalemia may precipitate digoxin toxicity. Hypokalemia is manifested by muscle weakness, confusion, lethargy, anorexia, nausea, and changes in ECG readings. Low levels of magnesium, or hypomagnesemia, may also precipitate digoxin toxicity. Hypomagnesemia is manifested by agitation, twitching, hyperactive reflexes, nausea, vomiting, and changes in ECG readings. Also closely assess digoxin levels once the drug has been administered because of its narrow therapeutic index (see Chapter 2). Measure and document baseline weight as well. Perform a careful assessment of the following systems: (1) Neurological system—Note any history of headaches, fatigue, confusion, or convulsions; assess level of alertness and orientation; (2) GI system—Document any changes in appetite (e.g., decrease) or reports of diarrhea, nausea, or vomiting; (3) Cardiac system—Note any pulse rate lower than 60 beats per minute or greater than 100 beats per minute, hypotension, abnormal heart sounds, abnormal ECG findings (if this test is ordered), and any history of irregularities; and (4) Visual and sensory systems—Document baseline vision as well as any changes in vision, such as green, yellow, or purple halos surrounding the peripheral field of vision. See Table 25-1 for more information on adverse effects of digoxin. Also assess for any cautions, contraindications, and drug interactions (see Table 25-2).

Nursing Diagnoses

- Ineffective peripheral tissue perfusion related to the pathophysiological influence of heart failure
- Deficient knowledge related to lack of information and experience with heart failure as well as first-time use of drugs indicated for heart failure
- Nonadherence with therapy regimen related to lack of information about the disease process as well as the drug(s) and adverse effects

Planning

Goals

- Patient will exhibit improved cardiac output with improved tissue perfusion once therapy is initiated.

- Patient will state use, action, adverse effects, and toxic effects of therapy.
- Patient will remain adherent to drug therapy regimen.

Outcome Criteria

- Patient experiences improved to strong peripheral pulses; pink, warm extremities; and an improved ability to carry out activities of daily living (ADLs).
- Patient demonstrates sufficient knowledge about disease process related to heart failure, stating the importance of the need for lifelong therapy, constant monitoring by the health care provider, energy conservation, and other measures to minimize oxygen demands.
  - Patient demonstrates proper technique for measuring radial pulse for 1 full minute before taking medication.
  - Patient states the most common adverse effects to expect with digoxin therapy, such as bradycardia or tachycardia (pulse rate lower than 60 beats per minute or greater than 100 beats per minute as indicated by the health care provider), headache, fatigue, confusion, halo vision, anorexia, nausea, and vomiting.
  - Patient states the importance of reporting to the health care provider any symptoms that are indicative of digoxin toxicity, specifically anorexia, nausea, vomiting, and loss of appetite.
- Patient's adherence to therapy results in improved heart function with subsequent heart rate greater than 60 beats per minute and lower than 100 beats per minute, with regular rhythm.
  - Patient reports improved ability to perform ADLs with minimal dyspnea and increased energy levels.
  - Patient reports taking medication consistently, at the same time every day, and recording daily weights.
  - Patient remains free from exacerbations of heart failure and states no severe adverse effects while taking medication exactly as ordered.

Implementation

Nursing interventions associated with the use of ACE inhibitors, ARBs, β-blockers, and adrenergic drugs are discussed further in Chapters 19, 20, and 23. Hydralazine and isosorbide dinitrate must also be used with extreme caution because of associated syncope. If syncope occurs, the drug will most likely be discontinued. Monitor blood pressure and other vital signs, especially with the first few doses of hydralazine and isosorbide dinitrate (because of the risk of syncope). Drug interactions, cautions, and contraindications have been previously discussed.

Always check for compatibility of solutions when giving the PDI milrinone. Record intake and output, heart rate, blood pressure, weight (daily), and respiration rate, as well as heart and breath sounds. Report any evidence of hypokalemia to the prescriber immediately, and monitor the patient's vital signs closely. When heart failure drugs such as digoxin, milrinone, and digoxin immune Fab are administered parenterally, use an infusion pump unless the order is to administer them as an intravenous push.

Before administering any dose of the cardiac glycoside digoxin, check serum potassium and magnesium levels to make sure they are within normal limits, to prevent toxicity. *Always* measure the patient's apical pulse rate (auscultate the apical heart rate, found at the apical impulse located at the left midclavicular, fifth intercostal space) for 1 full minute. If the pulse rate is 60 beats per minute or lower, or if it is greater than 100 beats per minute, generally the nurse will withhold the dose and notify the health care provider of the problem immediately. Although withholding the dose is usually indicated, health care facilities and health care providers often have their own protocols that apply to individual patients. In addition, contact the health care provider if a patient experiences any of the following signs and symptoms of digoxin toxicity: headache, dizziness, confusion, nausea, or visual disturbances (blurred vision or yellow–green halo). ECG findings in a patient with digoxin toxicity would show heart block, atrial tachycardia with block, or ventricular dysrhythmias. Remember that most institutions and nursing units follow protocols or policies on digoxin and its administration.

Other nursing interventions include checking the dosage form, prescribed amounts, and the health care provider's order carefully to make sure that the correct drug dosage ordered has been dispensed (e.g., 0.0625, 0.125, or 0.25 mg). Oral digoxin may be administered with meals but not with foods high in fibre (e.g., bran) because the fibre will bind to the digoxin and lead to altered absorption and bioavailability of the drug. If the medication is to be given intravenously, it is critical to patient safety that it be infused undiluted at approximately 0.25 mg per minute, over longer than a 5-minute period, or as per hospital protocol. Digoxin is incompatible with many other medications in solution or syringe; therefore, double-check compatibility before administering parenterally.

Consider the interventions for patients undergoing digitalization separately from those related to other drugs. Digitalization for the management of heart failure is often done in critical care units because cardiac monitoring is required. Rapid digitalization (to achieve faster onset of action) is generally reserved for patients with heart failure who are in acute distress. Such patients are hospitalized because digoxin toxicities can appear quickly in this setting and are directly correlated with the high drug concentrations used. If a patient undergoing rapid digitalization exhibits any of the manifestations of toxicity, contact the health care provider immediately. Continuously observe such patients, taking frequent measurements of vital signs and serum drug and potassium levels. Slow digitalization (rarely used) is generally performed on an outpatient basis in patients with heart failure who are not in acute distress. In such a situation, it takes longer for toxic effects to appear (depending on the drug's half-life) than with rapid digitalization. The main advantages of slow digitalization are that it can be performed on an outpatient basis, oral dosage forms can be used, and it is safer than rapid digitalization. The disadvantages are that it takes longer for therapeutic effects to occur, and the symptoms of toxicity are more gradual in onset and therefore more insidious.

If toxicity occurs and digoxin rises to a life-threatening level, administer the antidote, digoxin immune Fab, as ordered. It is given parenterally over 30 minutes, and in some scenarios as an intravenous bolus (e.g., if cardiac arrest is imminent). All vials of the drug should be refrigerated. The drug is stable for 4 hours after being mixed; use it immediately or discard if it is not used within 4 hours. One vial of digoxin immune Fab binds 0.5 mg of digoxin. Check compatible solutions for dilution prior to infusion of the antidote. Closely monitor blood pressure, apical pulse rate and rhythm, ECG, and serum potassium levels, and record findings. Document baseline data and begin to observe closely for changes in assessment findings, such as changes in muscle strength, occurrences of tremor and muscle cramping, changes in mental health status, and irregular heart rhythms (from hypokalemia), as well as confusion, thirst, and cold clammy skin (from hyponatremia). If the treatment does reduce the toxicity, these problems will decrease considerably, compared with the patient's baseline.

Evaluation

Monitoring patients after the administration of drugs to improve heart contractility is critical for identifying therapeutic effects and adverse effects. Because positive inotropic drugs increase the force of myocardial contractility; alter electrophysiological properties, leading to a decrease in heart rate (negative chronotropic effect); and decrease AV node conduction properties (negative dromotropic effect), their therapeutic effects include the following:

* Increased urinary output
* Decreased edema
* Decreased dyspnea and crackles
* Decreased fatigue
* Resolution of paroxysmal nocturnal dyspnea
* Improved peripheral pulses, skin colour, and temperature

For patients taking lisinopril, valsartan, metoprolol, dobutamine hydrochloride, or hydralazine and isosorbide dinitrate, therapeutic effects include improvement in symptoms of heart failure and improved cardiac function. During therapy, evaluation must include monitoring for the adverse effects of these medications, which have been discussed previously in the pharmacology section.

Therapeutic effects of milrinone include an improvement in heart function with a corresponding alleviation of the patient's heart failure. Monitor for the adverse effects of hypotension, dysrhythmia, headache, ventricular fibrillation, chest pain, and hypokalemia. Evaluate patients taking milrinone for significant hypotension.

CASE STUDY

Phosphodiesterase Inhibitor for Heart Failure

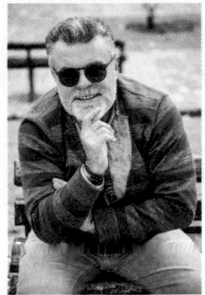

Devon, a 58-year-old retired bus driver, has been in the hospital for a week for treatment of heart failure. He had a myocardial infarction a year ago and tells the nurse that he "hasn't felt well for weeks." He is currently receiving carvedilol, lisinopril, furosemide, and potassium supplements (all orally), but he has had little improvement.

Today during morning rounds, the nurse notes that Devon is having increased difficulty with breathing, and his heart rate is up to 120 beats per minute. His weight has increased from 72 to 76 kg overnight, and his lower legs and ankles show edema rated as 3+. Crackles are heard over both lungs, and his pulse oximetry reading is 91% (down from 98% earlier). In addition, Devon is very restless. Oxygen is started, a Foley catheter is inserted, and Devon is transferred to the intensive care unit.

After examining Devon, the health care provider writes new medication orders as follows:
Change furosemide to 60 mg intravenously twice a day
Continue carvedilol and lisinopril
Start an infusion of milrinone as follows:
Loading dose: 50 mcg/kg over 10 minutes, followed by an infusion of 0.5 mcg/kg/min

1. Describe the drug effects of the medications Devon is receiving for his heart failure.
2. What laboratory values will you need to monitor while Devon is receiving the milrinone?
3. Identify the potential problem.
4. Are there any additional concerns? What will the nurse need to do at this point?
5. In addition to being given education regarding his medications, what should Devon be taught to monitor while recovering at home?

For answers, see http://evolve.elsevier.com/Canada/Lilley/pharmacology/.

If hypotension occurs, contact the health care provider, and discontinue the infusion or decrease the rate while waiting to hear from the health care provider.

While monitoring for the therapeutic effects of digoxin, assess patients for the development of toxicity because of the drug's low therapeutic index. Toxic effects associated with digoxin may include nausea, vomiting, and anorexia. Monitoring laboratory values such as serum creatinine, potassium, calcium, sodium, and chloride levels—as well as watching the serum levels of digoxin (normal levels between 0.8 and 2 ng/mL)—is important to ensure safe and efficacious treatment.

PATIENT TEACHING TIPS

❖ Hydralazine and isosorbide dinitrate combination may cause syncope; this needs to be explained to patients, along with instructions to change positions carefully.

❖ Instruct patients to take their radial pulse rate before each dose of digoxin or as indicated. Daily weights are important and need to be measured at the same time every morning and with the same amount of clothing. For older adults and for patients with cognitive impairments or complex physical disabilities, it is important that home health care personnel or a hospital-based heart failure clinic supervise the medication regimen. This is important because these individuals are at risk for adverse effects, toxicity, and drug interactions. If the pulse rate is lower than 60 beats per minute or is erratic; if the pulse rate is 120 beats per minute or greater; or if there is anorexia, nausea, or vomiting, the health care provider must be contacted. Emphasize to patients the importance of reporting any palpitations or feelings that the heart is racing, changes in heart rate or irregular heart rate, the occurrence of dizziness or fainting, any changes in visions, or weight gain (1 kg or more in 24 hours or 2 kg or more in 1 week).

❖ Advise patients to keep a daily journal with notation of medications, daily weights, dietary intake and appetite, any adverse effects or changes in condition, and a daily rating of how they are feeling.

❖ Instruct patients to wear a medical alert bracelet or necklace, as well as to keep a current medication and medical history that lists allergies, medical diagnoses, and medications (in either written or electronic form) and have it available at all times. This information needs to be updated frequently or with each visit to a health care provider.

❖ Digoxin is usually taken once a day. Encourage patients to take it at the same time every day. If a dose is missed, they may take the omitted dose if no more than 12 hours have passed from the time the drug was to have been taken. Instruct patients that if more than 12 hours have passed since the missed dose, they should not skip that dose, *not* double up on the next digoxin dose, and contact the health care provider immediately for further instructions.

❖ Instruct patients to *never* abruptly cease taking any of the medications being taken for heart failure. If problems occur, advise patients to always contact their health care provider.

❖ If potassium-depleting diuretics are being taken as part of therapy, encourage patients to consume foods high in potassium and to report any weakness, fatigue, or lethargy. In addition, any worsening of dizziness or dyspnea, or the occurrence of any unusual problems, should be reported immediately.

❖ With medication regimens for heart failure, most patients are encouraged to avoid using antacids or eating ice cream, milk products, yogourt, cheese, or bran for 2 hours before or 2 hours after taking medication, to avoid interference with the absorption of the oral dosage forms of these medications.

KEY POINTS

❖ Inotropic drugs affect the force of myocardial contraction; positive inotropics (e.g., digoxin) increase the force of contractions, and negative inotropics (e.g., β-blockers) decrease myocardial contractility. Chronotropics affect heart rate, with positive chronotropics increasing heart rate and negative chronotropics decreasing heart rate. Dromotropic drugs affect the conduction of electrical impulses through the heart; positive dromotropic drugs increase the speed of electrical impulses through the heart, whereas negative dromotropic drugs have the opposite effect.

❖ Know the protocol for heart failure management because digoxin, once the cornerstone of treatment for heart failure, is now used only after all other recommended drugs have been tried. The 2012 Canadian Cardiovascular Society Heart Failure Management Guidelines Update: Focus on Acute and Chronic Heart Failure (2013) provides protocol guidelines for treatment of heart failure, including the following: Drugs of choice to initiate treatment are the ACE inhibitors (e.g., lisinopril, enalapril, captopril) or the ARBs (valsartan, candesartan, losartan) and β-blockers (e.g., metoprolol, a cardioselective β-blocker; carvedilol, a nonspecific β-blocker). The loop diuretics (e.g., furosemide) are used to reduce the symptoms of heart failure secondary to fluid overload, and the aldosterone inhibitors (e.g., spironolactone, eplerenone) are added as the heart failure progresses. Only after these drugs are used is digoxin added. Hydralazine and isosorbide dinitrate in combination are approved for use particularly in patients who are Black. Supplementation with omega-3 polyunsaturated fatty acids is also recommended.

KEY POINTS—cont'd

❖ Be aware of important physiological concepts such as ejection fraction. A patient's ejection fraction reflects the contractility of the heart and is approximately 65% (0.65) in a normal heart. This value decreases as heart failure progresses; therefore, patients with heart failure have low ejection fractions because their hearts are failing to pump effectively.

❖ Recognize that hypotension, dysrhythmias, and thrombocytopenia are major adverse effects of milrinone use.

❖ Keep informed of the contraindications to the use of digoxin, which include a history of allergy to the digitalis medications, ventricular tachycardia and fibrillations, and AV block.

EXAMINATION REVIEW QUESTIONS

1. When teaching a patient about the signs and symptoms of cardiac glycoside toxicity, the nurse should alert the patient to watch for which of the following?
   a. Visual changes such as photophobia
   b. Flickering lights or halos around lights
   c. Dizziness when standing up
   d. Increased urine output

2. During assessment of a patient who is receiving digoxin, which findings would indicate an increased possibility of toxicity?
   a. Apical pulse rate of 62 beats/min
   b. Digoxin level of 1.5 ng/mL
   c. Serum potassium level of 2 mmol/L
   d. Serum calcium level of 4.8 mmol/L

3. When monitoring a patient receiving an intravenous infusion of milrinone, which adverse effect will the nurse look for?
   a. Anemia
   b. Proteinuria
   c. Thrombocytopenia
   d. Decreased blood urea nitrogen and creatinine levels

4. A patient is taking a β-blocker as part of the treatment plan for heart failure. The nurse knows that the purpose of the β-blocker for this patient is to do which of the following?
   a. Increase urine output
   b. Prevent stimulation of the heart by catecholamines
   c. Increase the contractility of the heart muscle
   d. Cause peripheral vasodilation

5. The nurse is assessing a patient who is receiving a milrinone infusion and checks the patient's cardiac rhythm on the heart monitor. What adverse cardiac effect is most likely to occur in a patient who is receiving intravenous milrinone?
   a. Tachycardia
   b. Bradycardia
   c. Atrial fibrillation
   d. Ventricular dysrhythmia

6. The nurse is administering an intravenous infusion of a phosphodiesterase inhibitor to a patient with heart failure. The nurse will evaluate the patient for which therapeutic effects? (Select all that apply.)
   a. Positive inotropic effects
   b. Vasodilation
   c. Decreased heart rate
   d. Increased blood pressure
   e. Positive chronotropic effects

7. The medication order for a 5-year-old child is to: "Give digoxin elixir, 15 mcg/kg, PO now." The child weighs 20 kg. How many milligrams will this child receive?

Answers: 1. b, **2.** c, **3.** c, **4.** b, **5.** d, **6.** a, b, e, **7.** 0.3 mg

CRITICAL THINKING ACTIVITIES

1. A nurse administered 125 mg of digoxin instead of 0.125 mg intravenously. The patient has developed a severe heart block dysrhythmia, and the slow heart rate has not responded to administration of atropine and other measures. The nurse stays with the patient while the charge nurse notifies the health care provider. What will be the priority in this situation? What will the nurse expect to give next? How could this situation have been prevented?

2. A nurse is making morning medication rounds. One patient, a 78-year-old-man, states that he has been nauseated and without an appetite and has experienced some diarrhea. He has been taking digoxin for the past few weeks for the treatment of recently diagnosed heart failure. What is the nurse's priority action? Explain your answer.

3. A patient is receiving an ACE inhibitor, a diuretic, and a β-blocker as treatment for mild heart failure. He has a history of hypothyroidism—which is controlled by thyroid replacement hormones—and chronic bronchitis. He states that he stopped smoking a year ago, after smoking two packs of cigarettes a day for 30 years. This morning, he reported a dry cough but said he does not feel short of breath, even when getting up to go to the bathroom. He is unable to produce any sputum. When the nurse listens to his lungs, his breath sounds are clear except for a few scattered rhonchi bilaterally. His weight is the same as the previous morning, and his ankles show only trace edema (2 days ago, he had 2+ edema on the edema scale). His temperature is 36.9°C (98.4°F), his pulse is 88 beats per minute, and his blood pressure is 124/86 mm Hg. He says to the nurse, "This cough is awful! I am so afraid that my heart failure is getting worse or that I'm getting pneumonia!" What is the nurse's priority action?

For answers, see http://evolve.elsevier.com/Canada/Lilley/pharmacology/.

Antidysrhythmic Drugs

Objectives

After reading this chapter, the successful student will be able to do the following:

1. Describe the anatomy and physiology of a normal heart as well as cardiac electrophysiology, including normal conduction patterns, rate, and rhythm.

2. Briefly discuss the various disorders of cardiac electrophysiology and their consequences to the patient.

3. Define the terms *dysrhythmia* and *arrhythmia*.

4. Identify the various causes of abnormal heart rhythms and their impact on the patient's health and activities of daily living.

5. Identify the most commonly encountered dysrhythmias.

6. Compare the various dysrhythmias pertaining to their basic characteristics, impact on the structures of the heart, and related symptoms.

7. Contrast the various classes of antidysrhythmic drugs, citing prototypes in each class and describing their mechanisms of action, indications, routes of administration, dosing, adverse effects, cautions, contraindications, and drug interactions, as well as any toxic reactions or related drug protocols.

8. Develop a collaborative plan of care that includes all phases of the nursing process for patients receiving each class of antidysrhythmic drug.

e-Learning Activities

Website
(http://evolve.elsevier.com/Canada/
Lilley/pharmacology/)

evolve

- Answer Key—Textbook Case Studies
- Answer Key—Critical Thinking Activities
- Chapter Summaries—Printable
- Review Questions for Exam Preparation
- Unfolding Case Studies

Drug Profiles

    adenosine, p. 509
▸▸ amiodarone (amiodarone hydrochloride)*, p. 507
▸▸ atenolol, p. 506
▸▸ diltiazem (diltiazem hydrochloride)*, p. 508
    esmolol (esmolol hydrochloride)*, p. 507
    flecainide (flecainide acetate)*, p. 505
    ibutilide (ibutilide fumarate)*, p. 508
▸▸ lidocaine (lidocaine hydrochloride)*, p. 505
▸▸ metoprolol (metoprolol tartrate)*, p. 507
    procainamide (procainamide hydrochloride)*, p. 505
    propafenone (propafenone hydrochloride)*, p. 506
    quinidine (quinidine sulfate)*, p. 505
▸▸ sotalol (sotalol hydrochloride)*, p. 508
▸▸ verapamil (verapamil hydrochloride)*, p. 509

▸▸ Key drug

*Full generic name is given in parentheses. For the purposes of this text, the more common, shortened name is used.

Key Terms

Action potential Electrical activity that consists of polarization and depolarization and that travels across the cell membrane of a nerve fibre during the transmission of a nerve impulse and across the cell membrane of a muscle cell during contraction. (p. 495)

Action potential duration (APD) The interval beginning with baseline (resting) membrane potential, followed by depolarization, and ending with repolarization to baseline membrane potential. (p. 497)

Arrhythmia Technically "without rhythm,"; absence of a heart rhythm (i.e., no heartbeat at all). More commonly used in clinical practice to refer to any variation from the normal rhythm of the heart. Also referred to as *dysrhythmia*, which is the primary term used in this chapter and book. (p. 494)

Asystole State of no cardiac electrical activity in the heart or no heartbeat. (p. 494)

Atrial fibrillation Rapid atrial contractions that incompletely pump blood into the ventricles. (p. 498)

Cardiac Arrhythmia Suppression Trial (CAST) A major research study conducted by the National Heart, Lung, and Blood Institute in the United States to investigate the possibility of eliminating sudden cardiac death in patients with asymptomatic ectopy after a myocardial infarction. (p. 506)

Cardioversion A procedure by which an abnormally fast heart rate (tachycardia) or cardiac dysrhythmia is converted to a normal rhythm using electricity or drugs. (p. 498)

Depolarization The movement of positive and negative ions on either side of a cell membrane across the membrane in a direction that brings the net charge to zero. (p. 495)

Dysrhythmia Any disturbance or abnormality in the rhythm of the heartbeat. (p. 494)

Effective refractory period (ERP) The period after the firing of an impulse during which a cell may respond to a stimulus but the response will not be passed along or continued as another impulse. (p. 497)

Internodal pathways (Bachmann's bundle) Special pathways in the atria that carry electrical impulses spontaneously generated by the sinoatrial node. These impulses cause the heart to beat. (p. 497)

Relative refractory period (RRP) The time after generation of an action potential during which a nerve fibre will show a (reduced) response only to a strong stimulus. (p. 497)

Resting membrane potential (RMP) The voltage that exists when the cell membranes of heart muscle (or other muscle or nerve cells) are at rest. (p. 494)

Sodium–potassium adenosine triphosphatase (ATPase) pump A mechanism for transporting sodium and potassium ions across the cell membrane against an opposing concentration gradient. Energy for this transport is obtained from the hydrolysis of adenosine triphosphate (ATP) by means of the enzyme ATPase. (p. 495)

Sudden cardiac death Unexpected, fatal cardiac arrest. (p. 506)

Threshold potential (TP) The critical state of electrical tension required for spontaneous depolarization of a cell membrane. (p. 497)

Torsades de pointes A rare ventricular dysrhythmia that is associated with long QT interval and can degenerate into ventricular fibrillation and sudden death without medical intervention; often simply referred to as *torsades*. (p. 501)

Vaughan Williams classification The system most commonly used to classify antidysrhythmic drugs. (p. 501; see also Table 26-2, p. 501)

Ventricular tachycardia A rapid heartbeat from impulses originating in the ventricles. (p. 498)

DYSRHYTHMIAS AND NORMAL CARDIAC ELECTROPHYSIOLOGY

A **dysrhythmia** is any deviation from the normal rhythm of the heart. Technically, the term *arrhythmia* (meaning "without rhythm") implies **asystole**, or no heartbeat. Thus, the more accurate term for an irregular heart rhythm is *dysrhythmia*. However, *arrhythmia* is commonly used synonymously with *dysrhythmia* in clinical practice. Dysrhythmias can develop in association with many conditions, such as after a myocardial infarction (MI) or heart surgery, or as the result of coronary artery disease (CAD). Dysrhythmias are usually serious and may require treatment with an antidysrhythmic drug or nonpharmacological therapies; not all dysrhythmias require medical treatment. A cardiologist is usually consulted to make the judgement.

Disturbances in heart rhythm are the result of abnormally functioning cardiac cells. Thus, an understanding of the mechanism responsible for dysrhythmias first requires review of the electrical properties of cardiac cells. Figure 25-1 on p. 478 illustrates the overall anatomy of the conduction system of the heart. Figure 26-1 illustrates some of the properties of this system based on a single cardiac cell. Inside a resting cardiac cell, a net negative charge exists relative to the outside of the cell. This difference in the electronegative charge exists in all types of cardiac cells and is referred to as the *resting membrane potential (RMP)*. The RMP results from an uneven distribution of ions (sodium, potassium, and calcium) across the cell membrane, known as *polarization*. Each ion moves through its own specific protein channel that sits across the cell membrane. These proteins work continuously to restore the specific intracellular and extracellular concentrations of each ion. At the RMP, the ionic concentration gradient (distribution) is such that potassium ions are more highly concentrated intracellularly, whereas sodium and calcium ions are more highly concentrated extracellularly.

The polarized distribution of extracellular sodium and calcium ions and intracellular potassium, chloride (Cl^-) and bicarbonate (HCO_3^-) ions is maintained by the

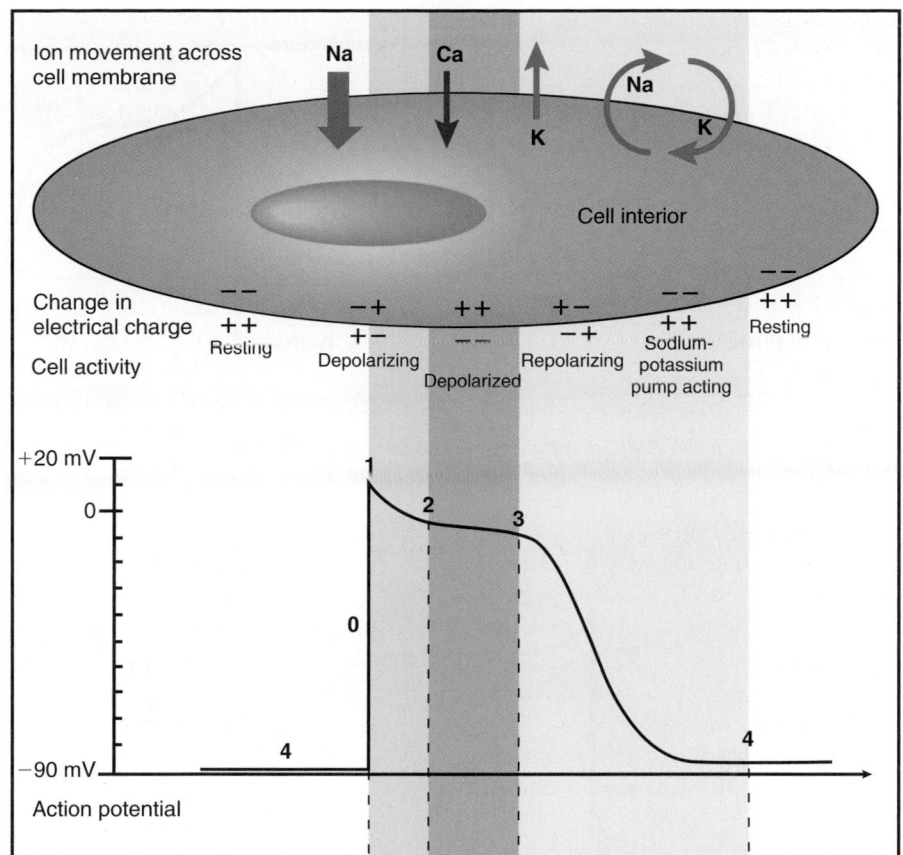

FIG. 26-1   Phases of the action potential of a cardiac cell. In resting phase (4), the cell membrane is polarized. The cell's interior has a net negative charge, and the membrane is more permeable to potassium ions (K) than to sodium ions (Na). When the cell is stimulated and begins to depolarize (0), sodium ions enter the cell, potassium leaves the cell, calcium (Ca) channels open, and sodium channels close. In its depolarized phase (1), the cell's interior has a net positive charge. In the plateau phase (2), calcium and other positive ions enter the cell and potassium permeability declines, which lengthens the action potential. Then (3) calcium channels close and sodium is pulled from the cell by the sodium-potassium pump. The cell's interior then returns to its polarized, negatively charged state (4). (Source: Monahan, F. D. (2007). *Phipps' medical-surgical nursing: Health and illness perspectives* (8th ed.). St Louis, MO: Mosby.)

sodium–potassium adenosine triphosphatase (ATPase) pump energized by adenosine triphosphate (ATP). Cardiac cells become excited when there is a change in the baseline distribution of ions across their membranes (RMP) that leads to the propagation of an electrical impulse. This change is known as an *action potential;* action potentials occur in a continuous and regular manner in the cells of the heart conduction system (i.e., the sinoatrial [SA] node, atrioventricular [AV] node, and His-Purkinje system). All of these tissues have the property of spontaneous electrical excitability known as *automaticity,* an excited state that creates action potentials that in turn generate electrical impulses that travel through the myocardium, ultimately to create the heartbeat via contraction of cardiac muscle fibres.

An action potential has five phases. Phase 0 is also called the *upstroke* because it appears as an upward line on the graph of an action potential, as shown in Figures 26-2. Both of these figures graphically illustrate the cycle of electrical changes that create an action potential. Note

the variation in the shape of the curve of the graph, depending on the relative conduction speed of the specific tissue involved (SA node versus Purkinje fibre). A faster rate of conduction corresponds to a steeper slope on the graph.

During phase 0, the resting cardiac cell membrane suddenly becomes highly permeable to sodium ions, which rush from outside of the cell membrane to inside (influx) through what are known as *fast channels or sodium channels.* This disruption of the earlier polarized state of the membrane is known as **depolarization**. Depolarization can be thought of as a temporary equalization of positive and negative charges across the cell membrane. This condition causes the release of electrochemical energy that drives the resulting electrical impulses through adjacent cells. Phase 1 of the action potential begins a rapid period of repolarization that continues through phases 2 and 3 to phase 4, which is the RMP. In phase 1, the sodium channels close and the concentrations of each ion begin to move back toward their

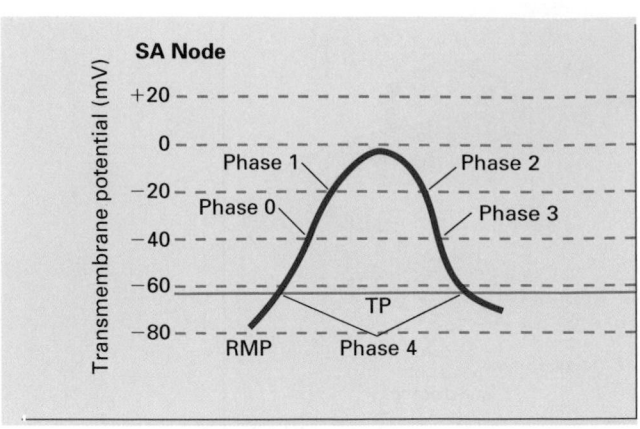

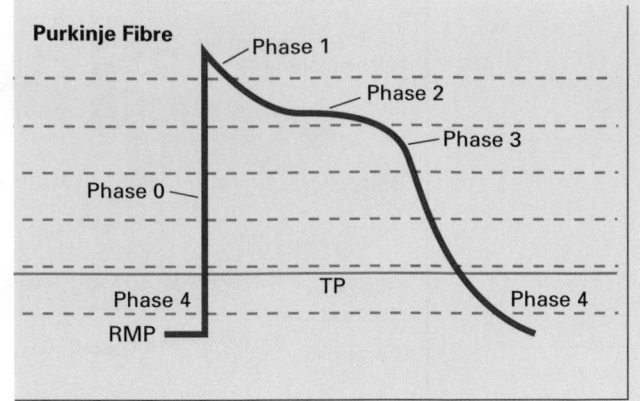

FIG. 26-2 Action potentials. *RMP*, resting membrane potential; *SA*, sinoatrial; *TP*, threshold potential.

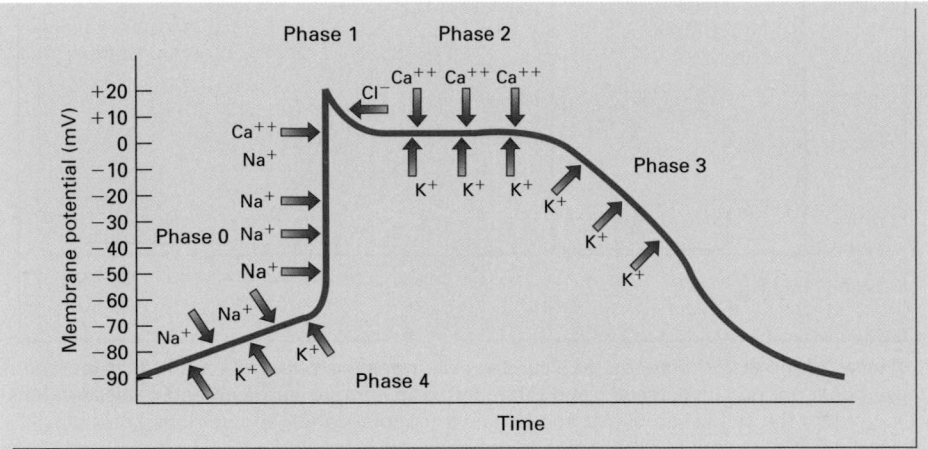

FIG. 26-3 Purkinje fibre action potential.

ion-specific RMP levels. During phase 2, calcium ion influx occurs through the slow channels or calcium channels. They are called *slow channels* because the calcium influx occurs relatively more slowly than the earlier sodium influx. Potassium ions then flow from inside of the cell to outside (efflux) through specific potassium channels. This is done to offset the elevated positive charge caused by the influx of sodium and calcium ions. In the case of the Purkinje fibres, this causes a partial plateau (flattening on the graph), during which the overall membrane potential changes only slightly, as seen in Figure 26-2, B. In phase 3, the ionic flow patterns of phases 0 to 2 are changed by the sodium–potassium ATPase pump (or, more simply, the *sodium pump*), which re-establishes the baseline polarized state by restoring both intracellular and extracellular concentrations of sodium, potassium, and calcium (see Figure 26-1). As a result, the cell membrane is ultimately repolarized to its baseline level or RMP (phase 4). Note that this entire process occurs over approximately 400 milliseconds—that is, four hundred thousandths (less than half) of 1 second.

There is some variation in this period between different parts of the conduction system. As an example, Figure

26-3 illustrates the pattern of movement of sodium, potassium, and calcium ions into and out of a Purkinje cell during the four phases of the action potential. Note that there are several differences in the action potentials of SA nodal cells and Purkinje cells. The level of the RMP for a given type of cell is an important determinant of the rate of its impulse conduction to other cells. The less negative (i.e., the closer to zero) the RMP is at the onset of phase 0 of the action potential, the slower is the upstroke velocity of phase 0. The slope of phase 0 is directly related to the impulse velocity. An upstroke with a steeper slope indicates faster conduction velocity. Thus, in the Purkinje cells, electrical conduction is relatively fast, and therefore electrical impulses are conducted quickly. These cells are referred to as *fast-response cells*, or *fast-channel cells*, and Purkinje fibres can therefore be thought of as fast-channel tissue. Many antidysrhythmic drugs affect the RMP and sodium channels, which in turn influences the rate of impulse conduction.

In contrast to Purkinje fibres, the cells of the SA node have a slower upstroke velocity, or a slower phase 0. This is illustrated in Figure 26-2, A, as an upstroke curve that is less steep, which indicates a relatively slower rate of electrical conduction in these cells.

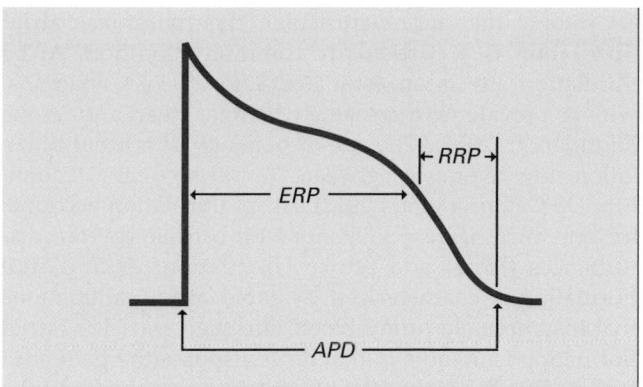

FIG. 26-4 Aspects of an action potential. *APD*, action potential duration; *ERP*, effective refractory period; *RRP*, relative refractory period.

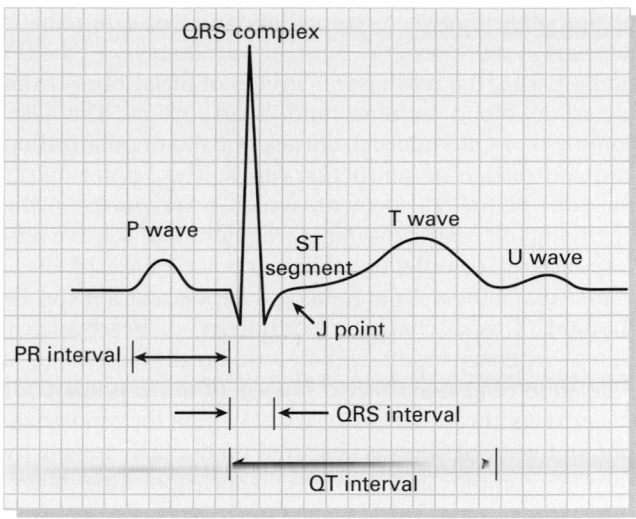

FIG. 26-5 The waves and intervals of a normal electrocardiogram. (Source: Goldberger, A. L. (2006). *Clinical electrocardiography: A simplified approach* (7th ed.). St. Louis, MO: Mosby.)

AV nodal cells are comparable to SA nodal cells in this regard. This slower upstroke in the SA and AV nodes is primarily dependent on the entry of calcium ions through the slow channels or calcium channels. This means that nodal action potentials are affected by calcium influx as early as phase 0. The nodes are therefore called *slow-channel tissue*, and conduction in these cells is slower than that in other parts of the conduction system. Drugs that affect calcium ion movement into or out of these cells (e.g., calcium channel blockers) tend to have significant effects on the SA and AV nodal conduction rates.

The interval between phase 0 and phase 4 is called the **action potential duration (APD**; Figure 26-4). The period between phase 0 and midway through phase 3 is called the *absolute* or **effective refractory period (ERP).** During the ERP, the cardiac cell cannot be stimulated to depolarize and generate another action potential. During the remainder of phase 3 until the return to the RMP (phase 4), the cardiac cell *can* be depolarized again if it receives a powerful enough impulse (such as one induced by drug therapy or supplied by an electrical pacemaker). This period is referred to as the **relative refractory period (RRP).** Figure 26-4 illustrates these aspects of an action potential. Again, the actual shape of the action potential curve varies in different parts of the conduction system.

The RMP of certain cardiac cells gradually decreases (becomes less negative) over time in ongoing cycles. This is due to small changes in the flux of sodium and potassium ions. Depolarization eventually occurs when a certain critical voltage is reached **(threshold potential [TP]).** This process of spontaneous depolarization is referred to as *automaticity*, or *pacemaker activity*. It is normal when it occurs in the SA node (see Figure 25-1 on p. 484), but when spontaneous depolarizations occur elsewhere, dysrhythmias often result.

The SA node, the AV node, and His-Purkinje cells all possess the property of automaticity. The SA node is the natural pacemaker of the heart because it spontaneously depolarizes the most frequently. The SA node has an intrinsic rate of 60 to 100 depolarizations or beats per minute; that of the AV node is 40 to 60 beats per minute;

and that of the ventricular Purkinje fibres is 40 or fewer beats per minute.

As the pacemaker of the heart, the SA node, located near the top of the right atrium, generates an electrical impulse that travels through the atria via specialized **internodal pathways (Bachmann bundle).** This impulse causes the atrial myocardial fibres to contract, creating the first heart sound. Next, the impulse reaches the AV node, situated near the bottom of the right atrium, which slows this fast-moving electrical impulse to allow the ventricles to fill with blood.

Next, the AV nodal cells generate an electrical impulse that passes into the *bundle of His*, a band of heart muscle fibres located between the right and left ventricles (ventricular septum). The bundle of His distributes the impulse into both ventricles via the right and left bundle branches, which terminate in the Purkinje fibres located in the myocardium. Stimulation of the Purkinje fibres causes ventricular contraction and ejection of blood from the ventricles. Blood from the right ventricle is pumped into the pulmonary circulation, whereas blood from the left ventricle is pumped into the systemic circulation. The bundle of His and Purkinje fibres are often referred to as the His-Purkinje system. Any abnormality in cardiac automaticity or impulse conduction often results in some type of dysrhythmia.

Electrocardiography

The electrophysiological cardiac events described thus far in this chapter correspond more simply to the tracings of an electrocardiogram (ECG; Figure 26-5). The P wave corresponds to spontaneous impulse generation in the SA node, followed immediately by depolarization of atrial myocardial fibres and their muscular contraction. This sequence normally determines the heart rate. It is affected by the balance between sympathetic and parasympathetic nervous system tone, the intrinsic automaticity of the SA nodal tissue, the mechanical stretch of atrial fibres from incoming blood volume, and heart drugs. The QRS complex (or QRS interval) corresponds to depolarization and contraction of ventricular fibres. The J point marks the start of the ST segment, which corresponds to the beginning of ventricular repolarization. The T wave corresponds to completion of the repolarization of these ventricular fibres. As an analogy, depolarization can be thought of as discharge or contraction of heart muscle fibres, whereas repolarization can be thought of as a relaxation of just-contracted muscle fibres to prepare for the next contraction (heartbeat). Note that the repolarization of the atrial fibres is obscured on the ECG tracing by the QRS complex and thus has no corresponding deflection in the tracing. The U wave is not always present, and its physiological basis is uncertain. When the U wave occurs, it is generally correlated with electrophysiological events such as repolarization of Purkinje fibres. These events may be a source of dysrhythmias caused by a triggered automaticity. Prominent U waves are often associated with sinus bradycardia, hypokalemia, use of quinidine and other class Ia antidysrhythmics, and hyperthyroidism. Abnormal U waves (inverted) are associated with serious conditions such as MI, acute angina, coronary artery spasms, and ischemic heart disease. The PR and QT intervals and the ST segment are parts of the ECG tracing that are often altered by disease or by the adverse effects of certain types of drug therapy or drug interactions, as discussed in later sections of this chapter.

Common Dysrhythmias

A variety of cardiac dysrhythmias are recognized. Some are easier to treat than others using drug therapy and interventional cardiology procedures, such as pacemaker implantation, catheter ablation, **cardioversion** (a procedure by which an abnormally fast heart rate [tachycardia] or cardiac dysrhythmia is converted to a normal rhythm using electricity or drugs), and implantable cardioverters–defibrillators. Dysrhythmias are subdivided into several broad categories depending on their anatomical site of origin in the heart. Supraventricular dysrhythmias originate above the ventricles in the SA or AV node or atrial myocardium. Ventricular dysrhythmias originate below the AV node in the His-Purkinje system or ventricular myocardium. Dysrhythmias that originate outside the conduction system (i.e., in atrial or ventricular cells) are considered ectopic, and their specific points of origin are called *ectopic foci*. Conduction blocks are dysrhythmias that involve disruption of impulse conduction between the atria and ventricles, through the AV node directly affecting ventricular function. They may also originate in the His-Purkinje system. Less commonly, impulse conduction between the SA and AV node is affected. Several of the most common dysrhythmias are described in Table 26-1, and corresponding ECG tracings are provided. They are also described further in the following text.

Among the supraventricular dysrhythmias, **atrial fibrillation** is a particularly common condition. Atrial fibrillation affects an estimated 1 to 2% of Canadians, with its prevalence increasing with age (Heart and Stroke Foundation, 2015). The age of patients with atrial fibrillation now averages between 75 and 85 years (Camm, Lip, De Caterina et al., 2012). Atrial fibrillation accounts for one third of hospitalizations for cardiac rhythm disturbances (Heart and Stroke Foundation, 2015). Atrial fibrillation is characterized by rapid atrial contractions that incompletely pump blood into the ventricles. Atrial fibrillation is notable in that it predisposes the patient to stroke. This is because the blood tends to stagnate in the incompletely emptied atria and is therefore more likely to clot. If such blood clots manage to make their way into the left ventricle, they may embolize to the brain and result in stroke. Although theoretically there would be a similar risk for pulmonary embolism, this is of less clinical concern with atrial fibrillation than is the risk for stroke. It is estimated that 20% of all strokes are caused by atrial fibrillation (Camm et al., 2012). Patients with ongoing atrial fibrillation are often given warfarin sodium as well as dabigatran, apixaban, or rivaroxaban for anticoagulant therapy (see Chapter 26) to reduce the likelihood of stroke.

AV nodal re-entrant tachycardia is a conduction disorder that often gives rise to a dysrhythmia known as *paroxysmal supraventricular tachycardia*. (The word *paroxysmal* means "sudden recurrence or intensification of symptoms.") AV nodal re-entrant tachycardia occurs when electrical impulse transmission from the AV node into the His-Purkinje system of the ventricles is disrupted. As a result, some of the impulses circle backward (retrograde impulses) and re-enter the atrial tissues to produce a tachycardic response. In Wolff–Parkinson–White syndrome, ectopic impulses that begin near the AV node actually bypass the AV node and reach the His-Purkinje system before the normal AV-generated impulses. This is one cause of ventricular tachycardia, although it is technically supraventricular in origin.

Varying degrees of AV block (often called heart block) involve different levels of disrupted conduction of impulses from the AV node and His-Purkinje system to the ventricles. Although first-degree AV block is often asymptomatic, third-degree block—or complete heart block—often requires use of a cardiac pacemaker to ensure adequate ventricular function. There can also be blocks within the His-Purkinje system of the ventricles, known as *bundle branch blocks*.

Premature ventricular contractions (PVCs) occur when impulses originate from ectopic foci within the ventricles (His-Purkinje system). PVCs probably occur periodically in many people, but they become problematic when they occur frequently enough to compromise systolic blood volume. **Ventricular tachycardia** refers to a rapid heartbeat from impulses originating in the ventricles. It can be nonsustained (brief) or sustained, requiring definitive treatment. Worsening ventricular

Continued

TABLE 26-1

Common Dysrhythmias

Dysrhythmia	Description	ECG Tracing
Atrial flutter (AF)	Often progresses to atrial fibrillation (F = flutter waves)	monitor F F F F atrial flutter
Atrial fibrillation (AF)	Rapid, ineffective atrial contractions (F = fibrillation waves)	f f f f f f f f atrial fibrillation
Paroxysmal supraventricular tachycardia (PSVT)	Heart rate of 180–200 beats/min or higher	II
Premature ventricular contractions (PVCs)	Contractions generated by impulses arising from ectopic foci within ventricular myocardium	VPB VPB aV$_R$ APB II

TABLE 26-1

Common Dysrhythmias—cont'd

Dysrhythmia	Description	ECG Tracing
Nonsustained ventricular tachycardia (NSVT)	Relatively brief period (20 sec or less) in which ventricles contract rapidly on their own as well as in response to AV impulses	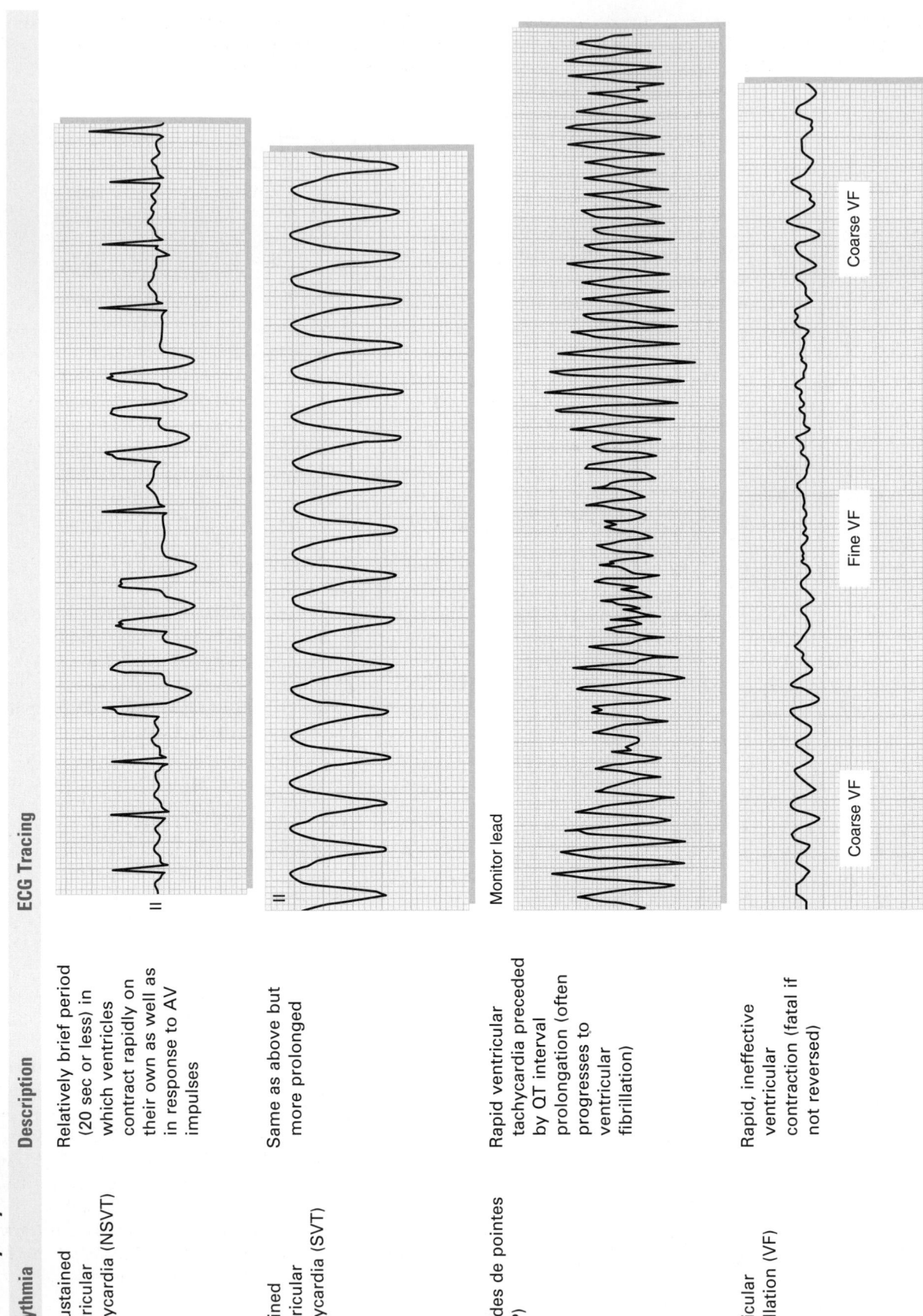
Sustained ventricular tachycardia (SVT)	Same as above but more prolonged	
Torsades de pointes (TdP)	Rapid ventricular tachycardia preceded by QT interval prolongation (often progresses to ventricular fibrillation)	
Ventricular fibrillation (VF)	Rapid, ineffective ventricular contraction (fatal if not reversed)	

APB, atrial premature beat; *AV*, atrioventricular; *ECG*, electrocardiogram; *VPB*, ventricular premature beat.

tachycardia can deteriorate into **torsades de pointes,** an intermediate dysrhythmia that often deteriorates into ventricular fibrillation. Ventricular fibrillation is fatal if not reversed, which most often requires electrical defibrillation. Interestingly, torsades de pointes often responds preferentially to intravenous magnesium sulfate.

ANTIDYSRHYTHMIC DRUGS

Numerous drugs are available to treat dysrhythmias. These drugs are categorized according to where and how they affect cardiac cells. Although other classifications are described in the literature, the most commonly used system is the **Vaughan Williams classification.** This system is based on the electrophysiological effect of particular drugs on the action potential. This approach identifies four major classes of drugs. Class I antidysrhythmics are considered membrane-stabilizing drugs: I (including Ia, Ib, and Ic), II, III, and IV. The drugs in these four classes are listed in Table 26-2.

There is currently a gradual trend away from the use of class Ia drugs. Class III drugs have emerged as being among the most widely used antidysrhythmics. Class IV drugs (calcium channel blockers) have limited usefulness in tachydysrhythmias (dysrhythmias involving tachycardia), unlike most of the other classes. The role of class II drugs (β-blockers) continues to grow in the field of cardiology, including in dysrhythmia management. Digoxin, the cardiac glycoside discussed in Chapter 24, still has

a place in dysrhythmia management, especially in the prevention of dangerous ventricular tachydysrhythmias secondary to atrial fibrillation.

Mechanism of Action and Drug Effects

Antidysrhythmic drugs work by correcting abnormal cardiac electrophysiological function. They do this to varying degrees and by various mechanisms. Class I drugs are membrane-stabilizing drugs and exert their actions on sodium (fast) channels. There are some slight differences in the actions of the drugs in this class, so they are divided into three subclasses. These subclasses are Ia, Ib, and Ic drugs and are based on the magnitude of the effects each drug has on phase 0, the APD, and the ERP. Class Ia drugs (quinidine, procainamide, and disopyramide) block the sodium channels; more specifically, they delay repolarization and increase the APD. Class Ib drugs (phenytoin sodium and lidocaine) also block the sodium channels, but unlike class Ia drugs, they accelerate repolarization and decrease the APD. Phenytoin sodium is more commonly used as an antiepileptic (Chapter 15) than as an antidysrhythmic drug. Class Ic drugs (flecainide and propafenone) have a more pronounced effect on the blockade of sodium channels but have little effect on repolarization or the APD.

Class II drugs are the β-adrenergic blockers (β-blockers, see Chapter 20) and they are commonly used as antihypertensives (see Chapter 23) and antianginal drugs (Chapter 24). They work by blocking sympathetic nervous system stimulation to the heart and, consequently, the transmission of impulses in the heart's conduction system. This results in depression of phase 4 depolarization. These drugs mostly affect slower-conducting cardiac tissues.

Class III drugs (amiodarone, dronedarone, sotalol, and ibutilide) increase the APD by prolonging repolarization in phase 3. The primary role of potassium channels in cardiac action potentials is cell repolarization; these drugs are also referred to as calcium channel blockers. They affect fast tissue and are most commonly used to manage dysrhythmias that are difficult to treat. They are usually reserved for patients for whom other therapies have failed. Sotalol has properties of both class II and class III drugs, and it may be listed as a member of either class.

Class IV drugs (verapamil, diltiazem) are the calcium channel blockers, which, similar to β-blockers, are also used as antianginal drugs (Chapter 24) and antihypertensives (Chapter 23). As their name implies, they act specifically by inhibiting the calcium channels, which reduces the influx of calcium ions during action potentials. This results in depression of phase 4 depolarization.

The mechanisms of action of the major classes of antidysrhythmics are summarized in Table 26-3. The effects of the various classes of drugs are summarized in Box 26-1.

Indications

Antidysrhythmic drugs are effective in treating a variety of cardiac dysrhythmias. The antidysrhythmic drugs and

---

| **TABLE** | **26-2** |

Vaughan Williams Classification of Antidysrhythmic Drugs

Functional Class	Drugs
Class I: Membrane-stabilizing drugs; fast sodium channel blockers	
Ia: ↑ blockade of sodium channel, delay repolarization, ↑ APD	quinidine sulfate, disopyramide, procainamide
Ib: ↑ blockade of sodium channel, accelerate repolarization, ± APD	lidocaine, phenytoin
Ic: ↑↑↑ blockade of sodium channel ± on repolarization; also suppress re-entry	flecainide, propafenone
Class II: β-blocking drugs	All β-blockers
Class III: Drugs whose principal effect on cardiac tissue is to ↑ APD	amiodarone dronedarone, sotalol,* ibutilide
Class IV: Calcium channel blockers	verapamil, diltiazem
Other: Antidysrhythmic drugs that have the properties of several classes and therefore cannot be placed in one particular class	digoxin, adenosine

APD, action potential duration; ↑, increase; ±, increase or decrease.
*Sotalol also has class II properties.

TABLE 26-3

Antidysrhythmic Drugs: Mechanisms of Action

Vaughan Williams Class	Action	Tissue	Effect on Action Potential
I	Blocks sodium channels, affects phase 0	Fast	
II	Decreases spontaneous depolarization, affects phase 4	Slow	
III	Prolongs APD	Fast	
IV	Blocks slow calcium channels	Slow	

APD, action potential duration.

BOX 26-1 Effects of Antidysrhythmic Drugs

Class Ia (disopyramide, quinidine, procainamide)

- Depress myocardial excitability
- Prolong the effective refractory period
- Eliminate or reduce ectopic foci stimulation
- Decrease inotropic effect
- Have anticholinergic (vagolytic [has inhibitory effects on the vagus nerve]) activity

Class Ib (lidocaine, mexiletine, phenytoin)

- Decrease myocardial excitability in the ventricles
- Eliminate or reduce ectopic foci stimulation in the ventricles
- Have minimal effect on the SA node and automaticity
- Have minimal effect on the AV node and conduction
- Have minimal anticholinergic (vagolytic) activity

Class Ic (flecainide, propafenone)

- Produce dose-related depression of cardiac conduction, especially in the bundle of the His-Purkinje system
- Have minimal effect on atrial conduction
- Eliminate or reduce ectopic foci stimulation in the ventricles
- Have minimal anticholinergic (vagolytic) activity

- Flecainide use now reserved for the most serious dysrhythmias

Class II (β-blockers [e.g., acebutolol, esmolol, metoprolol])

- Block β-adrenergic heart stimulation
- Reduce SA nodal activity
- Eliminate or reduce atrial ectopic foci stimulation
- Reduce ventricular contraction rate
- Reduce cardiac output and blood pressure

Class III (amiodarone, dronedarone, sotalol*, ibutilide)

- Prolong the effective refractory period
- Prolong the myocardial action potential
- Block both α- and β-adrenergic heart stimulation

Class IV (diltiazem, verapamil)

- Prolong AV nodal effective refractory period
- Reduce AV nodal conduction
- Reduce rapid ventricular conduction caused by atrial flutter

---

AV, atrioventricular; *SA*, sinoatrial.
*Sotalol also has class II properties.

---

the most common indications for their use are listed in Table 26-4.

Contraindications

As with all drugs, contraindications to the use of antidysrhythmic drugs include known drug allergy to a specific product. Other contraindications may include second- or third-degree AV block, bundle branch block, cardiogenic shock, sick sinus syndrome, or any other major ECG changes, depending on the clinical judgement of a cardiologist. The concurrent use of certain drugs that interact with antidysrhythmics is also considered. The reason for these concerns is that all antidysrhythmic drugs can

potentially worsen existing dysrhythmias (also termed *dysrhythmogenic*). The risk is greater in patients with structural heart damage (e.g., after MI). In patients with AV block and bundle branch block, there is a danger of drug-induced ventricular failure if a drug further compromises the already existing AV conduction delays. The safe prescribing of antidysrhythmic drugs is an area that requires strong clinical expertise and careful judgement on a case-by-case basis.

Adverse Effects

Adverse effects common to most antidysrhythmics include hypersensitivity reactions, nausea, vomiting, and

TABLE	26-4

Antidysrhythmic Drugs: Indications

Drug	Indications
CLASS Ia disopyramide procainamide hydrochloride quinidine sulfate	Atrial fibrillation, premature atrial contractions, premature ventricular contractions, ventricular tachycardia, Wolff–Parkinson–White syndrome
CLASS Ib lidocaine hydrochloride	Ventricular dysrhythmias only (premature ventricular contractions, ventricular tachycardia, ventricular fibrillation)
CLASS Ic flecainide acetate propafenone hydrochloride	Ventricular tachycardia and supraventricular tachycardia dysrhythmias, atrial fibrillation and flutter; Wolff–Parkinson–White syndrome
CLASS II β-blockers atenolol hydrochloride esmolol hydrochloride metoprolol hydrochloride	Both supraventricular and ventricular dysrhythmias (act as general myocardial depressants)
CLASS III amiodarone hydrochloride dronedarone hydrochloride ibutilide fumarate sotalol hydrochloride*	Life-threatening ventricular tachycardia or fibrillation Atrial fibrillation or flutter resistant to other drugs
CLASS IV calcium channel blockers diltiazem hydrochloride verapamil hydrochloride	Paroxysmal supraventricular tachycardia; rate control for atrial fibrillation and flutter

*Sotalol hydrochloride also has class II properties.

diarrhea. Other common effects include dizziness, headache, and blurred vision. In addition, many antidysrhythmic are capable of producing new dysrhythmias (prodysrhythmic effect). Prolongation of the QT interval is a potentially severe adverse effect shared by many antidysrhythmics. The concern with QT prolongation is the potential for induction of torsades de pointes. As with any drug class, there are also cases of unpredictable or idiosyncratic adverse effects (see Chapter 2) that are not related to drug concentration in the body. Idiosyncratic reactions are unpredictable; however, it is thought that such effects will eventually be explained by genetic variations. Table 26-5 summarizes the most commonly reported adverse effects by specific drug.

Toxicity and Management of Overdose

The main toxic effects of the antidysrhythmics involve the heart, circulation, and central nervous system (CNS). Specific antidotes are not available.

Interactions

Antidysrhythmics can interact with many different categories of drugs. The most serious drug interactions are those that result in dysrhythmias, hypotension or hypertension, respiratory distress, or excessive therapeutic or toxic drug effects. Drug interactions occur when the presence of one drug strengthens or weakens the pharmacological effects of another. This is most commonly seen when the first drug affects the activity of the enzymes that metabolize the second drug, either speeding or slowing its elimination. One particular interaction common to many antidysrhythmics is the potentiation of anticoagulant activity with warfarin sodium (Coumadin®; see Chapter 27). Because many patients receiving antidysrhythmic therapy also need warfarin sodium, the international normalized ratio (INR) must be monitored and necessary adjustments made to the warfarin sodium dosage. This is especially true with amiodarone. The INR will increase by 50% in almost 100% of patients receiving amiodarone and warfarin sodium. Grapefruit juice can also inhibit the metabolism of several antidysrhythmics, such as amiodarone, disopyramide, and quinidine. Other common interactions are summarized in Table 26-6. To explain the mechanism for each interaction is beyond the scope of this text; readers needing more detailed information are encouraged to consult the appropriate references.

Dosages

For dosage information on selected antidysrhythmic drugs, refer to the table on p. 511.

Text continued on p. 509

TABLE 26-5

Antidysrhythmic Drugs: Common Adverse Effects

Class	Drug	Adverse Effects
Ia	procainamide hydrochloride	Hypotension, rash, diarrhea, nausea, vomiting, agranulocytosis, SLE-like syndrome
	quinidine sulfate	Hypotension, QT prolongation, lightheadedness, diarrhea, bitter taste, anorexia, blurred vision, tinnitus, angina
Ib	lidocaine hydrochloride	Bradycardia, dysrhythmia, hypotension, anxiety, metallic taste
Ic	flecainide acetate	Dizziness, visual disturbances, dyspnea, palpitations, nausea, vomiting, diarrhea, weakness
	propafenone hydrochloride	Prodysrhythmic effect, angina, tachycardia, syncope, AV block, dizziness, fatigue, dyspnea
II	β-blockers	Bradycardia, hypotension, dizziness, fatigue, AV block, heart failure, hyperglycemia, mask the symptoms of hypoglycemia, bronchospasm, wheezing, dry mouth, erectile dysfunction
III	amiodarone hydrochloride	Pulmonary toxicity, thyroid disorders, bradycardia, hypotension, SA node dysfunction, AV block, ataxia, QT prolongation, torsades de pointes, vomiting, constipation, photosensitivity, abnormal liver function test results, jaundice, visual disturbances, hyperglycemia or hypoglycemia, and dermatologic reactions including rash, toxic epidermal necrolysis, vasculitis, blue–grey colouring of the skin (face, arms, neck)
	ibutilide fumarate	Nonsustained ventricular tachycardia, ventricular extrasystoles, tachycardia, hypotension, AV block, headache, nausea
	sotalol hydrochloride*	Bradycardia, chest pain, palpitations, fatigue, dizziness, lightheadedness, weakness, dyspnea
IV	Calcium channel blockers	Constipation, bradycardia, heart block, hypotension, dizziness, dyspnea

AV, atrioventricular; SA, sinoatrial; SLE, systemic lupus erythematosus.
*Sotalol also has class II properties.

TABLE 26-6

Selected Antidysrhythmic Drugs: Common Drug Interactions

Drug (Class)	Interacting Drugs	Effects*
quinidine sulfate (Ia)	amiodarone hydrochloride, dronedarone hydrochloride, amitriptyline hydrochloride, erythromycin, haloperidol, sotalol hydrochloride, moxifloxacin hydrochloride	Additive QT prolongation
	digoxin	Increase in digoxin levels by 50%
	HMG-CoA reductase inhibitors (statins)	Increased statin levels and toxicity
lidocaine hydrochloride (Ib)	amiodarone hydrochloride, azole antifungals, β-blockers, erythromycin, verapamil hydrochloride, cimetidine, tolvaptan	Increased serum levels of lidocaine
propafenone hydrochloride (Ic)	cimetidine, quinidine sulfate, pimozide	Increased propafenone levels; use is contraindicated
	digoxin, warfarin sodium, β-blockers	Increase in level of interacting drugs
	Class Ia and III antidysrhythmics, erythromycin	Prolonged QT interval
amiodarone hydrochloride (III)	Azole antifungals, clarithromycin, erythromycin, haloperidol, moxifloxacin, quinidine sulfate, procainamide hydrochloride	Prolonged QT interval
	digoxin, diltiazem hydrochloride, verapamil hydrochloride, β-blockers	AV block
	warfarin sodium, digoxin	Increase in INR by 50% in almost 100% of patients, increase in digoxin levels by 50%
	cyclosporine	Increased cyclosporine levels and toxicity
	HMG-CoA reductase inhibitors (statins)	Increased statin levels and toxicity
sotalol hydrochloride (III)†	Calcium channel blockers	Additive effects on AV conduction, bradycardia
	Class I antidysrhythmics, erythromycin, moxifloxacin, amiodarone hydrochloride	Prolonged QT interval, bradycardia
	Diuretics	Promote loss of K in the urine which increases the risk for sotalol toxicity, resulting in dysrhythmia
verapamil hydrochloride, diltiazem hydrochloride (IV)	amiodarone hydrochloride, β-blockers, flecainide acetate, digoxin	Bradycardia, decreased cardiac output, hypotension
	Azole antifungals, clarithromycin, erythromycin, isoniazid, HIV drugs	Increased verapamil effects
	HMG-CoA reductase inhibitors (statins)	Increased statin levels and toxicity

AV, atrioventricular; HIV, human immunodeficiency virus; HMG-CoA, hydroxymethylglutaryl-coenzyme A; INR, international normalized ratio.
*Note that enhanced activity of any antidysrhythmic drug may reach the level of drug toxicity, including potentially fatal cardiac dysrhythmias.
†Sotalol also has class II properties.

DRUG PROFILES

The four classes of antidysrhythmics produce a variety of effects on the action potential of the cardiac cell and exert a major effect on cardiac electrophysiological function. The diversity of therapeutic effects and adverse effects presents a special challenge to ensuring the safe and efficacious use of these drugs. Because the nursing process related to the administration of antidysrhythmics differs for each of the four classes of drug, each group is discussed separately.

CLASS IA DRUGS

Class Ia drugs are considered membrane-stabilizing drugs because they possess local anaesthetic properties. They stabilize the membrane and have depressant effects on phase 0 of the action potential. These drugs include procainamide, quinidine, and disopyramide.

procainamide hydrochloride

The electrophysiological effect of procainamide (Procan SR®) is similar to that of quinidine. Procainamide is useful in the management of atrial and ventricular tachydysrhythmias, although it is not used frequently. Significant adverse effects include ventricular dysrhythmias and blood disorders. It can cause a systemic lupus erythematosuslike syndrome, which occurs in approximately 30% of patients on long-term therapy. It can also cause gastrointestinal (GI) effects such as nausea, vomiting, and diarrhea. Other adverse effects include fever, maculopapular rash, flushing, and torsades de pointes resulting from prolongation of the QT interval. For a list of drugs that prolong the QT interval, refer to www.RxFiles.ca. Use of procainamide is contraindicated in patients with a known hypersensitivity to it and in those with heart block or systemic lupus erythematosus. Procainamide is available in both oral and parenteral forms.

PHARMACOKINETICS

Route	Onset of Action	Peak Plasma Concentration	Elimination Half-Life	Duration of Action
IV/IM	10–30 min	10–60 min	3 hr	3 hr
PO	0.5–1 hr	1–2 hr	3 hr	3–8 hr

quinidine sulfate

Quinidine sulfate has both a direct action on the electrical activity of the heart and an indirect (anticholinergic) effect. Significant adverse effects of quinidine include cardiac asystole and ventricular ectopic beats. Quinidine can cause cinchonism; symptoms of mild cinchonism include tinnitus, loss of hearing, slight blurring of vision, and GI upset. Contraindications to the use of the drug include hypersensitivity, thrombocytopenic purpura resulting from previous therapy, AV block, intraventricular conduction defects, and torsades de pointes. Quinidine is available in parenteral form.

PHARMACOKINETICS

Route	Onset of Action	Peak Plasma Concentration	Elimination Half-Life	Duration of Action
IV	Minutes	Immediate	Unknown	Short

CLASS IB DRUGS

Class Ib drugs share many characteristics with class Ia drugs but act preferentially on ischemic myocardial tissue. They have little effect on conduction velocity in normal tissue. Class Ib drugs have a weak depressive effect on phase 0 depolarization, the APD, and the ERP. They include lidocaine and phenytoin.

▶▶lidocaine hydrochloride

Lidocaine hydrochloride (Xylocaine®) is the prototypical class Ib drug. It is one of the most effective drugs for the treatment of ventricular dysrhythmias, but it can only be administered intravenously because it has an extensive first-pass effect (i.e., when taken orally, the liver metabolizes most of it to inactive metabolites). Because of its extensive liver metabolism, dosage reduction by 50% is recommended for patients with liver failure or cirrhosis. Dosage reductions may also be necessary in patients with kidney impairment because of extensive excretion of the drug and its metabolites by the kidney.

Lidocaine exerts its effects on the conduction system of the heart by making it difficult for the ventricles to develop a dysrhythmia. This action is known as raising the ventricular fibrillation threshold. It occurs by decreasing the sensitivity of the cardiac cell membrane to impulses and decreasing the cell's ability to depolarize on its own (decreasing automaticity). Many of these effects are accomplished by blocking the fast sodium channels.

Significant adverse effects include CNS toxic effects such as twitching, convulsions, and confusion; respiratory depression or arrest; and the cardiovascular effects of hypotension, bradycardia, and dysrhythmias. Use of the drug is contraindicated in patients who are hypersensitive to it, who have severe SA or AV intraventricular block, or who have Stokes–Adams or Wolff–Parkinson–White syndrome. Lidocaine is available only in parenteral form for intramuscular or intravenous administration. Lidocaine is commonly used as a local anaesthetic (see Chapter 12); a transdermal form is also available for analgesia (see Chapter 11).

PHARMACOKINETICS

Route	Onset of Action	Peak Plasma Concentration	Elimination Half-Life	Duration of Action
IV	2–15 min	5–10 min	8 min	20 min–1.5 hr

CLASS IC DRUGS

Class Ic drugs (flecainide, propafenone) produce a more pronounced blockade of the sodium channel than class Ia and Ib drugs but have little effect on repolarization or the APD. These drugs significantly slow conduction in the atria, AV node, and ventricles. Because of their marked effect on conduction, class Ic drugs strongly suppress PVCs, reducing or eliminating them.

flecainide acetate

Flecainide acetate (Tambocor®) is a chemical analogue of procainamide. Historically, clinicians have been hesitant to prescribe flecainide because of the findings of a large,

Continued

DRUG PROFILES—cont'd

multicentre study, the **Cardiac Arrhythmia Suppression Trial (CAST)**. This study showed that mortality and nonfatal cardiac arrest rates in patients treated with this drug were comparable with or higher than those seen in patients who received the placebo. Because of these findings, Health Canada required that the labelling of flecainide be revised to indicate that its use should be limited to the treatment of documented, life-threatening ventricular dysrhythmias. However, since the findings of the CAST were initially published in 1992, there have been numerous studies showing that flecainide is safe and effective for the treatment of atrial fibrillation. According to the most current practice guidelines, flecainide is considered a first-line drug (combined with an AV-blocking drug) in the treatment of atrial fibrillation. It is not to be used in patients with CAD.

Flecainide is better tolerated than quinidine or procainamide. It has a negative inotropic effect and depresses left ventricular function. Less serious but more common, noncardiac adverse effects include dizziness, visual disturbances, and dyspnea. Contraindications to its use include hypersensitivity, cardiogenic shock, second- or third-degree AV block, and non–life-threatening dysrhythmias. Flecainide is available only for oral use.

PHARMACOKINETICS

Route	Onset of Action	Peak Plasma Concentration	Elimination Half-Life	Duration of Action
PO	3 hr	1.5–3 hr	11–12 hr	12–27 hr

propafenone hydrochloride

Propafenone hydrochloride (Rythmol®) is similar in action to flecainide. It reduces the fast inward sodium current in Purkinje fibres and to a lesser extent in myocardial fibres. Unlike other class I drugs, propafenone has mild β-blocking effects. This may contribute to its overall effects on the conduction system. It is also believed to have calcium channel–blocking effects, which may contribute to its mild negative inotropic effects.

Until recently, propafenone's use was limited to the treatment of documented, life-threatening ventricular dysrhythmias such as sustained ventricular tachycardia, as was flecainide. Recent findings suggest that it has benefit in the treatment of atrial fibrillation as well. Treatment is initiated while the patient is in the hospital. Unlike flecainide, however, propafenone can be given to patients with depressed left ventricular function and may be a better drug than disopyramide, procainamide, and quinidine in these patients. However, it should be used with caution in patients with heart failure because it has some β-blocking properties and dose-dependent negative inotropic effects.

Propafenone is generally well tolerated. The most commonly reported adverse reaction is dizziness. Patients may also report a metallic taste, constipation, and headache, along with nausea and vomiting. These GI adverse effects may be reduced by taking the drug with food. Propafenone use is contraindicated in patients with a

known hypersensitivity to it, as well as in patients with bradycardia, bronchial asthma, significant hypotension, uncontrolled heart failure, cardiogenic shock, and various conduction disorders. It is available only for oral use.

PHARMACOKINETICS

Route	Onset of Action	Peak Plasma Concentration	Elimination Half-Life	Duration of Action
PO	2 hr	3–5 hr	2–10 hr	Unknown

CLASS II DRUGS

Class II antidysrhythmics are the β-blockers (see Chapter 23). They work by blocking sympathetic nervous system stimulation to the heart and the heart's conduction system, and consequently prevent catecholamine-mediated actions on the heart. This action is known as a *cardioprotective quality* of β-blockers. The resulting cardiovascular effects include a reduced heart rate, delayed AV node conduction, reduced myocardial contractility, and decreased myocardial automaticity. The pharmacological effects of the β-blockers are beneficial after an MI. Following an MI, numerous catecholamines are released that make the heart hyperirritable and predisposed to many types of dysrhythmias. β-blockers offer protection from these potentially dangerous complications. Several studies have demonstrated a significant reduction (on average 25%) in the incidence of **sudden cardiac death** after MI in patients treated with β-blockers on an ongoing basis.

Although there are several β-blockers, only a few are commonly used as antidysrhythmics. Those currently approved by Health Canada are acebutolol hydrochloride, esmolol, metoprolol, propranolol hydrochloride, and sotalol (which has class II and III properties). Selected drugs are described here. The class II drugs are recommended for use during pregnancy only when the benefit outweighs the risk to the fetus.

▶atenolol

Atenolol (Tenormin®) is a cardioselective β-blocker. It preferentially blocks the β₁-adrenergic receptors that are located primarily in the heart. Noncardioselective β-blockers block not only the β₁-adrenergic receptors on the heart but also the β₂-adrenergic receptors in the lungs and can potentially exacerbate pre-existing asthma or chronic obstructive pulmonary disease. In addition to having class II antidysrhythmic properties, atenolol is used in the treatment of hypertension and angina. Its use is contraindicated in patients with severe bradycardia, second- or third-degree heart block, heart failure, cardiogenic shock, or a known hypersensitivity. This drug is available in oral form.

PHARMACOKINETICS

Route	Onset of Action	Peak Plasma Concentration	Elimination Half-Life	Duration of Action
PO	1 hr	2–4 hr	6–7 hr	24 hr

DRUG PROFILES—cont'd

esmolol hydrochloride

Esmolol hydrocloride (Brevibloc®) is an ultra-short-acting β-blocker with pharmacological and electrophysiological effects on the heart's conduction system that are similar to those of atenolol. Esmolol is also a cardioselective β-blocker that preferentially blocks the β_1-adrenergic receptors in the heart. It is used in the acute treatment of supraventricular tachydysrhythmias or dysrhythmias that originate above the ventricles. It is also used to control hypertension and tachydysrhythmias that develop after an acute MI. Use of esmolol is contraindicated in patients with a known hypersensitivity to it or those with severe bradycardia, second- or third-degree heart block, heart failure, cardiogenic shock, or severe asthma. It is available only in injectable form.

PHARMACOKINETICS

Route	Onset of Action	Peak Plasma Concentration	Elimination Half-Life	Duration of Action
IV	Immediate	6 min	9 min	15–20 min

▶ metoprolol tartrate

Metoprolol tartrate (Lopresor®) is another cardioselective β-blocker commonly given after an MI to reduce the risk of sudden cardiac death. It is also used in the treatment of hypertension and angina. The contraindications to metoprolol use are the same as those to atenolol and esmolol. It is available in both oral and injectable forms.

PHARMACOKINETICS

Route	Onset of Action	Peak Plasma Concentration	Elimination Half-Life	Duration of Action
IV	1 min	20 min	3–8 hr	5–8 hr
PO	1 hr	2–4 hr	3–8 hr	10–20 hr

CLASS III DRUGS

Class III drugs include amiodarone, dronedarone hydrochloride, sotalol (which also has class II properties), and ibutilide. Amiodarone controls dysrhythmias by inhibiting repolarization and markedly prolonging refractoriness and the APD. Ibutilide is indicated for conversion of atrial fibrillation or flutter to a normal sinus rhythm. Amiodarone is indicated for the management of life-threatening ventricular tachycardia or ventricular fibrillation that is resistant to other drug therapy. This drug has also been effective in the treatment of sustained ventricular tachycardias. Amiodarone has recently been used more frequently to treat atrial dysrhythmias.

Dronedarone hydrochloride (Multaq®) is the newest antidysrhythmic drug. It is similar to amiodarone and is thought to have less potential for causing the classic amiodarone adverse effects and less potential for drug interactions. However, as with any newly marketed drug, the true incidence of toxicity is not known until it is used in numerous patients. In 2011, Sanofi, the manufacturer of dronedarone, worked with Health Canada and issued an advisory regarding the potential for hepatotoxicity related to dronedarone. Later that year, Health Canada also issued a safety communication regarding an increased risk of death and serious cardiovascular events associated with its use.

▶ amiodarone hydrochloride

Amiodarone hydrochloride (Cordarone®) markedly prolongs the APD and the ERP in all cardiac tissues. Besides exerting these dramatic effects, it is also known to block both the α- and β-adrenergic receptors of the sympathetic nervous system. Clinically, it is one of the most effective antidysrhythmic drugs for controlling supraventricular and ventricular dysrhythmias. It is indicated for the management of sustained ventricular tachycardia, ventricular fibrillation, and nonsustained ventricular tachycardia. It is reported to be effective in 40 to 60% of all patients with ventricular tachycardia. It is the drug of choice for ventricular dysrhythmias according to the Advanced Cardiac Life Support guidelines. Recently, it has shown promise in the management of atrial dysrhythmias that are difficult to treat with other less toxic drugs.

Amiodarone has many undesirable adverse effects, and these can be are attributed to its chemical properties. Amiodarone is *lipophilic*, or "fat loving." Therefore—because it crosses the phospholipid bilayer of the cell by passive diffusion—once absorbed, it can penetrate and concentrate in the adipose tissue of any organ in the body. For example, it can concentrate in the liver, resulting in hepatic cell injury. It also has iodine in its chemical structure. One organ that sequesters iodine from the diet is the thyroid gland. As a result, amiodarone can cause either hypothyroidism or hyperthyroidism. The package insert for amiodarone lists iodine allergy as a contraindication. However, evidence for avoiding amiodarone in patients with iodine hypersensitivity is extremely limited and does not appear to support its contraindication in patients with severe dysrhythmias.

Adverse reactions occur in approximately 75% of patients treated with this drug, but the incidence is higher and the severity greater with higher dosages (those exceeding 400 mg/day) and prolonged therapy. One of the most common adverse effects is corneal microdeposits, which may cause visual halos, photophobia, and dry eyes. These occur in virtually all adults who take the drug for longer than 6 months. Photosensitivity is also common, reported in 10 to 75% of patients taking amiodarone.

The most serious adverse effect of amiodarone is pulmonary toxicity, which is fatal in about 10% of patients and involves a clinical syndrome of progressive dyspnea and cough accompanied by damage to the alveoli. The result can be pulmonary fibrosis. Another serious complication of amiodarone is that it may not only treat dysrhythmias but also provoke them. Amiodarone has an exceptionally long half-life, approaching many days. As a result, the therapeutic as well as any adverse effects of amiodarone may linger long after the drug has been discontinued. In fact, it may take as long as 2 to 3 months after the drug has been discontinued for some adverse effects to subside. Therapy is usually started in the hospital and is closely monitored until the patient's serum levels are within a therapeutic range.

Continued

DRUG PROFILES—cont'd

Amiodarone has two significant drug interactions, namely with digoxin and warfarin sodium. It is reported that digoxin levels will increase by 50% and that the INR will increase by 50% in 100% of patients taking these drugs in combination with amiodarone. When the drug is started in patients who are already taking one of these drugs, it is recommended that the dose of digoxin or warfarin sodium be reduced by 50% at the start of therapy.

Use of amiodarone is contraindicated in patients who have a known hypersensitivity to it and in those with severe sinus bradycardia, or second- or third-degree heart block. Recommended conversions are available for cases in which the patient is maintained on long-term oral amiodarone therapy after intravenous amiodarone administration is discontinued. This drug is marketed in both oral and injectable forms.

PHARMACOKINETICS

Route	Onset of Action	Peak Plasma Concentration	Elimination Half-Life	Duration of Action
PO	1–3 wk	2–10 hr	15–100 days	10–150 days
IV	Minutes (bolus); 1 hr (IV)	10–15 minutes	30–45 minutes	short

ibutilide fumarate

Ibutilide fumarate (Corvert®) is a class III antidysrhythmic drug. Unlike the other two drugs in this class, ibutilide fumurate is indicated for atrial dysrhythmias. Atrial fibrillation and atrial flutter cause irregular contractions of the heart and can lead to serious outcomes, such as decreased cardiac output, heart failure, low blood pressure, and stroke. Although other pharmacological therapies are used to treat atrial fibrillation and flutter, ibutilide is the only drug available for rapid conversion of these two conditions to normal sinus rhythm. The only other treatment that can produce rapid conversion is electrical cardioversion. Although it is effective, electrical cardioversion carries the risk, expense, and inconvenience of both the procedure itself and the anaesthesia it requires.

Ibutilide is dosed based on patient weight. Use of ibutilide is contraindicated in patients who have previously demonstrated hypersensitivity to it. As with other antidysrhythmic drugs, ibutilide is to be used with caution because it can also produce dysrhythmias, most significantly ventricular tachycardia and torsades de pointes. Class Ia antidysrhythmic drugs (e.g., disopyramide, quinidine, and procainamide) and other class III drugs (e.g., amiodarone and sotalol) should not be administered with ibutilide, nor should they be given within 4 hours after infusion of ibutilide because of their potential to prolong refractoriness. Ibutilide is available only in the injectable form.

PHARMACOKINETICS

Route	Onset of Action	Peak Plasma Concentration	Elimination Half-Life	Duration of Action
IV	10 min	30 min	6 hr	4 hr

▶▶ sotalol hydrochloride

Sotalol hydrochloride (Rylosol®) is a selective β-blocker that is used to treat dysrhythmias. It is unique in that it possesses antidysrhythmic properties similar to those of the class III drugs (such as amiodarone), while simultaneously exerting β-blocker or class II effects on the conduction system of the heart. In addition, sotalol has prodysrhythmic properties similar to those of the class Ic drugs. This means that while patients are taking sotalol, it can cause serious dysrhythmias, such as torsades de pointes or a new ventricular tachycardia or fibrillation. Like flecainide and propafenone, sotalol was historically reserved for the treatment of documented, life-threatening ventricular dysrhythmias such as sustained ventricular tachycardia. However, recent data indicates it to be safe.

Contraindications to sotalol use include hypersensitivity to it, bronchial asthma, cardiogenic shock, and sinus bradycardia. Sotalol is available only in oral form.

PHARMACOKINETICS

Route	Onset of Action	Peak Plasma Concentration	Elimination Half-Life	Duration of Action
PO	1–2 hr	2.5–4 hr	12 hr	8–16 hr

CLASS IV DRUGS

Class IV antidysrhythmic drugs are the calcium channel blockers. Besides being effective antidysrhythmics, calcium channel blockers are useful in the treatment of hypertension (Chapter 23) and angina. Verapamil and diltiazem are the two most commonly used calcium channel blockers for (1) treating dysrhythmias, specifically those that arise above the ventricles (paroxysmal supraventricular tachycardia) and (2) controlling the ventricular response to atrial fibrillation and flutter by slowing conduction and prolonging refractoriness of the AV node (i.e., preventing the ventricles from beating as fast as the atria).

These drugs block the slow inward flow of calcium ions into the slow (calcium) channels in cardiac conduction tissue. The conduction effects of calcium channel blockers are limited to the atria and the AV node, where conduction is prolonged and the tissues are made more refractory to stimulation. These drugs have little effect on ventricular tissues.

▶▶ diltiazem hydrochloride

Diltiazem hydrochloride (Cardizem®, Tiazac®) is primarily indicated for the temporary control of a rapid ventricular response in patients with atrial fibrillation or flutter and paroxysmal supraventricular tachycardia. Its use is contraindicated in patients with hypersensitivity to it, acute MI, pulmonary congestion, Wolff–Parkinson–White syndrome, severe hypotension, cardiogenic shock, sick sinus syndrome, or second- or third-degree AV block. Diltiazem is available in both oral and parenteral forms.

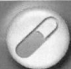
DRUG PROFILES–cont'd

PHARMACOKINETICS

Route	Onset of Action	Peak Plasma Concentration	Elimination Half-Life	Duration of Action
PO	0.5–1 hr	2–3 hr	3.5–9 hr	4–12 hr

▶▶ verapamil hydrochloride

Verapamil hydrochloride (Isoptin SR®) has actions similar to those of diltiazem in that it also inhibits calcium ion influx across the slow calcium channels in cardiac conduction tissue. This results in dramatic effects on the AV node. Verapamil is used to prevent and convert recurrent paroxysmal supraventricular tachycardia and to control ventricular response in atrial flutter or fibrillation. It can also temporarily control a rapid ventricular response to these frequent atrial stimulations, usually decreasing the heart rate by at least 20%. Verapamil is used not only for the management of dysrhythmias, but also to treat angina, hypertension, and hypertrophic cardiomyopathy. The contraindications that apply to diltiazem apply to verapamil as well. It is also available in both oral and parenteral forms.

PHARMACOKINETICS

Route	Onset of Action	Peak Plasma Concentration	Elimination Half-Life	Duration of Action
PO	1–2 hr	3 hr	4.5–12 hr	6–8 hr

UNCLASSIFIED ANTIDYSRHYTHMICS

adenosine

Adenosine (Adenocard®) is an unclassified antidysrhythmic drug. It slows the electrical conduction time through the AV node and is indicated for the conversion of paroxysmal supraventricular tachycardia to sinus rhythm. It is particularly useful when the paroxysmal supraventricular tachycardia has failed to respond to verapamil or when the patient has coexisting conditions such as heart failure, hypotension, or left ventricular dysfunction that limits the use of verapamil. Its use is contraindicated in patients with second- or third-degree heart block, sick sinus syndrome, atrial flutter or fibrillation, or ventricular tachycardia, as well as in those with a known hypersensitivity to it. It has an extremely short half-life of less than 10 seconds. For this reason, it is administered only intravenously and only by a fast direct intravenous injection followed by a fast direct intravenous saline flush. It commonly causes asystole for a period of seconds. All other adverse effects are minimal because of its short duration of action. Adenosine is available only in parenteral form. This drug would be given only with heart monitoring in a critical care setting.

PHARMACOKINETICS

Route	Onset of Action	Peak Plasma Concentration	Elimination Half-Life	Duration of Action
IV	Immediate	Immediate	Less than 10 sec	Extremely brief

NURSING PROCESS

▨ Assessment

Before any antidysrhythmic is administered to a patient, conduct a thorough nursing assessment and head-to-toe physical assessment, and complete a medical history and medication profile. Assess for contraindications, cautions, and drug interactions. Review any baseline ECGs and interpret the results, and measure the patient's vital signs, with attention to blood pressure; postural blood pressures; heart sounds; and heart rate, rhythm, and quality. Other signs and symptoms to assess that are related to decreased cardiac functioning (as a result of a dysrhythmia and decreased cardiac output) include apical-radial pulse deficits, jugular vein distention, edema, prolonged capillary refill (longer than 5 seconds), decreased urinary output, activity intolerance, chest pain or pressure, dyspnea, and fatigue. Document any changes in level of alertness, increase in anxiety levels, syncope, or dizziness.

Laboratory studies generally include kidney and liver function tests because abnormal functioning may call for a decrease in the drug dosage by the prescriber to prevent toxicity. Be sure to emphasize to the patient the interaction with grapefruit juice, which inhibits metabolism by cytochrome P450 3A4 hepatic enzymes (see Chapter 2 for a more in-depth discussion of this topic). The interaction of grapefruit juice with amiodarone, disopyramide, and quinidine leads to an increased risk of toxicity and cinchonism. Cinchonism results from an excessive dose of cinchonia bark used to manufacture quinine; it is characterized by headache, tinnitus, and vomiting. Other drug interactions with antidysrhythmics are presented in Table 26-6. Altering of dosages is necessary in these situations to help prevent excessive accumulation and toxicity. (See also Evidence in Practice: Antidysrhythmics and Older Adults).

With the use of lidocaine, assess the cardiovascular system, with attention to heart rate and blood pressure. With amiodarone, assess respiratory, thyroid, liver, dermatological, and hypertensive conditions due to possible drug-related pulmonary toxicity, exacerbation of thyroid disorders, abnormal liver function tests, and rash. Further assessment for drug interactions (see Table 26-6) as well as contraindications and cautions is also needed.

EVIDENCE IN PRACTICE

Antidysrhythmics and Older Adults

Background
A review article presented a thorough examination of research studies and clinical trials investigating the management of dysrhythmia in older adults. As noted in the article, the most interesting and recent application of pacemaker implantation has been for cardiac resynchronization in patients with advanced heart failure. Chronic heart failure is increasing in prevalence. Because older adults are more susceptible to atrial fibrillation, life-threatening ventricular dysrhythmias, and symptomatic bradycardia, it is very important for health care providers (HCPs) to be able to identify abnormal rhythms and initiate appropriate therapies to help prevent stroke and improve quality of life and survival. The article includes a review of the data, but it is the summary of the treatment modalities that is noteworthy.

Type of Evidence
The article provided a review of clinical trials and management of irregularities in heart rate in older adults. It also presented a review of treatment regimens.

Results of Study
Older adults are at increased risk for both atrial and ventricular irregularities even though they may be clinically healthy, and the occurrence of irregularities increases the risk of other problems in these patients. Discussed in this study were the options presented by a new generation of oral anticoagulants and percutaneously implanted devices that may soon play a more expanded role in the management of atrial fibrillation. Data from large clinical trials have shown that the use of automatic implanted cardioverter defibrillators (AICDs) to treat ventricular

tachydysrhythmias improves the survival of these patients. Biventricular pacing is also a treatment modality with an identifiable role in reducing morbidity in patients with heart failure. The article also reviews other studies and trials that evaluate the role of treatment modalities in the management of heart irregularities in older adults. The treatment methods examined have provided older adults with the possibility of improved quality of life, decreased morbidity, and longer survival.

Link of Evidence to Nursing Practice
Older adults are subject to a variety of insults to their physiological and psychological status, and even if they are in normal health for their age, the risk for abnormal heart conditions and rhythms is high. The studies reviewed in this article provide evidence of improved quality of life and reduced morbidity and mortality with the use of these treatment modalities. It is important for nurses to be aware of reliable, valid clinical trial data, such as those examined in the article, so that they can support patients and families throughout implementation of new treatment plans, including use of antidysrhythmics, anticoagulants, implanted pacemakers, cardioverters and defibrillators, and biventricular pacing. Research findings such as the trial data reviewed in this article may continue to improve patient care and lead to sound, evidence-informed medical and nursing practice.

Based on Wenger, N. K., Helmy, T., Patel, A. D., et al. (2005). Approaching cardiac arrhythmias in the elderly patient. *Medscape General Medicine*, 7(4). Retrieved from http://www.medscape.com/viewarticle/514471.

Pharmacokinetic Bridge to Nursing Practice

Amiodarone

A study of long-term oral amiodarone therapy for the treatment of dysrhythmias provides a different perspective on pharmacokinetics. To aid in evaluating the complex pharmacokinetic properties of amiodarone and developing an optimal dosing schedule for the drug in long-term oral drug therapy, serum concentrations of the drug and its metabolite, desethylamiodarone, were monitored in 345 Japanese patients receiving amiodarone. Serum concentrations of the drug and its metabolite were determined by an analysis called chromatography. In 245 participants who took fixed maintenance dosages of the drug for 6 months, there were small variations in the ratio of the serum level of the actual drug to the serum level of its metabolite. (The concept of metabolism as it relates to pharmacokinetics is discussed in Chapter 2). Other

pharmacokinetic properties of amiodarone included a slightly higher average clearance in women than in men, even though there were no differences between men and women in regard to age, dosage, or duration of action of the dose. Japanese patients showed little variation in the pharmacokinetics of the drug. From this study, one can see how important it is to understand basic pharmacokinetic parameters (e.g., dosing, clearance, drug metabolism, serum concentrations) and to recognize that they are critical components of drug therapy and the nursing process. It is also important to note that culture, gender, age, and racial or ethnic group have an impact on how each person responds to a drug and how each drug may vary in its action.

Nursing Diagnoses

- Decreased cardiac output related to the pathology of the dysrhythmia

DOSAGES   Selected Antidysrhythmic Drugs

Drug Name	Pharmacological Class	Usual Dosage Range
Class I		
quinidine sulfate	Class Ia antidysrhythmic	**Adults** IV: 200–750 mg infused at up to 10 mg/min
▶▶lidocaine hydrochloride (Xylocaine)	Class Ib antidysrhythmic	**Children** IV: bolus dose, 1 mg/kg; usual maintenance infusion rate, 20–50 mcg/kg/min **Adults** IV: Bolus dose 50–100 mg; may be repeated in 5 min; do not exceed 200–300 mg over 1 hr; usual maintenance infusion rate 1–4 mg/min
propafenone hydrochloride (Rythmol)	Class Ic antidysrhythmic	**Adults** PO: Start with 150 mg q8h and increase q3–4 days; usual range, 450–900 mg/day divided
Class II		
metoprolol tartrate (Lopresor)	β$_1$-blocker (class II antidysrhythmic)	**Adults** IV/PO: 3 bolus injections of 5 mg at 2-min intervals followed by 50 mg PO q6h for 48 h, thereafter 50–100 mg bid PO: 50–100 mg bid
Class III		
▶▶amiodarone hydrochloride (Cordarone)	Class III antidysrhythmic	**Adults** IV: 150 mg over 10 min, then 60 mg/h for 6 h, then 30 mg/h as maintenance dose PO: 800–1600 mg/day for 1–3 wk, reduced to 400–800 mg/day for 5 wk; usual maintenance dose 200–400 mg/day
ibutilide fumarate (Corvert)	Class III antidysrhythmic	**Adults** IV: 1-mg infusion over 10 min (if patient weighs less than 60 kg, then 0.1 mL/kg)
▶▶sotalol hydrochloride* (Rylosol)	Class III antidysrhythmic	**Adults** PO: 160–320 mg/day divided into 2–3 doses
Class IV		
▶▶diltiazem hydrochloride (Cardizem)	Calcium channel blocker (class IV antidysrhythmic)	**Adults** IV: Bolus dose 0.25 mg/kg over 2 min, second dose 0.35 mg/kg over 2 min after 15 min as needed, then 5–10 mg/h by continuous infusion PO: 120–360 mg daily
▶▶verapamil hydrochloride (Isoptin)	Calcium channel blocker (class IV antidysrhythmic)	**Children** IV: 0–1 yr: 0.1–0.2 mg/kg bolus over 2 min; 0.1–0.2 mg/kg repeat dose after 30 min; 1–15 yr: 0.1–0.3 mg/kg bolus over 2 min; do not exceed 5-mg dose; repeat dose not exceeding 10 mg may be given after 30 min **Adults** PO: Start with 80 mg tid–qid; daily range 240–480 mg IV: 5–10 mg bolus over 2 min; repeat dose of 10 mg may be given after 30 min
Unclassified		
adenosine (Adenocard)	Unclassified antidysrhythmic	**Adults** IV: 6-mg bolus over 1–2 sec; second rapid bolus of 12 mg as needed, which may be repeated a second time as needed

IM, intramuscular; IV, intravenous; PO, oral.
*Sotalol also has class II properties.

- Ineffective peripheral tissue perfusion related to the physiological impact of the dysrhythmia
- Deficient knowledge related to lack of experience with medication therapy

Planning

Goals

- Patient will experience improved cardiac output.
- Patient will experience improved peripheral perfusion/ circulation.
- Patient will demonstrate adequate knowledge about the medication therapy.

Outcome Criteria

- Patient's symptoms of dysrhythmia and subsequent decreased cardiac output are decreased and alleviated.
- Patient's peripheral pulses are bilaterally equal, strong, and regular; extremities are warm and pink.
- Patient states rationale for taking medication as prescribed, as well as its therapeutic effects and adverse effects.
- Patient experiences increase in energy and stamina and improved ability to carry out activities of daily living due to positive therapeutic outcomes from drug therapy.

Implementation

When antidysrhythmics are administered, monitor vital signs, especially pulse rate and blood pressure, before administering the drug; if pulse rate is lower than 60 beats per minute, notify the HCP. During the initiation of therapy, closely monitor the ECG and vital signs because of possible prolongation of the QT interval by more than 50%. The end result may be the occurrence of a variety of conduction disturbances. Advise patients that oral dosage forms are better tolerated if taken with food and fluids to help minimize GI upset, unless otherwise ordered. During treatment with quinidine (or with any of the antidysrhythmics), immediately report to the HCP any patient report of angina, hypotension, lightheadedness, loss of appetite, tinnitus, or diarrhea. An infusion pump is recommended for intravenous dosing of any of the classes of antidysrhythmics, with proper solution and dilution.

With lidocaine, vials of clear solution are labelled as either *for cardiac use* or *not for cardiac use*. This is important to remember when reading the vial's label so that the wrong drug is not given. It is also important to remember that lidocaine solutions need to be used with extreme caution and that it is the plain solution that is used to treat various cardiac conditions. Parenteral solutions of these drugs are usually stable for only 24 hours. Lidocaine is also used as an anaesthetic, so the different

concentrations of the drug need to be double-checked, if not triple-checked. In addition, lidocaine comes in a solution with epinephrine, a potent vasoconstrictor. This combined solution is indicated when the surgeon or physician is suturing or repairing wounds, with the lidocaine acting as an anaesthetic and the epinephrine causing vasoconstriction of the local blood vessels and helping to control bleeding of the area, or in dental or oral situations. The solution with epinephrine must *never* be used intravenously, but only as a topical anaesthetic. With lidocaine, document vital signs prior to initiation of and during therapy, and closely monitor the ECG. Often, when patients are receiving this drug, they are in a cardiac step-down unit, telemetry unit, or intensive care setting.

Amiodarone may lead to GI upset, which may be prevented or decreased by taking the drug with a meal or a snack. Photosensitivity (sunburn and other exaggerated skin reactions to the sunlight) and photophobia (light sensitivity) are other concerns with this drug. With photosensitivity, protective clothing, a hat and sunscreen are needed. Emphasize the importance of eye protection, such as with sunglasses or tinted contact lenses, to patients taking this medication. Encourage consumption of fluids and a high-fibre diet to minimize the constipation that is a common adverse effect of antidysrhythmic drugs. When β-blockers are used with an antidysrhythmic, any shortness of breath, weight gain, changes in baseline blood glucose levels, or excess fatigue (see Chapters 23 and 33) must be reported to the HCP immediately.

β-blockers, diltiazem, and verapamil may all be used to manage abnormal rhythms and are to be given only after checking and documenting pulse rates and blood pressures. Contact the HCP and withhold the drug—if supported by facility policy and the HCP's guidelines—if the pulse rate is 60 beats per minute or lower or 100 beats per minute or higher or if the systolic blood pressure is 90 mm Hg or lower.

Evaluation

It is important to monitor patients receiving all classes of antidysrhythmics to confirm the therapeutic effects as well as identify the adverse and toxic effects. Class I through class IV antidysrhythmics drugs have many overlapping therapeutic effects, adverse effects, and toxicities.

Therapeutic effects, in general, include improved cardiac output; decreased chest discomfort; decreased fatigue; improved vital signs, skin colour, and urinary output; and conversion of irregularities to normal rhythm. Adverse effects for the class I antidysrhythmics include hypotension, rash, diarrhea, drug-induced lupus erythematosuslike syndrome characterized by joint and muscle pain, fatigue, pericarditis, and pleuritis (with use of procainamide); ECG changes, bitter taste, anorexia, blurred vision, and tinnitus (with use of quinidine); and

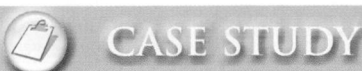

CASE STUDY

Antidysrhythmic Medications

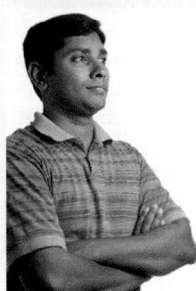

Vijay, a 46-year-old patient, is admitted to the emergency room after going to the hospital reporting chest pain. He is diagnosed with CAD with a partial block of one of his coronary arteries and is awaiting an angioplasty procedure. He has a history of alcoholism but states that he has not had a drink for 2 years, thanks to Alcoholics Anonymous. In the intensive care unit, Vijay's heart monitor indicates increased episodes of PVCs. When a 20-second run of ventricular tachycardia is noted, the nurse decides to implement the standing orders for a lidocaine infusion. The standing order reads: "For episodes of ventricular tachycardia, give a loading dose of 75 mg of lidocaine

intravenous (IV) push; repeat this dose in 5 minutes, and then begin a continuous infusion of 2 mg/min IV."
1. What factors will the nurse consider before beginning the lidocaine infusion?
2. What will the nurse monitor while Vijay is receiving this infusion?

Three days later, Vijay is ready for discharge. He has had the angioplasty procedure, which was deemed a success, and the lidocaine infusion was discontinued the previous day. He has been started on oral procainamide. Vijay asks the nurse, "What are the possible side effects of this drug? It seems that all drugs have bad side effects."
3. What is the nurse's best answer to this question?

_____

For answers, see http://evolve.elsevier.com/Canada/Lilley/pharmacology/.

gingival hyperplasia and decrease in blood pressure and pulse rate (with use of phenytoin sodium). Class II β-blockers may cause bradycardia, AV block, heart failure, bronchospasm, and changes in blood glucose levels. Amiodarone, a class III drug, may lead to

pulmonary toxicity, thyroid disorders, decrease in blood pressure and pulse rate, photosensitivity, and abnormal liver function. Calcium channel blockers, or class IV drugs, are associated with heart block, hypotension, constipation, dizziness, and dyspnea (see Table 26-6).

PATIENT TEACHING TIPS

❖ Instruct patients not to crush or chew any oral dosage form that is identified as sustained-release or extended-release and not to alter the original dosage form of the drug in any way.

❖ Some dosage forms are delivered in a sustained-released tablet or capsule that may be composed of a wax matrix, and this matrix may be visible in the patient's stool. This extended-release dosage form provides for a slow release of the medicine, and the wax substance may then be passed out of the body through the stool. Advise patients that the passing of the matrix through the stool occurs after the drug has been absorbed, and although the matrix is often visible to the naked eye, its presence in the stool is of no major concern.

❖ If the use of an oral preparation is associated with continual and moderate or severe GI distress, tell the patient to take the drug with food and to contact the HCP if nausea and vomiting worsen.

❖ If an antacid is needed, inform the patient that it must be taken either 2 hours before or 2 hours after the antidysrhythmic drug to avoid interference with drug absorption.

❖ Recommend a well-balanced diet and encourage an increase in fluid intake of up to 3 L of water a day, unless contraindicated.

❖ Educate the patient to limit or avoid caffeine and grapefruit intake. Caffeine-containing foods and beverages include coffee (decaffeinated coffee contains

2 to 4 mg caffeine per 240 mL, while caffeinated coffee contains 65 to 120 mg per 240 mL), tea, some soft drinks, chocolate, and energy drinks. Grapefruit can increase drug absorption and potential adverse effects.

❖ Instruct the patient to take medications exactly as prescribed, without doubling up or omitting doses. If the patient forgets a dose or is ill and cannot take a dose, contact the HCP for further instructions.

❖ Provide written and verbal instructions and demonstrations for measuring pulse and blood pressure.

❖ Advise the patient to use journalling to document how the patient feels each day. Recommend recording in the journal any worsening or improvement of symptoms, adverse effects, daily weights, activity tolerance, blood pressure readings, and pulse rate. (Daily weights need to be measured at the same time every day and with the same amount of clothing.)

❖ Tell the patient to contact the HCP immediately if there is a weight gain of 1 kg or more in 24 hours or 2.3 kg or more in 1 week.

❖ Inform the patient that changing positions purposefully and with caution is important because of the common adverse effect of orthostatic hypotension—moving too quickly may lead to dizziness, syncope, and subsequent injury or falls.

❖ At the beginning of therapy and after any dosage increase, encourage the patient to avoid driving and other hazardous activities until sedating adverse effects have resolved.

Continued

PATIENT TEACHING TIPS—cont'd

❖ Dry mouth may be helped by frequent mouth care, drinking fluids, chewing on sugarless gum, sucking on sugarless candy, and eating ice chips. Artificial saliva and special toothpaste made specifically for dry mouth and its management are available over the counter. Encourage frequent dental visits.

❖ Counsel the patient to avoid exertion, hot temperatures, saunas, and hot tubs because of heat-induced vasodilation, leading to orthostatic hypotension with dizziness or syncope and a subsequent risk for falls or injury. Alcohol intake may also lead to vasodilation and subsequent dizziness and syncope.

❖ Emphasize the need to wear a medical alert bracelet or necklace identifying the patient's specific medical diagnosis and provide a list of all medications and allergies. The patient needs to understand the importance of carrying this information (in either written or electronic form), having it available at all times, and updating it regularly and whenever there are major changes in the diagnosis and treatment regimen.

❖ Instruct the patient to report immediately to the HCP any dizziness, shortness of breath, chest pain, worsening of symptoms, or occurrence of new symptoms.

❖ The patient must *never* stop taking these medications without specific instructions to do so; an abrupt discontinuation of these drugs may lead to severe or life-threatening complications.

❖ With amiodarone, photosensitivity is an adverse effect; advise the patient to avoid sun exposure and to wear sun-protective clothing and dark glasses when outside. Sunblocks that block ultraviolet B light are recommended, such as those containing zinc or titanium chloride.

❖ With amiodarone, instruct the patient to immediately report any blue–grey discoloration of the skin (often after 1 year, and especially on the face, neck, and arms) as well as any jaundice, unusual rashes or skin reactions, nausea, vomiting, or dizziness.

KEY POINTS

❖ The SA node, AV node, and bundle of His-Purkinje cells are all areas in which there is automaticity (i.e., cells can depolarize spontaneously). The SA node is the pacemaker because it can spontaneously depolarize more easily and quickly than the other areas can.

❖ Any disturbance or abnormality in the pattern of the heartbeat and pulse rate is termed a *dysrhythmia*.

❖ Antidysrhythmic drugs are used to correct dysrhythmias; however, they may also cause dysrhythmias, and for this reason are said to be *prodysrhythmic*. The Vaughan Williams classification system is most commonly used to classify antidysrhythmic drugs. It classifies groups of drugs according to where and how they affect cardiac cells and what their mechanism of action is:

  • *Class I:* membrane-stabilizing drugs (e.g., class Ia: quinidine; class Ib: lidocaine; class Ic: flecainide)
  • *Class II:* β-adrenergic blockers that depress phase 4 depolarization (e.g., atenolol)

  • *Class III:* drugs that prolong repolarization in phase 3 (e.g., amiodarone, ibutilide)
  • *Class IV:* calcium channel blockers that depress phase 4 depolarization (e.g., verapamil)

❖ Nursing actions for the antidysrhythmic drugs include skillful nursing assessment and close monitoring of heart rate, blood pressure, heart rhythms, general well-being, skin colour, temperature, and heart and breath sounds. Some of the antidysrhythmics are administered in specialty areas (e.g., critical care units, coronary care units, emergency rooms) depending on the route (e.g., by IV) and the institution policy.

❖ Therapeutic responses to antidysrhythmics include a decrease in blood pressure in hypertensive patients, a decrease in edema, and restoration of a regular pulse rate without major irregularities or with improved regularity compared to before therapy.

EXAMINATION REVIEW QUESTIONS

1. A patient with a rapid, irregular heart rhythm is being treated in the emergency department with adenosine. During administration of this drug, the nurse will be prepared to monitor for which effect?
  a. Nausea and vomiting
  b. Transitory asystole
  c. Muscle tetany
  d. Hypertension

2. When assessing a patient who has been taking amiodarone for 6 months, the nurse monitors for which potential adverse effect?
  a. Hyperglycemia
  b. Dysphagia
  c. Photophobia
  d. Urticaria

EXAMINATION REVIEW QUESTIONS—cont'd

3. The nurse is assessing a patient who has been on quinidine and asks about adverse effects. Which of the following is an adverse effect associated with the use of this drug?
a. Muscle pain
b. Tinnitus
c. Chest pain
d. Excessive thirst

4. A patient calls the family medicine clinic to report that he saw his pills in his stools when he had a bowel movement. What will the nurse respond?
a. "The pills are not being digested properly. You should be taking them on an empty stomach."
b. "The pills are not being digested properly. You should be taking them with food."
c. "What you are seeing is the waxy matrix that contained the medication, but the drug has been absorbed."
d. "This indicates that you are not tolerating this medication and will need to switch to a different form."

5. The nurse is administering lidocaine and considers which condition, if present in the patient, a caution for the use of this drug?
a. Tachycardia
b. Hypertension
c. Ventricular dysrhythmias
d. Kidney dysfunction

6. When the nurse is teaching a patient about taking an antidysrhythmic drug, which statements by the nurse are correct? (Select all that apply.)
a. "Take the medication with an antacid if stomach upset occurs."
b. "Do not chew sustained-release capsules."
c. "If weight gain of 2.3 kg within 1 week occurs, notify your HCP at the next office visit."
d. "If you experience severe adverse effects, stop the drug and notify your physician."
e. "You may take the medication with food if stomach upset occurs."

7. A patient is in the emergency department with new-onset rapid-rate atrial fibrillation. The nurse is about to add a continuous infusion of diltiazem at 5 mg/hr, but must first give a bolus of 0.25 mg/kg over 2 minutes. The patient weighs 220 pounds. The medication comes in a vial of 5 mg/mL. How many milligrams will the patient receive, and how many millilitres will the nurse draw up for this dose?

Answers: 1. b, 2. c, 3. b, 4. c, 5. d, 6. b, e, 7. 25 mg; 5 mL.

CRITICAL THINKING ACTIVITIES

1. A patient who was admitted to the hospital for treatment of atrial fibrillation is about to go home with a new prescription for diltiazem (Cardizem). As the nurse goes over the patient's medication list, the patient reports, "I'm feeling very tired. And when I stand up, I can hardly walk because I'm so dizzy." What is the nurse's priority action?

2. A patient will be discharged from the hospital with a prescription for amiodarone (Cordarone). He has been ill for some time and tells the nurse, "I cannot wait to get to my beach house and relax outside by the ocean. I'm sure the fresh air will be good for me." What is the priority for patient teaching at this time?

3. A patient has been admitted to the emergency department and is experiencing paroxysmal supraventricular tachycardia that has not responded to treatment with calcium channel blockers. Immediately after the patient receives a dose of adenosine by intravenous push, the monitor shows asystole. What is the nurse's priority action in response to the asystole?

For answers, see http://evolve.elsevier.com/Canada/Lilley/pharmacology/.

CHAPTER 27

Coagulation Modifier Drugs

Objectives

After reading this chapter, the successful student will be able to do the following:

1. Briefly review the coagulation process and the impact of coagulation modifiers such as anticoagulants, antiplatelets, thrombolytics, and antifibrinolytics.

2. Compare the mechanisms of action, indications, cautions, contraindications, drug interactions, adverse effects, routes of administration, and dosages of the various anticoagulants, antiplatelets, thrombolytics, and antifibrinolytics.

3. Discuss the administration procedures and techniques as well as related standards of care for the various coagulation modifiers.

4. Identify any available antidotes for the coagulation modifiers.

5. Compare the laboratory tests used in conjunction with treatment with the various coagulation modifiers and their implications for therapeutic use of these drugs and monitoring for adverse reactions.

6. Develop a collaborative plan of care that includes all phases of the nursing process for patients receiving anticoagulants, antiplatelet drugs, thrombolytics, and antifibrinolytics.

e-Learning Activities

Website
(http://evolve.elsevier.com/Canada/Lilley/pharmacology/)

*e*volve

- Answer Key—Textbook Case Studies
- Answer Key—Critical Thinking Activities
- Chapter Summaries—Printable
- Review Questions for Exam Preparation
- Unfolding Case Studies

Drug Profiles

▸▸ alteplase, p. 532
  aminocaproic acid
  argatroban, p. 526
▸▸ aspirin, p. 530
▸▸ clopidogrel (clopidogrel bisulphate)*, p. 530
▸▸ dabigatran etexilate mesylate, p. 526
  desmopressin (desmopressin acetate)*, p. 533
▸▸ enoxaparin (enoxaparin sodium)*, p. 525
▸▸ eptifibatide p. 530
▸▸ fondaparinux sodium, p. 526
▸▸ heparin (heparin sodium)*, p. 525
▸▸ warfarin (warfarin sodium)*, p. 525

▸▸ Key drug

*Full generic name is given in parentheses. For the purposes of this text, the more common, shortened name is used.

Key Terms

Anticoagulants Substances that prevent or delay coagulation of the blood. (p. 518)

Antifibrinolytic drugs Drugs that prevent the lysis of fibrin and in doing so promote clot formation. (p. 520)

Antiplatelet drugs Substances that prevent platelet plugs from forming. (p. 518)

Antithrombin III (AT-III) A substance that inactivates three major activating factors of the clotting cascade: activated II (thrombin), activated factor X, and activated factor IX. (p. 521)

Clot Insoluble solid elements of blood (e.g., cells, fibrin threads) that have chemically separated from the liquid (plasma) component of the blood. (p. 517)

Coagulation The process of blood clotting; more specifically, the sequential process by which the multiple coagulation factors of the blood interact in the coagulation cascade (see below), ultimately forming an insoluble fibrin clot. (p. 517)

Coagulation cascade The series of steps beginning with the intrinsic or extrinsic pathways of coagulation and proceeding through the formation of a fibrin clot. (p. 517)

Deep vein thrombosis (DVT) The formation of a thrombus in one of the deep veins of the body; most commonly occurs in the iliac and femoral veins. (p. 521)

Embolus A blood clot (thrombus) that has been dislodged from the wall of a blood vessel and travels through the bloodstream; emboli that lodge in critical blood vessels can result in ischemic injury to a vital organ (e.g., heart, lung, brain) and result in disability or death. (p. 517)

Enzyme A protein molecule that catalyzes chemical reactions of other substances without being altered or destroyed in the process. (p. 523)

Fibrin A stringy, insoluble protein produced by the action of thrombin on fibrinogen during the clotting process; a major component of blood clots or thrombi (see thrombus). (p. 517)

Fibrin-specificity The property of some thrombolytic drugs of activating the conversion of plasminogen to plasmin only in the presence of established clots having fibrin threads, rather than inducing systemic plasminogen activation throughout the body. (p. 531)

Fibrinogen A plasma protein that is converted into fibrin by thrombin in the presence of calcium ions. (p. 523)

Fibrinolysis The continual process of fibrin decomposition produced by the actions of the enzymatic protein fibrinolysin; the normal mechanism for removing small fibrin clots, stimulated by anoxia, inflammatory reactions, and other kinds of stress. (p. 518)

Fibrinolytic system An area of the circulatory system undergoing fibrinolysis. (p. 518)

Hemophilia A rare, inherited blood disorder in which the blood does not clot normally. (p. 518)

Hemorheological drugs Drugs that alter the function of platelets without compromising their blood clotting properties. (p. 518)

Hemostasis The arrest of bleeding, either by the physiological properties of vasoconstriction and coagulation or by mechanical, surgical, or pharmacological means. (p. 517)

Hemostatic Referring to any procedure, device, or substance that arrests the flow of blood. (p. 520)

Plasmin The enzymatic protein that breaks down fibrin into fibrin degradation products; derived from plasminogen. (p. 518)

Plasminogen A plasma protein that is converted to plasmin. (p. 518)

Pulmonary embolus (PE) The blockage of a pulmonary artery by foreign matter such as fat, air, tumour cells, or a thrombus that has typically arisen from a peripheral vein. (p. 521)

Stroke Occlusion of the blood vessels of the brain by an embolus, thrombus, or cerebrovascular hemorrhage, resulting in ischemia to brain tissue (may be referred to as a *cerebrovascular accident*). (p. 520)

Thromboembolic events Events in which a blood vessel is blocked by an embolus carried in the bloodstream from the site of its formation; the tissue supplied by an obstructed artery may tingle and become cold, numb, cyanotic, and eventually necrotic (dead). (p. 521)

Thrombolytic drugs Drugs that dissolve thrombi by functioning similarly to tissue plasminogen activator (see below). (p. 520)

Thrombus Blood clot (plural: thrombi); an aggregation of platelets, fibrin, clotting factors, and the cellular elements of the blood that is attached to the interior wall of a vein or artery, sometimes occluding the lumen of the vessel. (p. 517)

Tissue plasminogen activator A naturally occurring plasminogen activator secreted by vascular endothelial cells in the walls of the blood vessels. Thrombolytic drugs are based on this blood component. (p. 517)

HEMOSTASIS AND COAGULATION

Hemostasis is a general term for any process that stops bleeding. This can be accomplished by mechanical means (e.g., compression to the bleeding site) or by surgical means (e.g., surgical clamping or cauterization of a blood vessel). When hemostasis occurs because of physiological clotting of blood, it is called *coagulation*, which is the process of blood clot formation. The technical term for a blood clot is *thrombus*. A thrombus that is not stationary but moves through blood vessels is an *embolus*. Normal hemostasis involves a complex interaction of substances that promote **clot** formation and substances that either inhibit coagulation or dissolve the formed clot. Substances that promote coagulation include platelets, von Willebrand factor, activated clotting factors, and tissue thromboplastin. Substances that inhibit coagulation include prostacyclin, antithrombin III, and proteins C and S. In addition, **tissue plasminogen activator** is a natural substance that dissolves clots that are already formed.

The coagulation system is illustrated in Figures 27-1 and 27-2. It is called a *cascade* (or *coagulation cascade*) because each activated clotting factor serves as a catalyst that amplifies the next reaction. The result is a large concentration of a clot-forming substance called *fibrin*. The

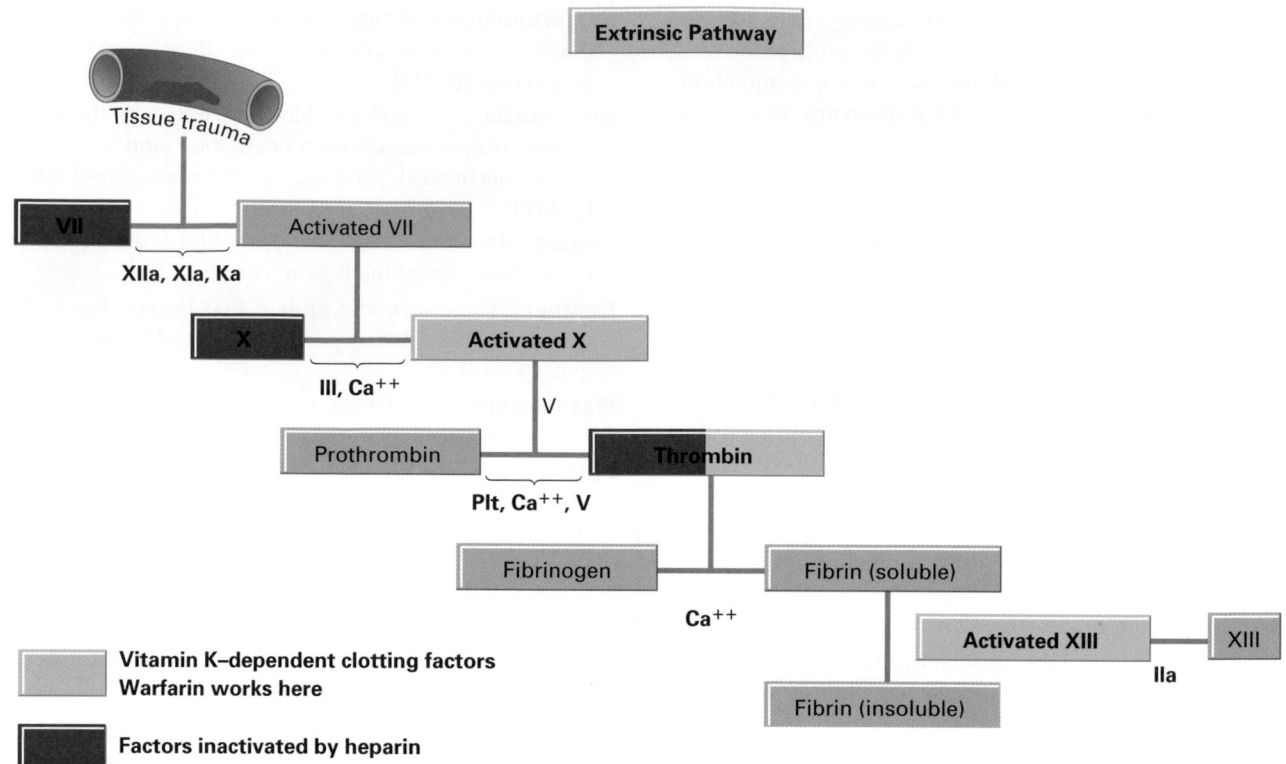

FIG. 27-1 Coagulation pathway and factors: extrinsic pathway. *Plt*, platelets.

coagulation cascade is typically divided into the intrinsic and extrinsic pathways, and these pathways are activated by different types of injury. When blood vessels are damaged by penetration from the outside (e.g., a knife or bullet wound), thromboplastin—a substance contained in the walls of blood vessels—is released. This release initiates the extrinsic pathway by activating factors VII and X (see Figure 27-1). The components of the intrinsic pathway are present in the blood in their inactive forms (see Figure 27-2). This pathway is activated when factor XII comes in contact with exposed collagen on the inside of damaged blood vessels. Figures 27-1 and 27-2 illustrate the steps that occur in the extrinsic and intrinsic pathways, respectively, and the factors involved. They also illustrate the sites of action of two commonly used anticoagulant drugs: warfarin and heparin.

Once a clot is formed and fibrin is present, the **fibrinolytic system** is activated. This system initiates the breakdown of clots and serves to balance the clotting process. **Fibrinolysis** is the reverse of the clotting process. It is the mechanism by which formed thrombi are lysed (broken down) to prevent excessive clot formation and blood vessel blockage. Fibrin in the clot binds to a circulating protein known as *plasminogen*. This binding converts plasminogen to plasmin. **Plasmin** is the enzymatic protein that eventually breaks down the fibrin thrombus into fibrin degradation products. This action keeps the thrombus localized, to prevent it from becoming an embolus that can travel and obstruct a major blood vessel

in the lungs, heart, or brain. Figure 27-3 illustrates the fibrinolytic system.

Hemophilia is a rare genetic disorder in which the previously mentioned natural coagulation and hemostasis factors are limited or absent. Hemophilia is categorized into two main types, depending on which of the coagulation factors is absent (factor VII, factor VIII, or factor IX). Patients with hemophilia can bleed to death if coagulation factors are not given.

COAGULATION MODIFIER DRUGS

Drugs that affect coagulation are some of the most dangerous drugs used today, and numerous factors can affect their action. These drugs are among those most commonly associated with adverse drug reactions. The drugs discussed in this chapter aid the body in reversing or achieving hemostasis, and they can be broken down into several main categories based on their actions. **Anticoagulants** inhibit the action or formation of clotting factors, thereby preventing clots from forming. **Antiplatelet drugs** prevent platelet plugs from forming by inhibiting platelet aggregation, which can be beneficial in preventing heart attacks and strokes. **Hemorrheological drugs** alter platelet function without preventing the platelets from working. Sometimes clots form and totally block a blood vessel. When this happens in one of the coronary arteries, a heart attack occurs, and the clot must be lysed to prevent or minimize damage to myocardial muscle.

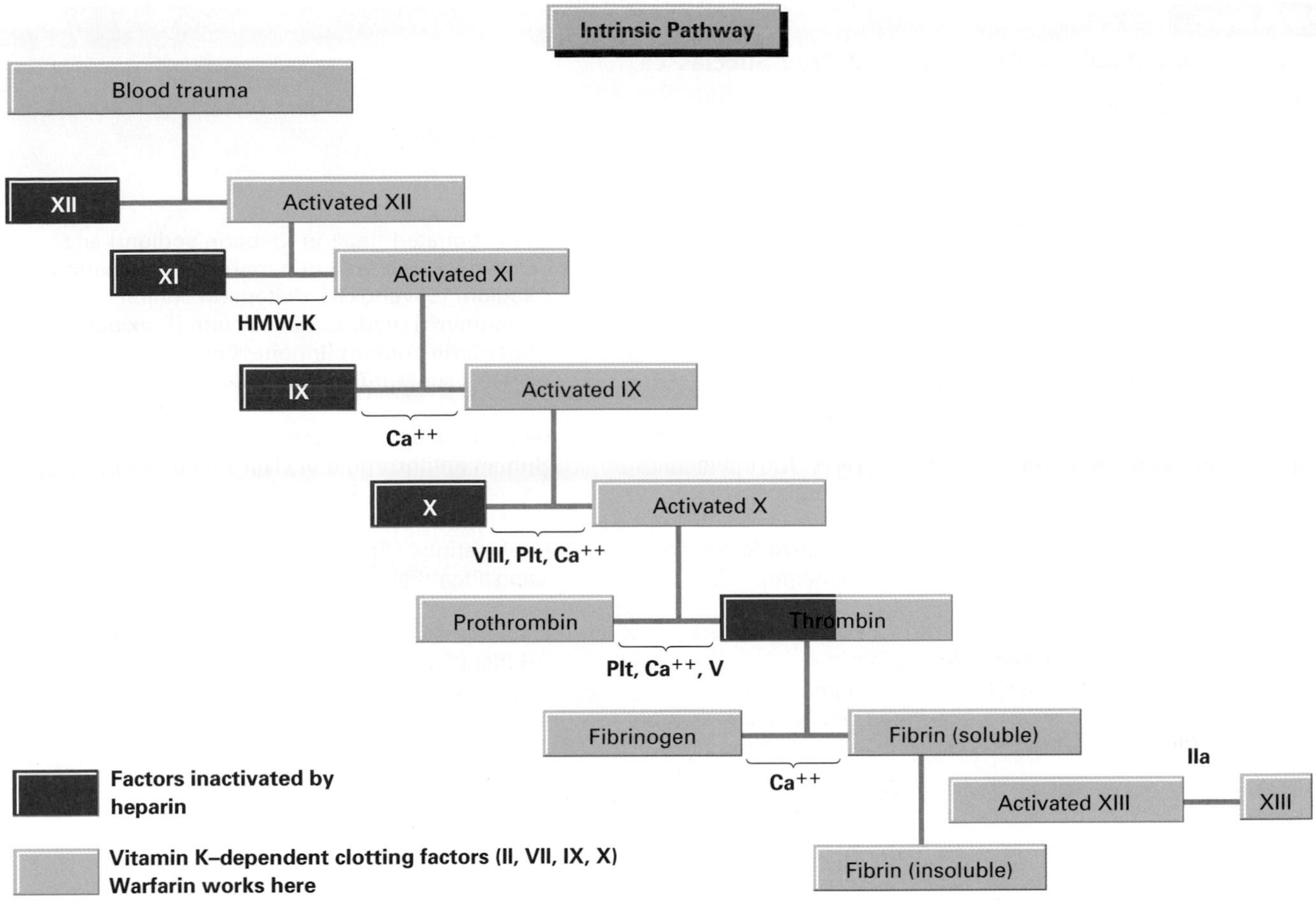

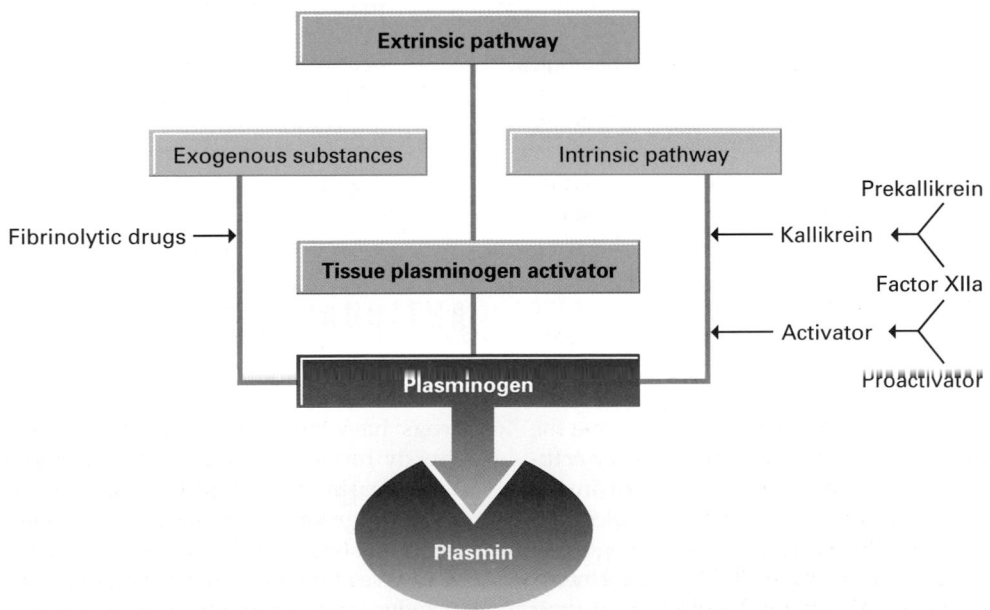

Intrinsic Pathway

Blood trauma

XII → Activated XII

XI → Activated XI

HMW-K

IX → Activated IX

Ca++

X → Activated X

VIII, Plt, Ca++

Prothrombin → Thrombin

Plt, Ca++, V

Fibrinogen → Fibrin (soluble)

Ca++

IIa

Activated XIII — XIII

Fibrin (insoluble)

■ **Factors inactivated by heparin**

▨ **Vitamin K–dependent clotting factors (II, VII, IX, X) Warfarin works here**

FIG. 27-2 Coagulation pathway and factors: intrinsic pathway. *HMW-K*, high-molecular-weight kininogen; *Plt*, platelets.

Extrinsic pathway

Exogenous substances   Intrinsic pathway

Prekallikrein

Fibrinolytic drugs →   Kallikrein ←

Factor XIIa

Tissue plasminogen activator

Activator ←

Proactivator

Plasminogen

Plasmin

FIG. 27-3 The fibrinolytic system.

TABLE 27-1

Coagulation Modifiers: Comparison of Drug Subclasses

Type of Coagulation Modifier and Mechanism of Action	Drug Class	Individual Drugs
PREVENT CLOT FORMATION		
Anticoagulants		
Inhibit clotting factors IIa (thrombin) and Xa	Heparins	Unfractionated heparin (heparin sodium) and low-molecular-weight heparins (enoxaparin sodium [Lovenox®], dalteparin sodium [Fragmin®], nadroparin calcium [Fraxiparine®], tinzaparin sodium [Innohep®])
Inhibit vitamin K–dependent clotting factors II, VII, IX, and X	Coumadins	warfarin sodium (Coumadin®)
Inhibit clotting factors IIa and Xa	Glycosaminoglycans	danaparoid sodium (Orgaran®)
Inhibit thrombin (factor IIa)	Direct thrombin inhibitors	Human antithrombin III (Thrombate III®), argatroban, bivalirudin (Angiomax®), dabigatran etexilate mesylate (Pradaxa®)
Inhibit factor Xa	Selective factor Xa inhibitor	fondaparinux (Arixtra®), rivaroxaban (Xarelto®), apixaban (Eliquis®)
Antiplatelet Drugs		
Interfere with platelet function	P2Y12 inhibitors	clopidogrel bisulphate (Plavix®), prasugrel (Effient®), ticagrelor (Brilenta®)
	Aggregation inhibitors/ vasodilators	treprostinil (Remodulin®)
	Glycoprotein IIb/IIIa inhibitors	abciximab (ReoPro®), eptifibatide (Integrilin®), tirofiban (Aggrastat®)
	Miscellaneous	anagrelide hydrochloride (Agrylin®), dipyridamole (Aggrenox®, Persantine®)
LYSE PREFORMED CLOTS		
Thrombolytics		
Dissolve thrombi	Tissue plasminogen activators	alteplase (Activase RT-PA®, Cathflo), tenecteplase (TNKase®)
PROMOTE CLOT FORMATION		
Antifibrinolytics		
Prevent lysis of fibrin	Systemic hemostats	tranexamic acid (Cyklokapron®), aprotinin (Trasylol®)
Reduce blood viscosity	Hemorrheological	pentoxifylline (Trental®)
REVERSAL DRUGS		
	Heparin sodium antagonist	protamine sulphate
	Warfarin sodium antagonist	vitamin K

Thrombolytic drugs lyse clots, or *thrombi*, that have already formed. This characteristic creates an important distinction between thrombolytics and anticoagulants, which can only prevent the formation of a clot. **Antifibrinolytic drugs,** also known as **hemostatic** *drugs,* have the opposite effect of these other classes of drugs—they actually promote blood coagulation and are helpful in the management of conditions in which excessive bleeding would be harmful. The various drugs in each category of coagulation modifiers are listed in Table 27-1. Understanding the individual coagulation modifiers and their mechanisms of action requires a basic working knowledge of the coagulation pathway and coagulation factors, which are described in the next section.

ANTICOAGULANTS

Drugs that prevent the formation of a clot by inhibiting certain clotting factors are called *anticoagulants*. These drugs have no direct effect on a blood clot that has already formed. They prevent intravascular thrombosis by decreasing blood coagulability. Their uses vary from preventing clot formation to preventing the extension of an established clot.

Once a clot forms on the wall of a blood vessel, it may dislodge and travel through the bloodstream. A dislodged clot is referred to as an *embolus.* If it lodges in a coronary artery, it causes a myocardial infarction (MI); if it obstructs a brain vessel, it causes a **stroke** (cerebrovascular accident [CVA]); if it travels to the lungs, it is a **pulmonary embolus (PE)**; and if it travels to a vein in the leg, it is a **deep vein thrombosis (DVT)**. Collectively, these complications are called **thromboembolic events** because they involve a thrombus that becomes an embolus and causes an adverse cardiovascular "event." Anticoagulants can prevent these from occurring if used in the correct manner. Both orally and parenterally administered anticoagulants are available, and each drug has a slightly different mechanism of action and indications. All of them have their own risks, mainly the risk of causing bleeding. The mechanisms of action of the anticoagulants vary depending on the drug. Drug classes of anticoagulants include older drugs such as unfractionated heparin and warfarin. There are also several newer drug classes, including low-molecular-weight heparins (LMWHs), direct thrombin inhibitors, and a selective factor Xa inhibitor. For dosage information refer to the table on p. 527.

Mechanism of Action and Drug Effects

Anticoagulants are also called *antithrombotic drugs* because they work to prevent the formation of a clot or thrombus, a condition known as *thrombosis*. All anticoagulants work in the clotting cascade but do so at different points. As shown in Figures 27-1 and 27-2, heparin *inhibits* circulating clotting factors. It binds to a substance called *antithrombin III (AT-III)*, which turns off three main activating factors: activated factor II (also called thrombin), activated factor X, and activated factor IX. (Factors XI and XII are also inactivated but do not play as important a role as the other three factors.) Of these, thrombin is the most sensitive to the actions of heparin. AT-III is the major natural inhibitor of thrombin in the blood. The overall effect of heparin is that it turns off the coagulation pathway and prevents clots from forming. However, it cannot lyse a clot. The drug name *heparin* usually refers to unfractionated heparin, which is a relatively large molecule and is derived from porcine intestine. In contrast, LMWHs are synthetic and have a smaller molecular structure. They include enoxaparin (Lovenox), dalteparin (Fragmin), nadroparin calcium (Fraxiparine), and tinzaparin sodium (Innohep). They all work similarly to heparin. Heparin binds primarily to activated factors II, X, and IX, whereas the LMWHs are much more specific for activated factor X (Xa) than for activated factor II (IIa, or thrombin). This property gives LMWHs a much more predictable anticoagulant response. As a result, frequent laboratory monitoring of bleeding times using tests such as activated partial thromboplastin time (aPTT), which is imperative with unfractionated heparin, is not required with LMWHs. When heparin is used for flushing catheters (10–100 units/mL), no monitoring is needed.

Warfarin (Coumadin) inhibits clotting factor synthesis. It works by inhibiting vitamin K synthesis by bacteria in the gastrointestinal (GI) tract. This action, in turn, inhibits production of clotting factors II, VII, IX, and X.

These four factors are normally synthesized in the liver and are known as *vitamin K–dependent clotting factors*. As with heparin, the final effect is the prevention of clot formation. Figures 27-1 and 27-2 show where in the clotting cascade this occurs.

Fondaparinux (Arixtra) inhibits thrombosis by its action against factor Xa alone. Rivaroxaban (Xarelto) and apixaban (Eliquis) are two new oral, direct-acting factor Xa inhibitors, approved for prophylaxis and treatment of DVT and treatment of atrial fibrillation. There are also currently five antithrombin drugs that inhibit thrombin molecules directly, one natural and four synthetic. The natural drug is human antithrombin III (Thrombate), which is isolated from the plasma of human donors. The synthetic drugs are argatroban (Argatroban), bivalirudin (Angiomax), and dabigatran (Pradaxa). Dabigatran is a new oral direct thrombin inhibitor. All of these drugs work similarly to inhibit thrombus formation by inhibiting thrombin.

Indications

The ability of anticoagulants to prevent clot formation is of benefit in certain conditions where there is a high likelihood of clot formation. These include MI, unstable angina, atrial fibrillation, presence of indwelling devices such as mechanical heart valves, and conditions in which blood flow may be slowed and blood may pool, such as major orthopedic surgery, prolonged periods of immobility, or even long plane rides. The ultimate consequence of a clot can be a stroke, an MI, a DVT, or a pulmonary embolism; therefore, the prevention of these serious events is the ultimate benefit of these drugs. Warfarin is indicated for *prevention* of any of these events, whereas unfractionated heparins, LMWHs, direct thrombin inhibitors, and the factor Xa inhibitor are used for both prevention and treatment. Patients at risk for clots are given DVT prophylaxis while in the hospital and after major surgery. LMWHs, are also routinely used as anticoagulant bridge therapy in situations in which a patient must stop warfarin for surgery or other invasive medical procedures. LMWH may also be contraindicated in patients with significant kidney disease; heparin would be preferred in this case. The term *bridge therapy* refers to the fact that heparins (unfractionated or LMWHs) act as a bridge to provide anticoagulation while the patient must be off of warfarin therapy. The remainder of the antithrombotic drugs have similar but more restricted indications, which are listed in the Dosages table on p. 527.

Contraindications

Contraindications to the use of anticoagulants are generally similar for all of the different drugs within this class. They include known drug allergy to a specific product and usually include any acute bleeding, as well as thrombocytopenia. Warfarin is strongly contraindicated in pregnancy, whereas the other anticoagulants are rated in lower pregnancy categories, where benefits of taking the drug during pregnancy may override potential risks.

LMWHs are contraindicated in patients with an indwelling epidural catheter; they can be given 2 hours after the epidural is removed. This is important to remember because giving an LMWH with an epidural has been associated with epidural hematoma.

Adverse Effects

Bleeding is the main complication of anticoagulation therapy, and the risk increases with increasing dosages. Such bleeding may be localized (e.g., hematoma at the site of injection) or systemic. It also depends on the nature of the patient's underlying clinical disorder and is increased in patients taking high doses of aspirin or other drugs that impair platelet function. One particularly notable common adverse effect of heparin is *heparin-induced thrombocytopenia (HIT)*, which is also called *heparin-associated thrombocytopenia (HAT)*. There are two types of HIT. Type I is characterized by a gradual reduction in platelets. In this type, heparin therapy can generally be continued. In contrast, in type II HIT there is an acute fall in the number of platelets (more than 50% reduction from baseline). Heparin therapy must be discontinued in patients with type II HIT. Thrombosis that occurs in the presence of HIT can be fatal. The greatest risk to the patient with HIT is the paradoxical occurrence of thrombosis, something that heparin normally prevents or alleviates. The incidence of this disorder ranges from 5 to 15% of patients and is higher with *bovine* (cow-derived) than with *porcine* (pig-derived) heparins. The direct thrombin inhibitors argatroban and bivalirudin as well as danaparoid sodium (Orgaran®, an anticoagulant/antithrombotic mixture), and fondaparinux are indicated for treating HIT. Warfarin can cause skin necrosis and "purple toes" syndrome. Other adverse effects are listed in Table 27-2.

Toxicity and Management of Overdose

Treatment of the toxic effects of anticoagulants is aimed at reversing the underlying cause. Although the toxic effects of heparin, LMWH, and warfarin are hemorrhagic in nature, the management is different for each drug. Symptoms that may be attributed to toxicity or an overdose of anticoagulants are hematuria, melena (blood in the stool), petechiae, ecchymoses, and gum or mucous membrane bleeding. In the event of heparin or warfarin toxicity, the drug is to be stopped immediately. In the case of heparin, simply stopping the drug may be enough to reverse the toxic effects because of the drug's short half-life (1 to 2 hours). In severe cases or when large doses have been given intentionally (i.e., during cardiopulmonary bypass for heart surgery), intravenous (IV) injection of protamine sulphate is indicated. This drug is a specific heparin antidote and forms a complex with heparin, completely reversing its anticoagulant properties. This occurs in as few as 5 minutes. In general, 1 mg of protamine sulphate can reverse the effects of 100 units of heparin. Protamine sulphate may also be used to reverse the effects of LMWHs. A 1-mg dose of protamine sulphate is administered for each milligram of LMWH given, (e.g., 1 mg protamine sulphate for 1 mg enoxaparin). If the heparin overdose has resulted in a large volume of blood loss, replacement with packed red blood cells may be necessary.

In the event of warfarin toxicity or overdose, the first step is to discontinue the warfarin. As with heparin, the toxicity associated with warfarin is an extension of its therapeutic effects on the clotting cascade. However, because warfarin inactivates the vitamin K–dependent clotting factors and because these clotting factors are synthesized in the liver, it may take 36 to 42 hours before the liver can resynthesize enough clotting factors to reverse the warfarin's effects. Giving vitamin K_1 (phytonadione) can hasten the return to normal coagulation. The dose and route of administration of the vitamin K depend on the clinical situation and its acuity (i.e., how quickly the warfarin-induced effects must be reversed and whether the patient is having significant bleeding). High doses of vitamin K (10 mg) given intravenously will reverse the anticoagulation within 6 hours. Current recommendations are to use the lowest amount of vitamin K possible, based on the clinical situation. This is because once vitamin K is given, warfarin resistance will occur for up to 7 days; thus, the patient cannot be anticoagulated by warfarin during this period. In such cases, either heparin or an LMWH may need to be added to provide adequate anticoagulation. In acute situations in which bleeding is severe and the time it would take for the vitamin K to take effect is too long, it may be necessary to administer transfusions of human plasma or clotting factor concentrates. Depending on the clinical situation, oral vitamin K is usually the preferred route. However, when the international normalized ratio (INR) is extremely elevated or the patient is bleeding, vitamin K is given intravenously. There is a risk of anaphylaxis when it is given by this route; the risk is diminished by diluting it and giving it over 30 minutes. Some institutions allow it to be given via IV push. Vitamin K is available in 5-mg tablets

---

TABLE	27-2

Anticoagulants: Common Adverse Effects

Drug Subclass	Adverse Effects
Heparins (unfractionated heparin, low-molecular-weight heparin)	Bleeding, hematoma, nausea, anemia, thrombocytopenia, fever, edema
Direct thrombin inhibitors (argatroban, bivalirudin, dabigatran etexilate mesylate)	Bleeding, dizziness, shortness of breath, fever, urticaria
Selective factor Xa inhibitors (fondaparinux, rivaroxaban)	Bleeding, hematoma, dizziness, rash, GI distress, anemia
warfarin sodium (Coumadin)	Bleeding, lethargy, muscle pain, purple toes

and in 10-mg and 1-mg injections. It is common to give the injectable form orally.

Transfusions may be indicated for overdoses of direct thrombin inhibitors and the selective factor Xa inhibitor fondaparinux, which both lack specific antidotes. These drugs may also be removed with hemodialysis.

Interactions

Drug interactions involving the oral anticoagulants are profound and complicated. The drugs and the results of an interaction are given in Table 27-3. The main interaction mechanisms responsible for increasing anticoagulant activity include the following:

- **Enzyme** inhibition of metabolism
- Displacement of the drug from inactive protein-binding sites
- Decrease in vitamin K absorption or synthesis by the bacterial flora of the large intestine
- Alteration in the platelet count or activity

The drugs that interact with warfarin and heparin are listed in Table 27-3. More specifics on significant drug interactions are discussed under the drug profiles. Although both aspirin and warfarin increase the risk of bleeding when given with heparin, they are commonly given together in clinical practice. In fact, when a patient is placed on IV heparin, it is recommended that warfarin be started at the same time. Heparin is continued until the warfarin effect is therapeutic, for at least 2 days.

Dosages

For dosage information on selected anticoagulants, refer to the table on p. 527.

ANTIPLATELET DRUGS

Another class of coagulation modifiers that prevent clot formation is that of the antiplatelet drugs. The anticoagulants work in the clotting cascade; in contrast, antiplatelet drugs act to prevent platelet adhesion at the site of blood vessel injury, which occurs before the clotting cascade.

Platelets normally flow through blood vessels without adhering to their surfaces. Blood vessels can be injured by a disruption of blood flow, trauma, or the rupture of plaque from a vessel wall. When such events occur, substances such as collagen and fibronectin, which are present in the walls of blood vessels, become exposed. Collagen is a potent stimulator of platelet adhesion, as it is a prevalent component of the platelet membranes called *glycoprotein IIb/IIIa* (GP IIb/IIIa). Once platelet adhesion occurs, stimulators (compounds such as adenosine diphosphate [ADP], thrombin, thromboxane A_2 [TXA_2], and prostaglandin H_2) are released from the activated platelets. These cause the platelets to *aggregate* (accumulate) at the site of injury. Once at the site of vessel injury, the platelets change shape and release their contents, which include ADP, serotonin, and platelet factor IV. The hemostatic function of these substances is twofold. First, they function as platelet recruiters, attracting additional platelets to the site of injury; second, they are potent vasoconstrictors. Vasoconstriction limits blood flow to the damaged blood vessel to reduce blood loss.

A platelet plug that has formed at a site of vessel injury is not stable and can be dislodged. The clotting cascade is therefore stimulated to form a more permanent fibrin plug (blood clot). The role of platelets and their relationship to the clotting cascade are illustrated in Figure 27-4.

Mechanism of Action and Drug Effects

Many of the antiplatelet drugs affect the cyclooxygenase pathway, which is one of the common final enzymatic pathways in the complex arachidonic acid pathway that operates within platelets and on blood vessel walls. This pathway as it functions in both platelets and blood vessel walls is illustrated in Figure 27-5.

Aspirin is widely used for its analgesic, anti-inflammatory, and antipyretic properties (see Chapter 49). It also has antiplatelet effects. Aspirin acetylates and inhibits cyclooxygenase in the platelet irreversibly so that the platelet cannot regenerate this enzyme. Therefore, the effects of aspirin last the lifespan of a platelet, or 7 days. This irreversible inhibition of cyclooxygenase within the platelet prevents the formation of TXA_2, a substance that causes blood vessels to constrict and platelets to aggregate. By preventing TXA_2 formation, aspirin prevents these actions, which results in dilation of blood vessels and prevention of platelets from aggregating or forming a clot.

Dipyridamole, another antiplatelet drug, also acts to inhibit platelet aggregation, by preventing the release of ADP, platelet factor IV, and TXA_2, all substances that stimulate platelets to aggregate or form a clot. Figure 27-4 shows how these substances accomplish this. Dipyridamole may also directly stimulate the release of prostacyclin and inhibit the formation of TXA_2 (see Figure 27-5).

Clopidogrel is a drug that belongs to the class of antiplatelet drugs called the *ADP inhibitors*. Its use has largely superseded that of the original ADP inhibitor ticlopidine hydrochloride. Clopidogrel's mechanism of action is entirely different from that of aspirin, as it inhibits platelet aggregation by altering the platelet membrane so that it can no longer receive the signal to aggregate and form a clot. This signal is in the form of **fibrinogen** molecules, which attach to glycoprotein receptors GP IIb/IIIa on the surface of the platelet. Clopidogrel inhibits the activation of this receptor. Clopidogrel has been shown to be somewhat better than aspirin at reducing the number of MIs, strokes, and vascular deaths in at-risk patients. The combination of aspirin and clopidogrel has been shown to be effective in patients with known cardiovascular disease, but not in patients who have only risk factors. Prasugrel hydrochloride (Effient) is a newer antiplatelet drug, similar to clopidogrel, that is used primarily after interventional cardiac procedures and in patients who do not respond to clopidogrel. The newest antiplatelet drug is ticagrelor (BRILINTA®). It is indicated for patients with acute coronary syndrome.

TABLE 27-3

Anticoagulants: Drug Interactions

Drug	Mechanism	Result
WARFARIN SODIUM		
acetaminophen (high doses) amiodarone hydrochloride bumetanide furosemide	Displacement from inactive protein-binding sites	Increased anticoagulant effect
aspirin/other NSAIDs Broad-spectrum antibiotics	Decreased platelet activity	
Barbiturates carbamazepine rifampin phenytoin	Enzyme induction	Decreased anticoagulant effect
amiodarone hydrochloride cimetidine ciprofloxacin erythromycin ketoconazole metronidazole omeprazole Sulfonamides Macrolides HMG-CoA reductase inhibitors (statins)	Enzyme inhibition	Increased anticoagulant effect
cholestyramine sucralfate	Impaired warfarin sodium absorption	Decreased anticoagulant effect
Natural Health Products: Dong quai Garlic Ginkgo St. John's wort	Unknown; case reports of increased INR	Increased bleeding risk from warfarin sodium
ginseng (alone and in Cold-FX)	Decreases INR	Increased risk of clotting
HEPARIN SODIUM		
aspirin/other NSAIDs	Decreased platelet activity	Increased bleeding risk
Oral anticoagulants Thrombolytics	Additive	Increased anticoagulant effect
ANTIPLATELETS		
Aspirin, NSAIDS	Decreased platelet activity	Increased bleeding risk
warfarin sodium, heparin sodium, thrombolytics rifampin	Additive	Increased bleeding risk
Natural health products: Garlic Ginkgo Kava	Increased effects	Increased bleeding risk

HMG-CoA, hydroxymethylglutaryl-coenzyme A; *INR*, international normalized ratio; *NSAIDs*, nonsteroidal anti-inflammatory drugs.

It must be avoided in patients taking more than 100 mg of aspirin daily.

Pentoxifylline, another antiplatelet drug, is a methylxanthine derivative with properties similar to those of other methylxanthines, such as caffeine and theophylline (see Chapter 38). It was one of the earliest antiplatelet drugs but is now much less commonly used. It reduces the viscosity of blood by increasing the flexibility of red blood cells and reducing the aggregation of platelets. It is sometimes referred to as a *hemorheological* drug, or a drug that alters the fluid dynamics of the blood. The antiplatelet effects of pentoxifylline are attributed to its inhibition

of ADP, serotonin, and platelet factor IV (see Figure 27-4). Pentoxifylline also stimulates the synthesis and release of prostacyclin (a natural occurring prostaglandin synthesized from arachidonic acid and a vasodilator) from blood vessels (see Figure 27-5). In addition, it may have effects on the fibrinolytic system by raising the plasma concentrations of tissue plasminogen activator (see Figure 27-3).

Another class of antiplatelet drugs is the GP IIb/IIIa inhibitors. They act by blocking the receptor protein by the same name that occurs in the platelet wall membranes. This protein plays a role in promoting the aggregation of platelets in preparation for fibrin clot formation.

DRUG PROFILES

Of the anticoagulants, warfarin, dabigatran etexilate mesylate, and rivaroxaban are used orally. The rest are given by IV or subcutaneous injection only. Intramuscular (IM) injection of these drugs is contraindicated because of their propensity to cause large hematomas at the site of injection.

warfarin sodium

Warfarin sodium (Coumadin) is a pharmaceutical derivative of the natural plant anticoagulant known as *coumarin*. Warfarin is the most commonly prescribed oral anticoagulant and is used exclusively in the oral form. Use of this drug requires careful monitoring of the prothrombin time (PT) and international normalized ratio (INR), which are standardized measures of the degree to which a patient's blood coagulability has been reduced by the drug. The PT and INR evaluate the extrinsic pathway of coagulation. The INR provides a standardized unit to report the results of the PT. A normal INR (without warfarin) is 0.8 to 1.2, whereas a therapeutic INR (with warfarin) ranges from 2 to 3.5, depending on the indication for use of the drug (e.g., atrial fibrillation, thromboprevention, prosthetic heart valve). Patients older than 65 years of age may have a lower INR threshold for bleeding complications and may need to be monitored accordingly. Older adult patients should be started on lower dosages initially. Recently, it has been shown that about one third of patients receiving warfarin metabolize it differently from the expected way, based on variations in certain genes, *CYP2CP* and *VKORC1*. Genetic testing for these genes is helpful in determining the appropriate initial dosage of warfarin. The maintenance dosage is still determined by the INR.

Warfarin has significant interactions with many drugs, including amiodarone hydrochloride, fluconazole, erythromycin, metronidazole, sulfonamide antibiotics, and cimetidine. Although many more drugs can interact with warfarin, the aforementioned are by far the most common. Combining warfarin and amiodarone hydrochloride will lead to a 50% increase in a patient's INR. When amiodarone hydrochloride is added to warfarin therapy, it is recommended that the warfarin dose be cut in half.

Because warfarin inhibits vitamin K–dependent clotting factors, foods that are high in vitamin K may reduce warfarin's ability to prevent clots. Common foods rich in vitamin K include leafy green vegetables (e.g., kale, spinach, collard greens). The most important aspect of these food–drug interactions is consistency in diet. Educate patients to maintain consistency in their intake of leafy green vegetables. Many patients are under the misconception that they must avoid all leafy green vegetables; however, this is not true. Once their maintenance warfarin dose is established, patients may still eat green vegetables, but they need to be consistent in their intake because increasing or decreasing it can affect their INR. Natural health products that interact with warfarin and result in increased risk of bleeding include dong quai, garlic, ginkgo, and St. John's wort.

PHARMACOKINETICS

Route	Onset of Action	Peak Plasma Concentration	Elimination Half-Life	Duration of Action
PO	24–72 hr	4 hr	0.5–3 days	2–5 days

enoxaparin sodium

Enoxaparin sodium (Lovenox) is the prototypical LMWH and is obtained by enzymatically cleaving large unfractionated heparin molecules into small fragments. These fragments of heparin have a greater affinity for factor Xa than for factor IIa and have a higher degree of bioavailability and a longer elimination half-life than unfractionated heparin. Laboratory monitoring, as is done with heparin therapy, is not necessary when enoxaparin is given because of its greater affinity for factor Xa. It is available only in injectable form. Other anticoagulants with comparable pharmacology and indications include danaparoid sodium and dalteparin sodium. Enoxaparin is a commonly used LMWH given for both prophylaxis and treatment. Dalteparin prefilled syringes are increasingly being used for the thromboprophylaxis in conjunction with surgery, and higher doses of the drug are used in the treatment of DVT and pulmonary embolism. All LMWHs have a distinct advantage over heparin in that they do not require any laboratory monitoring and can be given at home for the treatment of DVT or pulmonary embolism. This factor allows patients to be discharged from the hospital sooner. These drugs may also be used at home after major orthopedic surgery.

A potentially deadly medication error is to give heparin in combination with enoxaparin (or any LMWH, dabigatran sodium, or rivaroxaban). Always double-check that enoxaparin and heparin are never given to the same patient.

PHARMACOKINETICS

Route	Onset of Action	Peak Plasma Concentration	Elimination Half-Life	Duration of Action
Subcut	3–5 hr	4–5 hr	4–5 hr	12 hr

heparin sodium

Heparin sodium is a natural mucopolysaccharide anticoagulant obtained from porcine intestinal mucosa. Heparin Leo® is a brand name that refers only to small vials of aqueous heparin IV flush solutions used to maintain patency of heparin lock IV insertion sites. Because of the risk for the development of HIT, however, most institutions routinely use 0.9% normal saline as a flush for heparin-lock IV ports and have moved away from using heparin flush solutions for this purpose. Heparin flushes (100 units/mL) are still used for central catheters. When

Continued

DRUG PROFILES—cont'd

used for flushing purposes, there is no need for monitoring.

Heparin is commonly used for DVT prophylaxis in a dose of 5 000 units, two or three times a day, given subcutaneously, and it does not need to be monitored when used for prophylaxis. When heparin is used therapeutically, it is given by continuous IV infusion or, rarely, by subcutaneous injection. Most hospitals have weight-based protocols for heparin administration. Because the dosage is based on the patient's weight in kilograms, ensure that the appropriate weight is recorded and that only kilograms are used, not pounds. A potential double-dose medication error can occur if pounds and kilograms are mixed. This is also true for enoxaparin because it is also dosed on body weight when used therapeutically. When heparin is given by IV infusion, monitoring by frequent measurement of aPTT (usually every 6 hours until therapeutic effects are seen) is necessary. Because the required monitoring is time-consuming, many institutions now use enoxaparin in place of heparin.

Other drugs that affect the coagulation cascade can have additive effects with heparin, which may lead to bleeding.

Heparin is available only in injectable form in multiple strengths ranging from 10 to 10 000 units/mL. The vials of different strengths of heparin are similar and look alike. Indeed, they are available in strengths of 10, 100, 1 000, and 10 000 units/mL, so it is easy to mix up the vials. In fact, several newborns have died when a vial of more concentrated heparin was mistaken for a more dilute solution. Take great care in checking and double-checking the concentration of heparin before administering it.

PHARMACOKINETICS

Route	Onset of Action	Peak Plasma Concentration	Elimination Half-Life	Duration of Action
IV	Immediate	Immediate	1–2 hr	Dependent on infusion duration
Subcut	20–30 min	2–4 hr	1–2 hr	8–12 hr

dabigatran etexilate mesylate

Dabigatran etexilate mesylate (Pradaxa) is the first oral direct thrombin inhibitor approved for prevention of strokes and thrombosis in patients with nonvalvular atrial fibrillation. Dabigatran etexilate mesylate is a prodrug that becomes activated in the liver. It specifically and reversibly binds to both free and clot-bound thrombin. Dabigatran etexilate mesylate is excreted extensively in the kidneys, and the dose is dependent upon kidney function. The normal dose is 150 mg twice daily, but it must be reduced to 75 mg twice daily if creatinine clearance is less than 30 mL per minute. There is no antidote to dabigatran etexilate mesylate, and the most common and serious adverse effect is bleeding. No coagulation monitoring is required for dabigatran etexilate mesylate. Drug interactions include phenytoin (causing decreased effect) and amiodarone hydrochloride (causing increased effect). Information about storage and handling is discussed in the Nursing Process section later in the chapter.

PHARMACOKINETICS

Route	Onset of Action	Peak Plasma Concentration	Elimination Half-Life	Duration of Action
PO	2–3 hr	2 hr	12–17 hr	12 hr

fondaparinux sodium

Fondaparinux sodium (Arixtra) is a selective inhibitor of factor Xa, which is indicated for prophylaxis or treatment of DVT or PE. It is contraindicated with known allergy or in patients with a creatinine clearance less than 30 mL per minute or a body weight of less than 50 kg. Bleeding is the most common and serious adverse reaction. Thrombocytopenia has also been reported, and therapy should be stopped if platelet count falls below 100 000 platelets per microlitre. It should not be given for at least 6 to 8 hours after surgery and should be used with caution in conjunction with warfarin or other anticoagulants. Other adverse effects include anemia, increased wound drainage, postoperative hemorrhage, hematoma, confusion, urinary tract infection, hypotension, dizziness, and hypokalemia. There is no antidote for fondaparinux sodium, and its effect cannot be measured by standard anticoagulant tests. Fondaparinux sodium is given only by subcutaneous injection. The dose for prophylaxis is 2.5 mg daily. The dose for acute DVT or PE treatment is 5 to 10 mg daily, depending on body weight.

PHARMACOKINETICS

Route	Onset of Action	Peak Plasma Concentration	Elimination Half-Life	Duration of Action
Subcut	2 hr	2–3 hr	17–21 hr	24 hr

argatroban

Argatroban, which has the same trade name, is a synthetic direct thrombin inhibitor that is derived from the amino acid L-arginine. It is indicated both for treatment of active HIT (rather than heparin) and for percutaneous coronary intervention procedures in patients at risk for HIT (i.e., those with a history of the disorder). It is given only by the IV route. A lower dosage must be used in patients with severe liver dysfunction.

PHARMACOKINETICS

Route	Onset of Action	Peak Plasma Concentration	Elimination Half-Life	Duration of Action
IV	Immediate	1–3 hr	30–50 min	Dependent on infusion duration

DOSAGES Selected Anticoagulant Drugs

Drug	Pharmacological Class	Usual Dosage Range	Indications/Uses
argatroban	Synthetic thrombin inhibitor	*Adults* IV: 2–10 mcg/kg/min until aPTT 1.5 to 3 times baseline	Thromboprevention and treatment of HIT and with PCI in patients at risk for HIT
▸▸enoxaparin sodium (Lovenox)	LMWH	*Adults* Subcut: 30–40 mg every 12 hr for prophylaxis or 1 mg/kg every 12 hr for treatment	Prevention and treatment of thromboembolic and ischemic processes in unstable angina and in pre- and post-MI situations
heparin sodium	Natural anticoagulant	*Children* IV: Initial 75–100 units/kg, then 25–30 units/kg/hr; adjust to maintain aPTT of 60 to 85 seconds *Adults* Subcut: 333 units/kg followed by 250 units/kg every 12 hr IV: 10 000 units followed by 5 000–10 000 units every 4–6 hr IV infusion: 5 000 units followed by 20 000–40 000 units/day aPTT determines maintenance dose	Thrombosis/embolism, coagulopathies (e.g., DIC), DVT, and PE prophylaxis, clotting prevention (e.g., open heart surgery, dialysis)
dabigatran etexilate mesylate (Pradaxa)	Synthetic direct thrombin inhibitor	*Adults* PO: 110 mg bid (depending on kidney function)	Prevention of strokes and thrombosis in patients with nonvalvular atrial fibrillation; VTE prevention
fondaparinux (Arixtra)	Factor Xa inhibitor	Prophylaxis: 2.5 mg subcut daily Treatment: less than 50 kg: 5 mg daily; 50–100 kg: 7.5 mg daily; over 100 kg: 10 mg daily	Prevention and treatment of DVT and PE
▸▸warfarin sodium (Coumadin)	anticoagulant	*Adults* INR determines maintenance dose, usually 2–10 mg/day	Thromboprevention and treatment in DVT, PE, atrial fibrillation, post-MI

aPTT, activated partial thromboplastin time; *CVA*, cerebrovascular accident; *DIC*, disseminated intravascular coagulation; *DVT*, deep vein thrombosis; *HIT*, heparin-induced thrombocytopenia; *INR*, international normalized ratio; *IV*, intravenous; *LMWH*, low-molecular-weight heparin; *MI*, myocardial infarction; *PCI*, percutaneous coronary intervention; *PE*, pulmonary embolus; *PO*, oral; *PT*, prothrombin time; *Subcut*, subcutaneous; *VTE*, venous thromboembolism.

There are currently three available drugs in this class: tirofiban hydrochloride (Aggrastat), eptifibatide (Integrilin), and abciximab (ReoPro). The GP IIb/IIIa inhibitors are available only for IV infusion.

Indications

The therapeutic effects of antiplatelet drugs depend on the particular drug. Common indications for dual antiplatelet therapy (Aspirin and P2Y12 inhibitors) include post angioplasty and placement of a stent and 1 year post-MI). Aspirin has multiple therapeutic effects, but many of them vary depending on the dosage. Aspirin is recommended for stroke prevention in daily doses of 75 to 160 mg. (However, in clinical practice, dosages may vary.) Clopidogrel is also used for reducing the risk for fatal and nonfatal thrombotic stroke and is used for prophylaxis against transient ischemic attacks (TIAs) as well for post-MI prevention of thrombosis). Dipyridamole is used as an adjunct to warfarin in the prevention of postoperative thromboembolic complications. It is also used to decrease platelet aggregation in other thromboembolic disorders. GP IIb/IIIa inhibitors are used to treat acute unstable angina and MI and are also given during the endovascular procedure, coronary angioplasty. Their purpose is to prevent the formation of thrombi. This process is known as *thromboprevention*. This treatment approach is based on the fact that *prevention* of thrombus formation is easier and less risky overall from a pharmacological standpoint than is lysing a formed thrombus. Pentoxifylline is indicated for peripheral vascular disease.

Contraindications

Contraindications to the use of antiplatelet drugs include known drug allergy to a specific product, thrombocytopenia, active bleeding, leukemia, traumatic injury, GI ulcer, vitamin K deficiency, and recent stroke.

Adverse Effects

The potential adverse effects of the various antiplatelet drugs can be serious, and they all pose a risk for inducing a serious bleeding episode. The most common adverse effects are listed in Table 27-4.

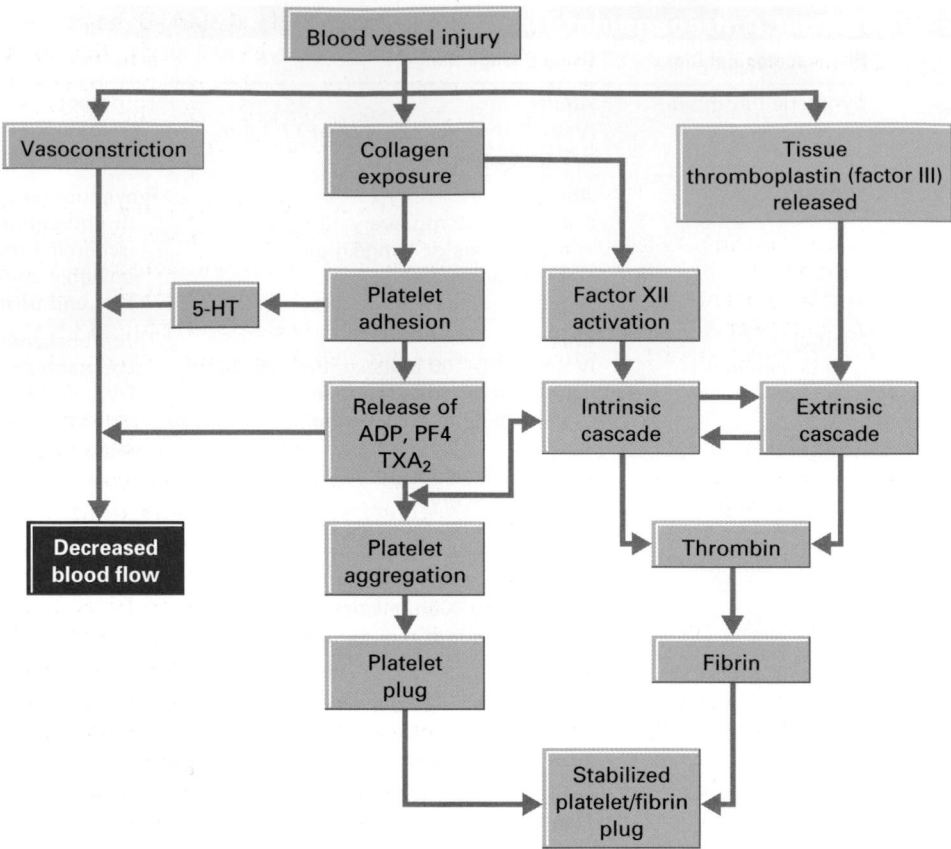

FIG. 27-4 Relationship between platelets and the clotting cascade. *ADP*, adenosine diphosphate; *5-HT*, serotonin; *PF4*, platelet factor 4; *TXA₂*, thromboxane A₂.

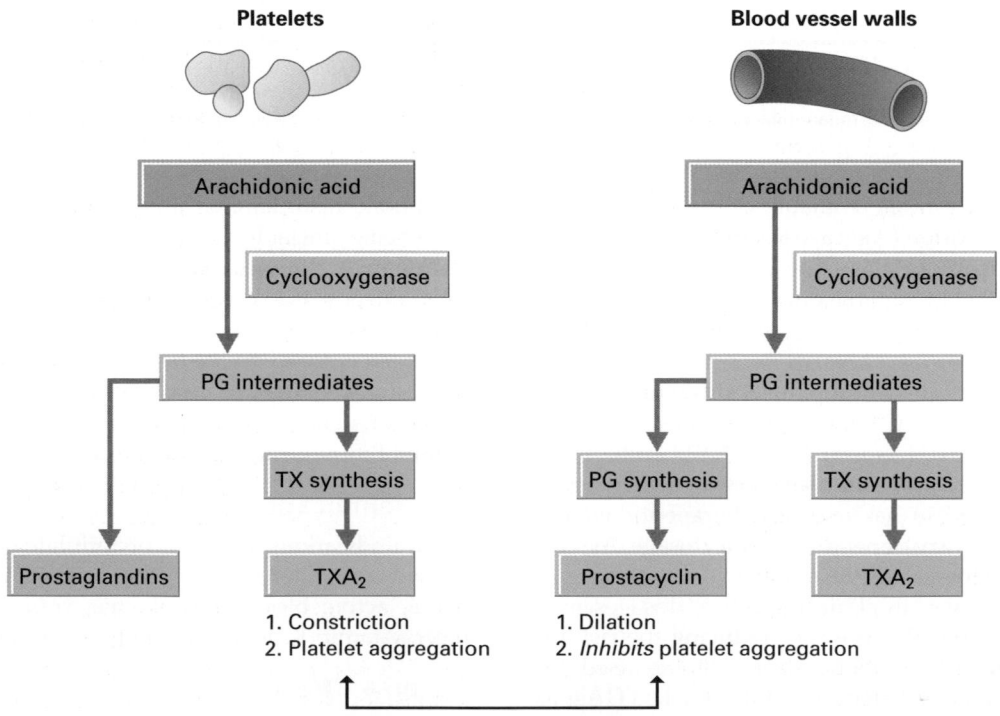

FIG. 27-5 Cyclooxygenase pathway. *PG*, prostaglandin; *TXA₂*, thromboxane A₂.

TABLE 27-4

Antiplatelet Drugs: Adverse Effects

Body System	Adverse Effects
ASPIRIN	
Central nervous	Drowsiness, dizziness, confusion, flushing
Gastrointestinal	Nausea, vomiting, GI bleeding, diarrhea
Hematological	Thrombocytopenia, agranulocytosis, leukopenia, neutropenia, hemolytic anemia, bleeding
CLOPIDOGREL	
Cardiovascular	Chest pain, edema
Central nervous	Flulike symptoms, headache, dizziness, fatigue
Gastrointestinal	Abdominal pain, diarrhea, nausea
Miscellaneous	Epistaxis, rash, pruritus
TICAGRELOR	
Respiratory	Dyspnea (on initiation)
Miscellaneous	Elevated uric acid levels
GP IIB/IIIA INHIBITORS	
Cardiovascular	Bradycardia, hypotension, edema
Central nervous	Dizziness
Hematological	Bleeding, thrombocytopenia

Interactions

Some potentially dangerous drug interactions can occur with antiplatelet drugs. The use of dipyridamole with clopidogrel, aspirin, or nonsteroidal anti-inflammatory drugs (NSAIDs) produces additive antiplatelet activity and increased bleeding potential. The combined use of steroids or nonaspirin NSAIDs with aspirin can increase the ulcerogenic effects of aspirin. The combined use of aspirin and heparin with GP IIb/IIIa inhibitors also further enhances antiplatelet activity and increases the likelihood of a serious bleeding episode. In spite of all of these potentially harmful interactions, it is not uncommon to see patients on daily maintenance doses of aspirin for thrombopreventive purposes, sometimes in combination with other antiplatelet drugs. The most commonly used dose in this situation is the "baby aspirin" dose of 81 mg (the standard adult dose is 325 mg). Even though GP IIb/IIIa and heparin have additive therapeutic effects when given concurrently and are listed as interacting drugs, it is common to see both used together. However, the therapeutic goal of heparin treatment, and thus the dose, is lower when used with a GP IIb/IIIa inhibitor.

Dosages

For dosage information on selected antiplatelet drugs, refer to the table on p. 530.

THROMBOLYTIC DRUGS

Thrombolytics are coagulation modifiers that lyse thrombi in the coronary arteries. This action re-establishes blood flow to the blood-starved heart muscle. If the blood flow is re-established early, the heart muscle and left ventricular function can be preserved. If blood flow is not re-established early, the affected area of the heart muscle becomes ischemic and eventually necrotic and nonfunctional.

Thrombolytic therapy made its debut in 1933, when a substance that broke down fibrin clots was isolated from a patient's blood. This substance was determined to be produced by certain bacteria growing in the patient's blood. The bacteria were found to be β-hemolytic streptococci (group A), and the substance was eventually called streptokinase (SK).

SK was first used in a patient in 1947 to dissolve a clotted hemothorax, but it was not until 1958 that it was given to a patient with an acute MI. In 1960, a naturally occurring human plasminogen activator called urokinase became available. Urokinase was found to exert fibrinolytic effects on pulmonary emboli. However, the results of the early thrombolytic trials conducted during the 1960s and 1970s involving patients who had had an acute MI were not taken seriously by the medical community. In the 1980s, the underlying cause of acute MI was determined to be due to coronary artery occlusion. This marked the start of rapid growth in the use of thrombolytic drugs for the early treatment of acute MI.

Since that time, several new thrombolytics have become available for this and other clinical uses. Tissue plasminogen activator (t-PA) and anisoylated plasminogen streptokinase activator complex (APSAC) are two of these drugs. Following the advent of these new thrombolytics came the results of several large, landmark thrombolytic research studies. These studies demonstrated that early thrombolytic therapy could produce a 50% reduction in mortality, a reduction in the infarct size, an improvement in left ventricular function, and a reduction in the incidence and severity of heart failure. These findings and developments, along with a better understanding of the pathogenesis of acute MI, have led the way to the advancements made in the treatment of acute MI. However, the use of thrombolytics has almost completely been replaced by interventional cardiologic procedures, such as percutaneous coronary intervention. Thrombolytics are still a viable option in hospitals that do not offer percutaneous coronary intervention. Currently available thrombolytic drugs include t-PAs (alteplase [Activase®] and tenecteplase [TNKase]). For dosage information on thrombolytics, see the table on p. 531.

Mechanism of Action and Drug Effects

There is a fine balance between the formation and dissolution of a clot. The coagulation system is responsible for forming clots, whereas the fibrinolytic system is responsible for dissolving clots. The natural fibrinolytic system within the blood takes several days to break down a thrombus. This is of little value in the case of a clotted blood vessel that supplies blood to the heart muscle. Necrosis of the myocardium would not be prevented by these natural means, but thrombolytic drug

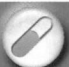

DRUG PROFILES

Antiplatelet drugs are extremely useful in the management of thromboembolic disorders. Each has unique pharmacological properties, and therefore they all are somewhat different from one another.

▶▶ aspirin

Aspirin is available in many combinations with other prescription and nonprescription drugs and has numerous product names. One unique contraindication for aspirin is its use in children and adolescents with flulike symptoms. The use of aspirin in such situations is associated with the occurrence of Reye's syndrome, a rare, acute, and sometimes fatal condition involving liver and central nervous system (CNS) damage (see Chapter 49). There is also allergic cross-reactivity between aspirin and other NSAIDs. Patients with documented aspirin allergy must not receive NSAIDs. Aspirin is available in both oral and rectal forms. A combination form of aspirin and dipyridamole (Aggrenox) is used for antiplatelet purposes.

PHARMACOKINETICS

Route	Onset of Action	Peak Plasma Concentration	Elimination Half-Life	Duration of Action
PO	15–30 min	0.25–2 hr	2–3 hr	4–6 hr

▶▶ clopidogrel bisulphate

Clopidogrel bisulphate (Plavix) is currently the most widely used ADP inhibitor. It has superseded ticlopidine hydrochloride because of the serious adverse reactions associated with the latter drug, including life-threatening neutropenia and agranulocytosis. It was initially believed that clopidogrel might be free from such adverse effects. However, some case reports of clopidogrel-associated hematological adverse effects are emerging. It is available only in oral form. Prasugrel hydrochloride (Effient) and ticagrelor (BRILINTA) are similar to clopidogrel.

PHARMACOKINETICS

Route	Onset of Action	Peak Plasma Concentration	Elimination Half-Life	Duration of Action
PO	1–2 hr	1 hr	8 hr	7–10 days

▶▶ eptifibatide

Eptifibatide (Integrilin) is a GP IIb/IIIa inhibitor, along with tirofiban hydrochloride (Aggrastat) and abciximab (ReoPro). These drugs are usually administered in critical care or cardiac catheterization laboratory settings where continuous cardiovascular monitoring is the norm. All are available only for IV use.

PHARMACOKINETICS

Route	Onset of Action	Peak Plasma Concentration	Elimination Half-Life	Duration of Action
IV	1 hr	Unknown	2–2.5 hr	4 hr

DOSAGES   Selected Antiplatelet Drugs

Drug	Pharmacological Class	Usual Dosage Range	Indications/Uses
▶▶ aspirin	Salicylate antiplatelet	*Adults* PO: 81–325 mg/day	MI prophylaxis TIA prophylaxis
▶▶ clopidogrel bisulphate (Plavix)	ADP inhibitor	*Adults* PO: 75 mg daily; 300 mg may be given as a one-time loading dose for patients with unstable angina, non–ST segment elevation	Reduction of atherosclerotic events; acute coronary syndrome without ST segment elevation
▶▶ eptifibatide (Integrilin)	GP IIb/IIIa inhibitor	*Adults Only* IV: Single bolus of 180 mcg/kg followed by continuous infusion of 2 mcg/kg/min; specific doses based on weight*	Unstable angina; Non–ST segment elevation MI coronary angioplasty

ADP, adenosine diphosphate; *GP*, glycoprotein; *IV*, intravenous; *MI*, myocardial infarction; *PO*, oral; *TIA*, transient ischemic attack.
*See manufacturer's directions for specific dose.

therapy activates the fibrinolytic system to break down the thrombus in the blood vessel quickly so that the delivery of blood to the heart muscle via the coronary arteries is quickly re-established. This prevents myocardial tissue (heart muscle) and heart function from being destroyed. Thrombolytics accomplish this by activating the conversion of plasminogen to plasmin, which breaks down, or lyses, the thrombus (see Figure 27-3). Plasmin is a *proteolytic* enzyme, which means that it breaks down proteins. It is a relatively nonspecific serine protease that

is capable of degrading proteins such as fibrin, fibrinogen, and other procoagulant proteins such as factors V, VIII, and XII. In other words, the substances that form clots are destroyed by plasmin. Essentially, thrombolytic drugs work by mimicking the body's own process of clot destruction. Although the individual thrombolytic drugs are somewhat diverse in their actions, they all have this common result.

SK, the original thrombolytic enzyme, and the naturally occurring urokinase have been removed from the

DOSAGES	Selected Thrombolytic Drugs		
Drug	**Pharmacological Class**	**Usual Dosage Range**	**Indications/Uses**
⊷alteplase (Activase)	t-PA	*Adults* IV: 0.9 mg/kg (total dose not to exceed 90 mg) over 60 min; 10% given as an IV bolus over 1 min; must be given within 3 hr of onset of symptoms	Acute ischemic stroke pulmonary embolism, myocardial infarction (STEMI)
Tenecteplase (TNKase)	t-PA	*Adults* IV: 30–50 mg (based on patient weight) bolus over 5 min	Myocardial infarction

CVA, cerebrovascular accident; *IV,* intravenous; *t-PA,* tissue plasminogen activator.

market, primarily because of their adverse effects—due to the fact that they are not fibrin specific. The newer thrombolytics have chemical specificity for fibrin threads **(fibrin-specificity)** and work primarily at the site of a clot. They still carry some bleeding risk, but much less than that of the thrombolytic enzymes.

t-PA is a naturally occurring plasminogen activator secreted by vascular endothelial cells (the walls of blood vessels). However, the amount secreted naturally is not sufficient to dissolve a coronary thrombus quickly enough to restore circulation to the heart and brain and reduce the severity of a myocardial infarction or ishemic stroke. Recombinant deoxyribonucleic acid (DNA) techniques are now used to produce t-PA, and thus it can be administered in quantities sufficient to dissolve a thrombus quickly. It is fibrin specific (clot specific); that is, only the fibrin clot stimulates t-PA to convert plasminogen to plasmin. Therefore, it has a lower propensity to induce a systemic thrombolytic state, compared to the thrombolytic enzymes.

Indications

The purpose of the thrombolytic drugs is to activate the conversion of plasminogen to plasmin, the enzyme that breaks down a thrombus. The presence of a thrombus that interferes significantly with normal blood flow on either the venous or the arterial side of the circulation is an indication for the use of thrombolytic therapy. An exception may be a thrombus that has formed in blood vessels that connect directly with the CNS. The indications for thrombolytic therapy include acute MI, arterial thrombosis, DVT, occlusion of shunts or catheters, pulmonary embolism, and acute ischemic stroke.

Contraindications

Contraindications to the use of thrombolytic drugs include known drug allergy to the specific product and any preservatives, as well as concurrent use of other drugs that alter clotting. Any history of recent major surgery, trauma, or bleeding (e.g., hemorrhagic stroke) are also contraindications to their use.

Adverse Effects

The most common undesirable effect of thrombolytic therapy is internal, intracranial, and superficial bleeding.

Other problems include hypersensitivity, anaphylactoid reactions, nausea, vomiting, and hypotension. These drugs can also induce cardiac dysrhythmias.

Toxicity and Management of Overdose

Acute toxicity primarily causes an extension of the adverse effects of the thrombolytic drug. Treatment is symptomatic and supportive, as thrombolytic drugs have a relatively short half-life and no specific antidotes.

Interactions

The most common effect of drug interactions is an increased bleeding tendency resulting from the concurrent use of anticoagulants, antiplatelets, or other drugs that affect platelet function.

A laboratory test interaction that can occur with thrombolytic drugs is a reduction in plasminogen and fibrinogen levels.

Dosages

For dosage information on alteplase, refer to the table above.

ANTIFIBRINOLYTIC DRUGS

Individual antifibrinolytic drugs have varying mechanisms of action, but all prevent the lysis of fibrin. Fibrin is the substance that helps make a platelet plug insoluble and anchors the clot to the damaged blood vessel (see Figures 27-1 and 27-2). The term *antifibrinolytic* refers to what these drugs do, which is to prevent the lysis of fibrin; in doing so, these drugs *promote* clot formation. For this reason, they are also called *hemostatic* drugs Their effects are opposite to those of anticoagulant and antiplatelet drugs, which *prevent* clot formation. Two synthetic antifibrinolytics are available—tranexamic acid and desmopressin—and one natural antifibrinolytic drug, aprotinin. Dosages, indications, and other information for desmopressin appear in the associated Dosages table on p. 533. There are also hemostatic drugs that are used *topically* (on the skin or tissue surface) in surgical settings to stop excessive bleeding. These include topical thrombin, microfibrillar collagen, absorbable gelatin, and oxidized cellulose.

DRUG PROFILES

All thrombolytic drugs exert their effects by activating plasminogen and converting it to plasmin, which is capable of digesting fibrin, a major component of clots.

▶▶ alteplase

Alteplase (Activase) is a pharmaceutically available rt-PA made through recombinant DNA techniques. It is fibrin specific and therefore does not produce a systemic lytic state. Tenecteplase (TNKase) is a newer form of alteplase that is given by IV push after MI. Because rt-PA is present in the human body in a natural state, its administration for therapeutic use does not induce an antigen–antibody reaction. The drug rt-PA has a short half-life of 5 minutes. It is believed to open the clogged artery rapidly, but its action is short-lived. Therefore, it is given with heparin to prevent reocclusion of the affected blood vessel. Alteplase is available only in parenteral form. There is also a smaller dosage form of alteplase, Cathflo® Activase, that is used to flush clogged IV or arterial lines. Alteplase is used specifically in ischemic stroke and tenecteplase is used specifically for lysis of suspected occlusive coronary artery thrombi associated with evolving transmural MI.

PHARMACOKINETICS

Route	Onset of Action	Peak Plasma Concentration	Elimination Half-Life	Duration of Action
IV	immediate	60 min	5 min	Dependent on infusion duration

TABLE 27-5

Antifibrinolytics: Mechanisms of Action

Antifibrinolytic Drug	Mechanism of Action
Synthetic drug: tranexamic acid (Cyklokapron®)	Forms a reversible complex with plasminogen and plasmin. By binding to the lysine binding site of plasminogen, tranexamic acid displaces plasminogen from the surface of fibrin. This prevents plasmin from lysing the fibrin clot. Therefore, the drug can work only if a clot has formed.
Natural drug: aprotinin (Artiss®, Trasylol®)	Inhibits the proteolytic enzymes trypsin, plasmin, and kallikrein, which lyse proteins that destroy fibrin clots. By inhibiting these enzymes, aprotinin prevents the degradation of the fibrin clot. It is also thought to inhibit the action of the complement system.
Other: desmopressin acetate (DDAVP)	Works by increasing von Willebrand factor, which anchors platelets to damaged vessels via the GP IIb platelet receptor. It appears that desmopressin acts as a general endothelial stimulant, stimulating factor VIII, prostaglandin I_2, and plasminogen-activated release.

GP, glycoprotein.

Although not technically antifibrinolytic drugs, there are three drugs used for the treatment of hemophilia. These are produced by recombinant DNA technology, which eliminates the risk associated with obtaining them from human blood. Products currently available include rVII, rVIII, and rIX. As mentioned earlier, factors VII, VIII, and IX are important in the coagulation pathway. Warfarin also inhibits these factors. These products are used in patients with hemophilia and are also used in patients with severe bleeding due to warfarin therapy.

Mechanism of Action and Drug Effects

Antifibrinolytic drugs vary in several ways. The various antifibrinolytic drugs and their proposed mechanisms of action are described in Table 27-5.

The drug effects of antifibrinolytics are specific and limited. They do not have many effects outside of their hematological ones. Tranexamic acid and aprotinin inhibit the breakdown of fibrin, which prevents the destruction of formed platelet clots. Desmopressin causes a dose-dependent increase in the concentration of plasma factor VIII (von Willebrand factor), along with an increase in the plasma concentration of rt-PA. The overall effect is increased platelet aggregation and clot formation. This drug is also an analogue of antidiuretic hormone and is discussed further in Chapter 31.

Indications

Antifibrinolytics are useful in both the prevention and treatment of excessive bleeding resulting from systemic hyperfibrinolysis or surgical complications. They have also proved successful in arresting excessive oozing from surgical sites such as chest tubes, as well as in reducing total blood loss and the duration of bleeding in the postoperative period.

Desmopressin may also be used in patients who have hemophilia A or type I von Willebrand's disease. As stated earlier, recombinant factors VII, VIII, and IX are used to treat hemophilia or to stop bleeding caused by excessive warfarin therapy.

DRUG PROFILES

desmopressin acetate

Desmopressin acetate (DDAVP®) is a synthetic polypeptide. It is structurally similar to vasopressin, or antidiuretic hormone, the natural human posterior pituitary hormone (see Chapter 31). Because of these physical characteristics, it is most often used to increase the resorption of water by the collecting ducts in the kidneys to prevent or control polydipsia, polyuria, and dehydration in patients with diabetes insipidus due to a deficiency of endogenous posterior pituitary vasopressin or in patients with polyuria and polydipsia resulting from trauma or surgery in the pituitary region.

Desmopressin also causes a dose-dependent increase in plasma factor VIII (von Willebrand factor), along with

an increase in t-PA, which results in increased platelet aggregation and clot formation; thus, it is often used to stop bleeding. Desmopressin is contraindicated in patients with a known hypersensitivity to it and in those with nephrogenic diabetes insipidus. It is available in both injectable and intranasal dosage forms as well as oral disintegrating tablets. Desmopressin nasal spray and tablets are used for primary nocturnal enuresis.

PHARMACOKINETICS

Route	Onset of Action	Peak Plasma Concentration	Elimination Half-Life	Duration of Action
IV	15–30 min	1–2 hr	2 hr	Unknown

DOSAGES   Selected Antifibrinolytic Drugs

Drug	Pharmacological Class	Usual Dosage Range	Indications/Uses
desmopressin acetate (DDAVP)	Synthetic posterior pituitary hormone	*Children and Adults* IV: 0.3 mcg/kg infused over 20–30 min; preoperative use: drug is administered 30 min before surgery	Surgical and postoperative hemostasis and management of bleeding in patients with hemophilia A or type I von Willebrand's disease

IV, intravenous.

TABLE   27-6

Antifibrinolytics: Adverse Effects

Body System	Adverse Effects
Cardiovascular	Dysrhythmias, orthostatic hypotension, bradycardia
Central nervous	Headache, dizziness, fatigue, hallucinations, convulsions
Gastrointestinal	Nausea, vomiting, abdominal cramps, diarrhea

Contraindications

Contraindications to the use of antifibrinolytic drugs include known drug allergy to a specific product and disseminated intravascular coagulation, which could be worsened by these drugs.

Adverse Effects

The adverse effects of antifibrinolytic drugs are infrequent and mild. However, there have been rare reports of these drugs causing thrombotic events, such as acute cerebrovascular thrombosis and acute MI. The common adverse effects of antifibrinolytics are listed in Table 27-6.

Interactions

When drugs such as estrogens or oral contraceptives are used concurrently with tranexamic acid or aprotinin, additive effects may occur, resulting in increased coagu-

lation. Few specific interactions have been reported for desmopressin, although caution should be used when giving it to patients receiving lithium carbonate, heparin, patients who have consumed alcohol or those receiving large doses of epinephrine. Drugs such as chlorpropamide and fludrocortisone-21-acetate may potentiate the antidiuretic response, which may lead to edema.

Dosages

For dosage information on desmopressin, refer to the table above.

NURSING PROCESS

Coagulation modifiers have a variety of uses, including the following: (1) prevention or elimination of clotting in a peripherally inserted catheter (PIC) (or peripherally inserted central catheter [PICC]), (2) maintenance of patency (without clotting) of a central venous catheter, (3) clot prevention in coronary artery bypass grafting, (4) prevention of clotting after major vessel injury, (5) treatment of thrombophlebitis to prevent venous or arterial thromboembolism, and (6) prevention of clotting with the use of prosthetics (e.g., heart valve replacements) and in atrial fibrillation. The drugs that are used for these different conditions are varied in their mechanisms of action, and the related general and specific nursing process issues will be discussed.

Assessment

Begin the nursing assessment associated with the use of all coagulation modifier drugs by taking a thorough patient health history, including the following: any drug or food allergies, current medical problems, underlying systemic disease processes, past and present medical history, family health history, dietary habits, changes in body weight over time, ability to perform activities of daily living, level of exercise or degree of sedentary lifestyle, employment activities, success of previous treatment regimens, blood pressure, pulse rate, respirations, body weight, height, recent dietary intake, and fluid intake. A medication history is also needed and should include a listing of all drugs the patient takes on a daily basis such as prescription drugs, over-the-counter medications, and natural health products, as well as any intake of nicotine, alcohol, or other substances.

Perform a thorough patient assessment to identify the presence of the following risk factors: immobility, history of limited activity or prolonged bed rest (i.e., generally for longer than 3 to 5 days); dehydration; obesity; smoking; heart failure; mitral or aortic stenosis; coronary heart disease with documented atherosclerosis or arteriosclerosis; peripheral vascular disease; pelvic, gynecologic, genitourinary (GU), abdominal, orthopedic, or major vascular surgery; history of thrombophlebitis, DVT, thromboembolism including pulmonary embolism, MI, or atrial fibrillation; peripheral edema; trauma to the lower extremities; use of oral contraceptives; and recent extended airline travel time. If the patient has a history of clotting disorders or thromboembolism, assess and document the following: presenting signs and symptoms of thrombophlebitis of the leg such as calf edema; pain, warmth, or redness directly over the vessel (more indicative of a superficial clot); increased diameter measurement of the calf of the affected leg; pain in the calf with dorsiflexion (often called Homan's sign; however, asking the patient to dorsiflex is a controversial method of assessment and is now discouraged, as the test may dislodge the clot) or pain upon gentle passive compression of the calf muscle against the tibia; and presenting signs and symptoms of pulmonary embolism such as chest pain, cough, dyspnea, tachypnea, drop in oxygen saturation (by oximetry or blood gas measurement), hemoptysis, tachycardia, drop in blood pressure, and possible shock. All contraindications, cautions, and drug interactions also need to be assessed (see pharmacology discussion) and documented.

Because of the effects of anticoagulants, it is also important to assess the skin, oral mucous membranes, gums, urine, and stool for any evidence of bleeding. Assess patients for any blood in the urine or stool, easy bruising, excessive bleeding from tooth brushing or shaving, or unexplained epistaxis while receiving these medications, and report any such findings. Laboratory tests performed before and during therapy with these drugs usually include, but are not limited to, baseline complete blood counts, hemoglobin level, hematocrit, lipoprotein fractionation, triglyceride and cholesterol levels, various clotting studies, and liver function tests. The serum laboratory tests that are usually ordered with anticoagulant therapy are presented in the Lab Values Related to Drug Therapy table.

With heparin and LMWHs, it is critical to patient safety to continuously assess the skin to identify potential subcutaneous injection sites. For these injection sites, *avoid* any area within 5 centimetres of the umbilicus, open wounds, scars, open or abraded areas, incisions, drainage tubes, stomas, or areas of bruising or oozing. These sites would be at higher risk for further tissue damage with injection of the anticoagulant. Appropriate sites for injection of subcutaneous heparin and LMWHs include the upper, outer area of the arms, the thigh, and the subcutaneous fatty area across the lower abdomen and between the iliac crests (see Chapter 10 for more information).

With use of the parenteral anticoagulant heparin, to ensure patient safety and prevent injury, assess for allergies, contraindications, cautions, and drug interactions (see pharmacology discussion). Severe hypertension, ulcer disease, ulcerative colitis, aneurysms, malignant hypertension, alcoholism, and traumatic brain injury are all conditions in which a bleed is potential and could be precipitated by parenteral anticoagulation. An important caution for heparin use is pregnancy or lactation; however, if there is a need for an anticoagulant during pregnancy, heparin is the drug of choice, not warfarin. Other information is shown in Table 27-1.

It is crucial to patient safety to remember that heparin is *not* interchangeable unit for unit with drugs in another class of anticoagulants, the LMWHs. Although the use of LMWHs leads to fewer adverse reactions in some patients, they are still associated with specific contraindications, cautions, and drug interactions (see previous discussion). When assessing the medication profile, remember that a potentially deadly medication error is to give heparin in combination with enoxaparin (or any LMWH). Always double-check that enoxaparin and heparin are never given to the same patient. The same assessment parameters discussed earlier for heparin are also appropriate for LMWHs. In addition, LMWHs contain sulfites and benzyl alcohol, and so assess patients for allergies to these substances. It is important to note again that the LMWHs differ from standard heparin and also from each other and, for this reason, they are not interchangeable. LMWHs may be used for outpatient anticoagulant therapy because these drugs usually require less close monitoring than standard heparin use. Assess the results of clotting studies prior to therapy.

The oral anticoagulant warfarin and its related contraindications, cautions, and drug interactions were discussed earlier in this chapter. All of the previously

LAB VALUES RELATED TO DRUG THERAPY

Anticoagulants

Laboratory Test	Normal Ranges	Rationale for Assessment
Activated partial thromboplastin time (aPTT), partial thromboplastin time (PTT)	With heparin therapy, aPTT values must fall between 1.5 and 2.5 times the control or baseline value. Normal control values are 25 to 35 seconds. Target therapeutic level of anticoagulation is between 45 and 70 seconds.	Therapeutic levels of aPTT indicate decreased levels of clotting factors and subsequent clotting activity; aPTT is the more sensitive part of PTT (and often replaces it). It is used to determine whether there are deficiencies in the patient's intrinsic coagulation pathway and to monitor heparin sodium therapy. aPTT is sensitive to changes in blood clotting factors, except for factor VII. Therefore, it is used to assess normal blood coagulation. With continuous IV infusions of heparin aPTT levels can be drawn at any time, but with intermittent infusions the aPTT should be drawn approximately 1 hour before a dose of heparin is scheduled to be given. Monitoring of aPTT is not done for prophylactic doses (i.e., 5 000 units every 12 hours subcut).
Prothrombin time (PT)	The normal control PT value ranges from 11 to 13 seconds; target therapeutic level of anticoagulation aimed at 1.5 times the control or about 18 seconds.	Prothrombin is a vitamin K–dependent protein and a major component of the clotting process. It reflects clotting activity and is used to monitor effectiveness of warfarin therapy. PT values vary for each laboratory centre and are based on the specifics of the testing procedure.
International normalized ratio (INR)	Target levels of INR range from 2 to 3 or an average of 2.5. For individuals taking warfarin for treatment of recurring systemic clots or emboli and those with mechanical heart valves, the target INR may be 2.5 to 3.5, with a middle value of 3.	INR determination is a routine test, based on a calculation of the PT, to evaluate coagulation while patients are taking warfarin. When the therapy is initiated, the INR and PT are measured daily until a stable daily dose is reached (i.e., the dose maintains the PT and INR within therapeutic ranges and does not cause bleeding). INR results actually reflect a dose of warfarin given 36 to 72 hours prior to the testing. Advantages of INR testing include the fact that there is more consistency among laboratories and a more consistent warfarin dosage. Some laboratories report INR and PT together.

mentioned assessment parameters are applicable to warfarin. Because of the drug's action, withdraw warfarin (as with all drugs altering bleeding or clotting), as ordered, before the patient undergoes any dental procedures or if there is any evidence of tissue necrosis, gangrene, diarrhea, intestinal flora imbalances, or steatorrhea. It is important to emphasize that this drug is indicated for prophylaxis and long-term treatment of a variety of thromboembolic disorders (see previous pharmacology discussion); constant and skillful assessment of the patient and clotting results is required. Most health care providers use standard protocols for warfarin to assist in dosing the drug based on PT and INR values. The most common starting dose for warfarin is 5 mg daily. However, the dose can range from 1 to 10 mg and may occasionally be even higher (e.g., 12 mg), depending on individual patient response. In most situations, dosage for adults is between 1 and 5 mg orally every day. In addition, it is important to understand the pharmacoki-

netics of warfarin because it takes about 3 days for the drug to reach a steady state. Patients taking heparin may receive warfarin before discontinuation of heparin for anticoagulation.

Dabigatran etexilate mesylate (Pradaxa), although an anticoagulant, is the first oral direct thrombin inhibitor. Additional assessment parameters include kidney function studies. No coagulation monitoring is needed for this drug. Assess for drug interactions with phenytoin and amiodarone. With fondaparinux sodium (Arixtra), carefully assess kidney function. As with dabigatran etexilate mesylate, its effect cannot be measured by standard anticoagulant tests.

With antiplatelet drugs, obtain a thorough nursing history and medication history as well as a physical assessment before beginning drug therapy. Possible drug interactions, cautions, and contraindications have been discussed, but close assessment of any bleeding is extremely important to patient safety. Because aspirin, other NSAIDs, and other antiplatelet drugs alter bleeding times, withhold these drugs as ordered for 5 to 7 days before the patient undergoes surgical procedures. Specific guidelines are generally given by the health care provider to avoid the concurrent use of other anticoagulants, antiplatelets, and fibrinolytics. See Chapter 49 for more information on aspirin. Perform a baseline cardiovascular assessment before beginning clopidogrel and document any pre-existing chest pain, edema, headache, dizziness, epistaxis, or flulike symptoms. Laboratory values usually include complete blood count, hemoglobin level and hematocrit, platelet counts, and PT and INR values. These laboratory values provide baseline levels with which therapy values can be compared. If platelet counts are at or fall below $80 \times 10^9/L$, notify the health care provider; antiplatelet therapy will most likely not be initiated (or will be discontinued).

In addition, it is important to patient safety to re-emphasize that aspirin must not be used in children and adolescents, patients with any bleeding disorder, pregnant or lactating women, or patients with vitamin K deficiency or peptic ulcer disease. Major consequences could occur if aspirin were used by such patients; for example, Reye's syndrome in children and adolescents, teratogenic effects in pregnant women, and ulcers or bleeding tendencies in patients with vitamin K deficiency or peptic ulcer disease. Know how each of the coagulation modifier drugs acts in the body to establish a sound knowledge base to support critical thinking and decision making; for example, such understanding would inform the decision to call the health care provider and not to administer two antiplatelets at the same time or the decision not to give a thrombolytic with heparin, warfarin, or aspirin or other NSAIDs. This type of critical drug information is important to ensure that patients receive the safest and most appropriate care during all phases of the nursing process.

The GP IIb/IIIa inhibitors (e.g., eptifibatide, tirofiban, and abciximab), require the same baseline assessment information (i.e., vital signs, medical history, history of chest pain and heart disease, complete blood cell counts, hemoglobin level, hematocrit, kidney function tests, and platelet counts) as well as assessment for any edema, bradycardia, or leg pain. Before or during therapy, should platelet counts fall below $90 \times 10^9/L$, contact the health care provider for further orders.

Thrombolytics require similar assessments, including attention to baseline complete blood counts and results of clotting studies. Additional concerns include a history of hypotension and cardiac dysrhythmias. The use of alteplase and other thrombolytics always carries the possibility of major concerns, cautions, contraindications, and drug interactions (see previous pharmacology discussion). Constantly assess any arterial punctures, venous cut-down sites, PICC sites, central infusion ports, or other possible sites for bleeding. Do not use IM injections in any situation, as they pose problems with bleeding. As with any drugs that alter clotting and platelet activity, the thrombolytics are associated with the risk of bleeding from wounds or from the GI, GU, or respiratory tract, so assess any drainage, urine, stool, emesis, sputum, and secretions for the presence of blood.

Antifibrinolytics require the same skillful assessment of baseline parameters and laboratory testing listed above; however, there are additional concerns for patients with dysrhythmias, hypotension, bradycardia, convulsive disorders, nausea, vomiting, abdominal pain, or diarrhea. These are possible adverse effects; thus in these situations, the health care provider may need to decrease the dosage of medication.

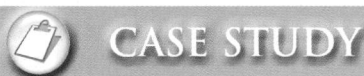

CASE STUDY

Heparin Therapy

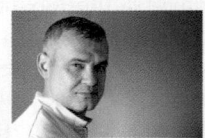

In the past 2 years, Maciej, a 56-year-old lawyer, has had three episodes of DVT. All occurred without complications, and all were treated successfully with anticoagulant therapy and bed rest. He has now arrived at the emergency department because of increased pain and swelling in his left calf that has lasted for the past 3 days. Initially, he is given 5 000 units subcut of heparin. On admission to the hospital for anticoagulant therapy, he is started on a continuous infusion of 25 000 units of heparin in 500 mL of 0.9% sodium chloride (prefilled bag).

1. What nursing actions should be implemented to ensure the accuracy and safety of the continuous heparin infusion?

2. What patient findings would indicate a therapeutic response to the heparin therapy?

Maciej suddenly reports numbness and tingling in his lower extremities with accompanying changes in muscle strength and sensation, 12 hours after the initiation and continuation of heparin therapy.

3. What would be the most appropriate nursing actions to implement?

DVT, deep vein thrombosis.

For answers, see http://evolve.elsevier.com/Canada/Lilley/pharmacology/.

Nursing Diagnoses

- Deficient knowledge related to new medication regimen and the need for altered lifestyle
- Risk for ineffective cerebral tissue perfusion related to the clotting disorder, such as thrombus and subsequent embolus formation
- Risk for injury related to possible adverse reactions to drugs altering blood clotting

Planning

Goals

- Patient will demonstrate adequate knowledge regarding medication therapy and its potential adverse effects, as well as the need for lifestyle changes.
- Patient will exhibit improved blood flow and tissue perfusion as a result of the therapeutic effects of the anticoagulant.
- Patient will remain free from injury resulting from either the disease or the medication being taken.

Expected Patient Outcomes

- Patient states the adverse effects of the drug therapy, ways to monitor for complications of the anticoagulants, the importance of scheduling follow-up appointments with the health care provider and of frequent laboratory studies, and the circumstances under which to contact the health care provider to prevent complications such as hemorrhage.
  - Patient states the nature of and rationale for the lifestyle changes needed, such as improved diet, exercise, and avoidance of smoking.
- Patient shows evidence of improved cerebral circulation while maintaining alertness, orientation, and stable neurological status.
  - Patient remains free of evidence of peripheral clotting with maintenance of pink, warm extremities with strong pedal pulses, or experiences a return to predisease state of maximal tissue perfusion.
- Due to safe medication use, patient is free from bruising, bleeding problems, and any other injury to self.

Implementation

Routinely monitor vital signs, heart sounds, peripheral pulses, and neurological status in all patients during and immediately after anticoagulant therapy. The various laboratory values to be monitored are presented in Laboratory Values Related to Drug Therapy on p. 527. If there is any change in pulse rate or rhythm, blood pressure, or level of consciousness, or unexplained restlessness occurs, contact the health care provider immediately. These changes may indicate bleeding or hemorrhage.

Knowledge of the proper techniques of administration is crucial for safe and effective use of heparin and the LMWHs (see Box 27-1 for other dosing and route information). Heparin is given by the subcutaneous or IV routes but not intramuscularly. Inadvertent IM injection can be easily avoided if only subcutaneous syringes that include a 1.5 cm, 25- to 28-gauge needle are used. No major harm would result if a subcutaneous dose was inadvertently administered intravenously. If rapid anticoagulation is needed, IV heparin, by continuous or intermittent infusion, may be prescribed. Whether the drug is given by IV infusion or subcutaneous injection, monitor daily clotting study results, and perform these studies as ordered for therapeutic doses (monitoring is not done for prophylactic treatment). The drug effects of heparin can be reversed with the IV administration of protamine sulphate. With subcutaneous heparin, several doses of protamine sulphate may be needed to reverse the anticoagulant effect because of the variable rates of absorption of this dosage form. See Box 27-1 for the procedure for the intermittent or continuous IV administration of heparin.

Administer LMWHs by subcutaneous injection deep into the injection site (see previous discussion), using the same techniques as for heparin. The abdomen is the preferred site. Rotate sites frequently. Avoid aspiration with subcutaneous injections to prevent hematoma formation and tissue injury. To avoid bruising, do not massage the site after the injection. Prefilled syringes of LMWHs are available for inpatient use and for at-home treatment. Solutions may be clear to pale yellow. The usual length of therapy is approximately 5 to 10 days, and it is important to be constantly aware of any bleeding problems while the patient is taking this or any other clot-altering drugs. Complete blood counts, platelet counts, and stool tests for occult blood will probably be performed during therapy for monitoring purposes. Tests for occult blood in the stool can be done if occult blood test paper and developer are available. Blood in the stool may occur as an adverse effect with LMWHs or any clot-altering drugs.

When the oral anticoagulant warfarin is prescribed, therapy is often initiated while the patient is still receiving heparin. This bridging or cross-over dosing is done purposely to allow time for the blood levels of warfarin to rise, so that when the heparin is eventually discontinued, therapeutic anticoagulation levels of warfarin will have been achieved. The full therapeutic effect of warfarin does not occur until 4 to 5 days after the first dose. Monitoring of the results of the various clotting studies is still of utmost priority, as is watching for any clotting or bleeding problems. The administration procedures for warfarin are outlined in Box 27-1.

For conversion from heparin to an oral anticoagulant such as warfarin, the dose of the oral drug is the usual initial dosage amount, with the health care provider using the PT and INR levels to determine the next appropriate dosage of warfarin. Once there is continuous therapeutic anticoagulation coverage and warfarin has reached therapeutic levels, the heparin or LMWH may then be discontinued without tapering. If uncontrolled bleeding

---

BOX 27-1 Anticoagulation Therapy and Related Nursing Considerations

---

Subcutaneous Heparin and Low-Molecular-Weight Heparin Injections

- After thoroughly checking the health care provider's order, assess the patient for any allergies, contraindications, cautions, or drug interactions.
- Always begin by performing hand hygiene, and maintain standard precautions. Gloves must be worn. Prefilled syringes are available. When the medication is not available in a prefilled or premeasured syringe, use a 1.5 to 2 cm, 25- to 28-gauge needle. Check the site for bleeding or bruising and do not massage or rub the site before or after the injection. *Do not aspirate* before injecting to prevent hematoma formation. See Chapter 10 for more information on the technique associated with heparin and LMWH injections.
- Make sure the patient is comfortable; then remove your gloves and wash your hands. Document the medication given on the medication record, and monitor the patient for a therapeutic response as well as for adverse reactions.

Intravenous Heparin Administration

- Always double-check the specific health care provider's order for dosage and rate of infusion before beginning therapy. Always follow the "rights" of medication administration to prevent overdosing or erroneous dosing. Make sure the proper diluent is used. Check the compatibility of solutions or other drugs before beginning the infusion.
- For continuous IV administration of heparin sodium, an IV pump must be used to ensure a precise rate of infusion.
- Continuous dosing is preferred over intermittent dosing because continuous dosing helps to maintain blood levels of the drug and because intermittent IV dosing is associated with a higher risk for bleeding abnormalities than continuous dosing.
- Treatment by continuous IV infusion generally begins with a loading dose and is followed by a maintenance dose. Be aware that dosage adjustments must be made exactly as ordered. The patient's activated partial thromboplastin time (aPTT) or results of other related clotting studies are used as parameters for dosing of standard heparin.
- In the past, for intermittent infusions, a heparin lock was used. Heparin locks are now referred to as *intermittent infusion locks* or *saline locks* (because the locks are flushed with isotonic saline and not heparin).

The exception is with PICC lines and central lines, in which heparin is still used as a flush.

- Intermittent infusions of heparin sodium are usually ordered to be given every 4 to 6 hours because of heparin's short half-life. Needleless systems are used for intermittent infusions and all other types of IV infusions.
- Regardless of the type of IV infusion (e.g., intermittent or continuous), it is crucial to check the site to determine whether infiltration has occurred so that hematoma formation may be prevented. If infiltration is suspected, remove the lock and replace it at a new site before the next scheduled infusion. Document appropriately.
- The therapeutic dosage of heparin is guided by aPTT with a targeted level of 1.5 to 2.5 times the control (normal) value. The aPTT is measured within 24 hours of beginning therapy, 24 to 48 hours after therapy starts, and 1 to 2 times weekly for about 3 to 4 weeks, on average. With long-term therapy, aPTT is monitored 1 to 2 times per month.

Oral Anticoagulant Administration

- It is important to recheck the health care provider's orders and the patient's medication and medical history before administering any coagulation modifier drug. Always check to make sure the patient has no known hypersensitivity to the drug.
- Scored tablets may be crushed and may be given with or without food.
- Many more drugs can interact with oral anticoagulants than with heparin, especially those that are highly protein bound (see Table 27-3). Always check the patient's medication list before initiating therapy with warfarin.
- Dosages of warfarin are calculated based on INR blood values. The INR is also used to monitor the effectiveness of therapy. Remember, however, that dosing is highly individualized. Warfarin therapy overlaps with heparin therapy (for about 5 days) until the INR is within therapeutic range for at least 24 hours at which time the heparin is discontinued. This is referred to as bridge therapy.
- Oral anticoagulants are to be administered at the same time every day to maintain steady blood levels.
- Document the dose, time of administration, and any other pertinent facts with these and all other medications.

---

occurs with any of these medications, take action to control bleeding, institute emergency measures to stabilize the patient's condition, and contact the health care provider immediately.

The anticoagulant dabigatran etexilate mesylate (Pradaxa) is given orally. It is packaged in aluminum blister strips and bottles. Dabigatran etexilate mesylate is

to be stored in and dispensed from its original container (e.g., blister pack or bottle). It is important to keep the bottle cap closed tightly after each use and keep the bottle away from excessive moisture, heat, or cold. If not stored properly and with the desiccant (drying agent to absorb moisture) in the packaging cap, the substance in the drug is easily broken down and potency is lost. This would result in less therapeutic effectiveness. This storage information is not widely disseminated and so it is important to be aware of these precautions. The drug can maintain its potency for up to 4 months if kept in the original bottle or blister package, not stored or placed in any other type of container, opened one bottle at a time, and closed tightly after the capsule is removed. The blister package is opened at time of use and the blister is not to be punctured prior to the use of the drug. Fondaparinux sodium (Aristra) is given subcutaneously and, as with dabigatran etexilate mesylate, has no standard anticoagulant tests for monitoring.

Of benefit to counter the toxic effects of anticoagulants is the use of antidotes. The antidote to hemorrhage or uncontrolled bleeding resulting from heparin or LMWH therapy is protamine sulphate. For heparin, 1 mg of protamine sulphate given intravenously neutralizes 100 units of heparin. For the LMWHs, 1 mg of protamine sulphate neutralizes each 1 mg of LMWH given. It is important to note that too-rapid infusion may lead to acute hypotensive episodes, bradycardia, dyspnea, and transient feelings of warmth and flushing. If the heparin overdose has resulted in a large blood loss, replacement with packed red blood cells may be necessary.

The aPTT ranges and hematocrit levels are generally used as ordered to monitor bleeding, clotting, and risk for bleeding. Always monitor patients receiving anticoagulant therapy, especially for any changes in blood pressure and pulse rate. The antidote to oral anticoagulant (warfarin) therapy is vitamin K. See the pharmacology section for more discussion on dosing and the impact of vitamin K on the effects of warfarin. When given intravenously, vitamin K may lead to anaphylaxis with resultant dyspnea, dizziness, rapid or weak pulse, chest pain, and hypotension, which may progress to shock and cardiac arrest. Always check facility policy and the health care provider's order for the specific dosage and route of administration. Continuous monitoring of the patient's vital signs, heart parameters, bleeding times, and clotting study results is important.

Constantly monitor the patient being treated with antiplatelet drugs (or any clot-altering drug) for signs and symptoms of bleeding during and after their use, including epistaxis, hematuria, hematemesis, easy or excessive bruising, blood in the stools, and bleeding of the gums. If invasive procedures must be performed or injections given, apply appropriate pressure to bleeding sites, and closely watch all areas of venous or arterial catheter insertion for bleeding. Advise patients to take extended-release dosage forms in their entirety and without chewing or crushing. Enteric-coated aspirin is best taken with 180 to 240 mL of water and with food to help reduce GI upset. To avoid irritation to the esophagus, instruct the patient to remain upright and not lie down for up to 30 minutes after each dose of aspirin. If aspirin has a strong, vinegar-like odour, discard the drug. Interventions with clopidogrel therapy are similar to those with aspirin. Advise the patient to report the following if they occur: aches in the joints, back pain, dizziness, severe headache, dyspepsia, flulike signs and symptoms, and epigastric pain.

Antiplatelet drugs are often discontinued for 7 days prior to surgery, as ordered. However, some surgical procedures (e.g., cardiovascular surgery) may warrant that the patient remain in an anticoagulated state intraoperatively. Oral forms of dipyridamole are recommended to be taken on an empty stomach; however, if this is not tolerated, the patient can take the drug with food. If nausea occurs, a carbonated beverage, unsalted crackers, or dry toast may help to alleviate this adverse effect. In addition, it may take up to 2 to 3 months of continuous therapy for the drug to reach therapeutic levels. Encourage patients to change positions slowly and take their time going from lying to sitting to standing because of the adverse effects of dizziness and orthostatic hypotension with antiplatelets.

Nursing considerations associated with GP IIb/IIIa inhibitors such as abciximab, eptifibatide, and tirofiban hydrochloride include some similar, yet different, nursing actions to antiplatelet drugs. Close monitoring of all vital signs, electrocardiogram readings, peripheral pulses, heart sounds, skin colour, and temperature are an important part of nursing care during and after the use of these drugs. Because GP IIb/IIIa inhibitors are used in combination with heparin to treat patients suspected of having acute coronary syndrome or those undergoing percutaneous transluminal coronary angioplasty (PTCA), there is always concern for the stability of the patient as well as a high risk for serious bleeding and extension of an acute MI. The patient in this situation is at risk for other medical complications, and this risk may be intensified by the drug. Avoid further invasive procedures while the patient is taking GP IIb/IIIa inhibitors to help prevent bleeding. If invasive procedures are required, continuously monitor for bleeding, and measure all vital parameters before, during, and after the procedure.

Protect IV tirofiban from light. Discard any unused solutions 24 hours after an infusion has been started. Do NOT give any other drugs with this drug except for heparin, which may be administered through the same IV line. For PTCA, abciximab, in particular, can be given by bolus or by continuous infusion; closely monitor infusion rates. Manufacturer guidelines call for the use of a sterile, nonpyrogenic, low protein–binding 0.2- or 0.22-micron filter, and while the vascular shield is in position, keep the patient on complete bed rest, with the head of the bed elevated at 30 degrees. Maintain the affected extremity in a straight position, and constantly monitor peripheral pulses and the colour and temperature of the distal extremities. Once the sheath is removed, apply pressure to the femoral artery for at least 30 minutes, either by manual or mechanical pressure. Apply a pressure dressing once bleeding has stopped. Closely monitor the site for any oozing or bleeding.

If serious bleeding occurs, discontinue the GP IIb/IIIa inhibitor and heparin (the usual protocol for PTCA) immediately, monitor the patient closely, and notify the health care provider immediately for initiation of emergency treatment. Always move and handle these patients with caution and avoid unnecessary trauma because of the risk for hematoma formation or bleeding. Do *not* take blood pressures in the lower extremities, but keep a close and constant watch on the patient's blood pressure (for hypotension) and pulse rate (for tachycardia). Also closely monitor the patient for any reports of abdominal or back pain, severe headache, and any other signs or symptoms of hemorrhage. When adhesive or sticky tape is removed, take care to avoid tearing or ripping the skin, which would lead to tissue trauma and further risk for bleeding. Monitor aPTT levels after the procedure and observe for bleeding, with attention to IM injection sites, arterial or venous puncture sites, and nasogastric tubes and urinary catheters. Avoid invasive procedures, if at all possible, during or immediately after the angioplasty.

Nursing considerations related to thrombolytics are quite similar to those for the other drugs already discussed. Specifically, carry out the preparation for their IV administration per manufacturer guidelines and per protocol. Avoid invasive procedures during the use of these drugs. Avoid simultaneous use of anticoagulants or antiplatelets. Frequently monitor IV infusion sites for bleeding, redness, and pain. IM injections of other drugs are contraindicated to prevent tissue damage and bleeding. Report any bleeding from gums or mucous membranes or the occurrence of epistaxis or increased pulse (higher than 100 beats per minute) to the health care provider immediately, and frequently monitor all vital signs. Other nursing considerations include monitoring for hypotension, restlessness, and a decrease in hemoglobin level or hematocrit, which are to be reported to the health care provider immediately (as they indicate possible shock). Advise patients to report pink, red, or cloudy urine; black, tarry stools or frank red blood in the stools; abdominal or chest pain; dizziness; or severe headache.

Thrombolytics require reconstitution for IV dosing with sodium chloride or 5% dextrose in water. Gently roll, don't shake, the solutions to mix and maintain a stable solution. Continually monitor the INR, aPTT, platelet counts, and fibrinogen levels, beginning no later than 2 to 3 hours after the administration of thrombolytics. Measure the patient's fibrinogen level to check for the occurrence of fibrinolysis. With the breakdown of fibrin (or fibrinolysis), INR will increase and aPTT will be prolonged. If bleeding occurs, the health care provider will most likely discontinue the drug and replace fibrinogen through infusions of whole blood plasma or cryoprecipitate. The antifibrinolytics aminocaproic acid or tranexamic acid may also be given. See Patient Teaching Tips.

With antifibrinolytics, it is important to understand the reasons for the use of these drugs, such as to stop bleeding from overdoses of thrombolytic drugs or to control bleeding during heart surgery. Tranexamic acid is usually given intravenously until bleeding is controlled.

Because of the possibility of drug-induced internal, intracranial, and superficial bleeding, closely monitor the patient, and if there is any change in motor strength or level of consciousness, notify the health care provider immediately. Nurses must apply their knowledge of certain adverse effects of drugs like these to prevent complications, maintain safety, and return patients to a healthier state. It is also important to monitor heart rate and blood pressure, with attention to quality and strength of peripheral pulses. For patients with hemophilia, tranexamic acid may be used to help decrease bleeding from dental extractions.

◪ Evaluation

Monitoring for the therapeutic and adverse effects of coagulation modifier drugs is crucial for their safe use. Because these drugs are used for a variety of purposes, therapeutic responses vary. Some of the therapeutic effects include decreases in chest pain, dizziness, and other neurological symptoms. Adverse effects of anticoagulants include bleeding and hematoma formation (heparin); thrombocytopenia (heparin and LMWHs); bleeding, dizziness, shortness of breath, and fever (direct thrombin inhibitors); bleeding, hematoma, dizziness, and GI distress (selective factor Xa inhibitors); and bleeding, lethargy, and muscle pain (warfarin). Early signs of drug overdose of any of the anticoagulant drugs include bleeding of the gums while brushing the teeth, unexplained nosebleeds or bruising, and heavier-than-usual menstrual bleeding. Abdominal pain, back pain, bloody or tarry stools, bloody urine, constipation, blood in the sputum, severe or continuous headaches, and vomiting of frank red blood or a coffee ground–like substance, indicating old blood, are all possible indications of internal bleeding.

Therapeutic effects of clopidogrel and other antiplatelet drugs include a decrease in the occurrence of clotting events such as TIAs and strokes. The adverse effects of aspirin, as an antiplatelet drug, include dizziness, confusion, nausea, vomiting, GI bleeding, diarrhea, thrombocytopenia, agranulocytosis, leukopenia, and neutropenia. Adverse effects of clopidogrel include chest pain, flulike symptoms, headache, dizziness, fatigue, abdominal pain, diarrhea, and epistaxis. Therapeutic levels of anticoagulants and other clot-altering drugs or coagulation modifier drugs are also monitored by laboratory studies such as aPTT, PT, and INR, described in Lab Values Related to Drug Therapy on p. 535. Remember, however, that aPTT levels are measured with heparin, whereas PT and INR are measured with warfarin. Once the level of the particular drug stabilizes and maintenance therapy is ongoing, the clotting studies may be performed at 1- to 4-week intervals, depending on the specific drug, the patient's responses, and the patient's overall physical condition. If a heparin or LMWH overdose occurs, the antidote is protamine ulfate, whereas vitamin K, or phytonadione, is the antidote to oral anticoagulant overdose.

Continuous monitoring of patients for signs and symptoms of internal or external bleeding is crucial during both the initiation and maintenance of therapy. Therapeutic effects of thrombolytics include improvement in cardiac status during an acute MI, improved blood flow from resolution of DVT, and improved neurological status. Adverse effects include bleeding, hypotension, and cardiac dysrhythmias. Therapeutic effects of antifibrinolytics include the arrest of oozing of blood from a surgical site or a decrease in blood loss. Adverse effects for which to monitor with the antifibrinolytics include orthostatic hypotension, dysrhythmias, headache, dizziness, fatigue, convulsions, nausea, vomiting, abdominal cramps, and diarrhea. Because of the complexity and life-threatening nature of the conditions for which these drugs are used, continuously monitor and re-evaluate the patient's response to the treatment, document this response accordingly, and always keep goals and outcome criteria in the plan of care to serve as benchmarks. Following the evaluation phase, the patient will hopefully emerge experiencing full therapeutic effects and minimal adverse and toxic effects related to drug therapy.

PATIENT TEACHING TIPS

❖ Coagulation modifier drugs are used in patients with heart valve replacements and to prevent serious complications related to clotting, such as strokes, MIs, clot formation (DVT of the legs), and TIAs. Their use necessitates frequent and close monitoring. Educate patients that a healthy lifestyle is an important part of therapy and includes eating the right foods, reducing weight if needed, ceasing smoking, controlling blood pressure, and reducing stress. Advise patients to provide a listing of all medications to all possible health care providers (e.g., dentists).

❖ Direct patients to take all of a clot-altering drug exactly as prescribed because too little of the drug may lead to clot formation and too much of the drug may lead to bleeding. Regular follow-up appointments are an important part of patient care, with frequent blood tests to monitor therapeutic effects and adverse effects of the medication. The results of blood tests will help health care providers determine proper dosage.

❖ At all times, patients must carry an identification card or wear a medical alert bracelet or necklace indicating allergies, medical diagnoses, drugs being taken, health care providers' names and telephone numbers, and an emergency contact name and number.

❖ Home heparin therapy may require that patients receive injections for a period of time, and LMWHs are generally used. If there is a switch from heparin to warfarin, there may be an overlap period of approximately 3 to 5 days during which both drugs are taken to allow therapeutic levels of the oral warfarin to be reached before the heparin is discontinued. Provide complete and thorough instructions to patients, and use return demonstrations to evaluate learning (see Chapter 7).

❖ Advise patients to report any unusual bleeding from anywhere on the body, including nosebleeds or excessive vaginal or menstrual bleeding, or any occurrence of blurred vision, severe headache, vomiting of blood, dizziness, fainting, fever, muscular or limb weakness, or rash.

❖ With dabigatran etexilate mesylate (Pradaxa), educate patients to protect the original bottle from moisture. Once a bottle is opened, it must be used within 4 months; this needs to be written on the bottle with the date of expiration. Instruct the patient to remove only 1 capsule from the opened bottle at the time of use and to immediately and tightly close the bottle. These capsules are *not* to be repackaged or placed in other pillboxes or organizers. Encourage patients to take the medication with food if dyspepsia occurs.

❖ To ensure safe, effective treatment, patients should be encouraged to keep a journal with daily notation of how they are feeling as well as how they are tolerating the medication and any adverse effects.

❖ To reduce risk factors for cardiovascular disease, the health care provider may recommend consumption of a low-fat, low-cholesterol diet; cholesterol-lowering drug therapy; weight reduction; control of blood pressure if hypertension is present; avoidance of smoking; management of stress; and regular exercise.

❖ Teach the patient about clot prevention measures to minimize sluggish circulation, (e.g., avoid tight-fitting clothing and socks, minimize sitting for prolonged periods of time, avoid crossing the legs at the knees, avoid prolonged bedrest, make stops during long trips every 1 to 2 hours to walk around, and keep well hydrated).

❖ When taking any of the anticoagulants (oral drugs, heparin, or LMWHs) or clot-altering drugs, encourage patients to avoid brushing the teeth with a hard-bristled toothbrush, shaving with a straight razor (instead, use an electric shaver), and engaging in any activity that would increase their risk of tissue injury. Always caution patients to be careful when shaving, trimming nails, gardening, or participating in rough or contact sports.

❖ Instruct patients to avoid ingesting large amounts of foods high in vitamin K (e.g., broccoli, Brussels sprouts, collard greens, kale, lettuce, mustard greens, tomatoes) while taking an anticoagulant, to minimize food–drug interactions. Also advise against fad diets as these can alter INR results.

❖ Capsicum (hot red pepper), feverfew, garlic, ginger, ginkgo, ginseng, and St. John's wort are some natural health products that have potential interactions with coagulation modifier drugs, especially with warfarin. Educate patients about these and other interactions.

❖ Patients should immediately report to their health care providers any decrease in urine output; constant ringing in the ears (tinnitus); swelling of the feet, ankles, or legs; dark urine; clay-coloured stools; abdominal pain; rash (medication use needs to be discontinued as ordered if rash occurs); or blurred vision.

Continued

PATIENT TEACHING TIPS—cont'd

❖ If doses of medications are omitted, advise patients to contact their health care providers for further instructions.

❖ Patients should be aware that oral dosage forms of any coagulation modifier medications are to be taken with at least 240 mL of water and with food to help minimize stomach upset.

❖ Patients should keep all medication containers out of the reach of children and use childproof caps. All syringes, needles, and other equipment must be kept out of the reach of children and other individuals.

KEY POINTS

❖ Coagulation modifiers act by preventing or promoting clot formation, lysing a preformed clot, or reversing the action of anticoagulants. Coagulation modifiers include anticoagulants, antiplatelets, thrombolytics, antifibrinolytics, and reversal drugs.

❖ Warfarin prevents clot formation by inhibiting vitamin K–dependent clotting factors (II, VII, IX, and X) and is used prophylactically to prevent clots from forming; it cannot lyse preformed clots.

❖ The degree of anticoagulation (for any of the medications) is monitored by the PT.

❖ Heparin, given intravenously or subcutaneously, prevents clot formation by binding to AT-III, which turns off certain activating factors. The overall effect is to inactivate the coagulation pathway and prevent clots from forming. Heparin does not lyse (break down) a clot. Antiplatelet drugs prevent clot formation by preventing platelet involvement in clot formation.

❖ Thrombolytic drugs are able to lyse preformed clots in blood vessels such as those that supply the heart with blood. Therapeutic effects for which to monitor include improved tissue perfusion, decreased chest pain, and prevention of further myocardial damage. Before giving these drugs, a thorough physical assessment should be performed and pertinent laboratory values (e.g., INR, aPTT, PT) should be checked.

❖ Antifibrinolytics prevent the lysis of fibrin, thus promoting clot formation, and have an effect opposite to that of the anticoagulants. Nursing care is individualized and is based on the characteristics of the patient, thorough assessment data, existing medical conditions, and the specific drug.

EXAMINATION REVIEW QUESTIONS

1. The nurse is monitoring a patient who is receiving antithrombolytic therapy in the emergency room because of a possible myocardial infarction. Which adverse effect would be of the greatest concern at this time?
   a. Dizziness
   b. Blood pressure of 130/98 mm Hg
   c. Slight bloody oozing from the IV insertion site
   d. Irregular heart rhythm

2. A patient is receiving instructions for warfarin therapy and asks the nurse about what medications she can take for headaches. The nurse will tell her to avoid which type of medication?
   a. Opioids
   b. Acetaminophen (Tylenol®)
   c. NSAIDs
   d. There are no restrictions while taking warfarin

3. The nurse is teaching a patient about self-administration of enoxaparin (Lovenox). Which statement should be included in this teaching session?
   a. "We will need to teach a family member how to give this drug in your arm."
   b. "This drug is given in the folds of your abdomen, but at least 5 centimetres away from your navel."
   c. "This drug needs to be taken at the same time every day with a full glass of water."
   d. "Be sure to massage the injection site thoroughly after receiving the drug."

4. A patient is receiving dabigatran etexilate mesylate (Pradaxa), 150 mg twice daily, as part of treatment for atrial fibrillation. Which condition, if present, would be a concern for a patient receiving this dose?
   a. Asthma
   b. Kidney impairment
   c. History of myocardial infarction
   d. Elevated liver enzymes

5. A patient has received a double dose of heparin during surgery and is bleeding through the incision site. While the surgeons are working to stop the bleeding at the incision site, the nurse will prepare to take what action at this time?
   a. Give IV vitamin K as an antidote
   b. Give IV protamine sulphate as an antidote
   c. Call the blood bank for an immediate platelet transfusion
   d. Obtain an order for packed red blood cells

6. A patient is starting warfarin (Coumadin) therapy as part of treatment for atrial fibrillation. The nurse will follow what principles of warfarin therapy? (Select all that apply).
   a. Teach proper subcutaneous administration
   b. Administer the oral dose at the same time every day
   c. Assess carefully for excessive bruising or unusual bleeding
   d. Monitor laboratory results for a target INR of 2 to 3
   e. Monitor laboratory results for a therapeutic aPTT value of 1.5 to 2.5 times the control value

EXAMINATION REVIEW QUESTIONS—cont'd

7. The order for enoxaparin (Lovenox) reads: Give 1 mg/ kg subcut every 12 hours. The patient weighs 242 lb, and the medication is available in an injection form of 120 mg/0.8 mL. How many milligrams will this patient receive? How many millilitres will the nurse draw up for the injection? (Round to hundredths.)

CRITICAL THINKING ACTIVITIES

1. After a patient undergoes total hip replacement, the nurse reviews the new postoperative orders and notes an order for dalteparin sodium (Fragmin) 2 500 International units subcutaneously 6 hours after surgery, then 5 000 international units daily for 7 days. When assessing the patient before administering the drug, the nurse sees that the patient has an epidural catheter for administration of pain medication. What is the nurse's priority action regarding the administration of the dalteparin sodium?

2. A patient is going home from hospital and will be taking warfarin (Coumadin). While discussing his medications just before his discharge, the patient says, "I want to get back to taking my vitamins with ginkgo. They really help my memory." What is the priority as the nurse answers the patient's question?

3. A patient who has been receiving a heparin infusion for DVT has a new order for warfarin (Coumadin). When the nurse explains that the warfarin is another drug to prevent blood clot formation, the patient asks if it is safe to be taking "two blood thinners at the same time." What is the nurse's best response to this patient's question?

For answers, see http://evolve.elsevier.com/Canada/Lilley/pharmacology/.

CHAPTER 28

Antilipemic Drugs

Objectives

After reading this chapter, the successful student will be able to do the following:

1. Explain the pathophysiology of primary and secondary dyslipidemia, including causes and risk factors.

2. Discuss the different types of lipoproteins and their role in cardiovascular diseases and in dyslipidemia.

3. List the drug classes with specific drugs that are used to treat dyslipidemia.

4. Compare the drugs used to treat dyslipidemia, including the rationale for their use in treatment as well as their indications, mechanisms of action, dosages, routes of administration, adverse effects, toxicity, cautions, contraindications, and associated drug interactions.

5. Develop a collaborative plan of care that includes all phases of the nursing process for patients receiving antilipemic drugs.

e-Learning Activities

Website
(http://evolve.elsevier.com/Canada/
Lilley/pharmacology/)

evolve

- Answer Key—Textbook Case Studies
- Answer Key—Critical Thinking Activities
- Chapter Summaries—Printable
- Review Questions for Exam Preparation
- Unfolding Case Studies

Drug Profiles

▸▸ atorvastatin (atorvastatin calcium)*, p. 552
▸▸ cholestyramine, p. 553
   ezetimibe, p. 556
   gemfibrozil, p. 556
▸▸ nicotinic acid, p. 554
▸▸ rosuvastatin, p. 552

▸▸ **Key drug**

*Full generic name is given in parentheses. For the purposes of this text, the more common, shortened name is used.

Key Terms

Antilipemic drugs Drugs that reduce lipid levels. (p. 545)

Apolipoproteins The protein components of alipoproteins. (p. 545)

Cholesterol A fat-soluble steroid alcohol found in animal fats, oils, and egg yolks and widely distributed in the body, especially in the bile, blood, brain tissue, liver, kidneys, adrenal glands, and myelin sheaths of nerve fibres. (p. 545)

Chylomicrons Microscopic droplets made up of fat and protein that are produced by cells in the small intestine and released into the bloodstream. Their main purpose is to carry fats to tissues throughout the body, primarily the liver. Chylomicrons consist of about 90% triglycerides and small amounts of cholesterol, phospholipids, and proteins. (p. 546)

Exogenous lipids Lipids originating outside the body or an organ (e.g., dietary fats). (p. 546)

Foam cells The characteristic initial lesion of atherosclerosis, also known as a *fatty streak*. (p. 547)

Hydroxymethylglutaryl–coenzyme A (HMG–CoA) reductase inhibitors A class of cholesterol-lowering drugs that act by inhibiting the rate-limiting step in cholesterol synthesis; also commonly referred to as *statins*. (p. 550)

Hypercholesterolemia   A condition in which higher than normal amounts of cholesterol are present in the blood. High levels of cholesterol and other lipids may lead to the development of atherosclerosis and serious illnesses such as coronary heart disease. (p. 547)

Lipoprotein   A conjugated protein synthesized in the liver that contains varying amounts of triglycerides, cholesterol, phospholipids, and protein; classified according to its composition and density. (p. 545)

Statins   A class of cholesterol-lowering drugs more formally known as *HMG–CoA reductase inhibitors.* (p. 549)

Triglycerides   Compounds that consist of fatty acids and a type of alcohol known as *glycerol.* Triglycerides make up most animal and vegetable fats and are the principal lipids in the blood, where they circulate bound to a protein, forming high-density and low-density lipoproteins (HDLs and LDLs). (p. 545)

OVERVIEW

Key to understanding the use of **antilipemic drugs** is a working knowledge of the pathophysiology of lipid abnormalities and their contribution to coronary artery disease (CAD). It is also important to understand, at the cellular level, the transport and use of **cholesterol** and **triglycerides** in the human body. Lipoproteins, apolipoproteins, receptors, and enzyme systems are all integral parts of these processes. Armed with this knowledge, clinicians can develop and implement a rational approach to treatment using both nonpharmacological and pharmacological interventions. See the Natural Health Products boxes on p. 548 and below for information on some common dietary products patients may use to control dyslipidemia.

LIPIDS AND LIPID ABNORMALITIES

Primary Forms of Lipids

Triglycerides and cholesterol are the two primary forms of lipids in the blood. Triglycerides function as an energy source and are stored in adipose tissue. Cholesterol is primarily used to make steroid hormones, cell membranes, and bile acids. Triglycerides and cholesterol are both water-insoluble fats that must be bound to specialized lipid-carrying proteins called **apolipoproteins**. This combination of triglycerides and cholesterol with an apolipoprotein is referred to as a **lipoprotein**. Lipoproteins transport lipids via the blood. They are made up of a lipid core of triglycerides, cholesterol esters, or both, which is surrounded by a thin layer of phospholipids, apolipoproteins, and cholesterol. The

---

 ## NATURAL HEALTH PRODUCTS

GARLIC (*Allium sativum*)

Overview
Garlic obtains its pharmacological effects from the active ingredient allicin.

Common Uses
Antispasmodic, antiseptic, antibacterial and antiviral, antihypertensive, antiplatelet, lipid reducer

Adverse Effects
Dermatitis, vomiting, diarrhea, anorexia, flatulence, antiplatelet activity

Potential Drug Interactions
May inhibit iodine uptake. May interact with warfarin, diazepam, and protease inhibitors. Use with nonsteroidal anti-inflammatory drugs may enhance bleeding.

Contraindications
Contraindicated in patients who will undergo surgery within 2 weeks and in patients with human immunodeficiency virus (HIV) infection or diabetes.
    Follow manufacturer directions on container for use of specific preparations.

FLAX (*Linum usitatissimum*)

Overview
Flax is a flowering annual found in the Europe and North America. Both the seed and the oil of the plant are used medicinally.

Common Uses
Treatment of atherosclerosis, hypercholesterolemia, hypertriglyceridemia, gastrointestinal distress (especially constipation), menopausal symptoms, bladder inflammation; among other uses

Adverse Effects
Diarrhea, allergic reactions

Potential Drug Interactions
Antihyperglycemic drugs: Theoretically can potentiate hypoglycemic effects
    Anticoagulant drugs: Theoretically can potentiate anticoagulant effects by reducing platelet aggregation and prolonging bleeding time

Contraindications
Pregnancy (more information needed); use with caution in diabetes and cardiovascular disease
    Follow manufacturer directions on container for use of specific preparations.

various types of lipoproteins are classified according to their density and the type of apolipoproteins they contain. The lipoproteins and their classifications are presented in Table 28-1.

Cholesterol Homeostasis

Cholesterol homeostasis involves a complex array of biochemical factors. Figure 28-1 summarizes the major concepts. Fats are taken into the body through the diet and are broken down in the small intestine to form triglycerides. These triglycerides are then incorporated into **chylomicrons** in the cells of the intestinal wall and are

absorbed into the lymphatic system. The primary purpose of chylomicrons is to transport lipids obtained from dietary sources (**exogenous lipids**) from the intestines to the liver to be used to make steroid hormones, lipid structural components for peripheral body cells, and bile acids.

The liver is the major organ where lipid metabolism occurs. The liver produces very-low-density lipoprotein (VLDL) from both endogenous and exogenous sources. The major role of VLDL is the transport of endogenous lipids to peripheral cells. Once VLDL is circulating, it is enzymatically cleaved by lipoprotein lipase and loses triglycerides. This creates intermediate-density lipoprotein (IDL), which is soon also cleaved by lipoprotein lipase to create low-density lipoprotein (LDL). Cholesterol is almost all that is left in LDL after this process. Any tissues that require LDL, such as endocrine cells, have LDL receptors. LDL and about half of IDL are reabsorbed from the circulation into the liver by means of LDL receptors on the liver.

High-density lipoprotein cholesterol (HDL-C) is produced in the liver and intestines and is also formed when chylomicrons are broken down. Lipids that are not used by peripheral cells are transferred as cholesterol esters to high-density lipoprotein (HDL). HDL then transfers the cholesterol esters to IDL to be returned to the liver. HDL is responsible for the "recycling" of

TABLE 28-1

Lipoprotein Classification

Lipoprotein Classification	Lipid Content	Protein Content
Chylomicron	Most	Least
VLDL	↑	↓
LDL		
IDL		
HDL	Least	Most

HDL, high-density lipoprotein; *IDL*, intermediate-density lipoprotein; *LDL*, low-density lipoprotein; *VLDL*, very-low-density lipoprotein.

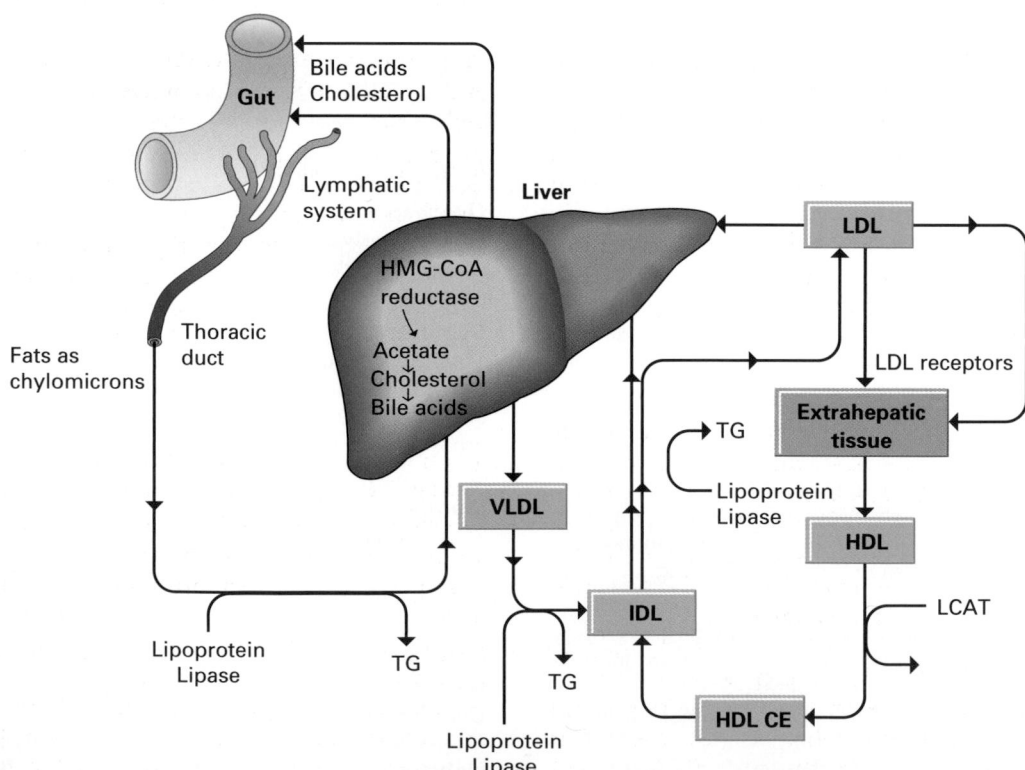

FIG. 28-1 Cholesterol homeostasis. *CE*, cholesterol ester; *HDL*, high-density lipoprotein; *HMG–CoA*, hydroxymethylglutaryl–coenzyme A; *IDL*, intermediate-density lipoprotein; *LCAT*, lecithin cholesterol acetyltransferase; *LDL*, low-density lipoprotein; *TG*, triglyceride; *VLDL*, very-low-density lipoprotein.

cholesterol. HDL is sometimes referred to as the *good lipid* (or *good cholesterol*) because it is believed to be cardioprotective.

If the liver has an excess amount of cholesterol, the number of LDL receptors on the liver decreases, resulting in an accumulation of LDL in the blood. One explanation for **hypercholesterolemia** (high levels of cholesterol in the blood), therefore, is down-regulation (reduced production) of liver LDL receptors. A major function of the liver is to manufacture cholesterol, a process that requires acetyl coenzyme A (CoA) reductase. Inhibition of this enzyme thus results in decreased cholesterol production by the liver.

Atherosclerotic Plaque Formation

Lipids and lipoproteins participate in the formation of atherosclerotic plaque, which subsequently leads to the development of CAD. The primary event that causes atherosclerosis appears to be repeated, subtle injury to the artery's wall through various mechanisms, including smoking, elevated blood pressure, diabetes, and elevated cholesterol. An ongoing inflammatory response plays a central role in all stages of the formation of an atherosclerotic plaque, also referred to as *atherogenesis*. When serum cholesterol levels are elevated, LDLs are oxidized by reactive oxygen free radicals produced by endothelial cells. In response to the injury, circulating monocytes adhere to the smooth endothelial surface of the coronary vasculature. These monocytes burrow into the next layer of the blood vessel (subendothelial tissue) and differentiate into macrophage cells, which then absorb the oxidized LDLs and slowly become large **foam cells**, the characteristic precursor lesion of atherosclerosis, also known as the *fatty streak*. Once this process is established, it is usually present throughout the coronary and systemic circulation. There is also smooth muscle proliferation and migration from the tunica media (middle layer of the artery) to the intima (inner layer of the artery) in response to cytokines secreted by damaged endothelial cells. This process eventually forms a fibrous capsule covering the fatty streak.

Cholesterol and Coronary Artery Disease

Numerous epidemiological trials have shown that as blood cholesterol levels increase, the incidence of death and disability related to CAD also increases. The risk for CAD in patients with cholesterol levels of 5.2 mmol/L is three to four times greater than that for patients with levels lower than 4 mmol/L. The incidence of CAD is lower in premenopausal women. This is thought to be secondary to the effects of estrogen because the risk of CAD climbs considerably in postmenopausal women. However, there is controversy in regard to this longstanding belief because two major trials of estrogen replacement therapy (ERT) did not demonstrate prevention of cardiovascular events in women receiving ERT. Other experimental studies that looked for any benefits of low-dose estrogen therapy in male patients also failed to demonstrate significant cardioprotective efficacy.

Heart disease is the second leading cause of death in Canada, with an estimated 16 000 related deaths occurring yearly, divided almost equally between men and women (Heart and Stroke Foundation, 2015). Thus, there are two goals of treatment: primary prevention in patients with risk factors, and secondary prevention of subsequent cardiac events in individuals who have CAD or have experienced a coronary event (e.g., myocardial infarction [MI]). The benefits of cholesterol reduction, specifically elevated low-density lipoprotein cholesterol (LDL-C) reduction, have been illustrated in a variety of trials. Results of some of the larger investigations support the view that, in patients with known risk factors for CAD, therapy with an antilipemic drug can reduce an individual's relative risk for CAD by 25 to 35%. Drug therapy can also reduce the incidence of first-time MIs and death caused by heart disease. Benefits of cholesterol reduction for secondary prevention have been illustrated in a variety of trials as well. In patients with documented CAD, treatment with a cholesterol-lowering drug has many positive outcomes—decreased coronary events, regression of coronary atherosclerotic lesions, reduced inflammation, and prolonged survival.

Measures taken early in life to reduce and maintain cholesterol levels within a desirable range can have dramatic effects in preventing CAD. These include lifestyle modifications in diet, weight, and activity level. The Heart and Stroke Foundation of Canada (2015) recommends following Canada's Food Guide for a healthy diet that reduces the risk of CAD. Diets lower in saturated fat and higher in fibre and plant chemicals known as *sterols* and *stanols*, and possibly the substitution of soy-based proteins for animal proteins, appear to promote healthier lipid profiles. The consumption of fatty fish or dietary supplements containing omega-3 fatty acids appears to have beneficial effects on triglyceride and HDL-C levels. Even modest weight reduction and exercise can have substantial therapeutic benefits in both the improvement of lipid profiles and reduction of the likelihood of heart disease.

Dyslipidemias and Treatment Guidelines

The decision to prescribe antilipemic drugs as an adjunct to diet therapy in patients with an elevated cholesterol level is based on the patient's clinical profile. This includes the patient's age, gender, menopausal status for women, family history, and response to dietary treatment, as well as the presence of risk factors (other than dyslipidemia) for premature CAD and the cause, duration, and phenotypic pattern of the patient's dyslipidemia.

A major source of guidance for antilipemic treatment in Canada has been the 2012 Update of the Canadian Cardiovascular Society Guidelines for the Diagnosis and Treatment of Dyslipidemia for the Prevention of Cardiovascular Disease in the Adult (Anderson et al., 2013). These recommendations are developed by a panel of

NATURAL HEALTH PRODUCTS

OMEGA-3 FATTY ACIDS (Fish Oil)

Overview
Omega-3 fatty acids are essential fatty acids, most commonly supplied as fish oil products. Several over-the-counter (OTC) products are available.

Common Uses
Cholesterol reduction

Adverse Effects
Rash, burping, allergic reactions, possible increase in total cholesterol or LDL levels in those patients with a combined dyslipidemia, weight gain

Potential Drug Interactions
Anticoagulant drugs: May prolong bleeding time. There is a theoretical risk of increased bleeding when omega-3 fatty acids are taken with anticoagulant drugs, but studies to date are inconclusive.

Contraindications
Pregnancy (more information is needed), allergy to fish oil
 Follow manufacturer directions on the bottle or box for use of specific preparations.

---

multidisciplinary Canadian experts, based on current evidence and practical experience. The focus of the most recent update continues to be cardiovascular risk assessment using the Framingham Risk Score (see http://www.palmedpage.com/Framingham/CCSFramingham.html for a risk calculator), based on conventional risk factors, to identify patients who will most benefit from primary prevention strategies. However, because risk is largely based on age, such that older individuals are more likely to be targeted for treatment, new to the guidelines is the addition of informing patients of their cardiovascular or "heart age" and assessing their risk of heart attack, stroke, or cardiovascular disease within the following 10 years (Anderson et al., 2013). The concept of heart age was created by a research team at McGill University Health Centre in Montreal. The Heart Age Calculator is a scientifically validated online tool, available to the public, that provides a personalized heart age and cardiovascular risk profile, as recommended by the Canadian Cardiovascular Society guidelines. Through knowing their heart age, patients will improve their management of blood pressure and elevated lipids, which can reduce apprehension regarding prescribed therapy. Health behaviour recommendations emphasize appropriate dietary intake of total cholesterol and saturated fat, weight control, physical activity, smoking cessation, and the control of other lifestyle risk factors such as stress. The other focus of the guidelines is on the management of individual patients who are at increased risk for CAD. LDL-C levels are the primary target in the guidelines.

The selection of diet and drug therapy options is determined by the presence of certain risk factors. The 2012 Canadian guidelines include CAD risk equivalents (low, intermediate, and high) and have been statistically calculated to equate 10-year risk for a major coronary event (e.g., MI) for patients who do not currently have CAD but may have other diseases such as diabetes. These risk factors are listed in Box 28-1.

When the decision to institute drug therapy has been made, the choice of drug should then be determined by

BOX 28-1

Coronary Artery Disease: Risk Factors

- Age: males over 40 years; females over 50 years or post-menopausal*
- Family history: History of premature CAD (e.g., MI or sudden death before 55 years of age in father or other male, first-degree relative, or before menopause in mother or other female, first-degree relative)
- Current cigarette smoker
- Hypertension: greater than 140/90 mm Hg or currently receiving antihypertensive drug therapy
- Low-density lipoprotein level: greater than 2 mmol/L; high-density lipoprotein level: lower than 1 mmol/L (men) or 1.3 mmol/L (women); cholesterol greater than 5 mmol/L; triglycerides: greater than 1.7 mmol/L; total cholesterol-to-HDL-C ratio: greater than 4.5 mmol/L
- Diabetes

---

*There are discrepancies in the literature regarding the ages for risk.
CAD, coronary artery disease; *HDL*, high-density lipoprotein; *MI*, myocardial infarction.

the specific lipid profile of the patient. Five patterns or phenotypes of dyslipidemia have been identified, and these are determined by the nature of the plasma (serum) concentrations of total cholesterol, triglycerides, and lipoprotein fractions (i.e., HDL-C, LDL-C, IDL-C, and VLDL-C). The various types of dyslipidemia are listed in Table 28-2. The process of characterizing a patient's specific lipid profile in this way is referred to as *phenotyping*.

TABLE 28-2

Types of Dyslipidemias

Phenotype	Lipoprotein Elevated	Lipid composition	
		Cholesterol (mmol/L)	Triglyceride (mmol/L)
I	Chylomicrons	Greater than 7.8	Greater than 34.2
IIa	LDL	Greater than 7.8	Normal equal to or about 1.7
IIb	LDL, VLDL	Greater than 7.8	Normal equal to or about 1.7
III	IDL	Greater than 10.6	Greater than 6.8 (1–3 times higher than cholesterol)
IV	VLDL	Normal or mildly elevated; approximately equal to 6.5	Greater than 4.6
V	VLDL, chylomicrons	Greater than 7.8	Greater than 22.8

IDL, intermediate-density lipoprotein; *LDL*, low-density lipoprotein; *VLDL*, very-low-density lipoprotein.

TABLE 28-3

Target Lipid Levels

Risk Categories and Target Lipid Levels

Risk Level	Initiate Therapy If	Primary Target LDL-C	Alternate Target
High FRS equal to or greater than 20%	Consider treatment for all	Equal to or less than 2 mmol/L or a greater than 50% reduction in LDL-C	• Apo B less than or equal to 0.8 mg/L • Non-HDL-C less than or equal to 2.6 mmol/L
Intermediate FRS 10–19%	• LDL-C equal to or greater than 3.5 mmol/L • For LDL-C less than 3.5 mmol/L, consider if: Apo B greater than or equal to 1.2 g/L or non-HDL-C is greater than or equal to 4.3 mmol/L.	Equal to or less than 2 mmol/L or a greater than 50% reduction in LDL-C	• Apo B less than or equal to 0.8 mg/L • Non-HDL-C less than or equal to 2.6 mmol/L
Low FRS under 10%	• LDL-C greater than or equal to 5 mmol/L • Familial hypercholesterolemia	Less than or 50% reduction in LDL-C	

Apo B, apolipoprotein B; *C*, cholesterol; *FRS*, Framingham Risk Scale; *HDL*, high-density lipoprotein; *LDL*, low-density lipoprotein, non-HDL-C, total cholesterol minus HDL-C.
Adapted from Anderson, T. J., Grégoire, J., Hegele, R. A., et al. (2013). 2012 update of the Canadian Cardiovascular Society Guidelines for the diagnosis and treatment of dyslipidemia for the prevention of cardiovascular disease in the adult. *Canadian Journal of Cardiology, 29*(2), 151–167. doi10.1016/j.cjca.2012.11.032

The Canadian Cardiovascular Society guidelines' focus is on cardiovascular risk assessment (Anderson et al., 2013). Very low-risk patients require no further testing or treatment with statins. A more liberal use of statins regardless of LDL-C is recommended for patients of intermediate risk. Statin treatment is indicated for all patients of high risk. One of the basic tenets of the Canadian guidelines is that health behaviour management is the cornerstone of all treatment, involving an approach that includes zero cigarette smoking, five daily servings of fruits and vegetables, and at least 150 minutes of moderate- to vigorous-intensity aerobic physical activity per week, in bouts of 10 minutes or more. A change in cardiovascular risk can encourage a patient when the positive benefits of a healthy diet, weight reduction, exercise, and smoking cessation are seen. Drug therapy for dyslipidemias entails a long-term commitment to the therapy.

Treatment decisions made based on the Framingham Risk Score and modified by family history, HDL-C and LDL-C levels are listed in Table 28-3. There is new information on the impact of unhealthy behaviours such as abdominal obesity, lack of regular exercise; diabetes; chronic kidney disease; and *cardiometabolic syndrome*. Features of cardiometabolic syndrome are listed in Box 28-2.

There are currently four established classes of drugs used to treat dyslipidemia: hydroxymethylglutaryl–coenzyme A (HMG–CoA) reductase inhibitors (statins), bile acid sequestrants, the B vitamin nicotinic acid (vitamin B3, also known as niacin), and the fibric acid derivatives (fibrates). In addition, a cholesterol absorption inhibitor, ezetimibe (Ezetrol®), is also available.

Cardiometabolic Syndrome: Identifying Features

- Waist circumference greater than 102 cm in men or 88 cm in women (North American); greater than 94 cm in men or 80 cm in women (Europod, Middle Eastern, sub-Saharan African, Mediterranean descent); greater than 90 cm in men or 80 cm in women (Asian, Japanese, South and Central American descent)
- Serum triglyceride level of 1.7 mmol/L or higher
- HDL-C level of less than 1 mmol/L in men or less than 1.3 mmol/L in women
- Blood pressure of 130/85 mm Hg or higher
- Fasting serum glucose level higher than 5.6 mmol/L

HYDROXYMETHYLGLUTARYL– COENZYME A REDUCTASE INHIBITORS

The rate-limiting enzyme in cholesterol synthesis is known as HMG–CoA reductase. Drugs in the class of medications that competitively inhibit this enzyme, the **hydroxymethylglutaryl–coenzyme A (HMG–CoA) reductase inhibitors**, are the most potent ones available for reducing plasma concentrations of LDL-C. Lovastatin was the first drug in this class to be approved for use. Since then, five other HMG–CoA reductase inhibitors have become available on the Canadian market: pravastatin sodium, simvastatin, atorvastatin, fluvastatin sodium, and rosuvastatin calcium. Because of the shared suffix of their generic names, these drugs are often collectively referred to as *statins*. Lipid levels may not be lowered until 6 to 8 weeks after the start of therapy. Few direct comparisons of the statins have been published. The following doses of drugs are considered "therapeutically equivalent," meaning they produce the same therapeutic effect: simvastatin, 20 mg; pravastatin sodium, 40 mg; lovastatin, 40 mg; atorvastatin, 10 mg; fluvastatin sodium, 80 mg; and rosuvastatin calcium, 5 mg.

Mechanism of Action and Drug Effects

Statins lower blood cholesterol level by decreasing the rate of cholesterol production. To produce cholesterol, the liver requires HMG–CoA reductase, which is the rate-limiting enzyme in the reactions. The statins inhibit this enzyme, thereby decreasing cholesterol production. When less cholesterol is produced, the liver increases the number of LDL receptors to recycle LDL-C from the circulation back into the liver, where it is needed for the synthesis of other needed substances such as steroids, bile acids, and cell membranes. Lovastatin and simvastatin are administered as inactive drugs or prodrugs that must be biotransformed into their active metabolites in the liver. In contrast, pravastatin sodium is administered in its active form.

Indications

The statins are recommended as first-line drug therapy for hypercholesterolemia (elevated LDL-C), the most common and dangerous form of dyslipidemia. More specifically, they are indicated for the treatment of type IIa and IIb dyslipidemia and have been shown to reduce the plasma concentrations of LDL-C. Their cholesterol-lowering properties are dose dependent; 5–80 mg/day of simvastatin lowers the LDL-C by 26 to 47% while 5–40 mg/day of rosuvastatin lowers the LDL-C by 45–63%. A 10 to 30% decrease in the concentrations of plasma triglycerides has also been observed in patients receiving these drugs. Another important therapeutic effect of the statins is an overall tendency for the HDL-C level to increase by 2 to 15%, a known beneficial factor that reduces the risk for cardiovascular disease.

These drugs appear to be equally effective in their ability to reduce LDL-C concentrations. However, rouvastatin is more potent on a per-milligram basis. Atorvastatin appears to be more effective at lowering triglycerides than other HMG–CoA reductase inhibitors. The statins are rarely combined with nicotinic acid or fibrates because of the statins superior efficacy and, the risk of adverse drug effects (see Adverse Effects). It should also be noted that rosuvastatin is often used to replace atorvastatin because of the associated adverse effects of atorvastatin. Rosuvastatin in thought to have fewer adverse effects and may improve the lipid profile compared to atorvastatin (Folse, Sternhufvud, Schuetz, et al., 2014).

Contraindications

Contraindications to the use of HMG–CoA reductase inhibitors (statins) include known drug allergy and pregnancy. Other contraindications may include liver disease or elevation of liver enzymes previous serious myopathy or rhabdomyolysis.

Adverse Effects

HMG–CoA reductase inhibitors are generally well tolerated, and significant adverse effects are fairly uncommon. However, mild and transient gastrointestinal (GI) disturbances, rash, and headache are the most common problems and tend to be under-reported in clinical trials. These and other less common adverse effects are listed in Table 28-4. Elevations in liver enzyme levels may also occur, and patients need to be monitored for excessive elevations, which may indicate the need for alternative drug therapy. Dose-dependent elevations in liver enzyme activity to values greater than three times the upper limit of normal have been noted in approximately 0.4% to 1.9% of patients taking HMG–CoA reductase inhibitors. The serum creatine phosphokinase concentrations may be increased by more than 10 times the normal level in patients receiving these drugs. Most of these patients have remained asymptomatic, however.

A clinically important adverse effect is myopathy, characterized by muscle pain, which may progress to a serious condition known as *rhabdomyolysis.* Health Canada (2012) has issued public health advisories regarding reports of myopathy and rhabdomyolysis cases associated with use of statins. Rhabdomyolysis is the breakdown of muscle protein accompanied by *myoglobinuria*, which is the urinary elimination of the muscle protein myoglobin. This abnormal urinary excretion of protein can place a severe strain on the kidneys, possibly leading to acute kidney injury and even death. It appears to be dose dependent. Advise patients receiving statin therapy to immediately report to the health care provider (HCP) any unexplained muscular pain or discomfort. When recognized reasonably early, rhabdomyolysis is usually reversible with discontinuation of the statin drug. Risk factors for myopathy include: age older than 65 years, hypothyroidism, renal insufficiency, and concurrent use of the antifungal drug gemfibrozil, the immunosuppressant cyclosporine, or macrolide antibiotics. In addition, the use of amiodarone hydrochloride, diltiazem hydrochloride, and amolopidine besylate is associated with an increased risk for myopathy. Patients of Asian descent (those of Filipino, Chinese, Japanese, Korean, Vietnamese, or South Asian origin) may be at greater risk of developing rhabdomyolysis. Although these adverse effects are relatively uncommon, and much benefit is often derived from statin use, HCPs are advised to use minimal effective doses, with baseline laboratory blood monitoring of liver function tests, lipid profile, and creatinine kinase and kidney function with repeat laboratory tests only if non-adherence, myopathy, or if manifestations of liver injury are suspected. Alternate day administration can be useful to reduce adverse effects and increase adherence. Educate patients about possible serious adverse drug effects, and instruct them to immediately report signs of toxicity, including muscle soreness, changes in urine colour (e.g., tea-coloured because of the presence of myoglobulin), fever, malaise, nausea, or vomiting. In 2012, Health Canada imposed new restrictions on simvastatin, which are discussed in detail in its Drug Profile. In 2013, Health Canada issued a label update for all statins, regarding the increased risk for elevated blood glucose levels with their use and a small elevated risk for the development of diabetes in patients with pre-existing risk factors. Health Canada also reaffirmed the position that the benefits of taking statins to reduce cholesterol levels outweighs associated risks. In 2012 (updated in 2015), the United States Food and Drug Administration (FDA) advised consumers and HCPs of information about statins, including the adverse effects of memory loss, forgetfulness and confusion; an increased risk of elevated blood glucose levels and the development of type 2 diabetes; and potential drug interaction with lovastatin resulting in myopathy. The FDA also advised that routine liver enzyme monitoring is no longer necessary.

Toxicity and Management of Overdose

Limited data are available on the nature of toxicity and overdose in patients taking HMG–CoA reductase inhibitors. Treatment, if needed, is supportive and based on the presenting symptoms.

Interactions

Drug interactions with the HMG–CoA reductase inhibitors are listed in Table 28-5. They are to be used cautiously in patients taking oral anticoagulants. In addition, the coadministration of the statins with drugs that are metabolized by cytochrome P450 enzyme 3A4 (CYP3A4; see Chapter 2) may lead to the development of rhabdomyolysis (see the section on adverse effects for the drugs). Patients taking statins are advised to limit their intake of grapefruit juice and grapefruits. Components in

TABLE	28-4

HMG–CoA Reductase Inhibitors: Adverse Effects

Body System	Adverse Effects
Central nervous	Headache, dizziness, blurred vision, fatigue, insomnia
Gastrointestinal	Constipation, diarrhea, nausea
Miscellaneous	Myopathy, skin rashes

HMG-CoA, hydroxymethylglutaryl–coenzyme A.

TABLE	28-5

HMG-CoA Reductase Inhibitors: Drug Interactions

Drug	Mechanism	Effect
warfarin sodium	Inhibit warfarin sodium metabolism	Increased risk of bleeding
erythromycin, azole antifungals, quinidine sulphate, verapamil hydrochloride, amiodarone hydrochloride, grapefruit juice, HIV and hepatitis C protease inhibitors, cyclosporine, clarithromycin, diltiazem hydrochloride, amlodipine besylate	Inhibit statin metabolism	Increased risk of myopathy
gemfibrozil	Potentiation	Increased risk of myopathy

grapefruit juice inactivate CYP3A4 in both the liver and intestines. This enzyme plays a key role in statin metabolism. The presence of grapefruit juice in the body results in sustained levels of unmetabolized statin drug, which increases the risk for major drug toxicity (e.g., rhabdomyolysis). Pravastatin sodium and fluvastatin sodium inhibit CYP3A4 to a much lesser degree than the other statins, whereas lovastatin and simvastatin are the most potent inhibitors of this enzyme.

Laboratory Test Interactions

Laboratory tests may be altered with the use of statins. Altered results may include increases in alanine transaminase (ALT) levels and activated clotting time, thrombocytopenia, and transient eosinophilia.

Dosages

For dosage information on atorvastatin, refer to the table on p. 556.

BILE ACID SEQUESTRANTS

Bile acid sequestrants, also called the *bile acid–binding resins* and *ion-exchange resins*, include cholestyramine resin, colestipol hydrochloride, and colesevelam. The first two of these drugs have been widely used for more than 20 years and have been evaluated extensively in well-controlled clinical trials. They have proven efficacy. The powdered form of cholestyramine resin is somewhat messy to use. Colestipol hydrochloride is available in granules and a tablet form. Colesevelam has a similar mechanism of action and is available only in tablet form. These drugs are considered second-line drugs after the more potent statins. They are suitable alternatives for patients intolerant of the statins. Generally, bile acid sequestrants lower the plasma concentrations of LDL-C by 15 to 30%. They also increase the HDL-C level by 3 to 8% and increase liver triglyceride and VLDL production, which may result in a 10 to 50% increase in triglyceride levels.

Mechanism of Action and Drug Effects

Bile acid sequestrants bind bile and prevent the resorption of bile acids from the small intestine. An insoluble bile acid and resin (drug) complex is formed and then excreted in the bowel movement. Bile acids are necessary for the absorption of cholesterol from the small intestine and are also synthesized from cholesterol

---

 ## DRUG PROFILES

The HMG–CoA reductase inhibitors are all potent inhibitors of the enzyme that catalyzes the rate-limiting step in the synthesis of cholesterol. Six statins are currently available in Canada: atorvastatin (Lipitor®), fluvastatin sodium (Lescol®), lovastatin, pravastatin sodium, rosuvastatin calcium (Crestor®), and simvastatin (Zocor®). There are some minor differences between drugs in this class of antilipemics; the most dramatic difference is that of potency. All six drugs are prescription only and are contraindicated in pregnant or lactating women and in those with active liver dysfunction or with elevated serum transaminase levels of unknown cause or who consume large quantities of alcohol. There have also been reports of elevations in fasting glucose and HbA1c levels. There is little evidence to recommend one drug over another although simvastatin is used less frequently because of its significant adverse effect profile, drug interactions, and lower potency when compared with atorvastatin or rosuvastatin.

▶▶atorvastatin calcium

Atorvastatin calcium (Lipitor) has become one of the most commonly 5, used drugs in this class of cholesterol-lowering drugs. It is used to lower total and LDL-C levels as well as triglyceride levels. Atorvastatin has also been shown to raise levels of "good" cholesterol, the HDL component. All statins are administered once daily, usually with the evening meal or at bedtime. One particular advantage of atorvastatin is that it can be dosed at any time of day. However, bedtime dosing provides peak drug levels in a time frame that correlates better with the natural diurnal (daytime) rhythm of cholesterol production in the body. Atorvastatin is available only in tablet form, in strengths of 10, 20, 40, and 80 mg.

PHARMACOKINETICS

Route	Onset of Action	Peak Plasma Concentration	Elimination Half-Life	Duration of Action
PO	0.5 hr	1–2 hr	7–14 hr	Unknown

▶▶rosuvastatin calcium

Rosuvastatin (Crestor) has also become a more popular statin and as with all statins, it is used primarily to lower total and LDL-C levels as well as triglyceride levels. It can also modestly raise levels of HDL, the "good" cholesterol. It is available only in tablet form, in strengths of 5, 10, 20, and 40 mg. The use of the 40-mg dose of rosuvastatin is contraindicated in the Asian population or in patients who have pre-disposing risk factors for myopathy/rhabdomyolysis. Rosuvastatin should not be taken concomitantly with ciclosporin and fusidic acid. In patients taking the protease inhibitors atazanavir/ritonavir or simeprevir, the dose of rosuvastatin is not to exceed 10 mg daily. In patients taking the protease inhibitors lopinavir/ritonavir, darunavir/ritonavir or tipranavir/ritonavir; gemfibrozil, clopidrogrel; eltrombopag; or dronedarone, the dose is not to exceed 20 mg. Decreased oral contraceptive efficacy is observed in doses greater than 40 mg.

PHARMACOKINETICS

Route	Onset of Action	Peak Plasma Concentration	Elimination Half-Life	Duration of Action
PO	3 days	3–5 hr	19 hr	Unknown

by the liver. This is one natural way that the liver excretes cholesterol from the body. The more that bile acids are excreted in the feces, the more the liver converts cholesterol to bile acids. This reduces the level of cholesterol in the liver and thus in the circulation as well. The liver then attempts to compensate for the loss of cholesterol by increasing the number of LDL receptors on its surface. Circulating LDL molecules bind to these receptors to be taken up into the liver, which has the benefit of reducing circulating LDL in the bloodstream.

Indications

Bile acid sequestrants may be used as primary or adjunct drug therapy in the management of type II hyperlipoproteinemia. A common strategy is to use them along with statins for an additive drug effect in reducing LDL-C levels. In addition, cholestyramine resin is also used to relieve the pruritus associated with partial biliary obstruction. Colesevelam may be better tolerated by higher-risk patients who are intolerant of other antilipemic therapy, including organ transplant recipients and those with serious liver or kidney disease. They may also be used in pregnant women if required for cholesterol control.

Contraindications

Contraindications to the use of bile acid sequestrants include known drug allergy, biliary or bowel obstruction, and phenylketonuria (PKU).

Adverse Effects

The adverse effects of colestipol hydrochloride, cholestyramine resin, and colesevelam are similar; however, colesevelam is reported to have fewer GI adverse effects and drug interactions. Constipation is a common problem and may be accompanied by heartburn, nausea, belching, and bloating. These adverse effects tend to disappear over time. Many patients require additional education and support to help them manage GI effects and adhere to their medication regimens. It is important that therapy be initiated with low doses and that patients be instructed to take the drugs with meals to reduce adverse effects. Patients may relieve constipation and bloating by increasing dietary fibre intake or taking a fibre supplement such as psyllium (e.g., Metamucil® or others), as well as increasing fluid intake. These drugs may cause mild increases in triglyceride levels. The most common adverse effects of the bile acid sequestrants are listed in Table 28-6.

Toxicity and Management of Overdose

Because bile acid sequestrants are not absorbed, an overdose can cause obstruction of the GI tract. Therefore, treatment of an overdose involves restoring gut motility.

Interactions

The significant drug interactions associated with the use of bile acid sequestrants are limited to effects on the absorption of concurrently administered drugs. All drugs should be taken at least 1 hour before or 4 to 6 hours after the administration of bile acid sequestrants. In addition, high doses of a bile acid sequestrant will decrease the absorption of fat-soluble vitamins (A, D, E, and K).

Dosages

For dosage information on a selected bile acid sequestrant, refer to the table on p. 556.

TABLE 28-6	
Bile Acid Sequestrants: Adverse Effects	
Body System	**Adverse Effects**
Gastrointestinal	Constipation, nausea, belching, bloating
Other	Headache, tinnitus, burnt odour of urine

 DRUG PROFILE

Bile Acid Sequestrants

The bile acid sequestrants cholestyramine resin, colestipol hydrochloride, and colesevelam are indicated for the treatment of type IIa and IIb dyslipidemia. They lower levels of cholesterol, particularly the LDL-C level, by increasing the destruction of LDL. However, their use may result in increases in the VLDL-C level. Because of the high incidence of GI adverse effects, adherence to prescribed dosage schedules is often poor. However, educating patients about the purpose and expected adverse effects of therapy can foster improve adherence. Warn patients not to take bile acid sequestrants concurrently with other drugs because of the consequence of reduced absorption. Other drugs must be taken at least 1 hour before or 4 to 6 hours after the bile sequestrant at other times of the day. This requirement cannot be overemphasized.

▶▶ *cholestyramine resin*

Cholestyramine resin (Olestyr®) is a prescription-only drug that is contraindicated in patients with a known hypersensitivity to it and in those who have complete biliary obstruction or PKU. It may interfere with the distribution of proper amounts of fat-soluble vitamins to fetuses of pregnant women or to nursing infants of nursing women taking the drug. Cholestyramine resin is now being used for its constipating effect, often given as needed for loose bowel movements.

NICOTINIC ACID

Nicotinic acid (niacin, Niaspan®) is not only a unique lipid-lowering drug, it is also a vitamin. Much larger doses of nicotinic acid are required for its lipid-lowering effects than are commonly given when it is used as a vitamin. Nicotinic acid is a B vitamin, specifically vitamin B_3. It is an effective and inexpensive medication that exerts favourable effects on plasma concentrations of all lipoproteins. Nicotinic acid is often given in combination with other antilipemic drugs to enhance their lipid-lowering effects.

Mechanism of Action and Drug Effects

Although the exact mechanism of action of nicotinic acid is unknown, its beneficial effects are believed to be related to its ability to inhibit lipolysis in adipose tissue, decrease esterification of triglycerides in the liver, and increase the activity of lipoprotein lipase. The drug's effects are primarily limited to reduction of the metabolism or catabolism of cholesterol and triglycerides. Nicotinic acid decreases LDL levels moderately (10 to 20%), decreases triglyceride levels (20 to 35%), decreases apolipoprotein B (Apo B), and increases HDL levels moderately (20 to 35%). Nicotinic acid is also a vitamin needed for many bodily processes. In large doses, it may produce vasodilation that is limited to the cutaneous vessels. This effect seems to be induced by prostaglandins. Nicotinic acid also causes the release of histamine, which results in an increase in gastric motility and acid secretion. Nicotinic acid may also stimulate the fibrinolytic system to break down fibrin clots.

Indications

Nicotinic acid has been shown to be effective in lowering lipid levels, including triglyceride, total serum cholesterol, apolipoprotein B, and LDL-C levels. It also increases HDL cholesterol levels. Nicotinic acid may also lower the lipoprotein(a) level, except in patients with severe hypertriglyceridemia. It has been shown to be effective in the treatment of types IIa, IIb, III, IV, and V dyslipidemia. Nicotinic acid's effects on triglyceride levels begin to be noticed after 1 to 4 days of therapy, with the maximum decrease seen after 3 to 5 weeks of continuous therapy.

Contraindications

Contraindications to the use of nicotinic acid include known drug allergy and may include liver disease, hypertension, peptic ulcer, and any active hemorrhagic process.

Adverse Effects

Nicotinic acid can cause flushing, pruritus, and GI distress. These undesirable effects can be minimized by starting patients on a low initial dosage and increasing it gradually, and by having patients take the drug with meals. Small doses of aspirin or nonsteroidal anti-inflammatory drugs (NSAIDs) may be taken 30 minutes before nicotinic acid to minimize cutaneous flushing. The most common adverse effects and those associated with nicotinic acid are listed in Table 28-7.

Interactions

Drug interactions associated with nicotinic acid are minimal. However, when nicotinic acid is taken with an HMG–CoA reductase inhibitor, the likelihood of myopathy development is greatly increased, although it is not uncommon to see these drugs used together.

Dosages

For dosage information on nicotinic acid, refer to the table on p. 556.

TABLE 28-7	
Nicotinic Acid: Potential Adverse Effects	
Body System	**Adverse Effects**
Gastrointestinal	Abdominal discomfort
Integumentary	Cutaneous flushing, pruritus
Other	Blurred vision, glucose intolerance, hepatotoxicity

DRUG PROFILES

▶▶ nicotinic acid

Used alone or in combination with other lipid-lowering drugs, nicotinic acid (niacin, vitamin B_3; Niaspan) is an effective, inexpensive medication that has beneficial effects on LDL-C, triglyceride, and HDL-C levels. Drug therapy is usually initiated at a small daily dose taken with or after meals to minimize the adverse effects. Liver dysfunction has been observed in individuals taking nicotinic acid. Niacin is contraindicated in patients who have shown a hypersensitivity to it; in those with peptic ulcer, liver disease, hemorrhage, or severe hypotension; and in lactating women. It is also not recommended for patients with gout.

PHARMACOKINETICS

Route	Onset of Action	Peak Plasma Concentration	Elimination Half-Life	Duration of Action
PO	Rapid	30–60 min	45 min	Unknown

FIBRIC ACID DERIVATIVES

Current fibric acid derivatives include bezafibrate, gemfibrozil and fenofibrate. These drugs primarily affect triglyceride levels but may also lower total cholesterol and LDL-C levels and raise HDL-C levels. They are often collectively referred to as *fibrates*.

Mechanism of Action and Drug Effects

Fibric acid drugs are believed to work by activating lipoprotein lipase, an enzyme responsible for the breakdown of cholesterol. This enzyme usually cleaves off a triglyceride molecule from VLDL or LDL, leaving behind lipoproteins. Fibric acid derivatives also suppress the release of free fatty acid from adipose tissue, inhibit the synthesis of triglycerides in the liver, and increase the secretion of cholesterol into bile. They have been shown to reduce triglyceride levels and serum VLDL and LDL concentrations. Independent of their lipid-lowering actions, fibric acid derivatives can also induce changes in blood coagulation; this involves a tendency toward a decrease in platelet adhesion. They can also increase plasma fibrinolysis, the process that causes fibrin, and therefore clots, to be broken down.

Indications

The fibric acid derivatives bezafibrate, gemfibrozil, and fenofibrate decrease triglyceride levels and increase HDL-C levels by as much as 25%. They decrease LDL concentrations in patients with type IIa and IIb dyslipidemias but increase LDL levels in patients with type IV and V dyslipidemias. They are indicated for the treatment of type III, IV, and V dyslipidemias and, in some cases, the type IIb form, although other classes of antilipemics are usually attempted first.

Contraindications

Contraindications to the use of fibrates include known drug allergy and may include severe liver or kidney disease, cirrhosis, or gallbladder disease.

Adverse Effects

The most common adverse effects of fibric acid derivatives are abdominal discomfort, diarrhea, nausea, headache, blurred vision, increased risk for gallstones, and prolonged prothrombin time. Liver function tests may also show increased enzyme levels. The more common adverse effects are listed in Table 28-8.

Toxicity and Management of Overdose

The management of fibrate overdose, which is uncommon, is supportive care based on presenting symptoms.

Interactions

Gemfibrozil can enhance the action of oral anticoagulants; thus, careful adjustment of the dosage of warfarin is required. The risk for myositis, myalgia, and rhabdomyolysis is increased when when either bezafibrate,

TABLE 28-8	
Fibric Acid Derivatives: Potential Adverse Effects	
Body System	**Adverse Effects**
Gastrointestinal	Nausea, vomiting, diarrhea, gallstones
Genitourinary	Impotence, decreased urine output, hematuria
Other	Drowsiness, dizziness, rash, pruritus, vertigo

gemfibrozil, or fenofibrate is given with a statin. Laboratory test interactions that can occur in patients taking gemfibrozil include a decrease in hemoglobin level, hematocrit value, and white blood cell count. In addition, aspartate aminotransferase (AST), activated clotting time, lactate dehydrogenase, and bilirubin levels can be increased. Fenofibrate may raise the blood level of ezetimibe if the two are taken concurrently.

Dosage

For dosage information on gemfibrozil, refer to the table on p. 556.

NURSING PROCESS

☑ Assessment

Before initiating therapy with any antilipemic drug, obtain a thorough health and medication history, with a listing of allergies and any prescription drugs, OTC drugs, and natural health products the patient is taking. Assess the patient's dietary patterns, stress levels, exercise program and frequency, weight, height, and vital signs, and document these parameters, especially food intake, over time, such as for several weeks. Also document the patient's use of tobacco, alcohol, and social drugs, along with information about frequency, amount, and duration of use. Some lipid disorders are hereditary; therefore, perform a thorough assessment of family history. Positive risk factors for CAD for which the patient needs to be assessed include the following. (1) males 40 years or older; females 50 years or older or postmenopausal (Anderson et al., 2013); (2) family history, including history of premature CAD (e.g., MI or sudden death before 55 years of age in father or other male, first-degree relative, or before menopause in mother or other female, first-degree relative); (3) cigarette smoking; (4) hypertension with a blood pressure higher than 140/90 mm Hg or current antihypertensive drug therapy; (5) low HDL cholesterol level (lower than 1 mmol/L in men or lower than 1.3 mmol/L in women); and (6) diabetes.

DRUG PROFILES

FIBRIC ACID DERIVATIVES (FIBRATES)

The fibric acid derivatives bezafibrate, gemfibrozil, and fenofibrate are prescription-only drugs. They are contra-indicated in patients with hypersensitivity, pre-existing gallbladder disease, significant liver or kidney dysfunc-tion, and primary biliary cirrhosis. Women of childbearing age must use birth control measures; if pregnancy occurs, the drugs must be discontinued. Fibrates decrease tri-glyceride levels and increase HDL levels by as much as 25%. They are effective for the treatment of mixed dyslipidemia.

gemfibrozil

Gemfibrozil is a fibric acid derivative that decreases the synthesis of Apo B and lowers the VLDL level. It can also increase the HDL level. In addition, it is highly effective for lowering plasma triglyceride levels. In a landmark study known as the Helsinki study, reported in 1987 in the *New England Journal of Medicine*, the triglyceride levels of the group receiving gemfibrozil were reduced by as much as 43% compared with those in the control group. Total cholesterol and LDL-C levels were reduced by 11% and 10%, respectively, and the HDL level was increased by 10%. Gemfibrozil is indicated for the treat-ment of type IV and V dyslipidemias and, in some cases, the type IIb form.

PHARMACOKINETICS

Route	Onset of Action	Peak Plasma Concentration	Elimination Half-Life	Duration of Action
PO	Several days	1–2 hr	1.3–1.5 hr	Unknown

CHOLESTEROL ABSORPTION INHIBITOR

ezetimibe

Ezetimibe (Ezetrol) is currently the only cholesterol absorp-tion inhibitor. Ezetimibe has a novel mechanism of action in that it selectively inhibits absorption of cholesterol and related sterols in the small intestine. The result is a reduc-tion in several blood lipid parameters: total cholesterol, LDL-C, Apo B, and triglyceride level. Serum levels of HDL-C have been shown to increase with the use of ezetimibe. Beneficial effects of ezetimibe appear to be further enhanced when it is taken with a statin drug. Ezetimibe may be used as monotherapy although it has the lowest potency. Recent studies have shown that, although the combination of ezetimibe and a statin is effective in reduc-ing LDL, the rate of atherosclerotic progression is no dif-ferent from when a statin is given alone. Use of ezetimibe and simvastatin is effective in reducing the risk of vascular events in patients with advanced chronic kidney disease.

Ezetimibe levels are increased by the fibric acid deriva-tives (fibrates). It is not known whether this is harmful, but concurrent use of ezetimibe and fibrates is not recom-mended. The use of ezetimibe with bile acid sequestrants has been shown to reduce the serum level of ezetimibe by 55% and 80% in two small studies. Ezetimibe is contra-indicated in those with a known hypersensitivity to it and in those with active liver disease or unexplained eleva-tions in serum liver enzymes. It may be taken with or without food, and for patient convenience it may be dosed at the same time as a statin drug, if prescribed.

PHARMACOKINETICS

Route	Onset of Action	Peak Plasma Concentration	Elimination Half-Life	Duration of Action
PO	Unknown	4–12 hr	22 hr	Unknown

DOSAGES   Selected Antilipemic Drugs

Drug	Pharmacological Class	Usual Dosage Range	Indications
▶atorvastatin calcium (Lipitor)	HMG–CoA reductase inhibitor	*Adults* PO: 10–80 mg/day	Dyslipidemia
▶cholestyramine resin (Olestyr)	Bile acid sequestrant	*Adults* PO: Powder, 4–24 g/day	
ezetimibe (Ezetrol)	Cholesterol absorption inhibitor	*Adults* PO: 10 mg 1 ×/day	
gemfibrozil	Fibric acid derivative	*Adults* PO: 600 mg bid 30 min before meals in a.m. and p.m.	
▶nicotinic acid (Niacin, Niaspan)	B vitamin	*Adults* PO: 1–2 g/day at bedtime	
simvastatin (Zocor)	HMG–CoA reductase inhibitor	*Adults* PO: 5–40 mg/day	

HMG–CoA, hydromethylglutaryl-coenzyme A; *PO*, oral.

Perform an assessment to identify any cautions, contraindications, and potential drug interactions before initiating use of any of the antilipemics. Also assess serum lipid values and lipoprotein levels (see Lab Values Related to Drug Therapy below). With the use of cholestyramine resin, which contains aspartame, a history of PKU is of particular interest. Patients with PKU cannot properly process the amino acid phenylalanine, a component of protein. High levels of phenylalanine lead to behavioural, cognitive, and learning dysfunction as early as at 3 weeks of age in such patients; dietary restrictions must continue throughout their lives. Adult patients with PKU require monthly testing of phenylalanine levels. Because of the aspartame in cholestyramine resin, another class of antilipemics would be indicated, as ordered, to prevent further complications from this disorder.

HMG–CoA reductase inhibitors (the statins) are not be used in patients who have liver disease or increased liver enzymes. Other contraindications, cautions, and drug interactions were previously discussed in the pharmacology section of this chapter. With the use of the statins and all antilipemics, assess patients' intake of alcohol, including the amount consumed and the period of time that alcohol has been used because of the potential for liver dysfunction associated with the majority of lipid-lowering drugs. The statins may have additional adverse effects on an already damaged liver. Monitor levels of liver enzymes that are indicative of liver function, AST, CPK, and ALT. Review lipid and lipoprotein levels before, during, and after drug therapy with statins, as well as with other antilipemic drugs. Assess patients for any musculoskeletal problems or concerns due to the possible adverse effect of myopathy. If AST or ALT blood levels increase or signs and symptoms of myopathy or rhabdomyolysis occur (i.e., muscle soreness, changes in urine colour, fever, malaise, nausea, or vomiting), the drug will most likely be discontinued by the health care provider. It is always important to determine if patients' cultural practices or beliefs will impact their adherence to dietary restrictions. Cultural practices may also include the use of natural health products that may constitute contraindications to the use of statins or other antilipemics.

Use of bile acid sequestrants requires careful assessment of possible contraindications such as a history of biliary or bowel obstructions and PKU. Drug interactions are numerous (see previous discussion) because of the decreased absorption of drugs caused by bile acid sequestrants. With nicotinic acid, patient assessment includes noting contraindications such as liver disease, peptic ulcer disease, gout, hypertension, and any active bleeding. Liver function studies are usually ordered for baseline and comparative levels with the majority of antilipemics. Fibric acid derivatives are not used in patients with liver, kidney, or gallbladder disease, and so assessment for these disorders is critical to patient safety. With ezetimibe, assess for liver disease and liver enzyme elevation before initiation of therapy.

 ## LAB VALUES RELATED TO DRUG THERAPY

Coronary Artery Disease

Laboratory Test	Normal Ranges	Rationale for Assessment
Lipid panel with serum cholesterol, triglycerides, and lipids	Serum cholesterol levels less than 5 mmol/L Triglyceride levels less than 1.7 mmol/L Low-density lipoprotein (LDL) cholesterol levels less than 2.5 mmol/L) High-density lipoprotein (HDL) cholesterol levels 1 mmol/L or greater for men; 1.3 mmol/L or greater for women Very-low-density lipoprotein (VLDL) cholesterol levels less than 3.4 mmol/L	A lipid panel is a serum test that measures lipids, fats, and fatty substances used as a source of energy in the body. Lipids include cholesterol, triglycerides, HDL, and LDL. When a lipid panel is ordered, the levels include all of the following: total cholesterol, triglycerides, HDL, LDL, VLDL, ratio of total cholesterol to HDL, and ratio of LDL to HDL. Lipid levels are important to health status and are indicators of health; if there are abnormalities (e.g., high cholesterol, triglycerides, HDL, VLDL and LDL levels), the individual is at increased risk for heart disease and stroke. Dietary and other lifestyle changes may be implemented to help decrease "bad" cholesterol levels (LDL and VLDL) and elevate "good" cholesterol levels (HDL). Medical treatment protocols may also be implemented to help prevent MI and stroke.

Based on Anderson, T. J., Grégoire, J., Hegele, R. A., et al. (2013). 2012 update of the Canadian Cardiovascular Society Guidelines for the diagnosis and treatment of dyslipidemia for the prevention of cardiovascular disease in the adult. *Canadian Journal of Cardiology, 29*(2), 151–167. doi:10.1016/j.cjca.2012.11.032

Nursing Diagnoses

- Imbalanced nutrition, more than body requirements, related to poor dietary habits including high fat intake
- Deficient knowledge related to a lack of knowledge about the disease, related complications, and drug therapy
- Risk for impaired liver function related to potential adverse and toxic effects of drug therapy

Planning

Goals

- Patient will maintain healthy nutritional intake with appropriate restrictions.
- Patient will demonstrate adequate knowledge of disease process and its associated drug therapeutic regimens.
- Patient will maintain baseline liver function during drug therapy.

Expected Patient Outcomes

- Patient states the importance of dietary restrictions, with emphasis on a low-fat, low-cholesterol, high-fibre, and low-calorie (if appropriate) diet, as prescribed.
  - Patient engages in a nutritional consultation to support implementation of changes in lifestyle and diet to help decrease cholesterol and triglyceride levels.
  - Patient follows guidelines in Canada's Food Guide, incorporating recommendations such as decreasing saturated and trans fat intake, boosting intake of polyunsaturated and monounsaturated fats, in-

creasing fruit and vegetable intake to a minimum of five servings per day, and consuming a low-carbohydrate or low-fat diet.
  - Patient implements regular aerobic exercise for 2 hours or more per week, as prescribed.
- Patient demonstrates adequate knowledge about disease processes and the need for lifelong treatment with drug therapy.
  - Patient states the rationale for antilipemic drug therapy (decrease in lipid levels).
  - Patient states the importance of taking the medication exactly as prescribed.
  - Patient states the various adverse effects, such as GI upset, changes in liver function tests, and belching, related to the specific drug prescribed.
  - Patient returns for follow-up care for monitoring of lipid levels and for adverse effects.
- Patient demonstrates knowledge of the risk for liver dysfunction associated with antilipemic therapy.
  - Patient states potential adverse effects to report to the health care provider, such as jaundice and abdominal pain.
  - Patient states the importance of follow-up care with the health care provider to monitor for changes in liver function and monitoring of liver function tests.

Implementation

Patients who are taking antilipemics for a long period may have altered levels of the fat-soluble vitamins and may then require supplementation of vitamins A, D, and K. Antilipemics may also cause problems with the liver and biliary systems and may cause GI problems such as constipation. Appropriate actions need to be taken to avoid or minimize constipation, such as increasing intake

CASE STUDY

Antilipemic Drug Therapy

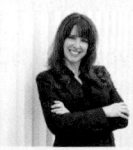

Sophie, a 49-year-old mayor, lives a busy life but manages to exercise regularly and tries to maintain a healthy lifestyle, including watching her diet. She is a nonsmoker and is not overweight. Recently, Sophie had a medical checkup and, to her surprise, was told that her lipid levels are elevated. She has no history of diabetes, and her blood pressure is within normal limits. Her nurse practitioner has recommended that she start the HMG–CoA reductase inhibitor (statin) drug atorvastatin (Lipitor) at a dosage of 20 mg every evening.

1. Sophie says, "Isn't there something else I can do instead of taking this medicine? I really don't like taking pills." What alternatives may be available to her?
2. After 4 months, Sophie's lipid levels have not improved. The nurse practitioner discusses Sophie's risk factors,

including the fact that her father died at 54 years of age of an MI. What other risk factors need to be considered?
3. Sophie agrees to take the medication and schedules a follow-up appointment in 3 months. Two months later, she wakes up with pain in her legs and feeling extremely tired. She thinks she is suffering the effects of a new workout program that she started the previous day. But when she goes to work, the pain gets worse, and she calls the nurse to describe her symptoms. What could be happening?
4. Sophie asks whether she will just be switched to another "statin" drug. How will the nurse respond?

_____

For answers, see http://evolve.elsevier.com/Canada/Lilley/pharmacology/.

of fibre and fluids. Monitoring the results of blood studies per the health care provider's instructions often includes noting levels of serum transaminases and results of other tests of liver function.

With the HMG–CoA reductase inhibitors, or statin drugs, serum levels of ALT, AST, and CK are often measured are usually measured for baseline and may be repeated if non-adherence is suspected (repeat lipid profile), if patient experiences myopathy (repeat CK) or if patient has manifestations of hepatic injury (repeat LFTs). If a lipid profile is ordered, instruct the patient to fast for 12 to 14 hours before the blood sample is drawn. Also, inform patients of the desired laboratory levels to be achieved (see Table 28-3). Because severe cardiovascular disease and strokes are associated with high cholesterol levels, it is critical to the maintenance of health and the prevention of complications that the patient continue with any prescribed nonpharmacological and pharmacological therapies, regardless of the specific antilipemic used. Another aspect to consider when administering these medications, specifically simvastatin (Zocor), is dosage amount. See the pharmacology discussion for prescribing restrictions on 80-mg dosage forms of simvastatin. There are additional concerns about simvastatin and other medications that were discussed in the pharmacology section of this chapter.

Bile acid sequestrants often come in powder form and should be mixed thoroughly with food or fluids (at least 120 to 180 mL of fluid). The powder may not mix completely at first, but patients need to be sure to mix the dose as much as possible and then dilute any undissolved portion with additional fluid. The powder should be dissolved for at least 1 full minute. Powder and granule dosage forms are *never* to be taken in dry form. It is important that bile acid sequestrants such as colestipol hydrochloride be taken 1 hour before or 4 to 6 hours after any other oral medication or meals because of the high risk for drug–drug or drug–food interactions. Bile acid sequestrants interfere with the absorption of other medications. Colestipol hydrochloride is also available in tablet form. Cholestyramine is to be taken just before meals or with meals, and it must never be given to a patient with PKU because it contains aspartame (see previous discussion). Constipation may be prevented with high fibre and increased fluid intake.

With nicotinic acid, flushing of the face may occur; educate patients regarding this adverse effect. To minimize GI upset, advise patients to take this medication with meals. Of the different dosage forms available, the extended-release dosage forms—which dissolve more slowly than the immediate-release forms but faster than the sustained-release forms—appear to be associated with less flushing of the skin. Other actions that may help to minimize flushing of the skin include titrating the drug dosage or taking a small dose of aspirin or an NSAID 30 minutes before the nicotinic acid, but only as ordered or recommended by the health care provider. Educate patients that fibric acid derivatives are to be taken as prescribed. Frequently monitor liver and kidney function tests and prothrombin times with these drugs. The cholesterol absorption inhibitor ezetimibe may be taken with or without food and may be taken with statin drugs.

Evaluation

Begin with evaluation of goals and outcome criteria when trying to evaluate the therapeutic versus adverse effects of these medications. In addition, cholesterol and triglyceride levels are used to monitor the patient's response to the medication regimen, and specific targets are listed in Table 28-3. While taking antilipemics, patients should remain on a low-fat, low-cholesterol diet as an integrated part of a change in lifestyle. Monitor patients receiving antilipemic drugs for therapeutic and adverse effects during their therapy. The therapeutic effects of both nonpharmacological and pharmacological measures are evidenced by a decrease in cholesterol and triglyceride levels to within normal levels (see previous serum laboratory values). Nonpharmacological measures include consumption of a low-fat, low-cholesterol diet; supervised, moderate exercise; weight loss; cessation of smoking and drinking; and relaxation therapy.

Adverse effects for which to monitor include GI upset, increased liver enzyme levels, hepatomegaly, myalgias, and other effects mentioned earlier in the chapter. Closely monitor patients' kidney and liver function before and throughout treatment to detect the development of liver or kidney dysfunction.

PATIENT TEACHING TIPS

❖ Advise patients to notify their HCPs if there are any new or troublesome symptoms or if there is persistent GI upset, constipation, gas, bloating, heartburn, nausea, vomiting, abnormal or unusual bleeding, muscle pain, or yellow discoloration of the skin.

❖ Advise patients to keep antilipemics and all medications out of the reach of children and protected with childproof lids.

❖ Encourage patients to maintain a diet that is rich in raw vegetables, fruit, and bran. Also encourage the consumption of fluids (up to 3 000 mL/day unless contraindicated) to help prevent the constipation associated with antilipemics.

❖ Advise patients to inform all HCPs about all medications being taken, including antilipemics. These drugs are highly protein-bound and are therefore associated with many drug interactions, including with drugs that a dentist might prescribe. In addition, antilipemics may alter clotting if taken on a long-term basis, so bleeding may occur during dental work.

❖ Educate patients that exercise is to be done in moderation and often with supervision, as indicated.

❖ Alert patients taking simvastatin to concerns regarding the use of 80-mg doses.

❖ Inform patients that when taking an HMG–CoA reductase inhibitor or statin drug, it is best to take the medication with at least 180 mL of water or with meals to help minimize GI upset. It takes several weeks before therapeutic results are seen. Monitor liver and kidney function laboratory studies every 3 to 6 months.

❖ Patients should be aware that drug and food interactions associated with statin drugs necessitate the avoidance of oral anticoagulants, erythromycin, verapamil hydrochloride, some antifungal drugs, and grapefruit products.

❖ Patients taking HMG–CoA reductase inhibitors need to know to report any muscle soreness, change in colour of the urine, fever, nausea, vomiting, or malaise to their HCPs immediately.

❖ Advise patients taking a bile acid sequestrant that the medication should be taken with meals to decrease GI upset. Other drugs must be taken 1 hour before or 4 to 6 hours after taking a bile acid sequestrant.

❖ Nicotinic acid is contraindicated in those with liver disease, peptic ulcer disease, gout, hypertension, or active bleeding. Instruct patients to take nicotinic acid with meals to decrease GI upset.

KEY POINTS

❖ There are two primary forms of lipids: triglycerides and cholesterol. Triglycerides function as an energy source and are stored in adipose tissue. Cholesterol is primarily used to make steroid hormones, cell membranes, and bile acids.

❖ Lipids and lipoproteins participate in the formation of atherosclerotic plaque, which leads to CAD, and it is important to understand the pathophysiology of this disease process so that appropriate patient education can be delivered.

❖ When plaque forms in the blood vessels that supply the heart with needed oxygen and nutrients, the lumens of these blood vessels will eventually decrease in size and the amount of oxygen and nutrients that can reach the heart (and major organs) will be reduced.

❖ Antilipemic drugs are used to lower high levels of lipids (triglycerides and cholesterol) in the blood.

❖ The major classes of antilipemics include HMG–CoA reductase inhibitors, bile acid sequestrants, nicotinic acid, fibric acid derivatives, and cholesterol absorption

inhibitors, with each having its own mechanism of action.

❖ While taking a history, it is important to assess patients for any possible cautions, contraindications, and drug interactions.

❖ Fat-soluble vitamins may need to be prescribed for patients taking antilipemics for long periods because these medications have long-term effects on the liver's production of these vitamins.

❖ When using the powder or granule, oral-based forms of these drugs, they must be mixed with noncarbonated liquids and *never* taken dry.

❖ Monitoring for adverse effects of antilipemics includes periodic liver and kidney function studies.

❖ Statins have gained much attention for their adverse effects of muscle aches and pain due to breakdown of muscle tissue. Some patients experience irreversible kidney damage and severe pain and may have to alter dosages or change drugs as ordered by the HCP.

EXAMINATION REVIEW QUESTIONS

1. A nurse administering nicotinic acid would implement which action to help to reduce adverse effects?
   a. Give the medication with grapefruit juice.
   b. Administer a small dose of aspirin or an NSAID 30 minutes before the niacin dose.
   c. Administer the medication on an empty stomach.
   d. Have the patient increase dietary fibre intake.

2. When administering nicotinic acid, the nurse needs to monitor for which adverse effect?
   a. Cutaneous flushing
   b. Muscle pain
   c. Headache
   d. Constipation

3. Which point will the nurse emphasize to a patient who is taking an antilipemic drug in the "statin" class?
   a. The drug needs to be taken on an empty stomach before meals.
   b. A low-fat diet is not necessary while taking these medications.
   c. It is important to report muscle pain immediately.
   d. Improved cholesterol levels should be evident within 2 weeks.

4. A patient is being assessed before a newly ordered antilipemic medication is given. Which condition would be a potential contraindication?
   a. Diabetes insipidus
   b. Pulmonary fibrosis
   c. Liver cirrhosis
   d. Myocardial infarction

5. A patient is currently taking a statin. The nurse considers that the patient may have a higher risk of developing rhabdomyolysis when also taking which product?
   a. NSAIDs
   b. A fibric acid derivative
   c. Orange juice
   d. Fat-soluble vitamins

6. The nurse is administering cholestyramine resin, a bile acid sequestrant. Which nursing interventions are appropriate? (Select all that apply.)
   a. Administering the drug on an empty stomach
   b. Administering the drug with meals
   c. Instructing the patient to follow a low-fibre diet while taking this drug
   d. Instructing the patient to take a fibre supplement while taking this drug
   e. Increasing fluid intake
   f. Not administering this drug at the same time as other drugs

7. The medication order reads: nicotinic acid, 1 g PO, every evening. The medication is available in 500-mg tablets. How many tablets will the patient receive per dose?

Answers: 1. b, **2.** a, **3.** c, **4.** c, **5.** b, **6.** b, d, e, f, **7.** 2 tablets

CRITICAL THINKING ACTIVITIES

1. A patient has started taking nicotinic acid as part of treatment for high cholesterol levels. After the first dose, he tells the nurse that he feels "hot" and that his face and neck are flushed. He says that he thinks he is having an allergic reaction. What is the nurse's priority action at this time?

2. While reviewing instructions for newly prescribed antilipemic medications, a patient informs the nurse that he "hates to mix powdered medicines" and plans to take his cholestyramine resin powder dry. What is the nurse's best response to this patient's comment?

3. A patient has been taking simvastatin for 6 months. Today he received a call that he needs to come to the office for a "laboratory check." What laboratory studies would need to be done at this time?

For answers, see http://evolve.elsevier.com/Canada/Lilley/pharmacology/.

CHAPTER 29

Diuretic Drugs

Objectives

After reading this chapter, the successful student will be able to do the following:

1. Describe the normal anatomy and physiology of the kidney.
2. Briefly discuss the impact of the kidney on blood pressure regulation.
3. Describe how diuretics work in the kidney and how they lower blood pressure.
4. Distinguish among the different classes of diuretics in regard to mechanisms of action, indications, dosages, routes of administration, adverse effects, toxicities, cautions, contraindications, and drug interactions.
5. Develop a collaborative plan of care that includes all phases of the nursing process for patients receiving diuretics.

e-Learning Activities

Website
(http://evolve.elsevier.com/Canada/
Lilley/pharmacology/)

evolve

- Answer Key—Textbook Case Studies
- Answer Key—Critical Thinking Activities
- Chapter Summaries—Printable
- Review Questions for Exam Preparation
- Unfolding Case Studies

Drug Profiles

acetazolamide, p. 565
amiloride (amiloride hydrochloride)* , p. 570
» furosemide, p. 567
» hydrochlorothiazide, p. 572
» mannitol, p. 568
metolazone, p. 572
» spironolactone, p. 570
triamterene, p. 570

» Key drug

*Full generic name is given in parentheses. For the purposes of this text, the more common, shortened name is used.

Key Terms

Afferent arterioles The small blood vessels approaching the glomerulus (proximal part of the nephron). (p. 563)

Aldosterone A mineralocorticoid steroid hormone produced by the adrenal cortex that regulates sodium and potassium balance. (p. 564)

Ascites Intraperitoneal accumulation of fluid (defined as a volume of 500 mL or more) containing large amounts of protein and electrolytes. (p. 570)

Collecting duct The most distal part of the nephron between the distal convoluted tubule and the ureters, which lead to the urinary bladder. (p. 564)

Distal convoluted tubule The part of the nephron immediately distal to the ascending loop of Henle and proximal to the collecting duct. (p. 564)

Diuretics Drugs or other substances that tend to promote the formation and excretion of urine. (p. 563)

Efferent arterioles The small blood vessels exiting the glomerulus; at this point blood has completed its filtration in the glomerulus. (p. 563)

Filtrate The material that passes through a filter; in the case of the kidney, the filter is the glomerulus, and the filtrate is the material extracted from the blood (normally liquid) that becomes urine. (p. 564)

Glomerular capsule The open, rounded, and most proximal part of the proximal convoluted tubule that surrounds the glomerulus and receives the filtrate from the blood. (p. 563)

Glomerular filtration rate (GFR) An estimate of the volume of blood that passes through the glomeruli of the kidney per minute. (p. 563)

Glomerulus The cluster of kidney capillaries that marks the beginning of the nephron and is immediately proximal to the proximal convoluted tubule. (p. 563)

Loop of Henle The part of the nephron that is immediately distal to the proximal convoluted tubules. (p. 564)

Nephron The functional filtration unit of the kidney, consisting of (in anatomical order from proximal to distal) the glomerulus, proximal convoluted tubule, loop of Henle, distal convoluted tubule, and collecting duct, which empties urine into the ureters. There are approximately 1 million nephrons in each kidney. (p. 563)

Open-angle glaucoma A condition in which pressure is elevated in the eye because of obstruction of the outflow of aqueous humour. (p. 565)

Proximal convoluted (twisted) tubule The part of the nephron that is immediately distal to the glomerulus and proximal to the loop of Henle. (p. 563)

OVERVIEW

Diuretics are drugs that accelerate the rate of urine formation through a variety of mechanisms. The result is the removal of sodium and water from the body. Diuretics were discovered accidentally when it was noticed that a mercury-based antibiotic had a potent diuretic effect. All the major classes of diuretic drugs in use today were developed between 1950 and 1970, and they remain among the most commonly prescribed drugs in the world.

The Canadian Hypertension Education Program recommends diuretics, especially the thiazides, as one option for first-line drug treatment of hypertension. The hypotensive activity of diuretics is due to many different mechanisms. They cause direct arteriolar dilation, which decreases peripheral vascular resistance. They also reduce extracellular fluid volume, plasma volume, and cardiac output, which may account for the decrease in blood pressure. They have long been the mainstay of therapy for not only hypertension, but also heart failure. Two of their advantages are their relatively low cost and their favourable safety profile. The primary disadvantage with their use is the metabolic adverse effects that can result from excessive fluid and electrolyte loss. These effects are usually dose related and are therefore controllable with dosage titration (careful adjustment).

This chapter reviews the essential properties and actions of the following important classes of diuretic drugs: carbonic anhydrase inhibitors, loop diuretics, osmotic diuretics, potassium-sparing diuretics, and thiazide and thiazide-like diuretics. Each class of diuretic acts on a different site (primarily within the kidney tubules) in the kidney.

The kidney plays an important role in the day-to-day functioning or homeostasis of the body. It filters out toxic waste products from the blood while simultaneously conserving essential substances. This delicate balance between elimination of toxins and retention of essential chemicals is maintained by the **nephron**. The nephron is the main structural unit in the kidney, and each kidney contains approximately 1 million nephrons. Diuretics exert their effect in the nephron. The initial filtering of the blood takes place in the **glomerulus**, a cluster of capillaries surrounded by the **glomerular capsule**. The rate at which this filtering occurs is referred to as the **glomerular filtration rate (GFR)**, and it is used as a gauge of how well the kidneys are functioning as filters. The GFR can be estimated mathematically by calculating creatinine clearance. A GFR below 60 for 3 months or more, or a GFR above 60 with kidney damage (marked by high levels of albumin in the urine), comprises the gold standard for determining chronic kidney disease. The GFR is used to determine necessary adjustment of drugs based on the patient's kidney function.

The GFR, which can also be thought of as the rate at which blood flows into and out of the glomerulus, is regulated by the small blood vessels entering the glomerulus (**afferent arterioles**), and exiting the glomerulus (**efferent arterioles**). Normally, about 180 L of blood is filtered through the nephrons every day. (A mnemonic [memory aid] that may help one to remember which arteriole is which is "A for *approach* and *afferent*" and "E for *exit* and *efferent*.") Alterations in blood flow such as those that occur in a patient in shock can therefore have a dramatic effect on kidney function. Diuretics may have diminished effects in situations of low blood flow, because the kidney receives less blood, and therefore less diuretic reaches the site of action.

The **proximal convoluted (twisted) tubule**, or, more simply, the *proximal tubule*, follows the glomerulus anatomically and returns 60 to 70% of the sodium and water from the filtered fluid back into the bloodstream. Blood vessels surround the nephrons and allow substances to be directly reabsorbed from or secreted into the bloodstream. This process is one of active transport that requires energy in the form of adenosine triphosphate (ATP) molecules. The active transport of sodium and potassium ions back into the blood causes the passive reabsorption of chloride and water. The chloride ions

(Cl⁻) and water passively follow the sodium ions (Na⁺) and, to a lesser extent, potassium ions (K⁺) by osmosis. Another 20 to 25% of sodium is resorbed back into the bloodstream in the ascending **loop of Henle**. Chloride is actively resorbed in the loop of Henle, and sodium passively follows.

The remaining 5 to 10% of sodium resorption takes place in the **distal convoluted tubule**, often called the *distal tubule*, which anatomically follows the ascending loop of Henle. In the distal tubule, sodium is actively filtered in exchange for potassium or hydrogen ions, a process regulated by the hormone **aldosterone**. The **collecting duct** is the final common pathway for the **filtrate** that started in the glomerulus. It is here that antidiuretic hormone acts to increase the absorption of water back into the bloodstream, thereby preventing it from being lost in the urine. The entire nephron, along with the sites of action of the different classes of diuretics, is shown in Figure 29-1.

DIURETIC DRUGS

The various diuretics are classified according to their sites of action within the nephron, their chemical structure, and their diuretic potency. The sites of action of diuretics are determined by the way in which they affect the solute (electrolyte) and water transport systems located along the nephron (see Figure 29-1). The commonly used classes of drugs and individual drugs in these classes are listed in Table 29-1. The most potent diuretics are the loop diuretics, followed by mannitol (an osmostic diuretic), metolazone (a thiazide-like diuretic), the thiazides, and the potassium-sparing diuretics. The potency of these diuretics is a function of where they act in the nephron to inhibit sodium and water resorption. The more sodium and water they inhibit from resorption, the greater the diuresis and, consequently, the greater the potency.

TABLE 29-1

Classification of Diuretics

Class	Drugs
Carbonic anhydrase inhibitors	acetazolamide, methazolamide
Loop diuretics	bumetanide, ethacrynic acid, furosemide
Osmotic diuretics	mannitol
Potassium-sparing diuretics	amiloride, eplerenone, spironolactone, triamterene (available only in combination with hydrochlorothiazide)
Thiazide and thiazide-like diuretics	chlorthalidone, hydrochlorothiazide, indapamide, metolazone

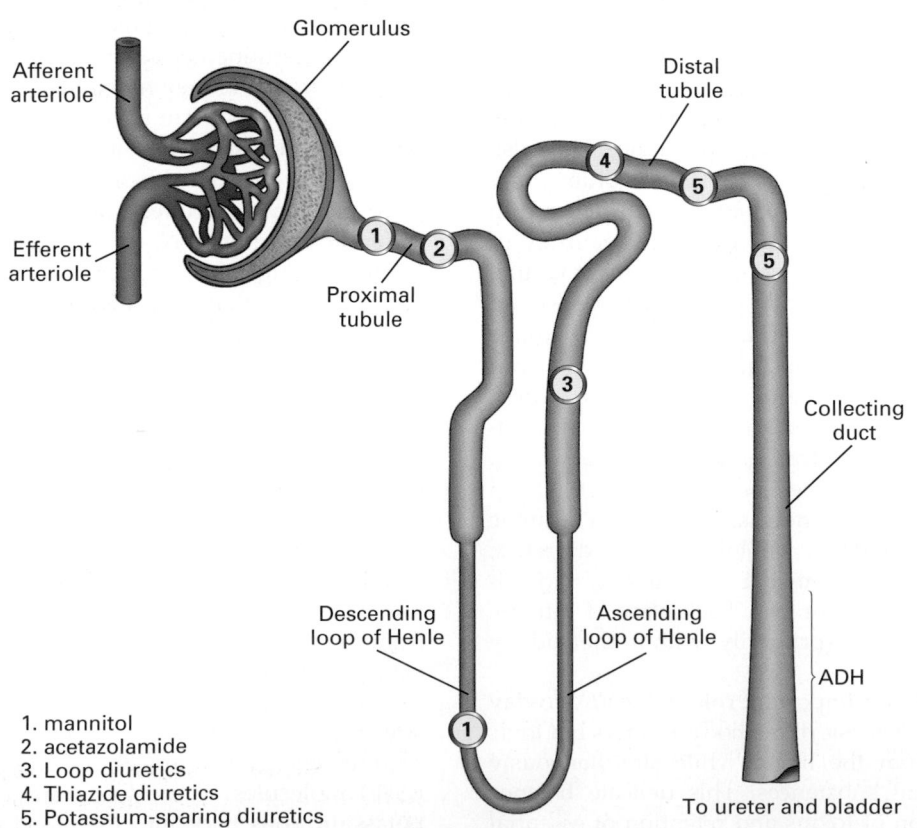

1. mannitol
2. acetazolamide
3. Loop diuretics
4. Thiazide diuretics
5. Potassium-sparing diuretics

FIG. 29-1 The nephron and diuretic sites of action. *ADH*, antidiuretic hormone.

CARBONIC ANHYDRASE INHIBITORS

Carbonic anhydrase inhibitors (CAIs) are chemical derivatives of sulfonamide antibiotics. As their name implies, CAIs inhibit the activity of the enzyme carbonic anhydrase, which is found in the kidneys, eyes, and other parts of the body. The CAIs act at the location of the carbonic anhydrase enzyme system along the nephron, primarily in the proximal tubule. Acetazolamide is the most commonly used CAI today.

Mechanism of Action and Drug Effects

The carbonic anhydrase system in the kidney is located just distal to the glomerulus in the proximal tubules, where approximately two thirds of all sodium and water are resorbed into the blood. In the proximal tubules, there is an active transport system that exchanges sodium for hydrogen ions. For sodium and water to be resorbed back into the blood, hydrogen must be exchanged for it. Without hydrogen, this cannot occur, and the sodium and water will be eliminated with the urine. Carbonic anhydrase makes hydrogen ions for this exchange. When its actions are inhibited by a CAI, such as acetazolamide, little sodium and water can be resorbed into the blood, and they are eliminated with the urine. CAIs reduce the formation of hydrogen (H^+) and bicarbonate ($HCO3^-$) ions from carbon dioxide and water through the noncompetitive, reversible inhibition of carbonic anhydrase activity. This action results in a reduction in the availability of the ions, primarily hydrogen, for use by active transport systems.

The reduction of the formation of bicarbonate and hydrogen ions can have effects on other parts of the body. CAIs can induce respiratory and metabolic acidosis. Both respiratory and metabolic acidosis can increase oxygenation during hypoxia by increasing ventilation and cerebral blood flow, and by the dissociation of oxygen from oxyhemoglobin, all of which are usually beneficial to the patient. An undesirable effect of CAIs is elevation of blood glucose levels, which causes glycosuria in patients with diabetes. This may be due in part to CAI-enhanced potassium loss through the urine.

Indications

Therapeutic applications of CAIs include the treatment of glaucoma, edema, epilepsy, and high-altitude sickness.

CAIs are used as adjunct drugs in the long-term management of acute **open-angle glaucoma** that cannot be controlled by topical miotic drugs or epinephrine derivatives alone (see Chapter 57). Glaucoma is caused by the obstruction of the outflow of aqueous humour. When CAIs are given, an increase in the outflow of the aqueous humour results. They are also used short term in conjunction with miotics to lower intraocular pressure in preparation for ocular surgery and as an adjunct in the treatment of secondary glaucoma.

Acetazolamide is also used to manage edema secondary to heart failure that has become resistant to other diuretics. However, as a class, CAIs are much less potent diuretics than loop diuretics or thiazides, and the metabolic acidosis they induce diminishes their diuretic effect in 2 to 4 days.

Acetazolamide is also effective in both the prevention and treatment of the symptoms of high-altitude sickness. These symptoms include headache, nausea, shortness of breath, dizziness, drowsiness, and fatigue.

Contraindications

Contraindications to the use of CAIs include known drug allergy, hyponatremia, hypokalemia, severe kidney or liver dysfunction, adrenal gland insufficiency, and cirrhosis.

Adverse Effects

Common undesirable effects of CAIs are metabolic abnormalities such as acidosis and hypokalemia. Drowsiness, anorexia, paresthesias, hematuria, urticaria, photosensitivity, and melena (blood in the stool) can also occur.

Interactions

Because CAIs can cause hypokalemia, an increase in digoxin toxicity may occur when they are combined with digoxin. Use with corticosteroids may also cause hypokalemia. The effects of amphetamines, carbamazepine, cyclosporine, phenytoin, and quinidine sulfate may be increased when these drugs are taken concurrently with CAIs.

Dosages

The usual dose of acetazolamide is 250 to 500 mg per day, which may be given orally or intravenously.

 DRUG PROFILE

acetazolamide

Use of acetazolamide (Acetazolam®) is contraindicated in patients who have a known hypersensitivity to it as well as in those with significant liver or kidney dysfunction, low serum potassium or sodium levels, acidosis, or adrenal gland failure. It is available in oral and parenteral forms. Potential benefits may warrant use of acetazolamide in pregnant women despite potential risks to the fetus.

PHARMACOKINETICS

Route	Onset of Action	Peak Plasma Concentration	Elimination Half-Life	Duration of Action
PO	1 hr	2–4 hr	10–15 hr	8–12 hr

LOOP DIURETICS

Loop diuretics (bumetanide, ethacrynic acid, and furosemide) are potent diuretics. Bumetanide and furosemide are chemically related to the sulfonamide antibiotics. They are therefore often listed as contraindicated in sulfa-allergic patients. However, analysis of the literature indicates that cross-reaction is unlikely to occur. Loop diuretics are commonly given to patients with sulfa allergy with no problems; however, always be aware of the possibility of allergy.

Mechanism of Action and Drug Effects

Loop diuretics have kidney, cardiovascular, and metabolic effects. These drugs act primarily along the thick ascending limb of the loop of Henle, blocking chloride and, secondarily, sodium resorption. They are also thought to activate kidney prostaglandins, which results in dilation of the blood vessels of the kidneys, the lungs, and the rest of the body (i.e., causing a reduction in kidney, pulmonary, and systemic vascular resistance). The hemodynamic effects of loop diuretics are a reduction in both the preload and central venous pressures (which are the filling pressures of the ventricles). These actions make them useful in the treatment of edema associated with heart failure, liver cirrhosis, and kidney disease.

Because of their rapid onset of action, loop diuretics are particularly useful when rapid diuresis is needed. The diuretic effect lasts at least 2 hours. Loop diuretics have a distinct advantage over thiazide diuretics in that their diuretic action continues even when the creatinine clearance decreases below 25 mL/min. This means that even when kidney function diminishes, loop diuretics can still work however, higher doses, administered by IV, may be required to achieve diuresis because of the decline in kidney function. Because of their potent diuretic effect and their duration of action, loop diuretics are usually effective when given in a single daily dose. This allows the kidney tubule time to partially compensate for the potassium depletion and other electrolyte derangements that often accompany around-the-clock diuretic therapy. Despite this, the major adverse effect of loop diuretics is electrolyte disturbance. Prolonged administration of high dosages can also result in hearing loss stemming from ototoxicity, although this is rare.

Summary of Major Drug Effects of Loop Diuretics

Loop diuretics produce a potent diuresis and subsequent loss of fluid. The resulting decreased fluid volume leads to a decreased return of blood to the heart, or decreased filling pressures. This has the following cardiovascular effects:

- Reduces blood pressure
- Reduces pulmonary vascular resistance
- Reduces systemic vascular resistance
- Reduces central venous pressure
- Reduces left ventricular end-diastolic pressure

The metabolic effects of loop diuretics are secondary to electrolyte losses resulting from potent diuresis. Major electrolyte losses include loss of sodium and potassium and, to a lesser extent, calcium. Changes in the plasma levels of insulin, glucagon, and growth hormone have been observed in association with loop diuretic therapy.

Indications

Loop diuretics are used to manage edema associated with heart failure and liver or kidney disease, to manage hypertension, and to increase the kidney excretion of calcium in patients with hypercalcemia. As with certain other classes of diuretics, they may also be indicated in cases of heart failure resulting from diastolic dysfunction.

Contraindications

Contraindications to the use of loop diuretics include known drug allergy, hepatic coma, and severe electrolyte loss. Although allergy to sulfonamide antibiotics is listed as a contraindication, analysis of the literature indicates that cross-reaction with the loop diuretics is unlikely to occur. Loop diuretics are commonly given to such patients in clinical practice.

Adverse Effects

Common undesirable effects of loop diuretics are listed in Table 29-2. Hypokalemia is of serious clinical importance. To prevent hypokalemia, patients often receive potassium supplements along with furosemide. Furosemide can produce erythema multiforme, exfoliative dermatitis, photosensitivity, and, in rare cases, aplastic anemia.

Toxicity and Management of Overdose

Electrolyte loss and dehydration, which can result in circulatory failure, are the main toxic effects of loop diuretics that require attention. Treatment involves electrolyte and fluid replacement.

Interactions

Loop diuretics exhibit both neurotoxic and nephrotoxic properties, and they produce additive effects when given in combination with drugs that have similar toxicities. Related drug interactions are summarized in Table 29-3.

TABLE 29-2

Loop Diuretics: Common Adverse Effects

Body System	Adverse Effects
Central nervous	Dizziness, headache, tinnitus, blurred vision
Gastrointestinal	Nausea, vomiting, diarrhea
Hematological	Agranulocytosis, thrombocytopenia, neutropenia
Metabolic	Hypokalemia, hyperglycemia, hyperuricemia, hyponatremia, hypochloremia, hypocalcemia, hypomagnesemia, metabolic alkalosis in severe cases

TABLE 29-3

Loop Diuretics: Common Drug Interactions

Interacting Drug	Mechanism	Results
Aminoglycosides, vancomycin	} Additive effect	Increased neurotoxicity, especially ototoxicity
Corticosteroids, digoxin	} Hypokalemia	Additive hypokalemia, increased digoxin toxicity
lithium carbonate	Decrease in kidney excretion	Increased lithium toxicity
NSAIDs	Inhibition of kidney prostaglandins	Decreased diuretic activity

NSAIDs, nonsteroidal anti-inflammatory drugs.

 ## DRUG PROFILE

The currently available loop diuretics are bumetanide, ethacrynic acid, and furosemide. Ethacrynic acid is rarely used clinically. As a class, they are potent diuretics, but the potency of each drug within this class varies. The equipotent doses for these drugs are as follows:

PHARMACOKINETICS

bumetanide	ethacrynic acid	furosemide
1 mg	50 mg	40 mg

▶▶*furosemide*

Furosemide (Lasix®) is by far the most commonly used loop diuretic in clinical practice and the prototypical drug in this class. The trade name Lasix was derived from the fact that the duration of action is 6 hours. It has all the therapeutic and adverse characteristics of the loop diuretics mentioned earlier. It is used in the management of pulmonary edema and the edema associated with heart failure, liver disease, nephrotic syndrome, and ascites. It has also been used in the treatment of hypertension, usually that caused by heart failure.

Furosemide use is contraindicated in patients who have shown a hypersensitivity to it or to the sulfonamides (see previous discussion in regard to sulfonamide allergy) and in patients with anuria, hypovolemia, and electrolyte depletion. It is available in oral form—as a solution and as tablets—and in parenteral form. Potential benefits may warrant use of the drug in pregnant women despite potential risks to the fetus.

PHARMACOKINETICS

Route	Onset of Action	Peak Plasma Concentration	Elimination Half-Life	Duration of Action
IV	5 min	15 min	1–2 hr	2 hr
PO	30–60 min	1–2 hr	1–2 hr	6–8 hr

Loop diuretics also affect certain laboratory results. They cause increases in serum levels of uric acid, glucose, alanine aminotransferase, and aspartate aminotransferase. Their combined use with a thiazide (particularly metolazone) results in the blockade of sodium and water resorption at multiple sites in the nephron, a property referred to as *sequential nephron blockade*, which increases their effects. Nonsteroidal anti-inflammatory drugs (NSAIDs) may diminish the reduction of vascular resistance induced by loop diuretics because these two drug classes have opposite effects on prostaglandin activity.

Dosages

For dosage information on loop diuretics, refer to the table on p. 568.

OSMOTIC DIURETICS

The osmotic diuretics include mannitol, urea, organic acids, and glucose. Mannitol, a nonabsorbable solute, is the most commonly used.

Mechanism of Action and Drug Effects

Mannitol works along the entire nephron. Its major site of action, however, is the proximal tubule and descending limb of the loop of Henle. Because it is nonabsorbable, it increases osmotic pressure in the glomerular filtrate, which in turn pulls fluid, primarily water, into the renal tubules from the surrounding tissues. This process also inhibits the tubular reabsorption of water and solutes, which produces a rapid diuresis. Ultimately, this action reduces cellular edema and increases urine production, causing diuresis; however, it produces only a slight loss of electrolytes, especially sodium. Therefore, mannitol is not indicated for patients with peripheral edema because it does not promote sufficient sodium excretion.

Mannitol may induce vasodilation and, when it does so, it increases both glomerular filtration and kidney plasma flow. This makes it an excellent drug for preventing kidney damage during acute kidney injury. It is also often used to reduce intracranial pressure and cerebral edema resulting from head trauma. In addition, mannitol treatment may be tried when elevated intraocular pressure is unresponsive to other drug therapies.

Indications

Mannitol is the osmotic diuretic of choice. It is commonly used in the treatment of patients in the early, oliguric phase of acute kidney injury. For it to be effective in this situation, however, enough blood flow to the kidney and glomerular filtration must still remain to enable the drug to reach the kidney tubules. Increased kidney blood flow resulting from the dilation of blood vessels supplying blood to the kidneys is another therapeutic benefit of mannitol therapy in such patients. It can also be used to promote the excretion of toxic substances, reduce intracranial pressure, and treat cerebral edema. In addition, it can be used as a genitourinary irrigant in the preparation of patients for transurethral surgical procedures and as supportive treatment in patients with edema induced by other conditions.

Contraindications

Contraindications to the use of mannitol include known drug allergy, severe kidney disease, pulmonary edema (in which case loop diuretics are used instead), and active intracranial bleeding.

Adverse Effects

Significant undesirable effects of mannitol include convulsions, thrombophlebitis, and pulmonary congestion. Other less significant effects are headaches, chest pain, tachycardia, blurred vision, chills, and fever.

Interactions

There are no drugs that interact significantly with mannitol.

Dosages

For the recommended dosages of mannitol, refer to the table below.

POTASSIUM-SPARING DIURETICS

The currently available potassium-sparing diuretics are amiloride, eplerenone, spironolactone, and triamterene. (In Canada, triamterene is available only in combination with hydrochlorothiazide.) These diuretics are also

DRUG PROFILES

▸▸ mannitol

Mannitol (Osmitrol®) is the prototypical osmotic diuretic. Its use is contraindicated in patients with hypersensitivity to it as well as in those with anuria, severe dehydration, pulmonary congestion, or cerebral hemorrhage. Treatment should be terminated if severe heart or kidney impairment develops after the initiation of therapy. It is available only in parenteral form as 5%, 10%, 20%, and 25% solutions for intravenous (IV) injection. The volume infused differs based on the concentration of mannitol provided. Calculations may need to be performed to determine the volume to be used. Mannitol may crystallize when exposed to low temperatures. This is more likely to occur when concentrations exceed 15%. For this reason, mannitol should always be administered intravenously through a filter, and vials of the drug are often stored in a warmer. The use of mannitol may have adverse effects on a fetus, but potential benefits may warrant use of the drug in pregnant women despite potential risks.

PHARMACOKINETICS

Route	Onset of Action	Peak Plasma Concentration	Elimination Half-Life	Duration of Action
IV	0.5–1 hr	0.25–2 hr	1.5 hr	6–8 hr

DOSAGES   Selected Loop Diuretics and Osmotic Diuretics

Drug	Pharmacological Class	Usual Dosage Range	Indications
▸▸ furosemide (Lasix)	Loop diuretic	*Children* IM/IV: 0.5–1 mg/kg; max 1 mg/kg/day PO: 0.5–1 mg/kg q4h; max 2 mg/kg/day divided *Adults* IM/IV: 20–40 mg/dose; max 100 mg/day: administer high-dose IV therapy as a controlled infusion at a rate not exceeding 4 mg/min or less (always refer to agency policy prior to administration) PO: 20–80 mg/day as a single dose; max 200 mg/day	Heart failure, hypertension, kidney failure, pulmonary edema, cirrhosis
▸▸ mannitol (Osmitrol)	Osmotic diuretic	*Adults* IV infusion: 50–200 g/day 1.5–2 g/kg over 30–60 min 50–200 g IV given at a rate to induce urine output of 100–500 mL/hr	Kidney failure; high intraocular and intracranial pressure; drug intoxication (to induce diuresis)

IM, intramuscular; *IV*, intravenous; *PO*, oral.

referred to as *aldosterone-inhibiting diuretics* because they block aldosterone receptors. Spironolactone is a competitive antagonist of aldosterone, and for this reason it causes sodium and water to be excreted and potassium retained. It is the most commonly used of the three drugs.

Mechanism of Action and Drug Effects

Potassium-sparing diuretics act in the collecting ducts and distal convoluted tubules, where they interfere with sodium–potassium exchange. Spironolactone competitively binds to aldosterone receptors and therefore blocks the resorption of sodium and water that is induced by aldosterone secretion. These receptors are found primarily in the distal tubule. Amiloride and triamterene do not bind to aldosterone receptors; however, they inhibit both aldosterone-induced and basal sodium reabsorption, working in the distal tubule as well as the collecting ducts. They are often prescribed for children with heart failure because pediatric heart problems are frequently accompanied by an excess secretion of aldosterone, and the loop and thiazide diuretics are often ineffective in their management (see also Special Populations: Children, on use of diuretics in children).

The potassium-sparing diuretics are relatively weak compared with the thiazide and loop diuretics. When diuresis is needed, they are generally used as adjuncts to thiazide treatment. This combination is beneficial in two respects. First, the drugs have synergistic diuretic effects; second, the two drugs counteract each other's adverse metabolic effects. Thiazide diuretics cause potassium, magnesium, and chloride to be lost in the urine, and the potassium-sparing diuretics counteract this effect by elevating potassium and chloride levels.

Indications

Therapeutic applications of potassium-sparing diuretics vary depending on the particular drug. Spironolactone and triamterene are used to treat hyperaldosteronism and hypertension and to reverse the potassium loss caused by the potassium-wasting (i.e., loop and thiazide) diuretics. One common feature of heart failure is a hyperactive renin–angiotensin–aldosterone system. Research has identified this hyperactivity as a causative factor in permanent ventricular myocardial wall damage, known as *remodelling*, following myocardial infarction. Clinical drug trials have demonstrated a cardioprotective benefit of spironolactone in preventing this remodelling process, due to its aldosterone-inhibiting activity. The uses for amiloride are similar to those for spironolactone and triamterene, but amiloride is less effective in the long term. It may be more effective than spironolactone or triamterene in the treatment of metabolic alkalosis. It is used primarily in the management of heart failure. As with certain other classes of diuretics, potassium-sparing diuretics may also be indicated in cases of heart failure due to diastolic dysfunction.

Contraindications

Contraindications to the use of potassium-sparing diuretics include known drug allergy, hyperkalemia (i.e., serum potassium level greater than 5.5 mmol/L), and severe kidney failure or anuria. Triamterene may also be contraindicated in cases of severe liver failure.

Adverse Effects

Potassium-sparing diuretics have several common undesirable effects, which are listed in Table 29-4. There are also some significant adverse effects specific to individual drugs. Spironolactone can cause gynecomastia,

SPECIAL POPULATIONS: CHILDREN

Diuretics

- Calculate pediatric dosages of diuretic medications carefully, regardless of whether the patient is in the hospital or in the home setting. Weight should be measured and recorded daily at the same time every day so that both therapeutic effects and adverse effects of diuretics can be assessed. Because children are at greater risk for adverse effects and toxicity, they require closer and more cautious daily assessment in order to avoid consequences such as excess fluid volume, electrolyte loss, hypotension, and shock.
- The half-life of furosemide is increased in neonates, so the interval between doses may need to be lengthened, as ordered by the health care provider.
- Oral forms of diuretics may be taken with food or milk and are to be taken early in the day and at the same time every day.

- Children taking diuretics should avoid lengthy exposure to either heat or sun because it may precipitate heat stroke, exhaustion, and fluid volume loss.
- Thiazide diuretics cross the placenta and pass through to the fetus. Small amounts are distributed in breast milk; thus, breastfeeding is not advised for mothers who are taking these drugs.
- Laboratory test results that may be altered by diuretics include serum levels of calcium, glucose, and uric acid, which may be increased.
- Loop diuretics may also interfere with urea nitrogen, chloride, magnesium, potassium, and sodium levels; therefore, perform frequent monitoring.

amenorrhea, irregular menses, and postmenopausal bleeding. Triamterene may reduce folic acid levels and cause the formation of kidney stones and urinary casts. It may also precipitate megaloblastic anemia. However, adverse effects from triamterene are rare. Hyperkalemia may occur when potassium-sparing diuretics are used in combination with each other or with other potassium-sparing drugs such as angiotensin-converting enzyme (ACE) inhibitors (see Chapter 23, as well as the Interactions section that follows).

Interactions

Concurrent use of potassium-sparing diuretics and lithium, ACE inhibitors, or potassium supplements can

result in significant drug interactions. The administration of ACE inhibitors or potassium supplements in combination with potassium-sparing diuretics can result in hyperkalemia, which can result in fatal cardiac dysrhythmias if not identified and treated promptly. When lithium and potassium-sparing diuretics are given together, lithium toxicity can result. NSAIDs can inhibit kidney prostaglandins, which decreases blood flow to the kidneys and therefore decreases the delivery of diuretic drugs to this site of action. This action, in turn, can lead to a diminished diuretic response.

Dosages

For the recommended dosages of potassium-sparing diuretics, refer to the table below.

THIAZIDES AND THIAZIDE-LIKE DIURETICS

Thiazide and thiazide-like diuretics are generally considered equivalent in their effects. Thiazide diuretics, like several of the loop diuretics, are benzothiadiazines, chemical derivatives of sulfonamide antibiotics. Thiazide diuretics include hydrochlorothiazide and trichlormethiazide; hydrochlorothiazide is the most commonly

---

TABLE	29-4

Potassium-Sparing Diuretics: Common Adverse Effects

Body System	Adverse Effects
Central nervous	Dizziness, headache
Gastrointestinal	Cramps, nausea, vomiting, diarrhea
Other	Urinary frequency, weakness, hyperkalemia

 DRUG PROFILES

amiloride hydrochloride

Amiloride hydrochloride (Midamor®) is generally used in combination with a thiazide or loop diuretic in the treatment of heart failure. Hyperkalemia may occur in approximately 10% of the patients who take amiloride alone. It should be used with caution in older adults and in patients with kidney impairment or diabetes mellitus. It has weak antihypertensive properties. Amiloride is available only in oral form. It is also available in combination with hydrochlorothiazide (Novamilor®).

PHARMACOKINETICS

Route	Onset of Action	Peak Plasma Concentration	Elimination Half-Life	Duration of Action
PO	2 hr	6–10 hr	6–9 hr	24 hr

▸▸*spironolactone*

Spironolactone (Aldactone®) is a synthetic steroid that blocks aldosterone receptors. It is used in high dosages for the treatment of ascites, a condition commonly associated with cirrhosis of the liver. Monitor serum potassium levels frequently in patients taking spironolactone who have impaired kidney function or who are currently taking potassium supplements because hyperkalemia is a common complication of spironolactone therapy. It is the potassium-sparing diuretic most commonly prescribed for children who have heart failure. Recently, spironolactone has been shown to reduce morbidity and mortality rates in patients with severe heart failure when added to standard therapy.

Of the three commonly used potassium-sparing diuretics, spironolactone has the greatest antihypertensive activity. It is available only in oral form. It is also available in combination with hydrochlorothiazide (Aldactazide®). There is positive evidence of human fetal risk with the use of spironolactone but potential benefits may warrant use of the drug in pregnant women despite potential risks.

PHARMACOKINETICS

Route	Onset of Action	Peak Plasma Concentration	Elimination Half-Life	Duration of Action
PO	1–3 days	2–3 days	13–24 hr	2–3 days

triamterene

The pharmacological properties of triamterene are similar to those of amiloride. Like amiloride, triamterene acts directly on the distal renal tubule of the nephron to depress the resorption of sodium and the excretion of potassium and hydrogen. It has little or no antihypertensive effect. It is available only in combination with hydrochlorothiazide. There is positive evidence of human fetal risk with the use of spironolactone but potential benefits may warrant use of the drug in pregnant women despite potential risks.

PHARMACOKINETICS

Route	Onset of Action	Peak Plasma Concentration	Elimination Half-Life	Duration of Action
PO	2–3 hr	6–8 hr	2–3 hr	12–16 hr

DOSAGES   Selected Potassium-Sparing Diuretic Drugs

Drug	Usual Dosage Range	Indications
amiloride hydrochloride (Midamor)	*Adults* PO: 5–20 mg/day	Edema, heart failure (as an adjunct to loop diuretics)
eplerenone (Inspar)	*Adults* PO: 25–50 mg/day	Heart failure, hypertension
➤➤spironolactone (Aldactone)	*Children* PO: 3 mg/kg/day single or divided; 1–2 mg/kg maintenance *Adults* PO: 25–200 mg/day	Edema, hypertension, heart failure, ascites
triamterene 50 mg/ hydrochlorothiazide 25 mg	*Adults* PO: 1–4 tablets daily after meals	Edema, hypertension, heart failure, ascites

PO, oral.

prescribed and the least expensive. Hydrochlorothiazide is included in numerous combination products with antihypertensive drugs. The thiazide-like diuretics are similar in action to the thiazides and include chlorthalidone, indapamide, and metolazone. Metolazone may be more effective than other drugs in this class in the treatment of patients with kidney dysfunction.

Mechanism of Action and Drug Effects

The primary site of action of thiazide and thiazide-like diuretics is the distal convoluted tubule, where they inhibit the resorption of sodium, potassium, and chloride. This action results in osmotic water loss. Thiazides also cause direct relaxation of the arterioles, which reduces peripheral vascular resistance, or afterload. Decreased preload and afterload are their beneficial hemodynamic effects; these make them effective for the treatment of both heart failure and hypertension.

As kidney function decreases, the efficacy of thiazides diminishes because delivery of the drug to the site of activity is impaired. Thiazides are not to be used if creatinine clearance is less than 30 to 50 mL/min. Normal creatinine clearance is 125 mL/min, depending on the age of the patient. However, metolazone remains effective to a creatinine clearance of 10 mL/min and is used for edema accompanying kidney failure, including nephrotic syndrome, and states of diminished kidney function. It is also used for the treatment of edema associated with heart failure. The major adverse effects of these drugs stem from the electrolyte disturbances they produce. They are noted for precipitating hypokalemia and hypercalcemia, as well as metabolic disturbances such as dyslipidemia, hyperglycemia, and hyperuricemia.

Indications

The thiazide and thiazide-like diuretics are used in the treatment of edema of various origins, idiopathic hypercalciuria, and diabetes insipidus, in addition to hypertension. Any of these drugs can be used either as monotherapy or in combination with other drugs. As with certain other classes of diuretics, they may be indicated in cases of heart failure due to diastolic dysfunction.

Contraindications

Contraindications to the use of thiazides and thiazide-like diuretics include known drug allergy, hepatic coma (for metolazone), anuria, and severe kidney failure.

Adverse Effects

Major adverse effects of thiazide and thiazide-like diuretics relate to the electrolyte and metabolic disturbances they cause, primarily reduced potassium levels and elevated levels of calcium, lipids, glucose, and uric acid. Other effects, such as gastrointestinal disturbances, skin rashes, photosensitivity, thrombocytopenia, pancreatitis, and cholecystitis are less common. Dizziness and vertigo are common adverse effects of metolazone therapy and are attributed to sudden shifts in the plasma volume brought about by the drug. Headache, erectile dysfunction, and reduced libido are other adverse effects of these drugs that are important to know. Thiazide diuretics are associated with a higher risk of falls in older adults, with the highest risk in the first 3 weeks after a prescription is given (Gribben et al., 2010). Many of these adverse effects are dose related and are seen at higher doses, especially those above 25 mg. For example, the metabolic adverse effect of hyperglycemia is dose dependent. Thiazide doses (e.g., hydrochlorothiazide) should be kept less than or equal to 25 mg daily as doses 50 mg or greater produce metabolic adverse effects. The more common adverse effects of thiazide and thiazide-like diuretics are listed in Table 29-5.

Toxicity and Management of Overdose

An overdose of these drugs can lead to an electrolyte imbalance resulting from hypokalemia. Symptoms include anorexia, nausea, lethargy, muscle weakness, mental confusion, and hypotension. Treatment involves electrolyte replacement.

Interactions

Thiazides and related drugs interact with corticosteroids, diazoxide, digoxin, and oral hypoglycemics. The mechanisms and results of these interactions are summarized in Table 29-6. Excessive consumption of licorice can lead to an additive hypokalemia in patients taking thiazides.

Dosages

For recommended dosages for thiazide and thiazide-like diuretics, refer to the table on p. 573.

TABLE 29-5

Thiazide and Thiazide-Like Diuretics: Potential Adverse Effects

Body System/ Process	Adverse Effects
Central nervous	Dizziness, headache, blurred vision
Gastrointestinal	Anorexia, nausea, vomiting, diarrhea
Genitourinary	Erectile dysfunction
Hematological	Jaundice, leukopenia, agranulocytosis
Integumentary	Urticaria, photosensitivity
Metabolic	Hypokalemia, glycosuria, hyperglycemia, hyperuricemia, hypochloremic alkalosis

---

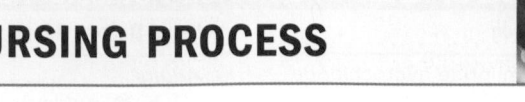

NURSING PROCESS

Assessment

Before giving a patient any type of diuretic, obtain a complete patient history and thorough medication history. Perform a physical assessment and document all findings, with emphasis on the body systems affected by the disease process or the indication for the diuretic, as well as on potential drug-related adverse effects. This would include assessing baseline breath sounds, heart sounds, and neurological status, as well as checking skin turgor and for pitting edema; moisture levels of mucous membranes and capillary refill are also important to assess with diuretic therapy. Because fluid volume levels and electrolyte concentrations are affected by diuretics, assess and document the patient's baseline fluid volume status (as indicated by vital signs, weight, and intake–output measurements). Assess postural blood pressures (e.g., lying, sitting, standing) before and during drug

---

TABLE 29-6

Thiazide and Thiazide-Like Diuretics: Common Drug Interactions

Drug	Mechanism	Result
Oral antihyperglycemic drugs	Antagonism	Reduced therapeutic hypoglycemic effect
Corticosteroids	Additive effect	Hypokalemia
digoxin	Hypokalemia	Increased digoxin toxicity
lithium	Decreased clearance	Increased lithium toxicity
NSAIDs	Inhibition of kidney prostaglandins	Decreased diuretic activity

---

 DRUG PROFILES

►►hydrochlorothiazide

Hydrochlorothiazide, (Urozide®) is a safe and effective diuretic. Hydrochlorothiazide is used in combination with many other drugs, including amiloride, angiotensin II receptor antagonists, the direct renin inhibitor aliskerin fumarate, spironolactone, ACE inhibitors, and β-blockers. Dosages exceeding 50 mg/day rarely produce additional clinical results and may only increase drug toxicity. This property is known as the *ceiling effect*. However, doses up to 100 mg/day are not uncommon. Hydrochlorothiazide is available only in oral form. Use in pregnancy poses no risk to the fetus.

metolazone

Metolazone (Zaroxolyn®) is a thiazide-like diuretic that appears to be more potent than the thiazide diuretics. This greater potency becomes important in patients with kidney dysfunction. It remains effective to a creatinine clearance as low as 10 mL/min. It may also be given in combination with loop diuretics to obtain a potent diuresis in patients with severe symptoms of heart failure. Its peak effect occurs much later than the effect of intravenous furosemide. Metolazone is available only in oral form. The administration of metolazone during pregnancy requires that the potential benefits of the drug be weighed against its possible hazards to the fetus.

PHARMACOKINETICS (HYDROCHLOROTHIAZIDE)

Route	Onset of Action	Peak Plasma Concentration	Elimination Half-Life	Duration of Action
PO	2 hr	4–6 hr	5–15 hr	6–12 hr

PHARMACOKINETICS

Route	Onset of Action	Peak Plasma Concentration	Elimination Half-Life	Duration of Action
PO	1 hr	1–2 hr	6–20 hr	24 hr

DOSAGES   Thiazide and Selected Thiazide-Like Diuretic Drugs

Drug	Pharmacological Class	Usual Dosage Range	Indications
▸▸hydrochlorothiazide (Urozide)	Thiazide diuretic	*Neonates and infants under 6 mo* PO: 1.5 mg/kg/day divided bid *Infants over 6 mo and children under 2 yr* PO: 12.5 mg/day divided bid *Children 2–12 yr* PO: 37.5–100 mg/day divided bid *Adults* PO: 25–200 mg/day, usually divided	Edema, heart failure as an adjunct to loop diuretics)
metolazone (Zaroxolyn)	Thiazide-like diuretic	*Adults* PO: 5–20 mg/day	

PO, oral.

therapy because of diuretic-induced fluid volume loss, which may lead to orthostatic hypotension (a drop in blood pressure of 20 mm Hg or more upon standing).

In addition, assess specific laboratory values associated with renal and hepatic functioning; for example, BUN level (normal range, 8 to 16.4 mmoL/L) and creatinine level (normal range, 50 to 100 micromoL/L) for kidney function, and ALP (normal range, 13 to 39 units/L), AST (normal range, 8 to 46 units/L in males; 7 to 34 units/L in females), and LDH (normal range, 45 to 90 units/L) for liver function. It is important to note, however, that normal ranges of these laboratory values may vary somewhat from facility to facility. Serum electrolyte levels are also crucial to assess before and during diuretic therapy because of the subsequent loss of electrolytes through the urine and their relationship to fluid volume status. Specifically, obtain and document serum potassium, sodium, chloride, magnesium, calcium, uric acid, and creatinine levels, as ordered. Arterial blood gas levels may also be ordered.

The use of CAIs requires close assessment of sodium and potassium levels. These drugs are not to be used in patients with a history of kidney or liver dysfunction. As with any diuretic that results in loss of potassium (excluding potassium-sparing diuretics), if these drugs are given concurrently with digoxin, there is increased risk for digoxin toxicity (because of hypokalemia).

Loop diuretics are more potent than thiazide diuretics, combination products, and potassium-sparing diuretics. These drugs may pose more problems for older adult patients or those with severe electrolyte loss and liver failure. An additional and significant concern for patients taking loop diuretics is their interaction with other medications that are neurotoxic or ototoxic (see Table 29-3). Cross-sensitivity has been documented in patients who are allergic to sulfonamide antibiotics. Loop diuretics may also cause severe skin reactions (e.g., exfoliative dermatitis with furosemide), so a thorough assessment of the patient's skin prior to administration is important. Additionally, with loop diuretics, potential drug–laboratory value interactions include increased serum uric acid and glucose levels. Cases of tinnitus and

reversible deafness have been reported with the use of IV furosemide.

With potassium-sparing diuretics, hyperkalemia may be an adverse effect; therefore, assess the patient's serum levels of potassium. Additionally, because of the potassium-sparing effect, contraindications include drugs or conditions that may result in hyperkalemia. Thus, potassium supplements, ACE inhibitors, and severe kidney failure are contraindications. Lithium toxicity may occur if given with these diuretics because of resultant hyperkalemia. See the previous discussion of additional cautions, contraindications, and drug interactions associated with diuretic use.

▨ Nursing Diagnoses

- Decreased cardiac output related to drug effects and adverse effects of diuretics (e.g., fluid and electrolyte loss)
- Deficient fluid volume related to drug effects and adverse effects of diuretics
- Risk for injury related to orthostatic hypotension and dizziness

▨ Planning

▰ Goals

- Patient will regain and maintain balanced cardiac output.
- Patient will regain and maintain balanced fluid volume status.
- Patient will remain free from injury.

▰ Expected Patient Outcomes

- Patient continues to show normal cardiac output while receiving diuretic therapy, as evidenced by vital signs, adequate intake, and output within normal limits (pulse between 60 and 100 beats per minute; blood pressure 120/80 mm Hg or within normal parameters for the patient; urine output 30 mL/h or higher).

CASE STUDY

Hydrochlorothiazide Therapy

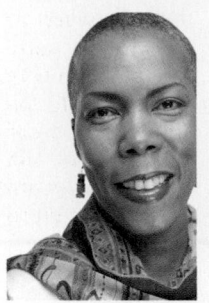

Glenda, a 62-year-old university professor, has been diagnosed with primary hypertension and will be taking 50 mg of hydrochlorothiazide (Urozide) daily. There is no evidence of renal insufficiency or cardiac damage at this time, nor is there evidence of retinopathy or other signs or symptoms of end-organ disease. She is anxious because the fall semester is starting and she has a heavy teaching load, but she is willing to take the steps needed for better health.

At her 1-month follow-up appointment, Glenda reports "feeling so tired" and asks whether the medication causes sleepiness. When questioned, she says that she takes the hydrochlorothiazide at dinnertime because she is afraid it will "interfere with her classes."

1. What do you suspect is happening with Glenda, and what would you recommend?

2. During this follow-up appointment, you ask Glenda if she is eating foods high in potassium. She looks embarrassed and answers, "I lost that pamphlet about the foods with potassium, but I try to drink orange juice every day." What foods should she eat for their potassium content?

3. The report on Glenda's potassium levels comes back from the laboratory, and the results are 3.4 mmoL/L. She asks, "Am I going to be put on a potassium pill, too?" What is your answer?

4. Six months later, Glenda is diagnosed with type 2 diabetes mellitus and is started on oral antihyperglycemic therapy. What will you teach her about managing her diabetes while taking the hydrochlorothiazide?

For answers see http://evolve.elsevier.com/Canada/Lilley/pharmacology/.

- Patient has strong pedal pulses and warm, pink extremities with rapid capillary refill.
- Patient regains balanced fluid volume status without dehydration or overhydration.
  - Patient's skin is pliable and with firm turgor.
  - Patient's laboratory values return within normal limits for urine specific gravity, serum sodium, chloride, and potassium.
- Patient takes diuretic therapy as directed and with adequate fluid intake, avoiding hypotensive episodes.
  - Patient changes positions slowly and with purpose while on diuretic therapy.
  - Patient reports any excessive dizziness, lightheadedness, palpitations, tingling of fingers and toes, confusion, disorientation, or fainting episodes.

Implementation

Measure and record blood pressure, pulse rate, intake and output, and daily weights during diuretic therapy. Changes from the initial assessment data that alert the nurse to potential problems with the drug therapy include the presence of dizziness, fainting, or lightheadedness on standing or changing positions; weakness; fatigue; tremor; muscle cramping; changes in mental health status; or cold clammy skin. Diuretic therapy may also precipitate heart irregularities or palpitations; therefore, continue to monitor heart rate and rhythm. Fluid loss from the action of the diuretic may lead to the adverse effect of constipation, so preventative measures are needed, such as increased intake of fluids and fibre (unless contraindicated). If constipation continues, the health care provider may need to provide alternatives such as psyllium-based, bulk-forming laxatives. Always give diuretics exactly as directed but with consideration of the patient's age and related needs. Appropriate dosing and timing of the drugs are often important to enhance therapeutic effects and minimize adverse effects. Because diuretics taken late in the afternoon or evening may lead to nocturia and subsequent loss of sleep, these medications are usually scheduled for morning dosing. Safety concerns exist with nocturia, especially with older adults, because possible confusion and dizziness associated with getting up in the middle of the night may create the potential for falls and injury (see also Special Populations: Older Adults: Diuretic Therapy).

Loop diuretics (if taken at high doses as ordered) may increase the risk for fluid volume and electrolyte depletion (e.g., hypokalemia, hyponatremia, dehydration). Monitoring of therapy includes frequent assessment of blood pressure and pulse rate—including orthostatic blood pressures and pulse rates (supine and standing)—hydration status, and capillary refill, as well as daily measurement of weight. Acute hypotensive episodes may occur with higher doses of loop diuretics and precipitate syncope and falls. Therefore, educate patients about safety measures to put in place to help prevent falls. Hypokalemia is the most commonly encountered electrolyte imbalance and may be very dangerous. Symptoms include anorexia, nausea, lethargy, muscle weakness, mental confusion, and hypotension. If IV dosage forms are given, it is crucial to check for diluents, drug incompatibilities, and intactness of the IV site. Double-check rates of infusion and use an infusion pump. With

SPECIAL POPULATIONS: OLDER ADULTS

Diuretic Therapy

- Before and during diuretic drug therapy, measure the patient's height, weight, intake and output, blood pressure, pulse rate, respiratory rate, and temperature. Assess breath and heart sounds and edematous areas. Monitor serum sodium, potassium, and chloride levels.
- Emphasize to older adult patients that diuretics need to be taken at the same time every day. These drugs are generally ordered to be taken in the morning to help prevent nocturia, which can result in lack of sleep. More importantly, nocturia can lead to injury if the individual needs to get out of bed to void and subsequently becomes dizzy or confused and falls. A bedside commode may be used to decrease the risk of injury.
- If an older adult patient is living alone and has minimal or no assistance with the medication regimen, visits from a home health provider or other health care provider may help ensure safety, efficacy, and adherence, not only in taking the medication but also in following all aspects of the therapeutic regimen.
- Exercise caution in administering diuretics to older adults because they are more sensitive to the therapeutic effects of these drugs (often reacting to smaller dosages of medication than are required by other patients) and may experience adverse effects such as dehydration, electrolyte loss, dizziness, and syncope.
- Encourage patients to change positions slowly because of the risk of orthostatic hypotension and subsequent falls and injury. Emphasize the importance of recording daily weights, blood pressures, and overall well-being.
- Advise patients that carrying a card or electronic device containing a brief medical history, blood pressure readings, names and telephone numbers for contact persons, and a list of medications is important to ensure safety and minimize complications. Many older adults are adept at using electronic devices, and information can be easily stored on a smartphone, tablet, or computer and changed as necessary. If a patient is not comfortable using a device, a physical card can be formatted to fit in a wallet, with a copy placed on the refrigerator door or in another visible location so that it will be easily available to emergency personnel should they need to visit the home. Such a card can be easily made using standard card stock or an index card.

Information can be entered using an erasable pen or pencil. Copies of the card should be given to caregivers, family members, significant others, health care providers, or dentists. The card then needs to be updated at regular intervals by the patient or another individual or health care provider involved in the patient's care. The following sample shows the headings and content for such a card (or the information to be made available on an electronic device):

1. Name: _____
2. Age: _____
3. Allergies (drug/food): _____ _____
4. Medical history (place an X to the left of all that apply; write in any not listed):

_Anemia	_Depression	_Nerve problems
_Asthma	_Diabetes	_Pacemaker or defibrillator device
_Bleeding problems	_Difficulty swallowing	_Recent weight gain
_Blood clots	_Heart problems	_Recent weight loss
_Breathing problems	_High blood pressure	_Stroke
_Cancer	_Low blood pressure	_Thyroid problems

   Others: _____
   _____
5. Surgeries (list all with date, type of surgery, purpose, any complications): _____
6. Prosthetics used: _____
7. Dentures/dental problems: _____
8. Assistive devices: Glasses _____ Hearing aids _____ Mobility assistance _____
9. Contact names and telephone numbers: _____
   _____
10. Current medications (prescription drugs; over-the-counter drugs; natural health products; others):
   Name of medication(s) _____
   Dosage(s) _____
   Frequency of doses _____
   Reasons for use of medications _____

potassium-sparing diuretics, potassium is reabsorbed and not excreted (as previously discussed), so hyperkalemia, rather than hypokalemia, may become problematic. Signs and symptoms of hyperkalemia include nausea, vomiting, diarrhea, and abdominal cramping (Chapter 30) and should be reported immediately. See Patient Education for more information.

▨ Evaluation

The therapeutic effects of diuretics include the resolution of or reduction in edema, fluid volume overload, heart failure, or hypertension (or the restoration of normal intraocular pressures, if used for such a purpose, as with the CAIs). Monitor patients for the occurrence of adverse reactions to diuretics, such as hypotension (from volume loss), electrolyte imbalances, metabolic alkalosis (arterial blood gas values may need to be measured), drowsiness (with CAIs), hypokalemia, tachycardia (less significant with mannitol), and hyperkalemia (with potassium-sparing diuretics). Review all goals and outcome criteria in the evaluation process.

PATIENT TEACHING TIPS

❖ Patients taking diuretics need to maintain proper nutritional intake and fluid volume and eat potassium-rich foods, except when contraindicated or when potassium-sparing diuretics are used. Foods high in potassium include bananas, oranges, apricots, dates, raisins, broccoli, green beans, potatoes, tomatoes, meats, fish, wheat bread, and legumes.

❖ Health care providers may recommend potassium supplementation, depending on the symptoms and serum levels of the individual patient. Continue to monitor potassium levels of those on potassium supplements. Normal serum potassium levels are 3.5–5 mmoL/L (see Chapter 30).

❖ Frequent laboratory tests may be indicated at the beginning of and throughout therapy with diuretics. These tests may include measurement of electrolytes, uric acid, and blood gases.

❖ Encourage patients to change positions slowly and to rise slowly after sitting or lying to prevent dizziness and possible fainting (syncope).

❖ Patients may need to be encouraged to increase their intake of fluids (if not contraindicated) to prevent dehydration and minimize constipation. Increased consumption of fibre may also help with constipation.

❖ Any unusual adverse effects or problems, such as excessive dizziness, syncope, weakness, or muscle aches, need to be reported immediately to the health care professional.

❖ Advise patients to keep a daily journal, in handwritten format or electronically; entries should include daily weights, how the patient feels each day, dosage of diuretic, and any other important information related to their diagnoses and medical treatment.

❖ Patients can prevent constipation with an increase in intake of fibre, bulk, roughage, and fluids, if not contraindicated.

❖ Educate patients about the signs and symptoms of hypokalemia, such as anorexia, nausea, lethargy, muscle weakness, mental confusion, and hypotension. In addition, emphasize the importance of being cautious regarding hot climates, excessive sweating, fevers, and the use of saunas or hot tubs. Heat raises core body temperature and causes further losses of potassium, sodium, and water through sweat, which may increase the risk of additional problems with hypotension and fluid–electrolyte imbalances. Fluid volume and electrolyte loss may also occur with vomiting or diarrhea.

❖ If a patient is taking a diuretic with digoxin, educate the patient, family members, and anyone involved in the patient's care about how to monitor pulse rate. The warning signs and symptoms of digoxin toxicity include headache, dizziness, confusion, nausea, visual disturbances, and bradycardia. A pulse rate of 60 beats per minute or lower is often used as a guideline, but always check facility policies or guidelines.

❖ Educate patients with diabetes mellitus who are also taking thiazide or loop diuretics about the need for close monitoring of blood glucose levels.

KEY POINTS

❖ The five main types of diuretics are CAIs and loop, osmotic, potassium-sparing, thiazide, and thiazide-like diuretics.

❖ The loop, potassium-sparing, thiazide, and thiazide-like diuretics are the most commonly used.

❖ Remember that loop diuretics are more potent than thiazides, combination diuretics, and potassium-sparing diuretics.

❖ It is important to have a thorough knowledge of kidney anatomy and physiology and how it relates to the action of the various diuretics; for example, if a loop diuretic is given, its site of action is the loop of Henle and it causes the excretion of sodium, potassium, and chloride into the urine.

❖ Methods for monitoring excess and deficit fluid volume include assessment of skin and mucous membranes, blood pressure, pulse rate, intake and output, and daily weights.

❖ With diuretics, always be concerned about members of more vulnerable patient populations, such as older adults, those with chronic illnesses, and patients with altered kidney or liver function.

EXAMINATION REVIEW QUESTIONS

1. The nurse is reviewing the medications that have been ordered for a patient for whom a loop diuretic has just been prescribed. The loop diuretic may have a possible interaction with which drug or class of drugs?
   a. Vitamin D
   b. warfarin sodium
   c. Penicillin
   d. NSAIDs

2. When monitoring laboratory test results for patients receiving loop and thiazide diuretics, the nurse knows to look for:
   a. Decreased serum levels of potassium
   b. Increased serum levels of calcium
   c. Decreased serum levels of calcium
   d. Increased serum levels of sodium

3. When the nurse is checking the laboratory data for a patient taking spironolactone, which result would be a potential concern?
   a. Serum sodium level of 140 mmoL/L
   b. Serum potassium level of 3.6 mmoL/L
   c. Serum potassium level of 5.8 mmoL/L
   d. Serum magnesium level of 0.8 mmoL/L

4. Which statement needs to be included when the nurse provides education for a patient with heart failure who is taking daily doses of spironolactone?
   a. "Be sure to eat foods that are high in potassium."
   b. "Avoid foods that are high in potassium."
   c. "Avoid grapefruit juice while taking this medication."
   d. "A low-fibre diet will help prevent adverse effects of this medication."

5. A patient with diabetes has a new prescription for a thiazide diuretic. Which statement will the nurse include when teaching the patient about the thiazide drug?
   a. "There is nothing for you to be concerned about when you are taking the thiazide diuretic."
   b. "Be sure to avoid foods that are high in potassium."
   c. "You need to take the thiazide at night to avoid interactions with your diabetes medication."
   d. "Monitor your blood glucose closely because the thiazide diuretic may cause the levels to increase."

6. An older adult patient has been discharged following treatment for a mild case of heart failure. He will be taking a loop diuretic. Which instruction(s) from the nurse are appropriate? (Select all that apply.)
   a. "Take the diuretic at the same time each morning."
   b. "Take the diuretic only if you notice swelling in your feet."
   c. "Be sure to stand up slowly because the medicine may make you feel dizzy if you stand up quickly."
   d. "Drink at least eight glasses of water each day."
   e. "Here is a list of foods that are high in potassium—you need to avoid these."
   f. "Please call your doctor immediately if you notice muscle weakness or increased dizziness."

7. The order reads: Give mannitol 0.5 g/kg IV now, over 2 hours. The patient weighs 165 lb, and you have a 100-mL vial of 20% mannitol. How many grams will the patient receive? How many millilitres of mannitol will you prepare for this infusion?

Answers: 1. d, 2. a, 3. c, 4. b, 5. d, 6. a, c, f, 7. 37.5 g, 187.5 mL

CRITICAL THINKING ACTIVITIES

1. While assessing a patient who is taking a diuretic, the nurse notes the following blood pressure readings:
   While lying in bed: 134/86 mm Hg
   While sitting on the side of the bed: 130/82 mm Hg
   While standing: 108/62 mm Hg
   In addition, the patient commented that he felt lightheaded while standing. What has happened, and what is the nurse's priority at this time?

2. A patient has been given a new order for spironolactone, 50 mg daily. While reviewing the patient's orders, the nurse notes that the patient has an existing order for potassium chloride (K-Dur®), 20 mmoL daily. The patient's potassium level is 3.9 mmoL/L. What is the nurse's priority action at this time?

3. The nurse is administering a thiazide diuretic to a patient who has been receiving digoxin for several months as part of treatment for a cardiac dysrhythmia. What is the priority for regular assessment, considering the use of these two drugs together?

For answers see http://evolve.elsevier.com/Canada/Lilley/pharmacology/.

CHAPTER 30

Fluids and Electrolytes

Objectives

After reading this chapter, the successful student will be able to do the following:

1. Review the function of fluid volume and compartments within the body as well as the role of each of the major electrolytes in maintaining homeostasis.

2. Identify the various electrolytes and give normal serum values for each.

3. Briefly discuss the various fluid and electrolyte disorders that commonly occur in the body, with attention to fluid volume or electrolyte deficits and excesses.

4. Identify the fluid and electrolyte solutions commonly used to correct states of deficiency or excess.

5. Discuss the mechanisms of action, indications, dosages, routes of administration, contraindications, cautions, adverse effects, toxicities, and drug interactions of the various fluid and electrolyte solutions.

6. Compare the various solutions used to expand or decrease a patient's fluid volume and electrolytes, considering how they work, why they are used, and specific antidotes available to counter any toxic effects.

7. Develop a collaborative plan of care that includes all phases of the nursing process for patients receiving fluid and electrolyte solutions.

e-Learning Activities

Website
(http://evolve.elsevier.com/Canada/
Lilley/pharmacology/)

evolve

- Answer Key—Textbook Case Studies
- Answer Key—Critical Thinking Activities
- Chapter Summaries—Printable
- Review Questions for Exam Preparation
- Unfolding Case Studies

Drug Profiles

albumin, p. 584
dextran, p. 584
fresh frozen plasma, p. 585
packed red blood cells, p. 585
potassium, p. 588
sodium chloride, pp. 582, 589
sodium polystyrene sulfonate (potassium exchange resin), p. 588
tolvaptan, p. 589

Key Terms

Blood The fluid that circulates through the heart, arteries, capillaries, and veins, carrying nutrients and oxygen to the body cells; consists of plasma—its liquid component—and three major solid components: erythrocytes (red blood cells or RBCs), leukocytes (white blood cells or WBCs), and platelets. (p. 579)

Colloids Protein substances that increase the colloid oncotic pressure. (p. 582)

Colloid oncotic pressure (COP) A form of osmotic pressure exerted by protein in blood plasma that tends to pull water into the circulatory system. (p. 580)

Crystalloids Substances in a solution that diffuse through a semipermeable membrane. (p. 581)

Dehydration Excessive loss of water from body tissues. It is accompanied by an imbalance in the concentrations of essential electrolytes, particularly sodium, potassium, and chloride. (p. 580)

Edema The abnormal accumulation of fluid in interstitial spaces. (p. 580)

Euvolemia The state of normal body fluid volume. (p. 579)

Euvolemic hyponatremia A normal body sodium level with increase in total body water. (p. 589)

Extracellular fluid (ECF)   The portion of the body fluid comprising the interstitial fluid and blood plasma. (p. 579)

Extravascular fluid (EVF)   Fluids in the body that are outside the blood vessels. (p. 579)

Gradient   A difference in the concentration of a substance on two sides of a permeable barrier. (p. 581)

Hydrostatic pressure (HP)   The pressure exerted by a liquid. (p. 580)

Hyperkalemia   A condition in which there is an abnormally high potassium concentration in the blood, most likely due to defective kidney excretion but also drugs. (p. 586)

Hypornatremia   A condition in which there is an abnormally high sodium concentration in the blood; more commonly results from excessive dietary sodium kidney disorders, or dehydration. (p. 587)

Hypokalemia   A condition in which there is an inadequate amount of potassium, the major intracellular cation, in the bloodstream. (p. 586)

Hyponatremia   A condition in which there is an inadequate amount of sodium, the major extracellular cation, in the bloodstream, caused by either inadequate excretion of water or excessive water intake or by drugs (e.., diuretics). (p. 587)

Interstitial fluid (ISF)   The extracellular fluid that fills in the spaces between most of the cells of the body. (p. 579)

Intracellular fluid (ICF)   The fluid located within cell membranes throughout most of the body. It contains dissolved solutes that are essential to maintaining electrolyte balance and healthy metabolism. (p. 579)

Intravascular fluid (IVF)   The fluid inside blood vessels. (p. 579)

Isotonic   Having the same concentration of a solute as another solution and thus exerting the same osmotic pressure as that solution, such as an isotonic saline solution that contains an amount of salt equal to that found in the intracellular and extracellular fluid. (p. 580)

Osmotic pressure   The pressure produced by a solution necessary to prevent the osmotic passage of solvent into it when the solution and solvent are separated by a semipermeable membrane. (p. 580)

Plasma   The watery, straw-coloured fluid component of lymph and blood in which leukocytes, erythrocytes, and platelets are suspended. (p. 579)

Serum   The clear, cell-free portion of the blood from which fibrinogen has been separated during the clotting process, as typically carried out with a laboratory sample. (p. 579)

OVERVIEW

Fluid and electrolyte management is one of the cornerstones of patient care. Most disease processes, tissue injuries, and surgical procedures greatly influence the physiological status of fluids and electrolytes in the body. Understanding fluid and electrolyte management requires knowledge of the extent and composition of the various body fluid compartments.

PHYSIOLOGY OF FLUID BALANCE

Approximately 60% of the adult human body is water. This is referred to as *total body water* (TBW), and it is distributed among the three main compartments in the following proportions: **intracellular fluid (ICF)**, 67%; **interstitial fluid (ISF)**, 25%; and plasma volume (PV), 8%. This distribution is illustrated in Figure 30-1. The actual volume of fluid that would normally be distributed in each compartment in an average 70-kg man with a TBW content of 60% is shown in Table 30-1. When the total body fluid content in the body is normal, it is referred to as **euvolemia**.

The terms used to identify the spaces within which the TBW is distributed can be quite confusing, and there are two basic approaches to distinguishing among the locations of the fluid. The TBW can be described as being inside or outside of the **blood** vessels (vasculature). If this point of reference is used, then the term *intravascular*

fluid (IVF) describes the fluid inside the blood vessels and the term *extravascular fluid (EVF)* refers to the fluid outside the blood vessels. Examples of EVF include lymph and cerebrospinal fluid. As these concepts are learned, it is important to remember the difference between the prefixes *intra-* (inside), *inter-* (between), and *extra-* (outside). The term *plasma* is used to describe the fluid that flows through the blood vessels (IVF). **Serum** is a closely related term (see Key Terms). The ISF is the fluid in the spaces between cells, tissues, and organs. When discussing blood vessels, the term *extravascular volume* is used; extravascular volume is made up of plasma and ISF. When discussing cells, the term *extracellular volume* is used; extracellular volume is composed of ISF and ICF. These terms are often confused and misused.

Extracellular fluid (ECF) consists of both plasma and ISF. There is one important difference between the plasma

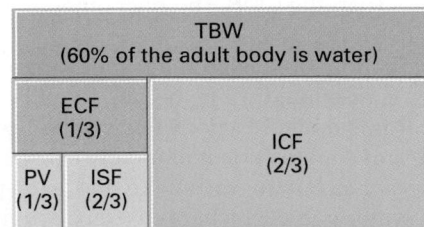

FIG. 30-1 Distribution of total body water (TBW). *ECF,* extracellular fluid; *ICF,* intracellular fluid; *ISF,* interstitial fluid; *PV,* plasma volume.

TABLE 30-1	
Types of Dehydration	
Type of Dehydration	**Characteristics**
Hypertonic	Occurs when water loss is greater than sodium loss, which results in a concentration of solutes outside the cells and causes the fluid inside the cells to move to the extracellular space, thus dehydrating the cells. Example: elevated temperature resulting in perspiration
Hypotonic	Occurs when sodium loss is greater than water loss, which results in higher concentrations of solute inside the cells and causes fluid to be pulled from outside the cells (plasma and interstitial spaces) into the cells. Examples: kidney insufficiency and inadequate aldosterone secretion
Isotonic	Caused by a loss of sodium and water from the body, which results in a decrease in the volume of extracellular fluid. Examples: diarrhea and vomiting

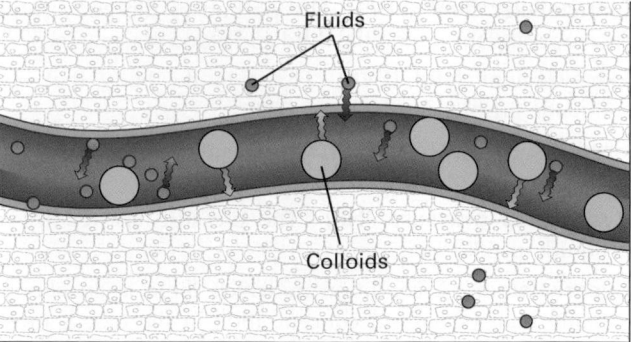

FIG. 30-2 Colloid osmotic pressure (oncotic pressure). As shown, the colloids inside the blood vessel are too large to pass through the vessel wall. The resulting oncotic pressure exerted by the colloids draws fluid from the surrounding tissues and other extravascular spaces into the blood vessels and keeps fluid inside the blood vessel.

TABLE 30-2	
Conditions Leading to Fluid Loss and Associated Symptoms*	
Condition	**Associated Symptoms**
Bleeding	Tachycardia and hypotension
Bowel obstruction	Reduced perspiration and mucous secretions
Diarrhea	Reduced urine output (oliguria)
Fever	Dry skin and mucous membranes
Vomiting	Reduced lacrimal (tears) and salivary secretions

*Note: There may be overlap involving more than one of the symptoms depending on the patient's specific condition.

and the ISF. Plasma has a protein concentration four times greater than that of ISF, of which albumin constitutes 80%. The reason for this higher intravascular concentration of protein is that these solutes (proteins) have a molecular weight, which makes them too large to pass through the walls of the blood vessels. Because of the difference in concentration, fluid flows from the area of low concentration in the interstitial compartment to the area of high concentration inside the blood vessel, trying to create an isotonic environment on either side of the blood vessel wall. (**Isotonic** means an equal concentration of solutes across a membrane.) The protein in the blood vessels exerts a constant **osmotic pressure** that prevents the leakage of too much plasma through the capillaries into the tissues (this creates a pulling pressure). Because proteins suspended in plasma are in a colloidal state, this particular pressure is called **colloid oncotic pressure (COP)**, and it is normally 24 mm Hg. The opposing, pushing pressure exerted by the ISF is called *hydrostatic pressure (HP)*; normally, it is 17 mm Hg, which is less than the COP. The phenomenon of COP is illustrated in Figure 30-2.

This regulation of the volume and composition of body water is essential for life, because it is the medium in which all metabolic reactions occur. The body keeps the volume and composition remarkably constant by preserving the balance between intake and excretion. The amount of water gained each day is kept roughly equal to the amount of water lost. When the body is unable to maintain this equilibrium, therapy with select agents becomes necessary. If the amount of water gained exceeds

the amount of water lost, a water excess, or overhydration, occurs. Such fluid excesses often accumulate in interstitial spaces, such as in the pericardial sac, intrapleural space, peritoneal cavity, joint capsules, and lower extremities. This is referred to as *edema*. In contrast, if the quantity of water lost exceeds that gained, a water deficit, or **dehydration**, occurs. Death may occur when 20 to 25% of TBW is lost.

Dehydration leads to a disturbance in the balance between the amount of fluid in the extracellular compartment and that in the intracellular compartment. Sodium is the principal extracellular electrolyte and plays a primary role in maintaining water concentration in the body because of its highly osmotic chemistry. In the initial stages of dehydration, water is lost first from the extracellular compartments. The amount of further fluid losses, COP changes, or both, determines the type of clinical dehydration that develops (Table 30-1). Clinical conditions that can result in dehydration and fluid loss, as well as the symptoms of dehydration and fluid loss, are presented in Table 30-2. When fluid that has been lost must be replaced, there are three categories of agents that can be used to accomplish this: crystalloids, colloids, and blood products. The clinical situation dictates which category of agents is most appropriate.

CRYSTALLOIDS

Crystalloids are fluids given by intravenous (IV) injection that supply water and sodium to maintain the osmotic **gradient** between the extravascular and intravascular compartments. Their plasma volume-expanding capacity is related to their sodium concentration. The different crystalloids are listed in Table 30-3.

Mechanism of Action and Drug Effects

Crystalloid solutions contain fluids and electrolytes that are normally found in the body. They do not contain proteins (colloids), which are necessary to maintain the colloid osmotic pressure and prevent water from leaving the plasma compartment. In fact, the administration of large quantities of crystalloid solutions for fluid resuscitation decreases the COP, attributable to a dilutional effect. Crystalloids are dispersed faster into the interstitial and intracellular compartments than colloids. This makes crystalloids a better choice for treating dehydration than for expanding the plasma volume alone, such as is used for hypovolemic shock.

Indications

Crystalloid solutions are most commonly used as maintenance fluids. They are used to compensate for insensible fluid losses, to replace fluids, and to manage specific fluid and electrolyte disturbances. Crystalloids also promote urinary flow. They are much less expensive than colloids and blood products. In addition, there is no risk of viral transmission or anaphylaxis and no alteration in the coagulation profile associated with their use, unlike with blood products. The choice of whether to use a crystalloid or colloid depends on the severity of the condition. The following are the common indications for either crystalloid or colloid replacement therapy:

- Acute liver failure
- Acute nephrosis
- Acute respiratory distress syndrome
- Burns
- Cardiopulmonary bypass
- Hypoproteinemia
- Reduction of the risk for deep vein thrombosis
- Hemodialysis
- Shock

Contraindications

Contraindications to the use of crystalloids include known drug allergy to a specific product or hypervolemia, and may include severe electrolyte disturbance, depending on the type of crystalloid used.

Adverse Effects

Crystalloids are a safe and effective means of replacing needed fluid. They do, however, have some unwanted effects. Because they contain no large particles, such as proteins, they do not stay within the blood vessels and can leak out of the plasma into the tissues and cells. This can result in edema anywhere in the body; peripheral edema and pulmonary edema are two common examples. Crystalloids also dilute the proteins that are in plasma, which further reduces the COP. To be effective, large volumes (multiple litres of fluid) are usually required. As a result, prolonged infusions may worsen acidosis or alkalosis, or adversely affect central nervous system function, due to fluid overload. Another disadvantage of crystalloids is that their effects are relatively short-lived.

Interactions

Interactions with crystalloid solutions are rare because they are similar if not identical to normal physiological substances. Certain electrolytes contained in lactated Ringer's solution may be incompatible with other electrolytes, forming a chemical precipitate (e.g., phenytoin sodium precipitates if mixed with dextrose).

TABLE	**30-3**

Crystalloids

Product	Osmolarity	Composition (mmol/L)						Volume (mL)
		Na	Cl	K	Ca	Mg	Lactate	
NS (0.9% isotonic)	308 mOsm	154	154	0	0	0	0	1 000
Hypertonic saline (3%)	154 mOsm	513	513	0	0	0	0	500
3.3% dextrose and 0.3% NS (⅔ and ⅓) (isotonic)*	259 mOsm	51	51	0	0	0	0	1 000
Lactated Ringer's (isotonic)	275 mOsm	130	109	4	3	0	28	1 000
D_5W (isotonic)*	260 mOsm	0	0	1	0	0	0	1 000
D_5W & 0.45% NS (hypertonic)	406 mOsm	77	77	0	0	0	0	1 000
Plasma-Lyte (isotonic)	294 mOsm	140	103	10	5	3	8	1 000

Ca, calcium; *Cl*, chloride; D_5W, 5% dextrose in water; *K*, potassium; *Mg*, magnesium; *Na*, sodium; *NS*, normal saline.
*D_5W alone in an IV bag is considered isotonic but acts as a hypotonic solution once in the bloodstream

Dosages

For the recommended dosages of crystalloids, refer to Table 30-4.

COLLOIDS

Colloids are protein substances that increase the COP and move fluid from the interstitial compartment to the plasma compartment by pulling the fluid into the blood vessels. Normally, this task is performed by the three blood proteins: albumin, globulin, and fibrinogen. The total protein level must be within the range of 74 g/L. If the protein level drops below 53 g/L, fluid shifts out of the blood vessels and into the tissues. When this happens,

colloid replacement therapy is required to reverse this process by increasing the COP. The COP decreases with age and also with hypotension and malnutrition. The commonly used colloids are listed in Table 30-5.

Mechanism of Action and Drug Effects

The mechanism of action of colloids is related to their ability to increase the COP. Because colloids cannot pass into extravascular space, there is a higher concentration of solutes (solid particles) inside the blood vessels (in intravascular space) than outside the blood vessels. Fluid moves from the extravascular space into the blood vessels in an attempt to make it isotonic. As such, colloids increase the blood volume, and they are often referred to

---

TABLE 30-4

Crystalloids and Colloids: Dosing Guidelines

	Crystalloids and Colloids			
	0.9% NS	**3% NS***	**5% Colloid†**	**25% Colloid‡**
TO RAISE PLASMA VOLUME BY 1 L, ADMINISTER:	5–6 L	1.5–2 L	1 L	0.5 L
FLUID COMPARTMENT DISTRIBUTED TO:				
Plasma	25%	25%	100%	200–300%
Interstitial space	75%	75%	0	Decreased fluid levels
Intracellular space	0	0	0	Decreased fluid levels

NS, normal saline.
*Hypertonic saline is a high-risk drug and should not be given faster than 100 mL/hr for short periods. Frequent monitoring of serum levels is required.
†Iso-oncotic solutions such as 5% albumin, dextran 70, and hetastarch.
‡Hyperoncotic solutions such as 25% albumin.

 DRUG PROFILE

The most commonly used crystalloid solutions are normal saline (NS or 0.9% sodium chloride) and lactated Ringer's solution. The available crystalloid solutions and their compositions are summarized in Table 30-3. Sodium chloride is also discussed briefly in the section on electrolytes and in the Nursing Process section.

sodium chloride

Sodium chloride (NaCl) is available in several concentrations, the most common being 0.9%. This is the physiologically normal concentration of sodium chloride, which is why it is referred to as *normal saline* (NS). Other concentrations are 0.45% (half-normal, hypotonic) and 3% (hypertonic saline). These solutions have different indications and are used in different situations, depending on how urgently fluid volume restoration is needed and the extent of the sodium loss.

Sodium chloride is a physiological electrolyte that is present throughout the body's water. Thus, there are no hypersensitivity reactions to it. It is safe to administer during any stage of pregnancy, but it is contraindicated in patients with hypernatremia or hyperchloremia. Hypertonic saline injection (3%) is contraindicated in the

presence of increased, normal, or only slightly decreased serum electrolyte concentrations. Correcting sodium too rapidly with hypertonic saline can lead to osmotic demyelination syndrome characterized by intramyelinitic splitting, vacuolization and myelin sheath rupture as well as brain shrinkage, which is potentially fatal. Conversely, infusing hypotonic saline is not recommended because it can cause hemolysis of the red blood cells (RBCs). Adding potassium to hypotonic solutions makes them isotonic and safe to give. Sodium chloride is also available as a 650-mg tablet.

The dose of sodium chloride administered depends on the clinical situation. The volume of crystalloid or colloid needed to expand the plasma volume by 1 litre (1 000 mL) is provided in Table 30-4, which can be used as a general guide to dosing.

PHARMACOKINETICS

Plasma Volume Expansion *	Colloid Oncotic Pressure	Duration of Expansion
60–70 mL	30 mm Hg	A few hours

*500 mL of normal saline will expand the plasma volume by 60 to 70 mL.

TABLE 30-5

Commonly Used Colloids

Product	Composition (mmol/L)		
	Na	Cl	Volume (mL)
Dextran 70†	154	154	500
Dextran 40†	154	154	500
Hetastarch	154	154	500
5% Albumin	145	145	500
25% Albumin	145	145	100

†Dextran is available in NaCl, which has 154 mmol/L of both Na and Cl. It is also available in 5% dextrose in water, which contains no Na or Cl.

TABLE 30-6

Blood Products

Product	Dosage
Cryoprecipitate	1 unit
Fresh frozen plasma	1 unit
Packed red blood cells	1 unit
Plasma protein fractions	1 unit
Whole blood	1 unit

as *plasma expanders*. They also make up part of the total plasma volume.

Colloids increase the COP and move fluid from outside the blood vessels to inside the blood vessels. They can maintain the COP for several hours. Colloids are naturally occurring products and consist of proteins (albumin), carbohydrates (dextran or starch), fats (lipid emulsion), and animal collagen (gelatin). Usually, they contain a combination of both small and large particles. The small particles are eliminated quickly and promote diuresis and perfusion of the kidneys; the larger particles maintain the plasma volume. Albumin is the one exception in that it contains particles that are all the same size.

Indications

Colloids are used to treat a wide variety of conditions. Clinically, colloids are superior to crystalloids because of their ability to maintain the plasma volume for a longer time. However, crystalloids are less expensive and are less likely to promote bleeding (see Adverse Effects discussion below). Conversely, crystalloids are more likely to cause edema because of the larger volumes needed to achieve the desired clinical effect. Crystalloids are better than colloids for emergency short-term plasma volume expansion.

Contraindications

Contraindications to the use of colloids include known drug allergy to a specific product or hypervolemia and may include severe electrolyte disturbance.

Adverse Effects

Colloids are relatively safe agents, although there are some disadvantages to their use. They have no oxygen-carrying ability and contain no clotting factors, unlike blood products. Because of this, they can alter the coagulation system through a dilutional effect, resulting in impaired coagulation and potential for bleeding. They may also dilute the plasma protein concentration, which in turn may impair platelet function. Rarely, dextran therapy causes anaphylaxis or kidney failure.

Interactions

No drug interactions occur with colloids.

Dosages

For the recommended dosages of colloids, refer to Table 30-4.

BLOOD PRODUCTS

Blood products can be considered biological drugs. RBC-containing products can improve tissue oxygenation and also augment plasma volume. Blood products are more expensive than crystalloids and colloids and are less available because they are natural products and require human donors. The available blood products are listed in Table 30-6. They are most often indicated when a patient has lost 25% or more blood volume.

Mechanism of Action and Drug Effects

The mechanism of action of blood products is related to their ability to increase COP and plasma volume. They achieve these outcomes in the same manner as colloids and crystalloids, by pulling fluid from the extravascular space to the intravascular space. Because of this property, they are also considered plasma expanders. RBC-containing products also have the ability to carry oxygen. They can maintain the COP for several hours to days. Because they come from human donors, they have all the benefits (and hazards) of human blood products. They are administered when a person's body is deficient in these products.

Indications

Blood products are used to treat a wide variety of clinical conditions, and the blood product used depends on the specific indication. The available blood products and the conditions they are used to treat are listed in Table 30-7.

Contraindications

There are no absolute contraindications to the use of blood products. However, because there is a risk for transfer of infectious disease, although remote, their use should be based on careful clinical evaluation of the patient's condition.

DRUG PROFILES

The specific colloid used for replacement therapy varies from institution to institution. The most commonly used are 5% albumin, dextran 40, pentaspan, and hetastarch. They have a rapid onset as well as a long duration of action. They are metabolized in the liver and excreted by the kidneys. Albumin is one exception; it is metabolized by the reticuloendothelial system and excreted by the kidneys and intestines. Hetastarch is a synthetic colloid with properties similar to those of albumin and dextran. Pentaspan is an artificial colloid derived from a waxy starch composed almost entirely of amylopectin.

albumin

Albumin is a natural protein that is normally produced by the liver. It is responsible for generating about 80% of the COP. Human albumin is a sterile solution of serum albumin that is prepared from pooled blood, plasma, serum, or placentas obtained from healthy human donors. It is pasteurized (heated at 60°C for 10 hours) to destroy any contaminants. Unfortunately, because it is derived from human donors, the supply is limited. Many institutions have specific indications for the use of albumin.

Albumin is contraindicated in patients with a known hypersensitivity to it and in those with heart failure, severe anemia, or kidney insufficiency. Albumin is available only in parenteral form in concentrations of 5% and 25%. For use during pregnancy, the potential benefits of albumin must be considered relative to the risk to the fetus. See Table 30-4 for the dosing guidelines.

PHARMACOKINETICS

Route	Onset of Action	Peak Plasma Concentration	Elimination Half-Life	Duration of Action
IV	Less than 1 min	Unknown	16 hr	Less than 24 hr

dextran

Dextran is a solution of glucose. It is available in two concentrations, dextran 40 and the more concentrated dextran 70, which has a molecular weight similar to that of albumin. Of the two, dextran 40 is more commonly used. Dextran is a derivative of sugar that has actions similar to those of human albumin in that it expands the plasma volume by drawing fluid from the interstitial space to the intravascular space.

Dextran is contraindicated in patients with hypersensitivity to it and in those with heart failure, kidney insufficiency, and extreme dehydration. It is available only in parenteral form in either a 5% dextrose solution or a 0.9% sodium chloride solution. For use during pregnancy, the potential benefits of dextran must be considered relative to the risk to the fetus. See Table 30-4 for the dosing guidelines.

PHARMACOKINETICS

Route	Onset of Action	Peak Plasma Concentration	Elimination Half-Life	Duration of Action
IV	5 min	Unknown	2–6 hr	4–6 hr

TABLE 30-7

Blood Products: Indications

Blood Product	Indications
Cryoprecipitate and plasma protein fraction	To manage acute bleeding (over 50% blood loss slowly or 20% rapidly)
Fresh frozen plasma	To increase clotting factor levels in patients with a demonstrated deficiency
Packed red blood cells	To increase oxygen-carrying capacity in patients with anemia, in patients with substantial hemoglobin deficits, and in patients who have lost up to 25% of their total blood volume
Whole blood	Same as for packed red blood cells, except that whole blood is more beneficial in cases of extreme (over 25%) loss of blood volume, because whole blood also contains plasma, the primary fluid volume of the blood; it also contains plasma proteins, the primary osmotic component, which help draw fluid back into blood vessels from surrounding tissues

Adverse Effects

Blood products can produce undesirable effects, some potentially serious. Because blood products come from other humans, they can be incompatible with the recipient's immune system. These incompatibilities are tested for before the products' administration by determining the respective blood types of the donor and recipient and by cross-matching to determine compatibility between selected blood proteins. This helps reduce the likelihood that the recipient will reject the blood product, which would precipitate transfusion reactions and anaphylaxis. Blood products can also transmit pathogens from the donor to the recipient; examples of such pathogens are hepatitis virus and HIV. Various preparation techniques are now used to reduce the risk for pathogen transmission, and these have resulted in a drastic reduction in the incidence of such problems.

Interactions

As with crystalloids and colloids, blood products are similar if not identical to normal physiological substances; therefore, they are involved in few interactions. Calcium and aspirin, which normally affect coagulation, may interact with these substances when infused in the body, in much the same way they interact with the body's blood products. Blood must not be administered with any solution other than normal saline.

Dosages

For the dosage guidelines pertaining to blood products, refer to Table 30-8.

PHYSIOLOGY OF ELECTROLYTE BALANCE

The chemical composition of the fluid compartments varies. The principal electrolytes in the ECF are sodium cations (Na^+) and chloride anions (Cl^-). The major electrolyte in the ICF is the potassium cation (K^+). Other important electrolytes are calcium (see Chapter 34), magnesium (see Chapter 53), and phosphorus (see Chapter 53). These different chemical components are vital to the normal function of all body systems. They are controlled by the renin–angiotensin–aldosterone system, antidiuretic hormone system, and sympathetic nervous system.

TABLE 30-8	
Suggested Guidelines for Blood Products: Management of Bleeding	
Amount of Blood Loss	**Fluid of Choice**
20% or less (slow loss)	Crystalloids
20–50% (slow loss)	Nonprotein plasma expanders (dextran, pentastarch, hydroxyethyl starch (Voluven®, Volulyte®), and hetastarch)
Over 50% (slow loss) or 20% (acutely)	Whole blood or packed red blood cells or plasmaprotein fraction and fresh frozen plasma
80% or more	As above, but for every 5 units of blood given, administer 1 to 2 units of fresh frozen plasma and 1 to 2 units of platelets to prevent the hemodilution of clotting factors and bleeding

DRUG PROFILES

Packed red blood cells and fresh frozen plasma are among the most commonly used blood products. All blood products are derived from pooled blood from human donors. Other less commonly used, but still important, blood products include whole blood, plasma protein fraction, cryoprecipitate, and platelets.

packed red blood cells

Packed red blood cells are obtained by centrifugation of whole blood and the separation of RBCs from plasma and the other cellular elements. The advantage of packed red blood cells is that their oxygen-carrying capacity is better than that of the other blood products, and they are less likely to cause cardiac fluid overload. Their disadvantages include high cost, limited shelf life, and fluctuating availability, as well as their ability to transmit viruses, trigger allergic reactions, and cause bleeding abnormalities. The Canadian National Advisory Committee on Blood and Blood Products (2014) recommends specific guidelines for the administration of RBCs. A restrictive transfusion strategy is recommended, for example, a hemoglobin of 70 to 80 g/L is recommended for hospitalized, stable patients; a hemoglobin of 70 g/L

or less for adult and pediatric intensive care patients; and a hemoglobin of 80 g/L or less for postoperative surgical patients or hospitalized, stable patients with pre-existing cardiovascular disease. Transfusions are considered for patients with specific symptoms (chest pain, orthostatic hypotension, tachycardia unresponsive to fluid resuscitation, heart failure). Always follow agency protocols for the administration of blood products. The suggested guidelines for their use in the management of blood loss are given in Table 30-8.

fresh frozen plasma

Fresh frozen plasma is obtained by centrifuging whole blood and removing the cellular elements. The resulting plasma is then frozen at –18°C. Fresh frozen plasma is not recommended for routine fluid resuscitation, but it may be used as an adjunct to massive blood transfusion in the treatment of patients with underlying coagulation disorders. The plasma-expanding capability of fresh frozen plasma is similar to that of dextran but slightly less than that of hetastarch. The disadvantage of fresh frozen plasma is that it can transmit pathogens. The suggested guidelines for its use are given in Table 30-8.

When these neuroendocrine systems are out of balance, adverse electrolyte imbalances commonly result. Patients who receive diuretics (see Chapter 29) are at risk for electrolyte abnormalities.

POTASSIUM

Potassium is the most abundant cationic (positively charged) electrolyte inside cells (the intracellular space), where the normal concentration is approximately 150 mmol/L. Approximately 95% of the potassium in the body is intracellular. In contrast, the amount of potassium outside the cells in the plasma ranges from 3.5 to 5.0 mmol/L. These plasma levels are critical to normal body function.

Potassium is obtained from a variety of foods, the most common being fruits and juices, vegetables, fish, and meats. Salt substitutes also contain potassium. It has been estimated that for normal body functions to be maintained, a person must consume 5 to 10 mmol of potassium per day. Fortunately, the average adult daily diet usually provides 35 to 100 mmol of potassium, which is well above the required daily amount. Excess dietary potassium is usually excreted by the kidneys in urine. However, if the kidneys lose their ability to filter and secrete waste products, potassium can accumulate. Excessive potassium can precipitate ventricular fibrillation and cardiac arrest. Hyperaldosteronism and the use of potassium-sparing diuretics can alter normal potassium balance as well. *Hyperkalemia* refers to a serum potassium level that exceeds 5.5 mmol/L. There are several causes of hyperkalemia, including the following:
- Angiotensin-converting enzyme (ACE) inhibitor use
- Burns
- Excessive loss from cells
- Infections
- Kidney failure
- Metabolic acidosis
- Potassium supplementation
- Potassium-sparing diuretic use
- Trauma

The opposite of hyperkalemia is **hypokalemia**, a deficiency of potassium. Hypokalemia is defined as a serum potassium level of less than 3.5 mmol/L. This condition is more often the result of excessive potassium loss than of poor dietary intake. As with hyperkalemia, there are many clinical conditions and other situations that can cause hypokalemia. These include the following:
- Alkalosis
- Increased secretion of mineralocorticoids (hormones of the adrenal cortex)
- Burns
- Corticosteroid use
- Diarrhea
- Diet extreme in nutritional deprivation
- Hyperaldosteronism
- Ketoacidosis
- Consumption of large amounts of licorice

BOX 30-1

Symptoms of Hypokalemia

Early	Late
Anorexia	Cardiac dysrhythmias
Hypotension	Neuropathy
Lethargy	Paralytic ileus
Confusion	Secondary alkalosis
Muscle weakness	
Nausea	

- Loop diuretic use
- Malabsorption
- Prolonged laxative misuse
- Thiazide or thiazide-like diuretic use
- Vomiting

A low serum potassium can increase the toxicity associated with digoxin, and this can precipitate serious ventricular dysrhythmias.

The early detection of hypokalemia is important to prevent serious, life-threatening consequences of this metabolic disturbance if it remains undetected. The key to early detection is recognizing its early symptoms, which are generally mild and can easily go unnoticed. Both the early (mild) symptoms and late (severe) symptoms of hypokalemia are listed in Box 30-1. Treatment involves both identifying and treating the cause and restoring serum potassium levels to normal (greater than 3.5 mmol/L). The consumption of potassium-rich foods can usually correct mild hypokalemia, but clinically significant hypokalemia requires the oral or parenteral administration of a potassium supplement, which usually contains potassium chloride.

Mechanism of Action and Drug Effects

The importance of potassium as the primary intracellular electrolyte is highlighted by the number of life-sustaining physiological functions that require it. Muscle contraction, the transmission of nerve impulses, and the regulation of heartbeats (the pacemaker function of the heart) are just a few of these functions.

Potassium is also essential for the maintenance of acid–base balance, isotonicity, and the electrodynamic characteristics of the cell. It plays a role in many enzymatic reactions, and it is an essential component of gastric secretions, kidney function, tissue synthesis, and carbohydrate metabolism.

Indications

Potassium replacement therapy is indicated in the treatment or prevention of potassium depletion in patients whose dietary measures prove inadequate. Potassium salts commonly used for this purpose include potassium chloride, potassium phosphate, and potassium acetate.

The chloride is necessary to correct the hypochloremia (low level of chloride in the blood) that commonly accompanies potassium deficiency, and the phosphate is used to correct hypophosphatemia. The acetate salt may be used to raise the blood pH in acidotic conditions.

Other therapeutic effects of potassium are related to its role in the contraction of muscles and the maintenance of the electrical characteristics of cells. Potassium salts may be used to stop irregular heartbeats (dysrhythmias) and to manage the tachydysrhythmias that can occur after heart surgery.

Contraindications

Contraindications to potassium replacement products include known drug allergy to a specific drug product, hyperkalemia from any cause, severe kidney disease, acute dehydration, untreated Addison's disease, severe hemolytic disease, and conditions involving extensive tissue breakdown (e.g., multiple traumas, severe burns).

Adverse Effects

The adverse effects of oral potassium therapy are primarily limited to the gastrointestinal (GI) tract and include diarrhea, nausea, and vomiting. More significant effects include GI bleeding and ulceration. The parenteral administration of potassium usually produces pain at the injection site. Cases of phlebitis have been associated with IV administration. This irritation may be intensified with the administration of IV antibiotics (e.g., cephalosporin). One option is to insert a peripherally inserted central catheter to prevent the IV line from going interstitial; this option also prevents phlebitis. The generally accepted maximum concentration for peripheral infusion is 20 to 40 mmol/L and up to 60 mmol/L for a central line. Excessive administration of potassium salts can lead to hyperkalemia and toxic effects. If IV potassium is administered too rapidly, cardiac arrest may occur. IV potassium must not be given faster than 10 mmol per hour to patients who are not on cardiac monitors. For critically ill patients on cardiac monitors, rates of 20 mmol per hour or more may be used.

Toxicity and Management of Overdose

The toxic effects of potassium are the result of hyperkalemia. Symptoms include muscle weakness, paresthesia, paralysis, cardiac rhythm irregularities that can result in ventricular fibrillation, and cardiac arrest. The treatment instituted depends on the degree of hyperkalemia and ranges from reversal of life-threatening problems to simple dietary restrictions. In the event of severe hyperkalemia, the IV administration of sodium bicarbonate, calcium gluconate or chloride, or dextrose solution with insulin is often required. These drugs correct severe hyperkalemia by causing a rapid intracellular shift of potassium ions, which reduces the serum potassium concentration. Such interventions are often followed with orally or rectally administered sodium polystyrene sulfonate (Kayexalate®) or hemodialysis to eliminate the extra potassium from the body. Less critical levels can be reduced with dietary restrictions.

Interactions

Concurrent use of potassium-sparing diuretics and ACE inhibitors can produce a hyperkalemic state. Concurrent use of non–potassium-sparing diuretics, amphotericin B, and mineralocorticosteroids can produce a hypokalemic state.

Dosages

Fluid and electrolyte therapy involves replacing any deficits or losses and providing maintenance levels for specific patient requirements. Accordingly, specific dosage amounts of fluids or electrolytes depend on several clinical factors, including the following:
- Specific patient losses
- Efficacy of patient physiological systems involved in fluid and electrolyte metabolism, especially adrenal, cardiovascular, and kidney functioning
- Current drug therapy for pathological conditions that complicate the amount and duration of replacement
- Selection of oral or parenteral replacement formulations

Suggested dosage guidelines for potassium with subsequent adjustments are 10 to 20 mmol administered orally several times a day or parenteral administration of 30 to 60 mmol every 24 hours.

SODIUM

Although sodium was discussed under crystalloids, it is also presented here in the electrolyte section because it is most commonly given for replenishing purposes. Sodium is the counterpart of potassium, in that potassium is the principal cation inside cells, whereas sodium is the principal cation outside cells. The normal concentration of sodium outside cells is 135 to 145 mmol/L, and it is maintained through the dietary intake of sodium in the form of sodium chloride, which is obtained from fish, meats, and other foods flavoured, seasoned, or preserved with salt.

Hyponatremia is a condition of sodium loss or deficiency and occurs when serum levels decrease to lower than 135 mmol/L. It is manifested by lethargy, hypotension, stomach cramps, vomiting, diarrhea, and seizures. Some of the same conditions that cause hypokalemia can also cause hyponatremia. Other causes of hyponatremia are excessive perspiration, occurring during hot weather or physical work; prolonged diarrhea or vomiting, especially in young children and older adults; kidney disorders; and adrenocortical impairment.

Hypernatremia is the condition of sodium excess and occurs when the serum levels of sodium exceed 145 mmol/L. The most common cause is poor kidney excretion stemming from kidney malfunction. Inadequate water consumption and dehydration are other causes. Symptoms of hypernatremia include red, flushed

DRUG PROFILES

potassium supplements

Potassium supplements (Odan K-20, Odan K-8, PMS oral solution) are administered to prevent or treat potassium depletion. The acetate, chloride, and citrate salts of potassium are available for oral administration. The parenteral salt forms of potassium for IV administration are acetate, chloride, and phosphate. The dosage of potassium supplements is usually expressed in millimoles (mmol; equal to milliequivalents [mEq]) of potassium and depends on the requirements of the individual patient. Different salt forms of potassium deliver varying milliequivalent amounts of potassium.

Potassium is contraindicated in patients with severe kidney disease, severe hemolytic disease, or Addison's disease and in those with hyperkalemia, acute dehydration, or extensive tissue breakdown stemming from multiple traumas. Potassium is safe for administration during pregnancy. Potassium is available in oral form as an extended-release tablet and oral solution. It is also available as an injection in many different formulations for IV use.

PHARMACOKINETICS

Route	Onset of Action	Peak Plasma Concentration	Elimination Half-Life	Duration of Action
IV	Immediate	Rapid	Variable	Variable

sodium polystyrene sulfonate (potassium exchange resin)

Sodium polystyrene sulfonate (Kayexalate, Solystat®) is a cation exchange resin and is used to treat hyperkalemia.

It is usually administered orally, via a nasogastric tube, or as an enema. Its action is in the intestine, where potassium ions from the body are exchanged for sodium ions in the resin. Most of this action occurs in the large intestine, which excretes potassium ions to a greater degree than the small intestine does. Although the drug effects in each case are unpredictable, approximately 1 mmol of potassium is lost from the body per gram of resin administered. It can cause disturbances in electrolytes other than potassium, such as calcium and magnesium. For this reason, patients' electrolytes are closely monitored during treatment with sodium polystyrene sulfonate. Kayexalate has been implicated in the development of intestinal necrosis, especially when used with the cathartic sorbitol. This condition may be fatal. Kayexalate should not be used in patients who do not have normal bowel function and should be discontinued in patients who develop constipation. Other adverse effects include hypernatremia, hypokalemia, hypocalcemia, hypomagnesemia, nausea, and vomiting. Drug interactions include antacids and laxatives, which should be avoided. It is typically dosed in multiples of 15 to 30 grams until the desired effect on serum potassium occurs. Onset of action varies from 2 to 12 hours and is generally faster with the oral route than with rectal administration. It is available in a powder for reconstitution, an oral suspension, and a rectal suspension. For use during pregnancy, the potential benefits of Kayexalate must be considered relative to the risk to the fetus.

skin; dry, sticky mucous membranes; increased thirst; temperature elevation; water retention (edema); hypertension; and decreased or absent urination.

Mechanism of Action and Drug Effects

As one of the body's electrolytes, sodium performs many physiological roles necessary for the normal functions of the body. It is the major cation in ECF and is principally involved in the control of water distribution, fluid and electrolyte balance, and osmotic pressure of body fluids. Sodium also participates along with both chloride and bicarbonate in the regulation of acid–base balance. Chloride, the major extracellular anion (negatively charged substance), closely complements the physiological action of sodium. Sodium is also capable of causing diuresis.

Indications

Sodium is administered primarily in the treatment or prevention of sodium depletion when dietary measures have proved inadequate. Sodium chloride is the primary salt used for this purpose. Mild hyponatremia is usually treated with the oral administration of sodium chloride tablets or fluid restriction. Pronounced sodium depletion is treated with IV sodium chloride or lactated

Ringer's solution. These drugs are discussed earlier in this chapter.

Hypertonic saline (3% NaCl) is sometimes used to correct severe hyponatremia. It is considered a high-risk drug because giving it too rapidly or in too high a dose can cause a syndrome known as *central pontine myelinolysis*, also known as *osmotic demyelination syndrome*. This syndrome can cause irreversible brain stem damage.

A new class of drugs for the treatment of euvolemic hyponatremia is the dual arginine vasopressin (AVP) V1A and V2 receptor antagonists. The drug in this class is tolvaptan (Samsca®). This class of drugs is often referred to as *vaptans*. Specific information on tolvaptan is listed under its drug profile.

Contraindications

The only usual contraindications to the use of sodium replacement products are known drug allergy to a specific product and hypernatremia.

Adverse Effects

The oral administration of sodium chloride can cause gastric upset consisting of nausea, vomiting, and cramps.

DRUG PROFILES

sodium chloride

Sodium chloride is primarily used as a replacement electrolyte for either the prevention or treatment of sodium loss. It is also used as a diluent for the infusion of compatible drugs and in the assessment of kidney function after a fluid challenge. Sodium chloride is contraindicated in patients who are hypersensitive to it. It is available in many IV preparations and in oral form as 650-mg tablets. For use during pregnancy, the potential benefits of sodium chloride must be considered relative to the risk to the fetus.

PHARMACOKINETICS

Route	Onset of Action	Peak Plasma Concentration	Elimination Half-Life	Duration of Action
IV	Immediate	Rapid	Unknown	Variable

tolvaptan

Tolvaptan (Samsca) is a nonpeptide dual arginine vasopressin (AVP) V1A and V2 receptor antagonist. It inhibits the effects of arginine vasopressin, also known as *antidiuretic hormone*, on receptors in the kidneys. It is specifically indicated for the treatment of hospitalized patients with **euvolemic hyponatremia**, or low serum sodium levels at normal water volumes. Adverse effects associated with the use of tolvaptan may include dry mouth, thirst, constipation, and polyuria. Closely monitor serum sodium levels during treatment, as overly rapid increases in serum sodium levels have been associated with potentially permanent adverse events, including osmotic demyelination syndrome. Several potential drug–drug interactions have been identified. Tolvaptan is metabolized by the hepatic enzyme CYP3A4; coadministration drugs that inhibit this enzyme (including but not limited to ketoconazole, itraconazole, clarithromycin, ritonavir, and indinavir) may increase serum levels. Tolvaptan is available as 15-mg and 30-mg tablets.

PHARMACOKINETICS

Route	Onset of Action	Peak Plasma Concentration	Elimination Half-Life	Duration of Action
PO	2–4 hr	4–8 hr	12 hr	24 hr

Venous phlebitis can be a consequence of its parenteral administration.

Toxicity and Management of Overdose

Hypernatremia leads to hypertension, edema, thirst, tachycardia, weakness, convulsions, and possibly coma. Treatment consists of increased fluid intake and dietary restrictions. In more serious cases, diuretics may be required to enhance urinary sodium excretion. IV administration of dextrose in water solution (e.g., 5% dextrose in water [D_5W] or 10% dextrose in water [$D_{10}W$]) may also be helpful by producing both intravascular sodium dilution and enhanced urine volume output.

Interactions

Sodium is not known to interact significantly with any drugs.

Dosages

Fluid and electrolyte therapy involves replacing any deficit losses and providing maintenance levels for specific patient requirements. Accordingly, specific dosage amounts of fluids or electrolytes depend on several clinical factors, as follows:

- Specific patient losses
- Efficacy of patient physiological systems involved in fluid and electrolyte metabolism, especially adrenal, cardiovascular, and kidney functioning
- Current drug therapy for pathological conditions that complicate the amount and duration of replacement
- Selection of oral or parenteral replacement formulations

Suggested dosage guidelines for sodium chloride with subsequent adjustments are 1 to 2 g administered orally several times a day or parenteral administration of 1 L of sodium chloride.

NURSING PROCESS

Assessment

For fluid replacement, patients' needs vary. Any medications or solutions ordered must be given exactly as prescribed and without substitution. However, never take an order from a health care provider at face value without confirming it against authoritative resources (e.g., current drug reference guides, *Compendium of Pharmaceuticals and Specialties* [CPS], a nursing pharmacology textbook, manufacturer's drug inserts) or speaking with a pharmacist. It is important to remember that the nurse is responsible for making sure that the drug therapy administration process—beginning with the assessment phase of the nursing process through to evaluation—is accurate and safe, meeting professional standards of care.

To assist in the development of a thorough assessment process, a brief review of the various solutions is needed. Parenterally administered hydrating and hypotonic solutions, such as 0.45% NaCl/D_5W, are used primarily for the prevention or treatment of dehydration. D_5W alone in an IV bag is considered isotonic but acts as a hypotonic solution once in the bloodstream. Isotonic solutions (e.g., 0.9% NaCl [normal saline]) are customarily used to augment extracellular volume in patients experiencing blood loss or severe vomiting. Isotonic NaCl is also used as diluting fluid for blood transfusions because D_5W results in hemolysis of RBCs (in transfusions). Hypertonic solutions (3% sodium chloride) are used for replacement of fluids and electrolytes in specific situations (see earlier discussion of hypertonic solutions).

After verifying all health care providers' orders and checking for accuracy and completeness (as with all drugs), assess the solution or product, the patient, and the IV site (if applicable). Also assess the following prior to administering IV infusions of fluids and electrolytes: the solution to be infused, infusion equipment, infusion rate of solution, concentration of parenteral solution, related mathematical calculations, laboratory values (e.g., sodium, chloride, potassium), and parenteral compatibilities. More specific assessment of the patient who is to receive a parenteral replacement solution needs to focus on gathering information about the patient's medical history, including diseases of the GI, kidney, cardiac, and liver systems. Obtain a medication history, including a list of prescription drugs, over-the-counter medications, and natural health products. Also take a dietary history including specific dietary habits and recall of all foods consumed during the previous 24 hours. Assess fluid volume and electrolyte status (through laboratory testing and measurement of urine specific gravity, vital signs, and intake and output). The skin and mucous membranes also reflect a patient's hydration status; assess skin turgor and rebound elasticity of skin on the glabella, the most prominent part of the forehead between the eyebrows, or under the clavicle. Well-hydrated skin in this area is resilient and returns quickly to its original position, while poorly hydrated skin retains the "tent" shape of the pinched skin. For infants, the area of the abdomen near the umbilicus is used to assess skin turgor. Document the findings as "immediate" rebound or "delayed" rebound. Count the number of seconds that the patient's skin stays in the pinched-up position; normal return is immediate; return within 2 seconds suggests moderate dehydration; more than 2 seconds before return indicates severe dehydration; and skin folding that persists for several seconds is described as *tenting*.

Essential to assessment is knowledge of the normal range for potassium, usually 3.5 to 5 mmol/L. Serum potassium levels below 3.5 mmol/L, or hypokalemia, may result in a variety of problems, such as heart irregularities and muscle weakness. Early symptoms of hypokalemia include anorexia, hypotension, lethargy, confusion, muscle weakness, and nausea. Late symptoms of hypokalemia include cardiac irregularities, neuropathies, and paralytic ileus. Avoid potassium supplementation or use it with extreme caution in patients taking ACE inhibitors or potassium-sparing diuretics (such as spironolactone). These drugs are associated with adverse effects of hyperkalemia and, if given with potassium supplementation, could worsen hyperkalemia and possibly result in severe heart dysrhythmias. Other concerns regarding contrain-

dications with potassium include severe kidney disease, untreated Addison's disease, severe tissue trauma, and acute dehydration. Oral potassium supplements are irritants and may be ulcerogenic; thus, perform a thorough GI tract assessment. If the patient has a history of ulcers or GI bleeding and oral supplementation is prescribed, contact the health care provider for further instructions.

The range of serum potassium levels defined as normal often varies depending on the institution and the health care provider. For identification and treatment of hyperkalemia, the normal range of potassium must be established. Realize that potassium levels of 5.3 mmol/L may be identified as the threshold for being considered abnormally high by some laboratories, whereas other laboratories may categorize 5 mmol/L as being abnormally high. Be sure to check hospital policy and laboratory guidelines for normal ranges and report any elevations (or decreases) in serum potassium. However, a serum level exceeding 5.5 mmol/L is considered by most sources to be toxic and dangerous to the patient; report this finding to the health care provider immediately. With close monitoring of patients, the dangerous effects of hyperkalemia (i.e., heart dysrhythmias) will be prevented or identified early and treated appropriately to prevent potentially life-threatening complications.

Venous access is an important issue with parenteral potassium supplementation because the vein can be irritated if infiltration occurs or if the solution has not been mixed thoroughly. The following are some important considerations regarding assessment and peripheral venous access (for potassium, sodium, fluid, and any other type of medication given by the IV route): (1) Assess the overall condition of the veins prior to selecting a site. (2) Try to use distal veins first. (3) Know the purpose of administering potassium and other electrolytes. (4) Calculate and set the rate, as ordered, for the infusion. (5) Know the anticipated duration of therapy. (6) Know any restrictions imposed by the patient's history. For example, in a patient who is postmastectomy with lymph node dissection, the affected arm must not be used. Likewise, the affected arm of a patient with a stroke must not be used. Limb circulation may be inadequate in these situations and lead to edema and other complications if it is used as a venous access site (see Lab Values Related to Drug Therapy: Serum Potassium).

Sodium is another electrolyte that is an ingredient in various IV replacement solutions. Hyponatremia, or serum sodium below 135 mmol/L, if not resolved with dietary or oral intake, may need to be treated with parenteral infusions. Signs and symptoms of hyponatremia include lethargy, hypotension, stomach cramps, vomiting, and diarrhea. Carefully assess venous access sites because of possible irritation of the vein and subsequent phlebitis. If replacement to correct hyponatremic states is overzealous, the result may be hypernatremia with fluid overload, edema, and dyspnea. Assess baseline vital signs, hydration status of the skin and mucous membranes, and level of consciousness for safe

LAB VALUES RELATED TO DRUG THERAPY

Serum Potassium

Laboratory Test	Normal Ranges	Rationale for Assessment
Serum potassium	3.5–5 mmol/L	The main function of potassium is the regulation of water and electrolyte content in the cell. Potassium also assists in the cellular metabolism of carbohydrates and proteins. A serum level less than 3.5 mmol/L is known as hypokalemia and a small decrease in potassium levels may have profound effects, including lethargy, muscle weakness, hypotension, and cardiac dysrhythmias. A serum potassium level greater than 5 mmol/L is known as hyperkalemia and is manifested by muscle weakness, paresthesia, paralysis, and cardiac rhythm abnormalities. Knowing normal ranges allows quicker identification of abnormalities and thus more timely management.

IV replacement and prevention of further complications. Contraindications to sodium replacement include elevated serum sodium levels, edema, and hypertension.

Hypernatremia also requires careful assessment. Manifestations of hypernatremia include red, flushed skin; dry, sticky mucous membranes; increased thirst; temperature elevation; water retention (edema); hypertension; and decreased or absent urination. Identifying any precipitating events, medical concerns, and risky situations is important to finding timely solutions. The populations at risk for hypernatremia include older adults, patients with kidney and cardiovascular diseases, those who are receiving sodium supplements or who have increased sodium intake, and those with decreased fluid intake. Perform an assessment of cautions, contraindications, and drug interactions.

Albumin and other colloids (e.g., dextran) have associated cautions, contraindications, and drug interactions that need to be assessed. Dextrans and other colloids are rarely used in practice anymore largely because there has been no demonstrated benefit over crystalloids and they are expensive to use. Contraindications include heart failure, severe anemia, and renal insufficiency. The rationale is that these products cause fluids to shift from interstitial to intravascular spaces. This shift places more strain on a patient's heart and respiratory systems. Assess the patient's hematocrit, hemoglobin levels, and serum protein levels. Assess the patient's blood pressure, pulse rate, respiratory status, and intake and output. Document and report any abnormal assessment findings (e.g., dyspnea, edema) immediately.

Fluid infusions may also include the giving of blood or blood components. Obtain a thorough history regarding any transfusions received previously and the patient's response. The patient's informed consent should be obtained prior to administering blood products (see Legal and Ethical Principles). Report any history of adverse reactions to transfusions or problems with packed red blood cells or fresh frozen plasma to the health care provider, and document the nature of these reactions. Assess the status and size of venous access areas. Check the patient's laboratory values (e.g., hematocrit, hemoglobin, white blood cells [WBCs], RBCs, platelets, clotting factors). Note baseline vital signs, blood pressure, pulse rate, respiratory rate, and temperature before infusing blood or blood products. Even the patient's general appearance, energy levels, ability to carry out activities of daily living (ADLs), and colour of extremities are important to note. Assess for any potential drug interactions, specifically with aspirin and calcium, as these may potentially alter clotting. During the infusion of blood components, constantly assess for the occurrence of a febrile nonhemolytic transfusion reaction. This occurs as a result of cytokines from leukocytes in RBCs or platelets, with the common symptoms of fever (defined as an elevation of 1°C), chills, or rigour. An allergic reaction is IgE mediated. It occurs because of a hypersensitivity to allergens in the transfused blood and manifests as a rash, urticaria, or pruritus. An anaphylactic reaction may also occur and is associated with anti-IgA in recipients who are IgA deficient. Acute hemolytic transfusion reaction is the most frequent and severe reaction and is most often the result of ABO incompatibility resulting in hemolysis of the RBCs. Assess for hemoglobinuria, hyperkalemia, hypocalcemia, hypothermia, and iron overload. Transfusion-related acute lung injury results in pulmonary edema in the absence of circulatory overload. Delayed immune-mediated reactions include a delayed hemolytic transfusion reaction, transfusion associated–graft-versus-host disease, and post-transfusion purpura.

Transfusion reactions require immediate recognition, laboratory investigation, and clinical management. When a transfusion reaction is suspected during blood administration, the best practice is to stop the transfusion and keep the IV line open with 0.9% normal saline. Then, check to make sure that the blood unit label and the patient's identification match to ensure that the "right" blood unit was administered to the "right" patient. In most cases, the residual contents of the blood component container should be returned the blood bank, together with a freshly collected blood sample from the patient, and a transfusion reaction investigation should

LEGAL & ETHICAL PRINCIPLES

Blood Transfusions and Informed Consent

In Canada, informed consent is required for the administration of all blood components and products and is required for hospital accreditation. The patient (or substitute decision maker) is to be informed of the type of blood component or blood product to be administered, the associated risks and benefits, as well as alternatives to transfusion if appropriate. The exception would be an emergency situation where treatment is necessary to preserve the life or health of the patient and consent cannot be obtained (if the patient is unconscious or otherwise unable to consent); in this type of case, the health care provider may administer blood products deemed essential to preserve the life or health of the patient.

The information should be presented in a language that the patient understands and in a way that allows for questions and provides the patient with sufficient time to assimilate all information and ask additional questions. Patients have the right to refuse blood products and should be informed of the risks of refusal. In Canada, where the population is culturally diverse, it is the ethical responsibility of health care providers to respect the cultural practices of patients while meeting legal and professional obligations.

Patients who are Jehovah's Witnesses are forbidden blood transfusions, based on their interpretation of the Bible. This stricture may include whole blood, RBCs, WBCs, platelets, and plasma, while other products such as albumin may be acceptable.

Always refer to the agency-specific policy about acquiring and documenting informed consent and also what to do if a patient refuses. Exact provisions will vary by province and territory.

---

be initiated. Always follow agency policy for the procedure following a suspected blood transfusion reaction.

In summary, safety and caution are top priorities when patients receive any blood product or fluid and electrolyte replacement. Deficient or excess fluid and electrolyte levels may pose tremendous risks to patients. Thorough assessment is crucial to patient safety. With many patients receiving therapies in the home setting, there is additional accountability and responsibility for performing skillful and thorough assessment before, during, and after therapy.

Nursing Diagnoses

- Risk for falls related to fluid and electrolyte losses
- Risk for imbalanced fluid volume related to drug-induced fluid deficits and excesses
- Risk for injury related to complications of the transfusion or infusion of blood products, blood components, or related agents

Planning

Goals

- Patient will remain free from falls and injury.
- Patient will regain balanced fluid volume status.
- Patient will remain free from injury related to complications of blood product infusion.

Expected Patient Outcomes

- Patient minimizes the risk for falls through careful actions.
  - Patient changes positions slowly and ambulates with assistance until symptoms (e.g., dizziness, lightheadedness) have subsided.

- Patient regains fluid volume status through replacement of up to 2 to 3 L/day of water, unless contraindicated.
  - Patient receives adequate fluid volume infusions with improvement of fluid and electrolyte status.
  - Patient's urinary output is at least 30 mL/hr.
  - Patient reports any dizziness, lethargy, confusion, disorientation, muscle weakness, irregular heart rhythm, or abdominal cramping.
- Patient remains free from injury during infusion of blood products or components.
  - Patient reports any shortness of breath, irregular heart rate or palpitations, or feelings of increased body temperature.
  - Patient's laboratory values (e.g., hemoglobin, hematocrit, RBCs) return to normal levels.

Implementation

Continued monitoring of the patient during fluid or electrolyte therapy is crucial to ensure safe and effective treatment. It is also important to continue monitoring to identify adverse effects early and to prevent complications related to either overzealous treatment or undertreatment. During replacement therapy, serum electrolyte levels need to remain within normal ranges. Educate patients at risk for volume deficits (especially older adults) about this risk and about the effect of a hot, humid environment on physiological functioning and the danger of exacerbation by excessive perspiration. Water is at the crux of every metabolic reaction that occurs within the body, and deficits will negatively impact physiological reactions and alter the composition of fluids and electrolytes. For any age group, staying hydrated at all times is a preventive measure.

With parenteral dosing, monitor infusion rates as well as the appearance of the fluid or solution (i.e., potassium and saline solutions should be clear, whereas albumin should be brown, clear, and viscous). Frequently monitor the IV site, as per agency policy and nursing standards of care, for evidence of infiltration (e.g., swelling, coolness to the touch around the IV site, no or decreased flow rate, and no blood return from the IV catheter) or thrombophlebitis (e.g., swelling, redness, heat and pain at the IV site). Volume overload, drug toxicity, fever, infection, and emboli are other complications of IV therapy.

With the administration of any of the discussed drugs per the IV route, maintain a steady and even flow rate to prevent complications. Infusion pumps are used for IV administration, particularly of potassium. Ensure that infusion rates follow the HCP's orders, and recheck all calculations for accuracy. Check the IV site, tubing, IV bag, and fluids or solutions as well as expiration dates. Always behave in a prudent, safe, and thorough manner when administering fluids and electrolyte solutions. Remember that older adults and children have an increased sensitivity to fluids and electrolytes.

With the various IV solutions, knowing their osmolality and concentrations is important to their safe use. Administration of isotonic solutions (e.g., 0.9% sodium chloride, lactated Ringer's solution) requires constant monitoring of vital signs and observation for possible fluid overload during and after therapy, especially in those at particular risk or those with heart failure. Hypertonic solutions are used rarely because of the risk of cellular dehydration and vascular volume overload. These solutions are also associated with phlebitis if IV infiltration or extravasation occurs in the peripheral veins. Therefore, if ordered, administer these solutions through a larger bore vein (e.g., central line), but only with close monitoring of the patient's vital signs and cardiac status.

For patients who are at risk for hypokalemia, provide educational materials and teaching to encourage consumption of certain foods high in potassium. The minimal daily requirement for potassium is 4 700 mg for adults and 3 000 to 4 500 mg for children between the ages of 1 and 14. Information on foods containing potassium should be shared with patients; these foods include some of the following: one medium-sized banana contains 422 mg of potassium, a 250 mL glass of orange juice contains 387 mg; and 177 mL of yogurt contains 362 mg. Conversely, if a patient is already hyperkalemic, advise the patient to avoid these food items (see Patient Teaching Tips for more information). If potassium levels do not increase with dietary changes, supplementation may be needed. Oral preparations of potassium, rather than parenteral dosage forms, are preferred whenever possible. Prepare the oral dosage forms per the manufacturer's insert or per policy and standard of care. Generally, oral forms of potassium (15 mL) should be dissolved completely in 100 to 250 mL of cold water, juice, or another liquid. Often, orange juice is used as the taste is bitter. Potassium should be taken with food or immediately after meals to minimize GI distress or irritation and to prevent too rapid absorption. Extended-release forms may still result in gastric upset and lead to ulcer development (being ulcerogenic). With oral supplementation, the safest and most effective intervention is frequent and close monitoring for reports of nausea, vomiting, abdominal pain, or bleeding (such as the occurrence of melena [blood in the stool] or hematemesis [blood in the vomitus]). If abnormalities are noted, continue to monitor vital signs and other parameters, and report findings to the HCP immediately. Monitor serum levels of potassium during therapy as well.

Hyperkalemia is treated with sodium polystyrene sulfonate (Kayexalate). It is used only in specific situations and under close monitoring of the patient and serum potassium, sodium, calcium, and magnesium levels. If it is given orally (or via nasogastric tube), elevate the head of the patient's bed to prevent aspiration. Each dose of sodium polystyrene sulfonate resin should be given as a suspension in a small quantity of water (20 to 100 mL depending on the dose, or 3 to 4 mL per gm of resin). There is potential for intestinal necrosis associated with the use of sodium polystyrene sulfonate (see earlier discussion of sodium polystyrene sulfonate). It is recommended that it not be administered with sorbitol because of the connection of these two drugs with the potentially fatal condition of colonic intestinal necrosis. If the oral form is given, do not give it with antacids or laxatives. If sodium polystyrene sulfonate is given by the rectal route, a retention enema is used. Follow the medication orders carefully, and expect that more than one dose may be needed. The enema must be retained as long as possible and followed by an HCP-prescribed cleansing enema. Usually, an initial cleansing enema is prescribed, and then the resin solution is administered. If leakage occurs, elevating the patient's hips on a pillow or placing the patient in a knee-chest position may be helpful.

Potassium chloride is the salt commonly used for IV infusions. Caution should be taken with potassium chloride use to avoid overdosage, as this can lead to cardiac arrest. IV dosage forms of potassium must always be given in a DILUTED form. There is no use or place for undiluted potassium because it is associated with cardiac arrest. Therefore, parenteral forms of potassium need to be diluted properly. Most potassium infusions are prepared by the manufacturer (e.g., 40 mmol/L potassium chloride in 0.9% sodium chloride injection); however, it is still imperative to double-check the order, amount of diluent, and concentration of potassium to diluent. Never assume that whatever was premixed is 100% correct, because the nurse is ultimately responsible for whatever is administered. Additionally, give diluted potassium only when there is adequate urine output of at least 30 mL/hr (to prevent toxicity). Manufacturer instructions and policy protocols generally recommend that IV solutions be given at concentrations of less than 40 mmol/L of potassium and at a rate not exceeding 20 mmol/hr. Toxicity or overdosage of potassium (hyperkalemia) is manifested by cardiac rhythm irregularities, muscle spasms, paresthesia, and possible cardiac arrest. As previously discussed, IV potassium is to be given no faster than 10 mmol/hr to those patients not on cardiac monitoring. In patients who are critically ill and on cardiac monitors, a rate of 20 mmol/hr or more may be used. Do not add potassium chloride to an already existing IV solution because the exact concentration cannot be accurately calculated and overdosage or toxicity may result. Make sure that all IV fluids are labelled appropriately and documented, as with any medication. An infusion pump or other rate-limiting device must always be used when administering IV solutions of potassium chloride to prevent unintentional bolus doses of potassium chloride. Potassium chloride must never be administered by IV push or IV bolus. Treatment of severe hyperkalemia caused by IV administration is through use of IV dextrose solution with insulin and possibly salbutamol. These drugs work by leading to a rapid shifting of potassium ions intracellularly, thereby reducing serum potassium concentration. Dialysis is also used to remove excess potassium.

Replacement of sodium is associated with similar concerns about dosing and route of administration to those of potassium chloride. When a patient is only mildly depleted, an increase in oral intake of sodium needs to be tried. Food items high in sodium include ketchup, mustard, cured meats, cheeses, potato chips, peanut butter, popcorn, and table salt. In some situations, salt tablets may be necessary. If the patient is given salt tablets, it is important to advise the patient to drink up to 3 000 mL/24 hr, unless contraindicated. If the sodium deficit requires IV replacement, venous access issues and drip rate are important (see previous discussion regarding IV infusion and IV sites). Hypertonic saline (3% NaCl) is sometimes used for severe hyponatremia but this use is considered a high risk due to the possible occurrence of osmotic demyelination syndrome. This occurs if the 3% NaCl is given too fast or in too high amounts; this results in irreversible brainstem damage. Other treatment of hyponatremia includes the use of orally administered tolvaptan (Samsca). This drug is indicated for euvolemic hyponatremia (see earlier discussion of sodium). Administer tolvaptan as ordered while monitoring serum sodium levels. Hypernatremia is treated with increased fluid intake and dietary restrictions, so the nurse must provide thorough and complete patient education. IV dextrose in water (D_5W or $D_{10}W$) may be indicated and helps by creating intravascular sodium dilution and enhanced urine volume output with sodium excretion.

Always carry out IV infusion of albumin and other colloids slowly and cautiously. Carefully monitor the patient to prevent fluid overload and possible heart failure, especially in patients at particular risk. Fluid overload is evidenced by shortness of breath, crackles at the bases of the lungs, decreased pulse oximeter readings, edema of dependent areas, and increase in weight (see previous parameters). Determine serum hematocrit and hemoglobin values in advance of therapy, as well as during and after therapy, so that any dilutional effects can be determined. For example, if a patient has received albumin and other colloids too quickly, and hypervolemia results, the patient's hemoglobin and hematocrit may actually be decreased. This decrease would be caused by dilutional factor because of too much volume in relation to the concentration of solutes. Clinically, the patient would appear to be anemic, but in fact the deficit would be attributed to the increase in volume. It is also important to remember that albumin needs to be given at room temperature.

For infusion of blood, always check the expiration date of the blood and blood components to make sure it is not outdated. Under NO circumstances should outdated blood be used. Blood is perishable, and has a 42-day "best before" date. Platelets are viable for 5 days. Policies at most health care agencies require that blood and blood products be double-checked by two registered nurses *before* the blood is hung and infused. This is important to prevent a mix-up in blood types. Blood types must always be a major concern because of the possible complications that can occur, some life threatening, if the wrong blood type is given or if the blood is given to the wrong person. The "rights" of drug administration are crucial in all that nurses do with medications, and administering blood is no exception.

When blood and blood products are infused, it is important to patient safety to document all vital signs and related parameters before, during, and after administration of the blood product component (e.g., packed red blood cells, fresh frozen plasma), or solution. Monitor vital signs, and frequently record these during and after administration. A transfusion reaction would most likely be manifested by the occurrence of the following: apprehension, restlessness, flushed skin, increased pulse and respirations, dyspnea, rash, joint or lower back pain, swelling, fever and chills (a febrile reaction beginning 1 hour after the start of administration and possibly lasting up to 10 hours), nausea, weakness, and jaundice. Report these signs and symptoms to the HCP immediately, and (regardless of when the reaction occurs) stop the blood or product, keeping the IV line patent with isotonic NS solution infusing at a slow rate. Always follow the facility's protocol for transfusion reactions.

In summary, encourage patients receiving any type of fluid or electrolyte substance, colloid, or blood component to immediately report unusual adverse effects to their HCPs. Reports may include chest pain, dizziness, weakness, and shortness of breath.

Evaluation

The therapeutic response to fluid, electrolyte, and blood or blood component therapy includes normalization of fluid volume and laboratory values, including RBCs, WBCs, and hemoglobin, hematocrit, and sodium and potassium levels. In addition to a review of these

CASE STUDY

Fluid and Electrolyte Replacement

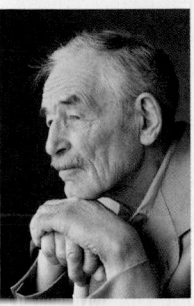

Ivan, an 85-year-old retired chemist, seems somewhat confused when his daughter comes home from work. When she brings him to the emergency department, his blood pressure is 90/62 mm Hg, his heart rate is 114 beats per minute, and his skin is dry but cool. His daughter says that he seems "much weaker" than usual, and he is unable to answer questions clearly. His daughter reports that he has "lost his appetite" lately and has not taken in much food or drink. The nurse starts an IV infusion of 0.9% sodium chloride (NS) at 100 mL/hr via a gravity drip infusion.

1. What do you think is Ivan's main medical problem at this time?

The emergency department is extremely busy, and when the nurse returns, she is shocked to see that almost the entire 500-mL bag of NS has infused within an hour's time.

2. What will the nurse do first? What will the nurse watch for at this time?

3. When monitoring Ivan's fluid status, which indicators will the nurse consider the most reliable?

Twenty-four hours after his admission, Ivan is much less confused and is able to transfer to a chair for lunch without much difficulty. He is receiving 5% dextrose/0.45% NS with 20 mmol of potassium chloride, at a rate of 75 mL/hr via an infusion pump. His daughter notices that the area above the IV insertion site is red, and Ivan reports that the area is "quite sore."

4. What is the possible problem with the IV line? What needs to be done at this time?

For answers, see http://evolve.elsevier.com/Canada/Lilley/pharmacology/.

laboratory values, evaluation of the patient's heart, respiratory, musculoskeletal, and GI functioning is also important. Therapeutic effects include improved energy levels, and tolerance for ADLs should return to normal. Skin colour will improve, and there will be improved shortness of breath as well as minimal to no dyspnea, chest pain, weakness, or fatigue. Correct treatment of blood volume problems will be evidenced by a return of laboratory values to normal, improved vital signs, an increase in energy, and near-normal oxygen saturation levels. The therapeutic response to albumin therapy includes an elevation of blood pressure, decreased edema, and increased serum albumin levels. Frequently monitor for adverse effects of any of these drugs and solutions, and check for distended neck veins, shortness of breath, anxiety, insomnia, expiratory crackles, frothy and blood-tinged sputum, and cyanosis (indicative of fluid volume overload).

PATIENT TEACHING TIPS

❖ As needed, educate patients about the differences in the signs and symptoms of hyponatremia and hypernatremia. Hyponatremia is manifested by lethargy, hypotension, stomach cramps, vomiting, diarrhea, and seizures. Some of the causes of hyponatremia include excessive perspiration, occurring during hot weather or physical work, and prolonged diarrhea or vomiting. Hypernatremia is associated with symptoms of water retention (edema); hypertension; red, flushed skin; dry, sticky mucous membranes; increased thirst; temperature elevation; and decreased or absent urination. The most common cause is poor renal excretion as a result of kidney malfunction. Inadequate water consumption and dehydration are other causes.

❖ Educate patients about the early symptoms of hypokalemia, such as anorexia, hypotension, lethargy, confusion, nausea, and muscle weakness. Late symptoms include cardiac dysrhythmias (the patient may feel palpitations or shortness of breath), neuropathies, and paralytic ileus.

❖ Share the symptoms of hyperkalemia with patients, including muscle weakness, paresthesia, paralysis, and cardiac rhythm abnormalities.

❖ Provide patients with adequate and appropriate information about how to take oral potassium chloride. Encourage patients to take oral doses with food or a snack, and tell them to report any GI upset or abdominal pain (indicative of gastric irritation from the oral potassium) to their health care providers immediately. Educate patients about potential drug interactions, such with as potassium-sparing diuretics and ACE inhibitors, because their concurrent use may produce hyperkalemia.

❖ Educate patients regarding foods high in potassium, including bananas, oranges, apricots, dates, raisins, broccoli, green beans, potatoes, tomatoes, meats, fish, wheat bread, and legumes.

Continued

PATIENT TEACHING TIPS—cont'd

❖ Advise patients that sustained-release capsules and tablets must be swallowed whole and should not be crushed, chewed, or allowed to dissolve in the mouth. Each prescribed dose is to be taken with a meal and a full glass of water. If a patient has difficulty swallowing the whole tablet, and if approved by the health care provider, the patient can break the tablet in half and take each half separately, drinking approximately half a glass of water (115 mL) with each half and taking the entire dose within a few minutes. The patient must take the full dose and not save partial dosages of potassium for later. Another option is to take the extended-release dosage form and place the whole tablet in 115 mL of water (recommended as the fluid for mixing this form). Instruct patients to allow 2 minutes for the tablet to disintegrate, stir for 30 seconds, and then drink the dose immediately. After this, adding 30 mL of water to the glass, swirling it, and then drinking the residual will allow adequate dosing. A straw may be used.

❖ Encourage patients to report any difficulty in swallowing, painful swallowing, or feeling as if the capsule or tablet is getting stuck in the throat. Other serious adverse effects that need to be reported include vomiting of coffee ground–like material, stomach or abdominal pain or swelling, and black tarry stools.

❖ Educate patients that salt substitutes contain potassium. Another alternative must be recommended if patients are hyperkalemic.

❖ If a patient is receiving IV potassium, tell the patient to report any feelings of irritation (e.g., burning) at the IV site.

❖ Educate patients about the safe use of salt tablets, and instruct them to take them as prescribed. Salt tablets must be taken with adequate fluid intake.

KEY POINTS

❖ Total body water is divided into intracellular (inside the cell) and extracellular (outside the cell) compartments. Fluid volume outside the cells is either in the plasma (intravascular volume) or between the tissues, cells, or organs.

❖ Colloids are large protein particles that cannot leak out of the blood vessels. Because of their greater concentration inside blood vessels, fluid is pulled into the blood vessels. Examples of colloids include albumin, hetastarch, and dextran. Administer albumin with caution because of the high risk for hypervolemia and possible heart failure. Monitor intake and output, weights, heart and breath sounds, and appropriate laboratory values.

❖ Blood products are the only fluids that are able to carry oxygen because they are the only fluids that contain hemoglobin. Patients will show improved energy and increasing tolerance for ADLs as a result of treatments with blood products. Pulse oximeter readings will also show improved readings.

❖ Dehydration may be hypotonic, resulting from the loss of salt; hypertonic, resulting from fever with perspiration; or isotonic, resulting from diarrhea or vomiting. Each form of dehydration is treated differently. Carefully assess intake and output as well as skin turgor, urine specific gravity, and blood values of potassium, sodium, and chloride.

❖ Hypertonic solutions must be used cautiously and given slowly because of the risk for hypervolemia from overzealous replacement.

❖ Early symptoms of hypokalemia include anorexia, hypotension, lethargy, confusion, nausea, and muscle weakness. Late symptoms include cardiac dysrhythmias (the patient may feel palpitations or shortness of breath), neuropathies, and paralytic ileus.

❖ Hyponatremia is manifested by lethargy, hypotension, stomach cramps, vomiting, diarrhea, and seizures. Hypernatremia is associated with symptoms of water retention (edema); hypertension; red, flushed skin; dry, sticky mucous membranes; increased thirst; temperature elevation; and decreased or absent urination.

❖ With administration of blood products, measurement of vital signs and frequent monitoring of the patient before, during, and after infusions are critical to patient safety. Blood products must be given only with normal saline (0.9% sodium chloride), because the solution of D_5W results in hemolysis of RBCs.

EXAMINATION REVIEW QUESTIONS

1. Which action by the nurse is most appropriate for the patient receiving an infusion of packed red blood cells?
a. Flush the IV line with normal saline before the blood is added to the infusion.
b. Flush the IV line with dextrose before the blood is added to the infusion.
c. Check the patient's vital signs once the infusion is completed.
d. Anticipate that flushed skin and fever are expected reactions to a blood transfusion.

2. When preparing an IV solution that contains potassium, which would the nurse know is a contraindication to the potassium infusion?
a. Diarrhea
b. Serum sodium level of 145 mmol/L
c. Serum potassium of 5.6 mmol/L
d. Dehydration

EXAMINATION REVIEW QUESTIONS—cont'd

3. When assessing a patient who is about to receive an albumin infusion, which would the nurse know is a contraindication for albumin?
a. Acute liver failure
b. Heart failure
c. Severe burns
d. Fluid-volume deficit

4. The nurse is preparing an infusion for a patient who has a deficiency in clotting factors. Which type of infusion is most appropriate for this patient?
a. Albumin 5%
b. Packed red blood cells
c. Whole blood
d. Fresh frozen plasma

5. While monitoring a patient who is receiving an infusion of a crystalloid solution, the nurse will monitor for which potential problem?
a. Bradycardia
b. Hypotension
c. Decreased skin turgor
d. Fluid overload

6. The nurse is administering an IV solution that contains potassium chloride to a patient in the critical care unit who has a severely decreased serum potassium level. Which action(s) by the nurse are appropriate? (Select all that apply.)
a. Administer the potassium by slow IV bolus.
b. Administer the potassium at a rate no faster than 20 mmol/h.
c. Monitor the patient's cardiac rhythm with a heart monitor.
d. Use an infusion pump for the administration of IV potassium chloride.
e. Administer the potassium IV push.

7. The order reads: "Infuse 1 000 mL of normal saline over the next 8 hours." The IV tubing has a drop factor of 15 gtt/mL. Calculate the mL/hr rate, and calculate the drops per minute setting for the IV tubing with this gravity infusion.

Answers: 1. a, 2. c, 3. b, 4. d, 5. d, 6. b, c, d, 7. 125 mL/hr; 31 gtt/min

CRITICAL THINKING ACTIVITIES

1. After having vomiting and diarrhea from the flu for the previous 24 hours, a patient is admitted for treatment of dehydration. The nurse knows that the priority action is to administer which type of fluid? Explain your answer.

2. During a transfusion of packed red blood cells, the patient reports that his back is starting to "hurt" and he feels anxious. His temperature is 37.1°C. What is the nurse's priority action?

3. The latest potassium level of a patient with hyperkalemia is 6.1 mmol/L, and the health care provider has ordered one 30-g dose of sodium polystyrene sulfonate via enema. The patient questions the nurse when he hears he is to receive an enema, saying, "How in the world is an enema going to help me?" What is the nurse's best answer?

For answers, see http://evolve.elsevier.com/Canada/Lilley/pharmacology/.

Drugs Affecting the Endocrine System

STUDY SKILLS TIP:
- QUESTIONING STRATEGY

QUESTIONING STRATEGY

One of the best ways to learn is to become actively involved with the text. The best way to get involved is to ask questions.

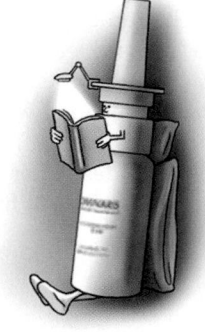

Part Title

As you begin each new part, ask a question to focus your attention. In Part Five, this question is: "What is the endocrine system?" This same question could be asked of Parts Two through Nine by simply replacing "endocrine" with the appropriate system for the specific part. Looking at the chapter titles in the part tells us that the endocrine system has to do with pituitary drugs, thyroid and antithyroid drugs, antidiabetic drugs, adrenal drugs, women's health drugs, and men's health drugs. Although this answer is general, it is a beginning and helps keep you aware of what you need to learn from each chapter.

Chapter Titles

Chapter titles provide the first mechanism to generate questions. The first question to ask is: "What is this chapter about?" That question is also answered immediately. "What is Chapter 31 about?" It is about pituitary agents.

The question to ask next is: "What do pituitary (Chapter 31), thyroid and antithyroid (Chapter 32), anti-diabetic and hypoglycemic (Chapter 33), adrenal (Chapter 34), women's health (Chapter 35), and men's health (Chapter 36) refer to?" Take the chapter title and state it as a question. What do you know about these subjects? Whether you know a lot, half of what there is to know, or just have familiarity with some aspects, this process allows you to focus your study technique.

Chapter Objectives

To enhance your study, turn each chapter objective into one or more questions. Here are some possible questions using the objectives from Chapter 33.

Objective 1

Discuss the normal actions and functions of the pancreas.
- Discuss the normal actions and functions of the pancreas.

Objective 2

Contrast age of onset, signs and symptoms, pharmacological and nonpharmacological treatment, incidence, and etiology of type 1 and type 2 diabetes.
- What is type 1 diabetes mellitus?
- What is type 2 diabetes mellitus?
- How do types 1 and 2 diabetes mellitus differ?

Since the objectives tell you what the authors expect you to know at the end of the chapter, starting out with questions based on the objectives will improve your learning and probably save you time.

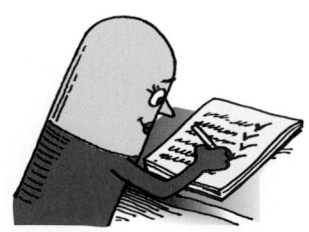

Chapter Headings

The same principle can be applied to each of the topic headings set out in the chapter. Continuing to use Chapter 33 as a model, here are some samples of questions that might be useful as preparation for reading.

Type 1 Diabetes Mellitus

- What is type 1 diabetes?
- What is mellitus?

As you start to process the chapter headings, you will also notice that they begin to answer some of the questions from the chapter objectives. This is a good time to begin setting up vocabulary cards.

Mechanism of Action and Drug Effects

- What is the mechanism of action of insulin?
- Is there more than one mechanism?
- What are the most important drug effects of insulin?
- Where do these effects take place?
- What is the evidence of these effects?

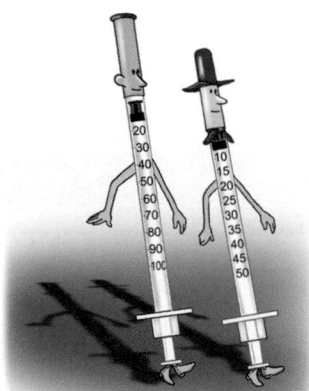

The idea is to focus on the major content of the chapter and establish a guide for learning as you read.

Print Conventions Within the Body of the Chapter

Print conventions are useful in this study skills strategy. The use of *italics*, **bold**, <u>underlining</u>, and multiple colours of ink are examples of print conventions. They are designed to catch your attention. Use them as a basis for questions.

Chapter 33

In the first paragraph of this chapter, the first obvious print convention is the word **insulin**. It is printed in bold. If you let your eyes float down the page and do not read anything, this word stands out. It must be important.

Now ask yourself:

- What is insulin?
- What is the relationship between insulin and type 1 diabetes mellitus?

There are more words on the first page of the chapter text that are in the same print style. Apply the same procedure to these terms. Also, note that two of the terms, *glycogen* and *glycogenolysis*, must have some direct relationship, since the second term contains the first word.

The basic question in each case is, "What does the term mean?" However, there should be more to your questions than just the basics. Glycogenolysis seems to mean that there is some operation or activity taking place. Ask yourself the following:

- What happens in glycogenolysis?
- Where does glycogenolysis occur?
- When does glycogenolysis occur?
- How does it relate to type 1 diabetes mellitus?

Chapter Tables

Tables give a summary of information discussed in the chapter. You can learn a great deal from tables if you take the time.

Look at Table 33-2. The table summarizes characteristics of type 1 and type 2 diabetes. There are two obvious questions for each type.

- What is type 1 (and type 2) diabetes?
- What are its characteristics?

Use these questions to study Table 33-2, and you will find that all the information you need to respond to these questions is found here. It may be useful to make a first pass through the chapter, focusing only on the tables before you begin to read. The table provides you with an overview on the topic. You will learn a great deal about some of the topics, and you will have established background information that will help you ask better questions and read with better understanding.

The time you spend asking questions makes the reading and learning go more quickly. Another benefit is that some of the questions you ask will appear on tests. These questions will be easy for you to answer, which will give you test-taking confidence and, in the end, better grades. After you use the strategy for two or three chapters, you will find that the benefits far outweigh the time it takes.

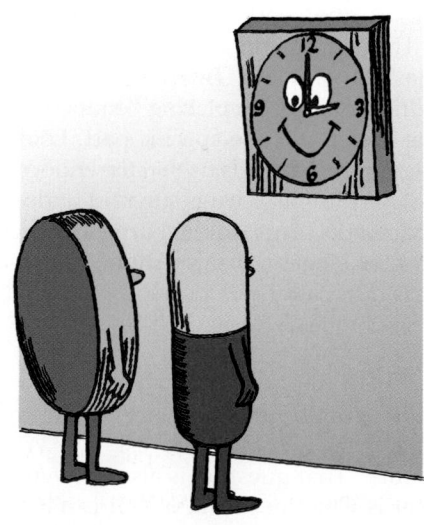

Pituitary Drugs

Objectives

After reading this chapter, the successful student will be able to do the following:

1. Describe the normal function of the anterior and posterior lobes of the pituitary gland and the impact of the pituitary gland on the human body.

2. Compare the various pituitary drugs in regard to their mechanisms of action, therapeutic effects, indications, contraindications, drug interactions, adverse effects, dosages, and routes of administration.

3. Develop a collaborative plan of care that includes all phases of the nursing process for patients receiving pituitary drugs.

e-Learning Activities

Website
(http://evolve.elsevier.com/Canada/Lilley/pharmacology/)

- Answer Key—Textbook Case Studies
- Answer Key—Critical Thinking Activities
- Chapter Summaries—Printable
- Review Questions for Exam Preparation
- Unfolding Case Studies

Drug Profile

▸▸ octreotide acetate, p. 606
▸▸ somatropin, p. 606
▸▸ vasopressin and desmopressin, p. 606

▸▸ Key drug

Key Terms

Hypothalamus The gland above and behind the pituitary gland and the optic chiasm. Both glands are suspended beneath the middle area of the bottom of the brain. The hypothalamus secretes the hormones vasopressin and oxytocin, which are stored in the posterior pituitary gland. The hypothalamus also secretes several hormone-releasing factors that stimulate the anterior pituitary gland to secrete a variety of hormones that control many body functions. (p. 602)

Negative feedback loop A system in which the production of one hormone is controlled by the levels of a second hormone in a way that reduces the output of the first hormone. A gland produces a hormone that stimulates a second gland to produce a second hormone. In response to the increased levels of the second hormone, the source gland of the first hormone reduces production of that hormone until blood levels of the second hormone fall below a certain minimum level needed; then, the cycle begins again. (p. 602)

Neuroendocrine system The system that regulates reactions to both internal and external stimuli, involving the integrated activities of the endocrine glands and nervous system. (p. 602)

Pituitary gland An endocrine gland that is suspended beneath the hypothalamus and supplies numerous hormones that control many vital processes. (p. 602)

ENDOCRINE SYSTEM

Maintenance of physiological stability is the primary goal of the endocrine system. The endocrine system must accomplish this task despite constant changes in the internal and external environments. Every cell and organ in the body comes under the influence of the endocrine system. It communicates with the approximately 50 million target cells in the body using a chemical "language" called *hormones*. Hormones are a large group of natural substances that cause highly specific physiological effects in the cells of their target tissues. They are secreted into the bloodstream in response to the body's needs and travel through the blood to their sites of action, the target cells.

For decades, the pituitary gland was believed to be the master gland that regulated and controlled the other endocrine glands. However, evidence now suggests that the central nervous system (CNS), specifically the **hypothalamus,** controls the pituitary gland. The hypothalamus and pituitary are now viewed as functioning together as an integrated unit, with primary direction coming from the hypothalamus. For this reason, these structures are now commonly referred to as the **neuroendocrine system**. In fact, understanding each of the systems can assist in the study of the other, as they are basically systems for signalling, each operating in a stimulus-and-response manner. Together, these two systems essentially govern all bodily functions.

The **pituitary gland** is made up of two distinct glands—the anterior pituitary gland (adenohypophysis) and the posterior pituitary gland (neurohypophysis). They are individually linked to and communicate with the hypothalamus, and each gland secretes its own distinct set of hormones. These various hormones are listed in Box 31-1 and shown in Figure 31-1.

Hormones are either water- or lipid-soluble. The water-soluble hormones are protein-based substances, such as the catecholamines norepinephrine and epinephrine. The lipid-soluble hormones consist of the steroid and thyroid hormones.

The activity of the endocrine system is regulated by a system of surveillance and signalling, usually dictated by the body's ongoing needs. Hormone secretion is commonly regulated by a **negative feedback loop.** This is best explained using a hypothetical example: When gland X releases hormone X, this stimulates target cells to release hormone Y. When there is an excess of hormone Y, gland X senses this excess and decreases its release of hormone X. A real example is the regulation of plasma glucose (see Chapter 33). As the plasma sugar level increases in the bloodstream, insulin sends a signal to the liver, muscles, and other cells to store excess glucose (e.g., as body fat and as glycogen in the liver and muscles).

PITUITARY DRUGS

A variety of drugs affect the pituitary gland. They are generally used either as replacement drug therapy to make up for a hormone deficiency or as diagnostic aids to determine the status of the patient's hormonal functions. The currently identified anterior and posterior pituitary hormones and the drugs that mimic or antagonize their actions are listed in Table 31-1.

The anterior pituitary drugs discussed in this chapter are cosyntropin, somatropin, and octreotide acetate; the posterior pituitary drugs discussed in this chapter are vasopressin and desmopressin.

Mechanism of Action and Drug Effects

The mechanisms of action of the pituitary drugs differ depending on the drug, but overall, they either augment or antagonize the natural effects of the pituitary hormones. Exogenously administered cosyntropin (Cortrosyn®) elicits all of the same pharmacological responses as those elicited by the endogenous corticotropin (also known as adrenocorticotropic hormone [ACTH]). Intravenous (IV) exogenous corticotropin is no longer manufactured; however, an intramuscular (IM) injection, known as Synacthen Depot®, is available. Cosyntropin travels to the adrenal cortex, located just above the kidney, and stimulates the secretion of the mineralocorticoid cortisol (the drug form of which is the steroid hydrocortisone sodium succinate [Solu-Cortef®]). Cortisol has many anti-inflammatory effects, including reduction of inflammatory leukocyte functions and scar tissue formation. Cortisol also promotes kidney retention of sodium, which can result in edema and hypertension.

The drug that mimics growth hormone (GH) is somatropin. This drug promotes growth by stimulating anabolic (tissue-building) processes, liver glycogenolysis (to raise blood sugar levels), lipid mobilization from body fat stores, and retention of sodium, potassium, and phosphorus. Somatropin promotes linear growth in children who lack normal amounts of the endogenous hormone.

BOX 31-1

Hormones of the Anterior and Posterior Pituitary Gland

Anterior Pituitary (Adenohypophysis)

Adrenocorticotropic hormone (ACTH)
Follicle-stimulating hormone (FSH)
Growth hormone (GH)
Luteinizing hormone (LH)
Prolactin (PH)
Thyroid-stimulating hormone (TSH)

Posterior Pituitary Gland (Neurohypophysis)

Antidiuretic hormone (ADH)
Oxytocin

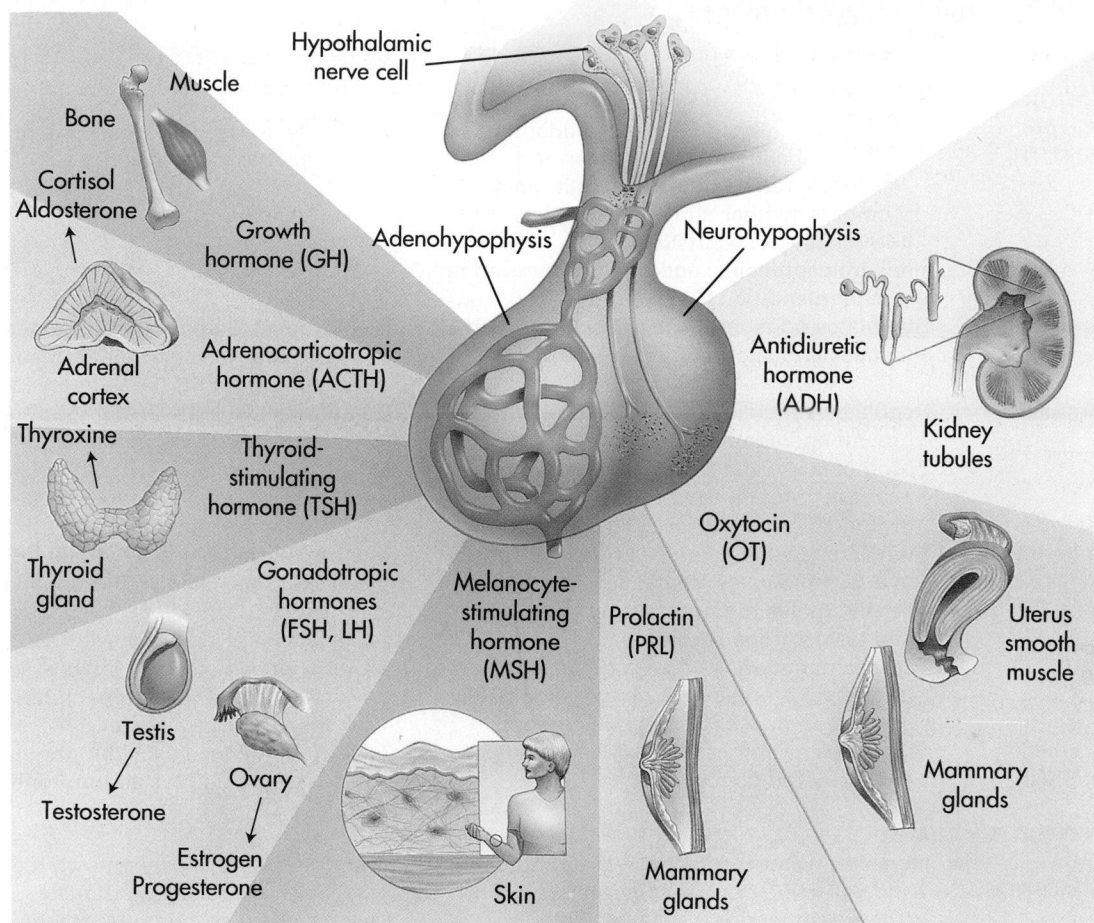

FIG. 31-1   Pituitary hormones and their target organs. *FSH*, follicle-stimulating hormone; *ICSH*, male analog of LH (interstitial cell–stimulating hormone); *LH*, luteinizing hormone. (Source: McCance, K. L., & Huether, S. E. (2014). *Pathophysiology: The Biologic basis for disease in adults and children* (7th ed.; p. 696). St. Louis, MO: Mosby; Modified from Patton, K. T., & Thibodeau, G. A. (2013). *Anatomy and physiology* (8th ed.) St. Louis, MO: Mosby.)

Octreotide acetate antagonizes the effects of the natural GH. It does so by inhibiting GH release. Octreotide acetate is a synthetic polypeptide that is structurally and pharmacologically similar to GH release–inhibiting factor, which is also called *somatostatin*. It also reduces plasma concentrations of vasoactive intestinal polypeptide (VIP), a protein secreted by a type of tumour known as a *VIPoma* that causes profuse watery diarrhea (see Chapter 53).

The drugs that affect the posterior pituitary gland, such as vasopressin and desmopressin, mimic the actions of the naturally occurring antidiuretic hormone (ADH). They increase water resorption in the distal tubules and collecting ducts of the nephrons and they concentrate urine, reducing water excretion by up to 90%. Vasopressin is also a potent vasoconstrictor in larger doses and is therefore used in certain hypotensive emergencies such as vasodilatory shock (septic shock). Desmopressin causes a dose-dependent increase in the plasma levels of factor VIII (antihemophilic factor), von Willebrand factor (acts closely with factor

VIII), and tissue plasminogen activator. These properties make it useful in treating certain blood disorders. The drug form of oxytocin mimics the endogenous hormone, thus promoting uterine contractions (see Chapter 35).

Indications

Cosyntropin is used in the diagnosis of adrenocortical insufficiency. Upon diagnosis, actual drug treatment generally involves replacement hormonal therapy using drug forms of the deficient corticosteroid hormones. These drugs are discussed in more detail in Chapter 34.

Somatropin is human GH produced by recombinant technology. It is effective in stimulating skeletal growth in patients with an inadequate secretion of normal endogenous GH, such as those with hypopituitary dwarfism.

Octreotide acetate is useful in alleviating certain symptoms of carcinoid tumours stemming from the secretion of VIP, including severe diarrhea and potentially life-threatening hypotension associated with a carcinoid crisis. It is also used for the emergency management

TABLE 31-1

Anterior and Posterior Pituitary Hormones

Hormone	Function and Mimicking Drug	Drugs
ANTERIOR PITUITARY GLAND		
Adrenocorticotropic hormone (ACTH)	Targets adrenal gland; mediates adaptation to physical and emotional stress and starvation; redistributes body nutrients; promotes synthesis of adrenocortical hormones (glucocorticoids, mineralocorticoids, androgens); involved in skin pigmentation	Cosyntropin: Used for diagnosis of adrenocortical insufficiency
Follicle-stimulating hormone (FSH)	Stimulates oogenesis and follicular growth in females and spermatogenesis in males	Menotropins: Same pharmacological effects as FSH; many of the other gonadotropins also stimulate FSH (see Chapter 35).
Growth hormone (GH)	Regulates anabolic processes related to growth and adaptation to stressors; promotes skeletal and muscle growth; increases protein synthesis; increases liver glycogenolysis; increases fat mobilization	Somatropin: Human GH for treatment of hypopituitary dwarfism
		Octreotide acetate: A synthetic polypeptide structurally and pharmacologically similar to GH release–inhibiting factor; inhibits GH
Luteinizing hormone (LH)	Stimulates ovulation and estrogen release by ovaries in females; stimulates interstitial cells in males to promote spermatogenesis and testosterone secretion	Mentropins, clomiphene citrate: Increase LH levels and the chance of pregnancy
Prolactin (PH)	Targets mammary glands; stimulates lactogenesis and breast growth in females; purpose in males is poorly understood	Bromocriptine mesylate: Inhibits action of prolactin and therefore inhibits lactogenesis (see Chapter 35)
Thyroid-stimulating hormone (TSH)	Stimulates secretion of thyroid hormones T_3 and T_4 by the thyroid gland	Thyrotropin α: Increases the production and secretion of thyroid hormones (see Chapter 32)
POSTERIOR PITUITARY GLAND		
Antidiuretic hormone (ADH)	Increases water resorption in distal tubules and collecting duct of nephron; concentrates urine; causes potent vasoconstriction	Vasopressin: ADH; performs all the physiological functions of ADH
		Desmopressin acetate: A synthetic vasopressin
Oxytocin	Targets mammary glands; stimulates ejection of milk and contraction of uterine smooth muscle (see Chapter 35)	

T_3, triiodothyronine; T_4, thyroxine.

of bleeding esophageal varices in patients with liver cirrhosis and for protection against rebleeding. Vasopressin and desmopressin are used to prevent or control polydipsia (excessive thirst), polyuria, and dehydration in patients with diabetes insipidus caused by a deficiency of endogenous ADH. Because of their vasoconstrictive properties, they are useful in the treatment of various types of bleeding, particularly gastrointestinal (GI) hemorrhage. The use of vasopressin is another strategy used to stop bleeding of esophageal varices. Vasopressin is also used in the Advanced Cardiac Life Support (ACLS) guidelines for treatment of pulseless cardiac arrest. Desmopressin is useful in the treatment of hemophilia A and type I von Willebrand's disease because of its effects on various coagulation factors.

Contraindications

Contraindications for the use of pituitary drugs vary with each individual drug and are listed in each of the drug profiles included in this chapter. Because even small

amounts of these drugs can initiate major physiological changes, all of them should be used with special caution in patients with acute or chronic illnesses, such as migraine headaches, epilepsy, and asthma.

Adverse Effects

Most of the adverse effects of the pituitary drugs are specific to the individual drug. Those drugs possessing similar hormonal effects generally have similar adverse effects. The most common adverse effects of the pituitary drugs described here are listed in Tables 31-2 to 31-4.

Interactions

Selected interactions involving pituitary drugs are summarized in Table 31-5.

Dosages

For dosage information on pituitary drugs, refer to the table on p. 607.

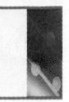

TABLE 31-2

Octreotide Acetate: Common Adverse Effects

Body System	Adverse Effects
Central nervous	Fatigue, malaise, headache
Endocrine	Increase or decrease in blood glucose levels
Gastrointestinal	Diarrhea, nausea, vomiting
Respiratory	Dyspnea
Musculoskeletal	Arthralgia
Cardiovascular	Conduction abnormalities

TABLE 31-3

Desmopressin and Vasopressin: Common Adverse Effects

Body System	Adverse Effects
Cardiovascular	Increased blood pressure
Central nervous	Fever, vertigo, headache
Gastrointestinal	Nausea, heartburn, cramps
Genitourinary	Uterine cramping
Other	Nasal irritation and congestion, tremor, sweating

TABLE 31-4

Somatropin: Common Adverse Effects

Body System	Adverse Effects
Central nervous	Headache
Endocrine	Hyperglycemia, hypothyroidism
Genitourinary	Hypercalciuria
Other	Rash, urticaria, development of antibodies to growth hormone, flulike syndrome

NURSING PROCESS

✍ Assessment

Before administering any of the pituitary drugs, perform a thorough assessment and document findings. Assess the patient's height, weight, and vital signs. Take a complete medication history with notation of allergies and use of prescription drugs, over-the-counter drugs, and natural health products. With octreotide acetate, the health care provider may order an electrocardiogram (ECG) prior to its use because of the adverse effect of conduction abnormalities. Assess baseline glucose levels and note respiratory status with octreotide acetate use. Extra caution and close monitoring of blood glucose is warranted in patients with diabetes as octreotide may affect insulin response (or response to other antidiabetic drugs). Patients taking octreotide acetate may require special dosing if they have decreased liver and kidney function; therefore, assess and record baseline liver and kidney function tests. It is also important that assessment includes steps to prevent medication errors and awareness of concerns regarding look-alike sound-alike drugs. Specifically, Sandostatin (octreotide acetate) should not be confused with Sandimmune® (cyclosporine).

With desmopressin, check vital signs and assess for a history of seizures, asthma, or cardiovascular disease. These conditions require cautious use with careful monitoring of vital signs, heart sounds, and breath sounds. If vasopressin is being administered for shock, close monitoring in an intensive care setting is needed, with ECG, vital signs, and other possibly invasive monitoring methods (e.g., arterial lines, central venous pressure lines, arterial blood gases). Obtain baseline thyroid, glucose, and calcium levels in patients receiving growth hormones due to the potential adverse effects of hyperglycemia, hypothyroidism, and hypercalciuria. Specifically, use of somatropin requires attention to the growth, motor skills, height, and weight of pediatric patients. Additionally, with all of the pituitary drugs, always perform a thorough assessment of cautions, contraindications, and drug interactions prior to their administration.

TABLE 31-5

Selected Drug Interactions Involving Pituitary Drugs

Pituitary Drug	Interacting Drug	Potential Result
desmopressin	carbamazepine	Enhanced desmopressin effects
	lithium carbonate, alcohol	Reduced desmopressin effects
octreotide acetate	cyclosporine	Case report of transplant rejection
	ciprofloxacin hydrochloride	Prolongation of QT interval
somatropin	Glucocorticoids	Reduction of growth effects
vasopressin	carbamazepine, fludrocortisone	Enhanced antidiuretic effect
	norepinephrine, lithium carbonate	Reduced antidiuretic effect

DRUG PROFILES

▶▶ octreotide acetate

Octreotide acetate (Ocphyl®, Sandostatin®) is useful in alleviating certain symptoms of carcinoid tumours stemming from the secretion of VIP, including severe diarrhea, flushing, and potentially life-threatening hypotension associated with a carcinoid crisis. It is also used for the treatment of esophageal varices (usually in combination with sclerotherapy). Octreotide acetate inhibits exocrine pancreatic secretion and reduces the incidence and severity of postoperative complications such as a fistula or abscess, which can lead to sepsis. It is contraindicated in patients who have shown a hypersensitivity to it or any of its components. Octreotide acetate may impair gallbladder function and needs to be used with caution in patients with kidney impairment. It may affect glucose regulation, and severe hypoglycemia may occur in patients with type 1 diabetes. It may cause hyperglycemia in patients with type 2 diabetes or in patients without diabetes. Octreotide acetate may enhance the toxic effects of drugs that prolong the QT interval. Ciprofloxacin may enhance the QT-prolonging effects of octreotide acetate. Octreotide acetate can be given intravenously, intramuscularly, or subcutaneously. It is available in prefilled syringes in 50-, 100-, and 500-mcg/mL dosages for subcutaneous injection. The drug is safe to use during pregnancy. Therapy with octreotide acetate is usually initiated at 50 mcg once or twice daily. The dosage is increased gradually based on tolerability, patient response, and the drug's effects on levels of tumour-producing hormones. Recommended dosages are given in the table on page 607.

PHARMACOKINETICS

Route	Onset of Action	Peak Plasma Concentration	Elimination Half-Life	Duration of Action
PO	Rapid	0.4–1 hr	1.7–1.9 hr	6–12 hr

▶▶ somatropin

Somatropin (Gentropin®, Humatrope®, Norditropin Simplex®, Nutropin®, Omnitrope®, Saizen®, Serostim®) is a GH that is indicated in the treatment of growth failure due to inadequate endogenous GH secretion. Serostim is limited to use in patients with HIV infection with wasting or cachexia in conjunction with antiviral therapy. It is not considered harmful to the fetus, but it is recommended to be discontinued during pregnancy. Somatropin is contraindicated in patients with hypersensitivity to any component of the product and in children with closed growth plates, patients with tumours, and patients with acute illnesses. Adverse effects include headache, injection site reactions, muscle pain, hypoglycemia, or hyperglycemia.

It is important not to shake the product. It is generally given subcutaneously; however, some manufactured products can be given intramuscularly. Check the specific prescribing information before administering. Somatropin is available in cartridges for use with pen delivery systems, disposable pens, as well as in prefilled syringes.

PHARMACOKINETICS

Route	Onset of Action	Peak Plasma Concentration	Elimination Half-Life	Duration of Action
Subcut or IM	Not available	2–6 hr	2–4 hr (Subcut)	18–20 hr

▶▶ vasopressin and desmopressin

Vasopressin (Pressyn®) is the exact synthetic protein form of the human antidiuretic hormone normally secreted by the pituitary gland while desmopressin (DDAVP®, Nocdurna®, Octostim®) is the synthetic structural analogue of the natural human hormone, arginine vasopressin. Desmopressin has 10 times the antidiuretic action of vasopressin, but 1500 times less vasoconstrictor action. Desmopressin is used to reduce the polyuria, nocturia, and polydipsia associated with vasopressin sensitive central diabetes insipidus as well as temporary polydipsia and polyuria after head injury or surgery in the area of the pituitary. It is also used for patients over 5 years of age with nocturnal enuresis. It is available in oral sublingual disintegrating and oral tablets, nasal spray or rhinyle, and parenterally. The Octostim injection and nasal spray forms are indicated for various types of bleeding (e.g., prevents bleeding in patients with mild hemophilia A and mild von Willebrand's disease Type I; the prevention of bleeding in patients with uremia during surgery and postoperatively). Vasopressin causes vasoconstriction and reduces portal blood flow, portal systemic collateral blood flow, and pressure on esophageal varices. It is also used for post-traumatic or post-operative diabetes insipidus in patients who are haemodynamically unstable, for hypotension associated with vasodilatory or septic shock unresponsive to catecholamines or who are acidotic or hypoxic, and increases myocardial oxygen delivery without increasing consumption. It may also be used during cardiac arrest (ventricular fibrillation or pulseless ventricular tachycardia) as an adrenergic agent equivalent to epinephrine. Vasopressin is available only as an injection for IM or IV use.

PHARMACOKINETICS (VASOPRESSIN)

Route	Onset of Action	Peak Plasma Concentration	Elimination Half-Life	Duration of Action
IV	Rapid	5–15 min	less than 10 min	10–20 min

DOSAGES   Selected Pituitary Drugs

Drug	Pharmacological Class	Usual Dosage Range	Indications/Uses
octreotide acetate (Ocphyl, Sandostatin)	Somatostatin (GH inhibitor) analogue	*Adults**	Acromegaly
		IV/Subcut/Depot IM: 100–600 mcg/day divided bid–qid	Metastatic carcinoid tumours (to control flushing and diarrhea symptoms)
		IV/Subcut/Depot IM: 200–300 mcg/day divided bid–qid	VIPomas
		IV/Subcut/Depot IM: 100–300 mcg/day divided bid–tid	Acromegaly
		Subcut: 100 mcg tid, for 7 days postsurgery	Prevention of fistula, abscess post-pancreatic surgery
		IV: 25 mcg/hr by continuous infusion × 48 h to 7 days	Bleeding esophageal varices
somatropin (Humatrope, others)	Anterior pituitary growth hormone	*Children* Subcut: 0.16–0.24 mg/kg divided into 6–7 doses	Growth failure
Somatrope (Serostim)	Anterior pituitary hormone	*Adults* Subcut: once daily at bedtime; dosage calculated by weight	HIV wasting associated with catabolism, weight loss or cachexia
vasopressin (Pressyn AR)	Natural or synthetic ADH	*Adults* IM/Subcut: 5–10 units bid–qid (max 60 units/day) *Children* IM/Subcut: 2.5–10 units bid–qid (max 60 units/day)	Diabetes insipidus
		Adults IV: 0.01–0.04 units/min *Children* IV: 0.3–0.4 milliunits/kg/min	Vasodilatory shock
		Adults IV: 0.2–0.4 units/min *Children* IV: 0.002–0.005 units/min	GI hemorrhage

ADH, antidiuretic hormone; *GH*, growth hormone; *GI*, gastrointestinal; *IM*, intramuscular; *IV*, intravenous; *Subcut*, subcutaneous; *VIPoma*, vasoactive intestinal peptide-producing tumour.
*Normally used only in adults.

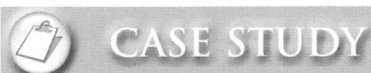
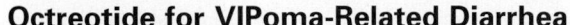

CASE STUDY

Octreotide for VIPoma-Related Diarrhea

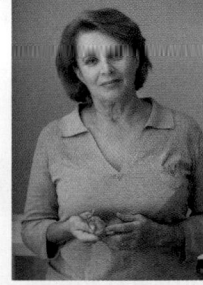

Josette, a 56-year-old aesthetician, has been diagnosed with a VIPoma (vasoactive intestinal peptide-producing tumour). She was scheduled for surgery but developed severe diarrhea. She has been hospitalized because she became dehydrated after 2 days of profuse, watery diarrhea. She has not eaten for several days. In addition to having diarrhea, she is nauseated, has facial flushing, and has lost 2.3 kg in 2 days. IV fluid replacement with normal saline has been started, and she will be receiving octreotide acetate (Sandostatin). She had her gallbladder removed 8 years ago but has no history of other illnesses.

1. How does the octreotide acetate work to control the VIPoma-related diarrhea?
2. As Josette begins therapy with octreotide acetate, the nurse should continue to assess what parameters?

After 2 days of treatment, Josette's episodes of diarrhea have become less frequent. However, the nurse notes that her blood glucose levels are elevated.

3. What is the best explanation for this elevation?

_____

For answers, see http://evolve.elsevier.com/Canada/Lilley/pharmacology/.

Nursing Diagnoses

- Disturbed body image related to specific disease processes or drug adverse effects and their influence on the patient's physical characteristics
- Acute pain related to GI adverse effects associated with the use of various pituitary drugs
- Deficient knowledge related to lack of information and experience with pituitary drug treatment

Planning

Goals

- Patient will maintain a positive body image while receiving drug therapy.
- Patient will experience little to no pain related to medication-induced GI upset or epigastric distress.
- Patient will gain increased knowledge about drug therapy.

Expected Patient Outcomes

- Patient openly verbalizes fears, anxieties, and concerns regarding changes in body image related to disease processes and the adverse effects of drug therapy to health care providers.
- Patient experiences minimal GI upset and gastric distress by taking medication with food or at mealtimes.
- Patient states specific rationale for drug therapy as well as adverse effects.
- Patient states the importance of keeping follow-up appointments with health care providers.

Implementation

Octreotide acetate must be given as ordered with attention to the route of administration. To avoid giving the incorrect medication, follow the "rights" consistently and the three checks of medication administration; be careful not to confuse octreotide acetate injection with the injectable depot suspension dosage form. Use only clear solutions and always check for incompatibilities. Mix injectable solutions by gently swirling the liquid. Make sure patients understand the importance of immediately reporting to the health care provider any abdominal distress such as diarrhea, nausea, or vomiting, if not manageable. Stress the importance of follow-up appointments for laboratory testing during treatment with this drug. Octreotide acetate cause alterations in blood glucose levels; closely monitor glucose levels during therapy, especially if patients have diabetes.

Administer desmopressin according to the health care provider's orders because dosage and route may vary with the indication. For desmopressin and somatropin, rotate subcutaneous injection sites (also given IM, in ventral gluteal site) to avoid tissue damage. Desmopressin dosage forms include sublingual disintegrating tablet, oral, IV, intranasal, and subcutaneous. Intranasal use may lead to changes in the nasal mucosa, leading to unpredictable absorption. Instruct patients to contact their health care providers immediately if the condition worsens. If used in patients diagnosed with diabetes insipidus, fluid intake may be adjusted according to the predicted risk of water intoxication and sodium deficit. See the Patient Teaching Tips for more information on dosage administration.

Vasopressin is available as an injection for IM/subcutaneous or IV use. Always check the clarity of parenteral solutions before administering the medication, and discard the solution if there are visible particles or there is any fluid discoloration. Be alert to the adverse effects of elevated blood pressure, fever, nausea, abdominal cramping, or diarrhea. If these worsen or persist, notify the health care provider immediately.

Evaluation

After goals and outcome criteria have been reviewed and treatment has begun, evaluate therapeutic responses to these drugs. With octreotide acetate, therapeutic effects include improvement of symptoms related to carcinoid tumours, VIPoma, or esophageal varices. With vasopressin, an improvement in diabetes insipidus, esophageal varices, or vasodilatory shock is expected. With somatropin, increased growth is expected for those for whom it is indicated. Adverse effects for which to evaluate include fatigue, headache, altered blood glucose levels, diarrhea, nausea, vomiting, conduction disorders, and dyspnea. Adverse effects associated with desmopressin and vasopressin include increased blood pressure, fever, headache, abdominal cramps, and nausea. Growth hormones may have the adverse effects of headache, hyperglycemia, hypothyroidism, hypercalciuria, and flulike syndrome.

PATIENT TEACHING TIPS

❖ Carefully discuss routes and techniques of administration with patients and anyone else involved in their care. With pediatric patients, demonstrate the technique of administration to family members or caregivers before discharge, and evaluate their comprehension with return demonstrations. Provide written instructions to patients, if age appropriate, but also to their family members or caregivers. A written or electronic journal about how the drug is being tolerated may prove to be beneficial. As for any medication or illness, patients should keep a medical alert bracelet, necklace, or wallet card with them at all times.

PATIENT TEACHING TIPS—cont'd

❖ Intranasal dosage forms of desmopressin are to be given only after the nasal passages have been cleared. The pump must be primed prior to use. Instruct patients to prime the nasal pump by pressing down the pump four times. The spray pump delivers 10 mcg of drug each time it is pressed. To administer a 10-mcg dose as ordered, place the spray nozzle in the nostril (for a child, have a parent, caregiver, or other adult administer the dose) and press the spray pump once. If a higher dose has been prescribed, half the dose is to be administered in each nostril. The pump cannot deliver doses smaller than 10 mcg. Once dosing is completed, replace the cap on the bottle. The pump will stay primed for up to 1 week. After 1 week, it will require repriming. The level of drug left in the pump should be carefully monitored so that there is always enough medication on hand. The pump may not have enough medication left after 25 doses (at 150 mcg per spray) or 50 doses (at 10 mcg per spray). Vasopressin is applied topically to the nasal membranes and is not to be inhaled.

❖ Somatropin is available in a variety of delivery forms. One is a disposable pen preloaded with a cartridge. One section of the cartridge contains the growth hormone in powder form, to be mixed with the diluent in the other section. Before the contents have been mixed, the syringe should be stored in the refrigerator. Educate patients or their parents, family members, or caregivers to attach the needle to the syringe by pushing it down onto the syringe and twisting it until it no longer turns. Hold the syringe with the needle pointing upwards and gently turn the plunger clockwise to mix the solution; do not shake. Administer by subcutaneous injection. Dispose of the syringe safely. Somatropin is also available in a multi dose prefilled pen with a variety of different dosages in mg/mL. The pen must be primed before the first use to ensure flow. The pen is dialed to get the correct dose (one click on the dose selector at the end of the pen). Inform patients that they must use a new needle with each injection.

❖ Educate parents about the fact that children with endocrine disorders may have an increased risk of bone problems. Instruct parents that if they notice their child limping, this needs to be evaluated by their health care provider. Closely monitor patients with diabetes for changes in serum glucose levels if taking octreotide acetate.

❖ Water intake amounts may need to be monitored closely in patients with diabetes insipidus. Exact amounts may be prescribed or determined for each patient.

KEY POINTS

❖ The pituitary gland is composed of two distinct glands: anterior and posterior. Each lobe secretes its own set of hormones: *anterior*—thyroid-stimulating hormone (TSH), GH, ACTH, prolactin, follicle-stimulating hormone (FSH), luteinizing hormone (LH); *posterior*—ADH, oxytocin.

❖ Pituitary drugs are used to either mimic or antagonize the action of endogenous pituitary hormones.

❖ Drugs that mimic the action of endogenous pituitary hormones include cosyntropin, somatropin, vasopressin, and desmopressin. A drug that antagonizes the actions of endogenous pituitary hormones is octreotide acetate.

❖ In the assessment of patients receiving pituitary hormones, record baseline vital signs, review blood glucose levels, and measure weight.

❖ For patients receiving somatropin, constantly monitor levels of thyroid hormones and growth hormones. Include measurement of vital signs, intake and output, and weight in the assessment.

EXAMINATION REVIEW QUESTIONS

1. A patient is experiencing severe diarrhea, flushing, and life-threatening hypotension associated with carcinoid crisis. The nurse will prepare to administer which drug?
a. octreotide acetate (Sandostatin)
b. vasopressin (Pressyn AR)
c. somatropin (Humatrope)
d. cosyntropin (Cortrosyn)

2. A patient is suspected of having adrenocortical insufficiency. The nurse expects to administer which drug to aid in the diagnosis of this condition?
a. octreotide acetate (Sandostatin)
b. vasopressin (Pressyn AR)
c. somatropin (Humatrope)
d. cosyntropin (Cortrosyn)

3. The nurse is reviewing the medication list for a patient who will be starting therapy with somatropin. Which type of drug would raise a concern that needs to be addressed before the patient starts the somatropin?
a. Nonsteroidal anti-inflammatory drug for arthritis
b. Antidepressant therapy
c. Penicillin
d. Glucocorticoid

Continued

EXAMINATION REVIEW QUESTIONS—cont'd

4. A patient who is about to be given octreotide acetate is also taking a diuretic, IV heparin, ciprofloxacin hydrochloride, and an opioid as needed for pain. The nurse will monitor for what possible interaction?
 a. Hypokalemia due to an interaction with the diuretic
 b. Decreased anticoagulation because of interaction with the heparin
 c. Prolongation of the QT interval due to an interaction with ciprofloxacin hydrochloride
 d. Increased sedation if the opioid is given

5. When monitoring for the therapeutic effects of intranasal desmopressin (DDAVP) in a patient who has diabetes insipidus, which assessment would the nurse look for as an indication that the medication therapy is successful?
 a. Increased insulin levels
 b. Decreased diarrhea
 c. Improved nasal patency
 d. Decreased thirst

6. Which drugs have an action similar to that of the naturally occurring hormone ADH? (Select all that apply.)
 a. cosyntropin (Cortrosyn)
 b. desmopressin (DDAVP)
 c. somatropin (Humatrope)
 d. vasopressin (Pressyn AR)
 e. octreotide acetate (Sandostatin)

7. The order reads: "Give octreotide acetate (Sandostatin) 50 mcg Subcut twice a day." The medication is available in an injectable form of 0.05 mg/mL. How many millilitres will the nurse draw up for the ordered dose?

Answers: 1. a, 2. d, 3. d, 4. c, 5. d, 6. b, d, 7. 1 mL.

CRITICAL THINKING ACTIVITIES

1. When the nurse checks the insertion site of a patient who is receiving an IV infusion of vasopressin, the site is swollen and cool to the touch. What is the nurse's priority action? Explain your answer.

2. A child is experiencing delayed growth due to an endocrine disorder. Which pituitary drug is used to treat this condition, and how does it work? What is the best way for the nurse to measure the patient's response to the drug therapy?

3. A patient will be receiving intranasal desmopressin (DDAVP), and the nurse is teaching the patient how to self-administer the drug. After the nurse explains how the pump works and how to prime the pump, what is important for the nurse to tell the patient to do just before taking the medication?

For answers see http://evolve.elsevier.com/Canada/Lilley/pharmacology/.

Thyroid and Antithyroid Drugs

Objectives

After reading this chapter, the successful student will be able to do the following:

1. Briefly describe the normal anatomy and physiology of the thyroid gland.
2. Discuss the various functions of the thyroid gland and related hormones.
3. Describe the differences in the diseases resulting from the hyposecretion and hypersecretion of the thyroid gland hormones.
4. Identify the various drugs used to treat the hyposecretion and hypersecretion states of the thyroid gland.
5. Discuss the mechanisms of action, indications, contraindications, cautions, drug interactions, adverse effects, dosages, and routes of administration of the various drugs used to treat hypothyroidism and hyperthyroidism.
6. Develop a collaborative plan of care that includes all phases of the nursing process for patients receiving thyroid replacement as well as for patients receiving antithyroid drugs.

e-Learning Activities

Website
(http://evolve.elsevier.com/Canada/
Lilley/pharmacology/)

evolve

- Answer Key—Textbook Case Studies
- Answer Key—Critical Thinking Activities
- Chapter Summaries—Printable
- Review Questions for Exam Preparation
- Unfolding Case Studies

Drug Profiles

▸▸ levothyroxine (levothyroxine sodium)*, p. 614
▸▸ propylthiouracil, p. 616

▸▸ Key drug

*Full generic name is given in parentheses. For the purposes of this text, the more common, shortened name is used.

Key Terms

Euthyroid   Referring to normal thyroid function. (p. 613)

Hyperthyroidism   A condition characterized by excessive production of the thyroid hormones. Also referred to as *thyrotoxicosis*. (p. 612)

Hypothyroidism   A condition characterized by diminished production of the thyroid hormones. (p. 612)

Thyroid-stimulating hormone (TSH)   An endogenous substance secreted by the pituitary gland that controls

the release of thyroid gland hormones and is necessary for the growth and function of the thyroid gland (also called thyrotropin). (p. 612)

Thyroxine (T₄)   The principal thyroid hormone that influences the body's metabolic rate. (p. 611)

Triiodothyronine (T₃)   A secondary thyroid hormone that also affects body metabolism. (p. 611)

THYROID FUNCTION

The thyroid gland lies across the larynx in front of the thyroid cartilage. Its lobes extend laterally on both sides of the front of the neck. The thyroid gland is responsible for the secretion of three hormones essential for the

proper regulation of metabolism: **thyroxine (T₄)**, **triiodothyronine (T₃)**, and calcitonin (see Chapter 35). It is located close to and communicates with the parathyroid glands, which lie just above and behind it. The parathyroid glands are two pairs of bean-shaped glands. These glands are made up of encapsulated cells, which are responsible for maintaining adequate levels of calcium in extracellular fluid, primarily by mobilizing calcium from bone (see Chapter 9).

Thyroxine (T_4) and triiodothyronine (T_3) are produced in the thyroid gland through the coupling of the amino acid tyrosine. The iodide (I^-, which is the ionized form of iodine) required for this process is acquired from the diet. One milligram of iodide is needed per week. This iodide is absorbed from the blood and then sequestered by the thyroid gland, where it is concentrated to 20 times its blood level. Here it is also converted to iodine (I_2), which is combined with tyrosine to make diiodotyrosine. The combination of two molecules of diiodotyrosine results in the formation of thyroxine, which therefore has four iodine molecules in its structure (T_4). Triiodothyronine is formed by the coupling of one molecule of diiodotyrosine with one molecule of monoiodotyrosine; thus, it has three iodine molecules in its structure (T_3). The biologic potency of T_3 is almost four times greater than that of T_4, but T_4 is present in much greater quantities. After these two thyroid hormones are synthesized, they are stored in the follicles in the thyroid gland in a complex with thyroglobulin (a protein that contains tyrosine and an amino acid), called the *colloid*. When the thyroid gland is signalled to do so, it breaks down the thyroglobulin–thyroid hormone complex enzymatically to release T_3 and T_4 into the circulation. This entire process is triggered by **thyroid-stimulating hormone (TSH)**, also called *thyrotropin*. Its release from the anterior pituitary is stimulated when blood levels of T_3 and T_4 are low.

The thyroid hormones are involved in a wide variety of bodily processes. They regulate the basal metabolic rate and lipid and carbohydrate metabolism; are essential for normal growth and development; control the heat-regulating system (thermoregulatory centre in the brain); and have several effects on the cardiovascular, endocrine, and neuromuscular systems. Therefore, hyperfunction or hypofunction of the thyroid gland can lead to a wide range of serious consequences.

HYPOTHYROIDISM

There are three types of **hypothyroidism.** Primary hypothyroidism stems from an abnormality in the thyroid gland. It occurs when the thyroid gland is not able to perform one of its many functions, such as releasing the thyroid hormones from their storage sites, coupling iodine with tyrosine, trapping iodide, converting iodide to iodine, or any combination of these defects. Primary hypothyroidism is the most common of the three forms of hypothyroidism. Secondary hypothyroidism begins at the level of the pituitary gland and results from reduced secretion of thyroid stimulating hormone (TSH). TSH is needed to trigger the release of the T_3 and T_4 stored in the thyroid gland. Tertiary hypothyroidism is caused by a reduced level of the thyrotropin-releasing hormone from the hypothalamus. This reduced level, in turn, reduces TSH and thyroid hormone levels. Symptoms of hypothyroidism include cold intolerance, unintentional weight gain, depression, dry and brittle hair and nails, and fatigue.

Hypothyroidism can also be classified by the point in the lifespan in which it occurs. Hyposecretion of thyroid hormones during youth may lead to *cretinism*. Cretinism is characterized by low metabolic rate, short stature, and severely delayed sexual development, and these features may be accompanied by intellectual disabilities. Hyposecretion of thyroid hormones as an adult may lead to myxedema. Myxedema is a condition manifested by decreased metabolic rate, but it also involves loss of mental and physical stamina, weight gain, hair loss, firm edema, and yellow dullness of the skin.

Some forms of hypothyroidism may result in the formation of a goitre, which is an enlargement of the thyroid gland resulting from its overstimulation by elevated levels of TSH. The TSH level is elevated because there is little or no thyroid hormone in the circulation.

Certain drugs can cause hypothyroidism. Amiodarone hydrochloride, an iodine-rich antidysrhythmic (see Chapter 26) has a wide range of effects on the thyroid. It acts as an enzyme inhibitor and decreases the peripheral conversion of T_4 to T_3 resulting in reduced T_3 levels. It also inhibits entry of T_4 and T_3 into the peripheral tissue with serum T_4 levels increasing; however, this does not create a state of hyperthyroidism (Gopalan, 2015). Amiodarone does have a direct cytotoxic effect on the follicular cells of the thyroid which can result in hyperthyroidism or thyrotosicosis.

HYPERTHYROIDISM

Excessive secretion of thyroid hormones, or **hyperthyroidism,** may be caused by several different diseases. Diseases known to cause hyperthyroidism include Graves' disease, which is the most common cause; Plummer's disease, also known as *toxic nodular disease*, which is the least common cause; multinodular disease; and thyroid storm, which is a severe and potentially life-threatening exacerbation of the symptoms of hyperthyroidism, often induced by stress or infection.

Hyperthyroidism can affect multiple body systems, resulting in an overall increase in metabolism. Commonly reported symptoms are diarrhea, flushing, increased appetite, muscle weakness, fatigue, palpitations, irritability, nervousness, sleep disorders, heat intolerance, and altered menstrual flow.

THYROID REPLACEMENT DRUGS

Hypothyroidism is treated with thyroid hormone replacement, using various thyroid preparations. These drugs can be either natural or synthetic in origin. The natural thyroid preparations are derived from the thyroid glands of animals such as cattle and pigs. Currently, only one natural preparation is available in Canada, called, simply, *thyroid* or *thyroid, desiccated*. *Desiccation* is the term for the drying process used to prepare this drug form. All natural preparations are standardized for their iodine content.

TABLE 32-1

Thyroid Drugs: Clinically Equivalent Doses

Thyroid Drug	Approximate Equivalent Dose
NATURAL THYROID PREPARATION	
thyroid	60–65 mg
SYNTHETIC THYROID PREPARATIONS	
levothyroxine	100 mcg or more
liothyronine	25 mcg

TABLE 32-2

Thyroid Drugs: Common Adverse Effects

Body System	Adverse Effects
Cardiovascular	Tachycardia, palpitations, angina, dysrhythmias, hypertension
Central nervous	Insomnia, tremors, headache, anxiety
Gastrointestinal	Nausea, diarrhea, cramps
Other	Menstrual irregularities, weight loss, sweating, heat intolerance, fever

TABLE 32-3

Thyroid Drugs: Interactions

Drug	Action
Insulin	Decreased efficacy of insulin (resulting in increased blood glucose levels)
Oral antihyperglycemics	Decreased efficacy of antidiabetic drugs (resulting in increased blood glucose levels)
Estrogen	Reduced thyroid drug activity
Digoxin	Decreased digoxin effectiveness
phenytoin and fosphenytoin	Reduced levothyroxine effectiveness
Phenobarbital	Reduced levothyroxine effectiveness

The synthetic thyroid preparations are levothyroxine (T_4) and liothyronine (T_3). The approximate clinically equivalent doses of the drugs are given in Table 32-1. This information is useful for guiding dosage adjustments when a patient is switched from one thyroid hormone to another. Monitoring of both serum TSH and free thyroid hormone levels is required to determine the appropriate dose of thyroid replacement drugs.

Mechanism of Action and Drug Effects

Thyroid drugs function in the same manner as endogenous thyroid hormones, affecting many body systems. At the cellular level, they act to induce changes in the metabolic rate, including the rate of protein, carbohydrate, and lipid metabolism, and to increase oxygen consumption, body temperature, blood volume, and overall cellular growth and differentiation. They also stimulate the cardiovascular system by increasing the number of myocardial β-adrenergic receptors. This, in turn, increases the sensitivity of the heart to catecholamines and ultimately increases cardiac output. In addition, thyroid hormones increase kidney blood flow and the glomerular filtration rate, which results in a diuretic effect.

Indications

Thyroid preparations are given to replace what the thyroid gland cannot produce to achieve normal thyroid levels (**euthyroid** condition). Levothyroxine is the preferred thyroid drug because its hormonal content is standardized and its effect is predictable. Thyroid drugs can also be used for the diagnosis of suspected hyperthyroidism (as a TSH-suppression test) and in the prevention or treatment of various types of goitre. They are also used for replacement hormonal therapy in patients whose thyroid glands have been surgically removed or destroyed by radioactive iodine in the treatment of thyroid cancer or hyperthyroidism. Hypothyroidism during pregnancy is treated with dosage adjustments every 4 weeks to maintain a TSH level at the lower end of the normal range. Fetal growth may be retarded if maternal hypothroidism remains untreated during pregnancy.

Contraindications

Contraindications to thyroid preparations include known drug allergy, recent myocardial infarction (MI), adrenal insufficiency, and hyperthyroidism. Levothyroxine contains cornstarch and lactose as fillers, and liothyronine sodium has modified food starch, which contains gluten. Many individuals with hypothyroidism have allergies to these ingredients.

Adverse Effects

The adverse effects of thyroid medications are usually the result of overdose. The most significant adverse effect is cardiac dysrhythmia, with the risk for life-threatening or fatal irregularities. Other more common undesirable effects are listed in Table 32-2.

Interactions

Thyroid drugs may enhance the activity of oral anticoagulants, the dosages of which may need to be reduced. Taking thyroid preparations concurrently with digoxin may decrease serum digoxin levels. Cholestyramine binds to thyroid hormone in the gastrointestinal (GI) tract, which possibly reduces the absorption of both drugs. Patients with diabetes taking a thyroid drug may require increased dosages of their hypoglycemic drugs. In addition, the use of thyroid preparations with epinephrine in patients with coronary disease may induce coronary insufficiency. See Table 32-3 for more drug interactions.

DRUG PROFILES

The most commonly used thyroid replacement drug is the synthetic drug levothyroxine. Some patients experience better results with the animal-derived products. Although the thyroid drugs differ chemically, their therapeutic actions are all the same. Factors to be considered before the initiation of drug therapy with a thyroid drug include the desired ratio of T_3 to T_4 (normal ratio is 1:17) to balance the cost, the risk for hyperthyroidism with clinical symptoms of hypothyroidism, and the desired duration of effect. Thyroid hormone replacement is safe for use during pregnancy. Thyroid replacement drugs are all contraindicated in patients who have had a hypersensitivity reaction to them in the past and in those with adrenal insufficiency, previous MI, or hyperthyroidism.

▸▸levothyroxine sodium

Levothyroxine sodium (Eltroxin®, Euthyrox®, Synthroid®), or T_4, is the most commonly prescribed synthetic thyroid hormone and is the drug of choice. One advantage it has over the natural thyroid preparations is that it is chemically pure, being 100% T_4 (thyroxine); this makes its effects more predictable than those of other thyroid

preparations. Levothyroxine's half-life is long enough that it is administered once a day. It is available in oral form and in parenteral form. Liothyronine sodium (Cytomel®) and desiccated thyroid (Thyroid®) are examples of similar drugs.

Switching between different brands of levothyroxine during treatment can destabilize the course of treatment. Thyroid function test results need to be monitored more carefully when switching products. Recommended dosages are given in the table on this page. Levothyroxine is dosed in micrograms. A common medication error is to interpret the intended dose in milligrams instead of micrograms. If not caught, this error would result in a thousandfold overdose. Doses higher than 200 mcg need to be questioned in case this error has occurred. The intravenous dose of levothyroxine is generally 50% of the oral dose.

PHARMACOKINETICS

Route	Onset of Action	Peak Plasma Concentration	Elimination Half-Life	Duration of Action
PO	3–5 days	3–4 days	6–10 days	1–3 wks

DOSAGES   Selected Thyroid Drugs

Drug	Pharmacological Class	Usual Dosage Range	Indications/Uses
▸▸levothyroxine sodium (Eltroxin, Euthyrox, Synthroid)	Synthetic levothyroxine (thyroid hormone T_4)	*Children 0–12 yr* PO: 3–15 mcg/kg/day *Adults* PO: 1–1.7 mcg/kg/day IM/IV: 50% of oral dose IV: 300–500 mcg in a single dose; then 75–100 mcg/day until thyroid levels improve	Congenital hypothyroidism Hypothyroidism Myxedema coma
liothyronine sodium (Cytomel)*	Synthetic liothyronine (thyroid hormone T_3)	*Adults* PO: 25–75 mcg/day PO: 50–100 mcg daily PO: 20–50 mcg daily	Hypothyroidism Myxedema Cretinism
desiccated thyroid (Thyroid)	Desiccated (dried) animal thyroid gland	*Children 0–12 yr* PO: 15–90 mg/day *Adults* PO: 15–120 mg/day	Congenital hypothyroidism Hypothyroidism

*Liothyronine is synonymous with triiodothyronine (T_3).
IM, intramuscular; *IV*, intravenous; *PO*, oral.

Dosages

For dosage information on the thyroid drugs, refer to the table above.

ANTITHYROID DRUGS

Treatment of hyperthyroidism is aimed at treating either the primary cause or the symptoms of the disease. Antithyroid drugs, iodides, ionic inhibitors, and radioactive isotopes of iodine are used to treat the underlying

cause, and drugs such as β-blockers are used to treat the symptoms. The focus of this discussion is on the antithyroid drugs called *thioamide derivatives*, thiamazole and propylthiouracil. In addition to the thioamides, radioactive iodine (iodine-131) may be used to treat hyperthyroidism. Radioactive iodine destroys the thyroid gland in a process known as *ablation*. It does this by emitting destructive β-rays once it is taken up into the follicles of the thyroid gland. Radioactive iodine is a commonly used treatment for both hyperthyroidism and thyroid cancer. Potassium iodide is also used as prophylaxis for radiation exposure. Thyroid surgery involves removal of part or all of the thyroid gland. It is usually an effective way to treat hyperthyroidism, but lifelong hormone replacement therapy is normally required after thyroid surgery.

Mechanism of Action and Drug Effects

Thiamazole and propylthiouracil act by inhibiting the incorporation of iodine molecules into the amino acid tyrosine, a process required to make the precursors of T_3 and T_4. This inhibition of iodine impedes the formation of thyroid hormones. Propylthiouracil has the added ability to inhibit the conversion of T_4 to T_3 in the peripheral circulation. Neither drug can inactivate already existing thyroid hormone.

The drug effects of thiamazole and propylthiouracil are limited primarily to the thyroid gland, and their overall effect is a decrease in the thyroid hormone level. Administration of these drugs to patients with hyperthyroidism lowers the high levels of thyroid hormone, thereby normalizing the overall metabolic rate.

Indications

Antithyroid drugs are used to treat hyperthyroidism and to prevent the surge in thyroid hormones that occurs during radioactive iodine therapy for or after the surgical treatment of hyperthyroidism or thyroid cancer. In some types of hyperthyroidism, such as that seen in Graves' disease, the long-term administration of these drugs (for several years) may induce a spontaneous remission. Surgical resection of the thyroid (thyroidectomy) is often used in patients who are intolerant of antithyroid drug therapy and in pregnant women, in whom both antithyroid drugs and radioactive iodine therapy are usually contraindicated.

Contraindications

The only usual contraindication to the use of the two antithyroid drugs is known drug allergy. Their use in pregnancy, though it may be necessary, is somewhat controversial. Propylthiouracil and thiamazole are effective drugs for the treatment of hyperthyroidism in pregnant women. However, the drug readily crosses the placenta and can cause goitre or cretinism in the fetus. Hyperthyroidism may be overcompensated by the metabolic demands of pregnancy; the lowest effective dose is recommended. However, there are case reports of scalp abnormalities when thiamazole is used. The choice of how to treat patients who are pregnant is specific to individual health care providers.

Adverse Effects

The most serious adverse effects of the antithyroid medications are liver and bone marrow toxicity. These and the more common adverse effects of thiamazole and propylthiouracil are listed in Table 32-4.

TABLE 32-4	
Antithyroid Drugs: Common Adverse Effects	
Body System	**Adverse Effects**
Central nervous	Drowsiness, headache, vertigo, paresthesia
Gastrointestinal	Nausea, vomiting, diarrhea, hepatitis, loss of taste
Genitourinary	Cloudy urine, decreased urine output
Hematological	Agranulocytosis, leukopenia, thrombocytopenia, hypothrombinemia, lymphadenopathy, bleeding
Integumentary	Rash, pruritus
Musculoskeletal	Myalgia, arthralgia
Renal	Increased blood urea nitrogen and serum creatinine levels
Other	Enlarged thyroid gland, nephritis

Interactions

Drug interactions that occur with antithyroid drugs include an increase in the activity of oral anticoagulants and additive leukopenic effects when they are taken in conjunction with other bone marrow depressants.

Dosages

For dosage information on propylthiouracil and thiamazole, refer to the table on p. 616.

PHARMACOKINETIC BRIDGE TO NURSING PRACTICE

Nurses must understand the pharmacokinetics of thyroid replacement drugs to think critically through clinical situations involving patients who are taking them. Thyroid replacement drugs possess specific pharmacokinetic characteristics.

For levothyroxine (Eltroxin®, Euthyrox®, Synthroid®), the pharmacokinetic characteristics include an onset of action of 3 to 5 days, peak plasma concentrations within 3 to 4 days, elimination half-life of 6 to 10 days, and a duration of action of 1 to 3 weeks. Levothyroxine has a narrow therapeutic margin. Due to its prolonged half life, there is an increased risk of toxicity. Toxicity is manifested by the following: weight loss, tachycardia, nervousness, tremors, hypertension, headache, insomnia, menstrual irregularities, and cardiac irregularities or palpitations. Clinical and laboratory evaluations are recommended at 6- to 8-week intervals (or 2- to 3-week intervals in patients who have severe hypothyroidism), and the dosage will need to be adjusted until the serum TSH concentration is normalized and signs and symptoms resolve. Once optimal replacement is achieved, evaluations are recommended at least annually, or whenever warranted by a change in patient status. Another

DRUG PROFILES

▶propylthiouracil

Propylthiouracil is a thioamide antithyroid drug. Approximately 2 weeks of therapy with propylthiouracil may be necessary before symptoms improve. It is available only in oral form. Thiamazole is the only alternative drug in this class and is rarely used clinically.

PHARMACOKINETICS

Route	Onset of Action	Peak Plasma Concentration	Elimination Half-Life	Duration of Action
PO	24–36 hr	1 hr	1.5–5 hr	2–3 hr

DOSAGES Selected Antithyroid Drugs

Drug	Pharmacological Class	Usual Dosage Range	Indications/Uses
thiamazole (Tapazole®)	Antithyroid	*Children* PO: 0.4 mg/kg/day; maintenance half of initial dose *Adult* PO: 15–60 mg/day	Hyperthyroidism
▶propylthiouracil* (generic only)	Antithyroid	*Children 6–10 yr* PO: 50–150 mg/day *Children over 10 yr* PO: 150–300 mg/day *Adults* PO: 300–900 mg/day	Hyperthyroidism

*Often abbreviated PTU.
PO, oral.

important pharmacokinetic property of levothyroxine is that the drug is highly protein bound. A protein-bound drug acts like a biological sustained-release drug and remains in the body longer, with increased risk of more interactions with other highly protein-bound drugs as well as greater risk for toxicity. Consumption of foods such as soybean flour (e.g., as found in infant formula), cottonseed meal, walnuts, calcium (e.g., as found in calcium-fortified orange juice), and dietary fibre may bind to and consequently decrease the absorption of levothyroxine sodium from the GI tract, thereby necessitating adjustments in dosing. This is yet another example of how important a current and thorough knowledge base about drugs—and specifically about their pharmacokinetics—is to their safe and efficient administration.

NURSING PROCESS

 Assessment

In assessing patients taking thyroid replacement drugs for hypothyroidism, record baseline vital signs for comparative purposes. Assess T_3, T_4, and TSH, before and during drug therapy, as ordered. It is important to thoroughly assess and document all past and present medical problems or concerns. Take a medication history that includes drug allergies and a list of all prescription drugs, over-the-counter drugs (OTC), and natural health products a patient is taking. Cautions, contraindications, and drug interactions associated with the use of thyroid hormone have been previously discussed; thoroughly assess patients for these prior to the initiation of therapy with these drugs. Review baseline vital signs, paying attention to any history of cardiac dysrhythmias because of the possible adverse effects of cardiac irregularities; these may be life-threatening. For female patients, perform a thorough assessment of the reproductive system due to the impact of thyroid hormones on this system.

It is also important to remember that certain thyroid hormones may work faster than others because of their dosage form and properties (see Pharmacokinetic Bridge to Nursing Practice). Drug interactions that deserve emphasis (because of their importance to patient safety and because they involve commonly used medications) include interactions with oral anticoagulants (leading to increased anticoagulant activity), digoxin (leading to a decrease in digoxin levels), cholestyramine, and oral antihyperglycemic drugs. See Table 32-3 for a more detailed listing of drug interactions. If the patient is taking an oral anticoagulant, monitor blood levels of the anticoagulant closely. Lifespan considerations include increased sensitivity to the effects of thyroid medications in older adults. Individualization of drug therapy is important with thyroid replacement because different patients may respond differently to the same drug or dosage (see Special Populations: Older Adults: Thyroid Hormones).

SPECIAL POPULATIONS: OLDER ADULTS

Thyroid Hormones

- Older adult patients are much more sensitive to thyroid hormone replacement drugs (as they are to most drugs). They are also more likely to experience adverse reactions to thyroid hormones than are patients in any other age group.
- Older adult patients experience more negative consequences related to drug therapy because their liver and kidney functioning is decreased.
- Thyroid hormone replacement requirements are approximately 25% lower in patients 60 years of age and older than in younger patients. Dosage in older adult patients may therefore need to be adjusted or titrated downward.

- Older adult patients must contact their health care providers immediately if they experience palpitations, chest pain, stumbling, falling, depression, incontinence, sweating, shortness of breath, symptoms of aggravated heart disease, cold intolerance, or weight gain.
- Drug therapy for older adult patients must be initiated with caution and with individualized dosages. If higher dosages are necessary, increases must be made with the health care provider's guidance and done gradually.

For antithyroid drugs, such as propylthiouracil and thiamazole, first measure vital signs and assess for signs and symptoms of thyroid crisis, or what is often called *thyroid storm*. Thyroid storm is manifested by exacerbation of the symptoms of hyperthyroidism (see previous discussion of hyperthyroidism symptoms on p. 612) and is potentially life-threatening.

Assessing for thyroid storm also means assessing for its potential causes, such as stress or infection. Related cautions and contraindications have been discussed previously, but some important drug interactions to re-emphasize include interactions with oral anticoagulants (which can cause an increase in anticoagulation and thus risk for bleeding) and any medications that may lead to bone marrow suppression or cause leukopenia (antithyroid drugs may cause additive effects or worsening of bone marrow suppression).

⬛ Nursing Diagnoses

- Nonadherance to drug therapy due to lack of experience or education related to thyroid hormone replacement and the need for daily self-administration
- Ineffective health management due to lack of experience or education related to the use of thyroid medication
- Risk for infection related to the bone marrow depression caused by antithyroid medication

⬛ Planning

⬛ Goals

- Patient will remain adherent to daily administration of thyroid hormone replacement therapy.
- Patient will demonstrate improvement in health management behaviours through more experience and education regarding the rationale for the use of the thyroid drug and its related adverse effects.

- Patient will remain free from infection while receiving antithyroid medication.

⬛ Expected Patient Outcomes

- Patient states the importance of taking thyroid hormone replacement therapy daily, as ordered.
  - Patient takes thyroid hormone replacement therapy upon awakening in the morning and on an empty stomach, to maximize therapeutic effects.
  - Patient takes medication in a single daily dose before breakfast and does not stop the medication without consulting a health care provider.
  - Patient understands that replacement therapy will be lifelong in most situations.
- Patient states the importance of taking the medication as prescribed as well as the rationale for its use.
  - Patient states the adverse effects associated with thyroid replacement therapy that need to be reported to a health care provider (e.g., cardiac dysrhythmias [felt as palpitations]).
  - Patient reports adverse effects that may indicate the need for re-regulation of dosage such as signs and symptoms of hyperthyroidism (e.g., irregular heartbeat, palpitations).
- Patient states ways to decrease the risk for infection while receiving an antithyroid medication, such as avoiding persons with infections, eating a nutritious diet, getting adequate rest, and increasing fluid intake.

⬛ Implementation

When thyroid drugs are administered, it is important that they are taken at the same time every day to maintain consistent blood levels of the drug. Emphasize to patients that it is best to take thyroid drugs once daily in the morning (e.g., 60 minutes before breakfast for optimum absorption) if possible, to decrease the likelihood of insomnia, which may result from evening dosing and the

CASE STUDY

Antithyroid Drug Therapy

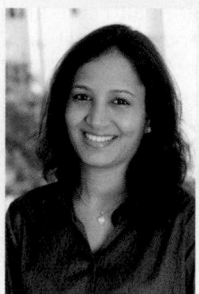

Rima, a 28-year-old restaurant manager, has been diagnosed with hyperthyroidism due to Graves' disease. Her health care provider has explained the proposed therapy with propylthiouracil to her and her husband. She has no other known health problems at this time.

1. What laboratory studies will be performed before drug therapy with propylthiouracil is started? Explain your answer.

2. Rima asks, "What do I need to know while I'm taking this drug?" List pertinent patient teaching points.

3. After 1 month of therapy, Rima comes into the health care provider's office for a follow-up visit. She is upset because a friend told her about a relative who had antithyroid therapy for cancer and said he was "radioactive." She is wondering if her medication has made her "radioactive." How will the nurse answer her question?

4. Six months later, Rima calls her health care provider's office and says, "I think I might be pregnant. What do I do about taking this drug?" What does the nurse need to tell her?

_____

For answers, see http://evolve.elsevier.com/Canada/Lilley/pharmacology/.

subsequent increase in energy level. Patients must also avoid interchanging brands because of problems with the bioequivalence of drugs from different manufacturers. If needed, patients may crush tablets. If a patient is scheduled to undergo radioactive isotope studies, thyroid medication is usually discontinued about 4 weeks before the test, but only as prescribed. Older adult patients may require alteration of the dosage amount, with a decrease of up to 25% for patients 60 years of age and older. Dosage is individualized and there is considerable variability in response, although improvement in symptoms is usually seen in 2 weeks, with good results seen within 4 to 8 weeks.

Educate patients taking the antithyroid drug propylthiouracil about taking the medication with meals to help decrease GI upset. Any fever, sore throat, mouth ulcers or sores, skin eruptions, or any unusual bleeding or bruising needs to be reported to the health care provider immediately. These symptoms may indicate liver and bone marrow toxicity and possible leukopenia. Further educate patients to avoid consuming iodized salt or shellfish because of their potential for altering the drug's effectiveness. Advise patients to be aware of the signs and symptoms of hypothyroidism, including unexplained weight gain, loss of mental and physical stamina, hair loss, edema (particularly around the face),

and yellow dullness of the skin (indicative of myxedema or a decrease in metabolic rate). If these symptoms occur, patients must report them immediately to the health care provider. Frequently monitor complete blood counts to watch for potential problems with leukopenia. It is also important to monitor the results of liver function studies during follow-up visits with the health care provider.

Evaluation

A therapeutic response to thyroid drugs is manifested by the disappearance of the symptoms of hypothyroidism; patients should demonstrate improved energy levels as well as improved mental and physical stamina. Monitor for the adverse effect of cardiac dysrhythmia (see Table 32-2). If a patient is receiving inadequate doses of the thyroid medication, a return of the symptoms of hypothyroidism may occur (see previous discussion).

Adverse effects include the possibility of leukopenia, which may be manifested by fever, sore throat, lesions, or other signs of infection. Symptoms indicating that a patient is not receiving adequate doses include tachycardia, insomnia, irritability, fever, and diarrhea, as well as continued signs and symptoms of hyperthyroidism (see previous discussion).

PATIENT TEACHING TIPS

❖ Patients should be aware that oral thyroid replacement drugs are best taken 1 hour before breakfast on an empty stomach to enhance their absorption, maintain constant hormone levels, and help prevent insomnia.

❖ Thyroid replacement medications are not to be abruptly discontinued; patients should know that lifelong therapy is usually the norm.

❖ Emphasize to patients the importance of keeping follow-up visits so the health care provider can monitor thyroid hormone levels, complete blood counts, and results of liver function studies.

❖ Brands of thyroid replacement drugs cannot be interchanged. Advise patients to always check that the

PATIENT TEACHING TIPS—cont'd

pharmacy has provided the correct brand of thyroid replacement drug.

❖ Signs and symptoms associated with hypothyroidism include myxedema with decreased metabolic rate, loss of mental and physical stamina, weight gain, hair loss, firm edema, and yellow dullness of the skin. Share this information with patients.

❖ Instruct patients taking thyroid replacement drugs to immediately report any of the following to the health care provider: chest pain, weight loss, palpitations, tremors, sweating, nervousness, shortness of breath, or insomnia, as these may indicate toxicity.

❖ Encourage patients to keep a daily journal with notations about how they are feeling, their energy levels and appetite, and any adverse effects.

❖ Advise patients that it may take up to 3 to 4 weeks to see the full therapeutic effects of thyroid drugs.

❖ Inform patients that all thyroid tablets must be protected from light.

❖ Signs and symptoms of hyperthyroidism include increased metabolic rate, diarrhea, flushing, increased appetite, muscle weakness, fatigue, palpitations, irritability, nervousness, sleep disorders, heat intolerance, and altered menstrual flow. Patients with

this disorder and those on drug therapy need to be aware of these signs and symptoms.

❖ Antithyroid medications are better tolerated when taken with meals or a snack. These drugs must also be given at the same time every day to maintain consistent blood levels of the drug. They must never be withdrawn abruptly.

❖ Instruct patients taking thyroid or antithyroid drugs to read all drug labels thoroughly and not to take any OTC medications without first consulting their health care provider or pharmacist.

❖ Patients taking antithyroid medications must avoid eating foods high in iodine, such as tofu and other soy products, turnips, seafood, iodized salt, and some breads. These foods may interfere with the effectiveness of the antithyroid drug.

❖ There are numerous drugs that interact with thyroid medications (e.g., antacids, digoxin, antidiabetic drugs (see Table 32-3). Provide a list of all medications to patients before and during therapy with thyroid medications.

❖ Provide patients with information on the Thyroid Foundation of Canada (http://www.thyroid.ca/).

KEY POINTS

❖ T_4 and T_3 are the two hormones produced by the thyroid gland; thyroid hormones are made by iodination and coupling with the amino acid tyrosine.

❖ Thyroid hormone replacement is generally carried out carefully by the health care provider, with frequent monitoring of serum levels until stabilization appears to have occurred. Monitor and review laboratory values to be sure that serum levels are within normal limits to avoid possible toxicity.

❖ Hyperthyroidism is caused by excessive secretion of thyroid hormone by the thyroid gland and may be caused by different diseases (Graves' disease, Plummer's disease, multinodular disease) or drugs. Always assess and document important information about the patient's medical history appropriately.

❖ Patients receiving levothyroxine need to report the occurrence of excitability, irritability, or palpitations to the health care provider because these symptoms may indicate toxicity.

❖ Adverse effects associated with thyroid drugs include tachycardia, palpitations, angina, dysrhythmias, hypertension, insomnia, tremors, headache, anxiety, nausea, diarrhea, cramps, menstrual irregularities, weight loss, sweating, fever, and heat intolerance.

❖ Adverse effects associated with antithyroid drugs include drowsiness, headache, vertigo, nausea, vomiting, diarrhea, loss of taste, bleeding, leukopenia, rash, myalgia, and arthralgia.

EXAMINATION REVIEW QUESTIONS

1. When monitoring the laboratory values of a patient who is taking antithyroid drugs, which values should the nurse know to watch for?
   a. Increased platelet counts
   b. Decreased white blood cell counts
   c. Decreased blood urea nitrogen level
   d. Increased blood glucose levels

2. The pharmacy has called a patient to notify her that her current brand of thyroid replacement hormone is on back order. The patient calls her clinic to ask what she

should do. What is the best response on the part of the nurse?
   a. "Go ahead and take the other brand that the pharmacy has available for now."
   b. "You can stop the medication until your current brand is available."
   c. "You can split the thyroid pills that you have left so that they will last longer."
   d. "You may require additional testing of thyroid hormone levels with a change in drug."

Continued

EXAMINATION REVIEW QUESTIONS—cont'd

3. When assessing an older adult patient, which nonspecific symptoms of hypothyroidism should the nurse keep in mind?
a. Leukopenia, anemia
b. Loss of appetite, polyuria
c. Weight loss, dry cough
d. Cold intolerance, depression

4. To help with the insomnia associated with thyroid hormone replacement therapy, which strategy should the nurse teach the patient to do?
a. Take half the dose at lunchtime and the other half 2 hours later.
b. Use a sedative to assist with falling asleep.
c. Take the dose upon awakening in the morning.
d. Reduce the dosage as needed if sleep is impaired.

5. The nurse is teaching a patient who has a new prescription for the antithyroid drug propylthiouracil. Which statement by the nurse is correct?
a. "There are no food restrictions while on this drug."
b. "You need to avoid foods high in iodine, such as iodized salt, seafood, and soy products."
c. "This drug is given to raise the thyroid hormone levels in your blood."
d. "Take this drug in the morning on an empty stomach."

6. When teaching a patient who has a new prescription for thyroid hormone, the nurse will instruct the patient to notify the health care provider if which adverse effects are noted? (Select all that apply.)
a. Palpitations
b. Weight gain
c. Angina
d. Fatigue
e. Cold intolerance

7. The nurse is giving an intravenous dose of levothyroxine (Synthroid). The order reads: "Give 0.1 mg IV push now." What is the ordered dose in micrograms?

Answers: 1. b, 2. d, 3. d, 4. c, 5. b, 6. a, c, 7. 100 mcg

CRITICAL THINKING ACTIVITIES

1. A patient has been taking thyroid drugs for about 16 months and has recently noted palpitations and some heat intolerance. What are the nurse's priority actions at this time?

2. A patient with a history of hypothyroidism is in her first trimester of pregnancy. She asks the nurse, "How often will they check my thyroid hormone levels? I'm very worried about how this medication will affect my baby." What is the nurse's best response?

3. A 33-year-old man, newly admitted to the medical–surgical unit from the step-down critical care unit, underwent a thyroidectomy 2 days earlier. While reviewing the orders, the nurse notices that the patient is to start receiving his thyroid medication upon transfer to the medical–surgical unit. The written orders specify that 25 mcg of levothyroxine is available in stock. However, the pharmacy has only 25 mcg of liothyronine in stock. What is the nurse's priority action at this time?

For answers see http://evolve.elsevier.com/Canada/Lilley/pharmacology/.

Antidiabetic Drugs

Objectives

After reading this chapter, the successful student will be able to do the following:

1. Discuss the normal actions and functions of the pancreas.

2. Contrast age of onset, signs and symptoms, pharmacological and nonpharmacological treatment, incidence, and etiology of type 1 and type 2 diabetes.

3. Differentiate gestational diabetes from type 1 and type 2 diabetes.

4. Discuss the various factors influencing plasma glucose levels in individuals without diabetes and in patients with diabetes.

5. Identify the drugs used to manage type 1 and type 2 diabetes.

6. Discuss the mechanisms of action, indications, contraindications, cautions, drug interactions, and adverse effects of insulin, oral antihyperglycemic drugs, and injectable antidiabetic drugs.

7. Compare rapid-, short-, intermediate-, and long-acting insulins in regard to their onset of action, peak effects, and duration of action.

8. Compare the signs and symptoms of hypoglycemia and hyperglycemia and their related treatments.

9. Develop collaborative plans of care that include all phases of the nursing process for patients with type 1 or type 2 diabetes, with a focus on drug therapies.

e-Learning Activities

Website
(http://evolve.elsevier.com/Canada/
Lilley/pharmacology/)

evolve

- Answer Key—Textbook Case Studies
- Answer Key—Critical Thinking Activities
- Chapter Summaries—Printable
- Review Questions for Exam Preparation
- Unfolding Case Studies

Drug Profiles

 acarbose, p. 637
▸▸ gliclazide, p. 637
▸▸ insulin glargine, insulin detemir, p. 631
▸▸ insulin isophane suspension (NPH), p. 631
 insulin lispro, p. 631
▸▸ metformin (metformin hydrochloride)*, p. 637
▸▸ pioglitazone, p. 638
▸▸ regular insulin, p. 631
▸▸ repaglinide, p. 638
▸▸ sitagliptin, p. 638

▸▸ Key drug

*Full generic name is given in parentheses. For the purposes of this text, the more common, shortened name is used.

Key Terms

Diabetes A complex disorder of carbohydrate, fat, and protein metabolism resulting from the lack of insulin secretion by the β-cells of the pancreas or from defects of the insulin receptors; sometimes referred to as *diabetes mellitus*. There are two major types of diabetes: type 1 and type 2. (p. 623)

Diabetic ketoacidosis (DKA) A severe metabolic complication of uncontrolled diabetes that, if untreated, may lead to serious hyperglycemic emergencies. (p. 626)

Gestational diabetes Diabetes that develops during pregnancy; it may resolve after pregnancy but may also be a precursor of type 2 diabetes in later life. (p. 626)

Glucagon A hormone produced by the α-cells in the islets of Langerhans; glucagon stimulates the conversion of glycogen to glucose in the liver. (p. 622)

Glucose One of the simple sugars that serves as a major source of energy. It is found in foods (e.g., fruits, refined sweets) and also is the final breakdown product of complex carbohydrate metabolism in the body; it is commonly referred to as *dextrose*. (p. 622)

Glycogen A polysaccharide that is the major carbohydrate stored in animal cells. (p. 622)

Glycogenolysis The breakdown of glycogen into glucose. (p. 622)

Hemoglobin A₁c (HbA₁c) Hemoglobin molecules to which glucose molecules are bound; also referred to as *glycosylated hemoglobin* and is most commonly referred to as A_{1C}. Blood levels of hemoglobin $A_{1}c$ are used to monitor and diagnose diabetes. (p. 628)

Hyperglycemia A fasting plasma glucose level of 7 mmol/L or higher or a nonfasting plasma glucose level of 11.1 mmol/L or higher. (p. 623)

Hyperosmolar hyperglycemic state (HHS) A metabolic complication that occurs in patients with type 2 diabetes, characterized by hyperglycemia, hyperosmolarity, and dehydration without significant ketoacidosis. (p. 626)

Hypoglycemia A plasma glucose level of less than 4 mmol/L with autonomic or neuroglycopenic symptoms that respond to the administration of a carbohydrate or the use of glucagon. (p. 639)

Impaired fasting glucose level A fasting glucose level of at least 6.1 mmol/L but lower than 6.9 mmol/L; it defines a prediabetic state often referred to as *prediabetes*. (p. 627)

Insulin A naturally occurring hormone secreted by the β-cells in the islets of Langerhans in the pancreas in response to increased levels of glucose in the blood. (p. 622)

Ketones Organic chemical compounds produced through the oxidation of secondary alcohols (e.g., fat molecules), including dietary carbohydrates. (p. 623)

Metabolic syndrome A cluster of risk factors including abdominal obesity, hypertension, dyslipidemia, and elevated plasma glucose that places individuals at significant risk of developing type 2 diabetes and cardiovascular disease. (p. 626)

Polydipsia Excessive intake of water; one of the common symptoms of uncontrolled diabetes. (p. 623)

Polyphagia Excessive hunger; one of the common symptoms of uncontrolled diabetes. (p. 623)

Polyuria Increased frequency or volume of urinary output; one of the common symptoms of uncontrolled diabetes. (p. 623)

Prediabetes A state in which one or more of the fasting glucose, glucose tolerance, or A_{1C} are higher than normal but not diagnostic; individuals with prediabetes are at high risk of developing diabetes and the resulting complications. (p. 627)

Type 1 diabetes Diabetes caused by an autoimmune disease resulting in β-cell destruction and that makes the individual prone to hyperglycemia and ketoacidosis; most commonly develops in children and adolescents. (p. 625)

Type 2 diabetes A type of diabetes that is most common in adults and is becoming increasingly common in children and adolescents; characterized by hyperglycemia that occurs as a result of predominant insulin resistance with relative insulin deficiency to a predominant secretory defect with insulin resistance. (p. 626)

PANCREAS

The pancreas is a large, elongated organ located behind the stomach. It functions as an exocrine gland (secreting digestive enzymes through the pancreatic duct) and a ductless endocrine gland (secreting hormones directly into the bloodstream). The endocrine functions of the pancreas are the focus of this chapter. **Insulin** and **glucagon** are the two main hormones produced by the pancreas. Both hormones play an important role in the regulation of glucose homeostasis, specifically the mobilization, use, and storage of glucose by the body. **Glucose** is one of the primary sources of energy for the cells of the body. It is also the simplest form of carbohydrate found in the body, and is often referred to as *dextrose*. There is a normal amount of glucose that circulates in the blood to meet body requirements for quick energy. Excess glucose is stored as **glycogen** in the liver and, to a lesser extent, in skeletal muscle tissue, where it remains until the body needs it. Glucose is also stored in adipose tissue as triglyceride body fat. When more circulating glucose is needed, glycogen—primarily that stored in the liver—is converted back to glucose through a process called **glycogenolysis.** The hormone responsible for initiating this process is glucagon. Glucagon has only minimal effects on muscle glycogen and adipose tissue triglyceride stores.

Glucagon is released from the α-cells of the islets of Langerhans in the pancreas. Glucagon is a protein hormone consisting of a single chain of amino acids (polypeptide chain). Its molecules are about half the size of those of insulin. Insulin is secreted from the β-cells of the islets. Insulin is a protein hormone composed of two amino acid chains (acidic A chain and basic B chain) joined by a disulfide linkage. There is a continuous homeostatic balance in the body between the actions of insulin and those of glucagon. This natural balance serves to maintain optimal plasma glucose levels, which normally range between 4 and 6 mmol/L. Because of the crucial role of the pancreas in producing and maintaining these two hormones, pancreatic or islet cell transplants are sometimes undertaken to treat type 1 diabetes that has not been successfully controlled by other means. Another common treatment is continuous insulin administration

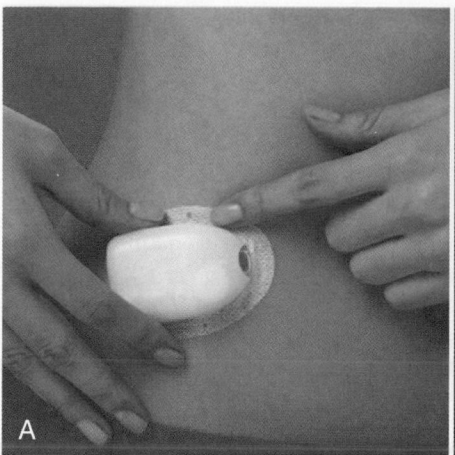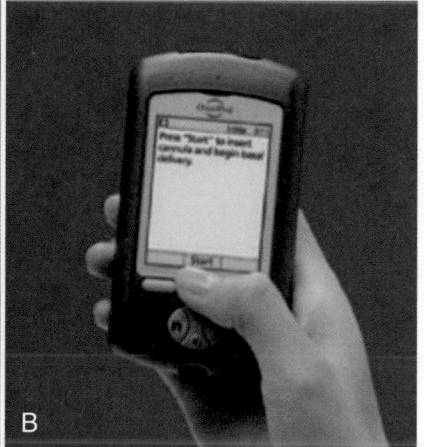

FIG. 33-1   A) OmniPod Insulin Management System. The Pod holds and delivers insulin. B) The Personal Diabetes Manager (PDM) wirelessly programs insulin delivery via the Pod. The PDM has a built-in glucose meter. (Source: Courtesy of Insulet Corporation.)

via a computerized insulin pump, which may be used to treat type 1 or type 2 diabetes. One of the newest advances in insulin delivery systems is the OmniPod system (see Figure 33-1), consisting of two parts. The Pod is a small, light, waterproof delivery system that attaches to the patient via a cannula. It delivers rapid-acting insulin continuously regulated by the patient's intake of carbohydrates. The Personal Diabetes Manager is a handheld remote that calculates the insulin doses and controls the Pod's insulin delivery. It also has the ability to determine the patient's plasma glucose. More information is available at http://www.myomnipod.ca/.

Insulin has several important metabolic functions in the body. It stimulates carbohydrate metabolism in skeletal and cardiac muscle and in adipose tissue by facilitating the transport of glucose into these cells. In the liver, insulin facilitates the phosphorylation of glucose to glucose-6-phosphate, which is then converted to glycogen for storage. By causing glucose to be stored in the liver as glycogen, insulin keeps the kidneys free of glucose. Without insulin, blood glucose levels rise; when the kidneys are unable to reabsorb this excess glucose, they excrete large amounts of glucose (a critical body nutrient and energy source), **ketones**, and other solutes into the urine. This loss of nutrient energy sources eventually leads to **polyphagia**, weight loss, and malnutrition. The presence of these solutes in the distal kidney tubules and collecting ducts also draws large volumes of water into the urine through osmotic diuresis, which leads to **polyuria**, **polydipsia**, and dehydration. These are all classic manifestations of type 1 diabetes.

Insulin also has a direct effect on fat metabolism. It stimulates lipogenesis and inhibits lipolysis and the release of fatty acids from adipose cells. In addition, insulin stimulates protein synthesis and promotes the intracellular shift of potassium and magnesium into the cells, thereby temporarily decreasing elevated blood concentrations of these electrolytes. Other substances such as cortisol, epinephrine, and growth hormone work synergistically with glucagon to counter the effects of insulin and cause increases in plasma glucose levels.

DIABETES

Hyperglycemia is a state involving excessive concentrations of glucose in the blood and results when the normal counterbalancing actions of glucagon and insulin fail to maintain normal glucose homeostasis (i.e., serum levels of 4 to 6 mmol/L). Complications in protein and fat metabolism (dyslipidemia; see Chapter 28) are also involved. The current key diagnostic criterion for diabetes is hyperglycemia with a fasting plasma glucose of higher than 7 mmol/L or a hemoglobin A_{1C} level greater than or equal to 6.5%. An A_{1C} level of 6.5% is the threshold for the development of microvascular disease and a predictor for the development of macrovascular disease. Diagnostic indicators are described in more detail in Box 33-1. Although there may be some variability in the diagnostic criteria for diabetes, this text uses the 2013 Canadian Diabetes Association (CDA) Clinical Practice Guidelines (updated in 2015) as a reference.

Diabetes is primarily a disorder of carbohydrate metabolism that involves either a deficiency of insulin, a resistance of tissue (e.g., muscle, liver) to insulin, or both. Whatever the cause of the diabetes, the result is hyperglycemia. Uncontrolled hyperglycemia correlates strongly with serious long-term macrovascular and microvascular complications. Macrovascular complications are usually secondary to large vessel damage caused by the deposition of atherosclerotic plaque. This compromises both central and peripheral circulation. In contrast, microvascular complications are secondary to damage to capillary vessels, which impairs peripheral circulation and damages eyes and kidneys. In addition, both autonomic and somatic nerve damage occur, caused primarily by metabolic changes and, to a lesser degree, by compromised circulation. Table 33-1 lists the common long-term complications of diabetes.

TABLE 33-1	
Major Long-Term Consequences of Diabetes (Type 1 and Type 2)	
Pathology	**Potential Consequences**
MACROVASCULAR (ATHEROSCLEROTIC PLAQUE)	
Coronary arteries	Myocardial infarction
Cerebral arteries	Stroke
Peripheral vessels	Peripheral vascular disease (e.g., neuropathies [see below], foot ulcers, possible amputations)
MICROVASCULAR (CAPILLARY DAMAGE)	
Retinopathy (retinal damage)	Partial or complete blindness
Neuropathy (autonomic and somatic nerve damage, due to both metabolic alterations and compromised circulation)	Autonomic nerve damage: Examples include diabetic gastroparesis, bladder dysfunction, unawareness of hypoglycemia, sexual dysfunction
	Somatic nerve damage: Examples include diabetic foot ulcer or leg or foot amputation (resulting from undetected injuries due to loss of sensation and from compromised circulation)
Nephropathy (kidney damage)	Proteinuria (microalbuminuria), chronic kidney failure (may require dialysis or kidney transplantation)

Source: Canadian Diabetes Association Clinical Practice Guidelines Expert Committee. (2013). Canadian Diabetes Association 2013 clinical practice guidelines for the prevention and management of diabetes in Canada. *Canadian Journal of Diabetes, 37*(Suppl. 1), S1–S212.

BOX 33-1

Criteria for Diagnosis of Diabetes

Fasting plasma glucose level equal to or higher than 7 mmol/L. ("Fasting" is defined as no caloric intake for at least 8 hours.)

OR

A_{1C} greater than 6.5% (in adults)

OR

Two-hour plasma glucose level of 11.1 mmol/L or higher during a 75 g oral glucose tolerance test (OGTT; Note that the OGTT is not recommended for routine clinical use.)

OR

Random plasma glucose level of 11.1 mmol/L or higher, measured at any time of day without regard to time since last meal

Diabetes has been recognized since 1550 BC, when Egyptians wrote of a malady they called *honeyed urine*. Not until the early 1920s was insulin finally isolated in Toronto, Ontario, by Nobel Prize–winners Frederick Banting and Charles Best. Its discovery is now considered one of the greatest triumphs of 20th-century medicine, and its use in the treatment of diabetes has proved to be lifesaving for millions of people affected by the disease.

Diabetes is not a single disease but a group of progressive diseases. For this reason, it is often regarded as a syndrome rather than a disease. In some cases, diabetes is caused by a relative or absolute lack of insulin that is believed to result from the destruction of β-cells in the pancreas, which leads to the inability to produce insulin. Hyperglycemia can also be caused by defects in insulin receptors that result in insulin resistance. The glycoproteins that serve as insulin receptors are attached to the surface of cells in the liver, muscle, and adipose tissue. These receptor proteins are stimulated by insulin molecules to move glucose from blood to cells. When insulin receptors become defective, they no longer respond normally to insulin molecules. Although serum insulin and glucose levels are both elevated in this situation, they do not respond and transport glucose into the cell where it is needed. The result is that glucose molecules remain in the blood, rather than being stored in the cells or tissues.

Two major types of diabetes are currently recognized and designated by the CDA: type 1 and type 2. The numerical designations for both conditions were adopted by the CDA as the preferred terms in 1995. Previous designations (e.g., insulin-dependent diabetes and noninsulin-dependent diabetes) were abandoned for several reasons: (1) many patients with type 2 diabetes do eventually become dependent on insulin therapy for control of their illness, and (2) the current epidemic of child and adult obesity in Canada is resulting in an increasing incidence of type 2 diabetes in children, adolescents, and young adults. Obesity is one of the major risk factors for the development of type 2 diabetes. Members of certain ethnic groups, including South Asian, Hispanic, and Indigenous individuals, are at higher risk for developing type 2 diabetes than are White people. The usual differences between type 1 and type 2 diabetes are listed in Table 33-2.

Approximately 10% of people with type 2 diabetes have circulating antibodies that suggest an autoimmune origin for the disease. This condition is known as *latent autoimmune diabetes in adults* (LADA) and is essentially a more slowly progressing form of type 1 diabetes.

TABLE 33-2

Characteristics of Type 1 and Type 2 Diabetes

Characteristic	Type 1	Type 2
Etiology	Autoimmune destruction of β-cells in the pancreas	Multifactorial genetic defects; strong association with obesity and insulin resistance resulting from a reduction in the number or activity of insulin receptors
Incidence	10% of cases	90% of cases
Onset	Usually younger than 20 yr	Age older than 40 yr; now increasingly seen in younger adults, adolescents, and children; attributed to rising prevalence of obesity
Endogenous insulin	Little or none	Normal levels in early disease; reduced later in disease
Insulin receptors	Normal	Decreased or defective
Body weight	Usually nonobese	Obese (80% of cases)
Treatment	Insulin	Weight loss, diet and exercise, and oral antihyperglycemics; earlier use of insulin is associated with improved outcomes

The most common signs and symptoms of type 1 diabetes are elevated plasma glucose levels (fasting glucose level higher than 7 mmol/L), polyuria, polydipsia, polyphagia, glucosuria, weight loss, blurred vision, and fatigue. These symptoms may also be observed in patients with type 2 diabetes, especially blurred vision and fatigue; however, other acute signs and symptoms may also occur (see Type 2 Diabetes, below).

Type 1 Diabetes

Type 1 diabetes is characterized by a lack of insulin production or by the production of defective insulin, which results in acute hyperglycemia. Affected patients require exogenous insulin to lower their plasma glucose level and prevent diabetic complications. It is believed that a genetically determined autoimmune reaction gradually destroys the insulin-producing β-cells of the pancreatic islets of Langerhans (see Figure 33-2). The preclinical phase of β-cell destruction may be prolonged, and can last up to several years. At some critical point, a rapid transition from preclinical to clinical type 1 diabetes occurs. This transition may be triggered by a specific event, such as an acute illness or major emotional stress. An unidentified viral infection is also strongly suspected to be an environmental trigger. Such stressors trigger the release of the counter-regulatory hormones cortisol and epinephrine. These hormones then mobilize glucagon to release glucose from the storage sites in the liver. This action further increases the already rising levels of glucose in the blood secondary to islet cell damage. At some point during this cascade of events, an autoimmune reaction may be initiated, destroying the insulin-producing β-cells of the pancreatic islets of Langerhans. The result is essentially a complete lack of endogenous insulin production by the pancreas, which necessitates long-term insulin replacement therapy. Fortunately, type 1 diabetes accounts for fewer than 10% of all diabetes cases. Patients with glucose variability have large fluctuations in their plasma glucose levels.

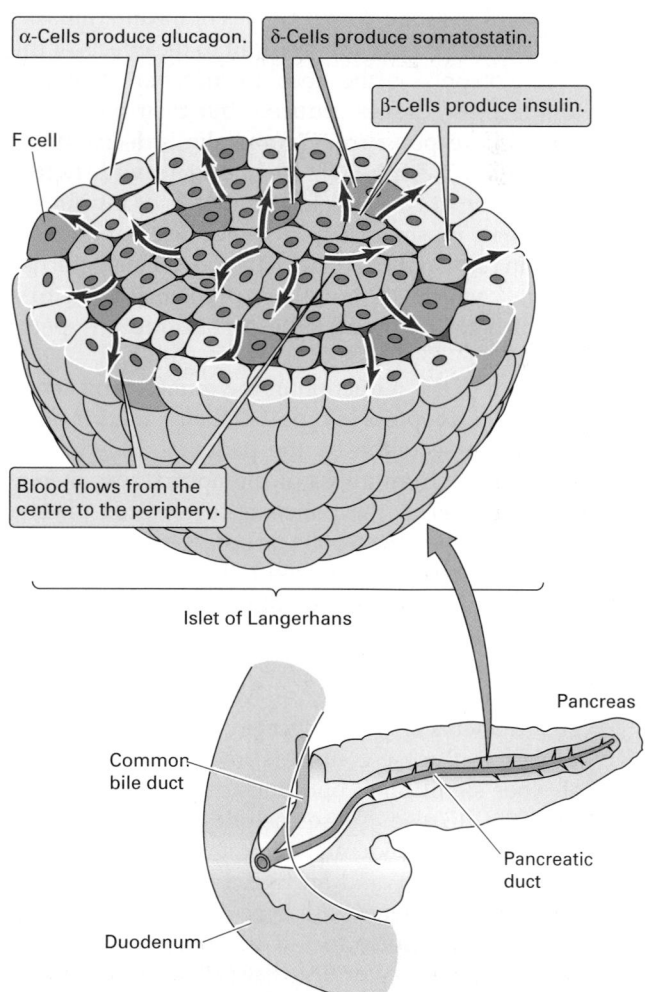

FIG. 33-2   The pancreas. A) Pancreas dissected to show main and accessory ducts. B) Exocrine glandular cells (around small pancreatic ducts) and endocrine glandular cells of the pancreatic islets (adjacent to blood capillaries). Exocrine pancreatic cells secrete pancreatic enzymes, α-endocrine cells secrete glucagon, and β-endocrine cells secrete insulin. (Source: Patton, K. T., & Thibodeau, G. A. (2010). *Anatomy and physiology* (7th ed.). St Louis, MO: Mosby.)

Type 2 Diabetes

Type 2 diabetes is by far the most common form of diabetes, accounting for at least 90% of all cases of diabetes; in 2010, it affected 2.5 million people in Canada. Because this form of diabetes does not always require insulin therapy, there are many common and dangerous misconceptions about type 2 diabetes: that it is a mild diabetes; that it is easy to treat; and that tight metabolic control is unnecessary because patients with this condition, who are mostly older adults, will die before diabetic complications develop. The clinical realities of this disease demonstrate otherwise.

Type 2 diabetes is caused by genetic and environmental factors that result in both insulin resistance and insulin deficiency; there is no absolute lack of insulin as in type 1 diabetes. One of the normal roles of insulin is to facilitate the uptake of circulating glucose molecules and movement into tissues to be used as energy. In type 2 diabetes, all of the main target tissues of insulin (muscle, liver, and adipose tissue) are resistant to the effects of the hormone. Not only is the absolute number of insulin receptors in these tissues reduced, but their individual sensitivity and responsiveness to insulin is decreased as well. Therefore, it is possible for a patient with type 2 diabetes to have normal or elevated levels of insulin yet still have high plasma glucose levels. These processes also result in impaired postprandial (after a meal) glucose metabolism, which is another problematic feature of type 2 diabetes that contributes to hazardous hyperglycemic states.

In addition to the reduction in the number and sensitivity of insulin receptors in type 2 diabetes, there is often reduced insulin secretion by the pancreas. This insulin deficiency results from a loss of the normal responsiveness of the β-cells in the pancreas to elevated plasma glucose levels. When the β-cells do not recognize glucose, they do not secrete insulin, and the normal insulin-facilitated transport of glucose into cells of muscle, liver, and adipose tissue does not occur. This situation is analogous to the loss of responsiveness of insulin receptors to insulin described earlier.

Type 2 diabetes is a multifaceted disorder. Although loss of plasma glucose control is its primary hallmark, several other significant conditions are strongly associated with the disease. These include obesity, coronary artery disease, dyslipidemia, hypertension, microalbuminuria (proteinuria), and an increased risk for thrombotic events. For patients with type 2 diabetes, the CDA recommends the regular use of aspirin (for secondary prevention of coronary artery disease), an angiotensin-converting enzyme inhibitor or an angiotensin receptor blocker, and antihyperlipidemic drug therapy (see Chapter 28), when indicated, in addition to any necessary antidiabetic drug therapy. **Metabolic syndrome** (or cardiometabolic syndrome) refers to a cluster of risk factors, including abdominal obesity, hypertension, dyslipidemia, and elevated plasma glucose; it places individuals at significant risk of developing type 2 diabetes and

cardiovascular disease. Approximately 80% of patients with diabetes are obese at the time of initial diagnosis. Obesity serves only to worsen insulin resistance because adipose tissue is often the site of a large proportion of the body's defective insulin receptors. The goal for patients with diabetes is a blood pressure less than 130/80 mm Hg and a low-density lipid (LDL) level of 2 mmol/L or less.

Acute Diabetic Complications: Diabetic Ketoacidosis and Hyperosmolar Hyperglycemic State

When plasma glucose levels are high but no insulin is present to allow glucose to be used for energy production, the body may break down fatty acids for fuel, producing ketones as a metabolic byproduct. If this occurs to a sufficient degree, **diabetic ketoacidosis (DKA)** may result. DKA is a complex, multisystem complication of uncontrolled diabetes. It occurs in 4.6 to 8 of 1 000 patients with diabetes. Without treatment, DKA will lead to unconsciousness and death. DKA is characterized by extreme hyperglycemia, the presence of ketones in the serum and urine, acidosis, dehydration, and electrolyte imbalances. Approximately 25 to 30% of patients with newly diagnosed type 1 diabetes present with DKA. Another complication of comparable severity that is triggered by extreme hyperglycemia is a **hyperosmolar hyperglycemic state (HHS)**. The most common precipitator of DKA and HHS is often emotional or physical (e.g., infection) stress. It was formerly believed that DKA occurred only in type 1 diabetes and HHS occurred only in type 2 diabetes. However, it is now recognized that both disorders can occur with diabetes of either type. This overlap is increasingly common, with the rapidly decreasing age of people with type 2 diabetes.

Table 33-3 describes the subtle differences between DKA and HHS. Treatment for either complication involves fluid and electrolyte replacement as well as intravenous (IV) insulin therapy (more common for DKA).

Gestational Diabetes

Gestational diabetes is a type of hyperglycemia that develops during pregnancy. It occurs in approximately 3.7% to 18% of Canadian pregnancies. Many patients control it well with diet, but the use of insulin may be necessary to decrease the risk of birth defects, hypoglycemia in the newborn, and high birth weight. In most cases, gestational diabetes subsides after delivery. However, an estimated 30% of patients who develop gestational diabetes develop type 2 diabetes within 5 to 15 years. This percentage is higher among women of Indigenous descent.

All pregnant women need to have plasma glucose screenings at regular prenatal visits. Women who develop gestational diabetes should be screened for lingering diabetes 6 to 8 weeks postpartum and be advised of their increased risk for recurrent diabetes and of the importance of regular medical checkups and weight control.

TABLE 33-3

Comparison of Features of Ketoacidosis and Hyperosmolar Hyperglycemic State Associated with Diabetes

Feature	Condition	
	Ketoacidosis	Hyperosmolar Hyperglycemic State
Age of patient	Younger than 65 yr	Older than 65 yr
Duration of symptoms	Less than 2 days	More than 5 days
Plasma glucose level	Equal to or greater than 14 mmol/L	Equal to or higher than 34 mmol/L
Plasma Na level	Within normal range (135–145 mmol/L) or less than 135 mmol/L	Within normal range (135–145 mmol/L) or greater than 145 mmol/L
Plasma K level	Less than 3.5 mmol/L (normal range 3.5–5 mmol/L	Less than 3.5 mmol/L (normal range 3.5–5 mmol/L
Plasma HCO_3 level	Low (equal to or less than 15 mmol/L [normal 21–28 mmol/L])	Normal
Ketone bodies in urine and plasma	Positive	
pH	Low (equal to or less than 7.3)	Normal
Serum osmolality	Less than 320 mOsm/kg	More than 320 mOsm/kg
Prognosis	3 to 10% mortality	10 to 20% mortality
Subsequent course	Insulin therapy required in all cases	Insulin therapy not required in many cases after initial treatment

Adapted from: Goguen, J., & Gilbert, J. (2013). Hyperglycemic emergencies in adults. *Canadian Journal of Diabetes, 37*(Suppl. 1), S72–S76; Lenahan, C. M., & Holloway, B. (2015). Differentiating between DKA and HHS. *Journal of Emergency Nursing, 41*(3), 201–207. doi:10.1016/j.jen.2014.08.015

Women who are known to have diabetes before pregnancy should have detailed prepregnancy counselling and prenatal care from a specialist experienced in managing pregnancies in women with diabetes. Specific issues pertaining to drug therapy for gestational diabetes are discussed further in the section on insulins.

Prevention and Screening

Both macrovascular and microvascular problems are now recognized at fasting plasma glucose (FPG) levels as low as 7 mmol/L. *Fasting* is defined as an 8-hour or overnight fast (no food from midnight until after the plasma sample is taken in the morning). The CDA guidelines identify **prediabetes** as impaired fasting glucose, impaired glucose tolerance, or an A_{1C} of 6 to 6.4%, each of which places individuals at high risk of developing diabetes and its complications. **Impaired fasting glucose** is defined as an FPG level higher than or equal to 6.1 mmol/L but less than 6.9 mmol/L. *Impaired glucose tolerance* is identified using an oral glucose challenge test (see Box 33 1). The CDA recommends that all adults 40 years of age and older be screened for elevated FPG or A_{1C} levels every 3 years. Several preventive measures are also recommended. Reducing alcohol consumption is helpful because alcohol is broken down in the body to simple carbohydrates, which leads to increases in plasma glucose levels. Regular exercise also lowers plasma glucose levels by increasing insulin receptor sensitivity.

Indigenous people in Canada have a high risk for the development of diabetes and its associated complications. Screening for risk factors should be initiated in early childhood, with prevention being a priority.

Screening should be undertaken every 1 to 2 years for adults who have one or more risk factors and every 2 years for children over 10 years of age or with established puberty who have one or more risk factors, including being exposed to diabetes in utero. A culturally appropriate comprehensive program of care, following the national guidelines, needs to be implemented. An available resource is the National Aboriginal Diabetes Association (www.nada.ca).

Nonpharmacological Interventions

For patients with new-onset type 2 diabetes, nonpharmacological lifestyle interventions are usually initiated as a first step in treatment. Weight loss not only lowers the plasma glucose and lipid levels of these patients, but it also reduces another common comorbidity, hypertension. Even a modest weight loss of 5% of initial body weight can reduce the risk of disease progression (from impaired glucose tolerance to type 2 diabetes) by 60%. Other recommended lifestyle changes include improvement of dietary habits (e.g., consumption of a diet higher in protein and lower in fat and carbohydrates), smoking cessation, reduced alcohol consumption, and regular physical exercise. Cigarette smoking is a known cause of type 2 diabetes, as there is a 30 to 40% higher risk of type 2 diabetes in smokers than nonsmokers (Tucker, 2014). A new study also pointed to an increased risk for developing type 2 diabetes in individuals exposed to secondhand smoke (Pan et al., 2015). Cigarette smoking doubles the risk of cardiovascular disease in patients with diabetes, largely because of its effects on peripheral vascular circulation and respiratory function.

Glycemic Goal of Treatment

The glycemic goal recommended by the CDA for patients with diabetes is a **hemoglobin A_{1C} (HbA_{1C})** level of less than 7%. The A_{1C} test measures the percentage of hemoglobin A that is irreversibly glycosylated. A_{1C} is an indicator of glycemic control in a patient over the preceding 2 to 3 months (the average lifespan of a red blood cell) and is not affected by recent fluctuations in plasma glucose levels. The mean level of plasma glucose in the 30 days immediately before the blood sampling contributes 50% of the A_{1C} level result, the period from 30 to 90 days prior contributes 40%, and the period from 90 to 120 days prior contributes 10%. The CDA recommends a fasting plasma glucose goal for patients with diabetes of 4 to 7 mmol/L and a 2-hour postprandial target of 5 to 10 mmol/L.

Antidiabetic Drugs

The two major classes of drugs used to treat diabetes are the insulins and oral antihyperglycemic drugs. Several new classes of injectable drugs with unique mechanisms of action have been developed that may be used in addition to insulins or oral antihyperglycemic drugs to treat resistant diabetes. All of these drugs are referred to as *antidiabetic drugs*, and they are aimed at producing what is known as a *normoglycemic* or *euglycemic* (normal plasma sugar) state.

INSULINS

Insulin is required in patients with type 1 diabetes. Patients with type 2 diabetes are not generally prescribed insulin until other measures (e.g., lifestyle changes and oral drug therapy) no longer provide adequate glycemic control. Currently, insulin is synthesized in laboratories with recombinant deoxyribonucleic acid (rDNA) technology and is referred to as *human insulin*. Insulin was originally isolated from cattle or pigs, but bovine (cow) and porcine (pig) insulins are associated with a higher incidence of allergic reactions and insulin resistance than is human insulin. Beef-derived insulin is no longer available on the Canadian market. To accommodate patients who still depend on animal-derived insulin, porcine insulins under the brand names of Hypurin Regular® and Hypurin NPH® continue to be available for purchase at Canadian pharmacies. Recombinant insulin is produced by bacteria or yeasts that have been altered to contain the genetic information necessary to reproduce an insulin that is like human insulin. The pharmacokinetic properties of insulin (onset of action, peak effect, and duration of action) can be altered by making various minor modifications to either the insulin molecule or the drug formulation (final product). This practice has led to the development of several different insulin preparations, including many combination insulin products that contain more than one type of insulin in the same solution. Such chemical manipulation of insulin activity helps

TABLE 33-4	
Insulin Mixing Compatibilities	
Type of Insulin	**Compatible With**
Regular insulin (Humulin R®, Novolin ge Toronto®)	All insulins except glargine and glulisine
Insulin glulisine (Apidra®)	NPH only
Insulin lispro (Humalog®), insulin aspart (NovoRapid®)	Regular, NPH insulins
Insulin detemir (Levemir®)	Must be given alone
Insulin glargine (Lantus®)	Must be given alone due to low pH of diluent
Regular insulin 30% and NPH 70% and (Humulin 30/70®, Novolin ge 30/70®); others	Premixed; do not mix with other insulins (e.g., regular, glulisine, lispro, aspart, detemir, glargine)

to meet the individualized meal-oriented metabolic demands for insulin of patients with diabetes. Further modifications can be accomplished by mixing compatible insulin preparations in a syringe before administration. The latest syringe compatibility data for currently available insulin products are given in Table 33-4. Thoroughly educate patients regarding how, when, and whether they can (or cannot) mix different types of insulin. Some combinations are chemically incompatible and can result in an undesirable alteration of glycemic effects.

Mechanism of Action and Drug Effects

Exogenous insulin functions as a substitute for the endogenous hormone. It serves to replace the insulin that is either not made at all or is made defectively in patients with diabetes. The drug effects of exogenously administered insulin involve many body systems, and these effects are the same as those of normal endogenous insulin. That is, exogenous insulin restores the patient's ability to metabolize carbohydrates, fats, and proteins; to store glucose in the liver; and to convert glycogen to fat stores. However, exogenous insulin does not reverse defects in insulin receptor sensitivity. Insulin pumps are an attractive way to administer insulin to patients, providing an alternative to multiple daily subcutaneous injections and allowing patients to match their insulin intake to their lifestyle. When an insulin pump is used, insulin is administered constantly over a 24-hour period, and the patient is then allowed to give bolus injections based on their food intake and activity level. Insulin pumps are described further in the Nursing Process section.

Indications

All insulin preparations can be used to treat both type 1 and type 2 diabetes, but each patient requires careful customization of the dosing regimen for optimal glycemic control. Additional therapeutic approaches indicated include lifestyle modifications (e.g., changes to dietary and exercise habits) and, for type 2 diabetes, oral drug therapy.

Contraindications

Contraindications to the use of all insulin products include known drug allergy to a specific product. Insulin is never to be administered to a patient who is already hypoglycemic. Plasma glucose must always be tested prior to administration.

Adverse Effects

Hypoglycemia resulting from excessive insulin dosing can result in confusion, coma, or seizure, as well as long-term complications of mild cognitive impairment. Hypoglycemia is the most immediate and serious adverse effect of insulin. Other adverse effects of insulin therapy include weight gain, lipodystrophy at the site of repeated injections, and, in rare cases, allergic reactions. Because weight gain is a common and often undesirable adverse effect, insulin therapy is usually delayed in type 2 patients until other drugs and lifestyle changes have failed to bring plasma glucose to target levels.

Interactions

Drug interactions that can occur with the insulins are significant; they are listed in Table 33-5.

Dosages

For dosage information on the various insulin products, refer to the table on p. 633. The concentration of insulin is expressed as the number of units of insulin per millilitre. For example, unit-100 insulin has 100 units in 1 millilitre. For this reason, insulin is a high alert medication; the consequences of an error in calculation and administration can have devastating consequences (see Chapter 6 for more information on high alert medications). Insulin is usually given by subcutaneous injection or via a subcutaneous infusion pump. In emergency situations requiring prompt insulin action, regular insulin can be given intravenously. Regular insulin is the only insulin that can be administered intravenously, and careful monitoring (e.g., of hourly plasma glucose levels) is required.

Insulin Use in Special Populations

Two special patient populations for whom careful attention is required during insulin therapy include children and pregnant women. Insulin dosages for members of both groups are calculated by weight, as they are for the general adult population. The usual range of a total daily dose is 0.5 to 1 unit/kg/day. Be aware that there are a few important differences regarding the use of some of the more unusual insulin products in children. The rapid-acting insulin lispro is approved for use in children older than 3 years of age. However, the combination lispro product Humalog® Mix25, which contains 75% insulin lispro protamine (an intermediate-acting insulin) and

---

TABLE	33-5

Selected Drug Interactions with Antidiabetic Drugs

Drug	Interacting Drug	Mechanism	Result
Insulin	Corticosteroids, niacin, diuretics, sympathomimetic drugs, thyroid drugs	Antagonizes insulin effect	Increased plasma glucose levels
	Alcohol, anabolic steroids, sulfa antibiotics, MAOIs, salicylates	Increases the hypoglycemic effects of insulin	Decreased plasma glucose levels
	Nonselective β-blockers	Masks the tachycardia from hypoglycemia	Risk of not noticing hypoglycemic symptoms
	Hypoglycemic drugs	Additive effects	Additive hypoglycemia
metformin hydrochloride	Cimetidine	Inhibits metabolism	Increased metformin effects
	Diuretics, steroids	Additive effects	Additive hypoglycemia
	Contrast media	Decreases excretion	Lactic acidosis
gliclazide	Long-acting sulfonamides, tuberculostatics, phenylbutazone, MAOIs, coumarin derivatives, salicylates, probenecid, propranolol hydrochloride, miconazole nitrate, cimetidine, disopyramide, ACE inhibitors	Enhanced effects	Increased hypoglycemia
	Diuretics (thiazides, furosemide), corticosteroids, oral contraceptives	Increases metabolism	Decreased effectiveness

MAOI, monoamine oxidase inhibitor; *ACE,* angiotensin-converting enzyme.

25% insulin lispro (a rapid-acting insulin), is not currently approved for use in children younger than 18 years of age. Glycemic targets are graduated with age; an A_{1C} of less than 8% is the target with children younger than 6 years of age. In addition, severe hypoglycemia must be minimized in this age group because of its association with later cognitive impairment. The target A_{1C} for children between the ages of 6 and 12 is 7.5% or less, and for adolescents, the target A_{1C} is the same as for adults. Children need age-appropriate education and supervision from health care providers and parents, which includes a safe and gradual transfer of responsibility to support a transition to self-management of their diabetes, as appropriate.

Women who are pregnant also require special care in regard to diabetes management. Although many such patients will return to a normal glycemic state after pregnancy, they also have a 30 to 60% risk of developing diabetes again in later life. Oral medications are generally not recommended for patients who are pregnant because of a lack of firm safety data. For this reason, insulin therapy is the only currently recommended drug therapy for pregnant women with diabetes. Approximately 15% of women who develop gestational diabetes require insulin therapy during pregnancy. Insulin does not normally cross the placenta. Effective glycemic control during pregnancy is essential because infants born to women with gestational diabetes have a twofold to threefold greater risk of congenital anomalies than those born to women without gestational diabetes. In addition, the incidence of stillbirth is directly related to the degree of maternal hyperglycemia. Weight reduction is generally not advised for pregnant women because it can jeopardize fetal nutritional status. Women with gestational diabetes tend to have babies that weigh more, and these children may have low plasma glucose postnatally. Insulin is excreted into human milk. It is currently unknown whether insulin glargine is excreted in breast milk, and thus it is to be avoided in breastfeeding women. It is important that insulin therapy and diet be well controlled for nursing mothers because inadequate or excessive glycemic control may reduce milk production.

There are currently four major classes of insulin, as determined by their pharmacokinetic properties: rapid acting, short acting, intermediate acting, and long acting. The duration of action ranges from several hours to over 24 hours, depending on the insulin class (Figure 33-3).

The insulin dosage regimen for all patients with diabetes is highly individualized and may consist of one or more classes of insulin administered at either fixed dosages or variable dosages in response to self-measurements of plasma glucose levels or the number of grams of carbohydrate consumed. With the use of insulins, clarity, colour, and appearance are important to understand for patient safety and for the prevention of adverse effects and complications. Several insulins are clear, colourless solutions. These include regular insulin, insulin lispro (Humalog), and insulin glargine (Lantus).

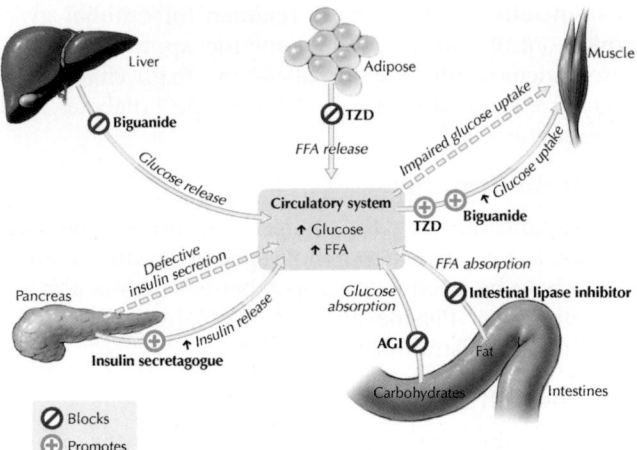

FIG. 33-3 Comparison of the pharmacokinetics of various insulins. (Source: Messinger-Rapport, B. J., Thomas, D. R., & Gammack, J. K. (2008). Clinical update on nursing home medicine. *Journal of the American Medical Directors Association, 9*(7), 460–475.)

Other insulins, such as NPH insulin (insulin isophane), are opaque (cloudy) white solutions. These differences are discussed further in the Implementation section under Nursing Process.

INHALED INSULIN

First introduced in the US market in 2006 and withdrawn in 2007 due to poor uptake by patients and health care providers, inhaled insulin (Afrezza®) was reintroduced in 2014 in the United States. Afrezza is a rapid-acting form of insulin delivered through an inhaler device. It reduces postprandial glucose levels and improves the A_{1C}. It is administered before each meal (or soon after starting a meal) and is rapidly absorbed from the lungs into the blood. It reaches peak plasma concentrations 12 to 14 minutes after administration, similar to the physiological mealtime response, and is eliminated within 2 to 3 hours. It is dosed in units and is delivered via cartridges.

Afrezza must be used in combination with a long-acting insulin in patients with type 1 diabetes. It is not recommended for the treatment of DKA or for patients who smoke. Afrezza appears to be less likely to cause weight gain and severe hypoglycemia than standard insulin. It is contraindicated in patients with asthma or chronic obstructive pulmonary disease. Afrezza does not currently have Health Canada approval for marketing.

ORAL ANTIHYPERGLYCEMIC DRUGS

Type 2 diabetes is a complex illness. Effective treatment involves several elements, including lifestyle modifications (e.g., diet control, exercise, smoking cessation, nutrition therapy), careful monitoring of plasma glucose

DRUG PROFILES

Rapid-Acting Insulins

▶▶ *insulin lispro*

There are currently three insulin products classified as rapid acting: insulin lispro (Humalog), insulin aspart (Novo-Rapid), and, more recently developed, insulin glulisine (Apidra). These products have the most rapid onset of action (approximately 15 minutes) as well as a shorter duration of action than insulins in other categories. The effect of insulin lispro is most like that of the endogenous insulin produced from the pancreas in response to a meal. After or during a meal, the glucose that is ingested stimulates the pancreas to secrete insulin. This insulin then facilitates the uptake of the excess glucose at hepatic insulin receptor sites for storage in the liver as glycogen. In individuals with diabetes, the insulin response to meals is often impaired; therefore, a rapid-acting insulin product is often used within 15 minutes of mealtime. This corresponds to the time required for the onset of action of rapid-acting insulins. It is essential that patients with diabetes eat a meal after an injection of rapid-acting insulin; otherwise, profound hypoglycemia may result. Insulin lispro was approved by Health Canada in 1998, becoming the first new insulin product to appear on the market in many years. Lispro 200 units/mL KwikPen® became available in 2015 and is used for patients with diabetes who require daily doses of more than 20 units of rapid-acting insulin.

PHARMACOKINETICS

Route	Onset of Action	Peak Plasma Concentration	Elimination Half-Life	Duration of Action
Subcut	10–15 min	1–1.5 hr lispro: 1–2 hr	60–80 min	3–5 hr lispro: 3.5–4.75 hr

Short-Acting Insulin

▶▶ *regular insulin*

Regular insulin (Humulin R, Novolin ge Toronto) is currently the only insulin that is classified as a short-acting insulin. Regular insulin can be administered via IV bolus, IV infusion, or even intramuscularly. These routes, especially the IV infusion route, are often used in cases of DKA or coma associated with uncontrolled type 1 diabetes. It also can be administered subcutaneously for the management of diabetes.

Regular insulin solution was the first medicinal insulin product developed. It was originally isolated from bovine and porcine sources, but it is now made primarily from human insulin sources, using rDNA technology.

There are some differences between regular insulin and the newer rapid-acting drugs. Both rapid-acting insulins, lispro and insulin aspart, are human insulin analogues. This means that they are insulin molecules with synthetic alterations to their chemical structures that change their onset or duration of action. Both of these insulins have a faster onset of action and take a shorter time to reach peak plasma level than regular insulin, but they also have a shorter duration of action.

PHARMACOKINETICS

Route	Onset of Action	Peak Plasma Concentration	Elimination Half-Life	Duration of Action
Subcut	30 min	2–3 hr	1.5 hr	6.5 hr

Intermediate-Acting Insulins

▶▶ *insulin isophane suspension (NPH)*

Insulin isophane suspension (Humulin N, Novolin ge NPH [also known as *NPH insulin*]) is the only available intermediate-acting insulin product. NPH is an acronym for *neutral protamine Hagedorn insulin*, the original name of this type of insulin. NPH insulin is a sterile suspension of zinc insulin crystals and protamine sulfate in buffered water for injection. The suspension appears cloudy or opaque (white). NPH insulin has a slower onset and a longer duration of action than regular insulin, but not as slow and long as the long-acting insulins. NPH insulin is often combined with regular insulin to reduce the number of insulin injections needed per day.

PHARMACOKINETICS

Route	Onset of Action	Peak Plasma Concentration	Elimination Half-Life	Duration of Action
Subcut	1–3 hr	4–10 hr	Unknown	Up to 18 hr

Long-Acting Insulins

▶▶ *insulin detemir and insulin glargine*

Two long-acting basal insulin products are now available: insulin glargine (Basaglar, Lantus) and insulin detemir (Levemir). Insulin glargine is normally a clear, colourless solution with a pH of 4. Once it is injected into subcutaneous tissue at a physiological pH of approximately 7.4, it forms microprecipitates that are slowly absorbed over the next 24 hours (for glargine, the duration is 24 hours, while for detemir the peak is 16 to 24 hours). It is an rDNA-produced insulin analogue and is unique in that it provides a constant level of insulin in the body. This enhances its safety because it does not cause blood levels to rise and fall, as do other insulins (i.e., there is no peak). Insulin glargine is usually dosed once daily, but it may be dosed every 12 hours, depending on the patient's glycemic response. Because insulin glargine provides a prolonged, consistent plasma glucose level, it is sometimes referred to as a *basal insulin*. Often, for those being switched from twice-daily NPH to insulin glargine, the initial daily glargine dose is reduced to 80% of the previous total NPH dose. Insulin detemir has a different mechanism of action from insulin glargine; these two insulins are not considered interchangeable. The duration of action of insulin detemir is dose dependent, so that lower doses require twice-daily dosing and higher doses may be given once daily.

Continued

DRUG PROFILES—cont'd

Insulin glargine recently became available in a 300 unit/mL disposable (pre-filled) pen (1.5 mL) as Touleo Solo-Star®. It contains three times as much insulin in 1 mL than standard insulin. Touleo has an onset of action over 6 hours following the injection, and its duration of action is up to 30 hours. It comes with a lower risk of hypoglycemia after transfer from other insulins, independent of time of injection, and is associated with less weight gain than other insulins. Touleo is not to be mixed with any other insulin products. The drug is indicated for once-daily subcutaneous administration in the treatment of patients over the age of 18 years with type 1 or type 2 diabetes who require basal (long-acting) insulin for glycemic control.

PHARMACOKINETICS

Route	Onset of Action	Peak Plasma Concentration	Elimination Half-Life	Duration of Action
Subcut	90 min	None	Unknown	Up to 24 hr

Fixed-Combination Insulins

Currently available fixed-combination insulin products include Humulin 30/70; Novolin 30/70, 40/60, and 50/50; NovoMix 30®; and Humalog Mix25 and Mix50. Each of these products contains two different insulins—one intermediate-acting type and either one rapid-acting type (Humalog, NovoLog) or one short-acting type (Humulin). The numeric designations indicate the percentages of each of the two components in the product. For example, Novolin 30/70 has 30% intermediate-acting insulin and 70% short-acting insulin. Notice that the numbers add up to 100 (percent). These products were developed to more closely simulate the varying levels of endogenous insulin that occur normally in people who do not have diabetes. In most insulin regimens, patients take a combination of a rapid-acting insulin to deal with the surges in glucose that occur after meals and an intermediate- or long-acting insulin for the periods between meals, when glucose levels are lower. However, this requires mixing and administering different types of insulins. Fixed-combination products were developed in an attempt to simplify the dosing process. The insulin lispro protamine component of Humalog Mix25 (25% insulin lispro injection, 75% insulin lispro protamine suspension) is a modified insulin lispro molecule with a longer duration of action. Combinations allow for twice daily dosing but often result in glycemic control that is not as tight as daily dosing with meals. Patients who cannot afford frequent glucose monitoring or who refuse more than two injections per day may insist on using a combination insulin with twice daily dosing.

Basal–Bolus and Sliding-Scale Insulin Dosing

Historically, sliding scale insulin was used to correct plasma glucose levels. In this method, subcutaneous doses of rapid-acting (lispro or aspart) or short-acting (regular) insulin are adjusted according to plasma glucose test results. This method was typically used in treating hospitalized patients with diabetes, whose insulin requirements may vary dramatically because of stress (e.g., infections, surgery, acute illness), inactivity, or variable caloric intake, including receipt of total parenteral nutrition (TPN) or time spent on a "nothing by mouth" (NPO) diet. Other hospital diets that result in high numbers of carbohydrates consumed are full liquid and clear liquid diets.

When an individual is on a sliding-scale insulin regimen, plasma glucose concentrations are determined several times a day (e.g., before meals and at bedtime) for patients on normal meal schedules, or every 4 to 6 hours around the clock for patients receiving TPN or enteral tube feedings. Subcutaneously administered regular insulin or rapid-acting insulin is then given in an amount that increases with the rise in plasma glucose. The disadvantage of sliding-scale dosing is that, because it delays insulin administration until hyperglycemia occurs, it does not meet basal insulin requirements and results in large swings in glucose control. Current research does not support the use of sliding scales or of insulin without concurrent use of basal insulin, and many institutions are moving away from sliding-scale coverage. Nonetheless, sliding-scale dosing is still commonly used.

Basal–bolus insulin therapy is now the preferred method of treatment for hospitalized patients with diabetes. Basal–bolus therapy involves attempting to mimic a healthy pancreas by delivering insulin constantly as a basal and then as needed as a bolus. The basal insulin is a long-acting insulin (insulin glargine), administered constantly to keep the plasma glucose from fluctuating due to the normal release of glucose from the liver. Bolus insulin (insulin lispro or insulin aspart) mimics the burst secretions of the pancreas in response to increases in plasma glucose levels. Bolus insulin is broken up into meal and correction boluses. Meal boluses are given to reduce plasma glucose with the intake of carbohydrates. Correction boluses are any boluses taken to bring plasma glucose back to normal. Plasma glucose levels are monitored frequently when using basal–bolus insulin. This method of treatment is far superior to the traditional sliding scale. Still, patients who need to receive nothing by mouth for therapeutic or diagnostic reasons are not good candidates for basal insulin due to the risk of hypoglycemia and the unpredictability of the insulin needed for glucose control while not eating.

levels, and therapy with one or more drugs. In addition, the treatment of associated comorbid conditions (such as high cholesterol and high blood pressure) can further complicate the entire process of treatment.

The 2013 CDA guidelines recommend that new-onset type 2 diabetes with an A_{1C} less than 8.5% be treated with lifestyle interventions for 2 to 3 months to achieve glycemic targets, with the addition of the oral biguanide drug metformin if lifestyle changes are not effective. The maximum effect of oral antihyperglycemic monotherapy is seen at 3 to 6 months. In patients with an A_{1C} of 8.5% or higher, metformin is initiated together with lifestyle

DOSAGES   Selected Human-Based Insulin Products

Drug	Pharmacological Class	Usual Dosage Range	Indications
Rapid-Acting			
⊪ insulin lispro (Humalog)	Human recombinant rapid-acting insulin analogue	Subcut: 0.5–1 unit/kg/day; doses are highly individualized to desired glycemic control; rapid-acting insulins are best given 15 min before a meal May be given per sliding scale or as basal–bolus; may also be given via continuous subcutaneous infusion pump	Diabetes, type 1 and type 2
Short-Acting			
⊪regular insulin (Humulin R, Novolin ge Toronto)	Human recombinant short-acting insulin	Subcut: Same dosage as insulin lispro; Subcut doses of regular insulin are best given 30 min before a meal Regular insulin may also be given per sliding scale and is the insulin usually given IV as a continuous infusion	Diabetes, type 1 and type 2
Long-Acting			
⊪insulin detemir (Levemir) insulin glargine (Lantus)	Human recombinant long-acting insulin analogues	Subcut only: Same dosage as others but approved only for once- or twice-daily dosage (basal dosing)	Diabetes, type 1 and type 2

IV, intravenous; *Subcut*, subcutaneous.

interventions, with consideration given to adding insulin to the regimen. A combination of oral antihyperglycemics and insulin often effectively controls glucose levels. Consideration is given to the chosen type of insulin when it is being added to oral drugs. Often, a lower dose of an intermediate-acting or a long-acting insulin combined with oral antihyperglycemics may result in better glycemic control, less weight gain, and less hypoglycemia than the use of a more typical dose of insulin alone. The use of bedtime insulin with metformin results in less weight gain than insulin therapy alone. DPP-4 inhibitors and glucagonlike peptide 1 (GLP-1) receptor agonists may also be combined with insulin and are effective at lowering plasma glucose levels. As type 2 diabetes progresses, insulin needs will probably increase, and the addition of short-acting or rapid-acting insulins may also need to be considered.

The initial use of combinations of submaximal doses of antihyperglycemics produces more rapid and improved glycemic control with fewer adverse effects, compared to monotherapy at maximal doses. Studies have shown that metformin and the sulfonylureas (available in generic form) were either similar to or superior to the more expensive thiazolidinediones, glinides, and α-glucosidase inhibitors. Numerous combined formulations of oral hyperglycemic drugs are available (e.g., Avandamet® [metformin and rosiglitazone]). Although not a traditional oral anthypoglycemic agent, bromocriptine mesylate (Cycloset®), a dopamine agonist (see Chapter 16), is now being marketed for the treatment of diabetes in the United States. Its exact mechanism of action is not known, but it has been shown to lower A_{1C} levels in patients with type 2 diabetes.

BIGUANIDE

Mechanism of Action and Drug Effects

Metformin is currently the only drug classified as a biguanide. It is considered a first-line drug, especially for patients with a body mass index over 25, and is the most commonly used oral drug for the treatment of type 2 diabetes. It is not used for type 1 diabetes. Metformin works by decreasing hepatic glucose production. It may also decrease intestinal absorption of glucose and improve insulin receptor sensitivity. This results in increased peripheral glucose uptake and use as well as decreased liver production of triglycerides and cholesterol. Unlike sulfonylureas, metformin does not stimulate insulin secretion and therefore is not associated with weight gain and significant hypoglycemia when used alone.

Indications

The CDA guidelines recommend metformin as the initial oral antihyperglycemic drug for treatment of newly diagnosed type 2 diabetes if no contraindications exist. Because it may also cause moderate weight loss, it is particularly useful for the many patients with type 2 diabetes who are overweight or obese. It is also used in patients who are prediabetic. Metformin may be used as monotherapy or in combination with other oral antihyperglycemic drugs if single-drug therapy is unsuccessful. For this reason, it is available in combination products containing either thiazolidinediones or incretin mimetics. Metformin may also be combined with insulin. The extended-release tablets can be used as montherpy or in combination with a sulfonylurea. It is not approved by Health Canada for use in children.

Contraindications

Metformin is contraindicated in patients with kidney disease or kidney dysfunction (creatinine clearance less than 30 mL/min). Because metformin is excreted primarily by the kidneys, it can accumulate in these individuals, increasing the risk of development of lactic acidosis. Other contraindications include alcoholism, metabolic acidosis, liver disease, heart failure, and other conditions that predispose patients to tissue hypoxia and increase the risk of lactic acidosis.

Adverse Effects

The most common adverse effects of metformin are gastrointestinal (GI). Metformin can cause abdominal bloating, nausea, cramping, a feeling of fullness, and diarrhea, especially at the start of therapy. Some research attributes the weight loss experienced early in the course of treatment to these adverse effects. These effects are all usually self-limiting and can be lessened by starting with low dosages, titrating up slowly, and taking the medication with food. Less common adverse effects with metformin are a metallic taste, hypoglycemia, and a reduction in vitamin B_{12} levels after long-term use. Metformin-associated lactic acidosis is an extremely rare complication with metformin, but the risk of this increases with extremely high plasma glucose levels or clinical conditions predisposing patients to hypoxemia. Metformin enhances anaerobic metabolism, which, with a lack of insulin, results in an increased lactic acid production. Lactic acidosis is lethal in up to 50% of cases. Symptoms of lactic acidosis include hyperventilation, cold and clammy skin, muscle pain, abdominal pain, dizziness, and irregular heartbeat.

Interactions

Drug interactions with metformin are listed in Table 33-5. In addition, the use of metformin with iodinated (iodine-containing) radiologic contrast media has been associated with both acute kidney injury and lactic acidosis. For these reasons, metformin therapy is to be discontinued the day of the test and for at least 48 hours after the patient undergoes any radiological study that requires the use of such contrast media.

Dosages

For dosage information on metformin, refer to the table on p. 640.

SULFONYLUREAS

Mechanism of Action and Drug Effects

The sulfonylureas comprise the oldest group of oral antihyperglycemic drugs. The drugs in this category that are currently used are considered second-generation drugs and have better potency and adverse effect profiles than first-generation drugs (e.g., acetazolamide and tolbutamide), which are no longer used clinically. Second-generation sulfonylureas include gliclazide (Diamicron®),

glyburide (Diabeta®), and glimepiride (Amaryl®). Sulfonylureas bind to specific receptors on β-cells in the pancreas to stimulate the release of insulin. In addition, sulfonylureas appear to secondarily decrease the secretion of glucagon. For this class of drugs to be effective, the patient must still have functioning β-cells in the pancreas. Thus, these drugs work best during the early stages of type 2 diabetes and are not used in type 1 diabetes.

Indications

The CDA guidelines currently recommend sulfonylureas as second-step drugs for patients with type 2 diabetes whose A_{1C} levels remain elevated after metformin is initiated. Because they have different mechanisms of action, sulfonylureas can be used in conjunction with metformin and thiazolidinediones. Sulfonylureas should not be used in patients with advanced diabetes dependent on insulin administration because the β-cells in such patients are no longer able to produce insulin. Once insulin is started, sulfonylureas are stopped.

Contraindications

Contraindications to the use of sulfonylureas include hypoglycemia or conditions that can predispose patients to hypoglycemia, such as reduced caloric intake (e.g., being made NPO), ethanol use, or advanced age. There is a potential for cross-allergy in patients who are allergic to sulfonamide antibiotics. Although such an allergy is listed as a contraindication by the manufacturer, most health care providers will prescribe sulfonylureas for such patients. However, be aware of the potential for cross-allergy, and inform patients of this possibility.

Adverse Effects

The most common adverse effect of the sulfonylureas is hypoglycemia, the degree of which depends on the dose, the patient's eating habits, and the presence of liver or kidney disease. Another predictable adverse effect is weight gain because of the stimulation of insulin secretion. Other adverse effects include skin rash, nausea, epigastric fullness, and heartburn.

Interactions

Drug interactions with the second-generation sulfonylureas are listed in Table 33-5.

Dosages

For dosage information on sulfonylureas, refer to the table on p. 640.

GLINIDES

Mechanism of Action and Drug Effects

Repaglinide (GlucoNorm®) and nateglinide (Starlix®) are the two drugs available in the glinide class. They are structurally different from the sulfonylureas but have a similar mechanism of action, in that they also increase insulin secretion from the pancreas. However, they have a much shorter duration of action and must be given with each meal.

Indications

Like the sulfonylureas, the glinides are indicated for the treatment of type 2 diabetes. They may be particularly useful for patients with diabetes who have high postprandial glucose levels and low levels of circulating insulin. The glinides can be used with metformin and thiazolidinediones, but cannot be combined with sulfonylureas because they share a similar mechanism of action.

Contraindications

Contraindications to the use of glinides are similar to those of the sulfonylureas.

Adverse Effects

The most commonly reported adverse effect of the glinides is hypoglycemia, which can occur if food is not eaten after a dose. Weight gain is also commonly reported.

Interactions

Drug interactions with the glinides are similar to those with the sulfonylureas.

Dosages

For dosage information on the glinides, refer to the table on p. 640.

THIAZOLIDINEDIONES (GLITAZONES)

Mechanism of Action and Drug Effects

The third major drug category to emerge for the oral treatment of type 2 diabetes is the thiazolidinediones, most commonly referred to as *glitazones*. This class of drugs acts by regulating genes involved in glucose and lipid metabolism. Glitazones are referred to as *insulin-sensitizing drugs*. They work to decrease insulin resistance by enhancing the sensitivity of insulin receptors. These drugs are also known to directly stimulate peripheral glucose uptake and storage, as well as to inhibit glucose and triglyceride production in the liver. Because glitazones affect gene regulation, they have a slow onset of activity over several weeks, and maximal activity may not be evident for several months. Some amount of preservation of β-cell function has also been reported with glitazone administration, thereby slowing disease progression in type 2 diabetes.

Indications

Thiazolidinediones are indicated for the management of type 2 diabetes. Because of their cost, adverse effect profile, and slow onset of action, they are usually reserved for patients who cannot tolerate or cannot achieve glucose control with metformin or the sulfonylureas.

Rosiglitazone mesylate (Avandia®) is associated with increased cardiovascular risk when compared to the other glitazone, pioglitazone hydrochloride (Actos®). These drugs may also be combined with metformin or a sulfonylurea for a synergistic effect. Pioglitazone hydrochloride can be used with insulin.

Contraindications

Thiazolidinediones are contraindicated for use in patients with New York Heart Association class III or IV heart failure and are to be used with caution in patients with liver or kidney disease.

Adverse Effects

The glitazones commonly cause peripheral edema and weight gain. This weight gain may be due to both water retention and an increase in adipose tissue. Their use has also been associated with reduced bone mineral density and an increased risk of fractures.

Interactions

Pioglitazone hydrochloride is partly metabolized by cytochrome P450 enzyme 3A4 (CYP3A4). Serum concentrations of pioglitazone hydrochloride may be increased if the drug is taken concurrently with a CYP3A4 inhibitor such as ketoconazole or erythromycin.

Dosages

For dosage information on thiazolidinediones, refer to the table on p. 640.

α-GLUCOSIDASE INHIBITORS

Mechanism of Action and Drug Effects

Among the less commonly used oral drugs is the α-glucosidase inhibitor acarbose (Glucobay®). As the category name implies, this drug works by reversibly inhibiting the enzyme α-glucosidase that is found in the small intestine. This enzyme is responsible for the hydrolysis of oligosaccharides and disaccharides to glucose. When this enzyme is blocked, glucose absorption is delayed. The timing of administration of α-glucosidase inhibitors is important, and they must be taken with food. When an α-glucosidase inhibitor is taken with a meal, excessive postprandial plasma glucose elevation (a glucose "spike") can be prevented or reduced, making this medication impractical for directly lowering fasting plasma glucose.

Indications

Alpha-glucosidase inhibitors are used to treat type 2 diabetes, usually in combination with another oral antihyperglycemic drug. Acarbose may be particularly effective in controlling high postprandial glucose levels.

Contraindications

Because of its adverse GI effects, acarbose is not recommended for use in patients with inflammatory bowel disease, malabsorption syndromes, or intestinal obstruction.

Adverse Effects

Acarbose can cause a high incidence of flatulence, diarrhea, and abdominal pain. At high dosages, it may also elevate levels of liver enzymes (transaminases). Unlike sulfonylureas, it does not cause hypoglycemia or weight gain. In the rare instance that a patient develops hypoglycemia from acarbose, complex carbohydrates cannot be used because α-glucosidase is blocked; IV or oral glucose must be administered.

Interactions

The bioavailability of digoxin, ranitidine hydrochloride, and propranolol hydrochloride may be reduced when they are taken with an α-glucosidase inhibitor.

Dosages

For dosage information on α-glucosidase inhibitors, refer to the table on p. 640.

DIPEPTIDYL PEPTIDASE 4 (DPP-4) INHIBITORS

Mechanism of Action and Drug Effects

Dipeptidyl peptidase-4 (DPP-4) inhibitors work by delaying the breakdown of incretin hormones (see Incretin Mimetics) by inhibiting the enzyme DPP-4. Incretin hormones are released throughout the day and are increased after a meal. When plasma glucose concentrations are normal or high, the incretin hormones increase insulin synthesis and lower glucagon secretion. By inhibiting the enzyme responsible for incretin breakdown (DPP-4), the DPP-4 inhibitors reduce fasting and postprandial glucose concentrations. Currently there are four DPP-4 inhibitors: sitagliptin phosphate monohydrate (Januvia®), alogliptin benzoate (Nesina®), saxagliptin hydrochloride (Onglyza®), and linagliptin (Tradjenta®). They are all available in combination formulations with metformin (e.g., Jentadueto® is the combination of linagliptin and metformin). There are several DPP-4 inhibitors currently under investigation. This class of drugs is commonly referred to as the *gliptins*.

Indications

The DPP-4 inhibitors are indicated as an adjunct to changes in diet and exercise habits to improve glycemic control in adults with type 2 diabetes.

Contraindications

The DPP-4 inhibitors are contraindicated in patients with known drug allergy.

Adverse Effects

The most common adverse effects of DPP-4 inhibitors are upper respiratory tract infection, headache, and diarrhea.

Hypoglycemia can occur and is more common if these drugs are used in conjunction with a sulfonylurea. Cases of pancreatitis have been reported.

Interactions

Sitagliptin phosphate monohydrate may increase digoxin levels. Concurrent use of sulfonylureas and insulin may increase the risk of hypoglycemia. The use of CYP3A4 inducers such as carbamazepine, dexamethasone, phenobarbital, phenytoin, and rifampin may decrease the glycemic lowering effect of saxagliptin. Rifampin may decrease the efficacy of linagliptin.

Dosages

The recommended dosage of sitagliptin phosphate monohydrate is 100 mg daily; for saxagliptin hydrochloride, it is 5 mg daily; for alogliptin benzoate, 25 mg daily; and for linagliptin, 5 mg daily.

SODIUM–GLUCOSE COTRANSPORTER 2 INHIBITOR

A new class of oral antihyperglycemic drugs, introduced in 2014, comprises the sodium–glucose cotransporter 2 inhibitors. There are currently two drugs available in this class: canagliflozin (Invokana®) and dapagliflozin (Forxiga®).

Mechanism of Action and Drug Effects

Sodium–glucose cotransporter 2 inhibitors block the tubular reabsorption of glucose in the kidney via the sodium–glucose cotransporter, a protein that facilitates 90% of glucose reabsorption in the proximal tubules of the kidneys. Selective inhibition of the sodium–glucose cotransporter results in a reduction of plasma glucose as kidney glucose excretion is increased. Consequently, glycemic control is improved. In addition, weight loss and a reduction in systolic blood pressure occur. They also raise the high-density lipoprotein cholesterol and the low-density lipoprotein cholesterol levels. The incidence of hypoglycemia related to sodium–glucose cotransporter 2 inhibitors is low, compared to that caused by the other oral antihyperglycemics.

Indications

Canagliflozin and dapagliflozin are recommended as an adjunct to changes in diet and exercise habits in combination with other glucose-lowering drugs (e.g., sulfonylurea, pioglitazone, insulin) and as a monotherapy for metformin-intolerant patients with type 2 diabetes.

Contraindications

The sodium–glucose cotransporter 2 inhibitors are contraindicated in patients with known drug allergy. These drugs are not to be used in patients with type 1 diabetes, in patients with kidney disease, or for the treatment of DKA.

Adverse Effects

The most frequently reported adverse effects of sodium–glucose cotransporter 2 inhibitors include vaginal yeast infections and urinary tract infections due to high concentrations of glucose in the urine. The greatest risk is in female patients and in male patients who are uncircumcised. Other adverse effects include diarrhea, constipation, and nausea. The use of canagliflozin or dapaglifozin creates osmotic diuresis, which may lead to intravascular volume depletion and associated manifestations (e.g., hypotension, dizziness, orthostatic hypotension, syncope, dehydration). Hyperkalemia may occur in individuals with kidney insufficiency. Elevated levels of LDLs, hemoglobin, serum creatinine, blood urea nitrogen, and serum phosphate, as well as a decrease in serum urate, have been reported. In 2015, Health Canada initiated a safety review for dapagliflozin and canagliflozin and the risk of DKA (Government of Canada, 2015). The symptoms of DKA occur unexpectedly and can occur with only slightly increased blood sugar levels in those with type 2 diabetes. There has been one known case of DKA related to sodium–glucose cotransporter 2 inhibitor use in Canada to date.

Interactions

Canagliflozin and dapagliflozin may increase the risk of hypoglycemia when combined with insulin or an insulin secretagogue. Use of the sodium–glucose cotransporter 2 inhibitors with insulin decreases efficacy and clinical benefit, requiring the dosage of the sodium–glucose cotransporter 2 inhibitors to be increased from 100 to 300 mg. Canagliflozin increases digoxin levels, requiring monitoring of digoxin levels. St. John's wort may reduce the clinical response to canagliflozin.

Dosages

The recommended initial dosage of canagliflozin is 100 mg once daily, preferably before breakfast. For those who are able to tolerate the 100 mg dose, require tighter glycemic control, and have adequate kidney function, the 300 mg dose may be considered. This class of drug's use during pregnancy is indicated only if the potential benefit justifies the potential risk to the fetus. The dosage of dapaglifloxin is 5 mg taken once daily at any time of the day, with or without food. It can be increased to 10 mg daily for patients requiring additional glycemic control.

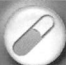 ## DRUG PROFILES

acarbose

Acarbose (Glucobay) is the only available α-glucosidase inhibitor. Acarbose works by blunting the elevation of blood glucose levels after a meal. In order for it to work optimally, it should be taken with the first bite of each meal. It may also be taken along with sulfonylureas or metformin. Use of acarbose is contraindicated in patients with a hypersensitivity to α-glucosidase inhibitors, as well as DKA, cirrhosis, inflammatory bowel disease, colonic ulceration, partial intestinal obstruction, or chronic intestinal disease.

PHARMACOKINETICS

Route	Onset of Action	Peak Plasma Concentration	Elimination Half-Life	Duration of Action
PO	1–1.5 hr	2 hr	2–3 hr	Unknown

▶▶ gliclazide

Gliclazide (Diamicron) is a second-generation sulfonylurea drug. In contrast to another second-generation sulfonylurea, glimepiride, it has a rapid onset and a short duration of action, with no active metabolites. This rapid onset of action allows it to function much like the pancreas normally does in response to meals, after which greater levels of insulin are required rapidly to deal with the increased glucose in the blood. When a patient with type 2 diabetes takes gliclazide, it rapidly stimulates the pancreas to release insulin. This, in turn, facilitates the transport of excess glucose from the blood into the cells of the muscles,

liver, and adipose tissues. Gliclazide also has antiplatelet and antioxidant properties.

Gliclazide use is contraindicated in cases of known drug allergy as well as in patients with type 1 diabetes or those with type 2 who experience variations in blood glucose levels. Unlike most other oral antihyperglycemic drugs, it is not contraindicated in patients with severe kidney failure. It works best if given 30 minutes before meals. This allows the timing of the insulin secretion induced by the gliclazide to correspond with the elevation in blood glucose level induced by a meal, in much the same way as endogenous insulin levels are raised in a person without diabetes. The extended-release dosage form of gliclazide can be given once daily, usually before breakfast.

PHARMACOKINETICS

Route	Onset of Action	Peak Plasma Concentration	Elimination Half-Life	Duration of Action
PO	1 hr	6 hr	16 hr	4–6 hr

▶▶ metformin hydrochloride

Metformin hydrochloride (Glucophage® Glumetza®) is currently the only biguanide oral antihyperglycemic drug. It works primarily by inhibiting hepatic glucose production and increasing the sensitivity of peripheral tissue to insulin. Because its mechanism of action differs from that of sulfonylurea drugs, it may be given along with these drugs.

Continued

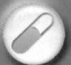
DRUG PROFILES—cont'd

Metformin use is contraindicated in patients with a known hypersensitivity to biguanides, liver or kidney disease, alcoholism, or cardiopulmonary disease.

PHARMACOKINETICS (IMMEDIATE RELEASE)

Route	Onset of Action	Peak Plasma Concentration	Elimination Half-Life	Duration of Action
PO	Over 6 hr	1–3 hr	1.5–5 hr	24 hr

▸▸pioglitazone hydrochloride

Pioglitazone hydrochloride (Actos) is classified as a glitazone or derivative. It is marketed for the treatment of patients with type 2 diabetes. Pioglitazone hydrochloride is used alone or with metformin, insulin, or a sulfonylurea. It works by decreasing insulin resistance. It can worsen or precipitate heart failure and is best avoided in patients with heart disease. The safety of this drug for use in pregnant women and children has not been established.

PHARMACOKINETICS

Route	Onset of Action	Peak Plasma Concentration	Elimination Half-Life	Duration of Action
PO	Delayed	2 hr	3–7 hr	Unknown

▸▸repaglinide

Repaglinide (GlucoNorm) is one of two antidiabetic drugs classified as *glinides*, the other being nateglinide (Starlix). These drugs have a mechanism of action similar to that of the sulfonylureas in that they also stimulate the release of insulin from pancreatic β-cells. They are especially helpful in the treatment of patients with erratic eating habits because the drug dose is skipped when a meal is missed. Contraindications include known drug allergy.

PHARMACOKINETICS

Route	Onset of Action	Peak Plasma Concentration	Elimination Half-Life	Duration of Action
PO	15–60 min	1 hr	2–3 hr	4–6 hr

▸▸sitagliptin phosphate monohydrate

Sitagliptin phosphate monohydrate (Januvia) was the first DPP-4 inhibitor approved by Health Canada. It is an oral drug that selectively inhibits the action of DPP-4, thereby increasing concentrations of the naturally occurring incretins GLP-1 and gastric inhibitory peptide (GIP). Sitagliptin phosphate monohydrate is indicated for the management of type 2 diabetes, either as monotherapy or in combination with metformin, a sulfonylurea, or a glitazone, but not with insulin. Clinical trials of sitagliptin phosphate monohydrate have demonstrated A_{1C} reductions of 0.6 to 0.8%, which is less than the reductions seen with traditional oral antihyperglycemic drugs. Significant hypoglycemia may occur when the drug is combined with a sulfonylurea. There have been no significant adverse effects documented. Because of postmarketing cases of acute pancreatitis, patients must be monitored closely for the development of pancreatitis after both initiation and dose increases. Sitagliptin phosphate monohydrate is given once daily as a 100-mg tablet with or without food. It is not recommended for use during pregnancy.

PHARMACOKINETICS

Route	Onset of Action	Peak Plasma Concentration	Elimination Half-Life	Duration of Action
PO	15–30 min	1 hr	12 hr	Unknown

Injectable Antihyperglycemic Drugs

INCRETIN MIMETICS

Mechanism of Action and Drug Effects

Incretins are hormones released by the GI tract in response to food. Incretins do the following:
1. Stimulate insulin secretion
2. Reduce postprandial glucagon production
3. Slow gastric emptying
4. Increase satiety

The most important incretin hormones identified to date are GLP-1 and GIP. These hormones are rapidly deactivated by the enzyme DPP-4. The incretin mimetics enhance glucose-dependent insulin secretion, suppress elevated glucagon secretion, and slow gastric emptying.

Currently, there are four incretin mimetics: albiglutide, dulaglutide, exenatide, and liraglutide.

Indications

Exenatide (Byetta®) was approved by Health Canada in 2010 as the first incretin mimetic drug. Exenatide is a long-acting analogue of GLP-1 that was initially derived from the salivary gland of the Gila monster. This drug is available only as a subcutaneous injection by prefilled pen and is indicated only for patients with type 2 diabetes who have been unable to achieve blood glucose control with metformin, a sulfonylurea, or insulin glargine. It is best given 60 minutes before a meal. Liraglutide (Victoza®) is similar to exenatide. At the time of writing, albiglutide (Eperzan®) had received a Notice of Compliance by Health Canada. Dulaglutide (Trulicity®), approved in January 2016, is another incretin mimetic available in a single use, pre-filled syringe or a pen. It is administered once weekly, at any time of day, with or without meals.

These drugs are not recommended for use during pregnancy.

Contraindications

Incretin mimetics are contraindicated in patients with known drug allergy. They should not be used in patients with end-stage kidney failure or severe kidney impairment.

Adverse Effects

Adverse effects of incretin mimetics include nausea, vomiting, and diarrhea. Rare cases of hemorrhagic or necrotizing pancreatitis after both initiation and dose increases have also been reported. Patients may experience rapid weight loss of more than 1.5 kg per week.

Interactions

Incretin mimetics can delay absorption of other orally administered drugs by slowing gastric emptying. In patients taking sulfonylurea drugs, the dose of the incretin mimetic may need to be reduced if hypoglycemia appears on initiation of exenatide therapy.

Dosages

The usual starting dosage of exenatide is 5 mcg within 1 hour of both the morning and evening meals. If necessary, the dosage may be increased after 1 month to 10 mcg twice daily before meals. The dose of liraglutide is initially 0.6 mg, and then it is titrated up to 1.2 or 1.8 mg daily. The recommended dosage of albiglutide is 30 mg once weekly given as a subcutaneous injection. The dosage may be increased to 50 mg once weekly if the glycemic response is inadequate. The recommended dosage of dulaglutide is 0.75 mg once weekly. The dose may be increased to 1.5 mg once weekly for additional glycemic control.

GLUCOSE-ELEVATING DRUGS

Hypoglycemia is an abnormally low blood glucose level (generally below 4 mmol/L). When the cause is organic and the effects are mild, treatment usually consists of dietary modifications (a higher intake of protein and lower intake of carbohydrates), to prevent a rebound postprandial hypoglycemic effect. Hypoglycemia is also a common adverse effect of many antihypoglycemic drugs when their pharmacological effects are greater than expected. The severity of hypoglycemia is determined by clinical manifestations. Initial manifestations are neurogenic from adrenergic mechanisms (related to the sympathetic nervous system) and include sweating, trembling, palpitations, anxiety, and a sensation of hunger. Because the brain needs a constant amount of glucose to function, neuroglycopenic manifestations include the central nervous system (CNS) manifestations of difficulty concentrating, confusion, weakness, drowsiness, vision changes, difficulty speaking, dizziness, and headache. Later symptoms include hypothermia and seizures. Without adequate restoration of normal plasma and CNS glucose levels (typically the plasma glucose is less than 2.8 mmol/L in hypoglycemia), coma and death will occur.

Oral forms of concentrated glucose are available for patients to use in the event of a hypoglycemic crisis. The CDA recommends the administration of 15 grams of glucose (e.g., glucose tablets, three packets of sugar dissolved in water, 8 Lifesavers, 175 mL of a regular soft drink or juice, or 15 mL of honey) to produce an increase in plasma glucose of approximately 2.1 mmol/L within 20 minutes. These fast-acting glucose sources are preferable to milk, orange juice, and glucose gels, which are slower to increase plasma glucose levels and provide symptom relief. Glucose gel acts quite slowly (less than 1 mmol/L increase at 20 minutes) and must be swallowed to have a significant effect. Plasma glucose should be retested 15 minutes after glucose administration, and if the level is less than 4 mmol/L, the individual should be retreated with an additional 15 grams of carbohydrate. When the hypoglycemia is reversed, a normal meal should be eaten; however, if the meal is longer than 1 hour away, a snack of 15 grams of carbohydrate and a protein should be consumed.

Table sugar (sucrose) will not produce as rapid an effect as the glucose products intended for use by patients with diabetes. This is because sucrose is a disaccharide (two-molecule sugar) that must first be digested in the body to yield glucose as a monosaccharide (one-molecule sugar) by-product. Commercially available, fast-acting glucose is available in gel, liquid, or tablet form. Because the α-glucosidase inhibitor acarbose interferes with the digestion of some carbohydrates, patients taking this drug must use glucose (dextrose) tablets or, if these are unavailable, milk or honey to treat hypoglycemia. In the hospital setting or when a patient is unconscious, IV glucose is an obvious option to treat hypoglycemia. Concentrations of up to 50% dextrose in water ($D_{50}W$) are most often used for this purpose.

In addition to oral or IV glucose, glucagon, a natural hormone secreted by the pancreas, is available as a subcutaneous injection to be given when a quick response to severe hypoglycemia is needed. Because glucagon injection may induce vomiting, roll an unconscious patient onto his or her side before injection. Glucagon is useful in treating the unconscious hypoglycemic patient without established IV access.

PHARMACOKINETIC BRIDGE TO NURSING PRACTICE

Continuous subcutaneous insulin infusion (CSII) has been used in patients with type 1 diabetes for over 25 years. Provision of insulin therapy by CSII is becoming an option for selected patients with diabetes in an attempt to minimize the risks and complications of the disease. Two options for achieving intensive diabetes

DOSAGES   Selected Oral Antihyperglycemic Drugs

Drug	Pharmacological Class	Usual Dosage Range	Indications
acarbose (Glucobay)	α-glucosidase inhibitor	PO: 50–100 mg tid, taken with first bite of meal	Type 2 diabetes
►►gliclazide (Diamicron, Diamicron MR)	Second-generation sulfonylurea	PO: 80–320 mg daily (doses above 160 mg divided, bid) MR: 30–120 mg once daily	
glimepiride (Amaryl)	Second-generation sulfonylurea	PO: 1–4 mg daily (max 8 mg daily)	
►►metformin hydrochloride (Glucophage)	Biguanide	PO: 500 mg bid–qid or 850 mg bid–tid daily; max daily dose 2550 mg	
►►pioglitazone (Actos)	Thiazolidinedione	PO: 15–45 mg once daily	
repaglinide (GlucoNorm)	Meglitinide	PO: 0.5–4 mg tid; best taken 15 min before a meal	
sitagliptin phosphate monohydrate (Januvia)	DPP-4 inhibitor	PO: 100 mg daily	
COMBINATION ORAL DRUGS			
rosiglitazone/metformin (Avandemet)	Combination thiazolidinedione/ biguanide	PO: 4 mg /500 mg–8 mg/2000 mg bid	
sitagliptin/metformin (Janumet®)	Combination incretin mimetic/biguanide	PO: 50 mg/500 mg–50 mg/850 mg –50 mg/1000 mg bid with meals	
Sitagliptin/metformin ER (JanumetXR®)	Combination incretin mimetic/biguanide modified release	PO: 50 mg/500 mg–50 mg/1000 mg –100 mg/1000 mg once daily with meals	
saxagliptin/metformin (Kombiglyze®)	Combination incretin mimetic/biguanide	PO: 2.5 mg/500 mg–2.5 mg/850 mg– 2.5 mg/1000 mg bid with meals	
linagliptin/metformin (Jentadueto®)	Combination incretin mimetic/biguanide	PO: 2.5/500 mg–2.5/ 850 mg–2.5/ 1000 mg bid	
alogliptin/metformin (Kazano®)	Combination incretin mimetic/biguanide	PO: 12.5 mg/500 mg–12.5 mg/850 mg –12.5 mg/1000 mg bid with meals	

MR, modified release; *PO*, oral.

management are used: basal–bolus regimens (long-acting basal insulin analogues and rapid-acting bolus insulin analogues) and CSII. With CSII, normal serum glucose levels are maintained by the continuous delivery of basal insulin, and then with food intake, primarily carbohydrate consumption, bolus doses of insulin are given. Use of an insulin pump (i.e., CSII) leads to a more rapid, consistent absorption of the drugs and a reduction in the occurrence of hypoglycemia. Research has also shown that use of an insulin pump helps to decrease the occurrence of elevated prebreakfast serum glucose levels, often called the *dawn phenomenon* (referring to the dawn of the day). The dawn phenomenon occurs when the counter-regulatory hormones (i.e., growth hormone, cortisol, and catecholamines) stimulate the liver to release glucose. By contrast, the Somogyi effect occurs when the same hormones are released in response to a low early morning plasma glucose level, which can result in an early morning hyperglycemia. In these instances, hyperglycemia is caused by an excess of insulin, poorly timed insulin (including inadvertent insulin administration), or missed meals or snacks. Because insulin pumps deliver insulin through the subcutaneous route and the infusion is a continuous one, fewer problems occur with the pump method than with once- or twice-daily injections. Patients using CSII achieve mean serum glucose and HbA$_{1C}$ levels that remain somewhat lower than those associated with basal–bolus therapy alone, so their risk for hypoglycemia is decreased. The use of CSII with a continuous glucose sensor results in improved plasma glucose control over basal–bolus therapy. Understanding new and different drugs and their pharmacokinetic properties allows the nurse to help patients achieve a better quality of life, minimize risks, and maximize wellness.

NURSING PROCESS

Assessment
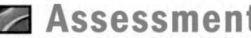

Before administering any type of antidiabetic drug, assess the patient's knowledge about the disease and recommended treatment. Complete a head-to-toe physical assessment, medication history, and nursing assessment, and document the findings. Prior to beginning treatment with insulin, as well as other with antidiabetic drugs, take a thorough medication history that includes a list of the patient's current medications, including over-the-counter (OTC) drugs and natural health products. Review the appropriate laboratory test results (e.g., plasma glucose, fasting plasma glucose level, A_{1C} level) for any abnormalities compared with baseline levels. Assess the health care provider's order for insulin so that the correct drug, route, type of insulin (e.g., rapid acting, short acting, intermediate acting, short- and intermediate-acting mixtures, long acting), and dosage are implemented correctly. Assess the specific insulin, paying additional attention to its unique pharmacokinetics, including onset of action, peak, and duration of action. Knowing this information prior to giving the insulin is crucial to patient safety because these drug properties actually define the parameters within which reactions, adverse effects, or therapeutic effects may potentially occur. If more than one insulin type is prescribed, mixing of insulins may be ordered. It is important for the nurse to know what combinations are chemically compatible (see Table 33-4) so as to avoid an undesirable altered glycemic effect. Additionally, with all insulin orders, perform a second check of the prepared insulin dosage against the medication order with another registered nurse, or perform checks per facility policy and document accordingly.

Assess blood glucose levels prior to administering insulin to avoid giving the drug to a patient who is already hypoglycemic. The CDA guidelines identify the key diagnostic criterion for diabetes as a fasting plasma glucose of greater than 7 mmol/L or a hemoglobin A_{1C} greater than 6.5% (see Box 33-1). Furthermore, the CDA recommends the following control criteria for patients with diabetes: fasting blood glucose within the range of 4 to 7 mmol/L or a hemoglobin A_{1C} of less than 7%. Keep in mind that allergic reactions are less likely to occur with recombinant human insulins because of their similarity to endogenous insulin; however, allergies may still occur and have to be considered in the assessment. Contraindications and cautions associated with insulin have been previously discussed. Significant drug interactions are presented in Table 33-5, but it is important to remember the drugs that work against the effect of insulin, including corticosteroids, thyroid drugs, and diuretics. Drugs that increase the hypoglycemic effects of insulin include alcohol, sulfa antibiotics, and salicylates.

Oral antihyperglycemic drugs also require close assessment for contraindications, cautions, and drug interactions, so obtain a thorough medication and patient history before administering these. Make sure to know each patient's history because type 2 diabetes can be treated with oral antihyperglycemic drugs, most of which require functioning β-cells in the pancreas. Functioning β-cells are not present in type 1 diabetes. With biguanides, be aware that older adults or malnourished patients may react adversely to this group of drugs. Contraindications, cautions, and interactions for this drug class have been previously discussed, but it is important to patient safety to emphasize the interaction between metformin and the iodine-containing radiologic contrast media used for certain diagnostic purposes (e.g., computed tomography with contrast). This interaction is associated with an increased risk for acute kidney injury and lactic acidosis. If a patient is taking metformin, closely assess and monitor for this scenario so that the metformin may be discontinued the day of the test and for at least 48 hours afterwards. See Table 33-5 for more drug interactions associated with the oral antihyperglycemic drugs.

With sulfonylureas, it is important to know baseline glucose levels as well as conditions that may predispose a patient to hypoglycemia, such as a drop in caloric intake, alcohol use, or advanced age. As well, assessment of allergic reactions to sulfonamide antibiotics is important because of the potential for cross-allergic reactions. With glinides, cautions, contraindications, and drug interactions are similar to those for sulfonylureas. With thiazolidinediones (glitazones), a major contraindication is class III or IV heart failure (as per the New York Heart Association classification). With α-glucosidase inhibitors (e.g., acarbose), assess for contraindications such as inflammatory bowel disease or malabsorption syndromes. With second-generation sulfonylureas, determine the patient's type of diabetes because these drugs are contraindicated in type 1 diabetes.

Exenatide, an incretin mimetic, requires assessment of the patient's diagnosis because the drug is used for patients with type 2 diabetes and an inability to control blood glucose levels with metformin, a sulfonylurea, or a glitazone. It should not be used with insulin.

For patients with diabetes, unstable serum glucose levels require immediate attention, so assess for any signs and symptoms of hypoglycemia (e.g., acute onset of confusion, irritability, tremor, and sweating, with progression to possible hypothermia and seizures, and blood glucose levels of less than 4 mmol/L) or of hyperglycemia (e.g., polyuria, polydipsia, polyphagia, glucosuria, weight loss, and fatigue, with plasma glucose levels of 14 mmol/L or higher). Assessment is even more critical for patients with diabetes who are also under stress, have an infection or are ill, are pregnant or lactating, or are experiencing trauma or any serious change in health status. With treatment, patients with hyperglycemia are at risk of hypoglycemia with the potential danger of loss of consciousness; therefore, constantly assess serum glucose levels and neurological status. Along with assessment of the therapeutic regimen and patient adherence to treatment, note any relevant ethnocultural factors, socioeconomic factors, and sources of social support, and continue to be aware of these throughout therapy.

Glucose-elevating drugs are to be given only after thorough assessment of a patient's presenting clinical picture and a thorough collection of data, including laboratory values, medication and health history, and a comprehensive list of current medications. Also assess for level of consciousness because glucagon injection may induce vomiting, and precautions must be implemented to prevent aspiration.

Nursing Diagnoses

- Imbalanced nutrition, less than body requirements, related to the body's inability to use glucose (for type 1 diabetes)
- Ineffective family therapeutic regimen management related to lack of experience with a significant daily treatment regimen for diabetes
- Risk for unstable glucose due to recent onset of possible signs and symptoms of diabetes

Planning

Goals

- Patient will maintain adequate and balanced nutrition, stabilizing weight and improving dietary habits, in support of the overall management of diabetes.
- Patient and family will state the importance of adherence to medication regimens, lifestyle changes, dietary restrictions, and avoidance of high-risk behaviours.
- Patient will begin to understand the etiology of unstable glucose levels and learn management strategies.

Expected Patient Outcomes

- Patient adheres to the diet recommended by the CDA or other dietary advisor per the orders of the health care provider or registered dietitian.
  - Patient eats a nutritious diet, gets sufficient rest and relaxation, and notifies a health care provider if any unusual problems occur when customary activities are changed.
- Patient and family report improvement in adherence to therapeutic regimen and disease management, demonstrating awareness of the potential complications and keeping all scheduled appointments with the health care provider to monitor therapeutic effectiveness of drug therapy, diet, and lifestyle changes.
- Patient takes medication as scheduled, monitors plasma glucose levels as prescribed, and watches for any signs and symptoms of hyperglycemia or hypoglycemia.
  - Patient's fasting plasma glucose (i.e., after 8 hours without food) goal is to be within the range of 4 to 7 mmol/L or hemoglobin A_{1C} less than 7%.

Implementation

With any patient who is taking insulin (or oral antihyperglycemic drugs), always check plasma glucose levels

(and other related laboratory values, as ordered) before giving the drug so that accurate baseline glucose levels are obtained and documented. Do not shake NPH (which appears cloudy) or premixed insulin mixtures, but roll them between the hands before administering the prescribed dose. Rolling helps to avoid air being trapped in the syringe and thus inaccurate dose administration. Administer insulins at room temperature. If insulin is to be used within 1 month, it may be stored at room temperature; otherwise, refrigeration is needed. Refrigeration is also recommended in warm or hot climates and during any major changes in environmental temperatures from hot to cold. Never use expired or discoloured insulin. For information about the handling, mixing, storage, and administration of insulin, refer to Box 33-2.

Administer insulin subcutaneously at a 90-degree angle unless the patient is emaciated, in which case it may be administered at a 45-degree angle. Only regular insulin may be administered intravenously; this method is often used in critical care settings. Use insulin syringes only for subcutaneous injections or when drawing up insulin dosage amounts. These syringes are easy to identify because of their orange caps and calibration in units, not millilitres. These syringes have preattached ultrafine needles that are 29 gauge and 12.7 millimetres in length (these are not changed after withdrawing the insulin). If mixed insulins are ordered, withdraw the regular or rapid-acting insulin (unmodified and clear) first, followed by the intermediate-acting or NPH insulin (modified and cloudy). Do this only after the appropriate amount of air has been injected into the vials. The amount of air to inject into the vials equals the prescribed number of units. Inject air into the intermediate-acting insulin vial first. Next, inject air into the regular, rapid-, or short-acting insulin vial. This technique helps keep the intermediate-acting insulin from contaminating the rapid-acting insulin vial. This contamination would lead to a change in the regular, rapid-, or short-acting, unmodified insulin by the NPH, intermediate-acting, modified insulin. The net effect is an interference with the activity of the regular insulin, thus impacting its effect in the patient (see Table 33-3 and Chapter 10).

Understanding the action of types of insulin and their related pharmacokinetics (e.g., onset, peak, duration) is critical for safe care and for patient education. For example, it is important to know that the rapid-acting insulins (insulin lispro, insulin aspart, insulin glulisine) have an onset of action of about 15 minutes and must be given 15 minutes before meals, compared with regular insulin or a short-acting insulin, which should be given 30 minutes before meals, as their onset of action is 30 to 60 minutes. If insulin lispro is to be mixed with NPH (intermediate-acting) insulin, give the combination 15 minutes before meals. Always double-check the health care providers' orders for clarification of the dosage and drug as well as of any dietary changes, such as a possible increase in carbohydrates and decrease in fat to avoid

BOX 33-2   Administration, Handling, and Storage of Insulin

Dosages, Storage, Handling, and Mixing

1. Individualize insulin dosages and monitor patients closely for adequate control of hypoglycemia and hyperglycemia. Follow guidelines for basal–bolus insulin therapy or sliding-scale dosing, depending on the specific regimen to be used in the hospital setting.
2. Adjust dosages, as ordered, to achieve the health care provider's specific fasting plasma glucose level for the patient. Using the CDA guidelines, this would be a fasting blood glucose level of 4 to 7 mmol/L or hemoglobin A_{1C} less than 7% for the patient with diabetes. Adjust dosages, as ordered, to achieve.
3. Store insulin for current use at room temperature. Avoid extreme temperatures and exposure to sunlight because these cause the insulin's protein structure to be permanently denatured. Extra vials not in use may be stored in the refrigerator. Vials being used in high environmental temperatures need to be stored in a refrigerator, but never give cold insulin. Never freeze insulin. To maintain drug stability, store insulin for only up to 1 month at room temperature or up to 3 months in the refrigerator.
4. Discard unused vials if they have not been used within several weeks (or follow hospital policy). Do not use any insulin that does not have the proper clarity or colour (e.g., clear for regular, cloudy for NPH).
5. Store prefilled insulin syringes in a refrigerator for up to 1 week.
6. Always check expiration dates of insulin and all equipment.

Administration

1. Administer insulin subcutaneously (see Chapter 10); however, regular insulin may be given intravenously in special situations (e.g., in postoperative patients, as a continuous infusion in a patient with DKA), if ordered.
2. Roll the drug vial gently between the hands without shaking to avoid bubble formation in the vial, which may lead to inaccurate dosage withdrawal. Give freshly mixed insulins within 5 minutes of mixing to avoid binding of the solution and subsequent altered activity of the drugs.
3. Administer insulin at the recommended times but always with meals or meal trays ready. Give insulin

lispro and other rapid-acting insulins approximately 15 minutes before meals (due to quick onset of action) and only after monitoring the patient's fasting serum glucose level (as with all insulin administration). Give regular insulin (short-acting insulin) 30 minutes before meals, and NPH insulin 30 to 60 minutes before meals.
4. When giving regular and NPH insulin at the same time (if ordered), mix the two appropriately (see discussion of mixing insulins in the Implementation subsection under Nursing Process). This mixture is usually given at least 30 minutes before mealtime.
5. Administer insulin subcutaneously at a 90-degree angle. However, if the patient is emaciated, a 45-degree angle may be more effective. Use only insulin syringes (see text discussion and Chapter 10).
6. Instruct patients using insulin injections to rotate sites within the same general location for about 1 week before moving to a new location (e.g., all injections for a week in the upper right thigh before moving a little lower on the right thigh). This technique allows for better insulin absorption and prevents the development of lipodystrophy (see below). Each injection site should be at least 1.25 to 2.5 centimetres away from the previous injection site. If this practice is followed, it will be approximately 6 weeks before the patient will have to rotate to a totally new area of the body. Note the following sites for subcutaneous insulin injections: thigh areas (front and back), outer areas of the upper arm (middle third of the upper arm between the shoulder and the elbow) and the abdominal area using the iliac crests as landmarks and using the fatty part of the abdomen, but not within 5 centimetres of the umbilicus or any incision or stoma (see Chapter 10).

   Lipodystrophy is characterized by small nodules (lipomas) or scar tissue within the skin. Lipodystrophy occurs less frequently with insulin analogues but can still occur. It is caused by the anabolic effect of insulin on fat and protein synthesis and is the result of injecting insulin in the same site rather than rotating sites. Insulin absorption will be altered in areas of lipodystrophy.
7. Continuous subcutaneous insulin infusion or multiple daily injections may be ordered for tight glucose control. Date the multiuse insulin vial when opened and refer to agency policies for expiration dates.

---

postprandial hypoglycemia). A meal high in fat can delay carbohydrate absorption, while rapid-acting insulin is already in its peak action.

Regardless of the specific type of recombinant human insulin used, understanding the peak, onset, and duration of action of the insulin (e.g., rapid acting versus short acting versus intermediate acting versus long acting) will help determine when food or meals are to be taken. The intermediate-acting insulin (NPH) has an onset of action of 1 to 2 hours, so serve meals at least 30 to 45 minutes

prior to its administration. Many combination products of rapid- or short-acting insulins with intermediate-acting insulin are available; give these combination insulins 15 to 30 minutes before meals. In the hospital setting, be sure that meal trays have arrived on the unit before giving insulin to avoid time lapses from unexpected delays and subsequent hypoglycemic episodes. Also be sure that other forms of allowed foods are available to patients in case meals are delayed and insulin has already been administered.

Patients may require dosing by the sliding-scale or a basal–bolus method in a hospital setting. Sliding scale has historically been the method for administering subcutaneous regular insulin doses adjusted according to serum glucose test results. Although controversial (see previous pharmacology discussion), sliding-scale dosing may be used for hospitalized patients with diabetes who are experiencing drastic changes in plasma glucose levels due to physical or emotional stress, infections, surgery, acute illness, inactivity, or variable caloric intake, as well as for patients needing intensive insulin therapy or patients—even those without diabetes—receiving total parenteral nutrition (TPN) with a high glucose concentration. When this insulin regimen is used, measure blood glucose levels several times per day (e.g., every 4 hours, every 6 hours, or at specified times such as 0700 hours, 1100 hours, 1600 hours, and midnight) to obtain fasting or preprandial blood glucose values. The newer method, basal–bolus insulin dosing, is now the preferred method of treatment for hospitalized patients with diabetes; orders for dosages and frequency will be issued by the health care provider. A long-acting insulin (insulin glargine) is used to mimic the basal secretion of a healthy pancreas and to create constant delivery of an amount of insulin, and then the bolus is used (insulin lispro or insulin aspart) to control increases in daily blood glucose levels. Bolus insulin is divided into meal and correction boluses (see pharmacology discussion). Monitor blood glucose levels frequently when using these methods.

Oral antihyperglycemic drugs are usually administered at least 30 minutes before meals, as ordered. With any antihyperglycemic drug or insulin, it is important for the nurse and patient to know what to do if symptoms of hypoglycemia occur; for example, the patient should take glucagon; eat glucose tablets, liquid, or gel; consume corn syrup or honey; drink fruit juice or a nondiet soft drink; or eat a small snack, such as crackers or half a sandwich (see previous discussion on hypoglycemia). If a patient receiving metformin is to undergo diagnostic studies with contrast dye, the health care provider will need to discontinue the drug prior to the procedure and restart it after the tests, only after re-evaluation of the patient's kidney status. During therapy with metformin, the risk of lactic acidosis is possible, so it is important to monitor for and then report any hyperventilation, cold and clammy skin, muscle pain, abdominal pain, dizziness, or irregular heartbeat. Some of the sulfonylureas are to be taken with breakfast; the α-glucosidase inhibitors are always taken with the first bite of each main meal, and the thiazolidinediones are given once daily or in two divided doses. Always check the exact timing of the dose against the health care provider's order and with consideration of the drug's onset of action.

It is critical to the safe and efficient use of oral antihyperglycemics to be certain, before the dose is given, that food will be tolerated or is being tolerated. If the oral drug is taken and no meal is consumed or it is consumed at a later time than usual, hypoglycemia may occur and result in negative health consequences and even unconsciousness. Because the glitazones (i.e., rosiglitazone maleate and pioglitazone) may both cause moderate weight gain and edema, it is important to weigh patients daily at a consistent time and with the same amount of clothing. Several combination oral antihyperglycemic drug products are available (see the pharmacology discussion) and need to be given exactly as prescribed. Exenatide is given by subcutaneous injection in patients with type 2 diabetes and cannot be used with insulin. Sitagliptin phosphate monohydrate is also not to be used with insulin and may be taken with or without food.

In special situations, such as when a patient has been ordered to have nothing by mouth (NPO status) and is taking either an oral antihyperglycemic drug or insulin, it is crucial to follow the health care provider's orders regarding drug administration. If there are no written orders related to this situation, contact the health care provider for further instructions. If a patient is on NPO status but is receiving an IV solution of dextrose, the health care provider may still order insulin, but always clarify this with the health care provider. Contact the health care provider if a patient becomes ill and unable to take the usual dosage of an oral antihyperglycemic drug (or insulin). Encourage patients to always wear a medical alert bracelet, necklace, or tag indicating their diagnoses, medications, and emergency contacts.

It is also important to stay informed and up to date about the latest research on diabetes and to keep patients and family members well informed, although many patients already will be. The patient needs to be considered a member of the team when making decisions about diabetes management. A knowledgeable patient will have better long-term glycemic control. See the Evidence In Practice box for more information on specific nursing research.

In summary, there are many nursing considerations related to drug therapy in patients with diabetes. Patient education is also important and needs to begin the moment the patient has entered into the health care system or upon diagnosis. Instruction that is tailored to each patient's educational level and that uses appropriate teaching–learning concepts and teaching aids is important to support patient adherence to the treatment regimen. In addition, be sure that all necessary resources are made available to patients (e.g., financial assistance, visual assistance, dietary plans, daily menus, CDA information, transportation assistance, Meals on Wheels, other community services). See Patient Teaching Tips for more information.

Evaluation

It is important to understand current therapeutic guidelines in the care of patients with diabetes. The prevailing key diagnostic criterion for diabetes is hyperglycemia with a fasting plasma glucose of 7 mmol/L or higher or a nonfasting blood glucose level of 11.1 mmol/L or

EVIDENCE IN PRACTICE

Sensor-Augmented Insulin Pump Therapy Trumps Multiple Daily Injections

Review

In patients with type 1 diabetes and poor glycemic control, the use of a sensor-augmented insulin pump significantly improves glycated hemoglobin levels as compared with regimens involving multiple daily insulin injections. Landmark research has confirmed that more effective glycemic control has been demonstrated with the use of these pumps than with the use of multiple daily injections.

Type of Evidence

Some 329 adults and 156 children were randomly assigned to either begin pump therapy with the MiniMed Paradigm REAL-Time system (Medtronic®) or continue with their regimen of multiple daily injections; patients were under close supervision for the duration of the study that lasted for one year. Patients in the study received intensive diabetes management education and training, including regarding carbohydrate counting and the administration of correction doses of insulin. Those who were randomized to insulin pump therapy were placed on it for 2 weeks. After they had become comfortable with the pump, the glucose sensor was added. This group used the insulin aspart, and the injection therapy group used both insulin aspart and insulin glargine. All patients were seen at 3, 6, 9, and 12 months and used Carelink, which is a diabetes-management software program. This program was used to relay the patients' glucose data to their health care providers from home. The patients needed to have computer access to participate in the study. It is important to know that the sensor-augmented pump therapy uses the two technologies of an insulin pump and continuous glucose monitoring all in one system. This pump allows patients and their health care providers to monitor treatment and their response through Internet-based software.

Results of Study

After 1 year, the researchers found that the patients on pump therapy had hemoglobin A$_{1C}$ levels that were significantly lower than those of the injection-therapy group. The baseline mean glycated hemoglobin level, which was initially 8.3% in the two groups, decreased to 7.5% in the pump therapy group as compared to 8.1% in the injection therapy group. Among the adults, the absolute reduction in the mean glycated hemoglobin level was 1.0 ± 0.7% in the pump-therapy group and 0.4 ± 0.8% in the injection-therapy group. The between-group difference in the pump-therapy group was –0.6%. The occurrence of hypoglycemia and DKA were similar in both groups. There was no significant weight gain in adult or child participants.

Link of Evidence to Nursing Practice

This study has been identified as one of the longest and largest randomized controlled studies of sensor-augmented insulin pump therapy in patients with type 1 diabetes. Another significant aspect of this study was its comparison of two therapeutic approaches. For nursing and for the care of patients with diabetes, the impact of this study is important, as it indicated that patients may be able to achieve better control of their diabetes, with improved outcomes and safety, through the use of pump therapy. Such favourable results, without the occurrence of increased hypoglycemia, represent an important breakthrough in the care of patients with type 1 diabetes. The possibility of improving patients' adherence to treatment and enhancing their quality of life is exciting; the results of this study hold great promise for enhancing evidenced-informed nursing practice and the treatment of type 1 diabetes.

Source: Bergenstal, R. M., Tamborlane, W. V., Ahmann, A., et al. (2010). Effectiveness of sensor-augmented insulin-pump therapy in type 1 diabetes. *New England Journal of Medicine, 363*(4), 311–320. doi:10.1056/NEJMoa1002853

CASE STUDY

Diabetes

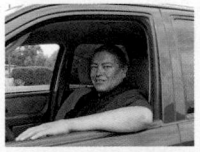

Joseph is a 58-year-old bus driver who received a diagnosis of type 2 diabetes 10 years ago; he has needed to take insulin for the last 2 years. He has been recovering, without complications, from a laparoscopic cholecystectomy; however, his plasma glucose levels have shown significant fluctuations over the last 24 hours. The health care provider has changed his insulin to lispro (Humalog) to evaluate whether this improves control of his plasma glucose levels.

1. What is the rationale for the use of oral antihyperglycemic drugs in a patient with type 2 diabetes? Why do some patients with type 2 diabetes need to begin taking insulin? What can be done to measure the control of a patient's diabetes over the short term and long term?
2. What are the pharmacokinetics of insulin lispro?
3. What special instructions, if any, should be given to Joseph about insulin lispro before he is discharged home from the hospital?

For answers, see http://evolve.elsevier.com/Canada/Lilley/pharmacology/.

higher. However, the therapeutic response to insulin and any of the oral antihyperglycemic drugs is a decrease in plasma glucose to the level prescribed by the health care provider or to near-normal levels. Most often, fasting plasma glucose levels are used to measure the degree of glycemic control achieved. Both fasting plasma glucose and postprandial plasma glucose are directly correlated to the risk of complications. The postprandial measure may indicate a stronger risk factor for cardiovascular complications than fasting levels. To estimate a patient's adherence to the therapy regimen for the previous several months, the level of A_{1C} is measured. This value reflects how well the patient has been managing diet and drug therapy. Patients with diabetes need to be monitored frequently by their health care providers (as well as at home)

to make sure they are adhering to their therapy regimens, evidenced by normalization of plasma test results. It is important to monitor patients for indications of hypoglycemia or hyperglycemia and insulin allergy as well. With short-acting insulins such as lispro, the onset of action is more rapid than with regular insulin and the duration of action is shorter, so monitor plasma glucose levels closely until the dosage is regulated and plasma glucose is at the level the health care provider desires. If a patient is switched from one insulin or oral antihyperglycemic drug to another, advise the patient that glucose levels must be monitored closely at home or by the health care provider. Always evaluate whether identified goals and expected outcome criteria are being achieved, and plan nursing care accordingly.

PATIENT TEACHING TIPS

❖ Encourage patients to wear medical alert jewellery, to carry a medical alert card at all times, and to keep medical information in clear view at home on the refrigerator.

❖ Provide instructions and demonstrations to patients regarding the proper storage of insulin, the equipment needed for administration, the drawing up and mixing of insulins (if ordered), correct technique for insulin injections, and the importance of rotation of subcutaneous insulin injection sites. Provide the opportunity for return demonstrations from patients, including of site rotation (see Chapter 10 for more information about insulin injections). Emphasize that insulin may be stored at room temperature unless heat is extreme or the patient is travelling. Encourage the patient to keep a daily dietary intake and blood glucose journal. Agency policy often includes the use of alcohol to cleanse the skin prior to injection for infection control purposes, although patients often do not use alcohol in their own environments.

❖ Educate patients about the need to have plasma glucose levels monitored. Emphasize instructions that are specific to the patient's glucometer. Stress the importance of exercise, hygiene, foot care, dietary plans, and weight control in the management of diabetes. Remind patients that illness can cause elevated plasma glucose levels; they should monitor levels closely and seek advice if unsure about managing the illness and the elevated plasma glucose levels but must not stop taking antidiabetic medications.

❖ Pay attention to and assess patients' financial situation when teaching about the frequency of blood glucose monitoring. Each blood glucose check costs over $1, and if patients must pay for supplies, this expense can add up quickly, especially for those who are economically disadvantaged. There is a wide variation in access to diabetes medications, supplies, and medical devices listed on federal, provincial and territorial formularies. Provincial or territorial drug plans provide Canadians with diabetes who are over

the age of 65 or receiving social assistance with access to diabetes mediations, devices, and supplies listed on provincial formularies. Many provinces and territories provide drug and supplies coverage through income-related deductibles and copayment programs. Provinces and territories may have financial assistance programs for diabetes-related expenses not otherwise covered.

❖ Advise patients to avoid smoking and alcohol consumption while using oral antihyperglycemic drugs, as well as to maintain strict adherence to dietary instructions. Instruct patients to avoid skipping meals or skipping doses of insulin or oral antihyperglycemic drugs and to contact a health care provider for further instructions when needed.

❖ Explain the difference between hypoglycemia and hyperglycemia (see earlier text discussion for specific signs and symptoms) to patients, with emphasis on the treatment of each (e.g., having on hand quick sources of glucose such as candy; sugar packets; OTC glucose tablets, liquid or gel; sugar cubes; honey; corn syrup; apple juice; or nondiet soft drinks for hypoglycemia, and having more insulin on hand for hyperglycemia, as ordered). Especially, encourage patients to have quick dosage forms of glucose available at all times.

❖ Educate patients about situations or conditions that lead to altered serum plasma glucose levels, such as fever, illness, stress, increased activity or exercise, surgery, and emotional distress. Encourage patients to contact their health care provider regarding any questions or concerns about maintaining glucose control.

❖ Educate patients about the importance of knowing preprandial plasma glucose levels prior to taking insulin and the importance of timing meals specifically, taking into account the type of insulin being used.

❖ Emphasize to patients the importance of having adequate supplies of insulin and equipment at all times and planning ahead for vacations. Instruct patients to keep all medications and related equipment out of the reach of children. If needed, magnifying attachments

PATIENT TEACHING TIPS—cont'd

are available for syringes and vials, and specialized syringes are available for people with vision impairments. Patients using these types of syringes learn to rely on the sound the syringe makes when a dosage is selected; for example, with a Novolog pen, 5 clicks equals 5 units.

❖ Encourage patients with diabetes to report any yellow discoloration of the skin, dark urine, fever, sore throat, weakness, unusual bleeding, or easy bruising.

❖ Emphasize to patients the importance of A_{1C} monitoring (e.g., at least two times per year for those with good glycemic control and quarterly for patients who are not at target values, have changed their therapy, or are not adhering to the therapy regimen). Review lifestyle modifications that support weight control and plasma glucose level maintenance, including changes in diet and exercise as well as drug therapy. Patients with type 2 diabetes have greater therapeutic responses to improvements in diet, exercise, and plasma glucose level control than patients with type 1 diabetes do. CDA recommendations for fasting plasma glucose level measurement need to be followed. Educate patients about the importance of engaging in supervised exercise as prescribed, as a lifelong lifestyle change. A registered dietitian is usually involved in patient care and assists with specific menu planning to help with changes in intake (e.g., implementing a low-fat diet with 160 to 300 g of carbohydrates). Nutrition therapy can reduce A_{1C} by 1 to 2% when combined with other aspects of diabetes management. Encourage patients to follow a healthy diet plan using Health Canada's publication, *Eating Well with Canada's Food Guide* (Health Canada, 2011). Educate patients about replacing high–glycemic index foods with low–glycemic index foods, and explain that, in doing, they will improve glycemic control. Examples of typical low–glycemic index food sources include beans, peas, lentils, pasta, pumpernickel or rye breads, parboiled rice, bulgur, barley, oats, quinoa, and fruits such as apples, pears, oranges, peaches, plums, apricots, cherries, or berries. Examples of higher–glycemic index foods include white or whole wheat bread, potatoes, highly extruded or crispy puffed breakfast cereals (e.g., corn flakes, puffed rice, puffed oats, puffed wheat), and fruits such as

pineapple, mango, papaya, cantaloupe, and watermelon. Educate patients that a higher intake of fibre, in particular cereal fibre, is associated with a decreased risk for cardiovascular disease and that a higher intake of soluble dietary fibre (e.g., eggplant, okra, oat products, beans, psyllium, barley) improves postprandial plasma glucose because it slows gastric emptying and delays the absorption of glucose in the small intestine.

❖ Emphasize the importance of CDA recommendations for patients with diabetes, including 150 minutes of moderate- to vigorous-intensity aerobic exercise each week, spread over at least 3 days of the week, with no more than 2 consecutive days without exercise. Resistance exercise should be included at least two times per week.

❖ Emphasize that therapy will be lifelong and that strict management of plasma glucose control, drug therapy, and lifestyle changes are critical to preventing and reducing the complications of diabetes.

❖ Stress the importance of strict foot care to patients and others involved in their care. Begin with discussing the need for a daily basic assessment of feet and toes to check for sores, lesions, cuts, bruises, ingrown toenails, and any other changes. Foot care is needed to enhance circulation and prevent infections. It may include soaking the feet daily or as ordered in lukewarm water (the temperature of the water must be checked), followed by adequate drying of the feet and application of moisturizing lotion. The feet and legs should be checked for abnormal changes in colour (e.g., purplish or reddish discoloration), swelling, the appearance of any drainage, or cool temperature of the feet to the touch. Emphasize the importance of contacting the health care provider for further instructions if there is suspicion of any type of wound or alteration in skin integrity. Frequent pedicures and nail trimming by a podiatrist or other licensed, certified individual may be indicated.

❖ Some of the oral antihyperglycemic drugs cause photosensitivity, so instruct patients to wear protective sunblock and appropriate clothing when exposed to the sun. Advise against the use of tanning beds.

KEY POINTS

❖ Insulin normally facilitates removal of glucose from the plasma and its storage as glycogen in the liver.

❖ Little or no endogenous insulin is produced by individuals with type 1 diabetes. It is much less common than type 2 diabetes and affects only about 10% of patients with diabetes. Patients with type 1 diabetes usually are not obese. Because insulin therapy is required for patients with type 1 diabetes, those who have the cognitive and financial ability should be encouraged to consider incorporating an insulin pump with continuous glucose monitoring as part of their

therapy. The CDA is advocating for public funding for insulin pumps because the use of insulin pump technology leads to improved health outcomes for people living with diabetes.

❖ The primary treatment for individuals with type 1 diabetes is insulin therapy. Patients with type 2 diabetes are initially managed with lifestyle changes (dietary changes, exercise, smoking cessation). If normal blood glucose levels are not achieved after 2 to 3 months of lifestyle changes, treatment with one or more oral antihyperglycemic drugs is often added to the regimen.

Continued

KEY POINTS—cont'd

❖ Insulin was originally isolated from cattle and pigs, but bovine and porcine insulins are associated with a higher incidence of allergic reactions and insulin resistance than human insulin. Porcine insulin is still available in Canada.

❖ Complications associated with diabetes include retinopathy, neuropathy, nephropathy, hypertension, cardiovascular disease, and coronary artery disease. Annual screening by an ophthalmologist specializing in retinopathies is needed in the care of patients with diabetes. Because of kidney complications (i.e., nephropathies), annual urinalysis screening and kidney function studies are also recommended for patients with diabetes.

❖ All rapid-acting, short-acting, and long-acting insulin preparations are clear solutions. Intermediate-acting

insulins are cloudy solutions. Mixtures of short- and intermediate-acting insulin still look uniformly cloudy. The cloudy appearance of these mixtures is due to the presence of the intermediate-acting insulin. When used, insulin vials are to be rolled in the hands instead of shaken.

❖ Always carefully check the exact timing of the dose of insulin or oral antihyperglycemic drug against the health care provider's order. Take into consideration the drug's pharmacokinetics, including onset of action, peak, and duration of action.

❖ Nursing care must be individualized, with patient education focused on the patient's needs and learning abilities. Include pertinent and age-appropriate information on the disease process, drug therapy, and lifestyle modifications.

EXAMINATION REVIEW QUESTIONS

1. Which is the most appropriate timing for the nurse's administration of a rapid-acting insulin to a hospitalized patient?
   a. Give it 15 minutes before the patient begins a meal.
   b. Give it ½ hour before a meal.
   c. Give it 1 hour after a meal.
   d. The timing of the insulin injection does not matter with a rapid-acting insulin.

2. Which statement is appropriate for the nurse to include in patient teaching regarding type 2 diabetes?
   a. "Insulin injections are never used with type 2 diabetes."
   b. "You don't need to measure your blood glucose levels because you are not taking insulin injections."
   c. "A person with type 2 diabetes still has functioning β-cells in the pancreas."
   d. "Patients with type 2 diabetes usually have better control over their diabetes than those with type 1 diabetes."

3. The nurse monitoring a patient for a therapeutic response to oral antihyperglycemic drugs will look for:
   a. fewer episodes of diabetic ketoacidosis (DKA)
   b. weight loss of 2.3 kg
   c. hemoglobin A_{1C} levels of less than 7%
   d. glucose levels of 9.5 mmol/L

4. A patient with type 2 diabetes is scheduled for magnetic resonance imaging (MRI) with contrast dye. The nurse reviews the orders and notices that the patient is receiving metformin (Glucophage). Which action by the nurse is appropriate?
   a. Proceed with the MRI as scheduled.
   b. Notify the radiology department that the patient is receiving metformin.
   c. Expect to hold the metformin the day of the test and for 48 hours after the test is performed.
   d. Call the health care provider regarding holding the metformin for 2 days before the MRI is performed.

5. A patient with type 2 diabetes has a new prescription for repaglinide (GlucoNorm). After 1 week, she calls the office to ask what to do because she keeps missing meals. "I work right through lunch sometimes, and I'm not sure whether I need to take it. What do I need to do?" What is the nurse's best response?
   a. "You need to try not to skip meals, but if that happens, you will need to skip that dose of repaglinide."
   b. "We will probably need to change your prescription to insulin injections because you can't eat meals on a regular basis."
   c. "Go ahead and take the pill when you first remember that you missed it."
   d. "Take both pills with the next meal, and try to eat a little extra to make up for what you missed at lunchtime."

6. When checking a patient's blood glucose level, the nurse obtains a reading of 2.3 mmol/L. The patient is awake but states he feels a bit "cloudy-headed." After double-checking the patient's glucose level and getting the same reading, which action by the nurse is most appropriate?
   a. Administer two packets of table sugar.
   b. Administer oral glucose in the form of a semisolid gel.
   c. Administer 50% dextrose IV push.
   d. Administer the morning dose of insulin lispro.

7. A patient is taking metformin for new-onset type 2 diabetes. When reviewing potential adverse effects, the nurse will include information about which of the following? (Select all that apply.)
   a. Abdominal bloating
   b. Nausea
   c. Diarrhea
   d. Headache
   e. Weight gain
   f. Metallic taste

Answers: 1. a, 2. c, 3. c, 4. c, 5. a, 6. b, 7. a, b, c, f

CRITICAL THINKING ACTIVITIES

1. A 25-year-old woman has been diagnosed with type 1 diabetes. She has been placed on a 1500-calorie diabetic diet and is to be started on insulin glargine. Today she received teaching about her diet, insulin injections, and management of diabetes. She received the first dose of insulin glargine at 9 PM; the next morning she reported feeling "dizzy." The nurse assesses that she is diaphoretic, weak, and pale, with a heart rate of 110 beats per minute. What is the nurse's priority action? What is the best explanation for these symptoms?

2. While making morning rounds, the nurse assesses a patient's ordered medications and finds that the patient is to be given NPH insulin each morning but is also on orders to receive nothing by mouth because of a scheduled surgical procedure. What is the nurse's priority action at this time regarding the administration of the insulin?

3. A patient with type 2 diabetes comes to the emergency department with an acute asthma attack and pneumonia. Her condition is stabilized, and she is admitted to the hospital to receive IV doses of antibiotics and corticosteroids. She says that, before this episode, she took oral drugs for diabetes and had her diabetes "under control," with fasting plasma glucose levels ranging from 5.6 to 5.9 mmol/L on most mornings. However, the next morning, her fasting plasma glucose level is 9.9 mmol/L, and her glucose levels remain elevated for the next few days. The patient is upset and declares, "I'm hardly eating anything extra. Why is my blood sugar so high?" What is the nurse's best answer to the patient's concerns?

For answers, see http://evolve.elsevier.com/Canada/Lilley/pharmacology/.

Adrenal Drugs

Objectives

After reading this chapter, the successful student will be able to do the following:

1. Discuss the normal anatomy, physiology, and related functions of the adrenal glands, including specific hormones released from the glands.

2. Briefly compare the hormones secreted by the adrenal medulla with those secreted by the adrenal cortex.

3. Contrast Cushing's syndrome, Addison's disease, and acute adrenal crisis (addisonian crisis).

4. Compare the glucocorticoids and mineralocorticoids in regard to the roles they perform in normal bodily functions, the diseases that alter them, how they are used in pharmacotherapy, and their basic properties.

5. Contrast the mechanisms of action, indications, dosages, routes of administration, cautions, contraindications, drug interactions, and adverse effects of glucocorticoids and mineralocorticoids.

6. Develop a collaborative plan of care that includes all phases of the nursing process for patients taking adrenal drugs.

e-Learning Activities

Website
(http://evolve.elsevier.com/Canada/
Lilley/pharmacology/)

evolve

- Answer Key—Textbook Case Studies
- Answer Key—Critical Thinking Activities
- Chapter Summaries—Printable
- Review Questions for Exam Preparation
- Unfolding Case Studies

Drug Profiles

▸▸ fludrocortisone 21-acetate, p. 656
    methylprednisolone, p. 656
▸▸ prednisone, p. 656

▸▸ Key drug

Key Terms

Addison's disease A potentially life-threatening condition caused by partial or complete failure of adrenocortical function, with resulting decrease in glucocorticoid, mineralocorticoid, and androgenic hormones; a chronic disease of hyposecretion of steroids. (p. 652)

Adrenal cortex The outer portion of the adrenal gland. (p. 651)

Adrenal crisis An acute, life-threatening state of profound adrenocortical insufficiency requiring immediate medical management; characterized by glucocorticoid deficiency, a drop in extracellular fluid volume, hyponatremia, and hyperkalemia. (p. 658)

Adrenal medulla The inner portion of the adrenal gland. (p. 651)

Aldosterone A mineralocorticoid hormone produced by the adrenal cortex that acts on the kidney tubules to regulate sodium and potassium balance in the blood. (p. 651)

Cortex The outer layers of a body organ or structure. (p. 651)

Corticosteroids Any of the natural or synthetic adrenocortical hormones, including those produced by the cortex of the adrenal gland (adrenocorticosteroids). (p. 651)

Cushing's syndrome A metabolic disorder characterized by abnormally increased secretion of the adrenocorticosteroids. (p. 652)

Epinephrine An endogenous hormone secreted into the bloodstream by the adrenal medulla; also a synthetic drug that is an adrenergic vasoconstrictor and also increases cardiac output. (p. 651)

Glucocorticoids A major group of corticosteroid hormones that regulate carbohydrate, protein, and lipid metabolism and inhibit the release of adrenocorticotropic hormone (corticotropin). (p. 651)

Hypothalamic–pituitary–adrenal (HPA) axis A negative feedback system involved in regulating the release of corticotropin-releasing hormone by the hypothalamus, adrenocorticotropic hormone (corticotropin) by the pituitary gland, and corticosteroids by the adrenal glands. Suppression of the HPA may lead to Addison's disease and possible adrenal crisis or addisonian crisis; this suppression results from chronic disease or exogenous sources, such as long-term glucocorticoid therapy. (p. 652)

Medulla The most interior portions of an organ or structure. (p. 651)

Mineralocorticoids A major group of corticosteroid hormones that regulate electrolyte and water balance; in humans, the primary mineralocorticoid is aldosterone. (p. 651)

Norepinephrine An adrenergic hormone, also secreted by the adrenal medulla, that increases blood pressure by causing vasoconstriction but does not appreciably affect cardiac output; the immediate metabolic precursor to epinephrine. (p. 651)

ADRENAL SYSTEM

The adrenal gland is an endocrine organ that sits on top of the kidneys like a cap. It is composed of two distinct parts called the *adrenal cortex* and the *adrenal medulla;* they are structurally and functionally different from one another. In general, the term *cortex* refers to the outer layers of various organs (e.g., cerebral cortex), while the term *medulla* refers to the most internal layers. The adrenal cortex comprises approximately 80 to 90% of the entire adrenal gland; the remainder is the medulla. The adrenal cortex is made up of regular endocrine tissue (hormone driven). The adrenal medulla is made up of neurosecretory endocrine tissue (driven by both hormones and peripheral autonomic nerve impulses). Therefore, the adrenal gland actually functions as two different endocrine glands, each secreting different hormones.

The adrenal medulla secretes two important hormones, both of which are catecholamines. These are **epinephrine,** which accounts for about 80% of the secretion, and **norepinephrine,** which accounts for the other 20%. (Both these hormones are discussed in Chapter 19 and are not described in any detail in this chapter.) Characteristics of the adrenal gland and the various hormones secreted by each type of tissue are presented in Table 34-1.

The hormones secreted by the adrenal cortex, which are the focus of this chapter, are broadly referred to as **corticosteroids.** They arise from the cortex and are made from the steroid known as *cholesterol.* There are two types of corticosteroids: **glucocorticoids** and **mineralocorticoids.** They are secreted by two different layers, or zones, of the cortex. The *zona glomerulosa,* the outer layer, secretes the mineralocorticoids, and the *zona fasciculata,* which lies under the zona glomerulosa, secretes the glucocorticoids. A third, inner layer, the *zona reticularis,* secretes small amounts of sex hormones. All the hormones secreted by the adrenal cortex are steroid hormones—that is, they have the steroid chemical structure.

The mineralocorticoids get their name from their important role in regulating mineral salts (electrolytes) in the body. In humans, the main physiologically important mineralocorticoid is **aldosterone.** Its primary role is to maintain normal levels of sodium in the blood (sodium homeostasis) by causing sodium to be resorbed from the urine back into the blood in exchange for potassium and hydrogen ions. In this way, aldosterone not only regulates blood sodium levels, but also influences potassium and pH levels of the blood.

The glucocorticoids have a broad range of effects and are necessary for many vital bodily functions. They are efficacious anti-inflammatory drugs as they suppress every component of the inflammatory process, play significant roles in carbohydrate, protein, and lipid metabolism, the immune response, and the response to stress. Natural glucocorticoids also have some mineralocorticoid activity and as a result affect fluid and electrolyte balance. Some of the more important functions are listed in Box 34-1. Without these hormones, life-threatening consequences may arise.

Adrenal corticosteroids are synthesized as needed; the body does not store them as it does other hormones.

TABLE	34-1

Adrenal Gland: Characteristics

Type of Tissue	Type of Hormone Secreted	Hormones Secreted and Related Drugs
ADRENAL CORTEX		
Endocrine	Glucocorticoids	Adrenocorticotropic hormone (ACTH), betamethasone valerate, cortisone acetate, dexamethasone, hydrocortisone acetate, triamcinolone acetonide
	Mineralocorticoids	Aldosterone
ADRENAL MEDULLA		
Neuroendocrine	Catecholamines	Epinephrine, norepinephrine

BOX 34-1

Adrenal Cortex Hormones: Biological Functions

Glucocorticoids

Anti-inflammatory actions
Carbohydrate and protein metabolism
Fat metabolism
Maintenance of normal blood pressure
Stress effects

Mineralocorticoids

Blood pressure control
Maintenance of serum potassium levels
Maintenance of pH levels in blood
Sodium and water resorption

Hypothalamic–Pituitary–Adrenal (HPA) Axis

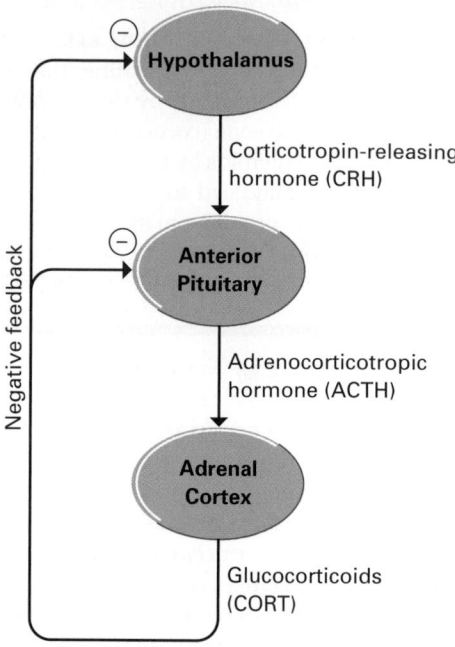

FIG. 34-2 Negative feedback control mechanism of adrenocortical hormones.

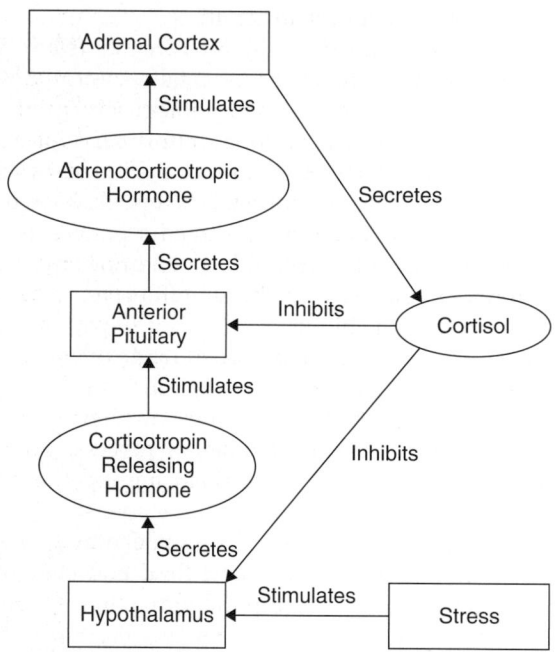

FIG. 34-1 Hypothalamic–pituitary–adrenal axis. (From Tucci , V., & Sokari, T. (2014). The clinical manifestations, diagnosis, and management of adrenal emergencies. *Emergency Medical Clinics of North America, 32*(2), 465–484. doi:10.1016/j.emc.2014.01.006.)

The body levels of these hormones are regulated by the **hypothalamic–pituitary–adrenal (HPA) axis** in much the same way that the levels of hormones secreted by the pituitary, thyroid, and pancreas are regulated. As the name implies, this axis consists of a highly organized system of communication between the adrenal gland, the pituitary gland, and the hypothalamus (see Figure 34-1). As is the case for the other endocrine glands, it uses hormones as the messengers and a negative feedback mechanism as the controller and sustainer of the process. This feedback mechanism operates as follows: When the

level of a particular corticosteroid is low, corticotropin-releasing hormone is released from the hypothalamus into the bloodstream and travels to the anterior pituitary gland, where it triggers the release of adrenocorticotropic hormone (ACTH; also called corticotropin). The ACTH is then transported in the blood to the adrenal cortex, where it stimulates the production of the corticosteroids. Corticosteroids are then released into the bloodstream. When they reach peak levels, a signal (negative feedback) is sent to the hypothalamus, and the HPA axis is inhibited until the level of corticosteroids again falls below the physiological threshold, whereupon the axis is stimulated once again (see Figure 34-2).

The oversecretion (hypersecretion) of adrenocortical hormones can lead to a group of signs and symptoms called **Cushing's syndrome**. This hypersecretion of glucocorticoids results in the redistribution of body fat from the arms and legs to the face, shoulders, trunk, and abdomen, which leads to the characteristic "moon face" (moon facies). Such a glucocorticoid excess can be due to several causes, including ACTH-dependent adrenocortical hyperplasia or tumour, ectopic ACTH-secreting tumour, or excessive administration of steroids. The hypersecretion of aldosterone, or primary aldosteronism, leads to increased retention of water and sodium, which causes muscle weakness due to the potassium loss.

The undersecretion (hyposecretion) of adrenocortical hormones causes a condition called **Addison's disease**. Patients with this disease often have vague, chronic, and nonspecific complaints. It is associated with abnormal laboratory values (e.g., hyponatremia, hyperkalemia, hypercalcemia, mild hypoglycemia, azotemia, anemia).

Clinical signs and symptoms include dehydration, hyperpigmentation, weakness and fatigue, nausea, vomiting, anorexia, and weight loss. The combination of a mineralocorticoid (fludrocortisone 21-acetate) and a glucocorticoid (prednisone or some other suitable drug) is used for treatment.

ADRENAL DRUGS

Most corticosteroids (naturally occurring or synthetic) have both glucocorticoid and mineralocorticoid properties. All of the naturally occurring corticosteroids are available as exogenous drugs. There are also higher-potency synthetic analogues. The adrenal glucocorticoids are an extremely large group of steroids and can be categorized in various ways. They can be classified by whether they are a natural or synthetic cortiosteroid, by their method of administration (e.g., systemic, topical), by their salt and water retention potential (mineralocorticoid activity), by their duration of action (i.e., short, intermediate, or long acting), or by some combination of these methods. The only corticosteroid drug with exclusive mineralocorticoid activity is fludrocortisone 21-acetate. Its uses are much more specific than those of the glucocortocoids and are discussed in the drug profile for fludrocortisone 21-acetate. The currently available synthetic adrenal hormones and adrenal steroid inhibitors are listed in Table 34-2.

Mechanism of Action and Drug Effects

The action of the corticosteroids is related to their involvement in the synthesis of specific proteins. There are several steps to this process. Initially, the steroid hormone binds to a receptor on the surface of a target cell to form a steroid–receptor complex, which is then transported through the cytoplasm to the nucleus of that target cell.

Once inside the nucleus, the complex stimulates the cell's deoxyribonucleic acid (DNA) to produce messenger ribonucleic acid (mRNA), which is then used as a template for the synthesis of a specific protein. It is these proteins that exert specific effects.

Most of the corticosteroids exert their effects by modifying enzyme activity; therefore, their role is more intermediary than direct. The naturally occurring mineralocorticoid aldosterone affects electrolyte and fluid balance by acting on the distal kidney tubules. It promotes sodium resorption from the nephrons into the blood, which pulls water and fluid along with it. In doing so, it causes fluid and water retention, which leads to edema and hypertension. It also increases urinary excretion of potassium and hydrogen via the kidney.

The glucocorticoid drug hydrocortisone (called cortisol in its naturally occurring form) has some mineralocorticoid activity and, therefore, has some of the same effects as aldosterone (i.e., fluid and water retention). However, its main effect is inhibition of inflammatory and immune responses. Glucocorticoids inhibit or help control the inflammatory response by stabilizing the cell membranes of inflammatory cells called *lysosomes*, decreasing the permeability of capillaries to the inflammatory cells and decreasing the migration of white blood cells into already inflamed areas. They may lower fever by reducing the release of interleukin-1 from white blood cells. They also stimulate the erythroid cells that eventually become red blood cells. The glucocorticoids also promote the breakdown (catabolism) of protein, the production of glycogen in the liver (glycogenesis), and the redistribution of fat from the peripheral to the central areas of the body. In addition, they have the following effects on various bodily functions: increasing levels of blood sugar, increasing the breakdown of proteins to amino acids, inducing lipolysis, stimulating bone

TABLE 34-2		
Available Synthetic Corticosteroids		
Type of Hormone	**Method of Administration**	**Individual Drugs**
Adrenal steroid inhibitor	Systemic	ketoconazole
Glucocorticoid	Topical	amcinonide, betamethasone dipropionate, betamethasone valerate, clobetasol propionate, desoximetasone, dexamethasone, diflucortolone valerate, fluocinolone acetonide, hydrocortisone acetate, mometasone furoate, prednicarbate, prednisolone acetate, triamcinolone acetonide
	Systemic	betamethasone, dexamethasone sodium phosphate, hydrocortisone sodium succinate, methylprednisolone sodium succinate, prednisolone sodium phosphate, prednisone, triamcinolone acetonide
	Inhaled	beclomethasone dipropionate, budesonide, fluticasone propionate, mometasone furoate
	Nasal	beclomethasone dipropionate, budesonide, flunisolide, fluticasone propionate, mometasone, triamcinolone acetonide
Mineralocorticoid	Systemic	fludrocortisone 21-acetate

demineralization, and stabilizing mast cells. The mechanism of bone demineralization is multifactorial but includes reduced calcium adsorption in skeletal cells, resulting in secondary hyperparathyroidism.

Indications

All of the systemically administered glucocorticoids have a similar clinical efficacy but differ in their potency, mineralocorticoid and glucocorticoid potency, and duration of action and in the extent to which they cause salt and fluid retention (see Table 34-3). Glucocorticoids have broad indications, including the following:

- Adrenocortical deficiency
- Adrenogenital syndrome
- Allergic disorders (e.g., anaphylaxis)
- Autoimmune blistering diseases
- Bacterial meningitis, particularly in infants
- Cancer
- Cerebral edema
- Collagen diseases (e.g., systemic lupus erythematosus)
- Chronic rhinosinusitis
- Dermatological diseases (e.g., exfoliative dermatitis, pemphigus, severe psoriasis)
- Endocrine disorders (e.g., thyroiditis)
- Gastrointestinal (GI) diseases (e.g., ulcerative colitis, regional enteritis)
- Exacerbations of chronic respiratory illnesses (e.g., asthma, chronic obstructive pulmonary disease)
- Hematological disorders (e.g., autoimmune hemolytic anemia, idiopathic thrombocytopenia; reduce bleeding tendencies)
- Nonrheumatic inflammation (e.g., acute or subacute bursitis, acute tendosynovitis)
- Ophthalmic disorders (decrease nonpyogenic inflammation)
- Organ transplant (decrease immune response to prevent organ rejection)
- Leukemias and lymphomas (palliative management)
- Nephrotic syndrome (remission of proteinuria)
- Rheumatic disorders (e.g., rheumatoid arthritis, psoriatic arthritis, acute gouty arthritis; adjunctive therapy in ankylosing spondylitis)

- Spinal cord injury
- Thyroiditis (e.g., nonsuppurative thyroiditis)

Glucocorticoids are also administered by inhalation for the control of steroid-responsive bronchospastic states. However, glucocorticoid inhalers are not used as rescue inhalers for acute bronchospasm but are for control. Nasally administered glucocorticoids are used to manage allergic rhinitis and to prevent the recurrence of polyps after surgical removal (see Chapter 37). Topical steroids are used in the management of inflammation of the eye, ear, and skin. Methylprednisolone sodium succinate is the most commonly used injectable glucocorticoid, followed by hydrocortisone sodium succinate and dexamethasone sodium succinate. Betamethasone or dexamethasone are the drugs of choice for women in premature labour (before 34 weeks gestation) to accelerate fetal lung maturation (Romejko-Wolniewicz, Teliga-Czajkowska, & Czajkowski, 2014). They promote the maturation of many vital fetal organs through the action of cortisol that binds to the glucocorticoid receptors of target cells, and therefore, help to decrease the incidence of respiratory distress syndrome and neonatal mortality associated with premature birth. They also increase the effectiveness of surfactant therapy (Msan, Usta, Mirza, et al., 2015).

Contraindications

Contraindications to the administration of glucocorticoids include drug allergy and may include cataracts, glaucoma, peptic ulcer disease, mental health concerns, and diabetes mellitus. The adrenal drugs may intensify these conditions. For example, one common adverse effect of these drugs seen in hospitalized patients is an increase in blood glucose levels, often requiring insulin. This is not to say that patients with diabetes who require glucocorticoids should not receive them, but it is important to be aware of the potential for increase in blood glucose levels. Because of their immunosuppressant properties, glucocorticoids are often avoided in the presence of any serious infection systemic fungal infections, and varicella. Exceptions to this rule are septic shock when low-dose hydrocortisone is added to the treatment

---

TABLE 34-3

Systemic Glucocorticoids: A Comparison

Drug	Origin	Duration of Action	Equivalent Dose (mg)*	Salt and Water Retention Potential
betamethasone	Synthetic	Long	0.75	Minimal
dexamethasone sodium succinate	Synthetic	Long	0.75	Minimal
hydrocortisone sodium succinate	Natural	Short	20	High
methylprednisolone sodium succinate	Synthetic	Intermediate	4	Low
prednisolone sodium phosphate	Synthetic	Intermediate	5	Low
prednisone	Synthetic	Intermediate	5	Low
triamcinolone acetonide	Synthetic	Intermediate	4	Minimal

*Drugs with higher potency require smaller milligram doses than those with lower potency. This column illustrates the approximate dose equivalency between different drugs that is expected to achieve a comparable therapeutic effect.

regimen for patients with septic shock that is unresponsive to IV fluids and vasopressor therapy and in tuberculous meningitis, for which glucocorticoids may be used to prevent inflammatory central nervous system damage. Caution is emphasized in treating any patient with gastritis, reflux disease, or ulcer disease because of the potential of these drugs to cause gastric perforation, as well as those with heart, kidney, or liver dysfunction because of associated alterations in elimination.

Adverse Effects

The potent metabolic, physiological, and pharmacological effects of corticosteroids can influence every body system, so these drugs can produce a wide variety of significant undesirable effects. The more common of these are summarized in Table 34-4. Moon facies is a common adverse effect of long-term use. Two of the adverse effects most commonly seen in hospitalized patients are hyperglycemia and psychosis. The most serious adverse effect of glucocorticoids is adrenal (HPA) suppression, which is discussed in the drug profiles. Due to their ability to cause fluid retention, glucocorticoids should be used with caution in patients with heart failure.

Interactions

Systemically administered corticosteroids can interact with many drugs:

- Their use with non–potassium-sparing diuretics (e.g., thiazides, loop diuretics) can lead to severe hypocalcemia and hypokalemia.
- Their use with aspirin, other nonsteroidal antiinflammatory drugs (NSAIDs), and other ulcerogenic drugs produces additive GI effects and an increased chance of gastric ulcer development.

- Their use with anticholinesterase drugs produces weakness in patients with myasthenia gravis.
- Their use with immunizing biologics inhibits the immune response to the biological agent.
- Their use with antidiabetic drugs may reduce the hypoglycemic effects of the latter and result in elevated blood glucose levels.

Many other drugs can interact with glucocorticoids, including thyroid hormones and antifungal drugs (such as fluconazole), which can decrease kidney clearance of the adrenal drug. Barbiturates and hydantoins can increase the metabolism of prednisone and similar drugs. Oral anticoagulants interact with adrenal drugs in ways that can affect the international normalized ratio. Oral contraceptives can increase the half-life of adrenal drugs. Various other drug interactions may be possible between adrenal drugs and over-the-counter (OTC) drugs and natural health products.

Dosages

For dosage information on adrenal drugs, refer to the table on p. 657.

NURSING PROCESS

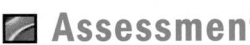 Assessment

Before administering any of the adrenal drugs, perform a thorough physical assessment to determine the patient's baseline nutritional, hydration, and immune status; baseline weight; intake and output; vital signs (especially

---

TABLE 34-4

Corticosteroids: Common Adverse Effects

Body System	Adverse Effects
Cardiovascular	Heart failure, edema, hypertension, all due to electrolyte imbalances (e.g., hyperkalemia, hypernatremia), impaired glucose intolerance, dysrhythmias, bradycardia, pulmonary edema, syncope, vasculitis
Central nervous	Convulsions; headache; vertigo; mental health status changes such as mood swings, nervousness, aggressive behaviours, or psychotic symptoms; neuritis peripheral neuropathy; paresthesia; arachnoiditis; meningitis; insomnia
Endocrine	Growth suppression, Cushing's syndrome, menstrual irregularities, carbohydrate intolerance, hyperglycemia, hypothalamic pituitary–adrenal axis suppression (particularly at times of stress as in trauma, surgery, or illness), hirsutism, hypertrichosis (abnormal growth of hair on the body), glycosuria
Gastrointestinal	Peptic ulcers with possible perforation, pancreatitis, ulcerative esophagitis, abdominal distension
Integumentary	Fragile skin, petechiae, ecchymosis, facial erythema, poor wound healing, urticaria, hypersensitivity reactions, acne, dry skin, skin hyperpigmentation, skin striae
Musculoskeletal	Myopathy, muscle weakness, loss of muscle mass, osteoporosis, osteonecrosis of femoral and humeral heads, pathological fracture, malaise
Reproductive	Irregular menstruation, sperm motility abnormalities, abnormal sperm concentration
Ocular	Increased intraocular pressure, glaucoma, cataracts
Other	Weight gain, leukocytosis, opportunistic infections, hypokalemia alkalosis, impaired healing

DRUG PROFILES

Corticosteroids

The systemic corticosteroids consist of seven chemically different but pharmacologically similar hormones. They all exert varying degrees of glucocorticoid and mineralocorticoid effects. Their differences are due to slight variations in their chemical structures.

Corticosteroids can cross the placenta and produce fetal abnormalities. For this reason, they are not recommended for use during pregnancy unless the potential benefits outweigh the risk. They can also be secreted in breast milk and cause abnormalities in the nursing infant. Their use is contraindicated in patients who have exhibited hypersensitivity reactions to them in the past, as well as in patients with fungal or bacterial infections. Short- or long-term use can lead to a condition known as *steroid psychosis*. One important point to know about long-term use of steroids is that they must not be stopped abruptly. These drugs require a tapering of the daily dose because their administration causes the endogenous (body's own) production of the hormones to stop. This is referred to as *HPA* or *adrenal suppression*. This suppression can cause impaired stress response and place the patient at risk of developing hypoadrenal crisis (shock, circulatory collapse) in times of increased stress (e.g., surgery, trauma). Adrenal suppression can occur as early as 1 week after a corticosteroid is started. HPA suppression typically does not occur in patients taking prednisone 5 mg/day (or equivalent) or less. Tapering of daily doses allows the HPA axis the time to recover and start stimulating the normal production of the endogenous hormones. Patients on long-term steroid therapy who are taking at least 10 mg/day (or equivalent) of prednisone and who undergo trauma or require surgery need additional doses of steroids (also known as *stress doses*).

It is important to differentiate between corticosteroids and anabolic steroids. Anabolic steroids are hormones, available for oral intake or by injection. These drugs are used for performance-enhancing purposes and to enhance muscle growth. Anabolic steroids act much like testosterone in the body. They increase muscle mass and masculine characteristics.

▸▸ fludrocortisone 21-acetate

Fludrocortisone 21-acetate (Florinef®) is the only available mineralocorticoid. It is used as partial replacement therapy for adrenocortical insufficiency in Addison's disease and in the treatment of salt-losing adrenogenital syndrome. It is contraindicated in cases of systemic fungal infection. Adverse effects generally pertain to water retention and include heart failure, hypertension, and elevated intracranial pressure (potentially leading to seizures). Other possible adverse effects involve several body systems and include skin rash, menstrual irregularities, peptic ulcer, hyperglycemia, hypokalemia, muscle pain and weakness, compression bone fractures, glaucoma, and thrombophlebitis, among others. Drugs with which fludrocortisone 21-acetate interacts include anabolic steroids (increased edema); barbiturates, hydantoins, and rifamycins (increased fludrocortisone 21-acetate clearance); estrogens (reduced fludrocortisone 21-acetate clearance); amphotericin B and thiazide and loop diuretics (hypokalemia); anticoagulants (enhanced or reduced anticoagulant activity);

antidiabetic drugs (reduced activity leading to hyperglycemia); digoxin (increased risk for dysrhythmias due to hypokalemia induced by fludrocortisone 21-acetate); salicylates (reduced efficacy); and vaccines (increased risk of neurological complications). Fortunately, adverse effects and serious drug interactions secondary to fludrocortisone 21-acetate therapy are uncommon because of the relatively small doses of the drug that are normally prescribed; fludrocortisone 21-acetate is preferably administered in conjunction with 10- to 20-mg daily doses of hydrocortisone sodium succcinate (10 to 20 mg daily in divided doses). Fludrocortisone 21-acetate is available only in oral form as a 0.1-mg tablet. Recommended dosages are given in the table on p. 657.

PHARMACOKINETICS

Route	Onset of Action	Peak Plasma Concentration	Elimination Half-Life	Duration of Action
PO	10–20 min	1.7 hr	18–36 hr	Unknown

▸▸ prednisone

Prednisone is one of the four intermediate-acting glucocorticoids; the others are methylprednisolone sodium succinate, prednisolone sodium phosphate, and triamcinolone acetonide. These drugs have half-lives that are more than double those of the short-acting corticosteroids (2 to 5 hours), and therefore they have longer durations of action. Prednisone is the preferred oral glucocorticoid for anti-inflammatory or immunosuppressant purposes. Along with methylprednisolone sodium succinate and prednisolone sodium phosphate, it is also used for exacerbations of chronic respiratory illnesses such as asthma and chronic bronchitis. Prednisone has minimal mineralocorticoid properties and therefore alone is inadequate for the management of adrenocortical insufficiency (Addison's disease). Prednisolone acetate, a prednisone metabolite, is the liquid drug form of prednisone. Prednisone is available in oral tablets. For recommended dosages, refer to the table on p. 657.

PHARMACOKINETICS

Route	Onset of Action	Peak Plasma Concentration	Elimination Half-Life	Duration of Action
PO	Unknown	1–2 hr	2–3 hr	8–36 hr

methylprednisolone sodium succinate

Methylprednisolone sodium succinate (Solu-Medrol®) is the most commonly used injectable glucocorticoid drug. It is used primarily as an anti-inflammatory or immunosuppressant drug (see Preventing Medication Errors box).

It is usually given intravenously. Like prednisone, it is not recommended for use during pregnancy. Most injectable formulations contain a preservative (benzyl alcohol) that cannot be given to children younger than 28 days of age.

PHARMACOKINETICS

Route	Onset of Action	Peak Plasma Concentration	Elimination Half-Life	Duration of Action
IV	Immediate	30 min	3–4 hr	24–36 hr

DOSAGES   Selected Antiadrenal and Corticosteroid Drugs

Drug	Pharmacological Class	Usual Dosage Range	Indications
▸▸fludrocortisone 21-acetate (Florinef)	Synthetic mineralocorticoid	*Children (including infants) and adults* PO: 0.1–0.2 mg daily	Addison's disease; salt-losing adrenogenital syndrome
methylprednisolone sodium succinate (Solu-Medrol)	Systemic corticosteroid	*Adults* IV: 10–500 mg depending on problem being treated	Wide variety of endocrine disorders (including adrenocortical insufficiency) and rheumatic, collagen, dermatologic, allergic, ophthalmic, respiratory, hematologic, neoplastic, gastrointestinal, and nervous system disorders; edematous states
▸▸prednisone (Winpred®)	Synthetic intermediate-acting glucocorticoid	*Children* PO: 0.05–2 mg/kg/ day divided daily qid *Adults* PO: 5–60 mg/day	Wide variety of endocrine (including adrenocortical insufficiency) and rheumatic, collagen, dermatological, allergic, ocular, respiratory, hematological, neoplastic, gastrointestinal, and nervous system disorders; edematous states

IV, intravenous; *PO*, oral.

PREVENTING MEDICATION ERRORS

Look-Alike Sound-Alike Drugs: Solu-Cortef® and Solu-Medrol®

Be careful about look-alike, sound-alike drugs. Medication errors often occur when drug names are similar.

Solu-Cortef is a trade name for hydrocortisone sodium succinate; Solu-Medrol is a trade name for methylprednisolone sodium succinate. Both are commonly used glucocorticoids and are given intravenously. However, 4 mg of Solu-Medrol is equivalent to 20 mg of Solu-Cortef; therefore, Solu-Medrol is five times stronger than Solu-Cortef. Despite their similar names, these drugs are not interchangeable!

blood pressure ranges); and skin condition, (noting bruising, fragility, turgor, and colour). Assess important baseline laboratory values including serum sodium, serum potassium, and serum glucose. These specific laboratory tests are important because of potential drug-related adverse effects (see Table 34-4). For instance, serum potassium levels usually decrease and blood glucose levels increase when a glucocorticoid (e.g., prednisone) is given. In addition, assess and document the patient's muscle strength and body stature. In the assessment, include the identification of potential contraindications, cautions, and drug interactions, including interactions with prescription drugs, OTC drugs, and natural health products.

For adrenal drugs, lifespan considerations include concern about their use during pregnancy and lactation. Growth suppression may occur in children receiving long-term adrenal drug therapy (e.g., glucocorticoids) if the epiphyseal plates of the long bones have not closed. However, there may be situations in which the benefits to the therapy outweigh the risks of the drug's adverse effects. Perform and document baseline height and weight measurements in children. Older adults are more prone to adrenal suppression with prolonged adrenal therapy and may require dosage alterations by the health care provider to minimize the impact of the drug on muscle mass, blood pressure, and serum glucose and electrolyte levels. Adrenal drugs may exacerbate muscle weakness; produce fatigue; worsen or precipitate osteoporosis, peptic ulcer disease, glaucoma, and cataracts; and increase intraocular pressure. Additionally, because the adrenal drugs are associated with the adverse effect of sodium retention, closely assess patients for exacerbation of any pre-existing edema or cardiac disease.

Nursing Diagnoses

- Disturbed body image related to the physiological effects of diseases of the adrenal gland on the body or the cushingoid appearance caused by glucoscorticoid therapy (e.g., prednisone)
- Excess fluid volume related to fluid retention associated with glucocorticoid and mineralocorticoid use
- Risk for infection related to the anti-inflammatory, immunosuppressive, metabolic, and dermatological effects of long-term glucocorticoid therapy
- Impaired skin integrity related to the adverse effects of glucocorticoids

Planning

Goals

- Patient will experience minimal body image disturbances.

- Patient will exhibit normal fluid volume status during treatment with glucocorticoid or mineralocorticoid therapy.
- Patient will remain free from infection during adrenal drug therapy.

■ Expected Patient Outcomes

- Patient openly verbalizes fears about body image disturbances and other changes to health care providers, family members, and significant others.
- Patient experiences minimal problems with fluid volume excess and experiences minimal to no edema.
  - Patient records daily weights.
  - Patient reports to the health care provider any increase in weight of more than 1 kilogram in 24 hours or 2.3 kilograms or more in 1 week.
- Patient notifies the health care provider if body temperature is higher than 38°C.
  - Patient performs frequent mouth and skin care to prevent infections.

■ Implementation

It is important to understand how glucocorticoids work in the body so that patients may receive adequate explanations and education to maximize the drug's therapeutic effects and minimize adverse effects. Remember the following points when giving these drugs: (1) Hormone production by the adrenal gland is influenced by time of day and follows a diurnal (daily or 24-hour) pattern, with peak levels occurring early in the morning between 0600 and 0800 hours, a decrease occurring during the day, and a lower peak in the late afternoon between 1600 and 1800 hours. (2) Cortisol levels increase in response to both emotional and physiological stress. (3) Cortisol levels increase when endogenous levels decrease due to a physiological negative feedback system. (4) When exogenous glucocorticoids are given, endogenous levels decrease; for endogenous production to resume, exogenous levels must be decreased gradually so that hormone output responds to the negative feedback system. (5) The best time to give exogenous glucocorticoids, if at all possible, is early in the morning (0600 to 0900 hours) to minimize adrenal suppression. It is important to remember, however, that patients must not alter dosing or abruptly discontinue medication without consulting a health care provider.

Prednisone, a synthetic glucocorticoid, and fludrocortisones 21-acetate, a synthetic mineralocorticoid, are given orally. It is recommended that oral dosage forms be given with milk or food to help minimize GI upset. Another option is for the health care provider to prescribe an H_2 receptor antagonist or a proton pump inhibitor to prevent ulcer formation because these drugs are ulcerogenic. Emphasize to patients to the importance of avoiding alcohol, caffeine, aspirin, and other NSAIDs to minimize gastric irritation and possible gastric bleeding

from compounding ulcerogenic effects. In long-term therapy, alternate-day dosing of glucocorticoids, if possible, will help minimize the adrenal suppression. Because of delayed wound healing, monitor patients taking these drugs for flulike symptoms, sore throat, and fever. Methylprednisolone sodium succinate, a systemic corticosteroid, is given intravenously. Mix all parenteral forms per manufacturer guidelines, with intravenous (IV) doses administered over the recommended time period and in the proper diluent.

With oral and all other forms of glucocorticoids that are given in the short or long term, abrupt withdrawal must be avoided. Abrupt withdrawal of adrenal drugs (e.g., prednisone, methylprednisolone sodium succinate) may lead to a sudden decrease in or no production of endogenous glucocorticoids, resulting in adrenal insufficiency. Signs and symptoms of partial or complete adrenal insufficiency or Addison's disease include fatigue, headache, confusion, fever, nausea, vomiting, abdominal pain, tachycardia, diaphoresis, dehydration, and hypotension. If left untreated, this condition could lead to an **adrenal crisis** or a life-threatening state of profound adrenocortical insufficiency requiring immediate medical management. Signs and symptoms of adrenal crisis, also referred to as *addisonian crisis*, include a severe drop in extracellular fluid volume with hypotension, hypoglycemia, hyponatremia, and hyperkalemia.

Other adrenal drug dosage forms include those for intra-articular, intrabursal, intradermal, intralesional, and intrasynovial administration. Administration of corticosteroids into these sites is done by an orthopedic or dermatology specialist, not by the nurse. Do not overuse intra-articular injections, and if a joint is injected with medication, the patient needs to rest that area for up to 48 hours after the injection is given. Application of cold packs over the injected area may be indicated for up to the first 24 hours to help minimize the discomfort associated with intra-articular injections. Topical dosage forms (e.g., for skin, eyes, or inhalation into the bronchial tree) are also available and must be administered as ordered. For dermatological use, clean and dry the skin before application. Wear gloves and apply the medication with either a sterile tongue depressor or a cotton-tipped applicator. Use sterile technique if the skin is not intact. Nasally administered glucocorticoids (e.g., beclomethasone dipropionate) must also be used exactly as ordered (see Chapter 37). Any written instructions that come with the product must be read and followed carefully. Before using nasal sprays, the patient needs to first clear the nasal passages and then use the spray exactly as per the instructions. After the nasal passages are cleared, the container is placed gently inside the nasal passage and the medication is released at the same time that the patient breathes in through the nose, one nasal passage at a time or as ordered.

Glucocorticoid inhalers (e.g., beclomethasone dipropionate, budesonide, fluticasone propionate, mometasone furoate) are to be used strictly as ordered; explain the negative consequences of overuse to the patient. Use of these inhaled glucocorticoids may lead to fungal infections (candidiasis) of the oral mucosa and oral cavity, larynx, and pharynx. Therefore, the patient must rinse the mouth and oral mucous membranes with lukewarm water after each use to prevent fungal overgrowth and further complications. In addition to fungal infections, hoarseness, throat irritation, and dry mouth are possible adverse effects associated with the use of inhaled corticosteroids. Occurrence of any of these conditions needs to be discussed with a health care provider. See Chapter 10 and Patient Teaching Tips for more information on inhaled dosage forms.

If a patient is receiving long-term maintenance glucocorticoid therapy and requires surgery, recognize the importance of reviewing the patient's medical records for laboratory values, cautions, contraindications, and drug interactions. If preoperative orders do not include the maintenance dosage of glucocorticoid therapy, contact the surgeon or another health care provider, and ensure that the situation is explained, including the possible need for a rapid-acting corticosteroid. After surgery, the dosage of the steroid may well be increased, with a gradual decrease in dosage over several days until the patient returns to baseline. In addition, be very aware of the decrease in wound healing in patients taking corticosteroids on a long-term basis.

In summary, because of their suppressed immune systems, patients taking corticosteroids need to avoid contact with people with known infections and report any fever, increased weakness, lethargy, or sore throat to a health care provider. Monitoring of nutritional status, weight, fluid volume, electrolyte status, blood pressure, skin turgor, and glucose levels during therapy is important to ensure safe and effective therapy. The health care provider needs to be notified if any of these symptoms occur: edema, shortness of breath (indicating possible heart failure), joint pain, fever, mood swings, or other unusual symptoms.

Evaluation

A therapeutic response to glucocorticoids includes a resolution of the underlying manifestations of the disease or pathology, such as a decrease in inflammation, increased feelings of well-being, less pain and discomfort in the joints, a decrease in lymphocytes, or other improvements in the condition for which the medication was ordered. Adverse effects include weight gain; increased blood pressure; sodium increase and potassium loss; mental health status changes such as mood swings, nervousness, aggressive behaviours, or psychosis; abdominal distension; ulcer-related symptoms; and changes in vision. Cushing's syndrome occurs with prolonged or frequent use of glucocorticoids and is characterized by moon facies, obesity of the trunk area (often referred to as belly fat), increase in blood glucose and sodium levels, loss of serum potassium, wasting of muscle mass, buffalo hump (accumulation of fat behind the neck), and other features previously discussed. Cataract formation and osteoporosis may also occur with long-term corticosteroid use. Rapid drops in cortisol levels (e.g., from abrupt withdrawal of medication) may lead to Addison's disease and addisonian crisis (see previous discussions).

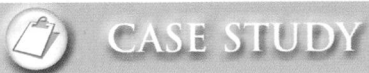

CASE STUDY

Glucocorticoid Drug Therapy

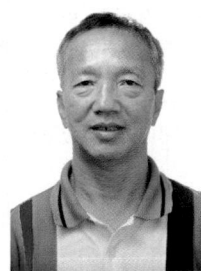

Jong-Ui, a 68-year-old factory worker, has been in the hospital for 1 week because of an exacerbation of chronic obstructive pulmonary disease, which was aggravated by drywall dust during home renovations. He has a history of type 2 diabetes. His current plasma glucose is 9.7 mmol/L. He says that he stopped smoking 4 years ago and tries to "watch what he eats" because he has gained weight recently. He also reports feeling more irritable than normal, and he has experienced difficulty sleeping. He has no history of drug allergies. He is receiving oxygen at 1 L/min through a nasal cannula. At this time, he is breathing more easily and hopes to be going home soon. His medication orders include the following, among others:

- metformin/sitagliptin phosphate monohydrate (Janumet®) 500 mg/50 mg twice a day by mouth (PO) with meals
- prednisone (Winpred), 20 mg, every morning PO

- salbutamol sulfate (Ventolin®) inhaler, 2 puffs every 4 hours

Jong-Ui is reporting a headache. When you check the medication sheet, you see two orders:

- acetaminophen (generic), 650 mg PO every 4 hours as needed for pain
- ibuprofen (generic), 200 mg PO every 6 hours as needed for pain

1. Which medication will you choose to give to Jong-Ui? Explain your answer.
2. Considering Jong-Ui's medications, what could be contributing to his elevated glucose level? What other laboratory values need to be monitored closely during this time?
3. What do you expect happened to cause Jong-Ui's report of weight gain, irritability, and difficulty sleeping?
4. What nursing diagnoses are appropriate for Jong-Ui?

For answers, see http://evolve.elsevier.com/Canada/Lilley/pharmacology/.

PATIENT TEACHING TIPS

❖ Patients should be aware that glucocorticoids are to be taken exactly as ordered and never abruptly discontinued. The health care provider should be contacted if there are situations that prevent proper dosing. Abrupt withdrawal may precipitate adrenal crisis, Addison's disease, or addisonian crisis.

❖ If a once-a-day dose of glucocorticoids is missed, the patient needs to take the dose as soon as possible after remembering that the dose was missed. If the patient does not remember until close to the time for the next dose, then the patient is usually instructed to skip the dose and resume the dosing on the next day without doubling up. If any questions arise, the patient should seek clarification from a health care provider. Educate patients about the adverse effects of long-term therapy, including changes in body appearance including acne, buffalo hump, truncal obesity, moon facies, and thinning of the extremities.

❖ For patients taking glucocorticoids, emphasize the importance of bone health and the use of fall prevention strategies, because long-term therapy with these drugs may lead to osteoporosis. The health care provider may suggest a daily supplement of oral calcium and vitamin D (see Chapter 9), and bisphosphonates (see Chapter 35) may also be considered. Foods high in vitamin D include cod liver oil (amount to be recommended by a health care provider) and salmon. Foods high in calcium include milk, cheese, yogourt, and ice cream. Fortified dairy products are high in both vitamin D and calcium.

❖ Glucocorticoid therapy involves a risk of vulnerability to infection. Educate patients taking them to avoid contact with people with known infections and report any fever, increased weakness, lethargy, or sore throat to a health care provider.

❖ Contact the health care provider immediately if any signs and symptoms of acute adrenal insufficiency appear, such as dehydration and weight loss.

❖ Patients taking fludrocortisone 21-acetate, a mineralocorticoid, should be aware that it is better tolerated if taken with food or milk to minimize GI upset. With any of the adrenal drugs, weight gain of 1 kg or more in 24 hours or 2.3 kg or more in 1 week needs to be reported to the health care provider immediately.

❖ Encourage patients to keep a journal to document responses to treatment, blood pressure readings, daily weight measurements, mood changes, and any adverse effects.

❖ Emphasize to patients the importance of follow-up appointments with the health care provider so that electrolyte levels and any adverse effects may be monitored. Also, stress the importance of maintaining a low-sodium and high-potassium diet, if ordered.

❖ Encourage patients to wear medical alert identification jewellery. A medical card or electronic device with important relevant information, including diagnoses, medications, and allergies, needs to be kept on their person at all times and updated frequently.

KEY POINTS

❖ The adrenal gland is an endocrine organ that is located on top of the kidneys and is composed of two distinct tissues: the adrenal cortex and the adrenal medulla. The adrenal medulla secretes two important hormones: epinephrine and norepinephrine; the adrenal cortex secretes two classes of hormones known as corticosteroids: glucocorticoids and mineralocorticoids.

❖ The biological functions of glucocorticoids include anti-inflammatory actions; maintenance of normal blood pressure; carbohydrate, protein, and fat metabolism; and stress effects. The biological functions of mineralocorticoids include sodium and water resorption, blood pressure control, and maintenance of potassium levels and blood pH.

❖ Patients taking adrenal drugs may receive them by various routes, such as orally, intramuscularly,

intravenously, intranasally, intra-articularly, and by inhalation.

❖ Glucocorticoid inhaled dosage forms are to be used only as prescribed and only after adequate patient education. Rinsing of the mouth after each use is needed to avoid oral fungal infections (oral candidiasis) and oral–pharyngeal irritation.

❖ Long-term or frequent glucocorticoid use produces increased levels of glucocorticoids, which can lead to Cushing's syndrome. Abrupt withdrawal of glucocorticoids leads to adrenal insufficiency and negative effects on a patient's homeostasis.

❖ When once-a-day dosing of corticosteroids is prescribed, adrenal suppression from corticosteroid therapy can be minimized if the dose is given between 0600 and 0900 hours, but it needs to be given only as ordered.

EXAMINATION REVIEW QUESTIONS

1. Which statement is correct regarding corticosteroids?
   a. They have few adverse effects.
   b. They are often used for their anti-inflammatory effects.
   c. They may be administered only by inhalant dosage forms.
   d. They may be used long term without major complications.

2. The nurse has provided teaching about oral corticosteroid therapy to a patient. Which statement from the patient shows a need for more teaching?
   a. "I will report any fever or sore throat symptoms."
   b. "I will stay away from anyone who has a cold or infection."
   c. "I can stop this medication if I have severe adverse effects."
   d. "I will take this drug with food or milk."

3. During long-term corticosteroid therapy, the nurse will monitor the patient for Cushing's syndrome, which is manifested by which symptoms?
   a. Weight loss
   b. Moon facies
   c. Hypotension
   d. Thickened hair growth

4. When teaching a patient who has been prescribed a daily dose of prednisone (Winipred), the nurse knows that the patient will be told to take the medication at which time of day to help reduce adrenal suppression?
   a. In the morning
   b. At lunchtime
   c. At dinnertime
   d. At bedtime

5. Which teaching is appropriate for a patient who is taking an inhaled glucocorticoid for asthma?
   a. "Exhale while pushing in on the canister of the inhaler."
   b. "Blow your nose after taking the medication."
   c. "Rinse your mouth thoroughly after taking the medication."
   d. "Do not eat immediately after taking the medication."

6. The nurse will monitor the patient's laboratory results for which adverse effects that can occur during long-term corticosteroid therapy? (Select all that apply.)
   a. Increased serum potassium levels
   b. Decreased serum potassium levels
   c. Increased sodium levels
   d. Decreased sodium levels
   e. Hyperglycemia
   f. Hypoglycemia

7. The order reads: "Give methylprednisolone sodium succinate (Solu-Medrol) 100 mg IV every 6 hours." The drug is available in vials of 80 mg/mL. How many millilitres will the nurse draw up for each dose?

Answers: 1. b, 2. c, 3. b, 4. a, 5. c, 6. b, c, e, 7. 1.25 mL.

CRITICAL THINKING ACTIVITIES

1. A patient with type 2 diabetes mellitus will be receiving IV doses of methylprednisolone sodium succinate (Solu-Medrol) to prevent cerebral edema after a head injury. A new nurse is working with you as you prepare to give this medication. The nurse asks, "Isn't this drug going to cause problems for this patient? Should we be giving it?" What is your best answer?

2. A patient has been taking high doses of oral prednisone for 1 week due to an exacerbation of asthma symptoms. He is about to go home and is given a prescription for another week of prednisone (Winpred) therapy, but with doses tapering downward before the medication is stopped. The patient asks, "Why do I need to bother with this drug if it's only for a week? Can't I just stop it now?" What is the priority when the nurse answers this patient's questions? Explain your answer.

3. Your patient is a 15-year-old male with a history of steroid-dependent asthma. He reports "always feeling tired and weak." He has been using inhaled bronchodilators for the past 5 years, and for the past 3 years, the doses have been increased. Over the previous 8 months, he has been hospitalized twice for severe asthma attacks (status asthmaticus), during which he was given IV and oral corticosteroid bursts (high doses over a few days). In addition, he has been taking daily oral steroids for the last 5 months. He has had a weight gain of 10 kg over the previous 3 months and an increased incidence of recent "colds," and his mother has expressed concern that he does not seem to be growing as quickly as his siblings did at this age. His mother also asks why if her son is getting "steroids," he looks as he does rather than like "all the bodybuilders on TV who are using steroids." What are the priority concerns for this patient? How would you respond to his mother's concerns? Explain your answer.

For answers, see http://evolve.elsevier.com/Canada/Lilley/pharmacology/.

Women's Health Drugs

Objectives

After reading this chapter, the successful student will be able to do the following:

1. Discuss the normal anatomy and physiology of the female reproductive system.

2. Discuss the normal hormonally mediated feedback system that regulates the female reproductive system.

3. Briefly describe the variety of disorders affecting women's health and the drugs used to treat them.

4. Discuss the rationales for use, indications, adverse effects, cautions, contraindications, drug interactions, dosages, and routes of administration of estrogen, progestins, uterine motility–altering drugs, and osteoporosis drugs.

5. Develop a collaborative plan of care that includes all phases of the nursing process for patients receiving any of the drugs related to women's health (estrogens, progestins, uterine mobility–altering drugs, and osteoporosis drugs).

e-Learning Activities

Website
(http://evolve.elsevier.com/Canada/Lilley/pharmacology/)

evolve

- Answer Key—Textbook Case Studies
- Answer Key—Critical Thinking Activities
- Chapter Summaries—Printable
- Review Questions for Exam Preparation
- Unfolding Case Studies

Drug Profiles

▸▸ alendronate (alendronate sodium)*, p. 674
clomiphene (clomiphene citrate)*, p. 676
contraceptive drugs, p. 670
▸▸ dinoprostone, p. 678
▸▸ estrogen, p. 668
▸▸ medroxyprogesterone (medroxyprogesterone acetate)*, p. 670
megestrol (megestrol acetate)*, p. 670
▸▸ menotropins, p. 675
▸▸ oxytocin, p. 678
raloxifene (raloxifene hydrochloride)*, p. 674

▸▸ Key drug

*Full generic name is given in parentheses. For the purposes of this text, the more common, shortened name is used.

Key Terms

Chloasma Hyperpigmentation due to an increase in melanin in the skin, characterized by brownish macules on the cheeks, forehead, lips, and neck; a common dermatological adverse effect of female hormonal medications (also called *melasma*). (p. 667)

Corpus luteum The structure that forms on the surface of the ovary after every ovulation and acts as a short-lived endocrine organ that secretes progesterone. (p. 664)

Endocrine glands Glands that secrete one or more hormones directly into the blood. (p. 663)

Estrogens   A major class of female sex steroid hormones; of the estrogens, estradiol is responsible for most estrogenic physiological activity. (p. 663)

Fallopian tubes   The passages through which ova are carried from the ovaries to the uterus. (p. 663)

Gonadotropin   The hormone that stimulates the testes and ovaries. (p. 663)

Hormone replacement therapy (HRT)   Any replacement of natural hormones with hormonal drug forms (also referred to simply as *hormone therapy [HT]*). Most commonly, HRT refers to estrogen replacement therapy for treating symptoms associated with menopause-related estrogen deficiency. (p. 666)

Implantation   The attachment to, penetration of, and embedding of the fertilized ovum in the lining of the uterine wall; one of the first stages of pregnancy. (p. 664)

Menarche   The first menses in a young woman's life and the beginning of cyclic menstrual function. (p. 664)

Menopause   The cessation of menses for 12 consecutive months that marks the end of a woman's childbearing capability. (p. 664)

Menses   The normal flow of blood that occurs during menstruation. (p. 663)

Menstrual cycle   The recurring cycle of changes in the endometrium in which the decidual layer is shed, regrows, proliferates, is maintained for several days, and is shed again at menstruation unless a pregnancy begins; also referred to as the *uterine cycle*. (p. 663)

Nucleic acids   Specific molecules in cells that are composed of strings of repeating units that serve to encode information; the two most common ones are DNA and RNA, whose functions have to do with the storage and expression of genetic information. (p. 665)

Osteoporosis   A condition characterized by the progressive loss of bone density and thinning of bone tissue and associated with an increased risk of fractures. (p. 672)

Ova   Female reproductive or germ cells (singular: *ovum*; also called *eggs*). (p. 663)

Ovarian follicles   The location of egg production and ovulation in the ovary; the follicle is the precursor to the corpus luteum. (p. 663)

Ovaries   The pair of female gonads located on each side of the lower abdomen beside the uterus; they store the *ova* (eggs) and release them during the ovulation stage of the menstrual cycle. (p. 663)

Ovulation   The rupture of the ovarian follicle, which results in the release of an unfertilized ovum into the peritoneal cavity, from which it normally enters the fallopian tube. (p. 663)

Progesterone   A sex hormone produced by the corpus luteum that serves to prepare the uterus for possible implantation. (p. 663)

Progestins   Synthetic or natural substances that have properties similar to progesterone but are not considered to be the naturally occurring progesterone that is present in the human female body. (p. 663)

Uterus   The hollow, pear-shaped female organ in which the fertilized ovum is implanted (see implantation) and the fetus develops. (p. 663)

Vagina   Part of the female genitalia that forms a canal from its external orifice through its vestibule to the uterine cervix. (p. 663)

OVERVIEW OF FEMALE REPRODUCTIVE FUNCTIONS

The female reproductive system consists of the **ovaries, fallopian tubes, uterus, vagina,** and the external structure known as the *vulva*. The development of these primary sex structures, initiation of their subsequent reproductive functions (starting at puberty), and their maintenance are controlled by pituitary **gonadotropin** hormones and the female sex steroid hormones, **estrogens** and **progestins.** Pituitary gonadotropins include follicle-stimulating hormone (FSH) and luteinizing hormone (LH). Both play a primary role in hormonal communication between the pituitary gland (see Chapter 31) and the ovaries in the continuous regulation of the **menstrual cycle** from month to month.

Estrogens are also responsible for stimulating the development of secondary female sex characteristics, including breast, skin, and bone development and distribution of body fat and hair. **Progesterone** helps create optimal conditions for pregnancy in the endometrium just after **ovulation** and also promotes the start of **menses** in the absence of a fertilized ovum.

The ovaries (female gonads) are paired glands located on each side of the uterus. They function both as **endocrine glands** and as reproductive glands. As reproductive glands, they produce within **ovarian follicles** mature **ova,** which are then ovulated or released into the space in the peritoneal cavity between the ovary and the fallopian tube. Fingerlike projections known as *fimbriae* lie adjacent to each ovary and serve to "catch" the released ovum and guide it into the fallopian tube. Once inside the fallopian tube, the ovum is moved through the lumen to the uterus. This movement is accomplished through the muscular contractions of the tube walls and the actions of ciliated cells inside the lumen of the tube, which "beat" in the direction of the uterus. Fertilization of the ovum, when it occurs, takes place in the fallopian tube.

As endocrine glands, the ovaries are responsible for producing the two types of sex steroid hormones, estrogens and progesterone. Chemically, the estrogens and progestational hormones include several distinct substances. However, only two of these hormones occur in significant amounts, and these have the greatest physiological activity. They are the estrogen estradiol and the progestational hormone progesterone. Estradiol is the principal secretory product of the ovary and has several estrogenic effects. One of these effects is the regulation of gonadotropin (FSH and LH) secretion via negative feedback to the pituitary gland. Others include promotion of the development of female secondary sex characteristics, monthly endometrial growth, thickening of the vaginal mucosa, thinning of the cervical mucus, and growth of the ductal system of the breasts. Progesterone is the principal secretory product of the **corpus luteum** and has progestational effects. These include promotion of tissue growth and secretory activity in the endometrium following the estrogen-driven follicular phase of the menstrual cycle. This important secretory process is required for endometrial egg **implantation** and maintenance of pregnancy. Other progestational effects include induction of menstruation when fertilization has not occurred and, during pregnancy, inhibition of uterine contractions, increase in the viscosity of cervical mucus (which protects the fetus from external contamination), and growth of the alveolar glands of the breasts.

The uterus consists of three layers: the outer protective *perimetrium*, the muscular *myometrium*, and the inner mucosal layer known as the *endometrium*. The myometrium provides the powerful smooth muscle contractions needed for childbirth. The endometrium is the site of the following:

- Implantation of a fertilized ovum and subsequent development of the fetus
- Initiation of labour and birthing of the infant
- Menstruation

The vagina serves as a common passageway for birthing and menstrual flow. In addition, it is a receptacle for the penis during sexual intercourse and the sperm after male ejaculation.

The menstrual cycle usually takes approximately 1 month to complete. Menstrual cycles begin during puberty with the first menses **(menarche)** and cease at **menopause**, which in most women occurs between 45 and 55 years of age. The hormonally controlled menstrual cycle consists of four distinct but interrelated phases that occur in overlapping sequence. Phase names correspond to activity in either the ovarian follicle or the endometrium (see Table 35-1).

- **Phase 1:** The *menstruation phase* (uterine cycle) initiates the cycle and lasts from 5 to 7 days.
- **Phase 2:** During the *follicular phase* (ovarian cycle), a mature ovum develops from an ovarian follicle. This phase is also called the *proliferative* or *preovulatory phase* and is characterized by rising estrogen secretion from the ovary and LH secretion from the pituitary gland. It terminates on or about day 14 of the cycle.
- **Phase 3:** The *ovulation phase* involves release of the unfertilized ovum from the ovary. This process occurs over an approximately 24- to 48-hour period starting at about day 14. Both estrogen and LH levels peak near this time.

TABLE 35-1

Phases of the Menstrual Cycle

Phase	Ovarian Follicle Activity	Endometrium Activity
Phase 1	Menstruation	Menstruation
Phase 2	Follicular phase (preovulatory)	Proliferative phase
Phase 3	Ovulation	Ovulation
Phase 4	Luteal phase (postovulatory)	Secretory phase

- **Phase 4:** The final phase of the cycle is the *luteal* or *postovulatory phase*. It is also known as the *secretory phase*. It occurs when the corpus luteum forms from the ruptured ovarian follicle. The corpus luteum is a mass of secretory cells on the surface of the ovary. Its primary function is to produce progesterone, which helps to optimize the endometrial mucosa for implantation of a fertilized ovum. The corpus luteum also serves as an initial source of progesterone needed during early pregnancy. This function is later assumed by the developing placenta. If fertilization does not occur, the corpus luteum then degenerates, causing a fall in progesterone levels. The menstrual cycle begins again on or about day 28.

Figure 35-1 illustrates the sequence of hormone secretions and related events that take place during the menstrual cycle.

Female Sex Hormones

ESTROGENS

There are three major endogenous estrogens: estradiol, estrone, and estriol. All are synthesized from cholesterol in the ovarian follicles and have the basic chemical structure of a steroid, known as the *steroid nucleus*. For this reason, they are sometimes referred to as *steroid hormones*. Estradiol is the principal and most active of the three and represents the end product of estrogen synthesis.

Exogenous estrogenic drugs, those used as drug therapy, were developed because most of the endogenous estrogens are inactive when taken orally. These synthetic drugs fall into two categories: steroidal and nonsteroidal. The estrogenic drugs currently in use are as follows:

- Conjugated estrogens (Premarin®)
- Esterified estrogens (Estragyn®)
- Estradiol transdermal (Climara®, Divigel®, Estrogel®, Sandoz Estradiol Derm®, Oesclim®)
- Estradiol vaginal ring (Estring®)
- Estradiol valerate
- Estrone (Folliculum®)
- Estropipate (Ogen®)

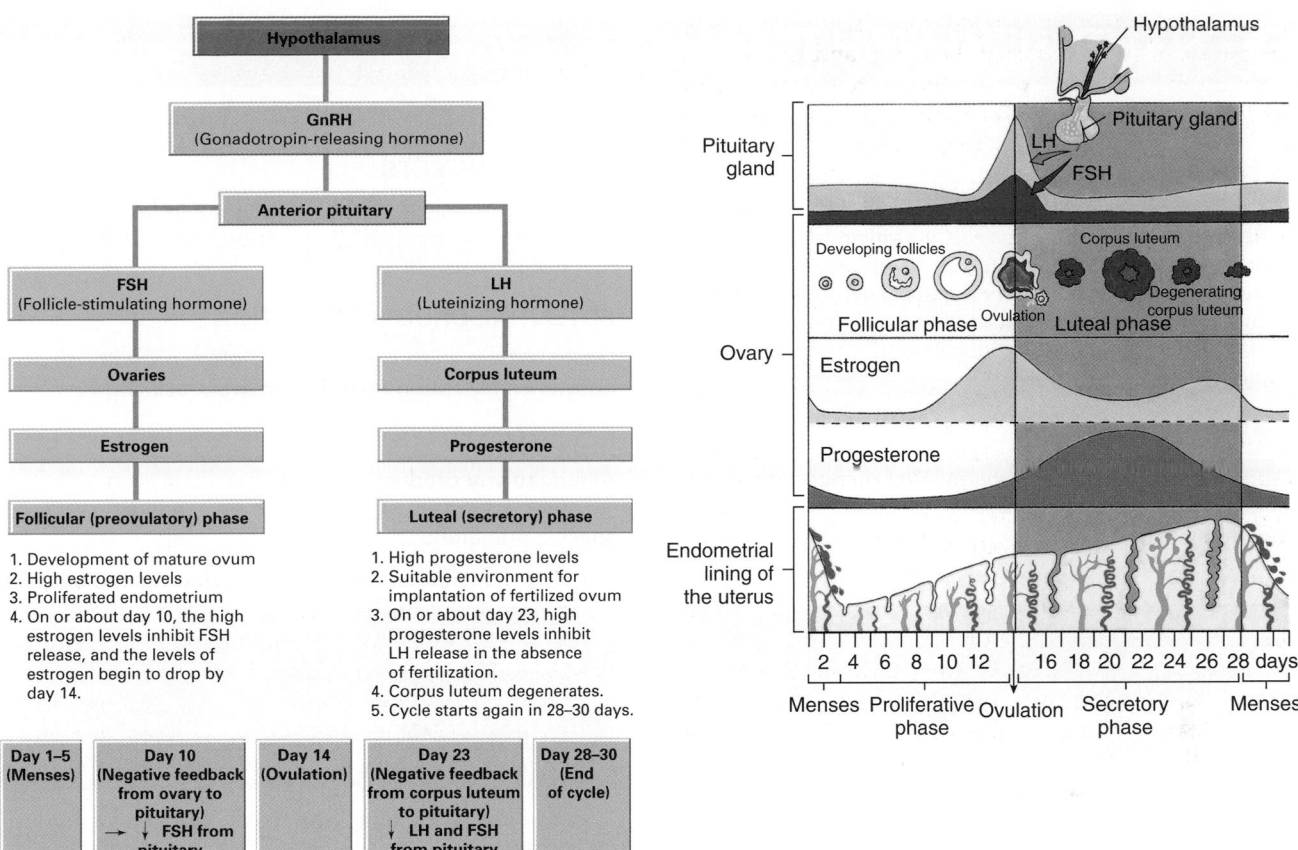

FIG. 35-1 Hormonal activity during the monthly menstrual cycle. Gonadotropin-releasing hormone (GnRH) from the hypothalamus stimulates the pituitary gland, causing it to secrete follicle-stimulating hormone (FSH) early in the cycle (coinciding with menses) and later luteinizing hormone (LH). FSH stimulates the ovaries to produce estrogen (primarily estradiol). Later in the cycle, the combined surges in the levels of estrogen, GnRH, FSH, and LH stimulate ovulation. The corpus luteum then secretes estrogen and progesterone, providing negative feedback to the hypothalamus and pituitary gland to reduce GnRH, FSH, and LH secretions. If the ovum (egg) is not fertilized by a spermatozoon, levels of estrogen and progesterone then fall to their monthly lows, GnRH and FSH rise again, and the onset of menses begins a new cycle. (Right; Source: Thibodeau, G. A., & Patton, K. T. (2010). *Anatomy and physiology* (7th ed.; p. 1055, Fig. 32-14). St. Louis, MO: Mosby.)

- Ethinyl estradiol (Alesse®, Alysena®, Aviane®, many others)
- Estradiol vaginal dose forms (Estring®, Premarin®, Vagifem®)
- Estrone (Estrone Vaginal Cream®)

The most widely used estrogen product is an estrogen mixture known as *conjugated estrogens*. This mixture contains a combination of natural estrogen compounds derived from and equivalent to the average estrogen composition of the urine of pregnant mares, hence its brand name of Premarin. A nonanimal source for this conjugated estrogen mixture is also available. The product Estrace is composed of various conjugated estrogens obtained from soybeans. This product was developed in response to consumer demand from women who wanted an alternative to animal-derived products (see the Natural Health Products box on p. 666). Some women obtain other natural estrogen products from naturopathic prescribers and prefer these to standard prescription drugs such as Premarin.

Patients report varying degrees of satisfaction with the numerous products available, and it can take both time and patience to find the best choice for a given individual. Ethinyl estradiol is one of the more potent estrogens and is most commonly found in oral contraceptive drugs. Another commonly used form of estrogen is the patch formulation. Several patches exist, all of which are dosed differently; thus patient education is necessary to ensure proper use. The most commonly used patch is Climara (estradiol).

Nonsteroidal estrogen products are no longer available for use in Canada for obstetric use because of major adverse effects with the use of diethylstilbestrol (DES). Box 35-1 describes this important episode in medical history.

Mechanism of Action and Drug Effects

The binding of estrogen to intracellular estrogen receptors stimulates the synthesis of **nucleic acids** (deoxyribonucleic acid [DNA] and ribonucleic acid [RNA]) and

NATURAL HEALTH PRODUCTS

Soy (Glycine Max)

OVERVIEW

Soy is a bean commonly grown throughout the world. The isoflavones in soy are chemically similar to the female hormone estradiol. Some studies have shown soy to be useful in the prevention of menopausal symptoms in peri-menopausal women. Other studies have found that soy reduces both low-density lipoprotein (LDL) and total cholesterol levels.

COMMON USES

Reduction of cholesterol level, relief of menopause symptoms (alternative to hormone therapy), osteoporosis prevention.

ADVERSE EFFECTS

Nausea, bloating, diarrhea, abdominal pain (ingested forms), and hypersensitivity reactions have been reported following the use of soy.

POTENTIAL DRUG INTERACTIONS

Orally administered soy may interfere with thyroid hormone absorption (avoid concurrent use).

CONTRAINDICATIONS

Allergy to soy products.
Follow manufacturer directions on the label for use of specific preparations.

BOX 35-1
Diethylstilbestrol

Between 1940 and 1971, an estimated 6 million mothers and their fetuses were exposed to diethylstilbestrol (DES). The drug was used to prevent reproductive problems such as miscarriage, premature delivery, intrauterine fetal death, and toxemia. This use resulted in significant complications involving the reproductive systems of both female and male offspring. Two large groups have been established to monitor these complications: the International Registry for Research on Hormonal Transplacental Carcinogenesis and the National Cooperative Diethylstilbestrol Adenosis (DESAD) Project.

BOX 35-2
Indications for Estrogen Therapy

- Atrophic vaginitis (shrinkage of the vagina or urethra)
- Hypogonadism
- Oral contraception (in combination with a progestin)
- Ovarian failure or castration (or removal of ovaries)
- Uterine bleeding
- Breast or prostate cancer (palliative treatment of advanced inoperable cases)
- Osteoporosis (treatment and prophylaxis)
- Cross-gender hormone treatment of male-to-female transgender individuals
- Vasomotor symptoms of menopause (e.g., hot flashes)
- Severe acne (in combination with cyproterone, an antiandrogen)

---

proteins, which are the building blocks for all living tissue. Estrogens are also required at puberty for the development and maintenance of the female reproductive system and the development of female secondary sex characteristics, a process known as *feminization*. Estrogens produce their effects in estrogen-responsive tissues, which have a large number of estrogen receptors, proteins that bind estrogens with high affinity and specificity. These tissues include the female genital organs, the breasts, the pituitary gland, and the hypothalamus. At the time of puberty, the production of estrogen increases greatly. This causes initiation of menses, breast development, redistribution of body fat, softening of the skin, and other feminizing changes. Estrogens play a role in the shaping of body contours and development of the skeleton. For instance, long bones are usually inhibited from growing, with the result that females are usually shorter than males. Estrogen receptors are found throughout the body and act on many other organ systems such as cardiovascular, skeletal, immune, gastrointestinal (GI), and neural sites. They have a significant role in health and disease. For example,

cardiovascular disease increases in women after menopause. It is believed that the decrease in estrogen levels is associated with the disruption of lipid or glucose regulation. Estrogen's cardioprotective effect may be due to the reduction of cholesterol levels through the elimination of LDLs from the circulating blood. Estrogen receptors are also expressed in endothelial and smooth muscle cells of vascular tissues and are thought to reduce the development of atherosclerosis.

Indications

Estrogens are used in the treatment or prevention of a variety of disorders that result primarily from estrogen deficiency. These conditions are listed in Box 35-2. **Hormone replacement therapy (HRT)** to counter such estrogen deficiency is most commonly known for its benefits in treating menopausal symptoms (e.g., vasomotor symptoms or hot flashes). Hot flashes result from ovarian follicular depletion and marked reduction in ovarian estrogen secretion. The thermoregulatory system in the hypothalamus is disrupted, with small changes in body temperature eliciting an exaggerated sweating (from vasodilation) and shivering response as well as an increase in heart rate. In combination with cyproterone, ethinyl estradiol is used to treat certain severe types of acne with associated symptoms of androgenization, including seborrhea and mild hirsutism in women who have been unsuccessfully treated with antibiotics and other treatments. This combination medication works by regulating hormones that affect the skin.

Contraindications

Contraindications for estrogen administration include known drug allergy, any estrogen-dependent cancer, undiagnosed abnormal vaginal bleeding, pregnancy, and active thromboembolic disorder (e.g., stroke, thrombophlebitis, active smokers) or a history of such a disorder.

Adverse Effects

Estrogens increase plasma fibrinogen and the activity of coagulation factors (e.g., factors VII and X) and decrease antithrombin III, the inhibitor of coagulation. Platelet activity is also enhanced, with the acceleration of aggregation. These changes create a state of hypercoagulability. Consequently, the most serious adverse effects of the estrogens are thromboembolic events such as deep vein thrombosis (DVT), stroke, and pulmonary embolism. The incidence of these effects is decreased with lower dose formulation of estrogens. The most common undesirable effect of estrogen use is nausea. Photosensitivity may also occur with estrogen therapy. One common dermatological effect of note is known as **chloasma**. Chloasma consists of brownish, macular spots that often occur on the forehead, cheeks, lips, and neck. This and other adverse effects are listed in Table 35-2.

TABLE 35-2

Estrogens: Common Adverse Effects

Body System	Adverse Effects
Cardiovascular	Hypertension, thrombophlebitis, edema
Gastrointestinal	Nausea, vomiting, diarrhea, constipation
Genitourinary	Amenorrhea, breakthrough uterine bleeding, enlarged uterine fibromyomas
Dermatological	Chloasma (facial skin discoloration; also called *melasma*) hirsutism, alopecia
Other	Tender breasts, fluid retention, decreased carbohydrate tolerance, headaches

Interactions

Estrogens can decrease the activity of oral anticoagulants, and the concurrent administration of rifampin and St. John's wort can decrease their estrogenic effect. Their use with tricyclic antidepressants may promote toxicity of the antidepressant. Smoking should be avoided during estrogen therapy because this, too, can diminish estrogenic effects and add to the risk for thrombosis.

Dosages

For dosage information on some of the many available estrogen products, refer to the table on p. 669.

PROGESTINS

Available progestational drugs, or progestins, include both natural and synthetic drugs. Progesterone is the most active natural progestational hormone and is the primary progestin component in most drug formulations. It is produced by the corpus luteum after each ovulation and during pregnancy by the placenta. In addition, there are two other major natural progestational hormones. The first is 17-hydroxyprogesterone, an inactive metabolite of progesterone. The second is pregnenolone, a chemical precursor to all steroid hormones that is synthesized from cholesterol in the ovary as was described for the estrogens. Because orally administered progesterone is relatively inactive and parenterally administered progesterone causes local reactions and pain, chemical derivatives were developed that are effective orally and are also more potent; their actions are also more specific and of longer duration. For example, Mirena® is a hormonal intrauterine device that is inserted into the uterus for long-term contraception. The following are some of the most commonly used progestins:

- levonorgestrel (Min-Ovral®, Minera®, Next Choice®, Norlevo®, Option 2®)
- medroxyprogesterone (Depo-Provera®, Medroxy®, Provera®)
- megestrol (Megace®)
- norethindrone acetate (Norlutate®); norethindrone (Micronor®)
- progesterone (Crinone®, Prometrium®)

Mechanism of Action and Drug Effects

All of the progestin products produce the same physiological responses as those produced by progesterone. These responses include induction of secretory changes in the endometrium, including diminished endometrial tissue proliferation; an increase in the basal body temperature; thickening of the vaginal mucosa; relaxation of uterine smooth muscle; stimulation of mammary alveolar tissue growth; feedback inhibition (negative feedback) of the release of pituitary gonadotropins (FSH and LH); and alterations in menstrual blood flow, especially in the presence of estrogen.

DRUG PROFILES

▶▶ *estrogen*

Estrogen is indicated for the treatment of many clinical conditions, primarily those resulting from estrogen deficiency (see Box 35-2). Many of these conditions occur around menopause, when the endogenous estradiol level is declining. Any estrogen capable of binding to the estrogen receptors in target organs can alleviate menopausal symptoms. As a general rule, the smallest dosage of estrogen that relieves the symptoms or prevents the condition is used. Although many women receive estrogen or estrogen–progestin therapy for many months or years, some health care providers (and patients) may prefer that patients be weaned from estrogen therapy because of known adverse effects. Two studies that were performed as part of the Women's Health Initiative (WHI), a large research program sponsored by the National Institute of Health (NIH) in the United States, demonstrated the detrimental effects of estrogen and combined estrogen–progestin therapy. Both studies attempted to determine the value of HRT, if any, in preventing diseases and conditions commonly affecting older women, including breast cancer, heart disease, stroke, and hip fracture. The WHI was launched in 1991 under the direction of the US National Heart, Lung, and Blood Institute (NHLBI). In one of the WHI studies of HRT, research subjects who took certain estrogen–progestin drugs were found to have an increased risk of breast cancer, heart disease, stroke, and blood clots, although their risks of hip fracture and colon cancer were reduced. These preliminary results were so alarming that this study of combined estrogen–progestin therapy was discontinued in 2002.

A part of the WHI investigation focusing on cognitive function, the WHI Memory Study, also identified adverse cognitive effects in women receiving combination estrogen–progestin therapy. These patients showed an increased risk of developing dementia and demonstrated reduced performance on tests of cognitive function. A second HRT study was begun in which women who had undergone hysterectomy received estrogen alone without progestin. In March 2004, however, these participants were advised to stop taking their assigned medications because the estrogen-only therapy appeared to be associated with an increased risk of stroke. The data also indicated that estrogen therapy had no effect on the rates of coronary artery disease or breast cancer but was associated with a reduced rate of hip fracture.

Since publication of the WHI studies, much confusion and controversy has arisen. One of the biggest challenges related to the WHI is that the majority of the women involved were at least 10 years postmenopause. Recent data have suggested that the use of estrogen in women who are younger is beneficial. Follow-up with the WHI study participants began in 2010. The North American Menopause Society (NAMS) also updated its position statement in 2012 regarding estrogen use in perimenopausal and postmenopausal women. The updated recommendations support the initiation of HT (hormone therapy) around the time of menopause to treat menopause-related symptoms and treat or reduce the risk of certain disorders, such as osteoporosis or fractures. The benefit–risk ratio for menopausal HT is favourable for women who initiate HT close to menopause but decreases in older women and with time since menopause. HRT is not recommended for women with histories of endometrial cancer. In women with breast cancer, estrogen therapy has not been proven safe and might raise recurrence risk. When hormone therapy is discontinued after several years of use, it is important to assess bone mineral density and begin treatment if indicated. Because HRT is a topic about which views are so rapidly changing, readers are referred to the website of the NAMS at www.menopause.org for the latest position statements. The Society of Obstetricians and Gynecologists of Canada supports the recommendations of the NAMS.

The pharmacological effects of all estrogens are similar because there are only slight differences in their chemical structure. These differences yield drugs of different potencies that in turn make them useful for a variety of indications. They also allow the drugs to be given by different routes of administration and often at highly customized doses.

Many fixed estrogen–progestin combination products have been developed over the years. Their use is commonly referred to as *continuous combined hormone replacement therapy*. The use of estrogen therapy alone has been associated with an increased risk of endometrial hyperplasia, a possible precursor of endometrial cancer. The addition of continuously administered progestin to an estrogen regimen reduces the incidence of endometrial hyperplasia associated with unopposed estrogen therapy. Examples of these fixed combinations are conjugated estrogens with medroxyprogesterone, norethindrone acetate with ethinyl estradiol, and estradiol with norethindrone acetate.

Indications

Progestins are useful in the treatment of functional uterine bleeding caused by a hormonal imbalance, fibroids, or uterine cancer; in the treatment of primary and secondary amenorrhea; in the adjunctive and palliative treatment of some cancers and endometriosis; and alone or in combination with estrogens in the prevention of conception. They may also be helpful in preventing a threatened miscarriage and alleviating the symptoms of premenstrual syndrome. Medroxyprogesterone is the most commonly used progestin. Norethindrone acetate is commonly used alone or in combination with estrogens as contraceptives. Megestrol is commonly used as adjunct therapy in the treatment of breast and endometrial cancers. When estrogen replacement therapy is initiated after menopause, progestins are

DOSAGES   Selected Estrogenic Drugs

Drug	Pharmacological Class	Usual Dosage Range	Indications
▶conjugated estrogens (C.E.S. Tablets, Congest, Premarin) and esterified estrogens (Estragyn)	Estrogenic hormone	PO: 0.3 mg/day cyclically, 3 wk on, 1 wk off or continuously PO: 0.3 mg/day; adjust to needs of patient PO: 0.3–0.625 mg/day cyclically, 3 wk on, 1 wk off or continuously PO: 1.25 mg/day cyclically, 3 wk on, 1 wk off or continuously; adjust to needs of patient	Atrophic vaginitis, vulvar atrophy Menopausal symptoms, osteoporosis Female hypogonadism Oophorectomy, primary ovarian failure
estradiol estradiol transdermal (Climara, Divigel, Estrogel, Sandoz Estradiol Derm, Oesclim)	Estrogenic hormone	Transdermal patch 0.05 mg, applied once a week on a clean, dry area of intact skin such as buttocks, lower abdomen or hip; adapted to patient needs	Vasomotor symptoms of menopause, osteoporosis prophylaxis
estradiol valerate	Estrogenic hormone	IM: Cyclic therapy schedule (28-day cycle; repeated every 4 weeks) Day 1 of each cycle: 20 mg; 2 wk after Day 1: 5 mg; 4 wk after Day 1: This is Day 1 of next cycle. Stop after 4 cycles	Amenorrhea, oophorectomy, primary ovarian failure, menopause, senile vaginitis, pruritus vulvae, palliation of inoperable progressing prostatic carcinoma in males

IM, intramuscular; *PO*, oral.

TABLE   35-3

Progestins: Common Adverse Effects

Body System	Adverse Effects
Gastrointestinal	Nausea, vomiting
Genitourinary	Amenorrhea, spotting
Other	Edema, weight gain or loss, rash, pyrexia, somnolence or insomnia, depression

often included to decrease the endometrial proliferation that can be caused by unopposed estrogen in women with an intact uterus. Formulations of progesterone are also used to treat female infertility (refer to the Dosages table on p. 670).

Contraindications

Contraindications for progestins are similar to those for estrogens.

Adverse Effects

The most serious undesirable adverse effects of progestin use include liver dysfunction, commonly manifested as jaundice, thrombophlebitis, and thromboembolic disorders such as pulmonary embolism. The more common adverse effects are listed in Table 35-3.

Interactions

There are reports of possible decreases in glucose tolerance when progestins are taken with antidiabetic drugs, and the dosage of the antidiabetic drug may need to be adjusted. The concurrent use of medroxyprogesterone or norethindrone or rifampin induces increased metabolism of the progestin.

Dosages

For recommended dosages of the progestins, refer to the table on p. 670.

SELECTIVE PROGESTERONE RECEPTOR MODULATOR

Ulipristal acetate (Fibristal®) is approved by Health Canada for treatment of moderate to severe signs and symptoms of uterine fibroids in adult women of reproductive age who are eligible for surgery. This is the first drug to be approved within a new class of drugs, that of the selective progesterone receptor modulators.

Uterine fibroids (leiomyomas) are benign, hormone-sensitive, smooth muscle tumours of the uterus. Fibroids are the most common tumours of the female reproductive tract in premenopausal women, with a prevalence of 40% in women between the age of 35 and 55 years (Health Canada, 2015). Fibroids occur more frequently and are more severe in Black women. The etiology of fibroids remains elusive and there are currently no long-term treatments available. Patients can be asymptomatic; however, symptoms may include heavy, prolonged menstrual bleeding and subsequent anemia; abdominal pressure; pelvic pain; increased urinary frequency; and infertility. Surgery includes myomectomy (surgical removal of fibroids) or a hysterectomy.

DRUG PROFILES

▶▶ medroxyprogesterone acetate

Medroxyprogesterone acetate (Depo-Provera®, Medroxy®, Provera®) inhibits the secretion of pituitary gonadotropins, which prevents follicular maturation and ovulation, stimulates the growth of mammary tissue, and has an antineoplastic action against endometrial cancer. Medroxyprogesterone is used to treat uterine bleeding, secondary amenorrhea, and endometrial cancer, and in combination with conjugated estrogens, is also used as a contraceptive. Its most common use is to prevent endometrial cancer caused by estrogen replacement therapy. It is sometimes used as adjunct therapy in certain types of cancer (Chapter 52). Medroxyprogesterone is available in oral and parenteral preparations. It is also available in a long-acting injection formulation called Depo-Provera. Depo-Provera is used for birth control, and one injection prevents conception for 3 months. There is concern about its use in women younger than 25 years of age and in its use for longer than 2 years due to the potential for bone density loss it creates.

PHARMACOKINETICS

Route	Onset of Action	Peak Plasma Concentration	Elimination Half-Life	Duration of Action
IM	Unknown	3 hr	50 days	3 mo

▶▶ megestrol acetate

Megestrol acetate (Megace®) is a synthetic progestin that is structurally similar to progesterone. Although megestrol shares the actions of the progestins, it is primarily used in the palliative management of recurrent, inoperable, or metastatic endometrial or breast cancer. Because it can cause appetite stimulation and weight gain, it is also used in the management of anorexia, cachexia, or unexplained substantial weight loss in patients with cancer. It is available only for oral use.

PHARMACOKINETICS

Route	Onset of Action	Peak Plasma Concentration	Elimination Half-Life	Duration of Action
PO	6–8 wk	1–3 hr	13–105 hr	4–10 mo

DOSAGES   Selected Progestational Drugs

Drug	Pharmacological Class	Usual Dosage Range	Indications
▶▶ medroxyprogesterone acetate (Depo-Provera, Medroxy, Premplus, Provera-Pak)	Progestin	PO: 5–10 mg/day for set number of days or cyclically (smaller doses may be given on a continuous daily basis)	Amenorrhea, uterine bleeding
		PO: 2.5–10 mg daily on last 10–14 days of each month to accompany estrogen dosing	Vasomotor symptoms of menopause
megestrol acetate (Megace)	Antineoplastic, hormone, apetite stimulant, progestin	PO: 400–800 mg/day	Anorexia, cachexia, or significant weight loss in patients with cancer
		PO: 160 mg/day	Palliative or adjunctive breast carcinoma
		PO: 80–320 mg/day divided	Endometrial carcinoma
		PO: 120 mg/day, single dose	Advanced hormone-responsive carcinoma of prostate

IM, intramuscular; *PO*, oral.

Ulipristal is a tissue-specific, partial progesterone antagonist. It reduces or eliminates uterine bleeding through its antiproliferative effect on endometrial tissue. It also reduces the size of fibroids by inhibiting cell proliferation and causing cell death. The usual dose is one 5-mg tablet per day, taken continuously for 3 months. Ulipristal should be initiated during the first 7 days of the menstrual period. The drug is contraindicated during pregnancy or in women who have a hypersensitivity to the drug.

CONTRACEPTIVE DRUGS

Contraceptive drugs are medications used to prevent pregnancy. Contraceptive devices are methods of pregnancy prevention such as reversible intrauterine devices,

male and female condoms, cervical diaphragms, and others, which are beyond the scope of a pharmacology text. However, it is important to note that long-acting reversible contraceptive methods (e.g., intrauterine devices and implants) are superior in preventing pregnancy when compared to other common contraceptive methods, including oral contraceptive pills, transdermal patch, contraceptive vaginal ring, and depot medroxyprogesterone acetate injection (Winner et al., 2012). Patients must be informed, for their own safety, of the fact that the use of contraceptive drug therapy only prevents pregnancy. These includes spermicidal drugs, such as the over-the-counter (OTC) foams for intravaginal use. These products most often contain the spermicide nonoxynol-9, which does kill sperm cells to prevent pregnancy but does not necessarily kill microbes capable of causing sexually transmitted infections, including HIV infection.

Estrogen–progestin combinations, often referred to as "the pill," are oral contraceptives that contain both estrogenic and progestational steroids. The most common estrogenic component is ethinyl estradiol, a semisynthetic steroidal estrogen. The most common progestin components are norethindrone and drospirenone.

The currently available oral contraceptives may be *biphasic*, *triphasic*, or *monophasic*, depending on the doses taken at different times of the menstrual cycle. The newest are the extended-cycle oral contraceptives. The biphasic drugs contain a fixed estrogen dose combined with a low progestin dose for the first 10 days and a higher progestin dose for the rest of the cycle; they are available in 21- or 28-day dosage packages. The triphasic products most closely duplicate the normal hormonal levels of the female cycle. There are also oral contraceptives that are progestin-only drugs. The monophasic and triphasic oral contraceptives are the most numerous on the market and the most widely prescribed. The extended-cycle oral contraceptives differ from the traditional 21 days on, 7 days off pills by decreasing or eliminating the hormone-free dosing interval. Consecutive days of hormone therapy may extend to between 84 and 365 days. Reasons for switching to an extended-cycle product include improved efficacy in women who forget to restart the pill and patient preference to decrease the frequency of menstrual bleeding. Some patients (e.g., those with menstrual irregularities) may require special assistance in selecting drug products with their health care providers. Three other important contraceptive medications are a long-acting injectable form of medroxyprogesterone, a transdermal contraceptive patch, and, most recently, an intravaginal contraceptive ring.

Mechanism of Action and Drug Effects

Oral contraceptive drugs have the same hormonal effects as the endogenous estrogen and progesterone. The drugs inhibit the release of gonadotropins by the hypothalamic-pituitary system, thus inhibiting ovulation. The exogenous hormones also directly increases uterine mucous viscosity, which results in (1) decreased sperm movement and fertilization of the ovum and (2) possible inhibition of implantation (nidation) of a fertilized egg (zygote) into the endometrial lining

Other incidental benefits to their use are that they improve menstrual cycle regularity and decrease blood loss during menstruation. A decreased incidence of functional ovarian cysts and ectopic pregnancies has also been associated with their use.

Indications

Oral contraceptives are used primarily to prevent pregnancy. In addition, they are used to treat endometriosis and hypermenorrhea and to produce cyclic withdrawal bleeding in patients with amenorrhea. Occasionally,

combination oral contraceptives are used to provide postcoital contraception. Postcoital contraception pills are not effective if the woman is already pregnant (i.e., egg implantation has occurred). They should be taken within 72 hours of unprotected intercourse with a follow-up dose 12 hours after the first dose. They are intended to prevent pregnancy after known or suspected contraceptive failure or unprotected intercourse. Ovral® is an ethinyl estradiol (50 mcg) and levonorgestrel (250 mcg) combination drug that is commonly used for this indication. It is taken orally and repeated 12 hours later. Levonorgestrel (Plan B®, NorLevo®, Next Choice®) is also used for postcoital contraception. Plan B and NorLevo consist of two tablets of levonorgestrel 750 mcg taken as a single dose. Next Choice consists of two tablets of levonorgestrel 750 mcg taken 12 hours apart.

One new oral contraceptive of note is Seasonale®, which includes both estrogen and progestin components. It is sold in packages containing 3 months of medication, including 1 week of nonhormonal tablets because Seasonale reduces a woman's menstrual cycles to once every 3 months.

Contraindications

Contraindications to the use of oral contraceptives include known drug allergy to a specific product, pregnancy, and known high risk for or history of thromboembolic events such as myocardial infarction (MI), venous thrombosis, pulmonary embolism, or stroke, history of current breast cancer. Women older than 35 years who smoke, patients with diabetes who have vascular disease, migraine headache in patients older than 35 years, and hypercoagulopathies.

Adverse Effects

Common adverse effects associated with the use of oral contraceptives are listed in Table 35-4. These effects include hypertension, thromboembolism, alterations in carbohydrate and lipid metabolism, increases in serum hormone concentrations, and alterations in serum metal

TABLE	35-4

Oral Contraceptives: Common Adverse Effects

Body System	Adverse Effects
Cardiovascular	Hypertension, edema, thromboembolism, pulmonary embolism, myocardial infarction
Central nervous	Dizziness, headache, migraines, depression, stroke
Gastrointestinal	Nausea, vomiting, diarrhea, anorexia, cramps, constipation, increased weight, cholestatic jaundice
Genitourinary	Amenorrhea, cervical erosion, breakthrough bleeding, dysmenorrhea, breast changes

DOSAGES Selected Contraceptive Medications

Drug	Pharmacological Class	Usual Dosage Range	Indications
Oral Contraceptives			
Levonorgestrel and ethinyl estradiol (Alesse, Alysena, Avian, Esme®, Min-Ovral®, Ovima®, Portia®)	Biphasic: fixed estrogen–variable progestin 21- or 28-day products	3 or 4 monthly phases of variable estrogen and progestin combinations; 21- or 28-day products; 28-day products contain 7 inert tabs	Prevention of pregnancy
norethindrone and ethinyl estradiol (Brevicon®, Loestrin®, Symphasic®)	Monophasic: fixed estrogen–progestin combinations; 21- or 28-day products	Monthly phase of 21-day or 28-day products; 28-day products contain 7 inert tablets	
levonorgestrel and ethinyl estradiol (Ortho 7/7/7®, Triquilar®)	Triphasic: 3 or 4 monthly phases of variable estrogen and progestin combinations	Monthly phase of 21-day or 28-day products; 28-day products contain 7 inert tablets	
levonorgestrel and ethinyl estradiol (Seasonale)	Extended-cycle products		
Injectable Contraceptives (Depot)			
⇥medroxyprogesterone acetate (Depo-Provera)	Progestin-only injectable contraceptive	IM: 150 mg q3 months	
Transdermal Contraceptives			
norelgestromin and ethinyl estradiol (Ortho Evra®)	Fixed-combination estrogen–progestin transdermal contraceptive	Transdermal patch: 1 patch applied weekly × 3 each month, scheduled around menses in week 4	
Intravaginal Contraceptives			
etonogestrel/ethinyl estradiol vaginal ring (NuvaRing®)	Fixed-combination estrogen–progestin intravaginal contraceptive	One ring inserted into vagina by patient and left in place for 3 weeks, followed by 1-week removal. A new ring is then inserted.	

IM, intramuscular.

ion concentrations (e.g., zinc, selenium, phosphorus, magnesium) and plasma protein levels. It is the estrogen component that appears to be the source of most of these metabolic effects.

Interactions

Several drugs and drug classes can potentially reduce the effectiveness of oral contraceptives, resulting in an unintended pregnancy. Educate patients about the need to use alternative birth control methods for at least 1 month during and after taking any of the following drugs: antibiotics (especially penicillins and cephalosporins), barbiturates, isoniazid, and rifampin. The effectiveness of other drugs, such as anticonvulsants, β-blockers, hypnotics, antidiabetic drugs, warfarin, theophylline, tricyclic antidepressants, and vitamins, may be reduced when they are taken with oral contraceptives.

Dosages

For the recommended dosages of oral contraceptives, refer to the table above.

Contraceptive Drugs

The Dosages table above provides selected examples of the many contraceptive drugs available. All work in similar fashion to prevent pregnancy. They are not to be used during pregnancy. Drugs that are intended for termination of pregnancy are known as *abortifacients* and are discussed later in this chapter.

DRUGS FOR OSTEOPOROSIS

Over their life time, 1 in 3 Canadian women and 1 in 5 men will experience a fracture as a direct result of **osteoporosis**, characterized by low bone density and deterioration of bone tissue. The majority of fractures (over 80%) occur in individuals over the age of 50 and are more prevalent than heart attacks, strokes and breast cancer combined. The annual cost to Canadian society is estimated at $2.3 billion (Osteoporosis Canada, 2015). Risk factors for postmenopausal osteoporosis include gender, age, a fragility fracture over the age of 40, a parent who has had a hip fracture, use of glucocorticoid drugs for more than 3 months, vertebral compression fracture, medical conditions in which absorption of nutrients is inhibited, and any other medical condition that may cause bone loss (Osteoporosis Canada, 2015). Additional risk factors include smoking, heavy alcohol consumption, particularly during adolescence and young adulthood, menopause before age 45, low estrogen levels, and weight under 60 kg. The emphasis of the most recent osteoporosis guidelines is on the need to assess for fracture risk with the goal of preventing the excess morbidity, mortality, and economic burden associated with osteoporosis and associated fragility fractures. Approximately 30 000 hip fractures occur annually in Canada, with 1 in 3 patients with hip fracture refracturing within 1 year and more than 1 in 2 within 5 years (Osteoporosis Canada, 2015).

Peak bone mass is achieved between the ages of 16 to 20 in girls and between the ages of 20 to 25 in young men. Bone loss begins in the mid-30s for both women and men, and at menopause, women begin to lose bone at a rate of between 2 and 3% per year (Osteoporosis Canada, 2015). Supplementation with calcium and vitamin D is thought to play a role in the prevention of osteoporosis. Current Canadian recommendations are that women older than age 50 have a daily intake of 1 200 mg of calcium through diet and supplements (those from 19 to 50 should have a daily intake of 1 000 mg). Also to support bone health, Osteoporosis Canada (2015) recommends daily supplementation with 800 to 2 000 units of vitamin D for adults over the age of 50 or young adults at high risk (and 400 to 1 000 units for adults between the age of 19 to 50).

Several drug classes are used for the treatment of existing osteoporosis: the bisphosphonates, the selective estrogen receptor modulators (SERMs), the hormones calcitonin and teriparatide, and, more recently, denosumab. Currently available bisphosphonates used for osteoporosis prevention and treatment include alendronate, etidronate disodium in combination with 500 mg of calcium carbonate (Didrocal® and Etidrocal® are the only forms used for the treatment of osteoporosis), risedronate sodium hemipentahydrate, (Actonel®, Actonel DR®) and once-a-year injection of zoledronic acid. Raloxifene and tamoxifen are the currently available SERMs. Tamoxifen is primarily used in oncology settings and is discussed further in Chapter 53. Raloxifene is indicated for use in the prevention and treatment of osteoporosis. Teriparatide stimulates bone formation, while denosumab (Prolia®, Xgeva®) prevents bone resorption.

Mechanism of Action and Drug Effects
Bisphosphonates

The bisphosphonates work by inhibiting osteoclast-mediated bone resorption, which in turn indirectly enhances bone mineral density. Osteoclasts are bone cells that break down bone, causing calcium to be reabsorbed into the circulation; this resorption eventually leads to osteoporosis if not controlled or countered by adequate

new bone formation. Strong clinical evidence indicates these drugs cause reversal of lost bone mass and reduction of fracture risk, and, as a result, they are considered drugs of choice for this condition.

Selective Estrogen Receptor Modulators

Raloxifene helps prevent osteoporosis by stimulating estrogen receptors on bone and increasing bone density in a manner similar to the estrogens.

Teriparatide

In contrast to the other therapies described thus far, which inhibit bone resorption, teriparatide is the first and currently only drug available that acts by stimulating bone formation. It is a derivative of parathyroid hormone and acts to treat osteoporosis by modulating the body's metabolism of calcium and phosphorus in a manner similar to that of the natural parathyroid hormone.

Denosumab

Denosumab (Prolia) is a monoclonal antibody that blocks osteoclast activation, thereby preventing bone resorption. It is given as a subcutaneous injection once every 6 months along with daily calcium and vitamin D supplementation. Denosumab is used in the treatment of osteoporosis and bone metastases.

Indications

Raloxifene is used primarily for the prevention of postmenopausal osteoporosis. The bisphosphonates and calcitonin are used in both the prevention and treatment of osteoporosis. Teriparatide is used mainly for the subset of osteoporosis patients at highest risk of fracture (e.g., those with prior fracture).

Contraindications
Bisphosphonates

Contraindications to bisphosphonate use include drug allergy, hypocalcemia, esophageal dysfunction, and the inability to sit or stand upright for at least 30 minutes after taking the medication (see further discussion below under adverse effects).

Selective Estrogen Receptor Modulators

Use of SERMs is contraindicated in women with a known allergy to these drugs, in women who are or may become pregnant, and in women with a history of or a current venous thromboembolic disorder, including DVT, pulmonary embolism, and retinal vein thrombosis.

Teriparatide

Contraindications to the use of teriparatide include known drug allergy.

Denosumab

Contraindications to the use of denosumab are hypocalcemia, kidney impairment or failure, and infection.

Adverse Effects

The primary adverse effects of SERMs are hot flashes and leg cramps. They can increase the risk of venous thromboembolism and are teratogenic. Leukopenia may also occur and predispose the patient to various infections. The most common adverse effects of bisphosphonates include headache, GI upset, and joint pain. However, the bisphosphonates are usually well tolerated. There is a risk of esophageal burns with these medications if they become lodged in the esophagus before reaching the stomach. For this reason, patients must take these medications with a full glass of water and must remain sitting upright or standing for at least 30 minutes afterward. Several case reports of osteonecrosis of the jaw in patients taking bisphosphonates have been released. Health Canada issued a public health advisory in 2011 alerting health care providers to the possible association between long-term bisphosphonate use and the development of severe (possibly incapacitating) bone, muscle, or joint pain, as well as low energy fractures. Intravenous (IV) bisphosphonates are often associated with an acute-phase reaction within 24 to 72 hours of the infusion, characterized by low grade fever, myalgias, and arthralgias. These symptoms subside with subsequent infusions. The risk of atypical fracture of the femur is reported to be less than 1%; this is thought to be the result of bone turnover suppression, during which old bone is replaced with new at a slow pace, resulting in microfractures and potential fracture. Common adverse effects of teriparatide include chest pain, dizziness, hypercalcemia, nausea, and arthralgia. Infections occur more frequently in those taking denosumab.

Interactions

Cholestyramine and ampicillin decrease the absorption of raloxifene, and raloxifene can decrease the effects of warfarin sodium. Calcium supplements and antacids can interfere with the absorption of the bisphosphonates, and therefore they need to be spaced 1 to 2 hours apart to avoid this interaction. Aspirin and other nonsteroidal anti-inflammatory drugs (NSAIDs) have the potential for additive GI irritation if taken with bisphosphonates.

Dosages

For the recommended dosages of osteoporosis drugs, refer to the table on p. 675.

DRUG PROFILES

▶▶ *alendronate sodium*

Alendronate sodium (Fosamax®) is an oral bisphosphonate and the first nonestrogen–nonhormonal option for preventing bone loss. This drug acts by inhibiting or reversing osteoclast-mediated born resorption. Recall that osteoclasts are the bone cells that cause breakdown or resorption of bone tissue as part of their normal physiological action. However, unchecked osteoclastic activity often leads to osteoporosis if not managed, so this drug represents a major breakthrough in the treatment of osteoporosis. It is indicated for the prevention and treatment of osteoporosis in men and in postmenopausal women. It is also indicated for the treatment of glucocorticoid-induced osteoporosis in men and for the treatment of Paget's disease in women. Data show that alendronate may reduce the risk of hip fracture by 51%, of spinal fracture by 47%, and of wrist fracture by 48%. Take precautions in patients with dysphagia, esophagitis, esophageal ulcer, or gastric ulcer because the drug can be extremely irritating to esophageal tissue. Case reports of esophageal erosions have been published. It is recommended that alendronate be taken with 240 mL of water immediately upon rising in the morning and that patients not lie down for at least 30 minutes after taking it. When patients whose condition has been stabilized on alendronate are hospitalized and cannot adhere to these recommendations, the medication is often withheld. Alendronate has an extremely long-term half-life, and so going several days without taking a dose will do little to reduce the therapeutic efficacy of the drug. There is debate on how long a woman should remain on bisphosphonate therapy, with most experts recommending a drug holiday after approximately 5 to 10 years.

Alendronate is available in tablet form combined with 2 800 and 5 600 units of vitamin D (Fosavance®). It can be taken daily (10 mg) or weekly (70 mg) for treatment of osteoporosis.

PHARMACOKINETICS

Route	Onset of Action	Peak Plasma Concentration	Elimination Half-Life	Duration of Action
PO	3 wk	Unknown	Longer than 10 yr due to storage in bone tissue	Unknown

raloxifene hydrochloride

Raloxifene hydrochloride (Evista®) is a SERM. It is used primarily for the prevention of postmenopausal osteoporosis. Interestingly, raloxifene has positive effects on cholesterol levels, but it is not normally used specifically for this purpose. It may not be the best choice for women near menopause because use of the drug is associated with the adverse effect of hot flashes. It is available only for oral use.

PHARMACOKINETICS

Route	Onset of Action	Peak Plasma Concentration	Elimination Half-Life	Duration of Action
PO	8 wk	Unknown	28 hr	Unknown

DOSAGES   Selected Drugs Used Specifically for Osteoporosis

Drug	Pharmacological Class	Usual Dosage Range	Indications
▸▸alendronate sodium (Fosamax)	Bisphosphonate	PO: 5 mg/day PO: 10 mg/day or 70 mg/wk	Osteoporosis prevention and treatment
etidronate disodium (Ditrocal, Etidrocal)	Biphosphonate and calcium	PO: cyclical regimen administered in 90-day cycles. Each white 400 mg etidronate disodium tablet is taken once daily × 14 days, followed by 76 blue calcium carbonate tablets to be taken once daily × next 76 days	Osteoporosis prevention and treatment
risedronate sodium (Actonel, Actonel DR)	Biphosphonate	PO: 5 mg/day; 35 mg/wk; 150 mg once monthly	Osteoporosis prevention and treatment
raloxifene hydrochloride (Evista)	Selective estrogen receptor modulator	PO: 60 mg daily	Osteoporosis prevention and treatment

PO, oral.

Drugs Related to Pregnancy, Labour, Delivery, and the Postpartum Period

FERTILITY DRUGS

Infertility in women is often the result of the absence of ovulation (anovulation), which is normally due to various imbalances in female reproductive hormones. Such imbalances can occur at the level of the hypothalamus, the pituitary gland, the ovary, or any combination of these. Exogenous administration of estrogens or progestins may be used to fortify the blood levels of these hormones when ovarian output is inadequate. The uses of the drug forms of these hormones were described earlier in this chapter.

Hormone deficiencies at the hypothalamic and pituitary levels are often treated with gonadotropin ovarian stimulants. These drugs stimulate increased secretion of gonadotropin-releasing hormone (Gn-RH) from the hypothalamus, which then results in increased secretion of FSH and LH from the pituitary gland. These hormones, in turn, stimulate the development of ovarian follicles and thus ovulation. They also stimulate ovarian secretion of the estrogens and progestins that are part of the normal ovulatory cycle. Proper selection and dosage adjustment of fertility drugs often requires the expertise of a fertility specialist. The various medical techniques used in the treatment of infertility, including drug therapy, are now collectively referred to as *assistive reproductive technology*. One common specific technique is in vitro fertilization, during which a woman's ovum is fertilized with her partner's sperm in a laboratory and the fertilized ovum is then medically implanted into the woman's uterus. The success of such fertilization techniques may be further encouraged with the use of medications such as those described earlier. Representative examples of ovulation-stimulant drugs include the drugs clomiphene, menotropins, and choriogonadotropin alfa.

Mechanism of Action and Drug Effects

Clomiphene is a nonsteroidal ovulation stimulant that works by blocking estrogen receptors in the uterus and brain. This action results in a false signal of low estrogen levels to the brain. The hypothalamus and pituitary gland then increase their production of Gn-RH (from the hypothalamus) and FSH and LH (from the pituitary), which stimulates the maturation of ovarian follicles. Ideally, this sequence of events leads to ovulation and increases the likelihood of conception in a previously infertile woman.

Menotropins is the drug name for a standardized mixture of FSH and LH that is derived from the urine of postmenopausal women. The FSH component stimulates the development of ovarian follicles, which leads to ovulation. The LH component stimulates the development of the corpus luteum, which supplies female sex hormones (estrogens and progesterone) during the first trimester of pregnancy. Choriogonadotropin alfa is a recombinant form (i.e., developed using recombinant DNA technology) of the hormone human chorionic gonadotropin. This hormone is naturally produced by the placenta during pregnancy and can be isolated from the urine of pregnant women. It is an analogue of LH and can provide a substitute for the natural LH surge that promotes ovulation. It does this by binding to LH receptors in the ovary and stimulating the rupture of mature ovarian follicles and the subsequent development of the corpus luteum. Human chorionic gonadotropin also maintains the viability of the corpus luteum during early pregnancy. This is crucial because the corpus luteum provides the supply of estrogens and progesterone necessary to support the first trimester of pregnancy until the placenta assumes this role. Choriogonadotropin alfa is often given in a carefully timed fashion following FSH-active therapy, such as with menotropins or clomiphene, when patient monitoring indicates sufficient maturation of ovarian follicles.

Indications

The drugs just discussed are used primarily for the promotion of ovulation in anovulatory female patients. They may also be used to promote spermatogenesis in infertile men. As was mentioned in the section on progestins, progesterone formulations are also used to treat female infertility.

Contraindications

Contraindications to the use of ovarian stimulants include known drug allergy to a specific product and may also include primary ovarian failure, uncontrolled thyroid or adrenal dysfunction, liver disease, pituitary tumour, abnormal uterine bleeding, ovarian enlargement of uncertain cause, sex hormone–dependent tumours, and pregnancy.

Adverse Effects

The most common adverse effects of the ovulation stimulants are listed in Table 35-5.

Interactions

The most notable drugs that interact with fertility drugs are the tricyclic antidepressants, the butyrophenones (e.g., haloperidol), the phenothiazines (e.g., promethazine hydrochloride), and the antihypertensive drug meth-

yldopa. When any of these drugs are taken with fertility drugs, prolactin concentrations may be increased, which may impair fertility.

Dosages

For recommended dosages of clomiphene, refer to the table below.

UTERINE STIMULANTS

A variety of medications are used to alter the dynamics of uterine contractions either to promote or prevent the start or progression of labour. In the immediate postpartum period, medications may also be used to promote rapid shrinkage (involution) of the uterus to reduce the risk of postpartum hemorrhage.

Three types of drugs are used to stimulate uterine contractions: ergot derivatives, prostaglandins, and the hormone oxytocin. These drugs all act on the uterus, a highly muscular organ that has a complex network of smooth muscle fibres and a large blood supply. They are often collectively referred to as *oxytocics*, after the naturally occurring hormone oxytocin, whose action they mimic. The uterus undergoes several changes during normal gestation and childbirth that at different times make it either resistant or susceptible to various hormones and drugs. Oxytocin is one of the two hormones secreted by the posterior lobe of the pituitary gland; the other is vasopressin, which is also known as *antidiuretic hormone* (see Chapter 31).

Mechanism of Action and Drug Effects

The uterus of a woman who is not pregnant is relatively insensitive to oxytocin, but during pregnancy, the uterus becomes more sensitive to this hormone and is most sensitive at term (the end of gestation).

During childbirth, oxytocin stimulates uterine contraction, and during lactation it promotes the movement of milk from the mammary glands to the nipples. Another class of oxytocic drugs is the prostaglandins, natural

TABLE 35-5

Fertility Drugs: Most Common Adverse Effects

Body System	Adverse Effects
Cardiovascular	Tachycardia, phlebitis, deep vein thrombosis, hypovolemia
Central nervous	Dizziness, headache, flushing, depression, restlessness, anxiety, nervousness, fatigue
Gastrointestinal	Nausea, bloating, constipation, vomiting, anorexia
Other	Urticaria, ovarian hyperstimulation, multiple pregnancies (twins or more), blurred vision, diplopia, photophobia, breast pain

DRUG PROFILES

clomiphene citrate

Clomiphene citrate (Clomid®, Serophene®) is used primarily to stimulate the production of pituitary gonadotropins, which in turn induces the maturation of the ovarian follicle and eventually ovulation. It is currently available only for oral use.

PHARMACOKINETICS

Route	Onset of Action	Peak Plasma Concentration	Elimination Half-Life	Duration of Action
PO	4–12 days	6 hr	5 days	30 days

DOSAGES   Selected Fertility Drugs

Drug	Pharmacological Class	Usual Dosage Range	Indications
clomiphene citrate (Clomid, Serophene)	Ovulation stimulant	PO: 50–100 mg daily for 5 days; cycle repeatable depending on response	Female infertility in selected patients

PO, oral.

hormones involved in regulating the network of smooth muscle fibres of the uterus. This network is known as the *myometrium*. Prostaglandins cause potent contractions of the myometrium and may also play a role in the natural induction of labour. When prostaglandin concentrations increase during the final few weeks of pregnancy, mild myometrial contractions, commonly known as Braxton Hicks contractions, are stimulated. The third major class of oxytocic drugs is the ergot alkaloids, which are also potent simulators of uterine muscle. These drugs increase the force and frequency of uterine contractions.

Indications

Oxytocin is available in a synthetic injectable form. This drug is used to induce labour at or near full-term gestation and to enhance labour when uterine contractions are weak and ineffective. Oxytocin is also used to prevent or control uterine bleeding after delivery, to induce completion of an incomplete abortion (including miscarriages), and to promote milk ejection during lactation.

The prostaglandins may be used therapeutically to induce labour by softening the cervix and enhancing uterine muscle tone. Cervical ripening (softening of the cervix) is determined by the Bishop score, a system used to determine the readiness of the cervix for induction of labour. The Bishop score is determined by assigning points to five measurements of the pelvic examination: dilation, effacement of the cervix, station of the fetus, consistency of the cervix, and position of the cervix.

The prostaglandins may also be used to stimulate the myometrium to induce abortion during the second trimester when the uterus is resistant to oxytocin. Examples of these drugs are dinoprostone and misoprostol. Misoprostol is an oral tablet and is also used as a stomach protectant (see Chapter 39). It is used off-label for cervical ripening and is administered orally or intravaginally. It offers the advantage of lower cost as opposed to the more expensive drug dinoprostone. Because of this, misoprostol is widely used in developing countries as well as in Canada. Be aware that the prescribing information states that misoprostol should not be used in this way; however, it is common to see it used thusly clinically.

Ergot alkaloids are used after delivery of the infant and placenta to prevent postpartum uterine atony (lack of muscle tone) and hemorrhage.

Mifepristone (Mifegymiso®) is a progesterone antagonist that stimulates uterine contractions and is used to induce elective termination of pregnancy at between 7 and 9 weeks. The drug is often given with the synthetic prostaglandin drug misoprostol for this purpose. Approved in 2015 by Health Canada, it will become available in 2016.

Contraindications

Contraindications to the use of labour-inducing uterine stimulants include known drug allergy to a specific product. Additional contraindications may include pelvic inflammatory disease, cervical stenosis, uterine fibrosis,

TABLE	35-6
Oxytocic Drugs: Most Common Adverse Effects	
Body System	**Adverse Effects**
Cardiovascular	Hypotension or hypertension, chest pain
Central nervous	Headache, dizziness, fainting
Gastrointestinal	Nausea, vomiting, diarrhea
Genitourinary	Vaginitis, vaginal pain, cramping
Other	Leg cramps, joint swelling, chills, fever, weakness, blurred vision

high-risk intrauterine fetal positions before delivery, placenta previa, hypertonic uterus, uterine prolapse, or any condition in which vaginal delivery is contraindicated (e.g., increased bleeding risk). Contraindications to the use of abortifacients include known drug allergy, the presence of an intrauterine device, ectopic pregnancy, concurrent anticoagulant therapy or bleeding disorder, inadequate access to emergency health care, or inability to understand or adhere to follow-up instructions.

Adverse Effects

The most common undesirable effects of oxytocic drugs are listed in Table 35-6.

Interactions

Few clinically significant drug interactions occur with the oxytocic drugs. The most common and important of these involve sympathomimetic drugs. Combining drugs that produce vasoconstriction, such as the sympathomimetics, with oxytocic drugs can result in severe hypertension.

Dosages

For the recommended dosages of selected oxytocic drugs, refer to the table on p. 678.

DRUGS FOR PRETERM LABOUR MANAGEMENT

Preterm labour is defined as substantial uterine contractions that could progress to delivery, occurring prior to the 37th week of pregnancy. When contractions of the uterus begin before term, it may be desirable to stop labour because premature birth increases the risk of neonatal death. Postponing delivery increases the likelihood of the infant's survival. However, this measure is generally employed only between weeks 20 to 37 of gestation because spontaneous labour occurring before the 20th week is commonly associated with a nonviable fetus and thus is usually not interrupted.

The nonpharmacological treatment of premature labour includes bedrest, sedation, and hydration. Drugs given to inhibit labour and maintain the pregnancy are called *tocolytics*. Tocolytics have generally been found

DRUG PROFILES

▸▸ dinoprostone

Dinoprostone (Prostin E$_2$®, Cervidil®, Prepidil®) is a synthetic derivative of the naturally occurring hormone prostaglandin E$_2$. It is used for ripening of an unfavourable cervix in pregnant women, at or near term, with a medical or obstetric need for labour induction. It is available for vaginal use as a gel in various dosage forms, a vaginal insert, and for oral use.

PHARMACOKINETICS

Route	Onset of Action	Peak Plasma Concentration	Elimination Half-Life	Duration of Action
Vaginal	10 min	2.5–5 min	Unknown	Not available

▸▸ ergonovine maleate

The ergot alkaloid ergonovine maleate is used primarily in the immediate postpartum period to enhance myometrial tone and reduce the likelihood of postpartum uterine hemorrhage. Its use is contraindicated in patients with a known hypersensitivity to ergot medications and in those with pelvic inflammatory disease. It should be used with caution in patients with hypertension. It is not to be used for augmentation of labour, before delivery of the placenta, or during a spontaneous abortion; it should also not be given to patients with pregnancy-induced hypertension. Ergonovine maleate is available for injection use.

PHARMACOKINETICS

Route	Onset of Action	Peak Plasma Concentration	Elimination Half-Life	Duration of Action
IM	2–5 min	30 min	0.5–2 hr	3 hr

▸▸ oxytocin

The drug oxytocin is the synthetic form of the endogenous hormone oxytocin and has all of its pharmacological properties.

PHARMACOKINETICS

Route	Onset of Action	Peak Plasma Concentration	Elimination Half-Life	Duration of Action
IV	Immediate	Immediate	3–5 min	1 hr

DOSAGES   Selected Uterine Stimulants

Drug	Pharmacological Class	Usual Dosage Range	Indications
▸▸ dinoprostone (Prostin E$_2$, Cervidil, Prepidil)	Prostaglandin E$_2$ abortifacient and cervical ripening drug	Vaginal insert (Cervidil): 10 mg (released at 0.3 mg/h over 12 hr) placed transversely into posterior vaginal fornix (the space behind the cervix)	Cervical ripening for induction of labour
		Cervical gel (Prostin E$_2$ gel): 1 mg in posterior fornix of vaginal canal; 1–2 mg repeated once in 6 hr	Cervical ripening for induction of labour
		PO: Tablets (Prostin E$_2$): 0.5 mg followed by 0.5 mg/hr × 8 hr	Elective and indicated induction of labour
		Vaginal gel (Prepidil): 0.5 mg into internal cervical os	Cervical ripening for induction of labour
▸▸ ergonovine maleate	Oxytocic ergot alkaloid	IM: 200 mcg after delivery of placenta, repeatable at 2- to 4-hr intervals, up to 5 doses	Postpartum uterine atony and hemorrhage
		IV: 200 mcg in 5 mL NS over 1 min	Emergency situations of excessive uterine bleeding
▸▸ oxytocin (X)	Oxytocic hypothalamic hormone	IV infusion: 1–2 microunits/min, titrated to effect	Labour induction
		IV: 10–40 units in 1 L of nonhydrating solution titrated to effect	Postpartum uterine atony and hemorrhage
		IM: 10 units in a single dose after delivery of placenta	

IM, intramuscular; *IV*, intravenous; *NS*, normal saline; *PO*, oral.

useful only in the short term to delay labour and allow for the administration of corticosteroids to accelerate the maturity of fetal lung development. Generally, tocolytics can delay labour for approximately 48 hours. Clear evidence that tocolytics reduce neonatal mortality or serious neonatal morbidity is limited. Currently available tocolytics, including the NSAIDs indomethacin and naproxen (considered prostaglandin synthesis inhibitors), the calcium channel blocker nifedipidine, and magnesium sulphate have not been shown to significantly improve outcomes. A Canadian-led study on nitroglycerin found that neonatal outcomes were improved but the overall effect was insignificant (Guo et al., 2011). Neonatal outcome improvement may be associated with the smooth muscle relaxation effect of nitroglycerin and improved placental blood flow. Because of the lack of evidence on the use of tocolytics in Canada, further discussion is not warranted here.

PHARMACOKINETIC BRIDGE TO NURSING PRACTICE

Estradot® is a form of estrogen that is approved to help ease the severity of postmenopausal hot flashes by increasing estrogen levels when these are found to be deficient in the patient. Estradot contains estradiol, which is identical to endogenous estrogen produced in women's bodies. The absorption of the topical emulsion dosage form results in measurable levels of estradiol on the skin for up to 8 hours after application. It is important to fully understand this pharmacokinetic property because the transfer of the drug to another individual may result. In fact, traces of Estradot have been found on other individuals from such transfer for up to a 2-day period. This transfer of medication to other individuals may be reduced by allowing the dosage form to fully dry and then covering it with clothing before having contact with another individual. Although no specific investigation of the tissue distribution of the estradiol absorbed from Estradot in humans has been conducted, it is known that the distribution of exogenous estrogens is similar to that of endogenous estrogens. The metabolism of exogenous estrogens is also similar to that of endogenous estrogens, with biotransformation taking place mainly in the liver and excretion in the urine. The specific dosage form of an emulsion is desirable because it may be applied easily, once daily to the thighs or calves. One dose is contained in two separate foil pouches, and patients need to be fully aware of the application instructions. For example, sunscreen products are not to be applied at the same time because sunscreen reduces the absorption of Estradot.

Knowing the pharmacokinetic properties of Estradot is necessary for safe and efficient administration of the drug. It is also important to understand all the pharmacokinetic properties of this drug to be able to thoroughly educate patients about the drug, its effect on the body, and subsequent implications for its absorption, distribution, metabolism, and excretion.

PITUITARY GONADOTROPIN INHIBITOR

Another drug used for women's health is the synthetic androgen, danazol (Cyclomen®). Danazol suppresses the pituitary–ovarian axis and inhibits the output of gonadotropins from the pituitary gland. It is used for the treatment of endometriosis and fibrocystic breast changes in women.

Endometriosis is an estrogen-dependent disorder in which endometrial tissue develops outside of the uterus on the ovaries, fallopian tubes, bowel, bladder, or tissue lining the pelvic cavity. It occurs in approximately 10% of women of reproductive age and causes severe pelvic pain and possible infertility. Danazol alters the endometrium so that it becomes inactive and atrophic. Danazol is administered in total daily doses ranging from 200 mg to 800 mg in 2 to 4 divided doses. It is given continuously for 3 to 6 months.

Fibrocystic breast changes are characterized by thickening, lumps, and cysts (fluid-filled sacs) in the breast tissues. These affect more than 50% of women between the ages of 30 and 50 during their lifetime. The action of danazol on the breasts is not known. The total daily dose of danazol is 100 mg to 400 mg given in 2 divided doses. Pain and tenderness usually respond to treatment after 30 to 40 days. However, breast lumps usually do not begin to regress until 60 to 90 days after the initiation of therapy.

Common adverse effects that can occur in patients receiving danazol are acne, edema (facial), mild hirsutism, decrease in breast size, deepening of the voice, oiliness of the skin or hair, weight gain, and seborrhea.

NURSING PROCESS

☑ Assessment

In this section, estrogenic and progestational (progestins or progesterone drugs) medications are discussed first, followed by the major drug classes used in the treatment of osteoporosis. Next, information on fertility drugs, uterine stimulants, and preterm labour management drugs is discussed. Before initiating therapy with any of the hormonal drugs (e.g., estrogens, progestins) or other women's health–related drugs, obtain the patient's blood pressure and weight and document the findings. Assess and document drug allergies, contraindications, cautions, and possible drug interactions. Include a thorough medication history, medical history, and menstrual history in the patient assessment. Note the results of the patient's last physical exam, clinician-performed breast exam, and gynecological exam as well.

Estrogen-only hormones are to be given only after the following disorders and conditions have been ruled out: any estrogen-dependent cancer, undiagnosed abnormal uterine bleeding, or active thromboembolic disorders such as stroke or thrombophlebitis or a history of these disorders. Include questions about breast examination, breast self-examination practices, and dates of last complete physical examination and Papanicolaou (Pap) smear in the assessment. It is important to assess for potential drug interactions such as with tricyclic antidepressants, which may reach toxic levels if given with estrogens. Advise patients to avoid smoking because of the risk of thrombosis. It has been documented that smoking also decreases the effectiveness of estrogen; hence, take a thorough smoking history. Ask about the number of packs smoked per day and the number of years the patient has smoked. Other drug interactions for which to assess include oral anticoagulants (because of decreased effectiveness) as well as rifampin and St. John's wort (because of decreased estrogen effectiveness). If being used for hormonal replacement therapy for menopausal symptoms, recent changes to older recommendations from the NAMS include the following: (1) hormone replacement is not recommended for women with histories of endometrial cancer; and (2) in women with breast cancer, estrogen therapy has not been proved safe and may raise recurrence risk. Therefore, perform a thorough assessment for history or diagnosis of endometrial or breast cancer. Bone density may also be impacted once hormone therapy is discontinued; further assessment is needed in patients with histories of endometrial or breast cancer.

Assess patients' knowledge about the use of hormones (e.g., estrogens and progestins), whether for contraception or replacement therapy. Also assess their readiness to learn, educational level, and degree of adherence to other medication regimens. The success of treatment with oral contraceptives, hormone replacement medications, and other therapies depends heavily on patients' understanding of instructions. With oral contraceptive drugs (e.g., combination estrogen–progestin drugs), perform a pregnancy test and assess for history of vascular or thromboembolic disorders (e.g., MI, venous thrombosis, stroke), malignancies of the reproductive tract, and abnormal vaginal bleeding. Closely monitor patients with the following: hypertension, migraine headaches, alterations in lipid or carbohydrate metabolism, fluid retention or edema, hair loss, amenorrhea, breakthrough vaginal or uterine bleeding, and uterine fibroids. The concern in the presence of any of these conditions is the potential for their exacerbation and for subsequent complications. Closely monitor patients who smoke because of their increased risk of complications (increased risk of thrombosis) with estrogens. Assess for drug interactions, such as with drugs leading to decreased effectiveness of oral contraception—antibiotics (especially penicillins and cephalosporins), barbiturates, isoniazid, and rifampin. Drugs that may have their therapeutic effects decreased if taken concurrently with oral contraceptives include antiepileptic drugs, β-blockers, hypnotics, antidiabetic drugs, warfarin sodium, theophylline, tricyclic antidepressants, and vitamins. When combination oral contraceptives are used for postcoital conception, the same contraindications, cautions, and drug interactions apply, even if the drug is for one-time use.

The chemically derived progestins, such as medroxyprogesterone and megestrol, have the same contraindications as estrogens. Additionally, with progestins, assess for a history of liver or gallbladder disease and thrombophlebitis. Be mindful that a significant drug interaction occurs with antidiabetic drugs. Thoroughly review the patient's medical history to be aware of the specific condition for which the progestin is ordered. Some of these include prevention of endometrial cancer caused by estrogen therapy, palliative management of recurrent endometrial or breast cancer, as well as management of anorexia and cachexia in those with cancer.

With the drug class of bisphosphonates, used in the treatment of osteoporosis, there are many contraindications, cautions, and drug interactions. Assessment of the following is therefore important to patient safety: drug allergy, esophageal dysfunction, hypocalcemia, and the inability to sit or stand upright for at least 30 minutes after taking the medication. SERMs are not to be used in patients who are or may become pregnant and in women with thromboembolic disorders including DVT. Assess for allergies to salmon with the use of the hormone calcitonin because the drug is derived from this fish. Drug interactions for which to assess include ampicillin and cholestyramine because they decrease the absorption of raloxifene. Raloxifene also decreases the effects of warfarin sodium. Assess patients for the drug interaction between bisphosphonates and calcium supplements or decreased absorption that occurs with the concurrent use of antacids as well as the potential for additive GI irritation with the concurrent use of aspirin and NSAIDs.

Use of clomiphene requires assessment of the patient's medical and medication history, with attention to the patient's menstrual history. Medical history is crucial to know, especially reproductive and uterine status because use of the drug may result in multiple pregnancy (twins or more) and compromise maternal health status. Patients are usually followed by a fertility specialist affiliated with a speciality clinic, where assessment of family stability and economic status will be undertaken because of the additional family and financial stressors associated with a multiple birth. Also include assessment of possible contraindications, such as primary ovarian failure (or primary ovarian insufficiency), when ovaries stop functioning before the age of 40, adrenal or thyroid dysfunction, liver disease, or abnormal uterine bleeding. Assess also for potential drug interactions with tricyclic antidepressants, haloperidol, phenothiazines, and methyldopa (an antihypertensive drug). Fertility may be impaired if clomiphene is given with these drugs.

Before administering uterine stimulants (e.g., oxytocin or prostaglandins), assess and document the patient's blood pressure, pulse, and respiration. Also determine fetal heart rate and contraction-related fetal heart rates and document findings. Contraindications to the use of labour-inducing uterine stimulants in early pregnancy include the presence of an intrauterine device for birth control, ectopic pregnancy, use of anticoagulants, bleeding disorders, and inability to understand and then comply with instructions. Assess for the concurrent use of sympathomimetics because of enhanced vasoconstrictive effects, possibly leading to severe hypertension. For labour and delivery, the patient's cervix must be ready for induction. (Consult a current maternal child health or obstetric nursing textbook for more information on the rating of the cervix.) Perform continuous monitoring of maternal blood pressure, pulse, contractions, and fluid status, as well as of fetal heart rate. Oxytocin is *not* used during the first trimester except in some cases of spontaneous or induced abortion.

With the ergot alkaloid methylergonovine maleate, assess the medication order after vital signs have been taken and note that the first dose is given after delivery of the placenta to help stimulate the uterus to contract and decrease blood loss after delivery in special situations. Continue to assess blood pressure during the drug's administration. Assess for contraindications such as pregnancy, labour, liver or renal disease, heart disease, and pregnancy-induced hypertension. Assess for any history of seizures. If this drug is given to women with hypertension, it may precipitate seizures or a stroke. The use of dinoprostone or other prostaglandin E_2 drugs is indicated in specific situations requiring termination of pregnancy. Ask the patient about the presence of any known contraindications, cautions, and drug interactions.

Nursing Diagnoses

- Decisional conflict related to the risks versus benefits of postmenopausal estrogen replacement therapy
- Acute pain related to adverse effects and improper dosing of a SERM
- Nonadherence related to lack of information and experience with daily dosing of oral contraceptives

Planning

Goals

- Patient will make an informed decision regarding the use of estrogen replacement therapy.
- Patient will experience minimal pain (epigastric) associated with SERMs.
- Patient will remain adherent to oral contraceptive therapy.

Expected Patient Outcomes

- Patient correctly self-administers estrogen replacement therapy daily after making the decision to opt for pharmacological treatment.
- Patient remains without esophageal pain after taking a SERM as ordered and with the full ability to sit or stand upright for at least 30 minutes after taking the oral dosage form to avoid esophageal irritation.
- Patient is adherent to oral contraceptive therapy, states rationale for daily use (effectiveness based on taking medication daily), and contacts a health care provider with any high incidence of adverse effects.

Implementation

When administering estrogens, directions need to be followed exactly. Provide precise and thorough instructions to patients when self-administration of the hormone is ordered. Oral dosage forms are best taken at the same time every day and with a meal or a snack to minimize GI upset.

It is also important to understand the indication and rationale for the use of estrogen so that you can give accurate facts about the drug to patients. If estradiol is being given, vasomotor symptoms of menopause are generally the indication, and the drug is to be given daily at the same time. If the estradiol transdermal patch is given, it is to be applied as ordered, usually with one patch applied once or twice weekly to the lower abdomen and not to the breast and chest areas. See the Patient Teaching Tips for more information.

Use of progestins is indicated for birth control, such as the use of Depo-Provera with one IM injection every 3 months. However, the use of Depo-Provera in women of reproductive age remains controversial because of associated bone density loss. Give Depo-Provera injections in deep muscle mass and rotate sites. Oral forms of medroxyprogesterone are used for amenorrhea and uterine bleeding. Doses are to be taken exactly as ordered, such as for a specific number of days or cyclically. Megestrol, a synthetic progestin, is often indicated for palliative reasons or for management of anorexia, cachexia, or weight loss in patients with cancer. It is given to maximize appetite, orally, as ordered. It is recommended, however, that the lowest dosage possible of either estrogens or progestins be used and titrated as needed, but only as ordered.

Oral contraception is available in various formulations based on doses that are taken at different times of the menstrual cycle (see Oral Contraceptives: Indications discussion above). Progestin-only oral contraceptive pills are taken daily. It is important for patients to take this oral contraceptive at the same time every day so that effective hormone serum levels are maintained. Use of the progestin-only pill leads to a higher incidence of ovulatory cycles if not taken as per instructions; therefore, there is an increased rate and risk of contraceptive failure, compared with estrogen–progestin drug therapy. Be aware that progestin-only drugs are usually prescribed for those women who cannot tolerate estrogens or for whom estrogens are contraindicated. Often, they are more effective in women who are older than 35 years of age and women who are breastfeeding. Combination estrogen–progestin pills contain low doses of estrogen. Biphasic forms contain fixed estrogen and variable progestin in 21 or 28 day products. The low-dose monophasic (fixed estrogen–progestin combination) forms are provided as 21 or 28 days of pills, with the 28-day products containing 7 inert tablets. Triphasic products offer 3 or 4 phases of variable estrogen and progestin combinations, and there are also new, extended-cycle products available. Make sure patients fully understand how to take the medication. Emphasize that the reduction in the level of estrogen has been associated with a decrease in adverse effects and a decrease in the risk for complications; however, more breakthrough bleeding will occur.

The success of therapy with bisphosphonates depends on providing thorough patient teaching and ensuring that patients understand all aspects of the drug regimen. With the use of oral bisphosphonates, emphasize the need to take the medication upon rising in the morning with a full glass (180 to 240 mL) of water, at least 30 minutes before the intake of any food, other fluids, or other medication. In addition, emphasize that patients must remain upright in either a standing or sitting position for approximately 30 minutes after taking the drug to help prevent esophageal erosion or irritation. Risedronate delayed-release tablets should be swallowed whole and should not be chewed, cut, or crushed. Inform the patient taking the SERM raloxifene that the drug must be discontinued 72 hours before and during prolonged immobility. Therapy may be resumed, as ordered, once the patient becomes fully ambulatory. See the Patient Teaching Tips for more information.

Fertility drugs (e.g., clomiphene) are often self-administered. Provide specific instructions on how to administer the drug at home and how to monitor drug effectiveness to improve the success of treatment. Journal tracking of the medication regimen is helpful to those involved in the care of infertile patients or couples. See the Patient Teaching Tips for more information.

Administer oxytocin only as ordered, and strictly follow any instructions or protocol. The cervix must be ripe (see earlier discussion). Prostaglandin E_2 may be instilled vaginally to help accomplish this if the patient's cervix is not ripe or at a Bishop score of 5 or higher. Because oxytocin has vasopressive and antidiuretic properties, the patient is at risk for hypertensive episodes as well as fluid retention; institute continuous monitoring of maternal blood pressure and pulse rate as well as fetal monitoring. Report any of the following to the health care provider if they occur: strong contractions, edema, or changes in fetal movement. Administer IV infusions (via infusion pump) of oxytocin with the proper dilutional fluid and at the proper rate. To minimize the adverse effects of the drug, IV piggyback dosing is often ordered so that the diluted oxytocin solution can be discontinued immediately if maternal or fetal decline occurs while an IV line with hydration is maintained. Doses are generally titrated as ordered and are based on the progress of labour and degree of fetal tolerance of the drug. If labour progresses at 1 centimetre per hour dilation, oxytocin may no longer be needed. The decision to stop the drug is made by the health care provider and on an individual basis. With oxytocin therapy, if there are hypertensive responses or major changes in the maternal vital signs *or* if the fetal heart rate shows any indication of fetal intolerance of labour, contact the health care provider immediately. Hyperstimulation may also occur. If contractions are more frequent than every 2 minutes and last longer than 1 minute (and are accompanied by changes in other parameters), stop the infusion and contact the health care provider immediately. If this does occur, place the patient in a side-lying position, maintain administration of IV fluids, and give oxygen as ordered (generally via tight face mask at 10 to 12 L/min), and monitor both the patient and fetus closely. If there is concern about overstimulation, discuss this with the health care provider and document actions thoroughly.

Dinoprostone is given by vaginal suppository to patients who are 12 to 20 weeks pregnant and are seeking termination and to patients in whom evacuation of the uterus is needed for the management of incomplete spontaneous abortion or intrauterine fetal death (up to 28 weeks). Give the drug exactly as ordered and monitor the patient closely.

Evaluation

Measure therapeutic responses to the various drugs discussed in this chapter by evaluating whether goals and outcome criteria have been met. Many drugs have been

---

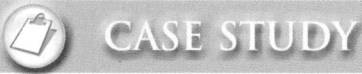 **CASE STUDY**

Bisphosphonate Drug Therapy for Osteoporosis

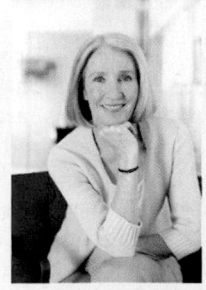

Janet is a relatively healthy 73-year-old retired law clerk who has recently been diagnosed with postmenopausal osteoporosis. She has been prescribed treatment with alendronate (Fosamax), 70 mg each month. She has many questions, and you review the drug and its use with her.

1. Janet tells you that she likes to have breakfast, take her morning medicines, and then lie down on the couch to read the morning newspaper. She asks whether the alendronate will fit into her routine. What will you tell her?

2. Janet calls the clinic to ask what to use for headaches. "I have several different types of headache pills, but aren't they all the same?" How will you respond?

3. A few months later, Janet comes in for a follow-up visit. She tells you that she is due for her next osteoporosis pill next week, but she has been having some jaw pain ever since she went to the dentist 2 weeks earlier to have a tooth pulled. She is worried that her osteoporosis has affected her jaw. What could be the reason for this pain? What do you think will be done about it?

For answers, see http://evolve.elsevier.com/Canada/Lilley/pharmacology/.

discussed, often with several indications for their use; thus, a therapeutic response would be occurrence of the indicated therapeutic effect. Monitor patients for adverse effects and toxicity as well.

Therapeutic responses to progestins include a decrease in abnormal uterine bleeding and the disappearance of menstrual disorders (e.g., amenorrhea). The adverse effects of progestins include edema, hypertension, cardiac symptoms, changes in mood and affect, and jaundice.

Therapeutic effects of estrogens may range from prevention of pregnancy, to a decrease in menopausal symptoms, to a reduction in the size of a tumour. Adverse effects of estrogens may include hypertension, thromboembolism, edema, amenorrhea, nausea, vomiting, facial skin discoloration, hirsutism, breast tenderness, and headache. Therapeutic responses to progestins include a decrease in abnormal uterine bleeding and the disappearance of menstrual disorders (e.g., amenorrhea). The adverse effects of progestins include jaundice, thrombophlebitis, liver dysfunction, and thromboembolic disorders. Adverse effects associated with oral contraceptives include hypertension, edema, thromboembolism, headaches, migraines, depression, stroke, nausea, vomiting, amenorrhea, and breakthrough bleeding.

Therapeutic effects of oxytocin and other uterine stimulants include stimulation of labour and control of postpartum bleeding. Adverse effects may include hypotension or hypertension, chest pain, nausea, vomiting, blurred vision, and fainting. The primary therapeutic effect of tocolytics is the absence of preterm labour. Adverse maternal effects may include vasodilation and increase in heart rate, and fetal side effects include possible intrauterine growth retardation.

The therapeutic effect of fertility drugs is successful conception. Adverse reactions include tachycardia, DVT, hypovolemia, central nervous system depression, nausea, vomiting, ovarian hyperstimulation, blurred vision, and photophobia. The therapeutic effects of osteoporosis drugs and related drugs include increased bone density and prevention or management of osteoporosis. Adverse effects of SERMs are hot flashes, leg cramps, leukopenia, headache, GI upset, joint pain, and esophageal burns if the drug is lodged in the esophagus before reaching the stomach.

PATIENT TEACHING TIPS

- Patients should be aware that hormonal drugs are better tolerated if taken with food or milk to minimize GI upset.
- With the use of oral contraceptives as well as any form of HRT with estrogens or progestins, encourage patients to openly discuss concerns about the medications. Assure patients that, although risks may be associated with HRT, the health care provider will weigh each case individually and make a recommendation based on the basis of benefits versus risks, but with the ultimate decision being the patient's.
- With estrogens and progestins, advise patients to report any of the following to a health care provider immediately: hypertension, edema, thromboembolism, migraines, depression, and breakthrough bleeding.
- Inform patients that treatment with ulipristal acetate often leads to a significant reduction in menstrual blood loss or amenorrhea within the first 10 days of treatment. If excessive bleeding persists, the patient should inform the health care provider. Menstrual periods should return within 4 weeks after the end of the treatment with ulipristal. The use of a nonhormonal contraceptive method is recommended during treatment.
- Advise patients to report any weight gain of 1 kg or more in 24 hours, as well as any breakthrough bleeding or change in menstrual flow.
- Instruct patients to take oral contraceptives exactly as ordered and to keep all appointments for follow-up examinations (e.g., pelvic examinations, Pap smears, health care provider–performed breast examinations).
- Teach patients the importance of and the correct technique for monthly breast self-examinations during the ideal time—that is, 7 to 10 days after the start of menstruation or 2 to 5 days after menses end. Stress the need for follow-up appointments and annual examinations by a health care provider.
- Hormones make patients sensitive to sunlight and tanning beds. Emphasize to patients that they must use appropriate sun protection at all times.
- If a patient is using progesterone-only intravaginal gel with other gels, advise the patient to insert the other gels at least 6 hours before or after the progesterone-based product.
- Slow-release progesterone intrauterine devices are placed in the uterine cavity by a health care provider. Provide thorough education about the fact that inserts are left in place for 5 years (after insertion) and then must be replaced. Advise patients to report abnormal uterine bleeding, cramping, abdominal pain, or amenorrhea immediately.
- Instruct patients using an estrogen–progestin vaginal ring for contraception regarding what to expect with its insertion. Use of this contraceptive device requires thorough teaching and follow-up, including instruction on insertion and removal techniques and a return demonstration, before the patient leaves the health care provider's office. Inform patients that menstruation will follow about 2 to 3 days after the ring is removed and instruct them to replace the used ring in its foil pouch and discard it in a waste receptacle. The ring should not be flushed down the toilet.
- Oral contraceptive hormones must be taken at the same time every day and exactly as prescribed. If one dose is missed, advise the patient to take the dose as soon as it is remembered; however, if it is close to the next dose time, advise the patient not to double up and to use a backup form of contraception in these

Continued

PATIENT TEACHING TIPS—cont'd

situations. Provide more specific instructions for the omission of more than 1 day's dose depending on the specific oral contraceptive drug prescribed. These specific instructions will most likely include the following: If the patient misses one "active" tablet in weeks 1, 2, or 3, the tablet needs to be taken as soon as she remembers. If the patient misses two "active" tablets in week 1 or week 2, the patient needs to take two tablets the day she remembers and two tablets the next day, and then continue taking one tablet a day until the pack is finished. The patient needs to be instructed to use a backup method of birth control, such as condoms, if she has intercourse in the 7 days after missing pills. If the patient misses two "active" tablets in the third week or misses three or more "active" tablets in a row, the patient needs to throw out the rest of the pack and start a new pack that same day. Instruct the patient to use a backup method of birth control if she has intercourse in the 7 days after missing pills.

❖ Emphasize to patients that OTC foams for intravaginal use do not prevent transmission of sexually transmitted infections or HIV.

❖ Stress to patients the importance of using condoms with hormonal contraception to prevent sexually transmitted infections.

❖ Emphasize to patients that backup contraception (e.g., condom use) is needed when antibiotics, barbiturates, griseofulvin, isoniazid, rifampin, or St. John's wort are taken with oral contraceptives, as these drugs and herbs diminish the effectiveness of oral contraception.

❖ Estradot is generally applied once daily to the thighs and calves, as ordered, with one dose provided in two separate pouches. Patients should be instructed not to apply sunscreen or other lotions at the same time because they interfere with the drug. To reduce the chance of transfer of this medication to other individuals, allow the areas to which it has been applied to dry completely before covering them with clothing. The drug contained in this dosage form, estradiol, has been found to be present on the skin up to 8 hours after application.

❖ Conjugated estrogens are used for menopausal symptoms and are given orally every day; however, other uses of these estrogens may require different doses and a different dosage schedule or regimen. Emphasize to patients the expected adverse effects such as edema, nausea, diarrhea, constipation, breakthrough uterine bleeding, chloasma (facial skin discoloration), hirsutism, tender breasts, and headaches. Encourage patients to report any of the following conditions: elevated blood pressure, severe headaches with changes in vision and vomiting, abdominal pain, and edema.

❖ Bisphosphonates (e.g., alendronate) are to be taken exactly as prescribed; that is, the drug is taken at least 30 minutes before the first morning beverage, food, or other medication and with at least 180 to 240 mL of water. Emphasize to patients the importance of remaining upright for at least 30 minutes after taking the medication to prevent esophageal and GI adverse effects. Esophageal irritation, dysphagia, severe heartburn, and retrosternal pain must be reported to the health care provider immediately to help prevent severe reactions.

❖ Patients taking bisphosphonates should be aware they may also require supplemental calcium and vitamin D, as ordered by the health care provider.

❖ Educate patients about making lifestyle changes as recommended, such as engaging in weight-bearing exercises (e.g., walking), stopping smoking, and limiting or eliminating alcohol intake. These measures will help minimize the adverse effects of oral contraception or drug therapy with hormones.

KEY POINTS

❖ Three major estrogens are synthesized in the ovaries: estradiol (the principal estrogen), esterone, and estriol. Exogenous estrogens can be classified into two main groups: steroidal estrogens (e.g., conjugated estrogens, esterified estrogens, estradiol) and the nonsteroidal estrogen diethylstilbestrol.

❖ Progestins have a variety of uses, including treatment of uterine bleeding, amenorrhea, and adjunctive and palliative treatment of some cancers.

❖ Oral contraceptives containing a combination of estrogens and progestins are the most commonly used form of reversible contraception currently available.

❖ Uterine stimulants (sometimes called *oxytocic drugs*) include ergot derivatives, prostaglandins, and oxytocin.

❖ Uterine relaxants (often called *tocolytic drugs*) are used to stop preterm labour and maintain pregnancy by halting uterine contractions.

❖ A thorough nursing assessment is necessary to ensure the safe and effective use of female reproductive drugs. Obtain information on the patient's past medical problems, history of menses and problems with the menstrual cycle, medications taken (prescribed and OTC), number of pregnancies and miscarriages, last menstrual period, and any related surgical or medical treatments.

❖ Several drug classes are used for the treatment of existing osteoporosis, including the bisphosphonates, the selective estrogen receptor modulators, the hormones calcitonin and teriparatide, and denosumab.

EXAMINATION REVIEW QUESTIONS

1. The nurse is assessing a patient who is to receive dinoprostone (Prostin E$_2$). Which condition would be a contraindication to the use of this drug?
   a. Pregnancy at 15 weeks' gestation
   b. GI upset or ulcer disease
   c. Ectopic pregnancy
   d. Incomplete abortion
2. The nurse is teaching a patient who is taking oral contraceptive therapy for the first time about possible adverse effects. Which adverse effects should the nurse discuss?
   a. Dizziness
   b. Nausea
   c. Tingling in the extremities
   d. Polyuria
3. The nurse is reviewing the use of obstetric drugs. Which situation is an indication for an oxytocin infusion?
   a. Termination of a pregnancy at 12 weeks
   b. Hypertonic uterus
   c. Cervical stenosis in a patient who is in labour
   d. Induction of labour at full term
4. The nurse has provided patient education regarding therapy with the SERM raloxifene (Evista). Which statement from the patient reflects a good understanding of the instruction?
   a. "When I take that long flight to Asia, I will need to stop taking this drug at least 3 days before I travel."
   b. "I can continue taking this drug even when travelling, as long as I take it with a full glass of water each time."
   c. "After I take this drug, I must sit upright for at least 30 minutes."
   d. "One advantage of this drug is that it will reduce my hot flashes."
5. The nurse is discussing therapy with clomiphene (Clomid) with a husband and wife who are considering trying this drug as part of treatment for infertility. It is important that they be informed of which possible effect of this drug?
   a. Increased menstrual flow
   b. Increased menstrual cramping
   c. Multiple pregnancy (twins or more)
   d. Sedation
6. A patient calls the clinic because she has realized that she missed one dose of an oral contraceptive. Which statement from the nurse is appropriate? (Select all that apply.)
   a. "Go ahead and take the missed dose now, along with today's dose."
   b. "Don't worry; you are still protected from pregnancy."
   c. "Please come to the clinic for a re-evaluation of your therapy."
   d. "Wait 7 days, and then start a new pack of pills."
   e. "You will need to use a backup form of contraception concurrently for 7 days."
7. The order reads: "Give calcitonin (Calcimar) 50 units Subcut daily." The medication is available in a vial that contains 200 units/mL. How many millilitres will the nurse draw up in the syringe for this dose?

Answers: 1. c, 2. b, 3. d, 4. a, 5. c, 6. a, e, 7. 0.25 mL

CRITICAL THINKING ACTIVITIES

1. A patient in her first pregnancy has spent 14 hours in labour and has made little progress. She is becoming exhausted, and her uterine contractions have decreased in strength. She is now receiving an oxytocin infusion. During this infusion, the nurse will perform many assessments. What are the priorities during the assessments?
2. The nurse is reviewing a cephalosporin prescription for a patient who has a severe sinus infection. The patient tells the nurse that she is taking a birth control pill and asks the nurse if there will be any problems with taking the antibiotic. What is the nurse's best answer?
3. A woman comes into the emergency department. She says that she is pregnant but that she is having contractions every 3 minutes and she is "not due yet." She is extremely upset. While assessing her vital signs and fetal heart tones, what is the most important question the nurse must ask the patient?

For answers see http://evolve.elsevier.com/Canada/Lilley/pharmacology/.

CHAPTER 36

Men's Health Drugs

Objectives

After reading this chapter, the successful student will be able to do the following:

1. Discuss the normal anatomy, physiology, and functions of the male reproductive system.

2. Compare various men's health drugs, with discussion of their rationales for use, dosages, and dosage forms.

3. Describe the mechanisms of action, dosages, adverse effects, cautions, contraindications, drug interactions, and routes of administration for the various men's health drugs discussed.

4. Develop a collaborative plan of care that includes all phases of the nursing process for patients receiving men's health drugs for treatment of benign prostatic hyperplasia, sexual dysfunction, hormone deficiency, or prostate cancer.

e-Learning Activities

Website
(http://evolve.elsevier.com/Canada/
Lilley/pharmacology/)

evolve

- Answer Key—Textbook Case Studies
- Answer Key—Critical Thinking Activities
- Chapter Summaries—Printable
- Review Questions for Exam Preparation
- Unfolding Case Studies

Drug Profiles

finasteride, p. 691
▸▸ sildenafil (sildenafil citrate)*, p. 691
▸▸ testosterone, p. 691

▸▸ Key drug

*Full generic name is given in parentheses. For the purposes of this text, the more common, shortened name is used.

Key Terms

Anabolic activity Any metabolic activity that promotes the building up of body tissues, such as the activity produced by testosterone that results in the development of bone and muscle tissue; also called *anabolism.* (p. 687)

Androgenic activity The activity produced by testosterone that causes the development and maintenance of the male reproductive system and male secondary sex characteristics. (p. 687)

Androgens Male sex hormones responsible for mediating the development and maintenance of male sex characteristics; chief among these are testosterone and its various biochemical precursors. (p. 687)

Benign prostatic hyperplasia (BPH) Nonmalignant (non-cancerous) enlargement of the prostate gland (also called *benign prostatic hypertrophy*). (p. 688)

Catabolism The opposite of anabolic activity; any metabolic activity that results in the breakdown of body tissues. Examples of conditions in which catabolism occurs are debilitating illnesses such as end-stage cancer and starvation. (p. 687)

Erythropoietic effect The effect of stimulating the production of red blood cells (erythropoiesis). (p. 687)

Prostate cancer A malignant tumour within the prostate gland. (p. 688)

Testosterone The main androgenic hormone. (p. 687)

OVERVIEW OF THE MALE REPRODUCTIVE SYSTEM

The male reproductive system consists of several structures; two of these structures, the testes and seminiferous tubules, produce the primary male hormones. The *testes*, a pair of oval glands located in the scrotal sac, are the male gonads. The *seminiferous tubules*, which are channels in the testes, are the site of spermatogenesis, which is the process by which mature sperm cells are produced.

Androgens comprise the group of male sex hormones (primarily testosterone) that mediate the normal development and maintenance of primary and secondary male sex characteristics (Figure 36-1). Secondary male sex characteristics include advanced development of the prostate, seminal vesicles (two glands adjacent to the prostate), penis, and scrotum, as well as male hair distribution, laryngeal enlargement, thickening of the vocal cords, and male body musculature and fat distribution. Androgens must be secreted in adequate amounts for these characteristics to appear. The most important androgen is **testosterone**, which is produced from clusters of interstitial cells embedded between the seminiferous tubules. Besides having **androgenic activity**,

testosterone is also involved in the development of bone and muscle tissue; inhibition of protein **catabolism** (metabolic breakdown); and retention of nitrogen, phosphorus, potassium, and sodium. These functions contribute to its **anabolic activity**. The hormone initiates the synthesis of specific proteins needed for androgenic and anabolic activity by binding to chromatin (strands of deoxyribonucleic acid [DNA]), in the nuclei of interstitial cells. In addition, testosterone appears to have an **erythropoietic effect**, in that it stimulates the production of red blood cells (see Chapter 55).

ANDROGENS AND OTHER DRUGS PERTAINING TO MEN'S HEALTH

Testosterone deficiency is treated with exogenous testosterone. There are several synthetic derivatives of testosterone that have improved pharmacokinetic and pharmacodynamic characteristics over the naturally occurring hormone. This is accomplished by combining various esters with testosterone, which prolong the duration of action of the hormone. For example, testosterone propionate is formulated as an oily solution, and its hormonal effects last for 2 to 3 days; the effects of testosterone cypionate and testosterone enanthate in oil last for up to 2 to 4 weeks. Orally administered testosterone has poor absorption because most of the dose is metabolized and destroyed by the liver before it can reach the circulation (first-pass effect; see Chapter 2). To circumvent this problem, researchers developed methyltestosterone and fluoxymesterone (both are controlled substances in Canada). A transdermal dosage gel and a metred-dose pump have provided another way to circumvent the first-pass effect that occurs with oral administration of this hormone.

There are other chemical derivatives of testosterone known as *anabolic steroids*. These are synthetic drugs that closely resemble the natural hormone but possess high anabolic activity. These drugs are no longer available in Canada by prescription. However, under Health Canada's Special Access Programme, health care providers can request medications that are not available for sale, such as the anabolic steroids oxandrolone and nandrolone deconate. Oxandrolone may be used to treat HIV-associated wasting syndrome (debilitation related to disease-induced nutritional malabsorption) and alcoholic hepatitis. Oxandrolone is also used in hospitalized patients to stimulate weight gain. Because of their muscle-building properties, anabolic steroids have a great potential for misuse by athletes, especially bodybuilders and weightlifters. Improper use of these substances can have many serious consequences, such as sterility, cardiovascular diseases, and even liver cancer. For this reason, anabolic steroids are currently classified as Schedule IV controlled substances by Health Canada. Misuse of these drugs can lead to psychological or physical dependence or both.

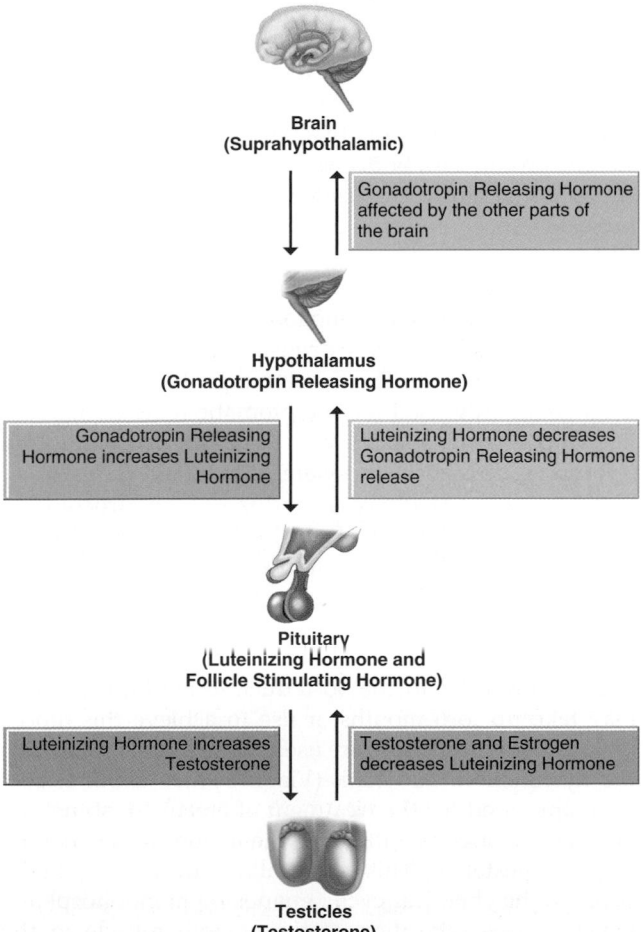

FIG. 36-1   Regulation of male characteristics by testosterone.

Mechanism of Action and Drug Effects

Natural and synthetic androgens have effects similar to those of the endogenous androgens. These include stimulation of the normal growth and development of the male sex organs (primary sex characteristics) and development and maintenance of secondary sex characteristics. Androgens stimulate the synthesis of ribonucleic acid (RNA) at the cellular level, thereby promoting cellular growth and reproduction. They also retard the breakdown of amino acids. These properties contribute to an increased synthesis of body proteins, which aids in the formation and maintenance of muscle tissue. Another potent anabolic effect of androgens is the retention of nitrogen, also essential for protein synthesis. Nitrogen promotes the storage in the body of inorganic phosphorus, sulfate, sodium, and potassium, all of which have important metabolic roles, including protein synthesis, nerve impulse conduction, and muscle contraction. All of these effects result in weight gain and an increase in muscular strength. Finally, androgens also stimulate the production of erythropoietin by the kidneys, which leads to enhanced erythropoiesis (red blood cell synthesis; see Chapter 55). However, the administration of exogenous androgens causes the release of endogenous testosterone to be inhibited as the result of feedback inhibition of the pituitary luteinizing hormone. Large doses of exogenous androgens may also suppress sperm production as a result of the feedback inhibition of pituitary follicle-stimulating hormone, which leads to infertility.

Androgen inhibitors block the effects of naturally occurring (endogenous) androgens. This is accomplished via inhibition of a specific enzyme, 5-α reductase. For this reason, these drugs are also called *5α-reductase inhibitors*. For unknown reasons, normal male physiology often results in a common enlargement of the prostate known as *benign prostatic hyperplasia (BPH)*. This process begins as early as 30 years of age and is present in at least 85% of men by 80 years of age. The most troubling symptom is usually varying degrees of obstructed urinary outflow; a digital rectal examination is recommended as part of yearly screening for men over the age of 50 to detect enlargement of the prostate. Although surgical treatment by transurethral resection of the prostate (TURP) is a common strategy, BPH is also treatable with a 5α-reductase inhibitors. There are currently two such drugs: finasteride and dutasteride. Finasteride (Proscar®), the prototypical drug for this class, works by inhibiting this enzyme, which normally converts testosterone to 5α-dihydrotestosterone (DHT). DHT is a more potent type of testosterone and is the principal androgen responsible for stimulating prostatic growth, as well as the expression of other male primary and secondary sex characteristics. Finasteride can dramatically lower prostatic DHT concentrations, which helps to reduce the size of the prostate to ease the passage of urine. Fortunately, finasteride does not cause antiandrogen adverse effects that might be expected, such as loss of muscle strength and fertility.

The effects of finasteride are limited primarily to the prostate, but this drug may also affect 5α-reductase–dependent processes elsewhere in the body, such as in the hair follicles, skin, and liver. Research has demonstrated that the pharmacological inhibition of 5α-reductase prevents the thinning of hair caused by increased levels of DHT. It has been noted that men taking finasteride experience increased hair growth. Therefore, finasteride is also indicated for the treatment of male pattern hair loss (Propecia®). Finasteride is indicated for treating hair loss only in men, not in women—finasteride can be teratogenic in pregnant women and its use in women of any age (pregnant or not) is still not recommended. Women need to wear gloves when handling finasteride. Another medication, minoxidil, can be used topically to treat hair loss in both men and women. It is discussed in more detail in Chapter 56.

There are also two other classes of androgen inhibitors. The first includes the androgen receptor blockers flutamide (Euflex®), nilutamide (Anandron®), and bicalutamide (Casodex®). These drugs work by blocking the activity of androgen hormones at the level of the receptors in target tissues (e.g., prostate). For this reason, these drugs are used in the treatment of **prostate cancer** (see Chapter 53). The second class is the gonadotropin-releasing hormone (Gn-RH) analogues, including leuprolide acetate (Eligard®, Lupron®), goserelin acetate (Zoladex®), and triptorelin pamoate (Trelstar®). These drugs work by inhibiting the secretion of pituitary gonadotropin, which eventually leads to a decrease in testosterone production. Both androgen receptor blockers and Gn-RH analogues are used most commonly to treat prostate cancer and are discussed in further detail in Chapter 53.

Another class of drugs that may be used to help alleviate the symptoms of obstruction due to BPH are the α_1-adrenergic blockers. These drugs are discussed in greater detail in Chapter 20. The α_1-adrenergic blockers that are most commonly used for symptomatic relief of obstruction secondary to BPH are terazosin hydrochloride (Hytrin®), doxazosin mesylate (Cardura®), tamsulosin hydrochloride (Flomax®), alfuzosin hydrochloride (Xatral®), and silodosin (Rapaflo®). Tamsulosin hydrochloride, alfuzosin hydrochloride, and silodosin appear to have a greater specificity for the α_1-receptors in the prostate and thus may cause less hypotension. These drugs have clinical effects of prostate shrinkage immediately, as opposed to the 5α-reductase inhibitors, which may take up to 6 months of use to achieve this. Phosphodiesterase inhibitors are used in the treatment of erectile dysfunction. Sildenafil (Viagra®) was the first oral drug approved for the treatment of erectile dysfunction. Sildenafil works by inhibiting the action of the enzyme phosphodiesterase. This in turn allows the buildup in the penis of the chemical cyclic guanosine monophosphate, which causes relaxation of the smooth muscle in the corpora cavernosa (erectile tubes) of the penis and permits the inflow of blood. Nitric oxide is also released

BOX 36-1   Currently Available Men's Health Drugs

α_1-Adrenergic–Blocking Drugs

doxazosin mesylate
tamsulosin hydrochloride
terazosin hydrochloride
alfuzosin hydrochloride

Anabolic Steroids

not available

Other Androgens

danazol (see Chapter 35)
testosterone

Antiandrogens

bicalutamide
flutamide
nilutamide

5α-Reductase Inhibitors

finasteride
dutasteride

Gonadotropin-Releasing Hormone Analogues

goserelin acetate
leuprolide acetate
triptorelin pamoate

Peripheral Vasodilator

minoxidil

Drugs for Erectile Dysfunction

sildenafil
tadalafil
vardenafil hydrochloride
alprostadil

---

inside the corpora cavernosa during sexual stimulation and contributes to the erectile effect. Two drugs that are similar but have a longer duration of action are vardenafil hydrochloride (Levitra®, Staxyn®) and tadalafil (Cialis®). Collectively, these drugs are referred to as *erectile dysfunction drugs*. Sildenafil and tadalafil are also used to treat pulmonary hypertension (see Chapter 23) under the trade names Revatio® and Adcirca®, respectively.

A second type of drug used to treat erectile dysfunction is the prostaglandin alprostadil (Calverject®, Muse®). This drug must be given by injecting it directly into the erectile tissue of the penis (Calverject) or pushing a suppository form of the drug (Muse) into the urethra.

A list of all of the drugs mentioned in the chapter used for men's health appears in Box 36-1. More information on selected drugs can be found in the Drug Profiles section.

Indications

The primary use for androgens is as hormone replacement therapy. Indications for other types of drugs discussed in this chapter are listed in Table 36-1.

Contraindications

Contraindications to the use of androgenic drugs include known androgen-responsive tumours. Use of sildenafil, vardenafil, and tadalafil hydrochloride is also contraindicated in men with major cardiovascular disorders, particularly if they use nitrate medications such as nitroglycerin. Concurrent use of erectile dysfunction drugs and nitrates may cause severe hypotension, which may not respond to treatment. Use of finasteride is contraindicated in women (especially pregnant women) and children.

TABLE 36-1

Men's Health Drugs: Indications

Drug	Indication
finasteride	Benign prostatic hyperplasia
	Male androgenetic alopecia
minoxidil	Hypertension
	Female and male androgenetic alopecia
oxandrolone, nandrolone deconate (available via Special Access)	HIV wasting syndrome, alcoholic hepatitis
sildenafil citrate, tadalafil, vardenafil hydrochloride	Erectile dysfunction
testosterone	Primary or secondary hypogonadism

Adverse Effects

Although rare, some of the most devastating effects of androgenic steroids occur in the liver, where they cause the formation of blood-filled cavities, a condition known as *peliosis of the liver*. This condition is a possible consequence of the long-term administration of androgenic anabolic steroids and can be life-threatening. Other serious liver effects are hepatic neoplasms (liver cancer), cholestatic hepatitis, jaundice, and abnormal liver function. Fluid retention is another undesirable effect of androgens and may account for some of the weight gain seen with their use. The serious adverse effects that can be caused by the androgens far outweigh the advantages

TABLE 36-2	
Men's Health Drugs: Selected Adverse Effects	
Drug Class	**Adverse Effects**
α_1-Adrenergic blockers	Tachycardia, hypotension, syncope, depression, drowsiness, rash, erectile dysfunction, increased urinary frequency, dyspnea, visual changes, headache
Androgens (including anabolic steroids)	Headache, changes in libido, anxiety, depression, acne, male pattern hair loss, hirsutism, nausea, abnormal liver function test results, priapism, elevated cholesterol level
5α-Reductase inhibitors	Reduced libido, hypotension, dizziness, drowsiness
Peripheral vasodilator (topical minoxidil)	With topical route, usually limited to localized dermatological reactions, including erythema, dermatitis, eczema, pruritus
Drugs for erectile dysfunction	Dizziness, headache, muscular pain, chest pain, hypertension or hypotension, rash, dry mouth, nausea, vomiting, priapism

to be gained from their use in those seeking improved athletic ability. Other less serious adverse effects of androgens are listed in Table 36-2.

Sildenafil, vardenafil, and tadalafil hydrochloride appear to have relatively favourable adverse effect profiles, with headache, flushing, and dyspepsia the most common adverse effects reported. However, in patients with pre-existing cardiovascular disease, especially those taking nitrates (e.g., nitroglycerin, isosorbide mononitrate, dinitrate), these drugs can lower blood pressure substantially, potentially leading to serious adverse events. *Priapism* or abnormally prolonged penile erection is a relatively uncommon, but possible, adverse effect of both the erectile dysfunction drugs and the androgens. This condition is a medical emergency and warrants urgent medical attention, though it is simply due to excess therapeutic response to the drug. Phosphodiesterase inhibitors can also cause unexplained vision loss.

Finasteride has been reported to cause loss of libido, loss of erection, ejaculatory dysfunction, hypersensitivity reactions, gynecomastia, and severe myopathy. The drug has also caused a 50% decrease in prostate-specific antigen (PSA) concentrations. Pregnant women must not handle crushed or broken tablets on a regular basis because of the possibility of topical absorption, which can lead to teratogenic effects.

Interactions

Androgens, when used with oral anticoagulants, can significantly increase or decrease anticoagulant activity (see Chapter 27). Concurrent use of androgens with ciclosporin (see Chapter 50) increases the risk of ciclosporin toxicity and is not recommended. Sildenafil, vardenafil, and tadalafil hydrochloride may cause severe hypotension when given together with nitrates such as nitroglycerin, isosorbide mononitrate, or isosorbide dinitrate (see Chapter 24). α-Blockers can cause additive hypotension when given with other drugs that lower blood pressure (see Chapter 23). Effects of tamsulosin may be increased when it is taken with azole antifungal drugs, erythromycin or clarithromycin (see Chapter 43),

cardiac drugs such as propranolol hydrochloride or verapamil hydrochloride (see Chapters 20 and 26), and protease inhibitors (see Chapter 45).

Dosages

For dosage information on men's health drugs, refer to the table on p. 692.

PHARMACOKINETIC BRIDGE TO NURSING PRACTICE

Drugs used to manage erectile dysfunction (e.g., sildenafil) essentially work in the same way as the body does to assist the patient in achieving an erection. The related pharmacokinetics must be understood so that the drug is taken safely and effectively. Sildenafil is a rapidly absorbed drug with onset of action within 1 hour, peak plasma concentrations within 1 hour, and a duration of action of up to 4 to 6 hours. If the drug is taken with a high-fat meal, absorption will be delayed, and it may take an additional 60 minutes for it to reach peak levels. This is yet another example of how specific drug pharmacokinetics can be affected by variables in a patient's everyday life, such as eating habits. Another pharmacokinetic consideration is that patients who are 65 years of age or older have reduced clearance of sildenafil and may experience increased plasma concentrations of free (or pharmacologically active) drug. This could possibly lead to drug accumulation and toxicity. (See Special Populations: Older Adults, Sildenafil: Use and Concerns.)

NURSING PROCESS

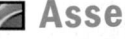 **Assessment**

Before any drug is given to a male patient for the treatment of the male reproductive tract, thoroughly assess

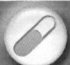 **DRUG PROFILES**

finasteride

Finasteride (Proscar) is available in tablet form in 1- and 5-mg strengths. The lower strength is indicated for androgenic alopecia in men. The higher strength is indicated for BPH, with clinical effects of prostate shrinkage occurring after approximately 3 to 6 months of continual therapy. A similar drug, dutasteride (Avodart®), is also indicated for BPH and is currently available in 0.5-mg capsule form. A combination of dutasteride and tamsulosin hydrochloride (Jalyn®) is available in a modified-release capsule for the treatment of moderate to severe BPH. Finasteride and dutasteride are contraindicated in patients who have shown hypersensitivity to them and in pregnant women and children. Both drugs are teratogenic. For recommended dosages, refer to the table on p. 692.

PHARMACOKINETICS

Route	Onset of Action	Peak Plasma Concentration	Elimination Half-Life	Duration of Action
PO	3–12 mo	8 hr	4–15 hr	14 days

▶▶ sildenafil citrate

Sildenafil citrate (Viagra) is approved for the treatment of erectile dysfunction. Other erectile dysfunction drugs with longer durations of action include vardenafil hydrochloride and tadalafil. Sildenafil potentiates the physiological sexual response, causing penile erection after sexual arousal by relaxing smooth muscle and increasing blood flow into the penis.

Sildenafil use is contraindicated in patients with a known hypersensitivity to it. Sildenafil can potentiate the hypotensive effects of nitrates, and its administration to patients who are using organic nitrates in any form, either regularly or intermittently, is contraindicated. For recommended dosages refer to the table on p. 692.

PHARMACOKINETICS

Route	Onset of Action	Peak Plasma Concentration	Elimination Half-Life	Duration of Action
PO	0.5–1 hr	1 hr	4 hr	2–4 hr

▶▶ testosterone

Testosterone (Androderm®) is a naturally occurring anabolic steroid. It is used for primary and secondary hypogonadism but may also be used to treat oligospermia in men as well as inoperable breast cancer in women, in which its purpose is to counteract tumour-enhancing estrogen activity. It is also used as replacement therapy for transgender individuals transitioning from female to male. When it is used as hormone replacement therapy, a transdermal product is desirable. There are presently two transdermal patch formulations. They attempt to mimic the normal circadian variation in testosterone concentration seen in young healthy men, in whom maximum testosterone levels occur in the early morning hours and minimum concentrations occur in the evening. Of the available transdermal delivery systems, Testoderm® is always applied to the scrotal skin, whereas Androderm and Androgel® are always applied to skin elsewhere on the body and never to the scrotal skin. Educate patients to wash their hands before application and then cover the area where testosterone has been applied, as transfer to others can occur. Axiron® is a topical solution in a metered-dose pump that is applied to the skin of the underarm.

Testosterone use is contraindicated in patients with hypersensitivity to it; severe kidney, heart, or liver disease; male breast cancer; prostate cancer; or genital bleeding, as well as in pregnant or lactating women. Testosterone is a Schedule IV controlled substance under the *Controlled Drugs and Substances Act*. It is available as an intramuscular injection, transdermal gel, transdermal patch, capsule, and pump. For recommended dosages refer to the table on p. 692.

PHARMACOKINETICS

Route	Onset of Action	Peak Plasma Concentration	Elimination Half-Life	Duration of Action
Topical	1–2 hr	8 hr	10–100 min	24 hr

---

presenting symptoms and obtain a complete history of past and present diseases or other medical conditions. In addition, assess the patient's urinary elimination patterns and any difficulties, and document the findings. The health care provider usually performs a rectal examination to palpate for enlargement of the prostate or other possible pathology. If enlargement exists, a serum PSA test will most likely be ordered, especially prior to any treatment, and this test may also be ordered during treatment. PSA levels may be increased in pathological conditions of the prostate; establish a baseline and monitor these levels for comparative purposes. PSA levels are expected to decrease with effective therapeutic regimens. PSA levels tend to increase with age as the prostate gland

grows. Recent research encourages the use of a PSA value of less than 4 mcg/L as the criterion for normal levels, although less than 2.5 mcg/L for patients under the age of 50 is recommended. (See also Evidence in Practice: Men's Health Concerns and Screening of Prostate Cancer.)

Prior to the administration of testosterone and related drugs, assess patients for liver disease, because peliosis (formation of blood-filled cavities) may occur. Peliosis is associated with long-term therapy and may be life-threatening. Perform liver function studies (e.g., LDH, CPK, bilirubin levels) as ordered, to monitor for the possible adverse effect of abnormal liver function and jaundice. Because edema is also a problem with these drugs,

DOSAGES Selected Men's Health Drugs

Drug	Pharmacological Class	Usual Dosage Range	Indications
finasteride (Propecia, Proscar)	5α-reductase inhibitor	*Adults* PO: 1 mg daily (Propecia) *Adults* PO: 5 mg daily (Proscar)	Androgenic alopecia (baldness; males only) Benign prostatic hyperplasia
sildenafil citrate (Viagra)	Phosphodiesterase inhibitor	*Adults (males only)* PO: 25–100 mg 1 hr before sexual intercourse; no more than once daily	Erectile dysfunction
tamsulosin hydrochloride (Flomax CR®)	Alpha 1 adrenoreceptor blocker	*Adults* PO: 0.4 mg	Benign prostatic hyperplasia
testosterone cypionate (Depo-Testosterone)	Androgenic hormone	*Adults and adolescents* IM: 50–400 mg q3–4 wk	Delayed puberty or hypogonadism (in males)
testosterone, transdermal (Androderm, AndroGel, Testim 1%)	Androgenic hormone	*Adults and adolescents* Androderm patch (applied to skin of back, abdomen, upper arms, or thighs): 2.5–5 mg/day AndroGel (applied to shoulders, arms, or abdominal skin): 5 daily (delivers 50 mg of testosterone)	Male hypogonadism Male hypogonadism

 # SPECIAL POPULATIONS: OLDER ADULTS

Sildenafil: Use and Concerns

- One in 10 men in the world has erectile dysfunction. Over 3 million men over the age of 40 are affected in Canada. It is one-and-a-half times more common among men with cardiovascular disease and three times more common among men with diabetes than among the general population. The incidence of erectile dysfunction increases with age, with 39% at 40 years of age and 65% in those older than 65 years of age.

- Sildenafil (Viagra) is a prescription medication that is commonly ordered to treat erectile dysfunction, but it is not without concerns and cautions for the patient. This is especially true for older adults, who generally have other medical conditions (e.g., kidney disorders, hypertension, diabetes) and are usually taking more than one other prescribed medication (e.g., nitrates).

- Liver function declines with age; therefore, drugs may not be metabolized as effectively in older adults as they are in younger adults. In addition, sildenafil is highly protein bound, which causes it to stay in the body longer and thus increases the possibility for drug interactions and toxicity.

- A decreased dosage of sildenafil is generally indicated for patients over 65 years of age and for those with liver or kidney impairment.

- Adverse effects to be concerned about in all patients, particularly older patients, include headache, flushing, and dyspepsia. Sildenafil must be used cautiously in patients who have heart disease and angina, because these patients are at greater risk for complications, especially if they are taking nitrates. Severe hypotension can occur. Sildenafil produces an 8 to 10 mm decrease in systolic blood pressure and a 5 to 6 mm decrease in diastolic blood pressure that begins 1 hour after taking a dose. The effect can last for approximately 4 hours.

- Discussing topics of a sexual nature may be comfortable for some patients but produce anxiety in others. Be aware of ethnocultural and gender differences in how individuals perceive their own sexuality, how they generally deal with sexual performance issues, and with whom they share this information. Be respectful of each individual's beliefs and feelings, including their sexual beliefs and practices. This requires knowledge, sensitivity, and objectivity.

recording baseline weights, intake and output, and history of any cardiovascular diseases is also important. Another contraindication for which to assess is that of a history of known androgen-responsive tumours.

Finasteride requires baseline assessment of urinary patterns with attention to frequency, urgency, and flow of urine with micturation. As the tissue responds to the drug and there is a reduction in the size of the prostate gland and thus improvement in the symptoms of BPH, urinary flow will be increased. With potentially teratogenic drugs such as finasteride, follow special handling precautions and advise any pregnant caregiver or partner to do the same. Finasteride is not to be given to women. Assessment of the patient's sexual functioning

EVIDENCE IN PRACTICE

Men's Health Concerns and Screening of Prostate Cancer

Review

Prostate cancer is the most common nonskin malignancy diagnosed in men and the third leading cause of cancer-related death in men in Canada. It is estimated that 24 000 men were diagnosed with prostate cancer in 2015 (representing 24% of the incidence of cancer in men) and 4 100 men died of this cancer (representing 10% of all cancer deaths). The lifetime risk of developing prostate cancer in Canadian men is 1 in 8, while the risk of dying from it is 1 in 27. The risk for developing prostate cancer increases after the age of 50, and it is most commonly diagnosed in men over the age of 65. Black men have a 60% higher incidence of prostate cancer than White men; they are often diagnosed at a younger age and the tumours tend to be more advanced and aggressive. Men of Asian ancestry tend to have a lower incidence of prostate cancer.

Screening with the prostate-specific antigen (PSA) may be done in men suspected of having prostate cancer. However, the use of the PSA test is controversial.

Types of Evidence

Hayes and Barry (2014) conducted a systematic review of the literature. Two trials dominated the literature: the Prostate, Lung, Colorectal and Ovarian screening trial and the European Randomized Study of Screening for Prostate Cancer. These trials examined whether PSA screening improved prostate cancer mortality when compared with no screening. The Prostate, Lung, Colorectal, and Ovarian trial randomized 76 685 men aged 55 to 74 years to annual PSA testing for 6 years and digital rectal examination for 4 years. The European trial randomized 182 160 men in 7 countries to PSA screening without digital rectal examination every 4 years.

Results

The European trial had an increase in the incidence of prostate cancer with PSA screening and a small survival benefit with PSA screening after an 11-year follow-up; however, aggressive management (e.g., radical prostatectomy) showed adverse outcomes of erectile dysfunction, urinary incontinence, and bowel problems. In addition, the Prostate, Lung, Colorectal, and Ovarian Cancer Screening Trial found an increased incidence of prostate cancer but no mortality benefit for yearly PSA screening after a follow-up of 13 years.

Link of Evidence to Nursing Practice

The current evidence is insufficient to clearly determine whether regular screening for prostate cancer using the PSA reduces mortality from prostate cancer. PSA screening tests detect prostate cancer at an early stage; however, early detection and early intervention may not alter overall outcomes. Approximately one in four men with an abnormal PSA result will actually have prostate cancer. In addition, potential harm, such as false positive results and complications of biopsy, may outweigh the benefit of screening. It is important for health care providers to discuss the potential risks and benefits of PSA screening with men aged 55 to 69 years who are at average risk of developing prostate cancer. A discussion of close surveillance and watchful waiting should also be included.

Sources: Canadian Cancer Society. (2015). *Prostate cancer statistics.* Retrieved from http://www.cancer.ca/en/cancer-information/cancer-type/prostate/statistics; Hayes, J. H., & Barry, M. J. (2014). Screening for prostate cancer with the prostate-specific antigen test: A review of current evidence. *Journal of the American Medical Association, 311*(11), 1143–1149. doi:10.1001/jama.2014.2085

and libido is important due to possible interference from the drug.

Before drugs for erectile dysfunction are given, the health care provider will perform a physical examination. Perform a thorough nursing assessment including vital signs, and obtain a thorough medication history, including whether the patient is on antihypertensives (e.g., diuretics such as hydrochlorothiazide and β-blockers such as atenolol), which may cause erectile dysfunction. Take a thorough cardiac history and assess for contraindications to the use of phosphodiesterase inhibitors (e.g., sildenafil, vardenafil hydrochloride [Levitra], and tadalafil [Cialis]), such as major cardiovascular disorders or the use of nitrate medications (nitroglycerin, isosorbide mononitrate, or dinitrate). The erectile dysfunction drugs and nitrates may lead to severe hypotension that may not respond to treatment.

Nursing Diagnoses

- Decreased cardiac output related to drug interaction between erectile dysfunction drug and nitrates
- Ineffective sexuality pattern related to the effects of treatment with androgens or therapy with phosphodiesterase inhibitors
- Deficient knowledge related to lack of information about the disease process of BPH and related drug therapy (including drug interactions with finasteride)

Planning

Goals

- Patient will maintain normal and adequate cardiac output.
- Patient will maintain or regain effective sexual patterns and functioning.
- Patient will display adequate knowledge regarding disease process and recommended drug therapy.

Expected Patient Outcomes

- Patient maintains blood pressure within normal limits with at least 120/80 mm Hg readings.
    - Patient experiences minimal drop in systolic and diastolic blood pressure during drug therapy with erectile dysfunction drugs or androgens.
    - Patient avoids potential interactions with medication regimen (e.g., nitrates not to be taken with erectile dysfunction drugs) as well as situations and substances that may exacerbate hypotension, such as saunas, alcohol, and hot climates.
    - Patient reports any repeated low blood pressure readings, dizziness, or feelings of lightheadedness to practitioner.
- Patient openly verbalizes feelings of inadequacy associated with changes in libido or sexual functioning and seeks out help from a health care provider.
    - Patient takes medication as prescribed to minimize adverse effects and maximize therapeutic effects.
    - Patient implements suggestions for improving libido and sexual functioning as recommended by the health care provider.
    - Patient verbalizes the ability to sustain and maintain an erection or complete the act of coitus.
- Patient states understanding of the rationale for drug therapy.

Implementation

The therapeutic effects of testosterone are maximized when the drug is taken as ordered and at regular intervals so that steady levels are maintained. If the drug is being used for hypogonadism or induction of puberty, dosages may be managed differently, so that at the end of the growth spurt the patient is placed on maintenance dosages. Instruct patients to apply Testoderm transdermal patches as ordered, which is usually to clean, dry scrotal skin that has been shaved for optimal skin contact, with daily replacement. Educate patients that Androderm patches should be placed on clean, dry skin on the back, abdomen, upper arms, or thighs; the scrotum and bony areas (shoulder, hip) are not to be used with this particular drug. Be sure the proper patch is being used and that drugs are not confused. AndroGel is to be applied to shoulders, arms, or abdominal skin as ordered. Axiron solution is applied to the underarm only, using a no-touch applicator. The pump should be primed prior to first use. One actuation delivers 30 mg of testosterone to the applicator. Once applied, educate the patient to let the application site dry for about 2 minutes before putting on clothing. If testosterone is being given intramuscularly, it is usually given every 2 to 4 weeks as prescribed. Mix the vial of medication thoroughly by agitating it before withdrawing the prescribed amount of medication.

Finasteride may be given orally without regard to meals. When used for treatment of the urinary symptoms of BPH, finasteride and related drugs may be ordered for approximately 3 to 6 months, with a re-evaluation of the condition following this period. Advise patients to protect the drug from exposure to light and heat. Due to the teratogenic effects of finasteride, emphasize that it must not be handled in any form by a pregnant woman. Recommend that female nurses and other female members of the health care team wear gloves when handling this medication. It is recommended that women of any age do not take this medication.

See the Natural Health Products box for a description of saw palmetto, a natural health product that is often taken to relieve symptoms of an enlarged prostate.

For patients taking erectile dysfunction drugs, alert them to the serious adverse effect of severe drops in blood pressure caused by interaction with nitrates. When taking sildenafil, vardenafil hydrochloride, or tadalafil, priapism (the abnormally prolonged erection of the penis), may occur; it is considered a medical emergency and requires immediate and urgent medical attention. See the Patient Teaching Tips for more information.

Evaluation

The therapeutic effects of drugs related to the male reproductive tract include improvement of the condition and symptoms for which the patient is being treated, such as hypogonadism, sexual dysfunction, erectile dysfunction, and urinary elimination problems caused by BPH. The therapeutic effects of some drugs (e.g., finasteride) may not be seen for 6 to 12 months, so it is important for the nurse to observe and monitor the patient for the intended effects of the drugs. In addition, evaluate for the adverse effects of these medications (see the Pharmacology section for specific adverse effects). Always evaluate goals and expected outcomes to see if the patient's needs have been met.

NATURAL HEALTH PRODUCTS

Saw Palmetto *(Serenoa repens, Sabul serrulata)*

OVERVIEW

Saw palmetto comes from a tree that is also known as the American dwarf palm. The therapeutically active part of the tree is its ripe fruit. Saw palmetto is believed to inhibit dihydrotestosterone and 5α-reductase. A prostatic-specific antigen test and digital rectal examination should be performed before initiation of treatment with saw palmetto for benign prostatic hyperplasia.

COMMON USES

Diuretic, urinary antiseptic, treatment of benign prostatic hyperplasia, treatment of alopecia

ADVERSE EFFECTS

Gastrointestinal upset, headache, back pain, dysuria

POTENTIAL DRUG INTERACTIONS

Nonsteroidal anti-inflammatory drugs (NSAIDs), hormones such as estrogen replacement therapy and oral contraceptives, immunostimulants

CONTRAINDICATIONS

None

CASE STUDY

Erectile Dysfunction Drugs

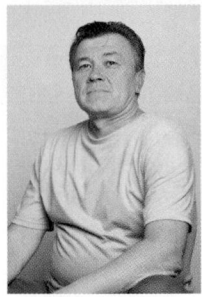

Yuri, a 63-year-old college instructor, is in the office for a yearly checkup. He feels he is generally healthy, and he does not take any medications. He says that he does have one problem that he wants to discuss with the health care provider. During his physical examination, he says, "I have something embarrassing to ask. I want to try one of those drugs that can help my sex life." The nurse practitioner reassures Yuri that he does not need to be embarrassed to ask about this. The nurse practitioner then assesses Yuri's sexual difficulties. At the end of the examination and assessment, Yuri is given a prescription for sildenafil (Viagra).

1. What teaching is important for Yuri before he starts this medication?
2. Eleven months later, Yuri is admitted to the emergency department with chest pains. After a thorough exami-

nation, including a cardiac catheterization, he is diagnosed with mild coronary artery disease and is started on an extended-release form of isosorbide-5-mononitrate, 60 mg every 12 hours. He is given a follow-up appointment with the nurse practitioner in 1 week. What specific teaching is important at this time?
3. Yuri comes to the office for the follow-up appointment and tells the nurse practitioner that he wants to try saw palmetto for his prostate health. He has a neighbour who takes it and has no problems with it, and he has noticed that he has had a slight increase in difficulty with urination. He is also upset about what he was told in the hospital about his medications. How will the nurse respond to Yuri and what assessments are needed at this time?

For answers, see http://evolve.elsevier.com/Canada/Lilley/pharmacology/.

PATIENT TEACHING TIPS

❖ Prior to the initiation of therapy with finasteride, provide education at the patient's educational level about the drug's therapeutic effects as well as adverse effects (see the previous discussion for more information). Educate female family members, significant others, and caregivers who are pregnant or of childbearing age about the need to avoid exposure during handling of this drug, including *not* touching any broken or crushed tablets, which could result in exposure to the drug and the risk of teratogenic effects. Emphasize the need to wear gloves when handling the medication. Finasteride may be given orally without regard to meals. Instruct patients to protect the drug from exposure to light and heat.

❖ Patients taking sildenafil should be aware that it is usually prescribed to be taken about 1 hour before sexual activity. This drug, and other drugs for erectile dysfunction, should not be taken with nitrates because this could lead to significant and potentially life-threatening hypotensive consequences.
❖ Inform patients that drug therapy for erectile dysfunction is not effective without sexual stimulation and arousal.
❖ Prior to therapy with testosterone, educate patients about all therapeutic and adverse effects. Emphasize the importance of follow-up appointments, which are crucial to evaluating the therapeutic effectiveness of the medication (as with any drugs discussed in this chapter).

Continued

PATIENT TEACHING TIPS—cont'd

❖ Patients should be informed that prolonged erections (i.e., longer than 4 hours) must be reported immediately to a health care provider and are considered a medical emergency.

❖ Educate patients that testosterone is not be withdrawn abruptly except under the supervision of the health care provider. Weaning is usually done over several weeks.

KEY POINTS

❖ The most commonly used drugs related to male health and the male reproductive tract are finasteride, sildenafil, and testosterone. It is important to know the ways these drugs work and their adverse effects, contraindications, cautions, and drug interactions to ensure their safe and effective use.

❖ Testosterone is responsible for the development and maintenance of the male reproductive system and secondary sex characteristics. Oral testosterone has poor pharmacokinetic and pharmacodynamic characteristics; thus, it is usually recommended that testosterone be administered parenterally or via a transdermal patch.

❖ Finasteride is usually indicated to stop growth of the prostate in men with BPH and to treat men with androgenic alopecia.

❖ Warn patients taking drugs for erectile dysfunction (e.g., sildenafil) about potential adverse effects, such as hypotension, headache, and heartburn.

❖ There are major concerns about deaths related to heart dysfunction associated with concurrent use of nitrates and drugs used for erectile dysfunction. Focus patient education on the prevention of drug interactions and related adverse effects and complications.

EXAMINATION REVIEW QUESTIONS

1. A patient has been taking finasteride (Proscar) for almost a year. The nurse knows that which of the following is important to monitor when a patient is taking finasteride (Proscar)?
a. Complete blood count
b. PSA levels
c. Blood pressure
d. Fluid retention

2. The nurse is performing an assessment of a patient who is asking for a prescription for sildenafil (Viagra). Which finding would be a contraindication to its use?
a. Age of 65 years
b. History of thyroid disease
c. Medication list that includes nitrates
d. Medication list that includes saw palmetto

3. During a counselling session for a group of adolescent athletes, the use of androgenic steroids is discussed. The nurse should explain that which problem is a rare but devastating effect of androgenic steroid use?
a. Peliosis of the liver
b. Bradycardia
c. Kidney failure
d. Tachydysrhythmias

4. The nurse is teaching a patient about the possible adverse effect of priapism, which may occur when taking erectile dysfunction drugs. What is the most important action for the nurse to emphasize if this occurs?
a. Stay in bed until the erection ceases.
b. Apply an ice pack for 30 minutes.
c. Turn toward the left side and rest.
d. Seek medical attention immediately.

5. The nurse is teaching a patient about the use of saw palmetto for prostate health. Which drugs that interact with saw palmetto include would the nurse include in the teaching?
a. Acetaminophen (Tylenol®)
b. Nitrates
c. NSAIDs
d. Antihypertensive drugs

6. When the Testoderm form of testosterone is ordered to treat hypogonadism in an adolescent boy, which instructions to be given by the nurse are correct? (Select all that apply.)
a. Place the patch on clean, dry skin on the back, upper arms, abdomen, or thighs.
b. Place the patch on clean, dry scrotal skin that has been shaved.
c. Place the patch on clean, dry scrotal skin, but do not shave the skin first.
d. Place the patch on any clean, dry, nonhairy area of the body.
e. Remove the old patch before applying a new patch.

7. A 16-year-old male is to receive testosterone cypionate (Depo-Testosterone), 50 mg IM every 2 weeks. The medication is available in 100-mg/mL vials. How many millilitres will the nurse draw up in the syringe to administer for each dose?

CRITICAL THINKING ACTIVITIES

1. During morning medication rounds, a nurse is about to give a dose of finasteride (Proscar) when the patient asks the nurse to crush the pill, which is not enteric coated. What is the nurse's priority action in response to his request?

2. A male patient calls the clinic to ask about topical testosterone gel. This morning, he applied the daily dose to his upper arms and, without thinking, picked up his young granddaughter soon afterward. He is upset because he thinks this will harm his granddaughter. What is the priority action at this time?

3. During an office checkup, a patient tells you, "Ever since I started that pill for my prostate gland I'm having trouble with sex. I just don't have the interest anymore. Could it be the pill?" When you check his medical record, you see that he started taking dutasteride (Avodart), a 5α-reductase inhibitor, 3 months ago. What is your best answer?

For answers, see http://evolve.elsevier.com/Canada/Lilley/pharmacology/.

PART SIX

Drugs Affecting the Respiratory System

STUDY SKILLS TIPS:
- STUDY ON THE RUN, PURR

STUDY ON THE RUN, PURR

Study on the Run (SOTR) is about making use of small blocks of time that pop up in your day. The steps Plan, Rehearse, and Review do not require that the entire chapter be covered in one study session. These steps benefit learning through repetition of material— the more you repeat something, the better you will recall it on a test.

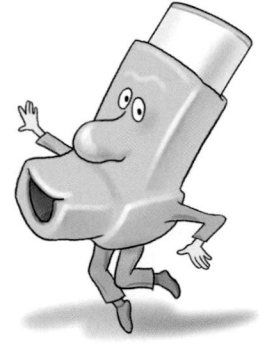

Where Is the Time?

Small blocks of time are everywhere in your day; it is just a matter of becoming aware of them. Finishing an exam early, standing in the checkout line, or even waiting for the washing machine to finish the last spin before you change loads can be time used for SOTR. Remember, every minute of time you use this way is a minute of time you will not have to find later.

SOTR and Plan

These study skills sections have repeatedly stressed the importance of questioning as an essential component of the Plan step. Look at the chapter objectives for Chapter 37. There are three objectives presented for this chapter. Work on the questions for as many of these objectives as you can in the time you have. If you complete questions for only two objectives, do not think that you are failing to complete something. Instead, learn to view what you

have done as that much less to do later. The time you spend now frees up that much more time during your large blocks of study time for intense study reading.

Will you forget the questions you generated before you have the opportunity to read the chapter? If you make it a habit to ask questions, you will find that you remember the focus questions well. If you have trouble remembering your questions, write them down in the margins of the text. Gradually, you will find that questioning has become such an automatic procedure that you will not need to write down the questions; you will remember them.

SOTR and Vocabulary

One of the most challenging aspects of a course like this is the almost overwhelming vocabulary load. As if the new vocabulary were not enough, you also need to keep reviewing previous parts and chapters because a term that was introduced three chapters ago has reappeared and you do not remember it clearly. Creating your own vocabulary cards is a perfect SOTR activity.

The basic card model is simple. The word, common form, prefix, or suffix appears on the card front. The back of the card may have just a little information, the minimum being a definition of what is on the front. Or the back of the card may contain considerable information. By including part, chapter, and page number on the back, you can locate the term quickly if the need arises. In addition, you may want to add a specific example from the text or one of your own creation to help clarify the term. Put as much information on the back as you find useful. It might also be helpful to colour code your cards. For example, all cards having to do with the cardiac system could be pink and all cards relating to the respiratory system, blue. Using these simple strategies makes your learning fun and effective.

Creating Vocabulary Cards With SOTR

Use the time between classes to create personal vocabulary cards. Grab your text and your blank note cards and open to the next chapter you will be studying. Flip over to the Key Terms section. Write the first key term on the front of a blank note card. Flip the card over. Write the part number, chapter number, and page number for the key term on the card. Pick a standard location for this—you can write these numbers in a top corner or a bottom corner, but make sure you put them in the same corner every time. Eventually, this practice will become a habit and make the preparation process faster. This consistency also helps when you are making use of the cards because you will know exactly what information you put on the card and where you put it. Put this card aside and repeat the process with the next key term. In those few minutes before you go to class, you can complete the basic preparation for a full set of cards, covering the 17 terms in the Chapter 37 Key Terms.

Note that the paragraph above did not suggest copying the definition from the Key Terms at this time. The term may be much easier to understand when used in the context of a sentence and a paragraph. If, as you read the chapter, you feel that the Key Terms definition is also useful to have on this card, you can always flip back, using the location information you put on the card.

SOTR and Vocabulary Review

Your vocabulary cards are ideal for SOTR action. Carry a deck of cards with you at all times. Whenever you have even a minute or two, you can pull out a stack of cards— cards from previous chapters or the current chapter. Use the oral ask-and-answer method discussed in the *Study Guide*. For instance, the first key term in Chapter 37 is *adrenergics*. Ask yourself aloud, "What is an *adrenergic*?" Then try to answer the question aloud. Answer: "An adrenergic is a drug that stimulates the sympathetic nerve fibres of the autonomic nervous system." It is not necessary to recall the exact definition presented in the

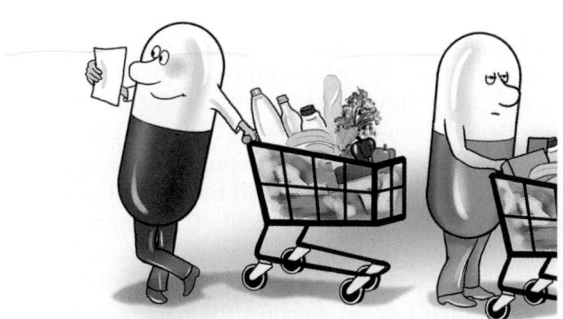

Key Terms or chapter. What is important is that you respond with a clear and meaningful answer. The answer given above is not exactly the same as that stated in the Key Terms, but the general concept is the same. Once you have stated your answer, turn the card over and check to make sure that you were correct. Each time you do this with a term, you are strengthening your long-term memory, and you will find that it takes less and less time to recall the terms you need.

SOTR and Chapter Review

It can be overwhelming if you think that review means rereading the material and that you therefore need large blocks of uninterrupted time. There is a much more efficient way to review, and it works well in short time blocks, making it a perfect technique for SOTR.

Look at the first page of Chapter 37. You should instantly see a number of visible structures that make it easy to review key terms and concepts without rereading the entire block of material. First, there is the chapter title: *Antihistamines, Decongestants, Antitussives, and Expectorants*. What are antihistamines? This is a question you would have generated when you were engaged in the Plan step of PURR. Now that you have read the chapter, repeat the question and answer it aloud. Answer aloud because you will hear what you say—you will either know the material or need to mark it to come back and reread. Now ask a more complex question: "What is the role of antihistamines? What do they do?" Now try to answer these questions. If you can, then you do not need to reread to find out what antihistamines are. Next, you will notice some words are in *italic*. Apply the same process. Using the boldface words and phrases as a stimulus, ask questions and try to answer them to your own satisfaction. If you cannot develop a satisfactory answer, then you know that some rereading is needed. But it is very focused. You are not trying to reread everything on the page, only the material right there, associated with the term.

Looking under the major heading Antihistamines, at the end of the first paragraph, you will read, "The release of excessive amounts of histamine can lead to anaphylaxis and severe allergic symptoms and may result in any or all of the following physiological changes." Ask questions. If you can answer them, no reading is necessary. If you cannot answer them, you know that the answers are found immediately after this sentence in the indented list. Use the structures in the chapter to accomplish focused review. Comprehension is improved, long-term memory is strengthened, and your test grades will reflect this.

The benefits of SOTR are enormous. There are no drawbacks. You are using time that otherwise would be "wasted." This time now becomes productive study time. The more active you become in looking for SOTR opportunities, the more you will find.

Antihistamines, Decongestants, Antitussives, and Expectorants

Objectives

After reading this chapter, the successful student will be able to do the following:

1. Provide specific examples of the drugs categorized as antihistamines (both sedating and nonsedating), decongestants, antitussives, and expectorants.

2. Discuss the mechanisms of action, indications, contraindications, cautions, drug interactions, adverse effects, dosages, and routes of administration for antihistamines, decongestants, antitussives, and expectorants.

3. Develop a collaborative plan of care that includes all phases of the nursing process for patients taking any of the antihistamines, decongestants, antitussives, and expectorants.

e-Learning Activities

Website
(http://evolve.elsevier.com/Canada/Lilley/pharmacology/)

evolve

- Answer Key—Textbook Case Studies
- Answer Key—Critical Thinking Activities
- Chapter Summaries—Printable
- Review Questions for Exam Preparation
- Unfolding Case Studies

Drug Profiles

codeine (codeine phosphate)*, p. 711
▸▸ dextromethorphan (dextromethorphan hydrobromide)*, p. 711
▸▸ diphenhydramine (diphenhydramine hydrochloride)*, p. 707
▸▸ guaifenesin, p. 712
▸▸ loratadine, p. 707
▸▸ oxymetazoline (oxymetazoline hydrochloride), p. 710

▸▸ Key drug

*Full generic name is given in parentheses. For the purposes of this text, the more common, shortened name is used.

Key Terms

Adrenergics (sympathomimetics) Drugs that stimulate the sympathetic nerve fibres of the autonomic nervous system that use epinephrine or epinephrinelike substances as neurotransmitters. (p. 708)

Antagonists Drugs that exert an action opposite to that of another drug or compete for the same receptor sites. (p. 703)

Anticholinergics (parasympatholytics) Drugs that block the action of acetylcholine and similar substances at ace-

tylcholine receptors, which results in inhibition of the transmission of parasympathetic nerve impulses. (p. 708)

Antigens Substances that are capable of inducing specific immune responses and reacting with the specific products of those responses, such as antibodies and specifically sensitized T lymphocytes. Antigens can be soluble (e.g., a foreign protein) or particulate or insoluble (e.g., a bacterial cell). (p. 704)

Antihistamines Substances capable of reducing the physiological and pharmacological effects of histamine. (p. 703)

Antitussives Drugs that reduce coughing, often by inhibiting neural activity in the cough centre of the central nervous system. (p. 710)

Corticosteroids Any of the hormones produced by the adrenal cortex, either in natural or synthetic form. They control many key processes in the body, such as carbohydrate and protein metabolism, the maintenance of serum glucose levels, electrolyte and water balance, and the functions of the cardiovascular system, skeletal muscle, kidneys, and other organs. (p. 708)

Decongestants Drugs that reduce congestion or swelling, especially of the upper or lower respiratory tract. (p. 708)

Empirical therapy A method of treating disease on the basis of observations and experience, rather than on knowledge of the precise cause for the disorder. (p. 702)

Expectorants Drugs that increase the flow of fluid in the respiratory tract, usually by reducing the viscosity of secretions, and facilitate their removal by coughing. (p. 711)

Histamine antagonists Drugs that compete with histamine for binding sites on histamine receptors. (p. 703)

Influenza A highly contagious infection of the respiratory tract caused by a myxovirus and transmitted by airborne droplets. (p. 702)

Non-sedating antihistamines Medications that work peripherally to block the actions of histamine and therefore do not generally have the central nervous system effects of many of the older antihistamines; also called *second-generation antihistamines* and *peripherally acting antihistamines*. (p. 707)

Reflex stimulation An irritation of the respiratory tract occurring in response to an irritation of the gastrointestinal (GI) tract. (p. 711)

Rhinovirus Any of approximately 100 serologically distinct ribonucleic acid (RNA) viruses that cause approximately 40% of acute respiratory illnesses. (p. 702)

Sympathomimetic drugs A class of drugs whose effects mimic those resulting from the stimulation of the sympathetic nervous system. (p. 709)

Upper respiratory tract infection (URI) Any infectious disease of the upper respiratory tract, including the common cold, laryngitis, pharyngitis, rhinitis, sinusitis, and tonsillitis. (p. 702)

COLD MEDICATIONS

Common colds result from a viral infection, most often infection with a **rhinovirus** or an **influenza** virus. These viruses invade the tissues (mucosa) of the upper respiratory tract (nose, pharynx, and larynx) to cause an **upper respiratory tract infection (URI)**. The inflammatory response elicited by these viruses stimulates excessive mucus production. This fluid drips behind the nose, down the pharynx, and into the esophagus and lower respiratory tract, which leads to symptoms typical of a cold: sore throat, coughing, and upset stomach. Irritation of the nasal mucosa often triggers the sneeze reflex and also causes the release of several inflammatory and vasoactive substances, which results in dilation of the small blood vessels in the nasal sinuses and leads to nasal congestion. Treatment of the common symptoms of URI involves the combined use of antihistamines, nasal decongestants, antitussives, and expectorants. In 2009, Health Canada issued recommendations that over-the-counter (OTC) cough and cold products not be given to children younger than 6 years of age. This recommendation followed numerous case reports of symptoms such as oversedation, seizures, hallucinations, tachycardia, and abnormal heart rhythms. There is also evidence that such medications are simply not effective in small children, and parents are advised to consult their pediatrician regarding the best ways to manage these illnesses in young children. The evidence for the effectiveness of antihistamine-decongestant-analgesic combinations in adults and older children is also limited although they may have some general benefit (De Sutter, van Driel, Kumar, & Skrt, 2012).

Many antihistamines, nasal decongestants, antitussives, and expectorants are available without a prescription. However, these drugs can only relieve the symptoms of a URI—they do nothing to eliminate the causative pathogen. Antiviral drugs are currently the only drugs that are effective; however, treatment with these medications is often hampered by the fact that the viral cause cannot be readily identified. Because of this, the treatment rendered can be based only on what is believed to be the most likely cause, given the presenting clinical symptoms. Such treatment is called **empirical therapy**. Some patients seem to gain benefit from the use of natural health products, such as vitamin C, preventing the onset of cold signs and symptoms or at least decreasing their severity. Natural health products commonly used for colds are echinacea and goldenseal (see Natural Health Products box on p. 703). There is limited research data on the efficacy of natural health products and some can have significant drug–drug or drug–disease interactions.

ANTIHISTAMINES

Histamine is a substance that performs many functions. It is involved in nerve impulse transmission in the central nervous system (CNS), dilation of capillaries, contraction of smooth muscle, stimulation of gastric acid secretion, and acceleration of the heart rate. There

NATURAL HEALTH PRODUCTS

ECHINACEA (Echinacea)

Overview

The three species of echinacea are *Echinacea angustifolia*, *Echinacea pallida*, and *Echinacea purpurea*. Echinacea has been shown in clinical trials to reduce cold symptoms and recovery time when taken early in the illness. This is believed to be due to its immunostimulant effects. At this time, there is no strong research evidence to warrant recommending echinacea for prevention of colds; further study is needed to show evidence of its therapeutic effects and indications.

Common Uses

Stimulation of the immune system, antisepsis, treatment of viral infections and influenzalike respiratory tract infections, promotion of healing of wounds, and treatment of chronic ulcerations

Adverse Effects

Dermatitis, upset stomach or vomiting, dizziness, headache, unpleasant taste

Potential Drug Interactions

Amiodarone hydrochloride, cyclosporine, phenytoin, methotrexate, ketoconazole, barbiturates; tolerance is likely to develop if used for more than 8 weeks

Contraindications

Contraindicated for patients with AIDS, tuberculosis, connective tissue diseases, multiple sclerosis

GOLDENSEAL (Hydrastis canadensis)

Overview

Goldenseal is native to wooded areas in Canada and the eastern United States. It is the dried root of a plant that is most commonly used for its biologically active alkaloids. These components have been shown to have antibacterial, antifungal, and antiprotozoal activity. The alkaloid berberine has both anticholinergic and antihistaminic activity.

Common Uses

Treatment of URIs, allergies, nasal congestion, and numerous genitourinary, skin, ophthalmic, and otic conditions

Adverse Effects

Gastrointestinal distress, emotional instability, mucosal ulceration (e.g., when used as a vaginal douche)

Potential Drug Interactions

Gastric acid suppressors (including antacids, histamine H_2 blockers [e.g., ranitidine hydrochloride], proton pump inhibitors [e.g., omeprazole]): theoretically reduced effectiveness because of acid-promoting effect of the herb

Antihypertensives: theoretically reduced effectiveness because of vasoconstrictive activity of the herb

Contraindications

Acute or chronic GI disorders; pregnancy (as it has uterine-stimulant properties); should be used with caution by those with cardiovascular disease

Source: Skidmore-Roth, L. (2010). *Mosby's handbook of herbs and natural supplements* (4th ed.). St. Louis, MO: Mosby.

---

are two types of cellular receptors for histamine. Histamine 1 (H_1) receptors mediate smooth muscle contraction and dilation of capillaries; histamine 2 (H_2) receptors mediate acceleration of the heart rate and gastric acid secretion. The release of excessive amounts of histamine can lead to anaphylaxis and severe allergic symptoms and may result in any or all of the following physiological changes:

- Constriction of smooth muscle, especially in the stomach and lungs
- Increase in body secretions
- Vasodilation and increased capillary permeability, which results in the movement of fluid out of the blood vessels and into the tissues, causing a drop in blood pressure and edema

Antihistamines are drugs that directly compete with histamine for specific receptor sites. For this reason, they are also called **histamine antagonists**. Antihistamines that compete with histamine for the H_2 receptors are called H_2 *antagonists* or H_2 *blockers* and include such drugs as cimetidine, ranitidine hydrochloride (Zantac®), famotidine (Pepcid AC®), and nizatidine (Axid®). Because they act on the GI system, they are discussed in

detail in Chapter 39. This chapter focuses on the H_1 antagonists (or H_1 blockers); they are the drugs commonly known as *antihistamines*. They are very useful drugs, as approximately 10 to 20% of the general population is sensitive to various environmental allergens. Histamine is a major inflammatory mediator in many allergic disorders, such as allergic rhinitis (e.g., hay fever, mold, and dust allergies), anaphylaxis, angioedema, drug fevers, insect bite reactions, and urticaria (pale red, raised, itchy bumps).

H_1 antagonists include drugs such as diphenhydramine (Benadryl®), chlorpheniramine maleate (generic; also found in Coricidin® in combination with acetaminophen, dextromethorphan hydrochloride, or both), fexofenadine hydrochloride (Allegra®), loratadine (Claritin®), desloratadine (Aerius®), and cetirizine hydrochloride (Reactine®). They are of greatest value in the treatment of nasal allergies, particularly seasonal hay fever. They are also given to relieve the symptoms of the common cold, such as sneezing and runny nose. When used in this way, they are palliative, not curative; that is, they can help alleviate the symptoms of a cold but can do nothing to destroy the virus causing it.

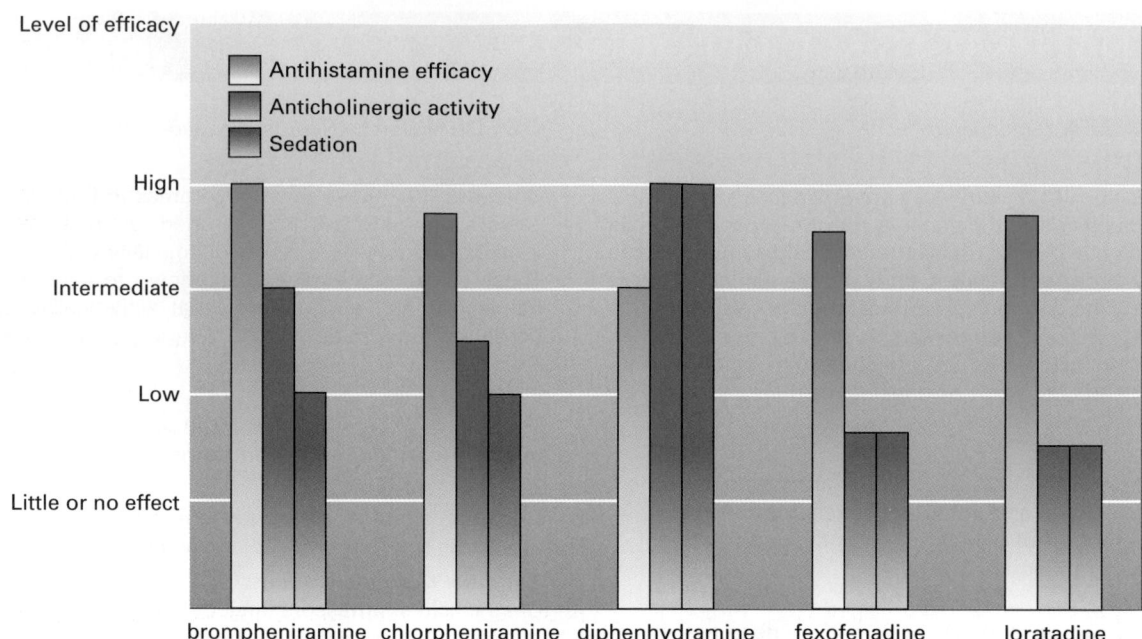

FIG. 37-1   Comparison of efficacy and adverse effects of selected antihistamines.

The clinical efficacy of the different antihistamines is similar, although they have varying degrees of antihistaminic, anticholinergic, and sedating properties. The actions and indications for a particular antihistamine are determined by its specific chemical makeup. All antihistamines compete with histamine for the H_1 receptors in the smooth muscle surrounding blood vessels and bronchioles. They also affect the secretions of the lacrimal, salivary, and respiratory mucosal glands, which are the primary anticholinergic actions of antihistamines. These drugs differ from each other in their potency and adverse effects, especially in the degree of drowsiness they produce. The antihistaminic, anticholinergic, and sedative properties of some of the more commonly used antihistamines are summarized in Figure 37-1. Because of their antihistaminic properties, they are indicated for the treatment of allergies. They are also useful for the treatment of problems such as vertigo, motion sickness, insomnia, and cough. Several classes of antihistamines are listed in Table 37-1, along with their various anticholinergic and sedative effects.

Mechanism of Action and Drug Effects

During allergic reactions, histamine and other substances are released from mast cells, basophils, and other cells in response to **antigens** circulating in the blood. Histamine molecules then bind to and activate other cells in the nose, eyes, respiratory tract, GI tract, and skin, producing the characteristic allergic signs and symptoms (see Figure 37-2). For example, in the respiratory tract, histamine causes extravascular smooth muscle (e.g., in the bronchial tree) to contract, whereas antihistamines cause it to relax. Also, histamine causes pruritus by stimulating

nerve endings. Antihistamines can prevent or alleviate this itching.

Circulating histamine molecules bind to histamine receptors on basophils and mast cells. This stimulates further release of histamine stored within these cells. Antihistamine drugs work by blocking the histamine receptors on the surfaces of basophils and mast cells, thereby preventing the release and actions of histamine stored within these cells. They do not push off histamine that is already bound to a receptor but compete with histamine for unoccupied receptors. Therefore, antihistamines are most beneficial when given early in a histamine-mediated reaction, before all of the free histamine molecules bind to cell membrane receptors. This binding of H_1 blockers to these receptors prevents the adverse consequences of histamine binding: vasodilation; increased GI, respiratory, salivary, and lacrimal secretions; and increased capillary permeability with resulting edema. The various drug effects of antihistamines are listed in Table 37-2.

Indications

Antihistamines are indicated for the management of nasal allergies, seasonal or perennial allergic rhinitis (e.g., hay fever), and some of the typical symptoms of the common cold. They are also useful in the treatment of allergic reactions, motion sickness, Parkinson's disease (because of their anticholinergic effects), and vertigo. In addition, they are sometimes used as sleep aids.

Contraindications

Use of antihistamines is contraindicated in cases of known drug allergy. They are not to be used as the sole drug therapy during acute asthmatic attacks. In such

TABLE 37-1

Effects of Selected Antihistamines

Chemical Class	Anticholinergic Effects	Sedative Effects	Comments
ALKYLAMINES			
brompheniramine maleate	Moderate	Low	Cause less drowsiness and more central nervous system stimulation; suitable for daytime use
chlorpheniramine maleate	Moderate	Low	
ETHANOLAMINES			
clemastine	High	Moderate	Substantial anticholinergic effects; commonly cause sedation; at usual dosages, drowsiness occurs in about 50% of patients; diphenhydramine and dimenhydrinate also used as antiemetics
dimenhydrinate	High	High	
diphenhydramine hydrochloride	High	High	
ETHYLENEDIAMINES			
pyrilamine	Low to none	Low	Weak sedative effects, but adverse GI effects are common
tripelennamine	Low to none	Moderate	
PHENOTHIAZINE			
promethazine hydrochloride	High	High	Drugs in this class are principally used as antipsychotics; some are useful as antihistamines, antipruritics, and antiemetics
PIPERIDINES			
cyproheptadine hydrochloride	Moderate	Low	Commonly used in the treatment of motion sickness; hydroxyzine hydrochloride is used as a tranquilizer, sedative, antipruritic, and antiemetic
hydroxyzine hydrochloride	Moderate	Moderate	
MISCELLANEOUS			
fexofenadine hydrochloride	Low to none	Low to none	Few adverse anticholinergic or sedative effects; almost exclusively antihistaminic effects, so can be taken during the day because no sedative effects occur; they are longer acting and have fewer adverse effects than other classes
loratadine	Low to none	Low to none	

TABLE 37-2

Antihistamines: Drug Effects

Body System	Histamine Effects	Antihistamine Effects
Cardiovascular (small blood vessels)	Dilates blood vessels, increases blood vessel permeability (allows substances to leak into tissues)	Reduces dilation of blood vessels and increases permeability
Immune (release of substances commonly associated with allergic reactions)	Released from mast cells along with several other substances, which results in allergic reactions	Does not stabilize mast cells or prevent the release of histamine and other substances, but does bind to histamine receptors and prevents the actions of histamine
Smooth muscle (on exocrine glands)	Stimulates salivary, gastric, lacrimal, and bronchial secretions	Reduces salivary, gastric, lacrimal, and bronchial secretions

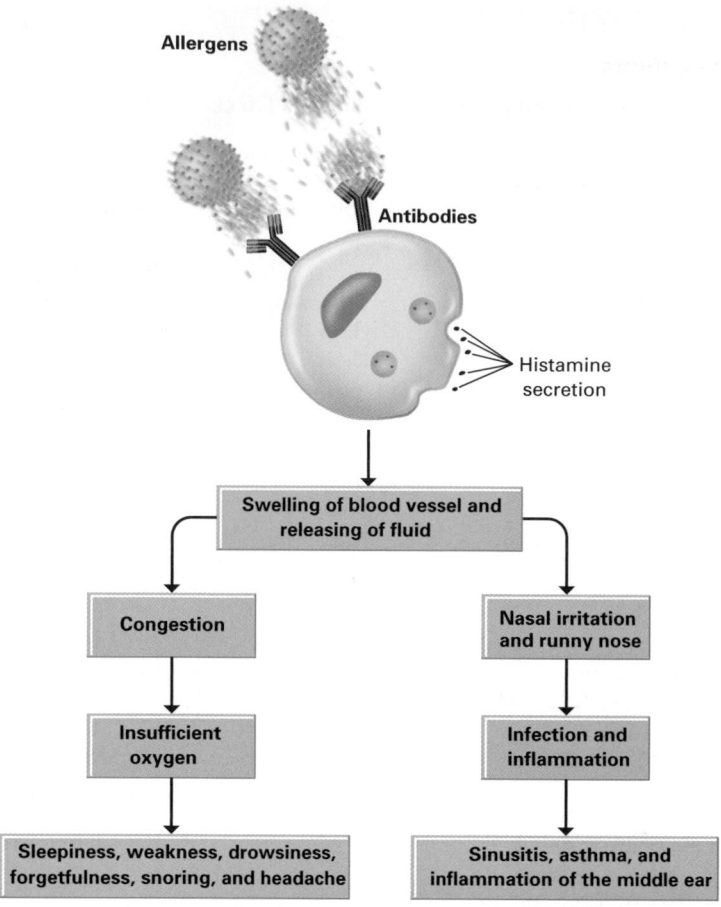

Allergens

Antibodies

Histamine
secretion

Swelling of blood vessel and
releasing of fluid

Congestion

Nasal irritation
and runny nose

Insufficient
oxygen

Infection and
inflammation

Sleepiness, weakness, drowsiness,
forgetfulness, snoring, and headache

Sinusitis, asthma, and
inflammation of the middle ear

FIG. 37-2 Mediation of the allergic response by histamine.

cases, a rapid-acting bronchodilator, such as salbutamol or, in extreme cases, epinephrine, is usually the most urgently needed medication. Other contraindications may include acute-angle glaucoma, heart disease, kidney disease, hypertension, bronchial asthma, chronic obstructive pulmonary disease (COPD), peptic ulcer disease, seizure disorders, benign prostatic hyperplasia (BPH), and pregnancy. Fexofenadine hydrochloride is not recommended for children under 6 years of age or those with kidney impairment. Desloratadine is not recommended for children. Loratadine is not recommended for children younger than 2 years of age. Antihistamines should be used with caution in patients with impaired liver function or kidney insufficiency, as well as in lactating mothers.

Adverse Effects

Drowsiness is usually the chief adverse effect of people who take antihistamines, but sedative effects vary among drugs in this class (see Table 37-1). Fortunately, sedative effects are much less common, although still possible, with newer "nonsedating" drugs. The anticholinergic (drying) effects of antihistamines can cause adverse effects such as dry mouth, changes in vision, difficulty urinating, and constipation. Reported adverse effects of antihistamines are listed in Table 37-3.

TABLE 37-3

Antihistamines: Reported Adverse Effects

Body System	Adverse Effects
Cardiovascular	Dysrhythmias, hypotension, palpitations, syncope,
Central nervous	Sedation, dizziness, muscular weakness, paradoxical excitement, restlessness, nervousness, seizures
Gastrointestinal	Nausea, vomiting, diarrhea, constipation, hepatitis
Other	Dryness of mouth, nose, and throat; urinary retention; vertigo; visual disturbances; tinnitus; headache

Interactions

Drug interactions of antihistamines are listed in Table 37-4. An allergist will usually recommend discontinuation of antihistamine drug therapy at least 4 days prior to allergy testing.

Dosages

For dosage information on selected antihistamines, refer to the table on p. 708.

TABLE	37-4		
Antihistamines: Drug Interactions			
Drug	**Interacting Drug**	**Mechanism**	**Result**
fexofenadine hydrochloride	Erythromycin and other cytochrome P450 inhibitors	Inhibited metabolism	Increased fexofenadine hydrochloride levels
	Phenytoin	Increased metabolism	Decreased fexofenadine hydrochloride levels
loratadine	Ketoconazole, cimetidine, erythromycin	Inhibited metabolism	Increased loratadine levels
diphenhydramine hydrochloride, cetirizine hydrochloride	Alcohol, monoamine oxidase inhibitors, central nervous system depressants	Additive effects	Increased central nervous system depression

DRUG PROFILES

Although some antihistamines are prescription drugs, most are available over the counter. Antihistamines are available in many dosage forms to be administered orally, intramuscularly, intravenously, or topically.

Nonsedating Antihistamines

A major advance in antihistamine therapy occurred with the development of the **nonsedating antihistamines** loratadine, cetirizine hydrochloride, and fexofenadine hydrochloride. These drugs were developed partly to eliminate many of the adverse effects (mainly sedation) of the older antihistamines. These drugs act peripherally to block the actions of histamine and therefore have significantly fewer of the CNS effects of many older antihistamines. For this reason, these drugs are also called *peripherally acting antihistamines* because they do not readily cross the blood–brain barrier, unlike their traditional counterparts. Another advantage of the nonsedating antihistamines is that they have longer durations of action, allowing for once daily dosing; this increases patient adherence to therapy.

▶▶ *loratadine*

Loratadine (Claritin) is a nonsedating antihistamine and is taken only once a day. It is structurally similar to cyproheptadine, but it does not readily distribute into the CNS, which diminishes the sedative effects associated with traditional antihistamines. However, at higher doses, central adverse effects such as drowsiness, headache, and fatigue can be seen. Loratadine is used to relieve the symptoms of seasonal allergic rhinitis (e.g., hay fever) as well as chronic urticaria. Loratadine and its primary active metabolite, desloratidine (Aerius), are both available over the counter.

Drug allergy is the only contraindication to the use of loratadine. The drug is available in oral form as a 10-mg tablet or soft gel capsule, as a 1-mg/mL syrup, as a 10-mg

rapidly disintegrating tablet, and in a combination tablet with the decongestant pseudoephedrine. For recommended dosages, refer to the table on p. 708.

PHARMACOKINETICS

Route	Onset of Action	Peak Plasma Concentration	Elimination Half-Life	Duration of Action
PO	1–3 hr	8–12 hr	8–24 hr	24 hr

Traditional Antihistamines

The traditional antihistamines are older drugs that work both peripherally and centrally. They also have anticholinergic effects, which in some cases make them more effective than nonsedating antihistamines. Some of the commonly used older drugs are diphenhydramine, brompheniramine maleate, chlorpheniramine maleate, dimenhydrinate, and promethazine hydrochloride. They are used either alone or in combination with other drugs for the symptomatic relief of many disorders ranging from insomnia to motion sickness. It is important to note that dimenhydrinate contains between 53 and 55.5% diphenhydramine, which causes the primary effect of drowsiness, and 8-chlorotheophylline, which counteracts drowsiness and causes a lower potency. However, drowsiness is still the primary effect.

Many patients respond to and tolerate these older drugs quite well, and because many are generically available, they are much less expensive. These drugs are available both over the counter and by prescription.

▶▶ *diphenhydramine hydrochloride*

Diphenhydramine hydrochloride (Aller-Aide®, Allernix®, Benadryl®, others) is a traditional antihistamine that acts both peripherally and centrally. It also has anticholinergic and sedative effects. In fact, it is used as a hypnotic drug because of its sedating effects. Its use is not generally advised in older adults because of the "hangover" effect and increased potential for falls. Diphenhydramine is one

Continued

DRUG PROFILES—cont'd

of the most commonly used antihistamines, in part because of its excellent safety profile and efficacy. It has the greatest range of therapeutic indications of any antihistamine available. It is used for the relief or prevention of histamine-mediated allergies, motion sickness, the treatment of Parkinson's disease (because of its anticholinergic effects; see Chapter 16), and the promotion of sleep (see Chapter 13). It is also used in conjunction with epinephrine in the management of anaphylaxis and in the treatment of acute dystonia reactions.

Diphenhydramine use is contraindicated in patients with a known hypersensitivity to it. It is to be used with caution in nursing mothers, neonates, and patients with lower respiratory tract symptoms. It is available in oral, parenteral, and topical preparations. In oral form,

diphenhydramine is available as caplets, capsules, chewable tablets, liquid, and in several combination products that contain other cough and cold medications. It is also available as an injection. In topical form, diphenhydramine is available as a spray. It is also available in combination with several other drugs that are commonly given topically as creams and lotions, such as calamine, camphor, and zinc oxide. For recommended dosages for the oral and injectable forms, refer to the table below.

PHARMACOKINETICS

Route	Onset of Action	Peak Plasma Concentration	Elimination Half-Life	Duration of Action
PO	15–30 min	2–4 hr	2–7 hr	4 hr

DOSAGES Selected Antihistamines

Drug	Pharmacological Class	Usual Dosage Range	Indications
Nonsedating Antihistamines			
▶loratadine (Claritin)	H₁ antihistamine	Children 2–9 yr (weighing less than 30 kg) PO: 5 mg (5 mL) once daily Children 10 yr and older (weighing more than 30 kg) PO: 10 mg (10 mL) once daily Children and adults 12 yr and older PO: 10 mg once daily Adult and pediatric 6 yr and older PO: 10 mg once daily Pediatric 2–5 yr PO: 5 mg once daily	Allergic rhinitis, chronic urticaria
Traditional Antihistamines (More Commonly Associated With Sedation)			
▶diphenhydramine hydrochloride (Allerdryl, Allernix, Benadryl)	H₁ antihistamine	Children equal to or more than 10 kg PO/IM/IV: 12.5–25 mg tid–qid Adults and children 12 yr and older PO: 25–50 mg hs Adults only PO/IM/IV: 25–50 mg tid–qid Adults only PO: 25–50 mg tid–qid	Allergic disorders, nighttime insomnia, motion sickness Nighttime insomnia Allergic disorders, PD symptoms Motion sickness

IM, Intramuscular; *IV*, Intravenous; *PD*, Parkinson's disease; *PO*, oral.

DECONGESTANTS

Nasal congestion is due to excessive nasal secretions and inflamed and swollen nasal mucosa. The primary causes of nasal congestion are allergies and URIs, especially the common cold. There are three separate groups of nasal **decongestants: adrenergics (sympathomimetics)**, which comprise the largest group; **anticholinergics (parasympatholytics)**, which are less commonly used; and selected topical **corticosteroids** (intranasal steroids).

Decongestants can be taken orally to produce a systemic effect, can be inhaled, or can be administered topically into the nose. Each method of administration has its advantages and disadvantages. Decongestants administered by the oral route include pseudoephedrine, which

is available over the counter. A commonly used nasal decongestant spray is phenylephrine hydrochloride, also available over the counter.

Drugs administered by the oral route produce prolonged decongestant effects, but their onset of action is more delayed and the effect less potent than for decongestants applied topically. However, the clinical problem of rebound congestion associated with topically administered drugs is almost nonexistent with oral dosage forms. Rebound congestion occurs because of the rapid absorption of drug through mucous membranes followed by a rapid decline in therapeutic activity. This rebound congestion can cause overuse of and dependence on the nasal spray, as patients take it frequently due to its rapid decline in activity. This is in contrast to oral dosage forms, which provide a more gradual increase and decline in pharmacological activity because of the time required for GI absorption. Nasal spray available in Canada contains oxymetazoline hydrochloride or xylometazoline, sympathomimetics associated with rebound congestion. Inhaled intranasal steroids and anticholinergic drugs are not associated with rebound congestion and are often used prophylactically to prevent nasal congestion in patients with chronic upper respiratory symptoms. Commonly used intranasal steroids include the following:

- beclomethasone dipropionate (Qvar®, Rivanase®)
- budesonide (Pulmicort®, Rhinocort®, Symbicort®)
- flunisolide (Rhinalar®)
- fluticasone furoate (Avamys®)
- fluticasone propionate (Flonase®)
- mometasone furoate (Nasonex®)
- triamcinolone acetonide (Nasacort®) (also now available OTC)

The only commonly used intranasal anticholinergic is ipratropium bromide nasal spray (Atrovent®). Other available nasal sprays are sodium cromoglycate (Rhinaris®-CS Anti-Allergic 2% Nasal Mist), a mast-cell stabilizer and a combination drug, Dymista®, which contains the antihistamine azelastine hydrochloride and the corticosteroid fluticasone propionate.

Mechanism of Action and Drug Effects

Nasal decongestants are most commonly used for their ability to shrink engorged nasal mucous membranes and relieve nasal stuffiness. Adrenergic drugs (e.g., oxymetazoline) accomplish this by constricting the small arterioles that supply the structures of the upper respiratory tract, primarily the blood vessels surrounding the nasal sinuses. When these blood vessels are stimulated by α-adrenergic drugs, they constrict. Once these blood vessels shrink, the nasal secretions in the swollen mucous membranes are better able to drain, either externally through the nostrils or internally through reabsorption into the bloodstream or lymphatic circulation. Because sympathetic nervous system stimulation produces the same effect, these drugs are sometimes referred to as *sympathomimetics*.

Nasal steroids target the inflammatory response elicited by invading organisms (viruses and bacteria) or other antigens (e.g., allergens). The body responds to these antigens by producing inflammation in an effort to isolate or wall off the area and by attracting various cells of the immune system to consume and destroy the offending antigens. Steroids exert their anti-inflammatory effect by causing these cells to be turned off or rendered unresponsive. The goal is *not* complete immunosuppression of the respiratory tract but rather to reduce the inflammatory symptoms to improve patient comfort and air exchange. The drug effects of intranasal steroids are also discussed in Chapter 34.

Indications

Nasal decongestants reduce the nasal congestion associated with acute or chronic rhinitis, the common cold, sinusitis, and hay fever or other allergies. They may also be used to reduce swelling of the nasal passages and to facilitate visualization of the nasal and pharyngeal membranes before surgery or diagnostic procedures.

Contraindications

Contraindications to the use of decongestants include drug allergy. Adrenergic drugs are contraindicated in acute-angle glaucoma, uncontrolled cardiovascular disease, hypertension, diabetes, hyperthyroidism, and prostatitis. They are also contraindicated in situations in which patients are unable to close their eyes (such as after a stroke) and in patients with a history of stroke or transient ischemic attacks, cerebral arteriosclerosis, longstanding asthma, BPH, or diabetes.

Adverse Effects

Adrenergic drugs are usually well tolerated. Possible adverse effects of these drugs include nervousness, insomnia, palpitations, and tremors. The most common adverse effects of intranasal steroids are localized and include mucosal irritation and dryness as well as epistaxis (which can be prevented by spraying away from the septum).

Although a topically applied adrenergic nasal decongestant can be absorbed into the bloodstream, the amount absorbed is usually too small to cause systemic effects in normal doses; excessive doses of these drugs are more likely to cause systemic effects elsewhere in the body. These may include cardiovascular effects such as hypertension and palpitations and CNS effects such as headache, nervousness, and dizziness. These systemic effects are the result of α-adrenergic stimulation of the heart, blood vessels, and CNS.

Interactions

There are few significant drug interactions with nasal decongestants. Systemic **sympathomimetic drugs** and sympathomimetic nasal decongestants are likely to cause drug toxicity when given together. Monoamine oxidase inhibitors (MAOIs) may result in additive pressor effects (e.g., raising of blood pressure) when given with sympathomimetic nasal decongestants. Other interacting drugs include methyldopa and urinary acidifiers and alkalinizers.

Dosages

For the recommended dosages of oxymetazoline hydrochloride, the only nasal decongestant profiled, refer to the table on p. 710.

ANTITUSSIVES

Coughing is a normal physiological function that serves the purpose of removing potentially harmful foreign substances and excessive secretions from the respiratory tract. The cough reflex is stimulated when receptors in the bronchi, alveoli, and pleura (lining of the lungs) are stretched. This causes a signal to be sent to the cough centre in the medulla of the brain, which in turn

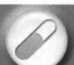
DRUG PROFILES

Many of the decongestants are OTC drugs, but the more potent drugs that can cause serious adverse effects are available only by prescription. Although nasal steroids are relatively safe, their use is also contraindicated in some circumstances, including in patients with nasal mucosal infections (because of their ability to depress the body's immune response as part of their anti-inflammatory effect) or known drug allergy.

Many inhaled corticosteroids (e.g., beclomethasone, dexamethasone, and flunisolide) are discussed in greater detail in Chapter 34. The adrenergic drug oxymetazoline hydrochloride is discussed in this chapter. Both these drug categories are generally first-line drugs for the treatment of chronic nasal congestion.

OXYMETAZOLINE HYDROCHLORIDE

Oxymetazoline hydrochloride (Claritin®, Dristan®, Drixoral®, Sinufrin®, Vicks®) is chemically and pharmacologically similar to the other sympathomimetic drug, xylometazoline hydrochloride (Balminil®, Otrivin®).

During a cold, the blood vessels that surround the nasal sinuses are dilated and engorged with plasma, white blood cells, mast cells, histamines, and many other blood components that are involved in fighting infections of the respiratory tract. This swelling, or dilation, blocks the nasal passages, which results in nasal congestion. When these drugs are administered intranasally, they cause dilated arterioles to constrict, which reduces nasal blood flow and congestion. Both drugs have the same contraindications as the other nasal decongestants. Oxymetazoline hydrochloride for nasal administration is available as a 0.05% solution and is meant to be instilled into each nostril. Common dosages for this drug are given in the Dosages table on p. 712.

PHARMACOKINETICS

Route	Onset of Action	Peak Plasma Concentration	Elimination Half-Life	Duration of Action
Intranasal	5–10 min	Unknown	Unknown	2–6 hr

stimulates the cough. Although coughing is primarily a beneficial response, there are times when it is not useful and may even be harmful (e.g., after a surgical procedure such as hernia repair, or in cases of nonproductive cough or "dry cough"). In these situations, the use of an **antitussive** drug may enhance patient comfort and reduce respiratory distress. There are two main categories of antitussives: opioid and nonopioid.

Although all opioid drugs have antitussive effects, only codeine and its semisynthetic derivative hydrocodone are used as antitussives. Both drugs are effective in suppressing the cough reflex and, if they are taken in the prescribed manner, their use does not generally lead to dependency. These two drugs are commonly incorporated into various combination formulations with other respiratory drugs and are rarely used alone for the purpose of cough suppression. There is increasing evidence that a single dose of honey might reduce mucus secretion and reduce cough in children.

Nonopioid antitussive drugs are less effective than opioid drugs. They are available either alone or in combination with other drugs in an array of OTC cold and cough preparations. Dextromethorphan is the most widely used of these antitussive drugs and is a derivative of the synthetic opioid levorphanol.

Mechanism of Action and Drug Effects

The opioid antitussives codeine and hydrocodone bitartrate, a semisynthetic opioid synthesized from codeine, suppress the cough reflex through direct action on the cough centre in the CNS (medulla). Opioid antitussives also provide analgesia and have a drying effect on the mucosa of the respiratory tract, which increases the viscosity of respiratory secretions. This helps to reduce symptoms such as runny nose and postnasal drip. The nonopioid cough suppressant dextromethorphan acts in the same way. Because it is not an opioid, however, it does not have analgesic properties, nor does it cause CNS depression.

Indications

Although they have other properties, such as analgesic effects in the case of opioid drugs, antitussives are used primarily to stop the cough reflex when the cough is nonproductive or harmful.

Contraindications

The only absolute contraindication to the antitussives is drug allergy. Relative contraindications include opioid dependency (for opioid antitussives) and high risk for respiratory depression (e.g., in frail older adults). Patients with these conditions are often able to tolerate lower drug dosages and still experience some symptom relief.

Additional contraindications and cautions include the following:
- dextromethorphan: contraindications of hyperthyroidism, advanced heart and vessel disease, hypertension, glaucoma, and use of MAOIs within the past 14 days
- diphenhydramine: see antihistamines
- codeine and hydrocodone bitartrate: contraindication with alcohol use; cautious use of codeine and hydrocodone required with patients with CNS depression, anoxia, high serum levels of carbon dioxide (hypercapnia), and respiratory depression; increased intracranial pressure, impaired kidney function, liver diseases, BPH, Addison's disease, and COPD.

DRUG PROFILES

Antitussives come in many oral dosage forms and are available both with and without a prescription. Most of the narcotic antitussives are available only by prescription because of their associated potential for misuse. Dextromethorphan is the most popular nonopioid antitussive available over the counter and is found in many trade name mixtures.

Illicit use and misuse of dextromethorphan is increasing (The Centre for Addiction and Mental Health, 2015). Consumption of large volumes of cough syrup results in vomiting. Therefore, the drug is being extracted from cough syrups and sold on the Internet in a tablet form that can be swallowed or a powder that can be snorted. Normal dosages are 15 to 30 milligrams. Illicit use may be 360 milligrams or more (Council on Drug Abuse, 2011). Dextromethorphan is a dissociative drug that causes a feeling of detachment, impaired motor coordination, and altered perception, impairing judgement as well as creating the potential for hallucinations and coma.

codeine phosphate

Codeine phosphate is a popular opioid antitussive drug. It is used in combination with many other respiratory medications to control coughs. Because it is an opioid, it is potentially addictive and can depress respiration as part of its CNS depressant effects. For this reason, codeine-containing cough suppressants are more tightly controlled than others (*Controlled Drugs and Substances Act*, Schedule I) but are commonly available by prescription. Cough suppressants containing codeine are also available behind the counter in the pharmacy. Cough suppressants are available in many oral dosage forms: solutions, tablets, capsules, and suspensions. Their use is contraindicated in patients with a known hypersensitivity to codeine and morphine (recall that codeine is metabolized to morphine) and in those suffering from respiratory depression, increased intracranial pressure, seizure disorders, or severe respiratory disorders. Common dosages are listed in the table on p. 712.

PHARMACOKINETICS

Route	Onset of Action	Peak Plasma Concentration	Elimination Half-Life	Duration of Action
PO	15–30 min	34–45 min	2.5–4 hr	4–6 hr

▶▶ dextromethorphan hydrobromide

Dextromethorphan hydrobromide is a nonopioid antitussive that is available alone or in combination with many other cough and cold preparations. It is widely used because it is safe and nonaddicting and does not cause respiratory or CNS depression when used in recommended dosages. Dextromethorphan has become a popular drug of misuse and is discussed in detail in Chapter 18. Its use is contraindicated in cases of drug allergy, asthma, emphysema, or persistent headache. Dextromethorphan is available as lozenges; solutions; liquid-filled capsules; granules; caplets; chewable, extended-release, or film-coated tablets; and an extended-release syrup. Benefits of this drug may warrant use in pregnant women despite potential risks. For recommended dosages, refer to the table on p. 712.

PHARMACOKINETICS

Route	Onset of Action	Peak Plasma Concentration	Elimination Half-Life	Duration of Action
PO	15–30 min	2.5 hr	Unknown	3–6 hr

Adverse Effects

The following are the common adverse effects of selected antitussive drugs:
- codeine and hydrocodone bitartrate: sedation, nausea, vomiting, lightheadedness, and constipation
- dextromethorphan: dizziness, drowsiness, and nausea
- diphenhydramine: sedation, dry mouth, and other anticholinergic effects

Interactions

Opioid antitussives (codeine and hydrocodone bitartrate) may potentiate the effects of other opioids, general anaesthetics, tranquilizers, sedatives, hypnotics, tricyclic antidepressants, alcohol, and other CNS depressants.

Dosages

For the recommended dosages of selected antitussive drugs, refer to the table on p. 712.

EXPECTORANTS

Expectorants aid in the expectoration (i.e., coughing up and spitting out) of excessive mucus that has accumulated in the respiratory tract, by breaking down and thinning out the secretions. They are administered orally either as single drugs or in combination with other drugs to facilitate the flow of respiratory secretions by reducing their viscosity. The clinical effectiveness of expectorants is somewhat questionable, however. Placebo-controlled clinical evaluations have failed to confirm that expectorants reduce the viscosity of sputum. Despite this, expectorants are popular drugs, are contained in most OTC cold and cough preparations, and provide symptom relief for many users. The most common expectorant in most OTC products is guaifenesin.

Mechanism of Action and Drug Effects

Expectorants have one of two different mechanism of actions, depending on the drug. The first is **reflex stimulation**, in which loosening and thinning of respiratory tract secretions occurs in response to an irritation of the GI tract produced by the drug. Guaifenesin is the only such drug currently available. The second mechanism of action is direct stimulation of the secretory glands in the respiratory tract.

DRUG PROFILES

▶▶ guaifenesin

Guaifenesin (Balminil®, Brochophan®, Robitussin®, others) is a commonly used expectorant that is available in several different oral dosage forms: capsules, tablets, and solutions. It is used in the symptomatic management of coughs of varying origins. It is beneficial in the treatment of productive coughs because it thins the mucus in the respiratory tract that is difficult to cough up. There are

few published pharmacokinetic data on guaifenesin, but its half-life is estimated to be approximately 1 hour. This short half-life helps explain why it is usually dosed several times throughout the day. However, although guaifenesin remains popular, there is some evidence to suggest that it has no greater therapeutic activity than water in terms of loosening respiratory tract secretions. For dosage information, refer to the table below.

DOSAGES   Selected Decongestant, Expectorant, and Antitussive Drugs

Drug	Pharmacological Class	Usual Dosage Range	Indication
codeine phosphate (as part of a combination product such as Dimetane-Expectorant-C®, Dimetapp-C®, CoActifed®, Robitussin AC®, others)	Opioid antitussive	*Adults and children over 12 yr* PO: 10 mL q4–6h	Cough suppression
▶▶ dextromethorphan hydrobromide (as part of a combination product such as Benylin DM-E®, Buckley's®, Dimetapp-DM®, Robitussin-DM®, Vicks, others)	Nonopioid antitussive	*Children 2–5 yr* PO: 2.5 mL q6h *Children 6–12 yr* PO: 5–10 mL q6h *Adults and children over 12 yr* PO: 10 mL q6h	Cough suppression
▶▶ guaifenesin (100 mg/mL) (Balminil, Robitussin, others)	Expectorant	*Children 2 yr to under 6 yr* PO: 2.5 mL q6h *Children 6 yr to under 12 yr* PO: 5 mL q6h PO: 10–20 mL q6h	Respiratory congestion, cough
▶▶ oxymetazoline hydrochloride (Claritin®, Drixoral, Sinufrin, Vicks, others)	Decongestant	*Adults and children over 12 yr* Nasally: 2–3 sprays each nostril q10–12h × 3 days	Nasal decongestant

PO, oral.

Indications

Expectorants are used for the relief of productive cough commonly associated with the common cold, bronchitis, laryngitis, pharyngitis, pertussis, influenza, and measles. They may also be used for the suppression of coughs caused by chronic paranasal sinusitis. By loosening and thinning sputum and bronchial secretions, they may also indirectly diminish the tendency to cough.

Contraindications

Guaifenesin is contraindicated in cases of known drug allergy.

Adverse Effects

The adverse effects of expectorants are minimal. Guaifenesin may cause nausea, vomiting, and gastric irritation.

Interactions

There are no known significant interactions involving guaifenesin.

Dosages

For dosage information on guaifenesin, the only expectorant profiled, refer to the table above.

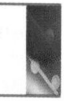

NURSING PROCESS

▨ Assessment

When a patient is to be given drugs to treat symptoms related to the respiratory tract, begin the assessment by gathering data about the condition and determining if symptoms are caused by an allergic reaction. Obtaining the patient's medical history and medication profile, completing a thorough head-to-toe physical assessment, and taking a nursing history are critical to understanding possible causes, risks, or links to diseases or conditions such as allergy, a cold, or influenza. For example, if an allergic reaction to a drug, food, or substance has occurred, the patient may be experiencing signs and symptoms such as hives, wheezing or bronchospasm, tachycardia, or hypotension (requiring immediate medical attention). However, if the cause is a cold or influenza, the symptoms would be different and would be treated completely differently. The drug of choice is then selected based on the type and severity of the symptoms.

Most nonsedating antihistamines (e.g., fexofenadine hydrochloride, loratadine, cetirizine hydrochloride) are contraindicated in those with known allergies to the drugs. Remember that the traditional, nonsedating antihistamines are usually discontinued at least 4 days before allergy testing is to be performed, but only on a health care provider's order and as directed. Assess for the following possible drug interactions that need to be avoided: fexofenadine hydrochloride given with erythromycin and other CYP450 inhibitors, leading to increased antihistamine levels; fexofenadine hydrochloride given with phenytoin, leading to decreased fexofenadine hydrochloride levels; loratadine given with some antifungals, cimetidine, and erythromycin, leading to increased antihistamine levels; and diphenhydramine and cetirizine hydrochloride given with alcohol, MAOIs, and CNS depressants, leading to increased CNS depression.

Before administering the traditional antihistamines such as diphenhydramine, chlorpheniramine maleate, or brompheniramine maleate, ensure that the patient has no allergies to this group of medications, even though these drugs are used for allergic reaction. Assess contraindications, cautions, and drug interactions with these and all other drugs. Use of these antihistamines is of concern in patients who are experiencing an acute asthma attack and in those who have lower respiratory tract disease or are at risk for pneumonia. The rationale for not using these drugs in these situations is that antihistamines (including nonsedating antihistamines) dry up secretions; if the patient cannot expectorate secretions, the secretions may become viscous (thick), occlude airways, and lead to atelectasis, infection, or occlusion of the bronchioles. It is also important to know that these drugs may lead to paradoxical reactions in older adults, with subsequent irritability as well as dizziness, confusion, sedation, and hypotension.

Use of decongestants requires assessment of contraindications, cautions, and drug interactions. Because decongestants are available in oral forms, nasal drops and sprays, and eye drop dosage forms, any condition that could affect the functional structures of the eye or nose may be a possible caution or contraindication. Decongestants may increase blood pressure and heart rate, so assess the patient's blood pressure, pulse, and other vital parameters. Patients with hypertension (controlled) can use topical decongestants short-term, but it is advised against using oral decongestants. If any patient has coronary artery disease, decongestants of any kind should be avoided. Because so many of these drugs are found in OTC cough and cold products and have been associated with numerous cases of oversedation, seizures, tachycardia, and even death, their use warrants extreme caution. Contraindications to the use of decongestants include drug allergy, acute-angle glaucoma, uncontrolled cardiovascular disease, hypertension, diabetes, and prostatitis. Topically applied adrenergic nasal decongestants may be absorbed into the circulation; however, the dosage amount absorbed is usually too small to cause systemic effects. If it is used too often, or excessive amounts are used, cardiovascular effects may be precipitated (e.g., increase in blood pressure) and there may be CNS stimulation (with headache, nervousness, or dizziness). Some drug interactions include the use of systemic sympathomimetics and sympathomimetic nasal decongestants together, which can create possible toxicity. Other drug interactions for which to assess with nasal decongestants include their use with MAOIs.

Inhaled intranasal steroids are contraindicated in situations in which the patient is experiencing a nasal mucosal infection or drug allergy. Chapter 34 discusses some of the inhaled corticosteroids. With the use of any decongestant, always perform a thorough assessment of signs and symptoms before and after use of these drugs. Include descriptions of cough, secretions, and breath sounds in this assessment.

With antitussive therapy, assessment is tailored to the patient and the specific drug. Most of these drugs result in sedation, dizziness, and drowsiness, so assessment of the patient's safety is important. Complete an assessment for allergies, contraindications, cautions, and drug interactions, and document the findings. In the respiratory assessment (as for all of the drugs in this chapter), include rate, rhythm and depth, as well as breath sounds, presence of cough, and description of cough and sputum if present. For individuals with chronic respiratory disease, the prescriber may order further studies to determine the safety of using these drugs without causing further respiratory concerns or depression. Pulse oximetry readings with measurement of vital signs may be used to provide more information. Assess for potential drug interactions such as those involving alcohol, MAOIs, and antihistamines. With use of codeine and hydrocodone bitratrate antitussives, there are contraindications with alcohol and other opioid drugs; these drugs must be used cautiously in those with CNS depression, anoxia, hypercapnia, respiratory depression, impaired renal function, or COPD. With the nonopioid antitussive dextromethorphan, monitor its use carefully because it is a popular drug of abuse (see Chapter 18).

Expectorants are generally well tolerated, and the only contraindication to their use is drug allergy. There are no known drug interactions for which to assess with use of the expectorant guaifenesin.

Nursing Diagnoses

- Impaired gas exchange related to the disorder, condition, or disease affecting the respiratory system and respiratory-related signs and symptoms
- Ineffective airway clearance related to diminished ability to cough or a suppressed cough reflex (with antitussives)

- Deficient knowledge related to the effective use of cold medications and other related products due to lack of information and patient teaching

Planning

Goals

- Patient will experience improved gas exchange with drug therapy.
- Patient will have improved airway clearance and relief of symptoms.
- Patient will display improved knowledge about drug therapy.

Expected Patient Outcomes

- Patient experiences improved oxygen exchange and breath sounds and a return to normal respiratory rate and rhythm.
- Patient takes medications exactly as prescribed to enhance airway clearance.
  - Patient increases fluid intake to thin secretions and increase expectoration of mucus.
  - Patient's breath sounds clear and there is expectoration of secretions as well as a return to a respiratory rate of 12 to 20 breaths/min.
  - Patient reports any of the following symptoms to the health care provider immediately: increase in cough, congestion, or shortness of breath; chest pain; fever (above 38°C); or any change in sputum production or colour (i.e., if not clear or if a change from baseline).
- Patient states rationale for therapy as well as adverse effects to expect while on drug therapy.
  - Patient remains adherent to the antihistamine, antitussive, decongestant, or expectorant medication regimen until symptoms are resolved or the health care provider orders discontinuation.

Implementation

If patients are receiving nonsedating antihistamines, advise them to take the drugs as directed. Reduced dosages may be needed for older adult patients or for patients with decreased kidney function. The H_1 receptor antagonist drugs do not cross the blood–brain barrier as readily as older antihistamines do and are therefore less likely to cause sedation. They are generally well tolerated with minimal adverse effects.

Instruct patients taking traditional antihistamines (e.g., diphenhydramine) to take the medications as prescribed. Most of these medications, including the OTC antihistamines, are best tolerated when taken with meals. Although food may slightly decrease absorption of antihistamines, it has the benefit of minimizing the GI upset these drugs may cause. Encourage patients who experience dry mouth to chew or suck on candy (sugarless if

needed) or OTC throat, cough, or cold lozenges, or to chew gum, as well as to perform frequent mouth care to ease the dryness and related discomfort. Because of the potential for serious drug interactions, other OTC or prescribed cold or cough medications must not be taken with antihistamines unless they were previously approved or ordered by the health care provider. Dosage amounts and routes may vary depending on whether the patient is an older adult, adult, or younger than 12 years of age, so encourage proper dosing and usage. Monitor blood pressure and other vital signs as needed. Monitor older adults and children for any paradoxical reactions, which are common with these drugs.

Patients taking decongestants are generally using the drugs for nasal decongestion. These drugs come in oral dosage forms, including sustained-release and chewable forms. Educate patients that all dosage forms are to be taken as instructed and encourage an increase in fluid intake of up to 3000 mL a day, unless contraindicated. Fluid helps liquefy secretions, assists in breaking up thick secretions, and makes it easier to cough up secretions. Counsel patients to use nasal decongestant dosage forms exactly as ordered and with no increase in frequency. Excessive use of decongestant nasal sprays or drops may lead to rebound congestion. See the Patient Teaching Tips for further information.

With antitussives, instruct patients that the various dosage forms of the drugs are to be used exactly as ordered. Drowsiness or dizziness may occur with the use of antitussives; therefore, caution patients against driving a car or engaging in other activities that require mental alertness until they feel back to normal. If the antitussive contains codeine, the CNS depressant effects of the narcotic opiate may further depress breathing and respiratory effort. Other antitussives, such as dextromethorphan, as well as codeine-containing drugs, are to be given at evenly spaced intervals so that the drug reaches a steady state.

Evaluation

A therapeutic response to drugs given to treat respiratory conditions, such as antihistamines, antitussives, decongestants, and expectorants, includes resolution of the symptoms for which the drugs were originally prescribed or taken. These symptoms may include cough; nasal, sinus, or chest congestion; nasal, salivary, and lacrimal gland hypersecretion; motion sickness; sneezing; watery, red, or itchy eyes; itchy nose; allergic rhinitis; and allergic symptoms. Some of the antihistamines, such as diphenhydramine, are also helpful as sleep aids, and a therapeutic response when they are taken for this purpose would be the successful induction of sleep. Monitor for the adverse effects of excessive dry mouth, nose, and throat; urinary retention; drowsiness; oversedation; dizziness; paradoxical excitement, nervousness, or restlessness; dysrhythmias; palpitations; nausea; diarrhea or constipation; and headache, depending on the drug prescribed.

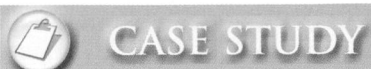

CASE STUDY

Decongestants

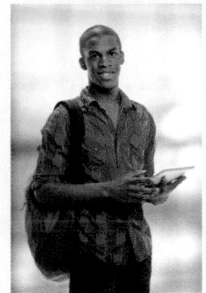

A 22-year-old male college student has had allergy symptoms since moving into his dormitory. When he calls the student health centre, he is told to try an OTC topical nasal decongestant. He tries one and is excited about the relief he experiences until 2 weeks later, when his symptoms return. He calls the student health centre again, upset because his symptoms are now worse.

1. What explanation do you have for the worsening symptoms?
2. What patient education should he have received about this type of drug?
3. What other OTC drugs and nonpharmacological measures could be suggested to improve this situation?

For answers, see http://evolve.elsevier.com/Canada/Lilley/ pharmacology/.

PATIENT TEACHING TIPS

❖ Provide patients with education about the sedating effects of traditional antihistamines. Patients need to avoid activities that require alertness until tolerance to sedation occurs or until they can accurately judge that the drug has no impact on motor skills or responses. Provide patients with a list of drugs that must be avoided, such as alcohol and CNS depressants.

❖ Suggest to patients that with traditional, nonsedating antihistamines, a humidifier may be needed to help liquefy sections, making expectoration of sputum easier. Encourage intake of fluids, unless contraindicated.

❖ Educate patients with upper or lower respiratory symptoms or disease processes about the impact of the environment on their symptoms or condition, and instruct patients to avoid dry air, smoke-filled environments, and allergens.

❖ Encourage patients to always check with a pharmacist for possible drug interactions because many OTC and prescription drugs could lead to adverse effects if taken concurrently with any of the antihistamines, decongestants, antitussives, or expectorants.

❖ Advise patients to take medication with food to avoid GI upset.

❖ Instruct patients to report any difficulty breathing, palpitations, or unusual adverse effects to a health care provider immediately.

❖ Instruct patients to take antitussives with caution and to report symptoms of pneumonia, such as fever, chest tightness, change in sputum from clear to coloured, difficult or noisy breathing, activity intolerance, or weakness.

❖ Prior to the use of decongestants, emphasize the importance of taking the medication as ordered and adhering to instructions regarding dose and frequency. Emphasize that frequent, long-term, or excessive use of decongestants (whether oral forms or nasal inhaled forms) may lead to rebound congestion, in which the nasal passages become more congested as the effects of the drug wear off. When this occurs, the patient generally uses more of the drug, precipitating a vicious cycle involving more congestion. Advise patients to report to a health care provider any heart palpitations, weakness, sedation, extreme dizziness, or excessive irritability.

❖ Advise patients taking expectorants to avoid alcohol and products containing alcohol and to not use these medications for longer than 1 week. If cough or other symptoms continue, the patient should contact the health care provider. Encourage intake of fluids, unless contraindicated, to help thin secretions for easier expectoration.

❖ Decongestants and expectorants are recommended to treat cold symptoms, but the patient must report a fever of higher than 38°C, cough, or other symptoms lasting longer than 3 to 4 days.

❖ Educate patients about the need for familiarity with the list of ingredients in combination drug mixtures to avoid using similar drugs groups. Many of the drugs used to manage colds, coughs, and sputum contain similar ingredients yet have different trade names.

KEY POINTS

❖ There are two types of histamine blockers: H_1 blockers and H_2 blockers. H_1 blockers are the drugs to which most people are referring when they use the term *antihistamine*. H_1 blockers prevent the harmful effects of histamine and are used to treat seasonal allergic rhinitis, anaphylaxis, reactions to insect bites, and so on. H_2 blockers are used to treat gastric acid disorders, such as hyperacidity or ulcer disease.

❖ Educate patients about the purposes of their medication regimens, the expected adverse effects, and any drug interactions. A list of all medications (prescription and OTC, as well as natural health products) needs to be provided to all health care providers.

❖ Decongestants act by causing constriction of the engorged and swollen blood vessels in the sinuses, which decreases pressure and allows mucous membranes to drain. It is important to understand the action of these drugs and know other important information such as significant adverse effects, including heart and CNS-stimulating effects that may result in palpitations, insomnia, restlessness, and nervousness.

❖ Nonopioid antitussive drugs may also cause sedation, drowsiness, or dizziness. Patients should not drive a car or engage in other activities that require mental alertness if these adverse effects occur. Codeine-containing antitussives may lead to CNS depression; these drugs are to be used cautiously and are not to be mixed with anything containing alcohol.

EXAMINATION REVIEW QUESTIONS

1. When assessing a patient who is to receive a decongestant, the nurse will recognize that a potential contraindication to this drug would be which condition?
   a. Glaucoma
   b. Fever
   c. Peptic ulcer disease
   d. Allergic rhinitis

2. When giving decongestants, the nurse must remember that these drugs have α-stimulating effects that may result in which effect?
   a. Fever
   b. Bradycardia
   c. Hypertension
   d. CNS depression

3. The nurse is reviewing the medication orders for prn (as necessary) medications that can be given to a patient who has bronchitis with a productive cough. Which drug will the nurse choose?
   a. An antitussive
   b. An expectorant
   c. An antihistamine
   d. A decongestant

4. The nurse knows that an antitussive cough medication would be the best choice for which patient?
   a. A patient with a productive cough
   b. A patient with chronic paranasal sinusitis
   c. A patient who has had recent abdominal surgery
   d. A patient who has influenza

5. A patient is taking a decongestant to help reduce symptoms of a cold. The nurse will instruct the patient to observe for which possible symptom, which may indicate an adverse effect of this drug?
   a. Increased cough
   b. Dry mouth
   c. Slower heart rate
   d. Heart palpitations

6. The nurse is giving an antihistamine and will observe the patient for which of the following adverse effects? (Select all that apply.)
   a. Hypertension
   b. Dizziness
   c. "Hangover" effect
   d. Drowsiness
   e. Tachycardia
   f. Dry mouth

7. The order for a 4-year-old patient reads: "Give guaifenesin, 80 mg PO, every 4 hours as needed for cough. Maximum of 600 mg/24 hours." The medication comes in a bottle that has 100 mg/5 mL. How many millilitres will the nurse give per dose?

Answers: 1. a, **2.** c, **3.** b, **4.** c, **5.** d, **6.** b, c, d, f, **7.** 4 mL.

CRITICAL THINKING ACTIVITIES

1. A patient calls the clinic to ask the nurse about taking an antihistamine for a "terrible cold." She says she is so tired of sneezing and blowing her nose. What are the priorities when the nurse assesses the patient's medical history before answering her about the use of antihistamines?

2. An older patient is discussing the use of guaifenesin with the nurse. He asks, "What else can I do to fight this terrible cold? I don't want to just take a pill." What is the nurse's best answer?

3. A patient is recovering from an emergency exploratory laparotomy. He had a cold before his surgery and is now coughing up large amounts of whitish yellow sputum. He is receiving intravenous fluids and antibiotics. He asks the nurse for something to make him stop coughing. The nurse reviews the medication sheet and sees both an expectorant and an antitussive ordered. Which medication would be the best choice at this time? Explain your answer.

For answers see http://evolve.elsevier.com/Canada/Lilley/pharmacology.

CHAPTER 38

Respiratory Drugs

Objectives

After reading this chapter, the successful student will be able to do the following:

1. Describe the anatomy and physiology of the respiratory system.
2. Discuss the impact of respiratory drugs on various upper and lower respiratory tract diseases and conditions.
3. List the classifications of drugs used to treat diseases and conditions of the respiratory system, and provide specific examples.
4. Discuss the mechanisms of action, indications, contraindications, cautions, drug interactions, dosages, routes of administration, adverse effects, and toxic effects of bronchodilators and other respiratory drugs.
5. Develop a collaborative plan of care that includes all phases of the nursing process for patients who use bronchodilators or other respiratory drugs.

e-Learning Activities

Website
(http://evolve.elsevier.com/Canada/
Lilley/pharmacology/)

evolve

- Answer Key—Textbook Case Studies
- Answer Key—Critical Thinking Activities
- Chapter Summaries—Printable
- Review Questions for Exam Preparation
- Unfolding Case Studies

Drug Profiles

fluticasone (fluticasone propionate)*, p. 732
ipratropium (ipratropium bromide)*, p. 726
methylprednisolone, p. 732
»» montelukast (montelukast sodium)*, p. 729
»» salbutamol (salbutamol sulphate)*, p. 725
»» salmeterol xinafoate, p. 723
»» theophylline, p. 728

»» Key drug

*Full generic name is given in parentheses. For the purposes of this text, the more common, shortened name is used.

Key Terms

Allergen Any substance that evokes an allergic response. (p. 720)

Allergic asthma Bronchial asthma caused by hypersensitivity to an allergen or allergens. (p. 720)

Alveoli Microscopic sacs in the lungs in which oxygen is exchanged for carbon dioxide; also called *air sacs*. (p. 719)

Antibodies Immunoglobulins produced by lymphocytes in response to bacteria, viruses, or other antigenic substances. (p. 720)

Antigen A substance (usually a protein) that causes the formation of an antibody and reacts specifically with that antibody. (p. 720)

Asthma Recurrent and reversible shortness of breath, resulting from narrowing of the bronchi and bronchioles. Key characteristics are inflammation, bronchial smooth muscle spasticity, and sputum production; inflammation is the most important characteristic. (p. 719)

Asthma attack Sudden onset of wheezing together with difficulty breathing. (p. 719)

Bronchodilators Medications that improve airflow by relaxing bronchial smooth muscle cells (e.g., xanthines, adrenergic agonists). (p. 723)

Chronic obstructive pulmonary disease (COPD) A chronic lung disorder characterized by persistent airflow obstruction that is partially reversible. It is usually progressive and is associated with an intensified chronic inflammatory response in the lungs. Formerly known as *chronic bronchitis* and *emphysema*. (p. 719)

Immunoglobulins Proteins belonging to any of five structurally and antigenically distinct classes of antibodies present in the serum and external secretions of the body. (p. 720)

Lower respiratory tract (LRT) The division of the respiratory system composed of organs located almost entirely within the chest. (p. 719)

Status asthmaticus A prolonged asthma attack; a medical emergency. (p. 719)

Upper respiratory tract (URT) The division of the respiratory system composed of organs located outside the chest cavity (thorax). (p. 719)

OVERVIEW

The main function of the respiratory system is to deliver oxygen to, and remove carbon dioxide from, the cells of the body. To perform this deceptively simple task requires an intricate system of tissues, muscles, and organs called the *respiratory system*. It consists of two divisions: the upper and lower respiratory tracts. The **upper respiratory tract (URT)** is composed of the structures located outside of the chest cavity, or thorax. These are the nose, nasopharynx, oropharynx, laryngopharynx, and larynx. The **lower respiratory tract (LRT)** is located almost entirely within the chest and is composed of the trachea, all segments of the bronchial tree, and the lungs. The URT and LRT have four main accessory structures that aid in their overall function. These are the oral cavity (mouth), the rib cage, the muscles of the rib cage (intercostal muscles), and the diaphragm. The upper and lower respiratory tracts together with the accessory structures make up the respiratory system. Elements of this system are in constant communication with each other as they perform the vital function of respiration and the exchange of oxygen for carbon dioxide.

The air we breathe is a mixture of many gases. During inhalation, oxygen molecules from the air diffuse across the semipermeable membranes of the **alveoli**, where they are exchanged for carbon dioxide molecules, which are then exhaled. The lungs also filter, warm, and humidify the air. Oxygen is then delivered to the cells by the blood vessels of the circulatory system, in which the respiratory system transfers the oxygen it has extracted from inhaled air to the hemoglobin protein molecules contained within red blood cells. Also within the circulatory system, the cellular metabolic waste product carbon dioxide is collected from the tissues by red blood cells. This waste is then transported back to the lungs via the circulatory system, where it diffuses back across the alveolar membranes and is then exhaled into the air. The respiratory system also plays a central role in speech, sense of smell, and regulation of pH (acid–base balance).

DISEASES OF THE RESPIRATORY SYSTEM

Several diseases impair the function of the respiratory system. Those that affect the URT include colds, rhinitis, and hay fever. These conditions and the drugs used to manage them are discussed in Chapter 37. The major diseases that impair the function of the LRT include asthma and **chronic obstructive pulmonary disease (COPD)**, formerly known as *emphysema* and *chronic bronchitis*. These diseases have one feature in common; they involve the obstruction of airflow through the airways. **Asthma** that is persistent and present most of the time despite treatment is also considered a COPD. Cystic fibrosis and infant respiratory distress syndrome are other disorders that affect the LRT, but they are not a focus of discussion in this chapter because treatment for them places more emphasis on nonpharmacological than on pharmacological measures.

ASTHMA

Bronchial asthma is defined as a

> heterogeneous disease, usually characterized by chronic airway inflammation. It is defined by the history of respiratory symptoms such as wheeze, shortness of breath, chest tightness and cough that vary over time and in intensity, together with variable expiratory airflow limitation (Global Initiative for Asthma [GINA], 2015, p. 1).

The alveolar ducts and alveoli distal to the bronchioles remain open, but the obstruction to the airflow in the airways prevents carbon dioxide from getting out of the air spaces and oxygen from getting into them. When an episode has a sudden and dramatic onset, it is referred to as an *asthma attack*. Most asthma attacks are short and respond to medication; normal breathing is subsequently recovered. However, an asthma attack may be prolonged and may not respond to typical drug therapy. When this happens, it is known as *status asthmaticus* and requires hospitalization. The onset of asthma occurs before 10 years of age in 50% of patients and before 40 years of age in approximately 80% of patients.

Asthma is characterized by chronic inflammation of the airways resulting in bronchial constriction (airflow limitation) and hyper-responsiveness to various exogenous and endogenous triggers; these triggers include allergens, exercise, viral respiratory infections, nasal and sinus difficulties, air pollutants, and drugs. Environmental triggers such as a viral infection, allergens, or irritants initiate an inflammatory cascade that involves a variety of chemical mediators and inflammatory cells. Typically,

---

BOX 38-1   Sequence of Events in the Early-Phase Response of Asthma

1. The offending allergen provokes the production of hypersensitive antibodies (most commonly immunoglobulin E [IgE]) that are specific to the allergen. This immunologic response initiates patient sensitivity.
2. The IgE antibodies are homocytotrophic (have an affinity for mast cells) and collect on the surface of mast cells, thus sensitizing the patient to the allergen.
3. Subsequent allergen contact provokes the antigen–antibody reaction on the surface of mast cells.

4. Mast cell integrity is then violated, and these cells release chemical mediators stored in the cell. They also synthesize and then release other chemical mediators. These mediators include bradykinin, eosinophil chemotactic factor of anaphylaxis (ECF-A), histamine, prostaglandins, and slow-reacting substance of anaphylaxis (SRS-A).
5. The released chemical mediators, especially histamine and SRS-A, trigger bronchial constriction and an asthma attack.

---

the response to environmental stimuli involves two asthmatic responses: an early-phase response and a late-phase response.

An **allergen** is any substance that elicits an allergic reaction. Exposure to inhaled allergens, such as pollen, dust mites, mould, or animal dander, can initiate an acute immune response in allergen-sensitive individuals (**allergic asthma**) that leads to airway inflammation. Exposure to the offending allergen causes an immediate reaction, called the *early-phase response*. This attack is mediated by antibodies already present in the patient's body that chemically recognize the allergen as a foreign substance, or **antigen**. These **antibodies** are specialized immune system proteins known as **immunoglobulins**. The antibody in individuals with asthma is usually immunoglobulin E (IgE), which is one of the five types of antibodies in the body (the others are IgG, IgA, IgM, and IgD). On exposure to the allergen, the patient's body responds by mounting an immediate and potent antigen–antibody reaction (immune response). This reaction occurs on the surfaces of cells that are rich in histamines, leukotrienes, and other substances involved in the immune response, such as mast cells. These substances are collectively known as inflammatory mediators, and they are released from mast cells as part of the immune response. This, in turn, as described in Chapter 37, triggers the mucosal swelling and bronchoconstriction that are characteristic of an allergic asthma attack. The sequence of events that occurs in a patient with allergic asthma is shown in Box 38-1.

The *late-phase response* peaks 5 to 12 hours after the initial response and may last from several hours to several days. It is thought that infiltration by neutrophils and eosinophils attract additional inflammatory mediators, especially leukotrienes, which create a self-sustaining cycle of inflammation and obstruction. The clinical symptoms are the same as during the early phase. However, as a result of the inflammation, airways become sensitized or hyper-responsive, such that subsequent episodes of asthma may be triggered not only by allergens but also by nonspecific stimuli such as strong odours, cold air, dust, and air pollution.

BOX 38-2

Classifications of Drugs Used to Treat Asthma

Controllers

Leukotriene receptor antagonists
Mast cell stabilizers
Inhaled and oral glucocorticosteroids
Anticholinergic drugs
Inhaled long-acting β_2-agonists (LABAs)
Combination inhaled glucocorticoid and inhaled long-acting β_2-agonist
theophylline
Long-acting β_2-agonists in combination with inhaled corticosteroids

Relievers

Inhaled short-acting β_2-agonists
Inhaled ipratropium (rarely used)
Inhaled corticosteroid and long-acting β_2-agonist, specifically budesonide and formoterol combination (to be used as relief for patients 12 years of age and older if using the combination as maintenance)

The Global Initiative for Asthma (GINA) is an initiative between the US National Heart, Lung, and Blood Institute; the US National Institutes of Health; and the World Health Organization to reduce world asthma prevalence, morbidity, and mortality. In 2012, the Canadian Thoracic Society produced and updated guidelines for the diagnosis and management of asthma. On the basis of these guidelines, drugs are classified as either for long-term symptom control or for rapid symptom relief. The specific drugs in each classification are listed in Box 38-2. Crucial to the management of asthma is patients' self-management, which should include a written individualized action plan. New to the guidelines is consideration of sputum cell counts of eosinophils, to determine

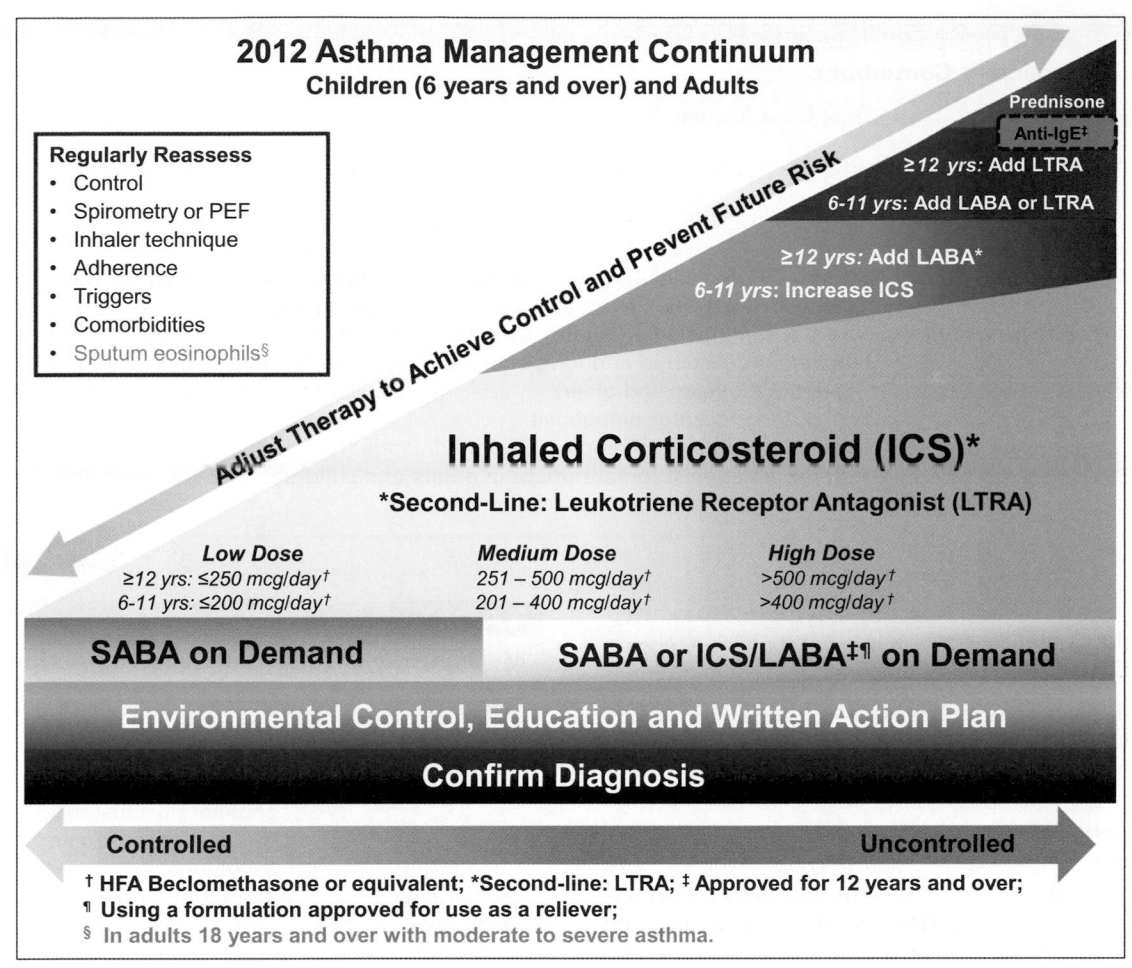

FIG. 38-1   The asthma management continuum. *HFA*, hydrofluoroalkane; *ICS*, inhaled corticosteroids; *IgE*, immunoglobulin E; *LABA*, long-acting β₂-agonist; *LTRA*, leukotriene receptor antagonist; *PEF*, peak expiratory flow. (Source: Lougheed, M. D., Lemiere, C., Ducharme, F. M., et al. (2012). Canadian Thoracic Society 2012 guideline update: Diagnosis and management of asthma in preschoolers, children and adults. *Canadian Respiratory Journal, 19*(2), p.162.)

the degree of inflammation and guide management for moderate-to-severe asthma (Lougheed et al., 2012). Asthma treatment for adults and children aged 6 years and older is based on the Asthma Management Continuum (Figure 38-1). The recommended drug classifications for treatment are listed in Table 38-1. Guidelines on the management and treatment of preschoolers were released in 2015 and are discussed in the Special Populations Box on p. 734.

CHRONIC OBSTRUCTIVE PULMONARY DISEASE

Chronic obstructive pulmonary disease (COPD) is a progressive respiratory disorder characterized by chronic airflow limitation with a range of pathological changes in the lung, systemic manifestations, and significant comorbidities that contribute to the severity of manifestations (Global Initiative for Chronic Obstructive Lung Disease [GOLD], 2015). GOLD's 2015 report on its global

strategy does not include the terms *emphysema* (damage to the lung parenchyma) or *chronic bronchitis* in the definition of COPD, as they do not adequately explain the numerous structural abnormalities involved in COPD. *Chronic bronchitis*, or the presence of cough and sputum for at least 3 months in each of 2 consecutive years, remains a useful term; however, chronic bronchitis is a separate disease.

When pulmonary tissues are exposed to inhaled smoke and other noxious particles, the physiological response in patients with COPD is an amplified chronic inflammation. The pathological changes that occur as a result of the inflammation are distributed throughout the pulmonary tissue, including the proximal airways, peripheral airways, lung parenchyma (respiratory bronchioles and alveoli), and pulmonary vasculature. The inflammatory cells in COPD are neutrophils, macrophages, and CD+8 lymphocytes. The inflammatory cells secrete numerous mediators, including tumour necrosis factor (TNF), interleukin 8 (IL-8), and leukotriene B4 (LT-B4). These mediators are believed to contribute to damage

TABLE 38-1	
Asthma Management Continuum	
Step	**Drug Classification**
Confirm diagnosis followed by environmental control, self-management education plus a written action plan.	
Step 1: Mild intermittent	Short-acting inhaled β_2-agonist as needed and early introduction of low-dosage inhaled glucocorticosteroid (in adults and children 6 years and older)
Step 2: Moderate persistent	Short-acting inhaled β_2-agonist as needed and medium-dosage inhaled corticosteroid Inhaled corticosteroid and long-acting β_2-agonist combination inhaler (in adults and children 12 years and older) Leukotriene receptor antagonist
Step 3–4 Severe uncontrolled	In addition to above therapies: Oral prednisone (FEV_1 less than 60%) Anti-IgE antagonist (omalizumab) in adults and children 12 years and over with atopic asthma

to lung structures. In addition, oxidative stress, produced by cigarette smoke and other inhaled particles, occurs when free radicals and other reactive species overwhelm the availability of antioxidants in the lungs. Free radicals further trigger damaging enzymes to be released from inflammatory cells and epithelial cells. Elevated levels of proteolytic (protein-destroying) enzymes then damage mucosal tissues of the airway.

The larger proximal airways (i.e., trachea, bronchi, bronchioles larger than 2 mm in diameter) respond by increasing mucus-secreting glands, increasing the number of goblet cells, and decreasing mucociliary function. These changes lead to hypersecretion of mucus, chronic cough, and increased susceptibility to bacterial infection. The peripheral airways (bronchioles smaller than 2 mm in diameter) also go through repeating cycles of injury and repair to the airway walls. This results in remodelling and eventually permanent scarring, thickening, and consolidation. Lung parenchyma (respiratory bronchioles and alveoli) is also affected, with resulting alveolar wall destruction and dilation and destruction of the respiratory bronchioles, resulting in hyperinflation and decreased gas exchange. Damage to the pulmonary vasculature leads to pulmonary hypertension, cor pulmonale, and the hypoxia and hypercapnia seen in patients with severe COPD. Assessment of COPD is based on the patient's level of symptoms, future risk of exacerbations, the severity of the spirometric abnormality, and the identification of comorbidities.

TREATMENT OF DISEASES OF THE LOWER RESPIRATORY TRACT

In the past, the treatment of asthma and other COPDs was focused primarily on the use of drugs that cause the airways to dilate. Now, there is a greater understanding of the pathophysiology of these diseases. The emphasis of research has shifted from the bronchoconstriction

TABLE 38-2	
Mechanisms of Antiasthmatic Drug Action	
Antiasthmatic	**Mechanism in Asthma Relief**
Anticholinergics	Block cholinergic receptors, thus preventing the binding of cholinergic substances that cause constriction and increase secretions
Leukotriene receptor antagonists	Modify or inhibit the activity of leukotrienes, which decreases arachidonic acid-induced inflammation and allergen-induced bronchoconstriction
β-Agonists and xanthine derivatives	Raise intracellular levels of cyclic adenosine monophosphate, which in turn produces smooth muscle relaxation and dilates the constricted bronchi and bronchioles
Corticosteroids	Prevent the inflammation commonly provoked by the substances released from mast cells
Mast cell stabilizers (sodium cromoglycate and nedocromil)	Stabilize the cell membranes of the mast cells in which the antigen–antibody reactions take place, thereby preventing the release of substances such as histamine

component of the disease to the role played by inflammatory cells and their mediators. Recent focus on inflammatory cells is also reflected in the various medication classes used to treat COPD, although bronchodilators still play an important role. A synopsis of the mechanisms of action of the classes of antiasthmatic drugs is provided in Table 38-2. Figure 38-2 provides an overview of the various drugs used to treat asthma.

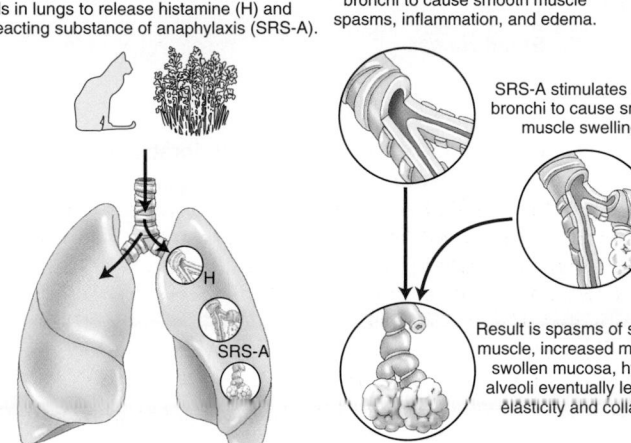

ALLERGENS such as dust, wool blankets, feather pillows, pollen, etc., in hypersensitive persons with IgE antibodies stimulate mast cells in lungs to release histamine (H) and slow-reacting substance of anaphylaxis (SRS-A).

HISTAMINE stimulates larger bronchi to cause smooth muscle spasms, inflammation, and edema.

SRS-A stimulates small bronchi to cause smooth muscle swelling.

Result is spasms of smooth bronchial muscle, increased mucus secretions, swollen mucosa, hyperinflation of alveoli eventually leading to loss of elasticity and collapsed alveoli.

LEUKOTRIENE ANTAGONISTS block the release of leukotrienes in the lungs. Inflammation causes an increase in leukotrienes, substances that constitute the slow-reacting substance of anaphylaxis (SRS-A).

THEOPHYLLINE increases cyclic AMP to inhibit breakdown of sensitized mast cells that stimulate the release of histamine, serotonin, and SRS-A.

MAST CELL STABILIZERS inhibit the release of histamine from mast cells to reduce allergic effects.

SYMPATHETIC AGONISTS stimulate sympathetic systems to decrease mucus secretions and relax bronchial muscle spasms.

CORTICOSTEROIDS produce an antiinflammatory effect and reduce mucus secretions and tissue histamine.

FIG. 38-2 Overview of the effects of various antiasthmatic medications. (Source: McKenry, L. M., Tessier, E., & Hogan, M. (2006). *Mosby's Pharmacology in Nursing* (22nd ed.). St. Louis, MO: Mosby.)

BRONCHODILATORS

Bronchodilators are an important part of pharmacotherapy for all respiratory diseases. Bronchodilators relax bronchial smooth muscle, which causes dilation of the bronchi and bronchioles that are narrowed as a result of the disease process. There are three classes of such drugs: β-adrenergic agonists, anticholinergics, and xanthine derivatives.

β-ADRENERGIC AGONISTS

The β-adrenergic agonists are a group of drugs that are commonly used during the acute phase of an asthmatic attack to reduce airway constriction and restore airflow to normal. They are agonists, or stimulators, of the adrenergic receptors in the sympathetic nervous system. The β- and α-adrenergic receptors are discussed in Chapters 19 and 20. The β-agonists imitate the effects of norepinephrine on β-receptors. For this reason, they are also called *sympathomimetic* bronchodilators. The β-agonists are categorized by their onset of action. Short-acting β-agonist (SABA) inhalers include salbutamol (e.g., Airomir®, Ventolin®) and terbutaline sulphate (Bricanyl®). Long-acting β-agonist (LABA) inhalers include formoterol (Foradil®, Oxeze®), indacaterol maleate (Onbrez® Breezhaler®), and salmeterol xinafoate (Serevent®). The LABAs are always prescribed with inhaled glucocorticosteroids. Traditionally, because the LABAs have a longer onset of action, they were not to be used for acute treatment; however, Health Canada has approved a combination glucocorticoid steroid and LABA, budesonide and formoterol fumarate dihydrate (Symbicort®), for use as a

reliever or rescue treatment for patients with moderate-to-severe asthma when asthma symptoms worsen.

Mechanism of Action and Drug Effects

The β-agonists dilate airways by stimulating the $β_2$-adrenergic receptors located throughout the lungs. There are three subtypes of β-agonists, based on their selectivity for $β_2$-receptors:

1. Nonselective adrenergic drugs, which stimulate the β-, $β_1$-(cardiac), and $β_2$-(respiratory) receptors. Example: epinephrine. Epinephrine is available as a prefilled syringe (Allerject®, EpiPen®) for self-administration by patients with severe allergic reactions (Figure 38-3).
2. Nonselective β-adrenergic drugs, which stimulate both $β_1$ and $β_2$ receptors. Example: isoproterenol hydrochloride.
3. Selective $β_2$ drugs, which primarily stimulate the $β_2$ receptors. Example: salbutamol.

These drugs can also be categorized according to their routes of administration as oral, injectable, or inhalational drugs. The various β-agonist bronchodilators are listed in Table 38-3.

The bronchioles are surrounded by smooth muscle. When the smooth muscle contracts, the airways are narrowed and the amount of oxygen and carbon dioxide exchanged is reduced. The action of β-agonist bronchodilators begins at the specific receptor stimulated and ends with the dilation of the airways. However, many reactions must take place at the cellular level for bronchodilation to occur. When a $β_2$-adrenergic receptor is stimulated by a β-agonist, adenylate cyclase is activated and produces cyclic adenosine monophosphate (cAMP). Increased levels of cAMP cause bronchial smooth muscles to relax,

TABLE 38-3

β-Agonist Bronchodilators

Drug	Type	Brand Names	Route of Administration
ephedrine	α-β		PO, IM, IV, Subcut
epinephrine	α-β	Adrenalin®	Subcut, IM, inhalation
fenoterol	β₂	Duovent UDV® (combined with ipratropium)	Inhalation
formoterol	β₂	Foradil, Oxeze	Inhalation
isoproterenol	β₁-β₂		IV, inhalation
salbutamol	β₂	Airomir, Ventolin	PO, inhalation
salmeterol	β₂	Serevent	Inhalation
terbutaline	β₂	Bricanyl	Inhalation

IM, intramuscular; *IV*, intravenous; *PO*, oral; *Subcut*, subcutaneous.

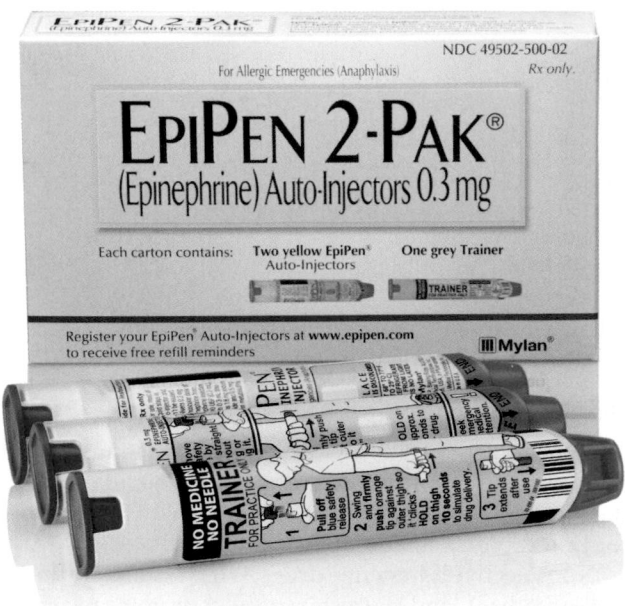

FIG. 38-3 The EpiPen Auto-Injector (epinephrine) is used for immediate treatment of anaphylaxis (allergic emergencies). The adult version is available in dosages of 0.3 mg for adults and for children weighing more than 30 kg. The EpiPen Junior is available in dosages of 0.15 mg for children weighing 15 to 30 kg. The EpiPen is given into the outer thigh, through the clothing. Anaphylactic emergencies also require emergency medical services in addition to the EpiPen. Additional information is available at www.epipen.ca. (© Mylan Specialty, L.P. Used with permission.)

which results in bronchial dilation and increased airflow into and out of the lungs. Nonselective adrenergic agonist drugs such as epinephrine also stimulate α-adrenergic receptors, causing constriction within the blood vessels. This vasoconstriction reduces the amount of edema or swelling in mucous membranes and limits the quantity of secretions normally produced by these membranes. In addition, these drugs also stimulate β₁-receptors, which results in cardiovascular adverse effects such as an increase in heart rate, force of contraction, and blood pressure, as well as central nervous system (CNS) effects such

as nervousness and tremor. Drugs such as salbutamol that predominantly stimulate the β₂-receptors have more specific drug effects and cause fewer adverse effects. By stimulating specifically the β₂-adrenergic receptors of the bronchial and vascular smooth muscles, they cause bronchodilation and may also have a dilating effect on the peripheral vasculature, which results in a decrease in diastolic blood pressure. In addition, the β₂-agonists are thought to stimulate the sodium–potassium adenosine triphosphatase ion pump in cell membranes. This action facilitates a temporary shift of potassium ions from the bloodstream into the cells, resulting in a temporary decrease in serum potassium levels. For this reason, β₂-agonists are also useful in treating patients with acute hyperkalemia. Finally, stimulation of β₂-receptors in uterine smooth muscle can cause beneficial uterine relaxation (see Indications).

Indications

The primary therapeutic effect of the β-agonists is the prevention or relief of bronchospasm related to bronchial asthma and COPD. However, they are also used for effects outside the respiratory system. Because some of these drugs have the ability to stimulate both β₁- and α-adrenergic receptors, they may be used to treat hypotension and shock (see Chapter 19).

Contraindications

Contraindications include drug allergy, uncontrolled cardiac dysrhythmias, and high risk of stroke (because of vasoconstrictive drug actions).

Adverse Effects

Mixed α- and β-agonists produce the most adverse effects because they are nonselective. These effects include insomnia, restlessness, anorexia, heart stimulation, hyperglycemia, tremor, and vascular headache. The adverse effects of the nonselective β-agonists are limited to β-adrenergic effects, including heart stimulation (tachycardia), tremor, anginal pain, and vascular headache. The β₂ drugs can cause both hypertension and hypotension, vascular headaches, and tremor. Overdose management may include careful administration of a β-blocker while

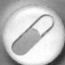 **DRUG PROFILES**

▸▸*salbutamol sulphate*

Salbutamol sulphate (Airomir, Ventolin) is a short-acting bronchodilating β-agonist. Other similar drugs include formoterol fumarate (Foradil, Oxeze), salmeterol xinaforte (Serevent), and terbutaline sulphate (Bricanyl). Salbutamol is the most commonly used drug in this class. If it is used too frequently, dose-related adverse effects may be seen because salbutamol loses its β₂-specific actions, especially at larger doses. As a consequence, the β₁-receptors are stimulated, which causes nausea, increased anxiety, palpitations, tremors, and an increased heart rate.

Salbutamol is available for oral, parenteral, and inhalational use. Inhalation dosage forms include metered-dose inhalers (MDIs) as well as solutions for inhalation (aerosol nebulizers). It is also available combined with ipratropium (Combivent®) for inhalations.

PHARMACOKINETICS

Route	Onset of Action	Peak Plasma Concentration	Elimination Half-Life	Duration of Action
Inhalation	Immediate	10–25 min	3–4 hr	3–4 hr

DOSAGES   Bronchodilators

Drug	Pharmacological Class	Usual Dosage Range	Indications
ipratropium bromide (Atrovent®, Ipravent®)	Anticholinergic	*Adults and children over 12 yr* MDI: 2 puffs tid–qid Nasal spray, 0.03%: 2 sprays bid–tid Nasal spray, 0.06%: 2 sprays bid–tid–qid *Children 5–12 yr* Inhalation solution: 125–250 mcg tid–qid *Adults* Inhalation solution: 250–500 mcg tid–qid	Asthma, bronchospasm
▸▸salbutamol sulphate (Airomir, Ventolin)	Short-acting β₂-agonist	*Children 2–6 yr* PO: 0.1 mg/kg tid–qid *Children 6–11 yr* PO: 2 mg tid–qid *Adults and children over 12 yr* PO: 2–4 mg tid–qid *Children 5–12 yr* Inhalation solution: 1.25–2.5 mg qid *Adults* Inhalation: 2.5–5 mg qid *Children 4 yr and over* MDI: 1 puff q3–4/day *Adults* MDI: 1–2 puffs qid *Adults* IV: 5 mcg/min–20 mcg/min diluted, continuous infusion	
▸▸salmeterol* (Serevent)	Long-acting β₂-agonist (LABA)	*Adults* 1 puff bid	Asthma, COPD

COPD, chronic obstructive pulmonary disease; *IV*, intravenous; *MDI*, metered-dose inhaler; *PO*, oral.
*Long-acting β-agonists are no longer to be used alone; they are combined with an inhaled glucocorticoid steroid (e.g., Advair® inhaler [fluticasone propionate and salmeterol]).

the patient is under close observation due to the risk of bronchospasm. Because the half-life of most adrenergic agonists is relatively short, the patient may just be observed while the body eliminates the medication.

Interactions

When nonselective β-blockers are used with the β-agonist bronchodilators, the bronchodilation from the β-agonist is diminished. The use of β-agonists with monoamine oxidase inhibitors (MAOIs) and other sympathomimetics

is best avoided because of the associated enhanced risk for hypertension. Patients with diabetes may require an adjustment in the dosage of their antihyperglycemic drugs, particularly patients receiving epinephrine, because of the increased blood glucose levels that can occur.

Dosages

For recommended dosages of selected β-agonists, refer to the table on p. 725.

ANTICHOLINERGICS

The anticholinergic (also called muscarinic antagonists) drugs used in the treatment of COPD are: ipratropium (Atrovent®) and tiotropium bromide monohydrate (Spiriva®) glycopyrronium bromide (Seebri Breezhaler®), aclidinium bromide (Tudorza Genuair®), and umeclidinium bromide (Incruse Ellipta®), glycopyrronium bromide (Seebri Breezhaler®), aclidinium bromide (Tudorza Genuair®), and umeclidinium bromide (Incruse Ellipta®). Three combinations of anticholinergics and long-acting β-agonists are currently available: aclidinium bromide and formoterol fumarate dihydrate (Duaklir Genuair®), tiotropium bromide and olodaterol hydrochloride (Inspiolto Respimat®), and umeclidinium bromide and vilanterol trifenatate (Anoro Ellipta®).

Mechanism of Action and Drug Effects

On the surface of the bronchial tree are receptors for acetylcholine (ACh), the neurotransmitter for the parasympathetic nervous system. When the parasympathetic nervous system releases ACh from its nerve endings, the neurotransmitter binds to the ACh receptors on the surface of the bronchial tree, which results in bronchial constriction and narrowing of the airways. Anticholinergic drugs block these ACh receptors to prevent bronchoconstriction. This action indirectly causes airway dilation. Anticholinergic drugs also help to reduce secretions in patients with COPD.

Indications

Because their actions are slow and prolonged, anticholinergics are used for prevention of bronchospasm associated with COPD and not for the management of acute symptoms. Tiotropium by inhaler is recommended as an add-on asthma control therapy that will improve outcomes for patients 18 years and older with asthma who remain symptomatic despite the use of inhaled corticosteroids and long-acting β-agonist maintenance therapy (GINA, 2015). This indication has not been approved in Canada.

Contraindications

The only usual contraindication to the use of bronchial anticholinergic drugs is drug allergy, including allergy to atropine sulphate. Caution is necessary in patients with acute angle-closure glaucoma or prostate enlargement.

Adverse Effects

The most commonly reported adverse effects of ipratropium and tiotropium bromide monohydrate therapy are related to the drugs' anticholinergic effects and include dry mouth or throat, nasal congestion, heart palpitations, gastrointestinal (GI) distress, urinary retention, increased intraocular pressure, headache, coughing, and anxiety. Ipratropium can be used during pregnancy; benefits of the use of tiotropium bromide monohydrate during pregnancy outweigh the potential risks.

Drug Interactions

Possible additive toxicity may occur when anticholinergic bronchodilators are taken with other anticholinergic drugs.

Dosages

For dosage information on anticholinergic drugs, refer to the table on p. 725.

XANTHINE DERIVATIVES

The natural xanthines consist of the plant alkaloids caffeine, theobromine, and theophylline, but only theophylline and caffeine are currently used clinically. There is one synthetic xanthine, aminophylline. Caffeine, which is actually a metabolite of theophylline, has other uses, described later.

Mechanism of Action and Drug Effects

Xanthines cause bronchodilation by increasing the levels of the energy-producing substance cAMP. They do this by competitively inhibiting phosphodiesterase, the enzyme responsible for breaking down cAMP. In patients with COPD, cAMP plays an integral role in the maintenance of

---

 DRUG PROFILES

ipratropium bromide

Ipratropium bromide (Atrovent) is the oldest and most commonly used anticholinergic bronchodilator. It is pharmacologically similar to atropine sulphate (see Chapter 22). It is available as a liquid aerosol for inhalation and as a multidose inhaler; both forms are usually dosed twice daily. Tiotropium bromide monohydrate (Spiriva) is a similar drug but is formulated for once-daily dosing (see Preventing Medication Errors Box). Many patients also benefit from taking both a β₂-agonist and an anticholinergic drug, with the most popular combination being salbutamol and ipratropium. Although many patients receive the two drugs separately, two combination products are available containing both of these drugs: Combivent (an MDI form) and Teva-Combo Sterinebs® (an inhalation solution).

PHARMACOKINETICS

Route	Onset of Action	Peak Plasma Concentration	Elimination Half-Life	Duration of Action
Inhalation	5–15 min	1–2 hr	1.6 hr	4–5 hr

PREVENTING MEDICATION ERRORS

Oral Ingestion of Capsules for Inhalation Devices

Some inhalation products use capsules and a device that pierces the capsules to allow the powdered medication to be inhaled with a special inhaler. Two products, Foradil Aerolizer® (formoterol fumarate inhalation powder) and Spiriva HandiHaler® (tiotropium bromide inhalation powder) contain such capsules. Even though these capsules are packaged with inhaler devices, they closely resemble oral capsules. The Institute for Safe Medication Practices Canada has received reports that the capsules have been taken orally by patients, which can potentially result in adverse effects. If the capsules are swallowed instead of taken using the inhalation device, the medication's onset of action may be delayed and its efficacy reduced, and as a result the patient receives inadequate drug delivery.

open airways. Higher intracellular levels of cAMP contribute to smooth muscle relaxation and inhibit IgE-induced release of the chemical mediators that drive allergic reactions (histamine, slow-reacting substance of anaphylaxis [SRS-A], others). Theophylline is metabolized to caffeine in the body, whereas aminophylline is metabolized to theophylline. Theophylline and other xanthines also stimulate the CNS, but to a lesser degree than caffeine. Stimulation of the CNS has the beneficial effect of acting directly on the medullary respiratory centre to enhance respiratory drive. In large doses, theophylline may stimulate the cardiovascular system, which results in both an increased force of contraction (positive inotropy) and an increased heart rate (positive chronotropy). The increased force of contraction raises cardiac output and, consequently, blood flow to the kidneys. This action, in combination with the ability of the xanthines to dilate blood vessels in and around the kidney, increases the glomerular filtration rate, which produces a diuretic effect.

Indications

Xanthines are used to dilate the airways in patients with asthma and COPD. They may be used in mild to moderate cases of acute asthma and as an adjunct drug in the management of COPD. Xanthines are now de-emphasized as treatment for milder asthma because of their potential for drug interactions and interpatient variability in therapeutic drug levels in the blood. Because of their relatively slow onset of action, xanthines are used more often for the prevention of asthmatic symptoms than for the relief of acute asthma attacks. However, they are also used as adjunct bronchodilators for patients with COPD. Caffeine is used without a prescription as a CNS stimulant, or analeptic (see Chapter 14), to promote alertness (e.g., for long-duration driving or studying). It is also used as a heart stimulant in infants with bradycardia and for enhancement of respiratory drive in infants in neonatal critical care units. It is not normally used clinically in adults for these purposes, although theoretically it would have similar effects.

Contraindications

Contraindications to therapy with xanthine derivatives include known drug allergy, uncontrolled cardiac dysrhythmias, seizure disorders, hyperthyroidism, and peptic ulcers.

Adverse Effects

The common adverse effects of the xanthine derivatives include nausea, vomiting, and anorexia. In addition, gastroesophageal reflux has been observed to occur during sleep in patients taking these drugs. Cardiac adverse effects include sinus tachycardia, extrasystole, palpitations, and ventricular dysrhythmias. Transient increased urination and hyperglycemia are other possible adverse effects. Overdose and other toxicity of xanthine derivatives are usually treated by the repeated administration of activated charcoal.

Interactions

The use of xanthine derivatives with any of the following drugs causes an increase in its serum level: allopurinol, cimetidine, macrolide antibiotics (e.g., erythromycin), quinolones (e.g., ciprofloxacin), influenza vaccine, rifampin, and oral contraceptives. Their use with sympathomimetics, or even caffeine, can produce additive heart and CNS stimulation. Rifampin increases the metabolism of theophylline, which results in decreased theophylline levels. St. John's wort (*Hypericum perforatum*) enhances the rate of xanthine drug metabolism; thus, higher dosages of theophylline and other xanthine derivatives may be needed. Cigarette smoking has a similar effect because of the enzyme-inducing effect of nicotine. Interacting foods include charcoal broiled, high-protein, and low-carbohydrate foods. These substances may reduce serum levels of xanthines through various metabolic mechanisms.

Dosages

For the recommended dosages of selected theophylline salts, refer to the table on p. 728.

NONBRONCHODILATING RESPIRATORY DRUGS

Bronchodilators (β-adrenergic agonists and xanthines) are just one type of drug used to treat asthma and COPD.

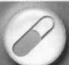

DRUG PROFILES

▶▶ theophylline

Theophylline (Theolair®, Uniphyl®) is the most commonly used xanthine derivative, although it has fallen out of favour due to its high adverse effect profile. It is available in oral and injectable (as aminophylline) dosage forms. Besides theophylline, which occurs in various salt forms, the other xanthine bronchodilator used clinically for the treatment of bronchoconstriction is aminophylline. Aminophylline is a prodrug of theophylline; it is metabolized to theophylline in the body. Aminophylline is sometimes given intravenously to patients with status asthmaticus who have not responded to fast-acting β-agonists such as epinephrine.

Theophylline has a narrow therapeutic index and the margin of safety above therapeutic doses is small. The beneficial effects of theophylline can be maximized by maintaining levels within a certain target range. If these levels become too high, unwanted adverse effects can occur. If levels become too low, the patient receives little therapeutic benefit. Although the optimal level may vary from patient to patient, most standard references have suggested that the therapeutic range for theophylline blood level is usually 55 to 110 micromol/L. Levels higher than 110 micromol/L are associated with toxic effects. The Canadian Thoracic Society guidelines (Lougheed et al., 2012) recommend that a serum concentration of 28 to 55 micromol/L will reduce adverse effects without loss of therapeutic benefit. Laboratory monitoring of drug blood levels is common to ensure adequate dosage, especially in the hospital setting.

PHARMACOKINETICS

Route	Onset of Action	Peak Plasma Concentration	Elimination Half-Life	Duration of Action
PO	Unknown	1–2 hr	7–9 hr	12 hr

DOSAGES	Theophylline Salts			
Drug	**Pharmacological Class**	**Usual Dosage Range**		**Indications**
▶▶theophylline (Theolair, Theo ER®, Uniphyl)	Xanthine-derived bronchodilator	*Adults* 400–600 mg/day in 1–4 divided doses		Asthma, COPD

There are also other drugs that are effective in suppressing underlying causes of some of these respiratory illnesses. These include leukotriene receptor antagonists (montelukast, zafirlukast), and corticosteroids (beclomethasone, budesonide, dexamethasone, flunisolide, fluticasone, ciclesonide, triamcinolone). Another drug class known as *mast cell stabilizers* is now rarely used and is no longer included in Canadian Asthma Management Continuum.

LEUKOTRIENE RECEPTOR ANTAGONISTS

When they became available in the 1990s, the leukotriene receptor antagonists (LTRAs) were the first new class of asthma medications to be introduced in Canada in more than 20 years.

Before the development of LTRAs, most asthma treatments focused on relaxing the contraction of bronchial muscles with bronchodilators. More recently, researchers have begun to understand how asthma symptoms are caused by the immune system at the cellular level. A chain reaction starts when a trigger allergen, such as cat hair or dust, initiates a series of chemical reactions in the body. Several substances are produced, including a family of molecules known as *leukotrienes*. In people with asthma, leukotrienes cause inflammation, bronchoconstriction, and mucus production; this, in turn, leads to coughing, wheezing, and shortness of breath.

Mechanism of Action and Drug Effects

The LTRAs montelukast (Singulair®) and zafirlukast (Accolate®) act directly by binding to the D4 leukotriene-receptor subtype (LTD4) in respiratory tract tissues and organs. The drug effects of LTRAs are limited primarily to the lungs. As their class name implies, LTRAs prevent leukotrienes from attaching to receptors located on circulating immune cells (e.g., lymphocytes in the blood) as well as local immune cells within the lungs (e.g., alveolar macrophages); this action alleviates asthma symptoms in the lungs by reducing inflammation. They prevent smooth muscle contraction of the bronchial airways, decrease mucus secretion, and reduce vascular permeability (which reduces edema) through their reduction of leukotriene synthesis. Other effects of LTRAs include prevention of the mobilization and migration of cells such as neutrophils and leukocytes into the lungs; this effect also serves to reduce airway inflammation.

Indications

The LTRAs montelukast and zafirlukast are used for the prophylaxis and long-term treatment and prevention of asthma in adults and children. Montelukast is considered safe in children 2 years of age and older and zafirlukast in children 12 years of age and older. Because it is dosed once daily, montelukast is the most widely used of these drugs and has also been approved for treatment of allergic rhinitis, a condition discussed in Chapter 37. These drugs are not intended for the management of acute asthmatic attacks. Improvement in asthma symptoms with their use is typically seen in about 1 week.

Contraindications

Known drug allergy or other previous adverse drug reaction is the primary contraindication to use of LTRAs. Allergy to povidone, lactose, titanium dioxide, or cellulose derivatives is also important to note, because these are inactive ingredients in these drugs.

Adverse Effects

The adverse effects of LTRAs differ depending on the specific drug. The most common adverse effects of zafirlukast include headache, nausea, and diarrhea. Both drugs may also lead to liver dysfunction. For this reason, monitor liver enzyme levels regularly in patients taking these drugs, especially early in the course of therapy.

Interactions

Montelukast has fewer drug interactions than zafirlukast. Phenobarbital and rifampin, both of which are enzyme inducers, decrease montelukast concentrations. For information on the drugs that interact with zafirlukast, see Table 38-4.

Dosages

For recommended dosages of montelukast, refer to the table on p. 730.

CORTICOSTEROIDS

Corticosteroids, also known as *glucocorticoids*, are either naturally occurring or synthetic drugs used in the treatment of pulmonary diseases because of their antiinflammatory effects. All have actions similar to those of the natural steroid hormone cortisol, which is chemically the same as the drug hydrocortisone. Synthetic steroids are more commonly used in drug therapy than naturally occurring ones. They can be administered by inhalation, orally, and intravenously (in severe cases of asthma when the drug cannot transfer to the airways because of airway obstruction). Corticosteroids administered by inhalation have an advantage over orally administered corticosteroids in that their action is limited to the topical site in the lungs. This generally limits, although does not completely prevent, systemic effects. The chemical structures of the corticosteroids given by inhalation have also been slightly altered to limit their systemic absorption from the respiratory tract. The corticosteroids administered by inhalation include the following:

- beclomethasone dipropionate (Qvar®)
- budesonide (Pulmicort Nebuamp®, Pulmicort Turbuhaler®, Rhinocort Aqua®, Rhinocort Turbuhaler®)
- fluticasone furoate (Avamys®)
- fluticasone propionate (Flovent Diskus®, Flovent HFA®)
- ciclesonide (Alvesco®, Omnaris®)
- mometasone (Asmanex Twisthaler®)

TABLE 38-4			
Drug Interactions: Leukotriene Receptor Antagonists			
Drug	**Interacting Drugs**	**Mechanism**	**Result**
montelukast sodium (Singulair)	phenobarbital, rifampin	Increased metabolism	Decreased montelukast levels
zafirlukast (Accolate)	aspirin	Decreased clearance	Increased zafirlukast levels
	erythromycin	Decreased bioavailability	Decreased zafirlukast levels
	warfarin sodium	Decreased clearance	Increased warfarin sodium levels

 ## DRUG PROFILES

Leukotriene receptor antagonists (LTRAs) are used primarily for oral prophylaxis and long-term treatment of asthma. The two drugs currently available are zafirlukast and montelukast. These drugs are not recommended for treatment of acute asthma attacks.

▸▸ *montelukast sodium*

Montelukast sodium (Singulair) belongs to the same subcategory of LTRAs as zafirlukast. Montelukast and zafirlukast act by blocking leukotriene D4 receptors to augment the inflammatory response. Montelukast offers the advantage of being Health Canada–approved for use in children

2 years of age and older (a chewable tablet is available for children). It also has fewer adverse effects and drug interactions than zafirlukast. Use of montelukast is contraindicated in patients with a known hypersensitivity to it. It is available only for oral use. Montelukast is reasonably safe to take during pregnancy.

PHARMACOKINETICS

Route	Onset of Action	Peak Plasma Concentration	Elimination Half-Life	Duration of Action
PO	30 min	3–4 hr	2.7–5 hr	24 hr

DOSAGES	Selected Leukotriene Receptor Antagonist		
Drug	**Pharmacological Class**	**Usual Dosage Range**	**Indications**
►►montelukast sodium (Singulair)	Leukotriene-receptor antagonist	*Children 2–5 yr* PO (chewable tablet): 4 mg daily in evening *Children 6–14 yr* PO (chewable tablet): 5 mg daily in evening	Prophylaxis and maintenance treatment of asthma
		Adults and adolescents over 15 yr PO: 10 mg daily in evening	Asthma and seasonal allergic rhinitis

PO, oral.

The systemic use of corticosteroids was described in Chapter 34. The systemic corticosteroids most commonly used include the following:

- prednisone (oral)
- methylprednisolone (intravenous [IV] or oral)

Mechanism of Action and Drug Effects

Although the exact mechanism of action of the corticosteroids has not been determined, it is conjectured that they have the dual effect of both reducing inflammation and enhancing the activity of β-agonists. The corticosteroids produce their anti-inflammatory effects through a complex sequence of actions. The overall effect is to prevent nonspecific inflammatory processes, including the accumulation of inflammatory mediators as well as altered vascular permeability (which causes edema).

Corticosteroids act by stabilizing the membranes of cells that normally release bronchoconstricting substances. These cells include leukocytes, or white blood cells (WBCs). There are five different kinds of WBCs, each with its own specific characteristics. Table 38-5 summarizes these five types of WBCs, their role in the inflammatory process, and the way in which corticosteroids inhibit their normal actions, combat inflammation, and produce bronchodilation. Inflammatory mediators are released primarily by lymphocytes in the circulation as well as by mast cells and alveolar macrophages. These latter two cell types are stationary inflammatory cells that remain localized in the tissues and organs of the respiratory tract.

Corticosteroids have also been shown to restore or increase the responsiveness of bronchial smooth muscle to β-adrenergic receptor stimulation, which results in more pronounced stimulation of the β₂-receptors by β-agonist drugs such as salbutamol. It may take several weeks of continuous therapy before the full therapeutic effects of the corticosteroids are felt.

Indications

Inhaled corticosteroids are used for the primary treatment of bronchospastic disorders to control the inflammatory responses that are believed to be the cause of these disorders; they are indicated for persistent asthma. Inhaled corticosteroids are often used concurrently with β-adrenergic agonists. In respiratory illnesses, systemic corticosteroids are generally used only for acute exacerbations, or severe asthma. Their long-term use is associated with adverse effects (see later). The Canadian Thoracic Society's guidelines (Lougheed et al., 2012) recommend the use of oral prednisone for short periods (usually 3 to 5 days) in children with a recent history of severe exacerbation of asthma and suboptimal response to SABAs during exacerbation, as well as in individuals older than 15 years of age with a history of severe acute loss of asthma control in the preceding year. When a more pronounced anti-inflammatory effect is needed, however, as in an acute exacerbation of asthma or other COPD, IV corticosteroids (e.g., methylprednisolone) may be used.

Contraindications

Drug allergy is the primary contraindication to corticosteroid use and is usually due to other ingredients in the drug formulation. Corticosteroids are not intended as sole therapy for acute asthma attacks. Inhaled corticosteroids are contraindicated in patients who are hypersensitive to glucocorticoids, in patients whose sputum tests positive for *Candida albicans* organisms, and in patients with systemic fungal infection, as the corticosteroids can suppress the immune system.

Adverse Effects

The main undesirable local effects of typical doses of inhaled corticosteroids include pharyngeal irritation, coughing, dry mouth, and oral fungal infections. Instruct patients to rinse their mouths after the use of an inhaled corticosteroid. Most of the drug effects of inhaled corticosteroids are limited to their topical site of action in the lungs. Because of the chemical structure of the inhaled dosage forms, there is relatively little systemic absorption of the drugs when they are administered by inhalation at normal therapeutic doses. However, the degree of systemic absorption is more likely to be increased in patients who require higher inhaled doses. When there is significant systemic absorption, which is most likely with high-dose IV or oral administration, corticosteroids can affect any of the organ systems in the body. Some of the possible systemic drug effects include adrenocortical insufficiency, increased susceptibility to infection, fluid and electrolyte disturbances, endocrine effects, CNS effects (e.g., insomnia, nervousness, seizures), and dermatological and connective tissue effects (e.g., brittle skin, bone loss, osteoporosis, Cushing's syndrome; see Chapter 34).

TABLE 38-5

White Blood Cells (Leukocytes)

Specific WBC*	Role in Inflammation	Corticosteroid Effect
GRANULOCYTES		
Neutrophils (65%)	Contain powerful lysosomes (tiny bodies that hold cellular digestive enzymes); release chemicals that destroy invading organisms and also attack other WBCs	Stabilize cell membranes so that inflammation-causing substances are not released
Eosinophils (2–5%)	Function primarily in allergic reactions and in protecting against parasitic infections; ingest inflammatory chemicals and antigen–antibody complexes	Little effect, if any
Basophils (0.5–1%)	Contain histamine, an inflammation-causing substance, and heparin, an anticoagulant	Stabilize cell membranes so that histamine is not released
AGRANULOCYTES		
Lymphocytes (25%)	Two types: T lymphocytes and B lymphocytes; T cells attack infecting microbial or cancerous cells; B cells produce antibodies against specific antigens	Decrease activity of lymphocytes
Monocytes (3–5%)	Produce macrophages, which can migrate out of the bloodstream to such places as mucous membranes, where they are capable of engulfing large bacteria or virus-infected cells	Inhibit macrophage accumulation in already inflamed areas, thus preventing more inflammation

WBC, white blood cell.
*Value in parentheses is the percentage of all leukocytes represented by the given type.

It is important to remember that when patients are switched to inhaled corticosteroids after receiving systemic corticosteroids, especially at high dosages for an extended period, adrenal suppression (addisonian crisis) may occur if the systemically administered corticosteroid is not tapered slowly. Patient deaths have been reported due to adrenal gland failure in cases when the switch to inhaled corticosteroids was made quickly and the dosage of systemic corticosteroids reduced too abruptly. Prevention of such an occurrence requires careful monitoring with slow tapering of systemic drug dosages. Patients who are dependent on systemic corticosteroids may need up to 1 year of recovery time after discontinuation of systemic therapy. There is evidence that bone growth is suppressed in children and adolescents taking corticosteroids. This suppression is more apparent in children receiving larger systemic (versus inhaled; children on inhaled corticosteroids reach their predicted adult height, but it may take them longer than other children not on inhaled corticosteroid treatment) dosages over long treatment durations. Growth needs to be tracked (e.g., with standardized charts) and medications re-evaluated should growth suppression become evident. In some cases, supplemental growth hormone may be prescribed.

Interactions

Drug interactions are more likely to occur with systemic (versus inhaled) corticosteroids. Corticosteroids may increase serum glucose levels, possibly requiring adjustments in dosages of antidiabetic drugs. Because of interactions related to metabolizing enzymes, they may also raise the blood levels of the immunosuppressants cyclosporine and tacrolimus. Likewise, the antifungal drug itraconazole may reduce clearance of the steroids, whereas phenytoin, phenobarbital, and rifampin may enhance clearance. There is also greater risk for hypokalemia with concurrent use of potassium-depleting diuretics such as hydrochlorothiazide and furosemide.

Dosages

For recommended dosages of selected corticosteroids, refer to the table on p. 732.

PHOSPHODIESTERASE-4 INHIBITOR

In 2010, Health Canada approved roflumilast (Daxas®), a selective inhibitor of the enzyme *phosphodiesterase type 4* (PDE4), the use of which results in decreased inflammation in the lungs. Decreasing inflammation helps to stop the narrowing of airways that occurs in COPD and also prevents excess mucus production from worsening, thus decreasing the frequency of life-threatening COPD exacerbations. It is not intended to treat acute bronchospasm. The most commonly reported adverse effects of roflumilast include nausea, diarrhea, headache, insomnia, dizziness, weight loss, and mental health symptoms such as anxiety and depression.

DRUG PROFILES

fluticasone propionate

Fluticasone propionate can be administered intranasally (Flonase®; one inhalation in each nostril daily) and by oral inhalation (Flovent Diskus, Flovent HFA; usually one inhalation by mouth twice daily). The lowest dose of fluticasone required to maintain good asthma control should be used. When a patient's asthma is well controlled, a reduction in the dose of fluticasone should be attempted in order to identify the lowest possible dose required to maintain control; such attempts at dose reduction should be carried out on a regular basis.

Fluticasone is also available in a combination formulation with the bronchodilator salmeterol xinaforte (Advair Diskus®, Advair® Inhalation Aerosol). Advair is one of the most commonly used inhalers and must never be used for acute treatment of asthma.

PHARMACOKINETICS

Route	Onset of Action	Peak Plasma Concentration	Elimination Half-Life	Duration of Action
Inhalation	Unknown	Unknown	3 hr	Up to 24 hr

methylprednisolone

Methylprednisolone is a systemic corticosteroid available in both oral (Medrol®) and injectable (Solu-Medrol®) forms.

PHARMACOKINETICS

Route	Onset of Action	Peak Plasma Concentration	Elimination Half-Life	Duration of Action
IV	Immediate	30 min	3–4 hr	24–36 hr

DOSAGES   Selected Corticosteroids

Drug	Pharmacological Class	Usual Dosage Range	Indications
fluticasone propionate (Flonase, Flovent Diskus, Flovent HFA)	Synthetic glucocorticoid	*Children 12 mo–4 yr* Flovent HFA: 100 mcg daily, bid, using a BABYHALER spacer device with a face mask *Children 4–16 yr* Flovent HFA, Diskus: 50–200 mcg bid *Adults and adolescents over 16 yr* Flovent HFA, Diskus: 100–400 mcg daily bid Flovent HFA, 3 strengths available: 50, 125, 250 mcg/actuation Flovent Diskus, inhalation powder, 4 strengths available: 50, 100, 250, 500 mcg/actuation *Children 4–11 yr* Flonase metered-dose nasal spray: 1–2 sprays (50 mcg/each metered dose) in each nostril bid (max 200 mcg daily)	Asthma (prophylaxis and maintenance treatment)
methylprednisolone (Solu-Medrol injection, Medrol tablets)	Synthetic glucocorticoid	Dose varies as above, but usually 40–120 mg IV over 30 min Oral taper: usually from 24–2 mg daily	Status asthmaticus Asthma

IV, intravenous.

MONOCLONAL ANTIBODY ANTIASTHMATIC

Omalizumab (Xolair®) is the newest asthma drug available. It is a monoclonal antibody that selectively binds to the immunoglobulin IgE, which in turn limits the release of mediators of the allergic response. Omalizumab is given by subcutaneous injection and has the potential for producing anaphylaxis. Anaphylaxis can be delayed from 2 hours to 4 days post injection. Patients receiving omalizumab must be monitored closely for hypersensitivity reactions.

NURSING PROCESS

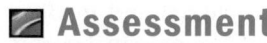 **Assessment**

The net drug effect of β-agonists, xanthine derivatives, anticholinergics, LTRAs, and corticosteroids is improved airflow in airway passages and increased oxygen supply. Thoroughly assess for cautions, contraindications, and drug interactions before administering these drugs, and assess the patient's skin colour; temperature; respiration rate, depth, and rhythm; breath sounds; blood pressure; pulse rate; and pulse oximetry readings (to determine oxygen saturation levels). Determine if the patient is having problems with cough, dyspnea, orthopnea, or hypoxia, or has other signs or symptoms of respiratory distress. If a cough is present, assess its character and frequency, the presence or absence of sputum, and the colour of any sputum. Assess the patient for the presence of any of the following: sternal retractions, cyanosis, restlessness, activity intolerance, heart irregularities, palpitations, hypertension, tachycardia, or use of accessory muscles to breathe, indicating significant respiratory compromise. Determine the anterior–posterior diameter of the thorax.

Obtain a complete medication history that includes information about prescription (e.g., questions about possible drug causes of respiratory distress in conjunction with asthma/COPD such as aspirin) and over-the-counter (OTC) drugs, natural health products, and alternative therapies. Also gather information on the use of nebulizers or humidifiers, the use of a home air conditioner, and the type and maintenance of heating and air conditioning systems, as forced-air systems can foster mould and dust mites. Collect information about environmental allergies such as to dust, mould, pollen, or mildew, as well as seasonal allergies and food allergies. Note the characteristics of any respiratory symptoms (e.g., seasonally induced, exercise- or stress-induced) and any family history of respiratory diseases. Identify any environmental exposures, such as to chemicals or irritants, as well as precipitating and alleviating factors for any respiratory symptoms and disease processes. Assess smoking habits because smoking exacerbates respiratory symptoms and because nicotine interacts with many respiratory drugs.

Cardiac status may be compromised because of respiratory distress or respiratory illnesses; thus, closely assess the patient's blood pressure, pulse rate, heart sounds, and electrocardiogram, as ordered. Blood gas analysis may be indicated, with attention to the patient's pH, oxygen, carbon dioxide, and serum bicarbonate levels. Assess nail beds for abnormalities (e.g., clubbing, cyanosis) and the area around the lips. Restlessness is often the first sign of hypoxia, so frequent assessment before, during, and after drug treatment is needed. If hypoxia is present, it needs to be reported to the health care provider. If chest radiographs, scans, or magnetic resonance images have been ordered, review the findings. Along with a physical assessment, perform a psychosocial and emotional assessment, because anxiety, stress, and fear may only further compromise the patient's respiratory status and oxygen levels. As well, assess patients' educational level and readiness to learn. Be sure to note the age of the patient because of increased sensitivity to drugs in older adults and children.

With the use of the β-agonists (e.g., salbutamol, salmeterol), cautions, contraindications, and drug interactions associated with these drugs must be noted. A respiratory assessment is needed to assess for allergies to the fluorocarbon propellant in inhaled dosage forms. Assess for contraindications in patients with dysrhythmias and those at risk for stroke. Assess patients' intake of caffeine (e.g., in chocolate, tea, coffee, candy, sodas) and any use of OTC medications containing caffeine (e.g., appetite suppressants, pain relievers). The intake of caffeine is important to determine because of its sympathomimetic effects and possible potentiation of adverse effects along with salbutamol and other β-agonists (e.g., restlessness, tachycardia, tremor, hyperglycemia, vascular headache, hypotension, or hypertension with β_2 drugs). Assess patients' medication history because β-agonists are not to be taken with MAOIs because of the associated enhanced risk for hypertension.

Specifically with the use of anticholinergics, include any history of heart palpitations, GI distress, benign prostatic hyperplasia, urinary retention, or glaucoma due to the adverse effects of these drugs, which can lead to potentiation of these conditions or symptoms. Ipratropium and its aerosol forms have been associated with bronchospasm, so assess patients for any pre-existing problems with the use of MDIs. If a combination product containing both ipratropium and fenoterol hydrobromide or salbutamol is prescribed, perform an assessment appropriate to the use of both of the drugs.

With corticosteroids (also known as glucocorticoids), perform a baseline assessment of vital signs, breath sounds, and heart sounds. Assessment for underlying adrenal disorders is crucial because of the adrenal suppression that occurs with the use of these medications. Age is important to consider because corticosteroids may be problematic for pediatric patients if long-term therapy or high dosage amounts are used. The systemic impact of corticosteroids on pediatric patients is suppressed growth (see the Adverse Effects section under Glucocorticoids for further discussion). As with the other drugs in this chapter, awareness of basic information about these drugs, especially their action, is important for safe use and prevention of medication errors. For example, glucocorticoids are used for their anti-inflammatory effects, β-agonists and xanthines for their bronchodilating effects, and anticholinergics for their blockage of cholinergic receptors. Knowing what drugs do and why they are used helps to prevent or decrease medication errors and adverse effects. Significant drug interactions for which to assess, especially with systemic versus inhaled corticosteroids, include antidiabetic drugs, antifungals, phenytoin, phenobarbital, rifampin, and potassium-sparing diuretics. See Chapter 34 for more information on these anti-inflammatory adrenal drugs.

In patients taking xanthine derivatives (e.g., theophylline), identify any contraindications and cautions. Perform a careful cardiovascular assessment, noting heart rate, blood pressure, and any history of cardiac disease; this is important because of the adverse effects of sinus tachycardia and palpitations. GI reflux may also occur with xanthines. Assess bowel patterns and for

SPECIAL POPULATIONS: CHILDREN

Asthma in Children Ages 1 to 5

- The Canadian Thoracic Asthma Clinical Society and the Canadian Pediatric Society jointly developed guidelines for the diagnosis and management of asthma in children 1 to 5 years of age.
- Asthma often begins prior to the age of 6 in children; early diagnosis and management of asthma in this age group is important to reduce both short- and long-term morbidity.
- Preschoolers have the highest rate of emergency room visits and hospitalizations for asthma-like symptoms.
- Wheezing in children under the age of 6 can lead to a reduction in the FEV1 at age 6 which persists into adulthood.
- Guidelines suggested for a diagnosis in this age group are: (1) documented wheezing, (2) improved airflow with therapeutic trial of SABA and inhaled corticosteroids.

- Daily long-term inhaled corticosteroids at the lowest dose are recommended first-line management once asthma is diagnosed and control achieved.
- The goal of long-term therapy is to prevent acute exacerbations. The patient should have a written action plan, adhere to medication regimen, use a spacer with inhaler correctly, and avoid exposure to environmental allergens and irritants that are identified during the evaluation.
- Encourage children to have normal activity levels; do not limit physical activity to control asthma symptoms.

From Ducharme, F.M., Dell, S.D., Radhakrishnan, D., et al., (2015). *Diagnosis and management of asthma in preschoolers: A Canadian Thoracic Society and Canadian Pediatric society position paper.* Canadian Respiratory Journal, 22(3), 135–143.

pre-existing disease such as gastroesophageal reflux or ulcers. Because of possible drug-induced transient urinary frequency, conduct a baseline assessment of urinary patterns. Assessment needs to also include the patient's medication history to assess for possible drug interactions such as with allopurinol, cimetidine, erythromycin, ciprofloxacin, oral contraceptives, caffeine, or sympathomimetics. Perform a dietary assessment, including questions about any consumption of a high-carbohydrate, low-protein diet. These dietary practices may lead to decreased theophylline elimination and increased serum theophylline levels, resulting in significant adverse effects in patients. A low-carbohydrate, high-protein diet, and intake of charbroiled meat, may increase theophylline elimination and decrease therapeutic serum theophylline levels. Note intake of any caffeine-containing foods, beverages, prescription drugs, OTC drugs, or natural health products because of additional interactions.

With LTRAs, assess for contraindications, cautions, and drug interactions. Determine liver functioning because of specific concerns about the use of these drugs in patients with altered liver function. As with other medications, older adults are more sensitive to these drugs.

With the PDE4 inhibitors, assess for presenting symptoms as well as any baseline psychiatric issues or disorders. Note that these drugs are not for acute bronchospasms. Omalizumab, a monoclonal antibody antiasthmatic drug, requires additional assessment of known risks associated with certain malignancies; taking a thorough nursing history will help identify any of these risks. Also be sure to assess for signs and symptoms of increased hypersensitivity, as omalizumab is a protein.

Nursing Diagnoses

- Impaired gas exchange related to pathophysiological changes caused by respiratory disease
- Fatigue related to the disease process and lack of oxygen saturation
- Nonadherence with the medication regimen related to undesirable adverse effects of drug therapy

Planning

Goals

- Patient will experience improved gas exchange due to improvement in disease process and symptomatology.
- Patient will exhibit improved energy and less fatigue.
- Patient will remain adherent with the medication regimen and with nonpharmacological therapies.

Expected Patient Outcomes

- Patient briefly describes measures to improve gas exchange such as use of deep breathing, use of medications as described, and avoiding precipitating factors.
  - Patient shows evidence of improved oxygen levels with a blood oxygen saturation level of 95% or higher (depending on pathology).
- Patient is well rested and allows time for frequent rest periods during activities of daily living while minimizing oxygen demands.
- Patient states the importance of taking medication as prescribed, the reasons for not increasing or decreasing the dosage of any drug, and the importance of not

stopping drug therapy abruptly, to prevent complications and exacerbations of the disease.
- Patient takes medication(s) as prescribed to improve oxygenation and prevent exacerbation of symptoms.

☑ Implementation

Nursing interventions that apply to patients with respiratory disease processes (e.g., COPD, asthma, other upper and lower respiratory tract disorders) include patient education and an emphasis on adherence and prevention, in addition to the specific actions related to the prescribed drug therapy. Emphasize measures that help to prevent, relieve, or decrease the manifestations of the disease. A resource that provides excellent information as well as photographs and slideshows can be found at http://www.asthma.ca/ (Asthma Society of Canada, 2016).

Bronchodilators and other respiratory drugs must be given exactly as prescribed and by the prescribed route (e.g., parenterally, orally, by intermittent positive pressure breathing, by inhalation). Demonstrate the proper method for administering the inhaled forms of these drugs to patients (see Chapter 10), who should then provide return demonstrations. Emphasize the importance of taking only the prescribed dose of β-agonists, anticholinergics, xanthines, LTRAs, or other respiratory drugs because of the possible adverse effects, such as tachycardia, hypertension or hypotension, vascular headaches, heart palpitations, GI distress, urinary retention, gastroesophageal reflux, dysrhythmias, nausea, and dizziness.

MDIs, dry powder inhalers, and nebulizers are popular methods of delivery for respiratory drugs. The use of MDIs often requires coordination to inhale the medication correctly and to obtain approximately 10 to 40% (Smith & Goldman, 2012) of drug delivery to the lungs. If a second puff of the same drug is ordered, instruct the patient to wait 1 to 2 minutes between puffs. If a second type of inhaled drug is ordered, instruct the patient to wait 2 to 5 minutes between medications or to take as prescribed. Use of a spacer, an external device attached to the MDI for improved drug delivery via enhanced actuation and inhalation coordination, may be indicated to increase the amount of drug delivered. For a small child or infant, a mask can be fitted to the spacer. Even small infants can use an MDI with spacer with effective drug delivery (DiBlasi, 2015). A dry powder inhaler (Diskus®) is a small, hand-held device that delivers a specific amount of dry micronized powder with each inhaled breath. A nebulizer dosage form delivers an aerosol of small amounts of misted droplets of the drug to the lungs through a small mouthpiece or mask. Although a nebulizer may take longer to deliver the drug to the lungs than any of the types of inhalers, the nebulizer dosage form may be more effective for some patients. When a nebulizer is used, some medications may be combined for administration (e.g., salbutamol and ipratropium). See Chapter 10 for more information. In many agencies, there is a trend to use the MDI method

of drug delivery over nebulizers. One Canadian study showed a reduction in hospitalizations and improved cost savings for children with mild-to-moderate asthma who used an MDI over a nebulizer (Doan, Shefrin, & Johnson, 2011). In addition, the use of nebulizers may increase the risk of pathogen transmission and thus increase the risk of nosocomial infections.

β-Agonists must be taken exactly as prescribed because overdosage may be life-threatening. Educate patients not to crush or chew oral sustained-release tablets and to take them with food to decrease GI upset. Instructions for inhaled dosage forms are presented in Chapter 10. See Figure 38-3 for instructions on the use of the EpiPen® Auto-Injector. Reassess respiratory status and breath sounds before, during, and after therapy with these drugs to determine therapeutic effectiveness.

Anticholinergic drugs used for respiratory diseases (e.g., ipratropium) are to be taken daily as ordered and with appropriate use of the MDI. See the Patient Teaching Tips for more information on the administration of these drugs. It is important for patients to wait from 1 to 2 minutes (or as prescribed) before inhaling the second dose of the drug to allow for maximal lung penetration. Encourage rinsing of the mouth with water immediately after the use of any inhaled or nebulized drug to help prevent mucosal irritation and dryness. Xanthine derivatives are also to be given exactly as prescribed. If they are to be administered parenterally, determine the correct diluent, compatibility, and rate of administration. Use IV infusion pumps to ensure dosage accuracy and help prevent toxicity. Too rapid an infusion may lead to profound hypotension with possible syncope, tachycardia, seizures, and even cardiac arrest. Oral forms should be taken with food to avoid GI upset. Continue to monitor patients for respiratory status and improvement in baseline condition during drug therapy.

The LTRAs, specifically montelukast and zafirlukast, are given orally. Of most concern are the montelukast chewable tablets, which contain aspartame and approximately 0.842 mg of phenylamine per 5-mg tablet. Some patients may need to avoid these substances. Emphasize that these drugs are indicated for treatment of chronic asthma, not acute asthma attacks. Stress that these drugs are to be taken as ordered and on a continuous schedule, even if symptoms improve. Encourage an increase in fluid intake, as with all the respiratory drugs, to help in decreasing the viscosity of secretions.

Inhaled corticosteroids (glucocorticoids) are yet another group of drugs that must be used as prescribed, and patients should be given cautions regarding overuse. Advise patients to take the medication as ordered every day, regardless of whether or not they are feeling better. Often these drugs (e.g., flunisolide) are used as maintenance drugs and are taken twice daily for maximal response. An inhaled β₂-agonist may be used before the inhaled glucocorticoid to provide bronchodilation before the administration of the anti-inflammatory drug. The inhaled bronchodilator is generally taken 2 to 5 minutes (or as ordered) before the corticosteroid aerosol. Stress the importance of keeping all equipment (inhalers or nebulizers) clean, including cleaning and changing filters (for nebulizers), and maintaining devices in good working condition. Use of a spacer may be indicated, especially if success with inhalation is limited. Recommend rinsing of the mouth immediately after use of inhaler or nebulizer dosage forms of corticosteroids to help prevent overgrowth of oral fungi and subsequent development of oral candidiasis (thrush). Children may need a health care provider's order to have these medications on hand at school and during athletic events or physical education. Peak flow meter use is also encouraged among patients of all ages to better regulate disease. A peak flow meter is a handheld device used to monitor a patient's ability to breathe out air; readings reflect the airflow through the bronchi and thus the degree of obstruction in the airways. Encourage patients to keep a record of peak flow levels, signs and symptoms of the disease, any improvement, and the occurrence of any adverse effects associated with therapy. In children, use of systemic forms of corticosteroids is of particular concern, because such use may lead to suppression of the hypothalamic–pituitary–adrenal axis and subsequent growth stunting. However, the benefits are considerable when compared with the risks. Inhaled forms are often combined with short-term systemic therapy in children. Continue to monitor every patient's condition during therapy, with a focus on the respiratory, cardiac, and central nervous systems.

With the use of PDE4 inhibitor drugs, educate patients about the importance of reporting any change in psychiatric status to their health care providers immediately. The monoclonal antibody antiasthmatic drug omalizumab is to be taken exactly as ordered. Since it is given as a subcutaneous injection, instruct the patient in self-injection, or alert the patient that frequent visits to a health care provider are necessary to receive the injection.

This drug is usually given every 2 to 4 weeks. Omalizumab is not indicated for acute asthma attacks, and it may be used in conjunction with other acute-acting asthma medications. Closely monitor patients for any allergic or hypersensitivity reactions.

Evaluation

The therapeutic effects of any of the drugs used to treat, prevent, or improve the control of acute or chronic respiratory symptoms and diseases include the following: decreased dyspnea, wheezing, restlessness, and anxiety; improved respiratory patterns with return to normal rate and quality; improved oxygen saturation levels; improved activity and arterial blood gas levels; improved quality of life; and decreased severity and incidence of respiratory symptoms. The therapeutic effects of bronchodilators (e.g., xanthines, β-agonists) include decreased symptoms and increased ease of breathing. Blood levels of theophylline should be between 55 and 110 micromol/L and need to be frequently monitored. Peak flow meters are easy to use and help reveal early decreases in peak flow caused by bronchospasm. They also aid in monitoring treatment effectiveness. Other respiratory drugs produce medication-specific therapeutic effects. Adverse effects for which to monitor during drug therapy include the following: β-agonists—headache, insomnia, tachycardia, and tremor; anticholinergics—headache, GI distress, urinary retention, and increased intraocular pressure; xanthines—nausea, vomiting, and palpitations; LTRAs—dyspepsia, headaches, and insomnia; and corticosteroids—adrenocortical insufficiency, increased susceptibility to infection, fluid and electrolyte disturbances, and insomnia. With corticosteroids, adrenal suppression may occur when high doses are received for an extended period of time. See the previous discussion for a complete listing of adverse effects.

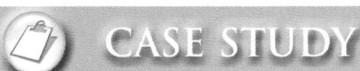 CASE STUDY

Chronic Obstructive Pulmonary Disease

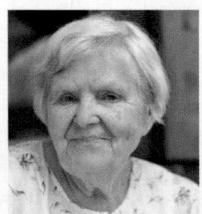

Hazel is a 73-year-old woman who has had chronic obstructive pulmonary disease (COPD) for approximately 10 years; it was caused by exposure to workplace environmental pollutants and by cigarette smoking. She is now retired and is frequently admitted to the hospital for treatment of her condition. She quit smoking 8 years ago. She is now in the hospital for treatment of an acute exacerbation of her COPD and an URT infection. The health care provider has ordered the following: ipratropium 2 puffs q3h and salbutamol 2 puffs q3h by MDI; chest physiotherapy bid and prn; levofloxacin 500 mg IV daily; measurement of intake and output; daily weight

measurement; assessment of vital signs, with breath sounds q2h and prn until stable; and salbutamol inhaler, 2 puffs q4h per respiratory therapy protocol.

1. What nursing interventions would be most appropriate for helping Hazel conserve energy while enhancing O_2 and CO_2 gas exchange?
2. What is the rationale for the use of salbutamol and ipratropium?
3. What is the rationale for the antibiotic? Be specific.
4. Would Hazel benefit from the use of systemic corticosteroids in the management of this exacerbation?

For answers, see http://evolve.elsevier.com/Canada/Lilley/pharmacology/.

PATIENT TEACHING TIPS

- ❖ Emphasize to patients that the sequence for the use of multiple inhaled medications is first, the long-acting β-agonist (alone or combined), followed by the long-acting anticholinergic, and, last, the corticosteroid. In general, the β-agonist, whether short- or long-acting, opens the airways and allows the corticosteroid and anticholinergic drugs to travel deeper into the lungs for improved therapeutic effect.
- ❖ Numerous devices exist for the delivery of respiratory drugs. New devices are constantly being made available. As each device is unique, educate patients on how to operate and maintain them and administer their medication. Provide resources that explain the use of inhalers.
- ❖ β-Agonists
  - Educate patients about any potential drug interactions.
  - Encourage patients with asthma or COPD to avoid precipitating events such as exposure to conditions or situations that may lead to bronchoconstriction and worsening of the disorder (e.g., allergens, stress, smoking, air pollutants).
  - Provide instructions about the proper use and care of MDIs, dry powder inhalers, and other such devices. See Chapter 10 for more specific information.
  - Emphasize the importance of not overusing the medication due to the risk of rebound bronchospasm.
- ❖ Xanthines
  - Educate patients about the interaction between smoking and xanthines (i.e., smoking decreases the blood concentrations of aminophylline and theophylline). Xanthines also interact with charcoal-broiled foods, and the consumption of these may lead to decreased serum levels of xanthine drugs.
  - Educate patients about food and beverage items that contain caffeine (e.g., chocolate, coffee, cola, cocoa, tea), because their consumption can exacerbate CNS stimulation.
  - Encourage patients to take the medication around the clock to maintain steady-state drug levels. Extended-release dosage forms and other oral dosage forms are not to be crushed or chewed. Advise patients that any worsening of adverse effects, such as epigastric pain, nausea, vomiting, tremor, and headache, must be reported immediately. Encourage patients to keep follow-up appointments because of the importance of monitoring therapeutic levels of medications and therapeutic effectiveness.
  - Some patients may need to learn to take their own pulse rate, so demonstrate to them the proper technique.
- ❖ Anticholinergics
  - Educate patients that ipratropium is used prophylactically to decrease the frequency and severity of asthma and must be taken as ordered and generally year round for therapeutic effectiveness.

- Encourage increased fluid intake unless contraindicated, to decrease the viscosity of secretions and increase the expectoration of sputum.
- When inhaled forms of these drugs (and other respiratory drugs) are used, instruct patients to take the prescribed number of puffs of the inhaler and no more than two puffs with one dosing, or as ordered. Educate patients about how to properly use an MDI with or without a spacer, how to use a dry powder inhaler, and how to properly clean and store the equipment (see Chapter 10). Instruct patients to wait 2 to 5 minutes (or as ordered) before using additional different inhaled medications.
- ❖ Leukotriene Receptor Antagonists
  - Educate the patient about the action and purpose of LTRAs and how they work by preventing leukotriene formation and thus preventing or decreasing inflammation, bronchoconstriction, and mucus production. Emphasize that these drugs are indicated for prevention, not treatment, of acute asthma attacks.
- ❖ Corticosteroids (Glucocorticoids)
  - In addition to adhering to the specified dosage and frequency of these drugs, if inhaled forms are used, patients must practise good oral hygiene (i.e., rinsing of the mouth) after the last inhalation. Rinsing the mouth with water is appropriate and necessary to prevent oral fungal infections. Instruct patients about how to keep inhalers clean. Every week, the canister should be removed from the plastic casing and the casing should be washed in warm, soapy water. Once the casing is dry, the canister and mouthpiece may be put back together and the cap applied. Glucocorticoids may predispose patients to oral fungal overgrowth. Provide explicit instructions for mouth care after each use.
  - Instruct patients to keep track of the doses left in each MDI. Many inhalers have built-in counters, but if one does not, the patient can do the following: Divide the number of doses in the canister by the number of puffs used per day to determine the number of days it will last. For example, if the patient takes 2 puffs, 4 times a day, this equals 8 inhalations per day. If there are 200 doses in a canister, dividing 200 by 8 gives the number of days the inhaler will last, 25 days. The MDI may then be marked with the date it will be empty and a refill then obtained a few days before that date. Note that using extra doses will alter the refill date. Advise the patient to always check expiration dates.
  - Stress to patients the importance of a written action plan, which is a personalized program developed by the health care provider and patient for managing asthma. Generally, those individuals who use individualized plans have better asthma control. An action plan should outline: (1) daily preventive management to maintain control; (2) when and how to adjust reliever and controller therapy to account for loss of control; and (3) clear

Continued

PATIENT TEACHING TIPS—cont'd

instructions regarding when to seek urgent medical attention. Adherence to maintenance therapy is a fundamental component of written action plans. In addition, the use of a peak flow meter on a daily basis will assist the patient to recognize early changes in expiratory airflow that may be signs of worsening asthma.

- Counsel patients to wear medical alert jewellery at all times and to carry a written or electronic medical record with all diagnoses and a list of medications and allergies. Emergency contact persons and phone numbers should also be listed.
- With the use of intranasal dosage forms, instruct patients on how to clear nasal passages before administration. The patient needs to tilt the head slightly forward, insert the spray tip into one nostril, and point the spray tip toward the inflamed nasal turbinates. Instruct the patient to pump the medication into the nasal passage while sniffing deeply and holding the other nostril closed. This procedure may then be repeated in the other nostril. It is recommended to discard any unused portion after 3 months or by the expiration date.
- Educate parents that adherence to inhaled corticosteroids will prevent asthma exacerbations.
- Educate patients about the fact that excess levels of systemic corticosteroids may lead to Cushing's syndrome, with symptoms such as moon facies, acne, increased fat pads, and swelling. Although use of inhaled forms helps to minimize this problem,

education on the subject remains important to patient safety. As noted previously, the risk of occurrence of these signs and symptoms is higher when these drugs are given systemically (i.e., orally or parenterally).

- Educate patients about the possibility of addisonian crisis, which may occur if a systemic corticosteroid is abruptly discontinued. These drugs require weaning prior to discontinuation. Addisonian crisis may be manifested by nausea, shortness of breath, joint pain, weakness, and fatigue. Patients must contact their health care providers immediately if these occur.
- Educate patients about the importance of reporting to a health care provider any weight gain of 1 kg or more in 24 hours or 2.3 kg or more in 1 week.

❖ Phosphodiesterase-4 Inhibitor
- Emphasize that patients taking roflumilast should report any notable changes in mood or emotions to a health care provider immediately.

❖ Monoclonal Antibody Antiasthmatic Drugs
- Omalizumab is used for the treatment of moderate to severe asthma and is not for aborting acute asthma attacks. Patients need to provide return demonstrations of subcutaneous injection techniques. Instruct patients to keep medications and needles, syringes, and other equipment out of the reach of children and to use puncture-proof needle waste containers. Each needle is used for only one injection.

KEY POINTS

❖ The β-agonists stimulate β₁- and β₂-receptors.

❖ Xanthines, such as theophylline, help to relax the smooth muscles of the bronchioles by inhibiting phosphodiesterase. Phosphodiesterase breaks down cAMP, which is needed to relax smooth muscles.

❖ Corticosteroids (e.g., beclomethasone, dexamethasone, flunisolide, triamcinolone) have many indications and work by stabilizing the membranes of cells that release harmful bronchoconstricting substances.

❖ The LTRAs, montelukast and zafirlukast, are given orally. Their adverse effects include headache, dizziness, insomnia, and dyspepsia.

❖ Omalizumab, a monoclonal antibody antiasthmatic drug, works by preventing the release of mediators that lead to allergic responses. It is given for preventative purposes.

EXAMINATION REVIEW QUESTIONS

1. A patient who has a history of asthma is experiencing an acute episode of shortness of breath and needs to take a medication for immediate relief. Which medication will the nurse choose for this situation?
   a. A β-agonist, such as salbutamol
   b. A leukotriene receptor antagonist, such as montelukast
   c. A corticosteroid, such as fluticasone
   d. An anticholinergic, such as ipratropium

2. After a nebulizer treatment with the β-agonist salbutamol, a patient reports feeling a little "shaky," with slight tremors of the hands. The patient's heart rate is 98 beats/min, increased from the pretreatment rate of 88 beats/min. The nurse knows that this reaction is a result of which effect?
   a. An expected adverse effect of the medication
   b. An allergic reaction to the medication
   c. An indication that he has received an overdose of the medication
   d. An idiosyncratic reaction to the medication

EXAMINATION REVIEW QUESTIONS—cont'd

3. A patient has been receiving an aminophylline (xanthine derivative) infusion for 24 hours. The nurse will observe for which adverse effect when assessing the patient during the infusion?
a. CNS depression
b. Sinus tachycardia
c. Increased appetite
d. Temporary urinary retention

4. During a teaching session for a patient who will be receiving a new prescription for the LTRA montelukast (Singulair), the nurse will tell the patient that the drug has which therapeutic effect?
a. Improves the respiratory drive
b. Loosens and removes thickened secretions
c. Reduces inflammation in the airway
d. Stimulates immediate bronchodilation

5. After a patient takes a dose of an inhaled corticosteroid such as fluticasone (Flovent), what is the most important action the patient needs to do next?
a. Hold the breath for 60 seconds.
b. Rinse out the mouth with water.
c. Follow the corticosteroid with a bronchodilator inhaler, if ordered.
d. Repeat the dose in 15 minutes if feeling short of breath.

6. The nurse is teaching a patient about the inhaler Advair (salmeterol and fluticasone). Which statements by the patient indicate a correct understanding of this medication? Select all that apply.
a. "I will rinse my mouth with water after each dose."
b. "I need to use this inhaler whenever I feel short of breath, but make sure it's not less than 4 hours between doses."
c. "This medication is taken twice a day, every 12 hours."
d. "I can take this inhaler if I get short of breath while exercising."
e. "I will call my doctor if I notice white patches inside my mouth."

7. A patient has been given an MDI of salbutamol and is instructed to take 2 puffs 3 times a day, with doses 6 hours apart. The inhaler contains 200 actuations, but does not have a dose counter. Calculate how many days the inhaler will deliver this ordered dose.

Answers: 1. a, 2. a, 3. b, 4. c, 5. b, 6. a, c, e 7. Approximately 33 days (200 divided by 6 puffs per day)

CRITICAL THINKING ACTIVITIES

1. A patient is taking a xanthine derivative and asks the nurse about drinking coffee with the medication. What is the nurse's best answer?

2. A patient was prescribed an oral LTRA 1 month ago. At today's follow-up appointment, he tells the nurse, "I don't think this pill works. I took it when I was short of breath, but it did not help." What is the priority when the nurse answers this patient's concerns?

3. A 13-year-old is taken to the clinic because he started to have an asthma attack while running outside in the cold air. He carries two metered-dose inhalers with him: fluticasone and salbutamol. Which inhaler is the priority at this time? Explain your answer.

For answers, see http://evolve.elsevier.com/Canada/Lilley/pharmacology/.

PART SEVEN

Drugs Affecting the Gastrointestinal System and Nutrition

STUDY SKILLS TIPS:

- ACTIVE QUESTIONING
- DETERMINING THE RIGHT QUESTIONS
- KINDS OF QUESTIONS
- QUESTIONING APPLICATION

ACTIVE QUESTIONING

One study technique whose benefits cannot be overemphasized is active questioning. In the PURR model, it is critical that you be able to generate questions in the Plan, Rehearse, and Review steps. The questions you generate will help maintain concentration as you study, improve your comprehension as you read assigned material, and develop long-term memory. Active questioning is a strategy that develops with practice. This approach keeps you on track, providing purpose and focusing your study on the questions you ask.

DETERMINING THE RIGHT QUESTIONS

Some questions generated during the Plan step will be useful in that they will focus on exactly the right issues for maximum learning. Some questions will seem logical and important when you are working with the limited amount of information available using the Plan step, but as you read the chapter, you will find that they miss the mark. Do not worry about whether each question you ask is perfectly focused. As you read, rehearse, and review the material, you can and should revise questions on the basis of your growing understanding of the material. Ask many questions to maintain active involvement in the learning process and anticipate questions that will appear on exams. The more questions you ask, the more effective

you will become as both an active questioner and an active learner. Consider writing your questions down to help guide you as you read, rehearse, and review.

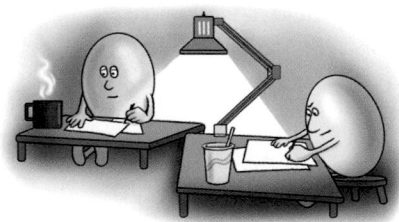

KINDS OF QUESTIONS

First, you must realize that more than one kind of question can be asked. Over the years, educators have proposed many questioning hierarchies, comprising three to eight different types of questions. Following is a simple approach that focuses on two types of questions.

Literal Questions

Literal questions are those that are answered directly and specifically by the text. If you were reading a Canadian history text and found a topic heading, "The First Prime Minister," an obvious question would be, "Who was the first prime minister?" The answer would be stated clearly and directly in the text under this heading. This is an example of a literal question. A literal question usually has a single correct response. The answer is stated directly in the text, and every reader will find the same information.

Interpretive Questions

Interpretive questions are more challenging because they require the reader to interpret, synthesize, evaluate, and analyze the material. They require not only knowledge of the literal information but also enough understanding to select several different bits of data and put them together. In Canadian history, an interpretive question might be, "Why was Lester Pearson considered an exemplary prime minister?" This question requires you to not only know the facts about Pearson but also evaluate and judge those facts in order to reach a conclusion that can be supported by the literal information. Some interpretive questions have only one correct response; others have more than one correct response. Both kinds of questions are essential in the learning process.

QUESTIONING APPLICATION

In Chapter 39, *pepsinogen* and *proenzyme* are terms the reader may not be familiar with. It is a strategy for success to emphasize unfamiliar concepts as a potential source of questions. What is pepsinogen? What is a proenzyme? Again, we can begin the questioning with simple, literal questions, but it is essential that interpretive questions also be asked. What do pepsinogen and proenzyme

have in common? How are the terms related in the broader topic of acid-related pathophysiology? These questions require that you read for broader general understanding.

At the end of each chapter, a section entitled "Critical Thinking Activities" is given. Even though this information is stated in question form, you should consider generating additional questions of your own. The first question in Chapter 39 is focused on a particular situation where the patient asks the question, "What does this drug do?" In answering it, some additional questions will help you focus your learning. What adverse effects are there with drugs used to treat gastrointestinal disorders? What is simethicone? To what class of drugs does it belong? What are its mechanisms of action and indications? The more active you become as a questioner, the easier it will become to ask the kinds of questions that are necessary for your learning.

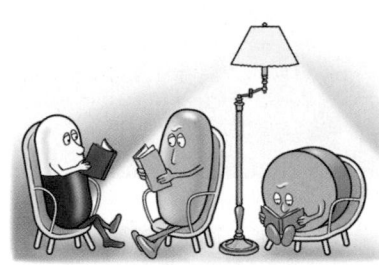

Acid-Controlling Drugs

Objectives

After reading this chapter, the successful student will be able to do the following:

1. Discuss the physiological influence of various pathologies, such as peptic ulcer disease, gastritis, spastic colon, gastroesophageal reflux disease (GERD), and hyperacidic states, on the health of patients and on their gastrointestinal (GI) tracts.

2. Describe the mechanisms of action, indications, cautions, contraindications, drug interactions, adverse effects, dosages, and routes of administration for the following classes of acid-controlling drugs: antacids, histamine-2–blocking drugs (H_2 receptor antagonists), proton pump inhibitors, and acid suppressants.

3. Develop a collaborative plan of care that includes all phases of the nursing process for patients receiving acid-controlling drugs.

e-Learning Activities

Website
(http://evolve.elsevier.com/Canada/Lilley/pharmacology/)

evolve

* Answer Key—Textbook Case Studies
* Answer Key—Critical Thinking Activities
* Chapter Summaries—Printable
* Review Questions for Exam Preparation
* Unfolding Case Studies

Drug Profiles

antacids, general, p. 746
▸▸ cimetidine, p. 750
▸▸ famotidine, p. 750
lansoprazole, p. 752
misoprostol, p. 753
▸▸ omeprazole (omeprazole magnesium)*, p. 752
pantoprazole, p. 752
ranitidine hydrochloride, p. 750
simethicone, p. 754
▸▸ sucralfate, p. 753

▸▸ Key drug

*Full generic name is given in parentheses. For the purposes of this text, the more common, shortened name is used.

Key Terms

Antacids Basic compounds composed of different combinations of acid-neutralizing ionic salts. (p. 746)

Chief cells Cells in the stomach that secrete the gastric enzyme pepsinogen (a precursor to pepsin). (p. 744)

Gastric glands Secretory glands in the stomach containing the following cell types: parietal, chief, mucous, endocrine, and enterochromaffin. (p. 744)

Gastric hyperacidity The overproduction of stomach acid. (p. 744)

Hydrochloric acid (HCl) An acid secreted by the parietal cells in the lining of the stomach that maintains the environment of the stomach at a pH of 1 to 4. (p. 744)

Mucous cells Cells whose function in the stomach is to secrete mucus that serves as a protective mucous coat against the digestive properties of HCl. Also called *surface epithelial cells*. (p. 744)

Parietal cells Cells in the stomach that produce and secrete HCl. These cells are the primary site of action for

many of the drugs used to treat acid-related disorders. (p. 744)

Pepsin An enzyme in the stomach that breaks down proteins. (p. 744)

OVERVIEW

One of the conditions of the stomach requiring drug therapy is hyperacidity, or excessive acid production. Left untreated, this condition can lead to such serious conditions as acid reflux, ulcer disease, esophageal damage, and, potentially, esophageal cancer. Overproduction of stomach acid is also referred to as *gastric hyperacidity*.

Hydrochloric Acid

The stomach secretes many substances with various physiological functions, including the following:

- Hydrochloric acid, an acid that aids digestion and serves as a barrier to infection
- Bicarbonate, a base that is a natural mechanism to prevent hyperacidity
- Pepsinogen, an enzymatic precursor to pepsin, an enzyme that digests dietary proteins
- Intrinsic factor, a glycoprotein that facilitates gastric absorption of vitamin B_{12}
- Mucus, which protects the stomach lining from both hydrochloric acid and digestive enzymes
- Prostaglandins, which have a variety of anti-inflammatory and protective functions (see Chapter 49)

The stomach, although one structure, can be divided into three functional areas. Each area is associated with specific glands. These glands are composed of different cells, and these cells secrete different substances. Figure 39-1 shows the three functional areas of the stomach and the distribution of the associated types of stomach glands.

The three primary types of glands in the stomach are the cardiac, pyloric, and gastric glands. These glands are named for their positions in the stomach. The cardiac glands are located around the cardiac sphincter (also known as the *gastroesophageal sphincter*); the gastric glands are in the fundus, also known as the *greater part of the body of the stomach*; and the pyloric glands are in the pyloric region and in the transitional area between the pyloric and the fundic zones.

The **gastric glands** are highly specialized secretory glands composed of several different types of cells: parietal, chief, mucous, endocrine, and enterochromaffin. Each cell secretes a specific substance. The three most important cell types are parietal cells, chief cells, and mucous cells. These cells are depicted in Figure 39-1.

Parietal cells produce and secrete **hydrochloric acid (HCl)**. They are the primary site of action of many of the drugs used to treat acid-related disorders. **Chief cells**

secrete pepsinogen. Pepsinogen is a proenzyme (enzyme precursor) that becomes **pepsin** when activated by exposure to acid. Pepsin breaks down proteins smaller polypeptides and amino acids and is therefore referred to as a *proteolytic* enzyme. **Mucous cells** are mucus-secreting cells that are also called *surface epithelial cells*. The secreted mucus serves as a protective coating against the digestive action of HCl and digestive enzymes. These three cell types play an important role in the digestive process. When the balance between these three cells and their secretions is impaired, acid-related diseases can occur. The most harmful of these involve acid hypersecretion and include peptic ulcer disease (PUD) and esophageal cancer. However, the most common acid-related condition is mild to moderate hyperacidity. Many lay terms (e.g., *indigestion, sour stomach, heartburn, acid stomach*) have been used to describe this condition of overproduction of HCl by the parietal cells. Hyperacidity is often associated with gastroesophageal reflux disease (GERD). According to the Canadian Digestive Health Foundation (2016), 5 million Canadians experience heartburn or acid regurgitation at least once each week. GERD is the tendency of excessive and acidic stomach contents to back up, or reflux, into the lower (and even upper) esophagus. Over time, this condition can lead to more serious disorders, such as erosive esophagitis and Barrett's esophagus, a precancerous condition. Therefore, to prevent serious disorders from occurring and to promote patient comfort, GERD is aggressively treated with one or more of the medications described in this section. HCl is secreted by the parietal cells in the lining of the stomach and maintains the environment of the stomach at a pH of 1 to 4. This acidity aids in the proper digestion of food and also serves as one of the body's defences against microbial infection via the GI tract. Many substances stimulate HCl secretion by the parietal cells, such as certain foods, including chocolate; caffeine; and alcohol. In moderation, any of these substances is usually not problematic. However, excessive consumption of large, fatty meals or alcohol, as well as emotional stress, may result in the hyperproduction of HCl and lead to hypersecretory disorders such as PUD.

The parietal cell is the primary target for many of the most effective drugs for the treatment of acid-related disorders. A closer look at how the parietal cell receives signals to produce and secrete HCl will enhance understanding of the mechanisms of action of many of the drugs used to treat acid-related disorders. The wall of the parietal cell has three types of receptors: acetylcholine

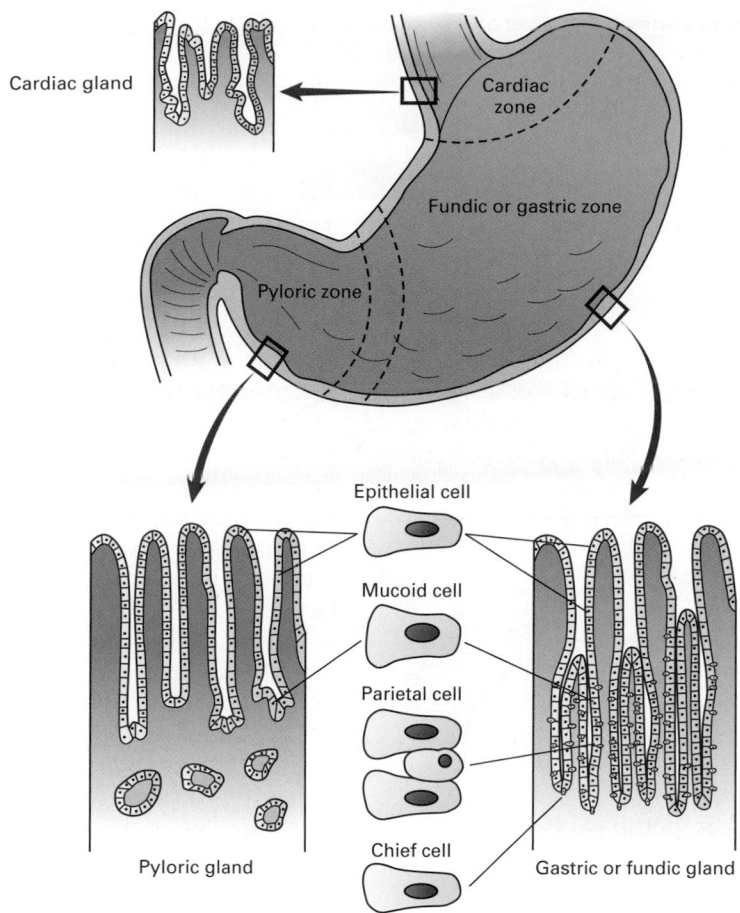

FIG. 39-1 The three specific zones of the stomach and the different glands.

(ACh), histamine, and gastrin. When any one of these is occupied by its corresponding chemical stimulant (ACh, histamine, or gastrin, which can all be considered first messengers), the parietal cell will produce and secrete HCl. Figure 39-2 shows the parietal cell with its three receptors. Once these receptors have become occupied, a second messenger is sent inside the cell. In the case of histamine receptors, occupation results in the production of adenylate cyclase. Adenylate cyclase converts adenosine triphosphate (ATP) to cyclic adenosine monophosphate (cAMP), which provides energy for the proton pump. The proton pump, or, more precisely, the hydrogen–potassium–adenosine triphosphatase (ATPase) pump, is a pump for the transport of hydrogen ions and is located in the parietal cells. The pump requires energy to work. If energy is present, the proton pump will be activated, and the pump will be able to transport hydrogen ions needed for the production of HCl.

In the case of both ACh and gastrin receptors, the second messenger that drives the proton pump is not cAMP, but calcium ions. Anticholinergic drugs (see Chapter 22) such as atropine sulphate block ACh receptors, which results in decreased hydrogen ion secretion from the parietal cells. However, these drugs are no longer used for this purpose and have been superseded by other drug classes discussed in this chapter. There is currently no drug to block the binding of the hormone gastrin to its corresponding receptor on the parietal cell surface.

In 1983, a certain gram-negative spiral bacterium, *Campylobacter pylori*, was isolated from several patients with gastritis. Over the next few years, this bacterium was studied further, and it became implicated in the pathophysiology of PUD. The official name of this bacterium was changed to *Helicobacter pylori* because it was felt to have more characteristics of the *Helicobacter* genus. The prevalence of *H. pylori* as measured by serum antibody tests is approximately 40 to 60% for patients older than 60 years of age and only 10% for those younger than 30 years of age. Although costly to administer, other available tests are the *H. pylori* fecal antigen test and the carbon 13 urea breath test. The bacterium is found in the GI tracts of approximately 90% of patients with duodenal ulcers and 70% of those with gastric ulcers; however, ulcers can occur without the presence of H. pylori. *H. pylori* is also found in many patients who do not have PUD, and its presence is not associated with acute, perforating ulcers. These latter observations suggest that more than one factor is involved in ulceration. Triple therapy includes a 7- to 14-day course of a proton pump inhibitor (discussed later in the chapter) and the antibiotics clarithromycin and either amoxicillin or metronidazole (see Chapters 43 and 44). Quadruple therapy is a

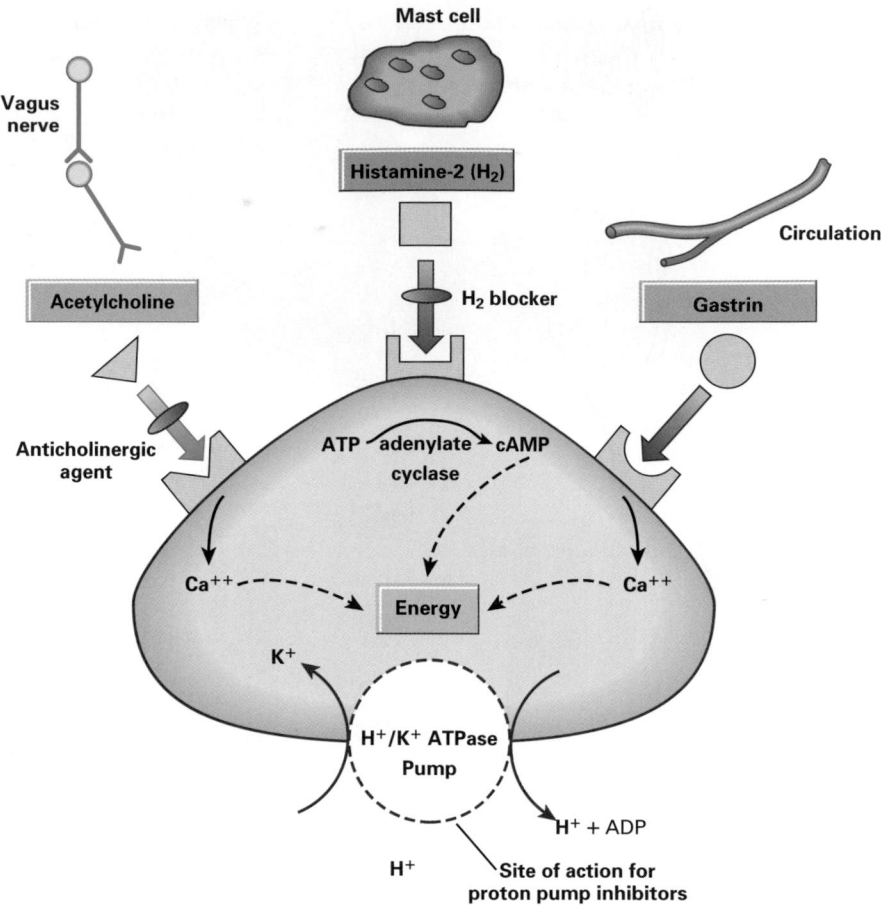

FIG. 39-2 Parietal cell stimulation and secretion. *ATP*, adenosine triphosphate; *cAMP*, cyclic adenosine monophosphate.

combination of a proton pump inhibitor, bismuth subsalicylate (this chapter), and the antibiotics tetracycline and metronidazole (see Chapters 43 and 44). Many different combinations are used, but all incorporate the aforementioned key drugs. Treatment with clarithromycin is the preferred first-line treatment because of high rates of metronidazole resistance. Optimum treatment remains controversial.

Stress-related mucosal damage is an important issue for critically ill patients. Stress ulcer prophylaxis (or therapy to prevent severe GI damage) is undertaken in almost every critically ill patient in a critical care unit (ICU) and for many patients on general medical surgical units. GI lesions are a common finding in ICU patients, especially within the first 24 hours after admission. The etiology and pathophysiology of physiological stress-related mucosal damage is multifactorial and is not fully understood. Factors include decreased blood flow, mucosal ischemia, hypoperfusion, and reperfusion injury. A common stress ulcer is the Curling ulcer, an acute peptic ulcer of the duodenum that occurs in patients with severe burns that occur when decreased blood volume leads to ischemia and cell necrosis of the gastric mucosa. Although the cause is unknown, a Cushing ulcer can occur after severe head trauma. Procedures performed

commonly in critically ill patients, such as passing nasogastric tubes, placing patients on ventilators, and others, predispose patients to bleeding of the GI tract. Coagulopathy, a history of peptic ulcer or GI bleed, sepsis, use of steroids, ICU stay of longer than 1 week, and occult bleeding indicate high risk of GI lesions. Guidelines suggest that all such patients receive either a histamine receptor–blocking drug or a proton pump inhibitor, both of which are discussed in detail in this chapter.

ANTACIDS

Antacids are basic compounds used to neutralize stomach acid. Antacids have been used for centuries in the treatment of patients with acid-related disorders. The ancient Greeks used crushed coral (calcium carbonate) in the first century AD to treat patients with dyspepsia. Antacids were the principal antiulcer treatment, along with anticholinergic drugs, until the introduction of histamine-2 (H_2) receptor antagonists in the late 1970s. The use of anticholinergic drugs has fallen out of favour because of poor efficacy and adverse effects. There is a wide variety of commercially available antacids that are over-the-counter (OTC) formulations and are still used extensively. They are inexpensive, available in a variety of dosage forms, and relatively safe, although not without some risk. Antacid tablet forms are slower acting than liquid formulations. They must be chewed thoroughly for effect.

Many formulations of antacids and a variety of combinations are available. Some effervescent antacids contain sodium bicarbonate, or baking soda. Alka-Seltzer®, which also contains acetylsalicylic acid, is an example. Bicarbonate reacts with stomach HCI to release carbon dioxide gas that is quickly absorbed but sometimes results in the release of the gas as a burp. In addition, many antacid preparations also contain the antiflatulent (antigas) drug simethicone (see the section, Miscellaneous Acid-Controlling Drugs, p. 752), a surfactant which reduces gas and bloating, but has no antacid effect. Some antacids are combined with an alginate, a tasteless substance derived from kelp or seaweed. It is not an antacid. Rather, it creates a physical gel barrier, actually floating between the gastric acids and the esophagus; the barrier prevents the acid from refluxing into the esophagus. Gaviscon® is one example of an antacid containing alginate sodium. Peppermint is the most common flavouring added to antacids, as it relaxes the lower esophageal sphincter so that gas can be released; however, it should not be used in patients with GERD as stomach acids would flow back into the esophagus.

Many aluminum- and calcium-based antacid formulations include magnesium, which not only contributes to the drug's acid-neutralizing capacity but counteracts the constipating effects of aluminum and calcium. There are multiple salts of calcium, with calcium carbonate being the most commonly used. However, calcium antacids may lead to the development of kidney stones and increased gastric acid secretion. Antacids containing magnesium must be avoided in patients with kidney failure. Sodium bicarbonate is a highly soluble antacid form with quick onset but a short duration of action.

Mechanism of Action and Drug Effects

Antacids work primarily by neutralizing gastric acidity. They do not prevent the overproduction of acid but instead help to neutralize acid secretions. It is also thought that antacids promote gastric mucosal defensive mechanisms, particularly at lower dosages. They do this by stimulating the secretion of mucus, prostaglandins, and bicarbonate from the cells inside the gastric glands. Mucus serves as a protective barrier against the destructive actions of HCl. Bicarbonate helps buffer the acidity of HCl. Prostaglandins prevent histamine from binding to its corresponding parietal cell receptors, which inhibits the production of adenylate cyclase. Without adenylate cyclase, no cAMP can be formed and no second messenger is available to activate the proton pump (see Figure 39-2). The primary drug effect of antacids is the reduction of the symptoms associated with various acid-related disorders, such as pain and reflux. A dose of antacid that raises the gastric pH from 1.3 to 1.6 (by only 0.3) reduces gastric acidity by 50%, whereas acidity is reduced by 90% if the pH is raised one entire point (e.g., 1.3 to 2.3).

Antacid-associated pain reduction is thought to be a result of base-mediated inhibition of the protein-digesting ability of pepsin, increase in the resistance of the stomach lining to irritation, and increase in the tone of the cardiac sphincter, which reduces reflux from the stomach.

Indications

Antacids are indicated for the acute relief of symptoms associated with peptic ulcer, gastritis, gastric hyperacidity, and reflux.

Contraindications

The only usual contraindication to antacid use is known allergy to a specific drug product. Other contraindications may include severe kidney failure or electrolyte disturbances (because of the potential toxic accumulation of electrolytes in the antacids themselves) and GI obstruction.

Adverse Effects

The adverse effects of the antacids are limited. Magnesium preparations, particularly milk of magnesia, can cause diarrhea. Aluminum- and calcium-containing formulations can result in constipation. Calcium products can also cause kidney stones. Excessive use of any antacid can theoretically result in systemic alkalosis. This adverse effect is more common with sodium bicarbonate than with other formulations. Another adverse effect that is more common with calcium-containing products is rebound hyperacidity, or acid rebound, in which the patient experiences hyperacidity when antacid use is discontinued. Long-term self-medication with antacids may mask symptoms of serious underlying diseases, such as bleeding ulcers or malignancy. Patients with ongoing symptoms need to undergo regular medical evaluations, because additional medications or other interventions may be needed. Box 39-1 lists several specific nursing concerns for patients taking antacids.

Interactions

Antacids are capable of causing several drug interactions when administered with other drugs (see Table 39-1). There are four basic mechanisms by which antacids cause interactions:

- *Adsorption* of other drugs to antacids, which reduces the ability of the other drug to be absorbed into the body
- *Chelation*, which is the chemical inactivation of other drugs that produces insoluble complexes
- *Increased stomach pH*, which increases the absorption of basic drugs and decreases the absorption of acidic drugs
- *Increased urinary pH*, which increases the excretion of acidic drugs and decreases the excretion of basic drugs

Most drugs are either weak acids or weak bases. Therefore, pH conditions in both the GI and urinary tracts will affect the extent to which drug molecules are absorbed. Ionized drug molecules are generally more water soluble and thus more likely to be excreted (at the

BOX 39-1   Nursing Concerns for Patients Taking Antacids

Aluminum, used to reduce gastric acid, binds to phosphate and may lead to hypercalcemia. Early hypercalcemia is characterized by constipation, headache, increased thirst, dry mouth, decreased appetite, irritability, and a metallic taste in the mouth. Later signs and symptoms of hypercalcemia include confusion, drowsiness, a rise in blood pressure, irregular heart rate, nausea, vomiting, and increased urination. Use of aluminum-based antacids may also produce hypophosphatemia, which is characterized by loss of appetite, malaise, muscle weakness, and bone pain. The use of calcium-containing antacids (e.g., calcium carbonate) may lead to milk-alkali

syndrome, which is associated with headache, anorexia, nausea, vomiting, and unusual tiredness. Use of sodium bicarbonate may lead to metabolic alkalosis if the drug is misused or used over the long term. Alkalosis is manifested by irritability, muscle twitching, numbness and tingling, cyanosis, slow and shallow respirations, headache, thirst, and nausea. Acid rebound occurs with the discontinuation of antacids that have high acid-neutralizing capacity and with overuse or misuse of antacid therapy. If acid neutralization is sudden and high, the result is an immediate elevation in pH to alkalinity and just as rapid a decline in pH to a more acidic state in the gut.

TABLE   39-1

Antacids: Drug Interactions

Interacting Drug	Mechanism	Result
Benzodiazepines	pH effects	Increased
Sulfonylureas		activity of
Sympathomimetics		interacting
valproic acid		drugs
Allopurinol	Decreased GI	Reduced
Tetracycline	absorption	effects of
Thyroid hormones		interacting
captopril		drugs
Corticosteroids		
Digoxin		
Histamine antagonists		
Phenytoin		
Isoniazid		
Ketoconazole		
Methotrexate		
Nitrofurantoin		
Phenothiazines		
Salicylates		
Quinolone antibiotics		

kidney) or not absorbed (from the GI tract). Common examples of drugs whose effects may be chemically enhanced by the presence of antacids (because of pH effects) include benzodiazepines, sulfonylureas (effects may also be reduced, depending on the drugs involved), sympathomimetics, and valproic acid. More commonly, the presence of antacids reduces the efficacy of interacting drugs by interfering with their GI absorption. Such drugs include allopurinol, tetracycline, thyroid hormones, captopril, corticosteroids, digoxin, histamine antagonists, phenytoin, isoniazid, ketoconazole, methotrexate, nitrofurantoin, phenothiazines, salicylates, and quinolone antibiotics. Advise patients to dose any interacting drugs at least 1 to 2 hours before or after antacids are taken. Significant patient harm may ensue when the quinolone antibiotics (ciprofloxacin, levofloxacin, moxifloxacin) are given with antacids. These antibiotics are

administered orally to treat serious infections. Antacids can reduce their absorption by more than 50%. Thus, antacids must be given either 2 hours before or 2 hours after the dose of a quinolone antibiotic.

Dosages

For information on dosages for selected antacid drugs, refer to the table on p. 749.

H_2 ANTAGONISTS

H_2 receptor antagonists, also called *H_2 receptor blockers*, are the prototypical acid-secretion antagonists. These drugs reduce but do not completely abolish acid secretion. They have become the most popular drugs for the treatment of many acid-related disorders, including PUD. This can be attributed to their efficacy, excellent safety profile, and acceptance by patients. This class includes cimetidine, ranitidine hydrochloride, famotidine, and nizatidine. There is little difference between the four available H_2 receptor antagonists in terms of efficacy. Ranitidine hydrochloride and famotidine are also available over the counter.

Mechanism of Action and Drug Effects

H_2 receptor antagonists competitively block the H_2 receptor of acid-producing parietal cells. This makes the cells less responsive not only to histamine but also to the stimulation of ACh and gastrin. This process is shown in Figure 39-2. Up to 90% inhibition of vagal- and gastrin-stimulated acid secretion occurs when histamine is blocked. However, complete inhibition has not been shown. The effect of H_2 antagonists is reduced hydrogen ion secretion from the parietal cells, which results in an increase in the pH of the stomach and relief of many of the symptoms associated with hyperacidity-related conditions.

Indications

H_2 receptor antagonists have several therapeutic uses, including the treatment of GERD, PUD, and erosive

DRUG PROFILES

Antacids, General

There are far too many individual antacid products on the market to mention all formulations. Briefly, OTC antacid formulations are available as capsules, chewable tablets, effervescent granules and tablets, soft chews, powders, suspensions, and plain tablets. This allows patients a variety of options for self-medication. Pharmacokinetic parameters are not normally listed for antacids, but these drugs are generally excreted quickly through the GI tract and the electrolyte homeostatic mechanisms of the kidneys. Antacids are considered safe for use during pregnancy if prolonged administration and high dosages are avoided. It is recommended that pregnant women consult their health care providers before taking an antacid. Many antacids available in Canada are combinations (e.g., aluminum hydroxide, magnesium hydroxide, and simethicone). One combination of aluminum hydroxide and magnesium hydroxide also contains a local anaesthetic (Mucaine®). Aluminum- and sodium-based antacids are often recommended for patients with kidney compromise because these antacids are more easily excreted than are antacids of other categories. Calcium-containing antacids are currently advertised as a source of calcium. Calcium carbonate neutralization will produce gas and possibly belching. For this reason, it may be combined with an antiflatulent drug such as simethicone (see the section, Miscellaneous Acid-Controlling Drugs). Calcium carbonate is also available combined with the biphosphonate etidronrate disodium. Magnesium-containing antacids commonly have a laxative effect; magnesium is always combined with other antacids. Both calcium- and magnesium-based antacids are more likely to accumulate to toxic levels in patients with kidney disease and are often avoided in this patient group.

DOSAGES   Selected Antacid Drugs*

Drug	Pharmacological Class	Usual Dosage Range	Indications
aluminum hydroxide and magnesium hydroxide and simethicone (Antacid Plus®, Diovol®, Gelusil®, Maalox Multiaction®)	Combination antacid	*Adults* PO: 400–2400 mg 3–6×/day	Hyperacidity
calcium carbonate and simethicone (Maalox®, Rolaids®)	Calcium-containing antacid	*Adults* PO: 0.5–1.5 g prn	Hyperacidity
Carbonic acid calcium salt and magnesium hydroxide (Rolaids®)	Magnesium- and calcium-containing antacid	*Adults* PO: 400 mg calcium and 84 mg magnesium (1–3 tablets daily)	Hyperacidity

*Many more antacid products are available than appear in this table. Dosages given are approximate dosages of active ingredients; there may be variations among different products and different dosage forms of the same product.
PO, oral.

esophagitis; adjunct therapy in the control of upper GI tract bleeding; and treatment of pathologic gastric hypersecretory conditions such as Zollinger-Ellison syndrome. This syndrome is one form of hyperchlorhydria, or excessive gastric acidity. H_2 receptor antagonists are commonly used for stress ulcer prophylaxis in critically ill patients. Because of their few adverse effects, these drugs may be administered preoperatively to raise gastric pH.

Contraindications

The only usual contraindication to the use of H_2 antagonists is known drug allergy. Liver and kidney dysfunction are relative contraindications that may warrant dosage reductions. Specific dose limitations and administration guidelines exist for OTC ranitidine and famotidine.

Adverse Effects

The H_2 receptor antagonists have a remarkably low incidence of adverse effects (less than 3% of cases). The four available H_2 antagonists are similar in many respects but have some differences in their adverse effect profiles. Table 39-2 lists the adverse effects associated with these drugs. Central nervous system adverse effects, such as confusion and disorientation, occur in less than 1% of patients taking H_2 receptor antagonists but are sometimes seen in older adults. Be alert for mental health status changes when giving these drugs, especially if they are new to the patient. Cimetidine may induce erectile dysfunction and gynecomastia, as a result of its inhibition of estradiol metabolism and displacement of dihydrotestosterone from peripheral androgen-binding sites. All four H_2 antagonists may increase the secretion of prolactin from the anterior pituitary. Thrombocytopenia has been reported with ranitidine hydrochloride and famotidine.

Interactions

Cimetidine carries a higher risk of drug interactions than the other three H_2 antagonists, particularly in older adults. These interactions may be of clinical importance.

TABLE 39-2

H₂ Antagonists: Adverse Effects

Body System	Adverse Effects
Cardiovascular	Hypotension (monitor for this effect with intravenous administration)
Central nervous	Headache, lethargy, confusion, depression, hallucinations, slurred speech, agitation
Endocrine	Increased prolactin secretion, gynecomastia (with cimetidine)
Gastrointestinal	Diarrhea, nausea, abdominal cramps
Genitourinary	Impotence, increased blood urea nitrogen and creatinine levels
Hematological	Agranulocytosis, thrombocytopenia, neutropenia, aplastic anemia
Hepatobiliary	Elevated liver enzyme levels, jaundice
Integumentary	Urticaria, rash, alopecia, sweating, flushing, exfoliative dermatitis

Cimetidine binds enzymes of the liver cytochrome P450 microsomal oxidase system. This is a group of enzymes in the liver that metabolize many different drugs. By inhibiting the oxidation (metabolism) of drugs metabolized via this pathway, cimetidine may raise the blood concentrations of such drugs. Ranitidine hydrochloride has only 10 to 20% of the binding action of cimetidine on the P450 system, and nizatidine and famotidine have essentially no effect on it. This interaction has little clinical significance for most drugs; however, significant interactions are more likely to arise with medications that have a narrow therapeutic range, such as theophylline, warfarin sodium, lidocaine, and phenytoin. All H₂ receptor antagonists may inhibit the absorption of certain drugs such as ketoconazole that require an acidic GI environment for gastric absorption. Smoking has been shown to decrease the effectiveness of H₂ receptor antagonists. For optimal results, H₂ receptor antagonists should be taken 1 hour before antacids.

Dosages

For dosage information for the H₂ antagonists, refer to the table on p. 751.

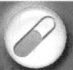

DRUG PROFILES

H₂ receptor antagonists are the prototypical acid-secretion antagonists. These drugs reduce acid secretion. They are among the most commonly used drugs in the world because of their efficacy, some availability over the counter, patient acceptance, and excellent safety profile. However, this drug class has been partially replaced by proton pump inhibitors (see the next section).

▸▸ cimetidine

Cimetidine was the first drug in this class to be released on the market. It is the prototypical H₂ receptor antagonist. Because of its potential to cause drug interactions, its use has been largely replaced by ranitidine hydrochloride and famotidine. Cimetidine is still used to treat certain allergic reactions.

PHARMACOKINETICS

Route	Onset of Action	Peak Plasma Concentration	Elimination Half-Life	Duration of Action
PO	15–60 min	1–2 hr	2 hr	4–5 hr

ranitidine hydrochloride

Ranitidine hydrochloride (Zantac®) was the second H₂ receptor antagonist introduced. Unlike cimetidine, it is not associated with concerns regarding drug interactions, and thus has become the most widely used H₂ receptor antagonist. It is available over the counter. It is also more potent,

specific, and longer acting than cimetidine. Administered parenterally, ranitidine can raise gastric pH in 1 hour, and its effects can last for up to 12 hours. It is available in oral and intravenous (IV) forms. Dosing is different for the different forms: oral ranitidine is dosed as 150 mg twice a day or 300 mg at bedtime, whereas the IV form is dosed at 50 mg every 8 hours.

PHARMACOKINETICS

Route	Onset of Action	Peak Plasma Concentration	Elimination Half-Life	Duration of Action
PO	1 hr	2–4 hr	2–3 hr	4–12 hr
IV	Immediate	Less than 15 min	2–3 hr	4–12 hr

▸▸ famotidine

Famotidine (Pepcid®) was the last H₂ receptor antagonist introduced and, like ranitidine hydrochloride, has minimal drug interaction concerns. It is available in oral and injectable forms. The dosing is the same for both forms.

PHARMACOKINETICS

Route	Onset of Action	Peak Plasma Concentration	Elimination Half-Life	Duration of Action
PO	1.4 hr	3 hr	2.6–4 hr	9–12 hr
IV	Immediate	Less than 15 min	2.6–4 hr	9–12 hr

DOSAGES	Selected Histamine-2 (H₂) Antagonists	
Drug	**Usual Dosage Range**	**Indications**
▶▶cimetidine (generic)	*Adults*	Dyspepsia, heartburn
	PO: 200 mg bid	
	PO: 300 mg qid or 400 mg bid and at bedtime or 800 mg at bedtime	Ulcers
	PO: 1 600 mg/day divided in 2 to 4 doses	GERD
	PO: 300 mg bid or 400 mg at bedtime	GERD
		Pathological hypersecretion
	PO: 300 mg tid and at bedtime; do not exceed 2 400 mg/day	Pathological hypersecretion
famotidine (Pepcid, Pepcid AC)	*Adults*	Dyspepsia, heartburn
	PO: 10 mg daily–bid	
	PO: 40 mg/day at bedtime or 20 mg bid	Ulcers
	PO: 20 mg q6h	Pathological hypersecretion
	IV: 20 mg q12h	
	PO: 20 mg bid	GERD
Ranitidine hydrochloride (Zantac)	*Adults*	Dyspepsia, heartburn
	PO: 75 mg bid	
	PO: 150 mg daily–bid or 300 mg at bedtime	Ulcers
	PO: 150 mg tid	
	PO: 150 mg qid	Erosive esophagitis

GERD, gastroesophageal reflux disease; *PO*, oral; *IV*, intravenous.

PROTON PUMP INHIBITORS

The newest drugs introduced for the treatment of acid-related disorders are the proton pump inhibitors (PPIs). These include lansoprazole (Prevacid®, Prevacid FasTab®), omeprazole (Losec®, Prilosec®), rabeprazole sodium (Pariet®), pantoprazole sodium (Panto®, Pantoloc®), dexlansoprazole (Dexilant®), and esomeprazole trihydrate (Nexium®). These drugs are more powerful than the H₂ receptor antagonists. The PPIs bind directly to the hydrogen–potassium–ATPase pump mechanism and irreversibly inhibit the action of this enzyme, which results in a total blockage of hydrogen ion secretion from the parietal cells.

Mechanism of Action and Drug Effects

The action of the hydrogen–potassium–ATPase pump is the final step in the acid-secretory process of the parietal cell (see Figure 39-2). If chemical energy is present to run the pump, it will transport hydrogen ions out of the parietal cell, which increases the acid content of the surrounding gastric lumen and lowers the pH. Because hydrogen ions are protons (positively charged atoms), this ion pump is also called the *proton pump*. PPIs bind irreversibly to the proton pump. This inhibition prevents the movement of hydrogen ions out of the parietal cell into the stomach, thereby blocking all gastric acid secretion. The PPIs stop more than 90% of acid secretion over 24 hours, which makes most patients temporarily achlorhydric (without acid). However, food absorption is not affected. For acid secretion to return to normal after a PPI has been stopped, the parietal cell must synthesize new hydrogen–potassium–ATPase. Although there are other proton pumps in the body, hydrogen–potassium–ATPase is

structurally and mechanically distinct from other hydrogen-transporting enzymes and appears to exist only in the parietal cells. Thus, the action of PPIs is limited to its effects on gastric acid secretion.

Indications

PPIs are currently indicated as first-line therapy for erosive esophagitis, symptomatic GERD that is poorly responsive to other medical treatment such as therapy with H₂ antagonists, short-term treatment of active duodenal ulcers and active benign gastric ulcers, gastric hypersecretory conditions (e.g., Zollinger-Ellison syndrome), and nonsteroidal anti-inflammatory drug (NSAID)-induced ulcers. They are also used for stress ulcer prophylaxis. Long-term therapeutic uses include maintenance of healing of erosive esophagitis and pathological hypersecretory conditions, including both GERD and Zollinger-Ellison syndrome. All of the PPIs can be used in combination with antibiotics to treat patients with *H. pylori* infections. The PPIs can be given orally or through a nasogastric or percutaneous enterogastric tube. For example, esomeprazole magnesium dehydrate capsules may be opened, the granules dissolved in 50 mL of water, and the solution given through the tube. Similar tubal administration is listed as an option by the manufacturer for lansoprazole capsules and tablets and omeprazole powder for oral suspension. Consult drug packaging for drug-specific instructions. Be aware of the particle size of the drug once it is in solution and the tube size being used. Several of the PPIs are now also available for IV use.

Contraindications

The only usual contraindication to the use of PPIs is known drug allergy.

Adverse Effects

PPIs are generally well tolerated. The frequency of adverse effects is similar to that for H₂ receptor antagonists. There was some early concern that long-term use of PPIs might promote malignant gastric tumours. This has not proven to be the case, however, and this initial concern has subsided. New concerns have arisen over the potential for long-term users of PPIs to develop osteoporosis. Researchers who conducted a Canadian population-based cohort study have cautioned health care providers to be alert to the possibility of an increased risk of acute kidney injury and interstitial nephritis in older patients on PPI therapy (Antoniou et al., 2015). This is thought to be due to the inhibition of stomach acid, and it is speculated that PPIs speed up bone mineral loss. Long-term use of high-dose PPIs has been associated with *Clostridium difficile* infections; risk of wrist, hip, and spine fractures; and pneumonia. Recently, depletion of magnesium was added to the risk profile.

Interactions

Few drug interactions occur with PPIs; however, they may increase serum levels of diazepam and phenytoin. There may be an increased chance of bleeding in patients who are taking both a PPI and warfarin sodium. Other possible interactions include interference with absorption of ketoconazole, ampicillin, iron salts, and digoxin. When given with clopidogrel, there is some concern of an increased risk of death if the patient has acute coronary syndrome; however, recent studies have not substantiated this concern. Sucralfate may delay the absorption of PPIs. Food may decrease absorption of the PPIs, and it is recommended that they be taken on an empty stomach usually before meals (usually breakfast) as it increases the effectiveness of the drug.

Dosages

For recommended dosages on selected PPIs, refer to the table on p. 753.

MISCELLANEOUS ACID-CONTROLLING DRUGS

There are a few other acid-controlling drugs that are unique in their mechanisms and other features. These include sucralfate and misoprostol. They are profiled individually in the following paragraphs. Other antacid drugs include bismuth subsalicylate (Pepto-Bismol®; see Chapter 40) and metoclopramide (see Chapter 41).

NURSING PROCESS

🖊 Assessment

Before an acid-controlling drug is given, perform a thorough patient assessment with attention to past and

---

💊 DRUG PROFILES

▸▸omeprazole magnesium

Omeprazole magnesium (Losec) was the first drug in this breakthrough class of antisecretory drugs. Orally administered PPIs (and H₂ receptor antagonists) often work best when taken 30 to 60 minutes before meals. Omeprazole was the first PPI to become available generically.

PHARMACOKINETICS

Route	Onset of Action	Peak Plasma Concentration	Elimination Half-Life	Duration of Action
PO	2 hr	3.5–5 hrs	0.5–1 hr	1–5 days

lansoprazole

Lansoprazole (Prevacid) is available in a sustained-release capsule and immediate-release tablets. The capsules can be opened and mixed (not crushed) with apple juice for administration via nasogastric tube. Lansoprazole is also available as HP-PAC®, a combination product with amoxicillin and clarithromycin for the treatment of *H. Pylori* infection.

PHARMACOKINETICS

Route	Onset of Action	Peak Plasma Concentration	Elimination Half-Life	Duration of Action
PO	Rapid	1.5–2 hr	1–2 hr	24 hr

pantoprazole sodium

Pantoprazole sodium (Pantoloc, Panto IV) is the only PPI available for IV use. Adding PPIs to endoscopic therapy has become a mainstay of treatment for peptic ulcer bleeding, with current consensus guidelines recommending high-dose IV PPI therapy (IV bolus followed by continuous therapy). IV pantoprazole has been shown to be significantly more effective than the H₂ receptor antagonists ranitidine and famotidine in preventing ulcer rebleeding after endoscopic hemostasis. It was also the first drug to be used as a continuous infusion for the treatment of GI bleeding. It is available as an oral tablet and an enteric-coated tablet.

PHARMACOKINETICS

Route	Onset of Action	Peak Plasma Concentration	Elimination Half-Life	Duration of Action
PO	2.5 hr	2–2.5 hr	1 hr	7 days
IV	End of infusion	End of infusion	1 hr	7 days

DOSAGES   Selected Proton Pump Inhibitors

Drug	Usual Dosage Range	Indications
lansoprazole (Prevasid, Prevasid FasTab)	*Adults* PO: 30 mg/day	Duodenal ulcer, gastric ulcer, esophagitis
omeprazole magnesium (Losec)	*Adults* PO: 20 mg/day for 4–8 wk PO: 60 mg once daily initially, then titrated and given in single or multiple daily doses, with dosage titration up to a maximum of 120 mg tid	Esophagitis, duodenal ulcer Hypersecretory conditions
pantoprazole sodium (Pantoloc, Panto IV)	*Adults* PO/IV: 20–80 mg/day depending on indication	GERD, ulcer, stress ulcer prophylaxis

GERD, gastroesophageal reflux disease; *PO*, oral; *IV*, intravenous.

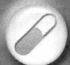

DRUG PROFILES

▶▶sucralfate

Sucralfate is a drug used as a mucosal protectant in the treatment of active stress ulcerations and in long-term therapy for PUD. Sucralfate acts locally, not systemically, binding directly to the surface of an ulcer. Sucralfate has as its basic structure a sugar, sucrose. Once sucralfate comes into contact with the acid of the stomach, it begins to dissociate into aluminum hydroxide (an antacid) and sulphate anions. The aluminum salt stimulates secretion of both mucus and bicarbonate base. The sulphated sucrose molecules of sucralfate are attracted to and bind to positively charged tissue proteins at the bases of ulcers and erosions, forming a protective barrier that can be thought of as a liquid bandage. By binding to the exposed proteins of ulcers and erosions, sucralfate also limits the access of pepsin. Pepsin is an enzyme that normally breaks down proteins in food but can have the same effect on GI epithelial tissue, either causing ulcers or making them worse. Sucralfate also binds and concentrates epidermal growth factor, present in the gastric tissues, which promotes ulcer healing. In addition, the drug stimulates the gastric secretion of prostaglandin molecules, which serve a mucoprotective function. Despite its many beneficial actions, sucralfate has fallen out of common use because its effects are transient and multiple daily doses (up to four) are therefore needed. It is indicated for stress ulcers, esophageal erosions, and PUD. The only usual contraindication to sucralfate use is known drug allergy. Adverse effects are uncommon but include nausea, constipation, and dry mouth. Only minimal systemic absorption occurs, and the drug is virtually inert. Sucralfate does not display typical pharmacokinetic parameters, and, as such, no pharmacokinetic table is provided. Drug interactions involve mainly physical interference with the absorption of other drugs. This can be alleviated by taking other drugs at least 2 hours ahead of sucralfate. Sucralfate is also best given 1 hour before meals and at bedtime. It can be used during pregnancy and is normally dosed at 1 g orally, 4 times daily.

misoprostol

Misoprostol (generic), a prostaglandin E analogue, has been shown to effectively reduce the incidence of gastric ulcers in patients taking NSAIDs (see Chapter 49). Prostaglandins have a wide variety of biological activities. They are thought to inhibit gastric acid secretion. They are also believed to protect the gastric mucosa from injury (cytoprotective function), possibly by enhancing the local production of mucus or bicarbonate, by promoting local cell regeneration, and by helping to maintain mucosal blood flow. Use of misoprostol is contraindicated in patients with known drug allergy and in pregnant women or women trying to become pregnant (see later in the chapter). Adverse effects include headache, GI distress, and vaginal bleeding. There are no major drug interactions, although antacids may reduce drug absorption. Although some studies show that synthetic analogues of prostaglandins promote the healing of duodenal ulcers, to accomplish this, the drugs must be used in dosages that usually produce disturbing adverse effects, such as abdominal cramps and diarrhea. Thus, they are not believed to be as effective as H_2 receptor antagonists and PPIs for this indication. Misoprostol induces uterine contractions and, therefore, has been used for its abortifacient properties. For this reason, it is not to be used during pregnancy. The usual dosage is 200 mcg, 4 times daily with meals, for the duration of NSAID therapy in patients at high risk for ulceration.

PHARMACOKINETICS

Route	Onset of Action	Peak Plasma Concentration	Elimination Half-Life	Duration of Action
PO	30 min	12 min	20–40 min	1–2 days

Continued

DRUG PROFILES—cont'd

simethicone

Simethicone (Ovol®, Pediacol®, Phazyme®) is used to reduce the discomfort of gastric or intestinal gas (flatulence) and aid in its release via the mouth or rectum. It is therefore classified as an antiflatulent drug. Gas commonly appears in the GI tract as a consequence of swallowing air as well as of normal digestive processes. Gas in the upper GI tract is composed of swallowed air and thus consists largely of nitrogen. It is usually expelled from the body by belching. The composition of flatus, however, is determined largely by the dietary intake of carbohydrates and the metabolic activity of the bacteria in the intestines.

Some foods, including legumes (beans) and cruciferous vegetables (e.g., cauliflower, broccoli), are well known for their gas-producing properties. Gas can also result from disorders such as diverticulitis, dyspepsia, peptic ulcers, and spastic or irritable colon; gaseous distention can also occur postoperatively. Simethicone works by altering the elasticity of mucus-coated gas bubbles, which causes them to break into smaller ones. This reduces gas pain and facilitates the expulsion of gas via the mouth or the rectum. Simethicone has no listed adverse effects, drug interactions, or pharmacokinetic parameters. It is available only for oral use. The usual simethicone dosage is 1 to 2 tablets, 4 to 6 times daily, as needed. A variety of different OTC products are available.

present medical history, with special focus on GI tract–related disorders and signs and symptoms of ulcer disease and GERD. Assess any foods and activities (e.g., smoking, stress) that may increase acid in the GI tract. Assess current bowel patterns, any changes in bowel patterns or GI tract functioning, and GI tract–related pain. Document all findings. Assess results of baseline serum chemistry laboratory tests, as ordered, with specific attention to liver function (e.g., serum ALP, ALT, AST levels) and kidney function (GFR, serum creatinine and BUN levels). As acid-controlling drugs have many interactions, close attention to all medications a patient is taking is required, and every medication history should include information about prescription drugs, OTC drugs, and natural health products.

Other components of assessment include performing a physical examination and taking a thorough cardiac history, with close attention to any history of heart failure, hypertension, or other heart diseases, and assessing for any presence of edema, fluid or electrolyte imbalances, or kidney disease. One reason it is important to assess for these conditions is that the high sodium content of various antacids may lead to exacerbation of heart problems, kidney dysfunction, and fluid–electrolyte concerns. When antacids are to be used, a medication history is essential regardless of the antacid being used. It is important to note that combination products containing both magnesium and aluminum may have fewer adverse effects than either antacid by itself. For example, aluminum-containing antacids are associated with constipation, whereas magnesium-containing antacids lead to diarrhea. The combination of these antacids is a balancing out of both adverse effects, leading to fewer problems with altered bowel patterns. Calcium-based antacids may also be used, especially as a source of calcium; however, they carry the risks of rebound hyperacidity, milk-alkali syndrome, and changes in systemic pH, especially if a patient has abnormal kidney function (see Box 39-1). Sodium bicarbonate is generally not recommended

as an antacid because of its associated high risk for systemic electrolyte disturbances and alkalosis. The sodium content of sodium bicarbonate is also high, which is problematic for patients who have hypertension, heart failure, or kidney insufficiency.

For patients using H_2 receptor antagonist drugs, assess kidney and liver function as well as level of consciousness because of possible drug-related adverse effects. Older adults are known to react to these drugs with more disorientation and confusion than younger adults. Do not administer drugs such as cimetidine and famotidine simultaneously with antacids. These drugs may be spaced 1 hour apart if both drugs need to be given. In patients taking nizatidine or ranitidine hydrochloride, assess baseline blood chemistry results with attention to levels of BUN, creatinine, bilirubin, ALP, AST, and ALT to document kidney and liver functioning before treatment is initiated. Before administering oral PPIs (e.g., lansoprazole, omeprazole, pantoprazole sodium), assess swallowing capacity because of the size of some of the capsules. Assess patients' medical history with an emphasis on any history of GI tract infections due to decreased acid-mediated antimicrobial protection. Since there are documented concerns about the use of PPIs and the development of osteoporosis, thoroughly assess patients for any history of this disorder. Also assess the length of time patients have been on PPIs. Drug interactions were discussed previously under PPIs, but important to mention are their interactions with diazepam, phenytoin, warfarin sodium, ampicillin, and iron salts. Always check the patient's medication list before these or any other type of medications are given.

Other GI-related drugs include sucralfate and simethicone. The use of simethicone (an antiflatulent) or sucralfate (an ulcer adherent) requires assessment of the patient's bowel patterns and bowel sounds. Assess for abdominal distention and rigidity, which may indicate a medical emergency. Treatment of PUD has become focused on the use of antibiotics (to attack the *H. pylori* bacteria), with frequent dosing of other drugs. Inquire also about the presence of any unusual signs and symptoms related to the GI tract.

Nursing Diagnoses

- Constipation related to the adverse effects of aluminum-containing antacids and other drugs used to treat hyperacidity
- Diarrhea related to the adverse effects of magnesium-containing antacids and other drugs used to treat hyperacidity
- Deficient knowledge related to lack of information about antacids, H_2 receptor antagonists, or PPIs, including their use and potential adverse effects

Planning

Goals

- Patient will experience minimal to no constipation while using antacids or other acid-controlling drugs.
- Patient will experience minimal to no diarrhea during antacid or acid-controlling medication regimen.
- Patient will demonstrate adequate knowledge about the use of antacid or acid-controlling medications and their expected adverse effects.

Expected Patient Outcomes

- Patient states measures to help prevent and minimize the adverse effect of constipation, including taking the antacid only as directed.
- Patient states measures to help prevent and minimize the adverse effect of diarrhea, such as avoiding magnesium-only antacids, especially milk of magnesia, and taking products that contain a combination of aluminum and magnesium.
- Patient states the purpose of taking antacids, H_2 receptor antagonists, or PPIs for management of gastric hyperacidity.
- Patient describes the various adverse effects associated with antacids, such as diarrhea, constipation, and acid rebound.
- Patient describes the expected adverse effects associated with other acid-controlling drugs, such as constipation, diarrhea, headache, and confusion, and seeks advice from a health care provider if adverse effects worsen or are not relieved after several days.

Implementation

When giving acid-controlling drugs, instruct patients to thoroughly chew chewable tablets and thoroughly shake liquid forms before they are taken. Antacids need to be given with at least 240 mL of water to enhance the absorption of the antacid in the stomach, except for newer forms that are rapidly dissolving drugs. If constipation or diarrhea occurs with single-component drugs, a combination aluminum-and-magnesium–based product may be preferred. Educate patients about the adverse effects of aluminum-only or magnesium-only products. It is also recommended that antacids be given as ordered but not within 1 to 2 hours of other medications because of the effect of antacids on the absorption of oral medications. Implement this dosing schedule without interrupting the safe dosing of the other medications. Dosing will differ if the health care provider has ordered the drug to be given with antacids. There may be serious harm if quinolone antibiotics are given with antacids because of a 50% reduction in antibiotic absorption. Serious infections may then go unsuccessfully treated due to altered absorption. Antacid overuse or misuse, or the rapid discontinuation of antacids with high acid-neutralizing capacity, may lead to acid rebound. Therefore, antacids should be used only as prescribed or as directed.

Because so many H_2 receptor antagonists and other acid-controlling drugs are now available over the counter, instruct patients about proper medication use (see the Patient Teaching Tips for more information). For example, ranitidine is to be taken 30 to 60 minutes before a meal, and antacids, if also used, need to be taken 1 hour before or after the cimetidine. Famotidine may be given orally without regard to meals or food. Give cimetidine with meals and, if it is administered with antacids, allow 1 to 2 hours before the antacid is given. Dilute IV forms of famotidine or ranitidine hydrochloride with appropriate solutions and infuse over the recommended time frame. With IV H_2 receptor antagonists, hypotension may occur with rapid infusion, so careful monitoring of the infusion and blood pressure is critical to patient safety. Refer to appropriate sources for information on other specific drugs and their IV administration. Monitor patients with diagnoses of ulcers or GI irritation for GI tract bleeding. Report any blood in the stools or the occurrence of black, tarry stools or hematemesis. Listen to bowel sounds and examine the abdomen to monitor for possible complications.

Regarding PPIs, give lansoprazole oral dosage forms as ordered. If a patient has difficulty swallowing these capsules, a capsule may be opened and the granules sprinkled over at least a tablespoon of applesauce, which then must be swallowed immediately. Administer omeprazole before meals, and educate patients that the capsule must be taken whole and not crushed, opened, or chewed. Omeprazole may also be given with antacids, if ordered. Always double-check the names and dosages of PPIs to ensure that they are not confused with similarly named drugs. Pantoprazole sodium may be given orally without crushing or splitting of the tablet form. Give IV dosage forms exactly as ordered, using the correct dilutional fluids. Infuse over the recommended time period. Other GI-related drugs, such as simethicone, may also be added to the oral medication protocol with PPIs. Simethicone is usually well tolerated. It is to be taken after meals and at bedtime. Instruct patients to

CASE STUDY

Proton Pump Inhibitors

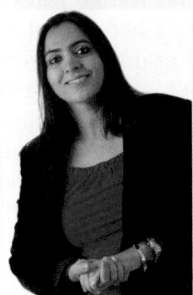

Gurmeet, a 50-year-old attorney, has self-treated for heartburn for years by drinking large amounts of antacids. She finally made an appointment with her health care provider, who referred her to a gastroenterologist. Her health care provider instructed her to stop taking the antacids.

1. Why did the health care provider ask her to stop taking the antacids?

A few weeks after her initial appointment, Gurmeet had an endoscopy, and it was discovered that she had gastroesophageal reflux disease (GERD) and gastritis secondary to stress-induced hyperacidity. The health care provider prescribed the PPI omeprazole (Prilosec, Losec) 20 mg once a day.

2. For what other conditions will the gastroenterologist test during this diagnostic stage?

3. What is the rationale for the use of PPIs to treat GERD?

4. What patient teaching is important for Gurmeet regarding the PPI?

_____

For answers, see http://evolve.elsevier.com/Canada/Lilley/pharmacology/.

thoroughly chew chewable tablets or shake suspensions well before use. Sucralfate is usually given 1 hour before meals and at bedtime, and tablets may be crushed or dissolved in water, if needed. Antacids are to be avoided for 30 minutes before or after administration of sucralfate. Misoprostol is to be given with food and is usually ordered to be taken with meals and at bedtime. Suggestions for patient education for all of these drugs are presented in Patient Teaching Tips.

✍ Evaluation

Therapeutic response to the administration of antacids, H_2 receptor antagonists, PPIs, and other GI-related drugs includes the relief of symptoms associated with peptic ulcer, gastritis, esophagitis, gastric hyperacidity, or hiatal hernia (i.e., decrease in epigastric pain, fullness, and abdominal swelling). Adverse effects for which to monitor include all of those listed for each of the drug categories and range from constipation or diarrhea to nausea, vomiting, abdominal pain, and hypotension. Milk-alkali syndrome, acid rebound, hypercalcemia, and metabolic alkalosis are known complications associated with various antacids; evaluate patients for these adverse effects and document measures taken to prevent or resolve them.

PATIENT TEACHING TIPS

❖ Patients should be aware that other medications should not to be taken within 1 to 2 hours after taking an antacid, unless prescribed, because of antacids' impact on the absorption of many medications in the stomach.

❖ Advise patients to contact a health care provider immediately if they experience severe or prolonged constipation or diarrhea, an increase in abdominal pain, abdominal distension, nausea, vomiting, hematemesis, or black and tarry stools (a sign of possible GI tract bleeding).

❖ If a patient is taking enteric-coated medications, tell the patient that the use of antacids may promote premature dissolution of the enteric coating. Enteric coatings are used to diminish the stomach upset caused by irritating medications, and if the coating is destroyed early in the stomach, gastric upset may occur.

❖ Encourage patients to take H_2 receptor antagonists exactly as prescribed. Inform patients that smoking decreases the drug's effectiveness. Advise the patient that H_2 antagonists are not to be taken within 1 hour of antacids.

❖ Advise patients to take omeprazole and other PPIs before meals. Inform the patient that if lansoprazole is being used, the granules in the capsule may be sprinkled in at least one tablespoon of applesauce if needed.

❖ Instruct patients to follow the manufacturer's directions when taking simethicone. Chewable forms must always be chewed thoroughly; liquid preparations need to be shaken thoroughly before administration. Encourage patients experiencing flatulence to avoid problematic foods (e.g., spicy, gas-producing foods) and carbonated beverages.

❖ Patients taking sucralfate should know that it must be taken on an empty stomach, and that antacids are to be avoided or, if indicated, taken 2 hours before or 1 hour after sucralfate administration.

❖ For a patient taking the drug regimen for the treatment of *H. pylori* infection, PUD, it is important to emphasize the need to take each drug, including the antibiotics, exactly as prescribed and without fail, to guarantee successful treatment. If treatment protocols are not followed appropriately, the condition may likely recur.

KEY POINTS

- ❖ The stomach secretes many substances, including HCl, pepsinogen, mucus, bicarbonate, intrinsic factor, and prostaglandins.
- ❖ Parietal cells are responsible for the production of acid.
- ❖ In acid-related disorders, there is an impairment of the balance among the substances secreted by the stomach.
- ❖ H_2 receptor antagonists are H_2 blockers that bind to and block histamine receptors located on parietal cells. This blocking renders these cells less responsive to stimuli, and thus decreases their acid secretion. Up to 90% inhibition of acid secretion can be achieved with the H_2 receptor antagonists.
- ❖ PPIs block the final step in the acid production pathway—the hydrogen–potassium–ATPase pump—and they block all acid secretion.
- ❖ Sucralfate is used for the treatment of PUD and stress-related ulcers. It binds to tissue proteins in eroded areas and prevents exposure of the ulcerated area to stomach acid.

- ❖ Misoprostol is a synthetic prostaglandin analogue that inhibits gastric acid secretion and is used to prevent NSAID-related ulcers.
- ❖ Cautious use of antacids is recommended in patients who have heart failure, hypertension, or other heart diseases or who require sodium restriction, especially if the antacid is high in sodium.
- ❖ Many drug interactions occur with acid-controlling drugs due to alteration of oral dosage forms, and so other medications are to be avoided within 1 to 2 hours of taking an antacid. Antacids are sometimes to be avoided when other acid-controlling drugs are taken.
- ❖ Magnesium–aluminum combination antacids are used to prevent the adverse effects of constipation and diarrhea. Some of the more serious concerns related to antacids include acid rebound, hypercalcemia, milk-alkali syndrome, and metabolic alkalosis.

EXAMINATION REVIEW QUESTIONS

1. A 30-year-old man is taking simethicone for excessive flatus associated with diverticulitis. During a patient teaching session, which statement by the nurse explains the mechanism of action of simethicone?
   - a. "It neutralizes gastric pH, thereby preventing gas."
   - b. "It buffers the effects of pepsin on the gastric wall."
   - c. "It decreases gastric acid secretion and thereby minimizes flatus."
   - d. "It causes mucus-coated gas bubbles to break into smaller ones."

2. When evaluating the medication list of a patient who will be starting therapy with an H_2 receptor antagonist, the nurse is aware that which drug may interact with it?
   - a. codeine sulphate
   - b. penicillin
   - c. ketoconazole
   - d. acetaminophen

3. When administering sucralfate, which action by the nurse is most correct?
   - a. Giving the drug with meals
   - b. Giving the drug on an empty stomach
   - c. Instructing the patient to restrict fluids
   - d. Waiting 30 minutes before administering other drugs

4. A patient with a history of kidney problems is asking for advice about which antacid he should use. The nurse will make which recommendation?
   - a. "Patients with kidney problems cannot use antacids."
   - b. "Aluminum-based antacids are the best choice for you."

   - c. "Calcium-based antacids are the best choice for you."
   - d. "Magnesium-based antacids are the best choice for you."

5. A patient who is taking oral tetracycline complains of heartburn and requests an antacid. Which action by the nurse is correct?
   - a. Give the tetracycline, but delay the antacid for 1 to 2 hours.
   - b. Give the antacid, but delay the tetracycline for at least 4 hours.
   - c. Administer both medications together.
   - d. Explain that the antacid cannot be given while the patient is taking the tetracycline.

6. When the nurse is administering a PPI, which actions by the nurse are correct? (Select all that apply.)
   - a. Giving the PPI on an empty stomach
   - b. Giving the PPI with meals
   - c. Making sure the patient does not crush or chew the capsules
   - d. Instructing the patient to open the capsule and chew the contents for best absorption
   - e. Administering the PPI only when the patient reports heartburn

7. The order reads: "Give ranitidine hydrochloride 50 mg in 100 mL normal saline IVPB tid and at bedtime. Infuse over 30 minutes." The infusion pump can be programmed to deliver only over 60 minutes (mL per hour). The nurse will set the pump to deliver how many mL/hour for each IVPB dose?

Answers: 1. d, 2. c, 3. b, 4. b, 5. a, 6. a, c, 7. 200 mL/hour

CRITICAL THINKING ACTIVITIES

1. A father brings his 2-month-old infant to the pediatric clinic and says, "He seems to have so much gas! Is there anything that can help?" The pediatrician suggests an infant formulation of simethicone. The father asks, "What does this drug do?" What is the nurse's best answer?

2. A patient with a history of decreased renal function tells the nurse, "I have finally found an antacid that gives me great relief!" The nurse checks the antacid's content and finds that the antacid is a combination of aluminum hydroxide and magnesium hydroxide. What is the nurse's priority action at this time? Explain your answer.

3. A patient tells the nurse, "I like taking antacids because they coat my stomach and protect my ulcer." What is the priority to consider when answering the patient's statement?

For answers, see http://evolve.elsevier.com/Canada/Lilley/pharmacology/.

CHAPTER 40

Antidiarrheal Drugs and Laxatives

Objectives

After reading this chapter, the successful student will be able to do the following:

1. Discuss the anatomy and physiology of the gastrointestinal (GI) tract, including the process of peristalsis.

2. Identify the various factors affecting bowel elimination and bowel patterns.

3. List the various groups of drugs used to treat alterations in bowel elimination, specifically diarrhea and constipation.

4. Discuss the mechanisms of action, indications, cautions, contraindications, drug interactions, dosages, routes of administration, and adverse effects of the various antidiarrheals, probiotics, and laxatives.

5. Develop a collaborative plan of care that includes all phases of the nursing process for patients taking antidiarrheals, probiotics, or laxatives.

e-Learning Activities

Website
(http://evolve.elsevier.com/Canada/Lilley/pharmacology/)

*e*volve

- Answer Key—Textbook Case Studies
- Answer Key—Critical Thinking Activities
- Chapter Summaries—Printable
- Review Questions for Exam Preparation
- Unfolding Case Studies

Drug Profiles

bisacodyl, p. 768
bismuth subsalicylate, p. 762
▸▸ diphenoxylate with atropine (diphenoxylate hydrochloride with atropine sulphate)*, p. 762
▸▸ docusate sodium, p. 767
▸▸ glycerin, p. 767
Lactobacillus, p. 762
▸▸ lactulose, p. 767
▸▸ loperamide (loperamide hydrochloride)*, p. 762
magnesium salts, p. 768
methylcellulose, p. 767
mineral oil, p. 767
polyethylene glycol (polyethylene glycol 3350)*, p. 768
▸▸ psyllium (psyllium hydrophilic mucilloid)*, p. 767
▸▸ senna, p. 768

▸▸ Key drug

*Full generic name is given in parentheses. For the purposes of this text, the more common, shortened name is used.

Key Terms

Antidiarrheal drugs Drugs that prevent or treat diarrhea. (p. 760)

Constipation A condition of abnormally infrequent and difficult passage of feces through the lower GI tract. (p. 761)

Diarrhea The abnormally frequent passage of loose stools. (p. 760)

Irritable bowel syndrome (IBS): A recurring condition of the intestinal tract characterized by bloating, flatulence, and often periods of diarrhea that alternate with periods of constipation. (p. 760)

Laxatives Drugs that promote bowel evacuation, such as by increasing the bulk of the feces, softening the stool, or lubricating the intestinal wall. (p. 761)

OVERVIEW

Diarrhea is the second leading cause of death in children under the age of 5, and is responsible for 760 000 deaths yearly. Globally, there are nearly 1.7 billion cases of diarrheal disease every year (World Health Organization, 2013). An average adult will experience diarrhea four times per year (Wanke, 2015).

Clostridium difficile is the most notable cause of health care–associated diarrhea and is becoming increasingly recognized as a community pathogen that is a significant threat. It is not discussed in this chapter as it is not treated with antidiarrheal drugs or laxatives. The key symptoms of GI disease are abdominal pain, nausea and vomiting, and diarrhea. **Diarrhea** is defined as the passage of stools with abnormally increased frequency, fluidity, and weight, or increased stool water excretion, and consists of three or more loose or liquid stools per day. Acute diarrhea refers to diarrhea of sudden onset in a previously healthy individual. It usually lasts from 3 days to 2 weeks and is self-limiting, resolving without sequelae. Chronic diarrhea lasts for longer than 3 to 4 weeks and is associated with recurrent passage of diarrheal stools, possible fever, nausea, vomiting, weight reduction, and chronic weakness.

The probable cause of diarrhea needs to be taken into consideration when designing a drug regimen to treat it. Causes of acute diarrhea include drugs, bacteria, viruses, nutritional factors, and protozoa. Causes of chronic diarrhea include tumours, AIDS, diabetes, hyperthyroidism, Addison's disease, and **irritable bowel syndrome (IBS)**. Treatment is aimed at decreasing stool frequency, alleviating abdominal cramps, replenishing fluids and electrolytes, and preventing weight loss and nutritional deficits from malabsorption. Often, replacement of fluids is the only treatment needed. Patients with diarrhea associated with a bacterial or parasitic infection must not use antidiarrheal drugs, because this will cause the organism to stay in the body longer and delay recovery.

ANTIDIARRHEALS

Drugs used to treat diarrhea are called **antidiarrheal drugs**. Based on their specific mechanisms of action, they are divided into different groups: adsorbents, antimotility drugs (anticholinergics and opiates), and probiotics (also known as intestinal flora modifiers and bacterial replacement drugs). These classes and the drugs in each class are listed in Table 40-1. Antidiarrheal and laxative drugs do not have the classic pharmacokinetics of other drugs, and thus pharmacokinetics tables such as those presented throughout the book are not included in this chapter.

Mechanism of Action and Drug Effects

Antidiarrheal drugs have various mechanisms of action. Adsorbents act by coating the walls of the GI tract. They

TABLE 40-1

Antidiarrheals: Drug Categories and Selected Drugs

Category	Antidiarrheal Drugs
Adsorbents	Activated charcoal, aluminum hydroxide, bismuth subsalicylate, cholestyramine, polycarbophil
Anticholinergics	Atropine sulphate, hyoscyamine
Opiates	Opium tincture, paregoric, codeine phosphate, diphenoxylate, loperamide hydrochloride
Probiotics and intestinal flora modifiers	*Lactobacillus acidophilus*, *Lactobacillus GG*, *Saccharromyces boulardii*

bind the causative bacteria or toxin to their adsorbent surface for elimination from the body through the stool. Adsorption is similar to absorption but differs in that it involves the chemical binding of substances (e.g., ions, bacterial toxins) onto the surface of an adsorbent. In contrast, *absorption* generally refers to the penetration of a substance into the interior structure of the absorbent or the uptake of a substance across a surface (e.g., the absorption of dietary nutrients into the intestinal villi). The adsorbent bismuth subsalicylate is a form of aspirin, or acetylsalicylic acid, and therefore it also has many of the same drug effects as aspirin (see Chapter 49). Activated charcoal is not only helpful in coating the walls of the GI tract and adsorbing bacteria but is also useful in cases of overdose because of its drug-binding properties activated charcoal should only be used under the supervision of a health care provider. The antilipemic drugs colestipol and cholestyramine (see Chapter 28) are anion exchange resins that are sometimes prescribed as antidiarrheal adsorbents and lipid-lowering drugs. Besides binding to diarrhea-causing toxins, they have the additional benefit of decreasing cholesterol levels.

Anticholinergic drugs work to slow peristalsis by reducing the rhythmic contractions and smooth muscle tone of the GI tract; they also have a drying effect and reduce gastric secretions. They are often used in combination with adsorbents and opiates (see later in the chapter). Anticholinergics are discussed in detail in Chapter 22. Probiotics are products obtained from bacterial cultures, most commonly *Lactobacillus* organisms, which make up the majority of the body's normal bacterial flora. These organisms are commonly destroyed by antibiotics. Probiotics work by replenishing these bacteria, which help to restore the balance of normal flora and suppress the growth of diarrhea-causing bacteria.

The primary action of opiates (see Chapter 11) often results in a decrease in bowel motility. A secondary effect of opiates is the reduction of the pain associated with diarrhea by relief of rectal spasms. Because they increase the transit time of food through the GI tract, they permit longer contact of the intestinal contents with the absorptive surface of the bowel, which increases the absorption of water, electrolytes, and other nutrients from the bowel and reduces stool frequency and net volume.

Indications

Antidiarrheal drugs are indicated for the treatment of diarrhea of various types and levels of severity. Adsorbents are more likely to be used in milder cases, whereas anticholinergics and opiates tend to be used in more severe cases. Probiotics are often helpful in patients with antibiotic-induced diarrhea.

Contraindications

Contraindications to the use of antidiarrheals include known drug allergy and any major acute GI condition, such as intestinal obstruction or colitis, unless the drug is ordered by the patient's health care provider after careful consideration of the specific case.

Adverse Effects

The adverse effects of the antidiarrheals are specific to each drug family. Most of these potential effects are minor and not life-threatening. The major adverse effects of specific drugs in each drug class are listed in Table 40-2. Probiotics do not have any listed adverse effects.

Interactions

Many drugs are absorbed from the intestines into the bloodstream, where they are delivered to their respective sites of action. A number of the antidiarrheals have the potential to alter this normal process, by either increasing or decreasing the absorption of these other drugs.

The adsorbents can decrease the effectiveness of many drugs, primarily by decreasing the absorption of certain drugs. Examples include digoxin, quinidine sulphate, and antihyperglycemic drugs. The oral anticoagulant warfarin sodium (see Chapter 27) is more likely to cause increased bleeding times or bruising when coadministered with adsorbents. This is thought to be because adsorbents bind to vitamin K, which is needed to make certain clotting factors. Vitamin K is synthesized by the normal bacterial flora in the bowel. The toxic effects of methotrexate are more likely to occur when it is given with adsorbents. The therapeutic effects of the anticholinergic antidiarrheals can be decreased by coadministration with antacids. Taking amantadine hydrochloride, tricyclic antidepressants, monoamine oxidase inhibitors, opioids, or antihistamines can result in increased anticholinergic effects when given with anticholinergics. The opiate antidiarrheals have additive central nervous system (CNS) depressant effects if they are given with CNS depressants, alcohol, opioids, sedative–hypnotics, antipsychotics, and skeletal muscle relaxants.

Bismuth subsalicylate can lead to increased bleeding times and bruising when administered with warfarin sodium, aspirin, or other nonsteroidal anti-inflammatory drugs. It can also cause confusion in older adults. Cholestyramine, when administered with glipizide, can result in decreased hypoglycemic effects. It is important not to give any drug within 2 hours before or 2 hours after cholestyramine as it decreases the absorption of that drug.

Dosages

For dosage information of antidiarrheal drugs, refer to the table on p. 672.

LAXATIVES

Laxatives are used for the treatment of **constipation**, which is defined as abnormally infrequent and difficult passage of feces through the lower GI tract. Constipation is a symptom, not a disease; it is a disorder of movement through the colon or rectum that can be caused by a variety of diseases, drugs, or lifestyles. Some of the more common causes of constipation are noted in Table 40-3.

The GI tract is responsible for the digestive process, which involves: (1) ingestion of dietary intake, (2) digestion of dietary intake into basic nutrients, (3) absorption of basic nutrients, and (4) storage and removal of fecal material via defecation (Figure 40-1).

Ingestion → Digestion → Absorption
→ Storage and removal

The usual time span between ingestion and defecation is 24 to 36 hours. The last segment of the GI tract, the large intestine (colon), is responsible for: (1) forming the stool by removing excess water from the fecal material, (2) temporarily storing the stool until defecation,

TABLE 40-2

Selected Antidiarrheals: Adverse Effects

Drug	Adverse Effects
bismuth subsalicylate	Increased bleeding time, constipation, dark stools, confusion, tinnitus, metallic taste, black tongue
atropine sulphate	Urinary retention, sexual dysfunction, headache, dizziness, anxiety, drowsiness, bradycardia, hypotension, dry skin, flushing, blurred vision
codeine phosphate, diphenoxylate hydrochloride	Drowsiness, dizziness, lethargy, nausea, vomiting, constipation, hypotension, urinary retention, flushing, respiratory depression

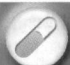

DRUG PROFILES

Drug therapy for diarrhea depends on the specific cause of the diarrhea, if it is known. All antidiarrheals are orally administered drugs available as suspensions, tablets, or capsules. Some antidiarrheals are available over the counter, whereas others require a prescription.

ADSORBENTS

bismuth subsalicylate

Bismuth subsalicylate is a salicylate by chemical structure. Even though it is available over the counter, it must be used with caution in children and adolescents who have or are recovering from chicken pox or influenza because of the risk of Reye's syndrome (see Special Populations: Children box). It can also cause all of the adverse effects associated with an aspirin-based product (see Chapter 49). Two alarming but harmless effects of bismuth subsalicylate are temporary darkening of the tongue and the stool. Bismuth subsalicylate is available for oral use.

ANTICHOLINERGICS

The anticholinergic atropine sulphate is used either alone or in combination with other antidiarrheals to slow GI tract motility. These drugs are referred to as *belladonna alkaloids* and are discussed in Chapter 22. Their safety margin is not as wide as that of many of the other antidiarrheals, because they can cause serious adverse effects if used inappropriately. For this reason, they are available only by prescription.

OPIATES

There are three opiate-related antidiarrheal drugs: codeine sulphate, diphenoxylate hydrochloride with atropine sulphate, and loperamide. The only opiate-related antidiarrheal available as an over-the-counter (OTC) medication is loperamide; all others are prescription-only drugs because of the risks of respiratory depression and dependency associated with opiate use.

▶▶diphenoxylate hydrochloride with atropine sulphate

Diphenoxylate hydrochloride with atropine sulphate is available as Lomotil®. Diphenoxylate hydrochloride is a synthetic opiate agonist that is structurally related to meperidine hydrochloride. It acts on the smooth muscle of the intestinal tract, inhibiting GI motility and excessive GI propulsion. It has little or no analgesic activity; however, because it is an opioid, misuse and chemical dependence can occur. Diphenoxylate hydrochloride is combined with subtherapeutic quantities of atropine sulphate to discourage its use as a recreational opiate drug. The amount of atropine sulphate present in the combination is too small to interfere with the conjugated diphenoxylate. When taken in large doses, however, the combination results in extreme anticholinergic effects (e.g., dry mouth, abdominal pain, tachycardia, blurred vision).

Use of the combination of diphenoxylate hydrochloride and atropine sulphate is contraindicated in patients experiencing diarrhea associated with pseudomembranous colitis or toxigenic bacteria. It is available only for oral use.

▶▶loperamide hydrochloride

Loperamide hydrochloride (Imodium®) is a synthetic antidiarrheal that is similar to diphenoxylate hydrochloride. The drug binds to opiate receptors in the intestinal wall; consequently, it inhibits the release of acetylcholine and prostaglandins, thereby reducing peristalsis and increasing intestinal transit time. Loperamide increases the tone of the anal sphincter and, in doing so, reduces incontinence and urgency. Therefore, it inhibits both peristalsis in the intestinal wall and intestinal secretion, thereby decreasing the number of stools and their water content. In addition, fluid and electrolyte loss diminishes. Although the drug exhibits many characteristics of the opiate class, physical dependence has not been reported with the use of loperamide. Because of its safety profile, it is the only opiate antidiarrheal drug available as an OTC medication. It is also available as a combination product with the antiflatulent simethicone. Loperamide use is contraindicated in patients with severe ulcerative colitis, pseudomembranous colitis, and acute diarrhea associated with *Escherichia coli*.

PROBIOTICS

Probiotics suppress the growth of diarrhea-causing bacteria and re-establish the normal flora that reside in the intestine. Most commonly, they are bacterial cultures of *Lactobacillus* organisms. Probiotics are often referred to as *intestinal flora modifiers*. Their mechanism of action is not completely understood, but their general benefits are suppression of growth or invasion by pathogenic bacteria, improvement of intestinal barrier function, modulation of the immune system, and modulation of pain perception.

Lactobacillus

The main types of probiotics in foods and supplements are *Lactobacillus* and *Bifidobacteria*. Most products are a combination of acid-producing bacteria prepared in a concentrated, dried culture for oral administration. They are normal inhabitants of the GI tract where, through the fermentation of carbohydrates (which produces lactic acid), they create an unfavourable environment for the overgrowth of harmful fungi and bacteria. *Lactobacillus acidophilus* has been used for more than 75 years for the treatment of uncomplicated diarrhea, particularly that caused by antibiotic therapy that destroys normal intestinal flora. Another commonly used probiotic is *Saccharomyces boulardii*.

SPECIAL POPULATIONS: CHILDREN

Antidiarrheal Preparations

- If diarrhea is accompanied by fever, malaise, or abdominal pain, contact a health care provider immediately because of the possibility of excessive fluid and electrolyte loss or possible infection. Dehydration and electrolyte loss occur rapidly in children because of their size and sensitivity to loss of fluid volume and electrolytes through the stool.
- Always contact a health care provider or pharmacist for the proper dosage of antidiarrheals if a child is 6 years of age or younger or if there is any doubt as to proper dosing. Never hesitate to contact a health care provider with any concern or question regarding any medication recommended for the child.
- Bismuth subsalicylate is a salicylate by chemical structure; therefore, it is to be used cautiously in children and adolescents who have been or are recovering from chicken pox or influenza because of the risk for Reye's syndrome (see Chapter 49).

- Immediately report to a health care provider any abdominal distention, abdominal firmness, abdominal pain, or worsening of or lack of improvement in diarrhea 24 to 48 hours after medication administration. Measurement of the amount of diarrhea by the number of soiled diapers or number of stools per day provides important information.
- Antidiarrheal preparations are always to be used cautiously in children. If symptoms persist or dehydration occurs (possibly evidenced by a lack of tears and decreased urine output), contact the health care provider.
- Always assess children and adolescents for the presence of an eating disorder such as bulimia or anorexia due to the use or misuse of laxatives associated with these conditions.

DOSAGES   Selected Antidiarrheal Drugs

Drug	Pharmacological Class	Usual Dosage Range	Onset of Action
bismuth subsalicylate (Bismuth®, Devron Chew®, Pepto-Bismol®)	Antimicrobial, antidiarrheal	Doses repeated q30–60 min, not to exceed 8/day; all doses PO *Children 3–5 yr** 5 mL or ⅓ tab *Children 6–9 yr** 10 mL or ⅔ tab *Children 10–12 yr** 15 mL or 1 tab *Adults* 30 mL or 2 tab	0.5–2 hr
⇥diphenoxylate hydrochloride with atropine sulphate (Lomotil)	Antidiarrheal	*Children 4–12 yr* PO: 0.3–0.4 mg/kg daily, divided tid–qid *Adults* PO: 20 mg/day, divided tid–qid	40–60 min
Lactobacillus acidophilus	Probiotic, dietary supplement	*Adults and children over 12 yr* PO: 1 cap bid	Unknown
⇥loperamide hydrochloride (Imodium)	Opiate antidiarrheal	*Children 6–12 yr* PO: 2 mg bid–tid *Adults and children over 12 yr* PO: 4 mg followed by 2 mg after each bowel movement (not to exceed 16 mg/day)	1–3 h

PO, oral.
*Used with caution in children and teenagers who have or are recovering from chicken pox or influenza because of the risk of Reye's syndrome.

and (3) extracting essential vitamins from the intestinal bacteria (particularly vitamin K). The type of stool depends on the time it spends in the colon and reflects diet, amount of fluid intake, medications, and activity. A common approach to determining the quality of the stool is the use of a stool chart. For example, the Bristol Stool Chart is one such aid that classifies stools into seven groups within the following categories: constipa-

tion, normal, and diarrhea and urgency. The colon is 120 to 150 cm long and is separated from the small intestine by the ileocecal valve. The colon extends into the rectum, which terminates at the anus. The rectum is the temporary storage site for the stool, which is composed of water and unabsorbed and indigestible material. Evacuation of the rectal contents is accomplished by bowel movements.

TABLE	40-3

Causes of Constipation

Causes	Examples
Adverse drug effects	Analgesics, anticholinergics, iron supplements, aluminum antacids, calcium antacids, opiates, calcium channel blockers
Lifestyle	Poor bowel movement habits: voluntary refusal to defecate resulting in constipation Diet: poor fluid intake and low-fibre diet or excessive consumption of dairy products Physical inactivity: lack of proper exercise, especially in older adults Psychological factors: anxiety, stress, hypochondria
Metabolic and endocrine disorders or conditions	Diabetes mellitus, hypothyroidism, hypercalcemia, hypokalemia, pregnancy
Neurogenic disorders	Autonomic neuropathy, intestinal pseudo-obstruction, multiple sclerosis, spinal cord lesions, Parkinson's disease, stroke

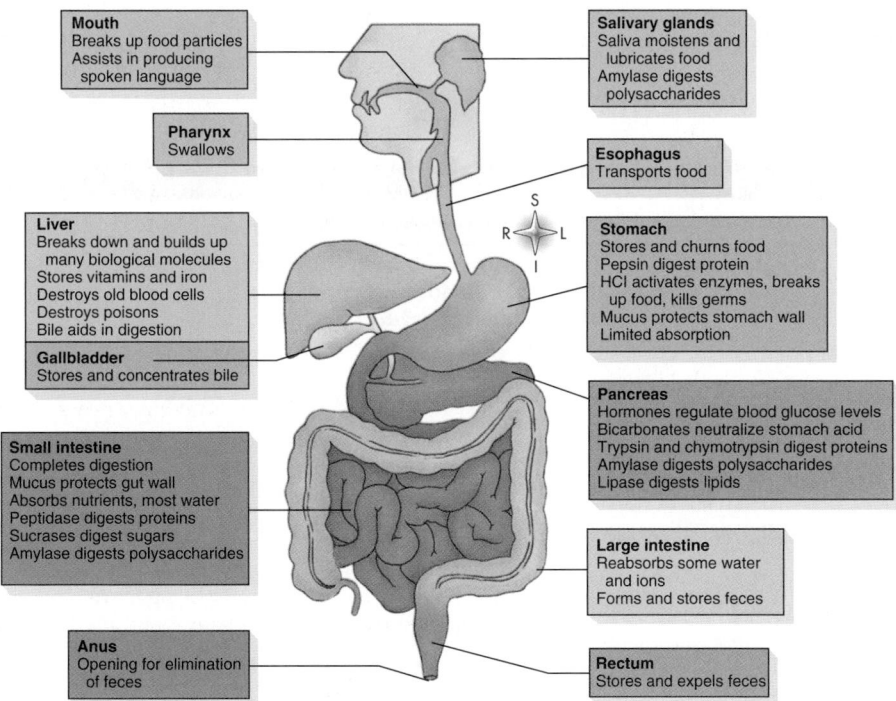

FIG. 40-1 The digestive system. (Source: Patton, K. T., & Thibodeau, G. A. (2014). *Mosby's Handbook of Anatomy and Physiology* (2nd ed.; p. 478). St. Louis, MO: Mosby.)

A bowel movement (defecation) is a reflex act that involves both smooth and skeletal muscles. The entry of feces into the rectum stimulates mass peristaltic movement that results in a bowel movement. However, voluntary initiation or inhibition of defecation is also possible via skeletal muscle pathways. Treatment of constipation is individualized, with consideration of the patient's age, concerns, and expectations; duration and severity of constipation; and potential contributing factors. Treatment can be either surgical (this is rare and is limited to extreme cases such as exploratory laparoscopy or bowel resection) or nonsurgical. Nonsurgical treatments can be separated into three broad approaches: dietary (e.g., fibre supplementation), behavioural (e.g., increased physical activity), and pharmacological. The focus in this chapter is on pharmacological treatment. Laxatives are among the most misused OTC medications. Long-term and often inappropriate use of stimulant laxatives may result in laxative dependence, produce damage to the bowel, or lead to previously nonexistent intestinal problems. With the exception of the bulk-forming type, laxatives are not to be used for long periods. Based on their mechanisms of action, laxatives are divided into five major groups: bulk-forming, emollient, hyperosmotic, saline, and stimulant. Table 40-4 lists the currently available laxative drugs categorized by drug family. The onset of action of laxatives is the most important pharmacokinetic feature of these drugs and is listed in the Dosages table on p. 767.

Mechanism of Action and Drug Effects

All laxatives promote bowel movements, but each class of laxative has a different mechanism of action. Laxatives may act by: (1) affecting fecal consistency, (2) increasing fecal movement through the colon, or (3) facilitating defecation through the rectum. Bulk-forming laxatives act in a manner similar to that of the fibre naturally contained in the diet. They absorb water into the intestine, which increases bulk and distends the bowel to initiate reflex bowel activity, thus promoting a bowel movement.

Emollient laxatives are also referred to as *stool softeners* (docusate sodium) and lubricant laxatives (mineral oil). Fecal softeners work by lowering the surface tension of GI fluids, so that more water and fat are absorbed into the stool and the intestines. The lubricant type of emollient laxatives works by lubricating the fecal material and the intestinal wall and preventing absorption of water from the intestines. Instead of being absorbed, this water content in the bowel softens and expands the stool. This promotes bowel distension and reflex peristaltic actions, which ultimately lead to defecation.

Hyperosmotic laxatives work by increasing fecal water content, which results in distention, increased peristalsis, and evacuation. Their site of action is limited to the large intestine. *Saline laxatives* increase osmotic pressure in the small intestine by inhibiting water absorption and increasing both water and electrolyte (salt) secretions from the bowel wall into the bowel lumen. This results in watery stool. Increased distention promotes peristalsis and evacuation. Rectal enemas of sodium phosphate, a saline laxative, produce defecation 2 to 5 minutes after administration.

As the name implies, *stimulant laxatives* stimulate the nerves that innervate the intestines, which results in increased peristalsis. They also increase fluid in the colon, which increases bulk and softens the stool. Table 40-5 summarizes the specific drug effects of the different classes of laxatives.

In 2009, a new class of drugs was approved for the treatment of specific types of constipation related to opioid use and bowel resection surgery. These peripherally acting opioid antagonists include methylnaltrexone bromide (Relistor®) and alvimopan (Enbereg®). These drugs block entrance of an opioid drug into the bowel cells, thus allowing bowels to function normally, even with continued opioid use. Methylnaltrexone bromide is approved only for advanced illness in palliative patients who have opioid-induced constipation. It is available only as an injection and is given once a day. Alvimopan is indicated to accelerate GI recovery time following partial large or small bowel resection surgery. Alvimopan has yet to be approved by Health Canada; however, it can be accessed through the Special Access Programme in some jurisdictions.

Indications

The following are some of the more common uses of laxatives:

- Facilitation of bowel movements in patients with inactive colon or anorectal disorders
- Reduction of ammonia absorption in hepatic encephalopathic conditions (lactulose only)
- Treatment of drug-induced constipation
- Treatment of constipation associated with pregnancy or the postobstetric period
- Treatment of constipation caused by reduced physical activity or poor dietary habits
- Removal of toxic substances from the body
- Facilitation of defecation in megacolon
- Preparation for colonic diagnostic procedures (e.g., colonoscopy) or surgery (e.g., bowel resection)

TABLE	40-4

Laxatives: Drug Categories and Selected Drugs

Category	Laxative Drugs
Bulk forming	psyllium, methylcellulose
Emollient	docusate sodium, mineral oil
Hyperosmotic	polyethylene glycol, lactulose, sorbitol, glycerin
Saline	magnesium sulphate, magnesium phosphate, magnesium citrate
Stimulant	senna, biscodyl

TABLE	40-5

Laxatives: Drug Effects

Drug Effect	Bulk	Emollient	Hyperosmotic	Saline	Stimulant
Increases peristalsis	Y	Y	Y	Y	Y
Causes increased secretion of water and electrolytes in small bowel	Y	Y	N	Y	Y
Inhibits absorption of water in small bowel	Y	Y	N	Y	Y
Increases wall permeability in small bowel	N	Y	N	N	Y
Acts only in large bowel	N	N	Y	N	N
Increases water in fecal mass	Y	Y	Y	Y	Y
Softens fecal mass	Y	Y	Y	Y	Y

TABLE 40-6	
Laxatives: Indications	
Category	**Indication**
Bulk forming	Acute and chronic constipation, irritable bowel syndrome, diverticulosis
Emollient	Acute and chronic constipation, fecal impaction, anorectal conditions requiring facilitation of bowel movements
Hyperosmotic	Chronic constipation, bowel preparation for diagnostic and surgical procedures
Saline	Constipation, bowel preparation for diagnostic and surgical procedures
Stimulant	Acute constipation, bowel preparation for diagnostic and surgical procedures

TABLE 40-7	
Laxatives: Adverse Effects	
Category	**Adverse Effects**
Bulk forming	Impaction above strictures, fluid disturbances, electrolyte imbalances, gas formation, esophageal blockage, allergic reaction
Emollient	Skin rashes, decreased absorption of vitamins, lipid pneumonia, electrolyte imbalances
Hyperosmotic	Abdominal bloating, rectal irritation, electrolyte imbalances
Saline	Magnesium toxicity (with kidney insufficiency), electrolyte imbalances, cramping, diarrhea, increased thirst
Stimulant	Nutrient malabsorption, skin rashes, gastric irritation, electrolyte imbalances, discoloured urine, rectal irritation

See Table 40-6 for specific therapeutic indications for each laxative drug class.

Contraindications

All categories of laxatives share the same general contraindications and precautions, including avoidance in the case of drug allergy and the need for cautious use in the presence of the following: acute surgical abdomen; appendicitis symptoms such as abdominal pain, nausea, and vomiting; fecal impaction (mineral oil enemas excepted); intestinal obstruction; as a weight loss aid; and undiagnosed abdominal pain.

Adverse Effects

The adverse effects of the various laxative drugs are specific to each group. Most of the adverse effects from laxatives are confined to the intestine; however, the overuse and misuse of laxatives can lead to many unwanted effects that are not expected or designed to occur with appropriate use. The major adverse effects of the laxative drugs are listed in Table 40-7. In addition, laxative dependency may occur when the colon stops reacting to usual doses of laxatives and larger amounts of laxatives are needed to produce bowel movements. Other serious effects may be a stretched or "lazy" colon, colon infection, and irritable bowel syndrome.

Interactions

Laxatives alter intestinal function; therefore, they can interact with other drugs, because many drugs are absorbed in the intestines. Bulk-forming laxatives can decrease the absorption of antibiotics, digoxin, salicylates, tetracyclines, and warfarin sodium. Mineral oil can decrease the absorption of fat-soluble vitamins (A, D, E, and K). Hyperosmotic laxatives can cause increased CNS depression if they are given with barbiturates, general anaesthetics, opioids, or antipsychotics. Oral antibiotics can decrease the effects of lactulose. Stimulant laxatives decrease the absorption of antibiotics, digoxin, nitrofurantoin, salicylates, tetracyclines, and oral anticoagulants.

Dosages

For dosage information on selected laxatives, refer to the table on p. 769.

NURSING PROCESS

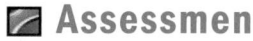 **Assessment**

Before administering antidiarrheal preparations, obtain a thorough history and perform an assessment of bowel patterns, general state of health, any recent illness, and any dietary changes. In the abdominal assessment, include auscultation of bowel sounds in all four quadrants *after* inspection of the entire abdomen but *before* percussion and palpation. Performing auscultation and inspection before percussion prevents any possible stimulation of peristalsis or bowel sounds that would not have otherwise occurred. When the frequency of bowel sounds ranges from 6 to 32 per minute, it is important to describe exactly what is heard and the amount of activity in each of the four quadrants. Terms such as *high-pitched, low-pitched, gurgling,* or *tinkling* may be used to describe the character or the sounds, whereas activity may be described as *hypoactive* (less than 6 sounds per minute), *normoactive* (between 6 and 32 sounds per minute), or *hyperactive* (more than the normal range). Bowel sounds

DRUG PROFILES

Laxatives are used for the treatment of constipation. Such treatment must involve an understanding of the whole patient. Many drugs in the five major groups of laxatives are available as OTC medications, whereas others require a prescription for use. The following profiles describe the prototypical drugs in each of the laxative groups.

BULK-FORMING LAXATIVES

Bulk-forming laxatives are composed of water-retaining (hydrophilic) natural and synthetic cellulose derivatives. Psyllium is an example of a natural bulk-forming laxative, and methylcellulose is an example of a synthetic cellulose derivative. Bulk-forming drugs increase water absorption, which results in greater total volume (bulk) of the intestinal contents. Bulk-forming laxatives tend to produce normal, formed stools. Their action is limited to the GI tract, so they cause few, if any, systemic effects. However, they need to be taken with liberal amounts of water to prevent esophageal obstruction and fecal impaction. Bulk-forming laxatives are all obtainable over the counter, are among the safest laxatives, and are the only ones that are recommended for long-term use.

methylcellulose

Methylcellulose is a synthetic bulk-forming laxative that attracts water into the intestine and absorbs excess water into the stool, stimulating the intestines and increasing peristalsis. Specific contraindications include GI obstruction and hepatitis. Methylcellulose is an oral drug available in powdered form that provides approximately 2 g of fibre per heaping tablespoon.

▶▶psyllium hydrophilic mucilloid

Psyllium hydrophilic mucilloid (Metamucil Preparations®) is a natural bulk-forming laxative obtained from the dried seed of the *Plantago psyllium* plant. It has many of the characteristics of methylcellulose. Psyllium is contraindicated in patients with intestinal obstruction or fecal impaction. Its use is also contraindicated in patients experiencing abdominal pain or nausea and vomiting. Psyllium is available for oral use in powder form.

EMOLLIENT LAXATIVES

Emollient laxatives either directly lubricate the stool and the intestines, as with mineral oil, or act as fecal softeners. By lubricating the fecal material and the intestinal walls lubricant emollient laxatives prevent water from moving out of the intestines, which softens and expands the stool. Stool softeners (docusate sodium) work by lowering the surface tension of fluids, which allows more water and fat to be absorbed into the stool and the intestines.

▶▶docusate sodium

Docusate sodium (Colace®) is a stool-softening emollient laxative that facilitates the passage of water and fats into the fecal mass, which softens the stool. This drug is used to treat constipation, soften fecal impactions, and facilitate

easy bowel movements in patients with hemorrhoids and other painful anorectal conditions. In addition to the docusate salt formulations, combination products are also available. They do not cause patients to defecate; they simply soften the stool to ease its passage. Docusate sodium use is contraindicated in patients with intestinal obstruction, fecal impaction, or nausea and vomiting.

mineral oil

Mineral oil eases the passage of stool by lubricating the intestines and preventing water from escaping the stool. Mineral oil is the only lubricant laxative in the emollient category. It is a mixture of liquid hydrocarbons derived from petroleum and is most commonly used to treat constipation associated with hard stools or fecal impaction.

Mineral oil use is contraindicated in patients with intestinal obstruction, abdominal pain, or nausea and vomiting. Mineral oil products are available for oral administration and as enemas.

HYPEROSMOTIC LAXATIVES

The hyperosmotic laxatives glycerin, lactulose, sorbitol, and polyethylene glycol (PEG) relieve constipation by increasing the water content of feces, which results in distention, peristalsis, and evacuation. They are most commonly used to treat constipation and to evacuate the bowels before diagnostic and surgical procedures.

▶▶glycerin

Glycerin promotes bowel movements by increasing osmotic pressure in the intestine, which draws fluid into the colon. Because it is a mild laxative, it is often used in children. Glycerin has properties similar to those of sorbitol, another hyperosmotic laxative. Glycerin use is contraindicated in patients who have shown a hypersensitivity reaction to it. It is available as rectal suppositories for both adults and children. A combination product of glycerin and mineral oil (Agarol®) is available for oral use.

▶▶lactulose

Lactulose is a synthetic derivative of the natural sugar lactose, which is not digested in the stomach or absorbed in the small bowel. It passes unchanged into the large intestine, where it is metabolized. Colonic bacteria digest lactulose to produce lactic acid, formic acid, and acetic acid; this process creates a hyperosmotic environment that draws water into the colon and produces a laxative effect. This drug-induced acidic environment also reduces blood ammonia levels by converting ammonia to ammonium. Ammonium is a water-soluble cation that is trapped in the intestines and cannot be reabsorbed into the systemic circulation. This effect has proved helpful in reducing serum ammonia levels in patients with hepatic encephalopathy. Lactulose use is contraindicated in patients on a low-galactose diet. It is available as a solution for either oral or rectal use.

Continued

DRUG PROFILES—cont'd

polyethylene glycol 3350

Polyethylene glycol (PEG 3350®) is most commonly used before diagnostic or surgical bowel procedures, because it is a potent laxative that induces total cleansing of the bowel. The 3350 designation refers to the osmolality of the drug. It is usually available in a powdered dosage form that contains a balanced mixture of electrolytes that also helps stimulate bowel evacuation (e.g., Clearlax®, Colyte®, Klean-Prep®, Pegalax®, PEGLYTE®, Restoralax®). The powder is reconstituted in a large volume of fluid (4 L) that is then gradually drunk by the patient on the afternoon of the day before the procedure. Use of PEG is contraindicated in patients with GI obstruction, gastric retention, bowel perforation, toxic colitis, toxic megacolon, or ileus.

Diarrhea usually occurs within 30 to 60 minutes after ingestion; complete evacuation and cleansing of the bowel is accomplished within 4 hours. MiraLax® is a PEG 3350 product that is available over the counter and can be used daily for constipation in much smaller amounts than those used for total bowel cleansing.

SALINE LAXATIVES

Saline laxatives consist of various magnesium or sodium salts. They increase osmotic pressure and draw water into the colon, producing a watery stool, usually within 3 to 6 hours of ingestion. Oral sodium phosphate–containing products used for bowel evacuation, such as Fleet Phospho-Soda®, were taken off the market because of concerns about acute phosphate nephropathy.

magnesium hydroxide

The magnesium saline laxative magnesium hydroxide (Phillips' Milk of Magnesia®) is an unpleasant-tasting OTC laxative preparation. It is to be used with caution in patients with kidney insufficiency, because it can be absorbed enough to cause hypermagnesemia. It is most commonly used to evacuate the bowel rapidly in preparation for endoscopic examination and to help remove unabsorbed poisons from the GI tract.

Use of magnesium hydroxide is contraindicated in patients with kidney disease, abdominal pain, nausea and vomiting, obstruction, acute surgical abdomen, or rectal bleeding. Magnesium hydroxide is available in oral liquid and tablet forms. It is also found in a variety of combination products, such as Diovol®, Maalox®, and Pepcid Complete®. Other magnesium products are listed in the discussion of saline laxatives earlier in this chapter. Note that magnesium *oxide* is used as a supplement, not as a laxative (see Chapter 9).

STIMULANT LAXATIVES

Stimulant laxatives induce intestinal peristalsis. In the past, several different stimulant laxatives were available; bisacodyl (Dulcolax®) and senna (Senokot®) are the remaining stimulants. Their site of action is the entire GI tract. The action of the stimulant laxatives is proportional to the dose. The stimulant class is the most likely of all laxative classes to cause dependence.

bisacodyl

Bisacodyl (Dulcolax) is the most commonly used stimulant laxative. It is available as an oral tablet and rectal suppository. It is used for constipation or for whole bowel evacuation prior to endoscopic examination. It is available over the counter.

▶▶senna

Senna (Senokot) is a commonly used OTC stimulant laxative. Senna is obtained from the dried leaves of the *Cassia acutifolia* plant. It may be used for relief of acute constipation or for bowel preparation for surgery or examination. Because of its stimulating action on the GI tract, it may cause abdominal pain. It can produce complete bowel evacuation in 6 to 12 hours. Senna is available orally as tablets and syrup. One product, Senokot-S®, includes both senna and the stool softener docusate sodium.

---

may also be absent. Perform a thorough abdominal assessment for any patient with GI concerns, including altered bowel status. Note the presence of tenderness, rigidity, changes in contour, bulges, and obvious peristaltic waves across the abdomen. Assess frequency, consistency, amount, colour, and odour (if present) of stools, and document the findings. In addition, it is critical to patient safety and health to be sure that the possibility of *Clostridium difficile* infection or other infectious diarrhea is ruled out. Assess for and document any contraindications, cautions, and drug interactions for all drugs. Report abdominal pain, bloody stools, confirmation of hypoactive to no bowel sounds, or fever to the health care provider immediately. When administering diphenoxylate hydrochloride with atropine sulphate, be wary of overuse because large amounts may result in dry mouth, abdominal pain, tachycardia, and blurred vision. Older adults are more

susceptible to fluid and electrolyte depletion associated with diarrhea; therefore, closely assess hydration status for such patients.

Laxative use requires further assessment in addition to the abdominal assessment and bowel pattern history described earlier. For example, focus questions on changes in bowel habits, long-term use of laxatives (because patients may become laxative dependent), and dietary and fluid intake. Assess vital signs, daily weights, intake and output, and fluid and electrolyte levels, and note the presence of any weakness because of the possibility of hypotension and volume or electrolyte depletion (with long-term laxative use). Another important area to assess is that of laxative misuse in older adults as well as in children and adolescents. Specifically, in children and adolescents, assess for eating disorders with concurrent use of laxatives.

DOSAGES   Selected Laxatives

Drug	Pharmacological Class	Usual Dosage Range	Onset of Action
bisacodyl (Dulcolax)	Stimulant laxative	*Children 6–12 yr* PO: 5 mg PR: 5 mg suppository *Adults and children over 12 yr* PO: 5–10 mg PR: 10 mg suppository	Oral: 6–12 h Rectal: 15–60 min
▸▸docusate sodium (Colace)	Stool softener, emollient laxative	*Children 3–12 yr** PO: 20–120 mg/day divided *Adults* PO: 100–200 mg/day divided	1–3 days
▸▸glycerin (Glycerin Suppository®)	Hyperosmotic laxative	*Children and adults* PR only: Insert one adult, child, or infant suppository PR daily–bid prn; attempt to retain 15–30 min; suppository does not have to melt to induce BM	15–30 min
▸▸**lactulose (generic)**	Disaccharide, hyperosmotic laxative	*Adults†* PO: 15–60 mL daily	24 hr
methylcellulose	Bulk-forming laxative	*Children 6–11 yr* ½ dose of that for 12 yr–adult dose *Adults and children over 12 yr* PO: 1 heaping teaspoon in 240 mL cold water daily–tid	12–24 hr
mineral oil (Mineral Oil®)	Emollient laxative	*Children 2–12 yr* PO: 5–15 mL PR: 59 mL × 1 *Children 12 yr and older/Adult* PO: 15–45 mL PR: 118 mL × 1	6–18 hr
polyethylene glycol (Klean-Prep, Pegalax)	Hyperosmolar laxative	*Adults* PO: 4 L solution, usually evening before procedure; patient needs to fast at least 4 hr before drinking solution	1 hr 1 hr
▸▸psyllium hydrophilic mucilloid (Metamucil Preparations)	Bulk-forming laxative	*Children 6–11 yr* ½ rounded tsp in water daily–tid *Adults and children over 12 yr* PO: 1 rounded tsp in 240 mL water or juice daily–tid	12–24 hr
▸▸senna (Senokot)	Stimulant-irritant laxative	*Children 2–5 yr†* PO: 2–5 mL at bedtime (max 2.5 mL bid) *Children 6–12 yr‡* PO (tabs): 1 tab daily (max 2 tabs bid) PO (liquid): 7.5–10 mL daily (max 5 mL bid) *Adults and children 12 yr and older* PO (tabs): 2–4 tabs daily (max 4 tabs bid) PO (syrup): 15 mL daily (max 30 mL bid)	6–24 hr

PO, oral; *PR*, rectal.

*Docusate sodium is available in both capsule and liquid forms.

†Rectal route is sometimes used to reverse hepatic coma.

‡There are many dosage forms; consult product labelling if in doubt. Most common dosage forms consist of 187 mg senna in tablet form and 1.7 mg/mL of sennosides in liquid form.

The type of laxative and its related mechanism of action dictate specific assessments because of differences in how strongly patients react to the various laxative drugs. Bulk-forming laxatives are often used to treat chronic constipation and have few adverse effects, but a basic abdominal and bowel pattern assessment and related history taking are still needed. Always assess and document contraindications, cautions, and drug interactions. Use docusate sodium or emollient laxatives cautiously in older adults.

Prior to the use of hyperosmotic laxatives (e.g., polyethylene glycol, lactulose, sorbitol, glycerin), assess baseline fluid and electrolyte levels to identify any deficits. All of the previously mentioned assessment measures regarding abdominal examination and bowel patterns are also appropriate for these drugs, with additional assessment for the presence of abdominal pain, the degree of peristalsis, and any history of recent abdominal surgery, nausea, vomiting, or weight loss. Older adults react more adversely to this class of laxatives, so their use in this group is to be avoided.

Saline laxatives (e.g., magnesium hydroxide) are to be used with caution in older adults because of possible dehydration and electrolyte loss. These drugs may also cause magnesium toxicity in those with compromised renal status. Kidney function studies are important to assess in those at risk. Senna and bisacodyl are examples of stimulant laxatives. They may also cause electrolyte imbalances, so baseline electrolyte levels are important to assess and monitor.

Nursing Diagnoses

- Constipation related to improper or inadequate diet
- Diarrhea related to GI irritation from food, bacteria, viruses, or pathology
- Deficit fluid volume related to loss of fluids and electrolytes caused by frequent, loose stools

Planning

Goals

- Patient will experience minimal constipation.
- Patient will experience minimal diarrhea.
- Patient will remain free from fluid and electrolyte disturbances related to changes in bowel patterns and lack of proper management of bowel alterations.

Expected Patient Outcomes

- Patient states measures to manage or prevent constipation such as increasing intake of fluids to 2 to 3 L per day, increasing intake of bulk and fibre (unless contraindicated), and increasing physical activity.
  - Patient takes recommended bulk-forming laxatives, stool softeners, as well as other approved laxatives, as prescribed and follows directions closely.
- Patient states measures to manage and prevent diarrhea such as increasing bulk; avoiding spicy, irritating foods and beverages; and avoiding caffeine.
  - Patient takes recommended antidiarrheal preparation as prescribed and instructed, with close attention to following directions on the medication.
- Patient reports to the health care provider any signs and symptoms of fluid and electrolyte loss, such as weakness, lethargy, decreased urinary output, or dizziness.
  - Patient implements measures to prevent fluid and electrolyte loss, including nonpharmacological and pharmacological therapies (see above).

Implementation

An effective and well-tolerated bowel protocol is an important component of care. Many agencies have developed specific protocols, requiring the least possible amount of intervention, that may be individualized for specific patients (e.g., increased fibre and fluid intake, rectal stimulation, establishing a daily predictable bowel care time, etc.) followed by pharmacological intervention.

Prior to the use of antidiarrheals, educate patients that the drugs must be taken *exactly* as directions indicate, with strict adherence to the recommended dose, frequency, and duration of treatment. Encourage patients to be aware of fluid intake and any dietary changes that would impact their health status or possibly exacerbate present symptoms. Instruct patients to be aware of the factors precipitating the diarrhea and, if symptoms persist, to contact their health care provider. Document any changes in bowel patterns, weight, intake and output, fluid volume, and mucous membrane status during and after the initiation of treatment, whether for constipation or diarrhea. Inform the patient that bismuth subsalicylate must be taken as directed and that this medication will turn the stool black or grey. If tablets are used, they must be chewed thoroughly before swallowing and with at least 180 mL of fluid. Bismuth subsalicylate is a salicylate-based product and is not to be taken with other salicylates to avoid the risk of toxicity. Encourage parents to check with their children's health care provider before giving bismuth subsalicylate to a child or adolescent with a viral infection, such as chicken pox or influenza, because of the risk for Reye's syndrome (see the Special Populations: Children box).

Diphenoxylate hydrochloride and loperamide may be given without regard to food intake but must be given with adequate fluid. Additionally, advise patients to follow the provided specific directions (e.g., the specific number of tablets recommended by the manufacturer after the first loose stool and the total number of tablets to be taken within a 24-hour period). Maximum amounts are not to be exceeded, and if diarrhea continues or other symptoms occur (e.g., fever, abdominal pain, bloody stools), instruct patients to contact a health care provider immediately. See Patient Teaching Tips for more information.

Probiotics may be recommended for a variety of altered bowel elimination patterns, whether diarrhea or constipation. Probiotics are available in foods and dietary supplements as well as in capsules, tablets, and powder dosage forms. Most of the probiotics are derived from *Lactobacillus* or *Bifidobacterium* bacteria. It is important to educate patients about probiotics and to emphasize their health benefits when administered in the proper amounts. Tell patients to take probiotics exactly as directed. Foods that contain probiotics include yogurt, fermented milk, miso, tempeh, and some juices and soy beverages. Bulk-forming laxatives such as methylcellulose must be administered as specified by the package insert, or as ordered. Methylcellulose is to be taken with at least 240 mL of liquid after the powder form has been thoroughly stirred into it. The fluid must be taken immediately because of a congealing effect; to avoid choking or swelling of the product in the throat or esophagus, the patient must swallow or receive the drug immediately upon stirring. The medication must never be taken or administered in its dry form. See the Patient Teaching Tips for more information.

Docusate sodium is available in a variety of oral dosage forms (e.g., capsules, tablets, syrups, elixir), and it is recommended to be taken with at least 180 mL of water or other fluid. An additional 1800 mL to 2400 mL of water per day is also suggested to help with stool softening. Bisacodyl, if ordered, is best taken on an empty stomach for faster action, and whole tablets must not be chewed or crushed. Advise the patient not to consume milk, antacids, or juices with the dose or within 1 hour of taking the medication. Rectal suppositories, if too soft, may be placed in a medicine cup with ice to harden before insertion. Once the wrapper is removed, apply a water-soluble lubricant to the suppository prior to insertion into the rectum. Use a glove or finger cot on the hand for insertion. For maximal effectiveness, encourage the patient to try to keep the suppository in place by lying still on the left side for at least 15 to 30 minutes to allow the drug to dissolve. Lactulose may be taken with juice, milk, or water to increase palatability. It is important to note that the normal colour of the oral solution is pale yellow. Administer rectal dosage forms as a retention enema with dilution as ordered, and instruct the patient to retain for 30 to 60 minutes. For proper insertion of a retention enema, lubricate the tip of the apparatus well and insert it carefully with the nozzle pointed toward the umbilicus of the patient, with the patient lying on the left side. Release the fluid gradually, and discontinue administration if the patient experiences severe abdominal pain. If long-term use of the drug is indicated, monitoring of serum electrolyte levels is needed.

Magnesium-based laxatives are generally used only in certain situations because they are potent. Encourage intake of fluids, and follow other instructions per the health care provider's order or the package instructions. Refrigeration may help increase the palatability of the oral solution. Emphasize the importance of taking these drugs exactly as prescribed for constipation, with consumption of a sufficient quantity of fluids and careful attention to adverse effects. Instruct the patient to mix a PEG-electrolyte solution with water or flavoured sports drink as directed and to shake well before drinking. Chilled solutions are tolerated better. Rapid drinking of each dose is recommended.

Evaluation

Therapeutic responses to any of the described medications include an improvement in the GI-related signs and symptoms reported by the patient (e.g., decrease in diarrhea or constipation), return to normal bowel patterns with normal bowel sounds, and absence of abnormal findings from an assessment of the abdomen and bowel patterns. Adverse effects for which to monitor patients vary according to each drug. Use goals and outcome criteria as a means to evaluate the collaborative plan of care related to each problem, whether constipation or diarrhea or both.

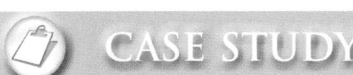 CASE STUDY

Long-Term Laxative Use

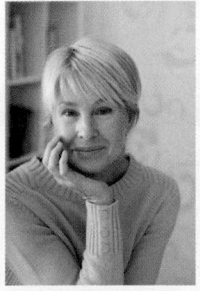

Gail is a 66-year-old retired teacher. She enjoys good health and exercises three times a week with a senior citizens' group in a supervised arthritis swim class at the local recreation centre. She arrives at the family practice office with reports of "constipation" and says that for the past 3 months she has had only one bowel movement every 3 days instead of one every day. In the assessment of this patient, the nurse discovers that Gail has been taking a stimulant laxative up to twice a day and is now also feeling "weak." Gail also says that she is experiencing "a lot of tummy cramping."

1. What are at least five questions the nurse should ask Gail? Provide reasons for each question.
2. What types of problems are generally related to long-term use of laxatives? Explain your answer.
3. What are some nonpharmacological ways Gail could prevent constipation?
4. What OTC drug is the best choice to help prevent constipation for Gail? Explain your answer.

For answers, see http://evolve.elsevier.com/Canada/Lilley/pharmacology/.

PATIENT TEACHING TIPS

❖ Instruct patients that antidiarrheals are to be taken exactly as prescribed, with close attention to indicated dosages with warnings of overuse.

❖ Counsel patients to take antidiarrheal drugs with caution when performing tasks that require mental alertness or precise motor skills until it is clear how the drug actually affects them. Advise patients to immediately report to a health care provider any abdominal distention, firmness or hardness of the abdomen, abdominal pain, worsening (or no improvement) of symptoms, rectal bleeding, unrelieved constipation, fever, nausea, vomiting or other GI-related signs and symptoms, dizziness, muscle weakness, or muscle cramping.

❖ To help patients with the adverse effect of dry mouth, encourage frequent mouth care, increased fluid intake, or the use of sugarless gum or candy.

❖ Bismuth subsalicylate may turn the stool tarry black, so warn patients that this may happen. Patients must avoid other drugs containing salicylates while taking bismuth subsalicylate. Always check for cautions and contraindications with this drug, especially for children.

❖ Patients should increase intake of fluids, preferably water, as well as of green leafy vegetables, fruits, whole grains, and other foods high in fibre to help minimize constipation. Exercise is also beneficial.

❖ Educate patients that what are normal bowel patterns for one person may not be normal for another. Assess previous normal bowel patterns with the patient.

❖ Keep all antidiarrheals and laxatives out of the reach of children.

❖ For patients taking powder forms of methylcellulose, emphasize the need to have the powder thoroughly mixed with at least 180 mL of liquid, which is stirred and then consumed immediately to avoid esophageal or throat obstruction.

❖ Probiotics are available over the counter in various dosages and under different product names. Advise patients to take them exactly as instructed and to be aware that adverse effects are generally not of concern. Cultured yogourt and cultured milk products provide probiotics.

❖ Inform patients taking senna to avoid other medications within 1 hour of taking it and that it often takes 6 to 12 hours for the laxative effect to occur.

KEY POINTS

❖ Diarrhea is a leading cause of morbidity and mortality in developing countries.

❖ Drugs used to treat diarrhea include adsorbents, anticholinergics and probiotics.

❖ Most acute diarrhea is self-limiting, subsiding in 3 days to 2 weeks.

❖ Fluid and electrolyte replacement is vital while a patient is experiencing diarrhea.

❖ Encourage patients to check and recheck dosage instructions before taking medications and to note any drug–food and drug–drug interactions.

❖ Anticholinergics work by decreasing GI peristalsis through their parasympathetic blocking effects. Adverse effects include urinary retention, headache, confusion, dry skin, rash, and blurred vision.

❖ Adsorbents work by coating the walls of the GI tract. They remain in the intestine and bind the causative bacteria or toxin to the adsorbent surface, so that it can be eliminated from the body through the stool. They may increase bleeding and cause constipation, dark stools, and black tongue.

❖ Probiotics are used to manage diarrhea and consist of bacterial cultures of *Lactobacillus*. They re-establish normal intestinal flora destroyed by infection or antibiotics and suppress the growth of diarrhea-causing bacteria.

❖ Opiates are used as antidiarrheals and help to decrease bowel motility, thus permitting longer contact of intestinal contents with the absorptive surface of the bowel. Opiates also help reduce the pain associated with rectal spasms.

❖ Laxatives, especially osmotic medications, may cause fluid and electrolyte loss.

❖ Alert patients to the misuse potential of laxatives and the problems associated with their misuse as well as laxative dependency issues.

❖ Stool softeners and bulk-forming drugs are often preferred to other drug classes in the treatment of constipation because they create fewer problems with fluid and electrolyte loss.

EXAMINATION REVIEW QUESTIONS

1. A patient is being prepared for a colonoscopy. The nurse expects which laxative to be used as preparation for this procedure?
a. methylcellulose
b. docusate sodium
c. PEG 3350
d. glycerin

2. The nurse is administering oral methylcellulose and keeps in mind that a potential concern with this drug is which of the following?
a. Dehydration
b. Tarry stools
c. Kidney calculi
d. Possible obstruction

EXAMINATION REVIEW QUESTIONS—cont'd

3. A 45-year-old woman has been diagnosed with irritable bowel syndrome (IBS) and has numerous bowel movements each day. She has been prescribed loperamide. What are the actions of this drug? Select all that apply.
   a. Reduces the daily fecal volume
   b. Increases viscosity and bulk of the bowel movements
   c. Reduces the loss of fluids and electrolytes associated with watery bowel movements
   d. Cures the disease process by eliminating the infection causing IBS
   e. Reduces bowel incontinence and urgency

4. When a nurse teaches a patient about taking bisacodyl tablets, which instruction is correct?
   a. "Take this medication on an empty stomach."
   b. "Chew the tablet for quicker onset of action."
   c. "Take this medication with juice or milk."
   d. "Take this medication with an antacid if it upsets your stomach."

5. A patient has been receiving long-term antibiotic therapy as part of treatment for an infected leg wound. He tells the nurse that he has had "spells of diarrhea" for the past week. Which medication is most appropriate for him at this time?
   a. bismuth subsalicylate
   b. *Lactobacillus acidophilus*
   c. diphenoxylate hydrochloride with atropine sulphate
   d. codeine sulphate

6. A parent calls to ask about giving a medication for diarrhea to his 12-year-old child, who is recovering from the flu. The nurse expects the health care provider to recommend which medication?
   a. bismuth subsalicylate
   b. *Lactobacillus GG*
   c. belladonna alkaloid and phenobarbital combination
   d. loperamide

7. A patient has been instructed to use an OTC form of the bulk-forming laxative methylcellulose to prevent constipation. The nurse will advise the patient of potential adverse effects, including which of the following? (Select all that apply.)
   a. Fluid and electrolyte disturbances
   b. Decreased absorption of vitamins
   c. Gas formation
   d. Darkened stools
   e. Discoloured urine

Answers: 1. c, 2. d, 3. a, b, c 4. a, 5. b, 6. d, 7. a, c

CRITICAL THINKING ACTIVITIES

1. The nurse is explaining to a group of older adults the importance of seeking treatment for diarrhea. During your discussion with the group, a member asks, "If I have eaten something 'bad,' does it matter if I take something to stop the diarrhea?" What is the nurse's best response, considering the age of the group?

2. A woman calls the clinic because her 4-month-old daughter, who is your patient, has had diarrhea for approximately 8 hours. What is the nurse's priority action at this time?

3. An 88-year-old patient is undergoing a bowel preparation for colonoscopy. What are the nurse's priorities regarding monitoring the patient during the bowel preparation?

For answers, see http://evolve.elsevier.com/Canada/Lilley/pharmacology/.

CHAPTER 41

Antiemetic and Antinausea Drugs

Objectives

After reading this chapter, the successful student will be able to do the following:

1. Discuss the pathophysiology of nausea and vomiting, including specific precipitating factors and diseases.

2. Identify the various antiemetic and antinausea drugs and their drug classification groupings.

3. Identify the mechanisms of action, indications for use, contraindications, cautions, and drug interactions of the antiemetic and antinausea drugs.

4. Develop a collaborative plan of care that includes all phases of the nursing process for patients taking antiemetic and antinausea drugs.

e-Learning Activities

Website
(http://evolve.elsevier.com/Canada/Lilley/pharmacology/)

evolve

- Answer Key—Textbook Case Studies
- Answer Key—Critical Thinking Activities
- Chapter Summaries—Printable
- Review Questions for Exam Preparation
- Unfolding Case Studies

Drug Profiles

aprepitant, p. 780
▸▸ metoclopramide (metoclopramide hydrochloride)*, p. 779
▸▸ ondansetron (ondansetron hydrochloride dihydrate)*, p. 780
▸▸ prochlorperazine, p. 779
promethazine hydrochloride, p. 780
scopolamine, p. 778

▸▸ Key drug

*Full generic name is given in parentheses. For the purposes of this text, the more common, shortened name is used.

Key Terms

Antiemetic drugs Drugs given to relieve nausea and vomiting. (p. 775)

Chemoreceptor trigger zone (CTZ) The area of the brain that is involved in the sensation of nausea and the action of vomiting. (p. 775)

Emesis The forcible emptying or expulsion of gastric and, occasionally, intestinal contents through the mouth; also called *vomiting*. (p. 775)

Nausea Sensation often leading to the urge to vomit. (p. 775)

Vomiting centre (VC) The area of the brain that is involved in stimulating the physiological events that lead to nausea and vomiting. (p. 775)

NAUSEA AND VOMITING

Nausea and vomiting are two gastrointestinal (GI) disorders that can not only be extremely unpleasant but can also lead to more serious complications if not treated promptly. **Nausea** is an unpleasant feeling that often precedes vomiting. If nausea does not subside spontaneously or is not relieved by medication, it can lead to vomiting. Vomiting, which is also called *emesis*, is the forcible emptying or expulsion of gastric and, occasionally, intestinal contents through the mouth. A variety of stimuli can induce nausea and vomiting, including foul odours or tastes, unpleasant sights, irritation of the stomach or intestines, and certain drugs (e.g., antineoplastic drugs, opioids).

The **vomiting centre (VC)** is an area in the brain that is responsible for initiating the physiological events that lead to nausea and vomiting. Neurotransmitter signals are sent to the VC from the **chemoreceptor trigger zone (CTZ)**, another area in the brain involved in the induction of nausea and vomiting. These signals alert these areas of the brain to the existence of nauseating substances (nauseous stimuli) that need to be expelled from the body. Once the CTZ and VC are stimulated, they initiate the events that trigger the vomiting reflex. The neurotransmitters involved in this process and their respective receptors are listed in Table 41-1. The various pathways and the areas of the body that send signals to the vomiting control are illustrated in Figure 41-1. Two specific types of nausea and vomiting, chemotherapy-induced and postoperative, produce much more intense symptoms and are treated much more aggressively than general nausea and vomiting.

ANTIEMETIC AND ANTINAUSEA DRUGS

Drugs used to relieve nausea and vomiting are called **antiemetic drugs**. All antiemetic drugs work at some site in the vomiting pathways. There are six categories of antiemetics, with varying mechanisms of action. When drugs from different categories are combined, antiemetic effectiveness is increased because more than one pathway becomes blocked. Some of the more commonly used antiemetics in the various categories are listed in Table 41-2. The sites at which antiemetics work in the vomiting pathway are shown in Figure 41-2.

Mechanism of Action and Drug Effects

Drugs used to prevent or treat nausea and vomiting have many different mechanisms of action. Most work by blocking one of the vomiting pathways, as shown in Figure 41-2. In doing so, they block the neurological stimulus that induces vomiting. The mechanisms of action of the drugs in the six antiemetic drug categories are summarized in Table 41-3.

Anticholinergic drugs (see Chapter 22) have several uses. As antiemetics, they act by binding to and blocking acetylcholine (ACh) receptors on the vestibular

TABLE	41-1

Neurotransmitters Involved in Nausea and Vomiting

Neurotransmitter	Site in the Vomiting Pathway
Acetylcholine (ACh)	VC in brain; vestibular and labyrinth pathways in inner ear
Dopamine (D_2)	GI and CTZ in brain
Histamine (H_1)	VC in brain; vestibular and labyrinth pathways in inner ear
Prostaglandins (PGs)	GI
Serotonin ($5\text{-}HT_3$)	GI; CTZ and VC in brain

ACh, acetylcholine; *CTZ*, chemoreceptor trigger zone; D_2, dopamine 2 receptor; *GI*, gastrointestinal; H_1, histamine 1 receptor; $5\text{-}HT_3$, 5-hydroxytriptamine 3; *VC*, vomiting centre.

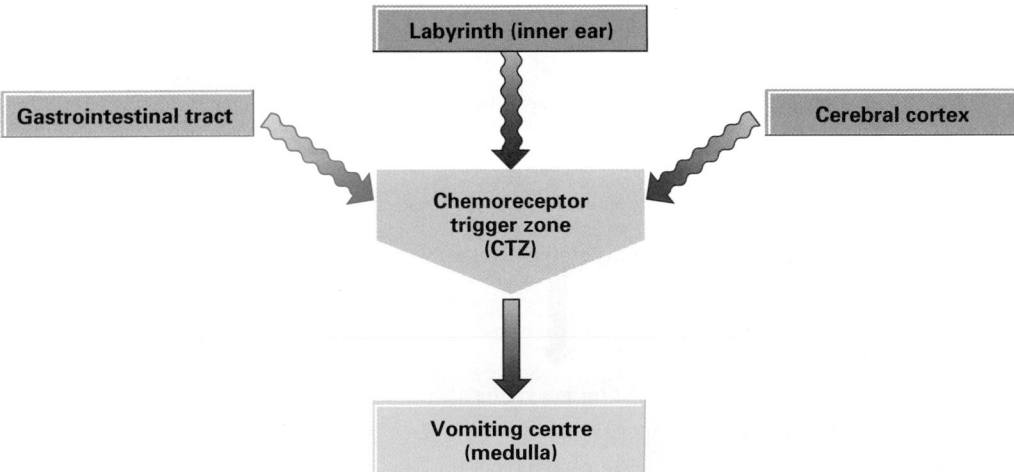

FIG. 41-1   Various pathways and areas in the body sending signals to the vomiting centre.

TABLE 41-2

Antiemetic Drugs: Common Drug Categories and Indications

Category	Antiemetic Drugs	Indications
Anticholinergics (ACh blockers)	scopolamine	Motion sickness, secretion reduction before surgery, nausea and vomiting
Antihistamines (H$_1$ receptor blockers)	dimenhydrinate, diphenhydramine, meclizine	Motion sickness, nonproductive cough, sedation, rhinitis, allergy symptoms, nausea and vomiting
Antidopaminergics	prochlorperazine hydrochloride, promethazine hydrochloride	Psychotic disorders (mania, schizophrenia, anxiety), intractable hiccups, nausea and vomiting
Prokinetics	metoclopramide hydrochloride	Delayed gastric emptying, gastroesophageal reflux, nausea and vomiting
Serotonin blockers	granisetron hydrochloride, ondansetron hydrochloride dihydrate, palonosetron hydrochloride	Nausea and vomiting associated with chemotherapy, postoperative nausea and vomiting
Tetrahydrocannabinol	Marihuana	Nausea and vomiting associated with chemotherapy, anorexia associated with weight loss in patients with AIDS and cancer

ACh, acetylcholine.

TABLE 41-3

Antiemetic Drugs: Mechanisms of Action

Category	Mechanism of Action
Anticholinergics	Block ACh receptors in the vestibular nuclei and reticular formation
Antihistamines	Block H$_1$ receptors, thereby preventing ACh from binding to receptors in the vestibular nuclei
Neuroleptics	Block dopamine in the CTZ and may also block ACh
Prokinetics	Block dopamine in the CTZ or stimulate ACh receptors in the GI tract
Serotonin blockers	Block serotonin receptors in the GI tract, CTZ, and VC
Tetrahydrocannabinol	Have inhibitory effects on the reticular formation, thalamus, and cerebral cortex

ACh, Acetylcholine; *H$_1$*, histamine-1; *CTZ*, chemoreceptor trigger zone; *GI*, gastrointestinal; *VC*, vomiting centre.

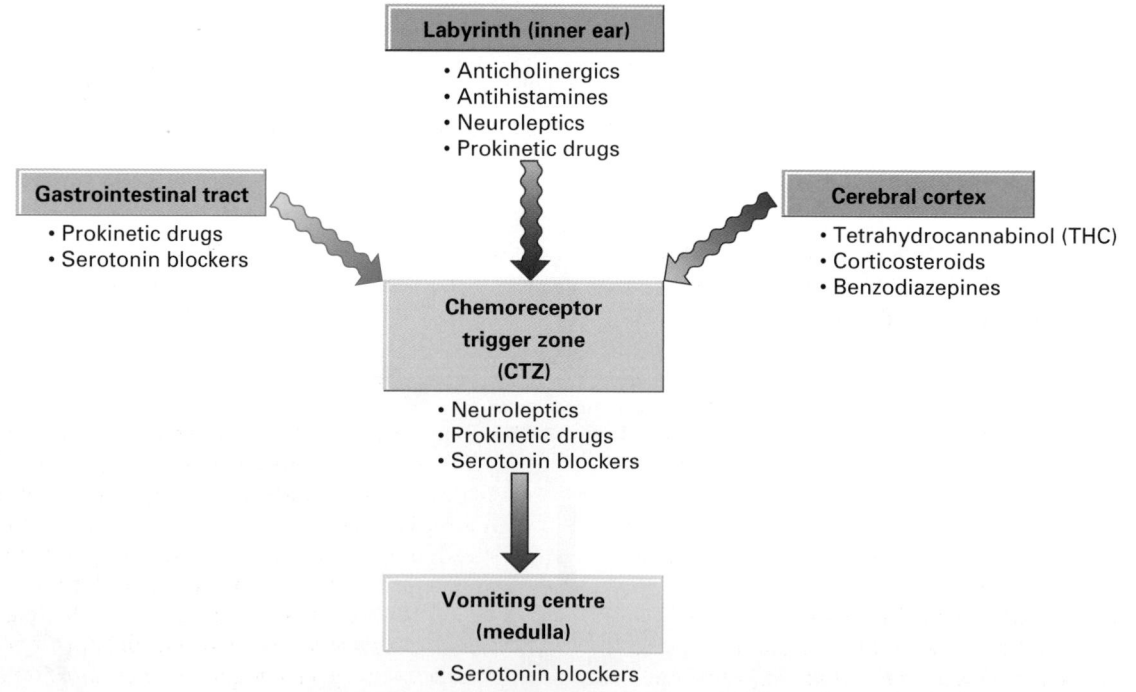

FIG. 41-2 Sites of action of selected antinausea drugs.

nuclei, which are located deep within the brain. When ACh is prevented from binding to these receptors, nausea-inducing signals originating in this area cannot be transmitted to the CTZ. Anticholinergics also block receptors located in the reticular formation and thus prevent ACh from binding to these receptors. This then prevents nausea-inducing signals originating in this area from being transmitted to the VC. Anticholinergics also tend to dry GI secretions and reduce smooth muscle spasms; both of these effects are often helpful in reducing acute GI symptoms, including nausea and vomiting.

Antihistamines (histamine-1 [H$_1$] receptor blockers) act by inhibiting vestibular stimulation in a manner similar to that of anticholinergics. Although they bind primarily to H$_1$ receptors, they also have potent anticholinergic activity, including antisecretory and antispasmodic effects. Thus the antihistamines (see Chapter 37) prevent cholinergic stimulation in both the vestibular and reticular systems. Nausea and vomiting occur when these systems are stimulated. Note that these drugs are not to be confused with histamine-2 (H$_2$) receptor blockers used for gastric acid control (see Chapter 39).

Antidopaminergic drugs, although they are traditionally used for their antipsychotic effects (see Chapter 17), also prevent nausea and vomiting by blocking dopamine receptors in the CTZ. Many of the antidopaminergics also have anticholinergic actions similar to those of anticholinergic drugs. In addition, antidopaminergic drugs calm the central nervous system (CNS).

Prokinetic drugs, in particular metoclopramide, act as antiemetics by blocking dopamine receptors in the CTZ, which desensitizes the CTZ to impulses it receives from the GI tract. Their primary action, however, is to stimulate peristalsis in the GI tract. This action enhances the emptying of stomach contents into the duodenum as well as intestinal movements.

Serotonin blockers work by blocking serotonin receptors located in the GI tract, CTZ, and vomiting centre. There are many subtypes of serotonin receptors, and these receptors are located throughout the body (CNS, smooth muscles, platelets, GI tract). The receptor subtype involved in the mediation of nausea and vomiting is the 5-hydroxytryptamine 3 (5-HT3) receptor. These receptors are the sites of action for the serotonin blockers such as ondansetron, palonosetron, and granisetron.

Tetrahydrocannabinol (THC), in a drug class by itself, is the major psychoactive substance in marihuana. The drug is occasionally used as an antiemetic because of its inhibitory effects on the reticular formation, thalamus, and cerebral cortex. These effects cause an alteration in mood and the body's perception of its surroundings, which may be beneficial in relieving nausea and vomiting. There are occasionally unusual cases of nausea and vomiting that respond well to THC; examples include patients being treated for cancer or AIDS who experience nausea and vomiting. In such patients, marihuana may also stimulate the appetite, as nutritional wasting syndromes are common in both diseases. The drug also demonstrates some benefit in controlling the symptoms of glaucoma. The pharmaceutical formation of THC, dronabinol and nabilone, is no longer available in Canada. There is a large, but highly controversial, political movement that is in favour of legalizing the marihuana plant for these uses. Currently, the federal government must provide reasonable access to a legal source of marijuana for medical purposes, including oils, fresh marihuana buds, and leaves, which are produced for sale by licensed medicinal producers. Medical marihuana may be delivered in a variety of methods that include smoking, vaporization, ingestion of marihuana-infused edibles, and hash oils. As discussed in Chapter 3, the main component responsible for the psychoactive effects is delta-9-tetrahydrocannabinol or THC. Other chemicals such as cannibal and cannabidol possess fewer mood-altering effects. When smoked or ingested, the psychoactive components attach to the cannabinoid receptors in the brain, CB1 and CB2, particularly in the areas involving body movement, memory, and vomiting. Peak effects after smoking marihuana occur in minutes and last for up to 2 hours; when ingested, its effects may linger for hours but the absorption may be unpredictable.

Indications

The therapeutic uses of antiemetic drugs vary depending on their drug category. There are several indications for the drugs in each class. These indications are listed in Table 41-2.

Contraindications

The primary contraindication for all antiemetics is known drug allergy. Other contraindications for specific drugs are mentioned in the drug profiles.

Adverse Effects

Most of the adverse effects of the antiemetics stem from their nonselective blockade of various receptors. Some of the more common adverse effects associated with the various categories of antinausea drugs are listed in Table 41-4.

Interactions

The drug interactions associated with the antiemetic drugs are specific to the individual drug categories. Anticholinergics have additive drying effects when given with antihistamines and antidepressants. Increased CNS effects are seen when antihistamine antiemetics are administered with barbiturates, opioids, hypnotics, tricyclic antidepressants, or alcohol. Increased CNS depression effects are seen when alcohol or other CNS depressants are given together with antidopaminergic drugs. Combining metoclopramide with alcohol can result in additive CNS depression. Anticholinergics and analgesics can block the motility effects of metoclopramide. Serotonin blockers and THC have no significant drug interactions.

Dosages

For dosage information on selected antiemetic drugs, refer to the table on p. 782.

NURSING PROCESS

◪ Assessment

Nurses play a crucial role in the assessment and management of nausea and vomiting. To improve the patient's

TABLE	41-4

Antinausea Drugs: Adverse Effects

Body System	Adverse Effects
ANTICHOLINERGICS	
Central nervous	Dizziness, drowsiness, disorientation
Cardiovascular	Tachycardia
Ears, eyes, nose, throat	Blurred vision, dilated pupils, dry mouth
Genitourinary	Difficult urination, constipation
Integumentary	Rash, erythema
ANTIHISTAMINES	
Central nervous	Dizziness, drowsiness, confusion
Ears, eyes, nose, throat	Blurred vision, dilated pupils, dry mouth
Genitourinary	Urinary retention
ANTIDOPAMINERGICS	
Cardiovascular	Orthostatic hypotension, tachycardia
Central nervous	Extrapyramidal symptoms, tardive dyskinesia, headache
Ears, eyes, nose, throat	Blurred vision, dry eyes
Gastrointestinal	Dry mouth, nausea and vomiting, anorexia, constipation
Genitourinary	Urinary retention
PROKINETICS	
Cardiovascular	Hypotension, supraventricular tachycardia
Central nervous	Sedation, fatigue, restlessness, headache, dystonia
Gastrointestinal	Dry mouth, nausea and vomiting, diarrhea
SEROTONIN BLOCKERS	
Central nervous	Headache
Gastrointestinal	Diarrhea
Other	Rash, bronchospasm, prolonged QT interval
TETRAHYDROCANNABINOL	
Central nervous	Drowsiness, dizziness, anxiety, confusion, euphoria
Ears, eyes, nose, throat	Visual disturbances
Gastrointestinal	Dry mouth

 DRUG PROFILES

Antiemetics are used to treat nausea and vomiting in a variety of clinical situations, including chemotherapy-induced and postoperative nausea and vomiting, both of which can be especially difficult to treat. The ultimate goals of antiemetic therapy are minimizing or preventing fluid and electrolyte disturbances and minimizing deterioration of the patient's nutritional status. Most of the antiemetics act by blocking receptors in the CNS, but some work directly in the GI tract. There are six major classes of antiemetic drugs, although there are other drugs that may also be used to treat nausea and vomiting, including corticosteroids such as dexamethasone (see Chapter 34) and anxiolytics such as lorazepam (see Chapter 17). Dexamethasone, lorazepam, and THC are beneficial in treating and preventing nausea and vomiting

caused by chemotherapy, especially when used in combination with the serotonin blockers. Lorazepam in particular is often used during chemotherapy because, in addition to its antiemetic effect, it also helps blunt the memory of the nausea and vomiting experience.

ANTICHOLINERGICS

scopolamine

Scopolamine hydrobromide is the primary anticholinergic drug used as an antiemetic. It has potent effects on the vestibular nuclei, which are within the area of the brain that controls balance. Scopolamine hydrobromide works by blocking the binding of ACh to the cholinergic receptors in this region, thereby correcting an imbalance between the

DRUG PROFILES—cont'd

neurotransmitters ACh and norepinephrine. Scopolamine hydrobromide is used to treat postoperative nausea and vomiting. Use of the drug is contraindicated in patients with glaucoma. Scopolamine is available in injectable form.

PHARMACOKINETICS

Route	Onset of Action	Peak Plasma Concentration	Elimination Half-Life	Duration of Action
IM	30–60 min	1–2 hr	9.5 hr	4–6 hr

ANTIHISTAMINES

Antihistamine antiemetics are some of the most commonly used and safest antiemetics. Two popular antihistamines are dimenhydrinate (Dinate®, Gravol®, Nauseatol®, others) and diphenhydramine hydrochloride (Aller-Aide®, Allernix®, Benadryl®, others). Many of the antihistamines are available over the counter. Hydroxyzine hydrochloride is used for antiemetic purposes and is available in oral and intramuscular formulations. Hydroxyzine hydrochloride must never be given by the intravenous (IV) route (see the Preventing Medication Errors Box on p. 781). Meclizine hydrochloride, another antihistamine, is no longer being manufactured in Canada.

ANTIDOPAMINERGIC

Prochlorperazine (Prochlorazine®) and promethazine hydrochloride (Histantil®) are the most commonly used antiemetics in the antidopaminergic class. These drugs have antidopaminergic as well as antihistaminergic and anticholinergic properties. Droperidol was one of the most commonly used drugs in the treatment and prevention of postoperative nausea and vomiting for several decades, until Health Canada called for a label warning and required continuous electrocardiographic monitoring with its use. These restrictions were in response to concerns over QT widening and possible ventricular dysrhythmias. Some institutions still use droperidol, whereas others have banned its use. Haloperidol, an antipsychotic, is a dopamine2-receptor antagonist that may also be used as an antiemetic, although data is limited about this area of use.

▶▶ *prochlorperazine*

Prochlorperazine (Proclorazine), particularly in its injectable form, is used frequently in the hospital setting. This drug is contraindicated in patients with hypersensitivity to phenothiazines, those in a coma, and those who have seizures, encephalopathy, or bone marrow depression. It is available for both injection and oral use.

PHARMACOKINETICS

Route	Onset of Action	Peak Plasma Concentration	Elimination Half-Life	Duration of Action
IM	30–40 min	2–4 hr	6–8 hr	3–4 hr

promethazine

Promethazine (Histanil®) is commonly used in hospitalized patients as an antiemetic. The preferred route is oral or intramuscular. The IV route is not a preferred route but is commonly used. However, extreme care must be taken to avoid accidental intra-arterial injection. If promethazine is inadvertently given intra-arterially instead of intravenously, severe tissue damage, often requiring amputation, can occur. The preferred parenteral route of administration for promethazine hydrochloride injection is by deep intramuscular injection. If administered intravenously, the drug is to be given in a concentration no greater than 25 mg per mL and at a rate not to exceed 25 mg per minute. It is best given in a running IV line at the port furthest from the patient's vein or through a large-bore vein (not a hand or wrist vein). Therapy must be discontinued immediately if burning or pain occurs with administration. Promethazine is contraindicated in children younger than 2 years of age. Sedation is the most common adverse effect and actually may be beneficial. Promethazine is not to be given subcutaneously. For more information, see the Preventing Medication Errors Box on p. 781.

PHARMACOKINETICS

Route	Onset of Action	Peak Plasma Concentration	Elimination Half-Life	Duration of Action
IM	20 min	4.4 hr	9–16 hr	2–6 hr

PROKINETICS

Prokinetic drugs promote the movement of substances through the GI tract and increase GI motility. The only prokinetic drug that is also used to prevent nausea and vomiting is metoclopramide.

▶▶ *metoclopramide hydrochloride*

Metoclopramide hydrochloride (Metonia®, Metoclopramide OMEGA®) is available only by prescription because it can cause some severe adverse effects if not used correctly. Metoclopramide is used for the treatment of delayed gastric emptying and gastroesophageal reflux and also as an antiemetic; specifically, metoclopramide OMEGA is indicated for prophylaxis of postoperative vomiting and vomiting associated with cancer chemotherapeutic regimens that include cisplatin as a component. Its use is contraindicated in patients with seizure disorders, pheochromocytoma, breast cancer, or GI obstruction, and also in patients with a hypersensitivity to it or to procaine or procainamide hydrochloride. Metoclopramide is available in both oral and parenteral formulations. Extrapyramidal adverse effects can occur with its use, especially in older adults, and older women in particular. In 2011, Health Canada informed health care providers and consumers of updated labelling for metoclopramide regarding its potential to cause the development of tardive dyskinesia with long-term use (longer than 12 weeks).

PHARMACOKINETICS

Route	Onset of Action	Peak Plasma Concentration	Elimination Half-Life	Duration of Action
PO	20–60 min	1–2.5 hr	2.5–6 hr	3–4 hr

SEROTONIN BLOCKERS

The serotonin blockers are also called *5-HT3 receptor blockers* because they block the 5-HT3 receptors in the GI

Continued

DRUG PROFILES—cont'd

tract, CTZ, and VC. (The chemical name for serotonin is 5-hydroxytryptamine [5-HT]). Drugs in this class have specific actions, and as a result they have few adverse effects. No significant drug interactions are known to occur with the use of serotonin blockers. These drugs are indicated for the prevention of nausea and vomiting associated with cancer chemotherapy and also for the prevention of postoperative or radiation-induced nausea and vomiting. Currently, there are three drugs in this category: granisetron hydrochloride (Kytril®), palonosetron (Aloxi®), and ondansetron (Zofran®). This class of drugs revolutionized the treatment of nausea and vomiting, especially in patients with cancer and postoperative patients. When used to prevent postoperative nausea and vomiting, a dose is usually given approximately 30 minutes before the end of the surgical procedure. When used to prevent or treat nausea and vomiting associated with cancer treatment, the drug is given in the first 24 to 48 hours of chemotherapy. In 2014, Health Canada issued a warning regarding ondansetron and its associated risk of dysrhythmias; this risk is expected to be greater when it is administered intravenously, with faster rates of infusion and larger doses. Efficacy and tolerance is similar in both older and younger adults; thus, there is no need to alter dosage schedules for older adult patients.

▶ondansetron hydrochloride dihydrate

Ondansetron hydrochloride dihydrate (Zofran) is the prototypical drug in its class. Approved in 1991, it represented a major breakthrough in treating chemotherapy-induced nausea and vomiting and, later, postoperative nausea and vomiting. It is also used for the treatment of hyperemesis gravidarum (nausea and vomiting associated with pregnancy). Its only listed contraindication is known drug allergy. It is available in both oral (tablets, solution, disintegrating tablet) and injectable forms. Doses up to 8 mg can be given by IV push over 2 to 5 minutes. Ondansetron was the first of the serotonin blockers to become available as a generic formulation, which significantly increased its use.

PHARMACOKINETICS

Route	Onset of Action	Peak Plasma Concentration	Elimination Half-Life	Duration of Action
IV	15–30 min	1–1.5 hr	3.5–5 hr	6–12 hr

TETRAHYDROCANNABINOL

THC is the major active substance in marihuana. It may be used for the treatment of nausea and vomiting associated with cancer chemotherapy and to stimulate appetite and weight gain in patients with AIDS.

PHARMACOKINETICS

Route	Onset of Action	Peak Plasma Concentration	Elimination Half-Life	Duration of Action
Inhaled	minutes	Unknown	Unknown	Unknown

MISCELLANEOUS ANTINAUSEA DRUGS

aprepitant

Aprepitant (Emend®) is the first in a new class of antiemetic drugs, approved in 2007. It is an antagonist of substance P–neurokinin-1 receptors in the brain. In contrast to other antiemetics, this drug has little affinity for 5-HT$_3$ (serotonin) and dopamine receptors. Studies show that aprepitant augments the antiemetic actions of both ondansetron and the corticosteroid dexamethasone. This drug is specifically indicated for the prevention of nausea and vomiting in highly and moderately emetogenic cancer chemotherapy regimens, including high-dose cisplatin, as well as postoperative nausea and vomiting. Common adverse effects include dizziness, headache, insomnia, and GI discomfort, but these are generally no more common than with other standard antiemetic regimens. Aprepitant may induce the metabolism of warfarin sodium, and the international normalized ratio (INR) needs to be checked before each cycle of aprepitant. The drug may reduce the effectiveness of oral contraceptives. Because aprepitant is a major inhibitor of the cytochrome P450 enzyme system, caution must be used in giving it together with drugs that are primarily metabolized by cytochrome P450 enzyme 3A4, including azole antifungals, clarithromycin, diltiazem, nicardipine, protease inhibitors, and verapamil. It may increase the bioavailability of corticosteroids, including dexamethasone and methylprednisolone, and dosages of these drugs may need to be adjusted by 25 to 50%.

doxylamine succinate and pyridoxine hydrochloride

Doxylamine succinate and pyridoxine hydrochloride (Diclectin®) delayed-release tablets combine the action of two unrelated compounds. Doxylamine succinate, an antihistamine, and pyridoxine hydrochloride (vitamin B6) provide both antinausea and antiemetic effects. The drug is indicated for the management of nausea and vomiting during pregnancy. Optimal effects of the drug occur when the drug is given 4 to 6 hours prior to the anticipated onset of symptoms. The delayed action of Diclectin permits the nighttime dose to be effective in the morning hours, when nausea occurs most frequently. The suggested recommended dosage for control of nausea is two tablets at bedtime, one tablet in the morning, and another mid-afternoon; however, this schedule should be individualized to each patient's requirements. The drug should be slowly tapered when discontinued to prevent return of symptoms.

This drug is contraindicated in patients who are hypersensitive to doxylamine succinate, other ethanolamine derivative antihistamines, pyridoxine hydrochloride, or any nonmedicinal ingredient in the formulation. It is also not recommended for those at risk for asthmatic attack, patients with narrow angle glaucoma, stenosing peptic ulcer, pyloroduodenal obstruction, or bladder-neck obstruction, or those who are taking monoamine oxidase inhibitors. It should not be taken concurrently with other medications or alcohol due to the antihistamine properties of doxylamine. This drug is also prone to misuse. Doxylamine may cause drowsiness as well as vertigo, nervousness, epigastric pain, headaches, palpitations, diarrhea, disorientation, irritability, convulsions, urinary retention, or insomnia. Pyridoxine is a vitamin and as such is well tolerated and has no adverse effects.

PREVENTING MEDICATION ERRORS

Right Route Is Essential

Two commonly used antiemetic drugs may have serious consequences for patients if they are given via the wrong route.

Hydroxyzine hydrochloride is an antihistamine-class antiemetic that is only to be given either by oral or intramuscular routes. However, as so many other antiemetics are given by the IV route, it may be easy to make the mistake of giving hydroxyzine hydrochloride intravenously. It is important to note that IV, intra-arterial, or subcutaneous administration of hydroxyzine hydrochlor-

ide may result in significant tissue damage, thrombosis, and gangrene.

Promethazine hydrochloride (Histantil) is another commonly used antiemetic. The oral and intramuscular routes are the preferred routes of administration for this drug; the IV route, while commonly used, is not the preferred route. If this drug is given intra-arterially, severe tissue damage, possibly leading to amputation, may occur.

These are just two examples that illustrate the importance of the "right route" with drug administration.

experience, nurses need to have the necessary instruments available to help them assess each symptom in a timely manner. Early and accurate assessment can promote the development of timely, patient-specific interventions and minimize the symptom experience.

Before any antinausea or antiemetic drug is administered, assess intake and output; examine the skin and mucous membranes, noting turgor and colour; and assess and document capillary refill (normal is less than 5 seconds). If laboratory tests are ordered (e.g., serum sodium, potassium, and chloride levels; hemoglobin level and hematocrit; red and white blood cell counts; urinalysis), assess and document the findings to establish baseline levels. Assess for any contraindications or cautions to the use of these drugs and for drug interactions, as well as any allergies. See Natural Health Products: Ginger.

Give the anticholinergic drug scopolamine only after careful assessment of a patient's health history and medication history. This drug is contraindicated in patients with a hypersensitivity to it and in those with glaucoma. If the patient has a history of narrow-angle glaucoma, use another antiemetic or antinausea drug. The same concern regarding use in patients with narrow-angle glaucoma applies to antihistamines; in addition, use antihistamines cautiously in children, who may have severe paradoxical reactions. Older adults may develop agitation, mental confusion, hypotension, and even psychotic-type reactions in response to these drugs. Other medications need to be considered for patients if these reactions occur.

Antidopaminergic drugs such as prochlorperazine are to be used only after cautious assessment for signs and symptoms of dehydration and electrolyte imbalance, through evaluation of skin turgor and of the tongue for the presence of longitudinal furrows. Monitor vital signs, especially blood pressure and pulse rate, due to this drug's adverse effects of orthostatic hypotension and tachycardia. CNS concerns for which to assess include any abnormal movements at baseline functioning, because these drugs can lead to adverse effects of extrapyramidal symptoms. Contraindications, cautions, and drug interactions for these drugs were discussed earlier.

Double-checking the name and mechanism of action is also important, as prochlorperazine may be confused with promethazine hydrochloride.

The prokinetic drug metoclopramide is often reserved for the treatment of nausea and vomiting associated with antineoplastic drug therapy or radiation therapy and for the treatment of GI motility disturbances. Metoclopramide is titrated to maximum benefit and tolerance. If the drug is not effective, add or switch to another dopamine antagonist (e.g., haloperidol). The action of this drug is decreased when it is taken with anticholinergics or opiates; therefore, assess for this interaction. Remember the Health Canada public health advisory regarding adverse reactions with long-term use (see previous discussion).

Give the serotonin blocker granisetron only after assessment of baseline vital signs and determination of age (its safety in children younger than 2 years of age has not been established). Ondansetron requires assessment for the signs and symptoms of dehydration and electrolyte disturbances. Assess skin turgor and examine mucous membranes for dryness and the tongue for longitudinal furrows.

Nursing Diagnoses

- Nausea related to disease pathology or adverse effects of specific groups of medications
- Impaired physical mobility related to adverse effects (e.g., sedation, lethargy, confusion) of antiemetics
- Risk for injury (falls) related to the adverse effects of the antiemetic medications (e.g., sedation and dizziness)
- Risk for deficient fluid volume related to nausea and vomiting and limited oral intake

Planning

Goals

- Patient will remain free from weakness and dizziness with use of pharmacological and nonpharmacological therapies.

DOSAGES	Selected Antiemetic and Antinausea Drugs		
Drug	**Pharmacological Class**	**Usual Dosage Range**	**Indications**
Anticholinergics			
scopolamine hydrobromide injection	Anticholinergic, belladonna alkaloid	*Children* IM, IV, Subcut: 0.006 mg/kg q6h *Adults* IM, IV, Subcut: 0.3–0.6 mg tid–qid	Antiemetic
Antihistamines			
▶meclizine hydrochloride (Bonamine®)	Anticholinergic, antihistamine	*Adults* PO: 25–50 mg 1 hr before travel and repeated daily during travel PO: 25–100 mg/day, divided	Motion sickness prophylaxis Treatment of vertigo
Antidopaminergics			
▶prochlorperazine (Prochlorazine)	Phenothiazine	*Children* Dosages vary based on weight and age *Adults* PO/rectal: 5–10 mg tid–qid IM/IV: 5–10 mg bid–tid	Antiemetic
promethazine hydrochloride (Histantil)	Phenothiazine	*Children over 2 yr* PO, IM, IV: 6.25–12.5 mg *Adults* PO, IM, IV: 12.5–25 mg	Antiemetic
Prokinetics			
▶metoclopramide hydrochloride (Metonia, metoclopramide OMEGA)	Dopamine antagonist	*Children 5–14 yr* IV: single dose 0.1 mg/kg *Adults* IV: 1–2 mg/kg (30 min before chemotherapy; repeat q2h × 2 doses, then q3h × 3 doses) IM: 10–20 mg × 1 dose near end of surgery	Chemotherapy antiemetic Chemotherapy antiemetic Prevention of postoperative nausea and vomiting
Serotonin Blockers			
▶ondansetron hydrochloride dihydrate (Zofran)	Antiserotonergic	*Children 4–12 yr* PO: 4 mg tid, after chemotherapy, × up to 5 days IV: 3–5 mg/m^2 over 15 min, immediately before chemotherapy, then oral as above *Adults* PO: 8 mg bid up to 5 days after the initial 24-hr IV dose IV: 8–16 mg over 15 min, given 30 min before chemotherapy, followed by 1 mg/hr continuous infusion up to 24 hr, or one dose of 32 mg over 15 min, given 30 min before chemotherapy PO: 16 mg, 1 hr before surgery IV: 4 mg over 2–5 min × 1 dose (second dose not shown to be effective in patients who fail first dose)	Chemotherapy antiemetic Chemotherapy antiemetic Prevention and treatment of postoperative nausea

IM, intramuscular; *IV*, intravenous; *PO*, oral; *Subcut*, subcutaneous.

- Patient will regain previous mobility status or maintain stable mobility during drug therapy.
- Patient will remain free from injury during drug therapy with antiemetics.
- Patient will maintain or regain fluid volume balance while undergoing treatment.

■ Expected Patient Outcomes Criteria

- Patient states specific rationales for reducing nausea and vomiting through use of antiemetic drug therapy as well as specific nondrug measures.
  - Patient states action of a specific antiemetic drug, its specific dosage, and the best time to take the

NATURAL HEALTH PRODUCTS

GINGER *(Zingiber officinale)*

Overview

Found naturally in the Asian tropics; now cultivated in other continents, including parts of the United States, and grown commercially in Canada; plant parts used are the rhizome and root; active ingredients include gingerols and gingerdione

Common Uses

Used as an antioxidant; also used for relief of various symptoms such as sore throat, migraine headaches, and nausea and vomiting (including that induced by cancer chemotherapy, morning sickness, and motion sickness); many other varied uses

Adverse Effects

Skin reactions, anorexia, nausea, vomiting

Potential Drug Interactions

Can increase absorption of all oral medications; may theoretically increase bleeding risk with anticoagulants (e.g., warfarin sodium [Coumadin®]) or antiplatelet drugs (e.g., clopidogrel [Plavix®])

Contraindications

Contraindicated in cases of known product allergy; may worsen cholelithiasis (gallstones); anecdotal evidence of abortifacient properties—some clinicians recommend avoiding use during pregnancy

Dosage

Available as a capsule; recommended dosage is 1 to 2 capsules per day or as recommended by a health care provider

drug; patient also identifies related adverse effects such as sedation, dizziness, and dry mouth.

- Patient states specific measures to decrease nausea and vomiting, such as avoiding irritating, spicy foods and beverages and possibly avoiding fluids and food until nausea and vomiting subside (but prior to becoming dehydrated).
- Patient states signs and symptoms of dehydration that should be reported to the health care provider if they occur, such as dry mouth, decrease in urinary output, decreased to no intake of fluids, lethargy, weakness, and dizziness.
- Patient increases physical mobility and activity, with assistance if needed, by 10 to 15 minutes per day with cautious movements, incorporating changing of positions, rising, walking, and performing activities of daily living.
- Patient states measures to implement to prevent injury, such as obtaining assistance while ill, rising slowly, changing positions slowly, taking medications as ordered, and initiating fluid intake once nausea and vomiting subside.
- Patient states measures to implement to prevent further fluid volume deficits, such as consumption of oral fluids (e.g., clear liquids) or chilled gelatin along with medications.

Implementation

Early intervention and prevention (avoiding triggers) are key approaches to managing nausea and vomiting. Nonpharmacological interventions can be used to supplement pharmacological treatment of nausea and vomiting. For example, patients should avoid foods that provoke nausea; avoid spicy, salty, and fatty foods or foods with a strong odour; eat small, frequent, bland meals every 1 to 2 hours; avoid mixing liquids and solid foods (e.g., eat a small portion of food, wait 20 to 30 minutes, then take

some liquid); try cool, carbonated drinks, and avoid lying flat after eating.

Many agencies follow a best practice algorithm to treat nausea and vomiting. In general, the effectiveness of antiemetic drugs varies among patients. Usually, antiemetics are selected according to etiology (e.g., postoperative, chemotherapy, palliation). If nausea is not controlled, the drug is individually titrated to its full dose (or smallest effective dose without adverse effects). If a drug is ineffective, another drug from another class that targets a different receptor is added. It is usual to add drugs, not substitute drugs, as there may be additive effects. Continuous medication may be more effective. For persistent nausea and vomiting, antiemetics should be prescribed on a regular dosing schedule with a breakthrough dose available. Multiple drug combinations in high doses may be needed. Antiemetics may also be administered prophylactically to prevent nausea related to the use of high dose opioids and chemotherapeutic drugs.

Undiluted forms of diphenhydramine hydrochloride must be cautiously administered intravenously, at the recommended rate of 25 mg/min. Intramuscular forms should be administered into large muscles (e.g., gluteus medius), and sites should be rotated if repeated injections are necessary. Promethazine hydrochloride may be given orally without regard to meals; parenteral doses should be given using the proper dilutional solutions and infusion rates. Measure vital signs and monitor patients for extrapyramidal symptoms throughout therapy. Encourage patients to avoid other CNS depressants and alcohol as well as to limit caffeine when this drug is used. Instruct patients taking promethazine to avoid driving and other activities that require mental alertness or precise coordination.

Metoclopramide should be given orally 30 minutes before meals and at bedtime. Infuse IV dosage forms over the recommended time period. For doses in excess of 10 mg, metoclopramide needs to be diluted in 50 mL of either 5% dextrose or 0.9% sodium chloride. Except for prophylaxis of vomiting induced by anticancer drugs, the total daily dosage must not exceed 0.5 mg/kg body weight. Inject the infusion slowly over a 15-minute period and repeat the dose every 2 hours for two doses, and then every 3 hours for three doses. In addition, keep solutions for parenteral dosing for only 24 hours and protect them from light. Metoclopramide should not be given to patients with epilepsy or in combination with any other medications such as phenothiazines that would lead to exacerbation of extrapyramidal reactions. Such reactions should be reported immediately to the health care provider. The development of tardive dyskinesia, an involuntary neurological movement disorder, has been associated with the long-term use of metoclopramide. Monitor for this potential problem and educate patients about it.

Granisetron hydrochloride may be given intravenously or orally. Infuse IV doses over the recommended time frame and dilute as appropriate. A transient taste disorder may occur, especially if the drug is taken with antineoplastic medications, but will diminish with continued therapy. Encourage the use of various relaxation techniques as complementary therapies. Ondansetron may be given orally, intramuscularly, or intravenously. Inject intramuscular doses into a large muscle mass. IV push is usually given over 2 to 5 minutes and infusions over 15 minutes, as ordered and per manufacturer guidelines. Oral forms are well tolerated regardless of the relation of dosing to meals. Encourage patients to avoid alcohol and other CNS depressants during this therapy and to avoid any activities requiring mental alertness or precise coordination. Antiemetics are usually given 30 to 60 minutes before chemotherapy, depending on the specific drug. Ondansetron is usually given 30 minutes before chemotherapy. Aprepitant is often used in combination with other medications to prevent nausea and vomiting associated with chemotherapy and is given, as ordered, for postoperative nausea and vomiting. The health care provider's orders may indicate other drugs to be administered as well as the timing of the dosage. Oral dosage forms are to be given as ordered.

▦ Evaluation

The therapeutic effects of antiemetic and antinausea drugs include a decrease in or elimination of nausea and vomiting, and avoidance or elimination of complications such as fluid and electrolyte imbalances and weight loss. Monitor patients for adverse effects such as GI upset, drowsiness, lethargy, weakness, extrapyramidal effects, and orthostatic hypotension during antiemetic treatment. Laboratory testing (e.g., electrolyte levels, blood urea nitrogen level, urinalysis with specific gravity) may be ordered for evaluation purposes. Defined goals and outcomes may also be used to evaluate therapeutic effectiveness.

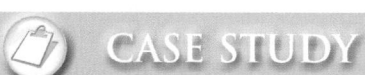 **CASE STUDY**

Nausea Associated With Chemotherapy

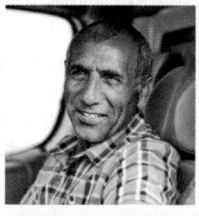 Scott, a 65-year-old retired bus driver, has started outpatient chemotherapy for a recent diagnosis of lung cancer. He has recovered well from a right lung lobectomy, the incisions are healing well, and he is now physically and emotionally ready for a 3-month regimen of chemotherapy. The premedication consists of a variety of drugs, including granisetron hydrochloride (Kytril). Scott has a prescription for oral ondansetron (Zofran) for use at home.

1. What is the mechanism of action of granisetron hydrochloride that makes it effective in the management of chemotherapy-induced nausea and vomiting?

2. What important patient teaching points regarding ondansetron should you emphasize to Scott?

3. After 2 weeks of therapy, the oncologist discontinues the ondansetron because Scott complains that it does nothing to help his nausea and vomiting. A friend suggests the use of marihuana but Scott expresses concern about this strategy. What would you explain to him?

For answers, see http://evolve.elsevier.com/Canada/Lilley/pharmacology/.

PATIENT TEACHING TIPS

❖ Warn patients using an antiemetic or antinausea drug about the adverse effect of drowsiness, and instruct the patient to use caution when performing hazardous tasks or driving while taking these drugs. Caution patients about taking antiemetic or antinausea drugs with alcohol and other CNS depressants because of possible toxicity and exacerbation of CNS depression.

❖ Educate patients about the possible adverse effects of ondansetron, including headache, which may be relieved with a simple analgesic (e.g., acetaminophen).

KEY POINTS

❖ Antiemetics help to control vomiting, or emesis, and are also useful in relieving or preventing nausea. Antiemetics are used to prevent motion sickness, reduce secretions before surgery, treat delayed gastric emptying, and prevent postoperative nausea and vomiting. Most of these drugs can cause drowsiness.

❖ Anticholinergics act by blocking ACh receptors in the vestibular nuclei and reticular formation. This blockade prevents areas in the brain from being activated by nauseous stimuli.

❖ Antihistamines act by blocking H₁ receptors, which produces the same effect as the anticholinergics do. Antidopaminergic antiemetics block dopamine receptors in the CTZ and may also block ACh receptors.

Prokinetic drugs also block dopamine receptors in the CTZ.

❖ Serotonin blockers (granisetron hydrochloride and ondansetron) may be highly effective antiemetics. They are most commonly used for the prevention of chemotherapy-induced nausea and vomiting.

❖ Antiemetics are often given 30 to 60 minutes before a chemotherapy drug is administered (time may vary depending on the specific drug) and may also be given during the chemotherapeutic treatment.

❖ Caution patients taking antiemetic or antinausea drugs that drowsiness and hypotension may occur and to avoid driving and using heavy machinery while taking these medications.

EXAMINATION REVIEW QUESTIONS

1. A 33-year-old patient is in an outpatient cancer centre for his first round of chemotherapy. The nurse knows that which schedule is the most appropriate timing for the IV antiemetic drug?
   a. 4 hours before the chemotherapy begins
   b. 30 minutes before the chemotherapy begins
   c. At the same time as the chemotherapy drugs
   d. At the first sign of nausea
2. When reviewing the various types of antinausea medications, the nurse recognizes that prokinetic drugs are also used for which disorder?
   a. Motion sickness
   b. Vertigo
   c. Delayed gastric emptying
   d. GI obstruction
3. A patient who has been receiving chemotherapy tells the nurse that he has been searching the Internet for antinausea remedies and that he found a reference to a product called aprepitant. He wants to know if this drug would help him. What would be the nurse's best answer?

   a. "This may be a good remedy for you. Let's talk to your health care provider."
   b. "This drug is used only after other drugs have not worked."
   c. "This drug is used only to treat severe nausea and vomiting caused by chemotherapy."
   d. "This drug may not help the more severe nausea symptoms associated with chemotherapy."
4. A patient is asking about using THC. Which statements about dried marihuana therapy are true? (Select all that apply.)
   a. It is useful for nausea and vomiting related to cancer chemotherapy.
   b. It is approved for the treatment of hyperemesis gravidarum.
   c. It is useful to help stimulate the appetite in patients with nutritional wasting.
   d. It may cause extrapyramidal symptoms.
   e. It may cause drowsiness or euphoria.
5. The order reads: "Give promethazine hydrochloride 12.5 mg IM q4h prn nausea/vomiting." The medication is available in 25-mg/mL vials. How many millilitres will the nurse draw up for this dose?

Answers: 1. b, 2. c, 3. d, 4. a, c, e, 5. 0.5 mL

CRITICAL THINKING ACTIVITIES

1. A patient who has received chemotherapy with a highly emetogenic drug has orders for both ondansetron (Zofran) and prochlorperazine hydrochloride. Which drug would be the best choice for the nurse to administer for the patient's nausea and vomiting, and how should it be administered for the best possible effects? Explain your answer.

2. The nurse is administering antiemetic drugs to a patient who has been vomiting. What is the priority for assessment at this time? Explain your answer.
3. The nurse has just given an 83-year-old patient a dose of an antinausea drug. Considering this patient's age, what is the nurse's priority action regarding evaluation of the drug's effects?

For answers see http://evolve.elsevier.com/Canada/Lilley/pharmacology/.

CHAPTER 42

Nutritional Supplements

Objectives

After reading this chapter, the successful student will be able to do the following:

1. Describe the various pathophysiological processes and disease states that may lead to nutritional deficiencies and require nutritional support.

2. Discuss enteral and parenteral nutrition used to treat the various nutritional deficiencies, including specific ingredients.

3. Describe the nurse's role in the process of initiating and maintaining continuous or intermittent enteral feedings, total parenteral nutrition, and other forms of nutrition.

4. Compare the various enteral feeding tubes, including their specific uses and the special needs of patients requiring this nutritional support.

5. Discuss the mechanisms of action, cautions, contraindications, routes of administration, drug interactions, adverse effects, and complications associated with enteral and parenteral nutrition.

6. Develop a collaborative plan of care that includes all phases of the nursing process for patients receiving enteral and parenteral nutrition.

7. Discuss the various laboratory values related to nutritional deficits or altered nutritional status and their impact on monitoring the therapeutic effects of the therapy.

e-Learning Activities

Website
(http://evolve.elsevier.com/Canada/
Lilley/pharmacology/)

evolve

- Answer Key—Textbook Case Studies
- Answer Key—Critical Thinking Activities
- Chapter Summaries—Printable
- Review Questions for Exam Preparation
- Unfolding Case Studies

Drug Profiles

amino acids, p. 793
carbohydrate formulation, p. 793
carbohydrates, p. 791
fat formulation, p. 791
lipid emulsions, p. 793
protein formulation, p. 791

Key Terms

Anabolism Metabolism characterized by the conversion of simple substances into the more complex compounds; tissue building. (p. 787)

Casein The principal protein of milk and the basis for curd and cheese. (p. 791)

Catabolism A complex metabolic process in which energy is liberated for use in work, energy storage, or heat production by the destruction of complex substances to form simple compounds. (p. 793)

Dumping syndrome A complex reaction to the rapid entry of concentrated nutrients into the jejunum of the small intestine; most commonly occurs with eating following partial gastrectomy or with enteral feedings that are administered too rapidly into the stomach or jejunum via a feeding tube. The patient may experience nausea, weakness, sweating, palpitations, syncope, sensations of warmth, and diarrhea. (p. 788)

Enteral nutrition The provision of food or nutrients via the gastrointestinal tract, either naturally by eating or through a feeding tube in patients who are unable to eat. (p. 787)

Essential amino acids Those amino acids that cannot be manufactured by the body. (p. 793)

Essential fatty acid deficiency A condition that develops if fatty acids that the body cannot produce are not present in the diet or in nutritional supplements. (p. 793)

Malnutrition Any disorder of undernutrition. (p. 787)

Multivitamin infusion (MVI) A concentrated solution that contains several water- and fat-soluble vitamins and is used as part of an intravenous (parenteral) nutritional source. (p. 792)

Nonessential amino acids Those amino acids that the body can produce without extracting them from dietary intake. (p. 793)

Nutrients Substances that provide nourishment and affect the nutritive and metabolic processes of the body. (p. 787)

Nutritional supplements Oral, enteral, or intravenous preparations used to provide optimal nutrients to meet the body's nutritional needs. (p. 787)

Nutritional support The provision of nutrients orally, enterally, or parenterally for therapeutic reasons. (p. 787)

Parenteral nutrition The administration of nutrients by a route other than through the alimentary canal, such as intravenously. (p. 787)

Pharmaconutrition The science elucidating the role nutrition plays in general health, as well as the key nutrients required by patients who are critically ill. (p. 787)

Semiessential amino acids Those amino acids that can be produced by the body but not in sufficient amounts in infants and children. (p. 793)

Total parenteral nutrition (TPN) The intravenous administration of the total nutrient requirements of patients with gastrointestinal dysfunction, accomplished via peripheral catheters, peripherally inserted central catheters, or central venous catheters. (p. 789)

Whey The thin serum of milk remaining after the casein and fat have been removed; it contains proteins, lactose, water-soluble vitamins, and minerals. (p. 791)

OVERVIEW

Nutrients are dietary products that undergo chemical changes when ingested (and metabolized) and cause tissue to be enhanced and energy to be liberated. Nutrients are required for cell growth and division; enzyme activity; protein, carbohydrate, and fat synthesis; muscle contraction; secretion of hormones (e.g., vasopressin, gastrin); wound repair; immune competence; gut integrity; and numerous other essential cellular functions. Providing for these nutritional needs is known as **nutritional support**. Adequate nutritional support is needed to prevent the breakdown of tissue proteins for use as an energy supply to sustain essential organ systems, which is what occurs during starvation. Malnutrition can decrease organ size and impair the function of organ systems (e.g., cardiac, respiratory, gastrointestinal [GI], liver, kidney). Nutritional support is a means of providing adequate nutrition to meet the body's nutritional needs.

Pharmaconutrition seeks to understand the ways in which nutrition affects health in general and specifically to understand the key nutrients that are required by patients who are critically ill.

Malnutrition is a condition in which the body's essential need for nutrients is not met by nutrient intake. The purpose of nutritional support is the successful prevention, recognition, and management of malnutrition. **Nutritional supplements** are dietary products used to provide nutritional support. Nutritional supplement products can be administered to patients in a variety of ways. They vary in the chemical complexity of their carbohydrates, proteins, and fats; electrolytes; vitamins and minerals; as well as in their amounts of these elements and their osmolality. These nutrients may be given in a digested form, a partially digested form, or an

undigested form. Nutritional supplements can also be tailored for specific disease states.

Patients' nutrient requirements vary according to age, gender, weight, level of physical activity, pre-existing medical conditions, nutrition status, and current medical or surgical treatment. Nutritional supplements are classified according to their method of administration as either enteral or parenteral. **Enteral nutrition** is the provision of food or nutrients through the GI tract. **Parenteral nutrition** is the intravenous (IV) administration of nutrients. Its purpose is to promote **anabolism** (tissue building), nitrogen balance, and maintenance or improvement of body weight. It is used when the oral or enteral feeding routes cannot be used (e.g., in postoperative patients or patients who are cachectic from advanced cancer or AIDS). The selection of either enteral or parenteral nutrition and the specific nutritional composition of the product used depend on the specific patient and the clinical situation.

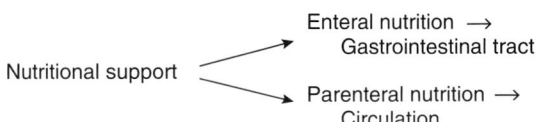

ENTERAL NUTRITION

Enteral nutrition is the provision of food or nutrients through the GI tract. The GI tract is the preferred route to deliver nutritional support (Marik, 2014). The most common and least invasive route of administration is the oral route. There are six enteral routes (Table 42-1) and five of these use a feeding tube (Figure 42-1).

Enteral nutrition formulas are designed to meet the basic macronutrient and micronutrient requirements of

TABLE	42-1

Routes of Enteral Nutrition Delivery

Route	Description
Esophagostomy	Feeding tube surgically inserted into the esophagus
Gastrostomy	Feeding tube surgically inserted directly into the stomach
Jejunostomy	Feeding tube surgically inserted into the jejunum
Nasoduodenal	Feeding tube placed from the nose to the duodenum
Nasojejunal	Feeding tube placed from the nose to the jejunum
Nasogastric	Feeding tube placed from the nose to the stomach
Oral	Nutritional supplements delivered by mouth

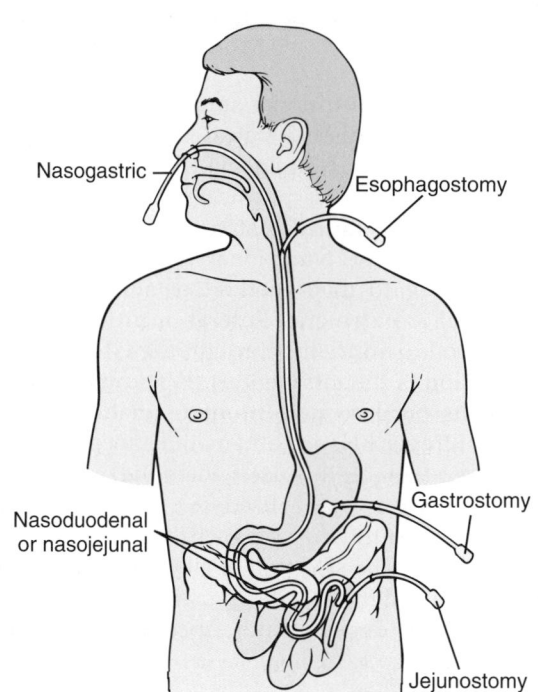

FIG. 42-1 Tube feeding routes. (Adapted from: Mahan, L. K., Escott-Stump, S., & Raymond, J. L. (2012). *Krause's food and the nutrition care process* (13th ed.; Figure 14-2). Philadelphia, PA: Saunders.)

individuals who are unable to meet their nutritional needs orally. Many specialty products have been developed to exhibit specific pharmacological properties, such as immune-enhancing formulas containing arginine, glutamine, nucleotides, and omega-3 fatty acids. Patients who may benefit from feeding tube delivery of nutrients include those with abnormal esophageal or stomach peristalsis, altered anatomy secondary to surgery, depressed consciousness, or impaired digestive capacity. The enteral route is considered superior to the parenteral route for the administration of nutritional

supplements. In patients who are critically ill, such as a patient with burns, early enteral nutrition within at least 24 to 72 hours is recommended. Early enteral nutrition has several advantages, such as protection of intestinal mucosal integrity, reduction of infection, and reduction of morbidity (Shankar, Daphnee, Ramakrishnan, et al., 2015).

Approximately 100 different enteral formulations are available. The enteral supplements have been divided into groups according to the basic characteristics of their formulations; these groups include elemental, polymeric, modular, altered amino acid, and impaired glucose tolerance formulations. These are described in Box 42-1.

Mechanism of Action and Drug Effects

The enteral formula groups provide the basic building blocks for anabolism. Different combinations and amounts of these nutrients are used based on the individual patient's anabolic needs. Enteral nutrition supplies complete dietary needs through the GI tract by the normal oral route or by feeding tube.

Indications

Enteral nutrition can be used to supplement an oral diet that is currently insufficient for a patient's nutrient needs or used alone to meet all of the patient's nutrient needs. Box 42-2 lists the main types of enteral nutritional supplements and their indications.

Contraindications

The usual contraindication to any kind of nutritional supplement is known drug allergy to a specific product or a genetic disease that renders a patient unable to metabolize certain types of nutrients.

Adverse Effects

The most common adverse effect of nutritional supplements is GI intolerance, manifesting as diarrhea. Infant nutritional formulations are often associated with allergies and digestive intolerance; other nutritional supplements are most commonly associated with osmotic diarrhea. Rapid feeding or bolus doses can result in **dumping syndrome**, which produces intestinal disturbances. In addition, tube feeding places patients at significant risk for aspiration pneumonia. This is especially true in patients in whom gag reflexes and general mobility are compromised.

Interactions

Various nutrients can interact with drugs to produce significant food–drug interactions. With some exceptions, food usually delays the absorption of drugs when administered simultaneously with them. High gastric acid content or prolonged emptying time can result in decreased effects of certain antibiotics (e.g., cephalosporins, erythromycin, penicillins). An increased absorption rate resulting in increased therapeutic effects

BOX 42-1

Enteral Formulations

Elemental Formulations

Peptamen®
Vital® HN

Contents: dipeptides, tripeptides, or crystalline amino acids, glucose oligosaccharides, and vegetable oil or medium-chain triglycerides (MCTs)

Vivonex®
  Plus

Comments: minimum digestion; residue is minimal

Vivonex®
  T.E.N.

Indications: partial bowel obstruction, irritable bowel disease, radiation enteritis, bowel fistulas, and short bowel syndrome

Polymeric Formulations

Complete

Contents: complex nutrients (proteins, carbohydrates, and fat)

Ensure®
Ensure
  Plus®
Isocal®
Osmolite®
Portagen®
Jevity®
Sustacal®

Indications: preferred over elemental formulations for patients with fully functional GI tracts and few specialized nutrient requirements

Modular Formulations

Carbohydrate

Contents: single-nutrient formulas (protein, carbohydrate, or fat)

Moducal®
Polycose®
Fat
MCT Oil®
Microlipid®
Protein
Beneprotein®
ProMod®

Indications: can be added to a monomeric or polymeric formulation to provide a more individualized nutrient formulation

Altered Amino Acid Formulations

Amin-Aid®

Contents: varying amounts of specific amino acids

Primene®
TwoCal®
TwoCal®
  HN
Travasol®

Indications: patients with diseases associated with altered metabolic capacities

Formulation for Impaired Glucose Tolerance

Glucerna®

Contents: protein, carbohydrate, fat, sodium, potassium

Indications: patients with impaired glucose tolerance (e.g., patients with diabetes)

---

can be seen when corticosteroids or vitamins A and D are given with nutritional supplements. The antibiotic effects of tetracyclines and quinolones are decreased when they are given with nutritional supplements as a result of chemical inactivation. These drugs must be given at least 2 hours before or after tube feedings.

Tube feedings can also reduce the absorption of phenytoin; this reduced absorption can result in seizures. It is recommended that tube feedings be held for at least 2 hours before and after the administration of phenytoin. However, doing so can be problematic, because the patient may not receive adequate nutrition if feedings are withheld. This issue is somewhat controversial, and some suggest that the interaction is more theoretical than actual. Thus, some institutions have opted to ignore the possible interaction and monitor phenytoin levels and patient status instead of withholding tube feedings; other institutions continue to withhold the tube feedings when phenytoin is administered. When continuous tube feedings are necessary, patients will often require phenytoin to be administered by IV.

Dosages

Because nutrient requirements vary greatly, dosages are individualized according to patient needs.

TOTAL PARENTERAL NUTRITION

Parenteral nutrition supplementation (IV administration) is the preferred method for patients who are unable to tolerate and maintain adequate enteral or oral intake. Instead of administration of partially digested nutrients into the GI tract (as in enteral nutrition), vitamins, minerals, amino acids, dextrose, and lipids are administered intravenously directly into the circulatory system. This effectively bypasses the entire GI system, which eliminates the need for absorption, metabolism, and excretion. Parenteral nutrition is also called **total parenteral nutrition (TPN)**.

TPN can supply all of the calories, carbohydrates, amino acids, fats, trace elements, vitamins, and minerals needed for growth, weight gain, wound healing, convalescence, immunocompetence, and other health-sustaining functions. TPN macronutrient calculators are available on the Internet and provide an empiric dose for the macronutrients included in a TPN formulation.

TPN can be administered through either a peripheral vein (usually via an 18-gauge catheter and with less than a 10% solution of dextrose), a peripherally inserted central catheter (PICC), or a central venous catheter. Each route of delivery of TPN has specific requirements and limitations. It is generally accepted that TPN is used only when oral or enteral support is impossible or when the GI absorptive or functional capacity is not sufficient to meet the nutrition needs of the patient. Some of the factors that must be considered in deciding whether to use a peripheral or central route for TPN for a given patient are listed in Table 42-2.

BOX 42-2 Enteral Nutrition Supplements: Indications

**Complete Nutritional Formulations
(i.e., for General Nutritional Deficiencies)**

- Inability to consume or digest normal foods
- Accelerated catabolic status
- Undernourished because of disease

**Incomplete Nutritional Formulations
(i.e., for Specific Nutritional Deficiencies)**

- Genetic metabolic enzyme deficiency
- Liver or kidney impairment

Infant Nutritional Formulations

- Sole nutritional intake for premature and full-term infants
- Supplemental nutritional intake for older infants receiving solid foods
- Supplemental nutrition for breastfed infants

TABLE 42-2

Peripheral and Total Parenteral Nutrition: Characteristics

Characteristic	Peripheral	Central
Goal of nutritional therapy (total versus supplemental)	Supplemental (total if moderate to low needs)	Total
Length of therapy	Short (fewer than 14 days)	Long (7 days or longer)
Osmolarity	Hyperosmolar (600–900 mOsm/L)	Hyperosmolar (600–900 mOsm/L)
Fluid tolerance	Must be high	Can be fluid restricted
Dextrose	Less than 10%	10–35%
Amino acids	Less than 3%	More than 3–7%
Fats	10–20%	10–20%
Calories/day	Less than 2 000 kcal/day	More than 2 000 kcal/day

PERIPHERAL TOTAL PARENTERAL NUTRITION

Peripheral TPN is one route of administration of TPN. A peripheral vein is used to deliver nutrients to the patient's circulatory system. Peripheral TPN is usually a temporary method of nutrition administration. The long-term administration of nutritional supplements via a peripheral vein may lead to phlebitis. It is considered a temporary measure to provide adequate nutrients in patients who have mild deficits or who are restricted from oral intake and have slightly elevated metabolic rates.

Peripheral TPN is valuable in patients who do not have large nutrition needs, can tolerate moderately large fluid loads, and need nutritional supplements only temporarily. Peripheral TPN may be used alone or in combination with oral nutritional supplements to provide the necessary fat, carbohydrate, and protein needed by the patient to maintain health.

Mechanism of Action and Drug Effects

Peripheral TPN provides the basic nutrient building blocks for anabolism. Different combinations and amounts of these supplements are used based on the individual patient's anabolic needs.

Indications

Peripheral TPN is used to provide complete daily nutrition or to administer nutrients to patients who need more nutrients than their current oral intake can supply. It is meant only as a temporary means (less than 2 weeks) of delivering TPN. Circumstances under which patients may benefit from the delivery of peripheral TPN are as follows:

- The patient must undergo a procedure that restricts oral feedings.
- The patient has anorexia caused by radiation or cancer chemotherapy.
- The patient has a GI illness that prevents oral food ingestion.
- The patient has undergone surgery of any type.
- The patient's nutritional deficits are minimal, but oral nutrition will not be reinstated for more than 5 days.

Contraindications

As mentioned previously regarding the enteral nutritional products, the only usual contraindication to nutritional supplements of any kind is known drug allergy to a specific product or a genetic disease that renders a patient unable to assimilate certain types of nutrients.

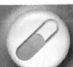 **DRUG PROFILES**

Enteral nutrition can be provided by a variety of supplements. Individual patient characteristics determine the appropriate enteral supplement. The four most commonly used enteral formulations are elemental, polymeric, modular, and altered amino acid.

ELEMENTAL FORMULATIONS

Elemental formulations are enteral supplements that contain dipeptides, tripeptides, or crystalline amino acids. Minimal digestion is required with elemental formulations. These supplements are indicated in patients with pancreatitis, partial bowel obstruction, irritable bowel disease, radiation enteritis, bowel fistulas, and short bowel syndrome. They are contraindicated in patients who have had hypersensitivity reactions to them. Elemental formulation supplements are available without a prescription.

POLYMERIC FORMULATIONS

Polymeric formulations are enteral supplements that contain complex nutrients derived from proteins, carbohydrates, and fat. The polymeric formulations are some of the most commonly used enteral formulations because they most closely resemble normal dietary intake. They are preferred over elemental formulations in patients who have fully functional GI tracts and have no specialized nutrient needs. Polymeric formulations are less hyperosmolar than elemental formulations and therefore cause fewer GI problems. They are contraindicated in patients who have had hypersensitivity reactions to them. They are available without a prescription.

The commonly used enteral supplement in the polymeric formulation category of enteral nutritional products is Ensure. It is lactose free and is also available in a higher-calorie formula called Ensure Plus. Other polymeric formulations are listed in Box 42-1. These supplements contain complex nutrients such as **casein** (the principal protein of milk) and soy protein for protein; corn syrup and maltodextrins for carbohydrates; and vegetable oil or milk fat for fat. They are available in liquid formulations only.

MODULAR FORMULATIONS

carbohydrate formulation

Moducal and Polycose are examples of commonly used enteral supplements in the carbohydrate modular formulation category. Both are carbohydrate supplements that supply carbohydrates only. They are intended as an addition to monomeric or polymeric formulations to provide a more individualized nutrient mix. They are available in liquid formulations only. These products are available without a prescription and are contraindicated only in patients who have had a hypersensitivity reaction to them.

fat formulation

Microlipid and MCT Oil are the formulations available in the fat category of enteral supplements. Microlipid is a fat supplement supplying only fats. It is a concentrated source of calories and contains 4.5 kcal/mL. These supplements are given to help individualize nutrient formulations. They may be used in patients with malabsorption and other GI disorders and in patients with pancreatitis. They are available in liquid formulations only. These products are obtainable without a prescription and are contraindicated only in patients who have had hypersensitivity reactions to them.

protein formulation

Beneprotein and ProMod are examples of protein modular formulations. They are used to increase patients' protein intake and provide additional proteins. They are derived from a variety of sources, such as **whey,** casein, egg whites, and amino acids. All of the available products are dried powders that must be reconstituted with water. They may sometimes be reconstituted by adding them to enteral nutrition formulations that are already in liquid form. They are indicated for patients with increased protein needs. They are contraindicated in patients who have had hypersensitivity reactions to them. Protein formulation supplements are available without a prescription.

ALTERED AMINO ACID FORMULATIONS

Amin-Aid is one of many amino acid formulation nutritional supplements available. Many of the nutritional supplements in this category are also listed as modular formulations because they can be used as both single-nutrient formulas and as nutritional formulations for patients with genetic errors of metabolism. Specialized amino acid formulations are used most commonly in patients who have metabolic disorders such as phenylketonuria, homocystinuria, or maple syrup urine disease. They are also used to supply nutritional support to patients with such illnesses as kidney impairment, eclampsia, heart failure, or liver failure.

Adverse Effects

The most severe adverse effect of peripheral TPN is phlebitis, which is vein irritation or inflammation of a vein. If phlebitis is severe and is not treated appropriately, it can lead to the loss of a limb, although this is rare. Another potential adverse effect is fluid overload. Peripheral TPN is limited to solutions with a lower dextrose concentration, generally less than 10%, to avoid sclerosis of the vein. Thus, large volumes are needed to meet a patient's daily nutritional requirements. Some patients, such as those with kidney or heart failure, cannot tolerate large fluid volumes. In these patients, fluid restriction may make it impossible to provide adequate calories through peripheral TPN.

CENTRAL TOTAL PARENTERAL NUTRITION

In central TPN, a large central vein is used to deliver nutrients directly into the patient's circulation. Usually, the subclavian or internal jugular vein is used. Central TPN is generally indicated for patients who require nutritional supplements for a prolonged period, usually longer than 7 to 10 days. It can also be used in the home care setting. There are a variety of indications for central TPN. The disadvantages of central TPN are the risks associated with venous catheter insertion and the use and maintenance of the central vein. There is a greater potential for infection, more serious catheter-induced trauma and related events, metabolic alterations, and other technical or mechanical problems than with peripheral TPN.

Mechanism of Action and Drug Effects

TPN is used to supply nutrients to patients who cannot ingest nutrients by mouth and cannot meet required daily nutritional needs by the enteral or peripheral parenteral routes. Like peripheral TPN, central TPN supplies the basic building blocks required for anabolism. It provides the necessary fat, carbohydrate, and protein that the patient needs to maintain health.

Indications

Central TPN delivers total dietary nutrients to patients who require nutritional supplementation. Circumstances under which patients may benefit from the delivery of central TPN include the following:
- The patient has large nutritional requirements (e.g., due to metabolic stress or hypermetabolism).
- The patient needs nutritional support for a prolonged period (longer than 7 to 10 days).
- The patient is unable to tolerate large amounts of fluid.

Contraindications

Central TPN is contraindicated in patients with known allergy to any of its components. Rarely, a patient who is allergic to eggs may have cross-sensitivity to lipid formulations. TPN is used only when the GI tract cannot be used (e.g., in postoperative patients or those who are otherwise unable to eat or digest and absorb nutrients).

Adverse Effects

The most common adverse effects of central TPN are those associated with the use of the central vein for delivery of the TPN. The risks associated with insertion of the infusion line, as well as the use and maintenance of the central vein for administration of TPN, can create some complications. Central TPN involves greater potential for infection, serious catheter-induced trauma and related events, and other technical or mechanical problems than are associated with peripheral TPN. Larger and more concentrated volumes of nutritional supplements are

TABLE 42-3		
Amino Acids: Recommended Daily Dosage Guidelines		
Healthy		**Malnourished or With Trauma or Burn**
Adult	**Infant or Child**	**Adult**
0.9 g/kg	1.5 to 3 g/kg	Up to 2 g/kg

being delivered with central TPN, and therefore there is also a greater chance for metabolic complications such as hyperglycemia.

Dosages

Dosage requirements vary from patient to patient. Age, gender, weight, and numerous other factors must be considered for proper administration of TPN. Guidelines for amino acids appear in Table 42-3.

TRACE ELEMENTS

Trace elements are available in individual solutions and in many different combinations. The following are considered trace elements:
- Chromium
- Copper
- Iodine
- Manganese
- Molybdenum
- Selenium
- Zinc

Specific dosages and frequencies depend on the individual patient's requirements, based on the current diet reference and determined by the health care provider. Vitamins and minerals may also be added accordingly. A common multivitamin combination is **multivitamin infusion (MVI)**.

NURSING PROCESS

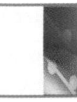

◢ Assessment

Perform a thorough nutritional assessment with attention to dietary history, weekly and daily food intakes, weight, and height before initiating any nutritional supplements. Conduct a thorough nursing history and survey of all systems, including questions about any unusual symptoms, possible nutritional concerns, nausea, vomiting, loss of appetite, and weight gain or loss. Focus other questions on past and present medical and health history; history of any difficulties with nutrition, GI

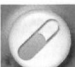

DRUG PROFILES

The individual components of peripheral and central TPN are the same. The differences lie in the concentrations and amounts of the components delivered per volume of nutritional supplement. The basic components of peripheral or central TPN are amino acids, carbohydrates, lipids, trace elements, vitamins, fluids, and electrolytes. Most of the electrolyte components are discussed in Chapter 30.

AMINO ACIDS

Amino acids have many roles in the maintenance of normal nutritional status. Their primary role is protein synthesis, or anabolism. Provision of adequate amino acids in nutritional supplements reduces the breakdown of proteins (**catabolism**) and also helps to promote normal growth and wound healing.

Amino acids are commonly classified as essential or nonessential, according to whether they can or cannot be produced by the body. **Nonessential amino acids** are those that the body produces and therefore need not be present in dietary intake. The body is able to manufacture, from nutritional nitrogen sources, all but eight of the available amino acids. **Essential amino acids** are those amino acids that cannot be produced by the body. Therefore, they must be included in daily dietary intake. Amino acids are used as building blocks for protein that is needed for normal growth and development. Two amino acids, histidine and arginine, are not manufactured by the body in large enough quantities during rapid growth periods such as infancy or childhood. Thus, they are referred to as **semiessential amino acids**. Box 42-3 lists amino acids according to their categories.

amino acids

Amino acid crystalline solutions (Aminosyn® 5%, 7%, 8.5%, and 10%, Primene® 10%) can be used in either peripheral or central TPN. Amino acids are a source of both protein and calories. They provide 4 kcal/g. The two currently available amino acid solutions differ only in their respective concentrations. The dosage of these solutions varies depending on the patient's weight and requirements. These supplements have no contraindications to their use.

carbohydrates

In nutritional support, carbohydrates are usually supplied to patients through dextrose. Dextrose is normally the greatest source of calories and provides 3.4 kcal/g. However, protein (amino acids) and lipids are also used as calorie sources (Figure 42-2). The concentration of dextrose in TPN is an important consideration. In peripheral TPN, dextrose concentrations are kept below 10% to decrease the possibility of phlebitis. In central TPN, dextrose concentrations can range from 10 to 50% but are commonly 25 to 35%. Because dextrose is a sugar, supplemental insulin may be given simultaneously with nutritional supplements. Use of a balanced nutritional supplement that contains dextrose and lipids as caloric sources decreases the need for large amounts of insulin.

fat

The average North American diet consists of 40% fat. This means that of the total calories supplied, 40 to 50% of the calories are obtained through fat grams. The ideal diet contains no more than 30% fat. IV fat emulsions serve two functions: they supply essential fatty acids and they are a source of energy or calories. As with the amino acids, certain fatty acids are essential because the body cannot produce them. Linoleic acid cannot be synthesized by the body. It is needed to produce linolenic and arachidonic acid. If these fatty acids are not present in dietary or nutritional supplements, an **essential fatty acid deficiency** may develop. Clinical signs of essential fatty acid deficiency are hair loss, scaly dermatitis, growth retardation, reduced wound healing, decreased platelets, and fatty liver (Figure 42-3).

lipid emulsions

The currently available lipid emulsions are Intralipid®, available as 10%, 20%, or 30% emulsions, and Liposyn® II, available as a 10% emulsion. They differ in fat origin. Intralipid is made from soybean oil, and Liposyn is made from safflower oil.

Lipid emulsions normally deliver 20 to 30% of total daily calories and must not exceed 60% of daily caloric intake. Fat emulsions are most beneficial when combined with dextrose solutions. The use of fat to meet caloric needs prevents potentially harmful conditions such as hyperglycemia, hyperinsulinemia, and hyperosmolarity, which can occur when a patient's entire caloric needs are being met solely by dextrose.

---

absorption, or food intolerance; stressors; and a complete medication profile, including a listing of all prescription drugs, over-the-counter (OTC) drugs, and natural health products. Consultation with a registered dietitian is crucial to help identify the nutrients that are missing in a particular patient's diet. Total body metabolic rate, body mass index, muscle mass, and other variables linked to nutritional status will most likely be assessed and are data that a nutritional consult may provide. Laboratory studies that may need to be assessed include the following: total protein, albumin, blood urea nitrogen (BUN), red blood cell (RBC), white blood cell (WBC), vitamin B_{12}, hemoglobin (Hgb), and hematocrit. Other laboratory studies may include cholesterol, electrolytes, total lymphocytes, serum transferrin, ferritin, urine creatinine clearance, lipid profile, and urinalysis. All of the described objective and subjective data will help the health care provider, dietitian, and other members of the health care team select the appropriate nutritional supplements for the patient.

BOX 42-3

Amino Acids: Classification

Essential	Nonessential	Semiessential
Isoleucine	Alanine	Arginine
Leucine	Asparagine	Histidine
Lysine	Aspartic acid	
Methionine	Cysteine	
Phenylalanine	Glutamine	
Threonine	Glutamic acid	
Tryptophan	Glycine	
Valine	Proline	
	Serine	
	Tyrosine	

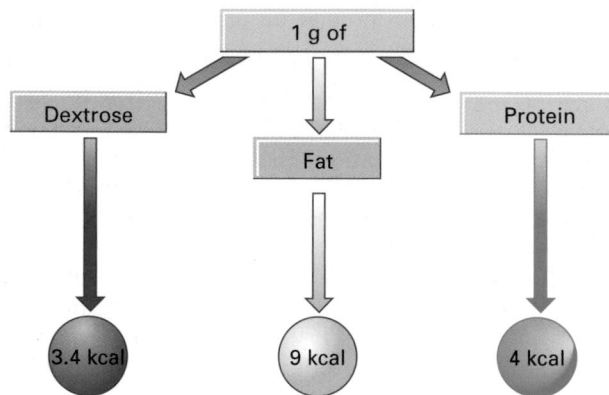

FIG. 42-2 One gram of dextrose, fat, or protein will provide varying amounts of energy as calories.

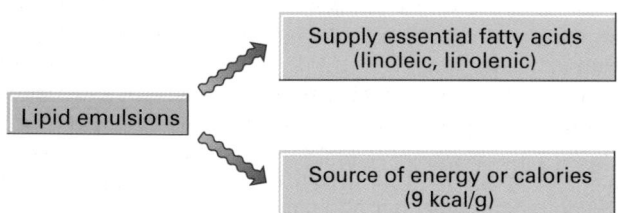

FIG. 42-3 Lipid emulsions supply essential fatty acids and energy.

Before administering an enteral nutrition supplement that is an elemental formulation, determine if the patient has a history of allergic reaction to any of the contents of the solution. Assess for contraindications and cautions and document the findings. Of most concern is assessing the patient's heart and kidney status and ensuring that the ingredients and the amount of solution will not be too taxing on these systems. In addition, because these solutions are given either by mouth or via tube feedings (see Chapter 10), it is important to assess the patient's ability to swallow, and bowel sounds, and to note any nausea or vomiting. Remember that protein-based formulations are to be avoided in patients with allergies to egg whites and whey.

Prior to the implementation of parenteral nutrition, assess for allergies to any of the ordered components of the IV solution and make note of the patient's age and metabolic needs. There are usually multiple combinations of products available; thus, it is important to assess the patient carefully for allergies to essential proteins, amino acids, carbohydrates, trace elements, minerals, vitamins, lipids, high concentrations of dextrose, and any other ingredients present. Assess your knowledge base about parenteral nutrition and situations that necessitate infusions through a central line, peripherally inserted central lines, or peripherally inserted midline catheters. (See http://evolve.elsevier.com/Canada/Lilley/pharmacology/ for more information.) Some of the complications of parenteral nutrition include pneumothorax, infection, air emboli or emboli related to protein or lipid aggregation (associated with central catheter IV lines), septicemia related to the nutrient-rich solutions with an invasive IV route of administration, metabolic imbalances because of the solution or ingredients, and vomiting (seen with lipid administration in parenteral nutrition). Also perform a complete baseline assessment and continuously monitor the following: (1) central line site, including patency, intactness, and appearance; (2) WBC and RBC counts as well as other laboratory values and parameters (listed earlier); (3) vital signs; (4) serum glucose; and (5) heart rhythm with electrocardiogram (ECG) readings (as prescribed).

Nursing Diagnoses

- Nutrition less than body requirements, related to inability to take in sufficient nutrients
- Diarrhea related to a decreased tolerance to enteral feedings and their ingredients
- Risk for infection (sepsis) related to parenteral infusions and use of central venous access line

Planning

Goals

- Patient will regain normal nutritional status through adequate dietary intake and supplemental feedings or nutrients.
- Patient will remain free from diarrhea related to enteral supplementation.
- Patient will remain free from infection during parenteral nutritional supplementation.

Expected Patient Outcomes

- Patient's nutritional status improves with enteral or parenteral nutritional supplementation as prescribed, as evidenced by proportional weight gain, adequate fluid volume status with improved skin turgor, improved urinary output to at least 30 mL/hr, and a return to normal of laboratory values such as total protein, albumin, ferritin, hematocrit, and hemoglobulin.

- Patient identifies measures to decrease diarrhea while receiving enteral feedings, such as use of prescribed drugs to decrease motility or use of OTC drugs or natural health products, as ordered.
- Patient states measures to minimize risk for infection at the TPN site (peripheral or central), such as checking the site frequently for redness, swelling, drainage, or abnormal warmth, and reporting these signs as well as fever or chills to the health care provider or home health care nurse immediately.

Implementation

Meeting a patient's nutritional needs relies on the implementation of agency-specific evidence-informed enteral or TPN feeding protocols and interprofessional collaboration, including the dietitian, nurse, pharmacist, and other health care providers. A health care provider's order must be complete and dated before enteral or total parenteral (peripheral or central) nutrition supplementation is started. In general, monitoring the status of the patient during and after enteral feedings is crucial to safe and prudent nursing care.

It is general practice with nasogastric feeding solutions to check for proper placement and detect gastric residuals to avoid pulmonary aspiration and other complications. A *gastric residual* refers to the volume of fluid remaining in the stomach at a point in time during enteral nutrition feeding. There is a wide range of residual volumes considered (from 150 to 500 mL); these volumes are often used to predict tube-feeding tolerance or pulmonary aspiration risk (Flynn Makic, Rauen, & VonRueden, 2013) or to confirm a decision to withhold feedings. According to Flynn Makic and colleagues, there is no evidence to support the use of residual volumes as markers to support withholding feedings or to prevent pulmonary aspiration, and this practice may, in fact, lead to underfeeding. Nonetheless, most agencies recommend checking for placement to ensure that the tube is in the stomach and has not passed through the larynx, through the trachea, and down into the bronchi of the lungs. One method of checking a nasogastric tube's placement involves aspirating fluid from the tube with a syringe and testing the pH to determine the acidity of the fluid. If the aspirate has a pH of 5.5 or lower, the tube is in the correct position. If these checks are not possible, a chest X-ray must be used. Measure gastric residual volumes and document these before each feeding as well as before administration of each medication. When checking gastric residual volumes, stop the tube feeding and then aspirate stomach contents using a syringe connected to the particular tube. If

the volume aspirated is more than the volume delivered over the previous 2 hours (of continuous feeding), return the aspirate, hold the feeding, and contact the health care provider while keeping the head of the patient's bed elevated. For intermittent bolus feedings, if the residual amount is more than 50% of the volume previously infused, it is the standard of care to return the aspirate, withhold the feeding, and contact the health care provider. A reduction in the tube feeding volume will probably then be ordered. Always check hospital or facility policy or protocol before the use of enteral feedings, and consistently check and manage residuals during therapy.

Newer tubes for nasogastric and other routes of enteral feeding have smaller diameters and are thinner (5 French to 10 French) and more pliable for better patient tolerance than older tubes. Small-bore tubes are more comfortable but have a greater likelihood of becoming clogged by medications or thick enteral formulations. Small-bore silastic feeding tubes with weighted ends are intended to float in the duodenum. Placement is verified by X-ray. However, the smaller-diameter tubes make gastric aspiration more difficult and their use is not recommended. Depending on agency policy, placement may be checked by auscultation of an air bolus. A forceful air bolus can remove the weighted end.

To prevent clogging of the feeding tube, it is often helpful to flush the tube with 30 mL of lukewarm water (per agency policy), using a gentle, back-and-forth motion with the plunger of the syringe. After instilling the water, if a stubborn clog does not immediately allow for back-and-forth motion, clamp the tube and let it soak for up to 20 minutes. Acidic juices and carbonated beverages should not be used because they may cause a protein precipitate that will result in further clogging. Itkin and colleagues (2011) documented that pancreatic enzymes and sodium bicarbonate have been successful in unclogging tubes and, if used prophylactically, will prolong the time to occlusion. Clog Zapper® is a food-grade powder referred to as an "enzyme cocktail" (with acids, buffers, antibacterial agents, and metal inhibitors) to clear blocked tubes. It is available premeasured and loaded in a ready-to-use system and is approved for use with gastric, jejunal, nasogastric, and nasojejunal tubes. Always follow agency-specific guidelines when using these strategies. Percutaneous enteral gastrostomy (PEG) tubes are also commonly used in many situations but do require surgical insertion by a gastroenterologist and are often inserted procedurally under procedural sedation. Their care includes performing dressing changes during the initial period and then checking for residuals regularly throughout their use. Placement need not be checked, but if it appears that the tube has come out of the opening and is longer than previously noted, stop the infusion and contact the health care provider.

Follow health care provider–ordered enteral feeding infusion rates and concentrations carefully. The patient should be in an upright position for enteral feeds. Usually, the initial rate is 50 mL/hr at one-half strength, but this can be increased per patient tolerance to a rate ordered by the health care provider. More rapid feeding increases the risk for hyperglycemia, dumping syndrome, and diarrhea. Infusion rates of enteral feedings may be adjusted by the health care provider as per the patient's tolerance of the feeding. Keep tube feeding formulas at room temperature and never administer them cold or warm. If all the necessary steps to decrease or prevent diarrhea have been taken and have failed, antidiarrheal medications may be needed. Lactose-free nutritional solutions are available and are recommended for patients who are lactose intolerant. Patients who have lactose intolerance may experience cramping, diarrhea, abdominal bloating, and flatulence with the ingestion of enteral milk-based feedings.

The preparation and administration of enteral medications requires a protocol for safe delivery. Drug absorption depends on the drug's solubility and ability to permeate the intestinal mucosa. The distal end of the feeding tube can be in the stomach, duodenum, or jejunum. Therefore, the position of the distal end should be determined prior to medication administration; consult with the pharmacist to ensure the medication will be properly dissolved and absorbed. The health care provider should always be cautious regarding medication compatibility with tube feeding. In general, the following are safe practices to follow when administering medications via enteral tubes: (1) prepare and administer medications one at a time; (2) open immediate-release gelatin capsules to remove the powder or to crush the solid contents, which are then diluted; (3) further dilute liquid forms of drugs; (4) crush tablets into a fine powder (using a self-contained crushing device to avoid mixing residues from other drugs) and dilute for administration; (5) use purified water for diluting to avoid the presence of chemical contaminants in tap water; and (6) avoid mixing drugs with the feeding formula—stop the formula and flush with at least 15 mL of purified water, follow with the medication using a clean 30 mL syringe, and flush with an additional 15 mL of purified water. The feeding can be resumed once the medication has been administered.

Assess parenteral nutrition infusions every hour or per the facility's policies and procedures. Document the status of the entire infusion system and equipment as well as the condition of the patient. The standard of care is to examine the patient first and then check the insertion site, infusion pump, and solution. To prevent infection, change parenteral nutrition tubing every time a new bag is added to the infusion or as per facility policy. It is also recommended that tubing changes occur daily with the beginning of each new infusion. A 1.2 micron filter is used to trap bacteria, including *Pseudomonas* species. Record the patient's temperature every 4 hours, or as ordered, during the infusion, and report any increase in temperature over 37.8°C to the health care provider immediately. Check the patient frequently for signs and symptoms of hyperglycemia, such as polydipsia, polyuria, headache, dehydration, nausea, vomiting, and weakness. Never accelerate infusion rates to increase plasma volume because the rapid increase of dextrose solution may precipitate hyperglycemia and other related complications. Insulin replacement may be needed with the increase in dextrose; therefore, measure serum glucose levels by glucometer (usually every 6 hours) so that hyperglycemia may be immediately recognized and treated.

Hypoglycemia is manifested by cold, clammy skin; dizziness; tachycardia; and tingling of the extremities. Hypoglycemia associated with parenteral nutrition may be prevented by gradual reduction of the IV feeding rate to allow the pancreas time to adapt to changing blood glucose levels. If parenteral nutrition is discontinued abruptly, rebound hypoglycemia may occur. This condition can be prevented by providing infusions of 5 to 10% glucose in situations in which parenteral nutrition must be discontinued immediately. Fluid overload may also occur with parenteral nutrition, manifested by weak pulse, hypertension, tachycardia, confusion, decreased urine output, and pitting edema; this problem may be prevented by maintaining infusion rates as ordered. If signs of fluid overload occur, slow the infusion rate, measure vital signs, contact the health care provider, and remain with the patient until the patient's condition has stabilized. Include auscultation of breath and heart sounds in the patient assessment, especially if additional therapies that may precipitate fluid overload are administered. Measurement of intake and output is usually indicated when parenteral nutrition is administered (and with enteral supplementation as well). See the Patient Teaching Tips for more information on the use of nutritional supplements.

▨ Evaluation

Therapeutic responses to nutritional supplementation include improved well-being, energy, strength, and performance of activities of daily living; an increase in weight; and laboratory test results that reflect improved nutritional status. Specific laboratory values may include some of the following: albumin, total protein, hematocrit, hemoglobin, RBC and WBC, electrolyte, blood glucose and insulin, and ferritin. Perform ongoing evaluation for adverse effects associated with all enteral or parenteral nutrition infusions during and after therapy, and complete nutritional re-evaluation periodically to ensure that the patient's nutritional needs are met. For outpatients, this may require frequent appointments with a health care provider or monitoring by a home health care nurse. Always refer to goals and outcome criteria to evaluate the effectiveness of therapy.

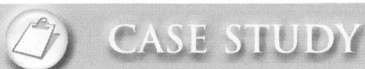

CASE STUDY

Total Parenteral Nutrition

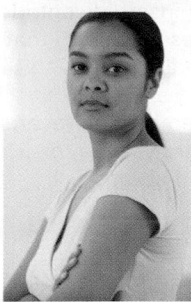

Lariba, a 28-year-old florist, has been unable to eat due to severe nausea and vomiting related to her pregnancy. She is at 13 weeks' gestation and has been admitted to the hospital because of dehydration and her inability to eat. The decision has been made to give her TPN for at least 1 week. After 1 week of therapy, her obstetrician will then decide whether to continue or stop the infusion, based on her response. She will be receiving the TPN infusion via a peripheral IV catheter, with infusion bags that will be changed every 24 hours.

1. Lariba is anxious about this infusion and asks the nurse, "Why is that bag so large? What is in the bag?" How will the nurse answer these questions?

2. The nurse explains to Lariba that her blood glucose levels will need to be monitored while she is receiving the TPN. Lariba begins to cry, saying, "This morning sickness is bad enough, but now I have diabetes too? How can that be?" What is the nurse's best response?

3. What potential complication will the nurse monitor for that can occur with peripherally administered TPN?

4. Before beginning the infusion, the nurse checks the ingredients of the TPN bag. The nurse notices that 20% dextrose is listed in the contents. Will the nurse add this bag to the patient's infusion? Explain your answer.

_____

For answers, see http://evolve.elsevier.com/Canada/Lilley/pharmacology/.

PATIENT TEACHING TIPS

❖ Patients are often discharged from a facility with the need for various types of tube feedings. In this situation, provide the patient, family members, and caregivers with education, instructions, and demonstrations about daily care of the tube, preparation of tube feedings, and related procedures. Present the education in a way that reflects the learning needs of the patient and those involved in the patient's care.

❖ Instruct patients, family members, and caregivers about the need for correct placement of the tube, which should be checked prior to each tube feeding if a nasogastric tube is used. Incorrect placement of a nasogastric tube would be manifested by coughing, choking, difficulty speaking, cyanosis, and subsequent respiratory distress. The head of the bed must remain elevated at 30 to 45° during infusions and for 1 hour afterwards to reduce gastroesophageal reflux and the probability for aspiration; this is more critical with nasogastric tube feedings than with tube feedings by other routes.

❖ Provide contact names and phone numbers of health care providers, home health care nurses, and other resources to patients, family members, and caregivers so that therapy can be monitored and problems and complications related to feeding averted. A fever, difficulty breathing, sounds of lung congestion, high amounts of residual, resistance to the flow of the feeding solution, and resistance when checking the residual all require additional monitoring. Appropriate interventions must be implemented, including seeking emergency medical care if needed.

❖ Patients who are discharged home and are receiving parenteral nutrition will need individualized education

as well as support from home health care or related health care services. Practice is critical to acquisition of skills by the patient, family members, or caregivers and must be an integral part of patient education. Before a patient is discharged, explain and demonstrate all procedures for storage, cleansing and care of the site, dressing changes, irrigation of the catheter, pump function and care, and changing of the bag, filters, and tubing; require return demonstrations by the patient. Advise the patient that parenteral nutrition in the home requires home health care services from a registered nurse to help prevent the complications of infection at the site, sepsis, fever, and pneumonia.

❖ Educate patients about the need to check serum glucose levels at home, as ordered by the health care provider if parenteral nutrition or other infused solutions high in dextrose are administered. Thoroughly explain the operation of a glucometer, with specific steps for its use included in a demonstration to the patient, family members, or caregivers. In addition, include and reinforce instructions for self-administration of insulin, if needed.

❖ Instruct patients to report to their health care provider any signs or symptoms of potential complications of parenteral nutrition, including fever, cough, chest pains, dyspnea, and chills (all of which are indicative of adverse reactions to lipid infusions). Restlessness, nervousness, fainting, and tachycardia are associated with hypoglycemia and must also be reported, as must the occurrence of polyuria, polydipsia, polyphagia, nausea, vomiting, headache, or weakness, which indicate hyperglycemia.

KEY POINTS

- ❖ A thorough nutritional assessment and consultation with a registered dietitian are essential to adequate interventions for malnourished patients.
- ❖ Various enteral feeding formulations with different nutritional content are available, including some that are lactose free.
- ❖ Enteral feedings may result in complications such as hyperglycemia, dumping syndrome, and aspiration of the nutritional supplement.
- ❖ Parenteral nutrition supplementation, intravenously administered, is total parenteral nutrition (TPN) or hyperalimentation. TPN may be administered through a central vein.
- ❖ TPN is administered through a central venous catheter because of the hyperosmolarity of the substances

used and the need for dilution provided by a larger-diameter vein to prevent venous damage. Parenteral nutrition given through a peripherally inserted central catheter line is another option but uses a solution that has a lower concentration of dextrose and other ingredients.

- ❖ Parenteral feedings may result in air embolism, fever, infection, fluid volume overload, hyperglycemia, or hypoglycemia. If they are discontinued abruptly, rebound hypoglycemia may result.
- ❖ Cautious and skillful nursing care may prevent or decrease the occurrence of complications associated with enteral or parenteral nutritional supplements.
- ❖ Always check the compatibility of putting medications in tube with the pharmacist.

EXAMINATION REVIEW QUESTIONS

1. The nurse is assessing an enteral feeding that is infusing via a nasogastric feeding tube. Which statement about this tube is accurate?
   a. It is surgically placed into the stomach.
   b. It is inserted through the nose into the jejunum.
   c. It is surgically inserted directly into the jejunum.
   d. It is inserted through the nose into the stomach.

2. When administering total parenteral nutrition (TPN), the nurse is aware that one purpose of IV fat (lipid) emulsions is to provide which nutrient?
   a. Calories
   b. Amino acids
   c. Minerals
   d. Immunoglobulins

3. The nurse is monitoring a patient who is receiving a TPN infusion and notes that the patient has cold, clammy skin; shows tachycardia; and is reporting feeling dizzy. What is the immediate action of the nurse?
   a. Stop the TPN infusion.
   b. Check the patient's blood glucose level.
   c. Order a stat (immediate) electrocardiogram.
   d. Obtain an order for blood cultures.

4. A patient has new orders for administration of peripheral TPN. The nurse knows that peripheral parenteral nutrition is most appropriate in which situation?
   a. Therapy is expected to last more than 14 days.
   b. Therapy is expected to last fewer than 14 days.
   c. A dextrose concentration of 20% is needed.
   d. Nutritional needs are 3 000 kcal/day.

5. During the night shift, a patient's infusion of TPN runs out, the pharmacy is closed, and a new bag of TPN will not be available for about 6 hours. Which action by the nurse would be the most appropriate action at this time?
   a. Hang a bottle of lipid solution.
   b. Hang a bag of normal saline.
   c. Hang a bag of 10% dextrose.
   d. Call the health care provider for stat TPN orders.

6. The nurse is assessing a patient who is receiving an enteral tube feeding. Which are possible adverse effects associated with enteral feedings? (Select all that apply.)
   a. Hypoglycemia
   b. Air embolism
   c. Aspiration
   d. Diarrhea
   e. Infection

7. A patient is receiving a tube feeding via a PEG tube of Glucerna at 50 mL/h. The orders also indicate to check the residual and flush the tubing every 4 hours with 30 mL of water. Calculate the total intake of fluid at the end of a 12-hour shift.

CRITICAL THINKING ACTIVITIES

1. A patient who is receiving enteral nutrition through a PEG tube is experiencing severe diarrhea. What is the nurse's priority action?

2. A patient has been receiving TPN with a 25% glucose content, and the nurse has just discovered that the central IV access line is clogged. What is of the most immediate concern, and what is the nurse's priority action at this time? Explain your answer.

3. At the beginning of the morning shift, the nurse is reviewing the medication orders for a patient who is receiving the impaired glucose tolerance formulation Glucerna through a nasogastric feeding tube. The patient has a history of seizures, and a dose of phenytoin (to be given via the tube) is due later in the morning. What is the nurse's priority action?

For answers, see http://evolve.elsevier.com/Canada/Lilley/pharmacology/.

PART EIGHT

Anti-infective and Anti-inflammatory Drugs

STUDY SKILLS TIPS:
- NURSING PROCESS
- ASSESSMENT
- NURSING DIAGNOSES
- EVALUATION

NURSING PROCESS

This study section focuses on the Nursing Process sections, using Chapter 43 as an example. Consider the following statement from Objective 11:

"Develop a collaborative plan of care that includes all phases of the nursing process for patients receiving drugs in each of the following classes of antibiotics: sulfonamides, penicillins, cephalosporins, macrolides, and tetracyclines."

The Nursing Process section focuses on major classifications, and you need to see both general and specific information about the classifications. Although the objective statement is only one sentence long, it clearly defines what you need to keep in mind as you study this section.

ASSESSMENT

When you read the Nursing Process section of a chapter, ask yourself. What do I need to learn? What do I need to know? What do I need to be able to do? Consider the following section from Chapter 43.

"To ensure effective treatment, in general, <u>before the administration</u> of any antibiotic, it is <u>crucial to gather data on a history of, or symptoms indicative of, hypersensitivity or allergic reactions (from mild reactions with rash, pruritus, angioedema, or hives to severe reactions with laryngeal edema, bronchospasm, hypotension, or possible cardiac arrest). Also determine the patient's age, weight, and baseline vital signs including body temperature. Examine the results of any laboratory tests that have been ordered, such as liver function studies (AST</u> <u>and ALT levels), kidney function tests (usually GFR, BUN, and creatinine levels), heart function tests (pertinent laboratory tests, electrocardiogram [ECG]), ultrasonography (if indicated), culture and sensitivity tests, and complete blood count (CBC) with hemoglobin/hematocrit (Hgb/Hct) levels and platelet and clotting tests.</u>"

In Chapter 43, you are assessing patients in relation to the pharmacological interventions discussed. Some underlining has been added here to bring focus to the points you need to be aware of as you study.

The word *crucial* tells you this is something that cannot be ignored. Before reading on, ask yourself, what crucial information should be considered before administering an antibiotic? As you keep reading, the answer is found in the sentence. You need to have data collected on the patient. The sentence goes on to identify the kind of data that should be available, and the sentence makes it clear that it has to be done "before the administration of any antibiotic."

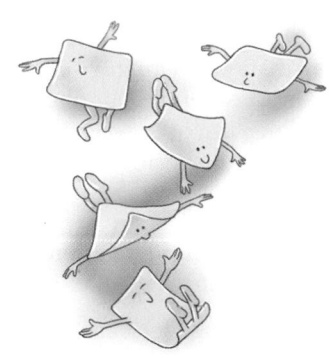

The first item is "hypersensitivities." Some individuals are allergic to certain antibiotics; it would be dangerous and possibly fatal to administer an antibiotic to a patient who is hypersensitive to it. Assessment for hypersensitivity also connects with effective treatment. As you consider each of the underlined elements in this sentence, keep in mind its relationship to effectiveness and appropriateness.

The patient's age should be known. Chapter 4 deals with concerns related to older adults and children. Patients in these age groups respond to drugs differently from the way young adults do. This response directly affects dosage and possibly even the choice of antibiotics to be administered. Again, this factor is directly related to the "effective treatment" referred to in this sentence.

Another part of the above section specifies liver, kidney, and heart functioning. Try to recall information that relates the specific antibiotics to these functions.

One more aspect of this sentence is the use of standard medical abbreviations. In earlier Study Skills Tips, it was suggested that you prepare vocabulary cards for these abbreviations. You need to know what CBC, Hgb, and Hct mean, what they measure, and how they relate to the appropriate administration of antibiotics. If these letters are not meaningful to you, then you will not be able to link what you know about the antibiotics with what you must know about administering them. Many test questions on nursing examinations use the standard abbreviations, and you must know them instantly and be able to relate them to the situation covered.

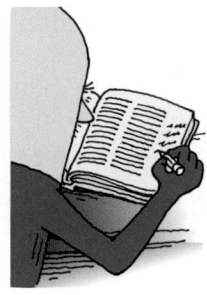

NURSING DIAGNOSES

Again, start with the question, "What am I supposed to learn?" The focus is on administration of antibiotics. What should you look for in working with patients that affects the administration of antibiotics?

This same procedure should be applied to the sections on Planning, Expected Patient Outcomes, and Implementation. Consider what each of these headings suggests about the nursing process, and read and evaluate the information, relating it to what you have already learned. Also, consider the implications of the information as possible test questions that may ask you to do more than recall specific facts. For example, consider the following case:

Patient A, age 23 years, has a temperature of 38.2°C. She was admitted yesterday and delivered a healthy infant 8 hours ago. She is breastfeeding her newborn.

What antibiotics might be administered? What specific antibiotics should be used with caution or eliminated from consideration?

This case demonstrates the need to read and think critically. You need to remember the specific facts from the chapter and be able to take a case study example and apply those facts to that specific situation. This process allows you to enhance your knowledge of antibiotics by understanding the general similarities and differentiating specifics that apply contextually.

EVALUATION

Evaluation is the final section under Nursing Process. What are you supposed to evaluate? Consider the second sentence under this section in Chapter 43.

"The therapeutic effects of antibiotics include a decrease in the signs and symptoms of infection; a return to normal vital signs, including temperature; negative results on culture and sensitivity tests; normal results for CBC; and improved appetite, energy level, and sense of well-being." This sentence makes it clear that you are evaluating the patient and the response to the antibiotics being administered. In evaluating the patient, what should you look for? Given that the focus of the nursing process is on contraindications, cautions, hypersensitivity, and reactions related to the administration of antibiotics, you should evaluate two aspects of the patient. Firstly, you should look for the positive responses indicating that the patient is responding well to treatment. When you read the next sentence in this section, you see: "Evaluation for adverse effects includes monitoring for …" This says that your role in evaluation is to monitor the patient for negative responses that occur once the treatment has been administered. Secondly, be prepared to educate the patient about these effects and possible steps to alleviate them.

Read the Nursing Process section in each chapter carefully and thoughtfully because it is in this section that you begin to see how the complex pharmacological material presented earlier in the chapter applies to your role as a nurse. Read this material with the same concern and care that you gave to the earlier part of the chapter; this is the section in which you think about *applying* all you have learned. Apply the PURR model, and be an active questioner and reader, and you will be successful in working with the Nursing Process in each chapter.

Antibiotics Part 1: Sulfonamides, Penicillins, Cephalosporins, Macrolides, and Tetracyclines

Objectives

After reading this chapter, the successful student will be able to do the following:

1. Discuss the general principles of antibiotic therapy.

2. Explain how antibiotics work to rid the body of infections.

3. Briefly compare the characteristics and uses of antiseptics and disinfectants.

4. List the most commonly used antiseptics and disinfectants.

5. Discuss any nursing-related considerations associated with the environmental use of antiseptics and disinfectants.

6. Discuss the benefits and risks of antibiotic use with attention to the overuse or misuse of antibiotics and the development of drug resistance.

7. Discuss the concept of superinfection, including its etiology and prevention.

8. Classify various antibiotics by their general category, including sulfonamides, penicillins, cephalosporins, macrolides, and tetracyclines.

9. Discuss the mechanisms of action, indications, cautions, contraindications, routes of administration, and drug interactions for the sulfonamides, penicillins, cephalosporins, macrolides, and tetracyclines.

10. Identify drug-specific adverse effects and toxic effects of each of the antibiotic classes listed earlier, and cite measures to decrease their occurrence.

11. Develop a collaborative plan of care that includes all phases of the nursing process for patients receiving drugs in each of the following classes of antibiotics: sulfonamides, penicillins, cephalosporins, macrolides, and tetracyclines.

e-Learning Activities

Website
(http://evolve.elsevier.com/Canada/
Lilley/pharmacology/)

evolve

- Answer Key—Textbook Case Studies
- Answer Key—Critical Thinking Activities
- Chapter Summaries—Printable
- Review Questions for Exam Preparation
- Unfolding Case Studies

Drug Profiles

▸▸ amoxicillin, p. 814
  ampicillin, p. 814
▸▸ azithromycin and clarithromycin, p. 820
  aztreonam, p. 818
▸▸ cefazolin (cefazolin sodium)*, p. 815
  cefepime (cefepime hydrochloride)*, p. 817
▸▸ cefoxitin (cefoxitin sodium)*, p. 816
  ceftazidime (ceftazidime pentahydrate)*, p. 816
▸▸ ceftriaxone (ceftriaxone sodium)*, p. 816
  cefuroxime (cefuroxime sodium)*, p. 816
▸▸ cephalexin, p. 815
  cloxacillin (cloxacillin sodium)*, p. 814
▸▸ doxycycline hyclate, p. 822
▸▸ erythromycin, p. 820
▸▸ imipenem/cilastatin, p. 817
  meropenem, p. 817
▸▸ penicillin G and penicillin V potassium, p. 814
  piperacillin (piperacillin sodium)*, p. 812
  sulfamethoxazole/trimethoprim (co-trimoxazole), p. 811
  tigecycline, p. 822

▸▸ Key drug

*Full generic name is given in parentheses. For the purposes of this text, the more common, shortened name is used.

Key Terms

Antibiotic Having the ability to destroy or interfere with the development of a living organism; most commonly refers to antibacterial drugs. (p. 805)

Antimicrobial stewardship An institutional activity that includes ensuring appropriate selection, dosing, choice of route, and duration of antimicrobial therapy. (p. 808)

Antiseptic One of two types of topical antimicrobial agents; a chemical that inhibits the growth and reproduction of microorganisms without necessarily killing them. Antiseptics are also called *static agents*. (p. 806)

Bactericidal antibiotics Antibiotics that kill bacteria. (p. 811)

Bacteriostatic antibiotics Antibiotics that do not kill bacteria but rather inhibit their growth. (p. 809)

β-Lactam A broad, major class of antibiotics that includes four subclasses: penicillins, cephalosporins, carbapenems, and monobactams, so named because of the β-lactam ring that is part of the chemical structure of all drugs in this class. (p. 810)

β-Lactamase Any of a group of enzymes produced by bacteria that catalyze the chemical opening of the crucial β-lactam ring structures in β-lactam antibiotics. (p. 811)

β-Lactamase inhibitors Medications combined with certain penicillin drugs to block the effect of β-lactamase enzymes. (p. 811)

Colonization The establishment and growth of microorganisms on skin, open wounds, or mucous membranes or in secretions without causing an infection. (p. 805)

Community-acquired infection An infection that is acquired by a person who has not recently been hospitalized or had a medical procedure (e.g., surgical procedure). (p. 805)

Definitive therapy The administration of antibiotics based on known results of culture and sensitivity testing identifying the pathogen causing infection. (p. 807)

Disinfectant One of two types of topical antimicrobial agents; a chemical applied to nonliving objects to kill microorganisms; also called *cidal agents*. (p. 806)

Empiric therapy The administration of antibiotics based on the health care provider's judgement of the pathogens most likely causing an apparent infection; it involves the presumptive treatment of an infection to avoid treatment delay, before specific culture information has been obtained. (p. 806)

Glucose-6-phosphate dehydrogenase (G6PD) deficiency An inherited disorder in which red blood cells are partially or completely deficient in glucose-6-phosphate dehydrogenase, a crucial enzyme in the metabolism of glucose. (p. 808)

Health care–associated infection An infection acquired during the course of receiving treatment for another condition in a health care facility. The infection is not present or incubating at the time of admission; also known as a *nosocomial infection*. (p. 805)

Host factors Factors that are unique to a particular patient that affect the patient's susceptibility to infection and response to antibiotic drugs; examples include a low neutrophil count or a lack of immunoglobulins in the blood that carry antibodies. (p. 808)

Infections Invasion and multiplication of microorganisms in body tissues. (p. 805)

Microorganisms Microscopic living organisms; also called *microbes*. (p. 805)

Prophylactic antibiotic therapy Antibiotics taken before anticipated exposure to an infectious organism in an effort to prevent the development of infection. (p. 807)

Pseudomembranous colitis A potentially necrotizing inflammatory bowel condition that is often associated with antibiotic therapy; often caused by the bacterium *Clostridium difficile*; also called by the more general term *antibiotic-associated colitis*. (p. 807)

Slow acetylation A common genetic host factor in which the rate of metabolism of certain drugs is reduced. (p. 808)

Subtherapeutic Generally refers to blood levels below therapeutic levels due to insufficient dosing. Also refers to antibiotic treatment that is ineffective in treating a given infection. Possible causes include inappropriate drug therapy, insufficient drug dosing, or bacterial drug resistance. (p. 807)

Superinfection (1) An infection occurring during antimicrobial treatment for another infection, resulting from overgrowth of an organism not susceptible to the antibiotic used. (2) A secondary microbial infection that occurs in addition to an earlier primary infection, often because of weakening of the patient's immune system function by the first infection. (p. 807)

Teratogens Substances that can interfere with normal prenatal development and cause one or more developmental abnormalities in the fetus. (p. 808)

Therapeutic Antibiotic therapy that is given in sufficient doses so that the concentration of the drug in the blood or other tissues renders it effective against specific bacterial pathogens. (p. 807)

MICROBIAL INFECTION

Microorganisms are everywhere, both in the external environment and in parts of the internal environment of our bodies. They can be harmful to humans, or they can be beneficial under normal circumstances but can become harmful when conditions are altered in some way. A person is normally able to remain healthy and resistant to infectious **microorganisms** because of the existence of certain host defences. These defences include actual physical barriers, such as intact skin or the ciliated respiratory mucosa, or physiological defences, such as the gastric acid in the stomach or immune factors such as antibodies. Other defences are the phagocytic cells (macrophages and polymorphonuclear neutrophils) that are part of the mononuclear phagocyte system.

Every known, major class of microbes contains organisms that can infect humans. This includes bacteria, viruses, fungi, and protozoa. The focus of this chapter is common bacterial **infections**.

Bacteria may take a number of different shapes. This property of bacteria is called their *morphology* (Figure 43-1), and they are often grouped based on this property. Bacteria may also be grouped according to other common recognizable characteristics. One of the most important ways of categorizing bacteria is on the basis of their response to the *Gram stain* procedure. Bacterial species that stain purple with Gram staining are classified as *gram-positive* organisms. Bacteria that stain red are classified as *gram-negative* organisms. This seemingly simple difference proves to be significant in guiding the choice of **antibiotic** therapy.

Gram-positive organisms have a thick cell wall, made of peptidoglycan; they also have a thick outer capsule. Gram-negative organisms have a cell wall structure that is more complex, with a smaller outer capsule, a peptidoglycan layer, and two cell membranes: an outer and inner membrane (Figure 43-2). These differences usually make gram-negative bacterial infections more difficult to treat, because drug molecules have a harder time penetrating the more complex cell walls of gram-negative organisms.

When normal host defences are somehow compromised, a person becomes susceptible to infection. Microorganisms invade and multiply in the body tissues, and if the infective process overwhelms the body's defence system, the infection becomes clinically apparent. The patient usually manifests some of the following classic signs and symptoms of infection: fever, chills, sweating, redness, pain and swelling, fatigue, weight loss, increased white blood cell (WBC) count, and the formation of pus. Not all patients will exhibit signs of the infection; this is especially true in older adults and patients who are immunocompromised.

To help the body and its normal host defences combat an infection, antibiotic therapy is often required. Antibiotics are most effective when their actions are combined with functioning bodily defence mechanisms. Oftentimes, patients will become colonized with bacteria. Although bacteria are present in open wounds, in secretions, on mucous membranes, or on the skin, such patients do not have any overt signs of infection; in older adults, confusion or altered orientation may be the only indicator. **Colonization** does not require antibiotic treatment. However, it is not uncommon for these colonizations to be treated, which may be one way in which drug-resistant organisms emerge.

Health Care–Associated Infection

A **community-acquired infection** is defined as one that is acquired by a person who has not recently (within the past year) been hospitalized or had a medical procedure (e.g., dialysis, surgery, catheterization). A **health care–associated infection**, previously known as a *nosocomial infection*, is defined as one that a patient acquires during the course of receiving treatment for another condition in a health care facility. The infection was not present or incubating at the time of admission but occurs more than

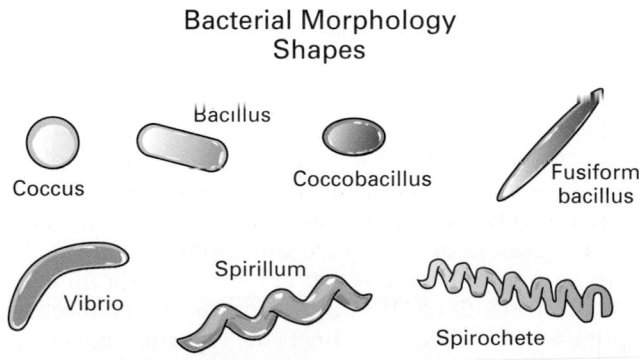

Bacterial Morphology Shapes

Coccus

Bacillus

Coccobacillus

Fusiform bacillus

Vibrio

Spirillum

Spirochete

FIG. 43-1 Morphology of bacteria. (Source: Murray, P. R., Rosenthal, K. S., Kobayashi, G. S., et al. (2009). *Medical microbiology* (6th ed.). St. Louis, MO: Mosby.)

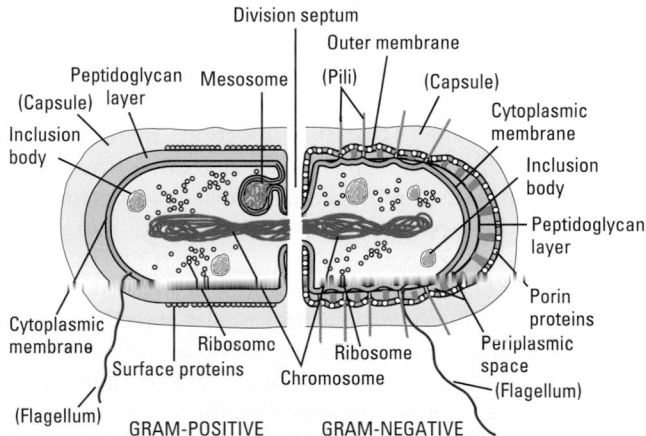

FIG. 43-2 Gram-positive and gram-negative bacteria. A gram-positive bacterium has a thick layer of peptidoglycan *(left)*. A gram-negative bacterium has a thin peptidoglycan layer and an outer membrane *(right)*. Structures in parentheses are not found in all bacteria. (Source: Murray, P. R., Rosenthal, K. S., Kobayashi, G. S., et al. (2009). *Medical microbiology* (6th ed.). St. Louis, MO: Mosby.)

48 hours after admission. Health care–associated infections are one of the top 10 leading causes of death in Canada. They tend to be more difficult to treat than community-acquired infections because the causative microorganisms have been exposed to strong antibiotics in the past and are the most drug resistant and the most virulent. The particular organisms that cause health care–associated infections have changed over time. Methicillin-resistant *Staphylococcus aureus* (MRSA) and vancomycin-resistant *Enterococcus* (VRE) (see Chapter 44) are currently two of the most important antibiotic-resistant organisms. Other serious pathogens include *Klebsiella, Acinetobacter*, and *Pseudomonas aeruginosa*. Most of these microorganisms are now resistant to many of the commonly used antibiotics. Gram-negative bacteria that produce the enzyme β-lactamase can break down commonly used antibiotics, making it difficult to treat infections with bacteria that produce extended spectrum β-lactamase (ESBL). Common producers of ESBL are *Enterobacteriaceae coli* and *Klebsiella pneumoniae*. Carbapenemase-producing *Enterobacteriaceae* (CPE) are resistant to the carbapenems.

Health care–associated infections develop in approximately 8% of children and 10% of adults in Canadian hospitals (Public Health Agency of Canada, 2013). The cost of treating such infections amounts to $1 billion annually. The majority (70% or more) of these infections are either urinary tract infections (UTIs) or postoperative wound infections. Often, they are acquired from various devices, such as mechanical ventilators, IV infusion lines, catheters, and dialysis equipment. Areas of the hospital associated with the greatest risk for acquiring a health care–associated infection are the critical care, dialysis, oncology, transplant, and burn units. This is because the host defences of the patients in these areas are typically compromised, which makes them more vulnerable to infection. Over 70% of health care–associated infections are preventable. The most common mode of transmitting them is by direct contact. Handwashing is the single most important activity that health care providers can do to prevent the spread of potentially deadly infections. Because health care–associated infections increase mortality, morbidity, and health care costs, one of Accreditation Canada's Required Organizational Practices focuses on patient safety, particularly infection control, as a priority area. The 2015 Required Organizational Practices are to identify and track health care–associated infections such as *Clostridium difficile*, surgical site infections, seasonal influenza, noroviruses, or UTIs, as well as other reportable diseases and antibiotic-resistant organisms. Other strategies for reducing health care–associated infections include the use of disinfectants and the use of antiseptics. A **disinfectant** is able to kill organisms and is used only on nonliving objects to destroy organisms that may be present. Disinfectants are sometimes called *cidal agents*. An **antiseptic** generally only inhibits the growth of microorganisms but does not necessarily kill them and is applied exclusively to living tissue. Antiseptics are also

TABLE 43-1

Antiseptics Versus Disinfectants

	Antiseptics	Disinfectants
Where used	Living tissue	Nonliving objects
Potency	Lower	Higher
Activity against organisms	Primarily inhibits growth (bacteriostatic)	Kills (bactericidal)

called *static agents*. The differences between antiseptics and disinfectants in a clinical sense are summarized in Table 43-1. Topical antimicrobial drugs are discussed further in Chapter 56.

GENERAL PRINCIPLES OF ANTIBIOTIC THERAPY

The selection of antimicrobial drugs requires clinical judgement and detailed knowledge of pharmacological and microbiologic factors. Antibiotics have three general uses: empiric therapy, definitive therapy, and prophylactic or preventative therapy. Antibiotic drug therapy begins with a clinical assessment of the patient to determine whether the patient has the common signs and symptoms of infection. The patient is assessed during and after antibiotic therapy to evaluate the effectiveness of the drug therapy, monitor for adverse drug effects, and make sure the infection is not recurring.

Often, the signs and symptoms of an infection appear long before an organism can be identified. When this happens and the risk of life-threatening or severe complications is high (e.g., suspected acute meningitis), an antibiotic is given to the patient immediately. The antibiotic selected is one that can best kill the microorganisms known to be the most common causes of infection. This is called **empiric therapy**. Before the start of empiric antibiotic therapy, specimens are obtained from suspected areas of infection to be cultured in an attempt to identify a causative organism. It must be emphasized that culture specimens must be obtained before drug therapy is initiated whenever possible. Otherwise, the presence of antibiotics in the tissues may result in misleading culture results. However, sometimes it is not possible to obtain a sample (especially sputum) in a reasonable amount of time, and antibiotic therapy is begun without a sample in such situations. If an organism is identified in the laboratory, it is then tested for susceptibility to various antibiotics. The results of these tests can confirm whether the empiric therapy chosen is appropriate for eradicating the organism identified. If not, therapy can be adjusted to optimize its efficacy against the specific infectious organism(s). Once the results of culture and sensitivity testing are available (usually in 48 to 72 hours), the antibiotic therapy is then tailored to treat the identified organism by using the most narrow-spectrum, least toxic drug based on sensitivity results. This is known as **definitive therapy**. Broad-spectrum antibiotics are those that are effective against numerous organisms (gram-positive, gram-negative, and anaerobic). Narrow-spectrum antibiotics are effective against only a few organisms. Once the results of culture and sensitivity testing are available, it is always better to use an antibiotic that targets the specific organism identified (i.e., a narrow-spectrum antibiotic). Overuse of broad-spectrum antibiotics contributes to resistance. The goal of therapy is to use the most narrow-spectrum drug possible, based on sensitivity results.

Antibiotics are also given for prophylaxis. This is often the case when patients are scheduled to undergo a procedure (e.g., surgery) during or after which the likelihood of microbial contamination is high. **Prophylactic antibiotic therapy** is used to prevent an infection. The risk of infection varies depending on the procedure being performed. For example, the risk of infection in a patient undergoing coronary artery bypass surgery (with standard preoperative cleansing of the body) is relatively low, compared with that in a person undergoing intra-abdominal surgery for the treatment of injuries sustained in a motor vehicle crash. In the latter case, the abdominal cavity is likely to be contaminated with bacteria from the gastrointestinal (GI) tract. This would constitute a contaminated or "dirty" surgical field, and thus the likelihood of clinically serious infection would be much higher than in the former case. Antibiotic therapy would likely be required for a longer period after the procedure. To be effective, prophylactic antibiotics need to be given before a procedure, generally 60 minutes before the incision, to ensure adequate tissue penetration. Prevent Surgical Site Infections is a national project of Safer Heathcare Now, the flagship program of the Canadian Patient Safety Institute, which provides hospitals with evidence-informed recommendations on the prioritization and implementation of surgical site infection prevention efforts, including the appropriate use of prophylactic antibiotics. Prophylactic antibiotics prior to dental procedures are recommended only for those at greatest risk of developing infective endocarditis, including individuals with a prosthetic heart valve; a history of infective endocarditis; certain specific, severe congenital heart conditions; or a heart transplant that has developed an issue with a heart valve (Canadian Dental Association, 2014). Furthermore, prophylaxis is recommended for the above patients who undergo procedures in which gingival tissues are manipulated or that perforate the oral mucosa.

To optimize antibiotic therapy, the patient is continuously monitored for both **therapeutic** efficacy and adverse drug effects. A therapeutic response to antibiotics is one in which there is a decrease in the specific signs and symptoms of infection compared with baseline findings (e.g., fever, elevated WBC count, redness, inflammation, drainage, pain). Antibiotic therapy is said to be **subtherapeutic** when these signs and symptoms do not improve. This can result from the use of an incorrect route of drug administration, inadequate drainage of an abscess, poor drug penetration to the infected area, insufficient serum levels of the drug, or bacterial resistance to the drug. Antibiotic therapy may result in an allergic or other major adverse reaction to the drug. These reactions can include rash, itching, hives, fever, chills, joint pain, difficulty breathing, or wheezing. Relatively minor adverse drug reactions such as nausea, vomiting, and diarrhea are quite common with antibiotic therapy and are usually not severe enough to require drug discontinuation.

Superinfection can occur when antibiotics reduce or completely eliminate the normal bacterial and fungal flora that are needed to maintain normal function in various organs. When these bacteria or fungi are killed by antibiotics, other bacteria or fungi are permitted to take over and cause infection. Another type of superinfection is the development of a vaginal or pharyngeal *Candida albicans* yeast infection. Antibiotic use is strongly associated with the potential for the development of diarrhea, a common adverse effect. However, antibiotic-acquired diarrhea becomes a serious superinfection when it causes antibiotic-acquired colitis, also known as **pseudomembranous colitis** or simply *C. difficile infection*. This happens because antibiotics disrupt the normal gut flora and can cause an overgrowth of *C. difficile.* The most common symptoms of *C. difficile* colitis are odorous watery diarrhea, abdominal pain, and fever. Whenever a patient who was previously treated with antibiotics develops watery diarrhea, the patient needs to be tested for *C. difficile* infection. If the results are positive, the patient will need to be treated for this serious superinfection. Infections with *C. difficile* are increasingly becoming resistant to standard therapy. For example, an emerging strain of *C. difficile*, NAP/0127, is more virulent than previous strains, with the ability to produce greater quantities of toxins. In addition, it is more resistant to the quinolones.

Yet another type of superinfection occurs when a second infection closely follows the initial infection and comes from an external source (as opposed to normal body flora), which may still be ongoing. A common example is a situation in which a patient who has a viral respiratory infection develops a secondary bacterial infection. This is likely due to weakening of the patient's immune system function by the primary viral infection. Although the viral infection will not respond to antibiotic therapy, antibiotics may be needed to treat the secondary bacterial infection. This situation calls for some diagnostic finesse on the part of the health care provider, who needs to avoid prescribing unnecessary antibiotics for a viral infection. The presence of coloured sputum (e.g., green or yellow) may or may not be a sign of a bacterial superinfection during a viral respiratory illness. Patients will often expect to receive an antibiotic prescription even when they show no signs of a bacterial superinfection. From their perspective, they know they are "sick" and want "some medicine" to expedite their recovery from illness. This expectation can create both diagnostic confusion and an emotional dilemma for the health care provider. In general, coughs, colds, and sore throats are usually viral. If a fever develops, suspect a bacterial secondary infection. Respiratory tract infections (e.g., otitis media, tonsillitis, pneumonia, bronchitis, sinusitis, pharyngitis, pertussis) are often caused by bacteria.

Over the decades, many easily treatable bacterial infections have become increasingly resistant to antibiotic therapy. One major cause of this phenomenon is the overprescribing of antibiotics, often in the clinical situations described earlier. Antibiotic resistance is now considered one of the world's most pressing public health problems. Another factor that contributes to antibiotic resistance is the tendency of many patients to not complete their antibiotic regimen. Individuals may also take antibiotics purchased abroad or on the Internet for self-diagnosed illnesses. Patients must be counselled to take the entire course of prescribed antibiotic drugs, even if they feel that they are no longer ill. As part of Accreditation Canada's Required Organizational Practices (2014), institutions that provide inpatient acute care, inpatient cancer care, inpatient rehabilitation, and complex continuing care must have a program in place for **antimicrobial stewardship**. Effective antimicrobial stewardship combined with a comprehensive infection control program will limit the emergence and transmission of antimicrobial-resistant bacteria.

Food–drug and drug–drug interactions are common problems when antibiotics are taken. Both tetracyclines and quinolone antibiotics have a common drug interaction with substances that chelate (e.g., calcium-containing substances such as milk, cheese, and antacids). They also chelate with vitamin/mineral supplements (e.g., iron, magnesium). This is especially important, as will be discussed later, because quinolone antibiotics are used orally to treat serious infections. If they are not absorbed, treatment failure is likely to ensue.

Other important factors that must be understood to use antibiotics appropriately are host-specific factors, or **host factors**. These are factors that pertain specifically to a given patient, and they can have an important impact on the success or failure of antibiotic therapy. Some of these host factors are age, allergy history, kidney and liver function, pregnancy status, genetic characteristics, site of infection, and host defences. Age-related host factors are those that apply to patients at either end of the age spectrum. For example, infants and children may not be able to take certain antibiotics such as tetracyclines, which affect developing teeth or bones; quinolones, which may affect bone or cartilage development in children; and sulfonamides, which may displace bilirubin from albumin and precipitate kernicterus (hyperbilirubinemia) in neonates. The aging process affects the function of organ systems. As individuals age, there is a gradual decline in the function of the kidneys and liver, the organs primarily responsible for metabolizing and eliminating antibiotics. Therefore, depending on an older adult's level of kidney or liver function, dosage adjustments may be necessary. Pharmacists often play a significant role in evaluating the dosages of antibiotics and other medications to ensure optimal dosing for a patient's level of organ function.

A patient's history of allergic reactions to an antibiotic is important in the selection of the most appropriate antibiotic for that patient. Penicillins and sulfonamides are two broad classes of antibiotics to which many people have allergic anaphylactic reactions. Symptoms of anaphylaxis include flushing; itching; hives; anxiety; fast, irregular pulse; and throat and tongue swelling. The most dangerous reaction is anaphylactic shock, in which a patient can suffocate from drug-induced respiratory arrest. Although this outcome is the most extreme, because it is a possibility, it is of utmost importance to consistently assess patients for drug allergies and document any known allergies clearly in medical records. All reported drug allergies are to be taken seriously and investigated further before making a final decision about administering a given drug. Many patients will say that they are "allergic" to a medication when in fact what they experienced was a common mild adverse effect such as stomach upset or nausea. Patients who report drug allergies need to be asked open-ended questions to elicit descriptions of prior allergic reactions, so that the actual severity of the reaction can be assessed. The most common severe reactions to any medication that need to be noted in the patient's chart include any difficulty breathing; significant rashes, hives, or other skin reactions; and severe GI intolerance. Although some antibiotics are ideally taken on an empty stomach, eating a small amount of food with the medication may be sufficient to help the patient tolerate it and realize its therapeutic benefits.

Pregnancy-related host factors are also important to the selection of appropriate antibiotics because several antibiotics can pass through the placenta and cause harm to the developing fetus. Drugs that cause development abnormalities in the fetus are called **teratogens**. Their use by women who are pregnant can result in birth defects.

Some patients also have certain genetic abnormalities that result in various enzyme deficiencies. These conditions can adversely affect drug actions in the body. Two of the most common examples of such genetic host factors are **glucose-6-phosphate dehydrogenase (G6PD) deficiency** and **slow acetylation**. The administration of antibiotics such as sulfonamides, nitrofurantoin, and dapsone to a person with G6PD deficiency may result in the *hemolysis*, or destruction, of red blood cells. Patients who are slow acetylators have a physiological makeup that causes certain drugs to be metabolized more slowly than usual in a chemical step known as *acetylation*. This can lead to toxicity from drug accumulation (see Chapter 2).

The anatomical site of the infection is an important host factor to consider when deciding not only which antibiotic to use but also the dosage, route of administration, and duration of therapy. Some antibiotics do not penetrate into certain sites of infection, such as the lungs, bone, or abscesses, which can lead to treatment failures.

Consideration of the discussed host factors, as well as drug pharmacokinetics, helps health care providers and pharmacists to ensure optimal drug selection for each individual patient. Continued patient assessment and proper monitoring of antibiotic therapy increase the likelihood that this therapy will be safe and effective. For example, in patients who are critically ill, their volume of distribution is generally larger and therefore water-soluble antibiotics require dosage increases; or in serious infections, antibiotics with shorter half-lives (i.e., cloxacillin) require more frequent dosing to endure adequate tissue penetration.

ANTIBIOTICS

Antibiotics are classified into broad categories based on their chemical structures. The common categories are sulfonamides, penicillins, cephalosporins, carbapenems, macrolides, quinolones, aminoglycosides, and tetracyclines. In addition to chemical structure, other characteristics that distinguish classes of drugs include antibacterial spectrum, mechanism of action, potency, toxicity, and pharmacokinetic properties. The four most common mechanisms of antibiotic action are: (1) interference with bacterial cell wall synthesis, (2) interference with protein synthesis, (3) interference with replication of nucleic acids (deoxyribonucleic acid [DNA] and ribonucleic acid [RNA]), and (4) antimetabolite action that disrupts critical metabolic reactions inside the bacterial cell. Figure 43-3 portrays these mechanisms in combating bacterial infections and indicates which mechanisms are used by several major antibiotic classes.

Perhaps the greatest challenge in understanding antimicrobial therapy is remembering the types and species of microorganisms against which a given drug can act.

The list of individual microorganisms against which a given drug has activity can be quite extensive and can seem daunting to inexperienced health care providers. Most antimicrobials have activity against only one *type* of microbe (e.g., bacteria, viruses, fungi, protozoa). However, a few drugs do have activity against more than one class of organisms.

The field of infectious disease treatment is continually evolving, largely because of the continuous emergence of resistant bacterial strains. For this reason, drug indications change frequently, often from year to year, as various bacterial species become resistant to previously effective anti-infective therapy. It is always appropriate to check the most current reference materials or consult with colleagues (e.g., nurses, pharmacists, other health care providers) when questions remain. Pharmacists are excellent resources regarding antibiotics. Many hospitals now have pharmacists who are specially trained in the treatment of infectious diseases.

SULFONAMIDES

Sulfonamides comprise one of the first groups of drugs used as antibiotics. Although there are many compounds in the sulfonamide family, only sulfamethoxazole combined with trimethoprim (a nonsulfonamide antibiotic)—known as Apo-Sulfratrim®, Protrim®, Septra® (available only as an injection), or Teva-Trimel®, and often abbreviated as SMX-TMP—is commonly used in clinical practice. Sulfisoxazole acetyl combined with erythromycin ethylsuccinate (a macrolide antibiotic) is occasionally used in pediatrics. Sulfasalazine, another sulfonamide, is used to treat ulcerative colitis and rheumatoid arthritis but is not used as an antibiotic.

Mechanism of Action and Drug Effects

Sulfonamides do not actually destroy bacteria but inhibit their growth. For this reason, they are considered **bacteriostatic antibiotics**. They inhibit the growth of susceptible bacteria by preventing bacterial synthesis of folic acid. Folic acid is a B-complex vitamin that is required for the proper synthesis of purines, one of the chemical components of nucleic acids (DNA and RNA). Chemical components of folic acid include para-aminobenzoic acid (PABA), pteridine, and glutamic acid. Specifically, in a process known as competitive inhibition, sulfonamides compete with PABA for the bacterial enzyme tetrahydropteroic acid synthetase, which incorporates PABA into the folic acid molecule. Because sulfonamides are capable of blocking a specific step in a biosynthetic pathway, they are also considered antimetabolites. Microorganisms that require exogenous folic acid (not synthesized by the bacterium itself) are not affected by sulfonamide antibiotics. Therefore, these drugs do not affect folic acid metabolism in human cells. Trimethoprim, although not a sulfonamide, works via a similar mechanism, inhibiting dihydrofolic acid reduction to tetrahydrofolate, which results in inhibition of the enzymes of the folic acid pathway.

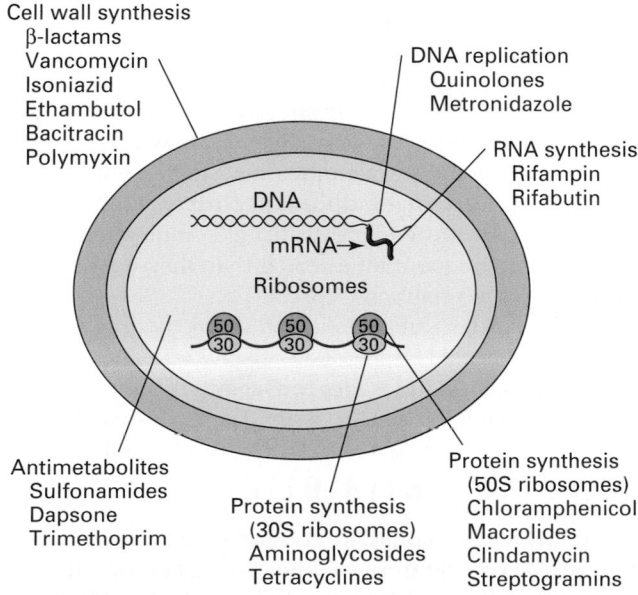

FIG. 43-3   Basic sites of antibiotic activity. *DNA*, deoxyribonucleic acid; *mRNA*, messenger ribonucleic acid; *RNA*, ribonucleic acid. (Source: Murray, P. R., Rosenthal, K. S., Kobayashi, G. S., et al. (2009). *Medical microbiology* (6th ed.). St. Louis, MO: Mosby.)

Indications

Sulfonamides have a broad spectrum of antibacterial activity, including activity against both gram-positive and gram-negative organisms. These antibiotics achieve high concentrations in the kidneys, through which they are eliminated. The combination of these two drugs allows for a synergistic (see Chapter 2) antibacterial effect. Commonly susceptible organisms include strains of *Enterobacter* species (spp.), *Escherichia coli, Klebsiella* spp., *Proteus mirabilis, Proteus vulgaris,* and *Staphylococcus aureus.* Unfortunately, however, resistant bacterial strains are a growing problem, as is the case with other antibiotic classes. Results of culture and sensitivity testing help optimize drug selection in individual cases. This combination drug is used for treating respiratory tract infections. However, it is now less effective against streptococci infecting the upper respiratory tract and the pharynx. Another specific use for SMX-TMP is prophylaxis and treatment of opportunistic infections in patients with pneumonia associated with HIV-associated infection, especially infection by *Pneumocystis jirovecii,* a common cause of HIV. SMX-TMP is also a drug of choice for infection caused by the bacterium *Stenotrophomonas maltophilia.* SMX-TMP has become common treatment for outpatient *Staphylococcus* infections, due to the high rate of community-acquired MRSA infections. MRSA and other resistant organisms are discussed in Chapter 44.

Contraindications

Use of sulfonamides is contraindicated in cases of known drug allergy to sulfonamides. Chemically related drugs such as the sulfonylureas (used to treat diabetes; see Chapter 33), thiazide and loop diuretics (see Chapter 29), and carbonic anhydrase inhibitors (see Chapter 29) are generally considered relatively safe in a patient with a sulfonamide allergy. However, the cyclooxygenase-2 inhibitors such as celecoxib (Celebrex®) should not be used (see Chapter 49) in patients with a known sulfonamide allergy. The use of sulfonamides is also contraindicated in pregnant women at term and in infants younger than 2 months of age.

Adverse Effects

Sulfonamide drugs are a common cause of allergic reactions. Patients will sometimes refer to this as "sulfa allergy" or even "sulfur allergy." Although immediate reactions can occur, sulfonamides typically cause delayed cutaneous reactions. Such reactions frequently begin with fever followed by a rash (morbilliform eruptions, erythema multiforme, Stevens-Johnson syndrome, toxic epidermal necrolysis). If severe allergic reactions occur, the drug should be discontinued. Photosensitivity reactions are another type of skin reaction, induced by exposure to sunlight during sulfonamide drug therapy. In some cases, such reactions can result in severe sunburn. Such reactions are also common with the tetracycline class of antibiotics discussed later in this chapter, as well as with other drug classes, and may occur immediately

TABLE	43-2
Sulfonamides: Reported Adverse Effects	

Body System	Adverse Effects
Hematological	Agranulocytosis, aplastic anemia, hemolytic anemia, thrombocytopenia
Gastrointestinal	Nausea, vomiting, diarrhea, pancreatitis, hepatoxicity
Integumentary	Epidermal necrolysis, exfoliative dermatitis, Stevens-Johnson syndrome, photosensitivity
Other	Convulsions, crystalluria, toxic nephrosis, headache, peripheral neuritis, urticaria, cough

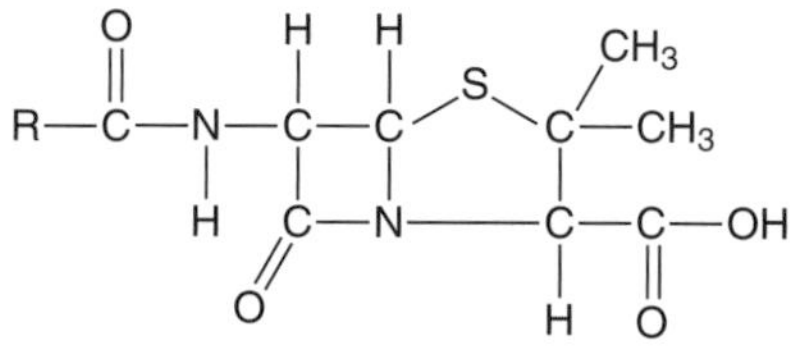

FIG. 43-4 Chemical structure of penicillins showing the β-lactam ring. *R,* variable portion of drug chemical structure.

or have a delayed onset. Other reactions to sulfonamides include mucocutaneous, GI, liver, kidney, and hematological complications, all of which may be fatal in severe cases. It is believed that sulfonamide reactions are immune mediated and involve the production of reactive metabolites in the body. Reported adverse effects to the sulfonamides are listed in Table 43-2.

Interactions

Sulfonamides can have clinically significant interactions with a number of other medications. Sulfonamides may potentiate the hypoglycemic effects of sulfonylureas in diabetes treatment, the toxic effects of phenytoin, and the anticoagulant effects of warfarin sodium, which can lead to hemorrhaging. Sulfonamides may increase the likelihood of cyclosporine-induced nephrotoxicity. Patients receiving any of the above drug combinations may require more frequent monitoring than they would if not taking the combinations.

Dosages

For recommended dosages on selected sulfonamides, refer to the table on p. 811.

β-LACTAM ANTIBIOTICS

The **β-lactam** antibiotics are commonly used drugs. They are so called because of the β-lactam ring that is part of the chemical structure (Figure 43-4). This broad group of drugs includes four major subclasses: penicillins, cephalosporins, carbapenems, and monobactams. They share a common structure and mechanism of

DRUG PROFILES

Sulfonamides act by interfering with bacterial synthesis of the essential nutrient folic acid. Most sulfonamide therapy today uses the combination drug sulfamethoxazole/trimethoprim.

sulfamethoxazole/trimethoprim

Sulfamethoxazole/trimethoprin (Apo-Sulfatrim, Protrim, Septra, Teva-Trimel) is a fixed-combination drug product containing a 5:1 ratio of sulfamethoxazole to trimethoprim. It is available in both oral and injectable dosage forms.

PHARMACOKINETICS

Route	Onset of Action	Peak Plasma Concentration	Elimination Half-Life	Duration of Action
PO	Variable	2–4 hr	7–12 hr	12 hr

DOSAGES   Selected Sulfonamides and Combination Drug Products

Drug	Pharmacological Class	Usual Dosage Range	Indications
sulfamethoxazole/trimethoprim (Apo-Sulfatrim, Protrim, Septra, Teva-Trimel)	Sulfonamide and folate antimetabolite	*Children* IV/PO: 5–10 mg/kg/day trimethoprim and 25–50 mg sulfamethoxazole divided bid–qid *Adults* IV/PO: 160–240 mg trimethoprim and 800–1 200 mg sulfamethoxazole bid–qid	Serious systemic infections, *Pneumocystis jirovecii*, pneumonia

IV, intravenous; *PO*, oral.

action—they inhibit the synthesis of the bacterial peptidoglycan cell wall.

Some bacterial strains produce the enzyme **β-lactamase**. This enzyme provides a mechanism for bacterial resistance to these antibiotics. The enzyme can break the chemical bond between the carbon (C) and nitrogen (N) atoms in the structure of the β-lactam ring. When this occurs, all β-lactam drugs lose their antibacterial efficacy. Because of this, additional drugs known as **β-lactamase inhibitors** are added to several of the penicillin antibiotics to make the drugs more powerful against β-lactamase–producing bacterial strains. Each of the four classes of β-lactam antibiotics is examined in detail in the following sections.

PENICILLINS

The penicillins are a large group of chemically related antibiotics that were first derived from a mould (fungus) often seen on bread or fruit. The penicillins can be divided into four subgroups based on their structure and the spectrum of bacteria they are active against: natural penicillins, penicillinase-resistant penicillins, aminopenicillins, and extended-spectrum penicillins. Examples of antibiotics in each subgroup and a brief description of their characteristics are given in Table 43-3.

Penicillins are **bactericidal antibiotics**, meaning they kill a wide variety of gram-positive and some gram-negative bacteria. However, some bacteria have acquired the capacity to produce β-lactamases capable of destroying penicillins. These enzymes can inactivate the penicillin molecules by opening the β-lactam ring. The β-lactamases that specifically inactivate penicillin mol-

ecules are called *penicillinases*. Bacterial strains that produce these drug-inactivating enzymes were a therapeutic obstacle until drugs were synthesized that inhibit these enzymes. Two of these β-lactamase inhibitors are clavulanic acid (also called *clavulanate*) and tazobactam. These drugs bind with β-lactamase to prevent the enzyme from breaking down the penicillin molecule, although they are not always effective. The following are examples of currently available combinations of penicillin and β-lactamase inhibitor:

- amoxicillin trihydrate/clavulanic acid (Amoxi-Clav®, Clavulin®)
- piperacillin/tazobactam sodium

Mechanism of Action and Drug Effects

The mechanism of action of penicillins involves the inhibition of bacterial cell wall synthesis. Once distributed by the patient's bloodstream to infected areas, penicillin molecules slide through bacterial cell walls to get to their site of action. Some penicillins, however, are too large to pass through these openings in the cell walls, and because they cannot get to their site of action, they cannot kill the bacteria. Some bacteria can make the openings in their cell walls small so that the penicillin cannot get through to kill them. The penicillin molecules that do gain entry into the bacterium must then find appropriate binding sites; these are known as *penicillin-binding proteins*. By binding to these proteins, the penicillin molecules interfere with normal cell wall synthesis, causing the formation of defective cell walls that are unstable and easily broken down (see Figure 43-3). Bacterial death usually results from lysis (rupture) of the bacterial cells because of this drug-induced disruption of cell wall structure.

TABLE 43-3

Classification of Penicillins

Subclass	Generic Drug Names	Description
Natural penicillins	penicillin G, penicillin V	Although many modifications of the original natural (mould-produced) structure have been made, these are the only two in current clinical use—penicillin G is the injectable form for IV or IM use; penicillin V is a PO dosage form (tablet and liquid)
Penicillinase-resistant drugs	cloxacillin sodium	Stable against hydrolysis by most staphylococcal penicillinases (enzymes that normally break down the natural penicillins)
Aminopenicillins	amoxicillin, ampicillin	Have an amino group attached to the basic penicillin structure that enhances their activity against gram-negative bacteria compared with natural penicillins
Extended-spectrum drugs	piperacillin sodium, clavulanic potassium/ticarcillin disodium, piperacillin sodium/tazobactam sodium	Have wider spectra of activity than do all other penicillins

IM, intramuscular; *IV*, intravenous; *PO*, oral.

Indications

Penicillins are indicated for the prevention and treatment of infections caused by susceptible bacteria. The micro-organisms most commonly destroyed by penicillins are gram-positive bacteria, including the *Streptococcus* spp., *Enterococcus* spp., and *Staphylococcus* spp. Most natural penicillins have little if any ability to kill gram-negative bacteria. However, the extended-spectrum penicillins have excellent gram-positive, gram-negative, and anaerobic coverage. Because of this, the extended-spectrum penicillins are used to treat many health care–acquired infections, including pneumonia, intra-abdominal infections, and sepsis. Piperacillin/tazobactam sodium is often used as an initial antibiotic when awaiting results of blood cultures.

Contraindications

Penicillins are usually safe and well-tolerated drugs. The only usual contraindication is known drug allergy. It is important to obtain an accurate history regarding the type of reaction that occurs in patients who state they are allergic to penicillins. It is also important to note that often drugs are referred to by their trade names, and these don't always end in "cillin" (e.g., Clavulin). Many medication errors have occurred when a penicillin drug called by its trade name is given to a patient with a penicillin allergy.

Adverse Effects

Allergic reactions to penicillin occur in 0.7 to 4% of treatment courses. The most common reactions are urticaria, pruritus, and angioedema. A wide variety of idiosyncratic (unpredictable) drug reactions can occur, such as maculopapular eruptions, eosinophilia, Stevens-Johnson syndrome, and exfoliative dermatitis. Maculopapular rash occurs in approximately 2% of treatment courses with natural penicillin and 5.2 to 9.5% of those with ampicillin. Between 1 and 5 incidents of anaphyl-axis occur in every 10 000 cases of penicillin therapy. Severe reactions are much more common with injected than with orally administered penicillin, as is the case with most other antibiotics. Patients who are allergic to penicillins have an increased risk of allergy to other β-lactam antibiotics. The incidence of cross-reactivity between cephalosporins and penicillins is reported as between 1 and 4%. Patients reporting penicillin allergy need to describe their prior allergic reaction; it is important to document the type of reaction. The decision to treat with cephalosporin therapy in such cases is often a matter of clinical judgement, based on the severity of reported prior reactions to penicillin drugs, the nature of the infection, the drug susceptibility of the infective organism if known, and the availability and patient tolerance of other alternative antibiotics. Generally speaking, only those patients with a history of throat swelling or hives from penicillin should not receive cephalosporins. Some patients may require skin testing and desensitization.

Penicillins are generally well tolerated and are associated with few adverse effects. As with many drugs, the most common adverse effects involve the GI system. Penicillins also disrupt the normal intestinal flora. The IV formulations of some penicillins contain large amounts of sodium or potassium. High doses may cause seizures. IV penicillins are often irritating to veins. It is important to monitor for extravasation or phlebitis and to be aware that pain can occur with infusion, and new sites may be needed. Doses must be adjusted for patients with kidney dysfunction. The most common adverse effects of the penicillins are listed in Table 43-4.

Interactions

Many drugs interact with penicillins; some have positive effects, and others have harmful effects. The most common and clinically significant drug interactions associated with penicillin use are listed in Table 43-5.

Dosages

For dosage information on selected penicillins, refer to the table on p. 815.

CEPHALOSPORINS

Cephalosporins are semisynthetic antibiotics widely used in clinical practice. They are structurally and pharmacologically related to penicillins. Similar to penicillins, cephalosporins are bactericidal and act by interfering with bacterial cell wall synthesis. They also bind to the same penicillin-binding proteins inside bacteria that were described earlier. Although there are a variety of such proteins, they are collectively referred to as *penicillin-binding* regardless of the type of β-lactam drug involved.

Cephalosporins can destroy a broad spectrum of bacteria, and this ability is directly related to the chemical changes that have been made to their basic cephalosporin structure. Modifications to this chemical structure by pharmaceutical scientists have given rise to five generations of cephalosporins. Depending on the generation, these drugs may be active against gram-positive, gram-negative, or anaerobic bacteria. They are not active against fungi and viruses. The different drugs of each generation have certain chemical similarities, and thus they can kill similar spectra of bacteria. In general, the level of gram-negative coverage increases with each successive generation. The first-generation drugs have the most gram-positive coverage, and the later generations have the most gram-negative coverage. Anaerobic coverage is found only with the second-generation drugs. Cefepime is the only fourth-generation cephalosporin available in Canada. Ceftaroline fosamil, the newest cephalosporin, often referred as the *fifth generation drug*, has a broad spectrum and covers gram-positive (including MRSA) and gram-negative organisms. It is not available in Canada; however, the drug manufacturer is seeking Health Canada approval for its use in Canada. The currently available parenteral and oral cephalosporin antibiotics are listed in Table 43-6. As is often the case, injectable drugs produce higher serum concentrations than drugs administered by the oral route and thus are used to treat more serious infections.

The safety profiles and contraindications of the cephalosporins are similar to those of the penicillins. The most commonly reported adverse effects are mild diarrhea, abdominal cramps, rash, pruritus, redness, and edema. Because cephalosporins are chemically similar to penicillins, someone with an allergic reaction to penicillin may also have an allergic reaction to a cephalosporin. This is referred to as *cross-sensitivity*. Investigators have observed that the incidence of cross-sensitivity between penicillins and cephalosporins is between 1 and 4%. However, only those patients who have had a serious anaphylactic reaction to penicillin must not be given cephalosporins. As a class, the cephalosporins are safe and effective antibiotics.

Penicillins and cephalosporins are practically identical in their mechanisms of action, drug effects, therapeutic effects, adverse effects, and drug interactions. For this reason, this information is not repeated for the cephalosporins, and the reader is referred to the pertinent discussion in the section on the penicillin drugs. Cephalosporins of all generations are safe drugs. Their use is contraindicated in patients who have shown a hypersensitivity to them and any patient with a history of life-threatening allergic reaction to penicillins. They are safe to use during pregnancy. Drug interactions are listed in Table 43-7.

Dosages

For the dosage information on selected cephalosporins, refer to the table on p. 818.

TABLE	43-4

Penicillins: Reported Adverse Effects

Body System	Adverse Effects
Central nervous	Lethargy, anxiety, depression, seizures
Gastrointestinal	Nausea, vomiting, diarrhea, taste alterations, oral candidiasis
Hematological	Anemia, bone marrow depression, granulocytopenia
Metabolic	Hyperkalemia, hypernatremia, alkalosis
Other	Pruritus, hives, rash

TABLE	43-5

Penicillins: Drug Interactions

Drug	Mechanism	Result
Aminoglycosides (IV) and clavulanic acid	Additive	More effective killing of bacteria
Methotrexate	Decreased kidney elimination of methotrexate	Increased levels of methotrexate
NSAIDs	Compete for protein binding	More free and active penicillin (may be beneficial)
Oral contraceptives	Uncertain	May decrease efficacy of the contraceptive
probenecid	Competes for elimination	Prolongs the effects of penicillins
rifampin	Inhibition	May inhibit the killing activity of penicillins
warfarin sodium	Reduced vitamin K from gut flora	Enhanced anticoagulant effect of warfarin sodium

IV, intravenous; *NSAIDs*, nonsteroidal anti-inflammatory drugs.

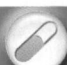

DRUG PROFILES

Penicillins are safe antibiotics and can be used during pregnancy if required. Their use is contraindicated in patients with a hypersensitivity to them, but because of their relatively good adverse effects profile, there are otherwise few contraindications to their use.

NATURAL PENICILLINS

▶▶*penicillin G and penicillin V potassium*

Penicillin G has three salt forms: benzathine, potassium, and sodium. All of these forms are given by injection, either intravenously or intramuscularly. The benzathine and procaine salts are used as longer-acting intramuscular (IM) injections. They are formulated into a thick, white, pastelike material that is designed for prolonged dissolution and absorption from the IM site of injection. Never give these preparations by the IV route, because their consistency is too thick for IV administration; such use can be fatal. The IM formulations can be especially helpful for treating the sexually transmitted infection syphilis because often only one injection is needed. Penicillin G potassium is formulated for IV use. Penicillin V potassium is available only for oral use.

PHARMACOKINETICS

Route	Onset of Action	Peak Plasma Concentration	Elimination Half-Life	Duration of Action
PO	Variable	30–60 min	30 min	4–6 hr
IV	Variable	30 min	24–54 min	4–6 hr

PENICILLINASE-RESISTANT PENICILLINS

cloxacillin sodium

Cloxacillin sodium is the only penicillinase-resistant penicillin currently available in Canada. This penicillinase-resistant penicillin is able to resist breakdown by the penicillin-destroying enzyme (penicillinase) commonly produced by bacteria such as staphylococci. For this reason, this drug may also be referred to as an *antistaphylococcal penicillin*. The chemical structure of cloxacillin features a large, bulky side chain near the β-lactam ring. This side chain serves as a barrier to the penicillinase enzyme, preventing it from breaking the β-lactam ring, which would inactivate the drug. There are, however, certain strains of staphylococci, specifically *Staphylococcus aureus*, that are resistant to cloxacillin. Such bacteria require alternative antibiotic regimens. Cloxacillin is available for oral and injectable use.

PHARMACOKINETICS

Route	Onset of Action	Peak Plasma Concentration	Elimination Half-Life	Duration of Action
IV	Variable	30–60 min	20–30 min	6 hr

AMINOPENICILLINS

There are two aminopenicillins: amoxicillin and ampicillin. They are so named because of the presence of a free amino group ($-NH_2$) in their chemical structure. This structural feature gives aminopenicillins enhanced activity against gram-negative bacteria, against which the natural and penicillinase-resistant penicillins are relatively ineffective. The aminopenicillins are also effective against some gram-positive organisms. Amoxicillin is an analogue of ampicillin.

▶▶*amoxicillin*

Amoxicillin (Moxilean®, Novamoxin®, others) is a commonly prescribed aminopenicillin. Amoxicillin is used to treat infections caused by susceptible organisms in the ears, nose, throat, genitourinary (GU) tract, skin, and skin structures. Pediatric dosages are sometimes higher than those used in the past because of the development of increasingly resistant *Streptococcus pneumoniae* organisms. The traditional adult dosage continues to be adequate in most cases. The drug is available only for oral use and can be given with or without food. It is also available in combination with clavulanic acid (Clavulin).

PHARMACOKINETICS

Route	Onset of Action	Peak Plasma Concentration	Elimination Half-Life	Duration of Action
PO	0.5–1 hr	1–2 hr	1–1.5 hr	6–8 hr

ampicillin

Ampicillin is available in two different salt forms: trihydrate and sodium. The different salt forms are administered by different routes. Ampicillin trihydrate is administered orally, whereas ampicillin sodium is given parenterally. This drug is still currently available, although it is used less frequently than in past years because of resistance.

PHARMACOKINETICS

Route	Onset of Action	Peak Plasma Concentration	Elimination Half-Life	Duration of Action
PO	Variable	1–2 hr	1–1.5 hr	4–6 hr
IV	Variable	5 min	1–1.8 hr	6–8 hr

EXTENDED-SPECTRUM PENICILLINS

By making a few changes in the basic structure of penicillin, drug developers produced another generation of penicillins that have a wider spectrum of activity than that belonging to either of the other two classes of semisynthetic penicillins (penicillinase-resistant penicillins and aminopenicillins) or to the natural penicillins. Currently, piperacillin sodium is the sole extended-spectrum penicillin available. Piperacillin is available in combination with tazobactam sodium. These β-lactamase–inhibiting products allow for enhanced multiorganism coverage, especially against anaerobic organisms that are common in intestinal infections and *Pseudomonas* spp., which are common in health care–acquired infections. Piperacillin/tazobactam is commonly used in hospitalized patients with suspected or documented serious infections. Because of its broad spectrum of activity (gram-positive, gram-negative, and anaerobic), it is often used as empiric therapy. This drug is available only by injection.

TABLE 43-6

Cephalosporins: Parenteral and Oral Preparations

First Generation		Second Generation		Third Generation		Fourth Generation		Fifth Generation
IV	PO	IV	PO	IV	PO	IV	PO	IV
cefazolin sodium	cephalexin	cefoxitin sodium	cefaclor	cefotaxime sodium	cefixime	cefepime hydrochloride		ceftaroline fosamil†
	cefadroxil	cefuroxime sodium	cefuroxime axetil*	ceftazidime				ceftolozane sulfate/ tazobactam sodium (Zerbaxa®)
			cefprozil	ceftriaxone				

IV, intravenous; *PO*, oral.
*Prodrug salts that aid in drug delivery into the gastrointestinal tract.
†Currently not available in Canada.

DOSAGES Selected Penicillins

Drug	Pharmacological Class	Usual Dosage Range	Common Indications
▸▸amoxicillin (Clavulin, Moxilean, Novamoxin, others)	Aminopenicillin	*Children less than 20 kg* PO: 20–40 mg/kg/day divided q8h *Adults* PO: 250–500 mg q8h	Otitis media; sinusitis; various susceptible respiratory, skin, and urinary tract infections
ampicillin (generic)	Aminopenicillin	*Children* PO/IV/IM: 25–50 mg/kg/day divided q6h (doses up to 300 mg/kg/day may be required for meningitis and other serious infections) *Adults* PO/IV/IM: 1–12 g/day divided q4–6h	Primarily infection with gram-negative infections such as *Shigella, Salmonella, Escherichia, Haemophilus, Proteus,* and *Neisseria* spp.; infection with some gram-positive organisms
cloxacillin sodium (generic only)	Penicillinase-resistant penicillin	*Children* PO/IM/IV: 25–50 mg/kg/day divided q6h *Adults* PO/IM/IV: 250–500 mg q6h	Infection with penicillinase-producing staphylococci
▸▸penicillin V potassium (Pen VK)	Natural penicillin	*Children and adults* PO: 125–500 mg (200 000–800 000 units) q6–8h	Primarily infection with gram-positive organisms such as *Streptococcus* (including *Streptococcus pneumoniae*)

IM, intramuscular; *IV*, intravenous; *PO*, oral; *spp.*, species.

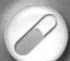 ## DRUG PROFILES

FIRST-GENERATION CEPHALOSPORINS

First-generation cephalosporins are usually active against gram-positive bacteria and have limited activity against gram-negative bacteria. They are available in both parenteral and oral forms. Currently available first-generation cephalosporins include cefazolin and cephalexin.

▸▸ *cefazolin sodium*

Cefazolin sodium is a prototypical first-generation cephalosporin. As with all first-generation cephalosporins, it provides excellent coverage against gram-positive bacteria but limited coverage against gram-negative bacteria.

It is available only for parenteral use. It is used commonly for surgical prophylaxis and for susceptible staphylococcal infections.

PHARMACOKINETICS

Route	Onset of Action	Peak Plasma Concentration	Elimination Half-Life	Duration of Action
IV	Variable	5 min	1.2–2.5 hr	8 hr

▸▸ *cephalexin*

Cephalexin (Keflex®) is a prototypical oral, first-generation cephalosporin. It also provides excellent coverage against

Continued

DRUG PROFILES—cont'd

gram-positive bacteria but limited coverage against gram-negative bacteria. It is available only for oral use.

PHARMACOKINETICS

Route	Onset of Action	Peak Plasma Concentration	Elimination Half-Life	Duration of Action
PO	Variable	1 hr	0.6–2 hr	6–12 hr

SECOND-GENERATION CEPHALOSPORINS

Second-generation cephalosporins have coverage against gram-positive organisms that is similar to that of the first-generation cephalosporins but have enhanced coverage against gram-negative bacteria. Both parenteral and oral formulations are available. Currently available second-generation cephalosporins include cefaclor, cefoxitin, cefuroxime, and cefprozil. These drugs differ slightly in their antibacterial coverage. Cefoxitin is often referred to as a *cephamycin* and has better coverage than the other drugs in this class against various anaerobic bacteria such as *Bacteroides fragilis*, *Peptostreptococcus* spp., and *Clostridium* spp.

▶▶ cefoxitin sodium

Cefoxitin sodium is a parenteral second-generation cephalosporin. It provides excellent gram-positive coverage and better gram-negative coverage than the first-generation drugs. Cefoxitin is used for gynecological infections, urinary tract infections, lower respiratory tract infections, bone and joint infections, and soft tissue infections. Normal intestinal flora include gram-positive, gram-negative, and anaerobic bacteria.

PHARMACOKINETICS

Route	Onset of Action	Peak Plasma Concentration	Elimination Half-Life	Duration of Action
IV	Variable	0.5 hr	1 hr	8 hr

cefuroxime sodium

Cefuroxime sodium is the parenteral form of this second-generation cephalosporin. The oral form is a different salt of cefuroxime, cefuroxime axetil (Ceftin®). It has more activity against gram-negative bacteria than first-generation cephalosporins but a narrower spectrum of activity against gram-negative bacteria than third-generation cephalosporins. It differs from the cephamycins such as cefoxitin in that it does not kill anaerobic bacteria. Cefuroxime axetil is a prodrug. It has little antibacterial activity until it is hydrolyzed in the liver to its active cefuroxime form. It is available only for oral use. Cefuroxime is available only in injectable form.

PHARMACOKINETICS

Route	Onset of Action	Peak Plasma Concentration	Elimination Half-Life	Duration of Action
PO	Variable	2–3 hr	1.3 hr	6–8 hr
IV	Variable	30 min	1–2 hr	6–8 hr

THIRD-GENERATION CEPHALOSPORINS

The available third-generation cephalosporins include cefotaxime sodium, cefixime, cefpodoxime proxetil, ceftazidime, and ceftriaxone. These are the most potent of the three generations of cephalosporins in fighting gram-negative bacteria, but they generally have less activity than first- and second-generation drugs against gram-positive organisms.

Because of specific changes in the basic cephalosporin structure, ceftazidime has significant activity against *Pseudomonas* spp. However, resistance is beginning to limit its usefulness. Cefixime and cefpodoxime proxetil are currently the only third-generation cephalosporins available for oral use. All the other third-generation drugs are available only in parenteral forms.

▶▶ ceftriaxone sodium

Ceftriaxone sodium is an extremely long-acting third-generation drug that can be given only once a day in the treatment of most infections. It also has the unique characteristic of being able to pass easily across the blood–brain barrier. For this reason, it is one of the few cephalosporins that is indicated for the treatment of meningitis, an infection of the meninges of the brain and spinal cord. The spectrum of activity of ceftriaxone is similar to that of the other third-generation drug cefotaxime sodium. It can be given both intravenously and intramuscularly. In some cases of infection, one IM injection can eradicate the infection. Ceftriaxone is 93 to 96% bound to plasma protein, a proportion higher than that of many of the other cephalosporins. This drug is also unique in that it is metabolized in the intestine after biliary excretion. Ceftriaxone is not given to neonates with hyperbilirubinemia or to patients with severe liver dysfunction. It should not be administered with calcium infusions. This drug is available only for injection.

PHARMACOKINETICS

Route	Onset of Action	Peak Plasma Concentration	Elimination Half-Life	Duration of Action
IV	Variable	1.5–4 hr	4.3–8.7 hr	24 hr

ceftazidime

Ceftazidime (Fortaz®) is a parenterally administered third-generation cephalosporin with activity against difficult-to-treat infections with gram-negative bacteria such as *Pseudomonas* spp. It is the third-generation cephalosporin of choice for many indications because of its excellent spectrum of activity and safety profile; however, resistance is beginning to limit its usefulness, and it is generally given in combination with an aminoglycoside (discussed in Chapter 44). Ceftazidime is available only in injectable form.

PHARMACOKINETICS

Route	Onset of Action	Peak Plasma Concentration	Elimination Half-Life	Duration of Action
IV/IM	Variable	1 hr	2 hr	8–12 hr

DRUG PROFILES—cont'd

FOURTH-GENERATION CEPHALOSPORINS

cefepime hydrochloride

Cefepime hydrochloride (Maxipime®) is the prototypical fourth-generation cephalosporin. Cefepime is a broad-spectrum cephalosporin that most closely resembles ceftazidime in its spectrum of activity. It differs from ceftazidime in that it has increased activity against many *Enterobacter* spp. (gram-negative) as well as gram-positive organisms. Cefepime is indicated for the treatment of uncomplicated and complicated UTIs, uncomplicated skin and skin structure infections, and pneumonia. It is available only in injectable form.

PHARMACOKINETICS

Route	Onset of Action	Peak Plasma Concentration	Elimination Half-Life	Duration of Action
IV	0.5 hr	0.5–1.5 hr	2 hr	8–12 hr

CARBAPENEMS

Carbapenems have the broadest antibacterial action of any antibiotics to date. They are bactericidal and inhibit cell wall synthesis. Because of this broad action, they are often reserved for complicated body cavity and connective tissue infections in acutely ill hospitalized patients. They are also effective against many gram-positive organisms. One hazard of carbapenem use is drug-induced seizure activity, which occurs in a relatively small percentage of patients. However, the risk of seizures can be reduced by proper dosage adjustment in susceptible patients. There is a small risk of cross-sensitivity in patients with penicillin allergies. Only those patients with anaphylactic-type reactions to penicillins must not receive a carbapenem. Currently available carbapenems include imipenem/cilastatin, meropenem, and ertapenem. Carbapenems must be infused over 60 minutes.

▶▶ imipenem/cilastatin

Imipenem/cilastatin (Primaxin®) is a fixed combination of imipenem, which is a semisynthetic carbapenem antibiotic similar to β-lactam antibiotics, and cilastatin sodium, an inhibitor of an enzyme that breaks down imipenem. Imipenem has a wide spectrum of activity against gram-positive and gram-negative aerobic and anaerobic bacteria. Cilastatin sodium is a unique drug in that it inhibits an enzyme in the kidneys called *dihydropeptidase*, which would otherwise quickly break down the imipenem. Cilastatin sodium also blocks the kidney tubular secretion of imipenem, which inhibits imipenem from being excreted from the kidneys, the drug's primary route of excretion.

Imipenem/cilastatin exerts its antibacterial effect by binding to penicillin-binding proteins inside bacteria, which in turn inhibits bacterial cell wall synthesis. Unlike many of the penicillins and cephalosporins, imipenem/cilastatin is resistant to the antibiotic-inhibiting actions of β-lactamases. Drugs with which it potentially interacts include cyclosporine, ganciclovir, and probenecid, all of which may potentiate the central nervous system (CNS) adverse effects (including seizures) of imipenem. Concurrent use with these drugs should be avoided whenever clinically feasible. The most serious adverse effect associated with imipenem/cilastatin therapy is seizures, which have been reported to occur in up to 1.5% of patients receiving less than 500 mg every 6 hours. In patients receiving higher dosages of the drug (more than 500 mg every 6 hours), however, there is about a 10% incidence of seizures. Seizures are more likely in older adults and in patients with renal disease. Seizures have been associated with all of the carbapenems, but the data suggest that they are less likely to occur with other members of this class than with imipenem/cilastatin.

Imipenem/cilastatin is indicated for the treatment of bone, joint, skin, and soft-tissue infections; bacterial endocarditis caused by *S. aureus*; intra-abdominal bacterial infections; pneumonia; UTIs and pelvic infections; and bacterial septicemia caused by susceptible bacterial organisms. The IM form of imipenem/cilastatin contains lidocaine, and its use is therefore contraindicated in patients with a known drug allergy to lidocaine or related local anaesthetics. All dosage forms contain the same number of milligrams of both imipenem and cilastatin.

meropenem and ertapenem

Meropenem (Merrem®) is the second drug in the carbapenem class of antibiotics. Compared with imipenem/cilastatin, meropenem appears to be somewhat less active against gram-positive organisms, more active against *Enterobacteriaceae*, and equally active against *Pseudomonas aeruginosa*. However, meropenem is the only carbapenem currently indicated for the treatment of bacterial meningitis. Ertapenem (Invanz®) has a spectrum of activity comparable to that of imipenem/cilastatin, although it is not active against *Enterococcus* or *Pseudomonas* spp.

PHARMACOKINETICS

Route	Onset of Action	Peak Plasma Concentration	Elimination Half-Life	Duration of Action
IV	Variable	2 hr	2–3 hr	6–8 hr

TABLE 43-7

Cephalosporins: Drug Interactions

Drug	Mechanism	Result
probenecid	Decreased kidney excretion	Increased cephalosporin levels
Oral contraceptives	Enhance oral contraceptive metabolism	Increased risk for unintended pregnancy

MONOBACTAMS

 DRUG PROFILE

aztreonam

Aztreonam (Clayston®) powder for aerosol use is the only monobactam antibiotic to be developed thus far. It is a synthetic β-lactam antibiotic that is active primarily against the aerobic gram-negative bacteria *Pseudomonas aeruginosa*. Aztreonam is a bactericidal antibiotic; it destroys bacteria by inhibiting bacterial cell wall synthesis, which results in lysis. Aztreonam is indicated for the management of cystic fibrosis in patients with chronic pulmonary *Pseudomonas aeruginosa* infections. It is to be used with the Altera® Nebulizer System. Its use is contraindicated in patients with a known drug allergy. The most common adverse effect is a cough. The recommended dosage for both adults and children 6 years of age and older is one single-use vial (75 mg not based on weight or adjusted for age) of aztreonam reconstituted with a 1 mL ampule of sterile diluent administered 3 times a day for a 28-day course. Each dose should be taken at least 4 hours apart. Aztreonam is taken in repeated cycles of 28 days on followed by 28 days off. The elimination half-life of the aerosol is 2.1 hours.

DOSAGES Selected Cephalosporins

Drug	Pharmacological Class	Usual Dosage Range	Indications
▸cefazolin sodium	First-generation cephalosporin	*Children* IM/IV: 25–100 mg/kg/day divided q6–8h *Adults* IM/IV: 250–1 000 mg q6–8–12h	Infections due to gram-positive organisms, some penicillinase-producing organisms, and some gram-negative organisms; preoperative and postoperative surgical prophylaxis
▸cefoxitin sodium	Second-generation cephalosporin	*Children* IV/IM: 80–160 mg/kg/day divided q4–6h, not to exceed 12 g/day *Adults* IM/IV: 3–12 g/day q6–8h; not to exceed 12 g/day	Infections; less coverage of gram-positive organisms, greater coverage of gram-negative and anaerobic organisms
cefuroxime sodium cefuroxime axetil* (Ceftin, tablet form)	Second-generation cephalosporin	*Children under 12 yr* PO: 20–30 mg/kg/day divided tid–qid IV/IM: 30–150 *Adults and children over 12 yr* PO (tabs): 250–500 mg bid IV/IM: 750–1 500 mg q8h	Comparable to those for cefazolin, and provides more coverage of gram-negative organisms
ceftazidime pentahydrate (Fortaz)	Third-generation cephalosporin	*Children* IM/IV: 25–50 mg/kg/day q8–12h *Adults* IM/IV: 250–2 000 mg q8–12h	Infections; more extensive coverage of gram-negative organisms, including *Pseudomonas* spp.
▸ceftriaxone sodium	Third-generation cephalosporin	*Children under 12 yr* IM/IV: 50–100 mg/kg/day once–bid *Adults and children over 12 yr* IM/IV: 1–2 g/day once–bid	Comparable to those for ceftazidime except that it does not cover *Pseudomonas spp.*
cefepime (Maxipime)	Fourth-generation cephalosporin	*Children 2 mo–12 yr* IV/IM: 50 mg/kg q8–12h *Adults and children over 12 yr* IV/IM: 500–2 000 mg daily–bid	Infections; provides more extensive coverage of gram-negative organisms and better gram-positive coverage than third generation, including organisms causing intra-abdominal infections

GI, gastrointestinal; *GU*, genitourinary; *IM*, intramuscular; *IV*, intravenous; *PO*, oral; *spp.*, species.
*Cefuroxime axetil is a prodrug for PO use that is hydrolyzed into the active ingredient in the fluids of the GI tract.

MACROLIDES

The macrolides are a large group of antibiotics that first became available in the early 1950s with the introduction of erythromycin. Macrolides are considered bacteriostatic; however, in high enough concentrations, they may be bactericidal to some susceptible bacteria. There are three macrolide antibiotics: azithromycin, clarithromycin, and erythromycin. Azithromycin and clarithromycin are currently the most widely used of the macrolides. Although the spectra of antibacterial activity of azithromycin and clarithromycin are similar to that of erythromycin, the former have longer durations of action, which allows them to be given less often. Azithromycin and clarithromycin produce fewer and milder GI tract adverse effects than erythromycin. Azithromycin is usually dosed over a shorter length of time than many of the erythromycin products. Azithromycin and clarithromycin also exhibit better efficacy in eradicating various bacteria and are capable of better tissue penetration than erythromycin. Because erythromycin has a bitter taste and is quickly degraded by the acidity of the stomach, several salt forms and many dosage formulations were developed to circumvent these problems. Fidaxomicin (Dificid®) is the newest macrolide antibiotic. It is indicated only for the treatment of diarrhea associated with *Clostridium difficile*. The most common adverse effects are nausea, vomiting, and GI bleeding. It is reasonably safe to use during pregnancy. It has minimal absorption and, as such, there are known drug interactions.

Mechanism of Action and Drug Effects

Macrolide antibiotics are bacteriostatic drugs that inhibit protein synthesis by binding reversibly to the 50S ribosomal subunits of susceptible microorganisms. Macrolides are effective in the treatment of a wide range of infections. These include various infections of the upper and lower respiratory tract, skin, and soft tissue caused by some strains of *Streptococcus* and *Haemophilus*; spirochetal infections such as syphilis and Lyme disease; gonorrhea; and *Chlamydia*, *Mycoplasma*, and *Corynebacterium* infections. Gonorrheal infections have become increasingly difficult to treat with macrolide monotherapy, so these drugs are sometimes used in combination with other antibiotics such as cephalosporins. Macrolides are also somewhat unique among antibiotics in that they are especially effective against several bacterial species that often reproduce inside host cells instead of in the bloodstream or interstitial spaces. Common examples of such bacteria, some of which were previously listed, are *Listeria*, *Chlamydia*, *Legionella* (one species of which causes Legionnaire's disease), *Neisseria* (one species of which causes gonorrhea), and *Campylobacter*.

Indications

Infections caused by *Streptococcus pyogenes* (group A β-hemolytic streptococci) are inhibited by macrolides, as are mild to moderate upper and lower respiratory tract infections caused by *Haemophilus influenzae*. Spirochetal infections treated with erythromycin and other macrolides are syphilis and Lyme disease. Various forms of gonorrhea and *Chlamydia* and *Mycoplasma* infections are also susceptible to the effects of macrolides.

A therapeutic effect of erythromycin outside its antibiotic actions is its ability to irritate the GI tract, which stimulates smooth muscle and GI motility. This action may be of benefit to patients who have decreased GI motility, such as delayed gastric emptying in patients with diabetes (known as diabetic gastroparesis). It has also been shown to be helpful in facilitating the passage of feeding tubes from the stomach into the small bowel. Azithromycin and clarithromycin are approved for the prevention and treatment of *Mycobacterium avium-intracellulare* complex infections. This is a common opportunistic infection often associated with HIV/AIDS (see Chapter 45). Clarithromycin also has been approved for use in combination with omeprazole for the treatment of patients with active ulcers associated with *Helicobacter pylori* infection.

Contraindications

The only usual contraindication to macrolide use is known drug allergy. Macrolides are often used as alternative drugs for patients with allergies to β-lactam antibiotics.

Adverse Effects

Erythromycin formulations cause many GI-related adverse effects, especially nausea and vomiting. Azithromycin and clarithromycin seem to be associated with a lower incidence of these GI tract complications. Reported adverse effects are listed in Table 43-8.

Interactions

There are a number of potential drug interactions with the macrolides. The macrolides possess two properties that can cause drug interactions: they are highly protein bound and they are metabolized in the liver. For drugs metabolized in the liver, drug interactions arise from competition between the different drugs for metabolic

TABLE 43-8	
Macrolides: Reported Adverse Effects	
Body System	**Adverse Effects**
Cardiovascular	Palpitations, chest pain, QT prolongation
Central nervous	Headache, dizziness, vertigo
Gastrointestinal	Nausea, hepatotoxicity, heartburn, vomiting, diarrhea, flatulence, cholestatic jaundice, anorexia, abnormal taste
Integumentary	Rash, urticaria, phlebitis at intravenous site
Other	Hearing loss, tinnitus

enzymes, specifically the enzymes known as the *cytochrome P450 complex* (see Chapter 2). Such enzymatic effects generally lead to more pronounced drug interactions than competition for protein binding. The result is a delay in the metabolic clearance of one or more interacting drugs and thus a prolonged and possibly toxic drug effect. Examples of some especially common drugs that compete for liver metabolism with the macrolides are carbamazepine, cyclosporine, theophylline, and warfarin sodium. When macrolides are given with these drugs, the results are enhanced effects and possible toxicity of the latter drugs. Therefore, patients must be monitored. Macrolides can also reduce the efficacy of oral contraceptives. Clarithromycin and erythromycin are not to be used with moxifloxacin, pimozide, thioridazine, or other drugs that prolong the QT interval, because malignant dysrhythmias can occur. Concurrent use of simvastatin or lovastatin with clarithromycin or erythromycin is not recommended. Azithromycin is not as prone to such interactions as are the other macrolides because of its minimal effects on the cytochrome P450 enzymes.

Dosages

For dosage information on selected macrolide antibiotics, refer to the table on p. 821.

TETRACYCLINES

The tetracyclines are bacteriostatic drugs that inhibit bacterial protein synthesis by binding to the 30S bacterial ribosome. The only available naturally occurring tetracycline is tetracycline hydrochloride. The two semisynthetic tetracyclines are doxycycline hyclate and minocycline hydrochloride. The newest tetracycline antibiotic is tigecycline (Tygacil®). Tigecycline is indicated for complicated infections, intra-abdominal infections, and community-acquired pneumonia. It is effective against many resistant bacteria. However, a warning of increased risk of all-cause mortality in patients treated

 DRUG PROFILES

Macrolide antibiotics are used to treat a variety of infections, ranging from Lyme disease to Legionnaire's disease. Of the three macrolide drugs currently available, erythromycin has been available for the longest period and has provided the anchor of treatment for various infections for more than four decades. Azithromycin and clarithromycin have fewer adverse effects and better pharmacokinetic profiles than erythromycin.

Macrolide use is contraindicated in patients with known drug allergy. Because macrolides are significantly protein bound and are metabolized in the liver, they may interact with other drugs that are also highly protein bound or hepatically metabolized.

▶▶ *erythromycin*

Erythromycin, which has many product names, was for many years the most commonly prescribed macrolide antibiotic; however, other macrolides are now more commonly used. The drug is available in several different salt and dosage forms for oral use that were developed to circumvent some of its chemical drawbacks. A parenteral form is available for IV use. Erythromycin is also available in topical forms for dermatological use (see Chapter 56) and in ophthalmic dosage forms (see Chapter 57). The absorption of oral erythromycin is enhanced if it is taken on an empty stomach, but because of the high incidence of stomach irritation associated with its use, many of its forms are taken with a meal or snack. With delayed-release capsules containing enteric-coated granules of the drug, maximum blood levels are obtained when administered at least 30 minutes and preferably 2 hours before or after a meal.

▶▶ *azithromycin and clarithromycin*

Azithromycin (Zithromax®) and clarithromycin (Biaxin®) are semisynthetic macrolide antibiotics that differ structurally from erythromycin and as a result have advantages over it. These include better adverse effect profiles, including less GI tract irritation, and more favourable pharmacokinetic properties. Both have a similar range of activity that differs only slightly from that of erythromycin. The two drugs are used for the treatment of both upper and lower respiratory tract and skin structure infections.

Azithromycin has excellent tissue penetration, so it can reach high concentrations in infected tissues. It also has a long duration of action, which allows it to be dosed once daily. It is usually given in a regimen of 500 mg on day 1 and then 250 mg per day for 4 days. The drug can be taken with or without food. It is available in oral and injectable forms.

Clarithromycin is given orally twice daily in adults and children older than 6 months of age. It can be given with or without food. The immediate-release oral formulations (tablets or oral suspension) are not bioequivalent and are not interchangeable with azithromycin sustained release due to a different pharmacokinetic profile. The extended-release preparation must not be crushed.

PHARMACOKINETICS (AZITHROMYCIN)

Route	Onset of Action	Peak Plasma Concentration	Elimination Half-Life	Duration of Action
PO	Variable	2.5–4 hr	60–70 hr	Up to 24 hr

PHARMACOKINETICS (CLARITHROMYCIN)

Route	Onset of Action	Peak Plasma Concentration	Elimination Half-Life	Duration of Action
PO	Variable	2–4 hr	3–7 hr	Up to 12 hr

DOSAGES   Selected Macrolides

Drug	Pharmacological Class	Usual Dosage Range	Indications
▸▸azithromycin (Zithromax)	Semisynthetic macrolide	*Children* PO: 30 mg/kg × 1 dose or 10 mg/kg/day × 3 days or 10 mg/kg × 1 dose, then 5 mg/kg/day × 4 days IV: 10 mg/kg × 1 day then 5 mg/kg/day × 4 days *Adults over 16 yr* PO: 500 mg × 1 dose, then 250 mg/day × 4 days PO: 500 mg daily × 3 days, or 2 g × 1 dose IV: 500 mg/day	Comparable to those for erythromycin, but especially GU and respiratory tract infections, including MAC infections
▸▸clarithromycin (Biaxin)	Semisynthetic macrolide	*Children* PO: 15 mg/kg/day bid (max 500 mg/dose) *Adults* PO: 250–500 mg q12h	Comparable with erythromycin, but especially for infections of the GI and respiratory tracts, including MAC infections
▸▸erythromycin (EES®, Erythro-EC®, many others)	Natural macrolide	*Children** 30–100 mg/kg/day divided q6h *Adults** PO: 250–500 mg q6h	Infections of respiratory and GI tracts and skin caused by gram-positive, gram-negative, and miscellaneous organisms

GI, gastrointestinal; *GU*, genitourinary; *IV*, intravenous; *MAC, Mycobacterium avium* complex; *PO*, oral.
*There are many types of dosage forms, and dosages may vary from those listed.

with tigecycline has been issued; the drug should be used only when other treatments are not available.

Tetracyclines are chemically and pharmacologically similar to one another. The most significant chemical characteristic of these drugs is their ability to bind to (chelate) divalent (Ca^{++}, Mg^{++}) and trivalent (Al^{+++}) metallic ions to form insoluble complexes. Therefore, their coadministration with milk, antacids, or iron salts causes a considerable reduction in the oral absorption of the tetracycline. In addition, their strong affinity for calcium usually precludes their use in children younger than 8 years of age because it can result in significant tooth discoloration. These drugs should also be avoided in pregnant women and nursing mothers. The drugs pass into breast milk, and this can be another route of exposure leading to tooth discoloration in nursing children.

Tetracyclines primarily differ from one another in the following ways:
- *Oral absorption:* All except tigecycline are adequately absorbed, but doxycycline and minocycline hydrochloride have the best absorption.
- *Body tissue penetration:* Doxycycline hyclate and minocycline hydrochloride possess the best penetration potential (brain and cerebrospinal fluid).
- *Half-life and resulting dosage schedule:* Refer to the Dosages table on p. 822 and the pharmacokinetics information in the Drug Profiles section.

Mechanism of Action and Drug Effects

Tetracyclines work by inhibiting protein synthesis in susceptible bacteria. They inhibit the growth of and kill a wide range of *Rickettsia*, *Chlamydia*, and *Mycoplasma* organisms, as well as a variety of gram-negative and gram-positive bacteria (see Indications). They are also useful in the treatment of spirochetal infections, such as syphilis and Lyme disease, and pelvic inflammatory disease.

Indications

Tetracyclines have a wide range of activity, and all drugs in this class are effective against essentially the same range of microbes. They inhibit the growth of many gram-negative and gram-positive organisms and even that of some protozoa. Traditionally used to treat acne in adolescents and adults, they are also considered the drugs of choice for the treatment of the following infections caused by susceptible organisms:
- *Chlamydia:* lymphogranuloma venereum, psittacosis, and nonspecific endocervical, rectal, and urethral infections
- *Mycoplasma: Mycoplasma* pneumonia
- *Rickettsia:* Q fever, rickettsial pox, Rocky Mountain spotted fever, and typhus
- *Other bacteria:* acne, brucellosis, chancroid, cholera, granuloma inguinale, shigellosis, spirochetal relapsing fever, Lyme disease, *H. pylori* infections associated with peptic ulcer disease (used as part of the treatment regimen), syphilis (used as an alternative drug to treat patients with penicillin allergy); tetracyclines are now unreliable in treating gonorrhea because of resistant bacterial strains.
- *Protozoa:* balantidiasis

Contraindications

The only usual contraindication to the use of tetracyclines is known drug allergy. However, tetracyclines must be avoided by pregnant and nursing women and should not be given to children under the age of 8 years.

Adverse Effects

All tetracyclines cause similar adverse effects. They can cause discoloration of the permanent teeth and tooth enamel hypoplasia in both fetuses and children, and they possibly stunt fetal skeletal development if taken during pregnancy. Other clinically significant undesirable effects include photosensitivity; alteration of the intestinal flora, which can result in diarrhea or vaginal candidiasis; reversible bulging fontanelles in neonates; thrombocytopenia, possible coagulation irregularities, and hemolytic anemia; and exacerbation of systemic lupus erythematosus. Other effects include GI upset, enterocolitis, and maculopapular rash.

Interactions

There are several significant drug interactions associated with the use of tetracyclines. When tetracyclines are taken with antacids, antidiarrheal drugs, dairy products, calcium, enteral feedings, or iron preparations, the oral absorption of the tetracycline is reduced. Tetracyclines can potentiate the effects of oral anticoagulants, which necessitates more frequent monitoring of their anticoagulant effects and possible dose adjustment. They can also antagonize the effects of bactericidal antibiotics and oral contraceptives. In addition, depending on the dosage, they can cause blood urea nitrogen levels to be increased.

Dosages

For dosage information on selected tetracyclines, refer to the table below.

The remaining antibiotic classes are discussed in Chapter 44.

 DRUG PROFILES

Tetracyclines were one of the first classes of antibiotics capable of providing coverage against a broad spectrum of microorganisms. Their use is contraindicated in patients who have had hypersensitivity reactions to them in the past and in lactating women. Resistance to one tetracycline implies resistance to all tetracyclines.

▸▸doxycycline hyclate

Doxycycline hyclate (Aprilon®, Atridox®, Doxycin®, Doxytab®, Periostat®, Vibramycin®) is a semisynthetic tetracycline antibiotic that was made by altering the naturally occurring tetracycline oxytetracycline. Doxycycline is available in Canada in the salt form hyclate. It is useful in the treatment of rickettsial infections, *C. difficile*, chlamydial and mycoplasmal infections, spirochetal infections, and many infections with gram-negative organisms. Doxycycline may also be used as a sclerosing drug in the treatment of pleural effusions. It is available in oral forms. Atridox is a controlled-release subgingival gel.

PHARMACOKINETICS

Route	Onset of Action	Peak Plasma Concentration	Elimination Half-Life	Duration of Action
PO	Variable	1.5–4 hr	14–24 hr	Up to 10–12 hr

tigecycline

Tigecycline (Tygacil) is the newest tetracycline, referred to as a *glycylcycline.* It differs from other tetracyclines in that it is effective against many organisms resistant to others in its class. It is indicated for the treatment of complicated skin and skin structure infections caused by susceptible organisms, including MRSA and vancomycin-sensitive *Enterococcus faecalis*, and for the treatment of complicated intra-abdominal infections. Tigecycline is given by injection only. Nausea and vomiting are the most common adverse effects, occurring in 20 to 30% of patients.

PHARMACOKINETICS

Route	Onset of Action	Peak Plasma Concentration	Elimination Half-Life	Duration of Action
IV	Immediate	Immediate after infusion	27 hr	12 hr

DOSAGES   Selected Tetracyclines

Drug	Pharmacological Class	Usual Dosage Range	Indications
▸▸doxycycline hyclate (Aprilon, Atridox, Doxycin, Doxytab, Vibramycin, others)	Tetracycline	*Adults* PO: 200 mg first day, then 100 mg daily thereafter	Broad antibacterial coverage, including treatment of skin infections and respiratory, GI, and GU tract infections
tigecycline (Tygacil)	Glycylcycline	*Adults* IV: 100 mg × 1, then 50 mg q12h	Skin and skin structure infections, MRSA infections, intra-abdominal infections

GI, gastrointestinal; *GU,* genitourinary; *IV,* intravenous; *MRSA,* methicillin-resistant *Staphylococcus aureus*; *PO,* oral.

NURSING PROCESS

Assessment

To ensure effective treatment, in general, before the administration of any antibiotic, it is crucial to gather data on a history of, or symptoms indicative of, hypersensitivity or allergic reactions (from mild reactions with rash, pruritus, angioedema, or hives to severe reactions with laryngeal edema, bronchospasm, hypotension, or possible cardiac arrest). Also, determine the patient's age, weight, and baseline vital signs including body temperature. Examine the results of any laboratory tests that have been ordered, such as liver function studies (AST and ALT levels), kidney function tests (usually GFR, BUN, and creatinine levels), heart function tests (pertinent laboratory tests, electrocardiogram [ECG]), ultrasonography (if indicated), culture and sensitivity tests, and complete blood count (CBC) with hemoglobin/hematocrit (Hgb/Hct) levels and platelet and clotting tests. Assess intake and output measurements, if appropriate, (e.g., urinary output of more than 30 mL/hr or 600 mL/24 hr). Recording a baseline neurological assessment (e.g., history of seizures) is important because of possible CNS adverse effects. Assess bowel sounds and patterns because of potential antibiotic-related GI tract adverse effects. Further assessment needs to include checking for contraindications, cautions, and drug interactions. Obtain a complete list of all medications, including over-the-counter (OTC) drugs and natural health products. Ethnocultural assessment is also important because of the well-documented variations in responses to antibiotics among different racial and ethnic groups, as well as some cultures' common use of folk remedies or alternative therapies to try to alleviate infections. Assess patients' learning preparedness, willingness to learn, and educational level because of the importance of patient education to safe medication administration. Note baseline findings from assessment of the oral mucosa, respiratory tract, GI tract, and GU tract because of the risk of superinfection in these areas. Superinfections are often evidenced by fever, lethargy, oral thrush, perineal itching, and other system-related symptoms. Because antibiotic resistance is so prevalent, ask the patient or caregiver questions about long-term use, overuse, or abuse of antibiotics. Assessment information related to each group of antibiotics is presented in the following paragraphs.

For patients taking sulfonamides, a careful assessment for drug allergies to sulfa-type drugs or sulfites, such as the oral sulfonylureas (antihyperglycemic drugs) and thiazide diuretics, is important to patient safety (see previous discussion on sulfonamides). Perform a thorough skin assessment during drug therapy because of the potential for occurrence of the adverse effect of Stevens-Johnson syndrome (see Table 43-2). Assess red blood cell count before beginning sulfonamide therapy because of the possibility of drug-related anemias. With frequent or long-term therapy, assess kidney function because of the potential for drug-related crystalluria. Check the patient's medication and medical history for any manifestations of G6PD and slow acetylation (see Chapter 2).

Before the initiation of therapy with penicillins, because of the high incidence of hypersensitivity, determine if there are drug allergies. Potential drug interactions are presented in Table 43-5. In addition, assess the patient for a history of asthma, sensitivity to multiple allergens, aspirin allergy, and sensitivity to cephalosporins because these are associated with a higher risk for penicillin allergy. If procaine penicillin is to be given, the patient should be assessed for procaine hypersensitivity. Note the results of culture and sensitivity testing as soon as they are available to confirm the appropriateness of therapy. Because of possible CNS and GI adverse effects, complete a thorough neurological, abdominal, and bowel assessment. Especially important for patients with electrolyte disturbances, heart disease, or kidney disease is assessment of serum sodium and potassium levels, primarily because of the high sodium and potassium ion concentrations in some penicillin preparations. For example, penicillin G contains 1.7 mmol of potassium ion per million units and 2 mmol of sodium ion per million units. With these particular preparations, if a patient has heart failure, fluid overload, or cardiac dysrhythmias, a high sodium or potassium level (hypernatremia or hyperkalemia) can lead to exacerbation of these problems. With any dosage forms of the penicillins, it is important to patient safety to assess for the possibility of an immediate, accelerated, or delayed allergic reaction.

Prior to the use of cephalosporins, conduct a thorough assessment of allergies, including allergy to penicillins, because of possible cross-sensitivity. Because of the similarity in their mechanism of action to penicillins, assessment data is also similar. Obtain information about the specific drug and note the generation of cephalosporins to which it belongs. Each of the drug generations has distinctive adverse effects and complications in addition to commonalities with the other groups.

Carbapenems are used when there are complicated connective tissue infections in acutely ill patients who are hospitalized. Assess patients for a history of seizure activity because of the potential for seizure-type, drug-induced reactions.

With macrolides, assessment of baseline heart function with documentation of vital signs is important because these drugs may lead to palpitations, chest pain, and ECG changes (QT prolongation). Note baseline hearing status because of drug-induced hearing loss and tinnitus. Assess liver function and determine if there is any history of liver disease due to possible hepatotoxicity and jaundice. Drug interactions have been discussed previously, but special consideration should be given to concurrent use of a macrolide with warfarin sodium, digoxin, or theophylline, resulting in possible toxicity of the latter drugs. Macrolides also reduce the effectiveness of oral contraceptives.

With the use of tetracyclines, as with all antibiotic therapy, carefully assess culture and sensitivity reports. There is concern regarding the use of these drugs in patients younger than 8 years of age because of the problem of permanent mottling and discoloration of the teeth. Use of these drugs in pregnancy may also pose problems for the fetus. Assess for any whitish sore patches on the oral mucosa (due to candidiasis or yeast infection) as well as any vaginal itching, pain, or cottage cheese–like discharge (because of vaginal candidiasis) for early identification and early treatment of superinfections (see previous discussion). Assess for significant drug interactions, including simultaneous use of antacids, antidiarrheal drugs, dairy products, calcium, enteral feedings, and iron preparations. These medications may lead to reduced absorption of the tetracycline. Tetracyclines may also decrease the effectiveness of oral contraceptives. Assess patients taking oral anticoagulants closely due to the possible potentiation of bleeding.

Antiseptics and disinfectants have also been discussed in this chapter.

Nursing Diagnoses

- Nonadherence with the treatment regimen related to lack of information or inability to pay for and obtain the necessary medication
- Deficient knowledge related to lack of information about the disease process and the medication regimen
- Risk for infection related to the patient's possible development of a compromised immune status (due to use of sulfonamides)

Planning

Goals

- Patient will remain adherent to the antibiotic therapy regimen for the full duration of treatment.
- Patient will demonstrate adequate knowledge about the disease process and related drug therapy.
- Patient will maintain homeostasis and a healthy immune system, as well as remain free from risk for infection.

Expected Patient Outcomes

- Patient describes the rationale for the specific antibiotic therapeutic regimen, associated adverse effects, and measures to decrease these adverse effects.
  - Patient takes a specific antibiotic with attention to instructions about whether to take it with meals or increased fluids, as well as foods, medications, and beverages to avoid while on the antibiotic regimen.
  - Patient briefly describes the importance to therapeutic effectiveness of taking the antibiotic exactly as prescribed and until the full prescription is taken.

- Patient takes medication exactly as prescribed and for the full time prescribed.
  - Patient reports any adverse effects that are unresolved and are of concern, such as jaundice, excessive fatigue, elevated temperature, increase in pain associated with the infection, or severe GI distress, nausea, or diarrhea.
- Patient remains free of elevated WBC counts and maintains temperature, pulse rate, and respiratory rate within normal ranges with negative culture and sensitivity reports.

Implementation

General nursing interventions that apply to antibiotics include the following: (1) Give oral antibiotics within the recommended time frames and with fluids or foods as indicated. (2) All medication is to be taken as ordered, in full, and around the clock to maintain effective blood levels, unless otherwise instructed by the health care provider. (3) Doses are not to be omitted or doubled up. (4) Oral antibiotics are not to be given at the same time as antacids, calcium supplements, iron products, laxatives containing magnesium, or some of the antilipemic drugs (see previous listing of drug interactions). (5) Natural health products are to be used only if they do not interact with the antibiotic. (6) Continuously monitor for hypersensitivity reactions after the initial assessment phase because immediate reactions may not occur for up to 30 minutes, accelerated reactions may occur within 1 to 72 hours, and delayed responses may occur after 72 hours. These reactions are characterized by wheezing; shortness of breath; swelling of the face, tongue, or hands (angioedema); itching; or rash. (7) If there are signs of a possible hypersensitivity reaction, stop the dosage form immediately (if IV, stop the infusion), contact the health care provider, and monitor the patient closely. (8) Results of a culture and sensitivity test must be obtained, if possible, before the first dose of antibiotic is given.

Sulfonamides need to be avoided in patients with G6PD and slow acetylation. Encourage increased intake of fluids (2 000 to 3 000 mL per day) to prevent drug-related crystalluria. Oral dosage forms are to be taken with food to minimize GI upset. Encourage patients to immediately report any of the following to the health care provider: worsening abdominal cramps, stomach pain, diarrhea, hematuria, severe or worsening rash, shortness of breath, or fever. These symptoms may indicate adverse reactions to these drugs; remember that the mucocutaneous, GI, hepatic, and hematologic complications may be fatal.

With penicillins, as with other antibiotics, the natural flora in the GI tract may be killed off by the antibiotic. Unaffected GI bacteria, such as *C. difficile*, may overgrow (see earlier discussion on penicillins for more information). This process may be prevented by the consumption of probiotics, such as products containing *Lactobacillus*, supplements, or cultured dairy products like yogourt, buttermilk, and kefir. Kefir is prepared using milk from sheep, goats, and cows. Soy milk kefirs are now also commercially available. Keep in mind the following important points when giving various penicillin formulations: (1) Advise patients to take oral penicillins with at least 180 mL of water (not juices, as they are acidic and may nullify the drug's antibacterial action). (2) Penicillin V, amoxicillin, and amoxicillin/clavulanate are given with water, 1 hour before or 2 hours after meals to maximize absorption; however, because of GI upset, these medications may need to be taken with a snack or meal. (3) Procaine and benzathine salt penicillins are thick solutions; give them as ordered, IM into a large muscle mass, using at least a 21-gauge needle, rotating sites as needed. (4) Reconstitute IM imipenem/cilastatin in sterile saline, with plain lidocaine—as ordered and if the patient has no allergy to it—and give into a large muscle mass. (5) With IV penicillins (e.g., ampicillin), as with any IV therapy, use the proper diluent and infuse the medication over the recommended time. Monitor the IV site frequently for swelling, tenderness, heat, redness, leaking, and pain. Calculate IV rates to deliver the prescribed amount per minute or hour. Change IV sites per facility protocol. (6) Check for compatibilities of IV fluids and drugs prior to infusion. (7) If the patient experiences an anaphylactic reaction to a penicillin (or any drug), give epinephrine and other emergency drugs as ordered, and have supportive treatment (e.g., oxygen) available at all times.

Orally administered cephalosporins may be given with food to decrease GI upset. Alcohol and alcohol-containing products are to be avoided because of the potentiation of a disulfiram-like reaction, known as *acute alcohol intolerance*, associated with some of the cephalosporins. Symptoms that may occur include stomach cramping, nausea, vomiting, headache, diaphoresis, pruritus, and hypotension. With the newer cephalosporins, as with many drug groups, check the drug names carefully to ensure patient safety because many drug names sound alike, and this can lead to medication errors.

Macrolides need to be administered with the same precautions as those used for other antibiotics. Macrolides are not to be given with or immediately before or after fruit juices to avoid interactions with the drug. Inform the patient about the many possible drug interactions (discussed previously), including those with OTC drugs and natural health products. Encourage patients to report any of the following to their health care provider immediately: chest pain, palpitations, dizziness, jaundice, rash, or hearing loss.

Tetracyclines cause photosensitivity, so advise patients to take precautions to avoid sun exposure and avoid tanning bed use. Encourage patients to take oral doses with at least 240 mL of fluids as well as food to minimize GI upset. However, warn patients *not* to take tetracyclines with calcium, magnesium, or iron. These chemicals chelate, or bind, with the tetracycline, leading to a significant reduction in the oral absorption, and thus the effectiveness, of this group of antibiotics. Therefore, concurrent use of dairy products, antacids, or iron needs to be avoided. Patients may consume these interacting foods and drugs 2 hours before or 3 hours after the tetracycline to avoid this interaction. Remember that tetracyclines can cause discoloration of the permanent teeth and tooth enamel in fetuses and children. They may also retard fetal skeletal growth if taken during pregnancy. Continuously monitor for diarrhea or vaginal yeast infections due to altered intestinal or vaginal flora.

Evaluation

Include monitoring of goals, outcome criteria, therapeutic effects, and adverse effects in the evaluation. Therapeutic effects of antibiotics include a decrease in the signs and symptoms of infection; a return to normal vital signs, including temperature; negative results on culture and sensitivity tests; normal results for CBC; and improved appetite, energy level, and sense of well-being. Evaluation for adverse effects includes monitoring for specific drug-related adverse effects (see each drug profile).

CASE STUDY

Antibiotic Therapy

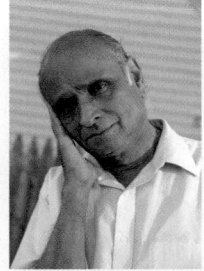

Rahul has been a resident of a complex continuing care facility since experiencing a left-sided stroke 5 years ago. Currently, his cardiovascular status and cerebrovascular status are stable. However, he has had a productive cough and a low-grade fever for 2 days. After physical assessment and chest radiographic examination, the heath care provider diagnoses him with pneumonia of the left lower lobe of the lung. The health care provider orders IV piperacillin/tazobactam sodium, 2.25 g every 8 hours, and oral theophylline, 300 mg every 12 hours. Rahul also takes warfarin sodium, 2 mg every evening. Maalox® 30 mL has been ordered as needed for GI upset and oral ibuprofen 400 mg to be given as needed for pain.

1. Explain the rationale behind the use of tazobactam sodium with piperacillin.
2. What assessments does the nurse need to undertake prior to starting the antibiotic?
3. What concerns or drug interactions should the nurse be aware of with the use of piperacillin/tazobactam and the other medications ordered for Rahul?
4. What parameters should be monitored to determine whether piperacillin/tazobactam is working? Explain your answer.

_____

_____

For answers see http://evolve.elsevier.com/Canada/Lilley/pharmacology/.

PATIENT TEACHING TIPS

❖ Provide patients with a list of foods and beverages that may interact negatively with antibiotics, such as alcohol, acidic fruit juices, and dairy products.

❖ Advise patients to report severe adverse effects to their health care providers and to keep any follow-up visits so that the effectiveness of therapy may be monitored. Laboratory tests (e.g., CBC) may also be performed at these visits.

❖ Foods that may help prevent superinfections (e.g., vaginal yeast infections) include yogourt, buttermilk, and kefir. Probiotic yogourt is now available for re-establishing the natural flora of the GI tract.

❖ Educate patients who are taking oral contraceptives for birth control about interactions between them and certain antibiotics; the effectiveness of oral contraceptives may be decreased with certain antibiotics. Reliable backup methods of contraception must be used in addition to oral contraceptives during antibiotic use.

❖ Recommend that patients wear medical alert jewellery if they have any drug allergies, especially if these are anaphylactic in nature. It is recommended that patients keep drug allergy information and a listing of medical diagnoses and medications on their person at all times.

❖ Sulfonamides are to be taken with plenty of fluids (2 000 to 3 000 mL per day), with food, to decrease GI effects.

❖ Penicillins are to be taken exactly as prescribed for the full duration indicated, as with all antibiotics. Doses are to be spaced at regularly scheduled intervals. Instruct patients to take oral dosage forms with water, avoiding the following: caffeine-containing beverages, citrus fruit, colas, fruit juices, and tomato juice (which decrease the effectiveness of the antibiotic). If a patient must take a penicillin drug four times a day, encourage the patient to set up a reminder system (with cell phone alarms or a watch) so that blood levels remain steady.

❖ Advise patients taking cephalosporins to report any unresolved GI upset, such as diarrhea and nausea, and to avoid alcohol.

❖ Warn patients taking tetracyclines to avoid exposure to tanning beds and direct sunlight or to use sunscreen and wear protective clothing because of drug-related photosensitivity. Photosensitive effects may be noticed from within a few minutes to hours after taking the drug and may last up to several days after the drug has been discontinued.

❖ Instruct patients taking macrolides to take the specific drug as directed, and check for interactions with other drugs being taken at the same time, especially interactions between erythromycin and other medications. For some drugs in this class (e.g., azithromycin), newer dosage forms are available in 3-day and 1-day dose packs rather than 5-day dose packs. Always be sure that patients know the proper dosages and instructions for the drugs they are taking.

KEY POINTS

❖ Antibiotics are either bacteriostatic or bactericidal. Bacteriostatic antibiotics inhibit the growth of bacteria but do not directly kill them. Bactericidal antibiotics directly kill the bacteria.

❖ Most antibiotics work by inhibiting bacterial cell wall synthesis in some way. Bacteria have survived over the ages because they can adapt to their surroundings. If a bacterium's environment includes an antibiotic, over time it can mutate in such a way that it can survive an attack by the antibiotic. The production of β-lactamases is one way in which bacteria can fend off the effects of antibiotics.

❖ Be aware of the most common adverse effects of antibiotics, which include nausea, vomiting, and diarrhea. Inform patients that antibiotics should be taken for the prescribed length of time.

❖ Each class of antibiotics is associated with specific cautions, contraindications, drug interactions, and adverse effects that must be carefully assessed for and monitored.

❖ Because normally occurring bacteria are killed during antibiotic therapy, superinfections may arise during treatment. These may be manifested by the following signs and symptoms: fever, perineal itching, oral lesions, vaginal irritation and discharge, cough, and lethargy.

EXAMINATION REVIEW QUESTIONS

1. A patient is scheduled for colorectal surgery tomorrow. He does not have sepsis, his WBC count is normal, he has no fever, and he is otherwise in good health. However, there is an order to administer an antibiotic on call before he goes to surgery. The nurse knows that which rationale explains this antibiotic order?
a. To provide empiric therapy
b. To provide prophylactic therapy
c. To treat for a superinfection
d. To reduce the number of resistant organisms

2. An adolescent patient is taking a tetracycline drug as part of treatment for severe acne. When the nurse teaches this patient about drug-related precautions, which is the most important information to convey?
a. When the acne clears up, the medication may be discontinued.
b. This medication needs to be taken with antacids to reduce GI upset.
c. The patient needs to use sunscreen or avoid exposure to sunlight, because this drug may cause photosensitivity.
d. The teeth should be observed closely for signs of mottling or other colour changes.

3. A newly admitted patient reports a penicillin allergy. The health care provider has ordered a second-generation cephalosporin as part of therapy. Which nursing action is appropriate?
a. Call the health care provider to clarify the order because of the patient's allergy.
b. Ask the pharmacy to change the order to a first-generation cephalosporin.
c. Give the medication and monitor for adverse effects.
d. Administer the drug with a nonsteroidal anti-inflammatory drug to reduce adverse effects.

4. During patient education regarding an oral macrolide such as erythromycin, the nurse will include which information?
a. If GI upset occurs, the drug will have to be stopped.
b. The drug needs to be taken with an antacid to avoid GI problems.
c. The patient needs to take each dose with a sip of water.
d. The patient may take the drug with a small snack to reduce GI irritation.

5. A woman who has been taking an antibiotic for a UTI calls the nurse practitioner to report severe vaginal itching. She has also noticed a thick, whitish vaginal discharge. Which explanation does the nurse practitioner suspect?
a. This is an expected response to antibiotic therapy.
b. The UTI has become worse instead of better.
c. A superinfection has developed.
d. The UTI is resistant to the antibiotic.

6. The nurse is reviewing orders for wound care, which include use of an antiseptic. Which statements best describe the use of antiseptics? (Select all that apply.)
a. Antiseptics are appropriate for use on living tissue.
b. Antiseptics work by sterilizing the surface of the wound.
c. Antiseptics are applied to nonliving objects to kill microorganisms.
d. The patient's allergies must be assessed before using the antiseptic.
e. Antiseptics are used to inhibit the growth of microorganisms on the wound surface.

7. The order for a child reads: "Give cefoxitin 160 mg/kg/day, IVPB, divided into doses given every 6 hours." The child weighs 55 lb. How much will the patient receive each day? For each dose?

Answers: 1. b, 2. c, 3. a, 4. d, 5. c, 6. a, d, e, 7. 4000 mg/day; 1000 mg/dose

CRITICAL THINKING ACTIVITIES

1. The nurse is reviewing a patient's medications that are due this morning and notes the following orders:
doxycycline, 200 mg, PO every morning
Multivitamin with iron, 1 tablet, PO every morning
Maalox, 30 mL, PO, twice a day
   What is the priority action when considering whether these medications can be given together?

2. The nurse is reviewing the orders for a patient who has been admitted for treatment of pneumonia. The antibiotic orders include an order for penicillin.

However, when the patient is asked about his allergies, he lists "penicillin" as one of his allergies. What will be the next action of the nurse?

3. A 79-year-old patient has been admitted for treatment of osteomyelitis. His orders include IV imipenem/cilastatin, oral lisinopril, oral phenytoin sodium, and a prn order for acetaminophen for a temperature over 38.3°C or for pain. The nurse is reviewing the patient's history and new orders. After reviewing the orders, what is the first action the nurse will take?

For answers see http://evolve.elsevier.com/Canada/Lilley/pharmacology/.

Antibiotics Part 2: Aminoglycosides, Fluoroquinolones, and Other Drugs

Objectives

After reading this chapter, the successful student will be able to do the following:

1. Apply the general principles of antibiotic therapy and all of the antibiotics covered previously in Chapter 43, in preparation for discussion of the following antibiotics or antibiotics classes: aminoglycosides, quinolones, clindamycin, metronidazole, nitrofurantoin, vancomycin hydrochloride, and several other miscellaneous antibiotics.

2. Describe the advantages and disadvantages associated with the use of antibiotics, including overuse and misuse of antibiotics, development of drug resistance, superinfections, and antibiotic-associated colitis.

3. Discuss the indications, cautions, contraindications, mechanisms of action, adverse effects, toxic effects, routes of administration, and drug interactions for the aminoglycosides, fluoroquinolones, clindamycin, metronidazole, nitrofurantoin, vancomycin hydrochloride, and miscellaneous antibiotics.

4. Develop a collaborative plan of care that includes all phases of the nursing process for the patient receiving antibiotics.

Drug Profiles

   amikacin (amikacin sulphate)*, p. 833
▸▸ ciprofloxacin (ciprofloxacin hydrochloride)*, p. 835
▸▸ clindamycin, p. 836
   colistimethate sodium, p. 838
   dapsone
   daptomycin
▸▸ gentamicin (gentamicin sulphate)*, p. 833
   levofloxacin, p. 835
   linezolid, p. 836
▸▸ metronidazole, p. 837
   nitrofurantoin, p. 837
   tobramycin, p. 833
▸▸ vancomycin hydrochloride, p. 838

▸▸ Key drug

*Full generic name is given in parentheses. For the purposes of this text, the more common, shortened name is used.

e-Learning Activities

Website
(http://evolve.elsevier.com/Canada/Lilley/pharmacology/)

evolve

- Answer Key—Textbook Case Studies
- Answer Key—Critical Thinking Activities
- Chapter Summaries—Printable
- Review Questions for Exam Preparation
- Unfolding Case Studies

Key Terms

Concentration-dependent killing A property of some antibiotics, especially aminoglycosides, whereby achieving high plasma drug concentration, even briefly, results in the most effective bacterial kill (compare *time-dependent killing*). (p. 830)

Extended-spectrum β-lactamases (ESBLs) A group of β-lactamase enzymes produced by some organisms that make the organism resistant to all β-lactam antibiotics (penicillins and cephalosporins) and aztreonam. Patients who are infected by such organisms must be in contact isolation; proper handwashing is key to preventing the spread of these organisms. (p. 829)

***Klebsiella pneumoniae* carbapenemase (KPC)** An enzyme first found in isolates of the bacterium *Klebsiella pneumoniae* that renders the organism resistant to all carbapenem antibiotics as well as β-lactam antibiotics and monobactams. Such organisms produce a serious resistant infection. (p. 829)

Methicillin-resistant *Staphylococcus aureus* (MRSA) A strain of *Staphylococcus aureus* that is resistant to the β-lactamase penicillin known as *methicillin*. Originally, the abbreviation *MRSA* referred exclusively to methicillin-resistant *S. aureus*. It is now used more commonly to refer to strains of *S. aureus* that are resistant to several drug classes, and therefore, depending on the context or health facility, it may also stand for *multidrug-resistant S. aureus*. (p. 829)

Minimum inhibitory concentration (MIC) A laboratory measurement of the lowest concentration of a drug needed to kill a certain standardized amount of bacteria. (p. 830)

Multidrug-resistant organisms Bacteria that are resistant to one or more classes of antimicrobial drugs. These include multidrug-resistant *Staphylococcus aureus*, extended-spectrum β-lactamase–producing organisms, and *Klebsiella pneumoniae* carbapenemase–producing organisms. (p. 829)

Nephrotoxicity Toxicity to the kidneys, often drug induced and manifesting in compromised kidney function;

usually reversible upon withdrawal of the offending drug. (p. 831)

Ototoxicity Toxicity to the ears, often drug induced and manifesting as varying degrees of hearing loss that is likely to be permanent. (p. 831)

Peak The highest concentration of a drug in the patient's bloodstream. (p. 830)

Postantibiotic effect (PAE) A period of continued bacterial suppression that occurs after brief exposure to certain antibiotic drug classes, especially aminoglycosides (discussed in this chapter) and carbapenems (see Chapter 43). The mechanism of this effect is uncertain. (p. 831)

Pseudomembranous colitis A necrotizing, inflammatory bowel condition that is often associated with antibiotic therapy. Some antibiotics (e.g., clindamycin) are more likely to produce it than others. More commonly referred to as *antibiotic-associated colitis* or *Clostridium difficile diarrhea* or *C. difficile infection*. (p. 836)

Synergistic effect Drug interaction in which the bacterial killing effect of two antibiotics given together is greater than the sum of the individual effects of the same drugs given alone. (p. 831)

Therapeutic drug monitoring Ongoing monitoring of plasma drug concentrations and dosage adjustment based on these values as well as on other laboratory indicators such as kidney and liver function tests; this monitoring is often carried out by a pharmacist in collaboration with medical, nursing, and laboratory staff. (p. 830)

Time-dependent killing A property of most antibiotic classes whereby prolonged high plasma drug concentrations are required for effective bacterial kill (compare *concentration-dependent killing*). (p. 830)

Trough The lowest concentration of a drug in the patient's bloodstream. (p. 831)

Vancomycin-resistant *Enterococcus* (VRE) *Enterococcus* species that are resistant to β-lactam antibiotics and vancomycin. Most commonly refers to *Enterococcus faecium*. (p. 829)

OVERVIEW

This chapter is a continuation of Chapter 43 and focuses on additional classes of antibiotics used for more serious and harder-to-treat infections. The majority of the drugs discussed in this chapter are administered by the *parenteral* (injection) route only, a route generally reserved for treating more clinically serious infections in the hospital setting. Also included in this chapter are miscellaneous drugs that are unique in their class, as well as newer drugs and drug classes. This chapter also focuses on multidrug-resistant organisms, specifically **methicillin-resistant *Staphylococcus aureus* (MRSA)**,

vancomycin-resistant *Enterococcus* (VRE), organisms producing **extended-spectrum β-lactamases (ESBLs)**, and organisms producing ***Klebsiella pneumoniae* carbapenemase (KPC)**.

Organisms that are resistant to one or more classes of antimicrobial drugs are referred to as *multidrug-resistant organisms*. These include MRSA, VRE, and ESBL- and KPC-producing organisms. MRSA has been around for many years, and, fortunately, new antibiotics have been developed to treat it. However, the threat of MRSA becoming resistant to all currently available antibiotics is all too real. MRSA is no longer seen just in hospitals; it has spread to the community setting, and approximately

50% of staphylococcal infections contracted in the community involve MRSA, depending on location; local community and hospital MRSA strains vary. VRE is usually seen in urinary tract infections. Some newer antibiotics have been developed to successfully treat VRE as well as MRSA. Unfortunately, ESBL- and KPC-producing bacteria are the newest players in this saga. Organisms that produce ESBL are resistant to all β-lactam antibiotics and aztreonam and can be treated only with carbapenems or sometimes quinolones. In the noble effort to treat infection with ESBL-producing organisms, the use of carbapenems has increased, and unfortunately, in response, bacteria have created a new means of resistance, namely, the ability to produce KPC. When patients become infected with KPC-producing bacteria, there are only two known antibiotics that can be used—tigecycline and colistimethate sodium. Reports of resistance to these antibiotics have been described; such resistance leaves patients with the infection untreatable. Multidrug-resistant organisms are one of the world's top health problems. When patients become infected with such organisms, they must be placed in contact isolation. VRE is no longer isolated in hospitals, whereas MRSA is isolated, although the two are often isolated together.

Many hospitals are placing all patients infected with KPC-producing bacteria in one area, and some hospitals have been shut down due to this organism. Proper handwashing is of the utmost importance. These organisms are spread by contact, so all health care providers must wash their hands before and after all patient contact. Some research indicates that patterns of antibiotic resistance for a certain class of antibiotics are influenced by the prescription of antibiotics in other, previously-assumed unrelated classes.

AMINOGLYCOSIDES

The aminoglycosides are a group of natural and semisynthetic antibiotics that are classified as bactericidal drugs (see Chapter 43). They are potent antibiotics, which makes them the drugs of choice for the treatment of virulent infections. The aminoglycoside antibiotics available for clinical use are listed in Table 44-1. These drugs can be given by several different routes, but they are not given orally because of their poor oral absorption.

The three aminoglycosides most commonly used for the treatment of systemic infections are gentamicin, tobramycin, and amikacin. Serum levels of these drugs are routinely monitored. Dosages are adjusted to maintain optimal levels that maximize drug efficacy and minimize the risk for toxicity. This process is known as *therapeutic drug monitoring*. Aminoglycoside therapy is monitored in this way because of the nephrotoxicity and ototoxicity associated with the use of aminoglycosides. Most commonly, dosing is adjusted to the patient's level of kidney function, based on estimates of creatinine clearance calculated from serum creatinine values. This task is often carried out by a hospital pharmacist, consulting for the health care provider. Not only are serum levels measured to prevent toxicity, but it has been shown that for the aminoglycosides to be effective, the serum level needs to be at least eight times higher than the **minimum inhibitory concentration (MIC)**. The MIC for any antibiotic is a measure of the lowest concentration of drug needed to kill a standard amount of bacteria. This value is determined in vitro (in the laboratory) for each drug. It has been shown that other classes of antibiotics, such as β-lactams, work on **time-dependent killing**, that is, the amount of time the drug is above the MIC is critical for maximal bacterial kill. However, aminoglycosides work primarily through **concentration-dependent killing**; that is, achieving a drug plasma concentration that is a certain level above the MIC, even for a brief period of time, results in the most effective bacterial kill. For this reason, although these drugs were originally given in three daily intravenous (IV) doses, the current predominant practice is once-daily aminoglycoside dosing in combination with other antibiotics for synergistic effects. Dosages of 5 to 7 mg/kg/day are used. Once-daily dosing provides a sufficient plasma drug concentration for bacterial kill, along with equal or lower risk for toxicity compared with multiple daily dosage regimens. Use of a once-daily regimen instead of the traditional three times daily regimen also reduces the nursing care time required and often allows for outpatient or even home-based aminoglycoside drug therapy.

Peak (highest) drug levels for once-daily regimens are usually not measured (this may vary among agencies) as it is assumed that the peak level for a single daily dose will be short lived and will drop within a reasonable time

TABLE	**44-1**			
Desired Traditional Serum Drug Levels of the Aminoglycoside Antibiotics				
	Peak		**Trough**	
Serum Drug Levels	**Multiple-Daily Dosing***	**Once-Daily Dosing**	**Multi-Daily Dosing**	**Once-Daily Dosing**
amikacin	20–30 mcg/mL†	Usually not measured	5–10 mcg/mL	Less than 10 mcg/mL
gentamicin and tobramycin	5–10 mcg/mL	Usually not measured	0.5–2 mcg/mL	0.5–2 mcg/mL

*q8h or q12h.
†mcg = microgram; note that one microgram = 1/1 000 (one thousandth) of a milligram or 1/1 000 000 (one millionth) of a gram. Also note that *microgram* is abbreviated *mcg*, whereas *milligram* is abbreviated *mg*.

frame. However, **trough** (lowest) levels are routinely measured to ensure adequate renal clearance of the drug and avoid toxicity. For dosage information on selected aminoglycosides, see the table on p. 833. Dosage regimens and ranges for serum levels may vary for different institutions.

With once-daily dosing, the blood sample for trough measurement is drawn 30 minutes prior to the next dose administration. The therapeutic goal is a trough concentration at or below 1 mcg/mL (which is considered undetectable). Trough levels above 2 mcg/mL are associated with greater risk for both ototoxicity and nephrotoxicity. **Ototoxicity** (toxicity to the ears) often manifests as some degree of temporary or permanent hearing loss. **Nephrotoxicity** (toxicity to the kidneys) manifests as varying degrees of reduced kidney function. This risk is generally indicated by laboratory test results such as serum creatinine level. A rising serum creatinine level suggests reduced creatinine clearance by the kidneys and is indicative of declining renal function. Trough levels are normally monitored initially and then once every 5 to 7 days until drug therapy is discontinued. The patient's serum creatinine level is measured at least every 3 days as an index of renal function, and drug dosages are adjusted as needed for any changes in renal function.

Traditional dosing of aminoglycosides (i.e., three times a day) can still be used. When an aminoglycoside is given in this manner, both peak and trough levels are measured. Samples for measurement of peak levels are drawn 30 minutes after a 30-minute infusion has ended, and samples for measurement of trough levels are drawn just before the next dose. The health care provider can adjust the dose based on a pharmacokinetic evaluation of these levels. When the drug is given in the traditional manner, the desired peak levels vary depending on the type of organism and the site of infection. Higher levels are needed when treating pneumonia than when treating a urinary tract infection—because aminoglycosides are eliminated by the kidney, the drug concentrates in the urine, so lower dosages can be used to treat urinary tract infections. Regardless of the infection being treated, however, it is desirable to keep the trough levels below 2 mcg/mL. Table 44-1 lists the traditional desired drug levels for these drugs.

Mechanism of Action and Drug Effects

Aminoglycosides work in a way that is similar to that of tetracyclines, in that they bind to ribosomes, specifically the 30S ribosome, thereby preventing protein synthesis in bacteria (see Figure 43-3). Aminoglycosides are most often used in combination with other antibiotics such as β-lactams or vancomycin in the treatment of various infections because the combined effect of the two antibiotics is greater than the sum of the effects of either drug acting separately. This is known as a *synergistic effect*. When aminoglycosides are used in combination with β-lactam antibiotics (i.e., penicillins, cephalosporins, monobactams [see Chapter 43]), the β-lactam

antibiotic is given first. This is because β-lactams break down the cell wall of the bacteria and allow the aminoglycoside to gain access to the ribosomes where they work. Aminoglycosides also have a property known as **postantibiotic effect (PAE)**. PAE is a period of continued bacterial growth suppression that occurs *after* short-term antibiotic exposure, as in once-daily aminoglycoside dosing (see earlier). Carbapenems are another antibiotic class with a PAE. The PAE is enhanced with higher peak drug concentrations and concurrent use of β-lactam antibiotics.

As is the case with most antibiotic drug classes, various bacterial mechanisms of resistance to aminoglycosides have emerged among gram-positive and gram-negative species that were previously more susceptible to these drugs. The prevalence and intensity of such resistance varies for the specific drugs, organisms, patient populations, disease states, and geographic prescribing patterns.

Indications

The toxicity associated with aminoglycosides limits their use to treatment of serious gram-negative infections and specific conditions involving gram-positive cocci, in which case gentamicin is usually given in combination with a penicillin. Gram-negative infections commonly treated with aminoglycosides include *Pseudomonas* spp. and several organisms belonging to the Enterobacteriaceae family (facultatively anaerobic gram-negative rods), including *Escherichia coli*, *Proteus* spp., *Klebsiella* spp., and *Serratia* spp. Such infections are often treated with a suitable aminoglycoside and an extended-spectrum penicillin, third-generation cephalosporin, or carbapenem. Gram-positive infections treated with aminoglycosides may include *Enterococcus* spp., *S. aureus*, and bacterial endocarditis, which is usually streptococcal in origin. A regimen of once daily doses is more common when treating gram-positive infections because this often enhances synergy with other antibiotics used. Aminoglycosides are never used alone to treat gram-positive infections. Aminoglycosides are also used for prophylaxis in procedures involving the gastrointestinal (GI) or genitourinary (GU) tract because such procedures carry a high risk for enterococcal bacteremia. They are also commonly given in combination with either ampicillin or vancomycin (for penicillin-allergic patients) for surgical patients with a history of valvular heart disease because diseased heart valves are more prone to enterococcal infection.

Aminoglycosides are to be administered with caution in neonates, whether premature or full term; because of the immaturity of the kidneys in newborns, prolonged actions of the aminoglycosides and a greater risk for toxicities may result. Serious infections in children for which aminoglycosides are used include pneumonia, meningitis, and urinary tract infections. Drug selection for both children and adults is based on the susceptibility of the causative organism. Refer to Table 44-2 for more

TABLE 44-2

Aminoglycosides: Comparative Spectra of Antimicrobial Activity

Aminoglycoside	Spectrum
amikacin sulphate	*Acinetobacter* spp., *Enterobacter aerogenes*, *Escherichia coli*, *Klebsiella pneumoniae*, *Proteus* spp., *Providencia* spp., *Pseudomonas* spp., *Serratia* spp., *Staphylococcus*
gentamicin sulphate	*E. aerogenes*, *E. coli*, *K. pneumoniae*, *Proteus* spp., *Pseudomonas* spp., *Salmonella* spp., *Serratia* spp. (nonpigmented), *Shigella* spp.
neomycin sulphate	Used as a topical antibacterial
paromomycin sulphate	Amebic dysentery
streptomycin sulphate	*Klebsiella granulomatis* (granuloma inguinale), *Yersinia pestis* (plague), *Francisella tularensis* (tularemia), *Mycobacterium tuberculosis* (tuberculosis), *Streptococcus* spp. (nonhemolytic endocarditis)
tobramycin sulphate	*Citrobacter* spp., *Enterobacter* spp., *E. coli*, *Klebsiella* spp., *Proteus* spp., *Providencia* spp., *P. aeruginosa*, *Serratia* spp.

information on the antibacterial spectra of specific amino-glycosides. A few aminoglycosides have more specific indications. Streptomycin sulphate is active against *Mycobacterium* spp. (see Chapter 46), whereas paromomycin sulphate is used to treat amebic dysentery, a protozoal intestinal disease (see Chapter 48). Aminoglycosides are inactive against fungi, viruses, and most anaerobic bacteria.

Contraindications

The only usual contraindication for aminoglycosides is known drug allergy. However, they have been shown to cross the placenta and cause fetal harm when administered to pregnant women. There have been several case reports of total irreversible bilateral congenital deafness in the children of women who received aminoglycosides during pregnancy. Therefore, aminoglycosides should be used in pregnant women only in the event of life-threatening infections when safer drugs are ineffective. These drugs are also distributed in breast milk. They should not be used by lactating women, to avoid the risk of drug toxicity in nursing infants.

Adverse Effects

Aminoglycosides are potent antibiotics and are capable of potentially serious toxicities, particularly to the kidneys (nephrotoxicity) and the ears (ototoxicity), in which they can affect hearing and balance functions. Duration of drug therapy needs to be as short as possible, based on sound clinical judgement and monitoring of the patient's progress. Nephrotoxicity typically occurs in 5 to 25% of patients and is usually manifested by urinary casts (visible remnants of destroyed kidney cells), proteinuria, and increased blood urea nitrogen (BUN) and serum creatinine levels. It is usually reversible, but patients' kidney function tests should be monitored throughout therapy. In contrast, ototoxicity is less common, occurring in 3 to 14% of patients, and often is not reversible. It can result in varying degrees of permanent hearing loss, depending on the dosage and duration of drug therapy. It is believed to result from injury

to the eighth cranial nerve (CN VIII, also called the *vestibulocochlear nerve*) and involves both cochlear damage (hearing loss) and vestibular damage (disrupted sense of balance). Other less common effects include headache, paresthesia, vertigo, skin rash, fever, overgrowth of non-susceptible organisms, and neuromuscular paralysis (very rare and reversible). The risk for these toxicities is greatest in patients with pre-existing kidney impairment, patients already receiving other renally toxic drugs, and patients receiving high-dose or prolonged aminoglycoside therapy.

Interactions

The risk for nephrotoxicity can be increased with concurrent use of other nephrotoxic drugs, such as vancomycin hydrochloride, cyclosporine, and amphotericin B. Concurrent use with loop diuretics increases the risk for ototoxicity. In addition, because aminoglycosides also kill normal intestinal bacterial flora, they also reduce the amount of vitamin K produced by these gut bacteria. These normal flora serve to balance the effects of oral anticoagulants such as warfarin sodium (Coumadin®). Therefore, aminoglycosides can potentiate warfarin sodium toxicity. Concurrent use with neuromuscular blocking drugs may prolong the duration of action of the neuromuscular blockade.

Dosages

For dosage information on selected aminoglycosides, refer to the table on p. 833.

QUINOLONES

Quinolones, sometimes referred to as *fluoroquinolones*, are potent, bactericidal, broad-spectrum antibiotics. Currently available quinolone antibiotics include norfloxacin hydrochloride, ciprofloxacin, levofloxacin, and moxifloxacin hydrochloride. With the exception of norfloxacin hydrochloride, these antibiotics have excellent oral absorption—in most cases, comparable to that of IV injection.

DRUG PROFILES

Historically, aminoglycoside antibiotics were used primarily to treat gram-negative infections. However, they are now used as a synergistic drug in the treatment of gram-positive infections as well. They are normally given intravenously or intramuscularly, but neomycin is administered only topically. Topical dosage forms of both gentamicin and tobramycin are available for dermatological (see Chapter 56) and ophthalmic (see Chapter 57) use. Currently available aminoglycosides include amikacin, gentamicin, paromomycin sulphate, streptomycin sulphate, and tobramycin. The variations in the suffixes of some of the drug names, in particular mycin versus–micin, denote different bacterial origins of the aminoglycosides.

amikacin sulphate

Amikacin sulphate is a semisynthetic aminoglycoside antibiotic that is often used for infections that are resistant to gentamicin or tobramycin. It is available only in injectable form.

PHARMACOKINETICS

Route	Onset of Action	Peak Plasma Concentration	Elimination Half-Life	Duration of Action
IV	Variable	1 hr	2–3 hr	8–12 hr
IM	Variable	30 min–2 hr	2–3 hr	8–12 hr

▸gentamicin sulphate

Gentamicin sulphate is the most commonly used aminoglycoside in clinical practice today. It is usually administered intramuscularly (according to the Health Canada monograph). The IV route is recommended for special indications when the intramuscular (IM) route is not feasible, such as in patients in shock, with severe burns, with hemorrhagic disorders or receiving anticoagulants, or with low muscle mass. The dosage is the same for both routes. It is indicated for the treatment of infection with several susceptible gram-positive and gram-negative bacteria. Gentamicin is available in several dosage forms, including injections, topical ointments, and ophthalmic drops and ointments.

PHARMACOKINETICS

Route	Onset of Action	Peak Plasma Concentration	Elimination Half-Life	Duration of Action
IV	Variable	30 min	2–3 hr	Up to 24 hr
IM	Variable	30–90 min	2–3 hr	Up to 24 hr

tobramycin

Tobramycin's dosages, routes of administration, and indications are comparable to those of gentamicin for generalized infections. In addition, it is commonly used to treat recurrent pulmonary infections in patients with cystic fibrosis, by both injectable parenteral and inhaled dosing. When used by inhalation, it goes by the trade name of TOBI. It is also available in topical and ophthalmic dosage forms.

PHARMACOKINETICS

Route	Onset of Action	Peak Plasma Concentration	Elimination Half-Life	Duration of Action
IV	Variable	30 min	2–3 hr	Up to 24 hr
IM	Variable	30–90 min	2–3 hr	Up to 24 hr

DOSAGES	Selected Aminoglycosides	
Drug	**Usual Dosage Range**	**Indications**
amikacin sulphate (generic)	*Neonates/Children/Adults* IM/IV: 15 mg/kg/day divided bid, administered over 30–60 min	Primarily gentamicin- and tobramycin-resistant gram-negative infections along with severe staphylococcal infections
▸gentamicin sulphate (generic)	*Neonates/Children/Adults* IM/IV: 3–5 mg/kg/day, divided 1–4 times daily	Primarily gram-negative infections along with severe staphylococcal infections
tobramycin (generic)	*Neonates* IV: 4 mg/kg q12h *Children* IV: 6–7.5 mg/kg/day, divided tid–qid *Adults* IV: 3–5 mg/kg/day, divided bid–tid or 2–3 mg/kg once daily	Primarily gram-negative infections along with severe staphylococcal infections

IM, intramuscular; *IV*, intravenous.

Mechanism of Action and Drug Effects

Quinolone antibiotics destroy bacteria by altering their deoxyribonucleic acid (DNA) (see Figure 43-3). They accomplish this by interfering with the bacterial enzymes DNA gyrase and topoisomerase IV. Quinolones do not inhibit the production of human DNA.

The quinolones kill susceptible strains of mostly gram-negative and some gram-positive organisms. Some quinolones are also believed to diffuse into and concentrate themselves in human neutrophils, killing bacteria such as *S. aureus*, *Serratia marcescens*, and *Mycobacterium fortuitum* that sometimes accumulate in these cells. Bacterial resistance to quinolone antibiotics has been identified among several bacterial species, including *Pseudomonas aeruginosa*, *S. aureus*, *Pneumococcus* spp., *Enterococcus* spp., and the broad Enterobacteriaceae family that includes *E. coli*.

Indications

Quinolones are active against a wide variety of gram-negative and selected gram-positive bacteria. Most are excreted primarily by the kidneys as unchanged drug. This characteristic, together with the fact that they have extensive gram-negative coverage, makes them suitable for treating complicated urinary tract infections. They are also commonly used to treat respiratory, skin, GI, bone, and joint infections.

Ciprofloxacin (Cipro®) was the first quinolone to enjoy widespread use. Resistance was soon seen in *Pseudomonas* and some *Streptococcus* spp. Ciprofloxacin and levofloxacin are available both orally and by injection and are both available in generic form, which means that they cost significantly less than brand name quinolones. Levofloxacin (Levaquin®) is somewhat more active than ciprofloxacin against gram-positive organisms such as *S. pneumoniae*, including penicillin-resistant strains, as well as *Enterococcus* and *S. aureus*. Moxifloxacin hydrochloride is also effective against *S. pneumoniae* as well as some strains of *S. aureus* and enterococci. However, MRSA and VRE are generally also resistant to moxifloxacin hydrochloride. The activity of moxifloxacin hydrochloride against many enteric gram-negative bacteria and *P. aeruginosa* is similar to that of levofloxacin and less than that of ciprofloxacin. Moxifloxacin hydrochloride often has stronger anaerobic bacterial coverage. Norfloxacin hydrochloride has limited oral absorption and is available only in oral form, so its use is limited to GU infections. Quinolones may be combined with aminoglycosides to treat *P. aeruginosa* infections; step-down to monotherapy is recommended once susceptibility results are confirmed. Moxifloxacin hydrochloride also has some in vitro activity against anaerobes. The use of quinolones in prepubescent children is not generally recommended because these drugs have been shown to affect cartilage development in laboratory animals. However, more recent evidence suggests that judicial use in children might be less of a risk than previously thought, and in fact these drugs are used commonly in children with cystic fibrosis. Box 44-1 lists selected microbes commonly susceptible to quinolone therapy in general, but there is some variation in spectra among drugs. Table 44-3 gives common indications for individual drugs.

Contraindications

The only true contraindication to quinolones is known drug allergy.

Adverse Effects

Quinolones are capable of causing a variety of adverse effects, the most common of which are listed in Table 44-4. Bacterial overgrowth is another possible complication of quinolone therapy, but this is more commonly associated with long-term use. More worrisome is a heart effect that involves prolongation of the QT interval on the

---

BOX 44-1

Overview of Quinolone-Susceptible Microbial Spectra

- **Gram-positive:** *Streptococcus* (including *S. pneumoniae*), *Staphylococcus*, *Enterococcus*, *Listeria monocytogenes*
- **Gram-negative:** *Neisseria gonorrhea*, *N. meningitidis*, *Haemophilus influenzae*, *H. parainfluenzae*, Enterobacteriaceae (including *Escherichia coli*, *Enterobacter*, *Klebsiella*, *Proteus mirabilis*, *Salmonella*, *Shigella*), *Acinetobacter*, *Pseudomonas aeruginosa*, *Pastorella multocida*, *Legionella*, *Mycoplasma pneumoniae*, *Chlamydia*
- **Anaerobes:** *Bacteroides fragilis*, *Peptococcus*, *Peptostreptococcus* (moxifloxacin hydrochloride is strongest)
- **Other:** *Rickettsia* (ciprofloxacin only)

TABLE 44-3

Quinolones: Common Indications for Specific Drugs

Generic Name (Brand Name)	Antibacterial Spectrum	Common Indications
ciprofloxacin (generic)	Extensive gram-negative and selected gram-positive coverage	Respiratory, skin and soft tissue, urinary tract, prostate, intra-abdominal, bone and joint infections; infectious diarrhea; meningococcal carriers; typhoid fever; uncomplicated gonorrhea
levofloxacin (Levaquin®)		Respiratory and urinary tract infections; skin and skin structure infections
moxifloxacin hydrochloride (Avelox®)		Respiratory and skin infections; intra-abdominal infections; community-acquired pneumonia
norfloxacin (Apo-Norflox®)		Urinary tract infections; sexually transmitted infections

electrocardiogram (ECG). Dangerous cardiac dysrhythmias are more likely to occur when quinolones are taken by patients who are also receiving class Ia and class III antidysrhythmic drugs, such as disopyramide and amiodarone hydrochloride. For this reason, such drug combinations are best avoided. A labelling warning is required by Health Canada for all quinolones because of the increased risk of tendinitis and tendon rupture with use of these drugs. This effect is more common in older adults, patients with kidney failure, and those on concurrent glucocorticoid therapy (e.g., prednisone). In addition, a second labelling warning was required concerning worsening symptoms such as muscle weakness and breathing difficulties in patients with myasthenia gravis. Central nervous system (CNS) stimulation in the form of seizures has been reported. Slow infusion of a dilute solution into a large vein will minimize patient discomfort and reduce the risk of venous irritation.

Interactions

There are several drugs that interact with quinolones. Their concurrent use with antacids, calcium, magnesium, iron, zinc preparations, or sucralfate causes a reduction in the oral absorption of the quinolone. Patients need to take the interacting drugs at least 1 hour before or after taking quinolones. Dairy products also reduce the absorption of quinolones and should be separated as stated previously for interacting drugs. Enteral tube feedings can also reduce the absorption of quinolones. Probenecid can reduce kidney excretion of quinolones. Nitrofurantoin (discussed later in this chapter) can antagonize the antibacterial activity of quinolones, and oral anticoagulants are to be used with caution in patients receiving quinolones because of the antibiotic-induced alteration of the intestinal flora, which affects vitamin K synthesis.

Dosages

For dosage information on selected fluoroquinolones, refer to the table on p. 836.

NURSING PROCESS

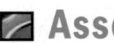 **Assessment**

Many of the antibiotics discussed in this chapter, in contrast to those in Chapter 43, are the types of drugs that

---

TABLE 44-4

Quinolones: Reported Adverse Effects

Body System	Adverse Effects
Central nervous	Headache, dizziness, insomnia, depression, restlessness, convulsions
Gastrointestinal	Nausea, constipation, increased AST and ALT levels, flatulence, heartburn, vomiting, diarrhea, oral candidiasis, dysphagia
Integumentary	Rash, pruritus, urticaria, flushing
Other	Ruptured tendons and tendonitis, worsening myasthenia gravis symptoms, fever, chills, blurred vision, phototoxicity, tinnitus

ALT, alanine aminotransferase; *AST*, aspartate aminotransferase.

 ## DRUG PROFILES

Two of the most commonly prescribed quinolones are ciprofloxacin and levofloxacin. Dosage information appears in the designated Dosages table on p. 836.

▶▶ *ciprofloxacin hydrochloride*

Ciprofloxacin hydrochloride was one of the first of the broad-coverage, potent quinolones to become available. It was first marketed in an oral form and is now available in injectable, ophthalmic (see Chapter 57), otic (see Chapter 58), and inhalation (TOBI) formulations. Because of its excellent bioavailability, it can work orally as well as many IV antibiotics. It is capable of killing a wide range of gram-negative bacteria and is effective against traditionally difficult-to-kill gram-negative bacteria such as *Pseudomonas*. Some anaerobic bacteria as well as atypical organisms such as *Chlamydia*, *Mycoplasma*, and *Mycobacterium* can also be killed by ciprofloxacin.

PHARMACOKINETICS

Route	Onset of Action	Peak Plasma Concentration	Elimination Half-Life	Duration of Action
IV	30 min	1 hr	3–4.8 hr	Up to 12 hr
PO	Variable	1–2 hr	3–4.8 hr	Up to 12 hr

levofloxacin

Levofloxacin (Levaquin) is one of the most widely used quinolones. It has a broad spectrum of activity similar to that of ciprofloxacin, but it has the advantage of once-daily dosing, as does gatifloxacin. Levofloxacin is available in both oral and injectable forms.

PHARMACOKINETICS

Route	Onset of Action	Peak Plasma Concentration	Elimination Half-Life	Duration of Action
IV	Variable	1–2 hr	6–8 hr	Up to 24 hr
PO	Variable	2 hr	6–8 hr	Up to 24 hr

DOSAGES Selected Quinolones

Drug	Pharmacological Class	Usual Dosage Range	Indications
▶▶ciprofloxacin hydrochloride	Fluoroquinolone	*Adults** IV: 200–400 mg q8–12h PO: 250–750 mg q12h	Broad gram-positive and gram-negative coverage for infections throughout the body
levofloxacin (Levaquin)		*Adults only* IV/PO: 250–750 mg once daily	Various susceptible bacterial infections

IV, intravenous; *PO*, oral.

*Not normally recommended for children under 18 years because of adverse musculoskeletal effects shown in studies of immature animals.

 DRUG PROFILES

MISCELLANEOUS ANTIBIOTICS

There are a number of antibiotics that do not fit into any of the previously described broad categories. Most have somewhat unique indications or are especially preferred for a particular type of infection. Although they may not be used as commonly as drugs from the other major classes, they are still of clinical importance. Several of these drugs are described individually in the following drug profiles. For dosage information on these drugs, refer to the table on p. 839.

▶▶*clindamycin*

Clindamycin (Dalacin C®) is a semisynthetic antibiotic. Clindamycin can be either bactericidal or bacteriostatic (see Chapter 43), depending on the concentration of the drug at the site of infection and on the infecting bacteria. It inhibits protein synthesis in bacteria (see Figure 43-3). Clindamycin is indicated for the treatment of chronic bone infections, GU tract infections, intra-abdominal infections, anaerobic pneumonia, septicemia caused by streptococci and staphylococci, and serious skin and soft-tissue infections caused by susceptible bacteria. Most gram-positive bacteria, including *Staphylococci*, *Streptococci*, and *Pneumococci*, are susceptible to clindamycin's actions. It also has the advantage of being active against several anaerobic organisms and is most often used for this purpose. However, resistant strains of gram-positive, gram-negative, and anaerobic organisms do occur. All Enterobacteriaceae strains are resistant to clindamycin. Clindamycin is contraindicated in patients with a known hypersensitivity to it, those with ulcerative colitis or enteritis, and infants younger than 1 month of age. GI tract adverse effects are the most common ones and include nausea, vomiting, abdominal pain, diarrhea, pseudomembranous colitis, and anorexia.

Pseudomembranous colitis (also known as *antibiotic-associated colitis*, *C. difficile* diarrhea, or *C. difficile* infection) is a necrotizing inflammatory bowel condition that is often associated with antibiotic therapy, especially clindamycin therapy. Clindamycin is available in oral, injectable, and topical (see Chapter 56) forms.

Clindamycin is also known to have some neuromuscular blocking properties that may enhance the action of neuromuscular drugs used in perioperative and critical care settings, such as vecuronium bromide (see Chapter

12). Patients receiving both drugs need to be monitored for excessive neuromuscular blockade and respiratory paralysis, and appropriate ventilatory support should be provided as needed.

PHARMACOKINETICS

Route	Onset of Action	Peak Plasma Concentration	Elimination Half-Life	Duration of Action
PO	30 min	45 min	2–3 hr	6 hr
IM/IV	Variable	IM: 3 hr IV: 10–45 min	2–3 hr	IM: 8–12 hr

linezolid

Linezolid (Zyvoxam®) is the first antibacterial drug in a new class of antibiotics known as oxazolidinones. This drug acts by inhibiting bacterial protein synthesis. Linezolid was originally developed to treat infections associated with VRE *faecium*, more commonly referred to as VRE. VRE is a notoriously difficult infection to treat and often occurs as a health care–associated infection. Linezolid has also received approval for the treatment of health care–associated pneumonia; complicated skin and skin structure infections, including cases caused by MRSA; and gram-positive infections in infants and children. MRSA is a virulent organism. However, methicillin, a penicillinase-resistant penicillin, has been removed from the Canadian market. Nonetheless, *MRSA* is still the term used, although oxacillin is now the test drug for this organism. To confuse things even further, oxacillin is rarely used for therapy, and oral linezolid is the most commonly used drug for methicillin-susceptible *S. aureus*. Linezolid is approved for treatment of community-acquired pneumonia and uncomplicated skin and skin structure infections.

The most commonly reported adverse effects attributed to linezolid are headache, nausea, diarrhea, and vomiting. It has also been shown to decrease platelet count. It is contraindicated in patients with a known hypersensitivity to it. It is available in oral and injectable forms. It has excellent oral absorption, which allows patients to continue oral therapy at home for serious infections that would otherwise require hospitalization. Linezolid has the potential to strengthen the vasopressor (prohypertensive) effects of vasopressive drugs (see Chapter 19) such as dopamine, by an unclear mechanism. Also, there have been postmarketing case reports of this drug causing

DRUG PROFILES—cont'd

serotonin syndrome when used concurrently with serotonergic drugs such as the selective-serotonin reuptake inhibitor (SSRI) antidepressants (see Chapter 17). It is recommended that the SSRI be stopped while the patient is receiving linezolid therapy; however, oftentimes this is not realistic and patients must be watched carefully for signs of serotonin syndrome. Finally, tyramine-containing foods, such as wine, aged cheese, soy sauce, smoked meats or fish, and sauerkraut, can interact with linezolid to raise blood pressure.

PHARMACOKINETICS

Route	Onset of Action	Peak Plasma Concentration	Elimination Half-Life	Duration of Action
PO	Variable	1–2 hr	5 hr	12 hr
IV	Variable	Immediate	6–7 hr	8–12 hr

▸▸ metronidazole

Metronidazole (Flagyl®) is an antimicrobial drug of the class nitroimidazole. It has good activity against anaerobic organisms and is widely used for intra-abdominal and gynecological infections caused by such organisms. Examples of the anaerobes against which it is active include *Peptostreptococcus* spp., *Bacteroides* spp., and *Clostridium* spp. Metronidazole is also indicated for treatment of protozoal infections such as amebiasis and trichomoniasis (see Chapter 48). It works by interfering with microbial DNA synthesis, and in this regard it is similar to the quinolones (see Figure 43-3). It is used orally to treat antibiotic-associated colitis; however, resistance has being noted. Metronidazole (given orally) is the treatment of choice in most cases of *C. difficile* colitis in children. Metronidazole is contraindicated in cases of known drug allergy. It is available in oral forms. The drug is not recommended for use during the first trimester of pregnancy. Adverse effects include dizziness, headache, GI discomfort, nasal congestion, and reversible neutropenia and thrombocytopenia. Drug interactions include acute alcohol intolerance when it is taken with alcoholic beverages, due to the accumulation of acetaldehyde, the principal alcohol metabolite. Patients must avoid alcohol for 24 hours before initiation of therapy and for at least 36 hours after the last dose of metronidazole. Metronidazole may also increase the toxicity of lithium, benzodiazepines, cyclosporine, calcium channel blockers, antidepressants (e.g., venlafaxine hydrochloride), warfarin sodium and other drugs. In contrast, phenytoin and phenobarbital may reduce the effects of metronidazole. These interactions occur because of various enzymatic effects involving the cytochrome P450 liver enzymes that result in altered metabolism when these drugs are taken concurrently with metronidazole.

PHARMACOKINETICS

Route	Onset of Action	Peak Plasma Concentration	Elimination Half-Life	Duration of Action
PO	Variable	1–2 hr	8 hr	Unknown
IV	Variable	1 hr	8 hr	Unknown

nitrofurantoin

Nitrofurantoin (Furantoin®, MacroBID®) is an antibiotic drug of the class nitrofuran. It is indicated primarily for urinary tract infections caused by *E. coli, S. aureus, Klebsiella* spp., and *Enterobacter* spp. It works by interfering with the activity of enzymes that regulate bacterial carbohydrate metabolism and by disrupting bacterial cell wall formation. It is contraindicated in cases of drug allergy and significant kidney function impairment because the drug concentrates in the urine. The drug is available only for oral use and is taken with food or milk to minimize gastric upset. Adverse effects include GI discomfort, dizziness, headache, skin reactions (mild to severe reactions have been reported), blood dyscrasias, ECG changes, possibly irreversible peripheral neuropathy, and hepatotoxicity. Although hepatotoxicity is rare, it is often fatal. Interacting drugs are few and include probenecid, which can reduce kidney excretion of nitrofurantoin, and antacids, which can reduce the extent of its GI absorption. The dose must be reduced for older adult patients and those with decreased renal function. Another drug that is approved for urinary tract infections is fosfomycin tromethamine (Monurol®). It is given as a one-time dose and maintains high concentrations in the urine for up to 48 hours.

PHARMACOKINETICS

Route	Onset of Action	Peak Plasma Concentration	Elimination Half-Life	Duration of Action
PO	2.5–4.5 hr	30 min	0.5–1 hr	5–8 hr

quinupristin/dalfopristin

Quinupristin and dalfopristin (Synercid®) are two streptogramin antibacterials marketed in a 30:70 combination. The combination drug is approved for IV treatment of bacteremia and life-threatening infection caused by VRE and for treatment of complicated skin and skin structure infections caused by *S. aureus* and *S. pyogenes,* including MRSA. This drug combination is available through the Special Access Programme, Health Canada.

Common adverse effects are arthralgias and myalgias, which may become severe. Adverse effects related to the infusion site, including pain, inflammation, edema, and thrombophlebitis, have developed in approximately 75% of patients treated through a peripheral IV line. The drug is contraindicated in patients with a known hypersensitivity to it. Drug interactions are limited; the most serious being potential increase in levels of cyclosporine. The drug is available only in injectable form. Quinupristin/dalfopristin must be infused with 5% dextrose in water (D5W) only and cannot be mixed with saline or heparin sodium, including heparinized flushes.

PHARMACOKINETICS (QUINUPRISTIN/DALFOPRISTIN)

Route	Onset of Action	Peak Plasma Concentration	Elimination Half-Life	Duration of Action
IV	1–2 hr	3–4 hr	1–3 hr	8–12 hr

Continued

DRUG PROFILES—cont'd

▶▶*vancomycin hydrochloride*

Vancomycin hydrochloride (Vancocin®) is a natural bactericidal antibiotic that is structurally unrelated to any other commercially available antibiotics. It destroys bacteria by binding to the bacterial cell wall, producing immediate inhibition of cell wall synthesis and death (see Figure 43-3). This mechanism differs from that of β-lactam antibiotics.

Vancomycin hydrochloride is the antibiotic of choice for the treatment of MRSA infection and infections caused by many other gram-positive bacteria. It is not active against gram-negative bacteria, fungi, or yeast. Oral vancomycin is indicated for the treatment of antibiotic-induced colitis (*C. difficile*) and for the treatment of staphylococcal enterocolitis. Because the oral formulation is poorly absorbed from the GI tract, it is used for its local effects on the surface of the GI tract. The parenteral form is indicated for the treatment of bone and joint infections and bacterial bloodstream infections caused by *Staphylococcus* spp. Resistance to vancomycin hydrochloride has been noted with increasing frequency in patients with infections caused by *Enterococcus* organisms. These strains have been isolated most often from GI tract infections but have also been isolated from skin, soft tissue, and bloodstream infections. Federal, provincial, territorial, and institution guidelines are available for the management and treatment of MRSA, VRE, *C. difficile*, and other superinfections.

Vancomycin hydrochloride is contraindicated in patients with known hypersensitivity to it. Because it is excreted rapidly by the kidneys, it should be used with caution in those with pre-existing kidney dysfunction, as blood levels can increase markedly, and with it, the risk of toxicity. Another adverse effect, nephrotoxicity, is more likely to occur with concurrent therapy with other nephrotoxic drugs such as aminoglycosides, cyclosporine, and contrast media used for CT scans. Vancomycin can also cause additive neuromuscular blocking effects in patients receiving neuromuscular blockers. Ototoxicity has occurred with serum levels above 80 mcg/mL, particularly in older adults. If the levels are too low (less than 5 mg/mL), the dosage may be subtherapeutic, with reduced antibacterial efficacy. Another common adverse effect that is bothersome but usually not harmful is known as *red man syndrome*. This syndrome is characterized by flushing, erythema, or itching of the head, face, neck, and upper trunk area. It is most commonly seen when the drug is infused too rapidly. It can usually be alleviated by giving the infusion of the dose over at least 1 hour. Rapid

infusions may also cause hypotension. Pains and muscle spasms in the back and chest may occur, as well as dyspnea. Optimal blood levels of vancomycin hydrochloride are a peak level of 18 to 50 mcg/mL and a trough level of 10 to 20 mcg/mL. Measurement of peak levels is no longer routinely recommended, and only trough levels are commonly monitored. There is a lack of clear evidence that nephrotoxicity and ototoxicity associated with vancomycin hydrochloride are prevented by adherence to specific concentration ranges. Vancomycin hydrochloride is poorly absorbed orally and is distributed slowly into peripheral tissues, so toxicity does not occur with oral doses. Blood samples for measurement of trough levels are drawn immediately before administration of the next dose. Because of the increase in resistant organisms, many clinicians use a trough level of 15 to 20 mcg/mL as their goal. Vancomycin hydrochloride is available in both oral and injectable forms.

PHARMACOKINETICS

Route	Onset of Action	Peak Plasma Concentration	Elimination Half-Life	Duration of Action
IV	Variable	1 hr	4–6 hr	Up to 24 hr; longer in those with kidney dysfunction

colistimethate sodium

Colistimethate sodium (Coly-Mycin®) is a polypeptide antibiotic that penetrates and disrupts the bacterial membrane of susceptible strains of gram-negative bacteria. It is an old drug that fell out of clinical use when newer, less toxic drugs became available. Unfortunately, due to the emergence of infections with KPC-producing organisms, it is now being used again, often as one of the only drugs available to treat KPC. Colistimethate sodium is available for IV, IM, and inhalational administration, commonly used in multi-drug resistant ventilator-associated pneumonias. It has serious adverse effects, including kidney failure and neurotoxic effects such as paresthesia, numbness, tingling, vertigo, dizziness, and impairment of speech. Colistimethate sodium crosses the placenta and needs to be used with caution in pregnant women. Colistimethate sodium is infused over 3 to 5 minutes.

PHARMACOKINETICS

Route	Onset of Action	Peak Plasma Concentration	Elimination Half-Life	Duration of Action
IV	Unknown	10 min	2–3 hr	8–12 hr

are often reserved for the treatment of more virulent infections and are mainly administered by parenteral routes; thus, they demand more skillful and thorough assessment of the patient and the specific drug. These antibiotics all require a crucial assessment on aa history of or symptoms indicative of hypersensitivity or allergic reactions, with symptoms ranging from mild reactions with angioedema, rash, pruritus, or hives to severe reactions with laryngeal edema, bronchospasm, or

possible cardiac arrest. Further assessment associated with these groups of antibiotics in general includes conducting a nursing physical examination and recording age, weight, and baseline vital sign values. Diagnostic and laboratory tests that may be ordered include some of the following: (1) AST and ALT levels (for assessing liver function); (2) urinalysis (glomerular filtration rate [GFR], BUN, and serum creatinine levels; for assessing kidney function); (3) ECG, echocardiogram, ultrasonography,

DOSAGES   Selected Miscellaneous Antibiotics

Drug	Pharmacological Class	Usual Dosage Range	Indications
▸▸clindamycin (Dalacin C)	Lincosamide	*Neonates under 1 mo* IM/IV: 5 mg/kg bid–tid *Children older than 1 mo* IM/IV: 20–40 mg/day, divided tid–qid PO: 8–20 mg/kg/day divided tid–qid *Adults* IM/IV: 600–2 700 mg/day, divided bid–tid–qid PO: 150–450 mg q6h	Anaerobes; streptococcal and staphylococcal infections of bone, skin, respiratory, and GU tract
colistimethate sodium (Coly-Mycin)	Polypeptide	*Adults* IV: 2.5–5 mg/kg/day; divided bid–qid; infuse over 3–5 min	Treatment of KPC-producing organisms
linezolid (Zyvoxam)	Oxazolidinone	*Adults only* IV/PO: 400–600 mg q12h	VRE; skin and respiratory infections caused by *Staphylococcus* and *Streptococcus* spp.
▸▸metronidazole (Flagyl)	Nitroimidazole	*Children* PO: 15–50 mg/kg/day divided tid *Adults* PO: 250–700 mg, divided bid–tid	Primarily anaerobic and gram-negative infections of abdominal cavity, skin, bone, and respiratory, and GU tracts
nitrofurantoin (Furantoin, MacroBID)	Nitrofuran	*Children/Adults* PO: 100 mg bid	Primarily UTIs caused by gram-negative organisms and *Staphylococcus aureus*
quinupristin/dalfopristin* (Synercid)	Streptogramins	*Children/Adults* IV: 7.5 mg/kg q8–12h	VRE; skin infections caused by streptococcal and staphylococcal infections
▸▸vancomycin (Vancocin)	Tricyclic glycopeptide	*Neonates, Infants, and Children* IV: 10–15 mg/kg q6–12h PO: 40 mg/kg *Adults* IV: 500–2 000 mg q12–24h PO: 125–500 mg tid–qid	Severe staphylococcal infections, including MRSA; other serious gram-positive infections, including *Streptococcus* spp.

GU, genitourinary; *IM*, intramuscular; *IV*, intravenous; *MRSA*, methicillin-resistant *S. aureus*; *PO*, oral; *spp.*, species; *UTIs*, urinary tract infections; *VRE*, vancomycin-resistant *Enterococcus*.
*Available through Special Access Programme, Health Canada.

and cardiac enzyme levels (for assessing cardiac function); (4) culture and sensitivity of the infected tissue or blood samples for assessing sensitivity of the bacteria to the antibiotic; (5) WBC count, hemoglobin level, hematocrit, RBC count, platelet count, and clotting values for baseline blood count levels. In the baseline neurological assessment, note sensory and motor intactness and assessment of any alterations in neurological functioning, for example, altered sensorium and level of consciousness, because of the potential for CNS adverse effects. Baseline abdominal and GI assessments are important, with a focus on bowel patterns and bowel sounds because of possible GI adverse effects. Note contraindications, cautions, and drug interactions, and obtain a complete list of the patient's medications, including over-the-counter drugs and natural health products. Perform an ethnocultural assessment because of the various responses of certain racial and ethnic groups to specific drugs as well as the potential use of alternative healing practices.

With any antibiotic, assess for superinfection, or a secondary infection that occurs with the destruction of normal flora during antibiotic therapy (see Chapter 43). Fungal superinfections may be evaluated by creamy white mouth lesions, fever, lethargy, or perineal itching. Assess the patient's immune system status and overall condition because if there is an immune deficiency (e.g., in patients with cancer, autoimmune disorders such as lupus erythematosus, AIDS, and any chronic illness), the patient's ability to physically resist infection may be diminished. Antibiotic resistance is a continual concern with antibiotic drug therapy, especially in children and in patients being treated in large health care institutions and long-term care facilities. Consider this possibility of resistance to certain antibiotics when assessing patients for symptoms of infection and superinfection. With aminoglycosides, assess for hypersensitivity and pre-existing conditions. Obtain a list of all medications the patient is taking because of the many cautions, contraindications, and drug interactions associated with these drugs.

The aminoglycosides are known for their ototoxicity and nephrotoxicity; therefore, if deemed appropriate, perform baseline hearing tests and assessment of vestibular function. There is an increased risk for nephrotoxicity with the use of other nephrotoxic drugs, such as cyclosporine and the IV contrast used for CT scans. For patients requiring a CT scan with contrast who are also on a nephrotoxic medication, alert the health care provider to the situation so that the dose may be adjusted and additional fluids or medications ordered. As well, perform kidney function studies (BUN level, urinalysis, and serum and urine creatinine levels) ordered, and document all results. If kidney baseline functioning is decreased, the health care provider may need to adjust the dosage amounts because of the risk of nephrotoxicity.

Complete a thorough neuromuscular assessment because of the possibility for drug-related neurotoxicity and higher risk for complications in those with impaired neurological functioning. For example, patients with myasthenia gravis or Parkinson's disease may experience worsening of muscle weakness because of the drug's neuromuscular blockade. Neonates (because of the immaturity of the nervous and kidney systems) and older adults (because of decreased neurological and kidney functioning) are also at highest risk for nephrotoxicity, neurotoxicity, and ototoxicity and require careful assessment before and during drug therapy. Assess hydration status. The toxicities of these drugs are greater in those with pre-existing renal impairment, those receiving other nephrotoxic drugs, and in those patients taking the aminoglycoside for a long period of time or on high-dose therapy.

Quinolones, such as ciprofloxacin, require careful assessment for pre-existing CNS conditions (e.g., seizures or stroke disorders) that may be exacerbated with the concurrent use of these drugs. Assess for a cardiac history, and note if the patient is taking certain antidysrhythmics because of the potential for dangerous cardiac irregularities. Significant drug interactions include antacids, iron, zinc preparations, and sucralfate, as they affect the absorption of the quinolone. Oral anticoagulants also interact with and alter the antibacterial activity of quinolones (see previous discussion).

If clindamycin is being used, assess for hypersensitivity to the drug or related compounds. Clindamycin is not to be used in patients with ulcerative colitis or in those younger than 1 month of age. Perform a thorough assessment of GI disorders because of the possibility of drug-induced pseudomembranous colitis, vomiting, and diarrhea (see previous discussion). Assess bowel sounds as well as bowel patterns prior to giving this drug. Preoperatively, or if patients are in an intensive care setting and receiving clindamycin, assess for the concurrent use of neuromuscular blocking drugs because of clindamycin's excessive blockade of neuromuscular functioning and respiratory paralysis. These patients, if in need of clindamycin, would need ventilator support.

Linezolid is used to treat health care–associated infections, pneumonia, and complicated skin infections, including MRSA. Use of methicillin (removed from the market) and oxacillin are no longer options for treatment, so this drug offers another pharmacotherapeutic option. Assess for the concurrent use of serotonergic drugs (e.g., SSRIs [antidepressants]) because of drug-induced serotonin syndrome (see Chapter 17). Additionally, assess for intake of tyramine-containing foods (e.g., wine, aged cheese, soy sauce, and smoked fish or meat) because of the risk of elevated blood pressure.

Assess patients taking metronidazole for allergy to the drug and to other nitroimidazole derivatives. As with all medications, assess for contraindications, cautions, and drug interactions, and document the findings (see previous discussion). It is important for patient safety to review culture and sensitivity reports before therapy is initiated. However, it may be necessary to start the medication regimen (due to clinical presentation) prior to results being obtained and then change medications as dictated by the culture and sensitivity results. Baseline assessments are needed of the neurological system (noting any dizziness, numbness, tingling, and other sensory or motor abnormalities), GI system (checking bowel sounds, bowel problems, and patterns), and GU system (documenting urinary patterns, colour of urine, and intake and output). Inquire about alcohol intake because of the interaction of alcohol with the drug and subsequent acute alcohol intolerance. Assess for potential drug interactions, such as with benzodiazepines, calcium channel blockers, various antidepressants, and warfarin.

Assessment of drug allergies is important with the use of nitrofurantoin. It is also important to assess kidney and liver function due to the possibility of hepatotoxic adverse effects as well as the need for a decrease in dosage amounts in older adults with kidney function impairment (creatinine clearance less than 60 mL/min). Complete a baseline assessment of any sensory or motor problems because of the possible adverse effect of peripheral neuropathy, which may be irreversible. Assess the patient's skin colour, turgor, intactness, and the presence of rash due to the possibility of drug-related, mild to severe skin reactions. With quinupristin/dalfopristin, assess vital signs as well as for any muscular aches and pains due to drug-induced arthralgia and myalgia.

For patients taking vancomycin, ask questions about other medications the patient is taking, especially drugs that are nephrotoxic or ototoxic. Assess the patient for a history of pre-existing kidney disease or hearing loss due to the possibility of nephrotoxicity or ototoxicity. Note the baseline hearing status because of the risk of hearing loss. Part of the health care provider's order will be to order trough levels of vancomycin. These labs will be drawn immediately before the next dose. Assessment of these levels is important to patient safety. Peak levels are used to calculate the exact dose that the patient needs to maintain therapeutic levels. It is important to assess the colour of the patient's skin because of the risk for red man syndrome. This syndrome is bothersome but usually not harmful, and is characterized by flushing of the face, head, neck, and upper trunk areas. Red man syndrome is seen when infusions are administered too rapidly, so always assess and monitor IV rates to be sure the drug is administered over at least 1 hour. Assess vital signs with attention to blood pressure because infusions that are too rapid may precipitate hypotension. Phlebitis may also occur, so assess for localized redness and swelling and pain or burning along the length of the vein. Because of multiple drug and diluent incompatibilities, as with several of the other parenteral antibiotics mentioned previously in this chapter, always assess for potential fluid and medication interactions.

With the emergence of multidrug-resistant organisms (e.g., MRSA, VRE, and ESBL- and KPC-producing organisms), ensure that proper handwashing techniques are used by health care providers and caregivers.

Nursing Diagnoses

- Deficient knowledge related to lack of information and experience with the medication regimen
- Risk for infection related to the patient's compromised immune status before and during treatment
- Risk for injury (compromised organ function) related to adverse effects of medications (e.g., ototoxicity and nephrotoxicity) and weakened physical state

Planning

Goals

- Patient will demonstrate adequate knowledge base about the antibiotic therapeutic regimen.
- Patient will remain free from infection and have improved immune status during antibiotic therapy.
- Patient will remain free from injury.

Expected Patient Outcomes

- Patient states action and rationale for use of antibiotic therapy.
  - Patient understands the need to take the antibiotic exactly as ordered and for the duration of therapy.
- Patient experiences an increased sense of well-being and improved immune status while taking antibiotics.
  - Patient remains without fever, pain, and malaise.
  - Patient experiences increased comfort and improved energy levels.
  - Patient experiences minimal adverse effects of antibiotic therapy.
- Patient remains free from injury in regard to adverse effects, such as minimal to no problems with GI upset, diarrhea, nausea, or hearing loss.
  - Patient states measures to minimize adverse effects associated with antibiotic therapy, such as taking medications with yogourt, increasing fluids, eating well-balanced meals, and following instructions associated with safe use of the specific antibiotic.

Implementation

Aminoglycosides, as well as any antibiotics, need to be given exactly as ordered and with adequate hydration. Encourage fluid intake up to 3000 mL/24 hours unless contraindicated. A culture and sensitivity test must be carried out, if possible, before the first dose of antibiotic. It is also important to identify the source of the infection, if possible. Parenteral dosage forms are most commonly used. Because of the potential for nephrotoxicity and ototoxicity, determine and monitor the patient's kidney function during therapy. Dosing is adjusted based on estimates of creatinine clearance calculated from the patient's serum creatinine level. This measurement assists in keeping a close watch on the patient's kidney function and thus helps to prevent toxicity. Also monitor BUN

 CASE STUDY

Vancomycin

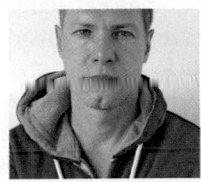

Greg, a 45-year-old graphic artist who is a quadriplegic, is being treated for an infected stage IV sacral pressure ulcer. The wound cultures have indicated the presence of multidrug-resistant *Staphylococcus aureus* (MRSA). The health care provider has ordered IV vancomycin to be given every 12 hours, application of dressings (twice a day) as part of the treatment, as well as a referral to the enterostomal therapist. In addition, Greg is placed on contact precautions because of the MRSA.

1. What will you assess before starting the vancomycin infusion?

2. Two days later, Greg reports feeling "hot" and itchy in his face and neck, and these areas are flushed. What do you suspect is happening?

3. What can you do to minimize complications during vancomycin infusions?

4. The health care provider orders measurement of vancomycin blood levels. What is the therapeutic goal when vancomycin levels are monitored?

5. What is the single best action you can take to prevent the spread of Greg's MRSA infection?

For answers, see http://evolve.elsevier.com/Canada/Lilley/ pharmacology/.

levels and GFR during therapy. Timing between doses and amount of drug are usually individualized. Alteration in auditory, vestibular, or kidney function may indicate the need for a possible dosage adjustment or withdrawal of the drug. Consumption of yogourt or buttermilk may help prevent antibiotic-induced superinfections (see Chapter 43).

With aminoglycosides, instruct the patient to report to the health care provider any changes in hearing, ringing in the ears (tinnitus), or a full feeling in the ears. Nausea, vomiting with motion, ataxia, nystagmus, or dizziness should also be reported immediately and may indicate problems with the vestibular nerve. With ophthalmic dosage forms, redness, burning, and itching of eyes may indicate an adverse reaction, and redness over the skin area may indicate an adverse reaction to topical forms. IM sites should be checked for induration. If noted, report it immediately to the health care provider, and do not reuse the site. Monitor IV sites for heat, swelling, redness, pain, or red streaking over the vein (sign of phlebitis), and initiate measures as per institutional protocol or policy. Keep in mind the following special considerations for gentamicin: (1) IM: Give deeply and slowly into muscle mass (ventrogluteal) to minimize discomfort; and (2) IV: Check for incompatibilities with other drugs, and give only clear or slightly yellow solutions that have been diluted with either normal saline (NS) or D_5W, infusing at the correct rate.

Quinolones, as with any self-administered antibiotics, are to be taken exactly as prescribed and for the full course of treatment. Instruct the patient not to take these medications with antacids, iron, zinc preparations, multivitamins, or sucralfate because the absorption of the antibiotic will be decreased. Instruct patients who need to take calcium or magnesium to take it 1 hour before or after the quinolone. Encouraging fluids is recommended, unless contraindicated. See Patient Teaching Tips for more information.

With clindamycin, instruct the patient to take the medication as ordered. Oral dosage forms are to be taken with 240 mL of water or other fluid. With topical forms, advise patients to avoid the simultaneous use of peeling or abrasive acne products, soaps, or alcohol-containing cosmetics to prevent cumulative effects; however, some products combine clindamycin with anti-acne medications (e.g., Benzaclin Topical Gel). Topical forms are to be applied in a thin layer to the affected area. Infuse IV dosage forms by piggyback technique and as ordered. Most resources state *never* to give these drugs via parenteral IV push. Dilute doses of the drug, and infuse per manufacturer guidelines. IV infusion that is too rapid can lead to severe hypotension and possible cardiac arrest. Give IM dosage forms deep into a large muscle mass (see Chapter 10).

Linezolid is generally given orally or intravenously, which makes it advantageous for those requiring an antibiotic with a spectrum similar to vancomycin for an extended period or on an outpatient basis. Oral dosages

are to be evenly spaced around the clock, as ordered, and given with food or milk to decrease the possibility of GI upset. Oral suspension forms must be given within 21 days of reconstitution. Protect IV doses from light, and infuse over 30 to 120 minutes; do not mix with any other medication. Foods that may increase blood pressure while taking linezolid need to be avoided; these include aged cheeses, wine, soy sauce, smoked meats or fish, and sauerkraut, due to their tyramine content (see Chapter 17).

Oral forms of metronidazole need to be given with food or meals to decrease GI upset. Educate patients not to chew extended-release dosages. It is recommended that intravaginal doses be administered at bedtime. Topical creams, ointments, or lotions are to be applied thinly to the affected area. An applicator should be used for intravaginal dosages. Gloves are worn to protect the hands from unnecessary exposure to medication and as part of standard precautions/routine practices. Do not apply topical forms close to the eyes, to avoid irritation. Store at room temperature IV dosage forms that are supplied in a ready-to-use infusion bag.

Nitrofurantoin is available in oral forms and must be given with sufficient fluids, food, or milk to reduce GI upset. To help prevent tooth staining and GI upset, do not crush tablets. Because of the risk for superinfection, hepatotoxicity, and peripheral neuropathy (which may be irreversible), closely monitor for signs and symptoms of these adverse effects and document the findings. Be aware that jaundice, itching, rash, and liver enlargement may indicate toxic effects to the liver, whereas numbness and tingling may occur with peripheral neuropathy.

For quinupristin/dalfopristin, only IV dosage forms are available. Reconstitute the drug using only D_5W. Use a gentle swirling action instead of shaking to mix the drug (to help minimize foaming). A diluted infusion bag of the drug is stable for up to 6 hours, or, if refrigerated, 54 hours. It is important to know these characteristics to help prevent untoward complications. Infusions are generally given over at least 60 minutes. Implement the same measures as with other antibiotics, to monitor for superinfection.

Vancomycin may be used orally but is poorly absorbed by this route and is used only to treat microbes in the GI tract (e.g., staphylococcal enterocolitis, C. *difficile*). Parenteral dosage forms must be used to treat infection outside of the intima of the GI tract. Reconstitute IV dosage forms as recommended (e.g., with either D_5W or NS) and infuse over at least 60 minutes. Too rapid an infusion of vancomycin or administration by IV push may lead to severe hypotension and red man syndrome. Extravasation may cause local skin irritation and damage, so frequently monitor the infusion and, in particular, the IV site. Constant monitoring for drug-related neurotoxicity, nephrotoxicity, ototoxicity, and superinfection remain crucial to patient safety. In addition, adequate hydration (at least 2 litres of fluids every 24 hours unless contraindicated) is important to prevent nephrotoxicity. Trough levels need to be ordered prior to the third or fourth dose; peak levels are no longer used (see the previous discussion for more information).

Because of the significant issue of multidrug-resistant organisms, encourage patients and family members not to abuse or overuse antibiotics and to report immediately to the health care provider any signs or symptoms of an infection that is not resolving or responding to antibiotic therapy. Regardless of drug management, in today's health care settings (e.g., acute and long-term facilities, medical offices, urgent care centres or walk-in clinics, emergency departments) as well as in the home setting and abroad, teach and demonstrate proper and thorough handwashing technique. The Centers for Disease Control and Prevention (CDC) and Health Canada recommend the following as the proper handwashing technique: Wash hands with warm running water and soap; lather well by rubbing hands vigorously for at least 15 to 20 seconds; pay attention to the wrist area, backs of the hands, areas between the fingers, and under the fingernails; and rinse well. Allow the water to run while drying hands with a paper towel and then use a dry paper towel as a barrier between the faucet and clean hands while turning off the water. If soap and water are not available and hands are not visibly soiled, gel hand sanitizers or alcohol-based hand wipes containing at least 60% ethyl alcohol or isopropanol may be used. Once the gel is applied and all surfaces covered, rub hands until gel is dry and do not towel gel off.

Evaluation

Once antibiotic therapy has been initiated, evaluation that is focused on goals, outcome criteria, therapeutic effects, and adverse effects must be ongoing. Ask patients to report any decrease in symptoms (e.g., associated with infection). Therapeutic goals include a return to normal of all blood counts and vital signs, negative results of culture and sensitivity testing, and improved appetite, energy level, and sense of well-being. Signs and symptoms of the infection will begin to resolve once therapeutic levels of antibiotics are achieved. Another aspect of evaluation is monitoring for adverse effects of therapy such as superinfections, antibiotic-associated colitis, nephrotoxicity, ototoxicity, neurotoxicity, hepatotoxicity, and other drug-specific adverse effects.

PATIENT TEACHING TIPS

❖ Aminoglycosides
- Educate patients about the drug, its purpose, and its adverse effects, including the risk of hearing loss, which may occur after completion of therapy. Advise them to report any change in hearing to the health care provider.
- Patients should be informed of the importance of drinking up to 3 000 mL/24 hours of fluids, unless contraindicated, with any medication but especially with antibiotics, to maximize absorption of oral doses, minimize some of the adverse effects, and ensure adequate hydration.
- Instruct patients to report to the health care provider any persistent headache, nausea, or vertigo. Educate them about the signs and symptoms of superinfection, such as diarrhea, vaginal discharge, stomatitis, loose and foul-smelling stools, or cough.

❖ Quinolones
- Educate patients about the importance of avoiding exposure to sun and tanning beds because of the risk of photosensitivity with these drugs. Recommend the use of sunglasses and sunscreen protection.
- Advise patients to report to the health care provider any headache, dizziness, restlessness, diarrhea, vomiting, oral candidiasis, flushing of the face, or inflammation of the tendons.
- Educate patients taking quinolones about drug interactions that may occur with the following drugs: calcium, magnesium, probenecid, nitrofurantoin, oral anticoagulants, iron, sucralfate, and zinc preparations. Instruct them to take calcium and magnesium supplements at least 1 hour before or after taking the quinolone. Probenecid may reduce the excretion of the antibiotic and cause toxicity. Since quinolones may alter the intestinal flora and thus vitamin K synthesis, oral anticoagulants must be used with caution in patients taking these antibiotics.
- Instruct patients taking ciprofloxacin or levofloxacin, both quinolones, to take the drug exactly as ordered.

❖ Clindamycin
- Instruct patients not to use topical forms of clindamycin near the eyes or near any abraded areas to avoid irritation.
- When vaginal dosage forms are used, patients need to be advised not to engage in sexual intercourse for the duration of the therapy. The full course of antibiotics is to be taken as ordered to obtain maximal therapeutic benefit.
- Instruct patients that, if topical dosage forms get into the eyes accidently, they should rinse the eyes immediately with copious amounts of cool tap water.

❖ Linezolid
- Instruct patients to continue therapy for the full prescribed length of treatment (as with all antibiotics).
- Educate patients to avoid tyramine-containing foods (e.g., red wine, aged cheeses) while taking the drug.
- Instruct patients to report to the health care provider any severe abdominal pain, fever, severe diarrhea, or worsening of signs and symptoms of infection.

❖ Metronidazole
- Caution patients taking metronidazole to avoid alcohol and any alcohol-containing products (e.g.,

Continued

PATIENT TEACHING TIPS—cont'd

cough preparations and elixirs) while taking the drug because of the risk for a disulfiram-like reaction (e.g., severe vomiting).
- Educate patients about the purpose of the drug, such as its use as either an antibacterial or an antifungal medication, because this knowledge is crucial to achieving therapeutic effects and preventing adverse effects.

❖ Nitrofurantoin
- Advise patients to report to the health care provider any abdominal cramping, dizziness, severe skin reactions, or jaundice.

❖ Vancomycin
- Instruct patients to report any changes in hearing, such as ringing in the ears or a feeling of fullness in the ears. Any nausea, vomiting, unsteady gait, dizziness, generalized tingling (usually after IV dosing), chills, fever, rash, or hives must also be reported.
- Monitor serum drug levels throughout therapy; this monitoring is key to prevention of toxicity. Trough levels are usually monitored throughout therapy. Stress to patients that follow-up appointments are important for monitoring serum drug levels and identifying possible toxic effects.

KEY POINTS

❖ Over the years, bacteria have developed enzymes and mechanisms to interact with antibiotics and render the antibiotic ineffective. Multidrug resistance is a significant health issue, and such resistant organisms include ESBL- and KPC-producing bacteria, MRSA, and VRE.

❖ The aminoglycosides are a group of natural and semisynthetic antibiotics that are classified as bactericidal drugs; they are extremely potent and are capable of potentially serious toxicities (e.g., nephrotoxicity, ototoxicity).

❖ Quinolones are extremely potent, bactericidal, broad-spectrum antibiotics and include norfloxacin hydrochloride, ciprofloxacin, levofloxacin, and moxifloxacin hydrochloride.

❖ Clindamycin is a semisynthetic derivative of lincomycin, an older antibiotic.

❖ Linezolid is an antibacterial drug used to treat infections associated with VRE *faecium*, more commonly referred to as VRE. VRE is a difficult infection to treat and often occurs as a health care–associated infection.

❖ Metronidazole (Flagyl) is an antimicrobial drug of the class nitroimidazole. It has good activity against anaerobic organisms and is widely used to treat intra-abdominal and gynecological infections; it is also

used to treat protozoal infections (e.g., amebiasis, trichomoniasis).

❖ Nitrofurantoin (MacroBID) is an antibiotic drug of the class nitrofuran. It is indicated primarily to treat urinary tract infections caused by *E. coli, S. aureus, Klebsiella* spp., and *Enterobacter* spp.

❖ Quinupristin/dalfopristin (Synercid) are two streptogramin antibacterials approved for IV treatment of bacteremia and life-threatening infection caused by VRE and for treatment of complicated skin and skin-structure infections caused by *S. aureus* and *S. yogenes*.

❖ Use of these antibiotics requires assessment for any history of or current symptoms indicative of hypersensitivity or allergic reactions (from mild reactions with rash, pruritus, and hives to severe reactions with laryngeal edema, bronchospasms, hypotension, and possible cardiac arrest).

❖ With the use of any antibiotic, it is important to assess for superinfection, or a secondary infection that occurs with the destruction of normal flora during antibiotic therapy. Superinfections may occur in the mouth, respiratory tract, GI tract, GU tract, or on the skin. Fungal infections are evidenced by fever, lethargy, perineal itching, and other anatomically related symptoms.

EXAMINATION REVIEW QUESTIONS

1. The nurse is assessing a woman who is receiving an antibiotic for community-acquired pneumonia, and the patient reports perineal itching. The nurse also notes that the patient has a thick, white vaginal discharge. What does the nurse suspect the patient is experiencing?
a. Resistance to the antibiotic
b. An adverse effect of the antibiotic
c. A superinfection
d. An allergic reaction

2. A patient has been admitted for treatment of an infected leg ulcer and will be started on IV linezolid. The nurse is reviewing the list of the patient's current medications. Which type of medication, if listed, would be of most concern if taken with the linezolid?
a. β-blocker
b. Oral anticoagulant
c. Selective serotonin reuptake inhibitor (SSRI) antidepressant
d. Thyroid replacement hormone

EXAMINATION REVIEW QUESTIONS—cont'd

3. While administering vancomycin, which of the following does the nurse know is the most important to assess before giving the medication?
a. Kidney function
b. WBC count
c. Liver function
d. Platelet count

4. During therapy with an IV aminoglycoside, the patient calls the nurse and says, "I am hearing some odd sounds, like ringing, in my ears." Which is the nurse's priority action at this time?
a. Reassure the patient that these are expected adverse effects.
b. Reduce the rate of the IV infusion.
c. Increase the rate of the IV infusion.
d. Stop the infusion immediately.

5. When giving IV quinolones, the nurse needs to keep in mind that these drugs may have serious interactions with which drugs?
a. Selective serotonin reuptake inhibitor (SSRI) antidepressants
b. Nonsteroidal anti-inflammatory drugs (NSAIDs)
c. Oral anticoagulants
d. Antihypertensives

6. The nurse is administering an IV aminoglycoside to a patient who has had gastrointestinal surgery. Which nursing measures are appropriate? (Select all that apply.)
a. Report a trough drug level of 0.8 mcg/mL, and hold the drug.
b. Enforce a strict fluid restriction.
c. Monitor serum creatinine levels.
d. Instruct the patient to report dizziness or a feeling of fullness in the ears.
e. Warn the patient that the urine may turn a darker colour.

7. The order reads: "Give vancomycin, 1250 mg in 250 mL NS, IVPB, every 12 hours. Infuse over 90 minutes." The nurse will set the infusion pump to what setting for mL/hour?

Answers: 1. c, 2. c, 3. a, 4. d, 5. c, 6. c, d, 7. 167 mL/hour

CRITICAL THINKING ACTIVITIES

1. A patient who has been receiving IV doses of metronidazole has been discharged and will continue therapy with oral doses of this medication. The patient remarks, "I'm so glad to be going home. Our annual office party is tomorrow night, and I've been looking forward to it all year long." What is the priority when teaching the patient regarding this drug?

2. A patient has been receiving therapy with the aminoglycoside tobramycin, and the nurse notes that the patient's latest trough drug level was 3 mcg/mL. This drug is given daily, and the next dose is to be administered now. Based on this trough drug level,

what is the nurse's priority action? Explain your answer.

3. A patient has a urinary tract infection caused by *Pseudomonas* spp. Two antibiotics have been ordered, both due at 0900 hr:
gentamicin, 300 mg, intravenously, daily (due at 0900 hr), infuse over 60 minutes
ceftazidime, 500 mg intravenously, every 12 hours (due at 0900 hr and 2100 hr), infuse over 30 minutes
Which antibiotic should the nurse infuse first? Explain your answer.

For answers, see http://evolve.elsevier.com/Canada/Lilley/pharmacology/.

CHAPTER 45

Antiviral Drugs

Objectives

After reading this chapter, the successful student will be able to do the following:

1. Discuss the effects of the immune system, paying attention to the different types of immunity.

2. Discuss the effects of viruses in the human body.

3. List specific drugs categorized as non-HIV antivirals and HIV antivirals or antiretrovirals.

4. Discuss the process of immunosuppression in patients with viral infections, specifically those with HIV infection.

5. Describe the stages of HIV/AIDS and various drugs used to manage the illness.

6. Discuss the mechanism of action, indications, contraindications, cautions, routes, adverse effects, and toxic effects of the various non-HIV and HIV antiviral drugs.

7. Develop a collaborative plan of care that includes all phases of the nursing process for patients receiving non-HIV and HIV antiviral drugs.

e-Learning Activities

Website
(http://evolve.elsevier.com/Canada/Lilley/pharmacology/)

evolve

- Answer Key—Textbook Case Studies
- Answer Key—Critical Thinking Activities
- Chapter Summaries—Printable
- Review Questions for Exam Preparation
- Unfolding Case Studies

Drug Profiles

▸▸ acyclovir, p. 854
    amantadine (amantadine hydrochloride)*, p. 854
    enfuvirtide, p. 860
▸▸ ganciclovir (ganciclovir hydrochloride)*, p. 854
▸▸ indinavir (indinavir sulphate)*, p. 860
▸▸ maraviroc, p. 860
▸▸ nevirapine, p. 860
    oseltamivir (oseltamivir phosphate)*, zanamivir, p. 854
▸▸ raltegravir (raltegravir potassium)*, p. 860
    ribavirin, p. 855
    tenofovir (tenofovir disoproxil fumarate)*, p. 861
▸▸ zidovudine, p. 861

▸▸ Key drug

*Full generic name is given in parentheses. For the purposes of this text, the more common, shortened name is used.

Key Terms

Acquired immune deficiency syndrome (AIDS) Infection caused by the human immunodeficiency virus (HIV), which weakens the host's immune system, giving rise to opportunistic infections. (p. 848)

Antibodies Immunoglobulin molecules that have an antigen-specific amino acid sequence and are produced by the humoral immune system (antibodies produced from B lymphocytes) in response to exposure to a specific antigen, the purpose of which is to attack and destroy molecules of this antigen. (p. 849)

Antigen A substance, usually a protein, that is foreign to a host and causes the formation of an antibody and reacts specifically with that antibody. Examples of antigens include bacterial exotoxins, viruses, and allergens. An allergen (e.g., dust, pollen, mould) is a specific type of antigen that causes allergic reactions (see Chapter 37). (p. 849)

Antiretroviral drugs A more specific term for antiviral drugs that work against retroviruses such as HIV. (p. 850)

Antiviral drugs Drugs that destroy viruses, either directly or indirectly, by suppressing their replication. (p. 849)

Cell-mediated immunity (CMI) One of two major parts of the immune system. CMI consists of nonspecific immune responses mediated primarily by T lymphocytes (T cells) and other immune system cells (e.g., monocytes, macrophages, neutrophils) but not antibody-producing cells (B lymphocytes). (p. 849)

Deoxyribonucleic acid (DNA) A nucleic acid composed of nucleotide units that contain molecules of the sugar deoxyribose, phosphate groups, and purine and pyrimidine bases. DNA molecules transmit genetic information and are found primarily in the nuclei of cells. (Compare with *ribonucleic acid [RNA]*). (p. 848)

Fusion The process by which viruses attach themselves to, or fuse with, the cell membranes of host cells, in preparation for infecting the cell for purposes of viral replication. (p. 848)

Genome The complete set of genetic material of any organism. The genome may consist of multiple chromosomes (groups of DNA or RNA molecules) in higher organisms; a single chromosome, as in bacteria; or one or two DNA or RNA molecules, as in viruses. (p. 848)

Herpesviruses Several different types of viruses belonging to the family Herpesviridae that cause various forms of herpes infection. (p. 849)

Host Any organism that is infected with a microorganism, such as bacteria or viruses. (p. 847)

Human immunodeficiency virus (HIV) The retrovirus that causes AIDS. (p. 848)

Humoral immunity One of two major parts of the immune system. Humoral immunity consists of specific immune responses in the form of antigen-specific antibodies produced from B lymphocytes (B cells). (p. 849)

Immunoglobulins Glycoproteins produced and used by the humoral immune system to attack and kill any substance (antigen) that is foreign to the body. An immunoglobulin with an antigen-specific amino acid sequence is called an *antibody* and is able to recognize and inactivate molecules of a specific antigen. (Also called *immune globulins*.) (p. 849)

Influenza viruses Viruses that cause influenza, an acute viral infection of the respiratory tract. There are three types of influenza virus: A, B, and C. Currently, medications are available to treat only types A and B. (p. 849)

Nucleic acids Complex biomolecules, including DNA and RNA, that contain the genetic material of all living organisms, which is passed to future generations during reproduction. (p. 848)

Nucleoside A structural component of nucleic acid molecules (DNA or RNA) that consists of a purine or pyrimidine base attached to a sugar molecule. (p. 850)

Nucleotide A nucleoside that is attached to a phosphate unit, which makes up the side chain "backbone" of a DNA or a RNA molecule. (p. 850)

Opportunistic infections Infections caused by any type of microorganism that occurs in an immunocompromised host but normally would not occur in an immunocompetent host. (p. 850)

Protease An enzyme that breaks down the amino acid structure of protein molecules by chemically cleaving the peptide bonds that link together the individual amino acids. (p. 852)

Replication Any process of duplication or reproduction, such as that involved in the duplication of nucleic acid molecules (DNA or RNA) during the reproduction processes of all living organisms; most commonly describes the entire process of viral reproduction, which occurs only inside the cells of an infected host organism. (p. 848)

Retroviruses Viruses belonging to the family Retroviridae. These viruses contain RNA (as opposed to DNA) as their genome and replicate using the enzyme reverse transcriptase. Currently, the most clinically significant retrovirus is HIV. (p. 849)

Reverse transcriptase An RNA-directed DNA polymerase enzyme. Reverse transcriptase promotes the synthesis of a DNA molecule from an RNA molecule, which is the reverse of the usual process. HIV replicates in this manner. (p. 852)

Ribonucleic acid (RNA) A nucleic acid composed of nucleotide units that contain molecules of the sugar ribose, phosphate groups, and purine and pyrimidine bases. RNA molecules transmit genetic information and are found in both the nuclei and cytoplasm of cells. (Compare with *deoxyribonucleic acid [DNA]*.) (p. 848)

Virion A mature virus particle. (p. 847)

Viruses The smallest known class of microorganisms; viruses can replicate only inside host cells. (p. 847)

GENERAL PRINCIPLES OF VIROLOGY

Viruses are tiny microorganisms, usually many times smaller than bacteria. Unlike bacteria, viruses can replicate only inside the cells of their **host**. In this respect, all viruses are obligate intracellular parasites. It must be emphasized that viruses are not cells, per se, but instead are particles that infect and replicate inside cells. A mature virus particle is known as a **virion**. Compared with other organisms, virions have a relatively simple structure that consists of the genome, the capsid, and the envelope. The **genome** is the inner core of the virion and is composed of single- or double-stranded **deoxyribonucleic acid (DNA)** or **ribonucleic acid (RNA)** molecules, but not both.

Viruses are the simplest of all organisms. The cells of more complex organisms have much larger strands of **nucleic acids**, or multiple strands, which make up chromosomes. The viral capsid is a protein coat that surrounds and protects the genome. It also plays a role in the **fusion** between virions and host cells. Fusion occurs when virions attach themselves to host cells in preparation for infecting the cells. The envelope is the outermost layer of the virion and is present in some, but not all, viruses. It has a lipoprotein structure containing viral antigens that are often chemically specific for various proteins on the surface of the host cell membranes. This biochemical specificity, when present, also facilitates the fusion process. The **human immunodeficiency virus (HIV)**, which causes **acquired immune deficiency syndrome (AIDS)**, functions in this manner.

Viruses can enter the body through at least four routes: by inhalation through the respiratory tract, by ingestion via the gastrointestinal (GI) tract, via the placenta from mother to infant, and through inoculation via skin or mucous membranes. Inoculation occurs in several ways, including sexual contact, blood transfusions, sharing of syringes or needles, organ transplants, or bites (including human, animal, insect, spider, and others). Once inside the body, the virus particles, or virions, begin to attach themselves to the outer membranes of host cells (cell membranes or plasma membranes), as illustrated in Figure 45-1.

The viral genome then passes through the plasma membrane into the cytoplasm of the host cell. It later enters the cell nucleus, where the **replication** process begins. The virion may use its own or the host's enzymes (or both) to direct the replication process. In the host cell nucleus, the viral genome uses the cell's genetic material (the nucleic acids RNA and DNA) to synthesize viral nucleic acids and proteins. These are then used to construct complete new virions. These new virions then exit the infected host cell by budding through the plasma membrane and go on to infect other host cells, where the replication process continues. The changes in the cell associated with viral replication are known as the *cytopathic effect* and usually result in the destruction of the host cell. Repeated over time, host cell destruction gives rise to the pathological effects of the virus, which can eventually impair or kill the host organism.

Although this cytopathic effect is the most common outcome, there are other possible outcomes of viral infection. One is viral transformation, which involves mutation of the host cell DNA or RNA and can result in malignant (cancerous) host cells. Viruses that can induce cancer in this way are known as *oncogenic viruses*. More common is latent, or dormant, infection, in which the virions remain inside host cells but do not actively replicate to any significant degree. For example, HIV infection may have a dormant phase of 10 years or more before giving rise to AIDS in an infected person. HIV infection is discussed in greater detail later in this chapter, in the section on retroviruses.

Viruses are widespread in the environment, and most viral infections may not be noticed before they are eliminated by the host's immune system. These are referred to as "silent" viral infections. Although the host's immune

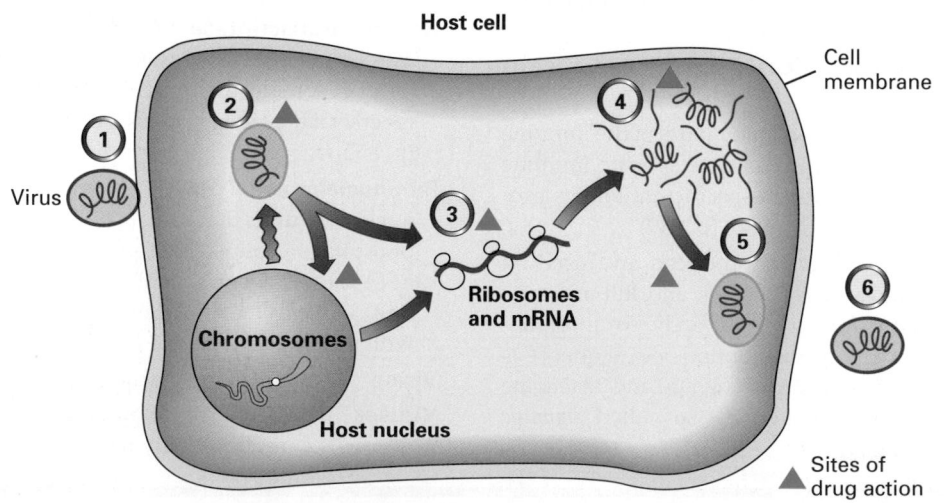

1. Attachment to host cell
2. Uncoating of virus and entry of viral nucleic acid into host cell nucleus
3. Control of DNA, RNA, and protein production
4. Production of viral subunits
5. Assembly of virions
6. Release of virions

FIG. 45-1 Virus replication. Some viruses integrate into host chromosomes and enter a period of latency. *mRNA*, messenger RNA. (Modified from Brody, T. M., Larner, J., & Minneman, K. P. (2010). *Human pharmacology: Molecular to clinical* (5th ed.). St. Louis, MO: Mosby.)

system acts to neutralize viral infection, it can become overwhelmed, depending on how virulent the virus is and how rapidly it replicates inside host cells. In most cases, however, a person's immune system is able to arrest and eliminate the virus. Host immune responses to viral infections are classified as either nonspecific or specific. Nonspecific immune responses include phagocytosis (the process of engulfing and killing) of viral particles by leukocytes such as neutrophils, macrophages, monocytes, and T lymphocytes (T cells). Another nonspecific immune response is the release of cytokines from these leukocytes. Cytokines are biochemical substances (e.g., histamine, tumour necrosis factor) that stimulate other protective immune functions. In addition, these activated immune system cells may also phagocytize infected host cells to curb the growth and spread of infection. These types of immune responses are collectively referred to as *cell-mediated immunity (CMI)*. Cell-mediated immunity is nonspecific in the sense that it does not involve **antibodies** that are specific for a given **antigen**. In contrast, specific immune responses include the production of antibodies from B lymphocytes (B cells). This type of immune response is called *humoral immunity.* Immune system function is discussed in more detail in Chapters 50 and 51.

OVERVIEW OF VIRAL ILLNESSES AND THEIR TREATMENT

There are at least six classes of DNA viruses and at least 14 classes of RNA viruses that are known to infect humans. Some of the more prominent viral illnesses include smallpox (poxviruses), sore throat and conjunctivitis (adenoviruses), warts (papovaviruses), influenza (orthomyxoviruses), respiratory infections (coronaviruses, rhinoviruses), gastroenteritis (rotaviruses, Norwalk-like viruses), HIV/AIDS (retroviruses), herpes (**herpesviruses**), and hepatitis (hepadnaviruses). Effective drug therapy is currently available for only a relatively small number of active viral infections. The drug therapy for hepatitis is discussed further in Chapter 54. HIV belongs to the relatively unique viral class known as **retroviruses** and is discussed in a separate section of this chapter.

Fortunately, many viral illnesses are survivable (e.g., chicken pox), albeit bothersome and uncomfortable. The incidence of some of these illnesses has been reduced by the development of effective vaccines (e.g., vaccines for polio, smallpox, measles, chicken pox). Vaccines are discussed in more detail in Chapter 51. However, many other viral illnesses are either fatal or have much more severe long-term outcomes (e.g., hepatitis, HIV infection).

Antiviral drugs are chemicals that kill or suppress viruses by either destroying virions or inhibiting their ability to replicate. The body's immune system has a better chance of controlling or eliminating a viral infec-

tion when the ability of the virus to replicate itself is suppressed. Drugs that destroy virions include disinfectants and immunoglobulins. Disinfectants such as povidone-iodine (Ovadine®) are virucides and are commonly used to disinfect medical equipment, as well as parts of the body during invasive procedures.

Immunoglobulins are concentrated antibodies that can attack and destroy viruses. They are isolated and pooled from human or animal blood. Their activity may be either nonspecific (e.g., human gamma globulin) or specific (e.g., rabies immunoglobulin, varicella-zoster immunoglobulin). Although such substances can technically be considered antiviral drugs, they are more commonly thought of as immunizing drugs and are therefore discussed in more detail in Chapter 51. A few antiviral drugs, such as interferons, stimulate the body's immune system to kill the virions directly. These drugs are discussed in Chapter 54.

The current antiviral drugs are all synthetic compounds that work indirectly by inhibiting viral replication as opposed to directly destroying mature virions. Relatively few of the known viruses can be controlled by current drug therapy. Some of the viruses in this group are the following:

- Cytomegalovirus (CMV)
- Hepatitis viruses
- Herpes viruses
- HIV
- **Influenza viruses** ("flu" viruses)
- Respiratory syncytial virus (RSV)

Active viral infections are usually more difficult to eradicate than those caused by bacteria. One reason is that viruses replicate only inside host cells rather than independently in the bloodstream or in other tissues. Most antiviral drugs must therefore enter these cells to disrupt viral replication. The need to develop antiviral drugs that are not overly toxic to host cells is one reason that there are relatively few effective antiviral medications on the market. However, the HIV/AIDS pandemic that began in the early 1980s strongly boosted antiviral drug research. This research has increased the number of available antiviral drugs to treat HIV and other viral infections such as influenza, CMV infection, and varicella-zoster virus (VZV) infection. Many drugs for the treatment of HIV are approved by Health Canada via an accelerated process, which means that they are approved faster than other drugs because of the nature of the illness. Because of the rapid addition of HIV drugs to the market, it is beyond the scope of this book to list every available drug.

Another reason viral illnesses are difficult to treat is that the virus has often replicated itself many thousands or possibly millions of times before symptoms of illness appear. Therefore, one goal in the field of infectious disease is to be able to diagnose viral illnesses before an infecting virus has undergone widespread replication in a human host. This would theoretically allow the dual benefit of both early drug therapy and easier elimination of the virus by the host's immune system. This has happened to some degree with HIV infection, with relatively early diagnosis made possible by blood tests to screen for HIV antibodies. Of course, the patient must also be alert to the need to seek medical care before serious illness develops. Recall that for a virus to replicate, virions must first attach themselves to host cell membranes in a process known as *fusion*. Once inside the cell, the viral genome makes nucleic acids and proteins, which are then used to build new viral particles, or virions (see Figure 45-1). All virions contain a genome that consists of either DNA or RNA, but not both. Antiviral drugs inhibit this replication in various ways. Most antiviral drugs enter the same cells that the viruses enter. Once inside, these antiviral drugs interfere with viral nucleic acid synthesis. Other antiviral drugs work by preventing the fusion process.

The best responses to antiviral drug therapy are usually seen in patients with competent immune systems. The immune system can work synergistically with the drug to eliminate or effectively suppress viral activity. Patients who are immunocompromised are at greater risk for **opportunistic infections,** which are infections caused by organisms that would not normally harm an immunocompetent person. The most common examples of immunocompromised patients are patients with cancer, organ transplant recipients, and patients with AIDS. These patients are prone to frequent and often severe opportunistic infections of many types, including those caused by other non-HIV viruses, bacteria, fungi, and protozoans. Such infections often require long-term prophylactic anti-infective drug therapy to control the infection and prevent recurrence because of compromised host immune functions.

Recall that there are two types of nucleic acids found in living organisms: DNA and RNA. There are also five organic bases that are major structural components of these nucleic acids. DNA consists of long chains of deoxyribose sugar molecules, phosphate groups, and purine (adenine or guanine) and pyrimidine (cytosine or thymine) bases. RNA consists of long chains of ribose sugar molecules linked to phosphate groups, together with purine (adenine or guanine) and pyrimidine (cytosine or uracil) bases. A **nucleoside** is a single unit, consisting of a base and its attached sugar molecule. Nucleosides have names similar to their bases, with minor spelling modifications (e.g., adenosine, guanosine, cytidine, thymidine). A **nucleotide** is a nucleoside plus its attached phosphate molecule. Most antiviral drugs are synthetic purine or pyrimidine nucleoside or nucleotide analogues. Some pharmacology texts categorize the antiviral drugs based on their nucleoside–nucleotide activity. However, for ease of learning, this book divides antiviral drugs into those that treat HIV infections and those that treat non-HIV viral infections. **Antiretroviral drugs** are indicated specifically for the treatment of infections caused by HIV, the virus that causes AIDS. The effectiveness of antiviral drugs varies widely among patients and even over time in the same patient.

HERPES SIMPLEX VIRUS AND VARICELLA-ZOSTER VIRUS INFECTIONS

The family of viruses known as Herpesviridae includes those viruses that cause all kinds of herpes infections. There are several specific types of such viruses. Herpes simplex virus type 1 (HSV-1) causes mucocutaneous herpes, usually in the form of perioral blisters ("fever blisters" or "cold sores"). Herpes simplex virus type 2 (HSV-2) causes genital herpes. Human herpesvirus 3 (HHV-3) causes both chicken pox and shingles. This virus is more commonly known as *herpes-zoster virus* or *varicella-zoster virus (VZV)*. Human herpes virus 4 (HHV-4), more frequently known as Epstein-Barr virus (EBV), is associated with illnesses such as infectious mononucleosis ("mono") and chronic fatigue syndrome. Human herpesvirus 5 (HHV-5) is more commonly known as *cytomegalovirus (CMV)* and is the cause of CMV retinitis (a serious viral infection of the eye) and CMV disease, which is most commonly seen in immunocompromised patients. Human herpesviruses 6 and 7 are not clinically significant, and infection with these viruses may be more likely to occur in immunocompromised patients. Human herpesvirus 8, also known as *Kaposi's sarcoma herpesvirus*, is an oncogenic virus believed to cause Kaposi's sarcoma, an AIDS-associated cancer. All of these viruses occur, often asymptomatically, in varying percentages of the population. Types 3 through 7 normally do not cause diseases that require medication, except in the case of immunocompromised patients. However, HSV-1 and HSV-2 and VZV (HHV-3) commonly cause illnesses that are now routinely treated with prescription medications.

Herpes Simplex Viruses

Although there can be anatomical overlap between the two types of herpes simplex virus, HSV-1 is most commonly associated with perioral blisters and is therefore often thought of as *oral herpes*. In contrast, HSV-2 is most commonly associated with blisters on both male and female genitalia and is therefore commonly referred to as *genital herpes*. Although they usually do not cause serious or life-threatening illness, both infections are annoying and highly transmissible through close physical contact (e.g., kissing, sexual intercourse). Outbreaks of painful skin lesions occur intermittently, with periods of latency (no sores or other symptoms) occurring between acute outbreaks. Although antiviral medications are not always required and are *not* curative, they can speed up the process of remission and reduce the duration of painful symptoms. This is particularly true if the medications are started early in an outbreak. Patients may be prescribed an ongoing lower dose of antiviral drug for prophylaxis of outbreaks. HSV infections can become serious, even life threatening, when the patient is immunocompromised or a newborn infant. Neonatal herpes is often a life threatening infection, and babies with this disease are often treated with intravenous (IV) antiviral drugs in neonatal critical care units. However, treatments may fail, causing infant death or permanent disability. Therefore, the best strategy is to prevent transmission to the newborn infant. For this reason, obstetricians will usually recommend delivery by Caesarean section for any mother with active genital herpes lesions.

Varicella-Zoster Virus

Varicella-zoster virus (VZV) is a type of herpesvirus (HHV-3) that most commonly causes chicken pox (varicella) in childhood, remains dormant for many years, and can then re-emerge in later adulthood as painful herpeszoster lesions, known as *shingles*.

Chicken pox is usually an uncomfortable but self-limiting disease of childhood. However, it is highly contagious and easily spreads by either direct contact with weeping lesions or via droplet inhalation. It can also lead to significant scarring. The serious condition *Reye's syndrome* (causing fatty liver damage with encephalopathy) may also complicate varicella, as can other viral infections such as influenza. Herpes zoster is caused by the reactivation of VZV from its dormant state, often decades after a case of childhood chicken pox. It is also referred to simply as *zoster*. Nearly one in three Canadians will develop shingles in their lifetime (Merck, 2012). Its most common manifestation is in the form of skin lesions that follow nerve tracts, known as *dermatomes*, along the skin surface. The most common site of these lesions is around the side of the trunk, although they can appear in other areas (e.g., along the trigeminal nerve dermatomes of the face). Zoster lesions are often extremely painful, and some patients require opioids for pain control and often anti-inflammatory drugs as well. In addition, postherpetic neuralgias (long-term nerve pain) remain following shingles outbreaks in as many as 50% of older adults. Early administration of antiviral drugs such as acyclovir may speed recovery, but this effect is usually not dramatic. Usually, the best results are seen when the antiviral drug is started within 72 hours of symptom onset; however, antivirals do not provide a cure.

Active childhood varicella (chicken pox) infections are usually self-limiting and are not normally treated with antiviral drugs, except in high-risk (e.g., immunocompromised) children. A univalent varicella virus vaccine is now routinely recommended for healthy children between 12 and 18 months of age who have not had chicken pox. A new combined multivalent vaccine (measles-mumps-rubella-varicella [MMRV]) is also available for healthy children aged 12 months to 12 years of age. A new vaccine, Zostavax®, is available for prevention of herpes shingles in patients 50 years of age or older (see Chapter 51).

In a small percentage of shingles cases, skin lesions may progress beyond the usual dermatome regions, and the virus can cause solid organ infections such as pneumonitis, hepatitis, encephalitis, and optic neuritis

(infection of the optic nerve). Such infections are uncommon, with older adults and immunocompromised patients being the most vulnerable. Rarely, these serious infections can be caused by first-time exposure to varicella (chicken pox). In general, these more serious infections require IV antiviral drugs, especially in high-risk patients. IV acyclovir is the most commonly used drug, and it may prevent fatalities or disability. Less serious infections are usually treated orally with acyclovir, valacyclovir, or famciclovir. Topical dosage forms of some of these drugs are also available and are discussed further in Chapter 56. Although VZV reactivation is comparable in pathology to that of HSV (i.e., oral or genital herpes lesions), VZV reactivation occurs much less regularly than HSV because of a lack of reactivation genes. Secondary bacterial infections (e.g., group A *Streptococcus* skin infection) are common with VZV exacerbations, so antibiotics may also be needed. This is especially true in cases of ophthalmic involvement.

ANTIVIRALS (NON-HIV)

The drugs discussed in this section include those used to treat non-HIV viral infections such as those caused by influenza viruses, HSV, VZV, and CMV. There are also antiviral drugs used for hepatitis A, B, and C viruses (HAV, HBV, and HCV). Hepatitis treatment is discussed in further detail in Chapter 54 because it involves some additional unique drug therapy.

Mechanism of Action and Drug Effects

Most of the current antiviral drugs work by blocking the activity of a polymerase enzyme that normally stimulates the synthesis of new viral genomes. The result is impaired viral replication, which results in viral concentrations low enough to allow elimination of the virus by the patient's immune system. If this does not occur, the virus may either enter a dormant state or remain at a low level of replication with continuous drug therapy.

Indications

The antivirals discussed in this section are listed in Table 45-1.

Contraindications

Most of the antiviral drugs used to treat non-HIV viral infections are surprisingly well tolerated. The only usual contraindication for most of these drugs is known severe drug allergy. However, a small number of contraindications are listed for a few of the antiviral drugs. Amantadine is contraindicated in lactating women, children younger than 12 months of age, and patients with an eczematous rash. Famciclovir is contraindicated in cases of allergy to it. Cidofovir has a strong propensity for renal toxicity, and it is contraindicated in patients who already have severely compromised renal function as well as those receiving concurrent drug therapy with other highly nephrotoxic drugs. It is also contraindicated in cases of allergy to probenecid because probenecid is recommended as concurrent drug therapy with cidofovir to help alleviate its nephrotoxicity. Ribavirin has additional specific contraindications besides drug allergy. Because of the drug's teratogenic potential, it is contraindicated in pregnant women as well as their male sexual partners. The aerosol form must not be used by pregnant women or by women who may become pregnant during exposure to the drug. This includes health care providers administering the drug in aerosol form because of the potential for second-hand inhalation by the health care provider.

Adverse Effects

The adverse effects of the antiviral drugs are as different as the drugs themselves. Each has its own specific adverse effect profile. Because viruses reproduce in human cells, selective killing is difficult, and consequently many healthy human cells, in addition to virally infected cells, may be killed in the process, resulting in more serious toxicities for these drugs. However, this effect is usually not as pronounced as in cancer chemotherapy, which often kills many more healthy cells. The more serious adverse effects are listed by drug in Table 45-2.

Interactions

Significant drug interactions that occur with the antiviral drugs arise most often when they are administered via systemic routes, such as intravenously and orally. Many of these drugs are also applied topically to the eye or body, however, and the incidence of drug interactions associated with these routes of administration is much lower. Selected common drug interactions for both antiviral and antiretroviral drugs are listed in Table 45-3.

Dosages

For dosage information on some of the commonly used nonretroviral antiviral drugs, refer to the table on p. 855.

HIV INFECTION AND AIDS

The retrovirus family got its name upon discovery of a unique feature of its replication process. Retroviruses are all RNA viruses and are unique in their use of the enzyme **reverse transcriptase** during their replication process. This enzyme promotes the synthesis of complementary (mirror image) DNA molecules from the viral RNA genome. A second enzyme, integrase, promotes the integration of this viral DNA into the host cell DNA. This hybrid DNA complex is known as a *provirus*. It produces new viral RNA genomes and proteins, which in turn combine to make mature HIV virions that infect other host cells. Another important enzyme is **protease**, which serves to chemically separate the new viral RNA from

---

TABLE   45-1

Examples of Antiviral Drugs (Non-HIV)

Drug	Indications
DRUGS TO TREAT HERPESVIRUSES	
acyclovir, famciclovir, valacyclovir hydrochloride	Herpes simplex types 1 and 2, herpes zoster, chicken pox
trifluridine	Herpes simplex keratitis
DRUGS TO TREAT INFLUENZA VIRUSES	
amantadine hydrochloride	Influenza A
zanamivir, oseltamivir phosphate	Influenza A and B
MISCELLANEOUS ANTIVIRALS	
ribavirin	Respiratory syncytial virus (RSV) infection
ganciclovir, valganciclovir, cidofovir, foscarnet sodium (available through Special Access Programme, Health Canada)	Cytomegalovirus infection, acyclovir-resistant herpes simplex infections

---

TABLE   45-2

Selected Antiviral Drugs: Adverse Effects

Antiviral Drug	Adverse Effects
abacavir	High risk for sensitivity reaction in patients who carry HLA-B*5701 allele
acyclovir	Nausea, vomiting, diarrhea, headache, burning when topically applied
amantadine hydrochloride	Insomnia, nervousness, lightheadedness, anorexia, nausea, anticholinergic effects, orthostatic hypotension, blurred vision
didanosine	Pancreatitis, peripheral neuropathies, seizures
foscarnet sodium (available through Special Access Programme, Health Canada)	Headache, seizures, electrolyte disturbances, acute kidney injury, bone marrow suppression, nausea, vomiting, diarrhea
ganciclovir	Bone marrow toxicity, nausea, vomiting, headache, seizures
indinavir sulphate	Nausea; abdominal, back, or flank pain; headache; diarrhea; vomiting; weakness; taste changes; acid regurgitation; nephrolithiasis
nevirapine	Rash, fever, nausea, headache, elevation in liver enzyme levels
ribavirin	Rash, conjunctivitis, anemia, mild bronchospasm
trifluridine	Ophthalmic effects: burning, swelling, stinging, photophobia, pain
zidovudine	Bone marrow suppression, nausea, headache

TABLE	45-3

Selected Antiviral Drugs: Interactions

Drug	Interacting Drugs	Interaction
NON-HIV DRUGS		
acyclovir	interferon	Additive antiviral effects
	probenecid	Increased acyclovir levels due to decreasing renal clearance
	zidovudine	Increased risk for neurotoxicity
amantadine hydrochloride	Anticholinergic drugs	Increased adverse anticholinergic effects
	CNS stimulants	Additive CNS stimulant effects
ganciclovir	foscarnet	Additive or synergistic effect against CMV and HSV-2
	imipenem	Increased risk for seizures
	zidovudine	Increased risk for hematological toxicity (i.e., bone marrow suppression)
ribavirin	Nucleoside reverse transcriptase inhibitors	Increased risk for hepatotoxicity and lactic acidosis
HIV DRUGS		
indinavir sulphate	Drugs metabolized by the CYP3A4 hepatic microsomal enzyme system (azole antifungals, clarithromycin, doxycycline, erythromycin, isoniazid, protease inhibitors, quinidine sulphate, statins, and verapamil hydrochloride)	Competition for metabolism resulting in elevated blood levels and potential toxicity
	rifabutin and ketoconazole	Increased plasma concentrations of rifabutin and ketoconazole
	rifampin	Increased metabolism of indinavir sulphate
nevirapine	Drugs metabolized by the CYP3A4 hepatic microsomal enzyme system (see indinavir sulphate)	Increased metabolism of these drugs
	Oral contraceptives	Decreased plasma concentrations of oral contraceptives
	Protease inhibitors	Decreased plasma concentrations of protease inhibitors
	rifampin and rifabutin	Decreased nevirapine serum concentration
tenofovir disoproxil fumarate	acyclovir, ganciclovir, valacyclovir	May increase serum concentrations of tenofovir disoproxil fumarate
	Protease inhibitors	Increased serum concentrations of tenofovir disoproxil fumarate
maraviroc	CYP3A4 inhibitors (see indinavir)	May increase maraviroc toxicity
	CYP3A4 inducers (phenytoin, carbamazepine, rifampin)	May decrease effects of maraviroc
	St. John's wort	May decrease effects of maraviroc
raltegravir	atazanavir sulphate (with or without ritonavir)	May increase effects of raltegravir
	rifampin	May decrease effects of raltegravir
zidovudine	acyclovir	Increased neurotoxicity
	interferon beta	Increased serum levels of zidovudine
	Cytotoxic drugs	Increased risk for hematologic toxicity
	didanosine	Additive or synergistic effect against HIV
	ganciclovir and ribavirin	Antagonized antiviral action of zidovudine

CMV, cytomegalovirus; *CNS*, central nervous system; *CYP3A4*, cytochrome P450 enzyme 3A4; *HIV*, human immunodeficiency virus; *HSV-2*, herpes simplex virus, type 2.

viral protein molecules. These components are initially synthesized into one large macromolecular strand, and the protease enzyme carefully breaks up this strand into its key components. Figure 45-2 illustrates the major structural features of the HIV virion, and Figure 45-3 illustrates the steps in its replication process.

Reverse transcriptase is not normally found in host cells; both reverse transcriptase and integrase are carried by the virus. "Reversal" of the usual replication processes led to the name *reverse transcriptase* for this enzyme and also to the name *retrovirus* for this family of viruses. Furthermore, the fact that retroviruses

DRUG PROFILES

amantadine hydrochloride

Amantadine hydrochloride (Dom-Amantidine®), one of the earliest antiviral drugs, has a narrow antiviral spectrum in that it is active only against influenza A viruses. It has been used both prophylactically and therapeutically. However, the most recent guidelines of the Association of Medical Microbiology and Infectious Disease (AMMI) Canada do not recommend the use of amantadine to prevent or treat influenza. The recommendations on the use of amantadine change yearly, based on the type of influenza that is prevalent. The reader is referred to the AMMI for the latest recommendations.

PHARMACOKINETICS

Route	Onset of Action	Peak Plasma Concentration	Elimination Half-Life	Duration of Action
PO	Within 48 hr	1–4 hr	17 hr	12–24 hr

▶▶ acyclovir

Acyclovir (Zovirax) is a synthetic nucleoside analogue that is used mainly to suppress the replication of HSV-1, HSV-2, and VZV. Acyclovir is considered the drug of choice for the treatment of both initial and recurrent episodes of these viral infections.

Acyclovir is available in oral, topical, and injectable formulations. Its topical use is discussed in Chapter 56. Other similar antiviral drugs include valacyclovir hydrochloride and famciclovir. However, these latter two drugs are currently available only for oral use and are indicated for the treatment of less serious infections. Note the slight inconsistencies in the spelling of these drug names. Valacyclovir is a prodrug that is metabolized to acyclovir in the body. It has the advantage of greater oral bioavailability and less frequent dosing (three times daily versus five times daily for acyclovir). It may also provide more effective relief of pain from zoster lesions.

PHARMACOKINETICS (ACYCLOVIR)

Route	Onset of Action	Peak Plasma Concentration	Elimination Half-Life	Duration of Action
PO	1.5–2 hr	1.5–2 hr	2–3 hr	10–15 hr
IV	Variable	1 hr	3 hr	8 hr

▶▶ ganciclovir hydrochloride

Like acyclovir, ganciclovir hydrochloride (Cytovene®, Valcyte®) is a synthetic nucleoside analogue of guanosine, but with a much different spectrum of antiviral activity. It is indicated for the treatment of infections caused by CMV. CMV is carried by up to 50% of the adult population and normally causes no harm. However, in immunocompromised patients (including premature infants), it can cause life-threatening or disabling opportunistic infections. Valganciclovir hydrochloride (Valcyte), foscarnet (Foscavir®), and cidofovir (Vistide®) are three other antiviral drugs that are used in the treatment of CMV infection. Of these three antiviral drugs, ganciclovir is the one most often used for this purpose. A common site of CMV infections in the immunocompromised patient is the eye, and it can result in CMV retinitis, a devastating viral infection that can lead to blindness. Ganciclovir is most commonly administered intravenously or orally. It is also administered to prevent CMV disease (generalized infection) in high-risk patients, such as those receiving organ transplants.

The dose-limiting toxicity of ganciclovir treatment is bone marrow suppression, whereas that of foscarnet and cidofovir is kidney toxicity. These toxicities must be kept in mind when deciding which drug is more appropriate in a particular patient. For example, a heart transplant recipient who contracts CMV retinitis is immunocompromised because of immunosuppressant drug therapy and is presumably taking cyclosporine, a nephrotoxic drug. Therefore, using foscarnet in this patient may be more dangerous than using ganciclovir. On the other hand, a patient who contracts a CMV infection and is immunocompromised because of a bone marrow transplant might be better treated using foscarnet.

Valganciclovir, a prodrug of ganciclovir formulated for oral use, is metabolized to ganciclovir in the body. As in the case described previously for valacyclovir hydrochloride and acyclovir, the prodrug provides greater oral bioavailability and allows less frequent daily dosing. Cidofovir and foscarnet are available only in injectable form.

PHARMACOKINETICS

Route	Onset of Action	Peak Plasma Concentration	Elimination Half-Life	Duration of Action
PO	Unknown	24 hr	4.8 hr	Variable

oseltamivir phosphate and zanamivir

Oseltamivir phosphate (Tamiflu®) and zanamivir (Relenza®) belong to one of the newest classes of antiviral drugs known as *neuraminidase inhibitors*. Both drugs are active against influenza virus types A and B. They are indicated for the treatment of uncomplicated acute illness caused by influenza infection in adults. They have been shown to reduce the duration of influenza infection by several days. The neuraminidase enzyme enables budding virions to escape from infected cells and spread throughout the body. Neuraminidase inhibitors are designed to stop this process in the body, speeding recovery from infection.

The most commonly reported adverse events with oseltamivir are nausea and vomiting; those with zanamivir are diarrhea, nausea, and sinusitis. Oseltamivir is available only for oral use. The drug is indicated for both prophylaxis and treatment of influenza infection. Zanamivir is available in blister packets of 5 mg of dry powder for inhalation. It is currently indicated only for treatment of active influenza illness. Treatment with oseltamivir and zanamivir needs to begin within 2 days of symptom onset.

PHARMACOKINETICS (OSELTAMIVIR)

Route	Onset of Action	Peak Plasma Concentration	Elimination Half-Life	Duration of Action
PO	Unknown	1–2 hr	1–3 hr	5–15 hr

DRUG PROFILES—cont'd

PHARMACOKINETICS (ZANAMIVIR)

Route	Onset of Action	Peak Plasma Concentration	Elimination Half-Life	Duration of Action
PO	Unknown	1–2 hr	2–5 hr	10–24 hr

ribavirin

Ribavirin (Virazole®) is a synthetic nucleoside analogue of guanosine, as are many of the other antiviral drugs, but it has a spectrum of antiviral activity that is broader than that of other currently available antiviral drugs. Ribavirin interferes with both RNA and DNA synthesis and as a result inhibits both protein synthesis and viral replication overall.

The inhalational form (Virazole) is used primarily in the treatment of hospitalized infants with severe lower respiratory tract infections caused by respiratory syncytial virus (RSV). This drug was first available only in inhalational form. More recently, oral dosage forms have become available for use in the treatment of hepatitis C; these are discussed in Chapter 54.

PHARMACOKINETICS

Route	Onset of Action	Peak Plasma Concentration	Elimination Half-Life	Duration of Action
Inhalation	Unknown	End of inhalation	1.4–2.5 hr	Variable
PO	Unknown	2–3 hr	120–170 hr	Unknown

DOSAGES   Antiviral Drugs (Non-HIV)

Drug	Usual Dosage Range	Indications
▸▸acyclovir (Zorvirax)	*Children 12 yr and under* IV: 250–500 mg/m² q8h × 7 days *Adolescents 12 yr and older/Adults* IV: 5 mg/kg q8h × 7 days *Children/Adults* PO: 200–800 mg q4h 5×/day × 7–10 days *Children/Adults* PO: 20 mg/kg (max 800 mg/dose) qid × 5 days	HSV-1 and HSV-2, including genital herpes, mucocutaneous herpes, and herpes encephalitis; herpes zoster (shingles); higher dose therapy for acute episodes; lower dose therapy for viral suppression Chicken pox (varicella)
amantadine hydrochloride (Dom-Amantidine)	*Children 9–12 yr/Adults* PO: 100 mg bid *Adults* PO: 200 mg divided once or twice daily	Influenza A virus
▸▸ganciclovir hydrochloride (Cytovene, Valcyte)	*Adults* IV: 5 mg/kg q12h × 2–3 wk PO: 900 mg once daily–bid with food	CMV retinitis; CMV prevention
oseltamivir phosphate (Tamiflu)	*Children 1–12 yr* PO: 30–75 mg bid *Adolescents 13 yr or over 40 kg/Adults* PO: 75 mg bid × 5 days	Influenza A or B
ribavirin (Virazole)	*Children* Aerosol: 6 g reconstituted to 20 mg/mL via continuous aerosol × 12 hr/day × 3–7 days	Severe RSV infection in hospitalized infants and toddlers
zanamivir (Relenza)	*Children 7 yr and older/Adults* Inhalation*: 10 mg (2 × 5-mg powder doses) bid; first day's doses must be at least 2 hr apart and q12h thereafter	Influenza A or B

*Use bronchodilator inhaler first if applicable.
HIV, human immunodeficiency virus; *HSV-1, HSV-2*, herpes simplex virus types 1 and 2; *IV*, intravenous; *PO*, oral; *RSV*, respiratory syncytial virus.

synthesize DNA from viral RNA molecules is also a reversal of the norm because in most other organisms, RNA molecules are synthesized from DNA molecules as part of the reproductive process. Reverse transcriptase has a high rate of errors when stringing together the purine and pyrimidine bases during transcription of the viral RNA genome into a DNA molecule in the replication process. This high rate of errors allows for more frequent genetic mutations among HIV virions and often results in viral strains that are resistant to both medications and the patient's immune system. Such mutations also hamper the development of an effective vaccine against the virus. Drugs used to treat HIV are called *antiretrovirals*.

The most common routes of transmission of HIV are sexual activity, IV drug use, and perinatal transfer from mother to child. Sexual intercourse, primarily receptive anal and vaginal intercourse, is the most common means of infection. Probability of transmission risk increases after seroconversion and if the partner is in the advanced disease stage (has a high viral load). According to the most recent data (World Health Organization, 2014), 36.9 million people worldwide are infected with HIV. Transmission was most common in homosexual or bisexual men, followed by high-risk heterosexual intercourse and IV drug use. Of the 71 300 Canadians living with HIV, 50% are men who have sex with men; 25% are women; and 12% are within the Indigenous population (Canadian Aids Treatment Information Exchange, 2015). Although HIV can be isolated from almost any bodily fluid, including tears, sweat, saliva, and urine, its concentrations in these fluids are much lower than those in blood and genital secretions. In approximately 6% of cases, specific risk factors cannot be determined. The risk of transmission to health care providers from percutaneous (needlestick) injuries is currently calculated at approximately 0.3%. Performing hand hygiene and maintaining standard precautions/routine practices to avoid contact with all body fluids during patient care dramatically reduces the risk of caregiver infection (see Box 10-1).

The rate of new infections is rising more rapidly in minority populations than in other groups, especially among Black and Indigenous people. Patients in developing countries often lack access to adequate drug therapy. Untreated HIV-infected pregnant women transmit the virus to their infants in 15 to 30% of pregnancies. This can occur transplacentally—causing infection in utero—or during birth. When the first antiretroviral drugs were developed in the 1980s, it was feared that they would be too toxic and teratogenic if given to pregnant women. However, prophylactic antiretroviral treatment of infected mothers has been shown to reduce infant infection by at least two thirds and is not normally harmful to either mother or infant. Medication may also be given prophylactically to the newborn infant, typically for the first 6 weeks of life. Infants and children with

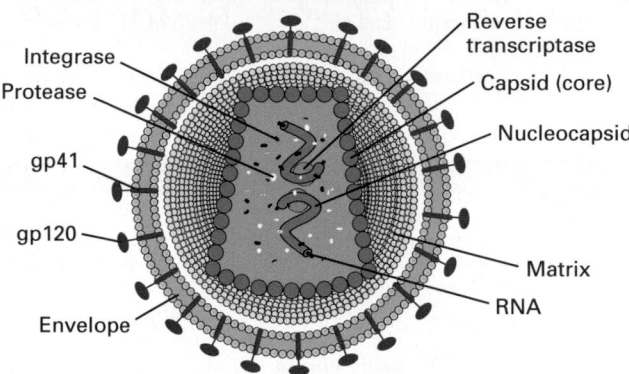

FIG. 45-2 HIV. Within the core capsid, the diploid, single-stranded, positive-sense RNA is complexed to nucleoprotein. *gp*, glycoprotein. (From Newman, W.A. (2012). *Dorland's illustrated medical dictionary* (32nd ed.). Philadelphia: Saunders.)

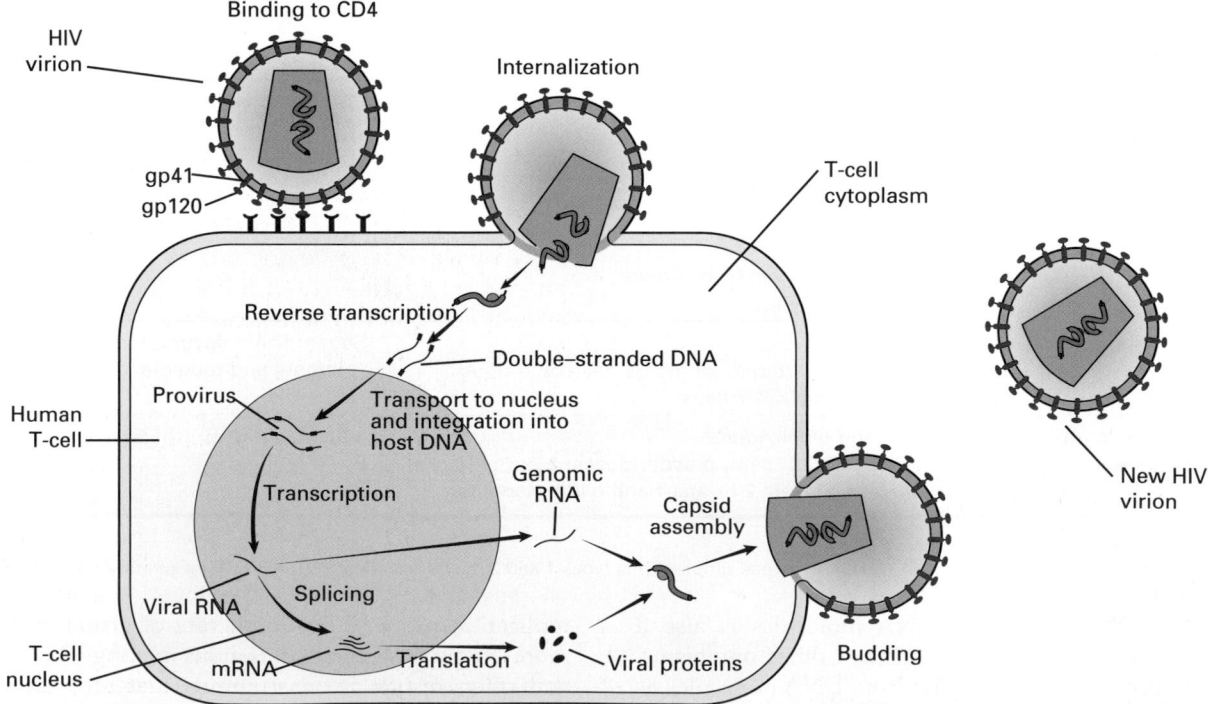

FIG. 45-3 Life cycle of the HIV virus. The extracellular envelope protein gp120 binds to CD4 on the surface of T lymphocytes or mononuclear phagocytes, while the transmembrane protein glycoprotein gp41 mediates the fusion of the viral envelope with the cell membrane. *gp*, glycoprotein; *mRNA*, messenger RNA. (From Newman, W.A. (2012). *Dorland's illustrated medical dictionary* (32nd ed.). Philadelphia: Saunders.)

established HIV infection must usually continue taking medication drugs indefinitely. Breast milk can transmit the virus to the infant in 10 to 20% of cases, and breastfeeding is contraindicated in developed countries. In those countries, however, breastfeeding may be the only available source of nutrition for the infant.

HIV infection that is untreated or treatment resistant eventually leads to immune system failure, with death occurring secondary to opportunistic infections. AIDS often progresses over a period of several years. Various health organizations, including the BC Centre for Disease Control and the World Health Organization (WHO), have published classification systems describing the various stages of this infection. The WHO system for adults sorts patients into one of four hierarchical clinical stages, ranging from stage 1 (asymptomatic) to stage 4 (AIDS).

Patients in stage 1 are asymptomatic or have persistent generalized lymphadenopathy (lymphadenopathy of at least two sites outside the inguinal for longer than 6 months). Stage 2 (mildly symptomatic stage) involves continued lymphadenopathy along with other symptoms, including fever, rash, night sweats, unexplained weight loss of less than 10% of total body weight and recurrent respiratory infections (such as sinusitis, bronchitis, otitis media, and pharyngitis), as well as a range of dermatological conditions. Stage 3 (moderately symptomatic stage) involves disease progression with the appearance of additional clinical manifestations, such as weight loss of greater than 10% of total body weight, prolonged (more than 1 month) unexplained diarrhea, and the development of opportunistic infections. Stage 4 (the severely symptomatic stage) includes AIDS-defining illnesses such as *Mycobacterium avium* complex infection and *Pneumocystis jirovecii* pneumonia.

Figure 45-4 illustrates events that roughly correlate with these four stages of HIV infection. This figure shows

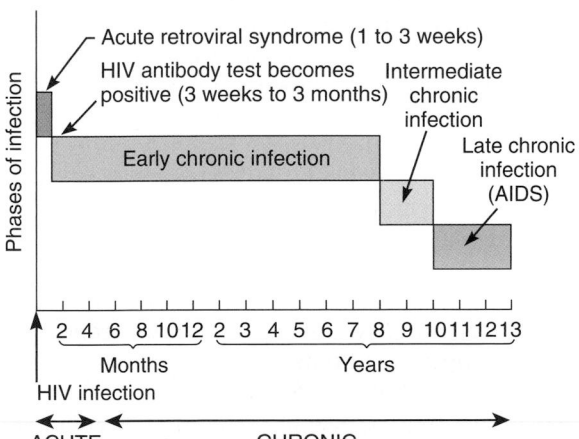

FIG. 45-4 Timeline for the spectrum of untreated HIV infection. The timeline represents the course of untreated illness from the time of infection to clinical manifestations of disease. (From Lewis, S. L., Dirksen, S. R., Heitkemper, M. M., et al. (2014). *Medical-surgical nursing: assessment and management of clinical problems* (9th ed.). Philadelphia: Elsevier.)

the hypothetical natural course of the disease through the stages in patients *without* treatment. Patients who are effectively treated with drug therapy usually do not progress through all of these stages, or at least such progression is slowed considerably (by years). In fact, treatment advances in antiretroviral drug therapy mean that HIV is now a chronic, manageable disease, and an individual who begins treatment today would live to the age of 70 or above (British Columbia Centre for Excellence in HIV/AIDS, 2013). *Antiretroviral therapy (ART)* refers to a combination of at least three antiretroviral drugs that provide maximal suppression of HIV and stop the progression of AIDS. ART is normally started immediately upon confirmation of HIV infection. Opportunistic infections are treated with infection-specific antimicrobial drugs (see corresponding chapters) as they arise. Prophylactic treatment for opportunistic infections is also common and is most frequently given when a patient's CD4+ count falls below 200 cells/mm^3. Opportunistic malignancies, such as Kaposi's sarcoma and lymphomas, are also treated with specific antineoplastic medications, which are discussed in Chapters 52 and 53, as well as with radiation and surgery, as indicated.

Research attempts to develop an effective anti-HIV vaccine are also underway throughout the world. Human clinical trials have been conducted since 1990, primarily in research volunteers who are not infected with HIV. However, vaccines are also being studied in patients who are HIV positive. Despite encouraging data regarding potential benefits, the design of an effective HIV vaccine continues to remain elusive.

DRUGS USED TO TREAT HIV INFECTION

Much has happened in medical science since HIV was first identified in the early 1980s. The increasing urgency and public awareness of the AIDS pandemic have stimulated much research in the fields of immunology and pharmacology. This wealth of research has resulted in the development of several increasingly effective antiretroviral drugs, as well as of antiviral drugs in general. Although new drug combinations have prolonged lives, these medications often carry significant toxicities. There are currently five classes of antiretroviral drugs: the reverse transcriptase inhibitors, the protease inhibitors, the fusion inhibitors, and the newest classes—the entry inhibitor–CCR5 co-receptor antagonists and the HIV integrase strand transfer inhibitors. There are currently two subclasses of reverse transcriptase inhibitors: nucleoside reverse transcriptase inhibitors (NRTIs) and the non-nucleoside reverse transcriptase inhibitors (NNRTIs). Drugs from many of these drug classes are combined together into a single drug dosage form for ease of use. Table 45-4 lists these drugs and their respective classes. In 2014, Health Canada approved Truvada® for the prevention of HIV in high-risk patients. HIV drug therapy

TABLE 45-4

Examples of Antiretrovirals Used to Treat HIV

Generic Name	Trade Name
NUCLEOSIDE REVERSE TRANSCRIPTASE INHIBITORS	
abacavir sulphate	Ziagen®
abacavir sulphate/lamivudine	Kivexa®
didanosine (enteric coated)	Videx EC®
emtricitabine	Emtriva®
lamivudine	3 TC®, Heptovir®
stavudine	Zerit®
tenofovir disoproxil fumarate	Viread®
tenofovir disoproxil fumarate/ emtricitabine	Truvada®
zidovudine	Retrovir®
NON-NUCLEOSIDE REVERSE TRANSCRIPTASE INHIBITORS	
delavirdine mesylate	Rescriptor®
efavirenz	Sustiva®
etravirine	Intelence®
nevirapine	Viramune®, Viramune XR®
PROTEASE INHIBITORS	
atazanavir sulphate	Reyataz®
darunavir ethanolate	Prezista®
fosamprenavir calcium	Telzir®
indinavir sulphate	Crixivan®
nelfinavir mesylate	Viracept®
ritonavir	Norvir®, Norvir Sec®
saquinavir mesylate	Invirase®
tipranavir	Aptivus®
FUSION INHIBITOR	
enfuvirtide	Fuzeon®
ENTRY INHIBITOR–CCR5 CO-RECEPTOR ANTAGONIST (ALSO KNOWN AS CCR5 ANTAGONIST)	
maraviroc	Celsentri®
HIV INTEGRASE STRAND TRANSFER INHIBITOR (ALSO KNOWN AS INTEGRASE INHIBITOR)	
raltegravir potassium	Isentress®
MULTICLASS COMBINATION PRODUCTS	
efavirenz/emtricitabine/tenofovir fumarate	Atripla®
abacavir/dolutegravir/lamivudine	Triumeq®
abacavir/lamivudine/zidovudine	Trizivir®
emtricitabine/rilpivirine hydrochloride/tenofovir disoproxil fumarate	Complera®
lamivudine/zidovudine	Combivir®
lopinavir/ritonavir	Kaletra®

CCR5, chemokine receptor 5; *HIV*, human immunodeficiency virus.

is rapidly changing. The reader is referred to various websites, including the Community AIDS Treatment Information Exchange, for updated information.

Mechanism of Action and Drug Effects

Although HIV/AIDS is a complex illness, the mechanisms of action of the drug classes are straightforward and distinct. The name of each drug class provides a reminder of its role in suppressing the viral replication process. For example, reverse transcriptase inhibitors act by blocking activity of the enzyme reverse transcriptase. Reverse transcriptase promotes the synthesis of new viral DNA molecules from the RNA genome. The protease inhibitors act by inhibiting the protease retroviral enzyme. This enzyme promotes the breakup of chains of protein molecules at designated points, a process necessary for viral replication. There is also one combination protease inhibitor that includes both lopinavir and ritonavir (Kaletra®). Both medications are protease inhibitors. The ritonavir component also serves to inhibit cytochrome P450–mediated enzymatic metabolism of the lopinavir component. There is currently one fusion inhibitor, enfuvirtide. This compound works by inhibiting viral fusion. This is the process by which an HIV virion attaches to (fuses with) the membrane of a host cell (T lymphocyte) before infecting it, in preparation for viral replication. The entry inhibitor–CCR5 co-receptor antagonists, or CCR5 antagonists, work by selectively and reversibly binding to the type 5 chemokine co-receptors located on the CD4 cells that are used by the HIV virion to gain entry to the cells. The integrase strand transfer inhibitors, also referred to as *integrase inhibitors*, work by inhibiting the catalytic activity of the enzyme integrase, thus preventing integration of the proviral gene into human DNA.

Single-drug therapy was most common in the early years of the HIV pandemic, partly because of a lack of treatment options. However, both the development of multiple antiretroviral drugs and the emergence of resistant viral strains have given rise to combination drug therapy as the current standard of care for ART and is the most effective treatment to date. ART usually includes at least three medications. The most commonly recommended drug combinations include two or three NRTIs; two NRTIs plus one or two protease inhibitors; or one NRTI plus one NNRTI, with one or two protease inhibitors. Despite the effectiveness of ART, health care providers may still need to alter a patient's drug regimen in cases of major drug intolerance (see Adverse Effects) or drug resistance. A patient's HIV strain can still evolve and mutate over time, which allows it to become resistant to any drug therapy, especially when that therapy is used for a prolonged period of time. Evidence of drug resistance includes a falling CD4+ count and increased viral load in a patient in whom a given drug regimen previously kept those symptoms under control.

All antiretroviral drugs have similar therapeutic effects in that they reduce the viral load. A viral load of less than 50 copies/mL is considered an undetectable viral load and is a primary goal of ART. HIV-infected patients need to be followed by health care providers with extensive training and specialization in drug therapy for infectious diseases. These health care providers must often make careful choices and changes in drug therapy over time, based on a patient's clinical response and the

TABLE 45-5			
Recommendation for Occupational HIV Exposure Chemoprophylaxis			
Type of Exposure	**Source**	**Prophylaxis**	**Therapy**
Percutaneous	Blood	Recommended	zidovudine + lamivudine + indinavir sulfate OR zidovudine + lamivudine ± indinavir sulfate
	Fluid containing visible blood or other potentially infectious fluid or tissue		
Mucous membrane	Blood	Offer	zidovudine + lamivudine
	Fluid containing visible blood or other potentially infectious fluid or tissue	Offer	zidovudine + lamivudine ± indinavir
		Offer	zidovudine ± lamivudine
Skin (i.e., prolonged contact, extensive area, area without skin integrity)	Blood	Offer	zidovudine + lamivudine ± indinavir sulfate

severity of any drug-related toxicities. When effective, treatment leads to a significant reduction in mortality and incidence of opportunistic infections, improves patients' physical performance, and significantly increases T-cell counts.

Indications

The only usual indication for all of the current antiretroviral drugs is active HIV infection. Prophylactic therapy is also administered as per agency protocol to individuals such as health care providers (e.g., via needle-stick injuries in hospitals) and high-risk infants with a known potential exposure to HIV (Table 45-5).

Contraindications

Because of the potentially fatal outcome of HIV infection, the only usual contraindication to a medication is known severe drug allergy or other intolerable toxicity. Most of the current antiretroviral drug classes have several alternative drugs to choose from if a patient is especially intolerant of a particular drug.

Adverse Effects

Common adverse effects of selected antiretroviral drugs are listed in Table 45-2. The need to modify drug therapy because of adverse effects is not uncommon. The goal is to find the regimen that will best control infection and that has as tolerable an adverse effect profile as possible. Different patients vary widely in their drug tolerance, and their drug tolerance may change over time. Thus, medication regimens often must be strategically individualized and evolve with the course of the patient's illness.

Approximately 20% of patients infected with HIV in Canada are also infected with hepatitis C virus (HCV), which tends to cause more severe disease in patients with HIV. Hepatitis C is the most important cause of chronic liver disease in Canada and is the most common reason for liver transplantation. Unfortunately, ART is strongly correlated with increased mortality from HCV-induced liver disease because the anti-HIV drugs produce strain on the liver, as these drugs are metabolized via the liver.

A major adverse effect of protease inhibitors is lipid abnormalities, including lipodystrophy, or redistribution of fat stores under the skin. This condition often results in cosmetically undesirable outcomes for the patient, such as a "hump" at the posterior base of the neck and also a skeletonized (bony) appearance of the face. In addition, dyslipidemias such as hypertriglyceridemia can occur, and insulin resistance and type 2 diabetes can result. It is reported that in these cases, switching a patient from a protease inhibitor to an NNRTI may help to reduce such symptoms without reducing antiretroviral efficacy.

The increase in long-term antiretroviral drug therapy because of prolonged disease survival has led to the emergence of another long-term adverse effect associated with these medication—bone demineralization and possible osteoporosis. When this condition occurs, it may require treatment with standard medications for osteoporosis, such as calcium, vitamin D, and bisphosphonates (see Chapter 35).

Interactions

Common selected drug interactions involving both antiretrovirals and other antivirals are listed in Table 45-3.

Dosages

Because of rapidly changing antiviral drug therapy and the complexity of dosing and the disease state, only selected dosages are listed in this book (refer to the Dosages table on p. 861). Refer to an up-to-date drug information handbook for specifics on dosing.

OTHER VIRAL ILLNESSES

There are numerous other viral infections; however, four of recent significance are avian influenza, West Nile virus

DRUG PROFILES

enfuvirtide

Enfuvirtide (Fuzeon) is the only medication in one of the newest classes of antiretroviral drugs called *fusion inhibitors*. It acts by suppressing the fusion process whereby a virion is attached to the outer membrane of a host T cell before entry into the cell and subsequent viral replication. This mechanism of action serves as yet another example of how antiretroviral drugs are strategically designed to interfere with specific steps of the viral replication process. The use of combinations of drugs that work by different mechanisms improves a patient's chances for continued survival by reducing the likelihood of viral resistance to the drug therapy regimen. Enfuvirtide is indicated for treatment of HIV infection in combination with other antiretroviral drugs. Adults and children have shown comparable tolerance of the drug in clinical trials thus far. Use of this drug in combination with other standard antiretroviral drugs has been associated with markedly reduced viral loads compared with drug regimens that did not include this drug. The drug is currently available only in injectable form.

PHARMACOKINETICS

Route	Onset of Action	Peak Plasma Concentration	Elimination Half-Life	Duration of Action
Subcut	Unknown	4–8 hr	4 hr	Unknown

▶indinavir sulphate

Indinavir sulphate (Crixivan) belongs to the protease inhibitor class of antiretroviral drugs. Others in this class include ritonavir (Norvir, Norvir Sec), saquinavir mesylate (Invirase), nelfinavir mesylate (Viracept), atazanavir sulphate (Reyataz), fosamprenavir calcium (Telzir), darunavir ethanolate (Prezista), tipranavir (Aptivus), and the combination product lopinavir/ritonavir (Kaletra®). Indinavir can be taken in combination with other anti-HIV therapies or alone. It is best dissolved and absorbed in an acidic gastric environment, and the presence of high-protein and high-fat foods reduces its absorption. Therefore, it is recommended that indinavir be administered in a fasting state. Indinavir therapy produces increases in CD4+ cell counts and significant reductions in viral load. Protease inhibitors are commonly given in combination with two reverse transcriptase inhibitors to maximize efficacy and decrease the likelihood of viral drug resistance. Indinavir is relatively well tolerated in most patients. Nephrolithiasis (kidney stones) occur in approximately 4% of patients. Patients who take indinavir are encouraged to drink at least 1.5 L of liquids every day to maintain hydration and help avoid nephrolithiasis. Indinavir and all other protease inhibitors are available only for oral use.

PHARMACOKINETICS

Route	Onset of Action	Peak Plasma Concentration	Elimination Half-Life	Duration of Action
PO	2 wk to therapeutic effect	0.5–1 hr	1.5–2.5 hr	6 mo

▶▶maraviroc

Maraviroc (Celesentri) is the only drug available in a new class of antiretrovirals called *CCR5 antagonists*. Maraviroc works by selectively and reversibly binding to the chemokine co-receptors located on the CD4 cells. It is used in treatment-experienced patients with evidence of viral replication and HIV-1 strains that are resistant to multiple antiretroviral therapies. It is used in combination with other antiretroviral drugs. Hepatotoxicity with allergic-type features has been reported. Drug interactions of significance include interactions with cytochrome P450 3A4 (CYP3A4) inhibitors (azole antifungals, clarithromycin, doxycycline, erythromycin, isoniazid, nefazodone, protease inhibitors, quinidine sulphate, and verapamil hydrochloride), which may increase maraviroc toxicity. CYP3A4 inducers, including phenytoin, carbamazepine, nafcillin, and rifampin, may decrease maraviroc's effects. Maraviroc is available only for oral use.

PHARMACOKINETICS

Route	Onset of Action	Peak Plasma Concentration	Elimination Half-Life	Duration of Action
PO	Unknown	0.5–4 hr	14–18 hr	Unknown

▶▶nevirapine

Nevirapine (Viramune) is an NNRTI. This is the second class of antiviral drugs indicated for the treatment of HIV infection. Other currently available NNRTIs include delavirdine mesylate (Rescriptor), efavirenz (Sustiva), and etravirine (Intelence). These drugs are often used in combination with NRTIs.

Nevirapine is well tolerated compared with other therapies for HIV. The most common adverse effects associated with nevirapine therapy are rash, fever, nausea, headache, and abnormal liver function tests. Nevirapine and the other NNRTIs are available only for oral use.

PHARMACOKINETICS

Route	Onset of Action	Peak Plasma Concentration	Elimination Half-Life	Duration of Action
PO	2 hr	2–4 hr	25–30 hr	24 hr

▶▶raltegravir potassium

Raltegravir potassium (Isentress) is one of two drugs in the new class called *integrase inhibitors*. Dolutegravir sodium (Tivicay®) is also available. Raltegravir works by inhibiting the activity of the integrase enzyme, thus preventing integration of the proviral gene into human DNA. Raltegravir is used in treatment-experienced patients with virus that shows multidrug resistance and active replication. Myopathy and rhabdomyolysis have been reported, as well as an immune reconstitution syndrome, which may result in an inflammatory response to a residual opportunistic infection. Raltegravir does not interact with CYP3A4 inducers or inhibitors (as many other AIDS drugs do).

PHARMACOKINETICS

Route	Onset of Action	Peak Plasma Concentration	Elimination Half-Life	Duration of Action
PO	Unknown	3 hr	9 hr	Unknown

DRUG PROFILES—cont'd

tenofovir disoproxil fumarate

Tenofovir disoproxil fumarate (Viread) is one of many NRTIs. Others in this class include emtricitabine (Emtriva), lamivudine (Epivir), stavudine (Zerit), and abacavir sulphate (Ziagen), as well as many combination products. Lactic acidosis and severe hepatomegaly have been reported with this drug and others in its class. Tenofovir is indicated for use against HIV infection in combination with other antiretroviral drugs. It is currently available only for oral use.

PHARMACOKINETICS

Route	Onset of Action	Peak Plasma Concentration	Elimination Half-Life	Duration of Action
PO	4–8 days for therapeutic effect	1 hr	10–14 hr	7 days

▶zidovudine

Zidovudine (Retrovir), also known as *azidothymidine* or *AZT*, is a synthetic nucleoside analogue of thymidine that

has had an enormous impact on the treatment and quality of life of people infected with HIV who have AIDS. It was the first and, for a long time, the only anti-HIV medication. Zidovudine, along with other antiretroviral drugs, is given to HIV-infected pregnant women and to newborns to prevent maternal transmission of the virus to the infant. The major dose-limiting adverse effect of zidovudine is bone marrow suppression, and this is often the reason a patient with HIV infection must be switched to another anti-HIV drug such as zalcitabine or didanosine. Some patients may receive a combination of two of these drugs, in lower doses, to maximize their combined actions. This strategy may reduce the likelihood of toxicity. Zidovudine is available in both oral and injectable formulations.

PHARMACOKINETICS

Route	Onset of Action	Peak Plasma Concentration	Elimination Half-Life	Duration of Action
PO	At least 6 mo for therapeutic effect	0.4–1.5 hr	0.8–2 hr	3–5 hr

DOSAGES   Antiretroviral Drugs

Drug	Pharmacological Class	Usual Dosage Range
enfuvirtide (Fuzeon)	HIV-1 fusion inhibitor	*Children 6–16 yr* Subcut: 2 mg/kg bid (max 90 mg/dose) *Adults* Subcut: 90 mg bid
▶indinavir sulphate (Crixivan)	Protease inhibitor	*Adults* PO: 800 mg q8h
maraviroc (Celsentri)	CCR5 antagonist	*Adults older than 18 yr* PO: 300 mg bid
▶nevirapine (Viramune)	Non-nucleoside reverse transcriptase inhibitor	*Adults* PO: 200 mg daily × 14 days, then bid
▶raltegravir potassium (Isentress)	Integrase strand transfer inhibitor	*Children 2 to younger than 12 yr* PO (Chewable tab): 50–300 mg bid *Adults & children older than 12 yr* PO: 400 mg bid
tenofovir disoproxil fumarate (Viread)	Nucleotide reverse transcriptase inhibitor	*Adults & adolescents 12 yr and older* PO: 300 mg once daily
▶zidovudine (Retrovir, AZT)	Nucleotide reverse transcriptase inhibitor	*Children 3 mo to 12 yr* IV: 120 mg/m² q6h (max 160 mg/dose) *Children 4 kg and above* PO: 18–24 mg/kg/day, divided bid–tid *Adults and adolescents 30 kg and above* PO: 600 mg/day divided bid–tid IV: 1–2 mg/kg q4h *Pregnant women* PO: 100 mg 5×/day until start of labour, then give IV bolus dose of 2 mg/kg over 1 hr, followed by an IV infusion of 1 mg/kg/hr until the umbilical cord is clamped *Newborn:* PO (oral solution): 2 mg/kg q6h starting within 12 hr of birth until 6 wk

IV, intravenous; *PO*, oral.

(WNv), severe acute respiratory syndrome (SARS), and H1N1.

In 2001, the first documented cases of WNv infection occurred in Canada, 2 years after it was identified in New York City. WNv is now endemic in all provinces in Canada and in the United States. WNv is a member of the arbovirus family and is transmitted to humans by mosquitoes. It also infects animals, primarily birds, and has been detected in horses and cows. In humans, WNv infection can lead to meningitis and encephalitis. It is currently being investigated to determine whether maternal–fetal transmission can occur during pregnancy. In the United States in 2001, an epidemic occurred with more than 4 000 documented human cases, including 284 deaths. Patients who had undergone organ transplants constituted one of the key groups infected. The virus can also be transmitted through blood transfusions, including platelets, red blood cells, and fresh frozen plasma, and has been detected in breast milk. There is new evidence that health care providers may develop WNv via needle sticks or cuts.

In June 2003, Health Canada began screening blood donations for WNv using a test developed by Canadian Blood Services. There are currently no specific antiviral medications or vaccines available for prevention or treatment of human WNv infection. Prevention focuses on reducing mosquito reproduction by eliminating unneeded pools of water near residential environments.

November 2002 marked the emergence of a new, serious viral infectious disease known as *SARS*. A large outbreak later occurred in Singapore in March 2003. This outbreak was eventually traced to a traveller returning from Hong Kong. Cases later appeared in Europe and North America. SARS can range from a mild to a life-threatening respiratory illness. The disease usually resolves on its own within 3 to 4 weeks. However, 10 to 20% of patients required mechanical ventilation and critical care support, and the overall fatality rate was 3%. Although standard antiviral drugs, including oseltamivir, have been used to treat SARS, no specific drug therapy has proved to be definitively helpful. The cause of SARS was determined to be a coronavirus, which was named the *SARS coronavirus*. Coronaviruses commonly cause mild to moderate upper respiratory tract illnesses in humans, including the common cold.

Avian influenza, or "bird flu," is an influenza virus infection that has been shown to infect birds in Europe as well as birds and humans in Asia. This disease is caused by an influenza A virus known as *avian influenza A, subtype H5N1*. The virus is carried in the intestines of many wild birds worldwide, often without causing any serious illness. However, more serious infections can be fatal and can spread rapidly among an entire flock of birds. Usually, these viruses do not infect humans. However, since 1997, there have been cases of human infection, mostly following contact with infected birds or their secretions or excrement (e.g., poultry workers). The majority of these cases have occurred in Europe and Asia. Human-to-human transmission has been especially rare. Symptoms have ranged from typical flulike symptoms such as fever, cough, sore throat, and muscle aches to eye infections and acute respiratory illness, even with life-threatening complications. This virus is resistant to amantadine, although it is believed (but remains to be confirmed) that zanamivir and oseltamivir would offer some therapeutic benefit for this condition.

Many health experts fear a flu pandemic caused by this virus if it mutates to a more easily transmissible form. This occurs frequently with influenza viruses in general, which is why a new seasonal flu vaccine must be developed each year. Although no one can predict if and when such a pandemic might occur with this virus, the WHO and other health agencies, including the BC Centre for Disease Control and the Public Health Agency of Canada, are continuously monitoring activity patterns as well as the virus's resistance to other antiviral drugs. Some countries have implemented a ban on the import of birds from countries where avian influenza has been shown to be prevalent.

In 2009, the WHO signaled that a pandemic was underway with the new influenza virus H1N1 (originally called *swine flu*). The H1N1 virus spreads person to person, much the same way the regular seasonal influenza virus spreads. Symptoms include fever, cough, sore throat, body aches, chills, and fatigue. Severe illness and death have occurred with H1N1. A vaccine was developed and made available in October 2009. Antiviral medications such as oseltamivir or zanamivir are recommended for all patients with suspected or confirmed influenza requiring hospitalization. Prophylactic treatment is considered for patients at high risk for complications.

The most recent significant outbreak is Ebola virus hemorrhagic disease, occurring in West Africa. Ebola was discovered in 1976, and several outbreaks have occurred in African countries since then. The most widespread epidemic of Ebola virus disease began in 2013 in Guinea and persisted for over 2 years. At the time of writing, the World Health Organization has not declared the epidemic over because of occasional outbreaks. Ebola is characterized by flulike symptoms that progresses to bleeding, organ failure, and death. It is spread via direct contact with blood or body fluids of an infected animal or human. There have never been any cases of Ebola in Canada, and Canada Border Services Agency assesses everyone arriving in Canada for signs of illness. All individuals from Sierra Leone, Guinea, and Liberia are screened and assessed. Canada was instrumental in developing a vaccine called rVSV-ZEBOV (see Chapter 51) at the Public Health Agency of Canada's National Microbiology Laboratory in Winnipeg.

NURSING PROCESS

▨ Assessment

Before administering an antiviral drug, perform a thorough head-to-toe physical assessment and take a medical and medication history. Document any known allergies. Assess the patient's nutritional status and baseline vital signs because of the profound effects of viral illnesses on physiological status, particularly if the patient is immunocompromised. Assess for any contraindications, cautions, and drug interactions.

When assessing the use of non-HIV antivirals, inquire about the patient's allergy to medications. Ask for a list of any prescription and over-the-counter drugs as well as natural health products. Before initiation of therapy, assess energy levels, any weight loss, vital signs, and the characteristics of any visible lesions. Document the findings for baseline comparison. It is also important to assess age because safety and efficacy of amantadine in neonates and infants less than 12 months of age have not been proven. Cidofovir requires assessment of renal function and is contraindicated in those with kidney compromise or with use of other nephrotoxic drugs. Ribavirin is contraindicated in pregnant women and in their male sexual partners due to its teratogenic properties; it must also not be handled by health care providers who are or might be pregnant. With ribavirin, analysis of respiratory secretions via sputum specimen will most likely be ordered for diagnostic purposes prior to initiation of drug therapy. With respiratory illness, also assess and document breath sounds, respiratory rate and patterns, cough, sputum production, and vital signs, including temperature. With foscarnet and cidofovir, assess kidney function because of the potential for renal toxicity.

Before giving acyclovir, assess vital signs and take a thorough medication history. Assess pain levels associated with the zoster lesions prior to giving the medication because relief of pain is expected with use of the drug. See Chapter 56 for more information on the topical form of acyclovir. Famciclovir also requires assessment of allergies. Oseltamivir and zanamivir, useful against influenza virus types A and B, must be given as ordered within 2 days of the onset of flu symptoms. Ganciclovir is associated with a dose-limiting toxicity of bone marrow suppression; therefore, assess blood counts prior to and during use.

With the use of HIV antivirals, or antiretrovirals, closely assess allergies, cautions, contraindications, and drug interactions. Because of the severity of HIV infections and potential for a fatal outcome, the main contraindication includes severe drug allergy and other toxicities. Use of protease inhibitors requires assessment of the patient's medical history, vital signs, baseline weight, allergies, medication history, and results of base-line laboratory tests, such as CBC and kidney and liver function studies. These laboratory tests are generally ordered during the different phases of treatment; document results appropriately. A major adverse effect of the protease inhibitors is lipid abnormalities, with redistribution of fat stores under the skin leading to undesirable cosmetic outcomes for the patient. Assess emotional status and support systems due to the impact of this adverse effect on body image. Bone demineralization is yet another adverse effect with long-term use, so assessment of calcium and vitamin D levels is crucial to patient safety before, during, and after therapy.

The antiretroviral drug maraviroc requires assessment of allergies and liver function as well as review of the list of medications the patient is taking because of many interacting drugs. Raltegravir is associated with myopathies and breakdown of muscle cells; thus, baseline notation of skeletal muscle functioning and pain level is crucial to patient safety. Perform a baseline measurement, and frequently monitor vital signs, including temperature, due to the possibility of opportunistic infections. The health care provider may also order CBCs and other laboratory studies before, during, and after therapy. Avoid tenofovir in patients with liver disorders. Bone marrow suppression is a dose-limiting adverse effect of zidovudine, so review blood cell counts and results of clotting studies before and during therapy.

With any of the drugs presented in this chapter, especially those used for the management of HIV infection, assessment of the patient's knowledge about the illness and the need for long-term and often lifelong therapy is crucial. In addition, assess the patient's knowledge about the illness as well as the patient's educational level and reading level and the way in which the patient learns best. Familiarity with community resources is important in implementing patient education effectively. Be sure to assess mental health status and emotional state because of the psychological impact and stigma associated with this chronic illness. Referrals to social work, counselling, and support groups may be appropriate. Value systems, social patterns, hobbies, support systems, and spiritual beliefs need to also be acknowledged and documented. Perform an assessment of financial status and resources as well. Many patients may need to be referred to social services because of lack of health care insurance and because many of these drugs need to be taken lifelong. For patients with chronic illnesses, the synthesis of this information will help ensure the development of a collaborative plan of care that is complete and holistic.

▨ Nursing Diagnoses

- Activity intolerance related to weakness secondary to decreased energy from pathology of viral infections
- Deficient knowledge related to the lack of information about and experience with long-term medication therapy and lack of information about the viral infection, its transmission, and its treatment

- Risk for injury related to the immunosuppressive effects of viral disease processes and their treatment

Planning

Goals

- Patient will experience improved energy and activity level while receiving therapy.
- Patient will demonstrate improved knowledge base about the disease process and the need for potential lifelong therapy.
- Patient will remain free from injury while taking medication for viral disease.

Expected Patient Outcomes

- Patient experiences increased periods of comfort, with greater participation in care and activities of daily living, as a result of successful treatment of viral infection.
  - Patient's energy levels improve to a level greater than what was experienced before antiviral therapy.
- Patient states the rationale for the treatment regimen and the possibility of lifelong therapy with HIV illnesses.
  - Patient understands the need for taking the medication exactly as prescribed.
  - Patient identifies possible adverse effects associated with the HIV antiviral drugs, such as GI upset.
  - Patient identifies financial resources to pay for lifelong medication therapy.
- Patient states the physical impact of a viral infection on the patient's overall state of health (e.g., compromised immune system) and the effect of appropriate therapy with either non-HIV antivirals or HIV antivirals (antiretrovirals).
  - Patient takes appropriate precautions during antiviral therapy such as avoiding others who are ill and staying away from crowds.

Implementation

Nursing interventions pertinent to patients receiving non-HIV antivirals include use of the appropriate technique when applying or administering ointments, aerosol powders, and IV or oral forms of medication. Wearing gloves and washing hands thoroughly before and after the administration of medication are necessary to prevent contamination of the site and spread of infection. It is important to both your safety and the safety of the patient to always begin by performing hand hygiene and maintain standard precautions/routine practices (see Box 10-1). The use of non-HIV antivirals or antiretrovirals may lead to superimposed infection or superinfections, so constantly monitor for such infections and implement measures for their prevention (see Chapters 52 and 53).

Instruct the patient to take oral antivirals with meals to help minimize GI upset. Also advise the patient to store capsules at room temperature and not to crush or break the capsules. Acyclovir is available in various dosage forms, and there are slight inconsistencies in the spelling of the drug names, so be sure to double-check the specific drug and dosage form ordered. Topical dosage forms (e.g., acyclovir) should be applied using a finger cot or gloves to prevent autoinoculation. Avoid eye contact with the drug. IV acyclovir is stable for 12 hours at room temperature and will often precipitate when refrigerated. Dilute IV infusions as recommended (e.g., with 5% dextrose in water or normal saline) and infuse with caution. Infusion over longer than 1 hour is suggested to avoid the kidney tubule damage seen with more rapid infusions. Be sure to refer to the manufacturer's guidelines for administration. Encourage adequate hydration during the infusion and for several hours afterwards to prevent drug-related crystalluria. Carefully monitor the IV site. Document and report to the health care provider any redness, heat, pain, swelling, or red streaks that may indicate possible phlebitis. Document the characteristics of any lesions. Implement appropriate isolation for individuals with chicken pox or herpes zoster, and give analgesics for comfort, as ordered. Some of the more common adverse effects of acyclovir include nausea, diarrhea, and headache. Comfort measures may need to be implemented.

Amantadine and other antivirals need to be taken for the entire course of therapy, and if a dose is missed, instruct the patient to take the dose as soon as it is remembered or contact the health care provider for further instructions. If dry mouth occurs due to anticholinergic effects, sucking on sugarless candy or chewing gum might be helpful. Encourage daily mouth care, including the use of dental floss, and regular preventive dental visits. Saliva substitutes may be needed, and if dry mouth continues for longer than 2 weeks, contact the health care provider for further management.

Orthostatic hypotension may occur, so it is important to monitor vital signs with postural blood pressures during therapy. If ganciclovir sodium is given intravenously, dilute it with 5% dextrose in water or normal saline to a concentration and in a time frame indicated by the drug monograph. Be sure to follow the manufacturer's guidelines for administration. Administration into large veins is recommended to provide the dilution needed to minimize the risk for vein irritation. When handling the solution of ganciclovir sodium, avoid exposure of eyes, mucous membranes, and skin to the drug, and use latex gloves and safety glasses for handling and preparation. If the drug comes in contact with the eyes, flush with plain water. If it comes in contact with mucous membranes or skin, thoroughly wash and rinse the affected areas with soap and water. Laboratory values including blood counts will most likely be monitored during therapy due to possible bone marrow toxicity. Ribavirin may be given by oral inhalation, but the drug is not to be administered to pregnant women or handled by health care providers who are (or may be) pregnant. Continually monitor for possible altered breath sounds, as wheezing may occur due to mild bronchospasm. Some antivirals are spelled similarly or sound alike; when these drugs are given, always check the order closely against the drug being administered. For example, acyclovir may be mistaken for valacyclovir hydrochloride or famciclovir. When the patient is taking oseltamivir and other non-HIV antivirals for influenza, it is important to remember that this medication must be prescribed and is most effective if started within 2 days of the onset of flu symptoms.

Aerosol generators are available from the drug manufacturer. Discard reservoir solutions if levels are low or empty, and change every 24 hours. For patients taking ribavirin and similar drugs for treatment of RSV via a small particle aerosol generator (SPAG) device, provide clear and precise instructions on how to properly mix and administer the drug. Be sure to reconstitute the drug (e.g., ribavirin powder) as instructed by the manufacturer's guidelines. Discard old solutions left in the equipment before adding fresh medication. Drugs administered using SPAG equipment are usually administered 12 to 18 hours daily for up to 7 days, beginning within 3 days of the onset of symptoms. There is much controversy about use of this drug in patients on ventilators, and it is to be administered only by health care providers who are specially trained in the use of the drug. Frequently empty any "rainout" in the tubing of the ventilator and continually monitor breath sounds in patients receiving inhaled forms of this drug, whether they are receiving artificial ventilation or not. Zanamivir is administered by inhalation using a Diskhaler® device. Be sure that the patient exhales completely first; then, while holding the mouthpiece between the teeth with lips snug around it and tongue down and out of the way, the patient needs to inhale deeply through the mouth and then hold the breath as long as possible prior to exhaling. Encourage rinsing of the mouth with water to prevent irritation and dryness, and instruct the patient never to exhale into the Diskhaler.

HIV antivirals, or antiretrovirals, include numerous drugs. There are special administration and handling guidelines for some of the dosage forms of these drugs. With zidovudine, monitor for the adverse effects of bone marrow suppression by checking the CBC. If the patient experiences signs and symptoms of an opportunistic infection (e.g., respiratory signs and symptoms, fever, changes in oral mucosa), contact the health care provider immediately. The patient may experience headaches; therefore, provide the appropriate form of analgesia, as ordered. See Table 45-2 for a listing of more adverse effects associated with the various antiviral drugs.

With the film-coated oral dosage forms, advise the patient not to alter the drugs in any way. Patients may improve the taste of ritonavir by mixing it with chocolate milk or a nutritional beverage within 1 hour of its dosing. Emphasize to the patient and the patient's family that ritonavir's dosage form needs to be protected from light. Absorption of oral dosages of zidovudine is not impeded by taking the drug with food or milk, but instruct the patient to remain upright or with the head of the bed elevated while administering the medication and for up to 30 minutes afterward to prevent esophageal ulceration. Give IV doses only if the solution is clear and does not contain any particulate matter. Be sure to use the appropriate dosage, diluents, and infusion time. Because these drugs often come in oral dosage forms, it is usually recommended that they be given with food. Generally, administer zidovudine and other antiretrovirals at evenly spaced intervals around the clock, as ordered, to ensure steady-state levels. With all oral and parenteral dosage forms of antiretrovirals, observe the patient for nausea and vomiting as well as any changes in weight, anorexia, or changes in bowel activities and patterns. Maraviroc and tenofovir are available for oral dosing and are to be given as prescribed.

Throughout therapy, always remember that the goal of treatment is to find the regimen that provides the best control of the individual patient's infection with the most tolerable adverse effects possible. Because patients vary greatly in their drug tolerance, carefully individualize medication regimens. Other nursing interventions associated with these drugs include the following: (1) Continually monitor for adverse effects throughout therapy, with a focus on the various organ systems, such as the GI, neurological, renal, and hepatic systems. (2) With oral forms of indinavir and nevirapine, encourage at least 6 to 8 glasses of water (unless contraindicated) daily to maintain adequate hydration and help prevent nephrolithiasis. (3) Nevirapine, zidovudine, and similar drugs may be associated with a rash; however, if the rash is accompanied by blistering, fever, malaise, myalgias, oral lesions, swelling or edema, or conjunctivitis, contact the health care provider immediately. (4) If drug therapy results in worsening of signs and symptoms, notify the health care provider immediately, who may discontinue the drug. (5) Continually monitor laboratory testing (e.g., CBC, kidney and liver function tests, and HIV RNA levels) and report any abnormalities to the health care provider. See the Patient Teaching Tips for more information.

Evaluation

The therapeutic effects of non-HIV antivirals and HIV antivirals (or antiretrovirals) include elimination of the virus or a decrease in the symptoms of the viral infections. There may be a delayed progression of HIV infection and AIDS as well as a decrease in flulike symptoms and the frequency of herpetic flare-ups and other lesion breakouts. With successful therapy, herpetic lesions will crust over, and the frequency of recurrence will decrease. In addition, constantly evaluate for the occurrence of adverse effects and toxicity associated with specific antiviral and antiretroviral drugs. These specific adverse effects are listed in Table 45-2. Continually reevaluate the collaborative plan of care to ensure that the goals and outcome criteria have been met. Remain constantly attentive in reviewing reports from the BC Centre for Disease Control, Health Canada, other provincial and territorial health care agencies, and public health care agencies on new strains of viruses and flu syndromes (see earlier discussion).

 CASE STUDY

Antiviral Therapy

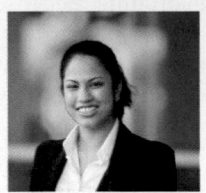 One of your patients, Suria, a 33-year-old biology professor, has just started therapy with tenofovir/emtricitabine and dolutegravir. She has many questions about this medication therapy, and you are meeting with her to review her questions.

1. She asks you why there are three drugs in this particular therapy. What is your explanation?

2. You are developing a patient teaching guide for Suria, emphasizing any specific cautions and symptoms to report to the health care provider. What instructions will you include?
3. At what level of platelets and white blood cells would there probably be a change or discontinuation of this drug?

_____

For answers, see http://evolve.elsevier.com/Canada/Lilley/pharmacology/.

PATIENT TEACHING TIPS

❖ Alert the patient to the adverse effect of dizziness while taking antiviral drugs, and instruct the patient to use caution while driving or participating in activities requiring alertness. Advise the patient to take all medications exactly as prescribed and for the full course of therapy.
❖ Patients should consult the health care provider before taking any other prescribed or over-the-counter drugs or natural health products.
❖ Inform the patient of all possible drug interactions, including with over-the-counter medications and natural health products.
❖ Advise patients who are immunocompromised to avoid crowds and persons with infections.
❖ Advocate for standard precautions/routine practices and safer sex practices for all patients but especially those with sexually transmitted viral infections, such as patients who are HIV positive. Condom use is a necessity in the prevention of these viral infections and other sexually transmitted infections. The presence of genital herpes requires sexual abstinence.
❖ It is generally recommended that female patients with genital herpes undergo a Papanicolaou (Pap) smear test every 6 months or as ordered by the health care provider to monitor the virus and effectiveness of treatment.
❖ Instruct the patient to report the following adverse reactions to the health care provider: decreased urinary output, seizure activity, syncope, jaundice, wheezing, abnormal sensations in the hands and feet, vomiting, or diarrhea.

❖ Provide the patient with adequate demonstrations, teaching aids, and instructions for special application procedures (e.g., instillation of ophthalmic drops, use of finger cots or gloves when applying medication to lesions, use of respiratory inhalation forms). Explain that gloves or finger cots are needed for medication application and cleansing to prevent the spread of lesions.
❖ Educate the patient that adherence to their medications is crucial to suppress viral replication and prevent opportunistic infections from occurring.
❖ Encourage fluids up to 3 000 mL/24 hr unless contraindicated.
❖ Educate the patient about the fact that antiviral drugs suppress but do not cure the viral infection.
❖ Instruct the patient to start valacyclovir or other antivirals as prescribed but at the first sign of a recurrent episode of genital herpes or herpes zoster. In addition, explain that early treatment within 24 to 48 hours is needed to achieve full therapeutic results.
❖ Instruct the patient to report to the health care provider immediately any difficulty breathing; drastic changes in blood pressure; bleeding; new symptoms; worsening of infection, fever, or chills; or other unusual problems.
❖ Emphasize the importance of follow-up appointments.

KEY POINTS

❖ Viruses are difficult to kill and to treat because they live inside human cells. Most antiviral drugs act by inhibiting replication of the virus. In this chapter, antiviral drugs are categorized as either non-HIV antivirals or HIV antivirals (antiretrovirals).

❖ Non-HIV antivirals include amantadine, acyclovir, ganciclovir, oseltamivir, and ribavirin. HIV antivirals include enfuvirtide, indinavir, maraviroc, nevirapine, raltegravir, tenofovir, and zidovudine.

❖ Administer antiretroviral drugs only after reading and understanding the orders from the health care provider and after performing a thorough nursing assessment that includes a review of the patient's nutritional status, weight, baseline vital signs, and kidney and liver functioning, as well as an assessment of heart sounds, neurological status, and GI functioning.

❖ Comfort measures and supportive nursing care are to accompany drug therapy. Patients need to drink plenty of fluids and to space medications around the clock, as ordered, to maintain steady blood levels of the drug.

EXAMINATION REVIEW QUESTIONS

1. During treatment with zidovudine, the nurse needs to monitor for which potential adverse effect?
 a. Retinitis
 b. Deep vein thrombosis
 c. Kaposi's sarcoma
 d. Bone marrow suppression

2. After giving an injection to a patient with HIV infection, the nurse accidentally receives a needle stick from a needle disposal box that was too full. Which of the following drugs might be included in recommendations for treating an occupational HIV exposure?
 a. didanosine
 b. lamivudine and enfuvirtide
 c. zidovudine, lamivudine, and indinavir
 d. acyclovir

3. When the nurse is teaching a patient who is taking acyclovir for genital herpes, which statement by the nurse is accurate?
 a. "This drug will help the lesions dry and crust over."
 b. "Acyclovir will eradicate the herpes virus."
 c. "This drug will prevent the spread of this virus to others."
 d. "Be sure to give this drug to your partner, too."

4. A patient who has been newly diagnosed with HIV has many questions about the effectiveness of drug therapy. After a teaching session, which statement by the patient reflects a need for more education?
 a. "I will be monitored for adverse effects and improvements while I'm taking this medicine."
 b. "These drugs do not eliminate the HIV, but hopefully the amount of virus in my body will be reduced."
 c. "There is no cure for HIV."
 d. "These drugs will eventually eliminate the virus in my body."

5. After surgery for organ transplantation, a patient is receiving ganciclovir sodium, even though he does not have a viral infection. Which statement best explains the rationale for this medication therapy?
 a. Ganciclovir sodium is used to prevent potential exposure to the HIV virus.
 b. This medication is given prophylactically to prevent influenza A infection.
 c. Ganciclovir sodium is given to prevent CMV infection.
 d. The drug works synergistically with antibiotics to prevent superinfections.

6. The nurse is reviewing the use of multidrug therapy for HIV with a patient. Which statements are correct regarding the reason for using multiple drugs to treat HIV? (Select all that apply.)
 a. The combination of drugs has fewer associated toxicities.
 b. The use of multiple drugs is more effective against resistant strains of HIV.
 c. Effective treatment results in reduced T-cell counts.
 d. The goal of this treatment is to reduce the viral load.
 e. This type of therapy reduces the incidence of opportunistic infections.

7. The order for an 11-year-old child who has chicken pox reads: "Give acyclovir (Zovirax) 20 mg/kg PO daily × 5 days. The child weighs 99 pounds. How much is each dose? Is this dose safe for this child?

Answers: 1. d, 2. c, 3. a, 4. d, 5. c, 6. b, d, e, 7. 900 mg; no, the dose exceeds the 800 mg maximum per dose

CRITICAL THINKING ACTIVITIES

1. A 19-year-old male college student was diagnosed with HIV approximately 7 months ago, and he has been going through several treatment regimens. The infectious disease specialist is planning this treatment regime again and will soon start treatment with didanosine. The student has experienced some bone marrow depression off and on during the last few months. He asks you, "Why is the doctor changing to didanosine therapy? What adverse effects does this new medicine have?" What are the nurse's best answers to his questions?

2. A young adult female patient underwent bone marrow transplantation, and less than 1 year later she contracted a cytomegalovirus (CMV) infection. She is concerned about the medications and asks, "Are these antiviral drugs going to be a problem? What if I get pregnant?" What is the nurse's priority when responding to her questions? Explain your answer.

3. A college student had symptoms of the flu since Friday, but she does not go to the student health office until the following Tuesday. She tells the nurse that she is "miserable" and that she heard about Tamiflu on the Internet. She wants to take it to "keep the flu from getting worse." What is the nurse's priority action at this time?

For answers, see http://evolve.elsevier.com/Canada/Lilley/pharmacology/.

CHAPTER 46

Antitubercular Drugs

Objectives

After reading this chapter, the successful student will be able to do the following:

1. Identify the various first-line and second-line drugs indicated for the treatment of tuberculosis.

2. Discuss the mechanisms of action, dosages, adverse effects, routes of administration, special dosing considerations, cautions, contraindications, and drug interactions of the antitubercular drugs.

3. Develop a collaborative plan of care that includes all phases of the nursing process for patients receiving antitubercular drugs.

4. Develop a comprehensive teaching guide for patients and families impacted by a diagnosis of tuberculosis or treatment with antitubercular drugs.

e-Learning Activities

Website
(http://evolve.elsevier.com/Canada/Lilley/pharmacology/)

evolve

- Answer Key—Textbook Case Studies
- Answer Key—Critical Thinking Activities
- Chapter Summaries—Printable
- Review Questions for Exam Preparation
- Unfolding Case Studies

Drug Profiles

ethambutol (ethambutol hydrochloride)*, p. 875
▸▸ isoniazid, p. 875
pyrazinamide, p. 875
rifabutin, p. 875
rifampin, p. 875
streptomycin (streptomycin sulphate)*, p. 876

▸▸ Key drug

*Full generic name is given in parentheses. For the purposes of this text, the more common, shortened name is used.

Key Terms

Aerobic Requiring oxygen for the maintenance of life. (p. 870)

Antitubercular drugs Drugs used to treat infections caused by *Mycobacterium* bacterial species. (p. 872)

Bacillus A rod-shaped bacterium. (p. 870)

Granulomas Small nodular aggregations of inflammatory cells (e.g., macrophages, lymphocytes); usually characterized by clearly delimited boundaries, as found in tuberculosis. (p. 870)

Interferon gamma release assays (IGRAs) Surrogate markers of *Mycobacterium tuberculosis* infection; indicate a cellular immune response to *M. tuberculosis*. (p. 870)

Isoniazid The primary and most commonly prescribed antitubercular drug. (p. 871)

Multidrug-resistant tuberculosis (MDR-TB) Tuberculosis that demonstrates resistance to two or more drugs. (p. 871)

Slow acetylator An individual with a genetic defect that causes a deficiency in the enzyme needed to metabolize isoniazid, the most widely used tuberculosis drug. (p.875)

Tubercle bacillus The characteristic lesion of tuberculosis; a small round grey translucent granulomatous lesion, usually with a caseated (cheesy) consistency in its interior. (See *granuloma*) (p. 870)

Tubercle bacilli Another common name for rod-shaped tuberculosis bacteria; essentially synonymous with *Mycobacterium tuberculosis*. (p. 870)

Tuberculosis (TB) Any infectious disease caused by species of *Mycobacterium*, usually *Mycobacterium tuberculosis* (adjectives: *tuberculous, tubercular*). (p. 870)

TUBERCULOSIS

Tuberculosis (TB) is the medical diagnosis of any infectious disease caused by a bacterial species known as *Mycobacterium*. TB is most commonly characterized by **granulomas** in the lungs. They are nodular accumulations of inflammatory cells (e.g., macrophages, lymphocytes) that are delimited ("walled off" with clear boundaries) and have a centre that has a cheesy, or caseated, consistency. (*Casein* is the name of a protein that is prevalent in cheese and milk.) Although there are two mycobacterial species that can cause TB, *Mycobacterium tuberculosis (MTB)* and *M. bovis*, infections caused by *M. tuberculosis* are the most common. There are also several other mycobacterial species, including *M. leprae*, which causes leprosy, and *M. avium-intracellulare* complex, which causes a disease that is similar to TB but often has gastrointestinal (GI) symptoms. Both of these latter diseases have varying susceptibility to different drugs used for TB. Infections with these bacteria are much less of a public health problem and hence are not the focus of this chapter.

MTB is an aerobic bacillus, which means that it is a long and slender, rod-shaped microorganism (**bacillus**) that requires a large supply of oxygen for it to grow and flourish (**aerobic**). This bacterium's need for a highly oxygenated body site explains why *Mycobacterium* infections most commonly affect the lungs. Early manifestations are often nonspecific and include a productive cough that lasts longer than 2 weeks and may contain blood, as well as weight loss, chest pain, weakness and fatigue, loss of appetite, fever, night sweating, and chills. Other common sites of infection are the growing ends of bones and the brain (cerebral cortex). Less common sites of infection include the kidney, liver, and genitourinary tract, as well as virtually every other tissue and organ in the body.

These **tubercle bacilli** (a common synonym for MTB) are transmitted from one of three sources: humans, cows (bovine; hence the species name *M. bovis*), or birds (avian), although bovine and avian transmission is much less common than human transmission. Tubercle bacilli are conveyed in droplets expelled by infected people or animals during coughing or sneezing and are then inhaled by the new host. After these infectious droplets are inhaled, the infection spreads to the susceptible organ sites by means of the blood and lymphatic system. MTB is a slow-growing organism, which makes it more difficult to treat than most other bacterial infections. Many of the antibiotics used to treat TB work by inhibiting growth (bacteriostatic) rather than by directly killing the organism. The reason microorganisms that grow slowly are more difficult to kill is because their cells are not as metabolically active as those of faster-growing organisms.

Most bactericidal (cell-killing) drugs work by disrupting critical cellular metabolic processes in organisms. Therefore, the most drug-susceptible organisms are those with faster (not slower) metabolic activity.

The first infectious episode is considered the primary TB infection; reinfection represents the more chronic form of the disease. However, TB does not develop in all people who are exposed to the bacteria. In some cases, the bacteria become dormant and are walled off by calcified or fibrous tissues. Patients with dormant bacteria may test positive for exposure, but are not necessarily infectious. In immunocompromised patients such as those with HIV, TB can inflict devastating and irreversible damage. The prevalence of HIV-TB co-infection is unknown. The steps for diagnosis of TB are listed in Box 46-1.

Canada has one of the lowest rates of active TB cases internationally. This is attributed to intensified public health efforts aimed at preventing, diagnosing, and treating TB as well as HIV infection, including more effective antiretroviral drug therapy (see Chapter 45). The reported number of new active and retreatment TB cases in 2013 was 1 640, for an incidence rate of 4.7 per 100 000. British Columbia, Manitoba, Saskatchewan, Nunavut, and the Northwest territories have incidence rates higher than the national rate. Nunavut reports the highest incidence

---

BOX 46-1

Diagnosis of Tuberculosis

Step 1: Perform tuberculin skin test (Tubersol®) or **interferon gamma release assay (IGRA)**. The tuberculin skin test is assessed for size of induration, positive predictive value, and risk of disease if the person is truly infected. IGRAs are more specific than the tuberculin skin test in populations vaccinated with Bacille Calmette–Guérin (BCG), especially if the BCG is given after infancy or multiple times.

  Step 2: If skin test results are positive, then perform chest X-ray.

  Step 3: If chest X-ray shows signs of TB, then perform culture of sputum* or stomach secretions.

---

*The acid-fast bacillus smear test is performed on sputum as a quick method of determining whether TB treatment and precautions are needed until a more definite diagnosis is made.

rate overall. The majority of reported TB cases are in foreign-born individuals; however, the incidence rate among Canadian-born Indigenous people remains the highest per 100 000 (Gallant, McGuire, & Ogunnaike-Cooke, 2015). Indigenous individuals face many health inequities, such as a higher incidence of diabetes and HIV/AIDS, crowded living conditions, and limited access to health care. Of increasing concern internationally is the number of cases of **multidrug-resistant tuberculosis (MDR-TB)**, posing a serious threat to TB prevention and control efforts. However, between 2002 and 2012, reported drug resistance in Canada remained consistently below international levels.

TB infects one third of the world's population. It is currently second only to HIV in the diseases with the greatest number of deaths caused by a single infectious organism. According to the World Health Organization, MDR-TB is defined as TB that is resistant to both isoniazid and rifampin (2012). Close contacts of patients with MDR-TB need to be treated as well, usually with isoniazid for 6 to 9 months.

Several factors have contributed to this TB crisis, but one important source of the problem is the increasing number of people who are members of groups that are particularly susceptible to the infection. These groups include people experiencing homelessness, those who are undernourished or malnourished, people infected with HIV, those who misuse drugs, patients with cancer, those taking immunosuppressant drugs, residents of correctional or long-term care facilities, and those who live in crowded housing with poor sanitation. Many factors affecting members of these groups also increase the likelihood that an acquired TB infection will be drug resistant. The majority of TB cases in Canada occur in new Canadians whose TB is reactivated either soon after their arrival in Canada or when they age (possibly due to a weakened immune system associated with the stressors of immigration or aging).

ANTITUBERCULAR DRUGS

The drugs used to treat infections caused by all forms of *Mycobacterium* are called *antitubercular drugs*, and these drugs fall into two categories: primary (first-line) and secondary (second-line) drugs. As these designations imply, primary drugs are those tried first, whereas secondary drugs are reserved for more complicated cases, such as infections resistant to primary drugs. Two effective drugs must be administered at all times. Therapy is given in two phases: the initial intensive and continuation. The initial intensive consists of drugs used in combination to achieve rapid destruction of the TB bacilli and rapid improvement in the patient's clinical condition. This phase results in reduced morbidity, mortality, and disease transmission. It lasts about 2 months, with drugs administered 5 days a week. A total of at least three effective drugs are recommended during this phase when bacillary load is high, to prevent drug resistance.

All patients in Canada with active TB that is potentially drug-resistant should be treated with a regimen of isoniazid, rifampin, pyrazinamide, and ethambutol for the initial 2 months. The second, or continuation, phase consists of the use of two drugs. The time frame for this phase is variable, depending on risk of relapse, the drugs given in the first phase, and drug susceptibility testing. During this phase, drugs may be given daily or intermittently. Intermittent administration is 3 days a week, and this approach is used with directly observed treatment (DOT). DOT is recommended for patients who have risk factors for nonadherence or who are members of population groups with historically high rates of treatment failure or relapse or poor rates of treatment completion. The antimycobacterial activity, efficacy, and potential adverse and toxic effects of the various drugs determine the class to which they belong. **Isoniazid** is a primary antitubercular drug and is the most widely used. It can be administered either as the sole drug in the prophylaxis of TB or in combination with other antitubercular drugs in the treatment of TB. The various first-line and second-line antibiotic drugs are listed in Box 46-2. There are also two miscellaneous TB-related injections—one diagnostic, the other a vaccine. These are described in Box 46-3.

Important considerations during drug selection are the likelihood of drug-resistant organisms and drug toxicity. The following are other key elements essential in the planning and implementation of effective therapy:

- Drug susceptibility tests are performed on the first *Mycobacterium* species that is isolated from a patient specimen (to prevent the development of MDR-TB).
- Before the results of the susceptibility tests are known, the patient is started on a four-drug regimen consisting of isoniazid, rifampin, pyrazinamide, and ethambutol, which together are 95% effective in combating the infection. The use of multiple medications reduces the possibility of the organism becoming drug

---

BOX 46-2

First-Line and Second-Line Antitubercular Drugs

First-Line Drugs

ethambutol hydrochloride (EMB)
isoniazid (INH)
pyrazinamide (PZA)
rifampin (RMP)

Second-Line Drugs

amikacin sulphate
levofloxacin hemihydrate
moxifloxacin hydrochloride

BOX 46-3

Miscellaneous TB-Related Injections

Purified protein derivative (PPD): A diagnostic injection given intradermally in doses of 5 tuberculin units (0.1 mL) to detect exposure to the TB organism. It is composed of a protein precipitate derived from TB bacteria. A positive result is actually indicated by induration (not erythema) at the site of injection and is also known as the Mantoux reaction, named for a physician who described it.

Bacillus Calmette–Guérin (BCG): A vaccine injection derived from an inactivated strain of *Mycobacterium bovis*. Although it is not normally administered in Canada because the risk of TB is not as high as elsewhere, it is given in some areas such as Indigenous communities in the Northwest Territories, where TB is endemic. BCG is part of the vaccination schedule for infants in these areas and is also offered to infants in the provinces of Ontario and Saskatchewan in communities where the risk of contracting TB is high. BCG is also used in much of the world to vaccinate young children against TB. Although it does not prevent infection, evidence indicates that it reduces active TB by 60 to 80% and is even more effective at preventing more severe cases involving dissemination of infection throughout the body. This vaccine can cause false-positive results on tuberculin skin tests.

resistant. These drugs are given for the first 2 months of treatment.

- Once drug susceptibility results are available, the regimen is adjusted accordingly. For example, if the tests reveal the disease is susceptible to all first-line drugs, then ethambutol can be stopped and pyrazinamide is then continued for the first 2 months. Then, isoniazid and rifampin are continued for the remaining 4 months. Treatment is continued for 9 months if there are risk factors for relapse, such as positive cultures or HIV co-infection.
- Patient adherence to the prescribed drug regimen needs to be monitored closely (e.g., by health units), because the incidence of both patient nonadherence and adverse effects is high.
- Despite the availability of many drugs to combat TB and the efforts mounted to detect and treat those infected with the disease, treatment has been made difficult by two previously mentioned problems: patient nonadherence with therapy and the growing incidence of drug-resistant organisms.

Mechanism of Action and Drug Effects

The mechanisms of action of the various antitubercular drugs vary depending on the drug. These drugs act on MTB by inhibiting protein synthesis, inhibiting cell wall synthesis, or by other mechanisms. The **antitubercular drugs** are listed in Table 46-1 by their mechanism of action. The major effects of drug therapy include reduction of cough and, therefore, reduction of the infectiousness of the patient. This reduction normally occurs within 2 weeks of the initiation of drug therapy, assuming that the patient's TB strain is drug sensitive.

TABLE 46-1

Antitubercular Drugs: Mechanisms of Action

Drugs	Description
INHIBIT PROTEIN SYNTHESIS	
rifabutin, rifampin, rifapentine, streptomycin	Streptomycin works by interfering with normal protein synthesis and causing the production of faulty proteins. Rifampin acts at a different point in the protein synthesis pathway than streptomycin. Rifampin inhibits RNA synthesis and may also inhibit DNA synthesis. Human cells are not as sensitive as mycobacterial cells and are not affected by rifampin except at high drug concentrations.
INHIBIT CELL WALL SYNTHESIS	
isoniazid	Isoniazid acts at least partly by inhibiting the synthesis of cell wall components, but the mechanism of this drug is still not clearly understood.
OTHER MECHANISMS	
ethambutol, isoniazid, pyrazinamide	Isoniazid is taken up by mycobacteria cells and undergoes hydrolysis to isonicotinic acid, which reacts with cofactor NAD to form a defective NAD that is no longer active as a coenzyme for certain life-sustaining reactions in the *Mycobacterium tuberculosis* organism. Ethambutol affects lipid synthesis, which results in the inhibition of mycolic acid incorporation into the cell wall and thus inhibits protein synthesis. The mechanism of action of pyrazinamide in the inhibition of TB is unknown. It can be either bacteriostatic or bactericidal, depending on the susceptibility of the particular *Mycobacterium* organism and the concentration of the drug attained at the site of infection.

NAD, nicotinamide adenine; *TB*, tuberculosis.

Indications

Antitubercular medications are indicated for the treatment of TB infections, including both pulmonary and extrapulmonary TB. Most antitubercular drug effects have not been fully tested in pregnant women. However, the combination of isoniazid and ethambutol has been used to treat pregnant women with clinically apparent TB, without teratogenic complications. Rifampin is another drug that is often safe during pregnancy; it is likely to be chosen to treat advanced TB.

Besides being used for the initial treatment of TB, antitubercular drugs have also proved effective in the management of treatment failures and relapses. Infection with species of *Mycobacterium* other than *M. tuberculosis* and atypical mycobacterial infections have also been successfully treated with these drugs. However, in general, antitubercular drugs are not as effective against other species of *Mycobacterium* as they are against MTB. Some of these other species that may be of particular concern in immunocompromised patients are *M. avium-intracellulare*, *M. flavescens*, *M. marinum*, and *M. kansasii*. Additional *Mycobacterium* infections that may respond to antitubercular drugs are those caused by *M. fortuitum*, *M. chelonae*, *M. smegmatis*, *M. xenopi*, and *M. scrofulaceum*. Treatment regimens for these non-TB mycobacterial infections often include the macrolide antibiotics clarithromycin or azithromycin (see Chapter 43), either alone or in combination with one or more antitubercular drugs.

In summary, antitubercular drugs are used primarily for the prophylaxis or treatment of TB. The effectiveness of these drugs depends on the type of infection, adequate dosing, sufficient duration of treatment, adherence to drug regimen, and the selection of an effective drug combination. The indications of the different antitubercular drugs are listed in Table 46-2.

Contraindications

Contraindications to the use of various antitubercular drugs include severe drug allergy and major kidney or liver dysfunction. However, it must be recognized that the urgency of treating a potentially fatal infection may have to be balanced against any prevailing contraindications. In extreme cases, patients are sometimes given a drug to which they have some degree of allergy, along with supportive care that enables them to at least tolerate the medication. Examples of such supportive care include treatment with antipyretics (e.g., acetaminophen), antihistamines (e.g., diphenhydramine hydrochloride), or even corticosteroids (e.g., prednisone or methylprednisolone).

One relative contraindication to ethambutol is optic neuritis. Chronic alcohol use, especially when associated with major liver damage, may also be a contraindication with any antitubercular drug. Other contraindications for specific drugs, if any, can be found in the drug profiles listed later in the chapter.

Adverse Effects

Antitubercular drugs are fairly well tolerated. Isoniazid, one of the mainstays of treatment, is noted for causing pyridoxine deficiency and liver toxicity. For this reason, supplements of pyridoxine (vitamin B_6; see Chapter 42) are often given concurrently with isoniazid, with a common oral dose being 25 mg daily. The most problematic drugs and their associated adverse effects are listed in Table 46-3.

Interactions

The drugs that can interact with antitubercular drugs can cause significant effects. See Table 46-4 for a listing of selected interactions. Besides these drug interactions,

---

TABLE 46-2

Antitubercular Drugs: Indications

Drug	Indications
amikacin sulphate	Used in combination with other antitubercular drugs in the treatment of clinical TB
ethambutol	First-line drug for treatment of TB
isoniazid	Used alone or in combination with other antitubercular drugs for treatment of pulmonary and extrapulmonary *M. tuberculosis* infection after failure of first-line drugs
pyrazinamide	Used with other antitubercular drugs in the treatment of clinical TB
rifabutin	Used to prevent or delay development of *M. avium-intracellulare* bacteremia and disseminated infections in patients with advanced HIV infection
rifampin	Used with other antitubercular drugs in the treatment of clinical TB
	Used in the treatment of diseases caused by mycobacteria other than *M. tuberculosis*
	Used for preventive therapy in patients exposed to isoniazid-resistant *M. tuberculosis*
	Used to eliminate meningococci from the nasopharynx of asymptomatic *Neisseria meningitidis* carriers when the risk of meningococcal meningitis is high
	Used for chemoprophylaxis in contacts of patients with Hib infection
	Used in the treatment of endocarditis caused by methicillin-resistant staphylococci, chronic staphylococcal prostatitis, and multiple-anti-infective–resistant pneumococci
streptomycin	Used in combination with other antitubercular drugs in the treatment of clinical TB and other mycobacterial diseases

Hib, *Haemophilus influenzae* type b; *HIV*, human immunodeficiency virus; *TB*, tuberculosis.

TABLE	46-3

Antitubercular Drugs: Common Adverse Effects

Drug	Adverse Effects
amikacin sulphate	Ototoxicity, nephrotoxicity
ethambutol	Retrobulbar neuritis, blindness
isoniazid	Peripheral neuropathy, hepatotoxicity, optic neuritis and visual disturbances, hyperglycemia
levofloxacin, moxiflozacin hydrochloride	Dizziness, headache, GI disturbances, visual disturbances, insomnia
pyrazinamide	Hepatotoxicity, hyperuricemia
rifabutin	GI tract disturbances, rash, neutropenia, red–orange–brown discoloration of urine, sweat, tears, sputum
rifampin	Hepatitis; hematological disorders; red–orange–brown discoloration of urine, tears, sweat, sputum
streptomycin	Ototoxicity, nephrotoxicity, blood dyscrasias

TABLE	46-4

Selected Antitubercular Drugs: Drug Interactions

Drug	Interacting Drugs	Mechanism	Results
isoniazid	Antacids	Reduce absorption	Decreased isoniazid levels
	rifampin	Has additive effects	Increased central nervous system and hepatotoxicity
	phenytoin, carbamazepine	Decrease metabolism	Increased phenytoin and carbamazepine effects
streptomycin	Nephrotoxic and neurotoxic drugs	Additive effects	Increased toxicity
	Oral anticoagulants	Alter intestinal flora	Increased bleeding tendencies
rifampin	β-Blockers, benzodiazepines, cyclosporine, oral anticoagulants, oral antihyperglycemics, oral contraceptives, phenytoin, quinidine sulphate, sirolimus, theophylline	Increase metabolism	Decreased therapeutic effects of these drugs

isoniazid can cause false-positive urine readings on urine glucose tests (e.g., Clinitest®) and an increase in the serum levels of the liver function enzymes alanine aminotransferase and aspartate aminotransferase.

Dosages

For the recommended dosages of selected antitubercular drugs, refer to the table on p. 876.

NURSING PROCESS

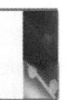 ## Assessment

Before administering any of the antitubercular drugs, to ensure the safe and effective use of these drugs, obtain a thorough medical history, medication profile, and nursing history. Perform a complete head-to-toe physical assessment. Note any specific history of diagnoses or symptoms of TB. Determine the results of the patient's last purified protein derivative (PPD), or tuberculin skin test, and the

reaction at the site of the intradermal injection. Review the most recent chest X-ray results. Assess the results of liver function studies (e.g., bilirubin level, liver enzyme levels) and kidney function studies (e.g., glomerular filtration rate, blood urea nitrogen [BUN], creatinine clearance). These values provide a comparative baseline throughout therapy. As noted earlier, major liver or kidney dysfunctions are contraindications to antitubercular drug therapy.

Because some drugs may lead to peripheral neuropathies, note baseline neurological functioning prior to therapy. Assess hearing status, especially when streptomycin is to be used, because of its drug-related ototoxicity. A gross eye examination is important due to the drug-induced adverse effects of visual disturbances and optic neuritis with isoniazid, and levofloxacin. Blindness may occur with the use of ethambutol.

Assessment of age is also important because the likelihood of adverse reactions and toxicity is increased in older adults due to age-related liver and kidney dysfunction. Additionally, the safety of antitubercular drugs in children 13 years of age or younger has not been established. Assess the patient's complete blood count before administering isoniazid, streptomycin, or rifampin because of

DRUG PROFILES

ethambutol hydrochloride

Ethambutol hydrochloride (Etibi®) is a first-line bacteriostatic drug used in the treatment of TB. It works by diffusing into the mycobacteria and suppressing ribonucleic acid (RNA) synthesis, which thereby inhibits protein synthesis. Ethambutol is included with isoniazid, pyrazinamide, and rifampin in many TB combination drug therapies. It may also be used to treat other mycobacterial diseases. It is contraindicated in patients with optic neuritis as it can both exacerbate and cause this condition, which can result in varying degrees of vision loss. Ethambutol is also contraindicated in children younger than 13 years of age. It is available only in oral form.

PHARMACOKINETICS

Route	Onset of Action	Peak Plasma Concentration	Elimination Half-Life	Duration of Action
PO	Variable	2–4 hr	3.5 hr	24 hr

▶▶isoniazid

Isoniazid (Isotamine®), abbreviated *INH*, is the mainstay in the treatment of TB and is also the most widely used antitubercular drug. It may be given as a single drug for prophylaxis or in combination with other antitubercular drugs for the treatment of active TB. It is a bactericidal drug that kills the mycobacteria by disrupting cell-wall synthesis and essential cellular functions. Isoniazid is metabolized in the liver through a process called *acetylation*, which requires a certain enzymatic pathway to break down the drug. However, some people have a genetic deficiency of the liver enzymes needed for this to occur. Such individuals are called **slow acetylators**. When isoniazid is taken by slow acetylators, the drug accumulates because there is not enough of the enzyme to break down the isoniazid. Therefore, the dosages of isoniazid may need to be adjusted downward in these patients.

Isoniazid is used in oral form. There is also a combination oral formulation of isoniazid, pyrazinamide, and rifampin (Rifater®). Isoniazid is contraindicated in those with previous isoniazid-associated liver injury or acute liver disease.

PHARMACOKINETICS

Route	Onset of Action	Peak Plasma Concentration	Elimination Half-Life	Duration of Action
PO	Variable	1–2 hr	1–4 hr	24 hr

pyrazinamide

Pyrazinamide (Tebrazid®) is an antitubercular drug that can be either bacteriostatic or bactericidal, depending on its concentration at the site of infection and the particular susceptibility of the mycobacteria. It is commonly used in combination with other antitubercular drugs for the treatment of TB. Its mechanism of action is unknown, but it is believed to work by inhibiting lipid and nucleic acid synthesis in the mycobacteria. Pyrazinamide is available in oral form. It is contraindicated in patients with severe liver disease or acute gout. In Canada, it is also not normally used in pregnant patients because of a lack of teratogenicity data, although it may be considered when there is resistance to isoniazid, rifampin, or ethambutol.

PHARMACOKINETICS

Route	Onset of Action	Peak Plasma Concentration	Elimination Half-Life	Duration of Action
PO	Variable	2 hr	9–10 hr	24 hr

rifabutin

Rifabutin (Mycobutin®) is the second drug discovered of three currently available rifamycin antibiotics, the others being rifampin and rifapentine. Rifabutin is a derivative of rifamycin. It is commonly used to prevent infections caused by *M. avium* complex, which includes several non-TB mycobacterial species; this is also the case with rifampin. A notable adverse effect of rifabutin is that it can turn urine, feces, saliva, skin, sputum, sweat, and tears a red–orange to red–brown colour. Rifabutin is currently available only for oral use. Rifapentine can be administered once a week because its half-life is five times longer than rifampin. However, its profile of effectiveness is not favourable and it is not recommended for treatment use in Canada. It is available only through Health Canada's Special Access Programme.

PHARMACOKINETICS

Route	Onset of Action	Peak Plasma Concentration	Elimination Half-Life	Duration of Action
PO	Variable	2–4 hr	16–69 hr	1 to several days

rifampin

Rifampin (Rifadin®, Rofact®) is the first drug discovered of the rifamycin class of synthetic macrocyclic antibiotics, which also includes rifabutin and rifapentine. The term *macrocyclic* connotes the large and complex hydrocarbon ring structure included in all the rifamycin compounds. Rifampin is the most potent antitubercular drug available. Its use shortens the length of the drug regimen to 9 months or less (if used in combination with pyrazinamide). Rifampin has activity against many *Mycobacterium* species, as well as against *Meningococcus*, *Haemophilus influenzae* type b, and *M. leprae*. It is a broad-spectrum bactericidal drug that kills the offending organism by inhibiting protein synthesis. Rifampin is available in oral formulations and, as previously mentioned, in combination with isoniazid and pyrazinamide (Rifater). Rifampin is contraindicated in patients with a known drug allergy to it or any other rifamycin. The drug is a potent enzyme inducer and is associated with many drug interactions (see Table 46-4). Rifampin may cause urine, saliva, tears, and sweat to be red–orange coloured.

PHARMACOKINETICS

Route	Onset of Action	Peak Plasma Concentration	Elimination Half-Life	Duration of Action
PO	Variable	2–4 hr	3.5 hr	Up to 24 hr

Continued

DRUG PROFILES—cont'd

streptomycin sulphate

Streptomycin sulphate is an aminoglycoside antibiotic. Introduced in 1944, it was the first drug that could effectively treat TB. Because of its toxicities and the pain associated with injections, it is used only as second-line therapy. Amikan sulphate is the preferred injectable drug and is recommended by the Canadian Thoracic Society. Streptomycin is currently available only in injectable form. It is usually not given to pregnant patients because of risk of fetal harm.

PHARMACOKINETICS

Route	Onset of Action	Peak Plasma Concentration	Elimination Half-Life	Duration of Action
IM	Variable	1–2 hr	2–3 hr	Up to 24 hr

DOSAGES   Selected Antitubercular Drugs

Drug	Pharmacological Class	Usual Dosage Range	Indications
ethambutol hydrochloride (Etibi)	Synthetic first-line antimycobacterial antibiotic	*Adults and adolescents over 13 yr* PO: 15–20 mg/kg/day; may also be divided in 2×/wk (max 2.5 g) and 3×/wk (max 2.5 g) dosage regimens with higher doses	Active TB
⇒isoniazid (Isotamine)	Synthetic first-line antimycobacterial antibiotic	*Children 12 yr and under or less than 35 kg* PO: 10–15 mg/kg/day (max 300 mg) or 20–30 mg/kg 3×/wk (max 600–900 mg/dose) *Adults* PO: 5 mg/kg daily (max 300 mg) or 10 mg/kg 3×/wk (max 600 mg/dose)	Active TB
pyrazinamide (Tebrazid)	Synthetic first-line antimycobacterial antibiotic	*Children and Adults* PO: 20–25 mg/kg/day (max 2 g) or 30–40 mg/kg 3×/wk (max 4 g) PO: 35 mg/kg/day (max 2 g) *Adults* PO: 20–25 mg/kg/day	Active TB
rifabutin (Mycobutin)	Semisynthetic second-line antimycobacterial antibiotic	*Adults* PO: 300 mg daily or 150 mg bid	Active TB
rifampin (Rifadin, Rofact)	Semisynthetic first-line antimycobacterial antibiotic	*Children* PO: 15 mg/kg daily (max 600 mg) or 10–20 mg/kg 3×/wk (max 600 mg) *Adults* PO: 10 mg/kg (max 600 mg) daily or 10 mg/kg 3×/wk (max 600 mg)	Active TB, latent TB in patients with advanced HIV

HIV, human immunodeficiency virus; *PO*, oral; *TB*, tuberculosis.

potential for drug-related hematological disorders. Kidney studies, such as creatinine clearance and BUN, may be ordered prior to therapy with streptomycin due to the nephrotoxicity associated with its use. Prior to the use of pyrazinamide, document uric acid baseline levels due to the possibility of the drug-induced adverse effect of hyperuricemia and subsequent symptoms of gout. Analysis of sputum specimens is usually ordered as well, to aid in determining the appropriate drug regimen. Contraindications, cautions, and drug interactions have been discussed previously.

🗹 Nursing Diagnoses

• Ineffective therapeutic regimen management by patient and family related to poor adherence with antitubercular drug therapy and lack of knowledge about long-term therapies

• Deficient knowledge related to the disease process and treatment protocol
• Risk for injury related to nonadherence with the drug therapy regimen and overall poor health status

🗹 Planning

🔳 Goals

• Patient will experience improved therapeutic regimen management and adherence.
  • Patient, patient's family, and others in the home environment will understand the disease process, methods of spread, and the need for the patient to remain on therapy, as prescribed.
• Patient will gain increased knowledge about antitubercular medication therapy and take medication regularly and for the length of time prescribed.

- Patient will remain free from injury related to nonadherence to antitubercular drugs.

■ Expected Patient Outcomes

- Patient shows improvement of disease state with adherence to the drug regimen, including a decrease in cough, fever, and sputum production; return of laboratory values to normal ranges; and no spread of infection to those in the home or surrounding environments.
  - Patient reports family support and lack of spread of infection to those in the home environment during antitubercular drug therapy.
- Patient states rationale for antitubercular drug therapy as well as anticipated adverse effects.
  - Patient takes medications as ordered and regularly, acknowledging that this will promote effective therapy and prevent complications, relapses, or recurrences.
  - Patient minimizes adverse effects by taking medication as prescribed.
  - Patient reports the following to the prescriber immediately: fever, increase in cough or sputum production, hearing loss, severe numbness or tingling of extremities, or altered vision.

■ Implementation

Because drug therapy is the mainstay of treatment for TB and often lasts for up to 24 months, patient education is critical, with special emphasis on adherence to the drug regimen. Provide simple, clear, and concise instructions to patients, with appropriate use of audiovisual aids and take-home information. Include in the education the fact that multiple drugs are often used to improve cure rates. Patients need to be able to state an understanding of all instructions. Because many patients affected by TB may be from other countries and cultures, it is important to have interpreter services available.

All antitubercular drugs need to be given exactly as ordered and at the same time every day. Consistent use and dosing around the clock are critical to maintaining steady blood levels and minimizing the chances of resistance to the drug therapy. Always emphasize to patients the need for strict adherence to the therapeutic regimen. Additionally, emphasize that the entire prescription must be finished over the prescribed time and as ordered by a health care provider, even if the patient is feeling better.

Although many drugs are given without food for maximum absorption, antitubercular drugs may need to be taken with food to minimize GI upset. Continuously monitor for any signs and symptoms of liver dysfunction, such as fatigue, jaundice, nausea, vomiting, dark urine, and anorexia; if any of these occur, notify the health care provider immediately. Also monitor kidney functioning (e.g., BUN, creatinine), and notify the health care provider if levels are altered. If vision changes occur (e.g., altered colour perception, changes in visual acuity),

in particular with ethambutol use, these changes must be reported immediately to the health care provider. Monitor uric acid levels during therapy, and advise patients to report any symptoms of gout such as hot, painful, or swollen joints of the big toe, knee, or ankle. In addition, the health care provider must be notified if there are signs and symptoms of peripheral neuropathy (e.g., numbness, burning, or tingling of extremities). Pyridoxine (vitamin B_6) may be beneficial for isoniazid-induced peripheral neuropathy. If the health care provider has ordered collection of sputum to test for acid-fast bacilli, it is best to obtain samples early in the morning. The most common order is for three consecutive morning specimens and a repeat specimen several weeks later. All drugs are to be taken as ordered and without any omission of doses for maximal therapeutic results.

Follow-up visits to the health care provider are important for monitoring therapeutic effects and observing for adverse effects and toxicity. If intravenous dosing of an antitubercular drug is ordered, use the appropriate diluent and infuse over the recommended time. Monitor the intravenous site every hour during the infusion for extravasation with possible tissue inflammation (e.g., redness, heat, swelling at the intravenous site). See the Patient Teaching tips for more information on antitubercular drugs.

Ethnocultural considerations associated with antitubercular drugs include those relating to patient and family education. When patients have active TB, thorough teaching of all family members is required and some family members may need prophylactic therapy with isoniazid for 9 months. Because some ethnocultural practices include living in tight-knit communities and close living quarters, this teaching is crucial to make sure the spread of this highly communicable disease is adequately prevented. All family members of patients with active TB, and others in close contact with them, must receive the same thorough instructions about maintaining their health and adhering to their medication regimens.

Health care facilities and individual health care workers are responsible for using effective TB infection prevention and control measures. Airborne precautions should be initiated immediately for suspected or confirmed TB. Respirators certified by the U.S. National Institute for Occupational Safety and Health (N95 or higher filter class) are to be used by health care providers who care for or transport patients with suspected or confirmed TB (Public Health Agency of Canada & Canadian Lung Association/Canadian Thoracic Society, 2014).

■ Evaluation

Always document a patient's response, or lack of response, to a therapeutic regimen. A therapeutic response to antitubercular therapy is reflected by a decrease in the symptoms of TB, such as cough and fever, and by weight gain. Along with improved clinical status, the results of laboratory studies (culture and sensitivity tests) and chest X-ray findings will aid in the confirmation of resolution of the infection. Goals and expected outcomes should continue to be monitored to confirm that the infection is being adequately treated and that the drug therapy is providing therapeutic relief without complications or toxicity and with minimal adverse effects. Also monitor patients for the occurrence of adverse reactions to antitubercular drugs, such as

hearing loss (related to ototoxicity); nephrotoxicity; seizure activity; altered vision or blindness; extreme GI upset; fatigue; nausea; vomiting; fever; jaundice; numbness, tingling, or burning of extremities; abdominal pain; and easy bruising. Family or others in close contact with patients with active TB should undergo further evaluation during and after the original patient's completion of therapy.

CASE STUDY

Antitubercular Drugs

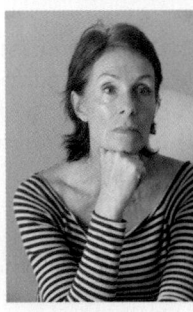

Monika, a 59-year-old homemaker, lives on a farm with her husband, Richard. Recently, she has been experiencing weight loss, night sweats, and a chronic cough. When she is given a purified protein derivative (PPD) test, the result is positive, and a chest X-ray indicates areas of consolidation characteristic of TB. She is hospitalized, and droplet transmission precautions are initiated to prevent the spread to others.

1. What is the next step in diagnosing the disease?

The physician orders that Monika be started on a four-drug regimen consisting of isoniazid, rifampin, pyrazin-

amide, and ethambutol until the final results of testing are obtained.

2. What is the purpose of the multiple drugs on this order?

3. What needs to be assessed before Monika begins this medication therapy?

Two weeks later, Monika is discharged. In addition to the current drug regime, she is given instructions to take pyridoxine (vitamin B₆).

4. Monika asks, "Can't I just take my regular multivitamin? Why do I need this one?" What is the nurse's best answer?

For answers, see http://evolve.elsevier.com/Canada/Lilley/pharmacology/.

PATIENT TEACHING TIPS

❖ During initial periods of the illness, instruct patients to make every effort to wash their hands frequently and cover their mouths when coughing or sneezing. Emphasize methods of proper disposal of secretions.

❖ Educate patients to take medications exactly as ordered by the health care provider, with attention to the need for long-term therapy and strict adherence to the drug regimen. Treatment may be ineffective if drugs are taken intermittently or stopped once the patient begins to feel better.

❖ Stress to patients the importance of follow-up appointments with the health care provider or health clinic so that the infection and therapeutic effectiveness of the drug regimen may be closely monitored.

❖ Instruct patients to avoid certain medications while taking antitubercular drugs, such as antacids, phenytoin, carbamazepine, β-blockers, benzodiazepines, oral anticoagulants, oral antihyperglycemic drugs, oral contraceptives, and theophylline. Inform the patient of all drug interactions prior to beginning therapy.

❖ Pyridoxine (vitamin B₆) may be indicated for patients taking isoniazid to prevent isoniazid-precipitated peripheral neuropathies and numbness, tingling, or burning of extremities.

❖ Educate patients taking isoniazid about the occurrence of the following adverse effects: numbness or tingling

of extremities, abdominal pain, jaundice, and visual changes.

❖ Advise patients taking rifampin to immediately report to a health care provider the occurrence of any of the following adverse effects: fever, nausea, vomiting, loss of appetite, jaundice, or unusual bleeding. These may indicate the possible occurrence of the adverse effects of hepatitis or various hematological disorders.

❖ Encourage patients to wear sunscreen and protective clothing during drug therapy to avoid ultraviolet light exposure. Drug-related photosensitivity reactions may be prevented by avoiding exposure to the sun.

❖ Women taking oral contraceptives who are prescribed rifampin should know that they must switch to another form of birth control. Oral contraceptives become ineffective when given with rifampin.

❖ Emphasize to patients the importance of proper rest, good sleep habits, adequate nutrition, and maintenance of general health.

❖ Advise patients to always keep antitubercular drugs and other medications out of the reach of children.

❖ Recommend that patients wear medical alert jewellery and carry a list at all times of allergies, medications, and medical conditions.

❖ Instruct patients to contact a health care provider immediately if they experience or observe any increase

PATIENT TEACHING TIPS—cont'd

in fatigue, cough, or sputum production; bloody sputum; chest pain; unusual bleeding; or yellowing of the skin or eyes.

❖ Patients taking rifampin or rifabutin may experience red–orange–brown discoloration of the skin, sweat,

tears, urine, feces, sputum, saliva, and tongue as an adverse effect of the drug. The discoloration reverses with discontinuation of the drug; however, contact lenses may be permanently stained.

KEY POINTS

❖ All antitubercular drugs are to be taken exactly as prescribed. Emphasize the importance of adherence to the therapeutic regimen and long-term dosing combined with healthy living practices.

❖ Therapeutic effects of antitubercular drugs include resolution of pulmonary and extrapulmonary MTB infections.

❖ Vitamin B_6 is needed to combat peripheral neuropathy associated with isoniazid.

❖ Counsel women taking oral contraceptive therapy who are prescribed rifampin about the need to use other forms of birth control.

❖ Educate patients about the importance of strict adherence to the drug regimen for improvement or cure of the condition. Provide instructions and education in various formats, including information about drug interactions and the need to avoid alcohol while taking any of the antitubercular medications.

EXAMINATION REVIEW QUESTIONS

1. The nurse is teaching a patient who is starting antitubercular therapy with rifampin. Which adverse effects would the nurse expect to see?
   a. Headache and neck pain
   b. Gynecomastia
   c. Red–brown urine
   d. Numbness or tingling of extremities

2. During antitubercular therapy with isoniazid, the patient receives another prescription for pyridoxine hydrochloride. Which statement by the nurse best explains the rationale for this second medication?
   a. "This vitamin will help to improve your energy levels."
   b. "This vitamin helps to prevent neurological adverse effects."
   c. "This vitamin works to protect your heart from toxic effects."
   d. "This vitamin helps to reduce GI adverse effects."

3. The nurse is counselling a woman who is beginning antitubercular therapy with rifampim. The patient also takes an oral contraceptive. Which statement by the nurse is most accurate regarding potential drug interactions?
   a. "You will need to switch to another form of birth control while you are taking rifampin."
   b. "Your birth control pills will remain effective while you are taking rifampin."
   c. "You will need to take a stronger dose of birth control pills while you are on rifampin."
   d. "You will need to abstain from sexual intercourse while on rifampin to avoid pregnancy."

4. When counselling a patient who has been newly diagnosed with TB, the nurse will make sure that the patient realizes that he is contagious for what period?
   a. During all phases of the illness
   b. Any time up to 18 months after therapy
   c. During the postictal phase of TB
   d. During the initial period of the illness until two consecutive culture specimens are negative

5. While monitoring a patient taking antitubercular drugs, the nurse knows that a therapeutic response to medication would be indicated by which improvement in the patient's condition?
   a. The patient states that she is feeling much better.
   b. The patient's laboratory test results show a lower white blood cell count.
   c. The patient reports a decrease in cough and night sweats.
   d. There is a decrease in symptoms, along with improved chest X-ray and sputum culture results.

6. The nurse is monitoring for liver toxicity in a patient who has been receiving long-term isoniazid therapy. Manifestations of liver toxicity include which of the following? (Select all that apply.)
   a. Orange discoloration of sweat and tears
   b. Darkened urine
   c. Dizziness
   d. Fatigue
   e. Visual disturbances
   f. Jaundice

7. The order for isoniazid reads: "Give 5 mg/kg PO daily." The patient weighs 275 lb. What is the amount per dose? Is this a safe dose?

CRITICAL THINKING ACTIVITIES

1. The nurse is reviewing medication therapy with a patient who has been newly diagnosed with TB. The patient asks, "How will the doctors know when I'm better? Will I have this disease forever?" What are the priorities when answering the patient's questions?

2. A 28-year-old health care worker has been diagnosed with active TB. She will be taking rifampin and is reviewing her current list of medications with the office nurse and asks, "I use birth control because we really don't want children right now. Can I still use 'the pill'?" What is the priority when answering her questions?

3. Peter, a 48-year-old businessman, has been taking rifampin as part of therapy for TB. He has been told that his bodily secretions will turn a red–orange–brown colour, and he asks, "What about my contact lenses? I can still wear them, right?" What is the nurse's best answer?

For answers, see http://evolve.elsevier.com/Canada/Lilley/pharmacology/.

CHAPTER 47

Antifungal Drugs

Objectives

After reading this chapter, the successful student will be able to do the following:

1. Identify the various antifungal drugs.

2. Describe the mechanisms of action, indications, contraindications, routes of administration, adverse and toxic effects, and drug interactions associated with the various antifungal drugs.

3. Develop a collaborative plan of care that includes all phases of the nursing process for patients receiving antifungal drugs.

e-Learning Activities

Website
(http://evolve.elsevier.com/Canada/Lilley/pharmacology/)

evolve

- Answer Key—Textbook Case Studies
- Answer Key—Critical Thinking Activities
- Chapter Summaries—Printable
- Review Questions for Exam Preparation
- Unfolding Case Studies

Drug Profiles

▸▸ amphotericin B, p. 886
  caspofungin (caspofungin acetate*), p. 886
▸▸ fluconazole, p. 886
  nystatin, p. 886
  terbinafine (terbinafine hydrochloride*), p. 886
  voriconazole, p. 886

▸▸ Key drug

*Full generic name is given in parentheses. For the purposes of this text, the more common, shortened name is used.

Key Terms

Antimetabolite A drug that either is a receptor antagonist or resembles a normal human metabolite and interferes with its function in the body, usually by competing for the metabolite's usual receptors or enzymes. (p. 882)

Dermatophytes Several fungi that are often found in soil and infect the skin, nails, or hair of humans. (p. 882)

Ergosterol The main sterol in fungal membranes (See *sterols*, below). (p. 883)

Fungi A large, diverse group of eukaryotic microorganisms that require an external carbon source and that form a plant structure known as a *thallus*. Fungi consist of yeasts and moulds. (p. 882)

Moulds Multicellular fungi characterized by long, branching filaments called *hyphae*, which entwine to form a complex branched structure known as a *mycelium*. (p. 882)

Mycosis Generally, any fungal infection. (p. 882)

Pathological fungi Fungi that cause mycoses. (p. 882)

Sterols Substances in the cell membranes of fungi to which polyene antifungal drugs bind. (p. 883)

Yeasts Single-celled fungi that reproduce by budding. (p. 882)

FUNGAL INFECTIONS

Fungi comprise a large and diverse group of microorganisms that includes all yeasts and moulds. **Yeasts** are single-celled fungi that reproduce by *budding* (in which a daughter cell forms by pouching out of and breaking off from a mother cell). These organisms have common practical uses in baking breads and preparing alcoholic beverages. **Moulds** are multicellular and are characterized by long, branching filaments. Some fungi are part of the normal flora of the skin, mouth, intestines, and vagina.

An infection caused by a fungus is called a **mycosis**. A variety of fungi can cause clinically significant infections or *mycoses*. These are called **pathological fungi**, and the infections they cause range in severity from infections with annoying symptoms (e.g., athlete's foot) to systemic mycoses that can become life-threatening. These infections are acquired by various routes—fungi can be ingested orally; can grow on or in the skin, hair, or nails; and, if the fungal spores are airborne, can be inhaled. There are four general types of mycotic infections: *systemic, cutaneous, subcutaneous,* and *superficial*. The latter three are infections of various layers of the *integumentary* system (skin, hair, and nails). Fungi that cause integumentary infections are known as **dermatophytes**, and such infections are known as *dermatomycoses*. The most severe systemic fungal infections generally affect people whose host immune defences are compromised. Commonly, these are patients who have received organ transplants and are taking immunosuppressive drug therapy, cancer patients who are immunocompromised as the result of chemotherapy, patients with autoimmune diseases receiving immunosuppressants, and patients with AIDS. In addition, the use of antibiotics, antineoplastics, or immunosuppressants such as corticosteroids may result in colonization by *Candida albicans*, followed by the development of a systemic infection. When the infection affects the mouth, it is referred to as *oral candidiasis*, or thrush. Thrush is common in newborns and patients who are immunocompromised. Vaginal candidiasis, commonly called a *yeast infection*, often affects women who are pregnant, have diabetes, are taking antibiotics, or are taking oral contraceptives. Most yeast infections are not contagious; however, *C. albicans* can be transmitted from mother to child during childbirth and occasionally during sexual intercourse. The characteristics of some of the systemic and cutaneous mycotic infections are summarized in Table 47-1.

ANTIFUNGAL DRUGS

Drugs used to treat fungal infections are called *antifungal drugs*. Systemic mycotic infections and some cutaneous or subcutaneous mycoses are treated with oral or parenteral drugs. Antifungals comprise a fairly small group of drugs. There are few such drugs because the fungi that cause these infections have proved to be difficult to kill, and research into new and improved drugs has occurred

at a slow pace. One difficulty is that often the chemical concentrations required for experimental drugs to be effective cannot be tolerated by humans. The drugs that have proved successful in the treatment of systemic mycoses as well as severe dermatomycoses include amphotericin B, caspofungin, clotrimazole, fluconazole, itraconazole, ketoconazole, micafungin sodium, miconazole, nystatin, posaconazole, anidulafungin, ravuconazole (in clinical III trials), terbinafine, and voriconazole. These drugs are the focus of this chapter.

Topical antifungal drugs are the most commonly used drugs in this class and are often administered without a prescription for the treatment of dermatomycoses as well as oral and vaginal mycoses. Although topical drug therapy is usually sufficient for these conditions, systemic oral medications are sometimes used, especially for more severe or recurrent cases. Antifungal drugs available for topical use are discussed further in Chapter 56. One antifungal drug, griseofulvin, is individually listed and is not specifically classified according to its chemical structures. The remaining drugs currently include four specific chemical classes: *polyenes* (amphotericin B and nystatin), *imidazoles* (ketoconazole), *triazoles* (fluconazole, itraconazole, voriconazole, and posaconazole), and the *echinocandins* (caspofungin, micafungin sodium, and anidulafungin). The imidazoles and triazoles are sometimes referred to by the more general term *azole antifungals*. Also included in some of these classes are drugs for topical use.

Mechanism of Action and Drug Effects

The mechanisms of action of the various antifungal drugs differ between drug subclasses. Flucytosine, also known as *5-fluorocytosine* (5-FC), available through the Special Access Programme, Health Canada, acts in much the same way as antiviral drugs. It is an **antimetabolite**, which is a drug that disrupts critical cellular metabolic pathways of the fungal cell. Once inside a susceptible fungal cell, the drug is deaminated by the enzyme *cytosine deaminase* to 5-fluorouracil (5-FU). Because human cells do not have this enzyme, they are not harmed by this antimetabolite. Once the 5-FU is generated inside the fungal cell, it interferes with fungal deoxyribonucleic acid (DNA) synthesis, which results in the inhibition of cell growth and reproduction and cell death. 5-FU is also available as an antineoplastic (anticancer) drug and is discussed in more detail in Chapter 52.

Griseofulvin, like flucytosine, is one of the older types of antifungal drugs. It works by preventing susceptible fungi from reproducing. It enters the fungal cell through an energy-dependent transport system and inhibits fungal mitosis (cell division) by binding to key structures known as *microtubules*. It has also been proposed that griseofulvin causes the production of defective DNA, which is then unable to replicate. Although griseofulvin and flucytosine are still currently available in the Canadian market, their clinical use has largely been supplanted by the newer antifungal drug classes.

TABLE 47-1

Mycotic Infections

Mycosis	Fungus	Endemic Location	Reservoir	Transmission	Primary Tissue Affected
SYSTEMIC INFECTION					
Aspergillosis	*Aspergillus* spp.	Universal	Soil	Inhalation	Lungs
Blastomycosis	*Blastomyces dermatitidis*	North America	Soil, animal droppings	Inhalation	Lungs
Candidiasis	*Candida albicans, glabrata, krusei, tropicalisis, parapsilosis*	Universal	Humans	Direct contact, overgrowth in response to treatment with antibiotic to which it is nonsusceptible	Blood, lungs
Coccidioidomycosis	*Coccidioides immitis*	Great Lakes, Canada	Soil, dust	Inhalation	Lungs
Cryptococcosis	*Cryptococcus neoformans*	Universal	Soil, birds, and chicken	Inhalation	Lungs, meninges of brain
Histoplasmosis	*Histoplasma capsulatum*	Universal	Soil, birds, and chickens	Inhalation	Lungs
CUTANEOUS INFECTION					
Candidiasis	*Candida albicans*	Universal	Humans	Direct contact, overgrowth in response to treatment with antibiotic to which it is susceptible	Mucous membrane, skin disseminated (may be systemic)
Dermatophytosis, tinea	*Epidermophyton* spp., *Microsporum* spp., *Trichophyton* spp.	Universal	Humans	Direct and indirect contact with infected persons	Scalp, skin (e.g., groin, feet)
Tinea versicolor	*Malassezia furfur*	Universal	Humans	Unknown*	Skin

Spp, species.
*Malassezia spp. are a usual part of the normal human flora and appear to cause infection only in select individuals.

The polyenes (amphotericin B and nystatin) act by binding to **sterols** in the cell membranes of fungi. The main sterol in fungal membranes is **ergosterol**. Human cell membranes have cholesterol instead of ergosterol. Because polyene antifungals have a strong chemical affinity for ergosterol instead of cholesterol, they do not bind to human cell membranes and therefore do not kill human cells. Once the polyene drug molecule binds to the ergosterol, a channel forms in the fungal cell membrane that allows potassium and magnesium ions to leak out of the fungal cell. This loss of ions causes fungal cellular metabolism to be altered, which leads to the death of the cell. Imidazoles and triazoles (ketoconazole, fluconazole, itraconazole, voriconazole, and posaconazole) act as either fungistatic or fungicidal drugs, depending on their concentration in the fungus. They are most effective in combatting rapidly growing fungi and work by inhibiting fungal cell cytochrome P450 enzymes. These enzymes are needed to produce ergosterol. The allylamine terbinafine is believed to act by a similar mechanism. When the production of ergosterol is inhibited, other sterols called *methylsterols* are produced instead, which results in a defect similar to that caused by the polyene antifungals, namely a leaky cell membrane that allows needed electrolytes to escape. The fungal cells die because they cannot carry on cellular metabolism. They are referred to as "hole-punchers" because of this mechanism of action.

The echinocandins (caspofungin, anidulafungin sodium, and micafungin) act by preventing the synthesis of *glucans*, essential components of fungal cell walls that are not present in mammalian cells. This also contributes to fungal cell death. Some of the fungi that are susceptible to these drugs are the pathogens involved in the mycoses listed in Table 47-1.

Indications

Indications for the use of the various antifungal drugs are specific to the drugs. The adverse effects of the newer antifungals are fewer and less serious than those of the older drugs. However, the drug of choice for the treatment of many severe systemic fungal infections remains one of the oldest antifungals, amphotericin B, which does have major adverse effects. Amphotericin B is effective against a wide range of fungi and is used to treat aspergillosis, blastomycosis, candidiasis, coccidioidomycosis, cryptococcosis, fungal endocarditis, histoplasmosis, zygomycosis, fungal septicemia, and many other systemic fungal infections. The activity of nystatin is similar to that of amphotericin B, but its usefulness is limited because of its toxic effects when given in the doses required to accomplish the same antifungal actions as amphotericin B. It is also not available in a parenteral form. Nystatin is most commonly used to treat oropharyngeal candidiasis, or thrush and candidal diaper dermatitis.

Fluconazole and itraconazole are synthetic azole antifungals. Fluconazole can pass into the cerebrospinal fluid (CSF) and inhibit the growth of cryptococcal fungi. This makes it effective in the treatment of cryptococcal meningitis. Both fluconazole and itraconazole are active against oropharyngeal and esophageal *Candida* infections. Itraconazole has poor CSF penetration but can be widely distributed throughout other areas of the body. It is indicated for the treatment of fungal infections in immunocompromised and nonimmunocompromised patients with disseminated candidiasis, histoplasmosis, blastomycosis, and aspergillosis. Ketoconazole inhibits many dermatophytes and fungi that cause systemic mycoses, but it is not active against *Aspergillus* organisms or *Phycomycetes* (common moulds) such as *Mucor* species (spp.). Fortunately, the newest triazole antifungal drug, voriconazole, does have activity against some of these more tenacious fungi, including *Aspergillus* spp. causing invasive infection, *Scedosporium* spp., and *Fusarium* spp.

Of the azole antifungals, fluconazole is the most effective for combating serious infections with *Candida*, *Cryptococcus*, *Blastomyces*, and *Histoplasma* organisms. Fluconazole is also used as prophylaxis to decrease the incidence of candidiasis in patients undergoing bone marrow transplantation who also receive cytotoxic chemotherapy or radiation therapy.

Griseofulvin inhibits dermatophytes of *Microsporum*, *Trichophyton*, and *Epidermophyton* spp. It has no effect on filamentous fungi such as *Aspergillus*, yeasts such as *Candida* spp., or dimorphic species such as *Histoplasma*. Terbinafine is a synthetic allylamine derivative used in an oral form for treatment of *onychomycoses*, fungal infections of the fingernails or toenails. The imidazole itraconazole is also sometimes used for this purpose. Topical forms of terbinafine are also used for various skin infections (see Chapter 56). The duration and frequency of topical treatment varies with the indication and is dependent on the severity of the infection.

Contraindications

Drug allergy, liver failure, kidney failure, and porphyria (for griseofulvin) are the most common contraindications for antifungal drugs. Itraconazole should not be used to treat onychomycoses in patients with severe heart problems. Prior treatment with itraconazole may reduce or inhibit the activity of polyenes such as amphotericin B. Voriconazole can cause fetal harm in pregnant women.

Adverse Effects

The major adverse effects caused by antifungal drugs are encountered most commonly in conjunction with amphotericin B treatment. Drug interactions and hepatotoxicity are the primary concerns in patients receiving other antifungal drugs, but the intravenous (IV) administration of amphotericin B is associated with a multitude of adverse effects. The most common and problematic of the adverse effects of the various antifungal drugs are listed in Table 47-2. With amphotericin B treatment in particular, health care providers commonly order various premedications (including antiemetics, antihistamines, antipyretics, and corticosteroids) to prevent or minimize infusion-related

---

TABLE 47-2

Selected Antifungal Drugs: Common Adverse Effects and Cautions

Body System	Adverse Effects	Caution
AMPHOTERICIN B (Systemic)		
Cardiovascular	Cardiac dysrhythmias	Recheck dosage and type of amphotericin B being administered
Central nervous	Neurotoxicity, tinnitus, visual disturbances, paresthesias, convulsions	
Kidneys	Kidney toxicity, potassium loss, hypomagnesemia	
Pulmonary	Pulmonary infiltrates	
Other (infusion related)	Fever, chills, headache, malaise, nausea, hypotension (occasionally), gastrointestinal upset, anemia	
CASPOFUNGIN (Systemic)		
Central nervous	Fever, chills, headache	Adjust dose for patients with liver dysfunction
Cardiovascular	Hypotension, peripheral edema, tachycardia	
Gastrointestinal	Nausea, vomiting, diarrhea, hepatotoxicity	
Hematologic	Decreased hemoglobin and hematocrit, leukopenia, anemia	
Integumentary	Rash, facial edema, itching	

TABLE 47-2

Selected Antifungal Drugs: Common Adverse Effects and Cautions—cont'd

Body System	Adverse Effects	Caution
VORICONAZOLE (Systemic)		
Central nervous	Hallucinations	
Gastrointestinal	Nausea, vomiting	
Hepatic	Increased liver enzyme levels	
Integumentary	Rash	
Other	Photophobia, hypokalemia	
FLUCONAZOLE (Systemic)		
Gastrointestinal	Nausea, vomiting, diarrhea, stomach pain	Use with caution in patients with kidney or liver dysfunction
Other	Increased liver enzymes, dizziness	
NYSTATIN (Topical)		
Gastrointestinal	Nausea, vomiting, anorexia, diarrhea, cramps	Local irritation may occur
Integumentary	Rash, urticaria	
TERBINAFINE (Systemic, Topical)		
Central nervous	Headache, dizziness	Rarely causes irritation
Gastrointestinal	Nausea, vomiting, diarrhea	
Integumentary	Rash, pruritus	
Other	Alopecia, fatigue	

TABLE 47-3

Antifungal Drugs: Drug Interactions

Drug	Possible Effects
AMPHOTERICIN B	
Digitalis glycosides	Amphotericin B–induced hypokalemia may increase the potential for digitalis toxicity
Nephrotoxic drug	Additive nephrotoxicity
Thiazide diuretics	Severe hypokalemia or decreased adrenal cortex response to corticotropin
FLUCONAZOLE, ITRACONAZOLE	
cyclosporine, phenytoin, sirolimus	Increased plasma concentrations of both drugs
Oral anticoagulants	Increased effects of anticoagulants
Oral antihyperglycemics	Reduced metabolism of antihyperglycemic drugs
Statins	Reduced metabolism of statins, increased toxicity
VORICONAZOLE	
quinidine sulphate	Prolongation of QT interval on electrocardiogram

reactions. The likelihood of such reactions can also be reduced by using longer-than-average drug infusion times (i.e., 2 to 6 hours) with this particular drug.

Interactions

There are many important drug interactions associated with antifungal drugs, some of which can be life-threatening. A common underlying source of the problem is that many of the antifungal drugs, as well as other drugs, are metabolized by the cytochrome P450 enzyme system. The result of the coadministration of two drugs that are both broken down by this system is that they compete for a limited number of enzymes, and one of the drugs ends up accumulating in the body. Key drug interactions for the systemic antifungal drugs are summarized in Table 47-3.

Dosages

For the dosage information on selected antifungal drugs, refer to the table on p. 887.

⇨ amphotericin B

Amphotericin B (Fungizone®) remains one of the drugs of choice for the treatment of severe systemic mycoses. The main drawback of amphotericin B therapy is that the drug causes many adverse effects. Almost all patients given the drug intravenously experience infusion syndrome often referred to as the "shake and bake" syndrome including fever, chills, hypotension, tachycardia, malaise, muscle and joint pain, anorexia, nausea and vomiting, and headache. For this reason, pretreatment with antipyretics, antihistamines, antiemetics, and corticosteroids is common to decrease the severity of the infusion-related reaction.

Lipid formulations of amphotericin B were developed in an attempt to decrease the incidence of adverse effects and increase its efficacy; however, lipid formulations may not achieve optimal concentrations within tissues due to its lower volume of distribution. There are currently three lipid preparations of amphotericin B: amphotericin B lipid complex (Abelcet®), amphotericin B cholesteryl complex (Fungizone), and liposomal amphotericin B (AmBisome®).

Amphotericin B is contraindicated in patients who have a known hypersensitivity to it and in those with severe bone marrow suppression or kidney impairment. However, patients who have life-threatening fungal infections may still be treated with this drug if cultures indicate that no other drug will kill the infection. The drug is available only in injectable form. Often a 1-mg test dose is given over 20 to 30 minutes to see if the patient will tolerate the drug. It has been used as a local irrigant (in the bladder) for the treatment of candidal cystitis and has been used intrapleurally and intraperitoneally for the treatment of fungal infections in these body cavities.

PHARMACOKINETICS

Route	Onset of Action	Peak Plasma Concentration	Elimination Half-Life	Duration of Action
IV	Variable	1 hr	1–15 days	18–24 hr

caspofungin acetate

Caspofungin acetate (Cancidas®) was the first echinocandin antifungal drug, approved in 2003. It is used for treatment of severe *Aspergillus* infection (invasive aspergillosis) in patients who are intolerant of or have infections refractory to other drugs. Caspofungin doses need to be reduced in patients with impaired liver function. This drug is available only in injectable form. Two additional echinocandins, micafungin sodium (Mycamine®) and anidulafungin (Eraxis®) have since been approved.

PHARMACOKINETICS

Route	Onset of Action	Peak Plasma Concentration	Elimination Half-Life	Duration of Action
IV	Unknown	1 hr	9–50 hr	Unknown

⇨ fluconazole

Fluconazole (Diflucan®) has proved to be a significant improvement in the area of antifungal treatment. It has a much better adverse-effect profile than that of amphotericin B, and it also has excellent coverage against many fungi. In fact, it is often preferred to amphotericin B because of these qualities. Since oral fluconazole has excellent bioavailability—which means that almost the entire dose administered is absorbed into the circulation—

the daily dose for oral tablets, suspension, and IV administration is the same. Administration of a loading dose on the first day of treatment, consisting of twice the usual daily dose, results in plasma concentrations that are close to a steady state by the second day.

PHARMACOKINETICS

Route	Onset of Action	Peak Plasma Concentration	Elimination Half-Life	Duration of Action
PO	1 hr	1–2 hr	22–30 hr	Variable

nystatin

Nystatin is a polyene antifungal drug that is often applied topically for the treatment of candidal diaper rash, taken orally as prophylaxis against candidal infections during periods of neutropenia in patients receiving immunosuppressive therapy, and used for the treatment of oral and vaginal candidiasis. It is not available in a parenteral form but is available as an oral suspension, topical cream, vaginal cream, and vaginal suppository. It is also available with metronidazole (Flagyl®) in a vaginal ovule or topical cream (Flagystatin®) for the treatment of mixed *Trichomonas vaginalis* and *C. albicans* infections. Nystatin ointments and creams are available over the counter.

PHARMACOKINETICS

Route	Onset of Action	Peak Plasma Concentration	Elimination Half-Life	Duration of Action
PO	24 hr	2 hr	Unknown	Unknown

terbinafine hydrochloride

Terbinafine hydrochloride (Lamisil®) is classified as an allylamine antifungal drug and is currently the only drug in its class. It is available in a topical cream and spray for treating superficial dermatological infections, including *tinea pedis* (athlete's foot), *tinea cruris* (jock itch), and *tinea corporis* (ringworm). A tablet form is also available for systemic use and is used primarily to treat onychomycoses of the fingernails or toenails.

PHARMACOKINETICS

Route	Onset of Action	Peak Plasma Concentration	Elimination Half-Life	Duration of Action
PO	Unknown	1–2 hr	22–26 hr	Unknown

voriconazole

Voriconazole (Vfend®) is used for treating severe fungal infections caused by *Aspergillus* spp. (invasive aspergillosis). It is also used for the treatment of systemic *Candida* in patients with normal neutrophil values as well as *Candida* infections of the skin, abdomen, kidney, bladder wall, and wounds. Therapy must be initiated with the specified loading dose regimen of either IV or oral voriconazole to achieve adequate plasma concentrations on the first day of therapy. Voriconazole is contraindicated in patients with a known drug allergy to it and in patients taking certain other drugs metabolized by the cytochrome P450 enzyme CYP3A4 (e.g., quinidine sulphate) because of the risk for induction of serious cardiac dysrhythmias. It is also the only antifungal drug contraindicated in pregnancy. The drug is available in oral and injectable forms.

PHARMACOKINETICS

Route	Onset of Action	Peak Plasma Concentration	Elimination Half-Life	Duration of Action
PO	Unknown	1–2 hr	Variable	Unknown

DOSAGES   Selected Antifungal Drugs

Drug	Pharmacological Class	Usual Dosage Range	Indications
▸amphotericin B (Fungizone)	Polyene antifungal	*Adults and children* IV: initial daily dose, 0.25 mg/kg; titrate up to 1–1.5 mg/kg/day	Broad spectrum of systemic fungal infections
amphotericin B lipid complex (ABLC); doses vary with product as follows: Abelcet AmBisome Amphotec	Polyene antifungal	*Adults and children* IV: 5 mg/kg once daily, infused at 2.5 mg/kg/hr IV: 3–6 mg/kg/day, infused over 1–2 hr IV: 3–4 mg/kg/day, infused at 1 mg/kg/ hr	Systemic fungal infections
caspofungin (Cancidas)	Echinocandin antifungal	*Adults* IV: 70 mg loading dose on day 1, followed by 50 mg/day thereafter; infuse doses over 1 hr	Invasive aspergillosis in patients who do not tolerate or respond to other drugs
▸fluconazole (Diflucan)	Synthetic triazole antifungal	*Children* IV/PO: 6–12 mg/kg/day 10–12 wk after negative CSF cultures *Adults* IV/PO: 200–400 mg daily × minimum of 10 wk after negative CSF culture results	Cryptococcal meningitis
		Children IV/PO: 3–12 mg/kg, (dose and duration depend on severity of infection) *Adults* IV/PO: 100–400 mg/day × 2–5 wk (dose and duration depend on severity of infection)	Oropharyngeal and esophageal candidiasis, systemic candidiasis
nystatin	Polyene antifungal	*Infants* PO: 100 000 units oral suspension dropped on tongue, held, and then swallowed tid–qid *Adults and children* PO: 400 000–600 000 units oral suspension (for children, dropped on tongue, held, and then swallowed) in oral cavity qid	Oral candidiasis, intestinal moniliasis
		Adults PO (tab): 500 000–1 000 000 units tid	Intestinal candidiasis
		Topical (cream, lotion, or powder): apply bid	Topical candidiasis
		Vaginal: insert one vaginal tablet or applicator of cream once to twice daily × 2 wk	Vaginal candidiasis
terbinafine hydrochloride (Lamisil)	Synthetic allylamine antifungal	*Adults* PO: 250 mg/day × 2–6 wk	Onychomycosis (fungal infection of finger- or toenails)
		Topical cream or solution: apply bid to affected area × 1–2 wk	Athlete's foot (tinea pedis), jock itch (tinea cruris), ringworm (tinea corporis)
voriconazole (Vfend)	Synthetic triazole antifungal	*Adults 40 kg and over* PO: loading dose of 400 mg × 2 doses q12h, then 200 mg bid maintenance *Adults less than 40 kg* PO: loading dose of 200 mg × 2 doses q12h, then 100 mg bid maintenance IV: loading dose of 6 mg/kg/ mL × 2 doses q12h, then 3–4 mg/kg bid	Invasive aspergillosis; candidemia and other invasive candidiasis

CSF, cerebrospinal fluid; *IV*, intravenous; *PO*, oral.

NURSING PROCESS

✐ Assessment

Although topical dosage methods are discussed in detail in Chapter 56, it is important to discuss all antifungal dosage forms and related nursing processes. Before initiation of therapy with antifungals, assess and document vital signs, weight, complete blood count (CBC) with differential, liver and kidney function tests, and culture and sensitivity test results.

Before administering amphotericin B (or any other antifungal drug), identify any contraindications, cautions, and drug interactions (see Tables 47-2 and 47-3). Baseline kidney function studies are generally ordered as well as liver function tests, due to adverse effects of nephrotoxicity and hepatotoxicity. Avoid any concurrent administration of nephrotoxic drugs if at all possible. There is a risk for severe adverse reactions (e.g., cardiac dysrhythmias, headache, chills, malaise, nausea, hypotension, anemia, gastrointestinal [GI] upset) with IV amphotericin B administration. Perform an assessment of any special premedication orders for the use of antiemetics, antihistamines, antipyretics, and anti-inflammatory drugs prior to giving amphotericin B. Bone marrow suppression is another contraindication to the use of amphotericin B.

Caspofungin requires careful assessment of blood pressure, pulse rate, liver function, red blood cell (RBC) counts, and white blood cell counts due to potential drug-induced adverse effects of hypotension, tachycardia, and hepatotoxicity. Fluconazole requires close assessment of pre-existing GI problems and kidney and liver functioning due to drug-induced adverse effects impacting these systems. See Tables 47-2 and 47-3 for more information about specific adverse effects and drug interactions for all antifungals.

✐ Nursing Diagnoses

- Acute pain related to symptoms of the infectious process
- Deficient knowledge related to a lack of information about and experience with antifungal drug therapy
- Risk for injury related to adverse effects of the medication regimen

✐ Planning

■ Goals

- Patient will have minimal to no pain after therapy has been initiated.
- Patient will gain increased knowledge about the antifungal drug, its use, and its adverse effects.

- Patient will experience minimal to no injury to self as related to the adverse effects of antifungal therapy.

■ Expected Patient Outcomes

- Patient is free of pain associated with the fungal infection once therapy is initiated.
  - Patient's fever and discomfort associated with the infection decreases with therapy.
  - Patient experiences improved health status, energy, and well-being.
- Patient demonstrates adequate knowledge about medication regimen by following directions about when and how to take the antifungal drug.
  - Patient experiences minimal to no adverse effects of drug therapy and reports to the health care provider any nausea, vomiting, or GI upset that becomes unmanageable.
  - Patient remains adherent with the medication regimen, not skipping doses while experiencing relief from the infection, and experiences a return to normal vital signs and negative findings on culture and sensitivity tests after the full course of therapy.
  - Patient experiences improved appetite, energy level, physical strength, and stamina after taking antifungal drugs for the prescribed period.
- Patient experiences minimal to no injury to self and is able to manage adverse effects or contacts the health care provider if they become problematic.
  - Patient takes medication as prescribed.
  - Patient returns to the health care provider regularly as recommended for monitoring of the infection and of drug therapy with various blood tests (e.g., CBC with differential, RBC count, hemoglobin level, hematocrit, kidney and liver function tests).

✐ Implementation

The nursing interventions appropriate for patients receiving antifungal drugs vary depending on the particular drug. With IV amphotericin B, do not administer solutions that are cloudy or have precipitates. Use of an IV infusion pump is recommended. Once the IV infusion has begun, monitor vital signs every 15 minutes, or as needed, to assess for adverse reactions, such as cardiac dysrhythmias, visual disturbances, paresthesias (numbness or tingling of the hands or feet), respiratory difficulty, pain, fever, chills, and nausea (see Table 47-2 for a listing of adverse effects). If a severe reaction occurs (e.g., exacerbation of adverse effects or a decline in vital signs), discontinue the infusion while continuing to closely monitor the patient, and contact the health care provider immediately. Monitor the IV site for signs of phlebitis (e.g., heat, pain, and redness over the vein). Continuously monitor all laboratory values during therapy (see earlier discussion). During long-term or at-home therapy, document weight frequently, as indicated. A gain of 1 kg or more in a 24-hour period or 2.3 kg or more in 1 week may indicate possible medication-induced kidney damage and the need for prompt medical attention. Follow manufacturer guidelines and the health care provider's orders for specific solutions and rates of IV administration. See the Patient Teaching Tips for further information.

Use only clear solutions of caspofungin, and dilute doses with the recommended amounts of normal saline. Liver toxicity may occur, so monitor liver function tests during therapy as ordered. In addition, monitor the patient for the occurrence of tachycardia, hypotension, fever, chills, or headaches. Hemoglobin and hematocrit levels must also be monitored frequently because of the possibility of drug-induced anemias. Fluconazole may be given either orally or intravenously, with IV dosage forms used if there is a specific indication or if the oral dosage forms are poorly tolerated. Administer IV dosage forms only if the solution is clear, and do not add other medications. If itching or a rash occurs, stop the infusion, take vital signs, and contact the health care provider. Nystatin is given orally as a suspension. For treatment of infections of the oral cavity, the nystatin should be dropped directly on the tongue using the calibrated dropper and held in the mouth for as long as possible and then swallowed. Instruct the patient to swish the medication solution thoroughly in the mouth for as long as possible before swallowing. For treatment of intestinal infections, nystatin may be dropped directly on the tongue by means of the calibrated dropper, or may be mixed with milk or lukewarm formula, honey, jelly, or peanut butter. Terbinafine may be given orally or topically. Local skin reactions that need to be reported include blistering, itching, oozing, redness, and swelling. Oral dosing of voriconazole is given 1 hour before or 1 hour after a meal. IV doses may be diluted with 5% dextrose in water or normal saline, with the accurate dose infused over the recommended time. Monitor visual acuity when this drug is given (especially if ordered for longer than 28 days); any visual changes should be reported to the health care provider.

Evaluation

The therapeutic effects of antifungals include improvement and eventual resolution of the signs and symptoms of fungal infection, if the patient has remained totally adherent to the therapy regimen. Increase in energy levels and improvement in overall sense of well-being, accompanied by a normal temperature and other vital sign values, also indicate a therapeutic response. Specific adverse effects for which to monitor in patients receiving antifungals are listed in Table 47-2. Evaluate goals and expected outcomes in the context of the collaborative plan of care.

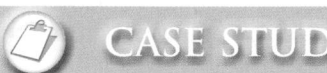 **CASE STUDY**

Amphotericin B

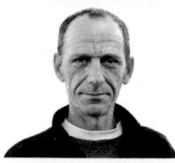 Albert, a 63-year-old retired delivery driver, has been hospitalized for pneumonia. Since his admission, he has been diagnosed with a severe systemic fungal infection, and an amphotericin B infusion will be started. Before beginning this medication, the nurse assesses the results of his kidney and liver function laboratory studies, as well as his CBC. The patency of the IV line is verified, and the nurse gives Albert a dose of oral acetaminophen (Tylenol®) as well as an antihistamine before starting the infusion.

1. What is the purpose of the acetaminophen and antihistamine?

2. The nurse stays with Albert for the first 15 minutes of the infusion and monitors his vital signs. Explain the rationale for these nursing actions.

3. One hour after the infusion is completed, Albert calls the nurse and says that he feels as if he may vomit, and he has chills, yet feels hot at the same time. What does the nurse need to do next?

4. Albert continues to feel "terrible" the rest of the night, and the next morning his health care provider changes the order to liposomal amphotericin B (AmBisome). Why did the health care provider continue an antifungal medication? What is the rationale behind this order change?

For answers see http://evolve.elsevier.com/Canada/Lilley/pharmacology/.

PATIENT TEACHING TIPS

❖ Instruct female patients taking antifungal medications for the treatment of vaginal infections to abstain from sexual intercourse (infection can be spread to the patient's partner via vaginal intercourse) until the treatment is completed and the infection is resolved, and advise patients to continue to take the medication even if actively menstruating. Tell patients to notify a health care provider if symptoms persist after treatment is completed.

Continued

PATIENT TEACHING TIPS—cont'd

❖ Some patients receiving amphotericin B may need long-term treatment (i.e., over weeks or months). If so, advise patients that possible adverse effects include tinnitus, blurred vision, burning and itching at the infusion site, headache, rash, fever, chills, hypokalemia, GI upset, and various anemias.

❖ Instruct patients taking caspofungin to immediately report to a health care provider any problems with shortness of breath, itching, facial swelling, or a rash.

❖ Encourage patients taking antifungals to practice good hand hygiene.

❖ Instruct patients regarding the proper dosing instructions for nystatin (e.g., for oral solutions, swish and swallow). If vaginal troches (small lozenges that dissolve in the vagina) are prescribed, use the appropriate applicator with a gloved hand and insert high into the vagina, and follow this with thorough handwashing (see Chapter 10).

❖ Yeast infections are common during pregnancy. Topical antifungals can be used for up to 7 days and are considered safe during pregnancy. Educate patients about the importance of using over-the-counter medications only when an infection is present; using these medications when there is no infection may contribute to the development of drug-resistant strains. Educate patients about the classic manifestations of a yeast infection (e.g., itching, burning, white discharge).

❖ Encourage patients to keep affected body areas clean and dry and to wear light and cool cotton underclothing, in the case of a vaginal infection. Avoid contact of the topical dosage form with the eyes, mouth, nose, or other mucous membranes.

❖ Voriconazole is to be taken 1 hour before or 1 hour after meals. Warn patients about the adverse effect of photophobia with the use of this drug.

KEY POINTS

❖ Fungi are a large and diverse group of microorganisms and consist of yeast and moulds. Yeasts are single-celled fungi that may be harmful (e.g., causing infections) or helpful (e.g., aiding in baking or brewing beer). Moulds are multicellular and are characterized by long, branching filaments called *hyphae*.

❖ Candidiasis is an opportunistic fungal infection caused by *Candida albicans* and occurs in patients taking broad-spectrum antibiotics, antineoplastics, or immunosuppressants, as well as in persons who are immunocompromised. When candidiasis occurs in the mouth, it is commonly termed *oral candidiasis* or *thrush*. Oral candidiasis is more commonly seen in newborns and individuals who are immunocompromised, such as with HIV/AIDS, than in the general population.

❖ Vaginal candidiasis is a yeast infection occurring primarily in women who have diabetes, are taking oral contraceptives, or are pregnant.

❖ Antifungals may be administered either systemically or topically. Some of the most common systemic antifungal drugs are amphotericin B and fluconazole; nystatin is an example of a topical antifungal.

❖ Before administering antifungals, thoroughly assess for allergies as well as determine what other drugs the patient is taking, including prescription drugs, over-the-counter drugs, and natural health products.

❖ Amphotericin B must be properly diluted according to manufacturer guidelines and administered using an IV infusion pump. Tissue extravasation of fluconazole at the IV infusion site leads to tissue necrosis; therefore, check the site hourly and document the assessment.

EXAMINATION REVIEW QUESTIONS

1. The nurse is assessing a patient who is about to receive antifungal drug therapy. Which problem would be of most concern?
   a. Endocrine disease
   b. Liver disease
   c. Heart disease
   d. Pulmonary disease

2. While monitoring a patient who is receiving IV amphotericin B, the nurse expects to see which adverse effect(s)?
   a. Hypertension
   b. Bradycardia
   c. Fever and chills
   d. Diarrhea and stomach cramps

3. When administering antifungal drug therapy, the nurse knows that which factor contributes to many drug interactions with antifungals?
   a. History of cardiac disease
   b. History of gallbladder surgery
   c. Ethnic background
   d. Cytochrome P450 enzyme system

4. During an infusion of amphotericin B, the nurse knows that which administration technique may be used to minimize infusion-related adverse effects?
   a. Encouraging fluids during the infusion
   b. Infusing the medication quickly
   c. Infusing the medication over an extended period of time
   d. Stopping the infusion for 2 hours after half of the bag has infused and then resuming 1 hour later

EXAMINATION REVIEW QUESTIONS—cont'd

5. When instructing a patient who is taking nystatin orally for oral candidiasis, which instruction by the nurse is correct?
   a. "Rinse for 5 minutes after meals and then spit out."
   b. "Rinse for 2 minutes after meals and then swallow."
   c. "Dissolve the medication in a glass of juice and then swallow."
   d. "The drug should be swallowed and followed by a glass of water."

6. When monitoring a patient who is receiving caspofungin, the nurse will look for which serious adverse effects? (Select all that apply.)
   a. Blood dyscrasias
   b. Hypotension
   c. Pulmonary infiltrates
   d. Tinnitus
   e. Hepatotoxicity

7. The order reads, "Give nystatin suspension, 500 000 units by mouth (swish and swallow) 4 times a day for 1 week." The medication is available in a suspension of 100 000 units per mL. How many millilitres will the nurse give per dose?

Answers: 1. b, **2.** c, **3.** d, **4.** c, **5.** b, **6.** a, b, e, **7.** 5 mL

CRITICAL THINKING ACTIVITIES

1. The nurse is reviewing newly written orders for a patient who has a vaginal yeast infection. One order reads, "Fluconazole, 150 mg, one tablet by mouth now for vaginal yeast infection." The unit secretary sees the order and asks, "Is that a mistake? How can one pill help that problem?" What is the nurse's best answer to this question?

2. A patient has severe respiratory aspergillosis and has not responded to antifungal therapy after 4 days. There is a new order for caspofungin (Cancidas). What is the most important assessment action by the nurse before administering this drug?

3. When the nurse is administering medications, the patient takes the oral nystatin suspension and says, "I know how to take this." He then swallows the liquid medication all at once. What is the nurse's priority action at this time?

For answers see http://evolve.elsevier.com/Canada/Lilley/pharmacology/.

CHAPTER 48

Antimalarial, Antiprotozoal, and Anthelmintic Drugs

Objectives

After reading this chapter, the successful student will be able to do the following:

1. Briefly discuss the infectious process associated with malaria, other protozoal infections, and helminthic infection processes.

2. Compare the signs and symptoms of malarial, other protozoal, and helminthic infection processes.

3. Identify the more commonly used antimalarial, antiprotozoal, and anthelmintic drugs.

4. Discuss the mechanisms of action, indications, cautions, contraindications, adverse effects, dosages, drug interactions, and routes of administration of the antimalarial, antiprotozoal, and anthelmintic drugs.

5. Develop a collaborative plan of care that includes all phases of the nursing process for patients receiving antimalarial, antiprotozoal, or anthelmintic drugs.

e-Learning Activities

Website
(http://evolve.elsevier.com/Canada/Lilley/pharmacology/)

evolve

- Answer Key—Textbook Case Studies
- Answer Key—Critical Thinking Activities
- Chapter Summaries—Printable
- Review Questions for Exam Preparation
- Unfolding Case Studies

Drug Profiles

atovaquone, p. 901
» chloroquine diphosphate and hydroxychloroquine, p. 896
» mefloquine hydrochloride, p. 897
» metronidazole, p. 901
pentamidine isetionate, p. 901
praziquantel, p. 904
» primaquine phosphate, p. 897
pyrantel pamoate, p. 904

» Key drug

Key Terms

Anthelmintic A category of drugs that destroy or prevent the development of parasitic worm (helminthic) infections. Also called *antihelmintic* or *vermicidal*. (Note that the terms for the drug categories are spelled with only one *h*, which appears in the second syllable of the term, whereas the term for worm infection (*helminthic*) is spelled with two *h*'s, appearing in both the first and third syllables of the term.) (p. 901)

Antimalarial drugs Drugs that destroy or prevent the development of the malaria parasite (*Plasmodium* sp.) in humans. Antimalarial drugs are a subset of the broader category of antiprotozoal drugs. (p. 894)

Antiprotozoal A type of drug that destroys or prevents the development of protozoa in humans. (p. 898)

Helminthic infections Parasitic worm infections. (p. 900)

Malaria   A widespread protozoal infectious disease caused by four species of the genus *Plasmodium*. (p. 893)

Parasite   Any organism that feeds on another living organism (known as a host) in a way that results in harm to the host organism. (p. 893)

Parasitic protozoa   Harmful protozoa that live on or in human beings or animals and cause disease. (Also called *parasitic protozoans*.) (p. 893)

Protozoa   Single-celled organisms that are the smallest and simplest members of the animal kingdom. (p. 893)

OVERVIEW

There are more than 28 000 known types of **protozoa,** which are single-celled organisms. Those that live on or in humans are termed *parasitic protozoa*. Billions of people worldwide are infected with these organisms, and as a result, these infections are considered a serious health problem. Some of the more common protozoal infections are malaria, leishmaniasis, trypanosomiasis, amoebiasis, giardiasis, and trichomoniasis. They are relatively uncommon in Canada but are becoming increasingly prevalent in immunocompromised individuals, including those with AIDS. Protozoal diseases are particularly prevalent among people living in tropical climates because it is easier for protozoa to survive and be transmitted in environments that are warm and humid year round. Although the population of Canada is relatively free from many of these protozoal infections, international travel and the immigration of people from other countries where such infections are endemic are providing opportunities for increased exposure of Canadians to protozoal infections.

MALARIA

The most significant protozoal disease in terms of morbidity and mortality is **malaria.** Worldwide, it is estimated that 350 to 500 million people are infected, with an annual death rate of 1 to 2 million people. In Africa alone, malaria accounts for more than 1 million infant deaths per year. The geographic areas with the highest prevalence of malaria are sub-Saharan Africa, Southeast Asia, and Latin America. Approximately 400 to 1 000 cases of malaria are reported to Health Canada annually, and these are seen mostly in people who have travelled to malaria-endemic countries. Malaria is caused by a particular genus of protozoa called *Plasmodium*, and there are four species of organisms in this genus, each with its own characteristics and its own ability to resist being killed by antimalarial drugs. These four species are *Plasmodium vivax*, *Plasmodium falciparum*, *Plasmodium malariae*, and *Plasmodium ovale*. Although *P. vivax* is the most widespread of the four species, *P. falciparum* is almost as widespread, causes significant morbidity and mortality, and is more drug resistant. The two remaining species are much less common and more geographically limited in their occurrence, but they can still cause serious malarial infections.

Most commonly, malaria is transmitted by the bite of an infected female *Anopheles* mosquito. This type of mosquito is endemic to many tropical regions of the world. Malaria can also be transmitted via blood transfusions, congenitally from mother to infant via an infected placenta, or through the use of contaminated needles. Despite the combined efforts of many countries to eradicate malaria, it remains one of the most devastating infectious diseases in the world. As is also the case with tuberculosis (see Chapter 46) and AIDS (see Chapter 45), many lives are lost to malaria, and the cost of treating and preventing the disease imposes a tremendous economic burden on the often poor countries where the disease is prevalent.

The *Plasmodium* life cycle is quite complex and involves many stages. The organism has two interdependent life cycles: the *sexual cycle*, which takes place inside the mosquito, and the *asexual cycle*, which occurs in the human host (Figure 48-1). In addition, the asexual cycle of the **parasite** consists of a phase outside the erythrocyte (primarily in liver tissues) called the *exoerythrocytic phase* (or the *liver phase*) and a phase inside the erythrocyte called the *erythrocytic phase* (or the *blood phase*). The malarial parasite undergoes many changes during these two phases (Figure 48-2).

Malaria signs and symptoms are often described in terms of the classic malaria paroxysm. A *paroxysm* is a sudden recurrence or intensification of symptoms. Symptoms include chills and rigour (violent shivering), followed by fever of up to 40°C and diaphoresis, often leading to extreme fatigue and prolonged sleep. This syndrome often repeats itself periodically in 48- to 72-hour cycles. Other common symptoms include headache, nausea, and joint pain.

ANTIMALARIAL DRUGS

Treatment for malaria is not initiated until the diagnosis has been confirmed by laboratory tests. Once confirmed, appropriate antimalarial treatment must be initiated immediately. Treatment is guided by three main factors: the infecting *Plasmodium* species, the clinical status of the patient, and the drug susceptibility of the infecting parasites as determined by the geographic area where the infection was acquired. Because resistance patterns are constantly changing, depending on geographic location, the reader is referred to the website of the US Centers for Disease Control and Prevention (CDC) for the most up-to-date information. People travelling to different parts of the world may require antimalarial prophylaxis, and they need to check with their health care providers or a

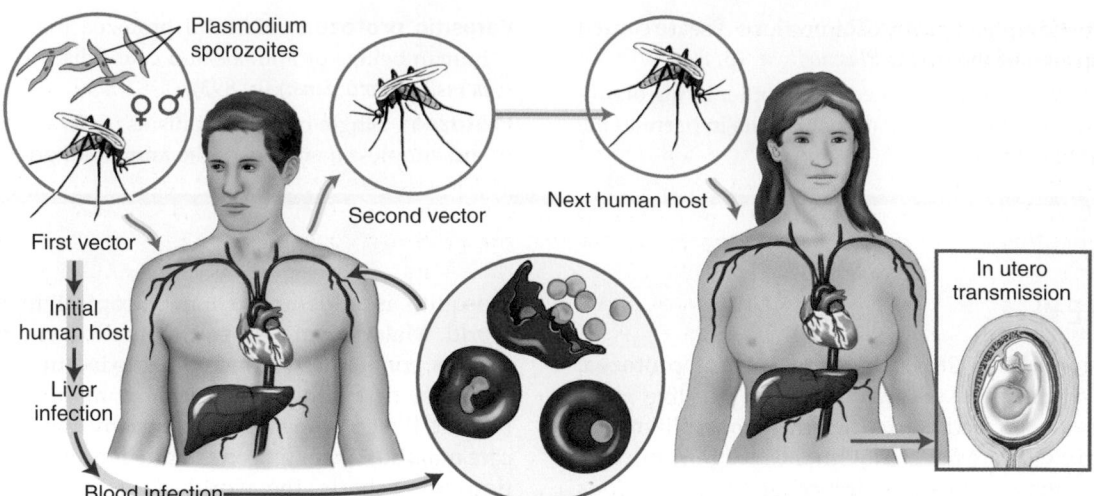

FIG. 48-1 An infected anopheles mosquito carries parasites to humans, causing malaria. These parasites mature in the liver before entering the bloodstream and rupturing red blood cells. A pregnant woman infected with malaria may transmit the disease to her unborn fetus.

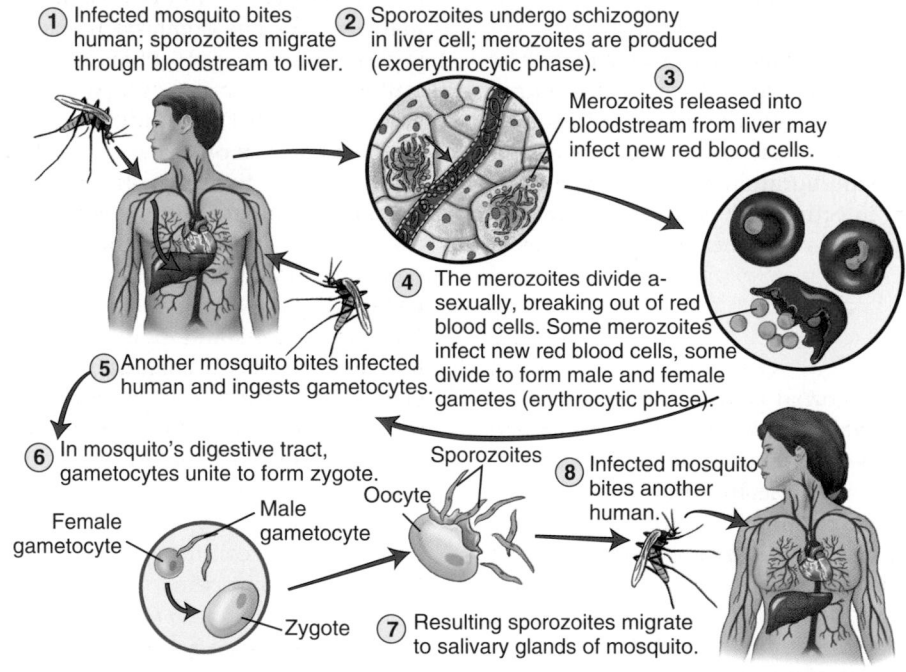

FIG. 48-2 Life cycle of the malarial parasite. (Source: Van Meter, K., & Hubert, R. (2010). *Microbiology for the healthcare professional.* St. Louis, MO: Mosby.)

travel clinic for specific drug therapy. The Public Health Agency of Canada's website provides a summary of information, including doses, for the antimalarial drugs routinely used in Canada. The Committee to Advise on Tropical Medicine and Travel (CATMAT), composed of experts, provides travel health–related advice for travellers and health care providers. CATMAT provides recommendations for the prevention and treatment of infectious diseases, strategies to disseminate this information, and priorities for research. **Antimalarial drugs** administered

to humans cannot affect the parasite during its sexual cycle when it resides in the mosquito. Instead, these drugs act against the parasite during its asexual cycle, which takes place within the human body. Often, antimalarial drugs are given in various combinations to achieve an additive or synergistic antimalarial effect. One example is the combination of the two antiprotozoal drugs atovaquone and proguanil hydrochloride (Malarone®). Malaria management is changing as the prevalence of drug-resistant malaria increases. For example, in Canada, doxycycline may be used to treat cases of drug-resistant malaria.

Mechanism of Action and Drug Effects

The mechanisms of action of the various antimalarial drugs differ depending on the chemical family of drugs to which they belong. The *4-aminoquinoline derivatives* (chloroquine diphosphate and hydroxychloroquine sulphate) act by inhibiting deoxyribonucleic acid (DNA) and ribonucleic acid (RNA) polymerase, enzymes essential to DNA and RNA synthesis by the parasite cells. Parasite protein synthesis is also disrupted, because protein synthesis is dependent on functioning nucleic acids (DNA and RNA). These drugs also raise the pH within the parasite, which interferes with the parasite's ability to metabolize and use erythrocyte hemoglobin; this is one reason these drugs are ineffective during the exoerythrocytic (liver) phase of infection. All of these actions contribute to the destruction of the parasite. Quinine sulphate, quinidine sulphate, and mefloquine are thought to be similar to the 4-aminoquinoline derivatives in their actions, in that all are believed to raise the pH within the parasite.

The *diaminopyrimidines* (trimethoprim [see Chapter 43]) act by inhibiting dihydrofolate reductase, an enzyme that is needed for the production of certain vital substances in malarial parasites. Specifically, inhibiting this enzyme blocks the synthesis of tetrahydrofolate, which is a precursor of purines and pyrimidines (nucleic acid components) and certain amino acids (protein components) that are essential for the growth and survival of plasmodia parasites. This drug is effective only during the erythrocytic phase. Trimethoprim is often used with a sulfonamide (sulfadoxine or dapsone) because of the resulting synergistic effects exerted by such drug combinations. Tetracyclines such as doxycycline (see Chapter 43) and lincomycins such as clindamycin hydrochloride (see Chapter 44) may also be used in combination with some of the other antimalarial drugs because of the synergistic effects resulting from these drug combinations.

Primaquine phosphate, an *8-aminoquinoline* that is structurally similar to the 4-aminoquinolines, has the ability to bind to and alter parasitic DNA. It is one of the few drugs effective in the exoerythrocytic phase. Atovaquone/proguanil also works by interfering with nucleic acid synthesis.

The drug effects of the antimalarial drugs are mostly limited to their ability to kill parasitic organisms, most of which are *Plasmodium* species (spp.). However, some of these drugs have other drug effects and therapeutic uses. Hydroxychloroquine also has anti-inflammatory effects and is sometimes used in the treatment of rheumatoid arthritis and systemic lupus erythematosus. Quinine sulphate and quinidine sulphate can decrease the excitability of both heart and skeletal muscles. Quinidine sulphate is currently used to treat certain types of cardiac dysrhythmias (see Chapter 26).

Indications

Antimalarial drugs are used to kill *Plasmodium* organisms, the parasites that cause malaria. The various antimalarial drugs act during different phases of the parasite's growth inside the human host. The antimalarials that exert the greatest effect on all four *Plasmodium* organisms during the erythrocytic or blood phase are chloroquine phosphate and hydroxychloroquine sulphate. Other drugs known to work during the blood phase are quinine sulphate, quinidine sulphate, and mefloquine hydrochloride. Because these drugs are ineffective during the exoerythrocytic phase, they cannot *prevent* infection. Health Canada, however, recommends the use of mefloquine hydrochloride for prevention and not as routine treatment for malaria because of the drug's adverse effect profile. The most effective antimalarial drug for eradicating the parasite during the exoerythrocytic phase is primaquine phosphate, which actually works during both asexual phases. Primaquine phosphate is indicated specifically for infection with *P. vivax*. Chloroquine and hydroxychloroquine (4-aminoquinolines) are the drugs of choice for the treatment of susceptible strains of malarial parasites. They are highly toxic to all *Plasmodium* spp., except resistant strains of *P. falciparum*.

Quinine sulphate is indicated for infection with chloroquine diphosphate–resistant *P. falciparum*, which can cause a type of malaria that affects the brain. Quinine sulphate can be used alone but is more commonly given in combination with a second drug such as a tetracycline (e.g., doxycycline hyclate). Other antimalarial drugs are generally preferred for the treatment of active disease. Mefloquine hydrochloride is a newer antimalarial drug that may be used for both prophylaxis and treatment of malaria caused by *P. falciparum* or *P. vivax*. The drug combination atovaquone/proguanil (Malarone) is also used for the prevention and treatment of *P. falciparum* infection.

Contraindications

Contraindications to various antimalarial drugs include drug allergy, tinnitus, and pregnancy (for quinine sulphate). Severe kidney, liver, or hematological dysfunction may also be a contraindication to the use of antimalarial drugs. Other drug-specific contraindications are noted in the drug profiles on pp. 896–897.

Adverse Effects

Antimalarial drugs cause diverse adverse effects, and these are listed for each drug in Table 48-1.

Interactions

Some common drug interactions associated with antimalarial drugs are listed in Table 48-2.

Dosages

For the recommended dosages for selected antimalarial drugs, refer to the table on p. 897.

TABLE 48-1

Antimalarial Drugs: Common Adverse Effects

Body System	Adverse Effects
CHLOROQUINE DIPHOSPHATE AND HYDROXYCHLOROQUINE SULPHATE	
Gastrointestinal	Diarrhea, anorexia, nausea, vomiting
Central nervous	Dizziness, headache, seizure, personality changes
Other	Alopecia, rash, pruritis
MEFLOQUINE HYDROCHLORIDE	
Central nervous	Headache, fatigue, tinnitus
Gastrointestinal	Stomach pain, anorexia, nausea, vomiting
Other	Fever, chills, rash, myalgia
PRIMAQUINE PHOSPHATE	
Gastrointestinal	Nausea, vomiting, abdominal distress
Other	Headaches, pruritus, dark discoloration of urine, hemolytic anemia due to G6PD deficiency
QUININE SULPHATE	
Central nervous	Visual disturbances, dizziness, headaches, tinnitus
Gastrointestinal	Diarrhea, nausea, vomiting, abdominal pain
Other	Rash, pruritus, hives, photosensitivity respiratory difficulties

G6PD, glucose-6-phosphate dehydrogenase.

TABLE 48-2

Antimalarial Drugs: Drug Interactions

Drug	Mechanism	Result
CHLOROQUINE DIPHOSPHATE		
divalproex sodium, valproic acid, anthelmintics, β-blockers, digoxin	Decreased serum levels of target drug	Treatment failures of target drugs
MEFLOQUINE HYDROCHLORIDE		
β-blockers, calcium channel blockers, quinidine sulphate, quinine sulphate	Unknown	Increased risk of dysrhythmia, cardiac arrest, seizures
PRIMAQUINE PHOSPHATE		
Other hemolytic drugs	Unknown	Increased risk for myelotoxic effects (monitor for muscle weakness)

DRUG PROFILES

The dosing instructions for several of the antimalarial drugs can be confusing because tablet strengths listed on the medication packaging often indicate the strength of the tablet in terms of the entire salt form of the drug, not just the active ingredient, which is referred to as the *base ingredient*. However, dosing guidelines often list recommended dosages for the base ingredient and not the entire salt. For example, as described later in the drug profile for chloroquine diphosphate, the tablets come in a 250-mg strength of the salt form of the drug, but these actually have only 150 mg of the active ingredient or base. Be mindful of this distinction.

▶▶*chloroquine diphosphate and hydroxychloroquine sulphate*

Chloroquine diphosphate is a synthetic antimalarial drug that is chemically classified as a 4-aminoquinoline derivative. It is also indicated for the treatment of other parasitic infections, such as amoebiasis. Hydroxychloroquine

sulphate (Plaquenil®) is another synthetic 4-aminoquinoline derivative that differs from chloroquine diphosphate by only one hydroxyl group (⁻OH). Its efficacy in treating malaria is comparable to that of quinine sulphate. Both medications also possess anti-inflammatory actions and have been used to treat rheumatoid arthritis and systemic lupus erythematosus since the 1950s. However, only hydroxychloroquine sulphate is now used for these indications.

Contraindications to the use of 4-aminoquinoline derivatives include visual field changes, optic neuritis, and psoriasis, but their use may still be warranted, based on sound clinical judgement.

Chloroquine diphosphate and hydroxychloroquine sulphate are available only for oral use. The use of these drugs during pregnancy may outweigh the potential harm, but it is recommended that they be used in pregnant women only in truly urgent situations. These drugs are also distributed into breast milk.

DRUG PROFILES—cont'd

PHARMACOKINETICS (CHLOROQUINE DIPHOSPHATE)

Route	Onset of Action	Peak Plasma Concentration	Elimination Half-Life	Duration of Action
PO	8–10 hr	1–2 hr	3–5 days	Variable

PHARMACOKINETICS (HYDROXYCHLOROQUINE SULPHATE)

Route	Onset of Action	Peak Plasma Concentration	Elimination Half-Life	Duration of Action
PO	4 hr	2–3 hr	32–50 days	Variable

mefloquine hydrochloride

Mefloquine hydrochloride is an analogue of quinine sulphate that is indicated for the management of mild to moderate acute malaria and for the prevention and treatment of malaria caused by chloroquine-resistant organisms. It is also used to treat multidrug-resistant strains of *P. falciparum*, which, as already noted, is a species of *Plasmodium* that is difficult to kill. The drug is commonly used prophylactically by travellers to prevent malarial infection while visiting malaria-endemic areas. The tetracycline antibiotic doxycycline hyclate (see Chapter 43) is also commonly used for this purpose. Mefloquine hydrochloride should not be used by patients with active depression or a history of mental health disturbances (e.g., depression, generalized anxiety disorder, psychosis, schizophrenia, other major mental health disorders) or a history of convulsions, as the drug may precipitate these conditions. Mefloquine hydrochloride is available only for oral use.

PHARMACOKINETICS

Route	Onset of Action	Peak Plasma Concentration	Elimination Half-Life	Duration of Action
PO	Less than 24 h	7–24 hr	21–22 days	Variable

primaquine phosphate

Primaquine phosphate is similar in chemical structure and antimalarial activity to the 4-aminoquinolines, but it is classified as an 8-aminoquinoline. It is one of the few antimalarial drugs that can destroy malarial parasites in their exoerythrocytic phase. Primaquine phosphate is indicated for curative therapy in acute cases of *P. vivax*, *P. ovale*, and, to a lesser degree, *P. falciparum* infection.

Primaquine phosphate is contraindicated in patients with known allergy or any disease states that may cause granulocytopenia, such as rheumatoid arthritis or systemic lupus erythematous. Primaquine phosphate must be used with caution in patients with methemoglobinemia, porphyria, methemoglobin reductase deficiency, and glucose-6-phosphate dehydrogenase (G6PD) deficiency (see Chapter 2). It is available only for oral use.

PHARMACOKINETICS

Route	Onset of Action	Peak Plasma Concentration	Elimination Half-Life	Duration of Action
PO	2 hr	1–3 hr	4–10 hr	24 hr

DOSAGES   Selected Antimalarial Drugs

Drug	Pharmacological Class	Usual Dosage Range	Indications
atovaquone/ proguanil hydrochloride* (Malarone)	Antimalarial	*Children* PO: Dosage varies depending on weight; 1–3 tab/day For all weights: start 1–2 days before entering endemic area and continue × 7 days after leaving endemic area† *Adults over 40 kg* PO: 1 tab/day; begin 1–2 days before entering endemic area and continue during exposure and × 7 days after leaving endemic area†	Malaria prophylaxis of *P. falciparum*
		Children PO: Dosage varies depending on weight; 1–tab/day × 3 days *Adults over 40 kg* PO: 4 tabs daily × 3 days	Malaria treatment of *P. falciparum*
chloroquine diphosphate (tablet: 155 mg chloroquine base (250 mg chloroquine diphosphate)	Synthetic antimalarial and antiamoebic	*Children* PO: 5 mg base/kg weekly; max 310 mg base weekly; begin 1 wk before entering endemic area and continue during exposure and × 4 wk after leaving endemic area *Adults* PO: 500 mg weekly, taken on exactly the same day every week, 2 wks before entering endemic area and × 4 wks after leaving endemic area	Malaria prophylaxis
		Children PO: 25 mg base/kg over 3 days; 10 mg base/kg on days 1 and 2 (do not exceed 620 mg base); 5 mg base/kg on day 3 *Adults* PO: 1000 mg followed by 500 mg after 6–8 hrs; followed by 500 mg on each of 2 consecutive days; 3-day total dose of 2.5 g.	Malaria treatment

Continued

DOSAGES Selected Antimalarial Drugs—cont'd

Drug	Pharmacological Class	Usual Dosage Range	Indications
▸▸hydroxychloroquine sulphate (Plaquenil) Tablet: 155 mg base	Synthetic antimalarial	*Children 6 yrs and older* PO: 5 mg base/kg (do not exceed adult dose) once weekly; on exactly the same day of each week beginning 2 wks before entering endemic area, continue during exposure and × 8 wk after leaving endemic area *Adults* PO: 400 mg on exactly the same day of each week beginning 2 wks before entering endemic area; continue during exposure and × 8 wk after leaving endemic area	Malaria prophylaxis
		Children 6 yrs and older PO: Total dose of 25 mg base/kg over 3 days: 10 mg base/kg (not to exceed 620 mg base) on day 1, 5 mg base/kg 4 hrs after first dose; 5 mg base/kg 18 hours after the second dose; 5 mg base/kg 24 hours after the third dose	Malaria treatment
		Adults PO: Loading dose of 800 mg, followed by 400 mg in 6–8 hrs; followed by 400 mg on each of the next 2 days for a total of 2 g of hydroxychloroquine sulphate or 1.55 g base; or single dose of 800 mg	Treatment of acute malaria attack
mefloquine hydrochloride (Lariam®)	Synthetic antimalarial	*Children* PO: Weekly dosing varies depending on weight *Adults and children over 45 kg* PO: 250 mg base weekly; begin 1 wk before entering endemic area and continue × 4 wk after leaving endemic area	Malaria prophylaxis
▸▸primaquine phosphate	Synthetic antimalarial	*Children* 0.5 mg base/kg/day; begin 1 day before entering endemic area and continue for 7 days after leaving endemic area *Adults* PO: 30 mg base daily; begin 1 day before entering endemic area and continue during exposure and for 7 days after leaving endemic area	Malaria prophylaxis

PO, oral.

*Each tablet of Malarone contains atovaquone 250 mg and proguanil hydrochloride 100 mg. Each Malarone Pediatric tablet contains atovaquone 62.5 mg and proguanil hydrochloride 25 mg.

†In addition to endemic areas, prophylaxis should be given for travel to any nonendemic area where prophylaxis for malaria is recommended by international travel health authorities.

OTHER PROTOZOAL INFECTIONS

There are several other common protozoal infections. These include amoebiasis (caused by *Entamoeba histolytica*), giardiasis (caused by *Giardia lamblia*), toxoplasmosis (caused by *Toxoplasma gondii*), amoebic dysentery or intestinal amoebiasis, and trichomoniasis (caused by *Trichomonas vaginalis*). These diseases are most prevalent in tropical regions. Pneumocystosis, which is caused by *Pneumocystis jirovecii* (formerly known as *Pneumocystis carinii*), used to be classified as a protozoal infection but is now classified as fungal infection. It is a common infection that complicates HIV and AIDS. Pneumocystosis is discussed in this chapter as opposed to the antifungal chapter (see Chapter 47) because it is treated with drugs discussed in this chapter.

These protozoal infections can be transmitted in a number of ways: from person to person (e.g., via sexual contact), through the ingestion of contaminated water or food, through direct contact with the parasite, or by the bite of an insect vector (mosquito or tick). Parasitic infections can be systemic and occur throughout the body, or they can be localized to a specific region. For example, amoebiasis most commonly affects the gastrointestinal (GI) tract (e.g., amoebic dysentery), whereas pneumocystosis is predominantly a pulmonary infection.

The more common protozoal infections are described briefly in Table 48-3, along with the **antiprotozoal** drugs commonly used in their treatment. Only selected drugs are discussed here. Patients whose immune systems are compromised are at particular risk for acquiring a protozoal infection; often, such infections are fatal in these patients.

NONMALARIAL ANTIPROTOZOAL DRUGS

Several drugs used to treat malaria are also used to treat nonmalarial protozoal infections, including chloroquine, primaquine, and atovaquone. Other antiprotozoal drugs

TABLE 48-3

Types of Protozoal Infections

Protozoal Infection	Description	Antiprotozoal Drug
Amoebiasis	Caused by the protozoal parasite *Entamoeba histolytica*; infection mainly resides in the large intestine but can also migrate to other parts of the body, such as the liver; usually transmitted in contaminated food or water	chloroquine, metronidazole, paromomycin sulphate
Giardiasis	Caused by *Giardia lamblia*; the most common intestinal protozoal infection, usually residing in the intestinal mucosa (most commonly the duodenum); may cause diarrhea, bloating, and foul-smelling stools; transmitted in contaminated food or water or by contact with stool from infected persons; in Canada, referred to as "beaver fever"	metronidazole, paromomycin sulphate
Pneumocystosis	Pneumonias caused by *Pneumocystis jirovecii* occur almost exclusively in immunocompromised people; always fatal if left untreated	atovaquone, dapsone, primaquine phosphate, pentamidine isethionate, sulfamethoxazole/ trimethoprim, trimetrexate
Toxoplasmosis	Caused by *Toxoplasma gondii*; can produce systemic infection in both immunocompetent and immunocompromised hosts; domesticated animals, usually cats, serve as the intermediate host for parasites, passing infective oocysts in their feces	Sulfonamides with pyrimethamine, clindamycin hydrochloride, metronidazole
Trichomoniasis	Sexually transmitted infection caused by *Trichomonas vaginalis*	metronidazole

TABLE 48-4

Antiprotozoal Drugs: Mechanisms of Action

Antiprotozoal Drug	Mechanism of Action
atovaquone	Atovaquone selectively inhibits mitochondrial electron transport, reducing synthesis of adenosine triphosphate (required for cellular energy); also inhibits nucleic acid synthesis
metronidazole	Interferes with DNA, resulting in inhibition of protein synthesis and cell death in susceptible organisms
pentamidine isethionate	Inhibits production of much-needed substances such as DNA and RNA. Can bind to and aggregate ribosomes; it is directly lethal to *Pneumocystis jirovecii* (now classified as a fungus), through inhibiting glucose metabolism, protein and RNA synthesis, and intracellular amino acid transport

DNA, deoxyribonucleic acid; *RNA*, ribonucleic acid.

normally used against nonmalarial parasites include metronidazole, paromomycin sulphate, and pentamidine isethionate.

Mechanism of Action and Drug Effects

Antiprotozoal drugs work by several different mechanisms. The most commonly used antiprotozoal drugs, together with brief descriptions of their mechanisms of action, are given in Table 48-4. Chloroquine was discussed earlier in this chapter in the section on malaria. The drug effects of antiprotozoal drugs are limited primarily to their ability to kill various forms of protozoal parasites.

Indications

Antiprotozoal drugs are used to treat various protozoal infections, ranging from intestinal amoebiasis to pneumocystosis. Indications for selected drugs are summarized in Table 48-5. Atovaquone and pentamidine isethionate

are used for the treatment of *P. jirovecii* infection. Metronidazole (effective for tissue amebicides in the bowel, liver, and extraintestinal tissues) and paromomycin sulphate (a luminal drug that acts on the bowel lumen to eradicate infection) are used to treat intestinal amoebiasis, the usual causative organism being *Entamoeba histolytica*. Metronidazole is also effective against several forms of bacteria, including anaerobic bacteria (see Chapter 44), as well as against protozoa and helminths (parasitic worms). Worm infection (helminthiasis) is discussed later in the chapter.

Contraindications

Contraindications to the use of antiprotozoal drugs include known drug allergy. Additional contraindications may include serious kidney or liver dysfunction or other illnesses, with the seriousness of the infection weighed against the patient's overall condition.

TABLE 48-5

Indications for Selected Antiprotozoal Drugs

Antiprotozoal Drug	Drug Effects
atovaquone	Indicated for treatment of acute mild to moderately severe *Pneumocystis jirovecii* (classified as a fungus) pneumonia in patients who cannot tolerate trimoxazole/sulfamethoxazole
metronidazole	Indicated for treatment of bacterial (including anaerobic), protozoal, and helminthic infections
pentamidine isethionate	Indicated for prevention and treatment of *P. jirovecii* pneumonia

TABLE 48-6

Selected Antiprotozoal Drugs: Adverse Effects

Body System	Adverse Effects
ATOVAQUONE	
Hematological	Anemia, neutropenia, leukopenia
Integumentary	Pruritus, urticaria, rash
Gastrointestinal	Anorexia, elevated liver enzymes, gastritis, nausea, vomiting, diarrhea, constipation
Central nervous	Headache
Metabolic	Hyperkalemia, hypoglycemia, hyponatremia
Other	Cough
METRONIDAZOLE	
Central nervous	Headache, dizziness, confusion, fatigue, peripheral neuropathy, weakness
Eyes, ears, nose, and throat	Blurred vision, sore throat, dry mouth, metallic taste, glossitis
Gastrointestinal	Nausea, vomiting, diarrhea, constipation
Genitourinary	Dysuria, cystitis
Hematological	Neutropenia
Integumentary	Rash, pruritus, urticarial
PAROMOMYCIN SULPHATE	
Gastrointestinal	Stomach cramps, nausea, vomiting, diarrhea
Central nervous	Hearing loss, dizziness, tinnitus
PENTAMIDINE ISETIONATE	
Cardiovascular	Hypotension, chest pain, dysrhythmias
Hematological	Leukopenia, thrombocytopenia, neutropenia
Integumentary	Pain at injection site, pruritus, urticaria, rash
Genitourinary	Nephrotoxicity
Gastrointestinal	Increased liver enzyme levels, pancreatitis, metallic taste, nausea, vomiting, diarrhea
Respiratory	Cough, wheezing, dyspnea, pharyngitis
Metabolic	Hypoglycemia followed by hyperglycemia
Other	Fatigue, chills, night sweats

Adverse Effects

The adverse effects of antiprotozoal drugs vary depending on the drug and are listed in Table 48-6.

Interactions

The common drug and laboratory test interactions associated with the use of antiprotozoal drugs are listed in Table 48-7.

Dosages

For dosage information on selected antiprotozoal drugs, refer to the table on p. 902.

HELMINTHIC INFECTIONS

Parasitic **helminthic infections** (worm infections) are a worldwide problem. It has been estimated that one third of the world's population is infected with these parasites, but persons living in developing countries where sanitary conditions are often poor are by far the most common victims. The incidence of worm infection in developed countries where sewage treatment is adequate is much lower, and usually only a few select helminthic diseases cause problems. The most prevalent helminthic infection in Canada is enterobiasis, caused by one genus of roundworm (also called pinworm), *Enterobius*.

TABLE 48-7

Antiprotozoal Drugs: Drug and Laboratory Test Interactions

Antiprotozoal Drug	Mechanism	Result
atovaquone	Compete for binding on protein, resulting in free, active atovaquone	Highly protein-bound drugs (e.g., warfarin sodium, phenytoin): may increase atovaquone drug concentrations and risk of adverse reactions
metronidazole	Decreased absorption of vitamin K from the intestines due to elimination of the bacteria needed to absorb vitamin K, increased plasma acetaldehyde concentration after ingestion of alcohol	Alcohol: causes a disulfiram-like reaction; action of warfarin sodium may be increased (increased bleeding risk)
pentamidine isethionate	Additive nephrotoxic effects	Use with an aminoglycoside, amphotericin B, colistimethate sodium, cisplatin, or vancomycin hydrochloride may result in nephrotoxicity

DRUG PROFILES

Antiprotozoal drugs are used for a number of infectious diseases, including infections with *Pneumocystis jirovecii* and *Trichomonas vaginalis*, amoebic dysentery (*Entamoeba histolytica*), toxoplasmosis, and giardiasis, among many others. All require a prescription and are available in either oral or injectable forms.

atovaquone

Atovaquone (Mepron) is a synthetic antiprotozoal drug indicated for the treatment of mild to moderate *P. jirovecii* pneumonia in patients who cannot tolerate sulfamethoxazole/trimethoprim (Chapter 43). It is available only for oral use.

PHARMACOKINETICS

Route	Onset of Action	Peak Plasma Concentration	Elimination Half-Life	Duration of Action
PO	8–24 hr	24–96 hr	2–3 days	Unknown

▸▸metronidazole

Metronidazole (Flagyl) is an antiprotozoal drug that also has fairly broad antibacterial activity as well as **anthelmintic** activity. The therapeutic uses of metronidazole are many and range from the treatment of trichomoniasis, amoebiasis, and giardiasis to the treatment of anaerobic bacterial infections and antibiotic-induced pseudomembranous colitis (see Chapters 43 and 44).

Metronidazole is believed to directly kill protozoa by causing free-radical reactions that damage their DNA and other vital biomolecules. Tinidazole is a newer, similar drug, available as Fasigyn® through Health Canada's Special Access Programme.

Metronidazole is contraindicated during the first trimester of pregnancy. Patients should avoid the use of alcohol (including drugs containing alcohol) while taking metronidazole because of the possibility of a disulfiram-like reaction (Antabuse® effect; e.g., flushing, vomiting, tachycardia). This reaction may occur due to the inhibition of the oxidation of acetaldehyde, the primary metabolite of alcohol. Metronidazole is available in oral and parenteral form as well as in topical preparations.

PHARMACOKINETICS

Route	Onset of Action	Peak Plasma Concentration	Elimination Half-Life	Duration of Action
PO	1 hr	1–2 hr	8 hr	Variable

pentamidine isetionate

Pentamidine isetionate is an antiprotozoal drug used mainly for the management of the fungal infection *P. jirovecii* pneumonia. It acts by inhibiting protein and nucleic acid synthesis. It is used for the treatment of active pneumocystosis and for prophylaxis of *P. jirovecii* pneumonia in patients at high risk for initial or recurrent *Pneumocystis* infection, such as patients with HIV infection and AIDS.

The only contraindication to pentamidine isethionate is known hypersensitivity to the drug. The drug needs to be used with caution in patients with blood dyscrasias, liver or kidney disease, diabetes mellitus, heart disease, hypocalcemia, or hypertension. Pentamidine isethionate is available solely for parenteral use. Intramuscular injections of this drug have been associated with pain, tenderness, redness, and induration at the site and should be used only when intravenous (IV) infusion is not feasible in patients with sufficient muscle mass.

PHARMACOKINETICS

Route	Onset of Action	Peak Plasma Concentration	Elimination Half-Life	Duration of Action
IV	0.5–1 hr	40 min	6 hr–4 wk	Variable

TABLE	48-8

Helminthic Infections

Infection	Organism and Other Facts
NEMATODES (INTESTINAL AND TISSUE ROUNDWORMS)	
Ascariasis	Caused by *Ascaris lumbricoides* (giant roundworm); worm resides in small intestine; treated with pyrantel pamoate or mebendazole
Enterobiasis	Caused by *Enterobius vermicularis* (pinworm); worm resides in large intestine; treated with pyrantel pamoate or mebendazole
PLATHELMINTHES (INTESTINAL TAPEWORMS OR FLATWORMS)	
Diphyllobothriasis	Caused by *Diphyllobothrium latum* (fishworm); acquired from fish; treated with paromomycin sulphate or praziquantel
Hymenolepiasis	Caused by *Hymenolepis nana* (dwarf tapeworm); treated with paromomycin sulphate or praziquantel
Taeniasis	Caused by *Taenia saginata* (beef tapeworm); acquired from beef; treated with paromomycin sulphate or praziquantel
	Caused by *Taenia solium* (pork tapeworm); acquired from pork; treated with paromomycin sulphate or praziquantel

DOSAGES	Selected Antiprotozoal Drugs		
Drug	**Pharmacological Class**	**Usual Dosage Range**	**Indications**
atovaquone* (Mepron®)	Synthetic antipneumocystis drug	*Adults* PO: 750 mg bid with meals × 21 days	Treatment of active PJP (now classified as a fungus)
▸▸metronidazole (Flagyl®)	Amoebicide, antibacterial, trichomonacide	*Children* PO: 35–50 mg/kg tid × 5–7 days *Adults* PO: 500–750 mg tid 3 × 5–10 days	Amoebiasis, including amoebic liver abscess
		Children PO: 25–35 mg/kg/day divided bid × 5–7 days *Adults* PO: 250 mg bid × 5–7 days	Giardiasis
		Adults: 1-day treatment PO: 2 g × 1 dose after a meal *Adults: 10-day treatment* PO: 250 mg tid × 10 days	Trichomoniasis
pentamidine isethionate	Synthetic antipneumocystis drug	*Adults and children:* IV/IM: 4 mg/kg/day by slow infusion × 14 days	Treatment of active PJP (now classified as a fungus)

IV, intravenous; *IM*, intramuscular; *PJP*, *Pneumocystis jirovecii* pneumonia; *PO*, oral.
*A combination product containing atovaquone and proguanil is also used against malaria.

Helminths that are parasitic in humans are classified in the following categories:
- Platyhelminthes (flatworms)
- Cestodes (tapeworms)
- Trematodes (flukes)
- Nematodes (roundworms)

The characteristics of a few of the most common of the many helminthic infections are summarized in Table 48-8. These usually first infect the intestines of their host and reside there, but they can sometimes also migrate to other tissues.

ANTHELMINTIC DRUGS

Unlike protozoa, which are the single-celled members of the animal kingdom, helminths are larger and have complex multicellular structures. Anthelmintic (also spelled *antihelmintic*) drugs work to destroy these organisms by disrupting their structures. The currently available anthelmintic drugs are specific to the worms they can kill. For this reason, the causative worm in an infected host must be accurately identified before treatment is started. This can usually be done by analyzing samples

TABLE	48-9	

Anthelmintics: Mechanisms of Action

Drug	Mechanism of Action	Indication
mebendazole	Selectively and irreversibly inhibits the uptake of glucose and other nutrients, which results in depletion of endogenous glycogen stores, eventual autolysis of the parasitic worm, and its death	Treatment of single or mixed helminthic infestations
praziquantel	Increases permeability of the cell membrane of susceptible worms to calcium, which results in the influx of calcium; this causes the worms to be dislodged from their usual site of residence in the mesenteric veins to the liver, where they are killed by host tissue reactions.	Schistosomiasis, opisthorchiasis (liver fluke infection), clonorchiasis (infection with clonorchis or Chinese or Oriental liver fluke), diphyllobothriasis (fish worm infection), hymenolepiasis (dwarf tapeworm infection), neurocysticercosis
pyrantel pamoate	Blocks acetylcholine at the neuromuscular junction, which results in paralysis of the worm; the paralyzed worm is expelled from the gastrointestinal tract by normal peristalsis.	Ascariasis, enterobiasis, other helminthic infections

of feces, urine, blood, sputum, or tissue from the infected host for the presence of ova or larvae of the particular parasite. Three anthelmintics are commercially available in Canada: mebendazole (Vermox®), praziquantel (Biltricide®), and pyrantel pamoate (Combantrin®, Jaa Pyral®).

Other drugs, such as niclosamide and piperazine, may be available either in other countries or by special request to Health Canada. Anthelmintics are specific in their actions. Mebendazole can be used to treat both tapeworms and roundworms. Praziquantel can kill flukes (trematodes). Pyrantel pamoate is effective against giant roundworms and pinworms.

Mechanism of Action and Drug Effects

The mechanisms of action of the various anthelmintics vary greatly from drug to drug, although there are some similarities among the drugs used to kill similar types of worms. The anthelmintic drugs and their respective mechanisms of action are listed in Table 48-9. The drug effects of anthelmintic drugs are limited to their ability to kill various forms of worms and flukes.

Indications

Anthelmintic drugs are used to treat roundworm, tapeworm, and fluke infections. Specific drugs are used to treat specific helminthic infections.

Contraindications

The only usual contraindication to a specific anthelmintic drug product is known drug allergy. Pyrantel pamoate is contraindicated in patients with liver disease. Praziquantel is also contraindicated in patients with ocular cysticercosis (tapeworm infection of the eye).

Adverse Effects

The anthelmintic drugs show a remarkable diversity in their drug-specific adverse effects. Common adverse effects are listed in Table 48-10.

TABLE	48-10

Anthelmintics: Common Adverse Effects

Body System	Adverse Effects
PRAZIQUANTEL	
Central nervous	Dizziness, headache, drowsiness
Gastrointestinal	Abdominal pain, nausea
Other	Malaise
PRIMAQUINE	
Gastrointestinal	Nausea, vomiting, abdominal distress
Other	Headaches, pruritus, dark discoloration of urine, hemolytic anemia due to glucose-6-phosphate dehydrogenase deficiency
PYRANTEL PAMOATE	
Central nervous	Headache, dizziness, insomnia
Gastrointestinal	Abdominal pain, nausea
Other	Malaise

Interactions

The concurrent use of pyrantel pamoate (an over-the-counter anthelmintic) with piperazine is not recommended, and pyrantel pamoate is used cautiously in patients with liver impairment. Pyrantel pamoate has also been shown to raise blood levels of theophylline in children. Dexamethasone and the anthelmintic praziquantel may raise blood levels of mebendazole. Histamine H_2 antagonists (e.g., cimetidine, ranitidine hydrochloride) may also raise blood levels of praziquantel.

Dosages

For dosage information for selected anthelmintic drugs, refer to the table on p. 904.

DRUG PROFILES

Anthelmintics are available only as oral preparations and, with the exception of pyrantel pamoate, all require a prescription. Different drugs are selected to treat infection by different helminthic species.

praziquantel

Praziquantel (Biltricide) is one of the primary anthelmintic drugs used for the treatment of various fluke infections. It is also useful against many species of tapeworm. It is contraindicated in patients with ocular worm infestation (ocular cysticercosis). It is available only for oral use.

PHARMACOKINETICS

Route	Onset of Action	Peak Plasma Concentration	Elimination Half-Life	Duration of Action
PO	1 hr	1–3 hr	4–5 hr	Variable

pyrantel pamoate

Pyrantel pamoate (Combantrin, Jaa Pyral) is a pyrimidine-derived anthelmintic drug indicated for the treatment of infection with intestinal roundworms, including ascariasis, enterobiasis, and other helminthic infections. It is available in Canada for oral use and is purchased over the counter.

PHARMACOKINETICS

Route	Onset of Action	Peak Plasma Concentration	Elimination Half-Life	Duration of Action
PO	1 hr	1–3 hr	Unknown	Unknown

DOSAGES	Selected Anthelmintic Drugs		
Drug	**Pharmacological Class**	**Usual Dosage Range**	**Indications**
praziquantel (Biltricide)	Trematode anthelmintic	*Adults and children over 4 yr* PO: approx. 25 mg/kg tid × 1 day	Fluke infections
pyrantel pamoate (Combantrin, Jaa Pyral)	Nematode anthelmintic	*Adults and children over 1 yr* PO: 11 mg/kg in a single dose (max dose 1 g)	Roundworm infections

PO, oral.

NURSING PROCESS

◾ Assessment

Before beginning treatment with an antimalarial drug, obtain a thorough travel and medication history, perform a head-to-toe physical assessment, and measure vital signs. Give special attention to assessment findings of any common manifestations of malaria, such as headache, nausea, and joint pain. Other symptoms include chills and rigour, followed by a fever of up to 40°C, frequently leading to extreme fatigue and prolonged sleep. Baseline visual acuity tests may be needed due to the contraindications of visual field problems and optic neuritis with chloroquine and quinine sulphate. Perform a skin assessment with the use of these drugs as well because of the contraindications affecting individuals with psoriasis. Other drugs, such as mefloquine hydrochloride and primaquine phosphate, require assessment of baseline hearing (with primaquine hydrochloride) and assessment for G6PD deficiency due to possible

drug-induced hemolytic anemia. Common drug interactions to assess for are listed in Table 48-2.

Antiprotozoal drugs and their contraindications, cautions, and drug interactions have been previously discussed. Assess baseline kidney and liver function as well as overall health status. Prior to the use of atovaquone, determine baseline blood counts due to the risk of drug-induced anemia, neutropenia, and leukopenia. Assess serum potassium, sodium, and glucose levels as ordered. Metronidazole requires assessment for allergy to any of the nitroimidazole derivatives as well as to parabens (for the topical dosage forms). Obtain appropriate specimens for analysis before treatment. Prior to use of metronidazole, assess blood counts, any central nervous system disorders or abnormalities, and bladder function. Pentamidine isethionate is associated with serious cardiac, hematological, skin, kidney, GI, and respiratory adverse effects; therefore, documentation of a thorough assessment of each of these systems is crucial to patient safety.

Prior to the administration of any of the anthelmintic drugs, obtain a thorough travel history and a history of foods eaten, especially meat and fish, and their means of preparation. Also assess other individuals in the patient's household for helminth infection. Obtaining stool specimens is indicated. Assess the patient's energy level, ability to perform activities of daily living, weight, and appetite, and document these findings. Assess for contraindications, such as liver disease and drug allergy, and any cautions. Assess for drug interactions, including with theophylline, antiepileptic drugs, and histamine H_2 antagonists.

Nursing Diagnoses

- Imbalanced nutrition, less than body requirements, related to the disease process and adverse effects of medication
- Deficient knowledge related to the infection and its drug treatment
- Ineffective therapeutic regimen management by patient and family, related to poor adherence to treatment and lack of knowledge about the infection and its treatment

Planning

Goals

- Patient will maintain balanced nutrition during drug therapy.
- Patient, family members, and significant others will demonstrate adequate knowledge regarding the infection and its treatment.
- Patient, family members, and others in the home environment will experience improved therapeutic regimen management and compliance.

Expected Patient Outcomes

- Patient states measures to enhance balanced nutrition, taking into account recommendations for increased caloric and protein intake.
  - Patient identifies menu planning strategies appropriate to meet increased nutritional demands.
  - Patient lists foods to be included in daily diet to improve overall nutritional status, incorporating recommendations from Canada's Food Guide along with prescribed dietary changes.
- Patient states the impact of infectious process on the human body and its functioning.
  - Patient states the various measures to prevent worsening of lesions and minimize tissue injury, such as washing hands thoroughly; reporting any worsening of lesions, drainage, fever, or joint pain; and taking medication as prescribed.
  - Patient states the importance of reporting the worsening of symptoms of the infection, including fever, lethargy, and loss of appetite.
  - Patient states the rationale for continuing with treatment for the prescribed length of time.

- Patient states the importance of effective therapeutic regimen management by and for the family, including adhering to therapy, returning for follow-up visits to the health care provider to monitor progress, being aware of any adverse drug reactions, and reporting any new symptoms in members of the family or household.

Implementation

With antimalarials, encourage adequate dietary and fluid intake while the patient is fighting the infection and taking medication. Take oral doses with at least 180 to 240 mL of water or other fluid, and increase fluid intake unless contraindicated. Because antimalarials concentrate in the liver first, emphasize to the patient the importance of follow-up visits to the health care provider so that liver function may be monitored during therapy.

Chloroquine and hydroxychloroquine are administered orally and are to be given exactly as prescribed. Follow dosing orders and instructions as prescribed, with specific attention to the loading doses, subsequent doses, and prophylactic dosing. Photosensitivity may occur with the use of quinine sulphate; provide adequate teaching about sun safety and the use of sunscreen. Sun protection must include protection from both UVA and UVB rays. See Patient Teaching Tips for more information. Most of the antiprotozoal drugs (e.g., atovaquone, metronidazole) are given with food when taken orally. Infuse IV doses of metronidazole as indicated in the manufacturer's instructions. During use of this drug, report to the health care provider any changes in neurological status (e.g., dizziness, confusion). All anthelmintic drugs are to be administered as ordered and for the prescribed length of time. Warn patients that the use of primaquine may lead to dark discoloration of the urine. Perform collection of stool specimens as ordered. The stool must not come in contact with water, urine, or chemicals because of the risk of destroying the parasitic worms or altering the test results. See Patient Teaching Tips for more information on anthelmintic drugs.

Evaluation

Monitor patients for the therapeutic effects of antimalarials, antiprotozoals, and anthelmintic drugs, such as improved energy levels and decrease in or eventual resolution of all symptoms. Evaluation of proper hygiene and prevention of the spread of the infestation or infection is also important. With these three groups of drugs, evaluate for the adverse effects associated with each type of drug (see Tables 48-1, 48-6, and 48-10). Some antimalarials and anthelmintics may precipitate hemolysis in patients with G6PD deficiency (mostly patients of African descent and those of Mediterranean ancestry); therefore, closely monitor these patients for this complication during the treatment protocol. See Chapter 2 for further discussion of G6PD deficiency.

CASE STUDY

Metronidazole

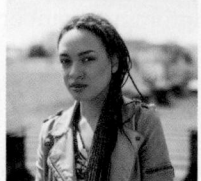

Kelis, a 28-year-old graduate student, just returned from an archeology internship in a developing country. She has had severe diarrhea for several days and has been diagnosed with intestinal amoebiasis. She will receive fluids for rehydration and metronidazole as part of her treatment.

1. What specific laboratory test must be ordered before the initiation of the metronidazole therapy? List other laboratory studies that will be performed.

2. Kelis is started on oral metronidazole treatment and after a day she reports that her diarrhea has decreased and that she feels a little better. During afternoon rounds, she tells the nurse that she has some nausea and feels dizzy and tired. She asks, "Is this because of my infection?" How will the nurse respond?

3. Kelis is discharged to home with a prescription to take the metronidazole for 8 more days (for a total of 10 days). The nurse knows that one serious adverse effect of this medication is leukopenia. What symptoms will the nurse tell Kelis to report?

4. A week later, Kelis calls to tell the nurse that she went out to a bar with some friends and became very ill after having one drink. Explain what happened.

For anwers, see http://evolve.elsevier.com/Canada/Lilley/pharmacology/.

PATIENT TEACHING TIPS

❖ Antimalarials are known to cause GI upset; however, this may be decreased if the medication is taken with food. Encourage patients to inform the health care provider if there is unresolved nausea, vomiting, profuse diarrhea, or abdominal pain. Patients should immediately report any visual disturbances, dizziness, or respiratory difficulties.

❖ Educate patients about the need for prophylactic doses of antimalarials, as prescribed, before visiting malaria-endemic countries, as well as the need to receive appropriate treatment upon return.

❖ As with other medications, patients should know to keep antimalarials out of the reach of children.

❖ Instruct patients to take the entire course of medication as directed.

❖ Patients should be aware that oral dosage forms of metronidazole are to be taken with food.

❖ Inform patients taking metronidazole for a sexually transmitted infection to avoid sexual intercourse until the health care provider indicates that it is safe.

❖ When a patient is taking metronidazole for amoebiasis, include in your instructions how to check stool samples correctly and safely, as well as how to dispose of samples properly.

❖ Apply topical forms of drugs with a finger cot or gloved hand, and caution patients to avoid contact of the drug with the eyes.

❖ Metronidazole may precipitate dizziness. Encourage patients to be cautious with all activities until response to the drug is noted and consistent.

❖ Anthelmintics are to be taken exactly as prescribed; emphasize to patients the importance of adherence to the drug regimen.

KEY POINTS

❖ Malaria is caused by *Plasmodium*, a particular genus of protozoa, and is transmitted through the bite of an infected female mosquito. The drug primaquine attacks the parasite when it is outside the exoerythrocytic (tissue) phase.

❖ Other common protozoal infections are amoebiasis, giardiasis, toxoplasmosis, and trichomoniasis. Protozoa are parasites that are transmitted by person-to-person contact, ingestion of contaminated water or food, direct contact with the parasite, or the bite of an insect (mosquito or tick). Pneumocystosis is now classified as a fungal infection, but it is treated with antiprotozoal drugs.

❖ Antiprotozoals include atovaquone and pentamidine isethionate. Metronidazole is an antibacterial, antiprotozoal, and anthelmintic. Paromomycin sulphate directly kills protozoa such as *Entamoeba histolytica*.

❖ Anthelmintics are drugs used to treat parasitic worm infections caused by cestodes (tapeworms), nematodes (roundworms), and trematodes (flukes).

❖ Nursing considerations with the use of any of the antimalarials, antiprotozoals, and anthelmintics include assessment for contraindications, cautions, and drug interactions.

EXAMINATION REVIEW QUESTIONS

1. The nurse is reviewing the medication history of a patient who is taking hydroxychloroquine. The patient's history does not reveal a history of malaria or travel out of the country. The patient is most likely taking this medication for which condition?
   a. *Plasmodium*
   b. A thyroid disorder
   c. Roundworms
   d. Rheumatoid arthritis

2. What teaching point would be appropriate for the nurse to include when informing a patient about the adverse effects of antimalarials?
   a. The skin may turn blotchy while these medications are taken.
   b. These medications may cause anorexia and abdominal distress.
   c. These medications may cause increased urinary output.
   d. You may experience periods of diaphoresis and chills.

3. When teaching a patient about potential drug interactions with antiprotozoal drugs, the nurse will include information about which drug or type of drug?
   a. acetaminophen
   b. warfarin sodium
   c. Decongestants
   d. Antibiotics

4. Before administering antiprotozoal drugs, the nurse will review which baseline assessment?
   a. Complete blood count
   b. Serum magnesium level
   c. Creatinine clearance
   d. Arterial blood gas concentration

5. The nurse knows that antimalarial drugs are used to treat patients with infections caused by which microorganism?
   a. *Plasmodium* spp.
   b. *Candida albicans*
   c. *Pneumocystis jirovecii*
   d. *Mycobacterium* spp.

6. When giving metronidazole, which of these appropriate administration techniques does the nurse implement? (Select all that apply.)
   a. Giving oral forms with food
   b. Giving oral forms on an empty stomach with a full glass of water
   c. Infusing IV doses over 30 to 60 minutes
   d. Administering IV doses by bolus over 5 minutes
   e. Obtaining ordered specimens before starting the medication

7. A 5-year-old patient has been diagnosed with malaria after returning from a trip. The patient is to receive one dose of mefloquine hydrochloride (Lariam), 25 mg/kg PO. The child weighs 44 pounds. How much mefloquine hydrochloride will this child receive? Is this a safe dose?

CRITICAL THINKING ACTIVITIES

1. You are preparing to give pyrantel pamoate (Combantrin) to a patient who is infected with intestinal roundworms. The patient is worried about this infection and its treatment and asks you, "What will this drug do to me? Does it have bad effects? I'm already sick enough!" What is your priority when answering the patient's questions?

2. Your friend is travelling to a country where there is high risk for malaria infection. The friend asks you what you think her nurse practitioner will order, if anything at all. What is your best response to this question?

3. A patient with a history of AIDS has severe *Pneumocystis jirovecii* pneumonia. As you prepare the ordered intravenous pentamidine, the patient asks you, "What are you doing? Why can't you give that to me in a pill?" What is your priority when answering the patient's questions?

For answers, see http://evolve.elsevier.com/Canada/Lilley/pharmacology/.

CHAPTER 49

Anti-inflammatory and Antigout Drugs

Objectives

After reading this chapter, the successful student will be able to do the following:

1. Discuss the inflammatory response and the role it plays in the generation of pain.

2. Compare disease processes (pathologies) that are inflammatory in nature.

3. Discuss the mechanisms of action, indications, adverse effects, dosage ranges, routes of administration, cautions, contraindications, drug interactions, and toxicities of the various anti-inflammatory and antigout drugs.

4. Develop a collaborative plan of care that includes all phases of the nursing process for patients receiving anti-inflammatory or antigout drugs.

e-Learning Activities

Website
(http://evolve.elsevier.com/Canada/
Lilley/pharmacology/)

evolve

* Answer Key—Textbook Case Studies
* Answer Key—Critical Thinking Activities
* Chapter Summaries—Printable
* Review Questions for Exam Preparation
* Unfolding Case Studies

Drug Profiles

▸▸ acetylsalicylic acid, p. 914
▸▸ allopurinol, p. 917
▸▸ celecoxib, p. 915
   colchicine, p. 917
▸▸ ibuprofen, p. 915
▸▸ indomethacin, p. 914
▸▸ ketorolac (ketorolac tromethamine)*, p. 915
   probenecid, p. 918

▸▸ Key drug

*Full generic name is given in parentheses. For the purposes of this text, the more common, shortened name is used.

Key Terms

Done nomogram A standard plot of graphic data, originally published in 1960 in the journal *Pediatrics*, for rating the severity of aspirin toxicity following overdose; serum salicylate levels are plotted against time elapsed since ingestion. (p. 913)

Gout Hyperuricemia (elevated blood uric acid level); the arthritis caused by tissue buildup of uric acid crystals. (p. 916)

Inflammation A localized protective response stimulated by injury to tissues that serves to destroy, dilute, or wall off (sequester) both the injurious agent and the injured tissue. (p. 909)

Nonsteroidal anti-inflammatory drugs (NSAIDs) A large, chemically diverse group of drugs that possess analgesic, anti-inflammatory, and antipyretic activity. (p. 909)

Salicylism The syndrome of salicylate toxicity, including symptoms such as tinnitus, nausea, and vomiting. (p. 912)

OVERVIEW

Inflammation is defined as a localized protective response stimulated by injury to tissues, which serves to destroy, dilute, or wall off (sequester) both the injurious agent and the injured tissue. Classic signs and symptoms of inflammation include pain, fever, loss of function, redness, and swelling. These symptoms result from arterial, venous, and capillary dilation; enhanced blood flow and vascular permeability; exudation of fluids, including plasma proteins; and leukocyte migration into the inflammatory focus. The inflammatory response is mediated by a host of endogenous compounds, including proteins of the complement system, histamine, serotonin, bradykinin, leukotrienes, and prostaglandins, the latter two being major contributors to the symptoms of inflammation.

Arachidonic acid is released from phospholipids in cell membranes in response to a triggering event (e.g., an injury). It is metabolized in either the prostaglandin pathway or the leukotriene pathway, both of which are branches of the arachidonic acid pathway, as shown in Figure 49-1. Both of these pathways lead to inflammation, edema, headache, and other pain characteristic of the body's response to injury or inflammatory illnesses such as arthritis.

In the prostaglandin pathway, arachidonic acid is converted by the enzyme cyclooxygenase into various prostaglandins. Prostaglandins mediate inflammation by inducing vasodilation and enhancing vasopermeability. These effects in turn potentiate the action of proinflammatory substances such as histamine and bradykinin in the production of edema and pain. These symptoms arise as a result of prostaglandin-induced hyperalgesia (excessive sensitivity). In this situation, stimuli that normally would not be painful, such as the movement of a joint through its natural range of motion, become painful because of the inflammatory process at work. Fever occurs when prostaglandin E_2 is synthesized in the preoptic hypothalamic region, the area of the brain that regulates temperature.

The leukotriene pathway utilizes lipoxygenases to metabolize the arachidonic acid and convert it into various leukotrienes. Although leukotrienes were discovered more recently than prostaglandins and are thus not as well studied, they are also mediators of inflammation, promoting vasoconstriction, bronchospasm, and increased vascular permeability with resultant edema (see Chapter 38).

NONSTEROIDAL ANTI-INFLAMMATORY DRUGS

Nonsteroidal anti-inflammatory drugs (NSAIDs) are among the most commonly prescribed drugs. Every year, over 10 million prescriptions are written for NSAIDs in Canada (Kümmerer, 2013). This figure represents over 4% of all prescriptions. Currently, more than 15 different NSAIDs are available in Canada; many of these are available to be purchased over the counter as well as by prescription. Some are used more commonly than others. Any one patient may respond better to one NSAID than to others, in terms of both symptom relief and adverse effects.

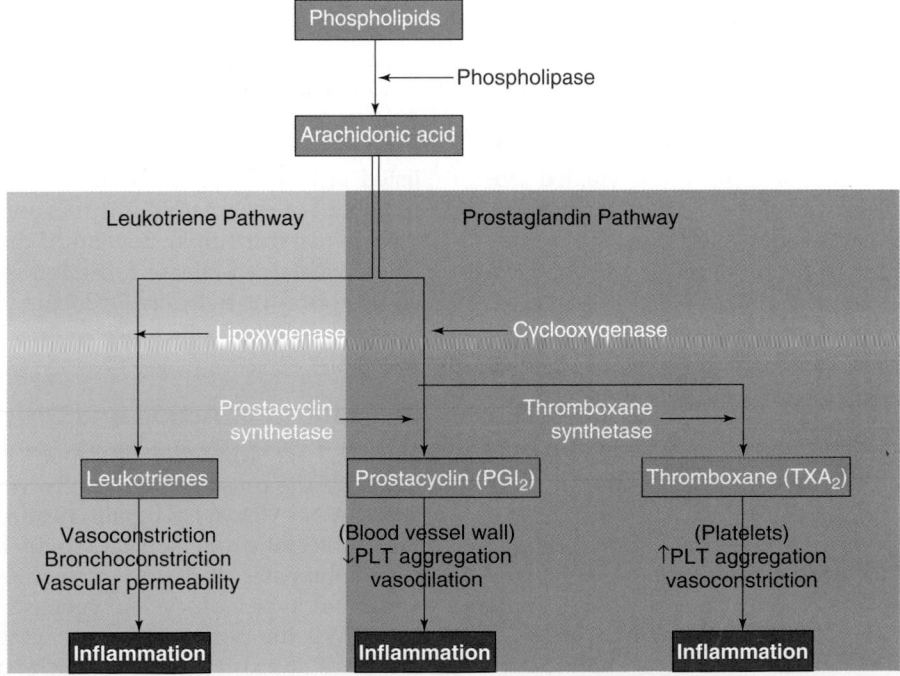

FIG. 49-1 Arachidonic acid pathway. *PGI$_2$*, Prostaglandin I$_2$; *PLT*, platelet; *TXA$_2$*, thromboxane A$_2$.

BOX 49-1 **Chemical Categories of NSAIDS**

Salicylates

aspirin
diflunisal

Acetic Acid Derivatives

diclofenac sodium (Voltaren®)
indomethacin sulindac
etodolac
ketorolac (Toradol®)
mefenamic acid (Ponstan®)

Cyclooxygenase-2 Inhibitors

celecoxib (Celebrex®)

Enolic Acid Derivatives

nabumetone
meloxicam (Mobicox®)
piroxicam

Propionic Acid Derivatives

flurbiprofen
ibuprofen (Advil®, Motrin®)
ketoprofen (Apo-Keto-E®)
naproxen (Naprolen®, Naprosyn®, Aleve®)
oxaprozin tiaprofenic acid

NSAIDs, nonsteroidal anti-inflammatory drugs.

NSAIDs comprise a large, chemically diverse group of drugs that possess analgesic, anti-inflammatory, and antipyretic activity. They are also used for the relief of mild to moderate headaches, myalgia, neuralgia, and arthralgia; alleviation of postoperative pain; relief of the pain associated with arthritic disorders such as rheumatoid arthritis, juvenile arthritis, ankylosing spondylitis, and osteoarthritis; and treatment of gout and hyperuricemia (discussed later in the chapter). Aspirin is an NSAID used for its effect in inhibiting platelet aggregation, which has been shown to have protective qualities against certain cardiovascular events such as myocardial infarction (MI) and stroke. Corticosteroid anti-inflammatory drugs (e.g., prednisone, dexamethasone) are also used for similar purposes and were discussed in Chapter 34. NSAIDs have generally more favourable adverse effect profiles than corticosteroidal anti-inflammatory drugs.

In 1899, acetylsalicylic acid (ASA; Aspirin) was marketed and rapidly became the most widely used drug in the world. The success of aspirin established the importance of drugs with antipyretic, analgesic, and anti-inflammatory properties, properties that all NSAIDs share. The widespread use of aspirin also yielded evidence of its potential for causing major adverse effects. Gastrointestinal (GI) intolerance, bleeding, and kidney impairment became major factors limiting its long-term administration. As a result, efforts were mounted to develop drugs that did not have the adverse effects of aspirin. This led to the discovery of other NSAIDs, which in general are associated with less serious adverse effects and a lower incidence for those effects; they are often better tolerated than aspirin in patients with chronic diseases. If aspirin were to be a newly discovered drug today, it would require a prescription.

As a single class, NSAIDs constitute an exceptional variety of drugs, and they are used for an equally wide range of indications. Box 49-1 categorizes these drugs into a number of distinct chemical classes. NSAIDs have been approved for a variety of indications and are considered the drug of choice for most of the conditions

---

BOX 49-2

NSAIDs: Health Canada–Approved Indications

- Acute gout
- Acute gouty arthritis
- Ankylosing spondylitis
- Bursitis
- Fever
- Juvenile rheumatoid arthritis
- Mild to moderate pain
- Osteoarthritis
- Primary dysmenorrhea
- Rheumatoid arthritis
- Tendinitis
- Various ophthalmic uses

NSAIDs, nonsteroidal anti-inflammatory drugs.

---

listed in Box 49-2. Almost all NSAIDs are used for the treatment of rheumatoid arthritis and degenerative joint disease (osteoarthritis). Several of these drugs are available in sustained-release formulations. This formulation allows once- or twice-daily dosing, which is known to improve patients' adherence to prescribed drug therapy regimens.

Mechanism of Action and Drug Effects

NSAIDs act through inhibition of the leukotriene pathway, the prostaglandin pathway, or both. More specifically, NSAIDs relieve pain, headache, and inflammation by blocking the chemical activity of the *cyclooxygenase* (COX) enzymes. It is now recognized that there are at least two types of cyclooxygenase. Cyclooxygenase-1 (COX-1) is the isoform of the enzyme that promotes the synthesis of prostaglandins, which have primarily beneficial effects on various body functions. One example is their role in maintaining an intact intestinal mucosa. In contrast, the cyclooxygenase-2 (COX-2) isoform promotes the synthesis of prostaglandins that are involved in inflammatory processes. In 1999, the newest class of NSAIDs, the COX-2 inhibitors, was approved. Drugs in this class work by specifically inhibiting the COX-2 isoform of cyclooxygenase and theoretically have limited or no effects on COX-1. Previous NSAIDs nonspecifically inhibited both COX-1 and COX-2 activities. This greater enzyme specificity of the COX-2 inhibitors allows for beneficial anti-inflammatory effects while reducing the prevalence of adverse effects associated with the nonspecific NSAIDs, such as GI ulceration. The leukotriene pathway is inhibited by some anti-inflammatory drugs, but not by salicylates.

All NSAIDs can be ulcerogenic and induce GI bleeding due to their activity against tissue COX-1. One notable effect of aspirin is the inhibition of platelet aggregation, also known as its *antiplatelet activity*. Aspirin has the unique property among NSAIDs of being an irreversible inhibitor of COX-1 receptors within platelets themselves. This in turn results in reduced formation by the platelets of thromboxane A$_2$, a substance that normally promotes platelet aggregation. This antiplatelet action has made aspirin, along with thrombolytic drugs (see Chapter 27), a primary drug in the treatment of acute MI and many other thromboembolic disorders. Other NSAIDs lack these antiplatelet effects.

Indications

Some of the therapeutic uses of this broad class of drugs are listed in Table 49-1; however, NSAIDs are used primarily for their analgesic, anti-inflammatory, and antipyretic effects, and for platelet inhibition.

NSAIDs are also widely used for the treatment of rheumatoid arthritis and osteoarthritis, as well as other inflammatory conditions, rheumatic fever, mild to moderate pain, and acute gout. They have proven beneficial

as adjunctive pain relief medications in patients with chronic persistent pain syndromes, such as pain from bone cancer and chronic persistent back pain. For the relief of pain, NSAIDs are sometimes combined with an opioid (see Chapter 11). They tend to have an opioid-sparing effect when given together with opioids because the drugs attack pain using two different mechanisms. This often allows less of the opioid to be used. Unlike opioids, NSAIDs show a ceiling effect that limits their effectiveness; that is, any further increase in the dosage beyond a certain level increases the risk of adverse effects without a corresponding increase in therapeutic effect. Refer to manufacturers' instructions for maximum dosages. In contrast, opioid doses may be titrated almost indefinitely to increasingly higher levels, especially in terminally ill patients with severe pain.

The appropriate selection of an NSAID is a clinical judgement based on consideration of the patient's history, including any previous medical conditions, the intended use of the drug, the patient's previous experience with NSAIDs, the patient's preference, and the cost.

Contraindications

Contraindications to NSAIDs include known drug allergy and conditions that place the patient at risk for bleeding such as rhinitis (due to possible epistaxis [nosebleed]), vitamin K deficiency, and peptic ulcer disease. NSAIDs should not be administered to a patient with a current hemorrhagic stroke. Patients with documented aspirin allergy must not receive NSAIDs. Other common contraindications are those that apply to most drugs and include severe kidney or liver disease. NSAIDs are considered relatively safe to use during pregnancy and do not increase the risk of spontaneous abortion (Daniel et al., 2014). Women who are pregnant should avoid using NSAIDs after 32 weeks' gestation, owing to the possibility of antiplatelet or prolonged bleeding effects. Although prenatal ductal constriction and closure have been described with

TABLE 49-1

Suggested NSAIDs for Patients with Various Medical Conditions

Medical Condition	Recommended NSAID
Ankylosing spondylitis	indomethacin, naproxen, sulindac, piroxicam
Dysmenorrhea	Fenamates, naproxen, ibuprofen
Gout	indomethacin, naproxen, sulindac
Headaches	aspirin, ibuprofen, naproxen
Hepatotoxicity	naproxen, ibuprofen, piroxicam, fenamates
History of aspirin or NSAID allergy	Avoid NSAIDs if possible; if deemed necessary, consider a nonacetylated salicylate
Hypertension	sulindac, nonacetylated salicylate, ibuprofen, etodolac
Osteoarthritis	diclofenac sodium, oxaprozin, indomethacin, piroxicam
Risk for gastrointestinal toxicity	celecoxib, nonacetylated salicylate, enteric-coated aspirin, diclofenac sodium, nabumetone, etodolac, ibuprofen, oxaprozin
Risk for nephrotoxicity	sulindac, nonacetylated salicylate, nabumetone, etodolac, diclofenac sodium, oxaprozin
warfarin sodium therapy	sulindac, naproxen, ibuprofen, oxaprozin

NSAIDs, Nonsteroidal anti-inflammatory drugs.

the maternal use of NSAIDs, frequently no clear underlying cause is found (Sridharan, Archer, & Manning, 2009). Interestingly, NSAIDs (ibuprofen or indomethacin) are used to close patent ductus arteriosus in neonates. NSAID use has also been associated with neonatal NSAID toxicity during the perinatal period. These drugs are also not recommended for nursing mothers because they are known to be excreted into human milk. Because of the potential of NSAIDs to increase bleeding, patients undergoing elective surgery need to stop taking NSAIDs at least 1 week prior to surgery.

Adverse Effects

Although NSAIDs are the most widely used class of drugs, and some are available without prescription, their potential for causing serious adverse effects has been underemphasized. Among the more common and potentially serious adverse effects of NSAIDs is their impact on the GI tract. Symptoms can range from mild, such as heartburn, to the most severe GI complication, GI bleeding. Most fatalities associated with NSAID use are related to GI bleeding. In addition, acute kidney injury is quite common with NSAID use, especially if the patient is dehydrated. The potential adverse effects of NSAIDs are listed in Table 49-2. Not all of the adverse effects necessarily apply to all drugs, but many do. In 2006, Health Canada began requiring warnings on all of the NSAIDs' packaging (see Box 49-3). In 2014, Health Canada updated its warning on diclofenac (based on a 2013 study by Bhala et al.) to include the increased risk of cardiovascular disease, particularly at higher doses (150 mg per day or more) and with longer duration of use. Patients with a history of or risk factors for heart disease, stroke, or uncontrolled high blood pressure may be at greater risk if they use diclofenac. This increased risk is also associated with high doses of ibuprofen (see discussion on ibuprofen).

Kidney function depends partly on prostaglandins; the use of NSAIDs can compromise existing kidney function. Disruption of prostaglandin function by NSAIDs is sometimes strong enough to precipitate acute kidney injury or chronic kidney failure, depending on the patient's current level of kidney function. Kidney toxicity can occur in patients who are dehydrated, those with heart failure or liver dysfunction, and those taking diuretics or angiotensin-converting enzyme (ACE) inhibitors.

Toxicity and Management of Overdose

Salicylate toxicity, usually from aspirin, is not as common as it once was; however, there are both chronic and acute manifestations of salicylate toxicity. Chronic salicylate intoxication is known as **salicylism** and results from either short-term administration of high dosages or prolonged therapy with high or even lower doses. The most common signs and symptoms of acute or chronic salicylate intoxication are listed in Table 49-3.

The most common manifestations of chronic salicylate intoxication in adults are tinnitus and hearing loss. Common manifestations in children are hyperventilation and central nervous system (CNS) effects such as dizziness, drowsiness, and behavioural changes. Metabolic

TABLE 49-2

NSAIDS: Adverse Effects

Body System	Adverse Effects
Cardiovascular	Moderate to severe noncardiogenic pulmonary edema
Gastrointestinal	Dyspepsia, heartburn, epigastric distress, nausea, vomiting, anorexia, abdominal pain, gastrointestinal bleeding, mucosal lesions (erosions or ulcerations)
Hematological	Altered hemostasis through effects on platelet function
Hepatic	Acute reversible hepatotoxicity
Renal	Reduction in creatinine clearance, acute tubular necrosis with acute kidney injury
Other	Skin eruption, sensitivity reactions, tinnitus, hearing loss

NSAIDs, nonsteroidal anti-inflammatory drugs.

BOX 49-3   Health Canada Required Warnings on All NSAIDs

The following warnings must now be included in the packaging for all NSAIDs:

Cardiovascular Risk

- NSAIDs may cause an increased risk of serious cardiovascular thrombotic events, MI, and stroke, which can be fatal. This risk may increase with duration of use. Patients with cardiovascular disease or risk factors for cardiovascular disease may be at greater risk.
- NSAIDs are contraindicated for the treatment of perioperative pain in the setting of coronary artery bypass graft surgery.

Gastrointestinal Risk

- NSAIDs cause an increased risk of serious GI adverse events, including bleeding, ulceration, and perforation of the stomach or intestines, which can be fatal. These events can occur at any time during use and without warning symptoms. Older adult patients are at greater risk for serious GI events.
- See Chapter 3 for more information on drug warnings.

GI, gastrointestinal; *MI*, myocardial infarction; *NSAIDs*, nonsteroidal anti-inflammatory drugs.

TABLE 49-3

Acute or Chronic Salicylate Intoxication: Signs and Symptoms

Body System	Signs and Symptoms
Cardiovascular	Increased heart rate
Central nervous	Tinnitus, hearing loss, dimness of vision, headache, dizziness, mental confusion, lassitude, drowsiness
Gastrointestinal	Nausea, vomiting, diarrhea
Metabolic	Sweating, thirst, hyperventilation, hypoglycemia or hyperglycemia

TABLE 49-4

Acute Salicylate Intoxication: Treatment

Severity	Treatment
Mild	1. Dosage reduction or discontinuation of salicylates 2. Symptomatic and supportive therapy
Severe	1. Discontinuation of salicylates 2. Intensive symptomatic and supportive therapy 3. Dialysis if high salicylate levels, unresponsive acidosis (pH less than 7.1), impaired kidney function or kidney failure, pulmonary edema, persistent CNS symptoms (e.g., seizures, coma), progressive deterioration despite appropriate therapy

CNS, central nervous system.

complications such as metabolic acidosis and respiratory alkalosis often occur to varying degrees in cases of chronic salicylate intoxication. Metabolic acidosis can also occur with acute intoxication, but it is usually less severe than that in patients with chronic intoxication. Hypoglycemia may also arise and can be life-threatening. The treatment of chronic salicylate intoxication is based on the presenting symptoms.

Serum salicylate concentrations may be determined but are not as useful in estimating the severity of toxicity because severe intoxication can occur with a concentration as low as 150 mg/kg.

The signs and symptoms of acute salicylate toxicity are similar to those of chronic intoxication, but the effects are often more pronounced and occur more quickly. Acute salicylate overdose usually results from the ingestion of a single toxic dose, and its severity can be judged based on the estimated amount ingested (in milligrams per kilogram of body weight), as follows:

- Little or no toxicity: less than 150 mg/kg
- Mild to moderate toxicity: 150 to 300 mg/kg
- Severe toxicity: 300 to 500 mg/kg
- Life-threatening toxicity: over 500 mg/kg

However, doses lower than 150 mg/kg have resulted in fatal toxicity. A serum salicylate concentration measured 6 hours or longer after the ingestion may be used in conjunction with the **Done nomogram** to estimate the severity of intoxication and help guide treatment. The Done nomogram is a graphic plot of serum salicylate level as a function of time since salicylate ingestion (Done, 1960). It was first published in a 1960 issue of the journal *Pediatrics* and is still widely used today for gauging acute salicylate toxicity. This nomogram is intended for estimating the severity only of acute intoxications and not chronic salicylate intoxication. Table 49-4 describes, in general terms, the treatment for cases of varying severity. Treatment goals include removing salicylate from the GI tract and preventing its further absorption; correcting fluid, electrolyte, and acid–base disturbances; and implementing measures to enhance salicylate elimination, including hemodialysis.

An acute overdose of nonsalicylate NSAIDs (e.g., ibuprofen) causes effects similar to those of salicylate overdose, but they are generally not as extensive or as dangerous. Symptoms include CNS toxicities such as drowsiness, lethargy, mental confusion, paresthesias (abnormal touch sensations), numbness, aggressive behaviour, disorientation, seizures, and GI toxicities such as nausea, vomiting, and GI bleeding. Intense headache, dizziness, cerebral edema, cardiac arrest, and death have also been known to occur in extreme cases. For suspected overdose, consultation with a poison control centre is recommended. Treatment consists of the administration of activated charcoal, with supportive and symptomatic treatment initiated thereafter. Unlike with salicylates, hemodialysis appears to be of no value in enhancing the elimination of nonsalicylate NSAIDs.

Interactions

Drug interactions associated with the use of salicylates and other NSAIDs can result in significant complications and morbidity. One significant drug interaction occurs between the use of NSAIDs and angiotensin-coverting enzyme inhibitors (ACEIs) and angiotensin-receptor inhibitors (ARBs). NSAIDs inhibit renal prostaglandins resulting in afferent arteriole vasoconstriction and ACEI/ARBs cause efferent arteriole vasodilation. The combination of both results in a drastic decrease in GFR which can lead to kidney failure (especially in patients with already compromised kidneys or in older adults). Some of the more common interactions are listed in Table 49-5.

NSAIDs can also interfere with laboratory test results. Specifically, salicylates can cause what are usually minor and transient elevations in liver enzymes (ALT, AST), but, unlike with acetaminophen (see Chapter 11), cases of severe hepatotoxicity are rare. Hematocrit, hemoglobin level, and red blood cell (RBC) count can drop if there is any drug-induced GI bleeding, and bleeding time may be prolonged. NSAID-induced hyperkalemia or hyponatremia can also occur.

Dosages

For the recommended dosages of selected NSAIDs, refer to the table on p. 916.

TABLE 49-5		
Salicylates and Other NSAIDs: Drug Interactions		
Drug	**Mechanism**	**Result**
Alcohol	Additive effect	Increased GI bleeding
Anticoagulants	Platelet inhibition, hypoprothrombinemia	Increased bleeding tendencies
ASA and other salicylates with NSAIDs	Reduce NSAID absorption, additive GI toxicities	Increased GI toxicity with no therapeutic advantage
Bisphosphonates	Additive GI effects	Increased GI bleeding risk
Corticosteroids and other ulcerogenic drugs	Additive toxicities	Increased ulcerogenic effects
ciclosporin	Inhibition of kidney prostaglandin synthesis	Increased nephrotoxic effects of cyclosporine; kidney failure
Diuretics and ACE inhibitors	Inhibition of prostaglandin synthesis	Reduced hypotensive and diuretic effects
lithium carbonate	Increased lithium absorption	Increased lithium concentrations
Protein-bound drugs	Compete for binding	More pronounced drug actions
Uricosurics	Antagonism	Decreased uric acid excretion
Natural health products: feverfew, garlic, ginger, gingko	Interference with platelet function	Increased bleeding risk

ACE, angiotensin-converting enzyme; *ASA*, acetylsalicylic acid; *GI*, gastrointestinal; *NSAIDs*, nonsteroidal anti-inflammatory drugs.

 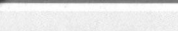

DRUG PROFILES

SALICYLATES

Aspirin is the most commonly used of all salicylates. Although aspirin is available over the counter (OTC), many of the other salicylate drugs, such as diflunisal, do require a prescription. Salicylates are most commonly used in solid oral dosage forms (e.g., tablets, capsules). Other available dosage forms include topical cream (Aspercreme®), oral liquids, and rectal suppositories. Aspirin is also contained in many combination products, including with antacids (e.g., Alka Seltzer®), with the antidyslipidemic pravastatin, and with the antiplatelet dipyridamole. Many of the available analgesic combinations contain caffeine, which provides an adjunctive analgesic effect. Aspirin is also available in special dosage forms, such as enteric-coated aspirin (Praxis ASA EC®), designed to protect the stomach mucosa by dissolving in the duodenum.

▶▶acetylsalicylic acid

Aspirin is known chemically as acetylsalicylic acid. It is the prototype salicylate and NSAID and is the most widely used drug in the world. A daily aspirin tablet (81 mg or 325 mg) is now routinely recommended as prophylactic therapy for adults who have strong risk factors for developing coronary artery disease or stroke, even if they have no prior history of such an event. The 81-mg (which is traditionally thought of as "children's" aspirin) effectively inhibits thromboxane A2 and the 325-mg strengths appear to be equally beneficial for the prevention of thrombotic events. For this reason, the lower strength is often chosen for patients who have any elevated risk of bleeding, such as those with prior stroke history, those with a history of peptic ulcer disease, or those taking the anticoagulant warfarin (Coumadin®). Aspirin is also often used to treat pain associated with headache, neuralgia,

myalgia, and arthralgia, as well as other pain syndromes resulting from inflammation, including arthritis, pleurisy, and pericarditis. The 81-mg dose, however, is not appropriate for treating pain in adults. Patients with systemic lupus erythematosus may benefit from aspirin therapy because of its antirheumatic effects. Aspirin is also used for its antipyretic action.

Aspirin and other salicylates all have one specific contraindication. This drug class is contraindicated in children with flulike symptoms because the use of these drugs has been strongly associated with Reye's syndrome. This is an acute and potentially life-threatening condition involving progressive neurological deficits that can lead to coma and may also involve liver damage. It is believed to be triggered by viral illnesses such as influenza as well as by salicylate therapy itself, in the presence of a viral illness. Survivors of this condition may or may not suffer permanent neurological damage.

PHARMACOKINETICS

Route	Onset of Action	Peak Plasma Concentration	Elimination Half-Life	Duration of Action
PO	15–30 min	1–2 hr	5–9 hr	4–6 hr

ACETIC ACID DERIVATIVES

There are several acetic acid derivatives, and they are listed in Box 49-1. Indomethacin and ketorolac are the most commonly used.

▶▶indomethacin

As with the other NSAIDs, indomethacin has analgesic, anti-inflammatory, antirheumatic, and antipyretic properties. Its therapeutic actions are of particular use in the

DRUG PROFILES—cont'd

treatment of rheumatoid arthritis, osteoarthritis, acute bursitis or tendinitis, ankylosing spondylitis, and acute gouty arthritis. The drug is available for both oral and rectal use.

PHARMACOKINETICS

Route	Onset of Action	Peak Plasma Concentration	Elimination Half-Life	Duration of Action
PO	30 min	2 hr	4.5 hr	4–6 hr

ketorolac

Ketorolac tromethamine (Toradol) is unique in that, although it does have some anti-inflammatory activity, it is used primarily for its powerful analgesic effects. Its analgesic effects are comparable to those of narcotic drugs such as morphine sulphate, which can make it a desirable choice for patients who are opiate-addicted and have acute pain control needs because ketorolac lacks the addictive properties of the opioids. Ketorolac is indicated for the treatment of moderate to severe acute pain such as that resulting from orthopedic injuries or surgery. Ketorolac can be given orally or by injection, and there is also a dosage form for ophthalmic use (see Chapter 57). It is available only by prescription. It is indicated for short-term use to manage moderate to severe acute pain. It is not indicated for treatment of minor pain or chronic pain. The most common adverse effects of ketorolac include kidney impairment, edema, GI pain, dyspepsia, and nausea. Ketorolac is not recommended for use in children under age 16, as safety and efficacy in children have not been established. It is important to note that the drug can be used only for up to 5 days for post-surgical patients and for up to 7 days for patients with musculoskeletal pain because of its potential adverse effects on the kidney and GI tract. If supplementary analgesia is required, a concomitant low dose of an opiate can be used.

PHARMACOKINETICS

Route	Onset of Action	Peak Plasma Concentration	Elimination Half-Life	Duration of Action
IV/IM	0.5 hr	1–2 hr	5–7 hr	4–6 hr

PROPIONIC ACIDS

▶▶ ibuprofen

Ibuprofen (Motrin, Advil) is the prototype NSAID in the propionic acid category, which also includes flurbiprofen, ketoprofen, naproxen, and oxaprozin. Ibuprofen is the most commonly used of the propionic acid drugs because of the numerous indications for its use and because of its relatively safe adverse effect profile. It is often used for its analgesic effects in the management of rheumatoid arthritis, osteoarthritis, primary dysmenorrhea, dental pain, and musculoskeletal disorders; in addition, it is used for its antipyretic actions. In 2015, Health Canada issued a warning about the risk of serious cardiovascular effects

(e.g., stroke, MI) associated with high doses of ibuprofen, at least 2 400 mg/day. The risk increases with dose size and duration of use.

Naproxen is the second most commonly used NSAID, with an adverse effect profile reported to be somewhat better than that of ibuprofen, as well as fewer drug interactions with ACE inhibitors given for hypertension. Evidence indicates that ibuprofen is more likely than naproxen to interact with these drugs and hinder their desired hypotensive effects. Both drugs are available for oral use in both OTC and prescription strengths. In 2011, an injectable form of ibuprofen became available.

PHARMACOKINETICS

Route	Onset of Action	Peak Plasma Concentration	Elimination Half-Life	Duration of Action
PO	30–60 min (analgesic); 7 days (anti-inflammatory)	1–2 hr	2–4 hr	4–6 hr

CYCLOOXYGENASE-2 INHIBITORS

The COX-2 inhibitors were developed primarily to decrease the GI adverse effects characteristic of other NSAIDs because of their COX-2 selectivity. However, they are not totally devoid of GI toxicity. Gastritis and upper GI bleeding have been reported with their use, although much less frequently than with the use of older NSAIDs. Originally, there were three COX-2 inhibitors; however, they were removed from the Canadian market because the use of rofecoxib (Vioxx®) and valdecoxib (Bextra®) was found to be associated with an increased risk of adverse cardiovascular events, including MI, stroke, and death.

▶▶ celecoxib

Celecoxib (Celebrex®) was the first COX-2 inhibitor and is the only one remaining on the market. It is indicated for the treatment of osteoarthritis, rheumatoid arthritis, acute pain symptoms, ankylosing spondylitis, and primary dysmenorrhea. Its use was recently approved by Health Canada for symptoms associated with ankylosing spondylitis. There is evidence that celecoxib use may pose a risk of cardiovascular events similar to that associated with rofecoxib and valdecoxib. However, there is inconsistency in the literature regarding the true potential for these effects. Other adverse effects associated with celecoxib include headache, sinus irritation, diarrhea, fatigue, dizziness, lower extremity edema, and hypertension. COX-2 inhibitors have little effect on platelet function. Celecoxib is not to be used in patients with known sulfa allergy.

PHARMACOKINETICS

Route	Onset of Action	Peak Plasma Concentration	Elimination Half-Life	Duration of Action
PO	1 hr	3 hr	11 hr	4–8 hr

Continued

DRUG PROFILES—cont'd

ENOLIC ACID DERIVATIVES

The enolic acid derivatives include piroxicam, meloxicam, and nabumetone. Piroxicam and meloxicam are potent drugs that are commonly used in the treatment of mild to moderate osteoarthritis, rheumatoid arthritis, and gouty arthritis. Both are available only in oral dosage formulations and have contraindications similar to those of the other NSAIDs.

Nabumetone is better tolerated than some of the other enolic acid derivatives in terms of GI adverse effects; it is relatively nonacidic compared with most of the other NSAIDs, which may account for its better GI tolerance. Currently, it is indicated only for the treatment of osteoarthritis and rheumatoid arthritis.

DOSAGES   Most Commonly Used NSAIDs

Drug	Pharmacological Class	Usual Dosage Range	Indications
▸▸acetylsalicylic acid (ASA, aspirin)	Salicylate	*Children 2–11 yr* PO/PR: 10–15 mg/kg q6h (max 65 mg/day) PO/PR: 60–90 mg/kg divided q4–6h (max 100 mg/kg) *Adults* PO/PR: 325–650 mg q4h (max 4 gm/day) PO: 3.6–5.4 gm/day, divided PO: 80–325 mg once daily	Analgesic, antipyretic Anti-inflammatory Fever, pain Anti-inflammatory Thromboprevention
▸celecoxib (Celebrex)	COX-2 inhibitor	*Adults over 18 yr* PO: 100–200 mg/day given in 1 or 2 doses PO: Initial 400 mg (day 1); then 200 mg/day × 7 days PO: 400 mg bid	Rheumatoid arthritis, osteoarthritis, ankylosing spondylitis Acute pain Reduction of number of hereditary colon polyps in familial adenomatous polyposis
▸ibuprofen (Motrin, Advil, others)	Propionic acid derivative	*Children under 2 yr* PO (drops): 5 mg/kg tid–qid *Children under 12 yr* PO (suspension): 120–375 mg q6–8h *Adults and children over 12 yr* 200–400 mg q4h (max 1 200 mg/day)	Fever, pain Arthritis, fever, pain, dysmenorrhea
▸indomethacin (Indocid P.D.A.®, Nu-Indo®)	Acetic acid derivative	*Adults and children over 14 yr* PO: 25–50 mg bid–tid (max 200 mg/day) PR: 50–100 mg bid (max 200 mg)	Arthritis including acute gouty arthritis, bursitis, or tendinitis
▸ketorolac tromethamine (Toradol)	Acetic acid derivative	*Adults* PO: 10 mg q4–6h (max 40 mg/day) × 5–7 days IM: 10–30 mg q4–6h (max 120 mg/day if under 65 yr; max 60 mg/day if older than 65 yr	Acute painful conditions that would otherwise require opioid-level analgesia

IM, intramuscular; *PO*, oral; *PR*, rectal.

ANTIGOUT DRUGS

Gout is caused by the overproduction of uric acid, decreased uric acid excretion, or both. This overproduction or decreased excretion can often result in hyperuricemia (too much uric acid in the blood). When the body contains too much uric acid, deposits of uric acid crystals, an end product of purine metabolism, collect in tissues and joints. This causes an inflammatory response and extreme pain because these crystals are like small needles that jab and stick into sensitive tissues

and joints. Purines are part of normal dietary intake and are used to make the essential structural units of deoxyribonucleic acid (DNA) and ribonucleic acid (RNA). During purine metabolism, they are converted from hypoxanthine to xanthine and eventually to uric acid. The normal pathway for purine metabolism is depicted in Figure 49-2. This pathway is overactive in patients with gout and is reduced by antigout drug therapy. The goals of gout treatment are to decrease the symptoms of an acute attack and prevent recurrent attacks.

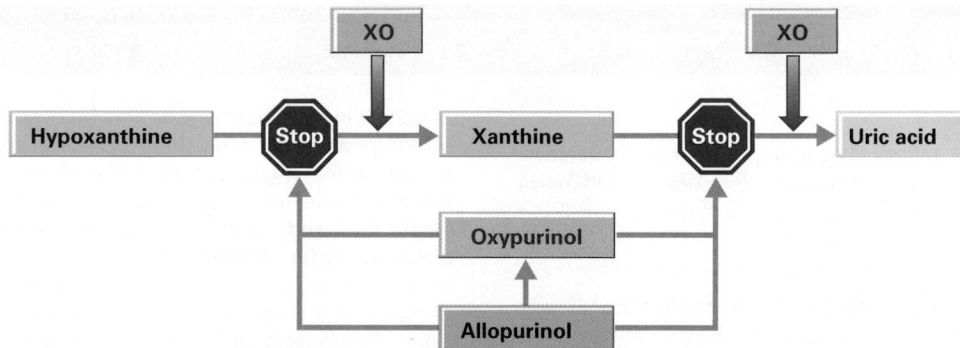

FIG. 49-2   Uric acid production. *XO*, xanthine oxidase.

 DRUG PROFILES

Although specific antigout drugs are available, the NSAIDs (described earlier) are considered first-line therapy for most patients with gout. The specific antigout drugs, allopurinol, febuxostat, colchicine, probenecid, and sulfinpyrazone, are targeted at the underlying defect in uric acid metabolism, which causes either overproduction or underexcretion of uric acid (see Figure 49-2). Both of these pathological processes lead to tissue accumulations of uric acid crystalline deposits (gouty deposits) and symptoms of gout. Not all gouty deposits occur within joints. Gouty arthritis is the condition in which one or more joints are inflamed due to the collection of gouty deposits inside the joint anatomy. This is also called *articular gout*, whereas gout that occurs in tissues outside of the joints is called *abarticular gout*.

allopurinol

The beneficial effect of allopurinol (Zyloprim®) in the relief of gout is the inhibition of the enzyme xanthine oxidase, which thereby prevents uric acid production. Allopurinol is indicated for patients whose gout is caused by excess production of uric acid (hyperuricemia). Allopurinol is also used to prevent acute tumour lysis syndrome (see Chapter 52).

Allopurinol is contraindicated in patients with a hypersensitivity to it. Significant adverse effects of the drug include agranulocytosis, aplastic anemia, and serious and potentially fatal skin conditions such as exfoliative dermatitis, Stevens-Johnson syndrome, and toxic epidermal necrolysis. Azathioprine and mercaptopurine both significantly interact with allopurinol, and as a result, their dosages may have to be adjusted. Allopurinol is available only for oral use. The usual recommended adult dosage is 200 to 800 mg/day, depending on the severity of the gout experienced by the patient, with the maximum dosage being 800 mg/day. Potential benefits of allopurinol may warrant the use of the drug in pregnant women despite potential risks. The new drug febuxostat (Uloric®) is a nonpurine selective inhibitor of xanthine oxidase. It is the first new drug approved for the treatment of gout since the 1960s. Febuxostat is more selective for xanthine oxidase than allopurinol and may pose a greater risk of cardiovascular events than allopurinol. It is not to be given

along with theophylline, azathioprine, or mercaptopurine. It is dosed as 80 mg/day.

PHARMACOKINETICS

Route	Onset of Action	Peak Plasma Concentration	Elimination Half-Life	Duration of Action
PO	1–2 wk	30–120 min	18–30 hr	Unknown

colchicine

Colchicine is the oldest available drug for the treatment of acute gout and is considered second-line therapy, after the NSAIDs. Colchicine appears to be effective in the treatment of gout by reducing the inflammatory response to deposits of urate crystals in joint tissue. Its mechanism of action is not clearly defined, but it is thought to inhibit the metabolism, mobility, and chemotaxis of polymorphonuclear leukocytes. Chemotaxis is the chemical attraction of leukocytes to the site of inflammation, which worsens an inflammatory response.

Colchicine is a powerful inhibitor of cell mitosis and can cause short-term leukopenia. For this reason, it is generally used for the short-term treatment of acute attacks of gout. However, it may be used for prophylaxis of acute attacks in dosages of 0.6 mg once or twice a day. The more severe adverse effects of colchicine can include bleeding into the GI or urinary tracts; the drug must be discontinued if such effects appear. Colchicine is contraindicated in patients with a known hypersensitivity to it and in those with blood dyscrasias or severe kidney, GI, liver, or cardiac disorders. There is no specific antidote for colchicine poisoning. The drug is available in oral forms only.

The usual adult dosage of colchicine for an acute gout flare is an initial dose of 1 to 1.2 mg initially, followed by 0.6 mg 1 hour later and every 2 hours until the gout pain disappears or until nausea, vomiting, or diarrhea develops. It is classified as pregnancy category D. The patient must wait 12 hours to resume prophylaxis (0.6 mg once or twice daily). When colchicine is used for the treatment of acute gout, 3 days must pass before a second course of therapy is initiated. Colchicine dosages must be reduced in patients with kidney impairment. There is evidence of fetal risk with the use of colchicine but the potential benefits of the drug may outweigh the risk.

Continued

DRUG PROFILES—cont'd

PHARMACOKINETICS

Route	Onset of Action	Peak Plasma Concentration	Elimination Half-Life	Duration of Action
PO	12 hr	0.5–2 hr	12–30 min	12 hr

probenecid

Probenecid (Benuryl®) inhibits the reabsorption of uric acid in the kidney and thus increases the excretion of uric acid. Drugs that promote uric acid excretion are known as *uricosurics*. Probenecid acts by binding to the special transporter protein in the proximal convoluted kidney tubule that takes uric acid from the urine and places it back into the blood. The probenecid is then reabsorbed back into the bloodstream while the uric acid remains in the urine, from where it is excreted. Besides being used to treat the hyperuricemia associated with gout and gouty arthritis, it also has the ability to delay the renal excretion of penicillin, which increases serum levels of penicillin and prolongs its effect (see Chapter 43). Probenecid is available as a 500-mg oral tablet. The usual adult dosage is 250 mg, twice a day, with food, milk, or antacids, for 1 week, followed by 500 mg twice daily thereafter. This dosage may be adjusted as needed to maintain desirable serum uric acid levels. Contraindications to the use of probenecid include peptic ulcer disease and blood dyscrasias. Probenecid is ineffective in patients with kidney impairment and is not to be used in these patients. There is no risk to the fetus if the drug is required during pregnancy.

PHARMACOKINETICS

Route	Onset of Action	Peak Plasma Concentration	Elimination Half-Life	Duration of Action
PO	1 hr	3 hr	3–17 hr	8 hr

NURSING PROCESS

Assessment

Prior to giving anti-inflammatory, antigout, and related drugs, it is crucial to patient safety and drug effectiveness to assess for drug allergies, contraindications, cautions, and drug interactions associated with each drug in these major groups. Before administering anti-inflammatory drugs, perform a thorough head-to-toe physical assessment, including a baseline pain assessment when appropriate; measure vital signs; and take a thorough medication history, noting any prescription medications, OTC medications, and natural health products the patient is taking (see Natural Health Products: Glucosamine and Chondroitin). Analyze results of laboratory tests reflecting hematological, kidney, and liver functioning, before initiation of therapy as ordered, especially if long-term use is indicated. These tests will include RBC count, hemoglobin level, hematocrit, white blood cell count, platelet count, blood urea nitrogen (BUN), and liver enzymes such as ALP, AST, and LDH. If NSAIDs are used in the short term for other conditions (e.g., fever, acute pain), laboratory studies are not usually indicated since these drugs are available over the counter and are self-administered.

Prior to the use of aspirin, NSAIDs, other anti-inflammatory drugs, and antigout drugs, assess and document the duration, onset, location, and type of inflammation and pain the patient is experiencing, as well as any precipitating, exacerbating, or relieving factors. Note any interference of the symptoms with the patient's ability to perform activities of daily living (ADLs). Inspect all joints with attention to deformities, immobility or limitations in mobility, overlying skin condition, and presence of any heat or swelling over the joint. Age is important to assess because aspirin and many of the other NSAIDs are not to be used in children and adolescents because of the associated increased risk of Reye's syndrome (see the Special Populations: Children box). These drugs are also to be used cautiously in older adults who have reduced liver and kidney function (See Special Populations: Older Adults: NSAIDs). Assessing the odour of aspirin is also important because a vinegary odour is associated with chemical breakdown of the drug. Prior to the use of aspirin, assess the patient for a history of asthma, wheezing, or other respiratory problems because of increased incidence of allergic reactions to aspirin in individuals with such a history. As well, identify patients who have been diagnosed with what is called the *aspirin triad*, which includes asthma, nasal polyps, and rhinitis; these conditions are considered to put the patient at risk for reactions to aspirin. Other contraindications, cautions, and drug interactions relevant to the use of aspirin and other NSAIDs have been discussed previously. Remember that acetylsalicylic acid (aspirin) and other NSAIDs have anti-inflammatory, antipyretic, analgesic, and antiplatelet activity but also carry a risk for ulcerogenic adverse effects and GI bleeding. NSAIDs carry the risk of acute reversible hepatotoxicity, kidney failure, hearing loss, and noncardiogenic pulmonary edema, so a review of patients' history of pre-existing medical conditions is important.

In addition to patient assessment, the use of ketorolac requires assessment of the drug order to ensure that the drug has been ordered for a short term (i.e., no more than 5 to 7 days) and only for patients experiencing moderate to severe acute pain. Assess patients for underlying signs of infection before the use of any NSAID or other anti-inflammatory drug because these drugs may mask symptoms. Prior to the use of celecoxib, document

NATURAL HEALTH PRODUCTS

Glucosamine and Chondroitin
OVERVIEW

Glucosamine is chemically derived from glucose. Its chemical name is *2-amino-2-deoxyglucose sulphate*. Glucosamine is thought to enhance the production of cartilage matrix components, increase hyaluronic production, and prevent collagen degeneration.

Chondroitin is a protein usually isolated from bovine (cow) cartilage. To date, there are no reports of disease transmission from cows to humans with chondroitin. It increases the hyaluronic production by human synovial cells, which maintains viscosity in synovial fluid.

COMMON USES

These two supplements are often used in combination for synergistic effect, and sometimes individually, to treat pain from osteoarthritis. Although most commonly taken orally, injectable forms are commercially available (e.g., for administration by a naturopathic health care provider).

ADVERSE EFFECTS

Glucosamine: Usually mild adverse effects that are comparable to those of a placebo in clinical studies, including GI discomfort, drowsiness, headache, and skin reactions.

Chondroitin: No major ill effects in studies lasting from 2 months to 6 years; GI discomfort is the most common adverse effect, but is usually well tolerated.

POTENTIAL DRUG INTERACTIONS

Both supplements: May enhance the anticoagulant effects of warfarin. (The patient's INR needs to be measured more frequently during glucosamine/chondroitin therapy and the warfarin dosage adjusted if indicated.)

Glucosamine: May cause an increase in insulin resistance, necessitating the need for higher dosages of oral hypoglycemics or insulin.

CONTRAINDICATIONS

Both supplements: No specific contraindications listed, but avoidance in pregnancy is recommended because of lack of firm safety data.

INR, international normalized ratio.

---

any cardiovascular disorders or symptoms because use of this drug carries a risk of cardiovascular events.

Prior to the use of antigout drugs, perform a thorough assessment of hydration status and baseline serum uric acid levels. Closely assess urinary output prior to and during drug therapy to ensure an output of at least 30 to 60 mL/hour. Determine and assess renal function through monitoring of glomerular filtration rate (GFR), BUN, and serum creatinine, as well as liver function through monitoring of ALP, AST, ALT, and LDH. If a patient is receiving febuxostat (Uloric), assess for any history of cardiovascular disease due to the risk of adverse effects linked to the cardiac system. Additionally, drug interactions may occur with theophylline, azathioprine, or mercaptopurine. If a patient is taking allopurinol, assess the integrity of the skin due to potentially life-threatening skin adverse effects, including exfoliative dermatitis, Stevens-Johnson syndrome, and toxic epidermal necrolysis. Assess blood counts because of the potential for aplastic anemia and agranulocytosis. Prior to the use of colchicine, conduct a thorough assessment for a history of GI distress; ulcers; or cardiac, kidney, or liver disease. Also worthy of mention regarding antigout drugs (e.g., allopurinol, colchicine, probenecid) is that these drugs may be used for either their short-term or long-term effects. Therefore, assess the order and indication for the antigout drug to ensure that the patient is receiving the appropriate treatment. Also assess for all contraindications, cautions, and drug interactions (see earlier discussion).

Nursing Diagnoses

- Acute pain related to disease process or injury to joints and other disease-affected areas
- Deficient knowledge related to first-time drug therapy for treatment of a disease process
- Risk for injury related to the effects of the disease and treatment on mobility and the performance of ADLs

Planning
Goals

- Patient will experience pain relief or relief of symptoms within the expected time frame.
- Patient will demonstrate increased knowledge about the disease process, medication regimen, and beneficial lifestyle changes.
- Patient will remain free from injury related to the disease process or drug regimen.

Expected Patient Outcomes

- Patient remains pain free or nearly pain free with adequate drug and nondrug therapy.

SPECIAL POPULATIONS: CHILDREN

Reye's Syndrome

Reye's syndrome is associated with the administration of aspirin to children and adolescents and is a potentially life-threatening illness. Encephalopathy and liver damage are two of the serious complications resulting from Reye's syndrome, which usually occurs after a viral infection, such as chicken pox or influenza B, during which aspirin is often given to decrease fever. To reduce the risk for Reye's syndrome, aspirin or medications that contain aspirin should not be given to children or adolescents to treat viral illnesses or fever. Other names for aspirin include acetyl-salicylic acid, acetylsalicylate, salicylic acid, and salicylate. Other drugs that can be used instead to reduce fever and relieve pain include acetaminophen and ibuprofen. Check the label on any medication that is to be given to a child because aspirin is contained in at least 50 OTC drugs, including, for example, Alka-Seltzer® and Anacin®. Aspirin is also found in numerous cold and flu preparations.

Signs and Symptoms of Reye's Syndrome

- Altered liver function
- Encephalopathy and fatty degeneration of the viscera, primarily in children and adolescents
- Changes in level of consciousness
- Coma, flaccid paralysis, loss of deep tendon reflexes
- Hypoglycemia
- Seizures
- Vomiting

Medical Management

- Provide supportive treatment in the Critical Care Unit
- Maintain life functions, restore metabolic balance, and control cerebral edema
- Administer intravenous glucose (10% or higher) for treatment of hypoglycemia
- Monitor blood glucose level; insulin may be needed
- Administer vitamin K for clotting problems

- Give fresh frozen plasma if needed for significant bleeding
- Provide prophylactic antiepileptic drugs
- Monitor intracranial pressure
- Initiate cautious fluid administration
- Administer osmotic diuretics with steroids if needed to treat cerebral edema

Nursing Management

- Critical care setting often indicated for care of these patients
- Assess neurological status, vital signs, and arterial and central venous pressures
- Monitor blood gas concentrations and intracranial pressure as ordered
- Control temperature to prevent elevations and increased O_2 demands
- Elevate the head of the bed
- Monitor intake and output
- Initiate hyperventilation (if patient is intubated and if ordered) to reduce intracranial pressure by lowering CO_2 levels and increasing O_2 levels
- Provide a quiet environment
- Handle gently
- Provide family support during critical phase of the illness
- Provide physical and emotional support for the child and family with recovery
- Ensure appropriate spiritual care is provided
- Educate the public about Reye's syndrome and its life-threatening complications

Source: Mayo Foundation for Medical Education and Research. (2014). *Reye's syndrome.* Retrieved from http://www.mayoclinic.org/diseases-conditions/reyes-syndrome/basics/definition/con-20020083.

- Patient states that pain and changes in joints and mobility are characteristic of inflammation, injury, or related disease processes and will decrease with effective therapy.
- Patient identifies factors that aggravate or alleviate pain, such as movement, activity, exercise, and changes in the weather or atmosphere.
- Patient states nonpharmacological measures to use to promote comfort, increase joint function and mobility, and improve performance of ADLs (e.g., biofeedback, imagery, massage, application of hot or cold packs, physiotherapy, relaxation therapy).
- Patient describes disease process requiring treatment with an NSAID or antigout drug therapy.
  - Patient states the expected impact of effective and consistent drug therapy in the prevention of

damage to the part of the musculoskeletal system being impacted by the disease process (of injury, gout, arthritis, etc.).
- Patient states adverse effects associated with NSAIDs or antigout drug therapy.
- Patient states symptoms that should be reported to the health care provider immediately, such as fever, increase in symptoms or joint pain, jaundice, changes in skin, or severe rash.
- Patient takes medication regimen as prescribed to prevent further damage and injury to self.
  - Patient contacts health care provider if there is a lack of improvement in injury or disease process.
  - Patient maintains follow-up appointments with health care provider to enhance therapeutic effectiveness and minimize injury.

SPECIAL POPULATIONS: OLDER ADULTS

NSAIDs

It is anticipated that, by 2036, there will be more than 10.4 million Canadians 65 years of age and older, exceeding 23% of the population. It is also anticipated that the use of OTC NSAIDs will be widespread and increasing in this population and requiring special attention and education to prevent or minimize adverse effects. Understanding the physiological changes that older adult patients experience will help ensure safe and effective use of these medications.

The underlying pharmacokinetic characteristics and physical and biological changes in older adult patients must be understood. Even if older adults have normal kidney and liver function, they have a reduced rate of drug metabolism and drug elimination compared with younger adults.

Patients 65 years of age and older do not have to be ill for NSAIDs to adversely affect them because of normal age-related physiological changes. The presence of chronic or multiple illnesses may result in an increased incidence of adverse reactions.

Some changes noted in older adult patients that effect drug treatment include changes in kidney elimination, protein binding, body composition, drug distribution, drug clearance, and sensitivity to drugs, as well as an increased incidence of adverse reactions to all types of medications.

Older patients who are at risk for kidney insufficiency because of natural physiological changes may experience changes in fluid balance as well as changes in drug reabsorption, excretion, and filtration processes; these changes may lead to drug toxicity.

Cardiac output decreases by 25% between the ages of 25 and 65, which results in decreased blood flow to the kidneys and, consequently, reduced GFR. There is also an overall decline in circulating blood volume, which may affect overall pharmacokinetics and lead to decreased drug absorption, distribution, metabolism, and excretion.

Many individuals older than 65 years of age become slow metabolizers of medications, which affects the way NSAIDs are handled by the liver. In addition, the liver decreases in size and weight with advancing age. Blood flow to the liver is also decreased. Drug metabolism is affected by these changes, resulting in the possible need to decrease drug dosages for older adults or monitor these patients closely for toxicity.

GI functioning is impacted by aging, with older adults having more acidic gastric juices and decreased gastric motility. These changes may lead to slower emptying of the stomach and result in decreased intestinal drug absorption. Serum levels of drugs, including NSAIDs, may be higher due to these factors, and overall drug dosages may need to be decreased. It has also been documented that older adults may be at increased risk for developing NSAID-related GI problems.

Interventions to help decrease NSAID-related adverse reactions include asking questions, listing all drugs, teaching about all medications, and assessing GI, cardiovascular, and neurological systems, based on patient concerns and symptoms. In addition, it is important to teach older adult patients about maximum doses of NSAIDs.

NSAID, Nonsteroidal anti-inflammatory drug.

Source: Wooten, J. M. (2012). Pharmacotherapy considerations in elderly adults. *Southern Medical Journal, 105*(8), 437–445. Retrieved from http://www.medscape.com/viewarticle/769412; Hunt, R. (2014). *The elderly patient taking NSAIDS and aspirin.* Retrieved from http://www.medscape.org/viewarticle/458018.

Implementation

If aspirin is used, the oral dosage forms are given with food, milk, or meals. Advise patients that sustained-released or enteric-coated tablets are not to be crushed or broken. Monitor serum levels of aspirin if aspirin therapy is used for its anti-inflammatory effect in the treatment of arthritis; however, this indication is rare. Because of its associated high risk of potentially severe adverse effects, aspirin is mainly used in lower doses (e.g., 81 mg) when it is indicated for cardioprotective reasons. If used in higher doses, monitor for clinical presentation as well as serum salicylate levels to help distinguish among mild, moderate, and severe toxicity (see pharmacology discussion). In such situations, it is important to be aware of signs and symptoms of toxicity, such as GI bleeding, other bleeding, and abdominal pain. If any of these occur, report the findings to the health care provider and ensure immediate treatment. If aspirin is used as an antipyretic, the patient's temperature generally begins to decrease within 1 hour. See the Patient Teaching Tips for more information on the safe use of aspirin.

Non-aspirin NSAIDs or other anti-inflammatory drugs may also come in enteric-coated or sustained-release preparations; stress to patients that these are not to be crushed or chewed. Oral dosage forms of these drugs, including ketorolac, may be taken with antacids or food to decrease GI upset or irritation. Instruct patients to report to the health care provider immediately any moderate to severe GI upset, dyspepsia with nausea, vomiting, abdominal pain, or blood in the stool or vomitus. During therapy with NSAIDs, continuously monitor the patient for bowel patterns, stool consistency, and any occurrence of GI symptoms or dizziness, and document the findings. Monitor laboratory tests during high-dose or long-term treatment, including complete blood count (CBC); BUN levels; platelet counts; and serum bilirubin, ALP, AST, and ALT levels. Emphasize safe ambulation with NSAID use as well as with the use of any other anti-inflammatory drugs or analgesics. With ketorolac, understand that dosing is not to exceed a 5- to 7-day time period with either the oral or intramuscular dosage forms. Administer intramuscular injections slowly into a large muscle mass. Educate patients prescribed celecoxib to take the drug only as ordered and, as with other NSAIDs, to avoid alcohol, aspirin, salicylates, and OTC drugs containing any of these drugs. Celecoxib may be taken without regard to meals; however, taking the drug with food and fluids may decrease GI upset. Instruct patients to report immediately to a health care provider any stomach or abdominal pain, other GI problems, unusual bleeding, blood in the stool or vomitus, edema, chest pain, or palpitations.

The antigout drugs are somewhat different from the NSAIDs, with different mechanisms of action and also different nursing considerations. Colchicine needs to be taken on an empty stomach for optimally complete absorption but is best tolerated if given with food. Educate the patient with gout on the importance of increasing fluid intake, up to 3 L/day, unless contraindicated. Advise patients to avoid alcohol and any OTC cold-relief products that contain alcohol while taking colchicine. In addition, inform patients with gout that adherence to the complete medical regimen, both pharmacological and nonpharmacological, is crucial to successful treatment. If allopurinol is prescribed, it is to be given with meals to minimize the occurrence of GI symptoms such as nausea, vomiting, and anorexia. If allopurinol is to be administered in conjunction with chemotherapy (in an attempt to decrease hyperuricemia associated with malignancy and cell death from successful treatment), it is recommended that it be given a few days before the chemotherapy. Patients taking allopurinol must also increase fluid intake to 3 L/day to maintain a urinary output of 2 L/day. This daily fluid intake will also assist in preventing the development of uric acid kidney stones. Patients need to avoid hazardous activities (e.g., driving) if dizziness or drowsiness occurs with the medication.

Alcohol and caffeine must also be avoided because these substances will increase levels of uric acid and decrease levels of allopurinol; the intake of even one to two alcoholic drinks per day is associated with higher levels of uric acid. A modified purine diet should be followed by patients with gout. Foods high in purine include seafood and red meats (especially organ meats), meat extracts, yeast, beer, beans, peas, oatmeal, lentils, spinach, asparagus, cauliflower, and mushrooms. Patients who are overweight or obese should be encouraged to lose weight, as they are at higher risk of developing gout.

Evaluation

Aspirin and NSAIDs may vary in their potency and anti-inflammatory and analgesic effects. Therapeutic responses to NSAIDs include the following: decrease in acute pain; decrease in swelling, pain, stiffness, and tenderness of a joint or muscle area; improved ability to perform ADLs; improved muscle grip and strength; reduction in fever; return to normal laboratory values for CBC and sedimentation rate; and return to a less inflamed state, as evidenced by sedimentation rates, X-ray examination, computed tomography scan, or magnetic resonance imaging. Monitoring for the occurrence of adverse effects and toxicity is essential to the safe and effective use of anti-inflammatory drugs (aspirin, celecoxib, other NSAIDs) and antigout drugs (see Box 49-3 and Tables 49-2 and 49-3).

Therapeutic responses to the antigout drug colchicine include decreased pain in affected joints and increased sense of well-being. Monitor patients taking this drug closely for any increased pain, blood in the urine, excessive fatigue and lethargy, or chills or fever, and contact the health care provider immediately should any of these occur. A therapeutic response to allopurinol includes a decrease in pain in the joints, a decrease in uric acid levels, and a decrease in stone formation in the kidneys.

CASE STUDY

NSAIDs

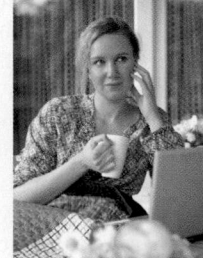

Jana, a 35-year-old writer, has developed severe pain in her right wrist and has been unable to make her publisher's deadlines because of the pain she is having. After magnetic resonance imaging and a physical examination, she is diagnosed with tendinitis and started on extended-release diclofenac (Voltaren®-XR), 75 mg twice a day. She is also given a wrist orthosis and instructed to resume work slowly once she is feeling better.

1. What instructions are important for Jana at this time?

2. After 1 week of therapy, Jana calls the office and says, "There has been no change! My wrist still hurts. I need to get better quickly!" What is the nurse's best response?

At her 1-month checkup, Jana is happy that her wrist has stopped hurting and that she has been able to resume her writing part time. She mentions, however, that she has felt extremely tired recently and has had increased abdominal discomfort. She also tells the nurse that her bowel movements have been darker and asks if that could be an adverse effect of the medicine.

3. Explain what is possibly happening, and what steps will be taken next.

For answers, see http://evolve.elsevier.com/Canada/Lilley/pharmacology/.

PATIENT TEACHING TIPS

❖ Instruct patients that anti-inflammatory drugs, if in sustained-release or enteric-coated forms, are not to be crushed or chewed. Educate patients that the full anti-inflammatory effect of the drug may not be apparent immediately, depending on the specific drug. For example, the onset of full therapeutic anti-inflammatory action of ibuprofen may take 7 days and its analgesic effects may take 30 to 60 minutes.

❖ Advise patients to provide a list of all medications to all health care providers, including dentists, especially if they are taking high dosages of aspirin or have been taking aspirin or another NSAID for prolonged periods. Aspirin and NSAIDs are generally discontinued 1 week prior to any type of surgery, including oral or dental surgery, per the health care provider's or surgeon's orders.

❖ Patients should know to always keep aspirin and other drugs out of the reach of children. If a child (or adult) has consumed large or unknown quantities of aspirin or another NSAID, contact a poison control centre and seek emergency medical attention immediately.

Children and adolescents must never take aspirin because of the risk of Reye's syndrome (see the Special Populations: Children box on p. 920). Acetaminophen in the recommended dosage range is usually preferred.

❖ Educate patients about the adverse effects of aspirin, such as GI upset, nausea, vomiting, diarrhea, dizziness, and tinnitus. Table 49-3 lists the signs and symptoms of acute or chronic salicylate intoxication. Instruct patients to report to a health care provider immediately any black or tarry stools, bleeding around the gums, petechiae, ecchymosis, or purpura.

❖ Inform patients about the most common adverse effects of NSAIDs (see Table 49-2). Advise patients to take NSAIDs with food, milk, or antacids to help minimize GI distress.

❖ Educate patients about the many drug interactions that can occur with aspirin, other NSAIDs, and antigout drugs.

❖ Alert the patient to look-alike sound-alike drugs, especially Celebrex (celecoxib), which may be confused with Celexa (citalopram) or Cerebyx (fosphenytoin).

KEY POINTS

❖ Anti-inflammatory drugs include aspirin, NSAIDs, and COX-2 inhibitors.

❖ NSAIDs are one of the most commonly prescribed categories of drugs. The first drug in this category to be synthesized was salicylic acid or aspirin. Aspirin is often included in the discussion of anti-inflammatory drugs and identified as such. NSAIDs have analgesic, anti-inflammatory, and antipyretic activities; aspirin also has antiplatelet activity. NSAIDs are thus often used in the treatment of gout, osteoarthritis, juvenile arthritis, rheumatoid arthritis, dysmenorrhea, and musculoskeletal injuries such as strains and sprains.

❖ The three main adverse effects of NSAIDs are GI intolerance, bleeding (often GI bleeding), and kidney impairment. Misoprostol may be given to prevent GI

intolerance and ulcers resulting from NSAID use. It is classified as a prostaglandin analogue. There are also many contraindications to the use of NSAIDs, such as GI tract lesions, peptic ulcers, and bleeding disorders.

❖ Most oral NSAIDs are better tolerated if taken with food to minimize GI upset.

❖ When NSAIDs are used to decrease joint inflammation in patients with arthritis, full therapeutic effects may not be experienced for 1 week or longer.

❖ Antigout drugs are indicated for either acute or chronic gout or gout prophylaxis. Diarrhea and abdominal pain are common adverse effects. Antigout drugs are often given to patients during cancer chemotherapy that causes cell death, to avoid goutlike syndromes and pain.

EXAMINATION REVIEW QUESTIONS

1. When a patient is receiving long-term NSAID therapy, which drug may be given to prevent the serious GI adverse effects of NSAIDs?
a. misoprostol
b. metoprolol tartrate
c. metoclopramide hydrochloride
d. magnesium sulphate

2. The nurse recognizes that manifestations of NSAID toxicity include which of these symptoms?
a. Constipation
b. Nausea and vomiting
c. Tremors
d. Urinary retention

3. During a teaching session about antigout drugs, the nurse tells the patient that antigout drugs act by which mechanism?
a. Increasing blood oxygen levels
b. Decreasing leukocytes and platelets
c. Increasing protein and rheumatoid factors
d. Decreasing serum uric acid levels

Continued

EXAMINATION REVIEW QUESTIONS—cont'd

4. Which statement by the nurse is accurate when teaching about antigout drugs?
   a. "Drink only limited amounts of fluids with the drug."
   b. "This drug may cause limited movement in your joints."
   c. "There are few drug interactions with this medication."
   d. "Colchicine is best taken on an empty stomach."

5. A mother calls the clinic to ask about what medication to give her 5-year-old child for a fever during a bout of chicken pox. The nurse's best response would be:
   a. "Your child is 5 years old, so it would be okay to use children's aspirin to treat his fever."
   b. "Start with acetaminophen or ibuprofen, but if these do not work, then you can try aspirin."
   c. "You can use children's dosages of acetaminophen or ibuprofen, but aspirin is not recommended."
   d. "It is best to wait to let the fever break on its own without medication."

6. A 49-year-old patient has been admitted with possible chronic salicylate intoxication after self-treatment for arthritis pain. The nurse will assess for which symptoms of salicylate intoxication?
   a. Tinnitus
   b. Headache
   c. Constipation
   d. Nausea
   e. Bradycardia

7. An order for a child reads: "Give ibuprofen suspension 30 mg/kg/day, divided into four doses, for pain." The child weighs 33 pounds. How many milligrams will this child receive per dose?

Answers: 1. a, 2. b, 3. d, 4. d, 5. c, 6. a, b, d, 7. 112.5 mg per dose

CRITICAL THINKING ACTIVITIES

1. A 68-year-old patient has been instructed to take aspirin, 81 mg every morning with breakfast, as part of treatment after having an MI. When discussing the aspirin therapy, he asks the nurse, "Will this also help my arthritis?" What is the nurse's best answer?

2. A patient has been taking ibuprofen (Motrin), 800 mg three times a day, for treatment of arthritis. She is scheduled for a laparoscopy. She asks you, "I hope I can continue the Motrin because I really ache if I don't take it. It's just minor surgery, right?" What is the nurse's priority when answering the patient's question?

3. A patient has been diagnosed with gout and will be taking colchicine. When reviewing the instructions for the medication, he asks, "I like to take my pills with breakfast." What is the nurse's priority when providing teaching?

For answers, see http://evolve.elsevier.com/Canada/Lilley/pharmacology/.

Immune and Biological Modifiers and Chemotherapeutic Drugs

TIME MANAGEMENT

The first step in preparing for a chapter or section exam is to plan for the time needed to study. Begin by assuming that your next test will cover the chapters in Part Nine. First, look at how much there is to cover. This will help you determine just how big a task you face. Also, consider how much study time you have been devoting to these chapters in the days before the exam. If you've been doing regular studying with frequent review sessions, the demand on your time in the day or two just before the exam will be less than if you have to do a major cram session to try to catch up on study that has been put off. The basic question to answer here is a simple one: "How much time do I need to schedule for exam preparation?" The answer varies for each student. Some will need 6, 8, or more hours of preparation time in the 2 to 3 days before the exam. Others will find that 3, 4, or 5 hours will be adequate. Assess your own learning and prior success to determine how much time is necessary for you.

One factor that should play a major role in determining how much time you need is your performance on prior exams. How have you been doing and how much time have you been spending to achieve that level? If you are not achieving according to your capabilities, then you should think about spending more time preparing for the next exam. If you are achieving at a satisfactory level, then plan on devoting about the same amount of time to test preparation as you did prior to the last exam.

The next step in preparing for an exam is to organize your time. Write down what you are going to study and when, as well as how much time you will spend doing so. Consider the following example based on the material in Chapters 50 and a Wednesday exam date:

1. Review Chapter 50 Objectives. Monday, 1600 to 1630 hours. Note objectives that are unclear for further review.
2. Examination and review questions. Monday, 1630 to 1715 hours. Break. 1715 to 1830.
3. Self-test using Chapter 50 Key Terms. Monday, 1830 to 1900 hours. Note terms that need further review for mastery.
4. Review Chapter 50 Objectives. Monday, 1900 to 1930 hours.
5. Question and answer review. Monday, 1930 to 2000 hours.
6. Self-test, Chapter 50 Key Terms. Monday, 2000 to 2030 hours.

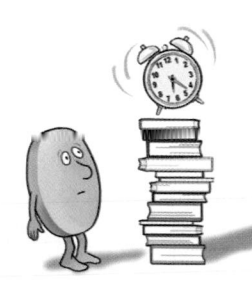

The advantage to this test preparation model is that it helps you to know where (and when) you must focus your attention in the days before the exam.

EVALUATE PRIOR PERFORMANCE

As you begin preparing to review for any exam, take some time to look back at previous exams. Evaluate your performance, and use your evaluation to improve on subsequent tests. As you look at prior tests, consider the following factors.

What Types of Errors Did I Make?

Students often find that they incorrectly answer certain types of questions. Assess your errors and try to pinpoint any recurring patterns in your mistakes. Did you miss multiple choice questions that contained an exemption in the stem? An exception stem asks for the response choice that is *wrong*. Questions that state "all of the following except" or ask "Which of the following would not be ..." are exemption questions. Students often choose one of the apparently correct responses. It is very important to pay close attention to the question in order to carefully see whether you are looking for a correct or an incorrect answer.

Did I Have Trouble With Questions That Required Mastery of Terminology?

Look at questions that demanded mastery of the terms from the chapters. If you missed more than one or two questions of that type, then you know you need to spend more time reviewing terminology.

Did I Miss Concept Questions?

If a question asks you to apply a principle, evaluate a drug response, or in some other way apply knowledge from the course, you are dealing with concepts rather than facts. If you missed a number of concept questions, then you should spend more of your review time studying applications and principles than memorizing facts and terms.

Did I Make Errors Because I Did Not Know the Material?

Some questions focus on the quality of your learning. If you miss one or two questions on an exam because you did not learn (or did not remember) the material, it is not a major problem. There will almost always be one or two questions that you do not know how to answer because you do not remember the material.

However, if you had to guess on several questions because you did not recall any information that seemed relevant, you may need to put more time into review. It is essential that you acknowledge to yourself that you have missed questions because you did not know the material so that you can take steps to correct the situation. You may need to do more oral rehearsal so that the material is stored in your long-term memory.

Did I Change My Answer After Selecting the Correct One?

When encountering a question for the first time, choose the best answer you can. Of course, there are times when you feel like changing your originally selected answer. If this is the case, consider your reason for changing the original response. Most often, test takers change their answer because they encountered a related idea in subsequent questions. If you feel that this is something you do, make sure to change your response only when you are absolutely sure. How do you know you are certain? You know when you can back up your changed response with factual information based on your studies. Changing your answer based on an emotional impulse can lead to changing your originally correct responses to incorrect ones. Remember that studying allows you to gain mastery with the factual information—so study with PURRpose!

ANTICIPATE THE TEST

Do not wait until exam time to find out what you should know. As you review, try to come up with questions you think might be on the test. This does not mean you need to try to write multiple-choice questions; just try to focus your review to help you keep the information in your long-term memory. Here are some examples of questioning that you might use, based on material found in Chapter 53:

1. What are immunomodulating drugs (IMDs)?
2. What is the role of IMDs in the care of patients with cancer?
3. What is the role of the immune system in treating cancer?

These sample questions were drawn from just the first few pages of the chapter. The first question focuses on literal comprehension. This type of question is easy to generate, and being able to answer this type of question is important, but if all of your questions are literal, it may be difficult for you to answer questions that require application of principles and concepts. It is essential that some questions require analysis, synthesis, and evaluation of the material. Question 3 is an example of this type of question.

PLAN FOR DISTRIBUTED STUDY

Many students wait too long to begin to review for a test and are forced into a pattern of long hours of intensive study all packed into the last day or two before the exam. Although cramming does work to some degree, it is not the most effective way to learn. It is better to distribute your review over a period of several days, with short, 30-minute to 1-hour study sessions several times each day. Distributing practice in this way allows time for you to think about what you have been learning, and it fosters encoding of material in long-term memory.

Spend more of your review time doing oral rehearsal (including asking and answering questions) than simply rereading material. Oral rehearsal encourages active learning, which enhances your ability to concentrate, improves comprehension and memory, and thus improves test performance.

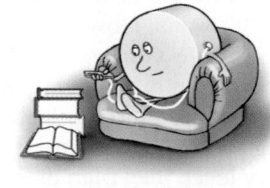

CHAPTER 50

Immunosuppressant Drugs

Objectives

After reading this chapter, the successful student will be able to do the following:

1. Discuss the role of immunosuppressive therapy in organ transplant recipients and in the treatment of autoimmune diseases.

2. Discuss the mechanisms of action, contraindications, cautions, adverse effects, routes of administration, drug interactions, and toxicities associated with the most commonly used immunosuppressants.

3. Develop a collaborative plan of care that includes all phases of the nursing process for patients receiving immunosuppressants after organ transplantation or for the treatment of autoimmune diseases.

e-Learning Activities

Website
(http://evolve.elsevier.com/Canada/
Lilley/pharmacology/)

evolve

- Answer Key—Textbook Case Studies
- Answer Key—Critical Thinking Activities
- Chapter Summaries—Printable
- Review Questions for Exam Preparation
- Unfolding Case Studies

Drug Profiles

▸▸ azathioprine (azathioprine sodium)*, p. 932
   basiliximab p. 932
▸▸ ciclosporin, p. 932
   glatiramer (glatiramer acetate)*, p. 932
   mycophenolate mofetil, p. 932
   sirolimus and tacrolimus, p. 932

▸▸ Key drug

*Full generic name is given in parentheses. For the purposes of this text, the more common, shortened name is used.

Key Terms

Autoimmune diseases A large group of diseases characterized by the alteration of the immune system's function in which immune response affects normal body tissue(s), resulting in pathological conditions. (p. 928)

Grafts Transplanted tissues or organs. (p. 932)

Immune-mediated diseases A large group of diseases that result when the cells of the immune system react to a variety of situations, such as transplanted organ tissue or drug-altered cells. (p. 928)

Immunosuppressants Drugs that decrease or prevent an immune response. (p. 928)

Immunosuppressive therapy Drug treatment used to suppress the immune system. (p. 928)

IMMUNE SYSTEM

The purpose of the immune system is to distinguish self from nonself and to protect the body from foreign material (antigens). There are three layers of barriers or lines of defence to protect the body (Figure 50-1). The first line of defence is a combination of physical (e.g., skin, mucous membranes, hair, and cilia) and chemical (e.g., gastric secretions, vaginal secretions, urine, tears, sweat, saliva, and cerumen). The second line of defence is the leukocytes. The third line of defence is the specific immune response. There are two types of immunity: humoral immunity, which is mediated by B lymphocytes, and cellular immunity, which is mediated by T lymphocytes. This chapter focuses on drugs that suppress the T lymphocytes.

The immune system defends the body against invading pathogens, foreign antigens, and its own cells that become cancerous, or neoplastic. Aside from performing this beneficial function, it can also attack itself and cause what are known as *autoimmune diseases* and *immune-mediated diseases.* The immune system also participates in hypersensitivity, or anaphylactic, reactions, which can be life-threatening. The rejection of kidney(s), lung(s), pancreas, liver, and heart (whole organ) transplants is directed by the immune system as well.

Drugs that decrease or prevent an immune response, and hence suppress the immune system, are known as *immunosuppressants.* Treatment with such drugs is referred to as *immunosuppressive therapy.* Immunosuppressants are used for many immune-related disorders, including rheumatoid arthritis, systemic lupus erythematosus, Crohn's disease, multiple sclerosis, myasthenia gravis, psoriasis, and others. Examples of these drugs include cyclophosphamide (see Chapter 52), glatiramer, fingolimod hydrochloride, and many immunomodula-

tors, which are discussed in Chapter 53. This chapter focuses on the drugs used in organ transplantation.

Transplantation is one of the most complex areas of modern medicine. Many different types of transplants are routinely performed, including, but not limited to, kidney, heart, liver, lung, pancreas, small bowel, bone marrow, and cornea transplantation. The primary concern with transplantation is rejection, which could necessitate that the transplanted organ be removed. Rejection occurs due to an immune response targeted against the transplanted organ. There are three categories of rejection. A hyperacute rejection (or antibody-mediated or humoral rejection) occurs within minutes to hours after a transplant, with an immediate systemic inflammatory response. An acute rejection can occur within the first 3 months mediated by macrophages and T cytotoxic lymphocytes. This type of rejection often occurs at least once after transplantation and is often reversible with an adjustment to immunosuppressant therapy or increased doses of corticosteroids. Chronic rejection occurs months to years post-transplantation and is considered irreversible. It is the result of a chronic, low-grade immune T cell– and B cell–mediated response. It is often not treatable. Immunosuppressants are used to inhibit the immune system and prevent organ rejection. Transplant patients remain on immunosuppressant therapy for the duration of their lives.

IMMUNOSUPPRESSANT DRUGS
Mechanism of Action and Drug Effects

All immunosuppressants have similar mechanisms of action in that they selectively suppress certain T lymphocyte cell lines. By suppressing the T lymphocyte cell lines, they prevent their involvement in the immune response. This suppression results in a pharmacologically immunocompromised state. Each drug differs in the

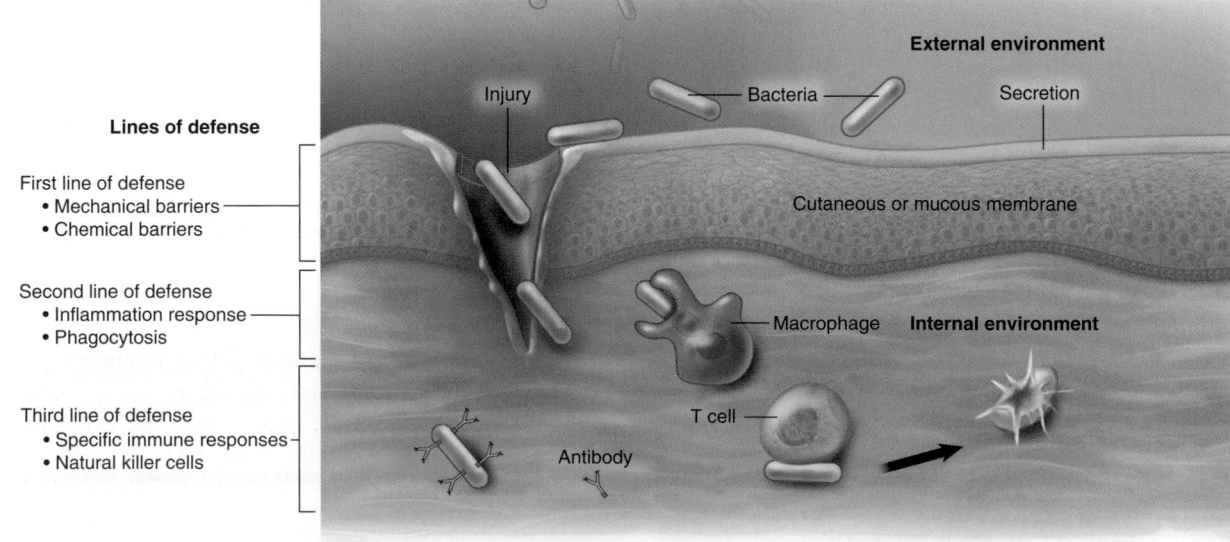

FIG. 50-1   A simplified depiction of the complicated immune system. (From: Patton, K. T., & Thibodeau, G. A. (2010). *Anatomy and physiology* (7th ed.). St. Louis, MO: Mosby.)

exact way in which it suppresses certain cell lines involved in an immune response. The major classes of immunosuppressant drugs used in preventing organ rejection include glucocorticoids, calcineurin inhibitors, mammalian target of rapamycin (mTOR) inhibitors, antimetabolites, and biologics. Corticosteroids inhibit all stages of T cell activation and are used for induction, maintenance immunosuppression, and acute rejection. Corticosteroids are discussed in depth in Chapter 34 and are not discussed further in this chapter. Calcineurin inhibitors (e.g., ciclosporin, tacrolimus) inhibit the action of phosphatase required for interleukin-2 production. Sirolimus does not inhibit calcineurin but instead forms a complex with an intracellular protein that binds to mTOR, which ultimately inhibits interleukin-2 communication. mTOR is a protein kinase that has a variety of functions related to the regulation of cell growth and proliferation. Antimetabolites (e.g., azathioprine, mycophenolate acetate) inhibit cell proliferation. Biologics (e.g., basiliximab) inhibit cytotoxic T-killer cell function.

Table 50-1 outlines the mechanisms of action and indications of the available immunosuppressant drugs.

Indications

The therapeutic uses of immunosuppressants are many and vary from drug to drug, as noted in Table 50-1. Two of these drugs, ciclosporin and tacrolimus, are indicated primarily for both prevention of rejection and treatment of organ rejection. Fingolimod hydrochloride and glatiramer are immunosuppressants that are indicated for the reduction of the frequency of relapses (exacerbations) in a type of multiple sclerosis known as *relapsing–remitting multiple sclerosis.*

Contraindications

The main contraindication for all immunosuppressants is known drug allergy. Relative contraindications, depending on the patient's condition, may include kidney or liver failure, hypertension, uncontrolled infection, and concurrent radiation therapy. While pregnancy

TABLE 50-1

Classification and Mechanisms of Action for Available Immunosuppressant Drugs

Drug Names	Mechanism of Action	Indications/Uses
azathioprine sodium (Imuran®)	Blocks metabolism of purines, inhibiting the synthesis of T cell DNA, RNA, and proteins, thereby blocking immune response	Prevention of organ rejection in kidney transplantation; treatment of rheumatoid arthritis
basiliximab* (Simulect®)	Suppresses T-cell activity by blocking the binding of the cytokine mediator IL-2 to a specific receptor	Prevention of organ rejection in kidney transplantation
ciclosporin (Sandimmune®, Neoral®, Cyclosporine®)	Inhibits synthesis of T cells by blocking the production and release of the cytokine mediator IL-2	Prevention of graft rejection following solid organ and bone marrow transplantation; treatment of rheumatoid arthritis and psoriasis
fingolimod hydrochloride (Gilenya®)	Decreases the amount of lymphocytes available to the CNS	Reduction of relapse frequency in patients with relapsing–remitting MS
glatiramer acetate (Copaxone®)	Precise mechanism unknown; believed to somehow modify immune system processes that are associated with symptoms of MS	Reduction of relapse frequency in patients with relapsing–remitting MS
mycophenolate mofetil (CellCept®), mycophenolate sodium (Myfortic®)	Prevents proliferation of T cells by inhibiting intracellular purine synthesis	Mycophenolate mofetil is indicated for the prevention of organ rejection in kidney, liver, and heart transplantation; mycophenolate sodium is indicated for the prevention of organ rejection in kidney transplantation
sirolimus (Rapamune®)	Inhibits T cell activation by binding to an intracellular protein known as *FK-binding protein 12* that subsequently prevents cellular proliferation	Prevention of organ rejection in kidney transplantation
tacrolimus (Advagraf®, Prograf®)	Inhibits T cell synthesis, possibly by binding to an intracellular protein known as *FK-binding protein 12*	Prevention of organ rejection in liver, kidney, and heart transplantation; unlabelled uses† include rejection in bone marrow, pancreas, pancreatic islet cell, and small intestine transplantation, as well as treatment of autoimmune diseases and severe psoriasis

*Note that "ab" in any drug name usually indicates that it is a monoclonal antibody synthesized using recombinant DNA technology.
CNS, central nervous system; *DNA*, deoxyribonucleic acid; *IL-2*, interleukin-2; *MS*, multiple sclerosis; *RNA*, ribonucleic acid.
†Use not approved by Health Canada but under investigation.

is not necessarily a contraindication to these drugs, immunosuppressants should be used in pregnant women only in urgent situations, under close care of a transplant team that includes pharmacists, nurses, and surgeons.

Adverse Effects

Immunosuppressant drugs have many significant adverse effects, which are listed in Table 50-2. Immunosuppressants place patients at increased risk of opportunistic infections. They may also increase the risk of certain types of cancers; for instance, patients on immunosuppressant therapy are at a greater risk of developing skin cancers than the general population. Other adverse effects are specific to the immunosuppressant drug. For example, ciclosporin and tacrolimus can cause nephrotoxicity. Corticosteroids, ciclosporin, and tacrolimus can cause post-transplant diabetes mellitus. Additionally, patients on immunosuppressant drugs need to avoid live vaccines.

Interactions

Transplant patients are placed on immunosuppressant drugs for their lifetime and are often on combination therapy, increasing their risk for drug interactions. Immunosuppressants have narrow therapeutic windows, and drug interactions can be significant. Drugs that cause

TABLE 50-2

Immunosuppressant Drugs: Common Adverse Effects

Body System	Adverse Effects
AZATHIOPRINE	
Hematological	Leukopenia, thrombocytopenia
Hepatic	Hepatotoxicity
CICLOSPORIN	
Cardiovascular	Moderate hypertension in as many as 50% of patients
Central nervous	Neurotoxicity, including tremors, in 20% of patients
Hepatic	Hepatotoxicity with cholestasis and hyperbilirubinemia
Renal	Nephrotoxicity is common and dose limiting
Other	Post-transplant diabetes mellitus, gingival hyperplasia, and hirsutism
TACROLIMUS	
Central nervous	Agitation, anxiety, confusion, hallucinations, neuropathy
Renal	Albuminuria, dysuria, acute kidney injury, kidney tubular necrosis
Other	Post-transplant diabetes mellitus
ANTIBODY IMMUNOSUPPRESSANTS (BASILIXIMAB)	
Multiple body systems	Cytokine release syndrome, which includes such immune-mediated symptoms as fever, dyspnea, tachycardia, sweating, chills, headache, nausea, vomiting, diarrhea, muscle and joint pain, and general malaise

increased levels of immunosuppressant drugs can cause toxicity, whereas drugs that reduce immunosuppressant drug levels may lead to organ rejection. The most significant drug interactions with immunosuppressant drugs are listed in Table 50-3. Many of these drugs are metabolized by the cytochrome P450 enzyme system, thus drug interactions are common and can be significant. Grapefruit can inhibit metabolizing enzymes and thus can increase the levels of ciclosporin, tacrolimus, and sirolimus. Foods that are high in potassium, such as bananas and tomatoes, can increase ciclosporin nephrotoxicity. Meals that have high fat content can increase sirolimus levels.

Ciclosporin, tacrolimus, and sirolimus can be involved in many drug interactions, several of which can be harmful. Drugs that may increase their actions are diltiazem, verapamil, fluconazole, itraconazole, clarithromycin, allopurinol, metoclopramide, amphotericin B, cimetidine, and ketoconazole. Grapefruit (including its juice), because of its inhibition of key metabolizing enzymes, can also increase the bioavailability of these three immunosuppressants. For example, ciclosporin can have a profound interaction with grapefruit juice; when they are taken together, there is an increase in the bioavailability of ciclosporin, from 20 to 200%. Drugs that may reduce the effects of these immunosuppressants include carbamazepine, phenobarbital, phenytoin, and rifampin; these interactions occur because some of the same cytochrome P450 metabolizing enzymes are shared among these drugs and the immunosuppressant drugs. Although these are the most significant interactions, there are many more of less significance.

Because of its antibodies, basiliximab is generally given in a relatively short, single course of therapy; it has a few recognized drug interactions. The potential for interactions between immunosuppressant drugs and natural health products also should not be overlooked. For example, the enzyme-inducing properties of St. John's wort have been demonstrated to reduce the therapeutic levels of ciclosporin and cause organ rejection. The immunostimulant properties of cat's claw and echinacea may be similarly undesirable in transplant recipients; these products have effects that are opposite those of the immunosuppressants.

Dosages

For the recommended dosages of selected immunosuppressants, see the table on p. 933. Immunosuppressants must be taken exactly as directed, at precise times and with a specific dietary plan. While adhering to dosage schedules can be a challenge for most patients, immunosuppressants should be taken continuously, with direct supervision from the transplant team. Ciclosporin and tacrolimus should not be taken at the same time. Sirolimus should be taken 4 hours after ciclosporin. If a dose is missed, it should be taken as soon as the patient remembers, unless it is close to the time the next dose is due; in this type of situation, patients must contact their transplant teams.

TABLE 50-3

Immunosuppressant Drugs: Selected Drug Interactions

Drug	Mechanism	Result
CICLOSPORIN		
clarithromycin	Inhibit metabolism of ciclosporin	Increased levels of ciclosporin and toxicity
fluconazole		
amiodarone hydrochloride		
verapamil hydrochloride		
allopurinol		
protease inhibitors		
phenytoin	Induce metabolism of ciclosporin	Decreased levels of ciclosporin and reduced effect
phenobarbital		
carbamazepine		
rifampin		
St. John's wort		
NSAIDs	Inhibit synthesis of renal prostaglandin	Increased nephrotoxic effects of ciclosporin; renal failure
Grapefruit juice	Increase absorption of ciclosporin	Increased levels of ciclosporin and toxicity
SIROLIMUS		
ciclosporin	Unknown	Increased concentration of sirolimus and nephrotoxic risk
fluconazole	Inhibit metabolism of sirolimus	Increased levels of sirolimus and toxicity
ketoconazole		
clarithromycin		
erythromycin		
Protease inhibitors		
verapamil hydrochloride		
Grapefruit juice		
rifampin	Induce metabolism of sirolimus	Decreased concentration and effect of sirolimus
phenytoin		
phenobarbital		
carbamazepine		
St. John's wort		
TACROLIMUS		
amphotericin	Increase nephrotoxicity of tacrolimus	Kidney failure
gentamicin		
tobramycin		
clarithromycin	Inhibit metabolism of tacrolimus	Increased levels of tacrolimus and toxicity
fluconazole		
ketoconazole		
voriconazole		
Protease inhibitors		
verapamil hydrochloride		
diltiazem		
Grapefruit juice		
rifampin	Induce metabolism of tacrolimus	Decreased effect of tacrolimus
phenytoin		
phenobarbital		
carbamazepine		
St. John's wort		
MYCOPHENOLATE		
Antacids	Reduce absorption of mycophenolate mofetil	Decreased effect of mycophenolate mofetil
Iron		
cholestyramine		
Oral contraceptives	Mycophenolate mofetil decreases progesterone levels	Possible pregnancy
rifampin	Induce metabolism of mycophenolate mofetil	Decreased effect of mycophenolate mofetil
AZATHIOPRINE		
allopurinol	Decrease metabolism of azathioprine	Bone marrow suppression

HMG-CoA, 3-hydroxy-3-methylglutaryl-coenzyme A; *NSAIDs*, nonsteroidal anti-inflammatory drugs.

▶▶*azathioprine*

Azathioprine (Imuran) is a chemical analogue of the physiological purines, such as adenine and guanine. It blocks T-cell proliferation by inhibiting purine synthesis, which in turn prevents deoxyribonucleic acid (DNA) synthesis. Azathioprine is used for prophylaxis of organ rejection concurrently with other immunosuppressant drugs, such as ciclosporin- and corticosteroids. It is available in both oral and injectable forms.

PHARMACOKINETICS

Route	Onset of Action	Peak Plasma Concentration	Elimination Half-Life	Duration of Action
PO	2–4 days*	1–2 hr	5 hr	Unknown

*6–8 wk for rheumatoid arthritis

basiliximab

Basiliximab (Simulect) is a monoclonal antibody that acts by inhibiting the binding of the cytokine mediator interleukin-2 (IL-2) to the high-affinity IL-2 receptor. Basiliximab is used to prevent rejection of transplanted kidneys (**grafts**) and is most often used as part of a multidrug immunosuppressive regimen that includes ciclosporin- and corticosteroids. It has a tendency to cause the allergiclike reaction known as *cytokine release syndrome*, which can be severe and involve anaphylaxis. Patients are often premedicated with corticosteroids (e.g., intravenous [IV] methylprednisolone), in an effort to avoid or alleviate this problem. Basiliximab is available only in injectable form.

PHARMACOKINETICS

Route	Onset of Action	Peak Plasma Concentration	Elimination Half-Life	Duration of Action
IV	1 day	3–4 days	7–9 days	Unknown

▶▶*ciclosporin*

Ciclosporin (Sandimmune, Cyclosporine, Neoral) is an immunosuppressant drug indicated for the prevention of organ rejection following solid organ transplantation and bone marrow transplantation. Ciclosporin is classified as a calcineurin inhibitor and works by inhibiting the production and release of IL-2. Similar to azathioprine, ciclosporin may also be used for the treatment of other autoimmune disorders, such as rheumatoid arthritis, nephrotic syndrome, psoriasis, and irritable bowel syndrome.

Ciclosporin is available in both oral and injectable forms. Neoral is available as an oral solution and capsules, while Sandimmune is the injectable form. Patients who are unable to take Neoral soft gelatin capsules or oral solution may be treated with Sandimmune intravenously at one-third of the oral dose. Ciclosporin has a narrow therapeutic range, and for this reason laboratory monitoring of drug levels may be implemented to ensure therapeutic plasma concentrations and to avoid toxicity.

PHARMACOKINETICS

Route	Onset of Action	Peak Plasma Concentration	Elimination Half-Life	Duration of Action
PO	1–3 hr	3.5 hr	1–2 hr (parent compound) 10–40 hr (metabolites)	Unknown

glatiramer acetate

Glatiramer acetate (Copaxone) is a mixture of random polymers of four different amino acids. This mixture results in a compound that is antigenically similar to myelin basic protein (a protein found on the myelin sheath of nerves). The drug is believed to work by blocking T-cell autoimmune activity against this protein, which reduces the frequency of the neuromuscular exacerbations associated with multiple sclerosis. Each 1 mL of Copaxone® solution contains 20 mg or 40 mg of glatiramer acetate and 40 mg of the inactive ingredient, mannitol. This drug is contraindicated in patients who have a sensitivity to glatiramer or to mannitol. It is available only in injectable form.

A new drug, fingolimod hydrochloride (Gilenya®), a sphingosine-1-phosphate receptor (S1PR) modulator, failed as an antirejection drug, but was approved for multiple sclerosis. It is an oral drug available for relapsing forms of multiple sclerosis. It has significant adverse effects, including headache, hepatotoxicity, flulike symptoms, back pain, atrioventricular block, bradycardia, hypertension, and macular edema. For these reasons, there is an extensive patient medication guide for all patients dispensed fingolimod hydrochloride.

▶▶*mycophenolate mofetil*

Mycophenolate mofetil (CellCept) is an antimetabolite and suppresses T cell proliferation. It is indicated for the prevention of organ rejection as well as the treatment of organ rejection. Mycophenolate mofetil is associated with an increased risk of congenital malformations and spontaneous abortions when used during pregnancy. It is available in oral and IV forms. Common adverse effects include hypertension (28 to 77% incidence), hypotension, peripheral edema, tachycardia, pain, headache, hyperglycemia, dyslipidemia, electrolyte disturbances, abdominal pain, leukopenia, thrombocytopenia, cough, and dyspnea.

PHARMACOKINETICS

Route	Onset of Action	Peak Plasma Concentration	Elimination Half-Life	Duration of Action
PO	4 wk	0.8–1.8 hr	8–16 hr	Unknown

▶▶*sirolimus and tacrolimus*

Sirolimus (Rapamune) is an immunosuppressant drug, similar in structure to tacrolimus (Prograf). Sirolimus is a macrocyclic immunosuppressive, antifungal, and antitumour drug, and tacrolimus is used to prevent organ rejection and to treat rejection once it occurs. Sirolimus works by inhibiting T lymphocyte activation in response to antigenic stimulation and inhibits antibody production, which in turn suppresses cytokine-mediated T cell proliferation. Sirolimus and tacrolimus are structurally related and act through similar mechanisms. Sirolimus is classified as an mTOR kinase inhibitor, whereas tacrolimus is classified as a calcineurin inhibitor. Sirolimus is available only for oral use, whereas tacrolimus is available in both oral and injectable forms. Sirolimus levels are increased when the drug is taken with high-fat meals.

Everolimus, an analogue of sirolimus, was originally approved for the treatment of certain forms of advanced cancer, such as advanced breast cancer, pancreatic neuroendocrine tumours, and renal cell carcinoma. It is available as Afinitor® and Afinitor Disperz™, which are not interchangeable drugs. Afinitor is used for the

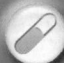 **DRUG PROFILES—cont'd**

treatment of patients 18 years of age and older with renal angiomyolipoma associated with tuberous sclerosis complex (TSC) who do not require immediate surgery, for hormone receptor-positive, HER2-negative advanced breast cancer, for differentiated neuroendocrine tumours of pancreatic origin, for metastatic kidney cancer, and for angiomyolipoma of the kidney associated with TSC. Both Afinitor® and Afinitor Disperz® are indicated for the treatment of patients with subependymal giant cell astrocytoma (SEGA) associated with TSC who are not candidates for surgical resection and who do not require immediate surgical intervention. Afinitor® is a tablet and Afinitor Disperz™ is a tablet for oral suspension.

PHARMACOKINETICS (Sirolimus)

Route	Onset of Action	Peak Plasma Concentration	Elimination Half-Life	Duration of Action
PO	Rapid	1–3 hr	60–80 hr	Unknown

PHARMACOKINETICS (Tacrolimus)

Route	Onset of Action	Peak Plasma Concentration	Elimination Half-Life	Duration of Action
PO	Variable	0.5–4 hr	21–61 hr	Unknown

DOSAGES   Selected Immunosuppressant Drugs

Drug	Pharmacological Class	Usual Dosage Range	Indications/Uses
⇥azathioprine (Imuran)	Antimetabolite	*Adults and children* IV/PO: 3–5 mg/kg/day to start, then 1–3 mg/kg/day maintenance	Prevention of rejection of kidney transplants
basiliximab (Simulect)	Monoclonal antibody	*Children 2–15 yr, less than 35 kg* IV: 10 mg within 2 hr of transplant surery, then 10 mg 4 days afterward *Adults* IV: 20 mg within 2 hr of transplant surgery, then 20 mg 4 days afterward	Prevention of rejection of kidney transplants
⇥ciclosporin (Sandimmune, Neoral)	Calcineurin inhibitor	*Adults* PO: 10–15 mg/kg as a single dose, 4–12 hr preoperatively; continue same dose daily postoperatively for 1–2 wk, then reduce by 5%/wk to a maintenance dose of 2–6 mg/kg/day IV: 3–5 mg/kg as a single dose, 4–12 hr preoperatively and continued daily postoperatively until patient can tolerate PO dosing	Prevention and treatment of rejection of kidney, liver, and heart transplants
glatiramer acetate (Copaxone)	Miscellaneous biologic	*Adults only* Subcut: 20 mg once daily	Treatment of RRMS
mycophenolate mofetil (CellCept)	Antimetabolite	*Children 2–18 yr* IV/PO: 600 mg/m² twice daily (maximum daily dose: 1.5–2 g daily) *Adults* IV/PO: 1–1.5 g twice daily	Prevention of rejection of kidney, liver, or heart transplants
mycophenolate sodium (Myfortic®)	Antimetabolite	*Adults* PO: 720 mg twice daily	Prevention of rejection of kidney transplants
sirolimus (Rapamune)	mTOR kinase inhibitor	*Children over 13 yr, less than 40 kg* IV/PO: 3-mg/m² loading dose on day 1, followed by maintenance of 1 mg/m²/day *Adults* IV/PO: 6-mg loading dose on day 1, followed by maintenance dose of 2 mg/day	Prevention of rejection of kidney transplants
tacrolimus (Advagraf, Prograf)	Calcineurin inhibitor	*Adults and children* IV: 0.01–0.05 mg/kg/day as continuous IV infusion; then PO: 0.1–0.2 mg/kg/day divided q12h	Prevention and treatment of rejection of liver, kidney, heart, lung, pancreas, and small bowel transplants

IV, intravenous; *PO*, oral; *RRMS*, relapsing–remitting multiple sclerosis; *Subcut*, subcutaneous.

NURSING PROCESS

☑ Assessment

Transplantation is a highly specialized area of medicine that brings forth complexity in both medical and ethical domains of health care. The primary concern for patients is organ rejection, which comes with the possibility of removal of the transplanted organ. Immunosuppressant therapy is used to inhibit the patient's immune system, to prevent organ rejection. Patients are placed on immunosuppressant drugs for the duration of the transplanted organ's life. Prior to any administration of immunosuppressants, perform a thorough patient assessment focused on obtaining baseline measurements that include vital signs and weight. Conduct a detailed health history, including past and present medical conditions, and document the following specific systemic information: (1) pre-existing diseases that impact the patient's immune status, such as diabetes, hypertension, and cancer; (2) urinary functioning and patterns; (3) presence of jaundice, edema, or ascites; (4) history of heart disease or dysrhythmias, chest pain, or heart failure; (5) level of central nervous system (CNS) functioning, with attention to any seizure disorders, alteration of motor or sensory function, paresthesias, or changing levels of consciousness; (6) respiratory status and baseline respiratory functioning, breath sounds, presence of asthma, pulmonary diseases, wheezing, cough, activity intolerance, dyspnea, or sputum production; (7) gastrointestinal (GI) functioning and patterns and bowel disease; (8) musculoskeletal intactness, with attention to range of motion, appearance of joints and any deformities, and ability to perform activities of daily living; and (9) presence and location of any inflammatory reactions as well as any pain, redness, or drainage. In addition, the following laboratory and diagnostic tests may be ordered: kidney function tests with glomerular filtration rate, blood urea nitrogen (BUN) and creatinine levels; liver function tests with ALP, AST, ALT, and bilirubin levels; and cardiovascular function with baseline electrocardiogram. See Table 50-2 for information on other systems affected by the immunosuppressant drugs. Assess for and document all cautions, contraindications, and drug interactions, as well as any concerns that the patient may have.

Azathioprine requires assessment of white blood cell (WBC) and platelet counts, noting any signs and symptoms of infection as well as any bleeding tendencies because of the risk of drug-related leukopenia and thrombocytopenia. Assess liver function prior to administering this drug. A significant drug interaction occurs between azathioprine and allopurinol; thus, it is important to assess for this interaction to avoid the resultant effect of bone marrow suppression. Prior to the use of ciclosporin, specifically assess the functional level of all organs as well as for any underlying cardiovascular, CNS, liver, or kidney disease because of potential drug-related toxicities involving these systems and the physiological impact of the organ transplant process on multiple systems. Perform a baseline oral assessment because of the possible adverse effect of drug-induced gingival hyperplasia with the use of this drug. Assess and document baseline blood pressures, because as many as 50% of patients on this drug experience subsequent moderate hypertension. Common drug interactions with ciclosporin for which to assess include protease inhibitors, HMG-CoA reductase inhibitors, clarithromycin, phenytoin, phenobarbital, St. John's wort, nonsteroidal anti-inflammatory drugs, and grapefruit juice (see Table 50-3).

Prior to the administration of tacrolimus, obtain a thorough patient history with attention to medication use, and perform a physical assessment with close attention to renal functioning through monitoring of BUN, serum creatinine, and serum electrolyte levels. When the drug is administered, closely assess the patient for the first 30 minutes following the first dose of the medication. Concern regarding anaphylactic reactions also continues past this first 30 minutes and the first dose. It is important to confirm that resuscitative equipment is accessible and functioning and that appropriate doses of epinephrine and oxygen are also readily available. Drug interactions with tacrolimus for which to assess are listed in Table 50-3. Prior to the use of basiliximab (an antibody immunosuppressant), complete a thorough documentation of baseline vital signs and other presenting manifestations because of the possible occurrence of cytokine release syndrome, with resultant fever, dyspnea, tachycardia, sweating, chills, vomiting, diarrhea, muscle or joint pain, and general malaise.

☑ Nursing Diagnoses

- Acute pain (e.g., joint and muscle aches, flu-like symptoms) related to adverse effects of immunosuppressant medications
- Risk for injury related to the physiological effects of the disease, overall weakness, and the adverse effects of immunosuppressants
- Risk for infection related to altered immune status caused by chronic disease, treatment with immunosuppressants, or the transplantation process

☑ Planning

■ Goals

- Patient will experience maximal comfort during drug therapy with immunosuppressants.
- Patient will remain free from injury.
- Patient will remain free from infection during therapy with immunosuppressants.

■ Expected Patient Outcomes

- Patient states measures to help maximize comfort and minimize adverse effects of drug therapy, such as taking acetaminophen for fever and joint pain; reporting unusually high blood pressure readings; and participating in relaxation therapy, massage, diversional activities, hypnosis, imagery, and biofeedback.
- Patient states measures to decrease injury to self, such as reporting to the health care provider the onset of fever, rash, sore throat, fatigue, breaks in skin (rashes, sores), or other unusual problems or symptoms that may develop during therapy.
- Patient maintains immune system and prevents infection with a healthy diet inclusive of an increase in caloric and protein intake, as deemed necessary during nutritional consultation, during drug therapy.
- Patient reports any fever, chills, increased malaise, productive cough, lethargy, fatigue, or confusion to the health care provider.
- Patient minimizes contact with large crowds and with individuals with known bacterial or viral infections while on immunosuppressive therapy.

◩ Implementation

Oral immunosuppressants need to be taken with food to minimize GI upset. It is also important, because of the immunosuppressed state of patients receiving immunosuppressants, that oral forms of the drugs be used whenever possible to decrease the risk of infection associated with parenteral injections and subsequent injury to the first line of defence (skin). An oral antifungal medication may be ordered to treat any oral candidiasis that occurs as a consequence of the treatment and the disease process; however, significant drug interactions may occur between the immunosuppressant and antifungal drug, so always check for drug interactions. Therefore, this possible interaction should be considered and avoided prior to giving the medications. With the use of any of the immunosuppressants, it is also important to be sure that supportive treatment equipment and related drugs are available in case of an anaphylactic or allergic reaction. Be aware of the high risk for such an occurrence, and be constantly prepared. The use of premedication protocols involving various antihistamines and anti-inflammatory drugs is also common. Depending on the immunosuppressant being administered, gloves, a mask, protective goggles or a gown may be worn by the nurse.

Ciclosporin is available in both oral and injectable formulations; do not refrigerate oral solutions. For the safe administration of oral liquid dosage forms, a graduated syringe for dispensing is provided with them. The oral solution may be mixed in a glass container with apple juice or orange juice and served at room temperature. The use of grapefruit juice as a diluent should be avoided, owing to its possible interference with the cytochrome P450 enzyme system. Once the solution is mixed, make sure that it is stirred well and the patient drinks it immediately. Other drinks, such as soft drinks, can be administered following administration of the drug. The syringe should not come into contact with the diluent. If the syringe is to be cleaned, do not rinse it, but wipe the outside with a dry tissue. Neoral soft gelatin capsules are to be swallowed whole. They are available in blister packs, which, when opened, have a characteristic normal odour. With intravenously administered ciclosporin, the dose must be diluted as recommended by the manufacturer and given according to standards of care and institutional policy. Always infuse this drug using an infusion pump and over the recommended period. Especially during the first 30 minutes, monitor the patient closely during the infusion for any allergic reactions manifested by facial flushing, urticaria, wheezing, dyspnea, or rash. Record vital signs frequently and document these. It is also important to closely monitor the patient's BUN, LDH, AST, and ALT during therapy, as ordered, to detect possible kidney and liver impairment. Oral hygiene may be performed frequently to prevent dry mouth and subsequent infections. The health care provider will also order blood tests to confirm therapeutic serum levels of ciclosporin.

Sirolimus and tacrolimus need to be administered as ordered by either the IV or oral route. If IV tacrolimus is to be discontinued and maintenance dosing is needed, oral tacrolimus is usually ordered to be given 8 to 12 hours after discontinuation of the IV drug. Do not store IV solution in polyvinyl chloride containers. It must be administered in appropriately designed containers and tubing. Oral dosages of tacrolimus are given on an empty stomach. As with ciclosporin, the oral dosage of tacrolimus are not to be put in Styrofoam containers. Inform patients to avoid the consumption of grapefruit while taking sirolimus or tacrolimus. Both drugs have long half-lives, so toxicity is a concern because of possible cumulative effects.

Because immunosuppressant therapy is lifelong and expensive, it is important for patients to receive adequate and appropriate emotional, spiritual, social, and financial support. Additionally, specifics of therapy must be emphasized with patients, family members, and significant others, such as the complexity of dosing and the need to always have a 1-week supply of medication available so that there is never a risk of running out. Continuous monitoring of drug serum levels is required.

◩ Evaluation

Continuously evaluate and re-evaluate goals and expected outcomes related to administration of immunosuppressants and the nursing process. In addition, evaluate therapeutic responses to immunosuppressants, including acceptance of the transplanted organ or graft and improved symptoms in those with autoimmune diseases. Complete blood count; erythrocyte sedimentation rate; C-reactive protein level; liver, kidney, and heart function tests; pulmonary function tests; chest X-ray; and analysis of T-lymphocyte surface phenotyping are a few of the tests performed to evaluate patients during and after drug therapy. Evaluation of drug-specific adverse effects and toxicities (see Table 50-2) and specific therapeutic drug levels (as indicated) should be ongoing.

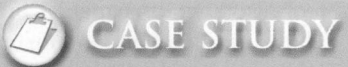

CASE STUDY

Ciclosporin

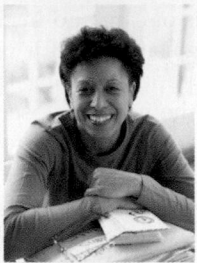

Valerie, a 62-year-old retired orchestra conductor, moved to another city after her husband died. Over the past few years she has developed kidney problems, and 3 years ago she was told that she needed a kidney transplant. After 3 years of waiting and undergoing hemodialysis, she was told that her niece was a match and was willing to donate a kidney. She has had the transplant, and after 1 week, the transplant seems to be successful so far.

Ciclosporin is one of the immunosuppressants she will be receiving. She was given her first dose of ciclosporin 12 hours before surgery and is now receiving oral doses. The nurse has provided instructions on how to take the oral doses at home.

1. The next day, when another nurse comes in with Valerie's morning medications, Valerie says, "You can't give me the medicine like that. Don't you know how to mix it?" What do you think the nurse did wrong?

2. What important measures will be taken to prevent toxicity?

3. Valerie tells the nurse that she can't wait to get home and relax by her pool. She is also looking forward to getting her strength back and going shopping with her friends. How will the nurse respond to these statements?

4. After Valerie gets home, she calls the office to ask about eating grapefruit. "The pill bottle says no grapefruit, but I thought the doctor said I could have a little bit. I bought some wonderful organic grapefruits, and I love fresh grapefruit juice. What should I do?" What is the nurse's best answer?

_____

For answers, see http://evolve.elsevier.com/Canada/Lilley/ pharmacology/.

PATIENT TEACHING TIPS

❖ Educate transplant patients about the need for lifelong immunosuppressant therapy with often complex therapeutic regimens.

❖ Emphasize to patients taking immunosuppressants the importance of avoiding situations that pose an increased risk of exposure to infection, such as being in crowds, malls, or movie theaters.

❖ Stress to patients the importance of reporting any headache, fever, sore throat, chills, joint pain, chest pain, dizziness, fatigue, problems with urination, or rash to the health care provider, as these may indicate infection and require immediate medical attention.

❖ Educate patients about signs of rejection such as flu-like symptoms, fever above 38°C, decreased urine output, weight gain, pain or tenderness over the transplant area, and fatigue. Patients must report these to the health care provider immediately, as rejection can often be managed with adjustments to dosages of immunosuppressant.

❖ Encourage patients to wear medical alert jewellery that clearly indicates what was transplanted and the time of transplantation.

❖ Educate female patients of childbearing age who are receiving immunosuppressants about the need to use some form of contraception during treatment and for up to 12 weeks after therapy ends.

❖ Advise patients to take most immunosuppressant drugs at the same time every day and, if a dose is omitted, to contact the health care provider for further instructions.

❖ Patients should be aware that follow-up appointments are important because of the need to monitor status through examinations and blood testing.

❖ Educate patients about the adverse effects of ciclosporin, (e.g., headache, tremor), and instruct patients to avoid consumption of grapefruit or grapefruit juice because of the related potential for an increase in blood concentrations of ciclosporin, tacrolimus, or sirolimus. This effect can last for over 24 hours and the effect can occur even when grapefruit juice is taken at a different time from the medication.

❖ Inform patients that gelatin capsules are to be stored in a cool, dry environment and must not be exposed to light. The dosage form must be kept in its original packaging.

❖ A possible adverse effect of ciclosporin is photosensitivity, which can cause patients to sunburn more easily. Instruct patients to avoid prolonged exposure to the sun, and encourage them to use sunscreen and wear protective clothing when outdoors.

PATIENT TEACHING TIPS—cont'd

❖ Inform patients who are to undergo transplant surgery that several days before surgery they may be told to take ciclosporin with corticosteroids. They may also be given an oral antifungal as prophylaxis for *Candida* infections.

❖ Encourage patients to inspect the oral cavity frequently for any white patches on the tongue, mucous membranes, or oropharynx; these patches may indicate oral candidiasis.

❖ Advise patients taking oral forms of ciclosporin to take the medication with meals or mixed with milk to minimize GI upset.

❖ Inform patients taking azathioprine that several days before transplant surgery they are to take all their medication by the oral route if possible and avoid

trauma as well as subcutaneous and intramuscular injections, which increase the risk for infection.

❖ Provide patients on tacrolimus or sirolimus with a list of foods, especially those high in fats and carbohydrates, that could negatively impact the absorption of the medication. Nutritional counselling can be extremely beneficial to patients and improve their understanding of food interactions as well as any concerns related to dyslipidemia and increased triglycerides associated with many of the immunosuppressive drugs.

❖ All immunosuppressants taken at home are to be taken exactly as ordered and at the same time every day. Educate patients about the adverse effects of the medication.

KEY POINTS

❖ Immunosuppressants decrease or prevent the body's immune response. Some of the clinical uses for immunosuppressants are suppression of immune-mediated disorders or malignancies and improvement of short-term and long-term allograft survival.

❖ Oral antifungals are generally given with immunosuppressant medications to treat oral

candidiasis that occurs as a result of immunosuppression and fungal overgrowth.

❖ Monitor the results of laboratory studies ordered by the health care provider, such as hemoglobin level and hematocrit, as well as red blood cell, WBC, and platelet counts. If values indicated in these tests drop below normal ranges, notify the health care provider.

EXAMINATION REVIEW QUESTIONS

1. A patient has a new order for glatiramer. The patient has not had an organ transplant. The nurse knows that the patient is receiving this drug for which condition?
   a. Psoriasis
   b. Rheumatoid arthritis
   c. Irritable bowel syndrome
   d. Relapse–remitting multiple sclerosis
2. When assessing a patient who is to receive ciclosporin, the nurse knows that which condition would be a contraindication for this drug?
   a. Acute myalgia
   b. Kidney disease
   c. Fluid overload
   d. Polycythemia
3. During therapy with azathioprine (Imuran), the nurse must monitor for which adverse effect?
   a. Bradycardia
   b. Diarrhea
   c. Vomiting
   d. Thrombocytopenia
4. During a teaching session for a patient receiving an immunosuppressant drug, the nurse will include which statement?
   a. "It is better to use oral forms of these drugs to prevent the occurrence of thrush."
   b. "You will remain on antibiotics to prevent infections."

   c. "It is important to use some form of contraception during treatment and for up to 12 weeks after the end of therapy."
   d. "Be sure to take your medications with grapefruit juice to increase absorption."
5. During drug therapy with basiliximab, the nurse monitors for signs of cytokine release syndrome, which results in which set of symptoms?
   a. Fever, dyspnea, and general malaise
   b. Neurotoxicity and peripheral neuropathy
   c. Hepatotoxicity with jaundice
   d. Thrombocytopenia with increased bleeding tendencies
6. When assessing a patient who is to begin therapy with an immunosuppressant drug, the nurse recalls that such drugs should be used cautiously in patients with which condition(s)? (Select all that apply.)
   a. Pregnancy
   b. Glaucoma
   c. Anemia
   d. Myalgia
   e. Kidney dysfunction
   f. Liver dysfunction
7. The order reads: "Give tacrolimus IV 0.03 mg/kg/day as a continuous IV infusion." The patient weighs 110 pounds. How many milligrams per day will this dose provide?

CRITICAL THINKING ACTIVITIES

1. The nurse is explaining the purpose of ciclosporin to a 58-year-old patient who has had a heart transplant. The patient asks, "How does this keep my immune system from attacking my new heart?" What is the nurse's best answer?

2. A patient is about to receive basiliximab as part of post-transplant drug therapy. Before the nurse administers the basiliximab, what action is most important to take in order to prevent adverse effects? Explain your answer.

3. A patient is on call for lung transplant surgery—she has been told the procedure could occur within 24 hours. The surgeon writes an order that says, "Avoid injections as much as possible." A new nurse questions this order, asking, "What does the surgeon mean by that?" What is the nurse's best answer?

For answers, see http://evolve.elsevier.com/Canada/Lilley/pharmacology/.

Immunizing Drugs and Pandemic Preparedness

Objectives

After reading this chapter, the successful student will be able to do the following:

1. Discuss the importance of immunity as it relates to immunizing drugs and their use in patients of all ages.

2. Identify the diseases that are treated or prevented with toxoids or vaccines.

3. Compare the mechanisms of action, indications, cautions, contraindications, adverse effects, toxicities, drug interactions, and routes of administration of various toxoids and vaccines.

4. Develop a collaborative plan of care that includes all phases of the nursing process related to the administration of immunizing drugs across the lifespan.

5. Develop a collaborative plan of care covering aspects of the nursing process related to pandemic preparedness, with emphasis on the nurse's role.

e-Learning Activities

Website
(http://evolve.elsevier.com/Canada/Lilley/pharmacology/)

evolve

- Answer Key—Textbook Case Studies
- Answer Key—Critical Thinking Activities
- Chapter Summaries—Printable
- Review Questions for Exam Preparation
- Unfolding Case Studies

Drug Profiles

diphtheria and tetanus toxoids and acellular pertussis vaccine tetanus (adsorbed), p. 946
Haemophilus influenzae type b conjugate vaccine, p. 946
▸▸ hepatitis B immunoglobulin, p. 950
▸▸ hepatitis B virus vaccine (inactivated), p. 947
herpes zoster vaccine, p. 950
▸▸ human papillomavirus vaccine, p. 949
▸▸ immunoglobulin, p. 950
▸▸ influenza virus vaccine, p. 947
▸▸ measles, mumps, rubella virus vaccine (live), p. 948
▸▸ meningococcal vaccine, p. 948
▸▸ pneumococcal vaccine, polyvalent and 13-valent, p. 948
▸▸ poliovirus vaccine (inactivated), p. 949
rabies immunoglobulin, p. 951
rabies virus vaccine, p. 949
$Rh_0(D)$ immunoglobulin, p. 950
▸▸ rotavirus oral vaccine, p. 950
tetanus immunoglobulin, p. 951
▸▸ varicella virus vaccine, p. 950
varicella-zoster immunoglobulin, p. 951

▸▸ Key drug

Key Terms

Active immunization A type of immunization that causes development of a complete and long-lasting immunity to a certain infection through exposure of the body to the associated disease antigen; it can be natural active immunization (i.e., having the disease) or artificial active immunization (i.e., receiving a vaccine or toxoid). (p. 941)

Active immunizing drugs Toxoids or vaccines that are administered to a host to stimulate host production of antibodies. (p. 944)

Antibodies Immunoglobulin molecules that have an antigen-specific amino acid sequence and are synthesized by the humoral immune system (B cells) in response to exposure to a specific antigen; their purpose is to attack and destroy molecules of this antigen. (p. 941)

Antibody titre The amount of an antibody needed to react with and neutralize a given volume of a specific antigen. (p. 944)

Antigens Substances, usually proteins and usually foreign to a host, that stimulate the production of antibodies and that react specifically with those antibodies; examples include bacterial exotoxins and viruses. An allergen (e.g., dust, pollen, mould) is an antigen that can produce an immediate-type hypersensitivity reaction or allergy. (p. 941)

Antiserum A serum that contains antibodies; it is usually obtained from an animal that has been immunized against a specific antigen. (p. 944)

Antitoxin An antiserum against a toxin (or toxoid); it is most often a purified antiserum obtained from animals (usually horses) by injection of a toxin or toxoid, so that antibodies to the toxin (i.e., antitoxin) can be collected from the animals and used to provide artificial passive immunity to humans exposed to a given toxin (e.g., tetanus immunoglobulin). (p. 944)

Antivenin An antiserum against a venom (poison produced by an animal) used to treat humans or other animals that have been envenomed (e.g., by snakebite or spider bite). (p. 944)

Biological antimicrobial drugs Substances of biological origin used to prevent, treat, or cure infectious diseases (e.g., vaccines, toxoids, immunoglobulins); these drugs are often simply referred to as *biologics*. (p. 941)

Bivalent vaccine A vaccine that stimulates an immune response against two different antigens (e.g., two different viruses or other microorganisms). (p. 949)

Booster shot A repeat dose of an antigen, such as a vaccine or toxoid, usually administered in an amount smaller than that used in the original immunization, given to maintain the immune response of a previously immunized patient at, or return the response to, a clinically effective level. (p. 944)

Cell-mediated immune system The immune response that is mediated by T cells (as opposed to B cells, which produce antibodies); T cells mount their immune response through activities such as the release of cytokines (chemicals that stimulate other protective immune functions) as well as through direct cytotoxicity (e.g., phagocytosis of an antigen). (p. 941)

Herd immunity Resistance to a disease on the part of an entire community or population because a large proportion of its members are immune to the disease. (p. 944)

Immune response A cascade of biochemical events that occurs in response to entry of an antigen (foreign substance) into the body; key processes of the immune response include phagocytosis ("eating of cells") of foreign microorganisms and synthesis of antibodies that react

with specific antigens to inactivate them. Immune response centres around the blood but may also involve the lymphatic system and the reticuloendothelial system (see later in Key Terms). (p. 941)

Immunization The induction of immunity by administration of a vaccine or toxoid (active immunization) or antiserum (passive immunization). (p. 941)

Immunizing biologics Toxoids, vaccines, or immunoglobulins that are targeted against specific infectious microorganisms or toxins. (p. 941)

Immunoglobulins Glycoproteins synthesized and used by the humoral immune system (B cells) to attack and kill all substances foreign to the body. (Synonymous with *immune globulins*.) (p. 941)

Passive immunization A type of immunization in which immunity to an infection occurs by injecting a person with antiserum or concentrated antibodies that directly give the host the means to fight off an invading microorganism (artificial passive immunization). The host's immune system therefore does not have to manufacture these antibodies. This process also occurs when antibodies pass from mother to infant during breastfeeding or through the placenta during pregnancy (natural passive immunization). (p. 941)

Passive immunizing drugs Drugs containing antibodies or antitoxins that can kill or inactivate pathogens by binding to the associated antigens. These are directly injected into a person (host) and provide that person with the means to fend off infection, bypassing the host's own immune system. (p. 944)

Quadrivalent vaccine A vaccine that stimulates an immune response against four different antigens (e.g., four different viruses or other microorganisms). (p. 949)

Recombinant Relating to or containing a combination of genetic material from two or more organisms. Such genetic recombination is one of the key methods of biotechnology and is often used to manufacture immunizing drugs and various other medications. (p. 944)

Reticuloendothelial system Specialized cells located in the liver, spleen, lymphatics, and bone marrow that remove miscellaneous particles from the circulation, such as aging antibody molecules. (p. 944)

Trivalent vaccine A vaccine that stimulates an immune response against three different antigens (e.g., three different viruses or other microorganisms). (p. 947)

Toxin Any poison produced by a plant, animal, or microorganism that is highly toxic to other living organisms. (p. 942)

Toxoids Bacterial exotoxins that are modified or inactivated (by chemicals or heat) so that they are no longer toxic but can still bind to host B cells in order to stimulate the formation of antitoxin; toxoids are often used in the same manner as vaccines to promote artificial active immunity in humans. They are one type of active immunizing drug (e.g., tetanus toxoid). (p. 941)

Vaccines   Suspension of live, attenuated, or killed microorganisms that can promote an artificially induced active immunity against a particular microorganism. They are

one type of active immunizing drug (e.g., tetanus vaccine). (p. 942)

Venom   A poison that is secreted by an animal (e.g., snake, insect, or spider). (p. 944)

IMMUNITY AND IMMUNIZATION

Centuries ago, it was noticed that people who contracted certain diseases acquired an immune tolerance to the disease so that, when exposed to the disease again, they did not experience a second incidence of the illness. This basic observation prompted scientists to investigate ways of artificially producing this tolerance. With this line of inquiry came insight into the way in which the immune system functions normally. Knowledge regarding how healthy immune systems work is essential to understanding how immunizing drugs work. Briefly, when the body first comes into contact with **antigens** (foreign proteins or polysaccharides) from an invading organism, specific information is imprinted into a cellular "memory bank" of the immune system. The body can then effectively fight any future invasion by mounting an **immune response.** This cellular memory bank consists of specialized immune cells known as *memory cells*. When an antigen presents itself to a person's humoral immune system (B lymphocytes or B cells) by binding to B cells, the B cells differentiate into two other types of cells— memory cells are one type, and the other is plasma cells. Plasma cells produce large volumes of antibodies against the antigen in question. **Antibodies** are immunoglobulin molecules that have antigen-specific amino acid sequences. **Immunoglobulins**, or immune globulins, are glycoprotein molecules synthesized by the humoral immune system for the purpose of destroying all substances that the body recognizes as foreign. Immunoglobulins can be general or specific. A general immunoglobulin lacks a specific amino acid sequence that allows it to recognize a specific antigen. An immunoglobulin with such a specific amino acid sequence is known as an *antibody*. It is because of this ability of the immune system to recognize specific antigens that individuals are rarely subjected twice to certain diseases, such as mumps, chicken pox, and measles. Instead, they have a complete and long-lasting immunity to those infections.

In contrast to the humoral immune system, which is the focus of this chapter, the **cell-mediated immune system** is the branch of the immune system that does not synthesize antibodies. Rather, it is driven by T cells (T lymphocytes) and works by the release of cytokines (chemicals that promote other immune system functions, e.g., inflammatory responses, runny nose) and by phagocytosis (engulfment and destruction of antigens by the T cells). The cell-mediated immune system is discussed in Chapter 54 because it is the target of immunosuppressant

drugs. To varying degrees, these two immune system branches work simultaneously, even interdependently. The humoral immune system is also activated and driven partly by cytokines from the cell-mediated immune system.

There are two ways of developing immunity to certain infections: **active immunization** and **passive immunization**. Each can be an artificial or natural process. In artificial active immunization, the body is clinically exposed to a relatively harmless form of an antigen that does not cause an actual infection. Information about the antigen is then imprinted into the memory of the immune system and the body's defences are stimulated to resist any subsequent exposure (by producing antibodies). In contrast, natural active immunization occurs when a person acquires immunity by surviving the disease and producing antibodies to the disease-causing organism. Artificial passive immunization involves clinical administration of serum or concentrated immunoglobulins. This directly gives the inoculated individual the substance needed to fight off the invading microorganism. This type of **immunization** bypasses the host's immune system. Finally, natural passive immunization occurs when antibodies are transferred from a mother to her infant through the bloodstream via the placenta during pregnancy. This protection is temporary and lasts for only a few weeks or months. The major differences between active and passive immunity are summarized in Table 51-1 and are discussed in greater depth in the following sections.

ACTIVE IMMUNIZATION

In general, **biological antimicrobial drugs** (also referred to simply as *biologics*) are substances such as antitoxins, antisera, toxoids, and vaccines that are used to prevent, treat, or cure infectious diseases. Toxoids and vaccines are known as *immunizing biologics*, and they target a particular infectious microorganism.

Toxoids

Toxoids are substances that contain antigens, most often in the form of bacterial exotoxins. These substances have been detoxified or weakened with chemicals or heat, which renders them nontoxic and unable to revert back to a toxic form. Nonetheless, they remain highly antigenic and can stimulate an artificial active immune response (production of antitoxin antibodies) when injected into a host patient. These antibodies can then neutralize the same exotoxin upon any future exposure.

TABLE 51-1

Active Versus Passive Immunity

Characteristic	Active	Passive
ARTIFICIAL		
Type of immunizing drug	Toxoid or vaccine	Immunoglobulin or antitoxin
Mechanism of action	Results from an antigen–antibody response similar to that after antigen exposure in the natural disease process	Results from direct administration of exogenous antibodies; antibody concentration will decrease over time, so if re-exposure is expected, it is good judgement to continue passive immunizations
Use	To prevent development of active disease in the event of exposure to a given antigen in individuals who have at least a partially functioning immune system	To provide temporary protection against disease in individuals who are immunocompromised, those for whom active immunization is contraindicated, and those who have been exposed to or anticipate exposure to the organism or toxin; an antibody response is not stimulated in the host
NATURAL		
Mechanism of action	Production of one's own antibodies during actual infection	Transmission of antibodies from mother to fetus through the placenta or from mother to infant during breastfeeding

Toxoids were first developed in 1923, at the Pasteur Institute, by Gaston Ramon and his associates, and modern versions are effective against diseases that are caused by **toxin**-producing bacteria, such as diphtheria and tetanus.

Vaccines

Vaccines are suspensions of live, attenuated (weakened), or killed (inactivated) microorganisms that can stimulate the production of antibodies against the particular organism. Subunit vaccines are similar to inactivated whole-cell vaccines but they contain only the antigenic parts of the vaccine. They can be protein-based (e.g., acellular pertussis, hepatitis B), polysaccharide (e.g., meningococcal disease caused by *Neisseria meningitidis* groups A, C, W135 and Y), or conjugate (e.g., *Haemophilus influenzae* type b (Hib) and pneumococcal). Most vaccines in the childhood immunization schedule require two or more doses in order to prompt the development of an adequate and persisting antibody response. The *Canadian Immunization Guide* recommends ages and the intervals between doses of the same antigen(s) that will offer optimal protection or have the best evidence of efficacy (Public Health Agency of Canada, 2015a). As with toxoids, slight alterations in the bacteria and viruses prevent the person injected from contracting the disease. They are still able to promote active immunization against the organism, including an antibody response. People vaccinated with live bacteria or viruses (as well as those who recover from an infection) may endure long-term immunity against that particular disease. However, protection provided by inactivated vaccines normally will diminish over time, and for this reason they must be given periodic booster shots to maintain immune system protection against infection with the specific organism.

It was Edward Jenner who noticed that milkmaids who had contracted cowpox infections were rarely victims of smallpox and was the first to study the relationship of cowpox to smallpox immunity. His observation led to the development of the smallpox vaccine, using the cowpox virus. With the help of the modern version of this vaccine, smallpox was considered to be eradicated by 1980. Routine smallpox vaccination of Canadians was discontinued in 1972. However, there is a Canadian Smallpox Contingency Plan that is updated as necessary by the Office of Emergency Preparedness, the Centre of Emergency Preparedness and Response, and the Public Health Agency of Canada, with recommendations for actions to be taken if a case of smallpox occurs in Canada or elsewhere in the world.

Today, there are vaccines available for more than 20 infectious diseases. Because of the complexities of developing a safe and effective vaccine, new vaccines appear periodically but not with the rapidity of other types of drugs. Most modern vaccines are produced in a laboratory by genetic engineering methods and contain some extract of the pathogen, or a synthetic extract, rather than the microbe itself. Some vaccines, such as the influenza vaccine, may contain actual whole or split virus particles. Most, however, contain a smaller fraction of the organism, such as the bacterial capsular polysaccharides that are used to make pneumococcal vaccine. The attenuating or killing agent is usually a chemical such as formaldehyde or a physical mechanism such as heat. Attenuation may also be accomplished with the repeated passage of the microbe through some medium, such as a fertile hen egg or a special tissue culture.

The search for new and better drugs will never end. Current goals include finding vaccines against HIV/

BOX 51-1   Available Immunizing Drugs

Active Immunizing Drugs

Bacille Calmette-Guérin vaccine (tuberculosis)

Cholera/traveler's diarrhea (oral)
Diphtheria and tetanus toxoids (adsorbed)
Diphtheria and tetanus toxoids, and acellular pertussis vaccine (adsorbed)
Diphtheria and tetanus toxoids, acellular pertussis, inactivated poliovirus, and *Haemophilus influenzae* type b conjugate vaccines
Diphtheria, tetanus, acellular pertussis (adsorbed), inactivated poliovirus, *Haemophilus influenzae* type b, hepatitis B (recombinant) vaccine, combined
Haemophilus influenzae type b conjugate vaccine
Hepatitis A virus vaccine (inactivated)
Hepatitis B virus vaccine (recombinant)
Hepatitis A virus vaccine (inactivated) and hepatitis B vaccine (recombinant)
Herpes zoster virus (live, attenuated)
Human papillomavirus vaccine (attenuated)
Influenza virus vaccine
Japanese encephalitis virus vaccine
rVSV-ZEBOV

Active Immunizing Drugs

Measles virus* vaccine (live, attenuated)
Measles, mumps, and rubella virus vaccine (live)
Meningococcal bacterial vaccine
Pneumococcal 13-valent conjugate vaccine
Pneumococcal 23-valent conjugate vaccine
Rabies virus vaccine
Rotavirus
Rubella virus vaccine (live)
Smallpox virus vaccine
Tetanus toxoid vaccine (adsorbed)
Tetanus immune globulin
Typhoid (oral and injection)
Varicella vaccine
Yellow fever virus vaccine

Passive Immunizing Drugs

Botulism antitoxin
Botulism immune globulin
Cytomegalovirus immunoglobulin
Diphtheria antitoxin
Hepatitis B immunoglobulin
Rabies immunoglobulin
$Rh_0(D)$ immunoglobulin
Tetanus immunoglobulin
Vaccinia immunoglobulin
Varicella-zoster immunoglobulin

*Also known as rubeola virus.

AIDS and malaria; the ultimate goal in the area of immunization is to develop an effective vaccine against all infectious diseases. A promising vaccine against *Ebolavirus*, developed in Canada (and supported by the World Health Organization), is the recombinant, replication-competent vesicular stomatitis virus–based vaccine expressing a surface glycoprotein of *Zaire Ebolavirus* (rVSV-ZEBOV®; Public Health Agency of Canada, 2015b). A single injection of the vaccine produces a rapid immune response against *Ebolavirus*. The currently available immunizing vaccines are listed in Box 51-1. Note that the drug given to prevent serious respiratory syncytial virus (RSV) infection is not an immunizing drug per se but is a specialized antiviral drug. It is discussed in Chapter 46. The RSV immunoglobulin is no longer available.

People who travel to different parts of the world may require specific vaccines. This information can be found on the US Centers for Disease Control and Prevention website. Individuals can also call or visit travel clinics that specialize in travel vaccination consultations. It is also important to recognize that many individuals who immigrate to Canada may have been vaccinated against diseases that are not part of the Canadian immunization schedule. They may also not have received vaccinations that those born in Canada typically receive in childhood, and may thus require a "catch-up" vaccination schedule.

The National Advisory Committee on Immunization (NACI) provides the Public Health Agency of Canada with ongoing medical, scientific, and public health advice regarding vaccines approved for use in humans in Canada and recommendations for immunization. All recommendations on vaccine use are published every 4 years in the *Canadian Immunization Guide,* which is available online. Within the immunization guide is detailed information about vaccines. There is also a catch-up schedule for people who may have missed immunizations as children.

PASSIVE IMMUNIZATION

In passive immunization, the host's immune system is bypassed, and the person is inoculated with serum containing immunoglobulins obtained from humans or animals. These substances provide the individual the means to fight off the invading organism. This is known as *artificially acquired passive immunity* and it confers temporary immunity against a particular antigen following exposure to the antigen. It differs from active immunization in that it produces a transitory (short-lived) immune state and the antibodies are already prepared for the host; the host's immune system does not have to synthesize its own antibodies. This allows for more rapid prevention or treatment of disease. Important examples include immunization with tetanus immunoglobulin, hepatitis immunoglobulin, rabies immunoglobulin, and snakebite antivenin.

Passive immunization occurs naturally between a mother and fetus or nursing infant, when the mother passes maternal antibodies directly, either through the placenta to the fetus or through breast milk to the nursing infant. This is called *naturally acquired passive immunity*.

There are specific populations that can benefit from passive immunization but not from active immunization (see Table 51-1). These include individuals who have been rendered immunodeficient for one reason or another (e.g., by drugs or disease) and who therefore cannot mount an immune response to a toxoid or vaccine injection because their immune systems are suppressed. **Passive immunizing drugs** are also used in individuals who already have the given disease, especially those with diseases that are rapidly harmful or fatal, such as rabies, tetanus, and hepatitis. Because these diseases can progress rapidly, the body does not have time to mount an adequate immune defence against them before death occurs. The passive immunization of such individuals confers a temporary protection that is usually sufficient to keep the invading organism from killing them, even though it does not stimulate an antibody response.

The passive immunizing drugs are divided into three groups: antitoxins, immunoglobulins, and snake and spider antivenins. An **antitoxin** is a purified **antiserum** that is usually obtained from horses inoculated with the toxin. An immunoglobulin is a concentrated preparation containing predominantly immunoglobulin G and is harvested from a large pool of blood donors. An **antivenin**, often referred to as an *antivenom*, is an antiserum containing antibodies against a **venom,** which is a poison secreted by an animal such as a reptile, insect, or other arthropod (e.g., spider). Most antivenins are obtained from animals (usually horses) that have been injected with the particular venom; however, the newer ones are produced by **recombinant** technology. The serum contains immunoglobulins that can neutralize the toxic effects of the venom.

IMMUNIZING DRUGS
Mechanism of Action and Drug Effects

Active immunizing drugs consist of vaccines and toxoids that may be administered either orally or intramuscularly and work by stimulating the humoral immune system. This system synthesizes immunoglobulins, of which there are five distinct types, designated as M, G, A, E, and D. These immunoglobulins attack and kill foreign substances that invade the body. When this occurs, the foreign substances are referred to as *antigens*, and the immunoglobulins are called *antibodies*.

Vaccines contain substances that trigger the formation of these antibodies against specific pathogens. They may contain the actual live or attenuated pathogen or a killed pathogen. The **antibody titre** is a measure of how many antibodies to a given antigen are present in the blood and

is used to assess whether enough antibodies are present to protect the body effectively against the particular pathogen. Sometimes levels of antibodies decline over time. When this happens, another dose of the vaccine is given to restore the antibody titres to a level that can protect the person against the infection. This repeat dose is referred to as a **booster shot**.

Toxoids are altered forms of bacterial toxins that stimulate the production of antibodies in the same way as vaccines. Because both toxoids and vaccines rely on the immunized host to mount an immune response, the host's immune system must be intact. Therefore, patients who are immunocompromised may not benefit from receiving vaccines or toxoids. Instead, their clinical situations may warrant giving them passive immunizing drugs such as immunoglobulins.

Passive immunizing drugs are the actual antibodies (immunoglobulins) that can kill or inactivate the pathogen. The process is called *passive* because the person's immune system does not participate in the synthesis of antibodies; the antibodies are provided by the immunizing drug. Immunity acquired in this way generally lasts for a much shorter time than that produced by active immunization. Passive immunization lasts only until the injected immunoglobulins are removed from the person's immune system by the **reticuloendothelial system**. The reticuloendothelial system is composed of specialized cells in the liver, spleen, lymphatics, and bone marrow.

Indications

Vaccines and toxoids are active immunizing drugs that have been developed for the prevention of many illnesses caused by bacteria and their toxins, as well as those caused by viruses. Antivenins, antitoxins, and immunoglobulins are passive immunizing drugs. Such drugs can inactivate spider and snake venom, bacterial toxins (exotoxins), and potentially lethal viruses, respectively. Box 51-1 lists the currently available immunizing drugs. The successful immunization of a high proportion of individuals within a population confers protection from infection on the remaining proportion of individuals who are nonimmune because the number of susceptible people is small. This type of protection is called *herd immunity*.

Antivenins, also known as *antisera*, are used to prevent or minimize the effects of poisoning by the venoms of crotalids (e.g., rattlesnakes, copperheads, cottonmouths, water moccasins), black widow spiders, and coral snakes. Of concern in Canada are the crotalids (rattlesnakes are found in northern Ontario, Manitoba, Alberta, and some parts of British Columbia) and black widow spiders, whose poison can be lethal. Most healthy adults do not die from the bites of spiders or snakes if they receive the appropriate treatment (i.e., administration of the appropriate antivenin). However, young children and older adults with health problems are particularly susceptible to the effects of the venom of some of these animals; for either group, an antivenin is needed to neutralize the venom following poisoning.

Contraindications

Contraindications to the administration of immunizing drugs include immediate or anaphylactic reaction to the vaccine or to any component of the vaccine or its container (e.g., latex). Live attenuated vaccines are generally contraindicated in individuals with severe asthma, immunocompromised persons, and pregnant women. Live and inactivated vaccines are also generally contraindicated in those who developed Guillain-Barre Syndrome within 6 weeks of receiving a vaccine. Anaphylactic reactions to vaccine components such as egg, gelatin, latex, thiomersol, are rare. Those with a proven anaphylactic reaction to these components may be vaccinated in a setting where appropriate management of the reaction can be under taken. In the case of a potentially fatal illness such as rabies, the drug may still need to be given and any allergic reaction controlled with other medications. Administration of some immunizing drugs is best deferred until after recovery from a febrile illness or a temporary immunocompromised state (e.g., following cancer chemotherapy), if possible. However, the decision about when to administer the drugs is often a matter of clinical judgement—the individual patient's condition and risk factors for serious illness may be arguments for or against administration of a given immunizing drug at a given time.

Adverse Effects

The undesirable effects of the various immunizing drugs can range from mild and transient to life-threatening and are listed in Table 51-2. The overwhelming majority of adverse effects are minor. Minor reactions can be treated with acetaminophen and rest. More severe reactions, such as fever higher than 39.4°C, can be treated with acetaminophen and tepid baths. Serum sickness sometimes occurs after repeated injections of equine-derived immunizing drugs. The signs and symptoms of serum sickness consist of edema of the face, tongue, and throat; rash; urticaria; arthritis; adenopathy; fever; flushing; itching; cough; dyspnea; cyanosis; vomiting; and cardiovascular collapse. Serum sickness is best treated with analgesics, antihistamines, epinephrine, or corticosteroids; hospitalization may be required.

Any serious or unusual reactions to immunizing drugs need to be reported to the Canadian Adverse Events Following Immunization Surveillance System (CAEFISS), a national vaccine safety surveillance program. There is also a collaboration between the Canadian Paediatric Society (CPS) and pediatric infectious disease specialists, called Immunization Monitoring Program ACTive (IMPACT), a pediatric hospital–based, national active surveillance system, to monitor serious adverse events following immunization, vaccination failures, and selected infectious diseases. IMPACT was established in 1990 to support the timely reporting of adverse events, particularly the most serious reactions in children. The Public Health Agency of Canada website provides extensive information on reporting systems and the data collected by these agencies. Such data are used to improve the quality of immunizing drugs and can even be possible grounds for a Health Canada recall of biologics that demonstrate adverse effects exceeding acceptable safety thresholds.

In the early 1980s, in response to vaccine-related injuries, many parents became reluctant to immunize their children against common, and even potentially fatal, childhood illnesses. There has also been controversy in the national news pertaining to a possible link between immunizations and autism in children. It was thought that thimerosal (a mercury-containing preservative used in vaccines) may have been a causative link. In Canada, the influenza vaccine and most hepatitis B vaccines are the only ones that contain thimerosal. In 2011, the medical community declared that the original study suggesting a link between vaccines and autism was fraudulent. It was suggested that the original author falsified the medical histories of the patients in his study and that he was "hoping to create a vaccine scare." Although there is no evidence to support a link between autism and vaccines, many parents are still reluctant to vaccinate their children.

Interactions

Drug interactions are not generally a problem with the majority of immunizing drugs, probably because immunizing drugs are normally given in a single dose or a relatively small number of doses. One drug class of note that can potentially reduce the efficacy of immunizing drugs is immunosuppressant drugs, including corticosteroids (see Chapter 34), transplant antirejection drugs (see Chapter 50), and cancer chemotherapy drugs (see Chapters 52 and 53). All of these drugs can, to varying degrees, hinder the generation of active immunity that would normally occur following vaccine or toxoid administration. The bacille Calmette-Guérin vaccine for tuberculosis (used in certain vulnerable groups in Canada and in developing countries) can cause false-positive results on the tuberculin skin test (see Chapter 46).

TABLE 51-2

Immunizing Drugs: Minor and Severe Adverse Effects

Body System	Adverse Effects
MINOR EFFECTS	
Central nervous	Fever, adenopathy, malaise, headache
Integumentary	Minor rash, soreness at injection site, urticaria, arthritis
SEVERE EFFECTS	
Central nervous	Fever higher than 39.4°C, encephalitis, convulsions, peripheral neuropathy, anaphylactic reaction, shock, unconsciousness
Integumentary	Rash
Respiratory	Dyspnea
Other	Cyanosis

Some vaccines are not to be given close in time to one another. For example, the meningococcal vaccine, whole-cell pertussis vaccine, and typhoid vaccine together have an undesirably large bacterial endotoxin content and should not be administered simultaneously. The effectiveness of measles, mumps, and rubella vaccines may be reduced by concurrent interferon therapy (see Chapter 54). Influenza vaccines may also theoretically lose efficacy if given while antiviral influenza drugs are being taken (see Chapter 45). It is recommended to give the influenza vaccine at least 48 hours after stopping such antiviral drug therapy. In general, immunizations requiring intramuscular (IM) injection are given with particular caution (and with appropriate monitoring) to patients receiving anticoagulant drugs such as warfarin sodium (see Chapter 27). Review the package inserts of any immunizing drugs given to obtain the latest information and identify other specific drug interactions that may occur. Hepatitis B immunoglobulin interacts with live vaccines; defer administration of such vaccines until 3 months after the dose of immunoglobulin is given.

Dosages

For the recommended dosages of selected immunizing drugs, refer to the appropriate drug profile. Readers are referred to the *Canadian Immunization Guide* for specifics.

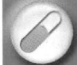

DRUG PROFILES

Some of the more commonly used vaccines, toxoids, and immunoglobulins are described in the following sections. The immunizing drugs currently available commercially in Canada, including several combination vaccines for the prevention of more than one disease, are listed in Box 51-1. Combination vaccines obviously reduce the number of injections that the patient receives, and thus their use is desirable when possible, especially in children.

ACTIVE IMMUNIZING DRUGS

diphtheria and tetanus toxoids, acellular pertussis vaccine (adsorbed)

The active immunizing drugs include diphtheria and tetanus toxoids and the acellular pertussis vaccine (adsorbed). *Adsorption* refers to the laboratory techniques used to make most vaccines and toxoids. The biological materials (i.e., virus or toxin particles) are adsorbed (separated out of solution and dried) onto carrier media such as alum, from which they are later removed for packaging into final dosage forms. Pertussis, also known as *whooping cough*, is highly contagious and is spread through contact with respiratory secretions. It has recently increased in incidence. Pertussis vaccine is available only as an acellular preparation in a combination vaccine, and the amount of acellular pertussis antigen present varies by product. Acellular pertussis consists of a single weakened toxoid, whereas previous pertussis vaccines contained multiple toxoids. Diphtheria toxoid is also available only in a combination vaccine. The vaccine combination *diphtheria and tetanus toxoids with acellular pertussis vaccine adsorbed* (DTaP®) was approved for the full childhood immunization series and has replaced the older tetanus, diphtheria, and pertussis vaccine, DPT. In Canada, a number of combination vaccines are available, including pentavalent and hexavalent vaccines. The pentavalent vaccine combines diphtheria, tetanus, pertussis, polio (inactivated polio virus [IPV]), and *Haemophilus influenzae* b conjugate (Hib; Pentacel®, Pediacel®, Infanrix-IPV/Hib®) while the hexavalent vaccine adds hepatitis B (HB) to the pentavalent combination (Infanrix-Hexa®).

Acellular pertussis vaccine is recommended for routine infant immunization, beginning at 2 months of age. DTaP-IPV (with or without Hib) vaccine is used for children under 7 years of age. DTaP-HB-IPV-Hib vaccine is used for children 6 weeks to 23 months of age and can be given to children aged 24 months to under 7 years, if necessary. DTaP-IPV or Tdap-IPV vaccine should be used as the booster dose for children at 4 to 6 years of age. Children 7 years of age and older receive the adult formulation of diphtheria-tetanus-pertussis–containing vaccine, with or without polio (Tdap or Tdap-IPV), for primary immunization or booster doses as it contains less diphtheria toxoid than preparations given to younger children and is less likely to cause reactions in older children. Tdap (Adacel®, Boostrix®) vaccine is administered to adolescents at 14 to 16 years of age as the first 10-year booster dose; Tdap-IPV (Adacel-Polio®, Boostrix-Polio®) vaccine should be used if IPV vaccine is also indicated. Infants and children receive a series of 0.5-mL injections at 2, 4, 6, and 18 months, followed by a booster of DTap-IPV or Tdap-IPV at 4 to 6 years and a booster of Tdap at 14 to 16 years.

These toxoids (DTaP, Tdap, Td [vaccine containing tetanus and diphtheria]) are available only as parenteral preparations to be given as deep IM injections. Their use is contraindicated in persons who have had a prior systemic hypersensitivity reaction or a neurological reaction to one of the ingredients. Some manufacturers indicate that use is contraindicated in cases of concurrent acute or active infections but not in cases of minor illness. Although there have been few, if any, studies documenting the safety of their use in pregnant women, it is generally considered safe to give diphtheria, tetanus, and pertussis toxoids after the first trimester.

Haemophilus influenzae type b vaccine

Haemophilus influenzae type b (Hib) vaccine (Act-HIB®) is a noninfectious, bacteria-derived vaccine. It is made by extracting *H. influenzae* particles that are antigenic and then chemically attaching these particles to a protein carrier medium for use in injections. All Canadian provinces and territories include Hib conjugate vaccine in their immunization programs for children. The vaccine is given by injection to previously unimmunized adults and children 5 years of age or older who are considered at high risk for acquiring *H. influenzae* infection. Conditions with increased risk of invasive Hib disease include

DRUG PROFILES—cont'd

the following: congenital (primary) immunodeficiency, malignant hematological disorders, HIV, anatomic or functional asplenia (including sickle cell disease), all transplant recipients, and recipients of cochlear implants. *H. influenzae* type b infection occurs worldwide and is most prevalent in children aged 2 months to 2 years. Before this vaccine was developed, infections caused by Hib were the leading cause of bacterial meningitis in children 3 months to 5 years of age; this form of bacterial meningitis has a mortality rate of 5 to 10%. This bacterium can also cause several other serious infections in children and adults. Severe neurological deficits occur in 10% to 15% of survivors and deafness in 15% to 20% (Public Health Agency of Canada, 2015). All Hib vaccine products are parenteral formulations that are administered intramuscularly. It is administered as part of the routine immunization of infants as discussed in the previous section. Hib-containing vaccine is not routinely indicated in children 5 years of age and older.

▶▶ *hepatitis B virus vaccine (inactivated)*

Hepatitis B virus vaccine (inactivated; Recombivax HB®, Engerix-B®) is a noninfectious viral vaccine containing hepatitis B surface antigen (HBsAg). It is made from viral particles and yeast, using recombinant deoxyribonucleic acid (DNA) technology. DNA from two or more organisms is combined, and yeast cells then produce this viral antigenic substance in mass quantities. The substance is attached to a carrier medium (alum) and made into a vaccine injection preparation. This antigenic HBsAg is used to promote active immunity to hepatitis B infection in persons considered at high risk for potential exposure to the hepatitis B virus (HBV) or HBsAg-positive materials (e.g., blood, plasma, serum). Health care providers, for example, are considered at high risk, and many hospitals require this vaccination upon employment. It is recommended that all children receive this vaccine, and it is usually started shortly after birth. It is also recommended that adults with diabetes receive hepatitis B vaccination because of defective phagocytic and neutrophil function. The vaccine does not interfere with insulin levels or control of plasma glucose. At the time of writing, NACI is reviewing the evidence for the use of the hepatitis B vaccine in adults with diabetes.

Use of the hepatitis B vaccine is contraindicated in individuals who have a history of anaphylactic hypersensitivity to the vaccine or any component of the vaccine (e.g., yeast). Pregnancy is not considered a contraindication to use. The vaccine is administered by IM injection and is given as a series of three injections (0.5 mL each). Hepatitis B vaccines are approved for use in Canada for preexposure and postexposure prophylaxis. Adults 19 years of age and older receive three 10-mcg doses of Energix-B on day 0, 1 month, and 6 months. A combination hepatitis A and hepatitis B vaccine (Twinrix®, Twinrix Junior®) is preferred for individuals travelling to countries where both hepatitis A and hepatitis B are endemic.

▶▶ *influenza virus vaccine*

The influenza virus vaccine is used to prevent influenza. Agriflu®, Fluad®, Fluviral®, Fluzone®, Influvac®, Intanza®, and Vaxigrip® are seasonal trivalent vaccines. Valent refers to the number of serotypes of viruses or bacteria included in the vaccine. Flulaval® and Fluzone® are quadrivalent vaccines. Agriflu, Fluviral, Fluzone, Influvac, and Vaxigrip are administered intramuscularly. Fluad is recommended for patients who are 65 years of age and older; it is administered intramuscularly. Intanza is administered intradermally. FluMist® is a live attenuated vaccine and is usually a **trivalent vaccine** (contains three virus strains). A new quadrivalent vaccine (FluMist Quadrivalent®) has been introduced and contains four vaccine virus strains: an A/H1N1 strain, an A/H3N2 strain, and two B strains. Both are administered intranasally. FluMist Quadrivalent is claimed to be 47% more effective in children aged 2 to 17 (according to the drug monograph). FluMist contains three live attenuated viruses, rather than killed viruses, as in the injectable influenza vaccine, and is recommended for healthy children between the ages of 2 to 17. Each dose is 0.2 mL, given as 0.1 mL in each nostril. Children 6 months to less than 24 months of age should be given 0.25 mL of Fluad Pediatric®, a trivalent vaccine, administered intramuscularly. NACI recommends that all individuals over the age of 6 months be vaccinated with the influenza vaccine, which is given each year prior to the beginning of the influenza season. Such inoculation is the single most important influenza control measure. Each year, a new influenza vaccine is developed by virology researchers. The vaccine usually contains three or, more recently, four different influenza virus strains. These strains are chosen from among the hundreds of influenza virus strains in the environment based on the latest epidemiological data indicating which influenza viruses will most likely circulate in North America in the upcoming winter. The effectiveness of a vaccine can vary considerably from season to season and depends on how well matched the vaccine is to the circulating viruses; in some years, there may be no benefit. Researchers attempt to determine the effectiveness of the vaccines in order to assess and confirm the value of influenza vaccination as a public health intervention. In addition, the effects of the vaccine can wear off, so a yearly vaccination is required. The vaccine is made from highly purified, egg-grown viruses that have been rendered noninfectious (inactivated). Influenza is characterized by abrupt onset of fever, myalgia, sore throat, and nonproductive cough. Severe malaise may last several days. More severe illness can occur in certain populations. Older adults, children, and adults with underlying serious health problems (e.g., HIV infection, asthma, cardiopulmonary disease, cancer, diabetes) are at increased risk for complications from influenza infections. Health care providers are also considered a high-risk group. The Canadian Nurses Association position is that all registered nurses should receive a yearly influenza vaccine. Many health care institutions strongly encourage influenza immunization, as health care providers are considered a high-risk group. In recent years, there has been a debate over whether receiving the influenza vaccine should be a mandatory requirement for employment. It is argued that such policies pressure nurses (and other health care providers) regarding their right to choose

Continued

DRUG PROFILES—cont'd

whether or not they are immunized (or should be forced to wear a mask if unvaccinated).

Mortality can result not only from influenza but also from cardiopulmonary and other chronic diseases that can be exacerbated by influenza. More than 90% of the deaths attributed to pneumonia and influenza occur among individuals 65 years of age or older. Another fairly unusual but important at-risk group is children and adolescents who are receiving long-term aspirin therapy (e.g., for juvenile arthritis) and who therefore might be at risk for developing Reye's syndrome after influenza (see Chapter 49).

Factors that may alter a vaccine's effectiveness are the age and immunocompetence of the vaccine recipient and the degree of similarity between the virus strains included in the vaccine and those that actually predominate during a given influenza season. Healthy individuals younger than 65 years of age have a 70% chance of avoiding illness caused by influenza when there is a good match between the vaccine and the circulating viruses.

Older adults, especially those residing in long-term care facilities, can avoid severe illness, secondary complications, and death by receiving the influenza vaccine. In older adults, the vaccine can prevent hospitalization and pneumonia up to 50 to 60% of the time and death up to 80% of the time. Achieving a high rate of vaccination among residents can reduce the spread of infection in a facility, thus preventing disease through herd immunity.

▶▶measles, mumps, and rubella virus vaccine (live, attenuated)

The measles, mumps, and rubella vaccine (M-M-R®, Priorix®) is virus preparation consisting of live measles, mumps, and rubella viruses that are weakened (attenuated). The vaccine promotes active immunity to these diseases by inducing the production of virus-specific immunoglobulin G and immunoglobulin M antibodies. The antibody response to initial vaccination resembles that caused by primary natural infection.

Administration of the measles vaccine or any of the combination products that include the measles virus is contraindicated in people with a history of anaphylactic reactions or some other immediate reaction to vaccine components. The measles and mumps component of the vaccine is prepared in chick embryo cell culture and may contain traces of egg protein. According to NACI, the trace amount of egg protein in the vaccine appears to be insufficient to cause an allergic reaction in egg-allergic individuals. Use of these vaccine products is also contraindicated in people who have had an anaphylactic reaction to topically or systemically administered neomycin because this antibiotic is used as a preservative in some preparations. These vaccines are not to be administered to pregnant women, and pregnancy needs to be avoided for 4 weeks following vaccination with a live virus. This precaution is based on the theoretical risk that the live virus vaccine may cause a fetal infection.

The measles vaccine is available in MMR or measles-mumps-rubella-varicella (MMRV) vaccines. Children receive a single dose subcutaneously at 12 to 15 months of age and a second dose at 18 months or any time thereafter, but should be given no later than around school entry.

meningococcal vaccine

There are three meningococcal vaccines in use in Canada: (1) monovalent conjugate meningococcal vaccines (Men-C-C, Mejugate®, NeisVac-C®), (2) quadrivalent conjugate meningococcal vaccines (Men-C-ACYW-135, Menactra®, Menveo®, Nimenrix®), and (3) a quadrivalent polysaccharide meningococcal vaccine (Men-P-ACYW-135) (Menomune®). These three vaccines are indicated for active immunization to prevent invasive meningococcal disease caused by *Neisseria meningitidis*. Men-C-C vaccine is recommended for all children at 12 to 23 months of age regardless of any doses given at less than 12 months of age. It is routinely given at 12 months and is recommended in unimmunized children less than 5 years of age. Men-C-C vaccine may be considered for children 5 to 11 years of age if not previously immunized as infants or toddlers. Men-C-C or Men-C-ACYW-135 vaccine is recommended for adolescents and young adults between 12 years and 24 years of age. The powder must be diluted with the included liquid conjugate component. Adverse effects include a 50% incidence of pain at the injection site and headache. Other adverse effects include myalgia, malaise, and nausea. Caution must be used to prevent sound-alike errors among the different brand names. The most current recommendations indicate a two-dose series should be given to individuals who are considered high risk because they are immunocompromised or have underlying medical conditions such as asplenia. All other patients receive a one-time dose.

Bexerso® is a new multicomponent meningococcal B vaccine indicated for active immunization of individuals from 2 months to 17 years of age against *Neisseria meningitidis* serogroup B strain. The number of injections given depends on the age of the patient. It is available as a suspension for IM injection provided in a prefilled glass syringe.

▶▶pneumococcal vaccine, polyvalent and 13-valent

Two forms of vaccine against pneumococcal pneumonia are available that also protect against any illness caused by *Streptococcus pneumonia*. *Pneumococcus* is the common name for the bacterium *S. pneumoniae*, the causative organism of this common bacterial infection. The polyvalent type of vaccine (Pneumovax 23®, Pneumo 23®, Pneu-P-23®) is used primarily in adults. (The term *polyvalent* refers to the fact that the vaccine is designed to be effective against the many [23] strains of pneumococcus most commonly implicated in adult cases of pneumonia.) This vaccine may also sometimes be recommended for children at higher risk for pneumonia as a result of serious chronic illnesses, especially those who are immunocompromised. However, the 13-valent conjugate vaccine is the pneumococcal vaccine that is routinely recommended for children. Its official full name is *thirteen-valent conjugate vaccine* (Pneu-C-13® or Prevnar 13®).

DRUG PROFILES—cont'd

The term *thirteen-valent* refers to the fact that the vaccine is designed to immunize against the top thirteen pneumococcal strains found in pneumonia cases in children. The pneumococcal 13-valent conjugate vaccine is included in the publicly funded immunization program of all provinces and territories in Canada. Routine infant immunization consists of the administration of three doses of Pneu-C-13 vaccine at a minimum of 8-week intervals, beginning at 2 months of age, followed by a fourth dose at 12 to 15 months of age. For healthy infants, a three-dose schedule may be used, with doses at 2 months, 4 months, and 12 months of age. It is recommended that healthy adults 65 years and older receive one dose of Pneu-P-23. Each dose is 0.5 mL, administered intramuscularly.

Contraindications to the use of either pneumococcal vaccine include known drug allergy to components of the vaccine itself, as well as the presence of current significant febrile illness or an immunosuppressed state as a result of drug therapy (e.g., cancer chemotherapy). The vaccine may sometimes still be given in such cases, if it is felt that withholding the vaccine poses an even greater risk to the patient.

poliovirus vaccine (inactivated)

The use of live oral polio vaccine (OPV) is no longer routine in Canada, due to case reports of vaccine-acquired polio. Since 1980, the only indigenous cases of poliomyelitis reported in Canada (11 cases) have been associated with use of the live OPV. Injected doses of inactivated polio vaccine (IPV) are instead recommended for routine use and are available in numerous preparations. All provinces and territories include IPV as part of routine immunization programs. It is administered intramuscularly (0.5 mL) as part of DTaP-IPV-Hib vaccine formulation at 2, 4, 6 and 18 months of age, or the DTaP-HB-IPV-Hib vaccine may be used to add protection against hepatitis B. A booster dose is administered at 4 to 6 years of age.

rabies virus vaccine

Vaccination against the rabies virus is not normally a routine immunization. Situations requiring this vaccine occur periodically in many practice settings. Rabies is a virus that can infect a variety of mammals, including skunks, foxes, raccoons, bats, dogs, and cats. The virus is usually transferred to humans by an animal bite and almost universally causes fatal brain tissue destruction if the patient is not treated with rabies vaccine and immunoglobulin (discussed later). Rabies virus vaccine (Imovax®, RabAvert®) is produced using laboratory techniques involving infected human cell cultures and selected antimicrobial drugs. Current recommendations call for a total of five IM injections of 1 mL on days 0, 3, 7, 14, and 28, following an animal bite that raises concern for rabies transmission. This includes a bite by any animal whose rabies immunization status is unknown or that escapes and cannot be observed for signs of rabies. This type of treatment is known as *postexposure prophylaxis*. Pre-exposure prophylaxis is recommended for people who are at high risk for exposure to the rabies virus (e.g.,

veterinarians). The pre-exposure course consists of only three injections (1 mL intramuscularly or 0.1 mL intradermally) on day 0, day 7, and between days 21 and 28. Periodic booster shots are also recommended for such individuals approximately every 2 to 5 years, or based on the levels of the patient's rabies virus antibody titres. Contraindications to the administration of rabies vaccine include a history of allergic reaction to the vaccine itself or to the drugs neomycin, gentamicin, or amphotericin B. However, given the life-threatening nature of rabies infection, treatment may still be required, with supportive therapy (e.g., epinephrine, diphenhydramine hydrochloride, corticosteroids) provided to minimize allergic reactions. Patients with any kind of febrile illness should delay occupational pre-exposure prophylaxis treatment until the illness has subsided.

human papillomavirus vaccine

Human papillomavirus virus (HPV) is a common cause of genital warts and cervical cancer. Genital HPV is a common virus that is transmitted through genital contact, most often during sex. Most sexually active people will get HPV at some time in their lives, although most will never even know it. It is most common in people in their late teens and early 20s. Every year, about 1 450 women are diagnosed with cervical cancer, and almost 380 women die from this disease in Canada. The papillomavirus vaccines (Gardasil®, Cervarix®) are the first and only vaccines known to prevent cancer. Cervarix is a **bivalent vaccine**, whereas Gardasil is a **quadrivalent vaccine**. Cervarix provides protection against two HPV types that cause approximately 70% of all cervical cancers—HPV-16 and HPV-18. Cervarix is approved only for use in females aged 10 to 25 and is not approved for use in males. Gardasil vaccine protects against four types of HPV—HPV-16 and HPV-18, as well as two types known to cause 90% of genital warts in females and males, HPV-6 and HPV-11. Gardasil is recommended for all females and males between the ages of 9 and 26. It is also approved for use in women up to the age of 46. Maximum benefit is achieved in females before they become sexually active. The vaccine is also beneficial in females aged 14 to 26 regardless of previous sexual activity, Pap abnormalities, cervical cancer, anogenital warts, or known HPV infection. In addition to being recommended for males between 9 and 26 years of age, Gardasil is also recommended for men of any age who have sex with men. In males, maximum benefit occurs between the ages of 9 and 13, prior to the onset of sexual activity. As with females, males between the ages of 14 and 26 who are sexually active benefit from Gardasil as they may not yet have HPV infection and it is unlikely that they have been infected with all four types of HPV present in the vaccine. The vaccine is given in three injections of 0.5 mL, administered intramuscularly. After the first dose, two more doses follow at 1 month and 6 months later. It is contraindicated in patients who show hypersensitivity to yeast or to their first injection of the vaccine. The Gardasil 9 vaccine is also now available in Canada. It helps to prevent against diseases associated with the HPV types 6, 11, 16, 18, 31, 33, 45, 52, and 58. These

Continued

DRUG PROFILES—cont'd

nine HPV types are known to cause approximately 90% of cervical cancers, 80% of cervical precancers, 75% of HPV-related vulvar, vaginal, and anal cancers and precancers, and over 90% of genital warts. The Society of Obstetricians and Gynecologists of Canada recommends HPV vaccination using Gardasil 9 for all girls and women aged 9 to 45 and for boys and men aged 9 to 26. The HPV vaccine is not recommended for pregnant patients, because appropriate studies have not been completed. Pain on injection is common.

herpes zoster vaccine

Zoster vaccine (Zostavax®) is a vaccine available for the prevention of herpes zoster. Herpes zoster, also known as *shingles*, is an extremely painful condition (also producing intense pruritus) caused by the varicella-zoster virus that also causes chicken pox. The vaccine is recommended for patients without complications who are 60 years of age or older and may be used in patients 50 years of age and older to prevent reactivation of the zoster virus that causes shingles. It is a one-time vaccine, and it can be given to patients who have already had shingles. The vaccine does not prevent postherpetic neuralgia. Herpes-zoster virus vaccine is a live attenuated vaccine. Its use is contraindicated in patients with hypersensitivity to neomycin, gelatin, or any component of the vaccine. It is also contraindicated in immunocompromised patients and those receiving immunosuppressant therapies, as well as in pregnant women. Because it is a live vaccine, there is a risk of transmission of the virus from the person who is vaccinated to other people. The vaccine is not to be used for the prevention of chicken pox and is not given to children. The drug must be stored in the freezer. Reactions at the injection site are usually mild and involves pain, swelling, or redness in 48% of recipients.

▶▶varicella virus vaccine

The live attenuated varicella virus vaccine (Varivax III®, Varilrix®) is used to prevent varicella (chicken pox). Varicella occurs primarily in children younger than 12 years of age or in individuals with compromised immune systems, such as older adults or patients with HIV. It is estimated that only 10% of children older than 12 years of age are still susceptible to varicella. Only 2% of adults develop varicella virus infections. However, 50% of the deaths associated with varicella infections are in adults. Half of these are in patients who are immunocompromised. The virus in varicella vaccine is attenuated by the passage of virus particles through human and embryonic guinea pig cell cultures. Varicella vaccine is stored in the refrigerator. It is not to be administered to patients who are immunocompromised or to patients who have received high doses of systemic steroids in the previous month. It is also recommended that salicylates be avoided for 6 weeks after administration of varicella vaccine because of the association between wild-type varicella, salicylate therapy, and Reye's syndrome (see Chapter 49). The varicella vaccine is given at 12 months of age, and then a second dose is given at 4 to 6 years of age. All patients receiving the vaccine need to receive a second dose. It is administered as a 0.5-mL dose subcutaneously.

rotavirus oral vaccine

There are two oral rotavirus vaccines available in Canada: RotaTeq®, a live pentavalent vaccine and Rotarix™, a live monovalent, attenuated human vaccine. Rotavirus is a highly infectious virus transmitted via the fecal-oral route and possibly the respiratory route. It survives on environmental surfaces and can be transmitted as fomites. The majority of cases occur during the winter and spring months. The rotavirus causes severe gastroenteritis with associated fever, vomiting, diarrhea, and electrolyte imbalance in children. The diarrhea can be so severe that it quickly leads to dehydration. Infants and children aged 3 months to 5 years of age are the most susceptible. Rotavirus vaccines are recommended for infants starting at 6 weeks to 14 weeks of age with the vaccination series complete before 8 months of age. RotaTeq requires three doses 4 to 10 weeks apart while Rotarix requires 2 doses with at least 4 weeks between doses.

PASSIVE IMMUNIZING DRUGS

The currently available antivenins, antitoxins, and immunoglobulins that comprise the passive immunizing drugs are listed in Box 51-1. Those that are commonly used are described in the following profiles.

▶▶hepatitis B immunoglobulin

Hepatitis B immunoglobulin (HBIg; HepaGam B®, Hyper-HEP B®) is used to provide passive immunity against hepatitis B infection in the postexposure prophylaxis and treatment of people exposed to HBV or HBsAg-positive materials (e.g., blood, plasma, serum). It is prepared from the plasma of human donors with high titres of antibody to HBsAg. All donors are tested for HIV antibodies to prevent HIV transmission.

Because of the possible devastating consequences of hepatitis B infection, pregnancy is not considered a contraindication to the use of hepatitis B immunoglobulin when there is a clear need for its use. All infants born to mothers infected with hepatitis B need to be given one dose (0.5 mL) HBIg intramuscularly within 12 hours after birth. Adults need to receive 0.06 mg/kg intramuscularly within 48 hours after exposure.

▶▶immunoglobulin

Immune globulin (GamaSTAN S/D®) is available in IM, subcutaneous, and intravenous dosage forms. It provides passive immunity by increasing antibody titre and antigen–antibody reaction potential. Immunoglobulin preparations contain immune antibodies directed against a broad range of pathogens and foreign antigens. Immunoglobulins are given to help prevent certain infectious diseases in susceptible persons or to ameliorate the diseases in those already infected. Immunoglobulins are pooled from the blood of several thousand human donors. This plasma is prepared by cold alcohol fractionation and usually washed with a detergent to destroy any harmful viruses, such

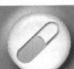

DRUG PROFILES–cont'd

as hepatitis or HIV. Health Canada–approved uses for immunoglobulins are primary humoral immunodeficiency syndrome, HIV in children, idiopathic thrombocytopenic purpura, B-cell chronic lymphocytic leukemia, and allogenic bone marrow transplant. Dosages vary widely.

Rh₀(D) immunoglobulin

$Rh_0(D)$ immunoglobulin (RhoGAM®, WinRho®) is used to suppress the active antibody response and the formation of anti-$Rh_0(D)$ antibodies in an $Rh_0(D)$-negative person exposed to Rh-positive blood. Because an $Rh_0(D)$-negative person reacts to Rh-positive blood as if it were a foreign, "nonself" substance, an immune response develops against it and an antigen–antibody reaction occurs. This reaction can be fatal. The administration of this immunoglobulin helps to prevent the reaction. The most common use of this product is in cases of maternal–fetal Rh incompatibility (postpartum). Only the mother is normally dosed. The objective is to prevent a harmful maternal immune response to a fetus during a future pregnancy if an Rh-negative mother becomes pregnant with an Rh-positive child.

$Rh_0(D)$ immunoglobulin is prepared from the plasma or serum of adults with a high titre of anti-$Rh_0(D)$ antibody to the red blood cell antigen $Rh_0(D)$. Administration of this immunoglobulin is contraindicated in people who have been previously immunized with this drug and in $Rh_0(D)$-positive or Du-positive patients. It is administered intramuscularly or intravenously at 28 weeks gestation, and 600 units are administered within 72 hours after delivery. After spontaneous or elective abortion of a pregnancy of 12 weeks gestation or less, 600 units is administered intramuscularly.

rabies immunoglobulin

Rabies immunoglobulin (Imogam Rabies Pasteurized®, HyperRab S/D®) is a passive immunizing drug that is administered concurrently with rabies virus vaccine following suspected exposure to the rabies virus. In humans, this usually occurs following an animal bite. Rabies immunoglobulin is derived from human cells that are harvested from people who have been immunized with rabies vaccine. The only contraindication to its use is drug allergy, although a patient with an allergy may still need to be dosed rather than face infection with the almost universally fatal rabies virus. The decision to dose a patient in such a case would be based on the probability

of rabies infection given the particular circumstances surrounding the animal bite. Rabies immunoglobulin is administered as a single dose (20 units per kg). Infiltrate as much of the dose as possible into the bite wound area and give the remainder intramuscularly in the gluteal region; do not administer into the same site as the rabies vaccine.

tetanus immunoglobulin

Tetanus immune globulin (Hypertet S/D®) is a passive immunizing drug effective against tetanus. It contains tetanus antitoxin antibodies that neutralize the bacterial exotoxin produced by *Clostridium tetani*, the bacterium that causes tetanus. The antitoxin neutralizes circulating toxins and competes with and partially binds with loosely bound toxin. However, the antitoxin has no effect on tissue-bound toxins. Optimum passive immunity occurs early in the disease process. Tetanus immunoglobulin is prepared from the plasma of adults who are hyperimmunized with the tetanus toxoid and is given as prophylaxis to people with tetanus-prone wounds (250 units intramuscularly as a single dose). It may also be used to treat active tetanus (3 000 to 6 000 units intramuscularly as a single dose).

varicella-zoster immunoglobulin

Varicella-zoster immunoglobulin (VZIG; VariZIG®) can be used to modify or prevent chicken pox in susceptible individuals who have had recent significant exposure to the disease. VZIG is best administered within 96 hours of exposure. Candidates for therapy with VZIG are those at high risk of serious disease or complications if they become infected with the varicella-zoster virus. Two examples are newborn children, including premature infants with significant exposure, and immunocompromised adults. If the infection manifests in a pregnant woman within 5 days of delivery, a dose of VZIG is recommended for the infant. It may also be beneficial to both mother and infant when given to the mother during pregnancy, preferably as soon as possible after diagnosis of infection. Healthy adults, including pregnant women, are evaluated on a case-by-case basis. The duration of protection against infection provided by VZIG is at least 3 weeks. VZIG is prepared from the plasma of normal blood donors with high antibody titres to varicella-zoster virus. It is administered intravenously or intramuscularly, 125 to 625 units within 96 hours of varicella exposure.

PANDEMIC PREPAREDNESS AND RESPONSE

In anticipation of an influenza pandemic in the near future, pandemic planning for the health care sector involves a federal, provincial, and territorial framework to provide a planned, coordinated, efficient, and effective public health response—the Canadian Pandemic Influenza Preparedness (CPIP): *Planning Guidance for the*

Health Sector. The plan is a collaborative effort put forth by public health and emergency preparedness and response experts from the government of Canada and provincial and territorial governments, as well as other expert stakeholders. The Canadian pandemic plan has two overall goals: (1) to minimize overall illness and deaths and (2) to minimize societal disruption associated with an influenza pandemic. The plan offers guidance and information to help support planning for and responding to an influenza pandemic. The original plan is regularly updated to reflect current thinking and new knowledge. Two key components to the plan are preparedness and response. *Preparedness* involves prevention strategies and activities to prepare for the pandemic, including guidelines for planning activities that would aid in managing an influenza pandemic. Surveillance, vaccine programs, the use of antivirals, health services, public health measures, and communication are all examples of such activities. *Response* involves high-level operational activities for an effective national health sector response, including roles and responsibilities for health care providers. A recovery plan would focus on the coordination of a postpandemic response for health care and emergency response sectors. Additional information about the CPIP is available at http://www.phac-aspc.gc.ca/cpip-pclcpi/.

NURSING PROCESS

✍ Assessment

Before administering a toxoid or vaccine, gather complete information about the patient's health history, including medications taken (prescription, over-the-counter, and natural health products), reactions to drugs, present and past health status, previous allergy test results, use of any immunosuppressants, presence of autoimmune or immunosuppressing diseases or infections, pregnancy and lactation status, and any unusual reaction to any substance. When children are to receive a vaccine or toxoid, assess and follow the prescribed immunization schedule and dose. The Public Health Agency of Health Canada (2015c) and the NACI provide the latest recommendations for adult and child immunizations in Canada. These recommendations, along with cautions, are easily accessible on the Internet and are available for referral to gain updated information prior to giving vaccines.

Because passive immunizing drugs may precipitate serum sickness, carefully assess patients who have chronic illnesses, are debilitated, or are older adults. This includes measuring vital signs, completing a physical assessment, and obtaining a medication history, as well as examining the results of any laboratory testing ordered by the health care provider. Document the patient's general health status with attention to overall well-being and any illnesses. See the discussion on passive vaccines as well as Box 51-1 and Table 51-1 for further information.

For the various active immunizing drugs, the Immunity and Immunization section and Tables 51-1 and 51-2 provide more specific insight and information, including contraindications, cautions, and drug interactions. It is also important to note that the use of these drugs in the following patient groups must be considered carefully: patients who are pregnant; those with active infection (especially infections caused by the same pathogen or an organism producing the same toxin); patients with severe febrile illnesses excluding minor illnesses such as a cold, mild infection, ear infection, or low-grade fever; and patients with a history of reactions or serious adverse effects related to the drug. In addition, research has shown that patients who are already immunocompromised (e.g., those with AIDS, older adults, those with chronic diseases or cancer, neonates) are at increased risk for serious adverse effects to toxoids or vaccines; therefore, use these drugs cautiously or not at all in such patients. Many adults assume that the vaccines they received as children will protect them for a lifetime. This is usually the case; however, many vaccines may require an additional dose of vaccine periodically to "boost" the immune system (e.g., every 10 years for the tetanus vaccine). Always check with a reliable source such as the public health unit or a family health care provider. Some adults, however, were never vaccinated as children, or newer vaccines were not available at the time they were vaccinated. In addition, immunity may fade over time, and as patients age, they may become more susceptible to serious diseases caused by common infections, such as *Pneumococcus* infections.

Tetanus, diphtheria, and pertussis vaccines are to be used in patients 6 weeks to 6 years of age and are contraindicated in those with previous vaccine reactions. In addition, the use of these toxoids is contraindicated in patients with any type of neurological reaction to the vaccine. Pertussis, or whooping cough, is contagious—spread through respiratory secretions—and can certainly become a widespread problem. Assess the age of the patient because DTaP is the preferred preparation in children from 6 weeks to 7 years of age unless the pertussis component is contraindicated. In adolescents and adults, Tdap is indicated.

The *H. influenzae* type b vaccine is administered to adults and children considered at high risk for acquiring *H. influenzae* infection, such congenital (primary) immunodeficiency; malignant hematological disorders; HIV; anatomic or functional asplenia (including sickle cell disease); all transplant recipients; and recipients of cochlear implants. In addition, the influenza vaccine should be administered yearly to adults and children over the age of 6 months. It is important to note that, each year, a new influenza vaccine is developed (see the earlier discussion on influenza vaccine). Assess whether the patient belongs in a high-risk group for exposure, such as health care providers. Assessment of age and medical history is important with these vaccines because individuals 65 years of age and older and those with chronic diseases are at risk for increased mortality from influenza. The influenza virus vaccine is contraindicated in those with a known hypersensitivity to it. Hepatitis B virus vaccines are indicated for those at high risk for exposure to the HBV or HBsAg-positive materials (e.g., blood, plasma, serum), such as health care providers. This vaccine is contraindicated in those allergic to yeast. Assess the needs of the patient receiving the vaccine because there are different formulations for children, adults older than 20 years of age, and individuals receiving dialysis or other immunocompromised patients.

The MMR vaccine is contraindicated in pregnant women, in persons with a history of anaphylactic reaction or other immediate reaction to egg ingestion, and in those with an anaphylactic reaction to topically or systemically administered neomycin. Prior to the administration of the meningococcal vaccine, gather data about any history of allergies. The pneumococcal vaccine is contraindicated in those with known allergy to the drug or its components or in those patients with significant febrile illness or an immunosuppressed state as a result of drug therapy (e.g., chemotherapy).

Do not give the papillomavirus vaccine (Gardasil, Cervarix) to patients with allergies to yeast or patients who have had a documented allergic reaction to the first injection of the vaccine. This vaccine is also contraindicated in pregnancy. The zoster vaccine (Zostavax) is for the prevention of herpes zoster. Assessment of age is an important factor in the administration of this vaccine. It is recommended for patients 50 years of age and older to prevent shingles and is not to be given to patients with a history of allergic reactions to neomycin, gelatin, or any component of the vaccine. Assessment of immune status is also important because it is not to be given to those who are pregnant, immunocompromised, or receiving immunosuppressant therapies. The varicella virus vaccine, Varivax, is used to prevent chicken pox, which occurs mainly in those younger than 8 years of age or in those who are immunocompromised. Assess the patient's medical and medication history because this vaccine should not be given to individuals who have received high doses of systemic steroids in the previous month. Advise patients receiving the vaccine to avoid salicylates for 6 weeks after its administration because of the risk of Reye's syndrome (see Chapter 49). Age of the patient is important because it is given at 12 months of age and then again at 4 to 6 years of age.

Nursing Diagnoses

- Acute pain related to local or systemic effects of the injection of a toxoid, vaccine, or passive immunizing drug
- Deficient knowledge related to the use of toxoids, vaccines, or passive immunizing drugs

Planning

Goals

- Patient will experience minimal pain associated with the injection of a toxoid, vaccine, or immunizing drug.

- Patient will demonstrate adequate and updated knowledge regarding the use of toxoids, vaccines, or immunizing drugs.

Expected Patient Outcomes

- Patient uses measures to increase comfort associated with injection, such as the application of warm packs to the site of injection, as indicated and as ordered by the health care provider, to help relieve localized discomfort or alleviate any localized reactions.
  - Patient uses additional comfort measures such as eating small meals, controlling the environmental temperature, decreasing stimuli, increasing opportunity for rest, and using analgesics and anti-inflammatory drugs as prescribed or recommended.
- Patient states rationale for and benefits versus risks of the use of toxoids, vaccines, or immunizing drugs.
  - Patient describes symptoms to report to the health care provider immediately should they occur, such as fever higher than 38.3°C, infection, wheezing, increasing weakness, or any other unusual reaction.

Implementation

When any immunizing drug is administered, always check and then recheck the specific protocols and schedules of administration to ensure accuracy and patient safety. Provide individuals receiving any immunizing drug with the proper instructions and updated written materials about the medication, technique and route of administration, adverse effects, and potential complications. Inform patients receiving vaccines that they will not "get" the disease in question from receiving the attenuated or dead virus. It is also important to follow the manufacturer's recommendations for storage and administration of the drug, routes and site of administration, and dosage, as well as precautions and contraindications pertaining to the drug's use. Always provide patients with a written record of immunization with the date of administration and a reminder of when a booster is needed. Encourage parents to keep and maintain an accurate journal of their child's immunization status, including dates of immunization and any reactions, if they occur. Canada is working toward the development of a national electronic Immunization Tracking System. Prior to giving a vaccine, always inquire about any previous reaction. Administer all immunizing drugs as prescribed, using the route specified. The midlateral muscle of the thigh is the preferred site for infants. The deltoid muscle is preferred for older children and adults. If a patient experiences discomfort at the injection site, apply warm compresses to the site, or administer an analgesic, antipyretic, or anti-inflammatory as ordered.

CASE STUDY

Varicella Vaccination

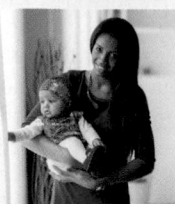

Alicia has taken her daughter, 12-month-old Jamie, for a well-baby checkup. Jamie has been healthy overall and is due for the varicella virus vaccination. The nurse reviews the vaccination process with Alicia and gives her information about what to expect after the vaccination.

1. Alicia looks at the information sheet and then asks, "This is just one shot, right? After this, she'll be immune to chicken pox. What a relief that will be!" What is the nurse's best response?

2. The nurse reviews the information with Alicia and tells her that a slight fever may develop. She asks Alicia what she has at home to give to Jamie if a fever or discomfort at the injection site develops. Alicia replies, "Oh, I have children's aspirin." What instructions will the nurse give regarding this?

3. The next morning, the skin around Jamie's injection site is slightly swollen, red, and warm to the touch. Alicia calls the office to "make sure everything is all right." What further assessment questions will the nurse ask Alicia?

4. Alicia's grandmother is visiting and tells Alicia, "Oh, I had that same vaccine 2 months ago! I don't ever want to get shingles." Is she correct? Did she receive the same vaccine that Jamie did?

_____

For answers, see http://evolve.elsevier.com/Canada/Lilley/pharmacology/.

Have epinephrine 1:1 000 readily available at the time of injection due to the risk of hypersensitivity reactions. Epinephrine is available in an autoinjector as 0.15 mg/0.15 mL (Allerject®) or in vials. Epinephrine solutions for injection (vials or autoinjectors) have a short shelf life of 12 to 18 months and, past this time, will start to break down to inactive substances. Replace epinephrine when outdated. Additionally, if fever (38.3°C or higher), convulsions with or without fever, altered consciousness, neurological symptoms, collapse, or somnolence occur, report them immediately to the health care provider, monitor the patient, and initiate emergency treatment as needed.

In regard to the possibility of an influenza pandemic, keep patients well informed and be aware of the need to minimize anxiety at all times. See the Patient Teaching Tips for more information.

Evaluation

The therapeutic response in patients receiving immunizing drugs is the prevention or amelioration of the specific disease being targeted. Adverse reactions for which to monitor in patients receiving immunizing drugs are specific to the drug, but there may be a localized reaction, including swelling, redness, discomfort, and heat at the site of injection or a more serious reaction that must be reported immediately to the health care provider (e.g., high fever, lymphadenopathy, rash, itching, joint pain, severe flulike symptoms, decreased level of consciousness, shortness of breath). For a complete list of expected reactions and adverse effects, both minor and severe, see Table 51-2. As immunizing drugs improve and newer ones are developed, it is hoped that fewer adverse effects and fewer adverse drug events and complications will be seen.

PATIENT TEACHING TIPS

❖ A localized reaction to the injection sometimes occurs when toxoids and vaccines are administered. Inform patients that the discomfort can be relieved by placing warm compresses on the injection site, resting, and taking acetaminophen or diphenhydramine hydrochloride, as directed by the health care provider. Instructions for the care of infants or children with such reactions are generally given by the child's health care provider when the immunizing drug is administered.

❖ Advise patients, parents, and caregivers to notify the health care provider if rash, itching, high or prolonged fever, or shortness of breath occurs after the vaccination.

❖ Stress that patients, parents, or caregivers should always keep a double record (two copies kept in separate places) of all medications being taken, including all vaccinations received.

❖ A vaccine adverse event reporting system is available through Health Canada (http://www.phac-aspc.gc.ca/im/aefi-essi-form-eng.php).

KEY POINTS

❖ A foreign substance in the body is termed an *antigen*; the body creates a substance called an *antibody* to specifically bind to it.

❖ B lymphocytes (B cells), when stimulated by the binding of an antigen molecule, begin to differentiate into memory cells and plasma cells.

❖ Memory cells remember what a particular antigen looks like in case the body is exposed to the same antigen in the future. Plasma cells manufacture antibodies and will mass-produce clones of antibodies upon re-exposure to a particular antigen.

❖ The two types of immunity are active and passive immunity. Different types of drugs are used to induce each, and these drugs are indicated for different populations, as follows:

• Active immunization involves administration of a toxoid or a vaccine that exposes the body to a relatively harmless form of the antigen (foreign invader) to imprint cellular memory and stimulate the body's defences to fight any subsequent exposure. It provides long-lasting or permanent immunity. The recipient must have an active, functioning immune system to benefit.

• Passive immunization involves the administration of immunoglobulins, antitoxins, or antivenins. Serum or concentrated immunoglobulins are obtained from humans or animals and, after screening and testing, are injected into the patient, directly giving the individual the ability to fight off the invading microorganism or inactivate a toxin. Passive immunization provides temporary protection and does not stimulate an antibody response in the host. It is used in patients who are immunocompromised or who have been exposed to, or anticipate exposure to, an organism or toxin.

❖ Patients who should not receive immunizing drugs include those with active infections, febrile illnesses, or history of a previous reaction to the drug. Use of these drugs in pregnant women is usually contraindicated.

❖ Patients who are immunocompromised are at greater risk of experiencing serious adverse effects from immunizing drugs.

❖ Encourage parents to keep updated records of their children's and their own immunizations with any toxoids or vaccines.

EXAMINATION REVIEW QUESTIONS

1. When assessing a patient who will be receiving a measles vaccine, the nurse will consider which condition to be a possible contraindication?
   a. Anemia
   b. Pregnancy
   c. Ear infection
   d. Common cold

2. When giving a vaccination to an infant, the nurse needs to tell the mother to expect which adverse effect?
   a. Fever over 38.3°C
   b. Rash
   c. Soreness at the injection site
   d. Chills

3. After a suspected hepatitis B exposure, prophylactic doses of which of the following would be given to the individual?
   a. Immune serum globulin
   b. Hepatitis B virus vaccine
   c. Hepatitis B immunoglobulin
   d. Rh₀(D) immunoglobulin

4. During a routine checkup, a 72-year-old patient is advised to receive an influenza vaccine injection. He questions this, saying, "I had one last year. Why do I need another one?" What is an appropriate response from the nurse?
   a. "The effectiveness of the vaccine wears off after 6 months."
   b. "Each year a new vaccine is developed on the basis of flu strains that are likely to be in circulation."

   c. "When you reach 65 years of age, you need boosters on an annual basis."
   d. "Taking the flu vaccine each year allows you to build your immunity to a higher level each time."

5. A 28-year-old is in the urgent care centre after stepping on a rusty tent nail. The nurse evaluates the patient's immunity status and notes that the patient thinks she had her last tetanus booster about 10 years ago, just before starting college. Which immunization would be most appropriate at this time?
   a. Immunoglobulin intravenous
   b. DTaP (diphtheria, tetanus, and acellular pertussis)
   c. Tdap (tetanus, diphtheria, and acellular pertussis)
   d. No immunizations are necessary at this time.

6. The nurse is providing teaching after an adult receives a booster immunization. Which adverse reactions should the patient report immediately to the health care provider? (Select all that apply.)
   a. Swelling and redness at the injection site
   b. Fever of 37.8°C
   c. Joint pain
   d. Heat over the injection site
   e. Rash over the arms, back, and chest
   f. Shortness of breath

7. The order for an adult who needs passive hepatitis B prophylaxis reads: "Give hepatitis B immunoglobulin, 0.06 mg/kg IM now and then again in 30 days." The patient weighs 176 pounds. How many milligrams will this patient receive per dose?

CRITICAL THINKING ACTIVITIES

1. A patient is in the emergency department after receiving a bite from a black widow spider (*Latrodectus mactans*). As you administer the antivenin for the black widow spider bite, he asks you, "Now will I be immune to black widow spiders after this shot? That's good, because we have a lot of them around the barn." What is the nurse's best response? Explain your answer.

2. Within 2 hours after a patient receives a tetanus booster vaccination, his wife calls the clinic. "He says that he is feeling weird and a little short of breath. You said to call if he is having a reaction, but it's hard to tell what is happening." What is the first instruction the nurse should give to this patient's wife?

3. You are working as a staff nurse on a medical–surgical unit in a suburban area. A coworker asks you, "What are we supposed to do if there is an influenza pandemic?" What is the nurse's best answer?

For answers, see http://evolve.elsevier.com/Canada/Lilley/pharmacology/.

Antineoplastic Drugs Part 1: Cancer Overview and Cell Cycle— Specific Drugs

Objectives

After reading this chapter, the successful student will be able to do the following:

1. Briefly describe concepts related to carcinogenesis.

2. Define the different types of malignancy.

3. Discuss the purpose and role of various treatment modalities in the management of cancer.

4. Define the term *antineoplastic*.

5. Discuss the role of antineoplastic therapy in the treatment of cancer.

6. Contrast the cell cycle of normal cells and malignant cells in regard to growth, function, and response of the cell to chemotherapeutic drugs and other treatment modalities.

7. Compare the characteristics of highly proliferating normal cells (including cells of the hair follicles, gastrointestinal tract, and bone marrow) with the characteristics of highly proliferating cancerous cells.

8. Briefly describe the specific differences between cell cycle–specific and cell cycle–nonspecific antineoplastic drugs (cell cycle–nonspecific drugs and miscellaneous other antineoplastics are discussed in Chapter 53).

9. Identify the drugs that are categorized as cell cycle–specific, including mitotic inhibitors, topoisomerase inhibitors, and antineoplastic enzymes.

10. Describe the common adverse effects and toxic reactions associated with the various antineoplastic drugs, including the causes for their occurrence and methods of treatment, such as antidotes for toxicity.

11. Discuss the mechanisms of action, indications, dosages, routes of administration, cautions, contraindications, and drug interactions of cell cycle–specific drugs, including mitotic inhibitors, topoisomerase inhibitors, and antineoplastic enzymes.

12. Apply knowledge about antineoplastic drugs to the development of a comprehensive collaborative plan of care for patients receiving cell cycle–specific drugs, mitotic inhibitors, topoisomerase inhibitors, and antineoplastic enzymes.

e-Learning Activities

Website
(http://evolve.elsevier.com/Canada/
Lilley/pharmacology/)

evolve

- Answer Key—Textbook Case Studies
- Answer Key—Critical Thinking Activities
- Chapter Summaries—Printable
- Review Questions for Exam Preparation
- Unfolding Case Studies

Drug Profiles

*Full generic name is given in parentheses. For the purposes of this text, the more common, shortened name is used.

Key Terms

Analogue A chemical compound with a structure similar to that of another compound but differing from it with respect to some component. (p. 967)

Anaplasia The absence of the cellular differentiation that is part of the normal cellular growth process (see *differentiation*; adjective: *anaplastic*). (p. 964)

Antineoplastic drugs Drugs used to treat cancer. Also called *cancer drugs, anticancer drugs, cancer chemotherapy,* and *chemotherapy*. (p. 964)

Benign Denoting a neoplasm that is noncancerous and therefore not an immediate threat to life. (p. 959)

Cancer A malignant neoplastic disease, the natural course of which is fatal (see *neoplasm*). (p. 959)

Carcinogen Any cancer-producing substance or organism. (p. 961)

Carcinomas Malignant epithelial neoplasms that tend to invade surrounding tissue and metastasize to distant regions of the body. (p. 959)

Cell cycle–nonspecific Denoting antineoplastic drugs that are cytotoxic in any phase of the cellular growth cycle. (p. 964)

Cell cycle–specific Denoting antineoplastic drugs that are cytotoxic during a specific phase of the cellular growth cycle. (p. 964)

Clone A cell (or group of cells) that is genetically identical to a given parent cell. (p. 959)

Differentiation An important part of normal cellular growth in which immature cells mature into specialized cells. (p. 959)

Dose-limiting adverse effects Adverse effects that prevent an antineoplastic drug from being given in higher dosages, often restricting the effectiveness of the drug. (p. 965)

Emetic potential The potential of a drug to cause nausea and vomiting. (p. 965)

Extravasation The leakage of any intravenously or intra-arterially administered medication into the tissue space surrounding the vein or artery. Such an event can cause serious tissue injury, especially with antineoplastic drugs. (p. 966)

Gene expression How a cell expresses a receptor or gene; the process in which information from a gene is used in the synthesis of a gene product. (p. 961)

Growth fraction The percentage of cells in mitosis at any given time. (p. 963)

Intrathecal A route of drug injection through the theca of the spinal cord and into the subarachnoid space. This route is used to deliver certain chemotherapy medications to kill cancer cells in the central nervous system. (p. 970)

Leukemias Malignant neoplasms of blood-forming tissues, characterized by the replacement of normal bone marrow cells with leukemic blasts, resulting in abnormal numbers and forms of immature white blood cells in the circulation. (p. 960)

Lymphomas Malignant neoplasms of lymphoid tissue. (p. 960)

Malignant Tending to worsen and cause death; anaplastic, invasive, and metastatic. (p. 959)

Metastasis The process by which a cancer spreads from the original site of growth to a new and remote part of the body (adjective: *metastatic*). (p. 959)

Mitosis The process of cell reproduction occurring in somatic (nonsexual) cells and resulting in the formation of two genetically identical daughter cells containing the diploid (complete) number of chromosomes characteristic of the species. (p. 962)

Mitotic index The number of cells per unit (usually 1 000) undergoing mitosis at a given moment. (p. 963)

Mutagen A chemical or physical agent that induces or increases genetic mutations by causing changes in deoxy-ribonucleic acid (DNA). (p. 961)

Mutation A permanent change in DNA that is transmissible to future cellular generations. Mutations can transform normal cells into cancer cells. (p. 959)

Myelosuppression Suppression of bone marrow function, which can result in dangerously reduced numbers of red blood cells, white blood cells, and platelets. (p. 965)

Nadir Lowest point in any fluctuating value over time; for example, the lowest white blood cell count measured after the count has been depressed by chemotherapy. (p. 966)

Neoplasm Any new and abnormal growth, specifically growth that is uncontrolled and progressive; a synonym for *tumour*; a malignant neoplasm or tumour is synonymous with *cancer*. (p. 959)

Nucleic acids Molecules of DNA and RNA in the nucleus of every cell (hence the name *nucleic acid*). Chromosomes are made up of DNA and encode all of the genes necessary for cellular structure and function. (p. 961)

Oncogenic Cancer producing; often applied to tumour-inducing viruses. (p. 961)

Paraneoplastic syndromes (PNSs) Symptom complexes arising in patients with cancer that cannot be explained by local or distant spread of their tumours. (p. 960)

Primary lesion The original site of growth of a tumour. (p. 959)

Sarcomas Malignant neoplasms of the connective tissues arising in bone, fibrous, fatty, muscular, synovial, vascular, or neural tissue; often first presenting as painless swellings. (p. 960)

Tumour A new growth of tissue characterized by a progressive, uncontrolled proliferation of cells. Tumours can be solid (e.g., brain tumour) or circulating (e.g., leukemia or lymphoma) and benign (noncancerous) or malignant (cancerous); circulating tumours are more precisely called *hematological tumours* or *hematological malignancies*; a tumour is also called a *neoplasm*. (p. 959)

Tumour lysis syndrome   A common metabolic complication of chemotherapy for rapidly growing tumours. It is characterized by the presence of excessive cellular waste products and electrolytes, including uric acid, phosphate, and potassium, and by reduced serum calcium levels. (p. 968)

OVERVIEW

Cancer is a broad term encompassing a group of diseases that are characterized by cellular transformation (e.g., by genetic **mutation**), uncontrolled cellular growth, possible invasion into surrounding tissue, and metastasis to other tissues or organs distant from the original body site. This cellular growth differs from normal cellular growth in that cancerous cells do not possess a growth control mechanism. Lack of cellular **differentiation** or maturation into specialized, productive cells is also a common characteristic of cancer cells. Figure 52-1 illustrates the multiple steps involved in the development of cancer.

Cancerous cells will continue to grow and invade adjacent structures. They may break away from the original tumour mass and travel by means of the blood or lymphatic system to establish a new clone of cancer cells and create a metastatic growth elsewhere in the body. A **clone** is a cell (or group of cells) that is genetically identical to a given parent cell. In the remainder of this chapter and the next chapter, the term *cancer* will be used to refer to any type of malignant neoplasm.

Metastasis refers to the spreading of a cancer from the original site of growth (**primary lesion**) to a new and remote part of the body (secondary or metastatic lesion). The terms *malignancy*, *neoplasm*, and *tumour* are often used as synonyms for *cancer*. A **neoplasm** (from Latin roots meaning new tissue) is a mass of new cells. It is another term for *tumour*. There are two types of tumours: benign and malignant. A **benign** tumour is of a uniform size and shape and displays no invasiveness (in terms of infiltrating other tissues) or metastatic properties. The terms *nonmalignant* and *benign* suggest that these tumours may be harmless, which is true in most cases. However, a benign tumour can be lethal if it grows large enough to mechanically interrupt the normal function of a crucial tissue or organ. **Malignant** neoplasms consist of cancer cells that invade (infiltrate) surrounding tissues and metastasize to other tissues and organs. Some of the various characteristics of benign and malignant neoplasms are listed in Table 52-1.

Various tumour types based on tissue categories include sarcomas, carcinomas, lymphomas, leukemias, and tumours of nervous tissue origin. Examples of these common malignant tumours are listed in Table 52-2. It is important to know the tissue of origin because this determines the type of treatment, the likely response to therapy, and the prognosis.

Carcinomas arise from epithelial tissue, which is located throughout the body. This tissue covers or lines

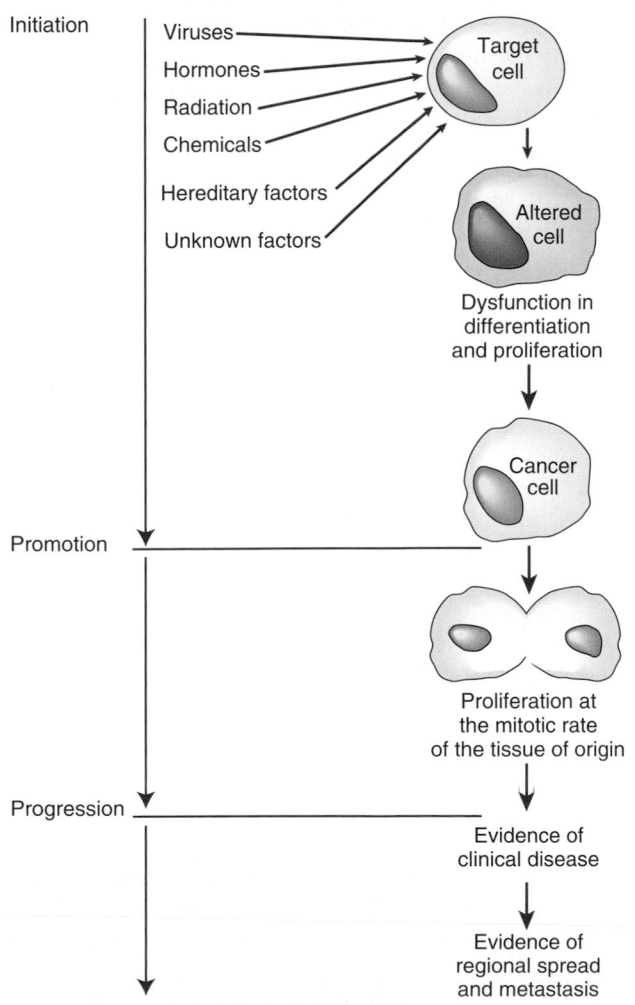

FIG. 52-1   Process of cancer development. (From Lewis, S. M., Dirksen, S. R., Heitkemper, M. M., et al. (2014). *Medical-surgical nursing in Canada: Assessment and management of clinical problems* (3ʳᵈ Canadian ed.: p. 350). Toronto, ON: Mosby.)

TABLE 52-1		
Tumour Characteristics: Benign and Malignant		
Characteristics	**Benign**	**Malignant**
Potential to metastasize	No	Yes
Encapsulated	Yes	No
Similar to tissue of origin	Yes	No
Rate of growth	Slow	Unpredictable and unrestrained
Recurrence after surgical removal	Rare	Common

TABLE 52-2

Tumour Classification Based on Specific Tissue of Origin

Tissue of Origin	Malignant Tissue
EPITHELIAL = CARCINOMAS	
Glands or ducts	Adenocarcinomas
Respiratory tract	Small and large cell carcinomas
Kidney	Kidney cell carcinoma
Skin	Squamous cell, epidermoid, and basal cell carcinoma; melanoma
CONNECTIVE = SARCOMAS	
Fibrous tissue	Fibrosarcoma
Cartilage	Chondrosarcoma
Bone	Osteogenic sarcoma (Ewing's tumour)
Blood vessels	Kaposi's sarcoma
Synovia	Synoviosarcoma
Mesothelium	Mesothelioma
LYMPHATIC = LYMPHOMAS	
Lymph tissue	Lymphomas (Hodgkin's, non-Hodgkin's)
Glia	Glioma
Adrenal medulla nerves	Pheochromocytoma
BLOOD AND BONE MARROW	
White blood cells	Leukemia
Bone marrow	Multiple myeloma

TABLE 52-3

Paraneoplastic Syndrome Associated With Some Cancers

Paraneoplastic Syndrome	Associated Cancer
Hypercalcemia, sensory neuropathies, syndrome of inappropriate antidiuretic hormone secretion (SIADH)	Lung
Disseminated intravascular coagulation	Leukemia
Cushing's syndrome	Lung, thyroid, testes, adrenal
Addison's disease	Adrenal, lymphoma

all body surfaces, both inside and outside the body. Examples are the skin, the mucosal lining of the entire gastrointestinal (GI) tract, and the lining of the bronchial tree (lungs). The purpose of these epithelial tissues is to protect the body's vital organs. **Sarcomas** are malignant tumours that arise primarily from connective tissues, although some sarcomas are tumours of epithelial cell origin. Connective tissue is the most abundant and widely distributed of all tissues and includes bone, cartilage, muscle, lymphatic, and vascular structures. Its purpose is to support and protect other tissues. **Lymphomas** are cancers within the lymphatic tissue. **Leukemias** arise from the bone marrow and are cancers of blood and bone marrow. Leukemias differ from carcinomas and sarcomas in that the cancerous cells do not form solid tumours but are interspersed throughout the lymphatic or circulatory system and interfere with the normal functioning of these systems. For this reason, they are sometimes referred to as *circulating tumours*, although *hematological malignancy* is a more precise term. Lymphomas can be quite bulky and are usually classified as solid tumours.

Patients with cancer may also experience various groups of symptoms that cannot be directly attributed to the spread of a cancerous tumour. Such symptom complexes are referred to as **paraneoplastic syndromes**

(PNSs). They are estimated to occur in up to 15% of patients with cancer and may even be the first sign of malignancy. *Cachexia* (general ill health and malnutrition) is the most common such symptom complex. Examples of other common PNSs are listed in Table 52-3. These syndromes are believed to result from the effects of biologically or immunologically active substances, such as hormones and antibodies, secreted by the tumour cells. Many patients also exhibit generalized symptoms such as anorexia, weight loss, fatigue, and fever.

ETIOLOGY OF CANCER

The etiology of cancer remains a mystery for the most part, and cancer researchers have made slow progress toward identifying possible causes. Certain etiological factors have been identified, and some of these factors and the cancers with which they are causally associated are listed in Table 52-4. Causative factors that have been identified include age-related and sex-related characteristics; genetic and ethnic factors; oncogenic viruses; environmental and occupational factors; radiation; and immunological factors.

AGE- AND GENDER-RELATED DIFFERENCES

The probability that a neoplastic disease will develop generally increases with advancing age. A number of rare cancers, such as acute lymphocytic leukemia and Wilms tumours, occur predominantly in children.

With the exception of cancers affecting the reproductive system, few cancers exhibit a sex-related difference in incidence. Lung and urinary cancers are more common in men than in women, but this may have more to do with exogenous factors such as smoking and occupational exposure to environmental toxins than to gender-related characteristics. The incidence of colon, rectal, pancreatic, and skin cancers, as well as leukemia, is comparable in men and women. A number of hematological cancers have a slight male predominance.

TABLE 52-4

Cancer: Proposed Etiological Factors

Risk Factor	Associated Cancer
ENVIRONMENT	
Radiation (ionizing)	Leukemia, breast, thyroid, lung
Radiation (ultraviolet)	Skin, melanoma
Viruses	Leukemia, lymphoma, nasopharyngeal
FOOD	
Aflatoxin	Liver
Dietary factors	Colon, breast, endometrial, gallbladder
LIFESTYLE	
Alcohol	Esophageal, liver, stomach, laryngeal
Tobacco	Lung, oral, esophageal, laryngeal, bladder
MEDICAL DRUGS	
Diethylstilbestrol	Vaginal in second generation, breast, testicular, ovarian
Estrogens	Endometrial, breast
Alkylating drugs	Leukemia, bladder
OCCUPATIONAL	
Asbestos	Lung, mesothelioma
Aniline dye	Bladder
Benzene	Leukemia
Vinyl chloride	Liver
REPRODUCTIVE HISTORY	
Late first pregnancy, early menses	Breast
Multiple sexual partners	Cervical, uterus
Nulliparity (no children)	Ovarian

GENETIC AND ETHNIC FACTORS

Few cancers have been confirmed to have a hereditary basis (some types of breast, colon, and stomach cancers are exceptions). Improved understanding of tumour biology has helped guide therapy tremendously. Two related advancements are determination of hormone receptor status and identification of specific **gene expression** in various types of tumour cells. For example, some tumour cells express themselves on their cell membrane surfaces, either estrogen receptors or progesterone receptors, and some tumour cells express specific genes such as the *HER2/neu* gene. Because these indicators aid in the classification of a patient's tumour, they also help in choosing appropriate drug therapy, predicting response to therapy and anticipating a prognosis. Discovery of the *BRCA1* and *BRCA2* genes has allowed identification of women who are at risk of breast cancer because they have a certain alteration in one of these *BRCA* genes. Many women with a family history of breast cancer choose to be tested for the presence of a *BRCA* gene mutation, which has led some women to undergo prophylactic breast removal. Tumours with identifiable gene expression patterns can show a familial pattern of inheritance. For example, Burkitt lymphoma is endemic in children aged 4 to 7 years in certain regions of equatorial Africa and other tropical locations. Outside Africa, adults with the sporadic form of this lymphoma are typically younger than 35 years. Another example of an ethnic predisposition is the high incidence of nasopharyngeal cancer in people of South Asian descent as well as among the Inuit population of Alaska and Canada. These associations with race are complicated by a well-recognized viral pathogenesis for both diseases.

ONCOGENIC VIRUSES

Extensive research has indicated that there are cancer-causing (**oncogenic**) viruses that can affect most mammalian species. Examples include human papilloma virus (HPV), feline leukemias, the Rous sarcoma virus in chickens, and the Shope papilloma virus in rabbits.

The herpesviruses are common examples of oncogenic viruses. Epstein–Barr virus is a type of herpesvirus. It is most commonly recognized as the cause of infectious mononucleosis (commonly referred to as *mono* or "the kissing disease"). However, it is also associated with the development of Burkitt lymphoma and nasopharyngeal cancer. Infection with HPV has been linked to cervical, anal, and oropharyngeal cancers.

OCCUPATIONAL AND ENVIRONMENTAL CARCINOGENS

A **carcinogen** is any substance that can cause cancer. In the nucleus of every cell are found molecules of **nucleic acids**, so named because of their location in the cell nucleus. The two types of nucleic acids are deoxyribonucleic acid (DNA) and ribonucleic acid (RNA). DNA molecules are the master molecules of genetic material within cells and contain the approximately 30 000 genes of the human genome. Genes are transcribed into messenger RNA molecules, which in turn are translated into protein molecules necessary for cellular structure and function. This process is discussed further in the section on alkylating drugs in Chapter 53. Environmental carcinogens include air and water pollution, pesticides, certain chemicals in foods, and many more. Occupational exposure is defined as any contact between the human body and a potentially harmful agent or environment in the workplace. Examples of such agents include asbestos, cadmium, benzene, radon, and vinyl chloride. A **mutagen** is any substance (e.g., chemicals in cigarette smoke, pesticides) or physical agent (e.g., radiation) that induces changes in DNA molecules. Mutations often transform normal cells into cancer cells.

RADIATION

Radiation is a well-known and potent carcinogenic agent. There are two basic types of radiation: (1) ionizing, or high-energy, radiation and (2) nonionizing, or low-energy, radiation. Both types can be carcinogenic. Ionizing radiation is potent and can penetrate deeply into the body. It is called *ionizing* because it causes the formation of ions within living cells. This type of radiation (used in X-ray studies) is also used to treat (irradiate) cancerous tumours (e.g., radium implants). Nonionizing radiation is much less potent and cannot penetrate deeply into the body. Ultraviolet light is an example of this type of radiation and is the cause of skin cancer. In contrast to chemotherapy, radiation therapy is considered a locoregional and not a systemic cancer treatment. Adverse effects of radiation therapy (e.g., radiation burns; nausea with GI tract irradiation) tend to be more localized to the site of treatment as well. Scientific specialists known as *radiation oncologists* are involved in the planning of radiation treatments, including calculation of the appropriate dose (dosimetry).

IMMUNOLOGICAL FACTORS

The immune system plays an important role in the body in cancer surveillance and in the elimination of neoplastic cells. Neoplastic cells are believed to develop in everyone; however, a healthy person's immune system recognizes them as abnormal and eliminates them through cell-mediated immunity (cytotoxic T lymphocytes; see Chapter 54). It has also been shown that the incidence of cancer is much higher in immunocompromised individuals. The relationship between cancer and a suppressed immune system has also been noted in patients with cancer being treated with immunosuppressive drugs after organ transplantation. The higher rates of cancers such as skin cancer and lymphoma in transplant patients are a result of this aggressive use of drugs to prevent organ rejection.

CELL GROWTH CYCLE

Normal cells in the body divide (proliferate) in a controlled and organized fashion. This growth is regulated by means of various mechanisms. In contrast, cancer cells lack regulatory mechanisms and divide uncontrollably. Often, the growth of cancer cells is also more constant or continuous than that of nonmalignant cells. Thus, one important growth index for malignant tumours is the time it takes for the tumour to double in size. This doubling time varies greatly for different types of cancers and is directly related to and important for determining the prognosis. Cancer treatment that cannot destroy every neoplastic cell does not prevent the regrowth of the tumour. The time it takes for regrowth to occur depends on the doubling time of the particular cancer. For example, Burkitt lymphoma has an extremely short doubling time. This shorter doubling time is associated with a tumour that, although it may be chemosensitive, is often difficult to cure due to rapid regrowth.

The cell growth characteristics of normal and neoplastic cells are similar. Both types of cells pass through five distinct growth phases: G_0, the resting phase, in which the cell is considered out of the cell cycle; G_1, the first gap phase; S, the synthesis phase; G_2, the second gap phase; and M, the **mitosis** phase (Figure 52-2).

During mitosis, one cell divides into two genetically identical daughter cells. Mitosis is further subdivided into four distinct subphases associated with the time periods before and during the alignment and separation of the chromosomes (DNA strands): prophase, metaphase, anaphase, and telophase. A complete cycle from one mitosis to the next is called the *generation time*. It is

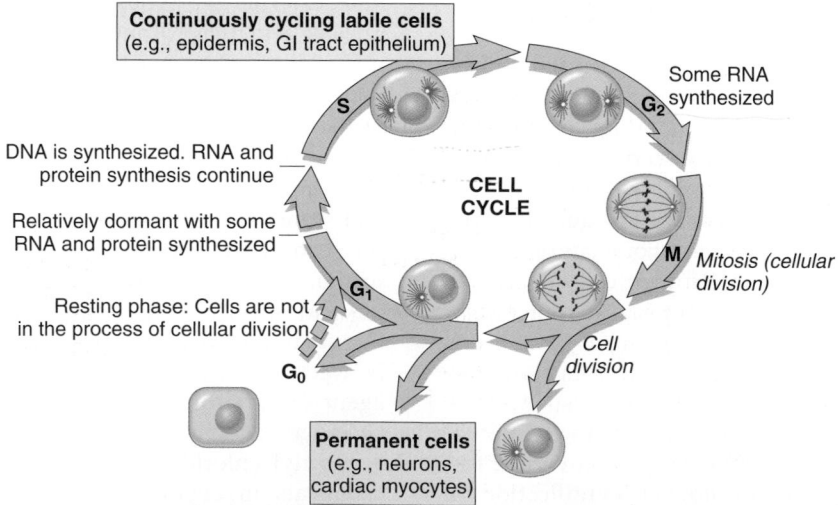

FIG. 52-2 Cell life cycle and metabolic activity. Generation time is the period from M phase to M phase. Cells not in the cycle but capable of division are in the resting phase (G_0). (Adapted from Kumar, V., Fausto, N. & Aster, J. C. (2010). *Robbins and Cotran pathologic basis of disease* (8th ed.; p. 86) Philadelphia, PA: Saunders.)

different for all tumours, ranging from hours to days. The cell growth cycle and the events that occur in the different phases are summarized in Table 52-5. Figure 52-3 shows at which points in the general phases of the cell cycle the cycle–specific chemotherapeutic drugs show their greatest activity.

The growth activity in a mass of tumour cells has an important bearing on the killing power of chemotherapy drugs. The percentage of cells undergoing mitosis at any given time is called the **growth fraction** of the tumour. The actual number of cells that are in the M phase of the cell cycle is called the **mitotic index**. Chemotherapy is

---

TABLE   52-5

Cell Cycle Phases

Phase	Description
G_0: Resting phase	Most normal human cells exist predominantly in this phase. Cancer cells in this phase are not susceptible to the toxic effects of cell cycle–specific drugs.
G_1: First gap phase or postmitotic phase	Enzymes necessary for deoxyribonucleic acid (DNA) synthesis are produced.
S: DNA synthesis phase	DNA synthesis takes place, from DNA strand separation to replication of each strand to create duplicate DNA molecules.
G_2: Second gap phase or premitotic phase	RNA and specialized proteins are made.
M: Mitosis phase	Divided into four subphases: prophase, metaphase, anaphase, and telophase; cell divides (reproduces) into two daughter cells.

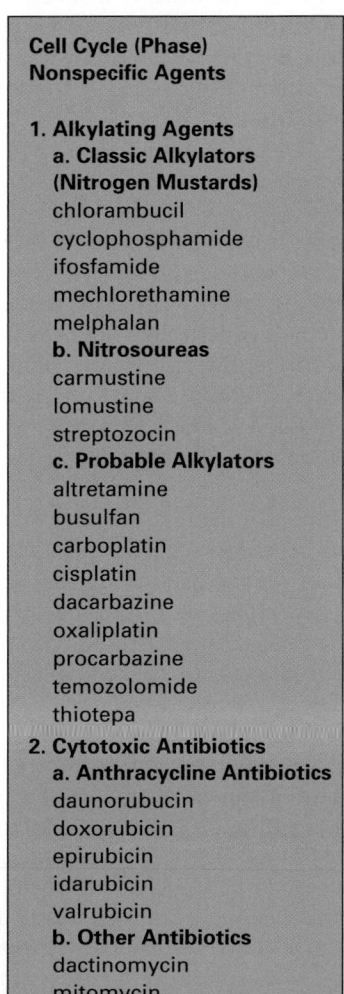

Cell Cycle (Phase) Nonspecific Agents

1. **Alkylating Agents**
   a. **Classic Alkylators (Nitrogen Mustards)**
   chlorambucil
   cyclophosphamide
   ifosfamide
   mechlorethamine
   melphalan
   b. **Nitrosoureas**
   carmustine
   lomustine
   streptozocin
   c. **Probable Alkylators**
   altretamine
   busulfan
   carboplatin
   cisplatin
   dacarbazine
   oxaliplatin
   procarbazine
   temozolomide
   thiotepa
2. **Cytotoxic Antibiotics**
   a. **Anthracycline Antibiotics**
   daunorubucin
   doxorubicin
   epirubicin
   idarubicin
   valrubicin
   b. **Other Antibiotics**
   dactinomycin
   mitomycin

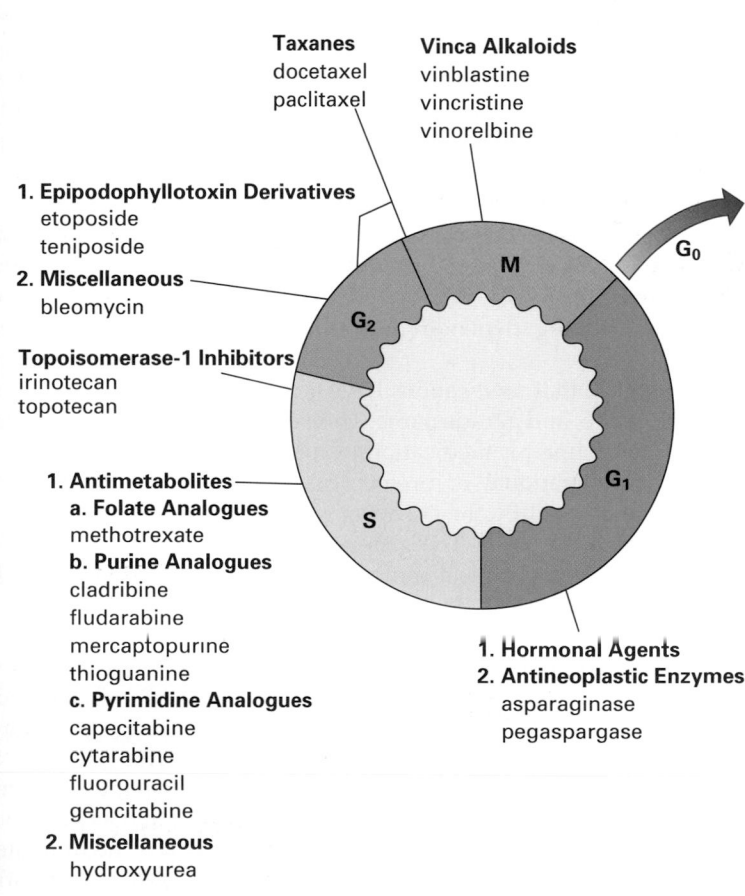

Taxanes
docetaxel
paclitaxel

Vinca Alkaloids
vinblastine
vincristine
vinorelbine

1. **Epipodophyllotoxin Derivatives**
   etoposide
   teniposide
2. **Miscellaneous**
   bleomycin

Topoisomerase-1 Inhibitors
irinotecan
topotecan

1. **Antimetabolites**
   a. **Folate Analogues**
   methotrexate
   b. **Purine Analogues**
   cladribine
   fludarabine
   mercaptopurine
   thioguanine
   c. **Pyrimidine Analogues**
   capecitabine
   cytarabine
   fluorouracil
   gemcitabine
2. **Miscellaneous**
   hydroxyurea

1. **Hormonal Agents**
2. **Antineoplastic Enzymes**
   asparaginase
   pegaspargase

FIG. 52-3   General phase of the cell cycle in which the cell cycle–specific chemotherapeutic drugs accomplish their greatest proportionate kill of cancer cells.

most effective in a rapidly dividing or highly proliferative tumour.

Hematopoietic stem cells are cells in bone marrow that have the capacity for self-renewal and repopulation of the different types of blood and bone marrow cells. In bone marrow, the hematopoietic stem cell divides asynchronously, regenerating itself while producing a cell that will go through a series of cell divisions to produce mature blood cells. Tumours in the bone marrow that affect a cell close to the stem cell are unable to mature and are considered poorly differentiated. The level of differentiation within a tumour, whether solid or circulating, becomes important in the treatment of neoplasms. This is because more highly differentiated tumours generally have a better therapeutic response (tumour shrinkage) to treatments such as chemotherapy and radiation. In contrast, some cancers, such as leukemia, involve proliferation of immature white blood cells (WBCs) known as *blast cells*. Cancers with a high proportion of such undifferentiated cells are less responsive to chemotherapy or radiation and are thus more difficult to treat. Lack of normal cellular differentiation is known as **anaplasia**, and such undifferentiated cells are said to be *anaplastic* cells.

CANCER DRUG NOMENCLATURE

The more technical term for cancer is *malignant neoplasm*. Drugs used to treat cancer are known as **antineoplastic drugs** but are also called *cancer drugs, anticancer drugs*, and, most commonly, *cytotoxic chemotherapy* or just *chemotherapy*. The nomenclature (naming system) of cancer drugs can be somewhat more complex and confusing than that of other drug classes. Cancer treatment is an intensively researched area in health care, with many active research protocols. Multiple names are often used for the same drug, depending on its stage of development.

Recall from Chapter 2 that medications have a chemical name, a generic name, and a trade name. This section introduces yet another name for medications, especially cancer drugs: the investigational or protocol name. A drug's chemical name is used by the chemists who first discover and work with the drug. The generic name is frequently first assigned to a chemical compound after a pharmaceutical manufacturer has determined that it is worthy of continued clinical research. It is often at this point that the chemical compound becomes an investigational drug. The trade name is a marketing name of a given drug used by the manufacturer primarily to market the drug. During the time before marketing and while a given medication is undergoing clinical research, it is frequently referred to by its protocol name. The protocol name is often a code name that consists of a combination of letters and numbers separated by one or more dashes. Although investigational drugs for all disease classes usually have some kind of protocol name, protocol names tend to be used more commonly in patient care settings

for cancer drugs than for other drug classes. Here are two typical examples that illustrate these concepts:

OTHER NAME	GENERIC NAME	TRADE NAME
STI-571 (protocol name)	imatinib mesylate	Gleevec®
5-fluorouracil* (chemical name)	fluorouracil	Same as generic

*The "5" refers to the position of a fluorine atom in the cyclic ring structure of the uracil molecule.

Because antineoplastic drugs can be carcinogenic, Health Canada mandates that carcinogenic studies be performed before any new drug is approved for use. However, no amount of clinical testing can fully reveal all of a drug's possible carcinogenic effects. Carcinogenic effects may not be observed in the laboratory animals on which the drug was tested but may become obvious only when the drugs are used in human subjects. Given the relatively small numbers of patients in clinical research trials, the carcinogenic potential of a given drug may not be observed until after the drug is marketed for use in the general population. If patterns of carcinogenicity begin to emerge during this period of postmarketing surveillance (or in postmarketing studies), the drug may be recalled from the market.

DRUG THERAPY

Cancer is normally treated with one or more of these major medical approaches: surgery, radiation therapy, targeted drug therapy, biologic therapy, and chemotherapy. *Chemotherapy* is a general term that technically can refer to chemical (drug) therapy for any kind of illness. In practice, however, this term usually refers to the pharmacological treatment of cancer. Figure 52-4 shows how various combinations of cancer treatment may succeed, or fail, over time.

Cancer chemotherapy drugs can be subdivided into two main groups based on where in the cell cycle they have their effects. Antineoplastic drugs that are cytotoxic (cell killing) in any phase of the cycle are called **cell cycle–nonspecific** drugs. Those drugs that are cytotoxic during a specific cell cycle phase are called **cell cycle–specific** drugs. These are broad categories that describe the activity of a drug within the cell cycle. Individual drugs may have actions that fall into both of these categories. Regardless of the cell cycle characteristics of a drug, it is more effective on rapidly growing tumours. This chapter discusses the cell cycle–specific drugs. Chapter 53 focuses on cell cycle–nonspecific drugs as well as various miscellaneous antineoplastic drugs.

The ultimate goal of any anticancer regimen is to kill every neoplastic cell and produce a cure, yet this goal is not achieved in most cases. Fortunately, some patients' immune systems may be able to clear any remaining tumour. Factors that affect the chances of cure and the

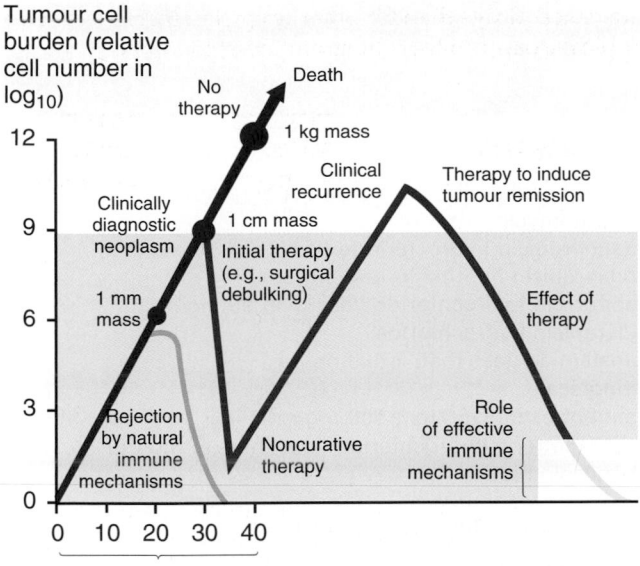

Tumour cell burden (relative cell number in log₁₀)

Time course of disease and therapy

FIG. 52-4 Relationship between tumour cell burden and phases of cancer treatment. (From McCance, K. L., & Heuther, S. (2006). *Pathophysiology: The biologic basis for disease in adults and children* (5th ed.). St Louis, MO: Mosby.)

length of patient survival include the cancer stage at time of diagnosis, the type of cancer and its doubling time, the efficacy of the cancer treatment, the development of drug resistance, and the general health of the patient. When a total cure is not possible, the primary goal of therapy is to control the growth of the cancer while maintaining the best possible quality of life for the patient, with the least possible level of discomfort and minimal adverse effects of treatment.

Cancer care and treatment involve many rapidly evolving medical sciences. Cancer is an intensively researched area, with the ultimate goals of research being to prevent cancer and prevent premature death. Chemotherapy medications are often dosed as part of complex, specific treatment protocols that are subject to frequent revision by oncology clinicians and researchers. For these reasons, the drug dosing information provided in this chapter is intended only to be representative of current cancer treatment and is not absolute or comprehensive. Furthermore, the indications listed for each specific drug are the primary current Health Canada approved indications. These, too, may change with time as a given drug is determined to be more (or less) effective for treating certain types of cancer. Also, in clinical practice, patients are often treated with one or more antineoplastic medications for "off-label" uses; that is, the drug is not currently approved for those particular uses by Health Canada.

No antineoplastic drug is effective against all types of cancer. Most cancer drugs have a low therapeutic index, which means that there is a narrow margin between the therapeutic effect and toxicity. Clinical experience has shown that a combination of drugs is usually more effective than single-drug therapy. Because drug-resistant cells often develop in tumours as a result of the tumour's genetic instability, exposure to multiple drugs with multiple mechanisms and sites of action will destroy more subpopulations of cells. The delayed onset of resistance to a particular antineoplastic drug is one benefit of combination drug therapy. To be most effective, however, the drugs used in such a combination regimen would ideally possess the following characteristics:

- Some efficacy even as single drugs in the treatment of the particular type of cancer
- Different mechanisms of action so that the cytotoxic effect is maximized; this includes differences in cell cycle specificity
- No or minimal overlapping toxicities

One major drawback to the use of antineoplastic drugs is that the majority cause adverse effects. These toxicities generally stem from the fact that chemotherapy drugs affect rapidly dividing cells—both harmful cancer cells and healthy, normal human cells. Three types of rapidly dividing human cells are the cells of hair follicles, GI tract cells, and bone marrow cells. Because most of today's antineoplastic drugs cannot differentiate between cancer cells and healthy cells, healthy cells are also destroyed, so hair loss, nausea and vomiting, and bone marrow toxicity are their undesirable consequences. Effects on the GI tract and bone marrow are often **dose-limiting adverse effects**; that is, the patient can no longer tolerate an increase in dosage that may be necessary to adequately treat the cancer and achieve good disease response.

Hair follicle cells are rapidly dividing cells. Cancer drugs that affect these cells often cause the adverse effect of *alopecia*, or hair loss. Many patients, particularly women, choose to wear wigs, hats, or scarves to disguise this adverse effect. Some antineoplastic drugs are harmful to the epithelial cells of the stomach and intestinal tract, which often leads to diarrhea and mucositis, and may also increase the risk of nausea and vomiting. The likelihood that a given drug will produce vomiting is known as its **emetic potential**. Anticancer drugs cause nausea and vomiting by stimulating the cells in the chemoreceptor trigger zone. Several antiemetic drugs are used to prevent these symptoms and are described in Chapter 41. Box 52-1 lists the relative emetic potential of selected chemotherapy drugs.

Myelosuppression, also known as *bone marrow suppression* or *bone marrow depression*, is another unwanted adverse effect of certain antineoplastics. It commonly results from drug- or radiation-induced destruction of certain rapidly dividing cells in the bone marrow, primarily the cellular precursors of WBCs, red blood cells (RBCs), and platelets. Myelosuppresion can also occur secondary to the disease processes of the cancer itself. It, in turn, leads to leukopenia, anemia, and thrombocytopenia. Cancer patients are often at great risk for infection because of leukopenia (reduced WBC count) secondary to chemotherapy. Patients often need antibiotics intravenously, either to prevent or treat bacterial infections.

| **BOX 52-1** | Relative Emetic Potential of Selected Antineoplastic Drugs* |

Low (Less Than 10 to 30%)

asparaginase
bleomycin
busulfan
capecitabine
chlorambucil
cladribine
cytarabine (less than 1 000 mg/m²)
daunorubicin, liposomal
docetaxel
doxorubicin hydrochloride (less than 20 mg/m²)
doxorubicin hydrochloride, liposomal
estramustine phosphate sodium
etoposide
fludarabine phosphate
fluorouracil (less than 1 000 mg/m²)
gefitinib
gemcitabine
hydroxyurea
imatinib mesylate
melphalan
mercaptopurine
methotrexate (less than 250 mg/m²)
mitomycin
paclitaxel
rituximab
teniposide
thioguanine
topotecan
trastuzumab
tretinoin
vinblastine sulphate
vincristine sulphate
vinorelbine tartrate

Moderate (30 to 60%)

cyclophosphamide (less than 750 mg/m²)
dactinomycin
daunorubicin hydrochloride (less than 50 mg/m²)
doxorubicin hydrochloride (20 to 60 mg/m²)
epirubicin hydrochloride (less than 90 mg/m²)
idarubicin hydrochloride
ifosfamide (less than 1 500 mg/m²)
irinotecan
methotrexate (250 to 1 000 mg/m²)
mitoxantrone hydrochloride (less than 15 mg/m²)
temozolomide

High (60 to More Than 90%)

carboplatin
carmustine
cisplatin
cyclophosphamide (750 to more than 1 500 mg/m²)
cytarabine (more than 1 000 mg/m²)
dacarbazine
dactinomycin
daunorubicin hydrochloride (more than 50 mg/m²)
doxorubicin hydrochloride (more than 60 mg/m²)
ifosfamide (more than 1 500 mg/m²)
lomustine
methotrexate (more than 1 000 mg/m²)
mitoxantrone hydrochloride (more than 15 mg/m²)
oxaliplatin
procarbazine hydrochloride
streptozocin

*Drugs in this list that are not covered in this chapter are described in Chapter 53.

Such patients are referred to as being neutropenic. Drug-induced anemia (reduced RBC count) often leads to hypoxia and fatigue, whereas thrombocytopenia (reduced platelet count) makes patients more susceptible to bleeding. The lowest level of WBCs in the blood following chemotherapy (or radiation) treatment is called the *nadir*. The time until the nadir is reached in a patient may become shorter and the recovery time for the bone marrow may become longer with multiple courses of antineoplastic treatment. The nadir normally occurs approximately 10 to 28 days after dosing, depending on the particular cancer drug or combination of drugs used to treat the patient. Anticipation of the nadir based on known cancer drug data can be used to guide the use of blood stimulants known as *hematopoietic growth factors* (see Chapter 54).

Common indications for various antineoplastic drugs classes are listed in the Dosages table. Also provided in various locations in this chapter and in Chapter 53 (Table 53-2 and Box 53-1) are drug-specific guidelines for the treatment of **extravasation**—unintended leakage of a chemotherapy drug (with vesicant potential) into the surrounding tissues outside of the intravenous line.

Because of the often severe toxicity of cancer medications, a current major focus of cancer drug research is the development of targeted drug therapy. Targeted drug therapy utilizes drugs that recognize a specific molecule involved in the growth of cancer cells while sparing healthy cells. Examples of targeted drugs include the following: imatinib (tyrosine kinase inhibitor), vorinostat (histone deactelyase inhibitors), temsirolimus (mTOR pathway inhibitors), erlotinib (EGFR inhibitors), sunitinib, sorafenib (multikinase inhibitors), bortezomib (proteasome inhibitors), crizotinib, and vismodegib. One example of biologic therapy is the class of cancer drugs known as *monoclonal antibodies* (see Chapter 54).

Pharmacokinetic data for antineoplastic medications is seldom used to guide dosing. Assay complexity coupled with a poor correlation between blood concentration and toxicity and efficacy limits its value. Only a handful of anticancer drugs benefit from therapeutic drug monitoring. For these reasons, pharmacokinetic data are not included with the drug profiles in this chapter. In spite of their notorious toxicity, given the often fatal outcome of neoplastic diseases, most cancer drugs are only rarely considered absolutely contraindicated. Even if a patient has a known allergic reaction to a given antineoplastic medication, the urgency of treating the patient's cancer still necessitates administering the medication and treating any allergic symptoms with premedications such as antihistamines, corticosteroids, and acetaminophen. For these reasons, no specific contraindications are listed for any of the drugs in this chapter.

Common relative contraindications for cancer drugs include weakened status of the patient as manifested by indicators such as extremely low WBC count, ongoing infectious process, severe compromise in nutritional and hydration status, reduced kidney or liver function, or a decline in function in any system that may be further affected by the toxic effects of the drug being administered. These are situations in which chemotherapy treatment is commonly delayed until the patient's status improves. In general, most chemotherapy is held when the patient's absolute neutrophil count (ANC) is less than 0.05×10^9 (severe neutropenia; see Chapter 53). Alternatively, dosages are often reduced for frail older adults or others with significantly compromised organ system function, depending on the drugs used.

Reduction in fertility is often a major concern in postpubertal patients. Cancer also complicates 1 in 1 000 pregnancies. All chemotherapy drugs are not recommended during pregnancy because of positive evidence of fetal risk. The choice to use chemotherapy in a pregnant woman is based on risk versus benefit. Both radiation and chemotherapy treatments can cause significant permanent fetal harm or death. The greatest risk is during the first trimester. Chemotherapy treatment during the second or third trimester is more likely to improve maternal outcome without significant fetal risk. However, radiation treatment poses great risk to the fetus throughout pregnancy and is reserved for the postpartum period if possible. Patients who are prepubertal are more resilient, however, and can have normal puberty and fertility following chemotherapy.

In older adults, *frailty* refers to loss of most of the patient's functional reserve and limited ability to tolerate even minimal physiological stress (e.g., chemotherapy treatment). More robust older adult patients are better candidates for cancer treatment, although frail patients often benefit as well, especially in terms of palliative (noncurative) symptom control.

CELL CYCLE–SPECIFIC ANTINEOPLASTIC DRUGS

Cell cycle–specific drug classes include antimetabolites, mitotic inhibitors, topoisomerase I inhibitors, and antineoplastic enzymes. These drugs are collectively used to treat a variety of solid and circulating tumours, although some drugs have much more specific indications than others.

ANTIMETABOLITES

A compound that is structurally similar to a normal cellular metabolite is known as an **analogue** of that metabolite. Analogues may have agonist or antagonist activity relative to corresponding cellular compounds. An antagonist analogue is also known as an *antimetabolite*.

Mechanism of Action and Drug Effects

Antineoplastic antimetabolites are cell cycle–specific analogues that work by antagonizing the actions of key cellular metabolites. More specifically, antimetabolites inhibit cellular growth by interfering with the synthesis or actions of several compounds crucial to cellular reproduction: the vitamin folic acid, purines, and pyrimidines. Purines and pyrimidines make up the bases contained in nucleic acid molecules (DNA and RNA). Antimetabolites work via two mechanisms: (1) by falsely substituting for purines, pyrimidines, or folic acid and (2) by inhibiting critical enzymes involved in the synthesis or function of these compounds. Thus, they ultimately inhibit the synthesis of DNA, RNA, and proteins, all of which are necessary for cell survival. Antimetabolites work primarily in the S phase of the cell cycle, during which DNA synthesis is most active. The available antimetabolites and the metabolites they antagonize are as follows:

Folate Antagonists

- methotrexate
- pemetrexed disodium
- raltitrexed disodium

Purine Antagonists

- cladribine
- fludarabine phosphate (F-AMP)
- mercaptopurine (6-MP)
- thioguanine (6-TG)

Pyrimidine Antagonists

- capecitabine
- cytarabine (ara-C)
- fluorouracil (5-FU)
- gemcitabine

Folic Acid Antagonism

The antimetabolite methotrexate is an analogue of folic acid. It inhibits dihydrofolate reductase, an enzyme responsible for converting folic acid to its active form, folate, which is needed for the synthesis of DNA. The result is that DNA is not produced and the cell dies. The drug also inhibits thymidine synthase and glycinamide ribonucleotide formultransferase that may assist to reduce the risk of drug resistance. In practice, the terms *folic acid* and *folate* are often used interchangeably. Pemetrexed disodium is a newer folate antagonist with a mechanism of action similar to that of methotrexate. Pralatrexate (Folotyn®) is the newest dihydrofolate reductase inhibitor, specifically indicated for T cell lymphoma. It is available in Canada through Health Canada's Special Access Programme.

Purine Antagonism

The purine bases present in DNA and RNA are adenine and guanine (see the discussion in Chapter 53). They are required for the synthesis of the purine nucleotides that are incorporated into nucleic acid molecules. Fludarabine phosphate is a synthetic analogue of adenine, while mercaptopurine and thioguanine are synthetic analogues of guanine. Cladribine is a more general purine antagonist. Cladribine is unique in that it actually lacks cell cycle specificity, unlike other drugs in its class. It is included in this section because of its similar pharmacology and mechanism of action. All of these drugs work by ultimately interrupting the synthesis of both DNA and RNA.

Although allopurinol is chemically similar to purines, it does not disrupt DNA synthesis. Instead, it inhibits xanthine oxidase, which reduces serum and urinary levels of uric acid. Rasburicase is an enzyme that degrades uric acid to more soluble end products. Uric acid is a common waste product that often accumulates in the blood following lysis of tumour cells, part of a condition known as **tumour lysis syndrome** (see Adverse Effects).

Pyrimidine Antagonism

The pyrimidine bases, cytosine and thymine, occur in the structure of DNA molecules. Cytosine and uracil are part of the structure of RNA molecules. These bases are essential for DNA and RNA synthesis. Fluorouracil is a synthetic analogue of uracil, and cytarabine is a synthetic analogue of cytosine. Capecitabine is actually a prodrug of fluorouracil and is converted to that drug in the liver and other body tissues. Because of its prodrug form, it can be given orally. Gemcitabine inhibits the action of two essential enzymes, DNA polymerase and ribonucleotide reductase. Overall, these drugs act in a way that is similar to that of the purine antagonists, incorporating themselves into the metabolic pathway for the synthesis of DNA and RNA, thereby interrupting synthesis of both of these nucleic acids.

Indications

Antimetabolite antineoplastic drugs are used for the treatment of a variety of solid tumours and some hematological cancers. They may also be used in combination chemotherapy regimens to enhance the overall cytotoxic effect. Methotrexate is also used to treat severe cases of psoriasis (a skin condition) as well as rheumatoid arthritis (see Chapter 54). Because some of these drugs are available in both oral and topical preparations, they are sometimes used for low-dose maintenance and palliative cancer therapy.

Allopurinol and rasburicase are both indicated for the hyperuricemia associated with tumour lysis syndrome and are usually given in anticipation of this condition during chemotherapy regimens associated with the syndrome. Allopurinol is also used commonly in oral form to treat gout (see Chapter 49). The commonly used drugs and their common specific therapeutic uses are listed in the Dosages table on p. 971.

Adverse Effects

As with most antineoplastic drugs, antimetabolites can cause hair loss, nausea, vomiting, diarrhea, and myelosuppression. The relative emetic potentials for some of these drugs are listed in Box 52-1. In addition, these drugs can cause other major types of toxicity, including neurological, cardiovascular, pulmonary, hepatobiliary, GI, genitourinary (GU), dermatological, ocular, otic, and metabolic toxicity. Common manifestations of these toxicities are listed in Table 52-6, approximately in order of increasing severity. Note that a single drug may not cause all of the specific symptoms that are listed for each toxicity category, and actual symptoms may vary widely in severity among patients. The most common general symptoms are fever and malaise. Metabolic toxicity also includes tumour lysis syndrome, a common postchemotherapy condition. This syndrome is often associated with induction (initial) chemotherapy for rapidly growing hematological malignancies. It may include hyperphosphatemia, hyperkalemia, and hypocalcemia. These electrolyte abnormalities are often treated with diuretics such as mannitol, IV calcium supplementation, oral or rectal potassium exchange resin, and oral aluminum hydroxide. Hyperuricemia can lead to nephropathy, and hemodialysis may be required in severe cases of tumour lysis syndrome.

A severe, but usually reversible, form of dermatological toxicity is known as *palmar–plantar dysesthesia* or paresthesia (also called *hand–foot syndrome*). It can range from mild symptoms such as painless swelling and erythema to painful blistering of the patient's palms and soles. Other severe, but fortunately uncommon, dermatological syndromes that can similarly affect the skin in more generalized regions include Stevens-Johnson syndrome and toxic epidermal necrolysis.

Interactions

As is true for cancer drugs in general, the administration of one antimetabolite drug with another that causes similar toxicities may result in additive toxicities. Therefore, the respective risks and benefits must be weighed carefully before therapy is initiated with either another antimetabolite or any other drug possessing a similar toxicity profile. Table 52-7 lists some known common examples of drugs that cause interactions with antimetabolites.

Dosages

For dosage information on selected antimetabolite chemotherapeutic drugs, refer to the table on p. 971. It is important to note that dosages of antineoplastics are highly variable, based on type of cancer, prior therapy, and planned coadministration of other agents.

TABLE 52-6

Common Manifestations of Antineoplastic Toxicity

Type of Toxicity	Common Manifestations
Neurological	Fatigue, weakness, depression, agitation, euphoria, insomnia, sedation, headache, reduced libido, confusion, amnesia, hallucinations (visual and auditory), dizziness, loss of taste or altered taste sensations, dysarthria (difficult articulation of speech), polyneuropathy (numbness in extremities), neuritis, paresthesia (abnormal touch sensations), facial paralysis, migraine, tremor, hemiplegia, loss of consciousness, seizures, ataxia, encephalopathy
Cardiovascular	Hot flushes, edema, thrombophlebitis and bleeding (e.g., near infusion site), chest pain, tachycardia, bradycardia, other dysrhythmias, angina, venous or arterial thrombosis, transient ischemic attacks, heart failure, myocardial ischemia, pericarditis, pericardial effusion, pulmonary embolism, aneurysm, cardiomyopathy, myocardial infarction, stroke, cardiac arrest, sudden cardiac death
Pulmonary–respiratory	Cough, rhinorrhea (runny nose), sore throat, sinusitis, bronchitis, pharyngitis, laryngitis, epistaxis (nosebleed), abnormal breath sounds, asthma, bronchospasm, atelectasis, pleural effusion, hemoptysis, hypoxia, respiratory distress, pneumothorax, diffuse interstitial pneumonitis, fibrosis, anaphylaxis, generalized allergic reactions
Hepatobiliary	Increased bilirubin and liver enzyme levels, jaundice, cholestasis, acalculic cholecystitis (inflamed gallbladder without stones), hepatitis, sclerosis, fibrosis, fatty liver changes, veno-occlusive liver disease, cirrhosis, hepatic coma
Gastrointestinal	Dyspepsia (heartburn), hiccups, gingivitis (inflamed gums), glossitis (inflamed tongue), abdominal pain, nausea, vomiting, diarrhea, constipation, gastroenteritis, stomatitis (painful mouth sores), oral candidiasis (thrush), ulcers, proctalgia (rectal pain), hematemesis, gastrointestinal hemorrhage, melena (blood in the stool), toxic intestinal dilation, ileus (bowel paralysis), ascites, necrotizing enterocolitis
Genitourinary	Oliguria, nocturia, dysuria, proteinuria, crystalluria, hematuria, urinary retention, abnormal kidney function test results, hemorrhagic cystitis, kidney failure
Dermatological	Rash, erythema, pruritus, ecchymosis, dryness, edema, photosensitivity, sweating, discoloration (pigmentation changes), freckling, petechiae, purpura, numbness, tingling, hypersensitivity, fissuring, scaling, seborrhea, acne, eczema, psoriasis, skin hypertrophy, subcutaneous nodules, alopecia, nail disorders including onycholysis (loss of nails), dermatitis, cellulitis, excoriation, maceration, ulceration, urticaria, abscesses, benign skin neoplasm, hemorrhage (at injection site), palmar–plantar dysesthesia–paresthesia, toxic epidermal necrolysis, Stevens-Johnson syndrome
Ocular	Eye irritation, increased lacrimation, nystagmus, photophobia, visual changes, conjunctivitis, keratitis, dacryostenosis (narrowing of lacrimal duct)
Otic	Hearing loss
Metabolic	Weight loss or gain, anorexia, dehydration, hypokalemia, hypocalcemia, hypomagnesemia, hypertriglyceridemia, hyperglycemia, syndrome of inappropriate secretion of antidiuretic hormone, hypoadrenalism, protein-losing enteropathy, hyperuricemia, tumour lysis syndrome
Musculoskeletal	Back pain, limb pain, bone pain, myalgia, joint stiffness, arthralgia, muscle weakness, fibromyositis

TABLE 52-7

Selected Antimetabolites: Common Drug Interactions

Antimetabolite	Interacting Drug	Observed and Reported Effects*
capecitabine	warfarin sodium	Altered coagulation test results with potential for fatal bleeding
	phenytoin	Reduced phenytoin clearance and toxicity
	leucovorin calcium	Potentiation of capecitabine with possible toxicity
cladribine	None listed	None listed
cytarabine	Digoxin	Reduced absorption likely due to cytarabine-induced damage to intestinal mucosa; elixir form may be better absorbed
	Aminoglycoside antibiotics	Reduced antibiotic efficacy against *Klebsiella pneumoniae* infections
fludarabine phosphate	Cytarabine	Increased antitumour activity of cytarabine
fluorouracil	warfarin sodium	Enhanced anticoagulant effects
	leucovorin calcium	Same as for capecitabine
	cimetidine	Increases toxicity of fluorouracil
gemcitabine	None listed	None listed

Continued

TABLE 52-7

Selected Antimetabolites: Common Drug Interactions—cont'd

Antimetabolite	Interacting Drug	Observed and Reported Effects*
mercaptopurine (6-MP)	allopurinol	Inhibition of 6-MP metabolism by inhibition of xanthine oxidase enzyme, with possible enhanced 6-MP toxicity; reduce dose to one third to one fourth
	warfarin sodium	6-MP reported to both enhance and inhibit effects of warfarin
	Hepatotoxic drugs	Increased risk of liver toxicity
methotrexate (MTX)	Protein-bound drugs and weak organic acids (e.g., salicylates, sulfonamides, sulfonylureas, phenytoin)	Possible displacement of MTX from protein-binding sites, enhancing its toxicity
	Penicillins, nonsteroidal anti-inflammatory drugs	Possible reduced renal elimination of MTX with potentially fatal hematological and gastrointestinal toxicity
	Live virus vaccines	Viral infection (true for any immunosuppressive drug)
	folic acid	Reduced MTX efficacy (theoretical only)
	theophylline	Reduced theophylline clearance
	Hepatotoxic drugs	Increased risk of liver toxicity
thioguanine	busulfan	Reports of hepatotoxicity, esophageal varices, and portal hypertension
	Other cytotoxic drugs in general	Reports of hepatotoxicity

*Not all mechanisms for these drug interactions have been clearly identified. The information in this table is based on reported clinical observations, with mention of known or theorized mechanisms when available.

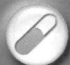 **DRUG PROFILES**

FOLATE ANTAGONISTS

▶▶ *methotrexate*

Methotrexate is the prototypical antimetabolite antineoplastic of the folate antagonist group and is currently one of three antineoplastic folate antagonists used clinically. It has proved useful for the treatment of solid tumours such as those found in breast, head and neck, and lung cancers and for the management of acute lymphocytic leukemia and non-Hodgkin's lymphomas. Methotrexate also has immunosuppressive activity, because it can inhibit lymphocyte multiplication. For this reason, it may be useful for the treatment of rheumatoid arthritis (see Chapter 54). Its combined immunosuppressant and anti-inflammatory properties also make it useful for the treatment of psoriasis.

High-dose methotrexate is associated with severe bone marrow suppression and is always given in conjunction with the "rescue" drug leucovorin. Leucovorin is an antidote for folic acid antagonists. The body produces active folic acid via metabolic steps utilizing the enzyme dihydrofolate reductase. Because methotrexate inhibits this enzyme, healthy cells die due to lack of folic acid. Giving leucovorin (which is rapidly converted to the active form of folic acid) provides the body with active folic acid, which prevents the death of normal cells. Methotrexate is available in both injectable and oral (tablet) form. A preservative-free injectable formulation is required for **intrathecal** administration (into the subarachnoid space), used in treatment of some cancers. One other folate antagonist is pemetrexed disodium, which acts similarly to methotrexate. However, it is used less commonly because its indication is limited to lung cancer.

raltitrexed disodium

Raltitrexed disodium (Tomudex®) is a quinazoline folate analogue that selectively inhibits a key enzyme (thymidylate synthase) required for the synthesis of DNA in cells, resulting in DNA fragmentation and cell death. It is actively transported into the cells via a reduced folate carrier and then extensively metabolized to polyglutamate forms without metabolic degradation. This particular property of raltitrexed facilitates a conventional dosing schedule of infusion every 3 weeks. Raltitrexed is cell cycle phase–specific for the S phase and is also a radiation-sensitizing agent. Raltitrexed is currently indicated for the treatment of advanced colorectal cancer.

PURINE ANTAGONISTS

The currently available purine antagonists are cladribine, fludarabine, mercaptopurine, and thioguanine. Mercaptopurine and thioguanine are administered orally, whereas the other two are available only in injectable form. These drugs are used primarily in the treatment of leukemia and lymphoma.

cladribine

Cladribine is indicated specifically for the treatment of a specific type of leukemia known as *hairy-cell leukemia*, so named because of the appearance of its cancerous cells under the microscope.

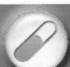 **DRUG PROFILES—cont'd**

fludarabine phosphate

Fludarabine phosphate (Fludara®), as with cladribine, also has a specific single indication, chronic lymphocytic leukemia. It is also commonly used in the treatment of follicular lymphoma and as part of salvage therapy in acute myelogenous leukemia.

PYRIMIDINE ANTAGONISTS

The currently available pyrimidine antagonists are capecitabine, cytarabine, fluorouracil, and gemcitabine. These drugs are used more commonly than the purine antagonists. They are available only in parenteral formulations, except for capecitabine, which is currently available only in tablet form. Dosage and other information appear in the table below.

capecitabine

Capecitabine (Xeloda®) is indicated primarily for the treatment of metastatic breast cancer and metastatic colorectal cancer.

▶▶cytarabine

Cytarabine (ara-C; Cytosar®) is used primarily for the treatment of leukemias (acute myelocytic, lymphocytic, and meningeal) and non-Hodgkin's lymphomas. It is available only in injectable form and may be administered intravenously, subcutaneously, or intrathecally. It is also now available in a special encapsulated liposomal form (Depocyt®), for intrathecal use only, in treating meningeal leukemia. Cytarabine has a unique set of adverse reactions, called "cytarabine syndrome." Cytarabine syndrome is characterized by fever, muscle and bone pain, maculopapular rash, conjunctivitis, and malaise. It usually occurs 6 to 12 hours following cytarabine administration. The syndrome may be treated or prevented with the use of corticosteroids.

fluorouracil

Fluorouracil (5-FU) is used in a variety of treatment regimens, including the palliative treatment of cancers of the colon, rectum, stomach, breast, and pancreas. It also is used in the adjuvant setting in the treatment of breast and colorectal cancers.

gemcitabine hydrochloride

Gemcitabine hydrochloride (Gemzar®) is an antineoplastic drug structurally related to cytarabine. Gemcitabine is believed to have antitumour activity superior to that of cytarabine. It is used as first-line therapy for locally advanced or metastatic cancer of the pancreas, for non–small cell lung cancer, and for advanced bladder cancer. Gemcitabine is increasingly used to treat other solid tumours, including breast cancer.

DOSAGES   Selected Antimetabolites**

Drug	Pharmacological Class	Usual Dosage Range*	Indications
capecitabine (Xeloda)	Pyrimidine antagonist (analogue)	PO: 1 250 mg/m² bid for 2 wk, followed by 1-wk rest period; this 3-wk cycle repeatable as ordered	Metastatic colorectal and breast cancer
cladribine	Purine antagonist (analogue)	IV: 0.09 mg/kg/day by continuous infusion for 7 consecutive days	Hairy-cell leukemia
▶▶cytarabine (Cytosar)	Pyrimidine antagonist (analogue)	IV: 100 mg/m²/day by continuous infusion for 7 days (other regimens as well)	Leukemias (several varieties), non-Hodgkin's lymphoma
fludarabine phosphate (Fludara)	Purine antagonist (analogue)	IV: 25 mg/m²/day for 5 consecutive days; repeatable every 28 days	Acute and chronic leukemias, non-Hodgkin's lymphoma
fluorouracil (5-FU)	Pyrimidine antagonist (analogue)	IV: short infusion (variable): 300–480 mg/m²; continuous infusion: 1 000–2 000 mg/m² over 24 hr, daily for 5 days; dosage varies afterward depending on patient response	Colon, rectal, breast, esophageal, head and neck, cervical, and kidney cancer
gemcitabine hydrochloride (Gemzar)	Pyrimidine antagonist (analogue)	IV: 1 000 mg/m² once weekly or as protocol dictates; cycle may be repeated or modified according to patient tolerance	Pancreatic, non–small cell lung, and bladder cancer
▶▶methotrexate (Metoject®)	Folate antagonist (analogue)	IV: 30–40 mg/m²/wk PO: 15–30 mg/day 5 days, repeated every 7 days, 3–5 courses	Acute lymphocytic† leukemia; gestational choriocarcinoma; breast, head and neck, and many other cancers

IV, intravenous; *PO*, oral.
*All dosages are for adults, unless indicated otherwise.
†The term *lymphocytic* is synonymous in the literature with the term *lymphoblastic*.
**Doses may vary depending on indication.

MITOTIC INHIBITORS

Mitotic inhibitors include natural products obtained from the periwinkle plant and semisynthetic drugs obtained from the mandrake plant (also known as the "may apple"). These vinca alkaloids include vinblastine, vincristine, and vinorelbine. Two newer plant-derived drugs are the *taxanes*. These include paclitaxel, once derived from the bark of the slow-growing Western (Pacific) yew tree, and docetaxel, a semisynthetic taxoid produced from the needles of the European yew tree. The current process of isolating the starting material for paclitaxel from the needles has made the drug supply more abundant than previously. Docetaxel is pharmacologically similar to paclitaxel. The newest taxanes are cabazitaxel (Jevtana®), which is indicated for prostate cancer, and eribulin mesylate (Halaven®), which is indicated for breast cancer.

Mechanism of Action and Drug Effects

Depending on the particular drug, these plant-derived compounds can work in various phases of the cell cycle (late S phase, throughout G_2 phase, M phase), but they all work shortly before or during mitosis, and thus they slow cell division. Each different subclass inhibits mitosis in a unique way.

The vinca alkaloids (vincristine, vinblastine, and vinorelbine) bind to the protein tubulin during the metaphase of mitosis (M phase). This action prevents the assembly of key structures called *microtubules*. This action, in turn, results in the dissolution of other important structures known as *mitotic spindles*. Without these mitotic spindles, cells cannot reproduce properly. This condition results in inhibition of cell division and cell death.

The taxanes paclitaxel, docetaxel, and cabazitaxel act in the late G_2 phase and M phase of the cell cycle. They promote the assembly of tubulin into stable microtubules, while simultaneously inhibiting their disassembly preventing anaphase.

Indications

Mitotic inhibitors are used to treat a variety of solid tumours and some hematological malignancies. They are often used in combination chemotherapy regimens to enhance the overall cytotoxic effect.

Adverse Effects

Like many of the antineoplastic drugs, mitotic inhibitor antineoplastic drugs can cause hair loss, nausea and vomiting, and myelosuppression (see Table 52-6). The emetic potential of some of the drugs is given in Box 52-1.

Toxicity: Management of Extravasation

Most of the mitotic inhibitor antineoplastics are administered intravenously, and extravasation of these drugs is potentially serious. Specific antidotes and additional

| TABLE | 52-8 |

Mitotic Inhibitor and Etoposide Extravasation: Listed Specific Antidote

Drug	Antidote Preparation	Method
etoposide teniposide vinblastine vincristine	hyaluronidase (Wydase®) 150 units/mL: add 1 mL NaCl (150 units/mL; available via the Special Access Programme)	1. Inject 1 to 6 mL into the extravasated site with multiple subcutaneous injections. 2. Repeat subcutaneous dosing over the next few hours. 3. Apply warm compresses.* No total dose established.

*Important: Administration of corticosteroids and topical cooling appear to worsen toxicity.

measures to be taken for the treatment of extravasation of the mitotic inhibitors are given in Table 52-8.

Interactions

A variety of drug interactions are possible with most antineoplastic drugs, some more significant than others. A few basic principles apply to all antineoplastic drug classes. Any drug that reduces the clearance of an anticancer drug also increases the risk of toxicity, whereas a drug that increases the elimination of an anticancer drug reduces its efficacy. The use of multiple antineoplastic drugs can cause severe neutropenia and infection, due to additive bone marrow suppression. Monitor and treat patients accordingly for hematological toxicity and infections. Observed drug interactions specific for mitotic inhibitor drugs are summarized in Table 52-9.

ALKALOID TOPOISOMERASE II INHIBITORS

Etoposide and teniposide are derivatives of epipodophyllotoxin. They exert their cytotoxic effects by inhibiting the enzyme topoisomerase II, which causes breaks in DNA strands. These drugs work during the late S phase and the G_2 phase of the cell cycle.

Dosages

For dosage information on selected mitotic inhibitors and topoisomerase II inhibitors, refer to the table on p. 974.

TABLE 52-9		
Selected Mitotic Inhibitors and Etoposide: Common Drug Interactions		
Drug	**Interacting Drug**	**Observed and Reported Effects***
etoposide	warfarin sodium	Enhanced anticoagulation
	ciclosporin	Reduced etoposide clearance
docetaxel	CYP3A4 inhibitors (e.g., azole antifungals, ciprofloxacin, clarithromycin, imatinib, verapamil, many others)	Enhanced docetaxel effect (possible toxicity)
	CYP3A4 inducers (e.g., carbamazepine, rifampin, phenytoin)	Reduced docetaxel effect
paclitaxel	doxorubicin hydrochloride	Increased cardiotoxicity
	CYP3A4 inhibitors and inducers	Same as for docetaxel
vincristine	phenytoin	Reduced phenytoin concentrations with consequent enhanced seizure risk
	asparaginase	Reduced vincristine clearance and increased neurotoxicity (give vincristine 12–24 hours before asparaginase)
	mitomycin	Increased risk of pulmonary toxicity
	CYP3A4 inhibitors and inducers	Same as for docetaxel

CYP3A4, cytochrome P450 subtype 3A4.

*Not all mechanisms for these drug interactions have been clearly identified. The information in this table is based on reported clinical observations, with mention of known or theorized mechanisms when available.

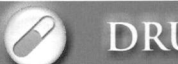 **DRUG PROFILES**

SELECTED MITOTIC INHIBITORS AND ETOPOSIDE

▶▶ etoposide

Etoposide (VePesid®) is a topoisomerase II inhibitor. Its structure, mechanism of action, and adverse effect profile are similar to those of teniposide. It is believed to kill cancer cells in the late S phase and the G_2 phase of the cell cycle. Etoposide is indicated for the treatment of non–small cell and small cell lung cancer, histiocytic lymphoma, and testicular cancer. It is available in oral and injectable forms. The oral form is poorly absorbed and has fallen out of favour because it produces significant toxicities without therapeutic benefit. The intravenous (IV) drug is formulated in a hydroalcoholic diluent, which can cause toxicity (hypotension) if administered in too high a concentration.

▶▶ paclitaxel

Paclitaxel (Abraxane®) is a natural mitotic inhibitor originally isolated from the bark of the Pacific yew tree. The European yew tree is the source of another mitotic inhibitor, docetaxel (Taxotere). Paclitaxel is currently approved for the treatment of breast cancer, non–small cell lung cancer, and Kaposi's sarcoma, among other cancers. Paclitaxel is extremely water insoluble (hydrophobic), and for this reason it is put into a solution containing oil rather than water. The particular oil is a type of castor oil called Kolliphor® EL (formerly known as Cremophor), the same oil with which ciclosporine is formulated. Many patients tolerate it poorly and show hypersensitivity associated with infusion. For this reason, before patients receive paclitaxel, they are premedicated with a steroid (dexamethasone), H_1 receptor antagonist (diphenhydramine hydrochloride), and H_2 receptor antagonist (ranitidine hydrochloride). Paclitaxel is available only in injectable form. There is an albumin-bound form of the drug (Abraxane®) that is not associated with severe infusion reactions.

▶▶ vincristine

Vincristine is an alkaloid isolated from the periwinkle plant and is indicated for the treatment of acute lymphocytic leukemia and other cancers. It is available only in a parenteral form. It is an M phase–specific drug that inhibits mitotic spindle formation. Vincristine is the most significantly neurotoxic of the cytotoxic drugs, but it continues to be used, in part because of its relative lack of bone marrow suppression. Special care must be taken not to inadvertently give vincristine via the intrathecal route. Several deaths have been reported due to this error. The World Health Organization (WHO) and the Institute for Safe Medication Practices suggest that vincristine be diluted in 25 mL of fluid and never dispensed via a syringe to prevent this lethal error from occurring. A special warning is required for all vincristine products dispensed that states "For Intravenous Use Only—Fatal If Given By Other Routes." (See the Preventing Medication Errors box.)

✋ PREVENTING MEDICATION ERRORS

Vincristine: Right Route Is Essential

For several years, the Institute for Safe Medication Practices has recommended changes in procedures to ensure that vincristine and other vinca alkaloids are not given intrathecally (via the spinal route) or by any route other than parenterally. Administering these drugs through the spinal route is almost always fatal, causing a slow and excruciating death. Mistakes occur when the drug is drawn up in a syringe for IV administration and then is inadvertently given via the intrathecal route. These errors are preventable. The WHO has suggested that pharmacies prepare vincristine in a diluted volume, such as in a 50-mL minibag of normal saline, to deter practitioners from

giving the drug intrathecally. Drugs given intrathecally are not normally dispensed in a minibag. Nurses, who may assist health care providers with intrathecal procedures, need to be aware of the potential fatal error that may occur if vincristine is given via the wrong route.

Data from: Institute for Safe Medication Practices. (2013). Death and neurological devastation from intrathecal vinca alkaloids: Prepared in syringes = 120; prepared in minibags = 0. Retrieved from https://www.ismp.org/newsletters/acutecare/showarticle.aspx?id=58.

DOSAGES   Selected Mitotic Inhibitors and Etoposide

Drug	Pharmacological Class	Usual Dosage Range*	Indications
Epipodophyllotoxin Derivative			
»etoposide (Etoposide Injection®, VePesid®)	Topoisomerase II inhibitor	IV: 50–100 mg/m²/day for 5 days PO: 100–200 mg/m²/day for 5 days	Testicular, small cell and non–small cell lung cancer, histiocytic lymphoma
Taxane			
»paclitaxel (Abraxane®)	Mitotic inhibitor	IV (Abraxane): 260 mg/m² q3wk	Metastatic breast cancer
Vinca Alkaloid			
»vincristine	Inhibitor of tubulin polymerization	*Children* IV: 2 mg/m² *Adults* IV: 1.4 mg/m²; fatal if given intrathecally	Acute leukemia, Hodgkin's lymphoma, rhabdosarcoma, breast cancer, small cell lung cancer, cervical cancer, malignant melanoma, colorectal cancer, non-Hodgkin's lymphoma, Wilms tumour

IV, intravenous; *PO*, oral.
*Note: Dosages may vary widely among treatment protocols.

TOPOISOMERASE I INHIBITORS

Topoisomerase I inhibitors comprise a relatively new class of chemotherapy drugs. The two drugs currently available in this class are topotecan and irinotecan. Both are semisynthetic analogues of the compound camptothecin, which was originally isolated in the 1960s from *Camptotheca acuminata*, a Chinese shrub. For this reason, they are also referred to as *camptothecins*.

Mechanism of Action and Drug Effects

The camptothecins inhibit proper DNA function in the S phase by binding to the DNA– topoisomerase I complex. This complex normally allows DNA strands to be temporarily cleaved and then reattached, in a critical step known as *relegation*. The binding of the camptothecin drugs to this complex slows this relegation process, which results in a DNA strand break.

Indications

The two currently available topoisomerase I inhibitors are used primarily to treat ovarian and colorectal cancer. Topotecan has been shown to be effective in metastatic cases of ovarian cancer that have failed to respond to platinum-containing regimens (e.g., cisplatin, carboplatin) and paclitaxel. Topotecan is also used to treat small cell lung cancer. Irinotecan is currently approved for the treatment of metastatic colorectal cancer, small cell lung cancer, and cervical cancer.

Adverse Effects

The main adverse effect of topotecan is bone marrow suppression. Topotecan is not to be given to patients with baseline neutrophil counts of less than 1.5×10^9/L. Other adverse effects are relatively minor compared with those of the other antineoplastic drug classes. These include mild to moderate nausea, vomiting, diarrhea, headache, rash, muscle weakness, and cough.

Irinotecan causes more severe adverse effects than topotecan. In addition to producing similar hematological adverse effects, it has been associated with severe diarrhea, known as *cholinergic diarrhea*. It is recommended that this condition be treated with atropine sulphate unless use of this drug is strongly contraindicated. Delayed diarrhea may occur 2 to 10 days after infusion of irinotecan. This diarrhea can be severe and even life-threatening due to dehydration and severe electrolyte imbalance. Delayed diarrhea should be treated aggressively with loperamide hydrochloride. There is a moderate risk of nausea and vomiting with irinotecan, which requires appropriate supportive care, such as IV rehydration and antiemetic drug therapy.

Interactions

Topotecan has a unique drug interaction involving the granulocyte colony–stimulating factor filgrastim (see Chapter 54). Filgrastim is commonly used to enhance neutrophil recovery after chemotherapy. When topotecan is given concurrently with filgrastim, myelosuppression has been shown to worsen. It is recommended that filgrastim be administered 24 hours after completion of a topotecan infusion. Laxatives and diuretics are not given with irinotecan because of their potential to worsen the dehydration resulting from the severe diarrhea that this drug can produce. Severe cardiovascular toxicity, including thrombosis, pulmonary embolism, stroke, and acute fatal myocardial infarction (MI), has been reported when irinotecan is given with fluorouracil and leucovorin. The role of irinotecan in this toxicity syndrome is unclear, because fluorouracil is a well-recognized cause of myocardial ischemia, including MI and sudden death. Such drug combinations are given with careful monitoring. Several additional recognized drug interactions occur with irinotecan, which are summarized in Table 52-10.

Dosages

For dosage information on selected topoisomerase I inhibitors, refer to the table on p. 976.

DRUG PROFILES

Selected Topoisomerase I Inhibitors

irinotecan hydrochloride

Irinotecan hydrochloride (Camptosar®) is often given with both fluorouracil and leucovorin. It is available only in injectable form.

topotecan hydrochloride

After initial therapy with other antineoplastics, cancer cells commonly become resistant to their effects. The use of topotecan hydrochloride (Hycamtin®) to treat ovarian cancer and small cell lung cancer has been studied extensively. As noted earlier, it produces therapeutic responses even in cases in which powerful drugs such as cisplatin and paclitaxel have failed. Topotecan is available only in injectable form.

TABLE 52-10

Irinotecan: Common Drug Interactions

Interacting Drug	Observed and Reported Effects*
CYP2B6 inhibitors (e.g., paroxetine hydrochloride, sertraline hydrochloride)	Increased effects and toxicity of irinotecan
CYP3A4 inhibitors (e.g., azole antifungals, ciprofloxacin hydrochloride, clarithromycin, imatinib, isoniazid, verapamil hydrochloride)	Increased effects and toxicity of irinotecan; concurrent use not recommended
CYP2B6 inducers (e.g., carbamazepine, phenytoin, nevirapine)	Reduced effects of irinotecan
CYP3A4 inducers (e.g., aminoglutethimide, carbamazepine, nevirapine, phenytoin)	Reduced effects of irinotecan
St. John's wort	Reduced effects of irinotecan; stop St. John's wort 2 wk before initiating irinotecan therapy

CYP2B6, cytochrome P450 liver enzyme subtype 2B6; *CYP3A4*, cytochrome P450 subtype 3A4.
*Note that not all mechanisms of these drug interactions have been clearly identified. The information in this table is based on reported clinical observations, with mention of known or theorized mechanisms when available.

TABLE 52-11

Selected Antineoplastic Enzymes: Common Drug Interactions

Enzyme	Interacting Drug	Observed and Reported Effects*
asparaginase	cyclophosphamide, mercaptopurine, vincristine	Interference with efficacy or clearance of asparaginase
	mercaptopurine, methotrexate, prednisone	Enhanced liver toxicity of asparaginase
	methotrexate	Reduced antineoplastic effect when given concurrently, but possibly enhanced antineoplastic effect when given 9 to 10 days before or shortly after methotrexate
	prednisone	Hyperglycemia (give asparaginase after prednisone)
	vincristine	Neuropathy (give asparaginase after vincristine)
	aspirin, nonsteroidal anti-inflammatory drugs, dipyridamole, heparin sodium, warfarin sodium	Use with caution due to possible coagulation abnormalities

*Note that not all mechanisms for these drug interactions have been clearly identified. The information in this table is based on reported clinical observations, with mention of known or theorized mechanisms when available.

DOSAGES   Selected Topoisomerase I Inhibitors

Drug	Pharmacological Class	Usual Dosage Range*	Indications
irinotecan hydrochloride (Camptosar)	Synthetic camptothecin	IV: 125 mg/m² on various days depending on protocol	Metastatic colorectal cancer
topotecan hydrochloride (Hycamtin)	Semisynthetic camptothecin	IV: 1.5 mg/m² once daily for 5 consecutive days on a repeatable 21-day course	Ovarian and small cell lung cancer

IV, intravenous.
*Dosages listed are for adults.

ANTINEOPLASTIC ENZYMES

Two antineoplastic enzymes are commercially available in Canada: pegaspargase and asparaginase. There are two asparaginase products: Kidrolase® and Erwinase®. Kidrolase is an *Escherichia coli*–based asparaginase. *Erwinia* asparaginase (Erwinase) is available for patients who have developed allergic reactions to Kidrolase. Pegaspargase and the two asparaginase drugs are synthesized from cultures of certain bacteria, using recombinant DNA technology.

Indications

The antineoplastic enzymes are approved exclusively for the treatment of acute lymphocytic leukemia.

Adverse Effects

Of particular note for the antineoplastic enzymes is a fairly unique adverse effect of impaired pancreatic function. This can lead to hyperglycemia and severe or fatal pancreatitis. Other types of adverse effects associated with these drugs involve the dermatological, liver, GU, neurological, musculoskeletal, GI, and cardiovascular systems.

Interactions

Commonly reported drug interactions involving antineoplastic enzymes are summarized in Table 52-11.

Dosages

For dosage information on antineoplastic enzymes, refer to the table on p. 977.

NURSING PROCESS

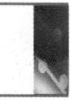 **Assessment**

With antineoplastic therapy, perform the following components of a thorough physical assessment: nursing history; past and present medical history; family history; medication profile with a notation of allergies as well as a listing of all prescription drugs, over-the-counter (OTC) drugs, and natural health products; height, weight, and vital signs; and baseline hearing and vision testing (as ordered). Also assess bowel and bladder patterns, neurological status, heart sounds, heart rhythm, breath sounds, and lung function. Examine the skin and mucosa, paying attention to turgor, hydration, colour, and temperature. Note any signs and symptoms of fear and anxiety with attention to reports of insomnia, irritability, shakiness, restlessness, and palpitations. Include an assessment of cultural, emotional, spiritual, sexual, and financial

DRUG PROFILES

▶▶ asparaginase

Asparaginase (Kidrolase) is for the treatment of acute lymphoblastic leukemia. Its mechanism of action is slightly different from that of traditional antineoplastics in that it is an enzyme that catalyzes the conversion of the amino acid asparagine to aspartic acid and ammonia. Leukemic cells are then unable to synthesize the asparagine required for synthesis of DNA and proteins needed for cell survival.

The only commercially available asparaginase products in Canada are Kidrolase and Erwinase. Kidrolase is derived from *E. coli* bacteria, and it is common for patients to develop allergic reactions to it. When this occurs, one alternative is to use the asparaginase synthesized from *Erwinia* bacteria, Erwinase. Another treatment alternative is pegaspargase, described in the following drug profile. All antineoplastic enzymes are available only in injectable form.

pegaspargase

Pegaspargase (Oncaspar®) has a mechanism of action, indications, and contraindications similar to those of asparaginase. It is essentially the same enzyme that has been formulated so as to reduce its allergenic potential. This process involves chemical conjugation of the enzyme with units of a relatively inert compound known as monomethoxypolyethylene glycol. Because polyethylene glycol is abbreviated PEG, this process is known as *pegylation*. Pegylation is a process that is increasingly used in formulating various drugs that are described in other chapters (e.g., see Chapter 54). These drugs are recognized by the prefix *peg* in their generic names. Pegaspargase is usually prescribed for patients who have developed an allergy to asparaginase, which is a common occurrence, especially with repeated treatment.

DOSAGES   Selected Antineoplastic Enzymes

Drug	Pharmacological Class	Usual Dosage Range*	Indications
▶▶asparaginase (Kidrolase)	*Escherichia coli*–derived L-asparagine amidohydrolase enzyme	IM/IV: 200–1 000 units/kg/day for 28 successive days; may continue for an additional 14 days if remission not induced	Acute lymphoblastic leukemia
pegaspargase (Oncaspar)	Pegylated version of asparaginase	IV/IM: 2 500 units/m² q14d	Acute lymphocytic leukemia (usually in patients who have developed an allergy to asparaginase)

IM, intramuscular; *IV*, intravenous.
*All dosages listed are for adults.

influences, concerns, and issues. Assess the patient's ability to perform activities of daily living (ADLs) and the patient's mobility status and gait. Perform a pain assessment using objective methods such as a numeric rating scale (e.g., 0 to 10, where 0 = no pain and 10 = worst pain ever). Note the pattern of pain, focusing on location, quality, onset, duration, and precipitating or alleviating factors. Document any oral, pharyngeal, esophageal, or abdominal pain; painful swallowing; epigastric or gastric pain, especially after eating spicy or acidic foods; achiness in joints or lower extremities; numbness or tingling; and any burning or sharp pain. Question the patient about past experiences with pain and about any drug, nondrug, or alternative therapies used, as well as about any previous successes or failures in pain management. Take into account cultural considerations relating to a cancer diagnosis.

Assess contraindications, cautions, and drug interactions; document the findings prior to the use of antineoplastic drugs. Laboratory tests that are usually ordered prior to their use include levels of electrolytes and

minerals, uric acid levels, complete blood count, platelet count, bleeding time, and cardiac enzyme levels, as well as tests of liver and kidney function (see the Lab Values box). Assays of tumour markers may also be ordered to establish baseline levels and determine the impact of the disease and subsequent therapeutic effectiveness. See Box 52-2 for more information about the specific adverse effects associated with destruction of populations of normal cells due to chemotherapy. Specific areas of assessment related to some of the more common adverse effects of chemotherapy on normal, rapidly dividing cells include the following:

- For altered nutritional status and impaired oral mucosa: Assess signs and symptoms of altered nutrition with a focus on weight loss, abnormal serum protein–albumin and blood urea nitrogen (BUN) levels (a negative nitrogen status due to low protein levels would be indicated by a decreasing BUN level), weakness, fatigue, lethargy, poor skin turgor, and pale conjunctiva. Assess oral mucosa for any signs and symptoms of stomatitis, such as pain or burning in the

LAB VALUES RELATED TO DRUG THERAPY

Rationales for Assessment and Monitoring of Blood Cell Counts With Antineoplastics

Antineoplastic drugs kill both normal and abnormal cells that are rapidly dividing, and thus the bone marrow and its rapidly dividing cellular constituents are negatively impacted. Because of this characteristic of chemotherapeutic drugs, RBCs, WBCs, and platelets are suppressed, and therefore their levels require frequent monitoring. Presented here is information specifically on RBCs and subsequent hemoglobin (Hgb) and hematocrit (Hct) levels as well as platelet levels. Chapter 46 contains more information on WBCs with neutrophil counts and nadir levels.

Laboratory Test	Normal Ranges	Rationale for Assessment
RBC count	M: $4.5–6 \times 10^{12}$/L F: $4.2–5.4 \times 10^{12}$/L	Bone marrow suppression from antineoplastics affects RBC values, leading to severe anemia. RBCs carry oxygen—attached to hemoglobin—from the lungs to the rest of the body. RBCs also help carry carbon dioxide back to the lungs for exhalation. Therefore, if RBC counts are low (e.g., with anemia), the body does not get the oxygen it needs, which leads to lack of energy, fatigue, intolerance of activity, shortness of breath, and hypoxemia. For patients with cancer who may already be experiencing the effects of bone marrow suppression from the disease and then from the treatment, this loss of oxygen saturation will be exacerbated, resulting in decreased ability to get up and about and perform activities of daily living.
Hct	M: 0.4–0.5% F: 0.38–0.47%	Hct measures the volume of RBCs in the blood, so if the RBC value is low, the Hct is also low. The impact of this low value is discussed above under RBCs.
Hgb level	M: 135–180 g/L F: 120–160 g/L	Hgb is the major substance in RBCs. It carries oxygen and is responsible for the red colour of the blood cell. With low levels of Hgb, the consequence to the patient is the same as noted with RBCs.
Platelets	$150–400 \times 10^9$/L	Platelets are the smallest type of blood cell and play a large role in the process of blood clotting. When bleeding occurs, the platelets swell, clump, and form a plug that helps stop the bleeding. Therefore, if platelet levels are lower than 10×10^9/L, the patient is at high risk for uncontrolled bleeding or hemorrhage. Some guidelines may use a platelet count of 5×10^9/L and above as the criterion. Seek out further information in policies and procedures, or contact the health care provider.

F, female; *M*, male; *RBCs*, red blood cells; *WBCs*, white blood cells.

BOX 52-2 Effects of Antineoplastic Drugs on Normal Cells and Related Adverse Effects

Antineoplastic drugs are designed to kill rapidly dividing *cancer* cells, but they also kill rapidly dividing *normal* cells. Such normal cells include cells of the oral and GI mucous membranes, hair follicles, reproductive germinal epithelium, and components of bone marrow (WBCs, RBCs, and platelets). The more common adverse effects of normal cell death are as follows:

- Killing of normal cells of the GI mucous membranes may result in adverse effects such as altered nutritional status, stomatitis with inflammation and ulceration of the mucosa throughout the GI tract, altered bowel function, poor appetite, nausea, vomiting (often intractable and requiring aggressive antiemetic treatment), and diarrhea.
- Killing of the normal cells of hair follicles leads to alopecia.
- Killing of normal cells in the bone marrow results in dangerously low (life-threatening) blood cell counts.

Because of the drugs' impact on these normal cells, the nurse must carefully assess patients' WBC counts (leukocytes, neutrophils, and band neutrophils), RBC counts, hemoglobin level, hematocrit, and platelet counts (see the Lab Values box). In addition, monitoring of patients' absolute neutrophil count (ANC) is needed (ANC = % of neutrophils + % bands × WBC). Monitoring ANC values allows nurses and other health care providers to identify the nadir, the lowest count, when the patient is most vulnerable. An ANC of 0.05 $\times 10^9$/L or lower indicates high risk for infection.

- Killing of germinal epithelial cells (also rapidly dividing) leads to sterility (irreversible) in males, damage to the ovaries with subsequent amenorrhea in females, and teratogenic effects with possible fetal death in pregnant women.

mouth, difficulty swallowing, taste changes, viscous saliva, dryness, cracking, and fissures with or without bleeding of the mucosa.

- For effects on the GI mucosa: Assess bowel sounds (hyperactive or hypoactive versus normoactive). Assess for signs and symptoms of diarrhea, such as frequent, loose stools (more than three stools per day), urgency, and abdominal cramping. Obtain information about the presence of blood in the stool as well as consistency, colour, odour, and amount. Assess for nausea and vomiting and determine whether symptoms are acute, delayed, or anticipatory; if vomiting occurs, determine the colour, amount, consistency, frequency, and odour, as well as whether blood is present. The severity of nausea and vomiting may be rated using a scale of 1 to 10 (where 10 indicates the worst symptoms) or using the terms *mild*, *moderate*, and *severe*.

- For alopecia: Assess the patient's views, concerns, and emotions about potential hair loss. Assess the patient's need to prepare for hair loss, either by leaving the hair as it is and allowing it to fall out on its own; having the hair cut short; or wearing a scarf, hat, bandanna, or hair wrap or purchasing a wig before the hair is actually lost. Purchasing a wig prior to chemotherapy will allow for a closer match to a patient's pre-chemotherapy hairstyle.

- For bone marrow suppression: Assess for signs and symptoms of anemia or decrease in RBCs, hemoglobin level, and hematocrit (e.g., pallor of the skin, oral mucous membranes, and conjunctiva; fatigue; lethargy; loss of interest in activities; shortness of breath; intolerance of activity; and inability to concentrate). Assess for signs and symptoms of leucopenia (decrease in WBCs [see Chapter 53] and an ANC below the normal range of $1.5 \times 10^9/L$, with severe neutropenia being less than $0.05 \times 10^9/L$), including fever; chills; tachycardia; abnormal breath sounds; productive cough with purulent, green- or rust-coloured sputum; change in the colour of urine; lethargy or fatigue; and acute confusion. (For more information, see Lab Values on p. 978). Assess for signs and symptoms of thrombocytopenia (decrease in thrombocytes [usually less than $100 \times 10^9/L$] and platelet clotting factors), including indications of unusual bleeding such as petechiae; purpura; ecchymosis; gingival (gum) bleeding; excessive or prolonged bleeding from puncture sites (e.g., intramuscular [IM] or IV sites or blood draw sites); unusual joint pain; blood in the stool, urine, or vomitus; and a decrease in blood pressure with elevated pulse rate (see the Lab Values box on p. 978 in this chapter as well as Chapters 27 and 28; see also Box 52-2). Always assess for the normal ranges of laboratory values.

- For possible sterility, teratogenesis, damage to ovaries with amenorrhea: In adult male patients, assess baseline reproductive history with attention to sexual functioning, fathering of children, and past and current reproductive or sexual problems or concerns. In adult female patients, in addition to the relevant aspects already mentioned, inquire about fertility, menstrual and childbearing history, and age of onset of menses and menopause, if applicable.

Prior to the use of cell cycle–specific drugs, document all allergies, cautions, contraindications, and drug interactions. Most antimetabolite drugs do not produce severe emesis for most patients (i.e., in fewer than 10% of cases). Some of the pyrimidine analogues have emetic potential, so perform an assessment of baseline GI functioning. In addition, the folate antagonists are not as likely as other drugs to cause emesis but may be associated with GI abnormalities, such as ulcers and stomatitis. Because these drugs are generally administered parenterally, assessing peripheral access areas or central venous sites is crucial to preventing risk of damage to surrounding tissue, joints, and tendons. Assess IV sites every hour, as needed or as per facility protocol, for redness, swelling, heat, and pain. One specific assessment consideration associated with use of the antimetabolite cytarabine is monitoring for the occurrence of cytarabine syndrome. This syndrome usually occurs within 6 to 12 hours after drug administration and is characterized by fever, muscle and joint pain, maculopapular rash, conjunctivitis, and malaise. Assessment and quick identification of this syndrome can lead to its prevention and appropriate treatment.

In patients receiving mitotic inhibitors (e.g., vinblastine, vincristine) and alkaloid topoisomerase II inhibitors (e.g., etoposide), perform baseline liver and kidney function studies as ordered. Serum uric acid levels are usually ordered because these levels rise with increased cell death from cancer or its treatment.

Other mitotic inhibitors, docetaxel and paclitaxel, are associated with severe neutropenia and a decrease in platelet counts (see the Lab Values box on p. 978 as well as Chapter 54); therefore, perform blood counts before, during, and after drug therapy. Constantly assess the patient for severe hypersensitivity reactions, characterized by dyspnea, severe hypotension, angioedema, and generalized urticaria (during treatments). Drops in blood cell counts may even occur before any clinical evidence is present. Note baseline neurological functioning as well as the presence of any peripheral neuropathies. Because these drugs have multiple incompatibilities and are irritants (irritating the IV site and vein) and vesicants (causing cell death with extravasation and necrosis with ulcerations), the nurse must be familiar with potential solution and drug interactions. It is appropriate to consult with the health care provider and pharmacist as well as refer to authoritative resources. Documentation must include initial and frequent follow-up assessments of the IV site.

Topoisomerase I inhibitors are associated with hematological adverse effects; thus, perform baseline WBC counts as ordered. Bone marrow suppression is predictable, noncumulative, reversible, and manageable;

therefore, do not give drugs such as topotecan to patients with baseline neutrophil counts of less than 1.5×10^9/L. Irinotecan causes more severe adverse effects than topotecan, so assess related systems and note the findings. The potential for irinotecan-related cholinergic diarrhea requires continuous assessment of the GI tract. Diarrhea may appear 2 to 10 days after the irinotecan infusion, and further medical treatment may be required if severe forms of diarrhea occur; the diarrhea can be life-threatening. There is only moderate risk of nausea and vomiting with irinotecan, which requires immediate and appropriate assessment and care. Drug interactions for which to assess include the concurrent administration of topotecan with filgrastim, which results in a worsening of myelosuppression. Do not give laxatives or diuretics with irinotecan due to the potential for severe diarrhea, fluid volume loss, and subsequent dehydration. When given with fluorouracil and leucovorin, severe cardiovascular toxicity (including thrombosis), pulmonary embolism, stroke, and acute fatal MI may occur. Perform a cautious and skillful assessment of related systems. See Table 52-10 for more drug interactions.

With the use of natural enzyme drugs (e.g., asparaginase, pegaspargase), assess pancreatic function because of the potential for severe or even fatal pancreatitis. Because of this risk of pancreatitis, assess the patient closely for moderate to severe abdominal pain (upper left quadrant), nausea, vomiting, and hyperglycemia. Serum alkaline phosphatase and WBC counts, if elevated, may indicate possible pancreatitis if also supported by clinical presentation. Additionally, assessment and documentation of dermatological, hepatic, GU, neurological, musculoskeletal, GI, and cardiovascular systems is important due to the impact of natural enzyme drugs on these systems.

Genetic considerations are an area of importance in the treatment of cancer with antineoplastics, as with all drug therapy. Assess individuals for the presence of the following characteristics before chemotherapy is initiated: (1) genetic markers for oral cancers, (2) genetic determinants of testosterone or estrogen metabolism, and (3) genetically linked enzyme system abnormalities such as those involving specific cytochrome P450 enzymes that metabolically convert nicotine to a carcinogenic substance. These genetic factors are extremely complex; nevertheless, be aware of the possible influence of genetic differences, and be forward thinking regarding the impact of drug research and genetics. See Chapter 5 for more information on genetics as related to drug therapy and the nursing process.

Nursing Diagnoses

- Diarrhea related to the adverse effects of antineoplastic drugs
- Acute pain related to the disease process and drug-induced joint pain, stomatitis, GI distress, and other discomforts associated with antineoplastic cell cycle–specific therapy
- Risk for infection related to drug-induced bone marrow suppression with possible leukopenia and neutropenia

Planning

Goals

- Patient will regain as near normal as possible bowel elimination patterns during antineoplastic therapy.
- Patient will achieve improved comfort levels with improved pain control and management of symptoms and adverse effects.
- Patient will remain free from infection.

Expected Patient Outcomes

- Patient states measures to minimize diarrhea.
  - Patient states foods and beverages to avoid, such as hot, spicy foods and beverages; alcohol; foods high in fibre; gaseous foods such as cruciferous vegetables; and raw seafood.
  - Patient takes antidiarrheal medication, as instructed and if indicated, to avoid dehydration and electrolyte loss.
- Patient experiences improved pain relief through use of pharmacological and nonpharmacological measures to manage chemotherapy-related adverse effects, such as joint pain, stomatitis, and GI distress.
- Patient requests medication(s) for comfort before pain is uncontrollable and severe.
- Patient uses a numeric scale of 0 to 10 for identification of pain level, with 0 being no pain and 10 representing the worst pain ever experienced.
- Patient uses nonpharmacological measures (e.g., relaxation, music therapy, pet therapy, biofeedback, massage, therapeutic touch, diversion) concurrently with drug therapy to increase comfort levels.
- Patient states measures to assist in supporting the immune system and preventing infection, such as frequent handwashing, performance of deep breathing exercises, increased intake of fluids, consumption of a well-balanced diet, avoidance of malls and other crowded places, and avoidance of people with colds, flu, or communicable respiratory illnesses.
  - Patient states ways to minimize oral mucosal breakdown and infection, such as frequent mouth care and dental hygiene measures; using mild toothpaste, gentle sponge toothettes, and non–alcohol-based mouthwash, as well as frequent fluid intake.
  - Patient demonstrates the use of various measures to enhance skin integrity, such as keeping skin clean, dry, and lubricated.
- Patient adheres to daily regimen for increasing urinary health, such increasing fluid intake and consuming fluids that minimize urinary infections (e.g., cranberry juice).

(Note that the nursing diagnoses, goals, and expected patient outcomes presented here are appropriate to treatment with many antineoplastic drugs.)

⬛ Implementation

Antineoplastic drugs are some of the most toxic medications given to patients because they cause the death of normal cells along with the death of cancer cells. The high potency of these drugs also places patients at higher risk for toxicity, serious complications, and adverse effects. The possibility of such adverse effects and toxicities require skillful nursing care based on cautious and thorough assessment and subsequent critical thinking. Consequently, chemotherapy administration requires specialized education. The Canadian Association of Nurses in Oncology had developed standards for the practice, education, and continuing competence of registered nurses. General considerations in nursing implementation applicable to most antineoplastic drugs, as well as some specific aspects of implementation related to cell cycle–specific drugs, are discussed in the following paragraphs. Other nursing process information related to cell cycle–nonspecific drugs is presented in Chapter 53.

For antineoplastic therapy in general, nursing considerations related to reducing fear and anxiety include establishing a therapeutic relationship, beginning with trust and empathy. Approach the patient in a warm, empathic, and supportive manner while projecting confidence in providing nursing care. Provide individualized explanations and teaching about the patient's illness, care, and treatments that are appropriate to the patient's educational level. Collaborate with all members of the health care team. Encourage patients to consider relaxation techniques such as listening to music, performing meditation, or engaging in guided imagery. To support the patient's emotional, mental, and physical health, it may be necessary to call on other sources of support, including social services, counselling services, financial assistance services, home support, and religious–spiritual support. Also necessary may be appropriate consults with other health care providers such as social workers, discharge planners, psychiatrists, mental health nurses, nurse practitioners, and oncology nurse specialists, as well as with support groups for the patient, family members, or significant others. A referral to palliative care may also be appropriate.

A variety of interventions that may be indicated for the management of stomatitis or excessive oral mucosa dryness and irritation include the following: (1) Instruct the patient to perform oral hygiene before and after eating or as needed to help provide cleanliness and comfort; also advise the patient to avoid lemon, glycerin, undiluted peroxide, or alcohol-containing products because they are drying and irritating to the oral mucosa. (2) Recommend that the patient use a soft-bristle toothbrush or soft-tipped toothette or swab with solutions of diluted, warm saline. (3) If dentures are used, encourage the patient to remove and clean them frequently and, if stomatitis is severe, to insert them only at mealtimes. (4) Advise the patient to use OTC saliva substitutes, keep the lips moist, and use sugarless candy or gum to stimulate saliva flow. (5) Stress to the patient that spicy, acidic, or hot foods; alcohol; and tobacco should be avoided because they are irritants. (6) Oral antifungal suspensions (e.g., nystatin) may be ordered if white patches are noted on the oral mucosa; the patient may use analgesic solutions (e.g., lidocaine swish and swallow), as ordered, to help manage discomfort.

Nausea and vomiting occur commonly with antineoplastic drugs. Emetic potential varies depending on the drug or treatment protocol (see earlier discussion and Box 52-1). Educate the patient on measures to enhance comfort during times of nausea and vomiting, including restricting oral intake as ordered; removing noxious odours or sights to avoid stimulating the vomiting centre; performing oral hygiene as needed; promoting relaxation through slow, deep breathing; consuming small, frequent meals and eating slowly; and consuming clear liquids and a bland diet. Use of IV fluids may be indicated for hydration purposes if nausea and vomiting are severe. Antiemetics are also a vital part of antineoplastic therapy (see Chapter 41 for a brief review of the pathophysiology of nausea and vomiting and more specific drug-related information). Premedication with antiemetics 30 to 60 minutes before administration of the antineoplastic(s) is the preferred treatment protocol to help reduce nausea and vomiting, prevent dehydration and malnutrition, and promote comfort. Combination antiemetic drug therapy may be more effective than single-drug therapy. An antiemetic may be given with the chemotherapeutic regimen as well as prescription medication for at-home use. Ginger ale and ginger-based teas may also be helpful.

Diarrhea is also a common adverse effect of antineoplastic therapy. Perform the following nursing interventions: (1) Advise patients to avoid or limit oral intake of irritating, spicy, and gas-producing foods; caffeine; high-fibre foods; alcohol; extremely hot or cold foods or beverages; and lactose-containing foods and beverages. (2) Consult appropriate personnel, as ordered, to help patients and family members plan meals and arrange ways to meet the patients' dietary and bowel elimination needs. (3) Administer opioids (e.g., paregoric), synthetic opioids (e.g., loperamide, diphenoxylate hydrochloride), or other antidiarrheals, as prescribed. Adsorbents–protectants and antisecretory drugs may also help reduce GI upset and diarrhea (see Chapter 40).

To address nutritional concerns, the following measures may prove beneficial in improving oral intake and nutritional status: (1) Perform a 24-hour recall of food intake, and report the typical week's diet for patients. (2) Use antiemetic therapy, pain management, mouth care, and hydration, as ordered, to reduce the adverse effects of therapy and improve appetite. (3) To ease taste alterations, advise patients to consume mild-tasting foods and to use chicken, turkey, cheese, Greek yogourt, nondairy yogourt or pudding, or tofu as protein sources, as tolerated. (4) Provide plastic rather than metal utensils if patients report a metallic taste. (5) Encourage patients to eat foods that are easy to swallow, such as custards; gelatins; puddings; milkshakes; eggnog; commercially prepared high-protein, high-calorie supplemental shakes; mashed white or sweet potatoes; blended drinks with crushed ice, fruit, and yogourt; nutritional supplement drinks and snacks; and lactose-free ice cream. (6) Instruct patients to avoid sticky or dry foods. (7) Encourage the consumption of small, frequent meals in environments that are conducive to eating (e.g., free of odours and excessive noise). (8) Appetite stimulants such as megestrol acetate or dronabinol may be used. (9) Encourage patients to practice energy conservation, including frequent rest periods before and after meals.

Alopecia is a common adverse effect of antineoplastics and is disturbing to patients regardless of age or gender. Warn patients and family members about the possibility of hair loss, and tell them when it will occur (usually 7 to 10 days after treatment begins, but this is dependent upon the specific drug used) and that it is reversible. Inform patients that new hair growth is often a different colour and texture from that of the hair lost. Provide information about the options of acquiring a wig or hairpiece, or wearing scarves or hats, before the actual hair loss. The Canadian Cancer Society may be a resource for items such as wigs, scarves, and hats.

Antineoplastic-induced bone marrow suppression leads to anemia, leukopenia, neutropenia, and thrombocytopenia (see previous discussion and Lab Values boxes in this chapter and Chapter 53). Anemia results in fatigue and loss of energy and is a common adverse effect of therapy and the disease process of cancer. Anemia may require blood transfusions, peripheral blood stem cell treatment, or treatment with prescribed medications such as iron preparations, folic acid, or erythropoietic growth factors (e.g., darbepoietin alfa). Injections of these substances may be given at home and may be administered at the first sign of a decrease in RBC levels. Conservation of energy and planning of care are very important in minimizing patient fatigue.

Risk of infection from leukopenia or neutropenia and immunosuppression is one of the more significant adverse effects of antineoplastic drugs and requires close attention. Inform the patient, family members, and caregivers that when WBC counts are low, the patient is at high risk for infection and that defences remain low until the counts recover. Following standard precautions/ routine practices and using good handwashing technique are essential in preventing transmission of infection in the hospital and home settings. Patients may also need to be placed on reverse isolation, especially if they have neutropenia. Because fever is a principal early sign of infection, take patients' oral or axillary temperature at least every 4 hours during periods in which they are at risk. Avoid taking the temperature rectally to minimize tissue trauma and breaks in skin integrity, and thus loss of the first line of defence and increased risk to infection. Encourage the patient to immediately report to the health care provider a temperature of 38.1°C or higher so that appropriate treatment may be initiated and complications avoided. Many facilities recommend taking special precautions during the care of a patient who is receiving chemotherapy (see Chapter 53 for details). If needed, and as ordered, administration of colony-stimulating factors may be beneficial. Filgrastim, pegfilgrastim, and sargramostim are examples of drugs given to accelerate WBC recovery during antineoplastic drug therapy. Use these drugs, as ordered, to minimize neutropenia. These medications act on the bone marrow to enhance neutrophil production and help decrease the incidence, severity, and duration of neutropenia. These drugs must be administered within a certain time frame (see Chapter 54). Encourage patients with immune suppression to be aware of environments and people to avoid, such as individuals who have recently been vaccinated (who may have a subclinical infection) or who have a cold or flu or other symptoms of an infection. Maintaining a "low-microbe" diet by washing fresh fruits and vegetables and making sure foods are well cooked is also recommended. Educate patients on the importance of performing oral care frequently (see discussion of stomatitis) and to turn frequently, cough, and breathe deeply to help prevent stasis of respiratory secretions.

Thrombocytopenia is also an adverse effect of antineoplastic therapy and puts patients at risk for bleeding. Monitor platelet counts, coagulation studies, RBC counts, hemoglobin levels, and hematocrit values and report any decreases (see the Lab Values box). Avoid injections if possible, and utilize alternative routes of administration. If injections or venipunctures are absolutely necessary, always use the smallest gauge needle possible and apply gentle, prolonged pressure to the site afterward. Monitor closely patients who have undergone bone marrow aspiration after the procedure for bleeding at the aspiration site. Perform blood pressure monitoring as needed. Be efficient and quick and do not overinflate the cuff to avoid bruising. Monitor patients for bleeding from the mouth, gums, and nose. Check for bleeding after tooth brushing and report excessive bleeding to the health care provider.

Inform patients that antineoplastics may have a negative impact on the reproductive tract, causing destruction of the germinal epithelium of the testes and damage to the ovaries and to a fetus (teratogenesis). Other problems may include sterility; amenorrhea; premature menopausal symptoms of hot flashes, decreased vaginal secretions, mood changes, or irritability; and decreased libido or sexual dysfunction. Counsel male patients about the risk for sterility, which may be irreversible. Discuss with male patients the option and topic of sperm banking before chemotherapy, if deemed appropriate. Stress that female patients of childbearing age who are sexually active need to protect themselves against pregnancy because of the risk of embryonic death. Encourage contraceptive measures during chemotherapy and for up to 8 weeks after discontinuation of therapy; however, some antineoplastic drugs require use of contraceptives for up to 2 years after completion of treatment because of the risk for genetic abnormalities.

With antimetabolites, always follow the practitioner's orders regarding premedication with antiemetics and antianxiety drugs. Follow orders or protocol for the use of other symptom-control medications, as prescribed. GI adverse effects are common with antimetabolites and usually occur on about the fourth day following their administration; these effects require preplanning for specific pharmacological interventions (e.g., antiemetics, antispasmodics, analgesics) and nonpharmacological measures (e.g., dietary changes, oral care). Antibiotic therapy may also be ordered prophylactically. See earlier discussion of nursing considerations associated with stomatitis, loss of appetite, diarrhea, nausea, vomiting, and anemia. For further discussion of the handling of antimetabolites and other IV antineoplastic drugs, see Box 53-2.

Use extreme caution in the handling and administration of cytarabine by the various routes (IV, subcutaneous, or intrathecal). Major concerns with cytarabine therapy include bone marrow suppression (see earlier discussion) and cytarabine syndrome (see the Assessment section). If high dosages are used, cytarabine may also cause central nervous system, GI, or pulmonary toxicity, so closely monitor these systems to ensure patient safety and comfort. For intrathecal administration, the drug may be reconstituted with sodium chloride, or the health care provider may use the patient's spinal fluid. Do not add fluorouracil to any other IV infusions; administer the drug by itself in the appropriate diluent. When an infusion port is not used, do not use IV sites over joints, tendons, or small veins, or in extremities that are edematous. Give IV dosages exactly as ordered, and constantly monitor the IV site, infusion port, and infusion solution and equipment. If IV infiltration occurs, follow the protocol for management of infiltration and contact the health care provider. Follow all hospital or infusion protocols without exception because treatment of extravasation is handled differently depending on the specific drug. If extravasation of a vesicant occurs, the drug is usually discontinued immediately; leave the IV cannula in place (for possible use of antidotes through the cannula to access the affected area), and follow facility protocol. The use of antidotes and other drugs, as well as hot or cold packs, is usually outlined in the protocol for managing extravasation (see Box 53-1). If topical forms of cytarabine are used, inform patients that it is important to apply the drug exactly as ordered, to the affected area only. Use gloves or a finger cot to apply the topical dosage form.

Gemcitabine, another antimetabolite, is dosed based on absolute granulocyte counts and platelet nadirs and is given if the counts exceed $1.5 \times 10^9/L$ and $1 \times 10^9/L$, respectively. Keep IV solutions at room temperature to avoid crystallization and use within 24 hours. Give infusions as ordered. Antiemetics and antidiarrheals may be needed. Mercaptopurine is available in oral dosage forms; give it as ordered. Finally, the antimetabolite methotrexate has numerous toxicities and adverse effects that may be minimized by appropriate medical treatment. For example, there may be orders for boosting immune status and blood cell counts before aggressive therapy is initiated. Cytoprotective drugs are used. Continue to monitor creatinine clearance, as ordered, to detect any nephrotoxicity. Nutritional status may be enhanced by increasing the intake of foods high in folic acid, including bran, dried beans, nuts, fruits, asparagus, and other fresh vegetables, if tolerated. Consumption of these foods is yet another measure to help minimize the possibility of methotrexate toxicity. If GI upset or stomatitis occurs, the patient may need to decrease any sources of irritation (e.g., high-fibre food). Methotrexate is usually given orally or intravenously. Wear gloves when giving the drug. If any of the solution comes in contact with the skin, wash the area immediately and thoroughly with soap and water. (See Box 53-2 for discussion of concerns in the handling and administration of vesicant drugs.)

For the mitotic inhibitors, specifically the taxane family of drugs, and docetaxel in particular, premedication protocols are usually specified and include administration of oral corticosteroids (e.g., dexamethasone) beginning several days before day 1 of therapy, to help decrease the risk of hypersensitivity. Closely monitor patients for the sudden onset of bronchospasms, flushing of the face, and localized skin reactions; these may indicate a hypersensitivity response requiring immediate treatment. In such situations, contact the health care provider immediately. These symptoms may occur within just a few minutes of beginning the infusion. In addition, any dyspnea, abdominal distension, crackles in the lungs, or dependent edema during therapy require immediate attention. Cutaneous reactions may also appear during therapy, such as rash on the hands and feet; these reactions also need immediate attention and treatment. With paclitaxel, the patient may also be premedicated with diphenhydramine hydrochloride, corticosteroids, and H_2 antagonist drugs. Take all measures to minimize tissue trauma (e.g., avoidance of IM injections and rectal temperature taking, if possible) to promote comfort and prevent bleeding and infection.

With the topoisomerase I inhibitors irinotecan and topotecan, monitor blood counts closely with every treatment. A drop in blood counts or severe diarrhea may cause a temporary postponement of therapy. Treat any extravasation of the solution immediately, and follow protocol. Ensuring that IV sites remain patent is crucial to the prevention of tissue damage secondary to extravasation of antineoplastic drugs that are considered irritants or vesicants. Nausea and vomiting may lead to dehydration and electrolyte disturbances. Advise patients and family members to report these symptoms immediately before adverse consequences occur (see previous discussion for specific interventions). IV incompatibilities are numerous for both these drugs and are of constant concern. With topotecan, IV extravasation is usually accompanied by a mild local reaction such as erythema or bruising. If these symptoms are noted, they must be managed immediately to avoid further trauma and risk for loss of skin integrity (the first line of defence against infection). Headache and difficulty breathing may be more common with topotecan than with irinotecan; therefore, closely and frequently monitor patients for these symptoms. The enzyme antineoplastics asparaginase and pegaspargase should be handled with extreme caution and care. Patients may receive an intradermal test dose of asparaginase before therapy begins or when a week or longer has passed between doses. With asparaginase and pegaspargase, if the solution comes in contact with the skin, thoroughly wash or rinse the area with copious amounts of water for a minimum of 15 minutes. During therapy, if there are signs and symptoms of oliguria, anuria (renal failure), or pancreatitis, the drug will most likely be discontinued. The IM route of administration is usually preferred because it carries a lower risk of causing clotting abnormalities, GI disorders, and kidney and liver toxicity. If solutions are cloudy, do not use them. If more than 2 mL is ordered or required for intramuscular dosing, use two injections. Pancreatitis is problematic with the use of these drugs and can be serious. Pay close attention to symptoms such as severe abdominal pain with nausea and vomiting. Constantly monitor serum lipase and amylase levels. If any signs or symptoms of pancreatitis occur, the health care provider will usually discontinue the drugs immediately. Use of cytoprotective drugs has been briefly discussed on p. 983, with further discussion provided in Chapter 53.

Evaluation

Focus evaluation of nursing care on reviewing whether goals and outcome criteria are being met, as well as on monitoring for therapeutic responses and adverse and toxic effects of antineoplastic therapy. Therapeutic responses may manifest as clinical improvement, decrease in tumour size, and decrease in metastatic spread. Evaluation of nursing care, with reference to goals and outcome criteria, may reveal improvements related to a decrease in adverse effects and a decrease in the impact of cancer on the patient's well-being. With therapeutic effectiveness, there will be increases in comfort, nutrition, hydration, energy levels, and ability to carry out ADLs, as well as improved quality of life. Revisit goals and outcome criteria to identify more specific areas to monitor. In addition, certain laboratory studies, such as tumour markers levels, levels of carcinoembryonic antigens, RBC and WBC counts, and platelet counts, may be performed to aid in determining how well the treatment protocol has worked and to monitor adverse effects of bone marrow suppression. Also, if ANC drops below 0.05×10^9, the health care provider may discontinue chemotherapy but then reinitiate it when the level is above 1×10^9, or as facility policy dictates. Other blood counts are considered, too. As part of the evaluation, health care providers may also order additional X-rays, computed tomographic scans, magnetic resonance images, tissue analysis, or other studies appropriate to the diagnosis both during and after antineoplastic therapy, at time intervals related to the anticipated tumour response.

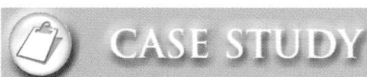

CASE STUDY

Facing Chemotherapy

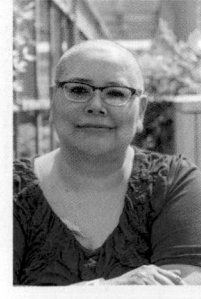

Phuong, a 48-year-old bank teller and mother of two adolescent daughters, has been diagnosed with breast cancer. She has undergone lumpectomy to remove the tumour and is about to start adjuvant chemotherapy. She states that she has "faced the facts" about her disease and the threat to her life but says, "I know this is silly, but I hate the thought of losing my hair to this disease."

1. What measures can be taken to help Phuong deal with her hair loss?

2. Ten days after her chemotherapy, Phuong's neutrophil count drops to 2×10^9/L. She has been hospitalized because she has developed a cough, and several of her friends have come in to visit and have brought a fresh fruit basket. What actions will be taken to protect her from infection?

3. During rounds, the nurse finds Phuong curled up in the bed and sobbing. Phuong says that she feels "so afraid" and is worried about who will care for her family if she dies. What actions will the nurse take at this time?

For answers, see http://evolve.elsevier.com/Canada/Lilley/pharmacology/.

PATIENT TEACHING TIPS

❖ Educate patients that GI adverse effects and irritation to the oral and GI mucosa may be decreased by avoiding intake of alcohol, tobacco, spicy and high-fibre foods, juices or foods containing citric acid, and foods that are very hot or cold or have a rough texture. Perishable foods that have been left out of refrigeration for more than 1 hour should not be consumed.

❖ Stress to patients that daily mouth care is important. Instruct them to report sores, pain, or white patches in the mouth to the health care provider immediately. Headache, fatigue, faintness, and shortness of breath (possibly indicative of anemia); bleeding and easy bruising (possibly indicative of a drop in platelet count); and sore throat and fever (possibly indicative of infection) also need to be reported immediately to the appropriate health care provider. Fever and chills may be the first signs of an oncoming infection.

❖ Discuss contraception, sperm banking, and other reproductive issues with postpubescent male patients and women of childbearing age.

❖ Emphasize to patients receiving antineoplastic drugs which OTC medications they should avoid (e.g., aspirin, ibuprofen, any combination products containing these drugs).

❖ Antineoplastics may cause alopecia. Before therapy, provide patients with the opportunity to discuss options for hair and scalp care. These options may include, but are not limited to, having the hair cut short before treatment; selecting, purchasing or renting a wig or hairpiece comparable to the patient's existing hair in colour, texture, length, and style; or having bandanas, scarves, or hats on hand before the hair is actually lost. Although hair loss is temporary, inform patients that it will occur and that hair will appear differently upon growing back. The Canadian Cancer Society may be a resource for wigs and hairpieces.

❖ The following websites are helpful online resources for patients and their family members and significant others: http://www.cancer.ca/, http://www.hc-sc.gc.ca/hc-ps/dc-ma/cancer-eng.php, http://www.wellspring.ca, http://www.bccancer.bc.ca, and http://www.oncolink.org/.

❖ With the use of cytarabine, encourage patients to increase fluid intake to help decrease the risk of dehydration and hyperuricemia.

❖ With the use of fluorouracil and gemcitabine, encourage patients to engage in frequent oral hygiene and to report to the health care provider immediately any bleeding, bruising, chest pain, diarrhea, nausea, vomiting, heart palpitations, infection, or changes in vision. Instruct patients to protect themselves from the sun while taking fluorouracil, including avoiding overexposure to sun or ultraviolet light and using protective clothing, sunscreen, and sunglasses.

❖ With the use of mercaptopurine, educate patients that alcohol must be avoided to help minimize drug toxicity.

❖ With the use of methotrexate, instruct patients to notify the health care provider if nausea and vomiting are problematic or uncontrollable, or if fever, sore throat, muscle aches and pains, or unusual bleeding occurs. Advise patients to avoid alcohol, salicylates, nonsteroidal anti-inflammatory drugs, and exposure to sunlight or ultraviolet light. Instruct both male and female patients to use contraceptive measures for up to 3 months or longer following drug therapy, if appropriate.

❖ With the use of taxanes, counsel patients to contact the health care provider immediately if any signs or symptoms of neuropathy (e.g., numbness or tingling of extremities) appear.

❖ If WBC counts are low during therapy with etoposide or teniposide, caution patients to avoid individuals who are ill. Additionally, advise them to report to the health care provider immediately any easy bleeding or bruising, difficulty breathing, fever, sore throat, or chills.

❖ With the use of the enzymes pegaspargase and asparaginase, encourage the patient to drink extra fluids and to report any severe nausea or vomiting, bleeding, excessive fatigue, fever, or other signs or symptoms of infection.

KEY POINTS

❖ Cancers are diseases that are characterized by uncontrolled cellular growth.

❖ *Malignancy* refers specifically to a neoplasm that is anaplastic, invasive, and metastatic, as opposed to benign.

❖ Tumours are generally classified by tissue of origin as follows: epithelial (carcinoma), connective (sarcoma), lymphatic (lymphoma), and leukocytic (leukemia).

❖ Antineoplastics are drugs used to treat malignancies. They may be either cell cycle–specific or cell cycle–nonspecific drugs or may have miscellaneous actions.

❖ Cell cycle–specific drugs kill cancer cells during specific phases of the cell growth cycle. Cell cycle–nonspecific drugs kill cancer cells during any phase of the cell growth cycle.

❖ Chemotherapy, or antineoplastic therapy, requires skillful and perceptive nursing care. It is important to act prudently and think critically when making decisions about the nursing care of patients receiving antineoplastic drugs.

❖ Cell cycle–specific drug classes include antimetabolites, mitotic inhibitors, alkaloid topoisomerase II inhibitors, topoisomerase I inhibitors, and antineoplastic enzymes.

Continued

KEY POINTS—cont'd

❖ Antineoplastic antimetabolites are cell cycle–specific antagonistic analogues that work by inhibiting the actions of key cellular metabolites.

❖ Two plant-derived antineoplastic drugs are the taxanes: paclitaxel, derived from the bark of the slow-growing Western (Pacific) yew tree, and docetaxel, a semisynthetic taxoid produced from the needles of the European yew tree. Docetaxel is pharmacologically similar to paclitaxel.

❖ The topoisomerase I inhibitors, topotecan and irinotecan, comprise a relatively new class of chemotherapy drugs.

❖ Antineoplastic enzymes include asparaginase and pegaspargase.

❖ Several drugs that are available are classified as cytoprotective and help to reduce the toxicity of various antineoplastics.

EXAMINATION REVIEW QUESTIONS

1. A patient is experiencing stomatitis after a round of chemotherapy. Which intervention by the nurse is correct?
   a. Clean the mouth with a soft-bristle toothbrush and warm saline solution.
   b. Rinse the mouth with commercial mouthwash twice a day.
   c. Use lemon glycerin swabs to keep the mouth moist.
   d. Keep dentures in the mouth between meals.

2. The nurse is caring for a patient who becomes severely nauseated during chemotherapy. Which intervention is most appropriate?
   a. Encourage light activity during chemotherapy as a distraction.
   b. Provide antiemetic medications 30 to 60 minutes before chemotherapy begins.
   c. Provide antiemetic medications only upon the request of the patient.
   d. Hold fluids during chemotherapy to avoid causing vomiting.

3. The nurse monitors a patient who is experiencing thrombocytopenia from severe bone marrow suppression by looking for which symptom(s):
   a. Severe weakness and fatigue
   b. Elevated body temperature
   c. Decreased skin turgor
   d. Excessive bleeding and bruising

4. A patient receiving chemotherapy is experiencing severe bone marrow suppression. Which nursing diagnosis is most appropriate at this time?
   a. Activity intolerance
   b. Risk for infection
   c. Disturbed body image
   d. Impaired physical mobility

5. If extravasation of an antineoplastic medication occurs, which intervention will the nurse perform first?
   a. Apply cold compresses to the site while elevating the arm.
   b. Inject subcutaneous doses of epinephrine around the IV site every 2 hours.
   c. Stop the infusion immediately, while leaving the catheter in place.
   d. Inject the appropriate antidote through the IV catheter.

6. The nurse is assessing a patient who has experienced severe neutropenia after chemotherapy and will monitor for which possible signs of infection? (Select all that apply.)
   a. Elevated WBC count
   b. Fever
   c. Nausea
   d. Sore throat
   e. Chills

7. The order for chemotherapy reads: "Give asparaginase IV 200 units/kg/day." The patient weighs 297 pounds. The pharmacy department will prepare the medication for IV infusion. How much drug will be given per dose? Is this a safe dose?

CRITICAL THINKING ACTIVITIES

1. A patient who has undergone three chemotherapy sessions is now experiencing stomatitis, and his wife exclaims, "He won't eat! What kinds of food can I give him? I'm concerned because he has no appetite and now he has these mouth sores." What is the nurse's priority response? Explain your answer.

2. A patient is receiving irinotecan as part of his chemotherapy regimen. He will be receiving the dose shortly and then will be sent home. The nurse is providing patient teaching before giving him the medication. What is one of the most important problems for which the patient will need to be ready once he is home? Explain the nurse's priority action.

3. A patient is receiving chemotherapy that includes the antimetabolite cytarabine. Several hours after the treatment, the patient reports shortness of breath. The nurse examines the patient and finds that his pulse rate is 118 beats/min, he has slight edema in his lower extremities, and crackles are audible over the bases of the lungs. In addition, his pulse oximetry reading is 92% on room air (previously it was 99%). What is the nurse's immediate priority action?

For answers see **http://evolve.elsevier.com/Canada/Lilley/pharmacology/**.

CHAPTER 53

Antineoplastic Drugs Part 2: Cell Cycle–Nonspecific and Miscellaneous Drugs

Objectives

After reading this chapter, the successful student will be able to do the following:

1. Review concepts related to carcinogenesis, types of malignancies and related terminology, and different treatment modalities, including the use of cell cycle–nonspecific and miscellaneous antineoplastic drugs.

2. Identify the various drugs that are classified as cell cycle–nonspecific or hormonal or that are considered miscellaneous drugs.

3. Discuss the common adverse effects and toxic effects of the cell cycle–nonspecific and miscellaneous antineoplastic drugs, including the reasons for their occurrence and methods of treatment, such as the use of any antidotes.

4. Describe the mechanisms of action, indications, dosages, routes of administration, cautions, contraindications, and drug interactions of the cell cycle–nonspecific drugs, hormonal drugs, and miscellaneous antineoplastic drugs.

5. Apply knowledge about the cell cycle–nonspecific, hormonal agonist–antagonist, and other miscellaneous antineoplastic drugs and their characteristics to the development of a comprehensive collaborative plan of care for patients with cancer who are receiving these drugs.

6. Briefly describe extravasation and other major adverse effects associated with the cell cycle–nonspecific and miscellaneous antineoplastics, including discussion of protocols and antidotes.

e-Learning Activities

Website
(http://evolve.elsevier.com/Canada/Lilley/pharmacology/)

evolve

- Answer Key—Textbook Case Studies
- Answer Key—Critical Thinking Activities
- Chapter Summaries—Printable
- Review Questions for Exam Preparation
- Unfolding Case Studies

Drug Profiles

bevacizumab, p. 994
▸▸ cisplatin, p. 992
▸▸ cyclophosphamide, p. 992
▸▸ doxorubicin (doxorubicin hydrochloride)*, p. 993
hydroxyurea, p. 994
imatinib (imatinib mesylate)*, p. 995
mitotane, p. 995
mitoxantrone (mitoxantrone hydrochloride)*, p. 993
octreotide, p. 995

▸▸ Key drug

*Full generic name is given in parentheses. For the purposes of this text, the more common, shortened name is used.

Key Terms

Alkylation   A chemical reaction in which an alkyl group is transferred from one molecule to another. In chemotherapy, alkylation leads to damage of cancer cell deoxyribonucleic acid (DNA) and cell death. (p. 989)

Bifunctional   Refers to alkylating drugs composed of molecules that have two reactive alkyl groups and are therefore able to alkylate at two sites on the DNA molecule. (p. 990)

Extravasation   The leakage of any intravenously or intra-arterially administered medication into the tissue space surrounding the vein or artery; such an event can cause

serious tissue injury, especially with antineoplastic drugs. (p. 991)

Mitosis   The process of cell reproduction occurring in somatic (nonsexual) cells and resulting in the formation of two genetically identical daughter cells, each containing the diploid (complete) number of chromosomes characteristic of the species. (p. 990)

Polyfunctional   Refers to the action of alkylating drugs that can engage in several alkylation reactions with cancer cell DNA molecules per single molecule of drug. (p. 990)

CELL CYCLE–NONSPECIFIC ANTINEOPLASTIC DRUGS

There are currently two broad classes of cell cycle–nonspecific cancer drugs: alkylating drugs and cytotoxic antibiotics.

ALKYLATING DRUGS

Records of the use of drugs to treat cancer date back several centuries. However, truly successful systemic cancer chemotherapy treatments are not documented until the 1940s. At that time, the first alkylating drugs were developed from mustard gas agents that were used for chemical warfare before and during World War I. The first drug to be developed was mechlorethamine hydrochloride, also known as *nitrogen mustard*. It is the prototypical drug of its class; however, it is no longer manufactured in Canada. Since its antineoplastic activity was discovered in the mid-twentieth century, many analogues have been synthesized for use in the treatment of cancer, and they are collectively referred to as *nitrogen mustards*.

The alkylating drugs commonly used in clinical practice in Canada today fall into three categories: classic alkylators (the nitrogen mustards); nitrosoureas, which have a different chemical structure from that of the nitrogen mustards but also work by **alkylation**; and miscellaneous alkylators, which also have a different chemical structure from the nitrogen mustards but are known to work at least partially by alkylation. These drugs are used to treat a wide spectrum of malignancies. The drugs in each category are as follows:

Classic alkylators (nitrogen mustards)
- chlorambucil
- cyclophosphamide
- ifosfamide
- melphalan

Nitrosoureas
- carmustine
- lomustine
- streptozocin

Miscellaneous alkylators
- busulfan
- carboplatin
- cisplatin
- dacarbazine
- oxaliplatin
- procarbazine hydrochloride
- temozolomide

Mechanism of Action and Drug Effects

The alkylating drugs act by preventing cancer cells from reproducing. Specifically, they alter the chemical structure of the cells' deoxyribonucleic acid (DNA), which is essential to the reproduction of any cell, by causing alkyl groups rather than hydrogen atoms to be attached to the nucleic acid. DNA molecules consist of two adjacent strands, each consisting of alternating sequences of phosphate and sugar molecules (Figure 53-1). These components make up the "backbone" of the DNA strands. These two strands are chemically linked to each other by the third DNA structural element—nitrogen-containing bases (adenine, guanine, thymine, and cytosine, abbreviated A, G, T, and C, respectively). These bases are bound to the sugar molecules of the DNA backbone, and two bases, linked to each other by hydrogen bonds, form the molecular bridges between the two DNA strands that bring them into the double helix structure. A nucleotide, which consists of one molecule each of base as well as sugar and phosphate that are bound together, is the structural unit of the molecules of both DNA and ribonucleic acid (RNA), another nucleic acid that is important in cellular reproduction. Messenger RNA (mRNA) molecules are produced by DNA molecules during the complex process of transcription. These mRNA molecules differ from DNA molecules in at least three ways: they are single stranded (versus double stranded); they do not include thymine but instead include another base, uracil (U); and their sugar molecules are ribose, which has a slightly different structure from that of the deoxyribose molecules of DNA.

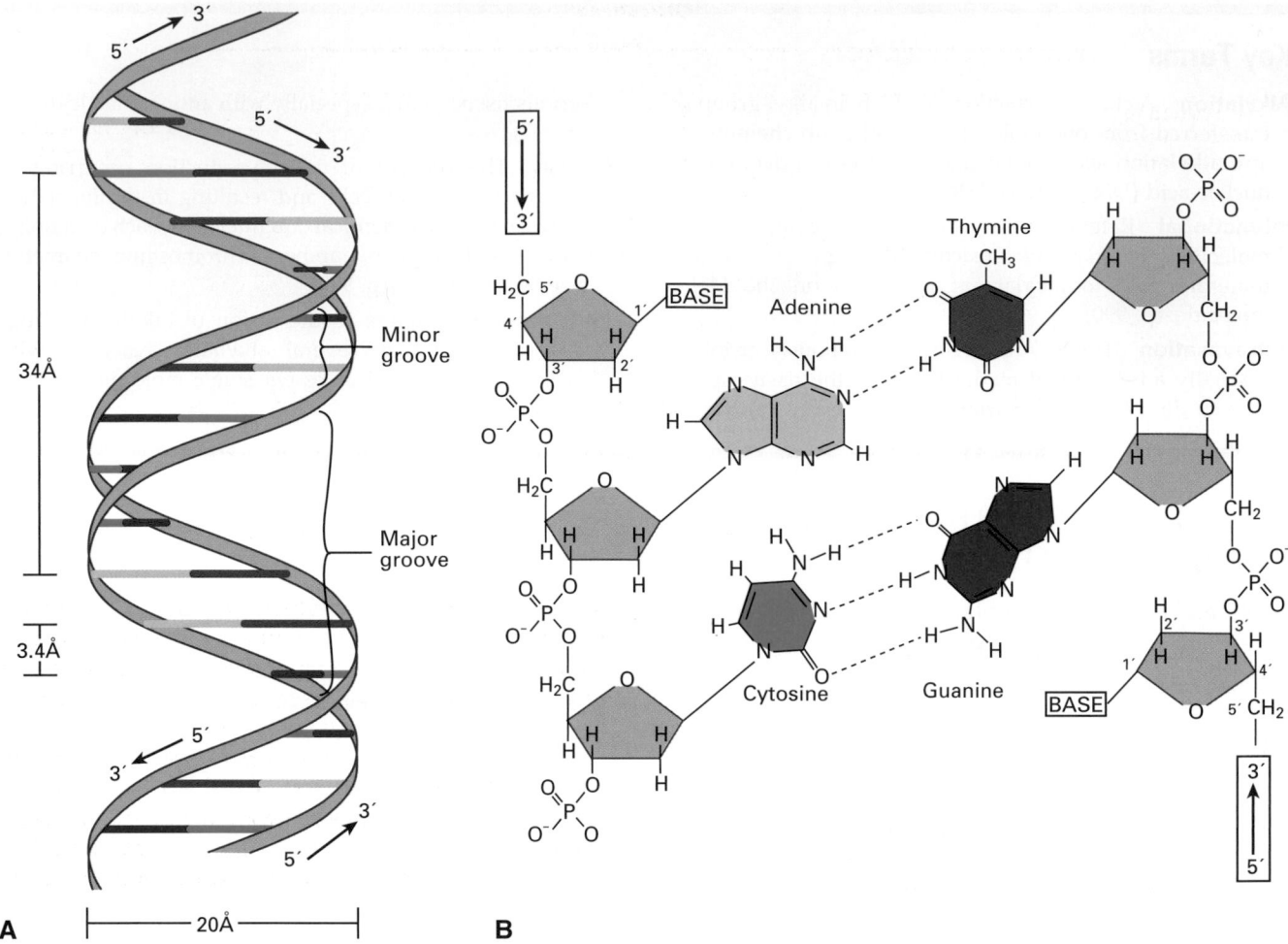

FIG. 53-1 Deoxyribonucleic acid (DNA) double helix. **A.** Diagrammatic model of the helical structure, showing its dimensions, the major and minor grooves, the periodicity of the bases, and the antiparallel orientation of the backbone chains (represented by ribbons). The base pairs (represented by rods) are perpendicular to the axis and lie stacked one on another. **B.** The chemical structure of the backbone and bases of DNA, showing the sugar–phosphate linkages of the backbone and the hydrogen bonding between the base pairs. There are two hydrogen bonds between adenine and thymine and three between cytosine and guanine. (From: Dorland, W. A. N. (2012). *Dorland's illustrated medical dictionary* (32nd ed.). Philadelphia, PA: Saunders.)

During the normal process of reproduction, the double helix uncoils and its two strands separate. A strand of RNA is then assembled next to each single DNA strand in a process known as *transcription*. RNA strands, in turn, are involved in both protein synthesis (translation) and replication of the original DNA structure before cell division, or **mitosis**. These processes ultimately result in the creation of a new cell with the same DNA sequence, and thus the same characteristics, as its parent cell.

Alkyl groups that are part of the structure of antineoplastic alkylating drugs attach to DNA molecules by forming covalent bonds with the bases described earlier. As a result, abnormal chemical bonds form between the adjacent DNA strands, which leads to the formation of defective nucleic acids that are then unable to perform the normal cellular reproductive functions mentioned previously. This leads to cell death.

Alkylating drugs can be characterized by the number of alkylation reactions in which they can participate.

Bifunctional alkylating drugs have two reactive alkyl groups that are able to alkylate two sites on the DNA molecule. **Polyfunctional** alkylating drugs can participate in several alkylation reactions. Figure 53-2 shows the location along the DNA double helix where the alkylating drugs work.

Indications

The most commonly used alkylating drugs today are effective against a wide spectrum of malignancies, including both solid and circulating tumours. Common examples of the various types of cancer that different alkylating drugs are used to treat are listed in the Dosages table on p. 992.

Adverse Effects

Alkylating drugs are capable of causing all of the dose-limiting adverse effects described in Chapter 44. Other adverse effects are described in Table 53-1. The relative

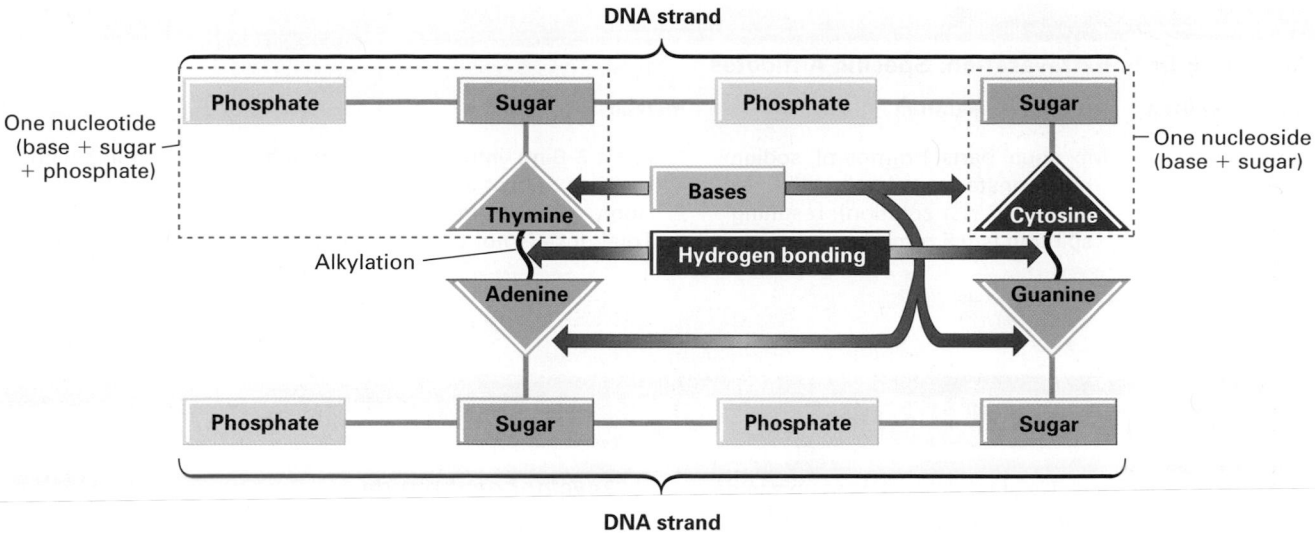

FIG. 53-2   Organization of deoxyribonucleic acid (DNA) and site of action of alkylating drugs.

TABLE	53-1

Commonly Used Alkylating Drugs: Severe Adverse Effects

Alkylating Drug	Severe Adverse Effects
busulfan	Pulmonary fibrosis
carboplatin*	Nephrotoxicity, neurotoxicity, bone marrow suppression
cisplatin	Nephrotoxicity, peripheral neuropathy, ototoxicity
cyclophosphamide	Hemorrhagic cystitis

*Carboplatin has less nephrotoxicity and neurotoxicity but more bone marrow suppression than cisplatin.

emetic potential of the alkylating drugs is given in Box 52-1. The adverse effects of these drugs are important because of their severity, but they can often be prevented or minimized by prophylactic measures. For instance, nephrotoxicity from cisplatin can often be prevented by adequately hydrating the patient with intravenous (IV) fluids.

Drug **extravasation** occurs when an IV catheter punctures the vein and medication leaks (infiltrates) into the surrounding tissues. With cancer chemotherapy drugs, in particular doxorubicin (a cytotoxic antibiotic), extravasation can cause severe tissue damage and necrosis (tissue death). Extravasation antidotes for select drugs are listed in Table 53-2.

Interactions

Only a few alkylating drugs are capable of causing significant drug interactions. The most important guideline for preventing such drug interactions is to avoid administering an alkylating drug with any other drug capable of causing similar toxicities. For example, a major adverse effect of cisplatin is nephrotoxicity. Therefore, if possible, do not administer it with a drug such

as an aminoglycoside antibiotic (gentamicin sulphate, tobramycin, or amikacin sulphate) because of the resulting additive nephrotoxic effects and hence the increased likelihood of kidney failure. Cyclophosphamide has a significant bone marrow–suppressing effect and ideally should not be administered with radiation therapy or with other drugs that suppress the bone marrow. In general, the nurse needs to work with available pharmacy and oncology staff to proactively anticipate (and avoid, if possible) undesirable drug and treatment interactions.

Dosages

For dosage information on selected alkylating drugs, refer to the Dosages table on p. 992. It is important to note that dosages are highly variable based on type of cancer, previous drugs used, and concurrent drug administration.

CYTOTOXIC ANTIBIOTICS

The cytotoxic antibiotics consist of natural substances produced by the mould *Streptomyces* as well as semisynthetic substances in which chemical changes have been made to the natural molecule. The most common toxicity of cytotoxic antibiotics is bone marrow suppression. The one exception is bleomycin, which instead causes pulmonary toxicity (pulmonary fibrosis and pneumonitis). Other severe toxicities associated with the use of cytotoxic antibiotics are heart failure (daunorubicin hydrochloride) and, in rare cases, acute left ventricular failure (doxorubicin). The available cytotoxic antibiotics, categorized according to the specific subclass to which they belong, are as follows:

Anthracyclines
- daunorubicin hydrochloride
- doxorubicin hydrochloride
- epirubicin hydrochloride

TABLE 53-2

Alkylating Drug Extravasation: Specific Antidotes

Alkylating Drug	Antidote Preparation	Method
carmustine	Mix equal parts 1 mmol/mL sodium bicarbonate (premixed) with sterile NS (1:1 solution); resulting solution is 0.5 mmol/mL	1. Inject 2–6 mL intravenously through the existing line with multiple Subcut injections into the extravasated site. 2. Apply cold compresses. 3. Total dose is not to exceed 10 mL of 0.5 mmol/mL solution.

NS, normal saline; *Subcut*, subcutaneous.

DRUG PROFILES

The most widely used alkylating drugs, based on standard treatment protocols, are profiled here. Information for drugs also appears in the Dosages table below.

▶▶ cisplatin

Cisplatin is an antineoplastic drug that contains platinum in its chemical structure. It is classified as a probable alkylating drug because it is believed to destroy cancer cells in the same way as the classic alkylating drugs, by forming crosslinks with DNA, thereby preventing its replication. It is also considered a bifunctional alkylating drug.

Cisplatin is used for the treatment of many solid tumours, such as bladder, testicular, and ovarian tumours. It is available only in injectable form.

▶▶ cyclophosphamide

Cyclophosphamide (Procytox®) is a nitrogen mustard derivative that was discovered during the course of research to improve mechlorethamine hydrochloride. It is a polyfunctional alkylating drug and is a prodrug requiring *in vivo* activation. It is used in the treatment of cancers of the bone and lymph nodes, as well as of other solid tumours. Cyclophosphamide is also used in the treatment of leukemias and multiple myeloma, as well as for non–cancer-related illnesses such as prophylaxis for rejection of kidney, heart, liver, and bone marrow transplants and the treatment of severe rheumatoid disorders. It is available in both oral and injectable dosage forms.

DOSAGES   Selected Alkylating Drugs

Drug	Pharmacological Subclass	Usual Dosage Range*	Indications
▶▶cisplatin	Platinum coordination complex	*Adults and children* IV: 50–75 mg/m² q3–4 wk or 15–20 mg/m² daily × 5 days q3–4 wk	Palliation for bladder cancer and for metastatic testicular and ovarian cancers
▶▶cyclophosphamide (Procytox)	Classic alkylator	IV: 10–20 mg/kg daily × 2–5 days (many other regimens as well)	HL, NHL; leukemia, breast and ovarian cancer; retinoblastoma; almost every solid tumour

HL, Hodgkin's lymphoma; *IV*, intravenous; *NHL*, non-Hodgkin's lymphoma.
*Note: Dosages are highly variable unless indicated otherwise.

- idarubicin hydrochloride
- valrubicin

Other cytotoxic antibiotics

- bleomycin sulphate (which is actually a cell cycle–specific drug)
- dactinomycin
- mitomycin hydrochloride
- mitoxantrone

Mechanism of Action and Drug Effects

Cytotoxic antibiotic antineoplastic drugs are cell cycle–nonspecific drugs. They interact with DNA through a process called *intercalation*, in which the drug molecule is inserted between the two strands of a DNA molecule, ultimately blocking DNA synthesis. These drugs inhibit the enzyme topoisomerase II, which leads to DNA strand breaks. Many of these drugs are able to generate free radicals, which also leads to DNA strand breaks and programmed cell death.

Indications

Cytotoxic antibiotics are used to treat a variety of solid tumours and some hematological malignancies as well. Commonly used examples of these drugs and the

TABLE   53-3

Cytotoxic Antibiotics: Severe Adverse Effects

Drug	Severe Adverse Effects
bleomycin sulphate	Pulmonary fibrosis, pneumonitis
dactinomycin, daunorubicin hydrochloride	Liver toxicity, tissue damage in the event of extravasation, heart failure
doxorubicin hydrochloride, idarubicin hydrochloride	Liver and cardiovascular toxicities
mitomycin hydrochloride	Liver, kidney, and lung toxicities
mitoxantrone	Cardiovascular toxicity

BOX 53-1

Treatment of Doxorubicin Hydrochloride Extravasation

1. Cool the site to patient tolerance for 24 hours.
2. Elevate and rest the extremity for 24 to 48 hours, and then have the patient resume normal activity as tolerated.
3. If pain, erythema, or swelling persists beyond 48 hours, discuss with the health care provider the need for surgical intervention or other treatment options.

Data from the US National Cancer Institute website, available at http://www.cancer.gov/, as well as the Health Canada Drug Database, http://www.hc-sc.gc.ca/dhp-mps/prodpharma/databasdon/index-eng.php, and http://www.bccancer.bc.ca. For additional information, see http://www.oncolink.com.

malignancies they are used to treat are given in the Dosages table on p. 994.

Adverse Effects

As with all of the antineoplastic drugs, cytotoxic antibiotics have the undesirable effects of hair loss, nausea and vomiting, and myelosuppression. The emetic potential of the drugs in this category is given in Box 52-1. Major adverse effects specific to the cytotoxic antibiotics are listed in Table 53-3.

Toxicity and Management of Overdose

Severe cases of cardiomyopathy are associated with large cumulative doses of doxorubicin. Routine monitoring of cardiac ejection fraction with multiple-gated acquisition (MUGA) scans, cumulative dose limitations, and the use of cytoprotectant drugs such as dexrazoxane can decrease the incidence of this devastating toxicity. Box 53-1 outlines the management of doxorubicin extravasation.

Interactions

The cytotoxic antibiotics that are used in chemotherapy interact with many drugs. They all tend to produce increased toxicities when used in combination with other chemotherapeutic drugs or with radiation therapy. Some drugs, most notably bleomycin sulphate and doxorubicin, have been known to cause serum digoxin levels to increase. Observe patients receiving one of these drugs along with digoxin for signs of digoxin toxicity. Dosage reduction or elimination of digoxin therapy may be indicated (see Chapter 25).

Dosages

For dosage information on selected cytotoxic antibiotics, refer to the Dosages table on p. 994.

 DRUG PROFILES

▸▸doxorubicin hydrochloride

Doxorubicin hydrochloride (Adriamycin PFS®) is used in many combination chemotherapy regimens. The drug is contraindicated in patients with a known hypersensitivity to it, patients with severe myelosuppression, and patients who are at risk for severe cardiac toxicity because they have already received a large cumulative dose of any of the anthracycline antineoplastics. It is available only in injectable form. Doxorubicin is also available in a liposomal drug delivery system (Caelyx®, Myocet®). In this dosage formulation, the drug is encapsulated in a lipid molecule bilayer called a *liposome*. The advantages of liposomal encapsulation are reduced systemic toxicity and increased duration of action. Liposomal encapsulation extends the biological half-life of doxorubicin to 50 to 60 hours and increases its affinity for cancer cells. The liposomal dosage formulation is currently indicated for the treatment of ovarian cancer, metastatic breast cancer, and AIDS-related Kaposi's sarcoma.

mitoxantrone hydrochloride

Mitoxantrone hydrochloride is indicated for the treatment of acute nonlymphocytic leukemia and metastatic carcinoma of the breast. It is also indicated for relapsed adult leukemia and for patients with lymphoma or hepatoma. It is available only in injectable form.

DOSAGES   Selected Cytotoxic Antibiotics

Drug	Pharmacological Subclass	Usual Dosage Range*	Indications
Anthracycline Antibiotics			
▸▸doxorubicin hydrochloride, conventional (Adriamycin®)	Anthracycline	IV: 60–75 mg/m² as a single injection given q21 days	Multiple cancers, including breast, bone, and ovarian, and leukemia, neuroblastoma, HL, NHL
doxorubicin hydrochloride, liposomal (Caelyx, Myocet®)	Anthracycline	IV: 20–50 mg/m² q3–4 wk for as long as tolerated and tumour is responsive to treatment	AIDS-related Kaposi's sarcoma when other chemotherapy drugs have failed or patient is intolerant of them; recurrent metastatic ovarian cancer
Anthracenedione Antibiotics			
mitoxantrone hydrochloride	Anthracenedione	IV: 14 mg/m² q3 wk	Metastatic breast cancer, acute myelocytic leukemia, lymphoma, hepatoma

AIDS, acquired immunodeficiency syndrome; *HL*, Hodgkin's lymphoma; *IV*, intravenous; *NHL*, non-Hodgkin's lymphoma.
*Dosages listed are for adults.

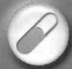

DRUG PROFILES

The various drugs in the miscellaneous category of antineoplastics are used to treat a wide range of cancers. Hydroxyurea and imatinib are administered orally. Bevacizumab and mitotane are available only in injectable form.

bevacizumab

Bevacizumab (Avastin®) was the first antineoplastic drug in a new category, that of the angiogenesis inhibitors. *Angiogenesis* is the creation of new blood vessels that supply oxygen and other blood nutrients to growing tissues. In the case of malignant tumours, angiogenesis that occurs within the tumour mass promotes continued tumour growth. As a tumour enlarges, its central tissues gradually die off (*necrosis*). However, its outer portion continues to grow, often to fatal proportions. Thus, inhibiting this process offers a promising new mechanism for antineoplastic drug action. Bevacizumab is a recombinant "humanized" monoclonal immunoglobulin G1 antibody derived from mouse antibodies. The scientific name for any compound derived from mouse tissue is *murine*. *Humanization* refers to the use of recombinant DNA techniques to make animal-derived antibody proteins more genetically similar to those of humans. It works by binding to and inhibiting the biological activity of human vascular endothelial growth factor (VEGF). VEGF is an endogenous protein that normally promotes angiogenesis in the body.

Bevacizumab is available only in injectable form. The only recognized contraindication is severe drug allergy or allergy to other murine products. It is approved for the treatment of metastatic colon cancer, rectal cancer in combination with 5-flurouracil (see Chapter 44), non–small cell lung cancer, and malignant glioblastoma. Bevacizumab was approved for the treatment of breast cancer; however, this indication was revoked by Health Canada.

Adverse reactions to bevacizumab include those affecting the cardiovascular system (hypertension or hypotension, deep vein thrombosis), central nervous system (CNS) pain (headache, dizziness, asthenia), skin (alopecia, dry skin), metabolism (weight loss, hypokalemia), gastrointestinal (GI) tract (nausea, vomiting, diarrhea, abdominal pain, constipation, GI hemorrhage), kidneys (nephrotoxicity with proteinuria), hematopoietic system (leukopenia [see Lab Values box]), and respiratory tract (infection). More severe effects can occur in any of these systems but are much less common than those listed. Drug interactions reported to date are limited but include potentiation of the cardiotoxic effects of the anthracycline antibiotics such as doxorubicin.

hydroxyurea

Hydroxyurea (Hydrea®) is an antimetabolite that interferes with the synthesis of DNA by inhibiting the incorporation of thymidine into DNA. More specifically, it

MISCELLANEOUS ANTINEOPLASTICS

The miscellaneous antineoplastic drugs are those that, because of their unique structure and mechanism of action, cannot be classified into the previously described categories. However, some drugs that are originally classified as miscellaneous drugs are later reclassified as more

is learned about their mechanisms of action and other characteristics. Drugs currently in the miscellaneous category include bevacizumab, everolimus, hydroxyurea (which is actually cell cycle–specific), imatinib, mitotane, ofatumumab, pazopanib hydrochloride, romidepsin, sorafenib tosylate, sunitinib malate, hormonal drugs, and radioactive and related antineoplastic drugs. Selected miscellaneous drugs are profiled in the following sections.

DRUG PROFILES—cont'd

inhibits ribonucleotide reductase, which is involved in conversion of ribonucleotides to deoxyribonucleotides. It works primarily in the S and G_1 phases of the cell cycle (refer to Figure 52-2 in Chapter 52), which makes it a cell cycle–specific drug. It is discussed in this chapter because it is included as a miscellaneous drug.

It is used in the treatment of squamous cell carcinoma together with radiation to take advantage of its radiosensitizing activity. It is also used in the treatment of various types of leukemia. The drug is available only in oral form. Adverse reactions include edema, drowsiness, headache, rash, hyperuricemia, nausea, vomiting, dysuria, myelosuppression, elevated liver enzyme levels, muscular weakness, peripheral neuropathy, nephrotoxicity, dyspnea, and pulmonary fibrosis. Hydroxyurea interacts with the anti-HIV drugs zidovudine and didanosine (see Chapter 45), which can actually have a synergistic effect with hydroxyurea. Concurrent use of hydroxyurea with fluorouracil increases the risk of neurotoxic symptoms. Because hydroxyurea can reduce the clearance of cytarabine, dosage reduction of cytarabine is recommended when the two are used concurrently.

imatinib mesylate

Imatinib mesylate (Gleevec®) is the standard of care for the treatment of chronic myeloid leukemia (CML). It works by inhibiting the action of a key enzyme (bcr-abl tyrosine kinase) responsible for causing CML. Although its name sounds similar to those of various monoclonal antibody drugs, imatinib is not a monoclonal antibody but rather a targeted therapy. It is available only in oral form. Common adverse reactions include fatigue, headache, rash, fluid retention, GI and hematological effects, musculoskeletal pain, cough, and dyspnea. Potential drug interactions are numerous and involve other drugs metabolized by cytochrome P450 liver enzymes. Examples include amiodarone hydrochloride, verapamil hydrochloride, warfarin sodium, azole antifungals, antidepressants, and antibiotics. A pharmacist may be needed to review the patient's medication regimen and adjust dosages or delete medications accordingly, in collaboration with the patient's health care provider.

mitotane

Mitotane (Lysodren®) is an adrenal cytotoxic drug that is indicated specifically for the treatment of inoperable adrenal corticoid carcinoma. Mitotane modifies the peripheral metabolism of steroids as well as directly suppressing the adrenal cortex. The drug alters the extra-adrenal metabolism of cortisol in humans, leading to a reduction in measurable 17-hydroxy corticosteroids, and causes increased formation of 6-β-hydroxy cortisol. It is available only in oral form. Adverse reactions include CNS depression, rash, nausea, vomiting, muscle weakness, and headache. Reported drug interactions include enhanced CNS depressive effects when taken concurrently with other CNS depressants (e.g., benzodiazepines). Mitotane may also increase the clearance of both warfarin sodium and phenytoin, reducing their effects. The potassium-sparing diuretic spironolactone may negate the effects of mitotane.

octreotide acetate

Octreotide acetate (Ocphyl®, Sandostatin®; see Chapter 31) is a unique medication used for the management of a cancer-related condition called *carcinoid crisis* and treatment of the diarrhea caused by vasoactive intestinal peptide–secreting tumours (VIPomas).

HORMONAL ANTINEOPLASTICS

Hormonal drugs are used in the treatment of a variety of cancers. The rationale is that sex hormones act to accelerate the growth of some common types of malignant tumours, particularly certain types of breast and prostate cancers. Therefore, therapy may involve administration of hormones with opposing effects (i.e., male versus female hormones) or drugs that block the body's sex hormone receptors. Some of the more commonly used hormonal drugs for cancers, such as breast cancer—which occur more commonly in women but also can occur in men—include the selective estrogen receptor modulator tamoxifen, the progestins megestrol acetate and medroxyprogesterone acetate, the aromatase inhibitors letrozole, anaztrozole, and exemestane, and the estrogen receptor antagonist fulvestrant. For cancers that occur in men, such as prostate cancer, the following drugs are used: the antiandrogens bicalutamide, abiraterone, cyproterone, enzalutamide, flutamide, and nilutamide; and the antineoplastic hormone estramustine phosphate sodium. The most common adverse effects of these drugs used to treat female and male cancers are listed in Table 53-4.

RADIOPHARMACEUTICALS AND RELATED ANTINEOPLASTICS

Antineoplastic drugs that are usually administered only by health care providers include porfimer sodium and various radioactive pharmaceuticals (radiopharmaceuticals). Porfimer sodium is used to treat esophageal or bronchial tumours that are present on the surface mucosa. The medication is given intravenously, and administration is followed by one or more sessions of laser light therapy to the esophageal or bronchial mucosa for direct tumour lysis and manual debridement. Radiopharmaceuticals are used to treat a variety of cancers and symptoms caused by cancers. Five commonly used radioisotopes are chromic phosphate P 32 (for cancer-induced peritoneal or pleural effusions),

TABLE 53-4

Hormonal Antineoplastics: Adverse Effects

Class	Drug	Adverse Effects
Aromatase inhibitors	anastrozole	Vasodilation, hypertension, hot flashes, mood disorders, weakness, arthritis
Selective estrogen receptor modulators	tamoxifen	Hypertension, peripheral edema, mood disorders, depression, hot flashes, nausea, weakness
Progestins	megestrol acetate, medroxyprogesterone acetate	Hypertension, chest pain, headache, weight gain, hepatotoxicity, dizziness, abdominal pain
Estrogen receptor antagonists	fulvestrant	Vasodilation, pain, headache, hot flashes, nausea, vomiting, pharyngitis
Antiandrogens	bicalutamide, flutamide, nilutamide	Peripheral edema, pain, hot flashes, gynecomastia, anemia, nausea, diarrhea
Gonadotropin-releasing hormone agonists	leuprolide, goserelin acetate	Rash, pain on injection, alopecia, body odour
Antineoplastic hormone	estramustine phosphate sodium	Edema, dyspnea, leg cramps, breast tenderness, nausea, anorexia, diarrhea

---

✎ LAB VALUES RELATED TO DRUG THERAPY

Rationales for Assessment and Monitoring of Blood Cell Counts With Antineoplastics

Laboratory Test	Normal Ranges	Rationale for Assessment
Leukocytes (WBCs)	$5–10 \times 10^9$/L	WBCs are protection against infection and, when an infection develops, the WBCs attack and destroy the causative bacteria, viruses, or other organisms. In response to the infection, WBCs increase in number dramatically. If WBCs are decreased from antineoplastic treatment and subsequent bone marrow suppression, and if they decrease to levels below 2×10^9/L (leukopenia), there is a high risk for severe infection and immunosuppression.
WBC components: Neutrophils	47–77% or above 1.5×10^9/L	The major types of WBCs are neutrophils, lymphocytes, monocytes, eosinophils, and basophils. Immature neutrophils are called *band neutrophils* and their number, along with neutrophil counts, provides a picture of the patient's immune system. If neutrophils are decreased to levels of less than 0.5×10^9/L (neutropenia), then there is risk for severe infection. If band neutrophils are included in the WBC differential count, then an abnormally low value reinforces the risk for severe infection (see Chapter 52).
Band neutrophils	0–3%	
Nadir	See normal range of each blood cell	*Nadir* refers to the lowest levels of bone marrow cells reached. The time to reach this nadir may become shorter and the recovery time longer with successive courses of antineoplastic treatment. A general estimate of the time to nadir is 10 to 28 days. Anticipation of the nadir allows the oncologist and health care team to develop a preventative treatment plan, which may include biological response modifiers and antibiotics.

WBCs, white blood cells.

Note: Similar information on red blood cells and platelet counts is given in Chapter 52. Also note that chemotherapy may be discontinued with anemia, leukopenia, neutropenia, or thrombocytopenia. Once counts recover (sometimes more quickly with certain drugs than with others), treatment is often reinitiated.

---

samarium SM 153 lexidronam (for bone cancer pain), sodium iodide I 131 (for thyroid cancer and hyperthyroidism), sodium phosphate P 32 (for various leukemias and palliative treatment of bone metastases), and strontium Sr 89 chloride (for bone cancer pain). One drug used in the treatment of various forms of non-Hodgkin's lymphoma is yttrium Y 90 ibritumomab tiuxetan (yttrium 90–labeled CD20 antibody [Zevalin®]). These medications are usually administered by nuclear medicine specialists.

NURSING PROCESS

Antineoplastics are some of the most toxic drugs given to patients (see Chapter 52) and because of their toxicities, serious complications and adverse effects may occur. Nursing care must be based on a thorough knowledge of cancer, its treatment, and the subsequent effects of different treatment modalities. The nurse should also bear in mind the potential of medication errors occurring with the administration of some of these drugs, such as errors that occur from confusing drugs with "sound-alike" names (see Preventing Medication Errors: Sound-Alike Drugs: "Rubicins"). This chapter presents information about cell cycle–nonspecific, hormonal, and miscellaneous antineoplastic drugs, whereas Chapter 52 covers cell cycle–specific antineoplastic drugs.

Assessment

Begin the overall assessment of patients taking any of the drugs discussed in this chapter with a thorough nursing history, medication profile, and past and present medical history. Measure and record vital signs. Document the presence of conditions that represent cautions or contraindications as well as potential drug interactions. Perform a head-to-toe physical assessment that includes attention to the following: skin turgor, including level of moisture and integrity of the skin and oral mucosa; baseline level of neurological functioning including level of consciousness, alertness, motor and sensory intactness, reflexes, and presence of any abnormal sensations; bowel sounds, bowel patterns, and inquiry into any problems such as diarrhea, constipation, nausea, vomiting, or reflux; urinary patterns and colour, amount, and odour of urine; breath sounds as well as respiratory rate, rhythm, and depth; and heart sounds. Laboratory tests that may be ordered include fluid and electrolyte levels (sodium, potassium, chloride, magnesium, calcium), red blood cell (RBC) and white blood cell (WBC) counts, hemoglobin, hematocrit, kidney and liver function tests, and serum protein–albumin levels.

For patients receiving alkylating drugs, bone marrow suppression (with carboplatin), pulmonary fibrosis (with busulfan), nephrotoxicity or neurotoxicity (more with cisplatin than carboplatin), and hemorrhagic cystitis (with cyclophosphamide) may occur; thus, perform an appropriate and thorough nursing assessment (see Assessment in Chapter 52). Assess deep tendon reflexes and baseline hearing level, and document the findings. Assess results of any baseline pulmonary function testing and perform a thorough respiratory assessment. High-dose cyclophosphamide may lead to hemorrhagic cystitis; therefore, document urinary patterns and any abnormal symptoms. Note hydration status before administering cyclophosphamide to avoid hemorrhagic cystitis.

One of the major adverse effects associated with the use of cytotoxic antibiotics (especially bleomycin) is pulmonary fibrosis. Medical testing (e.g., X-rays, pulmonary function tests, computed tomographic [CT] scans, magnetic resonance imaging [MRI] scans, arterial blood gas levels, and partial pressures of CO_2 and O_2) may be ordered to assess findings. When dactinomycin or daunorubicin hydrochloride are given intravenously, they are generally administered via a central line indwelling catheter device (e.g., Port-A-Cath® or MediPort®) because if they are given by peripheral IV line and extravasation occurs, there is a risk for necrosis with tissue sloughing that may erode through the layers of skin and underlying supportive structures (e.g., muscles, ligaments). See the previous discussion of extravasation as well as Table 53-2 and Box 53-2. In addition, in patients with documented cardiac disease or a history of thoracic irradiation, administer dactinomycin, daunorubicin hydrochloride, and doxorubicin with extreme caution due to cardiovascular toxicity. CT scans and ultrasound studies may be needed before and during treatment to assess cardiac ejection fraction because of the risk of cardiotoxicity, which is often associated with cumulative doses.

Prior to the use of hormonal antineoplastic drugs, obtain a thorough medical, nursing, and medication history. Many of the drugs included in this category are discussed in depth in Chapters 35 and 36, which also discuss aspects of the nursing process related to their use. Assessment associated with the use of estrogen antagonists, such as fulvestrant, tamoxifen, and andraloxifene hydrochloride, often begins with a review of the results of any tumour estrogen receptor assays, CT scans, X-rays, and other diagnostic testing. Perform a neurological assessment (see previous discussion and Chapters 35 and 52) with attention to baseline concerns of any pain, abnormal sensations, or headaches. Note any menopausal symptoms upon assessment because of the possible

PREVENTING MEDICATION ERRORS

Sound-Alike Drugs: "Rubicins"

The anthracycline chemotherapy drugs have the same sound-alike suffix and are often nicknamed the "rubicins." These drugs include daunorubicin hydrochloride, doxorubicin, epirubicin hydrochloride, idarubicin hydrochloride, and valrubicin. Even though these drugs are in the same class, their uses and drug effects are quite different. Medication errors have occurred because one "rubicin" was mistaken for another. It is important to refer to these drugs by their complete names rather than as a "rubicin."

BOX 53-2 **Concerns in the Handling and Administration of Vesicant Antineoplastic Drugs**

The handling and administration of antineoplastic drugs is of major concern because the nurse mixing and giving the drug may experience negative consequences. The pharmacy department is responsible for mixing these drugs, and preparation must be carried out carefully in an appropriate environment with use of a laminar airflow hood and personal protective equipment (mask, gown, gloves). All health care providers should also be familiar with their practice site policies as each institution may have slightly different protocols for handling and administering specific cytotoxic and non-cytotoxic hazardous medications. Many facilities recommend taking special precautions during the care of patients who are receiving chemotherapy, such as double-flushing patients' bodily secretions in the commode and using special hampers for the disposal of all items that come into contact with the patient. Special spill kits are employed to clean up the smallest chemotherapy spills. These precautions are necessary to protect health care providers from the cytotoxic effects of these drugs. In addition, appropriate and up-to-date knowledge about these drugs is important to safe and appropriate nursing care.

All nurses giving antineoplastic drugs must be certified to administer chemotherapy and must remain current in their scope of practice and secure in their competencies related to this treatment modality. All equipment and containers must be handled appropriately once infusion is completed. Hands and any exposed areas must be washed to ensure the safety of the health care provider. The British Columbia Cancer Agency (http://www.bccancer.bc.ca/) and the Canadian Association of Nurses in Oncology (http://www.cano-acio.ca/) offer exceptional resources for individuals involved in the care of patients receiving chemotherapy.

---

adverse effect of vasodilation and subsequent hot flashes. In addition, these drugs may cause nausea and vomiting, so a thorough GI assessment is beneficial.

Prior to the use of androgens (e.g., testosterone) in female patients, obtain a thorough gynecological history with attention to any menstrual issues or problems because of the adverse effect of menstrual irregularities. It is also important to assess the patient's body image and feelings of self-esteem because of the possible adverse effects of acne, hirsutism, and virilization in female patients as well as gynecomastia in male patients. See Chapter 36 for more information on the adverse effects of androgens.

Flutamide and nilutamide are antiandrogens and require thorough assessment of any heart diseases due to their potential to cause peripheral edema. This adverse effect could exacerbate any pre-existing heart disorder. Perform a thorough GI and gynecological assessment prior to the use of these drugs because of the possibility for nausea, diarrhea, and hot flashes. Documentation of the use of a reliable form of birth control is important because of teratogenic effects. Male sperm production may be affected (see Chapter 52), and a decline in sexual functioning or desire may occur because of these drugs' antiandrogenic effects. Before treatment, sperm can be frozen for future use in artificial insemination or other fertility treatments.

Prior to the use of gonadotropin-releasing hormone agonists, such as leuprolide and goserelin, assess patients for allergies to the drugs. Contraceptive history is important because women who are taking these drugs must use a nonhormonal contraceptive. Often, the health care provider will order laboratory tests for serum testosterone levels and prostatic acid phosphatase levels for male patients before and during therapy; an increase is normally noted during the initial week of therapy, and then levels return to baseline by 4 weeks from initiation.

For patients taking antiadrenal drugs (e.g., mitotane), in addition to performing a basic assessment, inquire about any GI disturbances because of the common adverse effects of nausea and vomiting. Miscellaneous antineoplastic drugs, glucocorticoids and mineralocorticoids may be given to prevent adrenal insufficiency and may also play a part in the therapeutic regimen. An understanding of baseline adrenal functioning through examination of laboratory test results is important.

With the miscellaneous drug hydroxurea, assessment of liver, kidney, neurological, and pulmonary function and baseline blood cell counts are important due to the adverse reactions associated with this drug. With use of bevacizumab, an angiogenesis inhibitor, assess cardiovascular, CNS, GI tract, and kidney functioning. Assess adverse effects of hypotension or hypertension, headache, pain, dizziness, nausea, vomiting, diarrhea, and nephrotoxicity.

☑ Nursing Diagnoses

- Decreased cardiac output related to the adverse effect of cardiotoxicity associated with cytotoxic antibiotics
- Diarrhea related to the adverse effects of antineoplastic drugs
- Imbalanced nutrition, less than body requirements, related to loss of appetite, nausea, and vomiting, as a result of antineoplastic therapy

☑ Planning

◼ Goals

- Patient's cardiac output will remain within normal limits while the patient is taking antineoplastics.
- Patient will experience minimal problems with alterations in bowel elimination (e.g., diarrhea).

- Patient will maintain adequate and balanced nutritional status while taking antineoplastics.

■ Expected Patient Outcomes

- Patient maintains normal blood pressure and heart rate while being monitored during therapy with cytotoxic antibiotics.
  - Patient demonstrates adequate knowledge for self-monitoring of daily blood pressure and pulse rate.
  - Patient understands the importance of taking daily weights.
  - Patient adheres to a daily heart-healthy regimen of conserving energy, planning activities, and asking for assistance with care and activities as needed.
- Patient or a family member or caregiver contacts health care providers immediately upon the occurrence of shortness of breath, high or low blood pressure or pulse rate, or chest pain.
- Patient states measures to prevent or decrease the occurrence of diarrhea during antineoplastic therapy, such as avoiding spicy foods, gas-producing foods, caffeine, high-fibre foods, alcohol, and extremely hot or cold foods and beverages.
  - Patient has preventative medication, as prescribed, such as synthetic opioids (e.g., loperamide hydrochloride) or adsorbents–protectants, to be taken to help with diarrhea.
- Patient maintains a daily regimen of healthy nutritional patterns, such as maintaining adequate fluid intake, maintaining a balanced diet as tolerated, avoiding foods that are irritating to the GI tract, and taking nutritional supplements as prescribed.

◢ Implementation

Before initiating drug therapy with the cell cycle–nonspecific drugs, hormonal antineoplastics, and miscellaneous antineoplastic drugs, the nurse must be completely knowledgeable about the given drug, its use, and its impact on all rapidly dividing cells, whether normal or malignant (see Chapters 52 and 53 for additional information).

Always handle alkylating drugs and all other antineoplastics with caution because of their possible carcinogenic, mutagenic, and teratogenic properties (see Box 53-2). Patients receiving alkylating drugs will more than likely experience problems related to bone marrow suppression, such as anemia, leukopenia, and thrombocytopenia (see Chapter 52 for specific interventions). Most nursing interventions are focused on preventing infection, conserving energy, preventing bleeding and injury, and reducing nausea. Other nursing considerations related to these drugs include taking vital signs every 1 to 2 hours or as needed during infusion, encouraging increased fluid intake, monitoring intake and output, following orders for IV therapy for hydration, and monitoring any vomiting. Contact the health care provider if vomiting is uncontrolled.

Monitor patients constantly for abnormal peripheral sensations, especially with the use of cisplatin. Report to the health care provider any numbness or tingling of extremities and any ringing or roaring in the ears or hearing loss. Encourage patients experiencing peripheral neuropathies to avoid extremely cold temperatures or the handling of cold objects. Cisplatin is particularly nephrotoxic, so monitor kidney function closely throughout therapy. IV hydration is often required at a rate of 100 to 200 mL/hr, starting before cisplatin administration with a total of 2000 to 3000 mL/day, depending on the dose of cisplatin and if not contraindicated. Do not use aluminum needles or administration sets with many of the alkylating-like drugs (e.g., cisplatin, olaxiplatin) because aluminum can degrade their platinum compounds; ensure that the proper infusion equipment is used. Because hemorrhagic cystitis is associated with cyclophosphamide use, make sure patients' hydration is maintained to minimize this adverse effect. Pulmonary toxicity may occur with some of the alkylating drugs, particularly busulfan; therefore, constantly monitor and be alert to cough, shortness of breath, and abnormal breath sounds. Immediately report these adverse effects to the prescriber. Other alkylating drugs may be given by various routes, such as intrapericardial, intratumoral, and intravesical. Be sure to perform appropriate interventions per the manufacturer's guidelines or facility policy. Reconstitute the parenteral formulations for any of these drugs according to the manufacturer's guidelines and suggestions. Not all diluents are compatible.

One important component of nursing care with alkylating drugs and their parenteral administration is continuous monitoring of the IV infusion site for signs and symptoms of infiltration. Infiltration could lead to extravasation of the medication into the surrounding tissue. To briefly review, IV infiltration is the leakage of fluids or blood from a dislodged catheter or needle cannula from the intima of the vein and into the surrounding tissue. Signs and symptoms of infiltration include inflammation at or near the insertion site, with swollen, taut, cool skin with pain and blanching; slowed or stopped IV infusion; and no backflow of blood into the IV tubing. The reason infiltration is of concern with alkylating drugs is that some of them are irritants and others are vesicants, carrying the potential of severe tissue damage. Therefore, if extravasation occurs with some of these drugs, the use of antidotes is required to try and prevent damage from leakage of the drug into the tissue. Specific antidotes for alkylating drugs are presented in Table 53-2. Always follow facility policy when treating extravasation of any medication. With IV infusions of antineoplastics, monitoring of the IV site and infusions is usually more frequent than with other medications, and some guidelines recommend hourly assessment. It is important to mention that the vast majority of chemotherapeutic drugs are administered via a central line indwelling catheter device (such as Port-A-Cath or MediPort). Check the device and its patency prior to the drug's administration.

Patients receiving cytotoxic antibiotics such as bleomycin may require very frequent monitoring of pulmonary function. Baseline chest X-rays may be obtained for comparison with subsequent X-rays if pneumonitis occurs. Monitor results of liver and kidney function tests throughout therapy with dactinomycin hydrochloride, daunorubicin, doxorubicin, or mitomycin hydrochloride. Assessing heart sounds, daily weights, blood pressure, and pulse rate, as well as monitoring for signs and symptoms of cardiovascular toxicities (e.g., alterations in vital signs, abnormal heart sounds, dyspnea, chest pain), is especially important with doxorubicin, idarubicin hydrochloride, and mitoxantrone. Additionally, if patients experience an increase of 1 kg or more in 24 hours or 2.3 kg or more in 1 week, notify the health care provider as this may reflect fluid retention related to heart failure. Mitomycin hydrochloride is associated with liver, kidney, and lung toxicities. Close monitoring of related systems during treatment is crucial to patient safety. As well, cytotoxic precautions (see previous discussion) and reverse isolation may be necessary, especially for patients who have neutropenia.

Use of hormone antagonists in the treatment of various cancers is common, particularly with breast and prostate cancer. Associated nursing interventions and patient education details related to the use of these hormone antagonists are discussed in depth in Chapters 35 and 36. Corticosteroid therapy and related nursing considerations are presented in Chapter 34.

Hydroxyurea is used sparingly but is a component of some treatment protocols. This drug is given orally. Monitor platelet and leukocyte counts of patients taking this drug due to the adverse effect of bone marrow suppression. Monitoring must be ongoing during therapy. If platelet count falls below $100 \times 10^9/L$ or leukocyte count falls below $2 \times 10^9/L$, therapy may need to be temporarily halted until counts rise toward normal values. See earlier discussion and Chapter 52 regarding nursing considerations associated with anemia, fatigue, weakness, bleeding tendencies, and infection. Additionally, hyperuricemia may precipitate gout-related symptoms (i.e., painful, swollen joints); report these to the health care provider so that the appropriate medication may be ordered. Often, a drug such as allopurinol is prescribed to help control high levels of uric acid caused by cell death from chemotherapy.

In addition to the nursing interventions discussed earlier and in Chapter 52, keep epinephrine, antihistamines, and anti-inflammatory drugs available in case of allergic or anaphylactic reactions. Each antineoplastic drug has its own peculiarities and its own set of cautions, contraindications, nursing implementations, and toxicities. Cytoprotective drugs are useful in reducing certain toxicities. For example, use of IV amifostine may help to

---

BOX 53-3

Indications of an Oncological Emergency

- Fever or chills with a temperature higher than 38.1°C
- New sores or white patches in the mouth or throat
- Swollen tongue with or without cracks and bleeding
- Bleeding gums
- Dry, burning, "scratchy," or "swollen" throat
- A cough that is new and persistent
- Changes in bladder function or patterns
- Blood in the urine
- Changes in GI or bowel patterns, including diarrhea lasting longer than 2 to 3 days, dyspepsia, nausea, vomiting, or constipation.
- Blood in the stool

_____

Note: The patient must contact the health care provider immediately if any of the listed signs or symptoms occurs. If the health care provider is not available, the patient must seek medical treatment at the closest emergency department.

---

reduce the kidney toxicity associated with cisplatin, and oral allopurinol may be given to reduce hyperuricemia (see Table 52-6 and Box 52-2). Other major concerns related to the care of patients receiving chemotherapy are the oncological emergencies that arise because of damage occurring to rapidly dividing normal cells as well as rapidly dividing cancerous cells. Some of the complications that are potential emergencies include infections, infusion reactions and allergies, stomatitis with severe ulceration, bleeding, metabolic aberrations, severe diarrhea, kidney failure, liver failure, and cardiotoxicity, including dysrhythmia or heart failure (Box 53-3).

Evaluation

Focus the evaluation of nursing care on determining whether goals and outcome criteria have been met, as well as on monitoring for therapeutic responses and adverse and toxic effects of antineoplastic therapy. Therapeutic responses may manifest as clinical improvement, decrease in tumour size, and decrease in metastatic spread. Evaluation of nursing care with reference to goals and outcomes may reveal improvements related to a decrease in adverse effects; decrease in the impact of cancer on the patient's well-being; increase in comfort, nutrition, and hydration; improved energy levels and ability to carry out activities of daily living; and improved quality of life. Goals and outcome criteria can be revisited to identify specific parameters to monitor. In addition, certain laboratory studies, such as measurement of tumour markers; levels of carcinoembryonic antigens; and RBC, WBC, and platelet counts may also be used to determine how well the goals and outcome criteria have been met. As part of the evaluation, health care providers may also order additional X-rays, CT scans, magnetic resonance imaging, tissue analyses, and other studies appropriate to the diagnosis, during and after antineoplastic therapy, at time intervals related to anticipated tumour response.

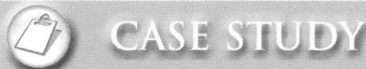 **CASE STUDY**

Chemotherapy With Alkylating Drugs

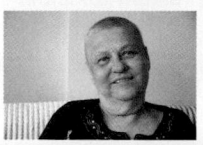 Antonia, a 50-year-old insurance auditor, is receiving cisplatin as part of treatment for ovarian cancer. She is receiving her third treatment today and has just arrived at the cancer treatment center for her outpatient infusion. Antonia says that she felt "okay" during the time between the last treatment and today but is not looking forward to today's treatment because of the adverse effects.

1. While the nurse prepares to start the infusion, what is important for the nurse to assess before beginning the chemotherapy?

2. What will the nurse do before the infusion to help reduce or prevent adverse effects?

3. During the infusion, Antonia mentions that she is hearing a slight "roaring" sound and that she feels a bit dizzy. What will the nurse do next?

4. After stopping the infusion, the nurse spills some of the chemotherapy solution on her arm and the floor. What is the nurse's priority action at this time?

_____

For answers, see http://evolve.elsevier.com/Canada/Lilley/pharmacology/.

PATIENT TEACHING TIPS

❖ Advise patients to avoid aspirin, ibuprofen, and products containing these drugs to help prevent excessive bleeding.

❖ Be open in discussion about the risk of alopecia (a complete discussion is presented in Chapter 52), an adverse effect of many of the antineoplastic drugs.

❖ Encourage patients to increase fluid intake up to 3 000 mL/day, if not contraindicated, to prevent dehydration and further weakening and, in the case of cyclophosphamide therapy, to prevent or help manage hemorrhagic cystitis.

❖ Constipation and diarrhea may be problematic, so educate patients about ways to help manage these alterations in bowel status that may be due to antineoplastic drugs or to opioids used for pain management. To help avoid constipation, increased intake of fluids and consumption of a balanced diet are important; however, oncologists often order either a stool softener or a mild noncramping laxative to prevent the problem. Diarrhea is generally treated with dietary restrictions and the use of antidiarrheals as ordered.

❖ The following are helpful online resources for patients and their family members and significant others: http://www.cancer.ca/en/, www.bccancer.bc.ca/, http://wellspring.ca/, http://www.hc-sc.gc.ca/hc-ps/dc-ma/cancer-eng.php, and www.oncolink.org/.

KEY POINTS

❖ Antineoplastics are drugs that are used to treat malignancies and are classified as cell cycle–specific drugs, cell cycle–nonspecific drugs, miscellaneous antineoplastics, and hormonal drugs.

❖ Cell cycle–specific drugs kill cancer cells during specific phases of the cell growth cycle, whereas the cell cycle–nonspecific drugs (discussed in this chapter) kill cancer cells during any phase of the growth cycle.

❖ Chemotherapy, or antineoplastic drug therapy, requires skillful and perceptive care, and the nurse must act prudently and make crucial decisions about the nursing care of patients receiving these drugs.

❖ Knowledge is important to ensure patient and health care provider safety and for protection from the adverse effects of antineoplastics.

❖ Always exercise extreme caution in the handling and administration of cell cycle–nonspecific (as well as cell cycle–specific) drugs.

❖ Hormonal drugs, both agonists and antagonists, are used to treat a variety of malignancies.

❖ Extravasation of strong vesicants (e.g., doxorubicin) may lead to severe tissue injury with complications such as permanent damage to muscles, tendons, and ligaments, and possible loss of a limb. Constantly monitor IV sites and infusions to prevent this possible complication. Checking the patency of central venous access devices is also important because the majority of chemotherapy drugs are given via this route.

❖ Oncological emergencies occur as a consequence of cell death and may be life-threatening. Skillful assessment and immediate intervention may help to decrease the severity of the problem or even reduce the occurrence of such emergencies.

EXAMINATION REVIEW QUESTIONS

1. A patient who is receiving chemotherapy with cisplatin has developed pneumonia. The nurse would be concerned about nephrotoxicity if which type of antibiotic was ordered as treatment for the pneumonia at this time?
   a. A penicillin
   b. A sulfa drug
   c. fluoroquinolone
   d. aminoglycoside

2. During treatment with doxorubicin (Adriamycin), the nurse must monitor closely for which potentially life-threatening adverse effect?
   a. Nephrotoxicity
   b. Peripheral neuritis
   c. Cardiomyopathy
   d. Ototoxicity

3. While teaching a patient who is about to receive cyclophosphamide (Procytox) chemotherapy, the nurse will instruct the patient to watch for which potential adverse effect?
   a. Cholinergic diarrhea
   b. Hemorrhagic cystitis
   c. Peripheral neuropathy
   d. Ototoxicity

4. When chemotherapy with alkylating drugs is planned, the nurse expects to implement which intervention to prevent nephrotoxicity?
   a. Hydrating the patient with IV fluids before chemotherapy
   b. Limiting fluids before chemotherapy
   c. Monitoring drug levels during chemotherapy
   d. Assessing creatinine clearance during chemotherapy

5. During therapy with the cytotoxic antibiotic bleomycin, the nurse will assess for a potentially serious adverse effect by what type(s) of monitoring?
   a. Blood urea nitrogen and creatinine levels
   b. Cardiac ejection fraction
   c. Respiratory function
   d. Cranial nerve function

6. While administering bevacizumab (Avastin), what will the nurse assess to monitor for drug-related toxicities? (Select all that apply.)
   a. Blood pressure
   b. Colour of the skin and sclera of the eye (for jaundice)
   c. Blood glucose level
   d. Urine protein level
   e. Hearing

7. The nurse is preparing to add a dose of bevacizumab (Avastin) to a patient's IV infusion. The dose is 70 mg of bevacizumab in 100 mL of normal saline, and it is to infuse over 90 minutes. The nurse will set the infusion pump to what rate for this dose?

Answers: 1. d, 2. c, 3. b, 4. a, 5. c, 6. a, d, 7. 67 mL/hour (66.66 rounds to 67)

CRITICAL THINKING ACTIVITIES

1. During an infusion of carmustine, a patient dislodges the IV catheter, and infiltration of the medication occurs. What is the nurse's priority action at this time? Explain your answer.

2. A patient has been receiving bleomycin irrigations through a chest tube for 3 days. Today he has begun to have an irregular and slow heart rhythm, as well as nausea, and says, "I'm seeing yellow hazy circles around the lights." He thinks the chemotherapy is causing these problems. The nurse reviews the patient's medications and notes that he is taking digoxin (Lanoxin®), lisinopril (Prinivil®), and simvastatin (Zocor®). What is the nurse's priority action at this time? Explain your answer.

3. During a prechemotherapy teaching session, a patient hears that she will be receiving a cytotoxic antibiotic as part of the medication regimen. The patient asks, "How can this drug help cancer? It's an antibiotic! Cancer is not an infection!" What is the nurse's best answer?

For answers, see http://evolve.elsevier.com/Canada/Lilley/pharmacology/.

CHAPTER 54

Biological Response–Modifying Drugs and Antirheumatic Drugs

Objectives

After reading this chapter, the successful student will be able to do the following:

1. Describe the basic anatomy, physiology, and functions of the immune system.

2. Compare the two major classes of biological response–modifying drugs: hematopoietic drugs and immunomodulating drugs.

3. Discuss the mechanisms of action, indications, dosages, routes of administration, adverse effects, cautions, contraindications, and drug interactions of the different biological response–modifying drugs.

4. Describe briefly the pathology associated with rheumatoid arthritis.

5. Discuss the mechanisms of action, indications, dosages, routes of administration, adverse effects, cautions, contraindications, and drug interactions of the different antirheumatic drugs.

6. Develop a collaborative plan of care that includes all phases of the nursing process for patients receiving biological response–modifying drugs and for those receiving antirheumatic drugs.

e-Learning Activities

Website
(http://evolve.elsevier.com/Canada/Lilley/pharmacology/)

evolve

- Answer Key—Textbook Case Studies
- Answer Key—Critical Thinking Activities
- Chapter Summaries—Printable
- Review Questions for Exam Preparation
- Unfolding Case Studies

Drug Profiles

abatacept, p. 1019
adalimumab, p. 1013
▸▸ aldesleukin, p. 1016
alemtuzumab, p. 1013
anakinra, p. 1016
belimumab, p. 1013
bevacizumab, p. 1013
canakinumab, p. 1010
certoizumab pegol, p. 1013
cetuximab, p. 1013
etanercept, p. 1019
▸▸ filgrastim, p. 1009
golimumab, p. 1013
infliximab, p. 1014
▸▸ interferon alfa-2b, interferon alfacon-1, peginterferon alfa-2a, peginterferon alfa-2b, p. 1011
▸▸ interferon beta-1a, interferon beta-1b, p. 1011
leflunomide, p. 1019
methotrexate, p. 1019
palivizumab, p. 1014
▸▸ rituximab, p. 1014
tofacitinib, p. 1019
trastuzumab, p. 1014
vedolizumab, p. 1010

▸▸ Key drug

Key Terms

Adjuvant A nonspecific immunostimulant that enhances overall immune function rather than stimulating the function of a specific immune system cell or cytokine through specific chemical reactions. (p. 1017)

Antibodies Immunoglobulin molecules (see Chapter 51) that have the ability to bind to and inactivate antigen molecules by forming an antigen–antibody complex; this process serves to inactivate foreign antigens that enter the body and are capable of causing disease. (p. 1006)

Antigen A biological or chemical substance that is recognized as foreign by the body's immune system. (p. 1005)

Arthritis Inflammation of one or more joints. (p. 1017)

Autoimmune disorder A disorder that occurs when the body's tissues are attacked by its own immune system. (p. 1017)

B lymphocytes (B cells) Leukocytes of the humoral immune system that develop into plasma cells and then produce the antibodies that bind to and inactivate antigens. B cells are one of the two principal types of lymphocytes; T lymphocytes are the other. (p. 1006)

Biological response–modifying drugs (BRMs) A broad class of drugs that includes hematopoietic drugs and immunomodulating drugs; often referred to as *biological response modifiers*, they alter the body's response to diseases such as cancer as well as autoimmune, inflammatory, and infectious diseases. Examples are cytokines (e.g., interleukin, interferons), monoclonal antibodies, and vaccines. They are also called *biomodulators* or *immunomodulating drugs*. Biological response–modifying drugs may be adjuvants, immunostimulants, or immunosuppressants. (p. 1005)

Cell-mediated immunity (CMI) All immune responses mediated by T lymphocytes (T cells); also called *cellular immunity*. Cell-mediated immunity acts in collaboration with humoral immunity. (p. 1006)

Colony-stimulating factors (CSFs) Cytokines that regulate the growth, differentiation, and function of bone marrow stem cells. (p. 1007)

Cytokines Nonantibody proteins released by specific cell populations (e.g., activated T cells) on contact with antigens. Cytokines act as intercellular mediators of an immune response. (p. 1006)

Cytotoxic T cells Differentiated T cells that can recognize and lyse (rupture) target cells that bear foreign antigens on their surfaces; also called *natural killer cells*. These antigens are recognized by the corresponding antigen receptors that are expressed (displayed) on the cytotoxic T cell surface. (p. 1006)

Differentiation The process of cellular development from a simplified into a more complex and specialized cellular structure; in hematopoiesis, the multistep processes involved in the maturation of blood cells. (p. 1008)

Disease-modifying antirheumatic drugs (DMARDs) Medications used in the treatment of rheumatic diseases that have the potential to arrest or slow the actual disease process instead of providing only anti-inflammatory and analgesic effects. (p. 1005)

Hematopoiesis All of the body's processes originating in the bone marrow that result in the formation of various types of blood components (adjective: *hematopoietic*); includes the three main processes of differentiation (see earlier): erythropoiesis (formation of red blood cells, or erythrocytes), leukopoiesis (formation of white blood cells, or leukocytes), and thrombopoiesis (formation of platelets, or thrombocytes). (p. 1005)

Humoral immunity All immune responses mediated by B cells, which ultimately work through the production of antibodies against specific antigens; humoral immunity acts in collaboration with cell-mediated immunity. (p. 1006)

Immunoglobulins Complex immune system glycoproteins that bind to and inactivate foreign antigens; synonymous with *immune globulins*. (p. 1006)

Immunomodulating drugs (IMDs) Various subclasses of biological response–modifying drugs that specifically or nonspecifically enhance or reduce immune responses; the three major types of immunomodulators, based on mechanism of action, are adjuvants, immunostimulants, and immunosuppressants (see Chapter 50). (p. 1005)

Immunostimulant A drug that enhances immune response through specific and nonspecific chemical interactions with particular immune system components; an example is interleukin-2. (p. 1016)

Immunosuppressant A drug that reduces immune response through specific chemical interactions with particular immune system components; an example is cyclosporine (see Chapter 50). (p. 1009)

Interferons One type of cytokine that promotes resistance to viral infections in uninfected cells and can also strengthen the body's immune response to cancer cells. (p. 1009)

Leukocytes All subtypes of white blood cells; leukocytes include granulocytes (neutrophils, eosinophils, and basophils), monocytes, and lymphocytes (B cells and T cells); some monocytes also develop into tissue macrophages. (p. 1006)

Lymphokine-activated killer (LAK) cells Cytotoxic T cells that have been activated by interleukin-2 and therefore have a stronger and more specific response against cancer cells than other cytotoxic T cells. (p. 1014)

Lymphokines Cytokines that are produced by sensitized T lymphocytes on contact with antigen particles. (p. 1006)

Memory cells Cells involved in the humoral immune system that remember the exact characteristics of a particular foreign invader or antigen for the purpose of an expediting immune response in the event of future exposure to this antigen. (p. 1006)

Monoclonal   A group of identical cells or organisms derived from a single cell. (p. 1006)

Plasma cells   Cells derived from B cells found in the bone marrow, connective tissue, and blood. They produce antibodies. (p. 1006)

Rheumatism   Any of several disorders characterized by inflammation, degeneration, or metabolic derangement of connective tissue structures, especially joints and related structures. (p. 1017)

T helper cells   Cells that promote and direct the actions of other cells of the immune system. (p. 1006)

T lymphocytes (T cells)   Leukocytes of the cell-mediated immune system; unlike B cells, they are not involved in the production of antibodies but instead occur in various cell subtypes (e.g., T helper cells, T suppressor cells, and cytotoxic T cells); they act through direct cell-to-cell contact or through production of cytokines that guide the functions of other immune system components (e.g., B cells, antibodies). (p. 1006)

T suppressor cells   Cells that regulate and limit the immune response, balancing the effects of T helper cells. (p. 1006)

Tumour antigens   Chemical compounds expressed on the surfaces of tumour cells. They signal to the immune system that these cells do not belong in the body, labelling the tumour cells as foreign. (p. 1005)

OVERVIEW OF IMMUNOMODULATORS

Over the last two decades, medical technology has developed a group of drugs whose primary site of action is the immune system. This has resulted in new additions to the class of drugs known as **biological response–modifying drugs (BRMs)**, or *biological response modifier(s)*. These drugs alter the body's response to diseases such as cancer and autoimmune, inflammatory, and infectious diseases. These drugs can enhance or restrict the patient's immune response to disease, can stimulate a patient's hematopoietic (blood-forming) function, and can prevent disease. *Hematopoiesis* is the collective term for all of the blood component–forming processes of the bone marrow. Two broad classes of BRMs are hematopoietic drugs and **immunomodulating drugs (IMDs)**. Subclasses of IMDs include interferons, monoclonal antibodies, interleukin receptor agonists and antagonists, and miscellaneous drugs. **Disease-modifying antirheumatic drugs (DMARDs)** are drugs used to treat rheumatoid arthritis, which is discussed later in the chapter.

IMDs therapeutically alter a patient's immune response. In cancer treatment, they make up the fourth type of cancer therapy, the others being surgery, chemotherapy, and radiation. The human immune system is most commonly viewed as the body's natural defence against pathogenic bacteria and viruses. However, it also has effective antitumour capabilities. An intact immune system can identify cells as malignant and destroy them. Normal cells are recognized as "self" and are not damaged, whereas tumour cells are recognized as "foreign" and are destroyed. People develop cancerous cells in their bodies on a regular basis. Normally, the immune system is able to eliminate these cells before they multiply to uncontrollable levels. It is only when natural immune responses fail to keep pace with these initially microscopic cancer cell growths that a person develops a true "cancer" that requires clinical intervention.

In terms of their activity against cancer cells, BRMs work by one of three mechanisms: (1) enhancement or restoration of the host's immune system defences against the tumour; (2) direct toxic effect on the tumour cells, which causes them to lyse, or rupture; or (3) adverse modification of the tumour's biology, which makes it difficult for the tumour cells to survive and reproduce.

Some IMDs are used to treat autoimmune, inflammatory, and infectious diseases. In these instances, the drug ideally functions either to reduce patients' inappropriate immune responses (in the case of inflammatory and autoimmune diseases, such as rheumatoid arthritis) or to strengthen the patient's immune response against microorganisms (especially viruses) and cancer cells. To better understand these complex drugs, a review of the physiology of the immune system is beneficial.

IMMUNE SYSTEM

The immune system is an intricate biological defence network of cells that are capable of distinguishing an unlimited variety of substances as being either foreign ("nonself") or a natural part of the host's or patient's body ("self"). When a foreign substance such as a bacterium or virus enters the body, the immune system recognizes it as being foreign and mounts an immune response to eliminate or neutralize the invader. Tumours are not truly foreign substances because they arise from cells of normal tissues whose genetic material (deoxyribonucleic acid [DNA] and ribonucleic acid [RNA]) has somehow mutated. Tumour cells express chemical compounds on their surfaces that signal to the immune system that these cells are a threat. These chemical markers are called *tumour antigens* or *tumour markers*, and they label the tumour cells as abnormal cells. An **antigen** is any substance that the body's immune system recognizes as foreign. Recognition of antigens varies among individuals, which is why some people are more prone than others to immune-related diseases such as allergies, inflammatory diseases, and cancer. The two major components of the body's immune system are **humoral immunity**, mediated by B cell functions (primarily antibody production), and **cell-mediated immunity (CMI)**, which is mediated by T cell functions. These two systems act together to recognize and destroy foreign particles and cells in the blood or other body tissues. Communication between these two divisions is vital to the success of the immune system as a whole. An attack against tumour cells by antibodies produced by the **B lymphocytes (B cells)** of the humoral immune system prepares those tumour cells for destruction by the **T lymphocytes (T cells)** of the cell-mediated immune system. This is just one example of the effective way that the two divisions of the immune system communicate with each other for a collaborative immune response.

Humoral Immune System

The functional cells of the humoral immune system are the B lymphocytes. They are also called *B cells* because they originate in the bone marrow. The B cells that are capable of generating a particular antibody normally remain dormant until the corresponding antigen is detected. When an antigen binds to receptors located on the B cells, a biochemical signal is sent to the B lymphocytes. These B cells then mature or *differentiate* into **plasma cells**, which in turn produce antibodies. **Antibodies** are **immunoglobulins** (large glycoprotein molecules; glyco = sugar; protein = amino acid chain) that bind to specific antigens, forming an antigen–antibody complex that inactivates disease-causing antigens.

The immune system in a healthy individual is genetically preprogrammed to be able to mount an antibody response against literally millions of different antigens. This ability results from the individual's lifetime antigen exposure and is further developed through exposure to new antigens and then passed down through many generations. Antibodies that a single plasma cell makes are all identical. They are therefore called **monoclonal** antibodies. Since the 1980s, monoclonal antibodies have also been prepared synthetically using recombinant DNA (rDNA) technology, which has resulted in new drug therapies.

There are five major types of naturally occurring immunoglobulins in the body: immunoglobulins A, D, E, G, and M. These unique types have different structures and functions and are found in various areas of the body. During an immune response, when B lymphocytes differentiate into plasma cells, some of these B cells become **memory cells**. Memory cells "remember" the exact characteristics of a particular foreign invader or antigen, which allows a stronger and faster immune response in the event of re-exposure to the same antigen. The cells of the humoral immune system are shown in Figure 54-1.

Cell-Mediated Immune System

The functional cells of the cell-mediated (as opposed to antibody-mediated) immune system are the T lymphocytes. They are also referred to as *T cells* because they

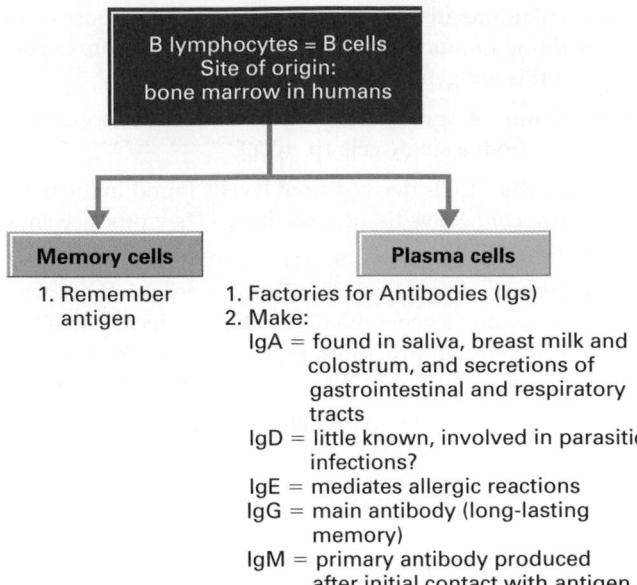

FIG. 54-1 Cells of the humoral (antibody-mediated) immune system. *Ig*, immunoglobulin.

mature in the thymus. There are three distinct populations of T cells: cytotoxic T cells, T-helper cells, and T-suppressor cells (Figure 54-2). They are distinguished by the different functions they perform. **Cytotoxic T cells** directly kill their targets by causing cell lysis or rupture. **T-helper cells** are considered the master controllers of the immune system—they direct the actions of many other immune components, such as lymphokines and cytotoxic T cells. **Cytokines** are nonantibody proteins that serve as chemical mediators of various physiological functions. **Lymphokines** are a subset of cytokines. They are released by T lymphocytes upon contact with antigens and serve as chemical mediators of the immune response. **T-suppressor cells** have an effect on the immune system that is opposite to that of T-helper cells, and they serve to limit or control the immune response. A healthy immune system has approximately twice as many T-helper cells as T-suppressor cells at any given time.

The major cells involved in the destruction of cancer cells are part of the cell-mediated immune system (see Figure 54-2). The cancer-killing cells of the cellular immune system are the macrophages (derived from monocytes), natural killer (NK) cells (another type of lymphocyte), and polymorphonuclear **leukocytes** (not lymphocytes), which are also called *neutrophils*. In contrast, T-suppressor cells have an important negative influence on antitumour actions of the immune system. Overactive T-suppressor cells may be responsible for clinically significant cancer cases by permitting tumour growth beyond the immune system's control.

BIOLOGICAL RESPONSE MODIFIERS

Therapy with BRMs combines the knowledge of several disciplines, including general biology, genetics,

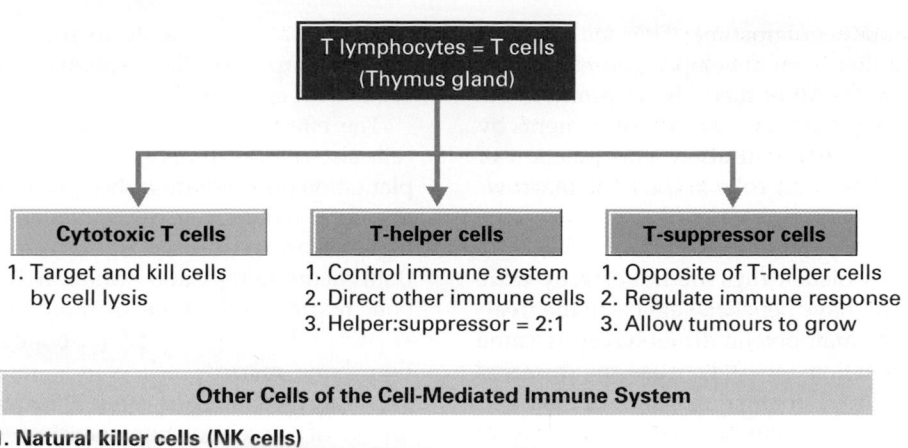

FIG. 54-2   Cells of the cellular immune system.

BOX 54-1   Biological Response Modifiers

Hematopoietic Drugs

Colony-Stimulating Factors
filgrastim (R-Methug-CSF)
pegfilgrastim

Other
darbepoetin alfa

Immunomodulating Drugs

Interferons
Interferon alfa-2a
interferon alfa-2b*
peginterferon alfa-2a
peginterferon alfa-2b
interferon beta-1a
interferon beta-1b

Monoclonal Antibodies
alemtuzumab
adalimumab
belimumab
bevacizumab
certolizumab
golimumab
infliximab
palivizumab

rituximab
trastuzumab

Interleukin Receptor Agonist and Antagonists
Agonist
aldesleukin (IL-2)

Antagonists
anakinra
tocilizumab

Miscellaneous Immunomodulators

Tumour Necrosis Factor Receptor Antagonist
etanercept

Retinoid Receptor Agonist
tretinoin

Adjuvants (Nonspecific Immunostimulants)
Bacille Calmette-Guérin vaccine
leflunomide
mitoxantrone
thalidomide
abatacept

_____

Il, interleukin.

immunology, pharmacology, medicine, and nursing. The general therapeutic effects of BRMs are as follows:
- Enhancement of hematopoietic function
- Regulation or enhancement of the immune response, including cytotoxic or cytostatic activity against cancer cells
- Inhibition of metastases, prevention of cell division, or inhibition of cell maturation

Box 54-1 lists the currently available BRM drugs used in the treatment of cancer and other illnesses that have

varying levels of immune system–related pathophysiology. The drugs are classified according to biological effects.

HEMATOPOIETIC DRUGS

Hematopoietic drugs include several medications developed over the past 10 to 15 years. Within this category are two erythropoietic drugs (epoetin alfa and darbepoetin alfa) and two **colony-stimulating factors**

(CSFs; filgrastim and pegfilgrastim). The one platelet-promoting drug that has been developed (oprelvekin) is not available in Canada. All of these drugs promote the synthesis of various types of major blood components by promoting the growth, **differentiation,** and function of their corresponding precursor cells in the bone marrow.

Mechanism of Action and Drug Effects

Although the hematopoietic drugs are not directly toxic to cancer cells, they do have beneficial effects in the treatment of cancer. All hematopoietic drugs have the same basic mechanism of action—they decrease the duration of chemotherapy-induced anemia and neutropenia and enable higher doses of chemotherapy to be given, decrease bone marrow recovery time after bone marrow transplantation or irradiation, and stimulate other cells in the immune system to destroy or inhibit the growth of cancer cells, as well as virus- or fungus-infected cells.

All of these drugs are produced by rDNA technology, which allows them to be essentially identical to their endogenously produced counterparts. These substances work by binding to receptors on the surfaces of specialized progenitor cells in the bone marrow. Progenitor cells are responsible for the production of three particular cell lines: red blood cells (RBCs), white blood cells (WBCs), and platelets. When a hematopoietic drug binds to a progenitor cell surface, the immature progenitor cell is stimulated to mature, proliferate (reproduce itself), differentiate (transform into its respective type of specialized blood component), and become functionally active. Hematopoietic drugs may enhance certain functions of mature cell lines as well. Epoetin alfa is a synthetic derivative of the human hormone erythropoietin, which is produced primarily by the kidneys. It promotes the synthesis of erythrocytes (RBCs) by stimulating RBC progenitor cells in the bone marrow. Darbepoetin alfa is a longer-acting form of epoetin alfa. These drugs are discussed in detail in Chapter 55. Filgrastim is a CSF that stimulates progenitor cells for the subset of leukocytes (WBCs) known as *granulocytes* (including basophils, eosinophils, and neutrophils). For this reason, it is also commonly called *granulocyte colony-stimulating factor* (G-CSF). Pegfilgrastim is a longer-acting form of filgrastim.

Indications

Neutrophils are the most important granulocytes for fighting infection. Infections often appear in patients who have experienced destruction of bone marrow cells as a result of cytotoxic chemotherapy. CSFs stimulate neutrophils to grow and mature and thus directly oppose the detrimental bone marrow actions of chemotherapy. Because these drugs reduce the duration of low neutrophil counts, they reduce the incidence and duration of infections. CSFs also enhance the functioning of mature cells of the immune system, such as macrophages and granulocytes. This effect increases the ability of the body's immune system to kill cancer cells, as well as virus- and fungus-infected cells. Ultimately, these

properties allow patients to receive higher dosages of chemotherapy. Similar benefits affecting RBC counts occur with epoetin alfa.

The effect of hematopoietic drugs on bone marrow cells also reduces recovery time after bone marrow transplantation and radiation therapy. Dosages of chemotherapy used in bone marrow transplantation are often much higher than those used in conventional chemotherapy. Both chemotherapy and radiation therapy are toxic to the bone marrow. When one or more CSFs are administered as part of the drug therapy for bone marrow transplantation, bone marrow cell counts return to normal in a significantly shortened time. This helps increase the likelihood of successful bone marrow transplantation and therefore patient survival. Specific drug indications are listed in the Dosages table on p. 1009.

Contraindications

Contraindications for all the hematopoietic drugs include drug allergy. Use of epoetin and darbepoetin is contraindicated in cases of uncontrolled hypertension. The initiation or intensification of antihypertensive therapy may be required during the early phase of treatment, when hemoglobin increases. Use of filgrastim and pegfilgrastim is contraindicated in the presence of more than 10% myeloid blasts (immature tumour cells in the bone marrow), because CSFs may stimulate malignant growth of these myeloid tumour cells.

Adverse Effects

Adverse effects associated with the use of hematopoietic drugs are mild. The most common are fever, muscle aches, bone pain, and flushing. Table 54-1 lists additional adverse effects.

Interactions

Filgrastim has significant drug interactions when given with myelosuppressive antineoplastic drugs. Remember that this drug is administered to enhance the production of bone marrow cells; therefore, when myelosuppressive antineoplastics are given with filgrastim, the drugs directly antagonize each other. Typically, filgrastim is not given within 24 hours of administration of myelosuppressive antineoplastics. However, it is often given soon after this time to help prevent the WBC nadir from

TABLE	**54-1**

Hematopoietic Drugs: Common Adverse Effects

Body System	Adverse Effects
Cardiovascular	Edema
Gastrointestinal	Anorexia, nausea, vomiting, diarrhea
Integumentary	Alopecia, rash
Respiratory	Cough, dyspnea, sore throat
Other	Fever, blood dyscrasias, headache, bone pain

reaching a dangerously low level and to speed WBC recovery. It is also recommended that filgrastim be used with caution or not be given with other medications that can potentiate their myeloproliferative (bone marrow–stimulating) effects; two examples of these are lithium carbonate and corticosteroids.

Dosages

For dosage information on hematopoietic drugs, refer to the table on p. 1009.

INTERFERONS

Interferons are proteins that have three basic properties: they are antiviral, antitumour, and immunomodulating. There are three different groups of interferon drugs: the alfa, beta, and gamma interferons, each with its own antigenic and biological activities. Interferons are most commonly used in the treatment of certain viral infections and certain types of cancer.

Mechanism of Action and Drug Effects

Interferons are recombinantly manufactured substances that are identical to the interferon cytokines naturally present in the human body. In the body, interferons are produced by activated T cells and by other cells in response to viral infection. Interferons protect human cells from attack by viruses by enabling the cells to produce enzymes that stop viral replication and prevent viruses from penetrating into healthy cells. Interferons prevent cancer cells from dividing and replicating and also increase the activity of other cells in the immune system, such as macrophages, neutrophils, and natural killer cells. Interferons also increase the expression of cancer cell antigens on cell surfaces, which enables the immune system to recognize cancer cells more easily and specifically mark them for destruction.

Overall, interferons have three different effects on the immune system. They can (1) restore its function if it is impaired, (2) augment its ability to function as the body's defence, and (3) inhibit it from working. This latter function may be particularly useful when the immune system has become dysfunctional, causing an autoimmune disease. This is believed to be the case in multiple sclerosis. Two interferons (interferon beta-1a and interferon beta-1b) are specifically indicated for treatment of multiple sclerosis. Inhibiting the dysfunctional immune system prevents further damage to the body from the disease process.

Indications

The beneficial actions of interferons (antiviral, antineoplastic, and immunomodulatory) make them excellent drugs for the treatment of viral infections, various cancers, and some autoimmune disorders. Currently accepted indications for interferons are listed in the Dosages table on p. 1012.

Contraindications

Contraindications to the use of interferons include known drug allergy and may include autoimmune disorders, hepatitis or liver failure, concurrent use of **immunosuppressant** drugs, AIDS-related Kaposi sarcoma, severe depression and severe liver disease.

DRUG PROFILES

▸▸*filgrastim*

Filgrastim (Neupogen®) is a synthetic analogue of human granulocyte CSF and is commonly referred to as *G-CSF*. Filgrastim promotes the proliferation, differentiation, and activation of the cells that make granulocytes. Granulocytes are the body's primary defence against bacterial and fungal infections. Filgrastim has the same pharmacological effects as those of endogenous human G-CSF, which is normally secreted by specialized leukocytes, known as *monocytes*, *macrophages*, and mature neutrophils. Filgrastim is indicated to prevent or treat febrile neutropenia in patients receiving myelosuppressive antineoplastics for nonmyeloid (non–bone marrow) malignancies. It must be given *before* a patient develops an infection, but not within 24 hours before or after myelo-

suppressive chemotherapeutic drugs, because administering it thusly tends to cancel out the therapeutic benefits of the filgrastim. Pegfilgrastim (Neulasta®) is a long-acting form of filgrastim that reduces the number of required injections. Both drugs are available for injection only. These drugs are usually discontinued when a patient's absolute neutrophil count (ANC) rises above 10×10^9/L. However, some health care providers will stop it when the ANC is between 1 and 2×10^9/L.

PHARMACOKINETICS

Route	Onset of Action	Peak Plasma Concentration	Elimination Half-Life	Duration of Action
Subcut or IV	1 hr	2–6 hr	3–5 hr	12–24 hr

DOSAGES   Hematopoietic Drug

Drug	Pharmacological Class	Usual Dosage Range	Indications
▸▸filgrastim (Neupogen)	Colony-stimulating factor	IV/Subcut: 5–10 mcg/kg/day	Chemotherapy-induced neutropenia

IV, intravenous; *Subcut*, subcutaneous.

Adverse Effects

The most common adverse effects of interferons can be broadly described as flulike symptoms: fever, chills, headache, malaise, myalgia, and fatigue. The major dose-limiting adverse effect of interferons is fatigue. Patients taking high dosages become so exhausted that they are often confined to bed. Antibodies may bind to interferons and neutralize their biological effects. Other adverse effects of interferons are listed in Table 54-2.

Interactions

Drug interactions are seen with interferon alfa-2b when it is used with drugs that are metabolized in the liver via the cytochrome P450 enzyme system. The combination results in decreased metabolism and increased accumulation of these drugs, which leads to drug toxicity. There is also some evidence that using interferons together with antiviral drugs such as zidovudine enhances the activity of both drugs but may lead to toxic levels of zidovudine. Live attenuated virus vaccines may carry a higher potential risk of infection and complication for patients on immunosuppressant medications. They may also be less effective following periods of immunosuppression and should not be administered for 3 months following treatment with immunosuppressant medications.

Dosages

For dosage information on interferons, refer to the table on p. 1012.

MONOCLONAL ANTIBODIES

Monoclonal antibodies are quickly becoming standards of therapy in many areas of medicine, including treatment of cancer, rheumatoid arthritis and other inflammatory diseases, and multiple sclerosis, as well as in organ transplantation. In cancer treatment, they have advantages over traditional antineoplastics in that they can specifically target cancer cells and have minimal effects on healthy cells. This characteristic reduces many of the adverse effects traditionally associated with antineoplastic drugs. There are several commercially available monoclonal antibodies used to treat cancer and rheumatoid arthritis; those most commonly used are listed in the Dosages table on p. 1015. The *mab* suffix in a drug name is usually an abbreviation for "monoclonal antibody." Muromonab is used in kidney transplantation. Canakinumab (Ilaris®) administered subcutaneously is used for the treatment of active systemic juvenile idiopathic arthritis in patients aged 2 years and older as well as cryopyrin-associated periodic syndromes. Vedolizumab (Entyvio®) is used to treat ulcerative colitis who have had an inadequate response, loss of response, or are intolerant to infliximab.

Mechanism of Action, Drug Effects, and Indications

Because these drugs are so diverse, specific information for each appears in the individual drug profiles provided later in this chapter.

Contraindications

The only clear contraindication to the use of monoclonal antibodies reported to date is drug allergy to a specific product. The use of monoclonal antibodies is usually contraindicated in patients with known active infectious processes because of their immunosuppressive qualities. Although known drug allergy is a contraindication, depending on the urgency of the clinical situation, a monoclonal antibody may be the only viable treatment option for a seriously ill patient. In such situations, allergic symptoms may be controlled with supportive medications such as diphenhydramine hydrochloride and acetaminophen (for fever control). All of the drugs that are tumour necrosis factor (TNF) antagonists are contraindicated in patients with active tuberculosis or other infections. Infliximab has been shown to worsen severe cases of heart failure and is dosed at no more than 5 mg/kg and only after considering other treatment options for its indications. Use of alemtuzumab is also contraindicated in patients with active systemic infections and immunodeficiency conditions, including AIDS.

Adverse Effects

Many, if not most, patients receiving these potent drugs manifest acute symptoms that are comparable with classic allergy or flulike symptoms, such as fever, dyspnea, and chills. The primary objective is to administer the medication and control such symptoms. Because the mechanisms of action of these drugs work through augmentation or inhibition of the human immune response, they can have a variety of adverse effects— some mild, some severe—that affect several body systems. Drug-specific adverse effects with the highest reported incidence (10 to 50% or more) are listed in Table 54-3. The risk of such adverse effects must be weighed against the severity of the patient's underlying illness. Many of these adverse effects may also be associated

TABLE 54-2	
Interferons: Adverse Effects	
Body System	**Adverse Effects**
General	Flulike syndrome, fatigue
Cardiovascular	Tachycardia, cyanosis, electrocardiogram changes, orthostatic hypotension
Central nervous	Confusion, somnolence, irritability, seizures, hallucinations
Gastrointestinal	Nausea, diarrhea, vomiting, anorexia, taste alterations, dry mouth
Hematological	Neutropenia, thrombocytopenia
Renal and hepatic	Increased blood urea nitrogen and creatinine levels, proteinuria, abnormal liver function test results

DRUG PROFILES

The three major classes of interferons are alfa, beta, and gamma (gamma products are not available in Canada), which are sometimes also written using the lowercase Greek letters α, β, and γ, respectively. The "alfa" designation is synonymous with the Greek letter "alpha," but the "alfa" spelling is now more commonly used clinically. Interferons vary in their antigenic makeup, biological actions, and pharmacological properties. Alfas comprise the most well-known class of interferons.

Interferon products are BRMs that can be broadly classified as cytokines. Cytokines are immune system proteins that serve two essential functions: they direct the actions of and communication between the cell-mediated and humoral divisions of the immune system, and they augment or enhance the immune response. Other cytokines include tumour necrosis factor, interleukins, and CSFs.

INTERFERON ALFA PRODUCTS

▶▶ *interferon alfa-2b, peginterferon alfa-2a*

The most commonly used interferon products are in the interferon alfa class. They are also referred to as *leukocyte interferons* because they are produced from human leukocytes. One newer type of interferon alfa is peginterferon alfa-2a. The *peg* refers to the attachment of a polymer chain of the hydrocarbon polyethylene glycol (PEG). This "pegylation" process increases the size of the interferon molecule. This increased size delays the drug's absorption, increases its half-life, and decreases its plasma clearance rate, which prolongs the drug's therapeutic effects. In addition, pegylation is believed to reduce the immunogenicity of the interferon and thus delay its recognition and destruction by the immune system. Similarly, pegfilgrastim, mentioned previously in this chapter, is a pegylated form of filgrastim and is also longer acting.

Interferon alfa-2a is indicated for use in patients with chronic active hepatitis B or chronic hepatitis C, chronic myelogenous leukemia, multiple myeloma, non-Hodgkin lymphoma, malignant melanoma, AIDS-related Kaposi sarcoma, hairy cell leukemia, basal cell carcinoma, or condylomata acuminate. Peginterferon alfa-2a is indicated for

use in patients with chronic active hepatitis B or chronic hepatitis C. Peginterferon alfa-2b is available in combination with the protease inhibitor boceprevir (see Chapter 45) and the nucleoside reverse transcriptase inhibitor ribavirin (Victrelis Triple®; see Chapter 45) for the treatment of chronic hepatitis C genotype 1 infection with compensated liver disease that has been previously untreated or treated unsuccessfully.

Interferons are indicated for use in patients over the age of 18 and are most commonly given by either intramuscular (IM) or subcutaneous injection, but intravenous (IV) and intraperitoneal routes have been used as well. Interferon alfa-2a is available in a multidose pen, and peginterferon alfa-2a is available in a prefilled syringe, single-use vial, and autoinjector. It is important to note that some interferons are dosed in millions of units. Although it is unacceptable to use the abbreviation MU for "millions of units," it may be written as such. It is imperative to double-check the dose, because the health care provider's writing of "MU" may be mistaken for "mg" or "mcg." If there is any question about the dose of any medication, double-check with the health care provider, the pharmacist, or another experienced colleague before administering the medication to the patient. Although this is true for all medications, it is a special consideration for interferons and other BRMs because of both their potency and their dosage variability.

INTERFERON BETA PRODUCTS

▶▶ *interferon beta-1a and beta-1b*

Interferon beta-1a and interferon beta-1b are the currently available interferon beta products. They interact with specific cell receptors found on the surfaces of human cells and possess antiviral and immunomodulatory activities. Both are produced by rDNA techniques and are indicated for the treatment of relapsing–remitting multiple sclerosis (to slow the progression of physical disability and decrease frequency of clinical exacerbations). Their only contraindication is drug allergy, including allergy to human albumin. Both drugs are available for injection only.

with the patient's disease process (e.g., infections) and even with other causes (e.g., headache, depression). This is especially true for the milder effects. The risk of acquiring an infection is a serious adverse effect of all of the BRM agents because they alter the normal immune response.

Interactions

Drug interactions associated with monoclonal antibodies are relatively few, and no major food interactions are listed. Administration of adalimumab with the antirheumatic drug anakinra (an interleukin) may increase the risk of serious infections secondary to neutropenia. The clearance of natalizumab may be reduced by concurrent administration of interferon beta-1a (both used for multiple sclerosis). Coadministration of anti-TNF drugs

(e.g., etanercept, anakinra) with infliximab may also increase the risk of neutropenia and infections. Etanercept is not to be given concurrently with varicella-zoster immunoglobulin (VZIG) because of undesirable drug interactions. However, etanercept may be resumed after completion of VZIG therapy. Bevacizumab is associated with increased risk of severe diarrhea and neutropenia when given concurrently with another drug used to treat colorectal cancer, irinotecan (see Chapter 52). Paclitaxel (see Chapter 52) has been shown to reduce the clearance of trastuzumab when the two are administered concurrently to treat breast cancer.

Dosages

For dosage information on the monoclonal antibodies, refer to the table on p. 1015.

DOSAGES Currently Available Interferons

Drug	Pharmacological Class	Usual Dosage Range	Indications
▸▸interferon alfa-2b (Intron A®)	Immunomodulator, antiviral, antineoplastic	IM/Subcut: 1–30 million units 3 ×/wk†	Chronic, active hepatitis B, chronic hepatitis C, chronic myelogenous leukemia, multiple myeloma, non-Hodgkin lymphoma, malignant melanoma, AIDS-related Kaposi sarcoma, hairy cell leukemia, basal cell carcinoma, condylomata acuminate
▸▸peginterferon alfa-2a (Pegasys®)	Immunomodulator, antiviral	Subcut: 180 mcg weekly for 48 wk	Chronic hepatitis C, chronic hepatitis B, HIV–HCV coinfection
▸▸interferon beta-1a (Avonex PEN®, Avonex PS®, Rebif®)	Immunomodulator	IM (Avonex): 30 mcg 1 ×/wk Subcut (Rebif): 22–44 mcg 3 ×/wk	Multiple sclerosis
▸▸interferon beta-1b (Betaseron®, Extavia®)	Immunomodulator	Subcut: 0.25 mg every other day	Multiple sclerosis

HCV, hepatitis C virus; *IM*, intramuscular; *PS*, prefilled syringe *Subcut*, subcutaneous.

TABLE 54-3

Common Adverse Effects Associated With Specific Immunomodulating Drugs

Drug	Adverse Effects
adalimumab	Localized inflammatory reaction at the injection site, infectious processes such as upper respiratory tract and urinary tract infections, higher rates of various malignancies
alemtuzumab	Rash, pruritus, nausea, vomiting, diarrhea, dyspnea, cough, muscle spasms, fever, fatigue, skeletal pain, myelosuppression
bevacizumab	Deep vein thrombosis, hypertension, diarrhea, abdominal pain, constipation, vomiting, gastrointestinal hemorrhage, leukopenia, asthenia, headache, dizziness, dry skin, proteinuria, hypokalemia, epistaxis, weight loss
cetuximab	Headache, insomnia, skin rash, conjunctivitis, gastrointestinal discomfort, anemia, leukopenia, dehydration, edema, weight loss, dyspnea, asthenia, back pain, fever
golimumab	Hypertension, increased liver function tests, infection
infliximab	Headache, rash, gastrointestinal discomfort, dyspnea, upper and lower respiratory tract infection
palivizumab	Upper respiratory infection, otitis media, rhinitis, rash, pain, hernia, increased aspartate aminotransferase, pharyngitis
rituximab	Fever, chills, headache; potentially fatal infusion-related events, including severe bronchospasm, dyspnea, hypoxia, pulmonary infiltrates, adult respiratory distress syndrome, angioedema. Tumour lysis syndrome (see Chapter 52) with acute kidney injury has also been reported; the drug must be stopped immediately and indicated supportive care provided if such a reaction appears imminent.
tocilizumab	Hypertension, rash, diarrhea, dizziness, anaphylaxis, infection, injection site reaction
tositumomab and iodine I-131 tositumomab	Headache, rash, gastrointestinal discomfort, muscle pains, dyspnea, pharyngitis, asthenia, fever, chills, infection
tofacitinib	Urinary tract infections, hypertension
trastuzumab	Fever, chills, headache, infection, nausea, vomiting, diarrhea, dizziness, headache, insomnia, rash, gastrointestinal discomfort, edema, dyspnea, rhinitis, asthenia, back pain, fever, chills, infection

INTERLEUKINS AND RELATED DRUGS

Interleukins are a natural part of the immune system and are classified as lymphokines. Lymphokines are soluble proteins that are released from activated lymphocytes such as natural killer cells. There are several known interleukins in the body (e.g., IL-1, IL-2, IL-3, IL-4, IL-5, IL-6, etc.). Currently, 36 interleukins have been identified. The pharmaceutical interleukin receptor agonists currently available are aldesleukin, tocilizumab (IL-6), and anakinra.

DRUG PROFILES

All the monoclonal antibodies are synthesized using rDNA technology. Because of the complexities of this technology, these drugs tend to be much more expensive than most other medications, with prices in the hundreds or thousands of dollars per single dose. Most of the monoclonal antibodies are used to treat various forms of cancer. Their advantage is that they offer excellent cell-killing specificity, aimed at cancer cells instead of all body cells. Nonetheless, these drugs are associated with significant adverse effects and therefore with risk, which must be weighed against their benefit using expert clinical judgement. Severe allergic inflammatory-type infusion reactions can occur, and patients may therefore be premedicated with acetaminophen or diphenhydramine hydrochloride to reduce the occurrence of such reactions. If reactions do occur, they may be treated with diphenhydramine hydrochloride and other drugs such as epinephrine and corticosteroids. Conventional pharmacokinetic data are not listed for most of these drugs because they do not follow standard pharmacokinetic models, owing to their unique behaviour in the body. It is known, however, that they may remain in cancerous tissues for weeks or months. Their elimination half-life is listed in the following profiles when known.

adalimumab

Adalimumab (Humira®) works through its specificity for human TNF alfa (TNFα). TNFα is a naturally occurring cytokine involved in normal inflammatory and immune responses. Adalimumab is indicated for the treatment of moderate to severe rheumatoid arthritis, alone or in combination with methotrexate or other DMARDs. In patients with rheumatoid arthritis, elevated levels of TNF are found in the synovial fluid in the spaces of affected joints. In addition to preventing TNFα molecules from binding to TNF cell surface receptors—part of the rheumatoid arthritis disease process—adalimumab also modulates the inflammatory biological responses that are induced or regulated by TNF. Adalimumab is also indicated for the treatment of psoriatic arthritis, ankylosing spondylitis, Crohn's disease, ulcerative colitis, and psoriasis. Use of adalimumab is contraindicated in patients with any active infectious process, whether localized or systemic, acute or chronic.

alemtuzumab

Alemtuzumab (MabCampath®) is approved to treat B cell–mediated chronic lymphocytic leukemia. It is classified as a recombinant humanized antibody that is directed against the CD52 glycoprotein that appears on the surfaces of virtually all B and T lymphocytes. Humanization involves the insertion of human DNA sequences during drug production to make the drug better tolerated by human patients. It is used specifically in patients for whom other first-line chemotherapy treatments, including treatment with alkylating drugs and the antimetabolite fludarabine (see Chapter 52), have failed. Its contraindications are drug allergy, active systemic infection, and documented immunodeficiency conditions such as HIV-positive status.

The half-life of alemtuzumab is 10 hours to 30 days. Alemtuzumab (Lemtrada®) is indicated for the management of adult patients with active relapsing–remitting multiple sclerosis who have had an inadequate response to interferon beta or other disease-modifying therapies.

belimumab

Belimumab (Benlysta®) is the first drug approved for the treatment of systemic lupus erythematosus in the past 40 years. It is a B lymphocyte stimulator–specific inhibitor. Its most common adverse effects include nausea, diarrhea, insomnia, bronchitis, migraine, and pain in the extremities. Its most serious adverse effects include infection (sometimes fatal), anaphylaxis, and depression. It is given via IV infusion.

bevacizumab

Bevacizumab (Avastin®) was approved for the treatment of metastatic colorectal cancer in combination with 5-fluorouracil (see Chapter 52), non–small cell lung cancer, and malignant glioblastoma. It is unique in that it binds to and inhibits vascular endothelial growth factor, a protein that promotes development of new blood vessels in tumours (as well as in normal body tissues). It has no listed contraindications but may complicate surgical wound healing because of its antivascular effects. The half-life of bevacizumab is 11 to 50 days.

certolizumab pegol

Certolizumab pegol (Cimzia®) is a TNF antagonist. It is used in combination with methotrexate for the treatment of rheumatoid arthritis, alone or in combination with methotrexate for psoriatic arthritis, and for active ankylosing spondylitis. Its most common adverse effects include headache, nausea, upper respiratory infection, hypertension, and infection. A patient medication guide must be dispensed with each prescription, warning patients of potential serious infections and possible lymphoma.

cetuximab

Cetuximab (Erbitux®) is approved for the treatment of metastatic colorectal cancer and squamous cell carcinoma of the head and neck. It is a recombinant monoclonal antibody made from both human and murine genetic material and is designed for concurrent use with the second-line antineoplastic drug irinotecan (see Chapter 52). It binds to epidermal growth factor on the surface of tumour cells, where it hinders cell growth through interference with cell metabolism. Cetuximab is used either in combination with irinotecan or alone in patients who are intolerant of the latter drug. It has no listed contraindications but is known to cause severe infusion reactions in up to 3% of patients receiving it. The half-life of cetuximab is 97 to 114 hours.

golimumab

Golimumab (Simponi®) is a TNF antagonist approved for the treatment of severe rheumatoid arthritis (in combination with methotrexate), psoriatic arthritis, and ankylosing

Continued

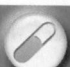
DRUG PROFILES—cont'd

spondylitis. It is also used in adult patients with moderately to severely active ulcerative colitis who have had an inadequate response to or contraindications with other treatments. Its most common adverse effects include hypertension, dizziness, high values on liver function tests, and infection. It is not to be given with other TNF antagonists. Patients taking golimumab must be monitored for infection, as with all TNF antagonists.

infliximab

Infliximab (Inflectra®, Remicade®, Remsima®) was one of the earliest monoclonal antibodies available. It antagonizes TNFα, similarly to adalimumab. It is approved for the treatment of ankylosing spondylitis, Crohn's disease, and rheumatoid arthritis (in combination with methotrexate). It is contraindicated in patients with severe heart failure (grade III or IV on the New York Heart Association scale) because it may worsen such heart failure. Health Canada also issued a warning regarding infliximab due to reported cases of fatal tuberculosis and fungal infections associated with use of this drug. It is recommended that patients be tested for latent tuberculosis before infliximab is administered. The half-life of infliximab is 8 to 9 days.

natalizumab

Natalizumab (Tysabri®) is approved for the treatment of relapsing–remitting multiple sclerosis. It is a humanized monoclonal antibody derived from murine myeloma cells. Natalizumab works by binding to the α4 subunits of integrins, proteins found on the surfaces of leukocytes (with the exception of neutrophils). These proteins are implicated in the multiple sclerosis disease process, but their exact mechanism has not been documented. However, the drug is known to inhibit the leukocyte adhesion that is mediated by these α4 protein subunits, also believed to be part of the disease process. Natalizumab has no listed contraindications. Its half-life is 11 days. Natalizumab is associated with multifocal leukoencephalopathy, a rare and serious viral infection of the brain. Patients receiving natalizumab must enrol in the Canadian Tysabri Care Program, a special distribution program. Only patients who are enrolled in the program are allowed to receive the drug.

palivizumab

Palivizumab (Synagis®) is a passive immunizing agent (humanized monoclonal antibody). It is indicated for the prevention of serious lower respiratory tract disease caused by the highly infectious respiratory syncytial virus in children who are at high risk of developing the disease. The recommended dose of palivizumab administered intramuscularly is 15 mg/kg of body weight. It is administered monthly during peak times (generally November to April). The first dose should be administered prior to the beginning of the infectious season, with subsequent doses administered monthly during the season. The mean half-life of pavlizumab is 20 days.

▶▶ rituximab

Rituximab (Rituxan®) specifically binds to antigen CD20. This antigen is a protein on the membranes of both normal and malignant B cells found in patients with non-Hodgkin lymphoma. Antigen CD20 is expressed in more than 90% of B cell non-Hodgkin lymphomas. Once rituximab binds to these B cells, a host immune response causes lysis of the cells. Rituximab has become a standard drug for the treatment of patients with follicular low-grade non-Hodgkin lymphoma for whom previous therapy has failed. It is recommended that patients be premedicated with acetaminophen and diphenhydramine hydrochloride before each infusion of the drug to reduce its well-known infusion-related adverse effects.

trastuzumab

Trastuzumab (Herceptin®, Kadcyla®) kills tumour cells by mediating antibody-dependent cellular cytotoxicity. It accomplishes this by inhibiting proliferation of human tumour cells that overexpress HER2 protein. The HER2 protein is overexpressed in 25 to 30% of primary malignant breast tumours and has been established as an adverse prognostic factor for early-stage breast cancer. Because of the relatively selective expression of HER2 on cancer cells, it has been an appealing target for antineoplastic therapy. The combination of trastuzumab and paclitaxel (Perjeta®/Herceptin) has produced encouraging results. Ventricular dysfunction and heart failure have been associated with trastuzumab. Monitor for signs and symptoms of heart failure and ventricular dysfunction before and during treatment. In addition, fatal hypersensitivity reactions, infusion reactions, and pulmonary events have occurred in association with it use; therefore, careful clinical judgement, risk evaluation, and informed patient consent are called for in its use. The half-life of trastuzumab is 10 to 30 days.

Mechanism of Action and Drug Effects

Interleukins cause multiple effects in the immune system, one of which is antitumour action. IL-2 is produced by activated T cells in response to macrophage-processed antigens and secreted interleukin (IL-1). It was formerly called *T-cell growth factor* because, among other actions, it aids in the growth and differentiation of T lymphocytes. The IL-2 derivative aldesleukin acts indirectly to stimulate or restore immune response. Aldesleukin binds to receptor sites on T cells, which stimulates the T cells to multiply. One type of cell that results from this multiplication are **lymphokine-activated killer (LAK) cells**. LAK cells recognize and destroy only cancer cells and ignore normal cells. Aldesleukin is currently the most widely used of the interleukin drugs. A detailed list of aldesleukin's specific immunomodulating effects appears in Box 54-2.

Anakinra is a recombinant form of the natural human IL-1 receptor antagonist. It competitively inhibits the binding of IL-1 to its corresponding receptor sites, which

DOSAGES   Monoclonal Antibodies

Drug	Pharmacological Class	Usual Dosage Range	Indications
adalimumab (Humira)	Anti–TNFα monoclonal antibody	*Adults only* Subcut: 40 mg every other week; may advance to 40 mg weekly if indicated	Moderate to severe rheumatoid arthritis, alone or in combination with methotrexate
alemtuzumab (MabCampath)	Anti–glycoprotein CD52	IV: 3–10 mg daily until maximum dose tolerated, then 30 mg 3 ×/wk (alternate days) for up to 12 wk	B cell chronic lymphocytic leukemia
alemtuzumab (Lemtrada)	Anti–glycoprotein CD52	IV: 12 mg daily for 2 treatment courses	Relapsing–remitting multiple sclerosis
belimumab (Benlysta)	B-lymphocyte stimulator-specific inhibitor	IV: 10 mg/kg at 2-week intervals	Systemic lupus erythematosus
certolizumab pegol (Cimzia)	Anti-TNF	Subcut: 400 mg at 2-week intervals × 2, then monthly	Rheumatoid arthritis, psoriatic arthritis, ankylosing spondylitis
bevacizumab (Avastin)	Anti–human vascular endothelial growth factor	IV: 5 mg/kg q14d	Metastatic colorectal cancer
cetuximab (Erbitux)	Anti–human epidermal growth factor	IV: 400 mg/m² loading dose, then 250 mg/m² weekly	Metastatic colorectal cancer, squamous cell carcinoma of head and neck
infliximab (Remicade)	Anti-TNF	*Adults* IV: 3–5 mg/kg at 0, 2, and 6 wk, then every 6 wk	Ankylosing spondylitis, Crohn's disease, rheumatoid arthritis, ulcerative colitis, psoriatic arthritis
natalizumab (Tysabri)	Anti–α⁴ integrin subunit	IV: 300 mg every 4 wk	Multiple sclerosis
▸▸rituximab (Rituxan)	Anti-CD20 surface antigen	IV: 375 mg/m² 1 ×/wk × 4 doses IV: 1 000 mg, 2 wk apart	Non-Hodgkin lymphoma Rheumatoid arthritis
trastuzumab (Herceptin)	Anti–HER2 protein monoclonal antibody	IV: Loading dose, 4–8 mg/kg IV: Maintenance dose, 2 mg/kg/wk	Breast cancer

IV, intravenous; *Subcut*, subcutaneous; *TNF*, tumour necrosis factor.

BOX 54-2

Interleukin-2: Drug Effects

Modulating Effects

Proliferation of T cells
Synthesis and secretion of cytokines
Increased production of B cells (antibodies)
Proliferation and activation of natural killer cells
Proliferation and activation of lymphokine-activated killer cells

Enhancing Effects

Enhancement of killer T-cell activity
Amplification of the effects of cytokines
Enhancement of the cytotoxic actions of natural killer cells and lymphokine-activated killer cells

are expressed in many different tissues and organs. Tocilizumab is a recombinant form of the natural IL-6 receptor antagonist.

Indications

Aldesleukin was previously indicated solely for metastatic kidney cell carcinoma, a malignancy that originates in the kidney tissues. It is now also approved for the treatment of metastatic malignant melanoma. Anakinra and tocilizumab are indicated for symptom control in patients with rheumatoid arthritis for whom other therapy has failed.

Contraindications

Contraindications to the administration of aldesleukin include drug allergy, organ transplantation, and abnormal results on thallium heart stress tests or pulmonary function tests. For anakinra and tocilizumab, the only usual contraindication is drug allergy.

Adverse Effects

Therapy with aldesleukin is commonly complicated by severe toxicity. A syndrome known as *capillary leak syndrome* is responsible for the severe toxicities of aldesleukin. As the name implies, capillary leak syndrome refers to a condition in which capillaries lose their ability to retain vital colloids, such as albumin and other essential components of blood vessels. Because the capillaries become "leaky," these substances migrate into surrounding tissues. This results in massive fluid retention (10 to 15 kg), which can lead to the life-threatening problems of respiratory distress, heart failure, dysrhythmias, and myocardial infarction. Fortunately, these effects are all reversible after discontinuation of the interleukin therapy. Close patient monitoring and vigorous supportive care are essential for patients receiving aldesleukin therapy. Other adverse effects that may be associated with aldesleukin are fever, chills, rash, fatigue, hepatotoxicity, myalgia, headache, and eosinophilia.

Anakinra has a much milder adverse effect profile than that of aldesleukin; it includes local reactions at the injection site, various respiratory tract infections, and headache. Tocilizumab has a high risk of causing anaphylaxis.

Interactions

Aldesleukin, when given with antihypertensives, can produce additive hypotensive effects. Coadministration of corticosteroids with aldesleukin can reduce its antitumour effectiveness and is to be avoided. Anakinra and tocilizumab are not to be used (or need to be used cautiously) with other immune modifiers due to the resultant increased risk of serious infections.

Dosages

For dosage information on the interleukin agonists and antagonists, refer to the table below.

MISCELLANEOUS IMMUNOMODULATING DRUGS

In addition to the drugs in the major classes discussed thus far, there are several additional medications can be broadly classified as miscellaneous IMDs. They work by various specific and nonspecific mechanisms. A special term used for **immunostimulant** drugs that work by a

---

 DRUG PROFILES

The interleukins are a group of naturally occurring cytokines in the body that were originally believed to be produced by and act primarily on WBCs. They are now recognized as multifunctional cytokines that are produced by a variety of cells but act at least partly within the lymphatic system.

▸▸*aldesleukin*

Aldesleukin (Proleukin®) is a human IL-2 derivative that is manufactured using rDNA technology. It is a cytokine that is produced by lymphocytes and is therefore classified as a lymphokine. Aldesleukin is currently approved only for the treatment of metastatic kidney cell carcinoma and metastatic melanoma, despite its activity against other cancers. Aldesleukin is contraindicated in patients with known drug allergy, abnormal thallium stress tests or pulmonary function tests (because of potential drug effects on cardiopulmonary function), and organ transplants (because of the immunostimulating qualities of the drug,

which may cause organ rejection). It is available only for injection.

anakinra

Anakinra (Kineret®) is an IL-1 receptor antagonist that is used to control the symptoms of rheumatoid arthritis. Its only current contraindication is known drug allergy. It is available for injection only.

tocilizumab

Tocilizumab (Actemra®) is an interleukin-6 antagonist approved for the treatment of severe rheumatoid arthritis. It is approved for patients who have not had an adequate response to other medications. It carries a significant risk of anaphylaxis, and premedication must be given. A medication guide must be given to all patients receiving tocilizumab. Its serious adverse effects include hepatotoxicity, infections, herpes zoster reactivation, and gastrointestinal (GI) perforation. Tocilizumab is not to be given with other BRM agents. It is given as an IV infusion.

DOSAGES	Interleukins and Related Drugs		
Drug	**Pharmacological Class**	**Usual Dosage Range**	**Indications**
▸▸aldesleukin (IL-2) (Proleukin)	Human recombinant IL-2 analogue	IV: 600 000 units/kg (0.037 mg/kg) q8h × 14 doses; rest for 9 days, repeat × 14 doses	Metastatic kidney cell carcinoma, metastatic malignant melanoma
anakinra (Kineret)	Interleukin-1 receptor antagonist	Subcut: 100 mg/day	Rheumatoid arthritis
tocilizumab (Actemra)	IL-6 antagonist	IV: 4–8 mg/kg monthly	Rheumatoid arthritis

IV, intravenous; *Subcut*, subcutaneous.

TABLE   54-4

Miscellaneous Immunomodulating Drugs

Drug (Trade and Other Names)	Classification	Indications	Mechanism of Action
abatacept (Orencia)	Selective costimulation modulator	Rheumatoid arthritis	Inhibits T cell activation
BCG vaccine (Immucyst®, OncoTICE®)	Live virus vaccine, adjuvant	Localized bladder cancer	Promotes local inflammation and immune response in bladder mucosa
etanercept (Enbrel)	Tumour necrosis factor receptor antagonist	Rheumatoid arthritis (including juvenile), active ankylosing spondylitis, plaque and psoriatic arthritis	Blocks effects of tumour necrosis factor, a major inflammatory mediator
leflunomide (Arava)	Antimetabolite	Rheumatoid arthritis	Exerts anti-inflammatory effects via inhibition of cellular DNA synthesis
mitoxantrone hydrochloride	Anthracycline antibiotic (also an antineoplastic drug)	Metastatic breast cancer, relapsed leukemia	Inhibits cellular RNA and DNA synthesis and alters chromosome structure
thalidomide (Thalomid®)	Immunostimulant	Multiple myeloma	Exact mechanism unclear, but may have anti-TNF properties, which counter the disease process
tretinoin† (Retin-A®, Vescanoid®)	Retinoid receptor agonist	Acute promyelocytic leukemia	Induces differentiation and maturation of leukemic cells, reducing proliferation of immature, disease-causing cells

BCG, bacille Camille-Guérin; *DNA*, deoxyribonucleic acid; *RNA*, ribonucleic acid; *TNF*, tumour necrosis factor.
†Available through Health Canada's Special Access Programme.

nonspecific mechanism is ***adjuvant***. These miscellaneous medications, including some that are classified as adjuvants, are outlined in Table 54-4.

RHEUMATOID ARTHRITIS

Rheumatism is a general term for any of several disorders characterized by inflammation, degeneration, or metabolic derangement of connective tissue structures, especially joints and related structures such as muscles, tendons, bursae, fibrous tissue, and ligaments. Rheumatoid **arthritis** is a chronic **autoimmune disorder** that commonly causes inflammation and tissue damage in joints. It can also cause anemia and diffuse inflammation in the lungs, eyes, and pericardium of the heart, as well as subcutaneous nodules under the skin (Figure 54-3). It is a painful and often disabling disease. It is diagnosed primarily based on symptoms and the results of a blood test for rheumatoid factor. Symptoms include pain, stiffness, and reduced range of motion. Treatment encompasses both pharmacological and nonpharmacological modalities, including physiotherapy and occupational therapy. There is no known cure for rheumatoid arthritis, and the goal of therapy is to alleviate current symptoms and to prevent further damage of the joints. Rheumatoid arthritis affects approximately 1 in 100 Canadians, or approximately 300 000 people in Canada (Arthritis Society, 2015) and usually appears between the ages of 25 and 50. Women are two to three times more likely than

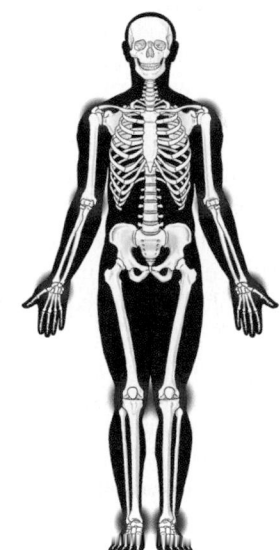

FIG. 54-3   Areas of the body affected by rheumatoid arthritis. Rheumatoid arthritis is most frequently seen in the shoulders, elbows, wrists, knees, and ankles, and it often affects the joints on both sides of the body equally.

men to have rheumatoid arthritis. Smokers and those with a family history are also at risk.

Early diagnosis and treatment of rheumatoid arthritis can prevent joint damage and make remission easier to achieve. Because rheumatoid arthritis is a disease characterized by inflammation, the nonsteroidal anti-inflammatory drugs (NSAIDs) are the most commonly used (see Chapter 49). Full dosages of NSAIDs are tried in the early stages of rheumatoid arthritis. Corticosteroids, also potent anti-inflammatory drugs (see Chapter 34), are also used to prevent inflammatory symptoms. These drugs, although they are effective in reducing inflammation, do not actually affect the disease itself. DMARDs not only provide anti-inflammatory and analgesic effects, but they can arrest or slow the disease processes associated with rheumatoid arthritis. Initiation of DMARDS in the first 6 months following diagnosis can reverse loss of function in 80% of patients and induce remission in 42 to 48% of patients.

DISEASE-MODIFYING ANTIRHEUMATIC ARTHRITIS DRUGS

DMARDs are drugs that modify the disease of rheumatoid arthritis. They exhibit anti-inflammatory, antiarthritic, and immunomodulating effects and work by inhibiting the movement of various cells into an inflamed, damaged area, such as a joint. These cells (neutrophils, monocytes, and macrophages) are responsible for causing many of the deleterious effects of chronic rheumatoid arthritis. By preventing the accumulation of these inflammatory cells in the area of the diseased joint, antiarthritic drugs prevent progression of the disease. DMARDs often have a slow onset of action of several weeks, versus minutes to hours for NSAIDs. For this reason, DMARDs are sometimes also referred to as *slow-acting antirheumatic drugs (SAARDs)*. They were previously thought of as second-line drugs for the treatment of arthritis because they can have much more toxic adverse effects than do the NSAIDs. However, the Canadian Rheumatology Association recommends the use of the combination of two DMARDs as first-line therapy in many patients (Bykerk et al., 2012). Its guidelines differentiate the two categories of DMARDs—nonbiological, or conventional, and biological. Nonbiological DMARDs include methotrexate, leflunomide, hydroxychloroquine sulphate, sodium aurothiomalate, cyclosporine, azathioprine, and sulfasalazine. The guidelines recommend starting with methotrexate alone or with another DMARD in most patients. Use of other drugs, including the biological DMARDs, is generally reserved for those patients who do not respond to methotrexate or combination DMARDs. The biological DMARDs include adalimumab, anakinra, certolizumab, etanercept, golimumab, infliximab, adalimumab, abatacept, rituximab, tocilizumab, and tofacitinib. Box 54-3 lists the DMARDs. Etanercept and abatacept are discussed in this section; the others were discussed in the section on monoclonal antibodies.

Mechanism of Action, Indications, and Adverse Effects

The mechanisms of action and adverse effects of the different DMARDs vary. The individual drug profiles

provide information on mechanism of actions and adverse effects. All of these drugs are indicated for the treatment of rheumatoid arthritis, and some have other uses, as previously mentioned.

Contraindications

DMARDs are not used in patients with active bacterial infection, active herpes zoster, active or latent tuberculosis, or acute or chronic hepatitis B or C. Etanercept, infliximab, and adalimumab are not to be used in patients with heart failure, lymphoma, or multiple sclerosis. Methotrexate, tofacitinib, and leflunomide are to be avoided during pregnancy and lactation. Tofacitinib (Xeljanz®) causes a decrease in heart rate and a prolongation of the PR interval and should not be used in individuals with heart failure, ischemic heart disease, heart block, or dysrhythmias.

NURSING PROCESS

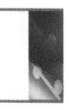

☑ Assessment

Prior to the administration of hematopoietic drugs, assess the medication order thoroughly, as well as the specific indication for each of the drugs prescribed. Once you understand the indication, specific laboratory value(s) may be easily determined for further assessment (e.g., WBC counts with filgrastim). After initial assessment and monitoring of baseline blood counts, measure drug response against these values. Additionally, prior to administering these medications, document baseline assessment of the following: vital signs, skin turgor and intactness, bowel sounds and patterns, and breath sounds. Assess also for any reports of pain and rate

DRUG PROFILES

methotrexate

Methotrexate is an anticancer drug that is commonly used for the treatment of rheumatoid arthritis in much lower dosages than those used for cancer. It is usually started at a dosage of 7.5 mg/wk but can be increased to 20 mg/wk. It is important to note that the drug is given once per week, not once per day. Serious medication errors, including deaths, have occurred when an order is mistranscribed and the drug is given daily instead of once a week. It is usually given orally for rheumatoid arthritis, but it can also be given by injection. Bone marrow suppression is the main adverse effect of methotrexate. Most patients are advised to take supplemental folic acid to lessen the likelihood of adverse effects. The onset of antirheumatic action is 3 to 6 weeks. The half-life of the drug is 3 to 10 hours.

Tofacitinib, another immunomodulatory drug used in the management of rheumatoid arthritis, is recommended to be used in combination with methotrexate in adult patients with moderately to severely active rheumatoid arthritis who have not responded adequately to methotrexate. Tofacitinib is thought to interfere with the activity of a specific enzyme (Janus kinase), which activates other cellular components that initiate the immune response. If methotrexate is not tolerated by a patient, tofacitinib may be used alone. The recommended dosage is 5 mg administered twice daily in combination with methotrexate.

leflunomide

Leflunomide (Arava®) is indicated for the treatment of active rheumatoid arthritis. It modulates or alters the response of the immune system to rheumatoid arthritis. It has antiproliferative, anti-inflammatory, and immunosuppressive activity. Its most common adverse effects are diarrhea, respiratory tract infection, alopecia, elevated liver enzyme levels, and rash. It is contraindicated in women who are or may become pregnant and is not to be used by nursing mothers or those with a hypersensitivity to it. Aspirin, other NSAIDs, or low-dose corticosteroids may be continued during leflunomide therapy. Leflunomide is available only for oral use. Its half-life is 14 to 15 days. Because of its long half-life, a loading dose of 100 mg per day is given for 3 days, followed by a maintenance dose of 20 mg per day.

etanercept

Etanercept (Enbrel®) is an rDNA-derived TNF-blocking drug. It binds to TNF and blocks its interaction with cell surface receptors. It is indicated for the treatment of rheumatoid arthritis (including juvenile rheumatoid arthritis) and moderate to severe chronic plaque psoriasis. It is contraindicated in patients with a known hypersensitivity to it and in those with sepsis or active infections (including chronic or local infections). It should be used with caution in patients with pre-existing demyelinating central nervous system (CNS) disorders, heart failure, or significant hematological abnormalities. Some dosage forms may contain latex, so screen patients for latex allergy. It has been reported to cause reactivation of hepatitis and tuberculosis. Live vaccines should not be given with etanercept. Common adverse effects include headache, reaction at the injection site, upper respiratory tract infection, dizziness, and weakness. The drug is administered subcutaneously. Drugs with which it interacts include anakinra, which may increase the risk of infection, and cyclophosphamide, which may increase the risk of malignancy. Etanercept has not been shown to be a risk to the fetus if used during pregnancy. It is not known if the drug is excreted in breast milk, and its use is not recommended in lactating women. Its onset of action is 1 to 2 weeks, and its half-life is 72 to 132 hours.

abatacept

Abatacept (Orencia®) is a selective co-stimulation modulator; it inhibits T cell activation. Abatacept is indicated for the treatment of rheumatoid arthritis. It is contraindicated in patients with a known hypersensitivity to it or any of its components. It should be used with caution in patients with a history of recurrent infections or chronic obstructive pulmonary disease. Bring patients up to date with all immunizations before starting abatacept therapy. Its adverse effects include headaches, upper respiratory tract infections, and hypertension. Abatacept may increase the risk of infections associated with live vaccines and may decrease the response to dead or live vaccines. Abatacept is not to be given with anakinra or TNF-blocking drugs because of the resultant risk of serious infections, or with the herb echinacea, which has immunostimulant properties. Abatacept is dosed according to body weight and is given at 4-week intervals. It is administered intravenously, and a filter must be used. Its half-life is 8 to 25 days. The recommended dosage is 50 mg subcutaneously, weekly.

accordingly (see discussion in Chapter 11). These areas are all important to assess when giving hematopoietic drugs because of the adverse effects of edema, nausea, vomiting, diarrhea, rash, cough, dyspnea, sore throat, fever, blood dyscrasias, headache, and bone pain. Assess potential IV and subcutaneous sites and, if appropriate, note chemotherapy-induced absolute neutrophil nadir (low point); this is important because timing of the dose is crucial in helping to boost blood cell counts. For example, with filgrastim, do *not* give the drug within 24 hours before or after chemotherapy. Also assess for any existing joint or bone pain because of the possible adverse effect of mild to severe bone pain with filgrastim. Specific information regarding assessment associated with use of epoetin alfa is found in Chapter 55.

Before administering any of the BRMs (and other drugs included in this chapter), assess your own knowledge about these medications, with attention to the drug's action, pharmacokinetic properties, associated cautions, contraindications, drug interactions, adverse effects, and toxicities. Assess patients for the presence of any conditions that represent contraindications or cautions to drug administration as well as possible interacting drugs. Assess for hypersensitivity to the drug, egg proteins, or immunoglobulin G. Furthermore, assess the following systems: (1) respiratory system, with attention to breath rate, rhythm, and depth as well as breath sounds, listening for any adventitious (abnormal) sounds; (2) cardiac system, with attention to vital signs, heart sounds, heart rate and rhythm, and oxygen saturation levels, as well as for edema or shortness of breath, presence of cyanotic discoloration around the mouth (circumoral cyanosis) or nail beds, and any chest pain; (3) CNS, with a focus on baseline mental status, as well as for any seizure-like activity or CNS abnormalities; and (4) immune system, noting ability to fight off infections and any history of chronic illnesses or suppressed immunity. Note nutritional status, height, and weight as well as results of any prescribed laboratory tests, such as complete blood count and especially hemoglobin and hematocrit levels, serum protein and albumin levels, and immunoglobulin levels (see Nursing Process in Chapters 52 and 53). Also document the presence or absence of underlying diseases or symptoms and the success or failure of medication regimens in the past. Assess patients' ability to carry out activities of daily living (ADLs), emotional and socioeconomic status, educational level, learning needs, desire and ability to learn, past coping strategies, and support systems. Before interferons (e.g., alfa-2b) are given, assess patients' history of drug allergies as well as any history of autoimmune disorders, hepatitis, liver failure, or AIDS. Contraindications to interferons include concurrent use of immunosuppressant drugs and Kaposi sarcoma. Determine baseline WBC and platelets counts prior to initiation of therapy due to the potential for drug-induced neutropenia and thrombocytopenia. Monitor other serum laboratory values such as blood urea nitrogen, creatinine, GFR, ALP, and AST before and during therapy due to the risk of problems with kidney and liver functioning. Document baseline neurological functioning, bowel status, heart sounds, pulse rate, and blood pressure (including postural readings). Significant drug interactions for which to assess include those drugs that are metabolized via the cytochrome P450 enzyme system in the liver because of the risk of subsequent drug toxicity.

With use of monoclonal antibody drugs (e.g., alemtuzumab, rituximab, trastuzumab), assess and document any history of allergic reactions. Assess for ranges of responses with these medications, including mild to severe reactions (see Table 54-3). Assessment of baseline vital signs and any signs of infection are important because of the risk of acquiring an infection when taking these drugs. Contraindications to their use include any active infectious process or HIV. There is a Health Canada warning that fatal tuberculosis or fungal infections have

been associated with the use of infliximab (Remicade), so any infectious process needs to be ruled out prior to its use. Trastuzumab also has a warning associated with it due to cases of ventricular dysfunction and heart failure. Fatal hypersensitivity and infusion reactions have occurred with this drug, so prior to administration there must be careful risk evaluation and subsequent prudent clinical decision making by the health care provider. Perform close monitoring and supervision before, during, and after the infusion of monoclonal antibody drugs. Table 54-3 provides a listing of common adverse effects associated with these drugs, indicating further areas and systems to be assessed.

Prior to the use of DMARDs, perform a close assessment of any past or present medical conditions as well as a thorough assessment of allergies. Compile a complete and thorough medication profile, listing prescription drugs, natural health products, and over-the-counter drugs. Assess the specific type of DMARD prescribed because there are nonbiological and biological DMARDS. Assess for contraindications to the use of DMARDs such as active bacterial infections, active herpes, active or latent tuberculosis, and acute or chronic hepatitis B or C. Additional contraindications are presented in the earlier discussion. Because bone marrow suppression is one of the main adverse effects of DMARDs, including methotrexate, assess and monitor baseline RBC, WBC, and platelet counts before, during, and after therapy. Another important area for assessment is the medication order by the health care provider, because serious medication errors have occurred when the order for this drug has been transcribed incorrectly and the drug has been given daily instead of once weekly, as recommended.

Before initiation of therapy with leflunomide, perform a complete assessment of liver functioning and obtain baseline blood cell counts. Because of the possible adverse effects of diarrhea and respiratory infections, assess respiratory and GI functioning. A thorough respiratory assessment includes obtaining a history of past and present respiratory disorders and infections as well as noting breath sounds, any presence of sputum, and baseline respiratory rate, rhythm, and depth. Assess bowel patterns and document findings. Etanercept is to be avoided in those with sepsis and active infections, so conduct a thorough assessment of WBC counts and of any signs, symptoms, or history of infection. Because some dosage forms may contain latex, it is crucial to also assess for latex allergy. The DMARD abatacept is given based on weight; thus, there is a need for an accurate weight to be taken before drug therapy. Additionally, assess the patient's immunization record because all immunizations must be current prior to beginning therapy with abatacept. Document the findings of baseline head-to-toe physical assessment, and note any musculoskeletal changes due to the pathology of arthritis and related changes in performance of ADLs before drug therapy is initiated as well as throughout the therapeutic regimen.

⬜ Nursing Diagnoses

- Risk for infection related to adverse effect of bone marrow suppression related to DMARDs and IMDs
- Imbalanced nutrition, less than body requirements, related to the adverse effects of BRMs
- Impaired skin integrity (rash) related to the adverse effects of BRMs

⬜ Planning

⬛ Goals

- Patient will remain free from infection or have minimal risk for infection during drug therapy
- Patient's nutritional status will return to as near normal as possible after initiation of drug therapy.
- Patient's skin and mucous membranes will remain intact.

⬛ Expected Patient Outcomes

- Patient states ways to minimize risk of infection such as through maintaining proper nutrition and adequate fluid intake, as well as identifying early signs and symptoms of infection.
  - Patient understands needed dietary adjustments (e.g., increase in protein) and uses Canada's Food Guide and advice from consultation with a dietitian to meet additional nutritional demands, thus preventing malnourishment and boosting nutritional status.
  - Patient knows to take temperature orally or via the axillary route every 4 hours during periods of increased risk of infection.
  - Patient states need to report temperature of 38.1°C or higher to the health care provider for appropriate and immediate treatment.

- Patient describes nutritional needs and daily meal planning reflecting dietary needs, such as consumption of a high-calorie, low-residue, high-protein diet, including high-energy foods with protein and complex carbohydrates, and increased intake of fluids.
  - Patient performs a 24-hour recall of food intake and can report a typical week's menus.
  - Patient understands the importance of consuming small, frequent meals in an environment conducive to eating.
  - Patient states measures to minimize GI adverse effects, such as eating small, frequent meals and avoiding spicy foods, and uses antiemetics as prescribed.
  - Patient understands the importance of energy conservation and takes frequent rests before and after meals while undergoing treatment.
- Patient's skin and mucous membranes remain intact and clean due to daily bathing, proper skin care with moisturizing products, and daily oral hygiene with gentle flossing as well as follow-up care with a dental professional.
  - Patient reports any breaks in skin, redness, irritation, areas of swelling, drainage, or pain to the health care provider.
  - Patient contacts a health care provider or dental professional with any concerns regarding poor dentition, sores in the mouth, bleeding in the mouth, or swelling of gums.

⬜ Implementation

Administer BRMs exactly as prescribed and in keeping with manufacturer guidelines to minimize adverse effects. It is important to acknowledge that infection is a serious adverse effect of these drugs and so this risk must always be weighed against the severity of the patient's underlying illness. Patients, especially those with a low neutrophil nadir, may be placed on reverse isolation. Appropriate

---

📋 CASE STUDY

Hematopoietic Biological Response Modifiers

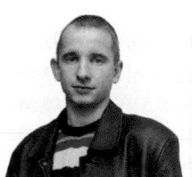

Pavel, a 38-year-old surveyor, is receiving a second round of chemotherapy as part of treatment for non-Hodgkin lymphoma. The oncologist is monitoring for signs of bone marrow suppression affecting the various blood cell components.

1. What symptoms would the nurse expect to see if Pavel had diminished production of platelets? White blood cells? Explain your answers.
2. Explain the purpose of an order for filgrastim for Pavel. The nurse will need to assess him for what conditions before beginning the filgrastim?

3. The nurse notices a woman with a baby about to enter Pavel's room. The baby is fussy, and the woman wipes the baby's nose after a sneeze. What does the nurse need to do at this time?
4. Pavel asks the nurse, "When can I stop having these injections? I hate having to have another shot!" What is the best answer to his question?

For answers, see http://evolve.elsevier.com/Canada/Lilley/pharmacology/.

cytotoxic precautions will be implemented by health care providers when handling and administering drugs. Measure vital signs with special attention to temperature. Premedication with acetaminophen and diphenhydramine hydrochloride to help minimize any allergic type of reaction may be necessary when administering any of the BRMs. With some of the BRMs, treatment with opioids, antihistamines, or anti-inflammatory drugs may be required for the management of bone pain and chills, if treatment with acetaminophen or diphenhydramine hydrochloride is not successful. Antiemetics may also be needed for any drug-related nausea or vomiting and may be administered prior to the administration of the BRM. Antiemetics may need to be dosed around the clock if nausea and vomiting are problematic. Encourage patients to rest when tired, not to overexert themselves, and to contact a health care provider if they experience profound fatigue or loss of appetite. Encourage patients to drink fluids, up to 2 to 3 litres per day (unless contraindicated), to promote excretion of the by-products of cellular breakdown and maintain cellular hydration. Consultation with a registered dietitian may help patients to learn about a nourishing diet to promote health and wellness (e.g., ensuring intake of foods high in protein and complex carbohydrates, as well as necessary minerals, vitamins, and natural health products). Discuss menu planning and grocery shopping and give specific individualized suggestions. Many grocery stores support online food shopping with pickup at the store on the same day, or home delivery options at no or minimal cost. Inform patients of community resources (e.g., Meals on Wheels, respite care organizations) as deemed appropriate and as needed.

With hematopoietic drugs, it is important to administer the drug as ordered. Determine and rotate subcutaneous and IV sites, as specified by facility policy. With filgrastim, administer the drug before a patient receiving myelosuppressive chemotherapy develops an infection, but not within 24 hours before or after a myelosuppressive chemotherapy drug is given. Once a patient's ANC reaches 1×10^9/L, discontinue the drug, as ordered and as recommended by the manufacturer. Give filgrastim and use 5% dextrose in water to dilute the product. When drugs are given subcutaneously, rotate injection sites. See the Patient Teaching Tips for more information.

When interferons are to be given, be sure to first read the order for correct spelling and be careful not to confuse the drug with any other sound-alike, look-alike drugs. Administer interferons parenterally by either the subcutaneous, IV, or IM route, depending on the drug. For example, interferon alfa-2b is given subcutaneously, intramuscularly, or subcutaneously. Be sure to rotate sites and use accurate technique (see Chapter 10). In the presence of concerns regarding infection, as occurs with many of the BRMs, monitor the patient's vital signs with attention to temperature and also for the occurrence of chills and headache. Electrocardiograms (ECGs) are generally prescribed before and during treatment, so monitor the results and report any chest pain, hypotension, hypertension, or dyspnea. Make sure to always check each brand of medication for dilution directions, as each brand has different directions. Read the package insert prior to giving any interferon. Acetaminophen may be prescribed to help with fever and headache. Encourage patients to increase their intake of fluids.

With the use of monoclonal antibodies, serious infections are a major concern, especially with belimumab, with which infection may sometimes be fatal. Constantly monitor for infection during therapy. Certolizumab, which is used for severe rheumatoid arthritis, is also associated with the risk of serious infections and possible lymphoma, which needs to be explained to patients. Continue to monitor blood counts during and after therapy with these drugs. Monitor patients for changes in blood pressure and pulse rate and for chest pain. Contact the health care provider immediately if there are significant changes in baseline parameters. Avoid infliximab in patients with severe heart failure. When giving this drug, it is important to monitor the patient for heart sounds, blood pressure, pulse rate, pulse oximetry reading, and ECG readings. If there are signs and symptoms of infection or changes in cardiac status, contact the health care provider immediately.

With the biological DMARD methotrexate, a test dose is usually administered to see how the patient reacts to the medication. Be aware of the warning about the need for cautious administration of this drug in those with kidney disease, infection, pulmonary disease, and stomatitis. Be sure that if methotrexate is ordered for rheumatoid arthritis, it is administered weekly as ordered. For more information on methotrexate, see Chapter 52. Give etanercept (yet another drug with specific warnings; see the previous discussion) subcutaneously into the thigh, abdomen, or upper arm, rotating injection sites. Give leflunomide cautiously while monitoring liver and kidney functioning; administer it orally with meals or food to minimize GI upset. Monitor daily weights due to possible edema.

▨ Evaluation

Therapeutic responses to BRMs include a variety of responses, such as a decrease in the growth of a lesion or mass, decreased tumour size, and an easing of symptoms related to a tumour or disease process. Other therapeutic responses are an improvement in WBC and platelet counts or a return of blood counts to normal levels, and absence of infection and hemorrhage. Encourage patients to keep a journal, as this may provide health care providers with more data from which to evaluate the patients' responses during and after therapy. Possible adverse effects for which to evaluate are presented in Tables 54-1 and 54-2. DMARDs are expected to have therapeutic results within a documented time frame (often weeks), with the patient experiencing increased ability to move joints, less discomfort, and an overall increased sense of improvement and well-being. Toxicity of these drugs may be manifested by liver, renal, and respiratory dysfunction and, for methotrexate, bone marrow suppression.

PATIENT TEACHING TIPS

- Advise patients to avoid hazardous tasks because of the CNS changes noted with several BRMs. Fatigue is also a common adverse effect; instruct patients to report excessive fatigue.
- Instruct patients to report to the health care provider immediately any signs of infection, such as sore throat, diarrhea, vomiting, or fever of 38.1°C or higher. Advise patients also to report excessive fatigue, loss of appetite, edema, or bleeding.
- Pregnancy is discouraged while patients are taking a BRM. Educate patients of childbearing age about contraceptive choices and the need to use contraception for up to 2 years after completion of therapy.
- Inform patients that adverse effects associated with BRMs usually disappear within 72 to 96 hours after therapy is discontinued.

- Interleukins may be self-administered; therefore, teach patients self-injection techniques and proper disposal of equipment (e.g., needles, syringes). Provide patients with corresponding written instructions. Encourage patients to keep a daily journal to record the site of injection and an overall rating of how they feel.
- Educate patients that bone pain and flulike symptoms often occur with some of the BRMs, and the use of nonopioid or, in some cases, opioid analgesics may be required. Some patients may find relief with acetaminophen or ibuprofen.
- With the use of DMARDs, patients will experience improved joint function and decreased pain. Encourage patients to report any bleeding, excess fatigue, fever, or respiratory symptoms to the health care provider.

KEY POINTS

- Cancer treatment has traditionally involved surgery, radiation, and chemotherapy. Surgery and radiation are usually local or regional therapies. Chemotherapy is generally systemic, but it often does not completely eliminate all of the cancer cells in the body. Adjuvant therapy is frequently used to destroy undetected distant micrometastases.
- The humoral and cellular immune systems act together to recognize and destroy foreign particles and cells. The humoral immune system is composed of lymphocytes known as B cells until they are transformed into plasma cells when they come in contact with an antigen (foreign substance). Plasma cells then manufacture antibodies to that antigen.
- BRMs provide another treatment option for patients who have malignancies or those who are receiving chemotherapy and have a need to boost blood cell counts. BRMs include hematopoietics, interferons, interleukins, monoclonal antibodies, and DMARDs. Use

of these drugs may augment, restore, or modify host defences against the tumour.
- Nursing management associated with the administration of BRMs focuses on the use of careful aseptic technique and other measures to prevent infection; proper nutrition, oral hygiene, and monitoring of blood counts; and management of adverse effects, including joint or bone pain and flulike symptoms.
- Do not administer filgrastim within 24 hours of a myelosuppressive antineoplastic, and follow the timeframe for its use (as prescribed), whether in an inpatient or home setting.
- The recommended therapy with nonbiological DMARDs usually begins with methotrexate or leflunomide for most patients. Biological DMARDs are generally reserved for those patients whose disease does not respond to methotrexate or leflunomide. The biological DMARDs include etanercept, infliximab, adalimumab, abatacept, and rituximab.

EXAMINATION REVIEW QUESTIONS

1. The nurse is conducting a class on drugs for malignant tumours for a group of new oncology staff members. Which best describes the action of interferons in the management of malignant tumours?
   a. Interferons increase the production of specific anticancer enzymes.
   b. Interferons have antiviral and antitumour properties and strengthen the immune system.
   c. Interferons stimulate the production and activation of T lymphocytes and cytotoxic T cells.
   d. Interferons help improve the cell-killing action of T cells because they are retrieved from healthy donors.

2. When planning care for a patient who is receiving interferon therapy, the nurse must keep in mind which major dose-limiting factor?
   a. Fatigue
   b. Bone marrow depression
   c. Fever
   d. Nausea

3. The nurse is administering methotrexate as part of the treatment for rheumatoid arthritis and will monitor for which sign of bone marrow suppression?
   a. Edema
   b. Tinnitus
   c. Increased bleeding tendencies
   d. Tingling in the extremities

Continued

EXAMINATION REVIEW QUESTIONS—cont'd

4. In caring for a patient receiving therapy with a myelosuppressive antineoplastic drug, the nurse notes an order to begin filgrastim (Neupogen) after the chemotherapy is completed. Which statement correctly describes when the nurse should begin the filgrastim therapy?
   a. It can be started during chemotherapy.
   b. It will begin immediately after chemotherapy is completed.
   c. It will be initiated 24 hours after chemotherapy is completed.
   d. It will not be started until at least 72 hours after chemotherapy is completed.

5. The nurse is monitoring a patient who has been receiving aldesleukin (IL-2; Proleukin) for the treatment of malignant melanoma. Which adverse effect, if noted on assessment, is of primary concern?
   a. Chills
   b. Fatigue
   c. Headache
   d. Fluid retention

6. The nurse is reviewing the medical history of a patient who is about to receive therapy with etanercept (Enbrel). Which conditions, if present, would be a contraindication or caution for therapy with this drug? (Select all that apply.)
   a. Urinary tract infection
   b. Psoriasis
   c. Heart failure
   d. Glaucoma
   e. Latex allergy

7. A patient is to receive filgrastim (Neupogen) after therapy with carmustine and radiation therapy for treatment of a brain tumour. The patient weighs 132 pounds. The protocol that the oncologist has written states that the filgrastim will be dosed at 5 mcg/kg. Filgrastim comes in a 300-mcg/mL vial. What dose will the patient receive? How many millilitres will the patient be given?

Answers: 1. b, 2. a, 3. c, 4. c, 5. d, 6. a, c, e, 7. 300 mcg; 1 mL

CRITICAL THINKING ACTIVITIES

1. A patient who has been receiving an alkylating chemotherapeutic drug is to receive the CSF filgrastim (Neupogen). A new nurse is preparing to start the filgrastim as soon as the chemotherapy is completed, and the charge nurse is reviewing the orders. What is the priority action of the charge nurse at this time? Explain your answer.

2. The nurse is monitoring a patient who is receiving the interleukin drug aldesleukin (Proleukin). The patient is experiencing fever, chills, fatigue, dyspnea, slight crackles, ankle edema rated as 2+, and headache. What is the nurse's priority action at this time?

3. The nurse is preparing to administer etanercept (Enbrel) to a patient with severe rheumatoid arthritis. During the assessment, the nurse notes that the patient has a history of moderate psoriasis, type 2 diabetes mellitus, and allergies to penicillin and latex. What is the nurse's priority action at this time?

For answers, see http://evolve.elsevier.com/Canada/Lilley/pharmacology/.

PART TEN

Miscellaneous Therapeutics: Hematological, Dermatological, Ophthalmic, and Otic Drugs

STUDY SKILLS TIPS:

- TIME MANAGEMENT
- PURR
- REPEAT THE STEPS

TIME MANAGEMENT

As you plan study time for Part Ten, it should be clear that Chapter 57 will take significantly more time to cover than the other chapters. Do not let the length of the chapter overwhelm you. Apply principles of time management to this chapter and you will succeed. The most important aspects of time management to apply to this chapter are the use of clear goal statements and action plan steps to achieve your goals.

Goal Statements

Remember SMART; goal statements must be **S**pecific, **M**easurable, **A**ttainable, **R**ealistic and **T**ime limited. For instance, saying to yourself, "I will study the chapter" is not a very specific goal; instead, saying "I will master the 30 terms in the Key Terms" is a more specific goal statement. Goal statements must be measurable. In the example of the goal of studying the key terms, including the number of terms contained in Chapter 57 helps clarify the goal. Your time is valuable, and you have a variety of competing priorities (e.g., other courses, family, friends, and other commitments). You must set a time limit on how long you will spend on this goal. Doing so allows you to be focused as you study, with a purpose-driven mentality.

Action Planning

The facet of time management that complements the creation of goal statements is the use of action

planning. An action plan is a series of small, specific activities that you will accomplish to meet the goals in your statements. Consider the example mentioned—your goal is to master the 30 terms. What will you do to meet that goal?

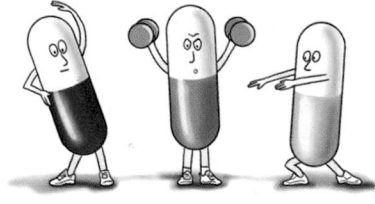

Action Steps Example

1. I will spend 1 hour making vocabulary drill cards for the terms found in the Key Terms in Chapter 57, from 1500 hours to 1600 hours on Monday.
2. I will spend 15 minutes on rehearsal and review of these cards every day until the exam on this chapter is over.
3. Each time I cannot define and explain a term, I will put an "x" on the card to identify it as a term needing more review.
4. I will spend 1 hour the night before the exam doing a comprehensive review of the terms in Chapter 57, with special emphasis on those cards that have one or more "x" marks. Action steps help ensure that you are spending your study time actively focusing on what you need to learn.

Notice the importance of having a SMART goal. Simply stating "I will study the chapter" makes the development of an action plan difficult. Revising this to satisfy SMART—"I will master the 30 terms in the Key

Terms"—facilitates the creation of a clear action plan that is well-defined and direct.

PURR

Prepare Example

Chapter 57, Objective 3: "Discuss the mechanisms of action, indications, dosage forms, application techniques, adverse effects, cautions, contraindications, and drug interactions of the various ophthalmic drugs."

- Question 1. What does *ophthalmic* mean? (literal question [LQ])
- Question 2. What are ophthalmic drugs? (LQ)
- Question 3. What is the mechanism of action of ophthalmic drugs? (LQ)
- Question 4. Do ophthalmic drugs have more than one mechanism of action? (LQ)
- Question 5. If ophthalmic drugs have more than one mechanism of action, how are their mechanisms similar, and how are they different? (interpretive question)

These questions are only suggestions for generated questions based on the chapter objectives. Many more questions can be asked about Objective 3. These questions are an essential part of the study process, as questions help make you an active reader and an active learner. The more questions you generate before reading, the easier it will be to understand the chapter.

Outline Example

1. *Looking through the chapter, decide how much material is appropriate for a single reading session.* The section headed Glaucoma is probably too much material. Guided by the chapter headings, this section could be broken down into six blocks of material. Block 1 would cover the introductory material under the main heading, as well as the material under the headings Antiglaucoma Drugs and Cholinergic Drugs. Block 2 would be the material under the heading Sympatho-mimetics (Mydriatics). The next four blocks would be β-Adrenergic Blockers, Carbonic Anhydrase Inhibitors, Osmotic Diuretics, and Prostaglandin Agonists.

2. *Apply the Prepare step to each block.* Beginning with the first block, generate some questions to guide your reading. Remember that it is important to ask questions that will focus on literal information as well as questions that will help you interpret, evaluate, and analyze as you read.

3. *Read the material.* As soon as you have completed generating questions for the first block of material, read the block immediately. Read for understanding. As you read, remember the questions you generated. This approach will help your concentration and comprehension.

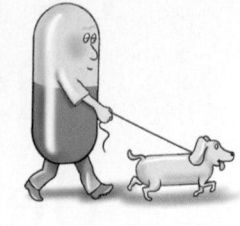

4. *Take a short break.* Once you have completed reading this section of the chapter, give your mind a chance to reflect and consolidate your learning. Limit the time you allow for a break and use the time for something pleasurable. Give yourself 5 or 10 minutes to read the newspaper, get a snack, or just take a short walk.

5. *Rehearse.* Before going on to the next section of the chapter, it is important to spend a few minutes in rehearsal. Using the questions from Step 2, go back over the material you read and try to respond to those questions. When you find yourself unable to answer a question, put a mark in the text beside the heading that caused the difficulty and move on. The mark will serve as a reminder for future review. At this point, your objective should not be to completely master the material but instead to see what you've learned, so that you can move smoothly into the next section. Breaking a chapter into blocks is useful, but it is also imperative to make links between sections as you study.

6. *Review.* After completing two or three major sections of the chapter, it is time to review. Start at the beginning of the chapter. Ask your questions; try to answer them. If you cannot formulate a clear answer, then some rereading is necessary. Also, pay attention to the marks you made during the Rehearse step. Those marks indicate areas you have already identified as needing review. When rereading, remember that your objective is to read only as much of the material as needed to be able to respond to self-generated questions. There simply is not enough time to read the entire chapter a second or third time.

REPEAT THE STEPS

Prepare, read for understanding, take a short break, and then rehearse the material you just read. It may seem that this process takes an excessive amount of time and involves a lot of repetition, but it will produce enhanced learning in the long run. The time spent in **Prepare**, **Under**-stand, and **Rehearse** will reduce the time needed to review. Frequent review as you move through the chapter will make the final Review stage at exam time go more quickly and will enable you to achieve mastery of the material.

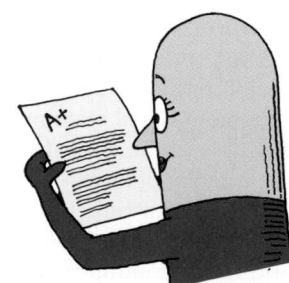

CHAPTER 55

Anemia Drugs

Objectives

After reading this chapter, the successful student will be able to do the following:

1. Discuss the importance of iron, vitamin B$_{12}$, and folic acid to the formation of blood cells.

2. Discuss the various types of anemia-related blood products.

3. Discuss the mechanisms of action, cautions, contraindications, drug interactions, uses, dosages, and special administration techniques of the various drugs used to treat anemia, as well as measures to enhance the effectiveness and decrease the adverse effects of these drugs.

4. Develop a collaborative plan of care that includes all phases of the nursing process for patients taking drugs used to treat anemia.

e-Learning Activities

Website
(http://evolve.elsevier.com/Canada/
Lilley/pharmacology/)

evolve

- Answer Key—Textbook Case Studies
- Answer Key—Critical Thinking Activities
- Chapter Summaries—Printable
- Review Questions for Exam Preparation
- Unfolding Case Studies

Drug Profiles

▸▸ epoetin alfa, p. 1030
     ferric gluconate, p. 1033
▸▸ ferrous fumarate, p. 1033
▸▸ folic acid, p. 1034
     iron dextran, p. 1033
     iron sucrose, p. 1033

▸▸ Key drug

Key Terms

Erythrocytes Another name for red blood cells (RBCs). (p. 1028)

Erythropoiesis The process of erythrocyte production. (p. 1028)

Erythropoietin A hormone secreted by the kidneys that increases the rate of production of red blood cells in the bone marrow in response to decreasing oxygen levels in the tissues. (p. 1028)

Globin The protein part of the hemoglobin molecule (see later); the four different structural chains most often found in adults are the α_1, α_2, β_1, and β_2 chains. (p. 1028)

Hematopoiesis The normal formation and development of all blood cell types in the bone marrow. (p. 1028)

Heme Part of the hemoglobin molecule; a nonprotein, iron-containing pigment. (p. 1028)

Hemoglobin (Hgb) A complex protein–iron compound in the blood that carries oxygen to the cells from the lungs and carbon dioxide away from the cells to the lungs. (p. 1028)

Hemolytic anemias Anemias resulting from excessive destruction of erythrocytes. (p. 1029)

Hypochromic Pertaining to less than normal colour; usually describes a red blood cell with decreased hemoglobin content and helps further characterize anemias associated with reduced synthesis of hemoglobin. (p. 1028)

Microcytic Pertaining to or characterized by smaller than normal cells. (p. 1028)

Pernicious anemia A type of megaloblastic anemia usually seen in older adults and caused by impaired intestinal absorption of vitamin B$_{12}$ (cyanocobalamin) due to lack of availability of intrinsic factor. (p. 1029)

Reticulocytes Immature erythrocytes characterized by a meshlike pattern of threads and particles at the former site of the nucleus. (p. 1028)

Spherocytes Small, globular, completely hemoglobinated erythrocytes without the usual central concavity or pallor. (p. 1029)

ERYTHROPOIESIS

The formation of new blood cells is one of the primary functions of bones. This process is known as *hematopoiesis*, and it includes the production of **erythrocytes** (red blood cells [RBCs]), as well as leukocytes (white blood cells) and thrombocytes (platelets). This process takes place in the myeloid tissue or bone marrow. This specialized tissue is located primarily in the ends, or epiphyses, of certain long bones and also in the flat bones of the skull, pelvis, sternum, scapulae, and ribs.

Erythropoiesis, the process of erythrocyte formation, is the focus of this chapter and involves the maturation of a nucleated RBC precursor into a hemoglobin-filled, nucleus-free erythrocyte. Erythropoiesis is driven by the hormone **erythropoietin**, which is produced by the kidneys. Erythropoietin is also produced commercially and is used to treat anemia in certain specific circumstances and is discussed in detail later in the chapter.

When RBCs are manufactured in the bone marrow by myeloid tissue, they are released into the circulation as immature RBCs called **reticulocytes**. Once in the circulation, reticulocytes undergo a 24- to 36-hour maturation process to become mature, fully functional RBCs. After this, they have a lifespan of approximately 120 days.

More than one third of an RBC is composed of hemoglobin. **Hemoglobin (Hgb)** is composed of two parts: heme and globin. **Heme** is a red pigment. Each heme group contains one atom of iron. **Globin** is a protein chain. The four different structural globulin chains most often found in adults are the α_1, α_2, β_1, and β_2. Together, four heme groups, each linked to one protein chain of globin, make one hemoglobin molecule (Figure 55-1).

TYPES OF ANEMIA

Anemias are classified into four main types, based on underlying causes (Figure 55-2). Anemias can be caused by maturation defects, or they can be secondary to excessive RBC destruction. Two types of maturation defects lead to anemias, categorized by the location of the defect within the cell: cytoplasmic maturation defects occur in the cell cytoplasm, and nuclear maturation defects occur in the cell nucleus. Factors responsible for excessive RBC destruction can be either intrinsic or extrinsic. Anemia of chronic disease is another common type of anemia.

Figure 55-3 summarizes the types of anemias arising from cytoplasmic maturation defects. Major examples include iron-deficiency anemia and genetic disorders such as thalassemia, which result in defective globin synthesis. In each of these anemias, RBCs appear **hypochromic** (lighter red than normal) and **microcytic** (smaller than normal) on a blood smear. Cytoplasmic maturation anemias occur as a result of reduced or abnormal hemoglobin synthesis. Because hemoglobin is synthesized

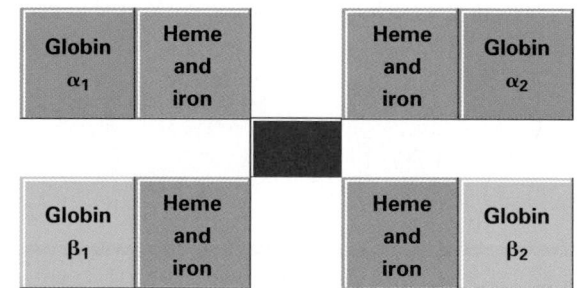

FIG. 55-1 Schematic structure of a hemoglobin molecule (α, alpha; β, beta).

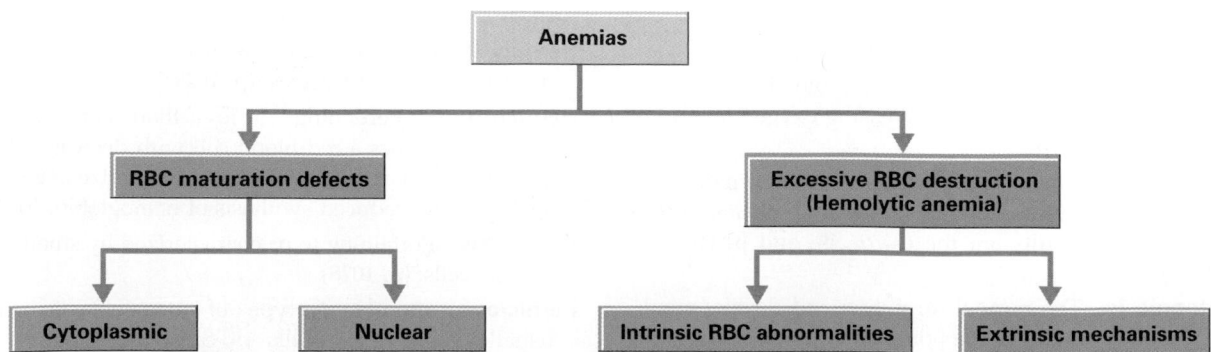

FIG. 55-2 Underlying causes of anemia are red blood cell (RBC) maturation defects and factors secondary to excessive RBC destruction.

from both iron and globin, a deficiency in either one can lead to a hemoglobin deficiency. Some common causes of iron-deficiency anemia are blood loss, surgery, childbirth, gastrointestinal (GI) bleeding (which can be caused by NSAID ingestion; see Chapter 49), menstrual blood flow, and bleeding hemorrhoids.

Figure 55-4 summarizes the types of anemias arising from nuclear maturation defects. These occur because of defects in deoxyribonucleic acid (DNA) or protein synthesis. Both DNA and protein require vitamin B_{12} and folic acid (B_9) to be present in normal amounts for their proper production. If either of these two vitamins is absent or deficient, anemias secondary to nuclear maturation defects may develop. RBCs actually appear to be normochromic (normal in colour) but are commonly macrocytic (larger than normal) on a blood smear. One example of this type of anemia is **pernicious anemia**, which results from a deficiency of vitamin B_{12}, used in the formation of new RBCs. The usual underlying cause is failure of the stomach lining to produce intrinsic

factor. Intrinsic factor is a gastric glycoprotein that allows vitamin B_{12} to be absorbed in the intestine (see Chapter 9). Another example of anemia arising from nuclear maturation defects is the anemia caused by folic acid deficiency. Both pernicious anemia and folic acid deficiency anemia are also known as types of *megaloblastic anemia*, because they are both characterized by large, immature RBCs. Megaloblastic anemias are not caused by a lack of intrinsic factor but are usually related to poor dietary intake. These types of anemia are most commonly seen in infancy, childhood, and pregnancy.

Figure 55-5 summarizes the types of anemias arising from excessive RBC destruction, or **hemolytic anemias**. These can occur because of abnormalities within the RBCs (intrinsic factors) or as a result of factors outside (extrinsic to) the RBCs. In both cases, the erythrocytes appear on a blood smear as **spherocytes**. RBC abnormalities caused by intrinsic factors are usually the result of a genetic defect. Examples include sickle cell

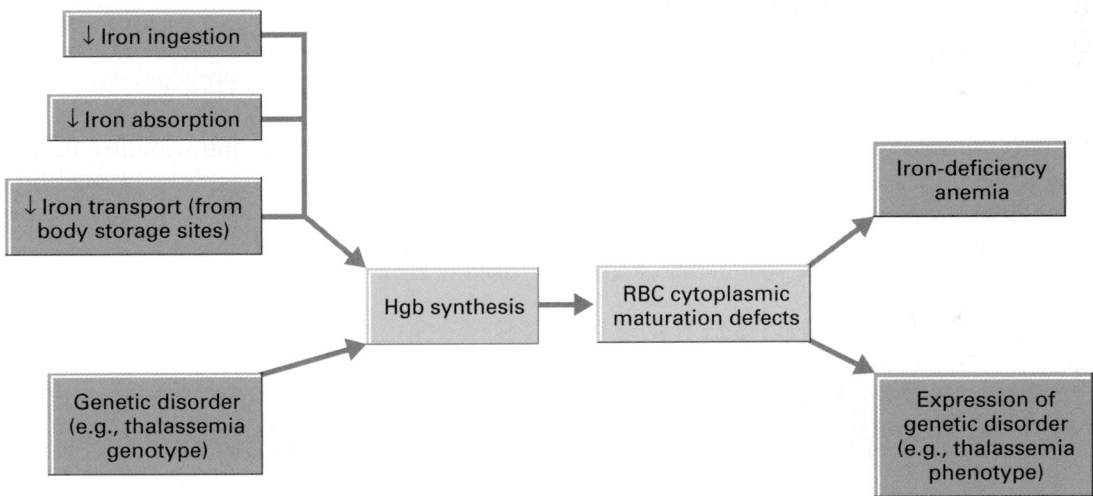

FIG. 55-3 Schematic showing common causes and results of red blood cell (RBC) cytoplasmic maturation anemia. ↓, decreased.

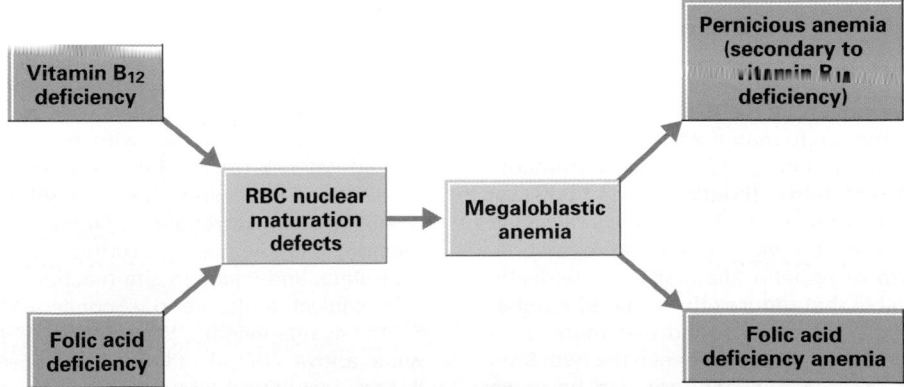

FIG. 55-4 Schematic showing common causes and results of red blood cell (RBC) nuclear maturation defects.

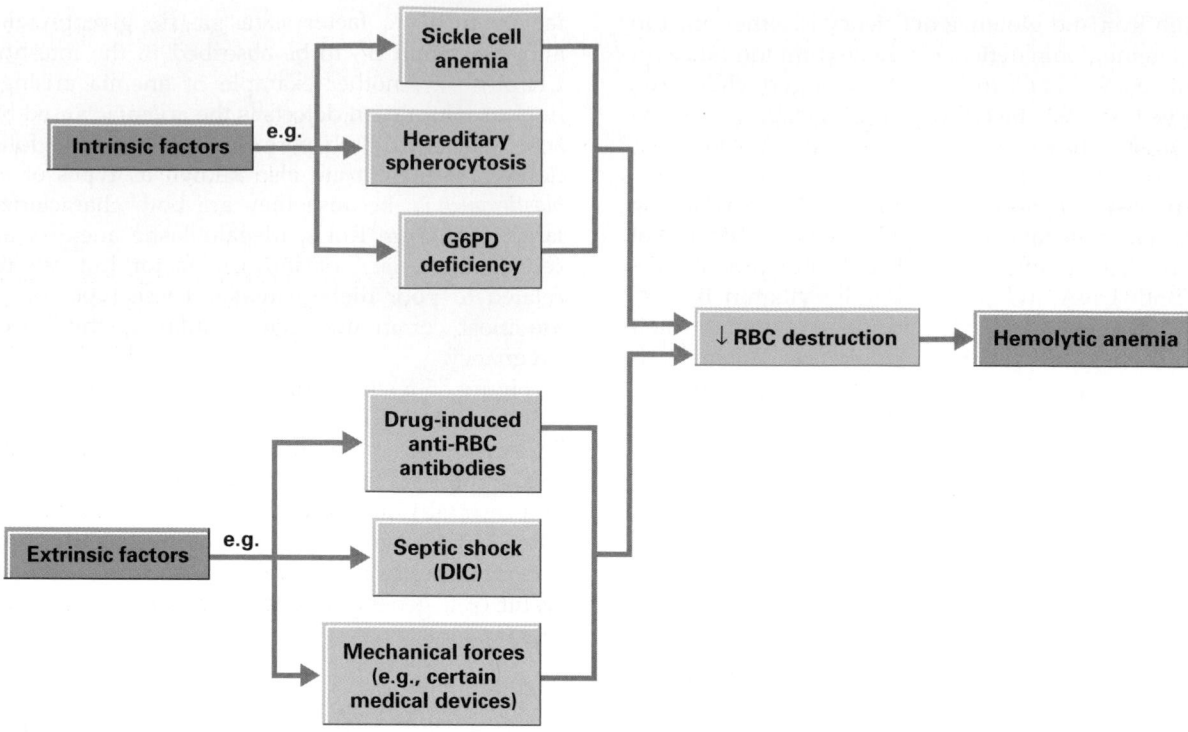

FIG. 55-5   Increased red blood cell (RBC) destruction occurs as a result of intrinsic and extrinsic factors. ↑, increased; *DIC*, disseminated intravascular coagulation; *G6PD*, glucose-6-phosphate dehydrogenase.

anemia, hereditary spherocytosis, glucose-6-phosphate dehydrogenase (G6PD) deficiency, and paroxysmal nocturnal hemoglobinuria. Examples of extrinsic mechanisms of excessive RBC destruction include drug-induced antibodies that target and destroy RBCs, septic shock that produces disseminated intravascular coagulation, and mechanical forces such as those created by intra-aortic balloon pumps, ventricular assist devices, and continuous venovenous hemodialysis (CVVHD), commonly used in critical care units.

ERYTHROPOIESIS-STIMULATING AGENTS

 DRUG PROFILES

▸▸*epoetin alfa*

Epoetin alfa (Eprex®) is a biosynthetic form of the natural hormone erythropoietin, which is normally secreted by the kidneys in response to a decrease in RBCs. It promotes the synthesis of erythrocytes (RBCs) by stimulating RBC progenitor cells in the bone marrow. Epoetin alfa and darbepoietin alfa are used to treat anemia that is associated with end-stage kidney disease, chemotherapy-induced anemia, and anemia associated with zidovudine therapy (see Chapter 45). Epoetin alfa causes the progenitor cells in the bone marrow to manufacture large numbers of immature RBCs and greatly speed up their maturation. This medication is ineffective without adequate body iron stores and bone marrow function. Most patients receiving epoetin alfa need to also receive an oral iron preparation. A longer-acting form of epoetin alfa, called darbepoetin (Aranesp®), is available that reduces the required number of injections, although one study found that there is no significant difference in overall cost between the two. Both drugs are available for injection only and can be given intravenously or subcutaneously. When they are given by the subcutaneous route, their onset of action is slower, and lower dosages can be used.

Contraindications to the use of erythropoiesis-stimulating agents (ESAs) include known drug allergy. Use of epoetin alfa and darbepoetin alfa is contraindicated in cases of uncontrolled hypertension and in patients who develop pure red cell aplasia following erythropoiesis regulating hormone. Hemoglobin levels above 100 g/L for cancer patients and 130 g/L for patients with kidney disease has been associated with harm and should be avoided. Use in patients with head or neck cancers or patients at risk for thrombosis is controversial as these medications increase tumour growth and risk for thrombosis. Their most frequent adverse effects include hypertension, fever, headache, pruritus, rash, nausea, vomiting, arthralgia, and injection site reaction.

In clinical trials, serious concerns about the use of ESAs became evident. When patients' hemoglobin levels were above 130 g/L, they experienced serious adverse events, including heart attack, stroke, and death. Individualized dosing is necessary to achieve and maintain

DRUG PROFILES—cont'd

hemoglobin levels within the range of 100 to 120 g/L. Patients with uncontrolled hypertension should not be treated with ESAs; blood pressure must be controlled prior to treatment with ESAs. They are to be used cautiously in patients with a history of seizures. Patients with cancer require a target hemoglobin of less than 120 g/L to minimize adverse effects associated with ESAs. Misuse of erythropoietin by athletes hoping to increase their oxygen-carrying capacity and improve their performance

places them at risk for diseases caused by increased blood viscosity (e.g., stroke, myocardial infarction). Erythropoietin is an illegal substance in the sports industry.

PHARMACOKINETICS

Route	Onset of Action	Peak Plasma Concentration	Elimination Half-Life	Duration of Action
Subcut or IV	7–10 days	5–24 hr	4–13 hr	Variable

TABLE 55-1

Ferrous Salts: Iron Content

Ferrous Salt*	Iron Content (in 300 mg)	Number of Tablets Taken Per Day (Adults)
Ferrous gluconate	35 mg or 11.6% iron	3–4 300-mg tablets
Ferrous sulphate	60 mg or 20% iron	3–4 324-mg tablets
Ferrous fumarate	100 mg or 33% iron	2–3 300-mg tablets

*Some patients may tolerate different formulations better; however, the number of tablets that must be consumed may decrease patient adherence.

IRON

Iron is a mineral that is essential for the proper function of all biological systems in the body. It is stored in many sites throughout the body (liver, spleen, bone marrow). Deficiency of this mineral is the principal nutritional deficiency resulting in anemia. Individuals who require the highest amount of iron are women (particularly pregnant and menstruating women) and children, and they are the groups most likely to develop iron-deficiency anemia. Most vitamin supplements for men contain little or no iron, because men are much less likely to develop iron-deficiency anemia. Nonetheless, dietary iron is usually sufficient for both men and women in developed countries. Dietary sources of iron include meats, certain vegetables and grains, beans, dried fruits, and eggs. These forms of iron must be broken down by gastric juices before the iron can be absorbed. Orange juice, veal, fish, and ascorbic acid may assist with iron absorption. Conversely, eggs, corn, beans, and many cereal products containing chemicals known as *phytates* may impair iron absorption. Oral iron preparations are available as ferrous salts. See Table 55-1 for a list of the currently available oral iron salts and their respective iron content. Proferrin® is a natural health product (NHP) and is the sole supplement in Canada that contains heme-iron polypeptide. This NHP preferentially absorbs heme-iron through specific receptors throughout the small intestine. FeraMax® is a polysaccharide-iron complex that has 150 mg of elemental iron available in one capsule.

Triferexx® is a NHP that contians vitamin C, vitamin B12, and folic acid as well as iron. When a patient cannot tolerate oral iron, intravenous (IV) iron may be administered. There are four injectable iron products available: iron dextran (Dexiron®, Infufer®), iron sucrose (Venofer®), ferric gluconate (Ferrlecit®), and ferumoxytol (Feraheme®).

Mechanism of Action and Drug Effects

Iron is an oxygen carrier in both hemoglobin and *myoglobin* (oxygen-carrying molecule in muscle tissue) and is critical for tissue respiration. Small quantities of iron are absorbed in the small intestine at a time, and non-heme iron needs to be transformed into its ferrous form and bound to a transporter to pass from the intestine into the bloodstream. Once in the bloodstream, iron is used in the bone marrow to make hemoglobin and the excess iron is stored as ferritin, primarily in the liver and some in the spleen. Iron is also a required component of a number of enzyme systems in the body and is necessary for energy transfer in the cytochrome oxidase and xanthine oxidase enzyme systems. Administration of iron corrects iron-deficiency symptoms such as anemia, dysphagia, dystrophy of the nails and skin, and fissuring or cracking of the angles of the lips, and also maintains the bodily functions described earlier.

Indications

Supplemental iron in multivitamins containing iron or iron supplements alone are indicated for the prevention or treatment of iron-deficiency anemia. In all cases of anemia, an underlying cause needs to be identified. After identification of the cause, treatment is aimed at attempting to correct the cause (e.g., chronic blood loss, such as from a peptic or duodenal ulcer, cancerous colon lesion, or Crohn's disease) rather than simply alleviating the symptoms. Iron supplementation is also used in erythropoietin therapy because it is essential for the production of RBCs.

Contraindications

Contraindications to the use of iron products include known drug allergy, hemochromatosis (iron overload), hemolytic anemia, and any other anemia not associated with iron deficiency.

TABLE 55-2	
Iron Preparations: Adverse Effects	
Body System	**Adverse Effects**
Gastrointestinal	Nausea, constipation, epigastric pain, black and tarry stools, vomiting, diarrhea
Integumentary	Temporarily discoloured tooth enamel and eyes, pain on injection

Adverse Effects

The most common adverse effects associated with oral iron preparations are nausea, vomiting, diarrhea, constipation, dark stools, stomach cramps, and stomach pain. Iron is a metal in its basic form and metals may carry a charge that is magnetic or electric, which can affect muscles and nerves in the bowel, resulting in constipation (slowing down peristalsis) or diarrhea (speeding up peristalsis). Iron supplements that work quickly add more of the metal to the body, so they may cause more constipation. Slow-release forms of iron may be easier on the digestive system but may not be absorbed as effectively. Dose is also important. Excess iron intake can lead to accumulation and iron toxicity. See Table 55-2 for a more complete listing of the undesirable effects associated with iron preparations. Older individuals tend to respond to lower doses of iron supplementation, and lower doses are associated with lower rates of adverse effects than higher doses.

Toxicity and Management of Overdose

Iron overdose is the most common cause of child poisoning deaths reported to Canadian poison control centres. Many iron supplements are enteric coated and resemble candy. Toxicity from iron ingestion results from a combination of corrosive effects on the GI mucosa and the metabolic and hemodynamic effects caused by the presence of excessive elemental iron.

Treatment of iron overdose is based on symptomatic and supportive measures, including suction and maintenance of the airway, correction of acidosis, and control of shock and dehydration with IV fluids, blood, oxygen, and vasopressors. Abdominal X-rays may be helpful because iron preparations are radiopaque and may be visualized on X-ray film. Serum iron concentrations may be helpful in establishing the amount ingested. A serum iron concentration of more than 54 micromol/L places the patient at serious risk for toxicity. In any case of iron overdose, consultation with a poison control centre is recommended. The GI tract is decontaminated via whole bowel irrigation. In patients with severe symptoms of iron intoxication, such as coma, shock, or seizures, chelation therapy with IV deferoxamine mesylate should be initiated.

Interactions

The absorption of iron can be enhanced when it is given with ascorbic acid or decreased when it is given with antacids and calcium. Iron preparations can decrease the absorption of certain antibiotics, including tetracyclines and quinolones.

Dosages

For dosage information on iron preparations, refer to the table on p. 1034.

FOLIC ACID

Folic acid is a water-soluble B-complex vitamin. It is also referred to as *folate*, the name of its anionic form. The human body requires oral intake of folic acid. Dietary sources of folic acid include dried beans, peas, oranges, and green vegetables. Several conditions can lead to folic acid deficiency. However, because folic acid is absorbed in the upper duodenum, malabsorption syndromes are the most common cause of deficiency.

Mechanism of Action and Drug Effects

Folic acid is used for erythropoiesis and for synthesis of nucleic acids (DNA and ribonucleic acid [RNA]). Dietary ingestion of folate is required for the production of DNA and RNA. It is also essential for normal erythropoiesis. Folic acid is not active in the ingested form. It must first be converted to tetrahydrofolic acid, which is a cofactor for reactions in the biosynthesis of nucleic acids.

Indications

Folic acid is used primarily to prevent and treat folic acid deficiency. Anemias caused by folic acid deficiency can be treated by exogenous supplementation of folic acid. There is also much evidence to support the use of folic acid in the prevention of neural tube defects such as spina bifida, anencephaly, and encephalocele. It is recommended that administration begin at least 1 month before pregnancy and continue through early pregnancy to reduce the risk for fetal neural tube defects. Folic acid is also indicated for the treatment of tropical sprue, a malabsorption syndrome.

Contraindications

Contraindications to the use of folic acid include known allergy to a specific drug product and any anemia not related to folic acid deficiency (e.g., pernicious anemia). Folic acid is not to be used to treat anemias until the underlying cause and type of anemia have been determined. For example, administering folic acid to a patient with pernicious anemia may correct the hematological changes of anemia (making the CBC normal), while deceptively masking neurological and other symptoms of pernicious anemia that result from B_{12} deficiency.

Adverse Effects

Adverse effects associated with folic acid use are rare. Allergic reaction or yellow discoloration of urine may occur.

DRUG PROFILES

Iron preparations are available by prescription and as over-the-counter (OTC) medications. They are contraindicated in patients with ulcerative colitis and regional enteritis, conditions involving excessive stores of iron in the body (e.g., hemosiderosis, hemochromatosis), peptic ulcer disease, hemolytic anemia, cirrhosis, gastritis, or esophagitis. Goals of therapy include maintenance of normal hemoglobin and hematocrit levels (see Box 55-1), as well as improved energy levels.

▶▶ferrous fumarate

The ferrous fumarate iron salts (Palafer®) contain the largest amount of iron per gram of salt consumed. Ferrous fumarate is 33% elemental iron; therefore, a 300-mg tablet of ferrous fumarate provides 100 mg of elemental iron. Ferrous fumarate is available only for oral use.

PHARMACOKINETICS

Route	Onset of Action	Peak Plasma Concentration	Elimination Half-Life	Duration of Action
PO	3–10 days	Unknown	6 hr	Variable

▶▶*ferrous sulphate*

Ferrous sulphate is the most frequently used form of oral iron. Ferrous sulphate ($FeSO_4$) is dosed at 300 mg two to three times a day for most adult patients. Confusion can arise with ferrous sulphate because while the typical dose is 300 mg, many commercially available products are 324 mg. The two doses are used interchangeably. To add to the confusion, each 324-mg tablet contains 65 mg of elemental iron. The adult dose of elemental iron is 50 to 100 mg given two to three times daily. Ferrous sulphate is also available as a syrup and as oral drops. Dosing for children is based on elemental iron.

PHARMACOKINETICS

Route	Onset of Action	Peak Plasma Concentration	Elimination Half-Life	Duration of Action
PO	1 wk	2 hr	6 hr	Variable

iron dextran

Iron dextran (Dexiron, Infufer) is a colloidal solution of iron (as ferric hydroxide) and dextran. It is intended for IV or intramuscular (IM) use for treatment of iron deficiency. Anaphylactic reactions to iron dextran, including major orthostatic hypotension and fatal anaphylaxis, have been reported in 0.3% of patients. Because of this, a test dose of 25 mg of iron dextran is administered before injection of the full dose. Because of the potential of iron dextran to cause anaphylaxis, its use has been replaced by use of the newer products, ferric gluconate and iron sucrose. Iron dextran is available only for injection.

PHARMACOKINETICS

Route	Onset of Action	Peak Plasma Concentration	Elimination Half-Life	Duration of Action
IM or IV	Unknown	24–48 hr	5–20 hr	3 wk

ferric gluconate

Ferric gluconate (Ferrlecit) is an injectable iron product that is indicated for repletion of total body iron content in patients with iron-deficiency anemia who are undergoing hemodialysis. The risk of anaphylaxis is much less with ferric gluconate than with iron dextran, and a test dose is not required. Doses higher than 125 mg are associated with increased adverse events, including abdominal pain, dyspnea, cramps, and itching.

PHARMACOKINETICS

Route	Onset of Action	Peak Plasma Concentration	Elimination Half-Life	Duration of Action
IV	End of infusion	7 min	1 hr	4 days

iron sucrose

Iron sucrose (Venofer) is another injectable iron product indicated for the treatment of iron-deficiency anemia in patients with chronic renal disease. It is also used for patients without kidney disease. The risk of its use precipitating anaphylaxis is much less than that associated with iron dextran, and a test dose is not required. Hypotension is its most common adverse effect and appears to be related to infusion rate. Large doses of iron sucrose are infused over 2.5 to 3.5 hours. Low-weight older adult patients appear to be at greatest risk of hypotension. The newest injectable iron product is ferumoxytol (Feraheme). Advantageously, it can be given undiluted as an IV push in 1 minute.

PHARMACOKINETICS

Route	Onset of Action	Peak Plasma Concentration	Elimination Half-Life	Duration of Action
IV	End of infusion	Unknown	6 hr	Unknown

BOX 55-1   Normal Hemoglobin and Hematocrit Values

Laboratory Test	Female	Male
Hemoglobin	120–160 g/L	140–180 g/L
Hematocrit	0.37–0.47 volume fraction	0.37–0.47 volume fraction

Interactions

No significant drug interactions occur with folic acid. However, oral contraceptives (see Chapter 35), corticosteroids (see Chapter 34), sulfonamides (see Chapter 43), and dihydrofolate reductase inhibitors (including the antineoplastic drug methotrexate [see Chapter 52] and the antibiotic trimethoprim [see Chapter 43]) can all cause signs of folic acid deficiency but are not affected by folic acid administration.

Dosages

For dosage information on folic acid, refer to the table on p. 1034.

OTHER ANEMIA DRUGS

Cyanocobalamin (vitamin B$_{12}$), which is discussed in Chapter 9, is used to treat pernicious anemia and other megaloblastic anemias. It can be given orally in a

---

 DRUG PROFILES

▶▶folic acid

Folic acid is a water-soluble B-complex vitamin used primarily in the treatment and prevention of folic acid deficiency and anemias caused by folic acid deficiency. Folic acid is available as an OTC medication in multivitamin preparations and by prescription as a single drug. It is contraindicated in patients with anemias that are neither megaloblastic nor macrocytic, including vitamin B$_{12}$ defi-

ciency anemia and uncorrected pernicious anemia. Folic acid is available for both oral and injectable use.

PHARMACOKINETICS

Route	Onset of Action	Peak Plasma Concentration	Elimination Half-Life	Duration of Action
PO	Unknown	60–90 min	Unknown	Unknown

DOSAGES   Selected Anemia Drugs

Drug (All Are Safe to Use During Pregnancy)	Pharmacological Class	Usual Dosage Range	Indications
▶▶epoetin alfa (Eprex)	Human recombinant hormone (erythropoietin) analogue	IV/Subcut: 2 000–40 000 units 1–3 × wk, depending on weight and indication	Chemotherapy-induced anemia; anemia associated with chronic kidney disease
ferric gluconate (Ferrlecit)	Parenteral iron salt	*Adults* IV: 10 mL (125 mg) diluted in 100 mL of 0.9% NS over 1 hr for 8 doses	Iron deficiency associated with hemodialysis
▶▶ferrous fumarate/ ferrous sulphate/ ferrous gluconate (as combination [Palafer])	Oral iron salt	*Adults and adolescents** PO: 1 capsule (300 mg with 100 mg elemental iron) daily	Iron-deficiency anemia
▶▶folic acid	Water-soluble B-complex vitamin	*Children†* PO/IV/IM: 0.1–0.4 mg/day *Adults†* PO/IV/IM/Subcut: Up to 1 mg/day	Folate deficiency; tropical sprue; nutritional supplementation; pregnancy-related supplementation
iron dextran (Dexiron, Infurer)	Parenteral iron salt	*Children and infants†* IM/IV: 5–10 kg: 25 mg/day elemental iron (0.5 mL/day); greater than 10 kg: 50 mg/day elemental iron (1 mL/day) *Adults†* IM/IV: 100 mg/day elemental iron (2 mL/day)	Iron deficiency when oral iron is unsatisfactory
iron sucrose (Venofer)	Parenteral iron salt	IV: 100 mg 1–3 times weekly to a cumulative dose of 1 000 mg; may give up to 500 mg as single dose on days 1 and 14	Iron deficiency in patients with chronic kidney failure

IM, intramuscular; *IV*, intravenous; *PO*, oral; *Subcut*, subcutaneous.
*Doses are in terms of elemental iron, not the salt itself.
†Expressed in milligrams of elemental iron. Dosages are calculated for each patient's weight according to manufacturer's label. Doses are approximate.

multivitamin preparation to treat vitamin B_{12} deficiency but is usually given by deep IM injection to treat pernicious anemia. Once remission of the anemia is seen, cyanocobalamin IM can be dosed once a month.

NURSING PROCESS

☑ Assessment

Before any drug is given to treat anemia, assess the patient's past and present medical history; compile a medication profile, including all prescription and OTC drugs and natural health products the patient is taking; also assess for drug allergies. It is important to assess for and document any signs and symptoms of anemia, such as fatigue, changes in nails and skin, and fissuring or cracking of the angles of the lips. It is also necessary to assess patients for contraindications, cautions, and drug interactions prior to beginning treatment with any of the drugs used to treat anemia. ESAs (epoetin alfa and darbepoetin alfa) are used to treat anemia associated with end-stage kidney disease and chemotherapy-induced anemia. Assessment of adequate body iron stores and bone marrow function is needed prior to administration of either of these drugs. Document baseline vital signs because blood pressure may elevate as hematocrit rises; medical intervention may be needed. Assess for allergies to ESAs as well as for other contraindications, such as uncontrolled hypertension and hemoglobin levels of greater than 100 g/L for patients with cancer and greater than 130 g/L for patients with kidney disease.

With iron products, significant contraindications include hemochromatosis, hemolytic anemia, and any other anemia that is not related to iron deficiency. Food and drug interactions affecting the absorption of iron preparations include ascorbic acid (increased absorption) and antacids (decreased absorption); iron preparations can decrease absorption of other drugs, such as tetracyclines and quinolones. Laboratory studies that may be ordered before, during, and after therapy include RBC counts, hemoglobin and hematocrit levels, reticulocyte counts, bilirubin levels, and baseline levels of folate or B-complex vitamins. Perform a nutritional assessment with a focus on the amount of iron in the patient's diet. A 24-hour recall of all food intake with serving sizes may be beneficial. A nutritional and dietary consultation may also be ordered. In addition, asking questions about the patient's energy levels, ability to carry out activities of daily living (ADLs), overall immunity to illnesses, and state of health may provide valuable information.

☑ Pharmacokinetic Bridge to Nursing Practice

Iron preparations provide perfect examples of how pharmacokinetic properties can impact drug dosing and efficacy. Oral iron is available in a variety of salt forms, such as ferrous fumarate, ferrous sulphate, and ferric gluconate. Although quite similar in mechanism of action, the specific salt forms are associated with different pharmacokinetics and offer varying amounts of elemental iron. The ferrous fumarate iron salts contain high proportions of iron per gram of salt consumed. For example, each 100 mg of ferrous fumarate provides 33 mg of elemental iron, whereas each 300-mg tablet of ferrous sulphate contains 65 mg of elemental iron. Even though the pharmacokinetics of the different oral iron salts are similar, the amount of elemental iron per 100 mg varies significantly. Because of these varying amounts of elemental iron, the iron salts must not be exchanged for one another and must be given with caution to avoid medication errors. Other pharmacokinetic properties of oral iron products, such as absorption and excretion, must be understood because unabsorbed iron—though harmless—turns the stool black and may mask melena (blood in the stool). It is recommended to take oral iron with juice (orange juice is preferred) or water but not with milk or antacids because of subsequent decreased drug absorption.

☑ Nursing Diagnoses

- Activity intolerance related to fatigue and lethargy associated with anemias
- Imbalanced nutrition, less than body requirements, related to inadequate food intake
- Constipation related to adverse effects of iron products

☑ Planning

■ Goals

- Patient will maintain or regain typical level of activity (as recommended by the health care provider).
- Patient will attain adequate nutritional status through the use of pharmacological and nonpharmacological measures.
- Patient will remain free from or will experience minimal constipation as an adverse effect of iron products.

■ Expected Patient Outcomes

- Patient is able to tolerate a gradual increase in activity as ordered (e.g., performing ADLs, walking 10 minutes per day with increases as tolerated) while on drug therapy for anemia.
  - Patient reports improved energy levels and decreased shortness of breath or activity intolerance during drug therapy.
- Patient improves dietary intake as recommended, with the help of Canada's Food Guide (http://www.hc-sc.gc.ca/fn-an/food-guide-aliment/index-eng.php) and its suggestions of appropriate amounts

of fruits and vegetables, grains and starches, and meats and other protein sources.

- Patient increases daily intake of iron through consumption of foods such as green leafy vegetables, eggs, and beans.
- Patient implements measures to minimize constipation, such as increasing intake of roughage, fibre, fruits, vegetables, and fluids.
  - Patient reports any unresolved constipation to health care provider once above measures have been implemented.
  - Patient takes medication for management of constipation, such as bulk-forming laxatives, as prescribed.

Implementation

Do not administer ESAs with any other product and do not shake the vial containing the drug. Prolonged, vigorous shaking may denature the glycoprotein, rendering it biologically inactive. During treatment, always monitor blood pressure and give vitamin B_{12} supplements orally as prescribed. Instruct the patient to dilute liquid dosage forms of iron products according to manufacturer instructions and to sip them through a plastic straw to avoid discoloration of tooth enamel. Other oral forms of iron need to be given with a large quantity of fluids but not with antacids or milk, and preferably not with meals because of the risk of decreased absorption of the drug. However, most individuals find that they do need to take oral iron products with meals or food because of the commonly encountered adverse effect of GI distress. If antacids or milk products are used, schedule them at least 1 to 2 hours before or after the oral dosage of iron. Iron products are generally packaged in a light-resistant, airtight container. Instruct patients to remain in an upright or sitting position for up to 30 minutes after taking oral dosage forms of iron products and related drugs to help minimize esophageal irritation or corrosion. Warn patients that the use of iron products will turn their stools from brown to a black, tarry colour. Patients taking epoetin alfa may also be taking oral iron preparations. See the Patient Teaching Tips for more information and the Special Populations: Older Adults: Iron Products box.

If a patient cannot tolerate oral iron, IV iron (e.g., iron dextran, iron sucrose, or ferric gluconate) may be prescribed. A test dose of iron dextran may be ordered, with the remaining dose given 1 hour later if no adverse reaction occurs. Intramuscularly administered iron must be given deep in a large muscle mass using the Z-track method (see Chapter 10). IV iron dextran must be given after the IV line has been flushed with 10 mL of normal saline and must be administered with the recommended amount of diluent and at the recommended drip rate. Keep epinephrine and resuscitative equipment available in case of an anaphylactic reaction (to iron or any drug that has an increased risk of causing anaphylaxis). In addition, it may be necessary for the patient to remain recumbent for 30 minutes after the IV injection to prevent drug-induced orthostatic hypotension. Encourage the patient to move slowly and purposefully during this time.

Evaluation

Focus the evaluation of therapeutic responses to drugs used for anemia on ensuring that goals and expected patient outcomes are met as well as on monitoring therapeutic and adverse effects. Therapeutic responses to ESAs may take 2 to 6 weeks, so monitor for increased energy, appetite, and sense of well-being. Adverse effects of ESAs may include heart attack, stroke, and possible death if ESAs are used in patients with a hemoglobin level greater than 130 g/L. Therapeutic responses to iron products include improved nutritional status, increased weight, increased activity tolerance and well-being, and absence of fatigue. Adverse effects of iron products include nausea, constipation, epigastric pain, black and tarry stools, and vomiting. Signs of toxicity include nausea, diarrhea, hematemesis, pallor, cyanosis, shock, and coma.

SPECIAL POPULATIONS: OLDER ADULTS

Iron Products

- Instructions on how to take oral forms of iron are crucial to safe administration. Implement a variety of teaching strategies to reinforce all verbal and written instructions. Make sure education is individualized, especially for patients with alterations in sensory perception. Caution patients not to make changes in their medication regimens, such as doubling doses or discontinuing a drug, without a health care provider's order.
- Provide older adults and their family members or caregivers with instructions about foods that are high in iron and how to include these foods in their menu planning. Instruct patients to preserve vegetables' content of vitamins and minerals by steaming them and not overcooking them through excessive boiling.
- Remind older patients that GI upset may occur with many drugs, including vitamins and iron. Iron products can be taken with food or a snack to help decrease GI upset.
- To facilitate proper diet, always educate older adults, as well as their spouses, family members, other significant others, and caregivers about appropriate community resources (e.g., Meals on Wheels, senior citizen community centres, public recreation centres).

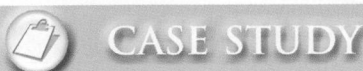

CASE STUDY

Erythropoiesis-Stimulating Agents

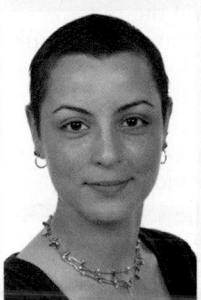

Justine, a 37-year-old homemaker, is receiving a second round of chemotherapy as part of treatment for ovarian cancer. Chemotherapeutic drugs may lead to the adverse effect of bone marrow suppression of various blood cell components.

Two weeks after this round of chemotherapy, Justine's hemoglobin level is 79 g/L (pretherapy value was 110 g/L), and her hematocrit is 0.28 (pretherapy value was 0.34). The following orders are received: epoetin alfa (Eprex) 150 units/kg subcutaneously three times a week; ferrous sulphate, 300 mg orally daily.

1. What is the purpose of the order for ferrous sulphate?

2. What conditions will the nurse assess for before beginning the epoetin alfa therapy?

3. The nurse needs to monitor Justine closely. What assessment findings would be of the most concern during this therapy?

4. After 5 weeks, Justine's hemoglobin level is 114 g/L and her hematocrit is 0.33. The next dose of epoetin alfa is due today. What action will the nurse take?

For answers, see http://evolve.elsevier.com/Canada/Lilley/pharmacology/.

PATIENT TEACHING TIPS

❖ Educate patients taking ESAs about the possible need to take oral iron supplements. These supplements are often needed to ensure adequate body iron stores, which are needed for the drug therapy to be effective.

❖ Encourage patients to take iron products cautiously and to be aware of the potential for poisoning if these drugs are taken in greater amounts than recommended. Patients should be aware that oral iron products need to be taken in their original dosage form and without alteration (e.g., without crushing).

❖ Instruct patients to take iron products exactly as ordered. Parenteral dosage forms may cause anaphylaxis and orthostatic hypotension. Recommend to patients that oral dosage forms of iron be taken with at least 120 to 180 mL of water or juice to help minimize GI upset and increase absorption.

❖ Patients should be aware that oral dosage forms of iron are not interchangeable, and prescription forms of these products may be different from one another. Products contain different iron salts and also come in different dose amounts.

❖ Instruct patients to remain upright for up to 30 minutes after taking an oral iron product to prevent esophageal irritation or corrosion. Remind patients that iron products may turn their stools a black, tarry colour.

❖ Encourage patients to maintain a diet high in iron, including foods such as dark green, leafy vegetables, dried fruits, beans, meats, and eggs.

❖ Remind patients to store iron tablets out of reach of children due to the risk of iron poisoning.

KEY POINTS

❖ Epoetin alfa (Eprex) is indicated for anemias associated with end-stage kidney disease and chemotherapy and requires careful use. Always check for route of administration, as this drug has a slower onset of action when given by the subcutaneous route as compared to the IV route.

❖ ESAs are ineffective without adequate body iron stores.

❖ Iron and folic acid are important in the treatment of many disorders and diseases (e.g., malignancies) to achieve RBC and hemoglobin formation that is as adequate as possible and to help prevent nutritional deficits that can affect all body systems, particularly the immune system.

❖ Drugs for anemia are often used in the treatment of pernicious anemia, malabsorption syndromes, hemolytic anemia, hemorrhage, and kidney and liver diseases.

EXAMINATION REVIEW QUESTIONS

1. When administering oral iron tablets, the nurse must keep in mind that which substance, other than water, is the most appropriate to give with these tablets?
   a. Pudding
   b. An antacid
   c. Milk
   d. Orange juice

2. The nurse is teaching a patient about oral iron supplements. Which statement is correct?
   a. "You need to take this medication on an empty stomach or else it won't be absorbed."
   b. "It is better absorbed on an empty stomach, but if that causes your stomach to be upset, you can take it with food."
   c. "Take this medication with a sip of water, and then lie down to avoid problems with low blood pressure."
   d. "If you have trouble swallowing the tablet, you may crush it."

3. The nurse is administering an IV dose of iron dextran. For which potential adverse effect is it most important for the nurse to monitor at this time?
   a. Anaphylaxis
   b. GI distress
   c. Black, tarry stools
   d. Bradycardia

4. The nurse is assessing a patient who is to receive folic acid supplements. It is important to rule out which condition before giving the folic acid?
   a. Malabsorption syndrome
   b. Pernicious anemia
   c. Tropical sprue
   d. Pregnancy

5. A patient with renal failure has severe anemia, and there is an order for darbepoetin alfa (Aranesp). Upon assessment, which condition listed will the nurse consider a contraindication to use of this medication?
   a. Uncontrolled hypertension
   b. Diabetes mellitus
   c. Hypothyroidism
   d. Angina

6. When iron sucrose is administered, which nursing interventions are correct? (Select all that apply.)
   a. Administer a test dose before giving the full dose.
   b. Give via deep IM injection into a large muscle mass using the Z-track method.
   c. Administer large doses over 2.5 to 3.5 hours, intravenously.
   d. Monitor the patient for hypertension.
   e. Monitor the patient for hypotension.

7. The order reads: "Give epoetin alfa (Eprex), 3 500 units Subcut, three times a week." The medication is available in a vial that contains 4 000 units/mL. How many millilitres will the nurse draw up for the ordered dose? Round to hundredths.

Answers: 1. d, 2. b, 3. a, 4. b, 5. a, 6. c, e, 7. 0.88 mL (rounded from 0.875)

CRITICAL THINKING ACTIVITIES

1. The nurse is administering an IV dose of iron dextran. A test dose has just been given. What important action will the nurse take next? Explain your answer.

2. A 27-year-old female patient has decided that she wants to start a family. She asks the nurse, "Are there any vitamins I need to take now to make sure I'm healthy?" What is the nurse's best answer?

3. A patient has been receiving epoetin alfa (Eprex) three times a week, during his dialysis treatments for chronic kidney failure. This morning, as the nurse prepares to give him a dose, he states, "I've felt strange today, and last night I had a little chest pain, but it went away after a few minutes so I didn't call the nurse." Will the nurse give the dose of epoetin alfa at this time? Explain your answer. What is the nurse's priority action at this time?

For answers, see http://evolve.elsevier.com/Canada/Lilley/pharmacology/.

CHAPTER 56

Dermatological Drugs

Objectives

After reading this chapter, the successful student will be able to do the following:

1. Discuss the normal anatomy, physiology, and functions of the skin.

2. Describe different disorders, infections, and conditions commonly affecting the skin.

3. Identify various dermatological drugs used to treat these disorders, infections, and conditions, and describe the various classifications of these drugs.

4. Discuss the mechanisms of action, indications, contraindications, cautions, other drug interactions, application techniques, and adverse effects associated with various topical dermatological drugs.

5. Develop a collaborative plan of care that includes all phases of the nursing process for patients using topical dermatological drugs.

e-Learning Activities

website
(http://evolve.elsevier.com/Canada/Lilley/pharmacology/)

evolve

- Answer Key—Textbook Case Studies
- Answer Key—Critical Thinking Activities
- Chapter Summaries—Printable
- Review Questions for Exam Preparation
- Unfolding Case Studies

Drug Profiles

*Full generic name is given in parentheses. For the purposes of this text, the more common, shortened name is used.

Key Terms

Acne vulgaris A chronic inflammatory disease of the pilosebaceous glands of the skin, involving lesions such as papules and pustules (pimples or comedones; referred to in this chapter as *acne*). (p. 1044)

Actinic keratosis A slowly developing, localized thickening of the outer layers of the skin resulting from long-term, prolonged exposure to the sun; also called *solar keratosis*. (p. 1050)

Atopic dermatitis A chronic skin inflammation seen in patients with hereditary susceptibility. (p. 1042)

Basal cell carcinoma The most common form of skin cancer; it arises from epidermal cells known as *basal cells* and is rarely metastatic. (p. 1042)

Carbuncles Necrotizing infections of skin and subcutaneous tissue caused by multiple furuncles (boils); they are usually caused by the bacterium *Staphylococcus aureus*. (p. 1043)

Cellulitis An acute, diffuse, spreading infection involving the skin, subcutaneous tissue, and sometimes muscle as well; it is usually caused by infection of a wound with *Streptococcus* or *Staphylococcus* species bacteria. (p. 1043)

Dermatitis Any inflammation of the skin. (p. 1042)

Dermatophytes Any of the common groups of fungi that infect skin, hair, and nails; these fungi are most commonly from the genera *Microsporum*, *Epidermophyton*, and *Trichophyton*. (p. 1045)

Dermatosis Any abnormal skin condition. (p. 1042)

Dermis The layer of the skin just below the epidermis, consisting of papillary and reticular layers and containing blood and lymphatic vessels, nerves and nerve endings, glands, and hair follicles. (p. 1040)

Eczema A pruritic, papulovesicular dermatitis occurring as a reaction to many endogenous and exogenous agents; characterized by erythema, edema, and an inflammatory infiltrate of the dermis and accompanied by oozing, crusting, and scaling. (p. 1042)

Epidermis The superficial, avascular layers of the skin, made up of an outer, dead, cornified portion and a deeper, living, cellular portion. (p. 1040)

Folliculitis Inflammation of a follicle, usually a hair follicle; a follicle is defined as any sac or pouchlike cavity. (p. 1043)

Furuncles Painful skin nodules caused by *Staphylococcus* organisms that enters the skin through the hair follicles; also called *boils*. (p. 1043)

Impetigo A pus-generating, contagious superficial skin infection, usually caused by *Staphylococci* or *Streptococci*; it generally occurs on the face, is most commonly seen in children, and may be recognized by honey-coloured crusts. (p. 1043)

Papules Small, circumscribed, superficial, solid elevations of the skin that are usually pink and less than 0.5 to 1 cm in diameter. (p. 1043)

Pediculosis An infestation with lice of the family *Pediculidae*. (p. 1049)

Pruritus An unpleasant cutaneous sensation that provokes the desire to rub or scratch the skin to obtain relief. (p. 1045)

Psoriasis A common, chronic squamous cell dermatosis with polygenic (multi-gene) inheritance and a fluctuating pattern of recurrence and remission. (p. 1042)

Pustules Visible collections of pus within or beneath the epidermis. (p. 1043)

Scabies A contagious disease caused by *Sarcoptes scabiei*, the itch mite, characterized by intense itching of the skin and injury to the skin (excoriation) resulting from scratching. (p. 1049)

Tinea A fungal skin disease caused by a dermatophyte and characterized by itching, scaling, and, sometimes, painful lesions; infections with any of various dermatophytes that occur on several sites; also called *ringworm*. (p. 1045)

Topical antimicrobials Substances applied to any surface that either kill microorganisms or inhibit their growth or replication. (p. 1043)

Vesicles Small sacs containing liquid; also called *cysts*. (p. 1043)

SKIN ANATOMY AND PHYSIOLOGY

The skin is the largest organ of the body. It covers the body and serves several functions, including protection, sensation, temperature regulation, excretion, absorption, and metabolism. It acts as a protective barrier for the internal organs. Without skin, harmful external forces such as microorganisms and chemicals would gain access to and damage or destroy many of the body's delicate internal organs. Part of this protection includes the skin's ability to maintain a surface pH of 4.5 to 5.5. This weakly acidic environment discourages the growth of microorganisms that thrive at a more alkaline pH. The skin also has the ability to sense changes in temperature, pressure, or pain—information that is then transmitted along nerve endings. The temperature of the environment changes continuously; despite this, the body maintains an almost constant internal temperature due in large part to the skin, which plays a major role in the regulation of body temperature. Heat loss and conservation are regulated in coordination with the blood vessels that supply blood to the skin and by means of perspiration. The skin is also able to excrete fluid and electrolytes through sweat glands. In addition, it stores fat, synthesizes vitamin D, and provides a site for drug absorption.

The skin is made up of two layers: the **dermis** and the **epidermis** (Figure 56-1). The outer skin layer, the epidermis, is composed of four layers. From the outermost to innermost layer, these are the stratum corneum, stratum lucidum, stratum granulosum, and stratum germinativum. The respective functions of these layers are described in Table 56-1.

None of these layers has a direct blood supply of its own. Instead, nourishment is provided through diffusion from the dermis below. The dermis lies between the epidermis and subcutaneous fat and differs from the epidermis in many ways. It is approximately 40 times thicker than the epidermis. Traversing the dermis is a rich supply of blood vessels, nerves, lymphatic tissue, elastic tissue, and connective tissue, which provide extra support and nourishment to the skin. Also contained in the dermis are the exocrine glands—the eccrine, apocrine, and sebaceous glands—and the hair follicles. The functions of the various types of exocrine glands are explained in Table 56-2.

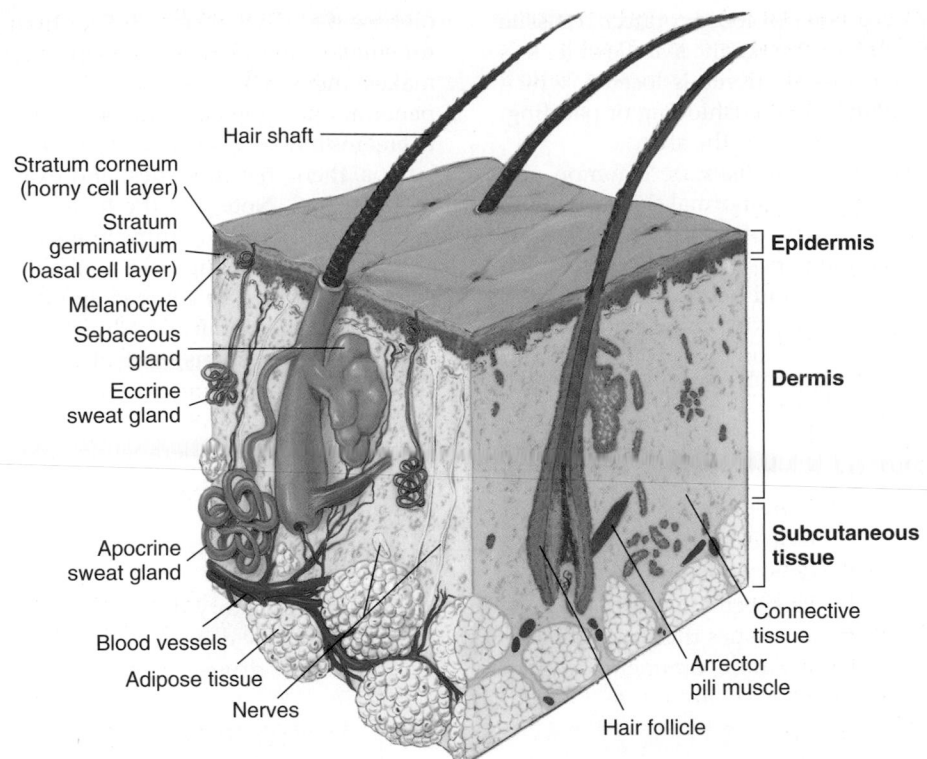

FIG. 56-1   Microscopic view of the skin. The epidermis, shown in longitudinal section, is raised at one corner to reveal the ridges in the dermis. (Source: Jarvis, C. (2008). *Physical examination and health assessment* (5th ed.) (p. 222). St. Louis, MO: Saunders.)

TABLE 56-1

Epidermal Layers

Layer	Description
Stratum corneum ("horny layer," so named because keratin is the same protein that makes up the horns of animals)	This is the outermost layer, consisting of dead skin cells that are made of a converted water-repellent protein known as *keratin*; it is the protective layer for the entire body. After it is desquamated, or shed, the layer is replaced by new cells from below.
Stratum lucidum ("clear layer")	This is the layer where keratin is formed; it is translucent and contains flat cells.
Stratum granulosum ("granular layer")	Cells die in this layer; granulated cells are located here, which gives this layer the appearance for which it is named.
Stratum germinativum ("germinative layer")	New skin cells are made in this layer; it contains melanocytes, which produce melanin, the skin colour pigment.

TABLE 56-2

Exocrine Glands of the Skin

Gland	Function
Sebaceous	Large, lipid-containing cells that produce oil or film that covers the epidermis; protects and lubricates skin, and is water repellent and antiseptic
Eccrine	Sweat glands that are located throughout the skin surface; help regulate body temperature and prevent skin dryness
Apocrine	Mainly in axillae, genital organs, and breast areas; emit an odour; believed to be scent or sex glands

Below the dermis is a layer of loose connective tissue called the *hypodermis*. It helps make the skin flexible. It is also here that subcutaneous fat tissue is located, which provides thermal insulation and cushioning or padding. It is also the source of nutrition for the skin.

Reactions or disorders of the skin are common and numerous. A **dermatosis** is any abnormal skin condition. Dermatoses include a variety of types of **dermatitis** (skin inflammation). Among these are conditions such as **atopic dermatitis, eczema,** and **psoriasis.** In addition, there are also a variety of skin cancers, including **basal cell carcinoma,** squamous cell carcinoma, and melanoma.

TOPICAL DERMATOLOGICAL DRUGS

Drugs that are administered directly to the site are called *topical dermatological drugs*. These drugs are available in a variety of prescription and over-the-counter (OTC) formulations that are suitable for specific indications. Each formulation has certain characteristics that make it beneficial for particular uses. For example, ointments have an oil base that makes them stickier than creams and better for smaller areas, whereas creams have a water base that makes them better for larger surfaces. Gels promote penetration of the active ingredient. Lotions are similar to creams but are lighter. More information on the formulations, their characteristics, and examples are provided in Table 56-3. Note that the focus of this chapter is primarily on topically administered medications. Because so many topical drugs are available, the scope of this chapter is limited to some of the more commonly used medications. Systemically administered drugs (transdermal delivery systems) are also used to treat several skin disorders and are cross-referenced throughout this chapter.

There are many therapeutic categories of dermatological drugs. Some of the most common ones are the following:
- Antibacterial drugs
- Antifungal drugs
- Anti-inflammatory drugs
- Antineoplastic drugs
- Antipruritic drugs (for itching)

TABLE 56-3

Dermatological Drug Formulations: Characteristics and Examples

Formulation	Characteristics	Examples
Aerosol foam	Can cover large area; useful for drug delivery into a body cavity (e.g., vagina, rectum) or hairy areas	Proctofoam®, contraceptive foams
Aerosol spray	Spreads thin liquid or powder film; covers large areas; useful when skin is tender to touch (e.g., burns)	Solarcaine®, Tinactin®
Bar	Similar to a bar of soap; useful as a wash with water	PanOxyl® (benzoyl peroxide)
Cleanser	Nongreasy; used as an astringent (oil remover) or wash with water	Neutrogena Ultra Sheer®
Cream	Contains water and can be removed with water; not greasy or occlusive; usually white semisolid; good for moist areas	hydrocortisone cream (Cortamed®), Benadryl® cream
Gel/jelly	Contains water and possibly alcohol; easily removed and good lubricator; usually clear, semisolid substance; useful when lubricant properties are desirable	K-Y® jelly, Benzamycin®, Erysol®
Lotion	Contains water, alcohol, and solvents; may be a suspension, emulsion, or solution; good for large or hairy areas	Calamine® lotion, Lubriderm® lotion, Kwellada-P® lotion
Oil	Contains little if any water; occlusive, liquid; not removable with water	Lubriderm® bath oil
Ointment	Contains no water; not removable with water; occlusive, greasy, and semisolid; desirable for dry lesions because of occlusiveness	petrolatum, (Vaseline®), zinc oxide ointment, A+D ointment
Paste	Similar properties to those of the ointments; contains more powder than ointments; excellent protectant properties	zinc oxide paste (Balmex®)
Pledget (pad)	Moistened pad is applied to or wiped over affected area	chlorhexidine gluconate
Powder	Slight lubricating properties; may be shaken on affected area; promotes drying of area where applied	Tinactin powder, Desenex® powder
Shampoo	Soapy liquid for washing hair and skin	ketoconazole (Nizoral®)
Solution	Nongreasy liquid; dries quickly	Various skin care products
Stick	Spreads thin chalky or viscous liquid film; often better for smaller areas	Benadryl Itch Relief
Tape	Moist occlusive formulation; consistent topical drug delivery; useful when small, straight areas require drug application	Various products

- Antiviral drugs
- Burn drugs
- Débriding drugs (promote wound healing)
- Emollients (skin softeners)
- Keratolytics (cause softening and peeling of the stratum corneum)
- Local anaesthetics
- Sunscreens
- Topical vasodilators

ANTIMICROBIALS

Topical antimicrobials are antibacterial, antifungal, and antiviral drugs that, as the name implies, are applied topically. Although topical antimicrobials have many of the same properties as systemic forms, there are differences in terms of their absorption, distribution, toxicities and adverse effects. Also, many topically administered drugs can have systemic effects, because they reach the circulation after being absorbed by the tissues.

GENERAL ANTIBACTERIAL DRUGS

Common skin disorders caused by bacteria are **folliculitis**, **impetigo**, **furuncles**, **carbuncles**, **papules**, **pustules**, **vesicles**, and **cellulitis**. The bacteria responsible are most commonly *Streptococcus pyogenes* and *Staphylococcus aureus*. Dermatological antibacterial drugs are used to treat or prevent these skin infections. The most commonly used drugs are bacitracin, polymyxin, and neomycin. Unfortunately, due to the high incidence of infection with methicillin-resistant *S. aureus* (MRSA), mupirocin is now also commonly used.

 DRUG PROFILES

▶▶*bacitracin*

Bacitracin (Baximycin®, Bioderm®) is a polypeptide antibiotic that is applied topically for the treatment or prevention of local skin infections caused by susceptible aerobic and anaerobic gram-positive organisms such as staphylococci, streptococci, anaerobic cocci, corynebacteria, and clostridia. It works by inhibiting bacterial cell wall synthesis, which leads to cell death. It can be either bactericidal or bacteriostatic, depending on the causative organism. Bacitracin's antimicrobial spectrum is broadened in several available combination drug products. Most of these contain neomycin or polymyxin B (see later in this chapter).

Adverse reactions to bacitracin are usually minimal; however, reactions ranging from skin rash to allergic anaphylactoid reactions have occurred. If itching, burning, inflammation, or other signs of sensitivity occur, discontinue bacitracin. This drug is available in ointment form and it is usually applied to the affected area one to three times daily. It is also available in systemic and ophthalmic (see Chapter 57) formulations.

neomycin and polymyxin B

Neomycin and polymyxin B are two additional broad-spectrum antibiotics that are available together in the nonprescription product known as Neosporin®. Neosporin cream is a combination of these two drugs alone, whereas Neosporin ointment also contains bacitracin. Several brand name and generic combinations of these three topical antibiotics are available, and all are commonly used as topical antiseptics for minor skin wounds. Although neomycin/polymyxin B is still a popular OTC product, there is evidence that use of the drug can increase the likelihood of future allergic reactions of the skin.

mupirocin

Mupirocin (Bactroban®) is an antibacterial product available only by prescription. It is used on the skin for treatment of staphylococcal and streptococcal impetigo. It is applied topically three times daily to treat colonization with MRSA. Adverse reactions are usually limited to local burning, itching, or minor pain.

silver sulfadiazine

Silver sulfadiazine (Flamazene®) has proved both effective and safe in the prevention and treatment of infections in burns. A major concern for individuals with burns is infection at the burn site. However, because increased systemic absorption of a drug can occur in compromised skin areas, to avoid causing dangerous systemic effects, topical burn drugs must not be too potent or toxic. This is especially true when large burned areas must be treated, because the drug may be applied over a large surface area of skin and therefore may be absorbed in high quantities. Conversely, the blood supply to burned areas is often drastically reduced, so systemically administered antibiotics either cannot reach the site or do so only in quantities too low to be effective. Therefore, the only way of administering these drugs to ensure that they reach the burn site is to apply them topically.

Silver sulfadiazine is a synthetic antimicrobial drug produced when silver nitrate reacts with the chemical sulfadiazine. It appears to act on the cell membranes and cell walls of susceptible bacteria and is used as an adjunct in the prevention and treatment of infection in second- and third-degree burns and less frequently for cellulitic or eczematous extremities. The adverse effects of silver sulfadiazine are similar to those of other topical drugs and include pain, burning, and itching. This drug should not be used in patients who are allergic to sulfonamide drugs. It is available only as a 1% cream and is applied topically to cleansed and débrided burned areas once or twice daily, using a sterile-gloved hand.

ANTIACNE DRUGS

Acne vulgaris is the most common skin infection. Its precise cause is unknown and somewhat controversial. Likely causative factors include heredity, stress, drug reactions, hormones, and bacterial infections. Common bacterial causes include *Staphylococcus* species (spp.) and *Propionibacterium acnes*. Some of the most commonly used antiacne drugs are benzoyl peroxide, clindamycin, eryth-romycin, tetracycline, isotretinoin, and the vitamin A acid known as *retinoic acid*. Many other drugs are also used in the treatment and prevention of acne, including systemic formulations of the antibiotics minocycline, doxycycline, and tetracycline (see Chapter 43). Some health care providers also prescribe oral contraceptives (see Chapter 35) for female patients with acne, because in some controlled studies estrogen has been shown to have beneficial effects against acne, especially hormone-driven acne.

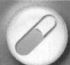 ## DRUG PROFILES

►►*benzoyl peroxide*

The microorganism that most commonly causes acne, *P. acnes*, is an anaerobic bacterium; that is, it needs an environment that is poor in oxygen to grow. Benzoyl peroxide is effective in combating such infection because it slowly and continuously liberates active oxygen in the skin, resulting in antibacterial, antiseptic, drying, and kera-tolytic actions. These actions create an environment that is unfavourable for the continued growth of the *P. acnes* bacteria, and they soon die. Drugs such as benzoyl peroxide that soften scales and loosen the outer horny layer of the skin are referred to as *keratolytics*.

Benzoyl peroxide generally produces signs of improvement within 8 to 12 weeks; clinical worsening may occur during the initial 2 to 4 weeks of use. Adverse effects tend to be related to dose (including overuse) and include peeling skin, red skin, or a sensation of warmth. Blistering or swelling of the skin is generally considered an allergic reaction to the product and is an indication to stop treatment. Overuse of this drug and also of tretinoin is common in adolescent patients who are attempting to quickly cure their acne. The result can be painful, reddened skin, which usually resolves upon return to use of these medications as prescribed.

Benzoyl peroxide is available in multiple topical dosage forms, including as a cleansing bar, liquid, lotion, mask, cream, gel, and cleanser. It is also available in various combination drug products. It is usually applied topically one to four times daily, depending on the dosage form and the health care provider's instructions. There have been no studies to determine the effects of benzoyl peroxide during pregnancy, but the benefits of using this drug during pregnancy are considered to outweigh the risk.

clindamycin phosphate

Clindamycin phosphate (Clindets®, Dalacin®) is a topical form of the systemic antibiotic clindamycin described in Chapter 44. It is most commonly prescribed for acne inflammatory lesions. Adverse reactions associated with this topical drug are usually limited to minor local skin reactions, including burning, itching, dryness, oiliness, and peeling. The drug is available in cream, gel, lotion, suspension, and pledget formulations. Clindamycin is usually applied once or twice daily. Combination therapy (e.g., benzoyl peroxide) may prevent bacterial resistance. It is safe to use during pregnancy.

►►*isotretinoin*

Isotretinoin (Accutane®, Clarus®, Epuris®) is an oral product indicated for the treatment of severe recalcitrant cystic acne. Isotretinoin inhibits sebaceous gland activity and has antikeratinizing (anti–skin-hardening) and anti-inflammatory effects. Isotretinoin is one of relatively few acne medications that are not to be used during pregnancy. This means that it is a proven human teratogen, or chemical that is known to induce birth defects. It is imperative that female patients of childbearing age be counselled and agree not to become pregnant during use of the drug. Because of these teratogenic effects, in 2005, the US Food and Drug Administration approved stringent guidelines regarding the prescription and use of this medication. Canada quickly followed the United States' lead with a risk management program called the Accutane Pregnancy Prevention Program (PPP). This program requires that women of childbearing age taking isotretinoin receive education about the teratogenicity of the drug and sign a form indicating that they have been educated through the PPP, understand the need for contraception, and will undergo pregnancy testing before, during, and after drug therapy. The risk management program features the following: a toll-free number that both patients and health care providers can call for information; suggestions for an expanded health care providers' checklist, including lists of potentially interacting medications and natural health products; a website with information regarding isotretinoin and contraception; improved education for health care providers and pharmacists; and information about the introduction of generic forms of isotretinoin. In addition, there have been case reports of suicide and suicide attempts in patients receiving isotretinoin. It has not been determined if the drug increases the risk for suicide or if psychosocial sequelae from severe acne are to blame for increased suicide risk. Advise patients to report any signs of depression to their health care providers. Follow-up treatment may be needed, and simply stopping the drug may be insufficient. The company that produced the drug under the brand name Accutane has withdrawn it from the market. Despite these rather strong concerns, this drug does prove to be helpful in treating severe cases of acne. Isotretinoin is available only for oral use.

tretinoin

Tretinoin (retinoic acid, vitamin A acid; Retin-A®, Stieva-A®) is a derivative of vitamin A that is used to treat acne and ameliorate dermatological changes (e.g., fine wrinkling, mottled hyperpigmentation, roughness) associated with photodamage (sun damage). The drug appears to act as an irritant to the skin, in particular the follicular epithelium. Specifically, it stimulates the turnover of epidermal cells, which results in skin peeling. While this is occurring,

DRUG PROFILES–cont'd

the free fatty acid levels of the skin are reduced, and horny cells of the outer epidermis cannot then adhere to one another. Without fatty acids and horny cells, comedones, or pimples, cannot exist.

Topically administered tretinoin has been shown to enhance the repair of skin damaged by ultraviolet radiation (e.g., sunlight, tanning beds, and tanning lights). It does this by increasing the formation of fibroblasts and collagen, both of which are needed to rebuild skin. The drug may also reduce collagen degradation by inhibiting the enzyme collagenase that breaks down collagen. Tretinoin's main adverse effects are local inflammatory reactions, which are reversible when therapy is discontinued. Common adverse effects are excessively red and edematous blisters, crusted skin, and temporary alterations in skin pigmentation. Tretinoin is available in many topical formulations, including creams, gels, and a liquid. Because of its potential to cause severe irritation and peeling, it may initially be applied only once every 2 or 3 days, in the evening due to photosensitivity. Treatment often starts with a low-strength product.

Retin-A Micro® is approved for the treatment of acne vulgaris. This particular acne product contains tretinoin inside a synthetic polymer called a *Microsponge delivery system*. This system is made of round microscopic particles of synthetic polymer. The microspheres act as reservoirs for tretinoin, allowing the skin to absorb small amounts of the drug over time. Retin-A Micro is currently available only in gel form. The potential benefits of all topical forms of tretinoin are considered to outweigh their risks when used during pregnancy. They are not to be confused with the oral capsule form of tretinoin (alitretinoin) used to treat leukemia, which is not to be used during pregnancy because of the risk of harm to the fetus. Another antiacne retinoid is adapalene, available in a topical gel or cream.

ANTIFUNGAL DRUGS

A few fungi produce keratinolytic enzymes, which allow them to live on the skin. Topical fungal infections are primarily caused by *Candida* spp. (candidiasis), **dermatophytes**, and *Malassezia furfur* (tinea versicolor). These fungi are found in moist, warm environments, especially in dark areas such as the feet or groin. Candidal infections are commonly caused by *Candida albicans*, a yeast-like opportunistic fungus present in the normal flora of the mouth, vagina, and intestinal tract. Two significant factors that commonly predispose a person to a candidal infection are immunodeficiency disorders and broad-spectrum antibiotic therapy, which promotes an overgrowth of nonsusceptible organisms in the natural flora of the body. Because these infections favour warm, moist areas of the skin and mucous membranes, they most commonly occur orally (e.g., thrush in infants), vaginally, and cutaneously, in sites such as beneath the breasts and in diapered areas. They may also cause nail infections.

Dermatophytes comprise a group of three closely related genera consisting of *Epidermophyton* spp., *Microsporum* spp., and *Trichophyton* spp. that use the keratin found on the skin to feed their growth. They produce superficial mycotic (fungal) infections of keratinized tissue (hair, skin, and nails). Infections caused by dermatophytes are collectively called **tinea**, or *ringworm*, infections. The name *ringworm* comes from the fact that the infection sometimes assumes a circular pattern at the site of infection. Tinea infections are further identified by the body location where they occur: tinea pedis (foot), tinea cruris (groin), tinea corporis (body), and tinea capitis (scalp). Tinea infections of the foot are also known as *athlete's foot* and those of the groin as *jock itch*.

Fungi usually invade the stratum corneum, which is the dead layer of desquamated (shed) cells. Inflammation occurs when fungi invade this layer; sensitivity (e.g., itching) occurs when they penetrate the epidermis and dermis.

Many of the fungi that cause topical infections are difficult to eradicate. The organisms are slow growing, and antifungal therapy may be required for periods ranging from several weeks to as long as 1 year. However, many topical antifungal drugs are available for the treatment of both dermatophyte infections and those caused by yeast and yeastlike fungi. Some of these drugs, their dosage forms, and their uses are listed in Table 56-4. Systemically administered antifungal drugs are sometimes used for skin conditions as well. These drugs were discussed in Chapter 47.

The most commonly reported adverse effects of topical antifungals are local irritation, **pruritus**, burning sensations, and scaling. Ciclopirox and clotrimazole are safe to use during pregnancy; ketoconazole and miconazole may have an adverse effect on the fetus but their benefits may outweigh the risks of use during pregnancy. Hypersensitivity is the one contraindication to the use of any of these drugs.

ANTIVIRAL DRUGS

Topical antivirals are now used less frequently than in years past, because systemic antiviral drug therapy has generally been shown to be superior for controlling such viral skin conditions. Nonetheless, two antiviral ointments are described here. As is the case with systemic drug therapy, these products are best used early in an outbreak of viral skin lesions. Topical antivirals are more likely to be used for acute outbreaks, whereas

DRUG PROFILES

▶▶*clotrimazole*

Clotrimazole (Canesten®) is available over the counter. It is available as a cream for the treatment of dermatophytoses (e.g., athlete's foot), superficial mycoses, and cutaneous candidiasis. Similar topical preparations (cream and vaginal tablets) are also available for intravaginal administration in the treatment of vulvovaginal candidiasis, commonly called a *yeast infection*, and vaginal trichomoniasis. Clotrimazole is available in many topical formulations: a 1% cream; 1%, 2%, and 10% vaginal creams; and 200- and 500-mg vaginal tablets. Different dosages and dosage forms are used for the treatment of different fungal infections. Clotrimazole is safe to use during pregnancy.

miconazole nitrate

Miconazole nitrate (Micatin®, Micozole®, Monistat®) is a topical antifungal drug that is available in several OTC products (e.g., cream, prefilled applicators or suppositories, ovules). It inhibits the growth of several fungi, including dermatophytes and yeast, as well as gram-positive bacteria, and is commonly used to treat dermatophytoses, superficial mycoses, cutaneous candidiasis, and vulvo-vaginal candidiasis. It is present in many remedies for athlete's foot, jock itch, and yeast infections.

For the treatment of athlete's foot, jock itch, ringworm, and other susceptible fungal infections, miconazole is applied sparingly to a cleansed, dry, infected area twice daily in the morning and evening. For the treatment of yeast infections, one 400-mg ovule suppository should be inserted in the vagina once daily at bedtime for 3 consecutive days. Also available is a dual pack, which contains one 100-mg suppository and 2% cream. The suppository is administered intravaginally once daily at bedtime for 7 days and the cream is applied to the itchy, irritated area. One-day regimens for vaginal candidiasis are also available (e.g., Monistat 1 Vaginal Ovule 1 200 mg × 1 day or Combi Pak 1 200 mg/2%cream × 1 day). The most common adverse effects of topically administered miconazole are vulvovaginal burning and itching, pelvic cramps and rash, urticaria, stinging, and contact dermatitis. Miconazole is available in a variety of topical formulations: a 2% cream; a 2% vaginal cream; and a 100- and 400-mg vaginal suppository. It is also available as a 1 200-mg vaginal suppository for one-time dosing. If used during pregnancy, miconazole may have adverse effects on the fetus; however, the benefits of its use may outweigh the risks.

TABLE 56-4

Topical Antifungal Drugs

Drug	Trade Names	Dosage Forms	Uses
ciclopirox	Loprox®, Stieprox Shampoo®)	1% cream and lotion, 1.5% shampoo, 8% lotion (for nails)	Candidiasis, dermatophytoses, tinea versicolor
clotrimazole	Canesten Combi-Pak	1% vaginal cream, 200- and 500-mg vaginal tabs	Candidiasis
	Clotrimaderm, Clotrimazole	1% and 2% topical creams	Candidiasis; dermatophytoses; tinea versicolor
	Lotriderm®	Cream (1% clotrimazole, 0.05% beclamethasone dipropionate)	Dermatophytoses
ketoconazole	Ketoderm cream®	2% cream	Candidiasis, dermatophytoses, tinea versicolor
	Nizoral®	2% shampoo	Dermatophytoses, tinea versicolor
miconazole nitrate	Micatin	2% cream, powder spray	Candidiasis, dermatophytoses, tinea versicolor
	Micozole	2% cream	Candidiasis, dermatophytoses, tinea versicolor
	Monistat	100-, 400-, and 1 200-mg vaginal ovules	Candidiasis
	Monistat Pak	2% cream; 100-, 400-, and 1 200-mg vaginal suppository	Candidiasis
nystatin	Flagylstatin® Nyaderm®	Cream, ovule	Candidiasis
terbinafine hydrochloride	Lamisil®	1% cream and spray	Dermatophytoses
tolnaftate	Tinactin, others	1% cream, solution, gel, powder, and spray	Dermatophytoses

systemic drugs are used for acute outbreaks and for ongoing prophylaxis against outbreaks. Viral infections are difficult to treat because they live in the body's healthy cells and use their cell mechanisms to reproduce; the same is also true for topical viral infections. Infections caused by herpes simplex types 1 and 2 and human papillomavirus (which causes anogenital warts) are particularly serious and are becoming more common.

The only topical antiviral drug currently available to treat such viral infections is acyclovir (Zovirax®). It works by comparable mechanisms as described for similar antiviral drugs in Chapter 45. Acyclovir acts by inhibiting the viral enzymes necessary for deoxyribonucleic acid synthesis. Acyclovir is available as a 5% topical cream, which is applied 4 to 6 times daily for up to 10 days. A finger cot or rubber glove should be worn for application of the ointment to prevent the spread of infection. The medication's most common adverse effects are stinging, itching, and rash. If used during pregnancy, acyclovir may have adverse effects on the fetus; however, the benefits of its use may outweigh the risks.

TOPICAL ANAESTHETICS

Topical anaesthetics are drugs that are used to numb the skin. They accomplish this by inhibiting the conduction of nerve impulses from sensory nerves, thereby reducing or eliminating the pain or pruritus associated with insect bites, sunburn, and allergic reactions to plants such as poison ivy, as well as many other uncomfortable skin disorders. They are also used to numb the skin before a painful injection (e.g., insertion of an intravenous line in a patient). Topical anaesthetics are available as ointments, creams, sprays, liquids, and gels, and are discussed in Chapter 12. A lidocaine/prilocaine combination drug (EMLA®) and lidocaine alone (Betacaine®, Lidodan®) are topical anaesthetic drugs that are used frequently, especially in pediatric patients. EMLA is applied 1 hour before a procedure, whereas lidocaine alone is effective within 30 minutes.

TOPICAL ANTIPRURITICS AND ANTI-INFLAMMATORIES

Topical antipruritic (anti-itching) drugs contain antihistamines or corticosteroids. Many exert a combined anaesthetic and antipruritic action when applied topically. The antihistamines and their therapeutic effects are covered in Chapter 37. Topical antihistamines are not be used to treat the following conditions because of systemic absorption and subsequent toxicity: chicken pox, widespread poison ivy lesions, and other lesions involving large body surface areas.

The most commonly used topical anti-inflammatories are the corticosteroids (see Chapter 34). They are generally indicated for the relief of inflammatory and pruritic dermatoses. When topically administered corticosteroids are used, many of the undesirable systemic adverse effects associated with the use of the systemically administered corticosteroids are avoided. The beneficial drug effects of topically administered corticosteroids are their anti-inflammatory, antipruritic, and vasoconstrictive actions.

The many different available dosage forms of the various corticosteroids vary in their relative potency, and this often guides their selection in the treatment of various conditions. For instance, corticosteroids that are fluorinated (which increases their potency) are used for the treatment of dermatological disorders such as psoriasis. Also, the vehicle in which the corticosteroid is contained may alter its vasoconstrictor properties and therapeutic efficacy. Ointments are generally the most penetrating, followed next by gels, creams, and lotions. Propylene glycol also enhances the penetration of a corticosteroid and its vasoconstrictor effects. Most corticosteroids are available in many topical formulations, which provides a variety of options. The currently available topical corticosteroids, along with their respective potencies, are listed in Table 56-5.

Adverse effects of topical corticosteroids include skin reactions such as acne eruptions, allergic contact dermatitis, burning sensations, dryness, itching, skin fragility, hypopigmentation, purpura, hirsutism (usually facial), folliculitis, roundness and swelling of the face, and alopecia (usually of the scalp). Another adverse effect is the

TABLE	56-5

Commonly Used Topical Corticosteroids (in Order of Decreasing Potency)

Range of Potency*	Corticosteroid
1. High potency	betamethasone dipropionate (cream, ointment, and lotion), clobetasol 17-propionate, halobetasol propionate (cream and ointment)
2. Moderate potency*	amcinonide, beclomethasone dipropionate (cream), betamethasone valerate (0.1% cream, ointment, and lotion), desoximetasone (0.05% cream) fluocinolone acetonide (cream and lotion), mometasone furoate, triamcinolone acetonide (0.5% cream and ointment)
3. Mild potency*	desonide, fluocinolone (0.01% solution), triamcinolone (0.1% cream), hydrocortisone

*Skin penetration and, thus, potency are enhanced by the vehicle containing the steroid. In decreasing order of effectiveness are ointments, gels, creams, and lotions.

opportunistic overgrowth of bacteria, fungi, or viruses as a result of the immunosuppressive effects of this class of drugs. *Tachyphylaxis* (weakening of drug effect over time) may also occur with these drugs, especially with long-term use or overuse. The usual adult dosage of these drugs is one or two applications daily as a thin layer over the affected area. Less potent topical corticosteroids are used in children, following the same dosing schedule. If used during pregnancy, corticosteroids may have adverse effects on the fetus; however, their benefits may outweigh the risk. They are contraindicated in patients with a hypersensitivity to them. Because many of these products are available orally as well as topically, the potential exists for both to be administered simultaneously. This is not recommended and is potentially harmful. The combined use of topical and oral preparations of the same drug can lead to toxicity.

ANTIPSORIATIC DRUGS

Psoriasis is a common skin condition in which areas of the skin become thick, reddened, and covered with silvery scales. Psoriasis is actually a result of a disordered immune system, although it is generally referred to as a skin condition. It is believed to involve *polygenic* (multi-gene) inheritance. Psoriasis has a fluctuating pattern of recurrence and remission. Flare-ups can be triggered by infection, stress, changes in climate, excessive alcohol intake, or dry skin. Although there are many subtypes, the most classic one is known as *plaque psoriasis* and typically manifests as large, dry, erythematous scaling patches of the skin that are often white or silver on top.

Commonly affected skin areas include the nails, scalp, genitals, and lower back. Treatment for mild to moderate cases usually begins with a topical corticosteroid. When this therapy is not successful, topical antipsoriatic drugs are used. In addition to these topical drugs, there are recently developed systemically administered antipsoriatic drugs. A thorough discussion of these drugs is beyond the scope of this chapter on topical medications, but those given by systemic injection include etanercept (Enbrel®) and adalimumab (Humira®), which are given subcutaneously. Etanercept is discussed in more detail in the chapter on biological response–modifying drugs (see Chapter 54). In addition, the antineoplastic antimetabolite methotrexate (see Chapter 52) may be used for its antipsoriatic properties. The newest injectable drug used to treat psoriasis, ustekinumab (Stelara®), is an interleukin-12 inhibitor and is indicated for plaque psoriasis. It is given subcutaneously, and its most serious adverse effect is increased risk of infection.

MISCELLANEOUS DERMATOLOGICAL DRUGS

There are many other topically applied drugs. Those discussed in this section are the topical ectoparasiticides (scabicides and pediculicides), hair growth drugs, antineoplastics, and immunomodulating drugs. Many of these drugs are available both over the counter and by prescription. Aloe vera and tea tree oil preparations (see the Natural Health Products box) are also available over the counter.

 DRUG PROFILES

tazarotene

Tazarotene is a receptor-selective retinoid. It is thought to normalize epidermal differentiation, reducing the influx of inflammatory cells into the skin. Synthetic retinoids are vitamin A analogues and are thought to play a role in skin cell differentiation and proliferation. Tazarotene is available in gel form and is approved for the treatment of stable plaque psoriasis and mild to moderately severe facial acne. Like isotretinoin, tazarotene is not recommended for use during pregnancy, and a negative pregnancy test 2 weeks before starting therapy is required for female patients.

tar-containing products

Drug products containing coal tar derivatives were among the first medications used to treat psoriasis and are still used today for this purpose. Tar derivatives are known to have antiseptic, antibacterial, and antiseborrheic properties, and they work to soften and loosen scaly or crusty areas of the skin. *Seborrhea* is excessive secretion of *sebum*, a normal skin secretion containing fat and epithelial cell debris. Tar-containing products are available in a variety of shampoo forms (for scalp psoriasis), as well as solution, oil, ointment, cream, lotion, gel, and even soap forms for bathing. These products typically contain 1 to 10% coal tar. Adverse reactions usually include minor skin burning, photosensitivity, and other irritations. These products may be applied from one to four times daily or once or twice weekly as prescribed.

calcipotriol

Calcipotriol (Dovonex®) is a synthetic vitamin D_3 analogue that works by binding to vitamin D_3 receptors in skin cells known as *keratinocytes*, the abnormal growth of which contributes to psoriatic lesions. Calcipotriol helps to regulate the growth and reproduction of keratinocytes. The most common adverse reaction to this drug is minor skin irritation. However, more serious reactions can occur in some cases, including worsening of psoriasis, dermatitis, skin atrophy, and folliculitis. Calcipotriol is usually applied twice daily. Its usefulness in pregnancy may outweigh its associated risks. Dovobet® is a combination product containing calcipotriene and betamethasone dipropionate, a topical steroid.

NATURAL HEALTH PRODUCTS

ALOE *(Aloe vera)*

Overview
The dried juice of the leaves of the aloe plant contain anthranoids, which give aloe a laxative effect when it is taken orally. For thousands of years, the topical application of the plant has been known to aid in wound healing.

Common Uses
Wound healing, treatment of constipation

Adverse Effects
Diarrhea, nephritis, abdominal pain, dermatitis when used topically

Potential Drug Interactions
Digoxin, antidysrhythmics, diuretics, corticosteroids

Contraindications
Contraindicated in patients who are menstruating or have kidney disease; can increase menstrual blood flow and also cause acute kidney injury

TEA TREE OIL *(Melaleuca alternifolia)*

Overview
Tea tree oil is extracted from the evergreen leaves of the *Melaleuca alternifolia* tree, a cultivated tea tree that is native to Australia, New Zealand, and Southeast Asia. The oil contains over 100 components. Tea tree oil is thought to disrupt the cell membranes of fungi. Its exact mechanism of action is not fully understood.

Common Uses
Treatment of minor cuts, burns, acne, athlete's foot, mild fungal nail infections

Adverse Effects
Dermatitis when used topically, eye irritant
Potential drug interactions
None well identified

Contraindications
Tea tree oil must not be taken orally.

DRUG PROFILES

ECTOPARASITICIDAL DRUGS

Ectoparasites are insects that live on the outer surface of the body. The drugs used to kill them are called *ectoparasiticidal drugs*. Lice are transmitted from person to person by close contact with infested individuals, clothing, combs, or towels. A parasitic infestation on the skin with lice is called **pediculosis**, and such infestations go by one of three different names, depending on the location of the infestation:
- Pediculosis pubis: pubic lice, or "crabs"; infestation by *Phthirus pubis*
- Pediculosis corporis: body lice; infestation by *Pediculus humanus corporis*
- Pediculosis capitis: head lice; infestation by *Pediculus humanus capitis*

Common findings in infested persons include itching; eggs of the lice (called nits) attached to hair shafts; lice on the skin or clothes; and, in the case of pubic lice, sky blue macules (discolored skin patches) on the inner thighs or lower abdomen. Pediculoses are treated with a class of drugs called pediculicides. A second common parasitic skin infection known as **scabies** is caused by the itch mite *Sarcoptes scabiei*. Scabies is transmitted from person to person by close contact, such as by sleeping next to an infested person. The scabies mite causes irritation and itching by boring into the horny layers of skin located in cracks and folds. Itching seems to occur most commonly in the evening. The drugs used to treat these infestations are called *scabicides*.

Treatment of these parasitic infestations should begin with identification of the source of infestation to prevent reinfestation. Next, the clothing and personal articles of the infested person must be decontaminated. This is best accomplished by washing them in hot, soapy water or by dry cleaning them. All close contacts of the person should also be treated to prevent reinfestation.

Many of the ectoparasiticidal drugs that have been used to treat lice have been removed from the market in Canada because of resistance, lack of efficacy, and potential for neurotoxicity. Crotamiton (Eurax®) is an ectoparasiticidal drug with an unclear mechanism of action; it is a scabicidal and also an antipruritic. It is applied to the entire body, with particular attention paid to skin folds and creases and under nailbeds; after 48 hours, the patient showers. Crotamiton produces a counterirritation; upon evaporation from the skin, the drug produces a cooling effect, which distracts the patient from the itching. Permethrin 5% (Kwellada-P® lotion, Nix® dermal cream) and 1% (Kwellada-P crème rinse, Nix crème rinse) as well as pyrethrins (e.g., piperonyl butoxide) are still in use (applied as directed and repeated in 7 to 10 days).

Another treatment for head lice is dimeticone 50% (Nyda®), a pediculicide that does not contain any neurotoxic chemicals and is effective in killing head lice and their eggs. It is safe for use in children 2 years and older. Dimeticone penetrates the tracheas of lice and the breathing holes of their eggs, blocking their oxygen supply and suffocating them through all stages of their development. Because of this mode of action, resistance to the drug does not occur. It is sprayed onto dry hair, massaged in, and left for 30 minutes. The dead lice are then removed with a lice comb. Once the hair dries (after 8 hours), it is shampooed.

HAIR GROWTH DRUGS

minoxidil

Minoxidil (Loniten®) is a vasodilating drug that is administered systemically to control hypertension (see

Continued

DRUG PROFILES—cont'd

Chapter 23). Topically, minoxidil (Rogaine®), has the same vasodilating effect, but when used in this way it is applied to the scalp to stimulate hair growth. The vasodilation it causes is one possible explanation for how it promotes hair growth. It may also act at the level of the hair follicle, possibly stimulating hair growth directly.

Minoxidil can be used in men who are experiencing baldness or hair thinning. It is not approved by Health Canada for use in women under 18 years of age or in women who are pregnant or breastfeeding. Treatment involves administering the drug to the affected (balding or thinning) area twice daily, usually morning and evening. It generally takes 4 months before results are seen. Systemic absorption of topically applied minoxidil may occur, with possible adverse effects, including tachycardia, fluid retention, and weight gain. Local effects may include skin irritation, and the drug is not be applied to skin that is already irritated, nor used concurrently with other topical medications applied to the same site. Note that the beneficial effects of this drug can be reduced by heat, including the use of a blow dryer.

The systemically administered drug finasteride (Proscar®, 5 mg) is used to treat benign prostatic hyperplasia, as discussed in Chapter 36. A lower-strength version known as Propecia® (1 mg) is also used to treat male pattern alopecia. Finasteride is not to be used during pregnancy because it is known to have adverse effects on the fetus, and women are not to handle this drug without gloves or crush this drug, thereby making it airborne.

SUNSCREENS

Sunscreens are topical products used to protect the skin from damage caused by the ultraviolet radiation of sunlight. There are numerous specific sunscreen products on the market. None requires a prescription for use. Each is composed of typically three to five various chemical ingredients that work together to provide ultraviolet protection and, usually, a moisturizing effect as well. Common examples of these ingredients are titanium dioxide, octyl methoxycinnamate, homosalate, and parabens. Sunscreens are rated with a sun protection factor (SPF) rating, which is a number ranging from 2 to 50 (and even higher in some newer products) in order of increasing potency of ultraviolet protection. Health Canada recommends the use of sunscreens with an SPF of 15 or greater to reduce the risk of skin cancer and early skin aging. Most sunscreens come in lotion, cream, or gel form. A smaller number of lip balms are also available. It is important for sunscreens to have both ultraviolet A and ultraviolet B protection. Sunscreen is not to be used on infants.

ANTINEOPLASTIC DRUGS

Skin cancer is the most common form of cancer. There are two types of nonmelanoma skin cancer: basal cell carcinoma and squamous cell carcinoma. Basal cell carcinoma is the most common and is rarely fatal, but it can be highly disfiguring. Squamous cell carcinoma, on the other hand,

can be fatal, with an estimated 500 deaths expected in 2015 in Canada (Canadian Cancer Society, 2016). The most aggressive skin cancer is melanoma; it accounts for only 3% of all skin cancers but is responsible for 75% of deaths associated with skin cancer. The most common cause of skin cancer is exposure to the sun and tanning beds. Early detection and prevention (with the use of sunscreen) are of the utmost importance.

fluorouracil

Various premalignant skin lesions and basal cell carcinomas may be treated with the topically applied form of the antineoplastic drug fluorouracil (Efudex®). As noted in Chapter 52, this drug is an antimetabolite that acts by interfering with key cellular metabolic reactions, destroying rapidly growing cells, such as premalignant and malignant cells. It is also used topically in the treatment of solar or **actinic keratosis** and superficial basal cell carcinomas of the skin, often in addition to local surgical excision. More aggressive skin cancers (squamous cell carcinoma and malignant melanoma) are not treated with fluorouracil but are usually treated with more aggressive interventions, such as surgery, radiation therapy, or systemic chemotherapy (see Chapters 52 and 53).

The adverse effects associated with the topical use of this antineoplastic drug are generally limited to local inflammatory reactions such as dermatitis, stomatitis, and photosensitivity. More serious effects include swelling, scaling, pain, pruritus, burning, soreness, tenderness, suppuration, scarring, and hyperpigmentation.

Fluorouracil is available as a topical cream. It can be applied with a nonmetalic applicator, clean fingertips, or gloved fingers. If the fingers are used, they need to be washed thoroughly immediately after application. The 1% fluorouracil cream is used for the treatment of multiple actinic keratoses of the head and neck. The cream is applied twice daily to the lesions. Superficial basal cell carcinoma may be treated with 5% fluorouracil, administered twice daily for at least 2 to 6 weeks. Another topical drug used for actinic keratoses and basal cell carcinomas is the immunomodulator imiquimod, discussed in the following section.

IMMUNOMODULATORS

▶▶*pimecrolimus*

Pimecrolimus (Elidel®) is available in a cream form for use in treating atopic dermatitis. Atopic dermatitis is caused by a hereditary susceptibility to pruritus and is often associated with allergic rhinitis, hay fever, and asthma. This drug works through a mechanism similar to that of the immunosuppressant drug tacrolimus (Advacraf®) used to prevent rejection of transplanted organs, which was discussed in Chapter 50. A topical form of tacrolimus (Protopic®) is also used and has similar actions and indications. Adverse reactions to both drugs are usually limited to minor skin irritations.

DRUG PROFILES—cont'd

imiquimod

Imiquimod (Aldara P®, Vyloma®) is an immunomodulating drug that has demonstrated efficacy in treating actinic keratoses, basal cell carcinoma, and anogenital warts. Its exact mechanism of action is unknown, but it is believed to somehow enhance the body's immune response to these conditions. It is applied two to five times per week, as prescribed, depending on the condition being treated. Adverse reactions to imiquimod include mild skin reactions such as burning, induration (hardness), irritation, pain, and bleeding, which can occur both locally (at the site of medication administration) and at skin areas remote from the site of administration. More severe adverse skin reactions include edema, erosion or ulceration, scaling, scabbing, exudation, and vesicle formation. Systemic reactions, likely related to systemic immunomodulating effects, include cough, upper respiratory infection, musculoskeletal reactions (e.g., back pain), and lymphadenopathy. This drug is available only in cream form.

WOUND CARE DRUGS

Although superficial skin wounds usually require minimal interventions, deeper skin wounds often require more deliberate care to promote optimal healing. Such care includes addressing systemic factors (e.g., body nutritional status) that are critical to tissue repair. Vitamin C (ascorbic acid) and zinc have been shown to improve wound healing when they are given orally. Topical wound care medications are one of the fundamental steps of wound care, referred to in the literature as *preparation of the wound bed*. When medications are required for wound care, consult with a wound care specialist. Wound *débridement* is removal of nonviable tissue and elimination of bacteria by suitable cleansing or surgical intervention. Drugs containing papain or a combination of papain and urea are commonly used as topical débriding drugs. Table 56-6 lists information regarding selected currently available wound care products.

TABLE 56-6

Selected Wound Care Products

Product Name	Advantages	Disadvantages	Contraindications
acetic acid (vinegar)	Low cost; antiseptic	Cytotoxic	Allergy
sodium hypochlorite (Clorox® bleach solution, 0.65%; Dakin's Solution®, 0.5%)	Aids débridement; reduces microbial count	Partly toxic and irritating to healing tissue	Clean, noninfected wounds
collagenase (Santyl®)	Good for patients taking anticoagulants or in whom surgery is contraindicated; selectively removes necrotic tissue; does not harm normal tissue; satisfactory for infected wounds	Requires health care provider's order; not for use with other common wound care products such as silver sulfadiazine; expensive	Clean wounds with granulation tissue and signs of healing but with limited areas of necrosis; product allergy
iodine (Iocidedosorb®)	Slow-release; safe for viable cells; absorbs exudates; promotes wound healing	Partly toxic to fibroblast cells; stains tissue	Iodine allergy

SKIN PREPARATION DRUGS

The skin must be disinfected before any invasive procedure. Isopropyl alcohol (70%) is most commonly used to prepare the skin before minor procedures such as drawing blood or giving injections. Isopropyl alcohol has been shown to lower the bacterial count on the skin for 20 to 40 minutes after application. Other drugs that are used to prepare the skin include povidone-iodine, chlorhexidine (Dexidin®, Hibitane®), and benzalkonium chloride (Agentquat®). Benzalkonium chloride is a surface-active drug that works by denaturing microorganisms or essentially destroying their proteins. Chlorhexidine acts by disrupting bacterial membranes and inhibiting cell wall synthesis. It is used primarily by health care providers as a surgical scrub or handwashing agent. Chorhexidine 2% and 70% alcohol swabs are also used to reduce skin microbial levels when used to cleanse an arterial or central line. Povidone-iodine is an antiseptic that kills bacteria, fungi, and viruses. It is used for the prevention or treatment of topical infections associated with surgery, burns, and minor cuts and scrapes, and for relief of minor vaginal infections. It is the most widely used antiseptic.

TABLE 56-7		
Skin Preparation Drugs		
Drug	**Effective Against**	**Adverse Effects**
isopropyl alcohol	Bacteria, fungi, virus	Excessive dryness of skin
chlorhexidine (Dexidin, Hibitane)	Bacteria, fungi	Central nervous system toxicity in neonates and burn patients
povidone-iodine	Bacteria, fungi, virus	Staining of skin, irritation and pain at wound sites; retards or reverses the granulation process
benzalkonium chloride (Agentquat)	Bacteria, fungi	Chemical burns if left in contact with skin for too long

There is no need to screen for iodine or shellfish allergies with its use—immunoglobulin E antibody–mediated seafood allergies are not linked to iodine; such allergies are to specific proteins in fish and shellfish, which do not contain iodine. Therefore, a fish or shellfish allergy does not automatically imply a sensitivity or allergy to iodine (Katelaris, 2009). Povidone-iodine is available in many different dosage forms. See Table 56-7 for more information on selected skin preparation drugs.

NURSING PROCESS

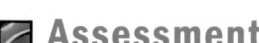 Assessment

Before administering any dermatological preparation, assess patients for any allergies (including allergies to all drug ingredients), contraindications, cautions, and drug interactions. Topical antibacterials are associated with a wide range of reactions because of the sensitivity of patients to antibiotics, even when in a different dosage form; therefore, if a patient is allergic to a systemic antibacterial, the patient will also be allergic to its topical dosage forms. Assess the results of any culture and sensitivity testing that was ordered before giving an antibacterial, to ensure appropriate identification of effective drugs. Before administering any type of topical medication (e.g., antimicrobial, corticosteroid, antiacne drug), always consider the concentration of the medication, length of exposure to the skin, condition of the skin, size of the affected area, and hydration of the skin. All of these factors have a significant influence on the action of the medication. Additionally, assess the medication order for not only the correct drug but also the prescribed route. Inspect the skin or affected area thoroughly under an adequate light source. Palpate the area with a gloved hand. In dark-skinned patients, an erythematous area may not be visible but may be palpated as an area of warmth. Accompany physical assessment of the skin with a documented assessment of surrounding structures, including lymph nodes.

Assess the patient's overall health status and hygiene practices, including whether the patient has experienced any trauma and whether there is any history of immunosuppression. Remember that the skin of young children and older adults is more fragile and permeable to certain topical dermatological preparations. These characteristics also lead to a higher risk of systemic absorption from the skin. It is important to note other possible situations that may result in a drug effect that is less than therapeutic, such as the use of topical drugs over an area containing pus or debris. Use of natural health products, such as topical aloe vera, also requires thorough assessment and notation of any allergies, contraindications, cautions, and drug interactions (see the Natural Health Products box on p. 1049).

Nursing Diagnoses

- Impaired skin integrity related to specific diseases, reactions, conditions, or breaks in skin barrier
- Deficient knowledge related to lack of experience with and exposure to use of topical drugs

Planning

Goals

- Patient's skin will remain intact and healed in appearance, and skin integrity will be maintained.
- Patient will demonstrate adequate knowledge about the use of dermatological medication.
- Patient will remain adherent to the drug regimen.

Expected Patient Outcomes

- Condition of patient's skin improves daily as stated by the patient, with less redness, drainage, discomfort, itching, or rash.
- Patient states the rationale for treatment, adverse effects of the specific dermatological preparation, and symptoms associated with the dermatological

preparation that should be reported to the health care provider.

- Patient demonstrates how to apply the medication in keeping with the health care provider's orders, with specific attention to the requirements for emollient, lotion, solution, spray, cream, gel, and ointment dosage forms.
- Patient experiences improvement in the condition of affected area(s) and demonstrates continued compliance with the medication regimen.
  - Patient applies or self-administers the medication, as prescribed or directed and at the recommended frequency.

Implementation

When a wound has been noted, a wound assessment and treatment flow sheet should be implemented and filled out each time wound care has been completed. In general, before any topical medication is applied, cleanse the affected site of any debris, drainage, and residual medication, taking care to follow any specific directions, such as removing water- or alcohol-based topical preparations with soap and water. Always begin (and end) by performing hand hygiene and maintain standard precautions/routine practices (see Box 10-1). Store all dosage forms of medication as recommended. Wear gloves, not only to prevent contamination from secretions but also to prevent absorption of the medication through the skin. Apply topical drugs using a gloved hand, tongue depressor, or cotton-tipped applicator. Shake or mix lotions and solutions thoroughly before use and apply them evenly (see Chapter 10). Wash hands before and after application of the medication. Apply any dressings as ordered, paying special attention to directions concerning occlusive, wet, or wet-to-dry dressing changes. It is important to note, however, that most topical dermatological drugs do not require the use of a dressing once the medication is applied. The medication order may also indicate that any dressing or coverage of the affected area is to be avoided. When medications are used for wound care, there is usually a step-by-step protocol for application of a cleansing agent, a possible débridement drug, and a rinsing solution, as well as final application of an antibacterial, antifungal, burn, antiseptic, or other solution that may have been ordered. Provide comprehensive patient education regarding wound care and use of topical dermatological drugs to ensure safe and effective treatment. If home health care is needed after discharge, arrangements need to be in place before the patient returns home. Document information about the site of drug application, including drainage (colour and amount), swelling, temperature, odour, skin colour, and pain or other sensations. Also record the type of treatment rendered and the response, with each treatment or application, as well as a comparative before-and-after assessment. Some health care agencies have procedures for taking pictures of wounds to assess for improvement in healing. Patients should be encouraged to continue this documentation when they are able to do so.

Follow the manufacturer's guidelines regarding the use of any dermatological preparation because each medication has a different type of base solution. Specific application procedures may be required for different dosage forms. It is also important to follow any instructions or orders regarding other treatments around the affected area, such as the use of an occlusive or wet dressing (see earlier in the chapter). Medicated areas may also need to be protected from exposure to air or sunlight. Strict adherence to the proper method of application and dosage of any dermatological preparation is important to its effectiveness. Doubling of the next dose following a missed dose is not recommended. After the medication administration process is complete, dispose of all contaminated dressings, gloves, and equipment properly. Maintain safety, comfort, and privacy for the patient at all times. See the Patient Teaching Tips for more information. Also see Table 56-6 for information about specific drugs for wound care and their advantages and disadvantages.

Evaluation

Begin evaluation by monitoring to ensure that goals and expected outcomes are being met. Therapeutic responses to the various dermatological preparations include improved condition of skin; healing of lesions or wounds; decrease in the size of the lesions with eventual resolution; and decrease in swelling, redness, weeping, itching, or burning in the affected area. Notify the health care provider if a therapeutic response is not observed within an appropriate time frame (anywhere from 48 to 72 hours or longer, depending on the drug, the disorder or skin problem, and the acute or long-term nature of the condition) or if signs and symptoms worsen or new ones appear. Adverse effects for which to evaluate include increased severity of symptoms, such as increased redness, swelling, pain, and drainage; fever; or any other unusual problems at the affected area. Adverse effects may range from slight irritation of the site where the topical drug has been applied, to an allergic reaction, to toxic systemic effects.

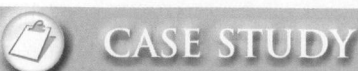

CASE STUDY

Medications for Wound Care

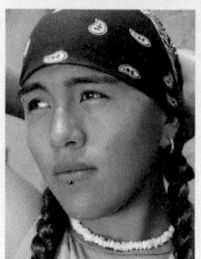

Akule, a 16-year-old student, was clearing brush with his father when he cut his hand. His mother washed the wound and told him to apply cream. Akule checked the family medicine cabinet and applied clotrimazole (Clotrimaderm) cream, the only cream in the cabinet.

Two days later, the wound is not better and is painful. Akule's mother takes him to the clinic to have the wound checked. The nurse finds that the laceration wound is deep but does not have any drainage. The wound is irrigated with normal saline, bacitracin is applied, and the wound is closed with adhesive strips and then covered with a loose gauze dressing. The nurse gives Akule instructions on how to care for the wound and tells him that this wound care is to be done twice a day for 1 week. In addition, the nurse suggests that Akule take vitamin C and zinc supplements for the next month and instructs him not to use the clotrimazole ointment on the wound.

1. Why did the nurse apply bacitracin instead of clotrimazole? Explain your answer.
2. What is the purpose of the vitamin C and zinc supplements?
3. The next day, Akule discovers a rash that covers both his arms and legs. The rash is itchy, and his skin is red with small bumps. He knows that there was poison ivy in the brush and wants something to stop the itching. What will be suggested?
4. The next evening, as he takes off the dressing to clean his wound, Akule finds that the area is swollen and more inflamed, with tiny red bumps around the wound. There is no drainage. What do you think has happened, and what will be done?

_____

For answers, see http://evolve.elsevier.com/Canada/Lilley/pharmacology/.

PATIENT TEACHING TIPS

❖ Advise patients to keep the skin clean and dry or clean and moist, as prescribed. Provide instructions to patients and caregivers about maintaining adequate general hygiene, cleanliness, and hydration, as well as proper nutrition, during drug therapy.

❖ Ensure that patients have a thorough understanding of how to prepare skin for the application of medication and any other instructions.

❖ Apply dressings to the affected area as directed, if indicated or ordered. Perform dressing application after medication use, and properly dispose of contaminated dressings or equipment. Emphasize the need for thorough handwashing before and after application of medication with a gloved hand, cotton-tipped applicator, or tongue depressor. Demonstrate proper techniques to all individuals involved in the care of patients. Always emphasize the importance of adherence to the drug regimen. Teach patients to use a thin layer of drug product; only the product that actually touches the skin has any benefit.

❖ Encourage patients to notify their health care providers of any unusual or adverse reactions or if the original condition worsens or fails to improve within a designated period of time.

❖ Counsel all female patients of childbearing age about the teratogenic hazards associated with fetal exposure to certain dermatological drugs. All sexually active women must use contraception during treatment with any teratogenic drug and for at least 1 month after its discontinuation.

❖ Educate patients about ways to prevent exposure to the sun through the use of sunscreen and protective clothing, as well as avoidance of overexposure. Tanning beds create risk for skin cancer as well, so share with patients appropriate and accurate information regarding their use and associated risk. Sunscreen must also be used with tanning beds in order to reduce the damage from the UV radiation.

❖ Vitamin D deficiency may be an issue for some sunscreen users and those who live at higher latitudes or are not exposed to sunlight. As adequate oral intake of Vitamin D is difficult to achieve without supplementation, many people with minimal exposure to sunlight do not activate vitamin D and are deficient in vitamin D.

❖ Patients should be taught how to self-assess all skin moles or lesions and monitor for any unusual changes in colour, size, texture, or shape, which should be reported to a health care provider.

KEY POINTS

- Dermatological drugs are used to treat topical infections.
- Common skin disorders caused by bacteria are folliculitis, impetigo, furuncles, carbuncles, and cellulitis.
- The bacterium most commonly responsible for acne is *Propionibacterium acnes*.
- The fungi that are responsible for causing topical fungal infections are *Candida* spp., dermatophytes, and *Malassezia furfur*.
- The most common topical fungal infections are *Candida* infections, for example, yeast infections.
- One of the most common topical viral infections is infection with herpes simplex virus types 1 and 2.
- Topical anaesthetics are used therapeutically to numb the skin. Indications for topical anaesthetics include insect bites, sunburn, poison ivy, and prevention of pain from injections.

- Corticosteroids are some of the most widely used topical drugs and are indicated for relief of topical inflammatory and pruritic disorders.
- Beneficial effects of corticosteroids include anti-inflammatory, antipruritic, and vasoconstrictor actions. Some of the negative effects of potent corticosteroid use or prolonged use of weaker corticosteroids include dermal atrophy and adrenal insufficiency.
- Adverse and toxic reactions to dermatological drugs can and do occur; therefore, administer these drugs cautiously and follow the health care provider's orders and manufacturer's guidelines. This is crucial to ensure safe and effective treatment.
- Patient education about each medication, its administration, and its effectiveness is important to ensure adherence with the treatment regimen.

EXAMINATION REVIEW QUESTIONS

1. The nurse is assessing the skin of an adolescent patient who has been using a benzoyl peroxide product for 2 weeks as part of treatment for acne. Which assessment findings indicate that the patient is having an allergic reaction and will need to stop treatment?
   a. Reddened skin over the treatment area
   b. Blistering skin over the treatment area
   c. Peeling skin over the treatment area
   d. Sensation of warmth when the product is applied

2. When considering the variety of OTC topical corticosteroid products, the nurse is aware that which type of preparation is generally most penetrating and effective?
   a. Gel
   b. Lotion
   c. Spray
   d. Ointment

3. The nurse is monitoring for an allergic reaction to topical bacitracin, which would be evident by the presence of which symptom(s)?
   a. Petechiae
   b. Thickened skin
   c. Itching and burning
   d. Purulent drainage

4. When the nurse is teaching a patient about the mechanism of action of tretinoin, which statement by the nurse is correct?
   a. "This medication acts by killing the bacteria that cause acne."
   b. "This medication actually causes skin peeling."
   c. "This medication acts by protecting your skin from ultraviolet light."
   d. "This medication has anti-inflammatory actions."

5. When the nurse is providing wound care with Dakin's Solution for a patient who has a stage III pressure ulcer, the patient exclaims, "I smell bleach! Why are

you putting bleach on me?" What is the nurse's best explanation?
   a. "This is a dilute solution and acts to reduce the bacteria in the wound so that it can heal."
   b. "This solution is used instead of medication to promote wound healing."
   c. "This solution is used to dissolve the dead tissue in your wound."
   d. "Don't worry; we would never use bleach on a patient!"

6. The nurse is instructing a parent on the use of dimeticone for treatment of a child's head lice. Which statement by the parent indicates a need for further education?
   a. "I will spray his hair, then rinse out the shampoo immediately."
   b. "I will leave the medication on his hair for 30 minutes before rinsing."
   c. "After the hair is dry, I will shampoo and dry his hair."
   d. "When the hair is dry, I will comb the hair to remove the nits."

7. The nurse is performing wound care on a burned area of a patient's arm using silver sulfadiazine cream. Which actions by the nurse are correct? (Select all that apply.)
   a. Applying the cream over the previous layer to avoid disturbing the wound bed
   b. Gently cleansing the wound to remove wound debris and the previous layer of cream
   c. Using clean gloves to apply the ointment
   d. Using sterile gloves to apply the ointment
   e. Always covering the wound with a dressing after applying the cream
   f. Washing hands before and after the procedure

CRITICAL THINKING ACTIVITIES

1. A 22-year-old woman with severe acne is receiving counselling before taking isotretinoin (Accutane) therapy. She has read the related warnings from Health Canada online and was shocked and concerned to learn that two negative pregnancy tests are required before starting therapy and that a pregnancy test must be performed monthly during therapy. What is the nurse's best answer to her concerns?

2. A child is being discharged after a minor surgical procedure. The child's mother has been instructed to use a povidone-iodine OTC antiseptic to cleanse the area. The mother expresses concern that her child has a sensitivity to shellfish and that she read on the Internet that this antiseptic should not be used in individuals who have an allergy or sensitivity to shellfish. What is the nurse's best response?

3. A 6-year-old child is sent home from school with head lice. His mother is worried that the lice will spread to her two younger children. You are her neighbour and a nurse. She asks what she can do to prevent the spread of lice.

For answers, see http://evolve.elsevier.com/Canada/Lilley/pharmacology/.

CHAPTER 57

Ophthalmic Drugs

Objectives

After reading this chapter, the successful student will be able to do the following:

1. Discuss the anatomy and physiology of the structures of the eye and the impacts of glaucoma and other disorders and disease processes on these structures.

2. List the various classifications of ophthalmic drugs, with examples of specific drugs in each class.

3. Discuss the mechanisms of action, indications, dosage forms, application techniques, adverse effects, cautions, contraindications, and drug interactions of the various ophthalmic drugs.

4. Develop a collaborative plan of care that includes all phases of the nursing process for patients receiving ophthalmic drugs.

e-Learning Activities

Website
(http://evolve.elsevier.com/Canada/Lilley/pharmacology/)

*e*volve

- Answer Key—Textbook Case Studies
- Answer Key—Critical Thinking Activities
- Chapter Summaries—Printable
- Review Questions for Exam Preparation
- Unfolding Case Studies

Drug Profiles

acetylcholine (acetylcholine chloride)*, p. 1064
apraclonidine (apraclonidine hydrochloride)*, p. 1064
▸▸ artificial tears, p. 1075
▸▸ atropine sulphate, p. 1074
▸▸ bacitracin zinc/polymyxin B sulphate, p. 1071
▸▸ betaxolol (betaxolol hydrochloride)*, p. 1067
▸▸ ciprofloxacin (ciprofloxacin hydrochloride)*, p. 1071
cromolyn (cromolyn sodium)*, p. 1075
cyclopentolate (cyclopentolate hydrochloride)*, p. 1074
▸▸ dexamethasone, p. 1073
▸▸ dipivefrin (dipivefrin hydrochloride)*, p. 1066
▸▸ dorzolamide hydrochloride, p. 1068
▸▸ erythromycin, p. 1071
fluorescein sodium, p. 1074
▸▸ gentamicin (gentamicin sulphate)*, p. 1071
glycerin, p. 1069
ketorolac (ketorolac tromethamine)*, p. 1073
▸▸ latanoprost, p. 1069
mannitol, p. 1069
olopatadine, p. 1075
▸▸ pilocarpine (pilocarpine hydrochloride)*, p. 1064
▸▸ sulfacetamide (sulfacetamide sodium)*, p. 1072
tetracaine (tetracaine hydrochloride)*, p. 1074
tetrahydrozoline (tetrahydrozoline hydrochloride)*, p. 1075
▸▸ timolol (timolol maleate)*, p. 1067
trifluridine, p. 1072

▸▸ Key drug

*Full generic name is given in parentheses. For the purposes of this text, the more common, shortened name is used.

Key Terms

Accommodation The adjustment of the lens of the eye for variations in distance. (p. 1061)

Anterior chamber The bubblelike portion of the front of the eye between the iris and the cornea. (p. 1060)

Aqueous humour The clear, watery fluid circulating in the anterior and posterior chambers of the eye. (p. 1060)

Canal of Schlemm A tiny, circular vein at the angle of the anterior chamber of the eye through which the aqueous humour is drained and ultimately funnelled into the bloodstream; also called *Schlemm's canal*. (p. 1060)

Cataract An abnormal, progressive condition of the lens of the eye, characterized by loss of transparency and resultant blurred vision. (p. 1060)

Ciliary muscles The circular muscles between the anterior and posterior chambers behind the iris; connected to the suspensory ligaments that control the lens curvature. (p. 1060)

Closed-angle glaucoma Glaucoma that occurs as a result of a narrowed anatomical angle between the lens and cornea; also called *narrow-angle glaucoma, congestive glaucoma*, and *pupillary closure glaucoma*. (p. 1061)

Cones Photoreceptive (light-receiving) cells in the retina of the eye that enable a person to perceive colours and play a large role in central (straight-ahead) vision. (p. 1061)

Cornea The convex, transparent, anterior part of the eye. (p. 1060)

Cycloplegia Paralysis of the ciliary muscles, which prevents the accommodation of the lens to variations in distance. (p. 1061)

Cycloplegics Drugs that paralyze the ciliary muscles of the eye. (p. 1061)

Dilator muscle A muscle that constricts *the iris* of the eye but dilates the pupil; also called *dilator pupillae*. (p. 1060)

Glaucoma An abnormal condition of elevated pressure within the eye because of obstruction of the outflow of aqueous humour. (p. 1061)

Intraocular pressure (IOP) The internal pressure of all fluids of the eye against the tunics (retina, choroid, and sclera). (p. 1060)

Iris The round, muscular portion of the eye that gives the eye its colour and serves as an aperture controlling the amount of light passing through the pupil. (p. 1059)

Lacrimal ducts Small tubes that drain tears from the lacrimal glands into the nasal cavity. (p. 1060)

Lacrimal glands Glands located at the medial corners of the eyelids that produce tears. (p. 1060)

Lens The transparent, curved structure of the eye that is located directly behind the iris and pupil and is attached to the ciliary body by ligaments. (p. 1060)

Lysozyme An enzyme with antiseptic actions that destroys some foreign organisms; it is normally present in tears, saliva, sweat, and breast milk. (p. 1060)

Miotics Drugs that constrict the pupils. (p. 1061)

Mydriatics Drugs that dilate the pupils. (p. 1061)

Open-angle glaucoma A type of glaucoma that is often bilateral, develops slowly, is genetically determined, and does not involve a narrowing of the angle between the iris and the cornea; also called *chronic glaucoma, wide-angle glaucoma*, and *simple glaucoma*. (p. 1061)

Optic nerve A major nerve that connects the posterior end of each eye to the brain, to which it transmits visual signals. (p. 1061)

Pupil A circular opening in the iris of the eye, located slightly to the nasal side of the centre of the iris; the pupil lies behind the anterior chamber of the eye and the cornea and in front of the lens. (p. 1060)

Retina The innermost layer of the eye, containing both rods and cones that receive visual stimuli and transmit them to the optic nerve. (p. 1061)

Rods Photoreceptive (light-receiving) elements arranged perpendicularly to the surface of the retina; rods are especially sensitive to low-intensity light and are responsible for black-and-white and peripheral (to-the-side) vision. (p. 1061)

Sphincter pupillae A muscle that expands the iris while constricting or narrowing the diameter of the pupil. (p. 1060)

Tears Watery saline or alkaline fluid secreted by the lacrimal glands to moisten the conjunctiva (see Figure 57-1). (p. 1060)

Uvea The fibrous tunic beneath the sclera that includes the iris, the ciliary body, and the choroid of the eye (see Figure 57-1); also called *tunica vasculosa bulbi* or the *uveal tract*. (p. 1060)

Vitreous humour A transparent, semigelatinous substance contained in a thin membrane filling the cavity behind the lens; also called the *corpus vitreum* or *vitreous body*. (p. 1060)

OCULAR ANATOMY AND PHYSIOLOGY

The eye is the organ responsible for the sense of sight. The structures of the eye are illustrated in Figure 57-1, all of which are needed for accurate eyesight. Each eyeball is nearly spherical and approximately 2.5 cm in diameter. Each eye is recessed into a small frontal skull cavity known as the *orbit*. The exposed anterior (front) portion of the eye is covered by three layers: the protective external layer (cornea and sclera), a vascular middle layer known as the *uvea* (includes the choroid, iris, and ciliary body), and the internal layer, known as the *retina*. All of these layers are protected by the eyelid, which serves as an external protection device.

Each eye is held in place and moved by six muscles controlled by cranial nerves III, IV, and VI. These muscles include the *rectus* and *oblique* muscles. There are four types of rectus muscles: inferior, superior, medial, and lateral. There are two types of oblique muscles: inferior and superior. These muscles are shown in Figure 57-2. (The medial rectus muscle is hidden from view in this figure but is directly across from the lateral rectus muscle.) The levator palpebrae superioris muscle opens the eyelid

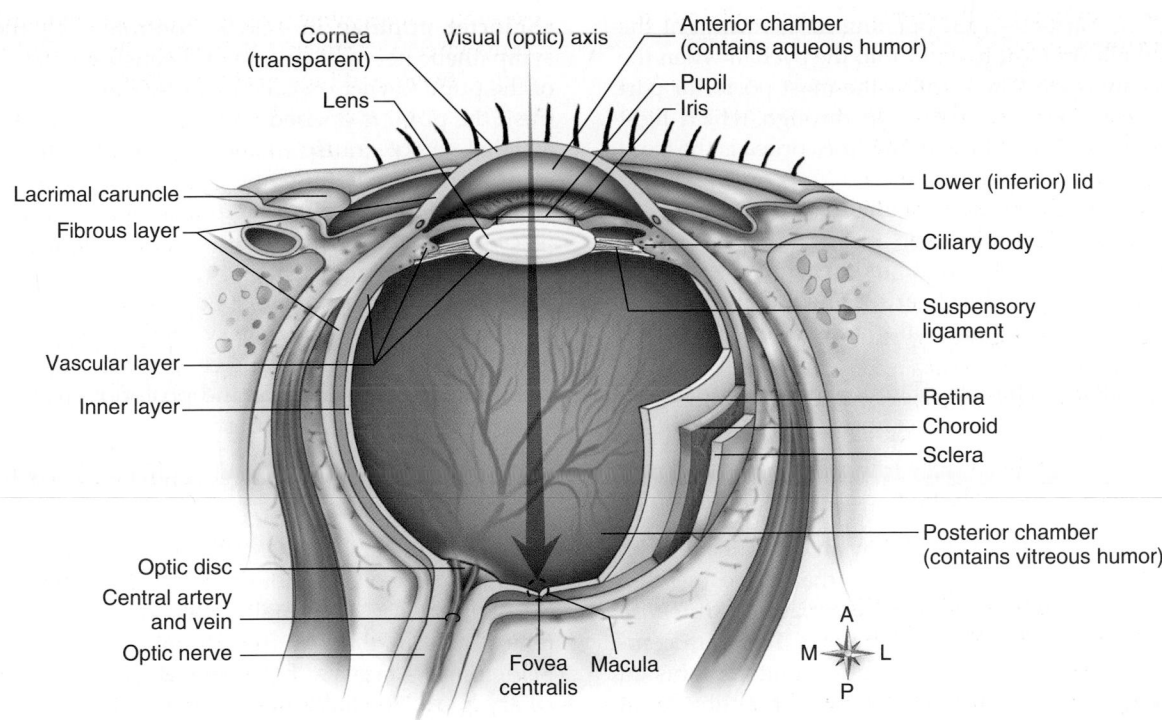

FIG. 57-1 Horizontal section through the left eyeball, looking from the top down. (Modified from: Patton, K. T., & Thibodeau, G. A. (2010). *Anatomy and physiology* (7th ed.). St. Louis, MO: Mosby.)

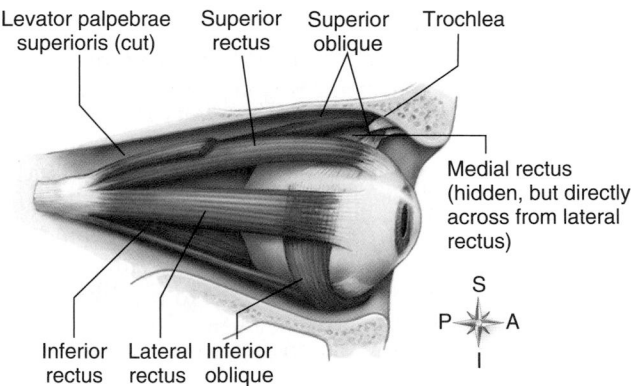

FIG. 57-2 Extrinsic muscles of the right eye, lateral view. (Modified from: Patton, K. T., & Thibodeau, G. A. (2010). *Anatomy and physiology* (7th ed.). St. Louis, MO, Mosby.)

(see later in this chapter). This muscle rests on top of the superior rectus muscle. There are several other important structures that are either part of or adjacent to the eye. The structures and the purpose of each are as follows:

- *Eyebrow:* Rows of short hairs above (superior to) the upper eyelid. The eyebrow protects the eye from direct light, falling dust or other small particles, and perspiration coming from the forehead.
- *Eyelid:* The layer of muscle and skin lined interiorly by the conjunctiva. The conjunctiva also covers the outer anterior surface of the eye, which includes the cornea. The eyelid is movable and can open or close. It

protects the eye when closed and allows vision when open. The eyelid is raised by contraction of the levator palpebrae superioris muscle and is lowered by relaxation of this muscle (see Figure 57-2).

- *Cornea:* The convex (outward-projecting), transparent, anterior portion of the eye. It can be thought of as a window that sits in front of the lens and allows the passage of light.
- *Eyelashes:* Two or three rows of hairs that are located on the edge (margin) of the eyelid. They help prevent small particles from falling into the eye when it is open.
- *Palpebral fissure:* The space between the upper and lower eyelids when the eyelids are open but relaxed.
- *Sclera:* A tough, white coat of fibrous tissue that surrounds the entire eyeball except for the cornea. It helps maintain the shape of the eye. Commonly called the *white* of the eye, the sclera is nonvascular and allows light to pass through it to the lens.
- *Choroid:* One of the middle-layer structures of the eyeball that contains the blood vessels supplying the eye; it also absorbs light.
- *Ciliary body:* The structure that supports the ciliary muscles that control the curvature of the lens via attached suspensory ligaments.
- *Conjunctiva:* The mucous membrane that lines the eyelids and also covers the exposed anterior surface of the eyeball.
- *Iris:* The coloured (pigmented) muscular apparatus behind the cornea.

- *Pupil*: The variable-sized opening in the centre of the iris that allows light to enter into the eyeball when the eyelids are open. The pupil is the most posterior part of the front portion of the eye through which light passes to the lens and the retina (the cornea is the front part of this window).
- *Medial canthus*: The site of union of the upper and lower eyelids near the nose.
- *Lacrimal caruncle*: A small, red, rounded elevation covered by modified skin at the medial angle of the eye; the site of the lacrimal glands (see later in the chapter).
- *Lateral canthus*: The site of union of the upper and lower eyelids away from the nose.

LACRIMAL GLANDS

The eye is kept moist and healthy by an intricate network of connected canals, ducts, and sacs that work together. The **lacrimal glands** produce tears that bathe and cleanse the exposed anterior portion of the eye. **Tears** are composed of an isotonic, aqueous solution that contains an enzyme called **lysozyme**, which acts as an antibacterial to help prevent eye infections. Tears drain into the nasal cavity through the **lacrimal ducts**.

LAYERS OF THE EYE

Overall, the eye can be thought of as having three separate anatomical layers. The fibrous outer layer of the eye has two parts that are continuous with each other: the sclera and the cornea. The sclera is a tough, fibrous layer that protects and maintains the shape of the eye. The **cornea** is a nonvascular, transparent portion of the outer layer that allows light to enter the eye. It is located at the extreme front of the eye and is continuous with the sclera. It is pain sensitive (a protective function) and obtains nutrition from **aqueous humour**, the clear, watery fluid that circulates in the anterior and posterior chambers of the eye. The vascular middle layer of the eye is composed of the iris (to the anterior), ciliary body, and choroid (to the posterior). These three structures are collectively called the *uvea*. The iris gives colour to the eye and has an adjustable opening in the centre called the **pupil**. The main function of the iris is to regulate the amount of light that enters the eye by causing the size of the pupil to vary. Pupil size is controlled by two smooth muscles. The

sphincter pupillae muscle is controlled by the parasympathetic nervous system and constricts the diameter of the pupil (an action called *miosis*; Figure 57-3). In contrast, the pupil is opened (an action called *mydriasis*) by a radial smooth muscle called the **dilator muscle**. It is composed of radiating fibres, like spokes of a wheel, which converge from the circumference of the iris toward its centre. Sympathetic nervous system impulses control this muscle (see Figure 57-3).

The anterior portions of both the retina and choroid merge to become the ciliary body, which produces aqueous humour. This is the clear, watery fluid that circulates in both the anterior and posterior chambers, and should not be confused with tears. Aqueous humour contributes, along with **vitreous humour**, to the **intraocular pressure (IOP)** of the eye. This is the internal pressure of all fluids against the tunics (retina, uvea, sclera) of the eye. Given the small size of the eye, any change in the volume of aqueous humour present can lead to increased or reduced IOP. Normally, the aqueous humour is removed from the **anterior chamber** via the **canal of Schlemm** at a rate that balances out its production by the ciliary body. The ciliary body also provides support for the suspensory ligaments to which the lens is attached. The **lens** is the transparent, crystalline structure of the eye, located directly behind the iris and the pupil. It has a biconvex (ellipsoid) shape and is held in place by suspensory ligaments that are attached to the **ciliary muscles**. Contraction of the ciliary muscles changes the shape of the lens. This function is important for visual accommodation (see below) as well as the focusing of light (and visual images) onto the retina. The ciliary muscle is controlled by the parasympathetic nervous system through the oculomotor nerve (cranial nerve III). The lens divides the interior of the eyeball into posterior (rear) and anterior (forward) chambers. The larger chamber behind the lens is filled with a jellylike fluid called the vitreous body. The lens is transparent to allow light to pass through it easily. A loss of lens transparency results in a visual condition called a *cataract*. A cataract is a grey–white opacity that can be seen within the lens. If cataracts are untreated, sight may eventually be completely lost. At the onset of a cataract, vision is blurred and may be further worsened by the glare of bright lights. *Diplopia*, or double vision, may also develop.

Before light rays reach the retina, they are focused into a sharp image by the lens of the eye. The elasticity of the

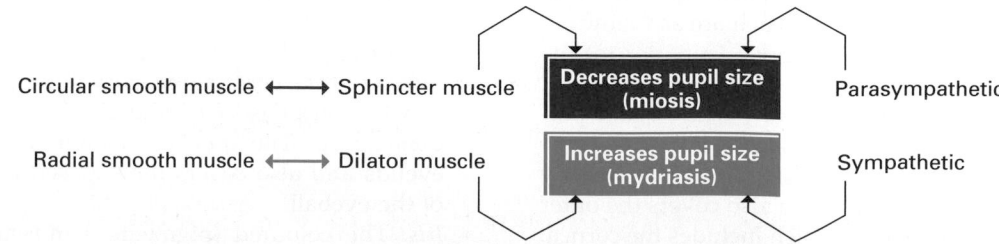

FIG. 57-3 Different nervous systems control pupil size.

lens enables it to change its shape and focusing power. This process is called *accommodation* and is facilitated by the ciliary body. Paralysis of accommodation is called **cycloplegia**. **Mydriatics** are drugs that dilate the pupil (e.g., apraclonidine). Drugs that constrict the pupil are called *miotics* (e.g., acetylcholine, pilocarpine). Drugs that paralyze the ciliary body are called *cycloplegics*, but they also have mydriatic properties (e.g., atropine sulphate, cyclopentolate) (Figure 57-4). All of these medications are used to facilitate visualization of the inner eye during ophthalmic examinations.

The third and inner layer of the eye is a thin, delicate layer known as the *retina*. It contains light-sensitive photoreceptors called *rods* and *cones*. The basic function of the retina is to receive the light image formed by the lens and to convert it via the rods and cones into the neural signals that support vision. **Rods** produce black-and-white vision, including shades of grey, and are especially sensitive in low light; **cones** are responsible for colour vision (Figure 57-5). In addition, rods are more active in providing peripheral (to-the-side) vision, whereas cones are more active in central (straight-ahead) vision. In the posterior central part of the retina, the nerve fibres of retinal cells join to form the **optic nerve**. The function of the optic nerve is to connect the retina with the visual centre of the brain, located within the occipital lobe that extends above and behind the cerebellum. It is this portion of the brain that interprets incoming visual stimuli.

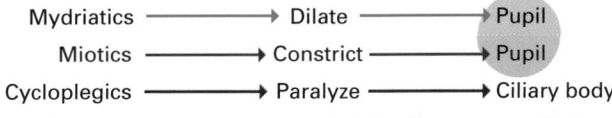

FIG. 57-4 Drug classes and their effects on pupil size.

TREATMENT OF EYE DISORDERS

Some of the minor ailments that affect the eye can be treated with over-the-counter (OTC) medications, but persistent, painful conditions generally require prescription medications. Medications used to treat disorders of the eye can be divided into several major drug groups: antiglaucoma drugs, antimicrobials, anti-inflammatory drugs, topical anaesthetics, diagnostic drugs, antiallergic drugs, and lubricants and moisturizers. There are also a variety of combination drug products that include two or more medications from different subclasses. The reader can assume the therapeutic indications for and drug effects of these combination products are the same as those of the single-ingredient drug products corresponding to their individual components. The focus of this chapter is on commonly used therapeutic medications.

A multitude of products is also available for use in the care of contact lenses, including contact lens–cleaning enzymes, irrigating solutions, and eye washes. Their use is fairly straightforward, and they carry limited risk. Complicated surgical drugs are beyond the scope of this chapter. The reader is advised to refer to manufacturer's packaging information for details about any unfamiliar product encountered in clinical practice.

GLAUCOMA

Glaucoma is a group of eye disorders that damage the optic nerve. In most cases, this is due to increased IOP that is caused by abnormally elevated levels of aqueous humour. Glaucoma occurs when the aqueous humour is not drained through the canal of Schlemm as quickly as it is formed by the ciliary body. The accumulated aqueous humour creates a backward pressure that pushes the vitreous humour against the retina. Continued pressure on the retina destroys its neurons, which leads to impaired vision and eventual blindness (Figure 57-6). Unfortunately, glaucoma is often without early symptoms, and many patients are not diagnosed until some permanent sight loss has occurred.

Two major types of glaucoma are discussed in this chapter: **closed-angle glaucoma** and **open-angle glaucoma**. Figure 57-7 shows the pathophysiology of each and provides an enlarged view of the involved eye structures. Table 57-1 lists additional characteristic features of each type. Glaucoma can be a primary illness (occurring on its own), or it can be secondary to another eye condition or injury (e.g., post-traumatic glaucoma). Congenital glaucoma can also occur in infants. The visual and optic

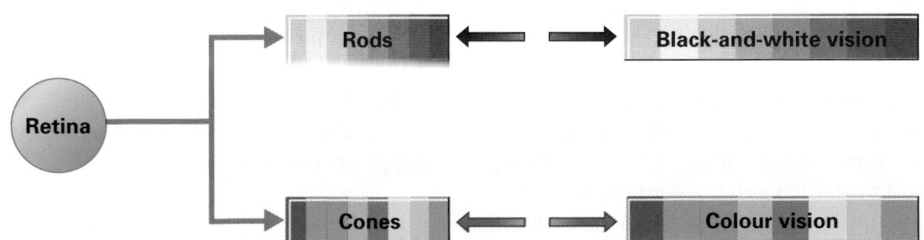

FIG. 57-5 Function of rods and cones in relation to colour vision.

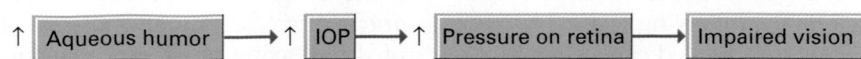

FIG. 57-6 How increased aqueous humour can result in impaired vision. *IOP*, intraocular pressure.

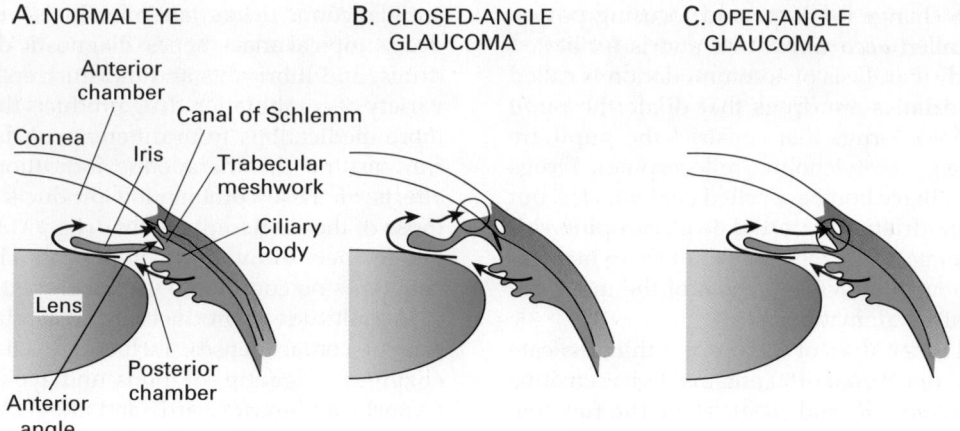

FIG. 57-7 Main structures of the eye and an enlargement of the canal of schlemm showing an aqueous flow. *A*, Flow in a normal eye. *B*, In closed-angle glaucoma, the closure of the anterior angle prevents aqueous humour from exiting through the canal of Schlemm, which leads to increased intraocular pressure. *C*, In open-angle glaucoma, the anterior angle remains open, but the canal of Schlemm is obstructed by tissue abnormalities. (Modified from: McKenry, L. M., Tessier, E., & Hogan, M. A. (2006). *Mosby's pharmacology in nursing—revised and updated* (22nd ed.). St. Louis, MO: Mosby.)

TABLE 57-1

Glaucoma: Types and Characteristics

	Closed-angle	**Open-angle**
Synonyms	Narrow-angle glaucoma, congestive glaucoma, and pupillary closure glaucoma	Chronic glaucoma, wide-angle glaucoma, and simple glaucoma
Chronicity	Acute (can cause rapid vision loss)	Chronic
Relative incidence	Less common	More common
Nature of angle	Narrow	Larger
Most common age of onset and race	30 yr or older, White	30 yr or older, Black
Major symptoms	Blurred vision, severe headaches, eye pain	Blurred vision, occasional headaches
Treatment	Topical or systemic drugs, surgery	Topical or systemic drugs, surgery

nerve changes typical of glaucoma can also occur in the absence of increased IOP (normotensive glaucoma). There are a few other less common forms of glaucoma (e.g., pigmentary glaucoma, pseudoexfoliative glaucoma) that are beyond the scope of this chapter.

ANTIGLAUCOMA DRUGS

Treatment of glaucoma involves reducing IOP by either increasing the drainage of aqueous humour or decreasing its production. Some drugs may do both. Drug therapy can delay and possibly even prevent the development of glaucoma. Glaucoma eye drops are colour-coded according to medication class to aid the patient in their identification. However, this may not be standard across Canada and may often change. Drug classes of eye drops used to reduce IOP include the following:

- Direct-acting cholinergics (also called *miotics* and *parasympathomimetic drugs*)
- Indirect-acting cholinergics (also called *miotics, cholinesterase inhibitors*, and *parasympathomimetic drugs*)
- Adrenergics (also called *mydriatics* and *sympathomimetic drugs*)
- Antiadrenergics (β-blockers; also called *sympatholytic drugs*)
- Carbonic anhydrase inhibitors
- Osmotic diuretics
- Prostaglandin agonists

See Table 57-2 for a comparison of the effects of these drugs on the aqueous humour.

CHOLINERGIC DRUGS

There are two categories of ophthalmic parasympathomimetic drugs, more concisely referred to as *cholinergic drugs*: direct-acting and indirect-acting. Some examples of direct-acting cholinergics include acetylcholine, carbachol, and pilocarpine. Indirect-acting cholinergics are also called *cholinesterase inhibitors*, and an example of this type of drug is echothiophate (currently not available in Canada). Because one primary drug effect of these drugs is pupillary constriction or miosis (see later), they are also commonly called *miotics*.

Mechanism of Action and Drug Effects

Acetylcholine is the neurochemical mediator of nerve impulses in the parasympathetic nervous system. It stimulates parasympathetic, or cholinergic, receptors located in the brain and throughout the body along parasympathetic nerve branches. This stimulation results in several effects on the eye: miosis (pupillary constriction), vasodilation of blood vessels in and around the eye, contraction of ciliary muscles, drainage of aqueous humour, and reduced IOP. Ciliary muscle contraction promotes aqueous humour drainage by widening the space where the drainage occurs. Miosis promotes aqueous humour drainage by causing the iris to stretch, which also serves to widen this space.

Both direct- and indirect-acting miotics have effects similar to those of acetylcholine, but their actions are more prolonged (Figure 57-8). The direct-acting miotics are able to directly stimulate ocular cholinergic receptors and mimic acetylcholine. Indirect-acting miotics work by binding to and inactivating the cholinesterases acetylcholinesterase and pseudocholinesterase, the enzymes that break down acetylcholine. As a result, acetylcholine accumulates and acts longer at cholinergic receptor sites. This action leads to drug effects that include miosis, ciliary muscle contraction, enhanced aqueous humour drainage, and reduced IOP by an average of 20 to 30% (Figure 57-9). Drug-induced miotic effects may be less pronounced in individuals with dark eyes (e.g., brown or hazel) than in those with lighter eyes (e.g., blue or green). This difference occurs because the pigment of the iris also absorbs the drug (which reduces its therapeutic effects), and dark eyes have more pigment.

Indications

The direct- and indirect-acting miotics are used for open-angle glaucoma, closed-angle glaucoma, and convergent strabismus ("cross-eye"; a condition in which one eye points toward the other) and in ocular surgery. They are also used to reverse the effect of mydriatic (pupil-dilating) drugs following ophthalmic examination. Specific indications may vary for different drugs, as shown in Table 57-3.

TABLE 57-2

Antiglaucoma Eye Drop Drug Effects on Aqueous Humour

Drug Class	Increased Drainage	Decreased Production
MIOTICS		
Direct-acting cholinergics	+++	0
Indirect-acting cholinergics (cholinesterase inhibitors)	+++	0
MYDRIATICS		
Sympathomimetics	++	+++
OTHERS		
β-Blockers	+	+++
Carbonic anhydrase inhibitors	0	+++
Osmotic diuretics	+++	0
Prostaglandin agonists	+++	0

TABLE 57-3

Miotics: Indications

Miotic Drug	Indications
acetylcholine	Need for complete and rapid miosis after cataract lens extraction, iridectomy
carbachol	Open-angle glaucoma
pilocarpine	Open-angle glaucoma, secondary glaucoma after iridectomy, cycloplegic reversal

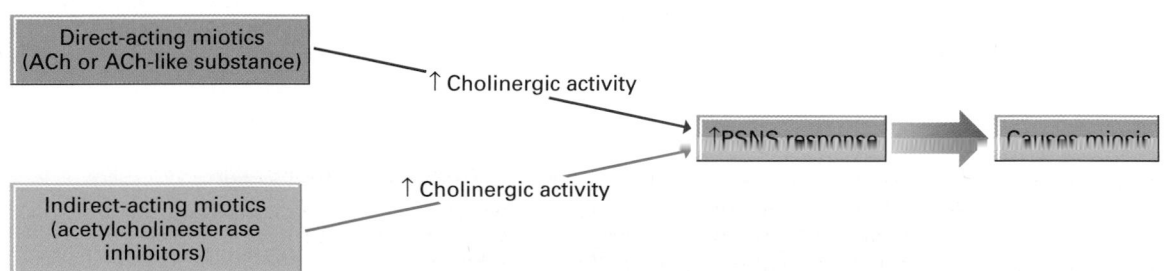

FIG. 57-8 Cholinergic response of miosis to parasympathomimetics. *ACh*, acetylcholine; *PSNS*, parasympathetic nervous system.

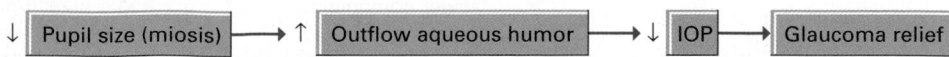

FIG. 57-9 The therapeutic effects of direct- and indirect-acting parasympathomimetics on glaucoma. *IOP*, intraocular pressure.

Contraindications

Contraindications to the use of miotics include known drug allergy and any serious active eye disorder in which induction of miosis might be harmful.

Adverse Effects

Most of the adverse effects associated with the use of cholinergics and cholinesterase inhibitors (miotics) are local and limited to the eye. Adverse effects are more likely to occur with indirect-acting miotics because they have longer-lasting effects. These effects include blurred vision, drug-induced myopia (nearsightedness), and accommodative spasms. Such effects are secondary to contraction of the ciliary muscle. Miotic drugs also cause vasodilation of blood vessels supplying the conjunctiva, iris, and ciliary body, which may lead to vascular congestion and ocular inflammation. Other undesirable effects include temporary stinging upon drug instillation, reduced nighttime or low-light vision, conjunctivitis, lacrimation (tearing), twitching of the eyelids (blepharospasm), and eye or brow pain. Systemic effects are uncommon with miotic drugs but are also more likely to occur with indirect-acting miotics (cholinesterase inhib-

itors). See Chapters 21 and 22 for more information on the systemic effects of these drugs.

Interactions

Drug interactions are unlikely with miotics because of the local actions of these drugs. When miotic drugs are given with topical adrenergics, antiadrenergics (e.g., β-blockers), or carbonic anhydrase inhibitors, additive lowering effects on IOP can be seen. Systemic cholinergic drugs can theoretically have additive cholinergic effects when given with miotics. Indirect-acting miotics may also potentiate the effects of the neuromuscular blocker succinylcholine (see Chapter 12).

Dosages

For recommended dosages of selected miotic drugs, refer to the table on p. 1064.

SYMPATHOMIMETICS (MYDRIATICS)

Sympathomimetic drugs are used for the treatment of glaucoma and ocular hypertension. These drugs include the α-receptor agonists brimonidine (Alphagan P®,

---

 DRUG PROFILES

DIRECT-ACTING MIOTICS

Direct-acting ophthalmic cholinergics include acetylcholine chloride (Miochol E®), carbachol (Miostat®), and pilocarpine (Akarpine®, Diocarpine®, Isopto Carpine®, Minims®). Indirect-acting drugs, which are also called *cholinesterase inhibitors*, are not available in Canada.

acetylcholine chloride

Acetylcholine chloride (Miochol E) is a direct-acting cholinergic drug that is used to produce miosis during ophthalmic surgery. It is a pharmaceutical form of the naturally occurring neurotransmitter in the body. It has a rapid onset and may begin to work almost immediately. It is administered directly into the anterior chamber of the eye before and after securing one or more sutures.

PHARMACOKINETICS

Route	Onset of Action	Peak Plasma Concentration	Elimination Half-Life	Duration of Action
Ocular	Instant (seconds)	Instant	3 min	10 min

▶▶*pilocarpine hydrochloride*

Pilocarpine hydrochloride (Akarpine, Diocarpine, Isopto Carpine, Minims) is a direct-acting cholinergic drug that is used as a miotic in the treatment of glaucoma. Pilocarpine is available in different strengths as an ophthalmic gel or solution.

PHARMACOKINETICS (IMMEDIATE-RELEASE FORMULATION)

Route	Onset of Action	Peak Plasma Concentration	Elimination Half-Life	Duration of Action
Ocular	10–30 min	75 min	Unknown	4–8 hr

DOSAGES	Selected Miotics		
Drug	**Pharmacological Class**	**Usual Dosage Range**	**Indications**
acetylcholine chloride (Miochol E)	Direct-acting cholinergic	0.5–2 mL preoperatively	Need for surgical miosis
▶▶pilocarpine hydrochloride (Akarpine, Diocarpine, Isopto Carpine, Minims)	Direct-acting cholinergic	Solution: 1–2 drops tid–qid Gel: 0.5 inch ribbon into lower conjunctival sac at bedtime (use any other eye drops at least 5 min before gel)	Chronic open-angle and closed-angle glaucoma; acute closed-angle glaucoma; preoperative and postoperative intraocular hypertension; need for reversal of drug-induced mydriasis

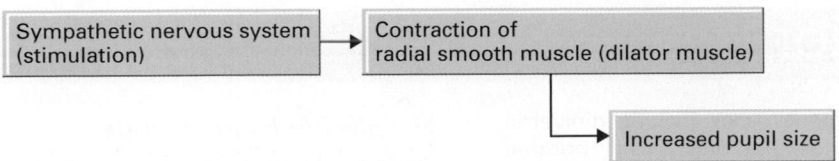

FIG. 57-10 Mechanism of mydriasis.

Combigan®, Onrel Tea®) and apraclonidine (Iopidine®), and the α- and β-receptor agonist dipivefrin.

Mechanism of Action and Drug Effects

Sympathomimetic drugs mimic the sympathetic neurotransmitters norepinephrine and epinephrine. They stimulate the dilator muscle to contract by means of α- or β-receptor interaction. This stimulation results in increased pupil size or *mydriasis* (Figure 57-10). Dilation is seen within minutes of instillation of the ophthalmic drops and lasts for several hours, during which time the IOP is reduced (Figure 57-11). α-Receptor stimulation reduces IOP by enhancing aqueous humour outflow through the canal of Schlemm. Production of aqueous humour by the ciliary body is also reduced. Both of these effects appear to be dose dependent.

Indications

Dipivefrin is used to reduce elevated IOP in the treatment of chronic, open-angle glaucoma, either as initial therapy or as long-term therapy. Increases in IOP during ophthalmic surgery are usually mediated via increased catecholamine stimulation of the sympathetic nervous system. Apraclonidine stimulates the α₂-receptors, which oppose these effects, and thus corrects the surgery-induced elevation in IOP. Brimonidine also has primarily α₂ activity but is used to lower IOP in patients with open-angle glaucoma or ocular hypertension.

Contraindications

Contraindications for the sympathomimetic ophthalmic drugs include known drug allergy.

Adverse Effects

Adverse effects of the sympathomimetic mydriatics are primarily limited to ocular effects and include burning, eye pain, and lacrimation. Such effects are usually temporary and may subside as the patient grows accustomed to the medication. Other ocular effects may include conjunctival hyperemia, localized melanin deposits in the conjunctiva, and release of pigment granules from the iris. Although systemic effects associated with the use of sympathomimetic mydriatics are uncommon, they are theoretically possible, especially with the use of larger doses or prolonged drug therapy. They include cardiovascular effects such as extrasystoles, tachycardia, and hypertension. Other effects that patients may experience are headache and presyncope.

Interactions

With sufficient topical absorption, sympathomimetic mydriatics have the potential to react with other drugs. Cardiac dysrhythmias are potentiated when mydriatic drugs are given with halogenated anaesthetics, cardiac glycosides, thyroid hormones, or tricyclic antidepressants. MAOIs are contraindicated with the use of apraclonidine.

Dosages

For dosage information on sympathomimetic drugs, refer to the table on p. 1066.

β-ADRENERGIC BLOCKERS

The antiglaucoma β-adrenergic blockers that reduce IOP include the β₁-selective blocker betaxolol, and nonselective β₁- and β₂-blockers levobunolol hydrochloride and timolol.

Mechanism of Action and Drug Effects

The ophthalmic β-blockers reduce both elevated and normal IOP. They do so by reducing aqueous humour formation. In addition, timolol may produce a minimal increase in aqueous outflow.

Indications

Ophthalmic β-blockers are used to reduce elevated IOP in various conditions, including chronic open-angle glaucoma and ocular hypertension. They may also be used alone or in combination with a topical miotic (e.g., pilocarpine), topical dipivefrin, or systemic carbonic anhydrase inhibitors. When used in combination, these drugs may have an additive intraocular

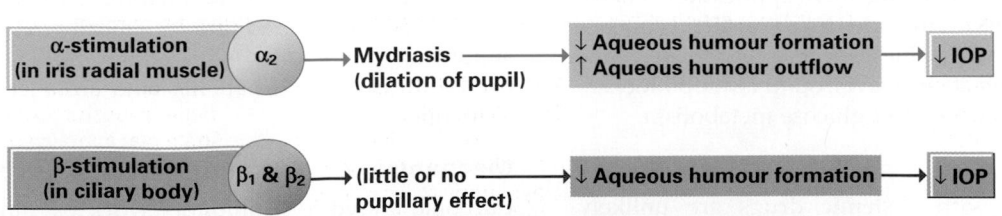

FIG. 57-11 Ocular effects of α- and β-stimulation. *IOP,* intraocular pressure.

DRUG PROFILES

Sympathomimetic ophthalmic drugs include dipivefrin, apraclonidine hydrochloride (Iopidine), and brimonidine tartrate (Alphagan, Alphagan P). These drugs are used for glaucoma, ocular hypertension, and ocular surgery.

apraclonidine hydrochloride

Apraclonidine hydrochloride (Iopidine) is structurally and pharmacologically related to the α_2-stimulant clonidine. It reduces IOP 23 to 39% by stimulating α_2- and β_2-receptors. It also prevents ocular vasoconstriction, which reduces ocular blood pressure as well as aqueous humour formation. Apraclonidine is used primarily to inhibit perioperative IOP increases, rather than to treat glaucoma. Brimonidine (Alphagan, Alphagan P) is a similar drug but is used primarily for glaucoma.

PHARMACOKINETICS (APRACLONIDINE)

Route	Onset of Action	Peak Plasma Concentration	Elimination Half-Life	Duration of Action
Ocular	1 hr	3–5 hr	8 hr	12 hr

▶▶ dipivefrin hydrochloride

Dipivefrin hydrochloride is a synthetic sympathomimetic miotic drug. It is a prodrug of epinephrine that has little or no pharmacological activity until hydrolyzed in the eye to two chemically modified forms of epinephrine. These chemical alterations account for the main advantage of this drug over epinephrine: it has enhanced lipophilicity (fat solubility) and can better penetrate into the tissues of the anterior chamber of the eye. This lipophilic quality also reduces the likelihood of any systemic adverse effects. Dipivefrin typically reduces mean IOP approximately 15 to 25%. On the basis of weight, dipivefrin is 4 to 11 times as potent as epinephrine in reducing IOP and 5 to 12 times as potent as epinephrine in terms of its mydriatic effects. Epinephrine eye drops are no longer used because there are newer drugs with better adverse effect profiles.

PHARMACOKINETICS

Route	Onset of Action	Peak Plasma Concentration	Elimination Half-Life	Duration of Action
Ocular	30 min	1 hr	1–3 hr	12 hr

DOSAGES Selected Ophthalmic Sympathomimetics

Drug	Pharmacological Class	Usual Dosage Range	Indications
apraclonidine hydrochloride (Iopidine)	Direct-acting	0.5% solution: 1–2 drops tid	Short-term adjunctive therapy for glaucoma not controlled by other drugs
▶▶ dipivefrin hydrochloride	Direct-acting	1 drop q12h	Chronic open-angle glaucoma

pressure–lowering effect. They may also be used to treat some forms of closed-angle glaucoma.

Contraindications

Contraindications for ophthalmic β-blockers include known drug allergy and any ocular condition in which β-receptor blockade might be harmful.

Adverse Effects

The adverse effects of antiglaucoma β-blockers are primarily limited to ocular effects. The most common ocular effects are transient burning and discomfort. Other adverse effects include blurred vision, pain, photophobia, lacrimation, blepharitis, keratitis (inflammation of the cornea), and decreased corneal sensitivity. Because these drugs are administered topically, few, if any, systemic effects are expected following their application. Theoretical systemic effects include bradycardia, bronchospasm, headache, and dizziness, as described for systemic β-blockers in Chapter 20. However, ophthalmic β-blockers have not been shown to affect glucose metabolism.

Interactions

Drug interactions with systemic drugs are unlikely because of the primarily localized nature of ophthalmically administered drugs. Theoretically, ophthalmic

β-blockers can have additive therapeutic or adverse effects when given with systemically administered β-blockers or other cardiovascular drugs (e.g., calcium channel blockers).

Dosages

For dosage information on β-adrenergic blockers, refer to the table on p. 1067.

CARBONIC ANHYDRASE INHIBITORS

Ophthalmic carbonic anhydrase inhibitors include brinzolamide (Azarga®, Azopt®) and dorzolamide (Cosopt®, Trusopt®). These two drugs are available only in topical ophthalmic form. Systemic carbonic anhydrase inhibitors are sometimes used as adjunct drug therapy for glaucoma and are described in Chapter 29. Both drugs are also sulfonamides and are chemically related to the sulfonamide antibiotics (see Chapter 43). They are to be used with caution in patients who are allergic to sulfa antibiotics.

Mechanism of Action and Drug Effects

Carbonic anhydrase inhibitors work by inhibiting the enzyme carbonic anhydrase, which results in decreased IOP by reduction of aqueous humour formation.

DRUG PROFILES

The currently available ophthalmic β-blocking drugs are betaxolol hydrochloride (Betoptic®), levobunolol hydrochloride (Betagan®), and timolol maleate (Timoptic®). These drugs are used for glaucoma and ocular hypertension.

▶▶ betaxolol hydrochloride

Betaxolol hydrochloride (Betoptic) is a β_1-selective β-blocker. It is one of the most potent and selective β-blocking drugs. Its ability to decrease aqueous humour formation and reduce IOP has made it an excellent drug for the treatment of ocular disorders such as open-angle glaucoma and ocular hypertension.

PHARMACOKINETICS

Route	Onset of Action	Peak Plasma Concentration	Elimination Half-Life	Duration of Action
Ocular	0.5–1 hr	2 hr	Unknown	More than 12 hr

▶▶ timolol maleate

Timolol maleate (Timoptic) differs slightly from the other ophthalmic β-blockers in that it may increase the outflow of aqueous humour as well as decrease its formation. The drug acts at both β_1- and β_2-receptors and is indicated for the treatment of open-angle glaucoma and ocular hypertension. It is available in various liquid forms, both with and without preservatives. Preservative-free products were developed for patients with allergies to benzalkonium chloride, a commonly used preservative. Timolol is also available in a gel-forming solution (with preservatives). These gel-forming products are longer acting and allow for once-daily dosing, a convenience over the twice-daily dosing that many patients require with the other timolol formulations.

PHARMACOKINETICS

Route	Onset of Action	Peak Plasma Concentration	Elimination Half-Life	Duration of Action
Ocular	15–30 min	1–2 hr	Unknown	12–24 hr

DOSAGES   Selected Ophthalmic β-Blockers

Drug	Pharmacological Class	Usual Dosage Range	Indications
▶▶betaxolol hydrochloride (Betoptic)	Direct-acting	1–2 drops bid	Chronic open-angle glaucoma; ocular hypertension
▶▶timolol maleate (Betimol®, Timoptic, Tim-AK®)	Direct-acting	Solution: 1 drop bid Gel-forming solution: 1 drop daily	Open-angle glaucoma; ocular hypertension

Indications

Ophthalmic carbonic anhydrase inhibitors are used primarily for the management of glaucoma, including both open-angle and closed-angle glaucoma; they may also be used preoperatively to control IOP.

Contraindications

Contraindications to the use of carbonic anhydrase inhibitors include known drug allergy and any ocular condition with which their use might be considered harmful in the judgement of an ophthalmologist. Allergy to sulfonamide antibiotics is a precaution, not a contraindication; however, patients need to be educated regarding the possibility of cross-reaction.

Adverse Effects

Systemic absorption of these drugs does occur (e.g., causing a bitter taste in 25%), although systemic adverse effects are rare. The same adverse effects listed for sulfonamide antibiotics in Chapter 43 can theoretically occur with these drugs. Patients with allergies to sulfonamides may develop cross-sensitivities to the carbonic anhydrase inhibitors.

Interactions

The systemic use of carbonic anhydrase inhibitors can result in several significant drug interactions, and the ophthalmic carbonic anhydrase inhibitors have a theoretical (but less likely) potential for these interactions. See Chapter 29 for information on systemic drug interactions.

Dosages

For dosage information on the carbonic anhydrase inhibitor dorzolamide, refer to the table on p. 1068.

OSMOTIC DIURETICS

Osmotic diuretic drugs may be administered intravenously, orally, or topically to reduce IOP. The osmotic diuretics that are most commonly used for this purpose are glycerin and mannitol.

Mechanism of Action and Drug Effects

Osmotic diuretics reduce ocular hypertension by causing the blood to become hypertonic in relation to both intraocular and spinal fluids. This creates an osmotic gradient that draws water from the aqueous and vitreous humours into the bloodstream, which causes a reduction in volume of intraocular fluid; the result is a decrease in IOP (Figure 57-12). Systemic (nonocular) effects of these drugs are discussed in Chapter 29.

DRUG PROFILE

There are currently two ophthalmic carbonic anhydrase inhibitors: brinzolamide (Azopt) and dorzolamide (Cosopt, Trusopt). Brinzolamide is available in combination with timolol (Azarga).

▸▸*dorzolamide*

Dorzolamide (Trusopt) is indicated for the treatment of elevated IOP associated with either ocular hypertension or open-angle glaucoma. Dorzolamide is available in com-

bination with timolol (Cosopt). It is available only as an ophthalmic solution. The other drug in this class, brinzolamide, has comparable indications, dosages, and pharmacokinetics.

PHARMACOKINETICS

Route	Onset of Action	Peak Plasma Concentration	Elimination Half-Life	Duration of Action
Ocular	Rapid	Variable	3–4 mo	Variable

DOSAGES Ophthalmic Carbonic Anhydrase Inhibitors

Drug	Pharmacological Class	Usual Dosage Range	Indications
▸▸dorzolamide (Trusopt)	Carbonic anhydrase inhibitor	1 drop tid	Open-angle glaucoma; ocular hypertension

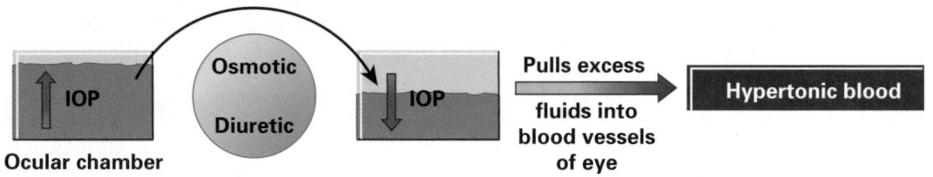

FIG. 57-12 Mechanism and ocular effects of osmotic diuretics. *IOP*, intraocular pressure.

Indications

Ocular uses for osmotic diuretics include treatment of acute glaucoma episodes and reduction of IOP before or after ocular surgery. Typically, glycerin is used first; if the treatment is unsuccessful, mannitol is tried.

Contraindications

Osmotic diuretics are contraindicated in patients with known drug allergy, significant anuria, acute pulmonary edema, cardiac decompensation, or severe dehydration, because they can worsen all of these conditions.

Adverse Effects

The most frequent adverse effects to osmotic diuretics are nausea, vomiting, and headache. The most significant adverse effects are fluid and electrolyte imbalances. Other effects are possible irritation and thrombosis at the injection site. Other potential adverse effects are listed in Table 57-4.

Interactions

The only significant drug interaction associated with osmotic diuretics is increased lithium excretion associated with mannitol.

Dosages

For dosage information on mannitol, refer to the table on p. 1069.

TABLE 57-4

Osmotic Diuretics (Mannitol): Adverse Effects

Body System	Adverse Effects
Cardiovascular	Edema, thrombophlebitis, hypotension, hypertension, tachycardia, angina-like chest pains, fever, chills
Central nervous	Dizziness, headache, convulsions, rebound increased intracranial pressure, confusion
Electrolytes	Fluid and electrolyte imbalances, acidosis, dehydration
Eyes, ears, nose, throat	Loss of hearing, blurred vision, nasal congestion
Gastrointestinal	Nausea, vomiting, dry mouth, diarrhea
Genitourinary	Marked diuresis, urinary retention, thirst

PROSTAGLANDIN AGONISTS

The newest class of drugs used to treat glaucoma is the prostaglandin agonists. There are currently three drugs in this class: latanoprost (Xalacom®, Xalatan®), travoprost (Travatan Z®), and bimatoprost (Lumigan®).

DRUG PROFILES

Osmotic diuretics include mannitol and glycerin. Mannitol is normally reserved for acute reduction of IOP during glaucoma crises and preoperative reduction of IOP in ophthalmic surgery. Glycerin is a component of OTC eye drops used to moisturize dry and irritated eyes.

mannitol

Mannitol (Osmitrol®) is used only by intravenous infusion to reduce elevated IOP when the pressure cannot be lowered by other treatments. Mannitol is effective in treating acute episodes of closed-angle, absolute, or secondary glaucoma and in lowering IOP before intraocular surgery. Mannitol does not penetrate the eye and may be used when irritation is present.

PHARMACOKINETICS

Route	Onset of Action	Peak Plasma Concentration	Elimination Half-Life	Duration of Action
IV	30–60 min	1 hr	15–100 min	6–8 hr

DOSAGES   Selected Osmotic Diuretics

Drug	Pharmacological Class	Usual Dosage Range	Indications
mannitol (Osmitrol)	Organic alcohol	IV: 1.5–2 g/kg infused over at least 30 min; for preoperative use give 1–1.5 hr before surgery	Acute reduction of elevated intraocular pressure

Mechanism of Action and Drug Effects

Prostaglandins reduce IOP by increasing the outflow of aqueous fluid between the uvea and sclera as well as via the usual exit through the trabecular meshwork (see Figure 57-7). A single dose of a prostaglandin agonist lowers IOP for 20 to 24 hours, which allows a regimen involving only a single daily dosage. Drug effects are primarily limited to these ocular effects.

Indications

Prostaglandin agonists are used in the treatment of glaucoma.

Contraindications

The only usual contraindication to the use of prostaglandin agonists is known drug allergy.

Adverse Effects

Prostaglandin agonists are generally well tolerated. Adverse effects include the sensation of a foreign body in the eye, punctate epithelial keratopathy (dotted appearance of cornea), stinging, conjunctival hyperemia ("bloodshot" eyes), blurred vision, itching, and burning. Systemic effects occur in a small percentage of patients and include skin reactions, upper respiratory infections, and headache. There is one unique adverse effect associated with all prostaglandin agonists: in some people with hazel, green, or bluish-brown eye colour, prostaglandin agonists will cause their eye colour to turn permanently brown, even if the medication is discontinued; as well, they can cause thickening, darkening, and lengthening of eyelashes. This adverse effect appears to be cosmetic only, with no known ill effects on the eye.

Interactions

Concurrent administration of prostaglandin agonists with any other eye drops containing the preservative thimerosal may result in precipitation. It is recommended that such medications be administered at least 5 minutes apart.

Dosages

For dosage information on the prostaglandin agonist latanoprost, refer to the table on p. 1070.

ANTIMICROBIAL DRUGS

A variety of infections can occur in the eye; many are self-limiting. However, some infections require the use of

DRUG PROFILE

▶▶latanoprost

Latanoprost is a prodrug of a naturally occurring prostaglandin known as *prostaglandin F$_{2\alpha}$*. When it is administered, it is converted by hydrolysis (with water from ocular fluids) to prostaglandin F$_{2\alpha}$, which in turn reduces IOP. Latanoprost is available only in eye drop form. About 3 to 10% of patients treated with latanoprost (Xalacom, Xalatan) have shown increased iris pigmentation after 3 to 4.5 months of treatment.

PHARMACOKINETICS

Route	Onset of Action	Peak Plasma Concentration	Elimination Half-Life	Duration of Action
Ocular	30–60 min	2 hr	17 min	24 hr

DOSAGES	Selected Prostaglandin Analogues		
Drug	**Pharmacological Class**	**Usual Dosage Range**	**Indications**
▶latanoprost (Xalacom, Xalatan)	Prostaglandin	1 drop every day in the evening	Open-angle glaucoma and ocular hypertension in patients who are intolerant of or whose condition is uncontrolled by other drugs

TABLE	57-5

Common Ocular Infections

Infection	Description
Blepharitis	Inflammation of the eyelids.
Conjunctivitis	Inflammation of the conjunctiva (the mucous membrane lining the back of the eyelids and the front of the eye except the cornea); it may be bacterial or viral and is often associated with common colds. When caused by *Haemophilus* organisms, it is commonly called *pink eye*; it is highly contagious but usually self-limiting.
Hordeolum (sty)	Acute localized infection of the eyelash follicles and the glands of the anterior lid; it results in the formation of a small abscess or cyst.
Keratitis	Inflammation of the cornea caused by bacterial infection; herpes simplex keratitis is caused by viral infection.
Uveitis	Infection of the uveal tract or the vascular layer of the eye, which includes the iris, ciliary body, and choroid.
Endophthalmitis	Inflammation of the inner eye structure caused by bacteria.

ophthalmic antimicrobials to be eliminated. Topical antimicrobials used to treat ocular infections include antibacterial, antifungal, and antiviral drugs. All require a prescription. Many of these drugs are also available for systemic administration for treatment of infections elsewhere in the body. The most commonly used antimicrobials from the main antimicrobial drug classes are discussed in this chapter. Some common eye infections may require antibiotic therapy and are listed in Table 57-5. The choice of a particular ophthalmic antimicrobial drug should be based on the following:

• Clinical experience
• Sensitivity and characteristics of the organisms most likely to cause the infection
• Characteristics of the infection
• Sensitivity and response of the patient
• Laboratory results (cultures and sensitivities)

Mechanism of Action and Drug Effects

Topical antimicrobials used to treat infections of the eye work to destroy the invading organism. Their specific antimicrobial actions are similar to those described for systemically administered drugs, which are discussed in Chapters 43, 44, 45, and 47. The effects of the drugs used to treat ocular infections are focused on the microorganism invading the eye. Some antimicrobials destroy the causative organism, whereas others simply inhibit the organism's growth, allowing the body's immune system to fight the infection.

Indications

The indication for ophthalmic antimicrobials is known or suspected infection with one or more specific micro-

organisms. Empirical treatment is based on reasonable clinical evaluation of presenting signs and symptoms. Topical use of antimicrobials helps prevent antimicrobial drug resistance that could arise from unnecessary systemic use. However, systemic antimicrobials may be administered to treat more severe ocular infections.

Contraindications

Contraindications to the use of antimicrobials include known drug allergy or a prior severe adverse drug reaction.

Adverse Effects

The most common adverse effects of ophthalmic antibiotics are local and transient inflammation, burning, stinging, urticaria, dermatitis, angioedema, and drug hypersensitivity. Topical application of antimicrobial drugs may also interfere with the growth of the normal bacterial flora of the eye, which may encourage the growth of other, more harmful organisms. If large doses are given, systemic adverse effects are possible.

Interactions

Systemic drug interactions with ophthalmic antimicrobials are unlikely because of their primarily local effects. One possible interaction involves the concurrent use of corticosteroids (e.g., dexamethasone). Corticosteroids have immunosuppressive effects that may impede the therapeutic effects of ophthalmic antimicrobials.

Dosages

For dosage information on ophthalmic antimicrobials, refer to the table on p. 1072.

DRUG PROFILES

AMINOGLYCOSIDES

Aminoglycosides (see Chapter 44) are antimicrobials that destroy bacteria by interfering with protein synthesis in bacterial cells, which leads to bacterial death. Aminoglycosides used to treat ocular infections include gentamicin (Diogent®) and tobramycin (Tobrex®). Adverse effects include swollen eyelids, mydriasis, and local erythema. Systemic reactions are rare because of poor topical absorption. Overgrowth of nonsusceptible organisms, which can lead to eye infections that are resistant to treatment, is a possibility with the use of aminoglycosides.

▶▶gentamicin sulphate

Gentamicin sulphate (Diogent, Gentak) is effective against a wide variety of gram-negative and gram-positive organisms. It is particularly useful against *Pseudomonas*, *Proteus*, and *Klebsiella* organisms. Gram-positive organisms that are effectively destroyed by gentamicin include staphylococci and streptococci that have developed resistance to other antibiotics. Gentamicin is available as an ophthalmic ointment and a solution.

PHARMACOKINETICS

Route	Onset of Action	Peak Plasma Concentration	Elimination Half-Life	Duration of Action
Ocular	Variable	Immediate	Unknown	6–12 hr

MACROLIDE ANTIBIOTICS

Macrolide antibiotics include erythromycin, azithromycin, and other drugs (see Chapter 43). Erythromycin is currently the only macrolide available for ophthalmic use.

▶▶erythromycin

Erythromycin is a macrolide antibiotic indicated for the treatment of various ophthalmic infections. Erythromycin eye ointment is indicated for the treatment of neonatal conjunctivitis caused by *Chlamydia trachomatis* and for the prevention of eye infections in newborns that may be caused by *Neisseria gonorrhoeae* or other susceptible organisms.

PHARMACOKINETICS

Route	Onset of Action	Peak Plasma Concentration	Elimination Half-Life	Duration of Action
Ocular	Variable	Immediate	Unknown	Variable

POLYPEPTIDE ANTIBIOTICS

Bacitracin and polymyxin B are polypeptide antibiotics. These drugs are rarely used systemically because of their potent nephrotoxic effects. They are bactericidal antimicrobials that inhibit protein synthesis in susceptible organisms, which leads to cell death. They are most commonly used in the treatment of surface infections caused by gram-positive bacteria.

▶▶bacitracin

Bacitracin is an ophthalmic antimicrobial drug used to treat various eye infections. It is available as a single-ingredient product and as a combination product with polymyxin. Such combination products have a broader spectrum of activity than the individual drugs on their own. Bacitracin is available in ointment form.

PHARMACOKINETICS

Route	Onset of Action	Peak Plasma Concentration	Elimination Half-Life	Duration of Action
Ocular	Variable	Immediate	Unknown	Variable

QUINOLONES

Quinolone antibiotics are effective broad-spectrum antibiotics. They are discussed in detail in Chapter 44. They are bactericidal, destroying a wide spectrum of organisms that are often difficult to treat. Currently, four ophthalmic quinolones are available: ciprofloxacin (Ciloxan®), gatifloxacin (Zymar®), moxifloxacin hydrochloride (Vigamox®), and ofloxacin (Apo-Ofloxacin®).

Significant adverse effects of ophthalmic quinolones include the formation of corneal precipitates during treatment for bacterial keratitis. Other reactions include corneal staining and corneal infiltrates. Systemic reactions are limited because of poor topical absorption; those that occur are usually taste disorders and nausea. Ophthalmic quinolones have no significant drug interactions with other drugs.

▶▶ciprofloxacin hydrochloride

Ciprofloxacin hydrochloride (Ciloxan) is a synthetic quinolone antibiotic. It is available in ointment and solution forms. Ciprofloxacin is indicated for the treatment of bacterial keratitis and conjunctivitis caused by susceptible gram-positive and gram-negative bacteria. One notable adverse reaction to ophthalmic ciprofloxacin is the appearance of white, crystalline precipitates within any corneal lesions. This has occurred in approximately 17% of patients, within 1 to 7 days of starting therapy. In all cases to date, the condition has been self-limiting, has not required drug discontinuation, and has not adversely affected clinical outcome.

PHARMACOKINETICS

Route	Onset of Action	Peak Plasma Concentration	Elimination Half-Life	Duration of Action
Ocular	Variable	Immediate	1–2 hr	Variable

SULFONAMIDES

Sulfonamides are synthetic bacteriostatic antibiotics that work by blocking the synthesis of folic acid in susceptible bacteria. Sulfacetamide sodium (AK-Sulf®) is used to treat conjunctivitis and other ocular infections caused by susceptible bacteria.

The adverse effects of ophthalmic sulfonamides are primarily limited to local reactions and include local irritation and stinging. Sulfonamide use can result in the overgrowth of nonsusceptible organisms. No significant topical toxic effects have been reported with its use.

Continued

DRUG PROFILES—cont'd

▸▸*sulfacetamide sodium*

Sulfacetamide sodium (AK-Sulf) is the most commonly used ophthalmic sulfonamide antibacterial drug. It is available in solution and ointment forms. It is also available in a combination with prednisolone acetate (AK-Cide®, Dioptimyd®).

PHARMACOKINETICS

Route	Onset of Action	Peak Plasma Concentration	Elimination Half-Life	Duration of Action
Ocular	Variable	Immediate	Unknown	Variable

ANTIVIRALS

The sole available antiviral ophthalmic drug is trifluridine (Viroptic®).

trifluridine

Trifluridine (Viroptic; 1% ophthalmic drops) is a pyrimidine nucleoside. Trifluridine inhibits viral replication by blocking the synthesis of viral deoxyribonucleic acid (DNA) by inhibiting viral DNA polymerase, an enzyme required for DNA synthesis. It is used for ocular infections (keratitis and keratoconjunctivitis) caused by types 1 and 2 of the herpes simplex virus. Significant adverse effects include secondary glaucoma, corneal punctate defects, uveitis, and stromal edema (edema in the tough, fibrous, transparent portion of the cornea known as the *stroma*). The drug exhibits no appreciable topical absorption, and no significant drug interactions have been reported.

DOSAGES   Selected Ophthalmic Antimicrobials

Drug	Pharmacological Class	Usual Dosage Range	Indications
Antibacterial Drugs			
▸▸bacitracin (AK-Tracin®)	Miscellaneous antibiotic	Solution: 1–2 drops every 1–4 hr	
▸▸ciprofloxacin (Ciloxan)	Quinolone	Solution: 1–2 drops every 2 hr for 2 days, and then 2 drops every 4 hr for 5 days Ointment: 12 mm ribbon tid for 2 days, then 12 mm ribbon daily for 5 days	Bacterial ocular infections
▸▸erythromycin (AK-Mycin®)	Macrolide	Ointment: 13 mm ribbon 2–6 times/day	
▸▸gentamicin (Diogent, Gentak)	Aminoglycoside	Solution: 1–2 drops every 2–4 hr Ointment: 13 mm ribbon 2–3 times/day	
▸▸sulfacetamide (AK-Sulf, Diosulf®)	Sulfonamide	Solution: 1–2 drops every 2–3 hr	
Antiviral Drug			
trifluridine (Viroptic)	Antiviral	Initially 1 drop every 2 hr while awake (max 9 drops/day); may later decrease to 5 drops/day	Viral ocular infections: keratitis, keratoconjunctivitis due to HSV types 1 and 2

HSV, herpes simplex virus.
Note: Dosages vary based on the type and severity of infection.

ANTI-INFLAMMATORY DRUGS

Many of the same anti-inflammatory drugs used systemically may also be used ophthalmically to treat ocular inflammatory disorders and ocular surgery–related pain and inflammation. These drugs include both nonsteroidal anti-inflammatory drugs (NSAIDs) and corticosteroids and are listed in Box 57-1.

Mechanism of Action and Drug Effects

Corticosteroids and NSAIDs, as discussed in Chapters 34 and 49, respectively, act to reduce inflammatory responses. When tissues are damaged, the membranes of affected cells release phospholipids, which are broken down by several different enzymes within the arachidonic acid metabolic pathway. Phospholipase is one of the first enzymes involved, and its activity is inhibited by corticosteroids. A second enzyme, cyclo-oxygenase, is the site of action of the NSAIDs (see Chapter 49); its inhibition reduces the pain, erythema, and other manifestations associated with inflammation.

Indications

Corticosteroids and NSAIDs are applied topically for the symptomatic relief of many ophthalmic inflammatory conditions. They may be used to treat corneal, conjunctival, and scleral injuries from chemical, radiation, or thermal burns or from the penetration of foreign bodies. They are used during the acute phase of the injury process to prevent fibrosis and scarring that results in visual impairment. Corticosteroids produce a greater immunosuppressant effect than the NSAIDs. Consequently, NSAIDs are often preferred as initial topical therapy for such injuries. NSAIDs are also used in the symptomatic treatment of seasonal allergic conjunctivitis.

Corticosteroids and NSAIDs are used prophylactically before ocular surgery to prevent or reduce intraoperative miosis. They are also used prophylactically after ocular surgeries, such as cataract extraction, glaucoma surgery, and corneal transplantation, to prevent inflammation and scarring.

Contraindications

Corticosteroids and NSAIDs are contraindicated in cases of known drug allergy. In addition, they are not to be used for minor abrasions or wounds because they may suppress the ability of the eye to resist bacterial, viral, or fungal infections. This is especially true of corticosteroids, which have stronger immunosuppressant effects than NSAIDs.

Adverse Effects

The most common adverse effect of corticosteroids is transient burning or stinging on application. The extended use of corticosteroids may result in cataracts, increased IOP, and optic nerve damage. If large doses are given, systemic absorption is possible. Systemic adverse effects of corticosteroids and NSAIDs are discussed in Chapters 34 and 49.

TOPICAL ANAESTHETICS

Topical anaesthetic ophthalmic drugs are local anaesthetics that are used to alleviate eye pain. The currently available topical anaesthetic used for ophthalmic purposes is tetracaine. Benoxinate hydrochloride is another topical anaesthetic available only in combination with fluorescein sodium (see later).

Mechanism of Action and Drug Effects

As described in Chapter 12, local anaesthetics stabilize the membranes of nerves, which results in a decrease in

---

BOX 57-1

Ophthalmic Anti-Inflammatory Drugs

NSAIDs	Corticosteroids
diclofenac sodium (Voltaren Ophtha®)	dexamethasone (AK-Dex®, Diodex, Dioptrol®, Maxidex)
flurbiprofen sodium (Ocufen®)	fluorometholone (Flarex®, FML®)
ketorolac tromethamine (Acular®)	loteprenol etabonate (Alrex®, Lotemax®)
	prednisolone acetate (Diopred®)
	rimexolone (Vexol®)

DRUG PROFILES

Corticosteroids and NSAIDs used to treat ophthalmic inflammatory disorders are listed in Box 57-1. The ophthalmic formulations of these drugs share many of the characteristics of their systemic drug counterparts. However, the ophthalmic derivatives have limited systemic absorption; therefore, the majority of their therapeutic and toxic effects are restricted to the eye. Potential benefits of the use of corticosteroids and NSAIDs during pregnancy may outweigh the possible risk to the fetus.

CORTICOSTEROID

▶▶*dexamethasone*

Dexamethasone (AK-Dex, Diodex, Dioptrol) is a synthetic corticosteroid that is available in many ophthalmic formulations. It is used to treat inflammation of the eye, eyelids, conjunctiva, and cornea, and it may also be used in the treatment of uveitis, iridocyclitis, allergic conditions, and burns, as well as in the removal of foreign bodies. Dexamethasone is available in ointment, suspension, and solution forms.

PHARMACOKINETICS

Route	Onset of Action	Peak Plasma Concentration	Elimination Half-Life	Duration of Action
Ocular	Variable	Immediate	Unknown	Variable

ketorolac tromethamine

Ketorolac tromethamine (Acular) is an NSAID used to reduce ocular inflammation caused by trauma, such as ocular surgery, as well as inflammation secondary to external agents, such as allergens and bacteria. Ketorolac is contraindicated in patients with known drug allergy. It is available in solution form. Ketorolac may delay eye wound healing and lead to corneal epithelial breakdown; therefore, consistently monitor the eye through the duration of therapy.

PHARMACOKINETICS

Route	Onset of Action	Peak Plasma Concentration	Elimination Half-Life	Duration of Action
Ocular	Rapid	Immediate	Unknown	4–6 hr

the movement of ions into and out of the nerve endings. When nerves are stabilized in this way, they cannot transmit signals about painful stimuli to the brain. Usually, the application of topical anaesthetic drugs to the eye results in local anaesthesia in less than 30 seconds.

Indications

Ophthalmic anaesthetic drugs are used to produce anaesthesia for short corneal and conjunctival procedures. They prevent pain during surgical procedures and certain painful ophthalmic examinations, including removal of embedded foreign objects. They are recommended only for short-term use and are not recommended for self-administration.

Contraindications

Contraindications to local ophthalmic anaesthetics include known drug allergy.

Adverse Effects

Adverse effects are rare with ophthalmic anaesthetic drugs and are limited to local effects such as stinging, burning, redness, lacrimation, and blurred vision. Systemic toxicity is rare but can theoretically lead to central nervous system (CNS) stimulation or CNS or cardiovascular depression.

Interactions

Because of their limited systemic absorption and short duration of action, ophthalmic anaesthetic drugs have no significant drug interactions.

 DRUG PROFILES

There is currently one drug available for this purpose: tetracaine hydrochloride (Minims®).

tetracaine hydrochloride

Tetracaine hydrochloride is a local anaesthetic of the ester type (see Chapter 12). It is applied as an eye drop to numb the eye for various ophthalmic procedures. Tetracaine begins to act in about 25 seconds and lasts for approximately 15 to 20 minutes. Additional drops are applied as needed. It is currently available only in solution form. Potential benefits of use during pregnancy may outweigh the possible risk to the fetus.

PHARMACOKINETICS

Route	Onset of Action	Peak Plasma Concentration	Elimination Half-Life	Duration of Action
Ocular	Less than 30 sec	1–5 min	Short	15–20 min

DIAGNOSTIC DRUGS

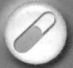 **DRUG PROFILES**

CYCLOPLEGIC MYDRIATICS

▸▸atropine sulphate

Atropine sulphate (Isopto Atropine 1%®, Dioptic's Atropine Solution®) solution is used as a mydriatic and cycloplegic drug. The drug dilates the pupil (mydriasis) and paralyzes the ciliary muscle (cycloplegic refraction), which prevents accommodation. It is used to assist in an eye examination or to treat uveal tract inflammatory states. The usual dose for uveitis (inflammation of the choroid, iris, or ciliary body) in children and adults is one to two drops of the solution 2 to 3 times daily. The dose for an eye examination is one drop of solution, ideally 1 hour before the procedure. Potential benefits of use during pregnancy may outweigh the possible risk to the fetus.

cyclopentolate hydrochloride

Cyclopentolate hydrochloride solution (Cyclogyl®) is used primarily as a diagnostic mydriatic and cycloplegic drug. Unlike atropine, it is not used to treat uveitis. The usual adult dose is one to two drops (0.5% or 1%). This is repeated in 5 to 10 minutes if needed. The dose for children is the same as that for adults. The drug effects usually subside within 24 hours. Other cycloplegic mydriatics are homatropine (Isopto Homatropine®) and tropicamide (Mydriacyl®). Both are topical ophthalmic solutions with indications similar to those of atropine and cyclopentolate, except that tropicamide, like cyclopentolate, is generally used for diagnostic purposes only and not for treatment of inflammatory states. Potential benefits of the use of cyclopegic mydriatics during pregnancy may outweigh the possible risk to the fetus.

OPHTHALMIC DYE

fluorescein sodium

Fluorescein sodium (AK-Fluor®) is an ophthalmic diagnostic dye used to identify corneal defects and to locate foreign objects in the eye. It is also used in fitting hard contact lenses. After the instillation of fluorescein sodium, various defects are highlighted in either bright green or yellow–orange, and foreign objects have a green halo around them. Dose determination and drug administration may be carried out by an ophthalmologist, an optometrist, or a health care provider in family practice. Potential benefits of the use of fluorescein sodium during pregnancy may outweigh the possible risk to the fetus.

ANTIALLERGIC DRUGS

DRUG PROFILES

ANTIHISTAMINES

olopatadine hydrochloride

Olopatadine hydrochloride (Patanol®) is an ophthalmic antihistamine used to treat symptoms of allergic conjunctivitis (hay fever), which can be seasonal or nonseasonal. It works by competing with histamine for receptor sites. Histamine normally produces ocular symptoms such as itching and tearing. Another ophthalmic antihistamine is ketotifen (Zaditor®). These drugs have mechanisms of action, therapeutic and adverse effects, and drug interactions similar to those of the systemic antihistamines described in Chapter 37, although systemic effects are less likely to occur with ophthalmic administration than with systemic administration. Recommended dosages for olopatadine hydrochloride are given in the Dosages table below. Potential benefits of its use during pregnancy may outweigh the possible risk to the fetus.

MAST CELL STABILIZERS

cromolyn sodium

Cromolyn sodium (Opticrom®) is an antiallergic drug that inhibits the release of inflammation-producing mediators from sensitized inflammatory cells called *mast cells*. It is used in the treatment of vernal keratoconjunctivitis (springtime inflammation of the cornea and conjunctiva). Other mast cell stabilizers with similar effects are nedocromil sodium (Alocril®) and lodoxamide (Alomide®). Recommended dosages for cromolyn can be found in the table below. There are no controlled studies in pregnant women that show that these drugs cause a risk to fetuses.

DECONGESTANTS

tetrahydrozoline hydrochloride

Tetrahydrozoline hydrochloride (Allergy Eye Drops®, Visine®) is an ophthalmic decongestant. It works by promoting vasoconstriction of blood vessels in and around the eye. This reduces the edema associated with allergic and inflammatory processes. It is specifically indicated to control redness, burning, and other minor irritations. Other ophthalmic decongestants include phenylephrine hydrochloride, oxymetazoline hydrochloride (Visine Workplace®), and naphazoline (Clear Eyes®). Recommended dosages for tetrahydrozoline are given in the table below. Potential benefits of its use during pregnancy may outweigh the possible risk to the fetus.

LUBRICANTS AND MOISTURIZERS

▸▸artificial tears

An array of products is available over the counter to provide lubrication or moisture for the eyes. These products are helpful to patients with dry or otherwise irritated eyes. Artificial tears are isotonic and contain buffers to adjust pH. In addition, they contain preservatives for microbial control and may contain viscosity agents. Corneal contact time of topical ophthalmic solutions increases with the viscosity of the formulations. Selected OTC brand names include GenTeal®, Isopto Tears®, Murine®, Akwa Tears®, Refresh®, and Tears Plus®. Many similar products are also available on the market, as solutions (eye drops) and as lubrication ointments. They are often dosed to patient comfort as needed. Restasis® is an ophthalmic form of the immunosuppressant drug ciclosporin (see Chapter 50). It is also used to promote tear production in those with the condition technically known as *keratoconjunctivitis sicca* (dry eyes). It can be used together with artificial tears if the drugs are given 15 minutes apart. There are no controlled studies in pregnant women that show that this drug causes a risk to fetusus.

DOSAGES	Ophthalmic Antiallergics		
Drug	Pharmacological Class	Usual Dosage Range	Indications
cromolyn sodium (Opticrom)	Mast cell stabilizer	1–2 drops in affected eye(s) 4–6 times daily	Vernal (springtime) conjunctivitis and keratitis (corneal inflammation)
olopatadine (Patanol 0.1%) (C)	Antihistamine	1–2 drops in affected eye(s) 2 times per day at an interval of 6–8 hours	Allergic conjuctivitis
olopatadine (Patanol 0.2%) (C)	Antihistamine	1 drop in affected eye(s) once a day	Allergic conjuctivitis
tetrahydrozoline (Murine Plus®, others)	Decongestant	1–2 drops in affected eye(s) up to 4 times daily	Redness, burning, or other minor irritation

NURSING PROCESS

✍ Assessment

Before administering an ophthalmic drug according to the health care provider's orders, perform a baseline assessment of the patient's eye and its structures. Document normal and abnormal findings, including any redness, swelling, pain, excessive tearing, eye drainage or discharge, decrease in visual acuity, or other unusual symptoms. Assess patients for any hypersensitivity to medications or chemicals and for any drug- or disorder-related contraindications, as well as possible drug interactions. It may be necessary to perform a visual acuity test (e.g., using a Snellen chart) after a suspected injury and subsequent treatment. Focus the nursing history on past or present systemic disease processes and exposure to any chemicals that could be topical irritants to the eye, skin, or mucous membranes, including past and present work-related and environmental exposures. Also, complete a medical history to identify all medications the patient is taking.

✍ Nursing Diagnoses

- Acute pain related to an eye disorder, infection, or inflammatory eye condition
- Deficient knowledge related to lack of information about the eye disorder and associated medication therapy
- Risk for injury (to eyes) related to improper use of medication or improper instillation procedures

✍ Planning

◗ Goals

- Patient will remain free from eye pain.
- Patient will demonstrate adequate knowledge related to the use of ophthalmic medication, including its application and side effects.
- Patient will remain free from injury (to eyes) related to therapy.

◗ Expected Patient Outcomes

- Patient minimizes eye pain related to the eye disorder by applying warm or cold compresses as prescribed, using nonaspirin analgesics as directed, and properly applying prescribed ophthalmic medication.
- Patient identifies rationale for use of ophthalmic medication and adverse effects associated with each medication, as well as signs and symptoms to be reported to the health care provider, such as drainage,

redness, increase in eye pain, or decrease in visual acuity.
- Patient minimizes self-injury related to the adverse effects of therapy by creating a safe environment in the home, including reducing clutter and removing any unused rugs or furniture; installing more lighting, especially night lights; and using assistive devices as needed, if vision is altered.

✍ Implementation

Always inspect ophthalmic solutions, and administer only clear, unexpired products (e.g., drops, ointments, solutions) to eyes. Shake all solutions and mix their contents thoroughly. Do not use any solutions with particulate matter. One of the most important standards to follow during the instillation of drops or ointment is to avoid touching the eye with the tip of the dropper or container to prevent contamination of the product. Remove any excess medication promptly and apply pressure to the inner canthus for 1 minute (or other specified duration). Applying pressure to the inner canthus after the instillation of medication is needed to prevent or decrease systemic absorption and subsequent systemic adverse effects. Apply ointments and any other ophthalmic topical drug dosage forms to the conjunctival sac and never directly onto the eye (cornea). To facilitate the instillation of ophthalmic medication, tilt the patient's head back and have the patient look up at the ceiling during administration. Several ophthalmic drugs with different actions may be ordered; give each drug exactly as prescribed and within the specified time period. Ointments may cause a temporary blurring of vision because of the film that bathes the eye. This film will decrease once the drug is absorbed, and vision will then become clearer. Always refer to the medication order, as well an authoritative drug resource, for specific instructions and guidelines about application techniques, the length of time to apply pressure to the inner canthus, and any other specific instructions. See Chapter 10 regarding ophthalmic drug administration. Follow directions for the use of antiviral ophthalmic preparations closely. Administer topical anaesthetics (for use in removal of a foreign body or treatment of eye injury) as ordered. Repeated and continuous use of such medications is not recommended because of the related risk of delayed wound healing, corneal perforation, permanent corneal opacification, and vision loss. When there is an abrasion or other injury to the eye and appropriate medications are ordered, patching of the affected eye is recommended. This helps prevent further injury resulting from loss of the blink reflex due to overuse of topical anaesthetics. Include education regarding any possible change in eye colour caused by medication. For example, latanoprost can change hazel, green, or bluish-brown eyes permanently to brown. See the Patient Teaching Tips for more information regarding ophthalmic medications.

Evaluation

Therapeutic responses to miotics include decreased aqueous humour of the eye with resultant decreased IOP and decreased signs, symptoms, and long-term effects associated with glaucoma. β-Adrenergic blockers are therapeutic if their use produces a decrease in IOP. Possible adverse effects for which to assess with their use include weakness, eye irritation, rash, bradycardia, hypotension, and dysrhythmias (see Chapter 20). Therapeutic responses to antibiotic and antiviral ophthalmic drugs include elimination of an infection or condition and reso-

lution of symptoms, as well as prevention of complications. Therapeutic responses to ophthalmic anaesthetics include prevention or relief of pain associated with an injury; their adverse effects may include CNS excitation (e.g., dizziness, tremors, restlessness, nervousness) if they are systemically absorbed. Anti-inflammatory ophthalmic solutions result in a decrease in allergic reactions, including a decrease in itching, tearing, redness, and eye discharge. A potential complication related to the use of these solutions is swelling of the conjunctiva (chemosis). Further monitoring of patients taking these medications includes re-evaluation of goals and expected outcomes.

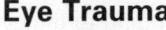 ## CASE STUDY

Eye Trauma

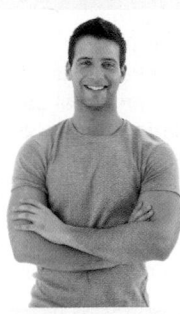

Paul, a 31-year-old construction worker, is being seen in the emergency department because of a possible eye injury. He was working without eye protection, and a gust of wind sprayed metal shavings into his face. The health care provider has instilled fluorescein sodium and has noted areas in the eyeball with green halos around them.

1. What is the purpose of the fluorescein sodium, and what is indicated by the green halos?

2. Paul is sent to an ophthalmologist for further treatment. What eye medication do you expect will be used for the next procedure?
3. After the procedure, Paul receives a prescription for dexamethasone ophthalmic ointment, which is to be administered three times a day. What specific patient teaching will the nurse share with Paul?
4. How could this injury have been prevented?

For answers, see http://evolve.elsevier.com/Canada/Lilley/pharmacology/.

PATIENT TEACHING TIPS

❖ Educate patients about the correct administration technique for the drugs they are taking. A recommended teaching strategy involves conducting a demonstration and requiring return demonstrations by patients.

❖ Encourage patients to use solutions only if they are clear and unexpired. Patients should keep solutions in containers for direct application and should keep eyedroppers sterile by avoiding touching the tip of the eyedropper or container to the surface of the eye.

❖ Educate patients receiving indirect-acting cholinergics about their adverse effects, such as blurred vision, bronchospasm, nausea, vomiting, bradycardia, hypotension, and sweating.

❖ With the use of any ophthalmic drug, instruct patients to report to the health care provider any severe stinging, burning, itching, or redness of the eye; excessive tearing or excessive dryness of the eye; puffiness of the eye or eyelids; discharge from the eye; fever; eye pain; or loss of or change in vision.

❖ Antiadrenergic drugs should be instilled as ordered. Once these drugs (and many other drugs used in the eye) are instilled, instruct patients to apply pressure to

the inner canthus with a tissue or 2 × 2 gauze pad for 1 full minute or as directed. Application of pressure to the inner canthus helps minimize systemic drug absorption and decrease the risk of systemic adverse effects. Advise patients to report to their health care providers immediately any blurred vision, difficulty breathing, wheezing, sweating, flushing, or loss of sight.

❖ Photosensitivity is an expected adverse effect of mydriatics; therefore, when these drugs are administered, encourage patients to wear sunglasses while in sunlight to help minimize eye discomfort and headaches.

❖ With the use of topical anaesthetics, advise patients to avoid rubbing or touching the eye while it is numb, because eye damage may result. An eye patch may be worn, if prescribed, to protect the eye because of loss of the blink reflex.

❖ Instruct patients to use ophthalmic drugs as prescribed and never to overuse them. Stress that products with expiration dates that have passed are not to be used and are to be discarded appropriately. Advise patients never to stop medications without consulting their

Continued

PATIENT TEACHING TIPS—cont'd

health care providers first because of the possibility of adverse reactions.

❖ Inform patients that contact lenses must not be worn while ophthalmic drugs are being instilled and for the duration of therapy, as the lenses may lead to further irritation.

❖ Ophthalmic ketorolac, an anti-inflammatory drug, may delay eye wound healing and lead to corneal epithelial breakdown. Instruct patients to report these problems if present or suspected.

KEY POINTS

❖ Glaucoma is a disorder of the eye caused by inhibition of the normal flow and drainage of aqueous humour. Treatment helps reduce IOP either by increasing the drainage of aqueous humour or decreasing its production.

❖ Drugs that increase aqueous humour drainage are direct-acting cholinergics, indirect-acting cholinergics, and β-blockers.

❖ A large proportion of inflammatory diseases of the eye are caused by viruses, and many ophthalmic antimicrobials are available to treat bacterial and viral infections of the eye. Common ocular infections include conjunctivitis, hordeolum (sty), keratitis, uveitis, and endophthalmitis.

❖ Anti-inflammatory ophthalmic drugs include corticosteroids and are used to inhibit inflammatory

responses to mechanical forces, chemicals, and immunological reactions.

❖ Topical anaesthetics are used to prevent pain to the eye and are beneficial during surgery, ophthalmic examinations, and removal of foreign bodies.

❖ Administer all ophthalmic preparations exactly as ordered. Always apply them into the conjunctival sac. Safe and accurate application or instillation technique also includes avoiding contact of the eyedropper or tube with the eye, to prevent contamination of the drug.

❖ Patients need to report to their health care providers any increase in symptoms, such as fever or eye pain or drainage.

EXAMINATION REVIEW QUESTIONS

1. The ophthalmologist has given a patient a dose of ophthalmic atropine drops before an eye examination. Which statement by the nurse accurately explains to the patient the reason for these drops?
   a. "These drops will cause the surface of your eye to become numb so that the doctor can do the examination."
   b. "These drops are used to check for any possible foreign bodies or corneal defects that may be in your eye."
   c. "These drops will reduce your tear production for the eye examination."
   d. "These drops will cause your pupils to dilate, which makes the eye examination easier."

2. When assessing a patient who is receiving a direct-acting cholinergic eye drop as part of treatment for glaucoma, the nurse anticipates that the drug affects the pupil in which way?
   a. It causes mydriasis, or pupil dilation.
   b. It causes miosis, or pupil constriction.
   c. It changes the colour of the pupil.
   d. It causes no change in pupil size.

3. During patient teaching regarding self-administration of ophthalmic drops, which statement by the nurse is correct?
   a. "Hold the eye dropper over the cornea and squeeze out the drop."
   b. "Apply pressure to the lacrimal duct area for 5 minutes after administration."
   c. "Be sure to place the drop in the conjunctival sac of the lower eyelid."
   d. "Squeeze your eyelid closed tightly after placing the drop into your eye."

4. When a nurse is providing teaching about eye medications for glaucoma, the nurse tells the patient that miotics help glaucoma by which mechanism of action?
   a. Decreasing intracranial pressure
   b. Decreasing intraocular pressure
   c. Increasing tear production
   d. Causing pupillary dilation

EXAMINATION REVIEW QUESTIONS—cont'd

5. Following assessment of a patient with glaucoma who has newly prescribed carbonic anhydrase inhibitor eye drops, the nurse would report to the health care provider a history of which condition?
a. Allergy to sulfa drugs
b. Decreased kidney function
c. Diabetes mellitus
d. Hypertension

6. The nurse is preparing to administer ketorolac (Acular) eye drops. The patient asks, "Why am I getting these eye drops?" Which is the correct answer by the nurse?
a. "These drops will reduce the pressure inside your eye as part of treatment for glaucoma."
b. "These drops are for a bacterial eye infection."
c. "These drops will relieve your dry eyes."
d. "These drops work to reduce the inflammation in your eyes."

7. A patient has undergone an eye procedure during which ophthalmic mydriatics and anaesthetic drops were used. The nurse gives which instructions to the patient prior to discharge? (Select all that apply.)
a. "Do not rub or touch the numb eye."
b. "You may reinsert your contact lenses before you leave."
c. "Be sure to wear sunglasses when you go outside."
d. "Your pupils will appear very tiny until the medication wears off."
e. "Report any increase in eye pain or drainage to the ophthalmologist immediately."

Answers: 1. d, 2. b, 3. c, 4. b, 5. a, 6. d, 7. a, c, e.

CRITICAL THINKING ACTIVITIES

1. A patient has a prescription for latanoprost (Xalatan). What is the most important piece of information that the nurse needs to tell the patient *before* the patient starts taking this medication?

2. A patient with type 2 diabetes has a new prescription for an ophthalmic β-blocker for treatment of glaucoma. Two days later, the patient calls the office and tells the nurse, "I looked up this drug on the Internet, and it says that this type of drug can mess up my blood sugar levels. I don't want to take the drops if that happens." What is the nurse's best response?

3. The nurse is assessing the eyes of a patient who had ocular surgery a week earlier. The patient has been receiving ketorolac tromethamine (Acular) ophthalmic solution. What is the priority action when the nurse assesses the eyes of this patient?

For answers, see http://evolve.elsevier.com/Canada/Lilley/pharmacology/.

CHAPTER 58

Otic Drugs

Objectives

After reading this chapter, the successful student will be able to do the following:

1. Describe the anatomy of the ear, including the outer, middle, and inner ear.

2. Name the various categories of ear disorders and explain their causes and signs and symptoms.

3. List various types of otic preparations and their indications.

4. Discuss the mechanisms of action, dosage, cautions, contraindications, drug interactions, and specific application techniques related to each of the otic drugs.

5. Develop a collaborative plan of care that includes all phases of the nursing process for patients receiving otic drugs.

e-Learning Activities

Website
(http://evolve.elsevier.com/Canada/
Lilley/pharmacology/)

evolve

- Answer Key—Textbook Case Studies
- Answer Key—Critical Thinking Activities
- Chapter Summaries—Printable
- Review Questions for Exam Preparation
- Unfolding Case Studies

Drug Profiles

» carbamide peroxide, p. 1083

» Key drug

Key Terms

Cerumen A yellowish or brownish waxy excretion produced by modified sweat glands in the external auditory canal; also called *earwax*. (p. 1083)

Otitis externa Inflammation or infection of the external auditory canal. (p. 1081)

Otitis media Inflammation or infection of the middle ear. (p. 1081)

OVERVIEW OF EAR ANATOMY

The ear is made up of three parts: the outer, middle, and inner ear. The outer ear is composed of the pinna (outer projecting part of the ear, also called the *auricle*) and the external auditory (or acoustic) meatus (also called the *external auditory canal* or simply the *ear canal*), which is the passageway to the tympanic membrane (or *eardrum*). The middle ear is composed of the tympanic cavity, the space enclosed by the tympanic membrane at one end and the oval window at the other. Within the middle ear are three tiny bones—the malleus (from the Latin for hammer), incus (anvil), and stapes (stirrup)—which together create a connection from the tympanic membrane to the oval window of the inner ear. Also within the middle ear is the auditory tube, or eustachian tube, which connects the middle ear to the nasopharynx. The inner ear includes the *cochlea*—the sensory organ for hearing—and the *semicircular canals*—the sensory organ for balance. The ear and its associated structures are illustrated in Figure 58-1.

Disorders of the ear can be categorized according to the portion of the ear affected. Outer ear disorders are generally the result of physical trauma or infection. Physical trauma usually consists of localized infections of the hair follicles, often causing the development of boils, and lacerations or scrapes to the skin. Foreign objects and infection or inflammation associated with

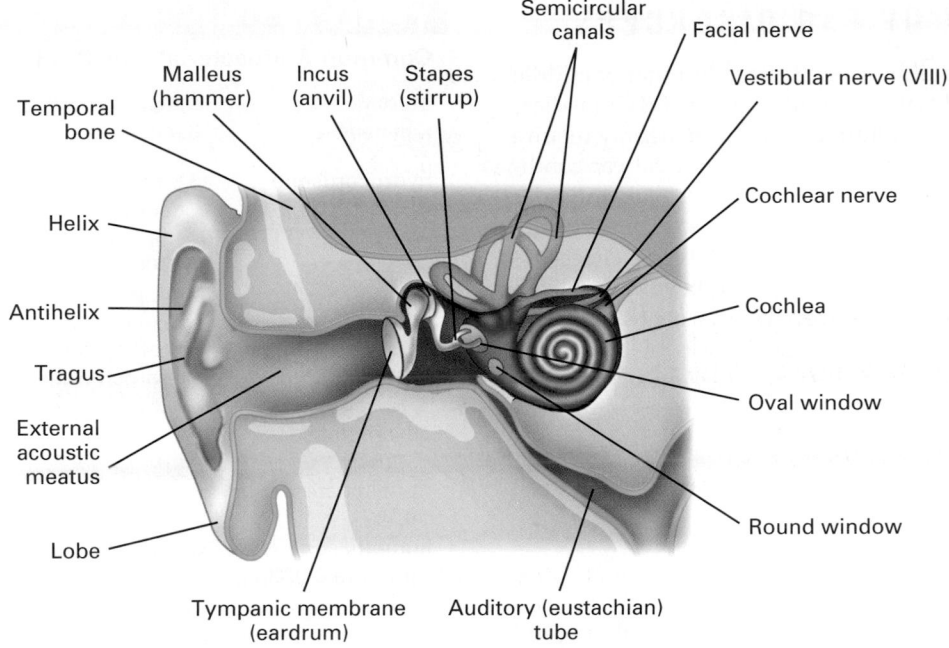

FIG. 58-1 Structure of the ear.

water sports are the usual sources of such trauma. In adults, the condition is also more likely to manifest as otitis externa involving the ear canal and external tympanic membrane. These disorders tend to be self-limiting and heal with time. Other examples of outer ear disorders are bacterial and fungal infections, earwax accumulation, contact dermatitis, seborrhea, and psoriasis, as evidenced by itching, local redness, inflammation, weeping, or drainage. Infections affecting the external auditory canal are known as *otitis externa*. (See otitis media below for symptoms.) These conditions usually respond to the same topical medications used for any other localized skin disorders, as discussed in Chapter 56. However, symptoms such as drainage, pain, and dizziness are sometimes also the first signs of a more serious underlying condition (e.g., head trauma, meningitis) and warrant prompt medical evaluation. Medications for disorders affecting the outer ear (ear canal) and middle ear are the focus of this chapter. Diseases of the inner ear can necessitate highly specialized medical practices that are beyond the scope of this chapter.

The most common disorders affecting the middle ear are bacterial and fungal infections and inflammation. Such disorders are often self-limiting, and treatments are usually successful. If problems persist or are left untreated, however, more serious problems such as hearing loss may result. Infections affecting the middle ear are known as *otitis media*. Otitis media is a common disease of infancy and early childhood. Children younger than 2 years are physiologically predisposed to acute otitis media because their eustachian tubes are shorter, of smaller calibre, and more horizontal compared with those of adults. Otitis media is often preceded by an upper respiratory tract infection. It may

also occur in adults, but it is then generally associated with trauma to the tympanic membrane. Common symptoms of both otitis media and otitis externa are pain, fever, malaise, pressure, a sensation of fullness in the ears, and impaired hearing. If the condition is left untreated, tinnitus (ringing in the ears), nausea, vertigo, mastoiditis, and temporary or permanent hearing loss may occur.

Otitis media is the second most common infection in children. Approximately 75% of children will have an episode of otitis media by 1 year of age, accounting for an estimated 1.8 million visits to health care providers annually. Medical management of otitis media is debated among the medical community, primarily due to the increased incidence of antibiotic resistance. Because of these concerns, treatment of otitis media has significantly changed over the last decade. The most recent Canadian guidelines were published in 2016 by the Infectious Diseases and Immunization Committee of the Canadian Paediatric Society. A growing number of health care providers do not recommend antibiotic treatment in children with mild otitis media with no fever or under 39°C for 24 hours. More emphasis is now given to observation, close follow-up, and use of analgesics, as otitis media usually resolves spontaneously. Many parents have concerns regarding treatment with only these components. If a decision is made to treat with an antibiotic, amoxicillin should be the first-line drug for most children as it has excellent middle ear penetration. If a patient fails to respond to treatment within 48 to 72 hours, the patient must be reassessed. If no antibiotics were given initially, they should be started or the initial antibiotic may need to be changed. Antibiotics are discussed in Chapters 43 and 44.

TREATMENT OF EAR DISORDERS

Some of the minor ailments that affect the outer or middle ear can be treated with over-the-counter (OTC) medications, but persistent, painful conditions generally require prescription medications. Drugs used to treat ear conditions are known as *otic drugs*, and most are topically applied to the ear canal. Because of this, they generally are not involved in drug interactions. Adverse effects are uncommon and usually do not extend beyond localized irritation. Otic drugs are normally only contraindicated in cases of known drug allergy. Classes of otic drugs include the following:

- Antibacterials (antibiotics)
- Antifungals
- Anti-inflammatory drugs
- Local analgesics
- Local anaesthetics
- Corticosteroids
- Wax emulsifiers

More serious cases of ear disorders may require treatment with systemic drugs such as antimicrobial drugs, analgesics, anti-inflammatory drugs, and antihistamines. These medications have been discussed in detail in previous chapters dealing with the respective drug classes.

ANTIBACTERIAL AND ANTIFUNGAL OTIC DRUGS

Antibacterial and antifungal otic drugs are often combined with steroids to take advantage of the anti-inflammatory, antipruritic, and antiallergic effects of the latter drugs. These drugs are used to treat outer and middle ear infections. Because they all work and are dosed similarly, available products are profiled together below. Systemic antibiotics are also commonly prescribed for these conditions (e.g., amoxicillin; see Chapter 43), either alone or in addition to the otic drugs described in the following sections. Tables 58-1 and 58-2 list several commonly used products and their component amounts. These drugs are used during pregnancy when potential benefits outweigh the risks to the fetus.

NURSING PROCESS

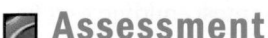 Assessment

Before administering any of the otic preparations, assess baseline hearing or auditory status, if deemed appropriate, and document the findings. Assessment of the outer and middle ear via otoscope can be undertaken to detect infection, cerumen buildup, or the presence of a foreign

TABLE	58-1

Common Antibacterial Otic Products

Steroid Component	Antibiotic Component	Trade Name
hydrocortisone acetate 1%	3.5 mg/mL of neomycin sulphate and 10 000 units/mL polymyxin B sulphate	Spor-HC Otic® Suspension
dexamethasone 0.1%	ciprofloxacin hydrochloride 0.3%	Ciprodex® Ciloxan®
dexamethasone sodium phosphate 0.1%		AK-Dex®, Diodex® solution 0.1%
flumethasone pivalate 0.02%	clioquinol 1%	Locacorten Vioform® ear drops

TABLE	58-2

Common Antifungal Otic Products

Ingredients	Trade Name
clioquinol 1%, flumethasone pivalate 0.02%	Locacorten Vioform ear drops

Neomycin, polymixin B, and hydrocortisone otic preparations are contraindicated in patients with a perforated eardrum.

body. Certified practice registered nurses can also follow decision support tools to diagnose and treat acute otitis media. Assess the patient's symptoms, past and present medical history, and use of prescription drugs, OTC drugs, and natural health products. Document any drug or food allergies. A baseline understanding of the anatomy of the ear, especially anatomical variations in patients of different age groups, is needed to ensure proper application technique is used. Contraindications, cautions, and drug interactions for otic drugs, chemicals, or solutions have been discussed previously in the treatment section; always assess the patient for these and document the findings. In addition, if the patient has a perforated eardrum, this is a contraindication to the use of otic drugs.

Nursing Diagnoses

- Acute pain related to ear infection or ear disorder
- Deficient knowledge related to lack of experience with otic drugs and their method of administration
- Nonadherence related to a lack of motivation or lack of understanding for the need of frequent ear drop instillation, as ordered

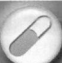

DRUG PROFILES

ANTIBACTERIAL PRODUCTS

Spor-HC Otic Suspension® is a three-drug combination that includes hydrocortisone and two antimicrobials: neomycin sulphate (an aminoglycoside; see Chapter 44) and polymyxin B sulphate. Hydrocortisone is the steroid most commonly used in otic drugs, although there is one preparation (Ciprodex®) containing both ciprofloxacin (a fluoroquinolone; see Chapter 44) and dexamethasone sodium phosphate. There is also a single-drug dexamethasone sodium phosphate (AK-Dex®) formulation. The purpose of the steroid component is to reduce the inflammation and itching associated with ear infections. An additional combination product comprises flumethasone pivaleate and clioquinol (Locacorten®). All of these products are used for the treatment of bacterial otitis externa or otitis media caused by susceptible bacteria, such as *Staphylococcus aureus*, *Escherichia coli*, *Klebsiella* species, and others. Neomycin sulphate, polymyxin B sulphate, and hydrocortisone acetate otic preparations are contraindicated in patients with a perforated eardrum because of the related risk of ototoxicity; ciprofloxacin and dexamethasone can be used with perforated eardrums. Their usual dosage is 4 drops, 3 to 4 times daily. With some otic drugs, as a means of dosing, it is recommended to saturate a retrievable cotton or tissue wick with the drug and let this wick soak inside the ear canal. The wick can be periodically remoistened with additional drug or removed and followed by further ear drops inserted directly into the ear canal. Follow specific instructions on drug packages or use the method recommended by the health care provider or pharmacist.

ANTIFUNGAL PRODUCTS

Fungal infections account for about 4% of ear infections. Antifungal otic drugs are used primarily for otitis externa. These drugs may also have antibacterial and antiviral properties. The preparation used as an antifungal in Canada is clioquinol 1%, flumethasone pivalate 0.02% (Locacorten Vioform ear drops). Flumethasone pivalate is a corticosteroid with anti-inflammatory, antipruritic, and vasoconstrictive properties and clioquinol is an antimicrobial. Polyethylene glycol is the vehicle that softens the cerumen and ensures prolonged contact of the active ingredients with the surface of the ear canal. It is contraindicated for use in patients with a perforated eardrum.

EARWAX EMULSIFERS

An additional common ear problem is the accumulation and eventual impaction (hardening) of earwax, or **cerumen,** which can also contribute to or complicate the infectious and inflammatory conditions described earlier. Products that soften and help to eliminate earwax are referred to as *earwax emulsifiers.* Cerumen is a natural product of the ear and is produced by modified sweat glands in the ear canal. It can vary in form and appearance from patient to patient, from almost liquid, to firm and solid, to dry and flaky. Its colour varies depending upon its composition and can vary from dark brown to light yellow. Glandular secretions, sloughed skin cells, normal bacteria present on the surface of the ear canal, and water may all be present in earwax. Ears are considered to be self-cleaning. Once earwax dries, the movement of the jaw helps to move the cerumen out. However, it can occasionally build up and become impacted, which results in pain and temporary partial hearing loss. As we know from chemistry, a non-polar substance is one that is not water soluble. Such a substance is said to be emulsified when it is chemically or physically converted to a more water-soluble form. *Earwax emulsifiers* loosen impacted cerumen, which allows it to be flushed out of the ear canal through irrigation with water. Often the simple application of olive, mineral, or almond oil is sufficient to soften wax.

▶▶ *carbamide peroxide*

Carbamide peroxide (Murine® Ear Wax Removal System Otic) is a commonly used earwax emulsifier. It is combined with other components (e.g., glycerin, a lubricant) that help soften and lubricate cerumen prior to irrigation. Carbamide peroxide slowly releases hydrogen peroxide and oxygen when exposed to moisture. The release of oxygen imparts a weak antibacterial action to this otic drug. In addition, the *effervescence* (foaming) resulting from the release of oxygen has the mechanical effect of emulsifying impacted cerumen to release it from the walls of the ear canal. Earwax emulsifiers are not to be used without a health care provider's recommendation when ear drainage, tympanic membrane rupture, or significant pain or other irritation is present. After allowing the drug to dissolve the earwax, one can remove the cerumen by gently flushing the ear canal with warm water from a bulb syringe. Some earwax removal products include such a syringe in the package. This drug is used during pregnancy when potential benefits outweigh the risks to the fetus.

▨ Planning

▩ Goals

- Patient will remain free from pain and other symptoms related to the ear disorder.
- Patient will demonstrate adequate knowledge about the treatment regimen and the use, application, and adverse effects of otic drugs.
- Patient will remain adherent to the medication regimen, as prescribed.

▩ Expected Patient Outcomes

- Patient experiences minimal to no discomfort with the use of prescribed medication.

- Patient uses measures to enhance comfort such as the use of warm compresses, as prescribed, as well as of non-narcotic analgesics, as directed.
- Patient reports immediately to the health care provider any increase in ear pain and other symptoms once therapy is initiated.
- Patient states rationale for the use of otic medication and ways to increase the drug's effectiveness, such as ensuring accurate application or instillation and afterward remaining supine or sitting with the affected ear upward for a short period. (See Chapter 10).
- Patient instills medication as prescribed, as related to dosage, frequency, and duration of therapy.

Implementation

Instill otic preparations only after the ear has been thoroughly cleansed and all cerumen has been removed (by irrigation if necessary, or as ordered). Ear drops, solutions, and ointments need to be at room temperature prior to instillation. Administration of solutions that are too cold may cause a vestibular type of reaction involving vomiting and dizziness. If a solution has been refrigerated, allow it to warm to room temperature. Higher temperatures may affect the potency of these solutions. When administering ear drops to adults, hold the pinna *up* and back; when administering them to children younger than 3 years of age, hold the pinna *down* and back. Allow a period of time for adequate coverage of the ear once the medication has been administered. Gentle massage to the tragus area of the pinna may also help increase coverage of the medication after the solution is given. See the Patient Teaching Tips and also Chapter 10 for more information on ear drop instillation.

Evaluation

The therapeutic effects of otic drugs are gauged by evaluating whether goals and objectives have been met. Therapeutic effects of otic drugs include a decrease in pain, redness, and swelling in the ear; a reduction in fever; and resolution of any other signs and symptoms associated with the ear disorder. Improvement in hearing may also be an anticipated therapeutic effect. Monitor the ear canal for the occurrence of rash or any signs of local irritation, such as redness and heat at the site. Evaluate the patient for adverse effects with each application or instillation, and report any unusual appearance of the pinna and ear canal immediately to the health care provider.

CASE STUDY

Ear Medications

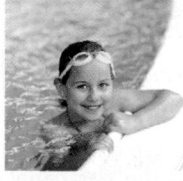 Raluca is eight years old and loves to swim in the neighbourhood pool. Lately, she has had a feeling of fullness in her left ear, and yesterday she told her mother that her ear is hurting and itching and that she feels "awful." Her mother took her temperature and found that it was 38.3°C. She called the pediatrician's office for an appointment, and Raluca is seen the next morning. After examining Raluca, the pediatrician says that Raluca has otitis media in her left ear and some earwax buildup in both ears. The pediatrician removes some of the earwax manually, writes a prescription for oral antibiotics for Raluca, and gives instructions to use an earwax emulsifier. The nurse meets with Raluca and her mother to review the instructions.

1. Raluca's mother asks, "Why is the antibiotic a suspension? It seems to me that if she has an ear infection, she should take ear drops!" What is the nurse's best response?
2. Raluca's mother also asks, "What will happen if this ear infection does not get better?" What is the nurse's best response?
3. Raluca reports that her ear "really hurts and itches." What can be given to her for this problem? How will it be given?

_____

For answers, see http://evolve.elsevier.com/Canada/Lilley/pharmacology/.

PATIENT TEACHING TIPS

❖ Provide thorough instructions to patients about the proper use of ear drops and the instillation of any medication into the ear. Warn patients that dizziness may occur after application of the medication, requiring the patient to remain supine or sitting during instillation and for a few minutes thereafter.

❖ Medication to be applied to the ear must be at room temperature. This may be achieved by running warm water over the medication bottle, but care must be taken to prevent getting water in the container, damaging the label so that the directions become unreadable, or making the solution too warm to use.

PATIENT TEACHING TIPS—cont'd

Advise patients not to heat the medication; for example, a microwave oven must not be used for warming because ear drops that are overheated may lose potency. If the pharmacy indicates that the drug should be kept in a refrigerator, instruct the patient to take it out of the refrigerator up to 1 hour before it is to be instilled so that it can warm up to room temperature. Most otic medications are stored at room temperature.

❖ Instruct patients to lie on the side opposite to that of the affected ear for about 5 minutes after instillation of otic drugs. A small cotton ball may be inserted gently into the ear canal to keep the drug in place, but it should not be forced into the ear or jammed down into the ear canal.

❖ Instruct patients to avoid the use of Q-tips® or cotton swabs to clean the ears (except for the outer margins of the outer ear), as well as to refrain from undergoing ear candling procedures and from using an oral jet irrigator in the ears. These practices can push cerumen deeper into the ear canal from where it cannot be removed. This can result in the accumulation of fungi, bacteria, and viruses, leading to pain and infection, hearing loss, or a ruptured eardrum.

KEY POINTS

❖ Otic drugs may include the following ingredients, either alone or in combination (depending on the health care provider's order): corticosteroids, antibacterials, antifungals, anti-inflammatories, and wax emulsifying compounds. Many of the anti-infective drugs are combined with corticosteroids (in solution) to take advantage of the additional anti-inflammatory, antipruritic, and antiallergic effects of the steroids.

❖ Some ear infections require additional drug therapy with systemic dosage forms of corticosteroids, antibiotics, antifungals, and anti-inflammatory drugs.

❖ Some disorders of the ear are self-limiting to a degree, but appropriate treatment is important to prevent local and systemic complications. If left untreated, ear infections and disorders may lead to partial or complete hearing loss.

❖ Cerumen, or earwax, is a natural product of the ear and is normally produced by modified sweat glands in the auditory canal; emulsifying otic drugs (such as carbamide peroxide) loosen and help remove this wax.

❖ Single drugs and combination drug products are used to treat many ear conditions, and it is important to know the indications for and specific information about these drugs to ensure their safe use.

EXAMINATION REVIEW QUESTIONS

1. While teaching a patient about treatment of otitis media, the nurse should mention that untreated otitis media may lead to which condition?
a. Mastoiditis
b. Throat infections
c. Fungal ear infection
d. Decreased cerumen production

2. During a teaching session about ear drops, the patients tells the nurse, "I know why an antibiotic is in this medicine, but why do I need to take a steroid?" Which is the nurse's best answer?
a. "The steroid will help to soften the cerumen."
b. "The steroid reduces itching and inflammation."
c. "The steroid also has antifungal effects."
d. "This medication helps to anaesthetize the area to decrease pain."

3. The nurse is preparing to administer ear drops. Which technique for administering ear drops is correct?
a. Warm the solution to 37.7°C before using.
b. Position the patient so that the unaffected ear is accessible.
c. Massage the tragus before administering the ear drops.
d. Gently insert a cotton ball into the outer ear canal after the drops are given.

4. The nurse is discussing treatment of earwax buildup with a patient. Which statement about earwax emulsifiers is true about these drugs?
a. They are useful for treatment of ear infections.
b. They loosen impacted cerumen so that it may be removed by irrigation.
c. They are used to rinse out excessive earwax.
d. They enhance the secretion of earwax.

5. During an examination, the nurse notes that a patient has a perforated tympanic membrane. There is an order for ear drops. Which action by the nurse is most appropriate?
a. Give the medication as ordered.
b. Check the patient's hearing, and then give the drops.
c. Hold the medication, and check with the health care provider.
d. Administer the drops with a cotton wick.

Continued

EXAMINATION REVIEW QUESTIONS—cont'd

6. The nurse is preparing to administer ear drops and finds that the bottle has been stored in the medication room refrigerator. Which is the best action by the nurse?
   a. Remove the bottle from the refrigerator, and administer the drops.
   b. Heat the bottle for 5 seconds in a microwave oven before administering the drops.
   c. Let the bottle sit in a cup of hot water for 15 minutes before administering the drops.
   d. Remove the bottle from the refrigerator 1 hour before the drops are due to be given.

7. The nurse is preparing to administer carbamide peroxide to an adult patient with impacted cerumen. Which actions by the nurse are correct? (Select all that apply.)
   a. Have the patient lie on his side with the affected ear up.
   b. Chill the medication before administering it.
   c. Pull the pinna of the ear down and back.
   d. Pull the pinna of the ear up and back.
   e. Gently irrigate the ear with warm water to remove the softened earwax.

Answers: 1. a, 2. b, 3. d, 4. b, 5. c, 6. d, 7. a, d, e

CRITICAL THINKING ACTIVITIES

1. A nurse is explaining about wax emulsifiers to a patient who has decreased hearing because of impacted cerumen. The patient asks, "How can this help me? What will this medication do for me?" What is the nurse's best answer?

2. When discussing ear drop administration with a patient, the patient says, "I'll keep these in the refrigerator so that they'll be cold when I give them to myself." What is the nurse's best response?

3. The nurse is observing while the mother of an infant administers ear drops for the first time. The mother says, "When I give the drops, I will pull the ear up and back like this, give the drops, and then massage the earlobe." What is the nurse's priority action at this time?

For answers, see http://evolve.elsevier.com/Canada/Lilley/pharmacology/.

Appendix
Pharmaceutical Abbreviations

Abbreviation	Translation
DRUG DOSAGE	
g or Gm	Gram
gtt	Drop
L	Litre
mEq	Milliequivalent
min	Minute
mL	Millilitre
tbsp	Tablespoon
tsp	Teaspoon
mcg	Microgram
DRUG ROUTE	
ID	Intradermal
IM	Intramuscular
IV	Intravenous
NG	Nasogastric
PO	Per os (orally; by mouth)
subcut	Subcutaneous
SL	Sublingual

Abbreviation	Translation
DRUG ADMINISTRATION	
ac	Before meals
ad lib	As desired, freely
bid	Twice a day
hr	Hour
NPO	Nothing by mouth
pc	After meals
prn	Pro re nata (when needed)
qh	Every hour
qid	Four times a day
Rx	Prescribe or take
stat	Immediately
tid	Three times a day

Case Study
Photo Credits

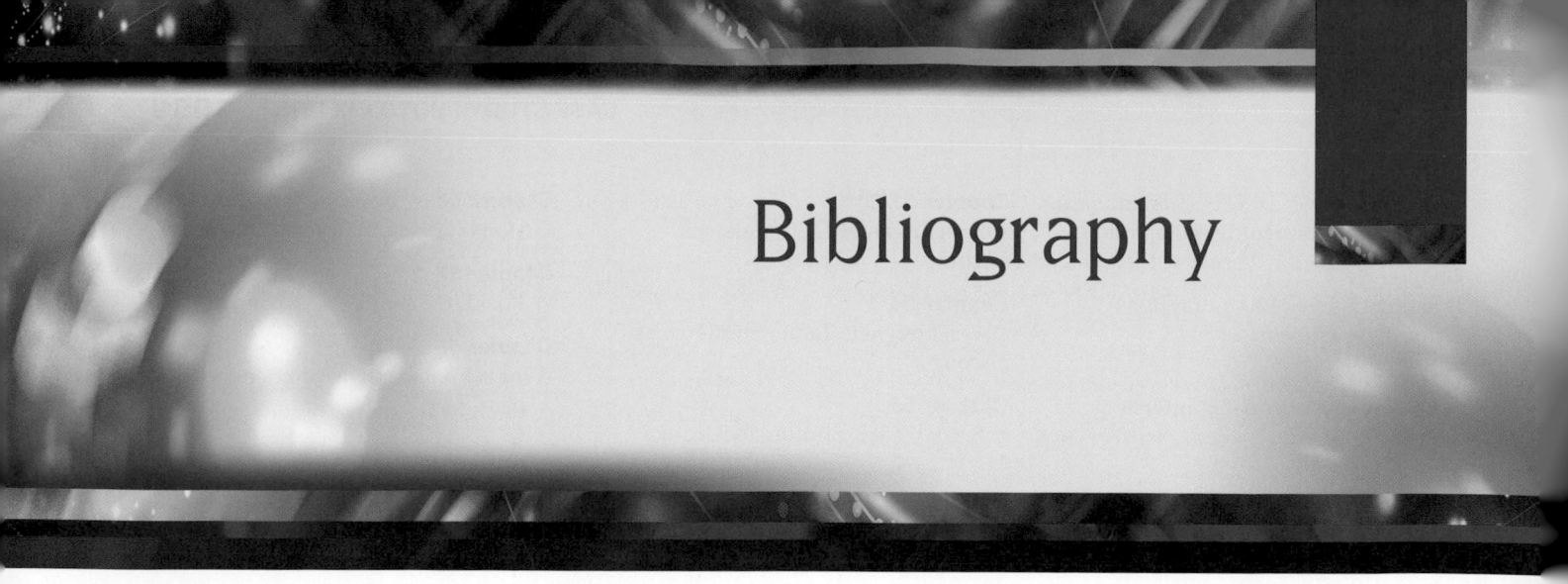

Bibliography

General References

Canadian Pharmacists Association. (2013). *Compendium of pharmaceuticals and specialties. The Canadian drug reference for health professionals.* Ottawa, ON: Author. The subscription based e-CPS is available at <http://www.pharmacists.ca/index.cfm/function/store/PublicationDetail.cfm?pPub=5>.

DiPiro, J. T., Talbert, R. L., Yee, G. C., et al. (2014). *Pharmacotherapy: A pathophysiological approach* (9th ed.). New York: McGraw-Hill.

Halter, M. J. (2013). *Varcarolis's Canadian psychiatric mental health nursing, a clinical approach* (1st Canadian ed.). Toronto, ON: Mosby.

Health Canada. (2013). *Drug product database.* Retrieved from <http://www.hc-sc.gc.ca/dhp-mps/prodpharma/databasdon/index-eng.php>.

Lewis, S. M., Dirksen, S. R., Heitkemper, M. M., et al. (2014). *Medical-surgical nursing in Canada: Assessment and management of clinical problems* (3rd Canadian ed.). Toronto, ON: Mosby.

Mosby. (2013). *Mosby's drug reference for health professions* (4th ed.). St. Louis, MO: Mosby.

NANDA International. (2014). *Nursing diagnoses 2015–17: Definitions and classification.* Hoboken, NJ: Wiley-Blackwell.

Part 1

Diekelmann, S., & Born, T. (2010). The memory function of sleep. *Nature Reviews. Neuroscience, 11,* 114–126. doi:10.1038/nrn2762.

Stickgold, R., & Walker, M. P. (2013). Sleep-dependent memory triage: Evolving generalization through selective processing. *Nature Neuroscience, 16,* 139–145. doi:10.1038/nn.3303.

Trockel, M. T., Barnes, M. D., & Egget, D. L. (2000). Health-related variables and academic performance among first year college students: Implications for sleep and other behaviors. *Journal of American College Health, 49*(3), 125–131.

Chapter 1

Brown, M. T., & Bussell, J. K. (2011). Medication adherence: WHO Cares? *Mayo Clinical Proceedings, 86*(4), 304–314. doi:10.4065/mcp.2010.0575.

Canadian Association of Physician Assistants. (2015). *Frequently asked questions.* Retrieved from <https://capa-acam.ca/features/faq>.

Canadian Nurses Association. (2008). *Code of ethics for registered nurses (2008 centennial edition).* Retrieved from <https://www.cna-aiic.ca/~/media/cna/page-content/pdf-fr/code-of-ethics-for-registered-nurses.pdf>.

Canadian Nurses Association. (2010). *Position statement. Evidence-based decision making and nursing practice.* Retrieved from <http://www.nanb.nb.ca/PDF/CNA-Evidence_Informed_Decision_Making_and_Nursing_Practice_E.pdf>.

College & Association of Registered Nurses of Alberta. (2014). *Medication guidelines.* Retrieved from <http://www.nurses.ab.ca/content/dam/carna/pdfs/DocumentList/Guidelines/MedicationGuidelines Jan2014.pdf>.

College of Nurses of Ontario. (2009). *Confidentiality and privacy – Personal health information.* Retrieved from <http://www.cno.org/Global/docs/prac/41069_privacy.pdf>.

College of Nurses of Ontario. (2015). *Practice standard: Medication.* Retrieved from <http://www.cno.org/Global/docs/prac/41007_Medication.pdf>.

College of Registered Nurses of British Columbia. (2013). *Practice standard. Nursing documentation.* Retrieved from <https://www.crnbc.ca/standards/lists/standardresources/151nursingdocumentation.pdf>.

College of Registered Nurses of British Columbia. (2015). *Dispensing medications.* Retrieved from <https://www.crnbc.ca/Standards/PracticeStandards/Pages/dispensing.aspx>.

Herdman, T. H. (Ed.), (2012). *NANDA International nursing diagnoses: Definitions and classifications, 2012–2014.* Hoboken, NJ: Wiley.

Herdman, T. H., & Kamitsuru, S. (Eds.), (2014). *NANDA International nursing diagnoses: Definitions and classification, 2015–2017.* Oxford, GB: Wiley Blackwell.

Ho, M. P., Bryson, C. L., & Rumsfield, J. S. (2009). Key issues in outcomes research. Medication adherence. Its importance in cardiovascular outcomes. *Circulation, 119,* 3028–3035. doi:10.1161/CIRCULATIONAHA.108.768986.

Indiana State Nursing Association. (2014). Developing a nursing IQ—Part 1. Characteristics of critical thinking: What critical thinkers do, what critical thinkers do not do. *ISNA Bulletin, 41*(1), 6–14.

Information and Privacy Commissioner of Ontario. (2009). *Innovative wireless home care services: Protecting privacy and personal health information.* Toronto: Author. Retrieved from <https://www.ipc.on.ca/images/Resources/wireless-homecare.pdf>.

Institute for Safe Medication Practices Canada. (2011). *Guidelines for timely medication administration; Response to the CMS "30-minute rule."* Retrieved from <http://www.ismp.org/news-letters/acutecare/articles/20110113.asp>.

International Council of Nurses. (2014) *International classification for nursing practice.* Retrieved from <http://www.icn.ch/what-we-do/international-classification-for-nursing-practice-icnpr/>.

Jones, D., Lunney, M., Keenan, G., et al. (2010). Standardized nursing languages: Essential for the nursing workforce. *Annual Review of Nursing Research, 28,* 253–294.

Jones, K. W. (2010). Medication risk must be balanced with benefit, not fear. *Annals of Pharmacotherapy, 44*(4), 737–739. doi:10.1345/aph.1M614.

Koharchik, L., Caputi, L., Robb, M., et al. (2015). Fostering clinical reasoning in nursing students. *American Journal of Nursing, 115*(1), 58–61. doi:10.1097/01.NAJ.0000459638.68657.9b.

Macdonald, M. (2010). Patient safety: Examining the adequacy of the 5 rights of medication administration. *Clinical Nurse Specialist, 24*(4), 196–201. doi:10.1097/NUR.0b013e3181e3605f.

NANDA International. (2014). *Nursing diagnoses 2015–2017: Definitions and classification* (10th ed.). Hoboken, NJ: Wiley.

Stokowski, L. (2012). *Timely medication administration guidelines for nurses: Fewer wrong-time errors?* Retrieved from <http://www.medscape.com/viewarticle/772501_5>.

Chapter 2

Leonti, M., & Casu, L. (2013). Traditional medicines and globalization: Current and future perspectives in ethnopharmacology. *Frontiers in Pharmacology, 4*(92), doi:10.3389/fphar.2013.00092.

Nkhoma, E. T., Poole, C., Vannappagari, V., et al. (2009). The global prevalence of glucose-6-phosphate dehydrogenase deficiency: A systematic review and meta-analysis. *Blood Cells, Molecules and Diseases, 42*(3), 267–278. doi:10.1016/j.bcmd.2008.12.005.

Chapter 3

Amir Raz, A., Campbell, N., Guindi, G., et al. (2011). Placebos in clinical practice: Comparing attitudes, beliefs, and patterns of use between academic psychiatrists and nonpsychiatrists. *Canadian Journal of Psychiatry, 56*(4), 198–208.

Canadian Nurses Association. (2007). *Framework for the practice of nurses in Canada.* Retrieved from <http://www.cnaiic.ca/~/media/cna/page%20content/pdf%20en/2013/07/25/13/53/rn_framework_practice_2007_e.pdf> (Framework is currently under revision (<https://www.cna-aiic.ca/en/becoming-an-rn/the-practice-of-nursing>)).

Canadian Nurses Association. (2008). *Code of ethics for registered nurses.* Ottawa, ON: Author. Retrieved from <http://www.cna-aiic.ca/en/on-the-issues/best-nursing/nursing-ethics>.

Government of Canada. (2015). *New rules will enhance oversight of marijuana for medical purposes authorizations—Increasing information sharing by licensed producers with Canadian healthcare licensing bodies.* Retrieved from <http://news.gc.ca/web/article-en.do?nid=986469&tp=1>.

Health Canada. (2015a). *Medical use of marihuana.* Retrieved from <http://www.hc-sc.gc.ca/dhp-mps/marihuana/index-eng.php>.

Health Canada. (2015b). *Special Access Programme—Drugs.* Retrieved from <http://www.hc-sc.gc.ca/dhp-mps/acces/drugs-drogues/sapfs_pasfd-eng.php>.

International Council of Nurses. (2012). *The international code of ethics for nursing.* Geneva, CH: Author. Retrieved from <http://www.icn.ch/who-we-are/code-of-ethics-for-nurses/>.

Klaus Linde, K., Fässler, M., & Meissner, K. (2011). Placebo interventions, placebo effects and clinical practice. *Philosophical Transactions of the Royal Society, 366*(1572), 1905–1912. doi:10.1098/rstb.2010.0383.

Law, M. R., Cheng, L., Dhalla, I. A., et al. (2012). The effect of cost on adherence to prescription medications in Canada. *Canadian Medical Association Journal, 184*(3), 297–302. doi:10.1503/cmaj.111270.

Office of the Privacy Commissioner of Canada. (2014). *Fact sheet. Privacy legislation in Canada.* Retrieved from <https://www.priv.gc.ca/resource/fs-fi/02_05_d_15_e.asp>.

Chapter 4

Alberta Health Services. (2009). *Health and Black Canadians.* Retrieved from <http://www.crha-health.ab.ca/programs/diversity/diversity_resources/health_div_pops/black.htm>.

Alzheimer Society Canada. (2013). *Risk factors.* Retrieved from <http://www.alzheimer.ca/en/About-dementia/Alzheimer-s-disease/Risk-factors?gclid=CJLOx6WCwLsCFahDMgodj2oAQQ>.

Alzheimer Society of Canada. (2015a). *The 72%.* Retrieved from <http://www.alzheimer.ca/en/the72percent>.

Alzheimer Society of Canada. (2015b). *Latest information and statistics.* Retrieved from <http://www.alzheimer.ca/en/Get-involved/Raise-your-voice/Latest-info-stats>.

Andrews, M., & Boyle, J. S. (Eds.), (2008). *Transcultural concepts in nursing care* (5th ed.). Philadelphia, PA: Wolters Kluwer/Lippincott Williams & Wilkins.

Bacchus, B., & Esmail, N. (2013). *Federal delays in approving new medicines 2013.* Retrieved from <http://www.fraserinstitute.org/uploadedFiles/fraser-ca/Content/research-news/research/publications/federal-delays-in-approving-new-medicines-2013.pdf>.

Beckett, V. L., Tyson, L. D., Carroll, D., et al. (2012). Accurately administering oral medication to children isn't child's play. *Archives of Disease in Childhood, 97*(9), 838–841. doi:10.1136/archdischild-2012-301850.

Brown, M. T., & Bussell, J. K. (2011). Medication adherence: WHO cares? *Mayo Clinic Proceedings, 86*(4), 304–314. doi:10.4065/mcp.2010.0575.

Canada Health Infoway. (2013). *2013–2014 summary corporate plan*. Retrieved from <https://www.infoway-inforoute.ca/index.php/about-infoway/what-we-do>.

Canada Trials. (2014). *What is clinical research*. Retrieved from <http://www.canadatrials.com/AboutClinicalResearch.php>.

Canadian Institute for Health Information. (2010). *Seniors and prescription drug use*. Retrieved from <http://www.cihi.ca/CIHI-ext-portal/pdf/internet/seniors_drug_info_en>.

Canadian Institute for Health Information. (2013). *Drug expenditure in Canada, 1985 to 2012*. Retrieved from <https://secure.cihi.ca/free_products/Drug_Expenditure_2013_EN.pdf>.

Charles, C. E., & Daroszewski, E. B. (2012). Culturally competent nursing care of the Muslim patient. *Issues in Mental Health Nursing, 33*(1), 61–63. doi:10.3109/01612840.2011.596613.

Clyne, B., Bradley, M. C., Hughes, C., et al. (2012). Electronic prescribing and other forms of technology to reduce inappropriate medication use and polypharmacy in older people: A review of current evidence. *Clinics in Geriatric Medicine, 28*(2), 301–322. doi:10.1016/j.cger.2012.01.009.

Duthley, B. (2013). *Update on 2004 background paper, BP 6.11 Alzheimer Disease*. Retrieved from <http://www.who.int/medicines/areas/priority_medicines/BP6_11Alzheimer.pdf>.

Editorial. (2013). The three stages of Alzheimer's disease. [Editorial]. *The Lancet, 377*, April 30, 2011. Retrieved from <www.thelancet.com>.

Employment and Social Development Canada. (2015). *Canadians in context—Aging population*. Retrieved from <http://www4.hrsdc.gc.ca/.3ndic.1t.4r@-eng.jsp?iid=33>.

Esmail, N. (2013). *Cutting Canada's drug approval delay while improving safety. Fraser Forum*. Retrieved from <http://www.fraserinstitute.org>.

Forgie, S., Zhanel, G., & Robinson, J. (2009). Management of acute otitis media. *Paediatric and Child Health, 14*(7), 457–460.

Fraller, D. B. (2013). State of the science: Use of biomarkers and imaging in the diagnosis and management of Alzheimer disease. *Journal of Neuroscience Nursing, 45*(2), 63–70.

Friedman, M., Bowles, V., & Jones, E. (2003). *Family nursing: Theory and practice* (3rd ed.). Upper Saddle River, NJ: Prentice Hall.

Giger, J. N., & Davidhizar, R. (2002). The Giger and Davidhizar transcultural assessment model. *Journal of Transcultural Nursing, 13*(3), 185–188.

Institute for Safe Medications Practices Canada. (2014). *Safe medication use in older persons information page*. Retrieved from <http://www.ismp-canada.org/beers_list/>.

Law, M. R., Cheng, L., Dhalla, I. A., et al. (2012). The effect of cost on adherence to prescription medications in Canada. *Canadian Medical Association Journal, 184*(3), 297–302. doi:10.1503/cmaj.111270.

Law, R., Bozzo, P., Koren, G., et al. (2011). FDA pregnancy risk categories and the CPS. Do they help or are they a hindrance? *Canadian Family Physician, 56*(3), 239–241.

Malenfant, É. C., & Morency, J.-D. (2011). *Population projections by aboriginal identity in Canada, 2006 to 2031*. Retrieved from <http://www.statcan.gc.ca/pub/91-552-x/91-552-x2011001-eng.htm>.

Matlow, A. G., Baker, G. R., Flintoft, V., et al. (2012). Adverse events among children in Canadian hospitals: The Canadian paediatric adverse events study. *Canadian Medical Association Journal, 184*(13), E709–E718. doi:10.1503/cmaj.112153.

McPherson, M., Ji, H., Hunt, J., et al. (2012). Medication use among Canadian seniors. *Healthcare Quarterly, 15*(4), 15–18. doi:10.12927/hcq.2012.23192.

Mikkonen, J., & Raphael, D. (2010). *Social determinants of health: The Canadian facts*. Retrieved from <http://www.thecanadianfacts.org/of-the-canadian-pop.pdf>.

Morgan, S., Hanley, G., Cunningham, C., et al. (2011). Ethnic differences in the use of prescription drugs: A cross-sectional analysis of linked survey and administrative data. *Open Medicine, 5*(2), e87–e93. Retrieved from <http://www.open-medicine.ca/article/view/428/405>.

Nestel, S. (2012). *Colour coded health care. The impact of race and racism on Canadians' health*. Retrieved from <http://www.wellesleyinstitute.com/wp-content/uploads/2012/02/Colour-Coded-Health-Care-Sheryl-Nestel.pdf>.

Public Health Agency of Canada. (2014). *The chief public health officer's report on the state of public health in Canada, 2014: Public health in the future*. Retrieved from <http://www.phac-aspc.gc.ca/cphorsphc-respcacsp/2014/chang-eng.php>.

Purnell, L. D., & Paulanka, B. J. (1998). *Transcultural health care: A culturally competent approach*. Philadelphia: F.A. Davis.

Querforth, H., & LaFerla, F. (2010). Mechanisms of disease: Alzheimer's disease. *New England Journal of Medicine, 362*(4), 329–344. doi:10.1056/NEJMra0909142.

Raphael, D. (2009). *Social determinants of health: Canadian perspectives*. Toronto, ON: Canadian Scholars Press.

Reason, B., Terner, M., Moses McKeag, A., et al. (2012). The impact of polypharmacy on the health of Canadian seniors. *Family Practice, 29*(4), 427–432. doi:10.1093/fampra/cmr124.

Rieder, M. J. (2011). Drug research and treatment for children in Canada. A challenge. *Paediatric and Child Health, 16*(9), 560.

Srivastava, R. (2006). *The healthcare professional's guide to clinical cultural competence*. Toronto, ON: Elsevier Canada.

Statistics Canada. (2012). *Definitions, data sources and methods. Previous standard—race (ethnicity)*. Retrieved from <http://www.statcan.gc.ca/concepts/definitions/previous-anterieures/ethnicity-ethnicite-pre-eng.htm>.

Statistics Canada. (2013). *Health trends*. Retrieved from <http://www12.statcan.gc.ca/health-sante/82-213/index.cfm?Lang=ENG>.

Statistics Canada. (2014). *Immigration and ethnocultural diversity in Canada*. Retrieved from <http://www12.statcan.gc.ca/nhs-enm/2011/as-sa/99-010-x/99-010-x2011001-eng.cfm>.

University of Ottawa. (2009). *Aboriginal medicine and healing practices*. Retrieved from <http://www.med.uottawa.ca/sim/data/Aboriginal_Medicine_e.htm>.

University of Ottawa. (2015). *Historical determinants of health status of aboriginal people in Canada*. Retrieved from <http://www.med.uottawa.ca/sim/data/Aboriginal_Health_Determinants_e.htm>.

Votova, K., Blais, R., Penning, M. J., et al. (2013). Polypharmacy meets polyherbacy: Pharmaceutical, over-the-counter, and natural health product use among Canadian adults. *Canadian Journal of Public Health, 104*(3), e222–e228.

Wong, S., Ordean, A., Kahan, M., et al. (2011). Substance use in pregnancy SOGC clinical practice guideline. *Journal of Obstetricians & Gynaecologists Canada, 33*(4), 367–384.

Wooten, J. M. (2012). Pharmacotherapy considerations in elderly adults. *Southern Medical Journal, 105*(8), 437–445. Retrieved from <http://www.medscape.com/viewarticle/769412_2>.

Chapter 5

Blix, A. (2014). Personalized medicine, genomics, and pharmacogenomics: A primer for nurses. *Clinical Journal of Oncology Nursing, 18*(4), 437–441. doi:10.1188/14.CJON.437-441.

Cheek, D. J. (2013). What you need to know about pharmacogenomics. *Nursing, 43*(3), 44–49.

Fabbri, C., Porcelli, S., & Serretti, A. (2014). From pharmacogenetics to pharmacogenomics: The way toward the personalization of antidepressant treatment. *Canadian Journal of Psychiatry, 59*(2), 62–75.

Hawcutt, D. B., Thompson, B., Smyth, R. L., et al. (2013). Paediatric pharmacogenomics: An overview. *Archives of Disease in Childhood, 98*(3), 232–237. doi:10.1136/archdischild-2012-302852.

Kaufman, A. L., Spitz, J., Jacobs, M., et al. (2015). Evidence for clinical implementation of pharmacogenomics in cardiac drugs. *Mayo Clinic Proceedings, 90*(6), 716–729. <http://dx.doi.org/10.1016/j.mayocp.2015.03.016> doi.

Mele, C., & Goldschmidt, K. (2014). Pharmacogenomics in pediatrics: Personalized medicine showing eminent promise. *Journal of Pediatric Nursing, 29*(4), 378–382. <http://dx.doi.org/10.1016/j.pedn.2014.04.005> doi.

Pereira, N. L., & Stewart, A. K. (2015). Clinical implementation of cardiovascular pharmacogenomics. *Mayo Clinic Proceedings, 90*(6), 701–704. doi:10.1016/j.mayocp.2015.04.011.

Reynolds, G. P. (2012). The pharmacogenetics of symptom response to antipsychotic drugs. *Psychiatry Investigation, 9*(1), 1–7. doi:10.4306/pi.2012.9.1.1.

Chapter 6

Accreditation Canada, the Canadian Institute for Health Information, the Canadian Patient Safety Institute, et al. (2012). *Medication reconciliation in Canada: Raising the bar—Progress to date and the course ahead.* Ottawa, ON: Accreditation Canada. Retrieved from <http://www.accreditation.ca/sites/default/files/med-rec-en.pdf>.

Antonio Ariza-Montes, A., Muniz, N. M., Montero-Simó, M. J., et al. (2013). Workplace bullying among healthcare workers. *International Journal of Environmental Research and Public Health, 10*(8), 3121–3139. doi:10.3390/ijerph10083121.

Baker, G. R., Norton, P. G., Flintoft, V., et al. (2004). The Canadian adverse events study: The incidence of adverse events among hospital patients in Canada. *Canadian Medical Association Journal, 170*(11), 1678–1686. doi:10.1503/cmaj.1040498.

Canadian Medical Association. (2013). *CMPA takes aim at disruptive behaviour by MDs.* Retrieved from <http://www.cma.ca/cmpa-takes-aim-disruptive-behaviour>.

Canadian Medical Protective Association. (2010). *Just culture of safety: Why protecting quality improvement reviews is important for everyone.* Retrieved from <http://fhs.mcmaster.ca/pediatrics/documents/QIImportant.pdf>.

Canadian Medication Incident Reporting and Prevention System (CMIRPS). (2014). *Canadian medication incident reporting and prevention system.* Retrieved from <http://www.cmirps-scdpim.ca/?p=14>.

Canadian Patient Safety Institute. (2013). *Canadian paediatric adverse events study.* Retrieved from <http://www.patientsafetyinstitute.ca/English/research/commissionedResearch/PaediatricAdverseEvents/Pages/default.aspx>.

Cooper, E. (2014). Nursing student medication errors: A snapshot view from a school of nursing's quality and safety officer. *Journal of Nursing Education, 53*(3S), S51–S54. doi:10.3928/01484834-20140211-03.

Cloete, L. (2015). Reducing medication errors in nursing practice. *Nursing Standard, 29*(20), 50–51.

Disclosure Working Group. (2011). *Canadian disclosure guidelines: Being open and honest with patients and families.* Edmonton, AB: Patient Safety Institute. Retrieved from <http://www.patient-safetyinstitute.ca/en/toolsResources/disclosure/Documents/CPSI%20Canadian%20Disclosure%20Guidelines.pdf>.

Einarsen, S., Hoel, H., Zapf, D., et al. (2011). The concept of bullying at work: The European tradition. In S. Einarsen, H. Hoel, D. Zapf, et al. (Eds.), *Bullying and harassment in the workplace: Developments in theory, research, and practice* (2nd ed., pp. 3–40). New York: CRC Press.

Federwisch, M., Ramos, H., & Adams, S. (2014). The sterile cockpit: An effective approach to reducing medication errors? *American Journal of Nursing, 114,* 47–55. doi:10.1097/01.NAJ.0000443777.80999.5c.

Feldman, L. S., Costa, L. L., Feroli, E. R., et al. (2012). Nurse-pharmacist collaboration on medication reconciliation prevents potential harm. *Journal of Hospital Medicine, 7,* 396–401. doi:10.1002/jhm.1921.

Fernandes, O., & Shojania, K. G. (2012). Medication reconciliation in the hospital: What, why, where, when, who and how? *Healthcare Quarterly, 15,* 42–49. doi:10.12927/hcq.2012.22842.

Gill, F., Corkish, V., Robertson, J., et al. (2012). An exploration of pediatric nurses' compliance with a medication and administration protocol. *Journal for Specialists in Pediatric Nursing, 17,* 136–146. doi:10.1111/j.1744-6155.2012.00331.x.

Greenall, J., Santora, P., Koczmara, C., et al. (2009). Enhancing safe medication use for pediatric patients in the emergency department. *The Canadian Journal of Hospital Pharmacy, 62*(2), 150–153.

Hutchinson, M., Vickers, M., Wilkes, L., et al. (2010). A typology of bullying behaviours: The experiences of Australian nurses. *Journal of Clinical Nursing, 19,* 2319–2328. doi:10.1111/j.1365-2702.2009.03160.x.

Institute for Safe Medication Practices. (2014a). *ISMP's list of high-alert medications.* Retrieved from <http://www.ismp.org/tools/institutionalhighAlert.asp>.

Institute for Safe Medication Practices. (2014b). *Canadian pharmaceutical bar coding project.* Retrieved from <http://www.ismp-canada.org/barcoding/>.

Institute for Safe Medication Practices Canada. (2013). Implementation planning for a medication bar code system. *ISMP Canada Safety Bulletin, 13*(13), 1–6. Retrieved from <http://www.ismp-canada.org/download/safetyBulletins/2013/ISMPCSB2013-13_ImplementationBarCodeSystem.pdf>.

Kovacs Burns, K. (2008). Involving patients and families. Canadian Patient Safety Champions: Collaborating on improving patient safety. *Healthcare Quarterly, 11*, 95–100. doi:10.12927/hcq.2008.19657.

Maaskant, J. M., Eskes, A., van Rijn-Bikker, P., et al. (2013). High-alert medications for pediatric patients: An international modified Delphi study. *Expert Opinion in Drug Safety, 12*(6), 805–814. doi:10.1517/14740338.2013.825247.

Manias, E., Kinney, S., Cranswick, N., et al. (2014). Medication errors in hospitalised children. *Journal of Paediatrics & Child Health, 50*(1), 71–77. doi:10.1111/jpc.12412.

Matlow, A. G., Baker, G. R., Flintoft, V., et al. (2012). Adverse events among children in Canadian hospitals: The Canadian Paediatric Adverse Events Study. *Canadian Medical Association Journal, 184*(13), E709–E718. doi:10.1503/cmaj.112153.

O'Hagan, J., MacKinnon, N. J., Persaud, D., et al. (2010). Self-reported medical errors in seven countries: Implications for Canada. *Healthcare Quarterly, 12*(Spec. Iss.), 55–61.

Patients for Patient Safety Canada. (2012). *Global patient safety alerts. Sharing for learning.* Retrieved from <http://www.patientsforpatientsafety.ca/>.

Potter, P. A., Griffin Perry, A., Ross-Kerr, J. C., et al. (2014). *Canadian fundamentals of nursing* (5th ed.). Toronto, ON: Mosby Canada.

Rogers-Clark, C., Pearce, S., & Cameron, M. (2009). Management of disruptive behaviour within nursing work environments: A comprehensive systematic review of the evidence. *JBI Library of Systematic Reviews, 7*(15), 615–678.

Sears, K., O'Brien-Pallas, L., Stevens, B., et al. (2013). The relationship between the nursing work environment and the occurrence of reported paediatric medication administration errors: A pan Canadian study. *Journal of Pediatric Nursing, 28*(4), 351–356. doi:10.1016/j.pedn.2012.12.003.

Stromquist, L. (2012). *Paediatric opioid safety resource kit. Consensus guidelines.* Retrieved from <http://ken.caphc.org/xwiki/bin/view/PaediatricOpioidSafetyResourceKit/Consensus+Guidelines>.

Wilkins, K., & Shields, M. (2008). Correlates of medication error in hospitals. *Health Reports, 192*, 1–12.

Wittich, C. M., Burkle, C. M., & Lanier, W. L. (2014). Medication errors: An overview for clinicians. *Mayo Clinic Proceedings, 89*(8), 1116–1125. doi:10.1016/j.mayocp.2014.05.007.

World Health Organization. (2016). *A taxonomy for patient safety.* Retrieved from <http://www.who.int/patientsafety/implementation/taxonomy/en/>.

Wright, W., & Khatri, N. (2015). Bullying among nursing staff: relationship with psychological/behavioral responses of nurses and medical errors. *Health Care Management Review, 40*(2), 139–147. doi:10.1097/HMR.0000000000000015.

Zed, P. J., Abu-Laban, R. B., Balen, R. M., et al. (2008). Incidence, severity and preventability of medication-related visits to the emergency department: A prospective study. *The Canadian Medical Association Journal, 178*(12), 153–1569. doi:10.1503/cmaj.071594CMAJ.

Chapter 7

Balestra, M. (2013). Clinical patient education challenges and risks. *Nurse Practitioner, 38*(12), 8–11. doi:10.1097/01.NPR.0000437580.06519.74.

Canadian Literacy and Learning Network. (2015). *Literacy statistics.* Retrieved from <http://www.literacy.ca/literacy/literacy-sub/>.

Canadian Nurses Association. (2015). *Health literacy.* Retrieved from <https://www.nurseone.ca/en/knowledge-features/health-literacy>.

Conn, V. S. (2015). Shifting the patient education paradigm. *Western Journal of Nursing Research, 37*(5), 563–565. doi:10.1177/0193945914568271.

Fitch, M. I., McAndrew, A., & Harth, T. (2013). Measuring trends in performance across time: Providing information to cancer patients. *Canadian Oncology Nursing Journal, 23*(4).

Gattullo, B. A., & McDevitt, D. (2013). On the horizon. Take the patient education challenge. *Nursing Made Incredibly Easy, 11*(3), 8–11.

Kececi, A., & Bulduk, S. (2012). *Health education for the elderly.* Retrieved from <http://cdn.intechopen.com/pdfs-wm/29304.pdf>.

Kelo, M., Martikainen, M., & Eriksson, E. (2013). Patient education of children and their families: Nurses' experiences. *Pediatric Nursing, 39*(2), 71–79. Retrieved from <http://www.pediatricnursing.net/ce/2015/article39011010.pdf>.

Life Literacy Canada. (2015). *Adult literacy facts.* Retrieved from <http://abclifeliteracy.ca/adult-literacy-facts>.

Mullen, E. (2013). Health literacy challenges in the adult population. *Nursing Forum, 48*(4), 248–255. doi:10.1111/nuf.12038.

Okoniewska, B., Santana, M. J., Groshaus, H., et al. (2015). Barriers to discharge in an acute care medical teaching unit: A qualitative analysis of health providers' perceptions. *Journal of Multidisciplinary Healthcare, 8*, 83–89. doi:10.2147/JMDH.S72633.

Polster, D. (2015). Patient discharge information. *Nursing, 45*(5), 42–49.

Public Health Agency of Canada. (2014). *Health literacy.* Retrieved from <http://www.phac-aspc.gc.ca/cd-mc/hl-ls/index-eng.php>.

Reddick, B., & Holland, C. (2015). Reinforcing discharge education and planning. *Nursing Management, 46*(5), 10–14. doi:10.1097/01.NUMA.0000463887.70222.50.

Remshardt, M. A. (2011). The impact of patient literacy on healthcare practices. *Nursing Management, 42*(11), 24–29. doi:10.1097/01.NUMA.0000406576.26956.53.

Roter, D. L., Rude, R. E., & Comings, J. (1998). A barrier to quality of care. *Journal of General Internal Medicine, 13*(12), 850–851. doi:10.1046/j.1525-1497.1998.00250.x.

Shah, R., Desai, S., Gajjar, B., et al. (2013). Factors responsible for noncompliance to drug therapy in the elderly and the impact of patient education on improving compliance. *Drugs & Therapy Perspectives, 29*(11), 360–366. doi:10.1007/s40267-013-0075-3.

Speros, C. I. (2009). More than words: Promoting health literacy in older adults. *The Online Journal of Issues in Nursing, 14*(3), doi:10.3912/OJIN.Vol14No03Man05.

Speros, C. (2011). Promoting health literacy: A nursing imperative. *Nursing Clinics of North America, 46*(3), 321–333.

Tamura-Lis, W. (2013). Teach-back for quality education and patient safety. *Urologic Nursing, 33*(6), 267–298.

VonHoltz, L. A., Hyolite, K. A., Carr, B. G., et al. (2015). Use of mobile apps: A patient-centered approach. *Academic Emergency Medicine : Official Journal of the Society for Academic Emergency Medicine, 22*(6), 765–768. doi:10.1111/acem.12675.

Chapter 8

Bailey, D. G., Dresser, G., & Arnold, J. M. O. (2013). Grapefruit–medication interactions: Forbidden fruit or avoidable consequences? *Canadian Medical Association Journal, 185*(4), doi:10.1503/cmaj.120951.

Benzie, I. F. F., & Wachtel-Galor, S. (Eds.), (2011). *Herbal medicine: Biomolecular and clinical aspects* (2nd ed.). Boca Raton, FL: CRC Press.

Canadian Institute for Health Information. (2014). *Prescribed drug spending in Canada, 2013: A focus on public drug programs.* Retrieved from <https://secure.cihi.ca/free_products/Prescribed%20Drug%20Spending%20in%20Canada_2014_EN.pdf>.

Chen, X. W., Sneed, K. B., Pan, S. Y., et al. (2012). Herb-drug interactions and mechanistic and clinical considerations. *Current Drug Metabolism, 13*(5), 640–651. doi:10.2174/1389200211209050640.

Do, T. T. (2015). *Medical marijuana legal in all forms, Supreme Court rules.* Retrieved from <http://www.cbc.ca/news/politics/medical-marijuana-legal-in-all-forms-supreme-court-rules-1.3109148>.

Goldman, R. (2011). Treating cough and cold: Guidance for caregivers of children and youth. *Paediatrics and Child Health, 16*(9), 564–566.

Hampton, L. M., Nguyen, D. B., Edwards, J. R., et al. (2013). Cough and cold medication adverse events after market withdrawal and labeling revision. *Pediatrics, 132*(6), 1047–1054. doi:10.1542/peds.2013-2236.

Health Canada. (2012). *About natural health products.* Retrieved from <http://www.hc-sc.gc.ca/dhp-mps/prodnatur/about-apropos/cons-eng.php>.

Health Canada. (2015a). *Natural and non-prescription health products.* Retrieved from <http://www.hc-sc.gc.ca/dhp-mps/prodnatur/index-eng.php>.

Health Canada. (2015b). *Guidance document questions and answers: Plain language labelling regulations.* Retrieved from <http://www.hc-sc.gc.ca/dhp-mps/prodpharma/applic-demande/guide-ld/pll_qa_fin_qr_elc-eng.php>.

Institute for Safe Medication Practices Canada. (2013). *Labelling and packaging: An aggregate analysis of medication incident reports.* Retrieved from <https://www.ismp-canada.org/download/LabellingPackaging/ISMPC2013_Labelling-Packaging_FullReport.pdf>.

Khajuria, H., & Navak, B. P. (2014). Detection of Δ9-tetrahydrocannabinol (THC) in hair using GC–MS. *Egyptian Journal of Forensic Sciences, 4*(1), 17–20. doi:10.1016/j.ejfs.2013.10.001.

Natural Health Products Directorate. (2011). *Health Canada Natural health product tracking survey—2010 final report. Ipsos-Reid; 2011.* Retrieved from <http://www.hc-sc.gc.ca/dhp-mps/prodnatur/index-eng.php>

Necyk, C., Barnes, J., Tsuyuki, R. T., et al. (2013). How well do pharmacists know their patients? A case report highlighting natural health product disclosure. *Canadian Pharmacists Journal, 146*(4), 202–209. doi:10.1177/1715163513493387.

Ramsay, C. (2009). *Unnatural regulation: Complementary and alternative medicine policy inCanada.* Studies in Health Care Policy. Retrieved from <https://www.fraserinstitute.org/sites/default/files/UnnaturalRegulation.pdf>.

Romanoa, B., Borrelli, F., Paganoa, E., et al. (2014). Inhibition of colon carcinogenesis by a standardized Cannabis sativa extract with high content of cannabidiol. *Phytomedicine: International Journal of Phytotherapy and Phytopharmacology, 21*, 631–639. doi:10.1016/j.phymed.2013.11.006.

Seden, K., Dickinson, L., Khoo, S., et al. (2010). Grapefruit-drug interactions. *Drugs, 70*(18), 2373–2407.

Sharma, P., Murthy, P., & Bharath, M. M. S. (2012). Chemistry, metabolism, and toxicology of cannabis: Clinical implications. *Iran Journal of Psychiatry, 7*(4), 149–156.

Shaw, D., Ladds, G., Duez, P., et al. (2012). Pharmacovigilance of herbal medicine. *Journal of Ethnopharmacology, 140*(3), 513–518. doi:10.1016/j.jep.2012.01.051.

Shehab, N., Schaefer, M. K., Kegler, S. R., et al. (2010). Adverse events from cough and cold medications after a market withdrawal of products labeled for infants. *Pediatrics, 126*(6), 1100–1107. doi:10.1542/peds.2010-1839.

Sullivan, J. E., & Farrar, H. C. (2011). Fever and antipyretic use in children. *Pediatrics, 127*(3), 580–587. doi:10.1542/peds.2010-3852.

Tachjian, A., Vigar, M., & Jahangir, A. (2010). Use of herbal products and potential interactions in patients with cardiovascular disease. *Journal of the American Association of Cardiology, 55*(6), 515–525. doi:10.1016/j.jacc.2009.07.074.

Walji, R., Boon, H., Barnes, J., et al. (2010). Consumers of natural health products: Natural-born pharmacovigilantes? *BMC Complementary and Alternative Medicine, 10*(8), doi:10.1186/1472-6882-10-8.

World Health Organization. (2015). *Essential medicines and health products. Traditional medicine: Definitions.* Retrieved from <http://www.who.int/medicines/areas/traditional/definitions/en/>.

Chapter 9

Barnes, J. L., Tian, M., Edens, N. K., et al. (2014). Consideration of nutrient levels in studies of cognitive decline. *Nutrition Reviews, 72*(11), 707–719. doi:10.1111/nure.12144.

Chan, T. H. (2015). *Vitamin E and health.* Retrieved from <http://www.hsph.harvard.edu/nutritionsource/vitamin-e/>.

Health Canada. (2010). *Canadian nutrient file.* Retrieved from <http://www.hc-sc.gc.ca/fn-an/nutrition/fiche-nutri-data/index-eng.php>.

Health Canada. (2013). *Dietary reference intakes.* Retrieved from <http://www.hc-sc.gc.ca/fn-an/nutrition/reference/index-eng.php>.

Health Canada. (2015). *Listing of monographs.* Retrieved from <http://webprod.hc-sc.gc.ca/nhpid-bdipsn/monosReq.do?lang=eng>.

Heart and Stroke Foundation. (2015). *Food for your brain.* Retrieved from <http://www.heartandstroke.com/site/apps/nlnet/content2.aspx?c=ikIQLcMWJtE&b=4869055&ct=11767301>.

Langella, C., Naviglio, D., Marino, M., et al. (2015). Study of the effects of a diet supplemented with active components on lipid and glycemic profiles. *Nutrition, 31*(1), 180–186.

Mackawy, A. M. H., Al-ayed, B. M., & Al-rashidi, B. M. (2013). Vitamin D deficiency and its association with thyroid disease. *International Journal of Health Sciences, 7*(3), 267–275.

Paganini-Hill, A., Kawas, C. H., & Corrada, M. M. (2015). Antioxidant vitamin intake and mortality: The Leisure World Cohort Study. *American Journal of Epidemiology, 181*(2), 120–126. doi:10.1093/aje/kwu294.

Podszun, M., & Frank, J. (2014). Vitamin E–drug interactions: molecular basis and clinical relevance. *Nutrition Research Reviews, 27*(2), 215–231. doi:10.1017/S0954422414000146.

Rosenbloom, M. (2014). *Vitamin toxicity.* Retrieved from <http://emedicine.medscape.com/article/819426-overview>.

Simon, K. C., Munger, K. L., & Ascherio, A. (2012). Vitamin D and multiple sclerosis: Epidemiology, immunology, and genetics. *Current Opinion in Neurology, 25*(3), 246–251. doi:10.1097/WCO.0b013e3283533a7e.

Wang, L., Sesso, H. D., Glynn, R. J., et al. (2014). Vitamin E and C supplementation and risk of cancer in men: Posttrial follow-up in the Physicians' Health Study II randomized trial. *American Journal of Clinical Nutrition, 100*(3), 915–923. doi:10.3945/ajcn.114.085480.

Yusuf, S., Dagenais, G., Pogue, J., et al. (2000). Vitamin E supplementation and cardiovascular events in high-risk patients. *New England Journal of Medicine, 342*, 154–160.

Chapter 10

Avşar, G., & Kaşikçi, M. (2013). Assessment of four different methods in subcutaneous heparin applications with regard to causing bruise and pain. *International Journal of Nursing Practice, 19*(4), 402–408. doi:10.1111/ijn.12079.

Bartley, N. (2012). Administering intramuscular and subcutaneous injections in children. *World of Irish Nursing & Midwifery, 20*(8), 39–42.

Beckett, V. L., Tyson, L. D., Carroll, D., et al. (2012). Accurately administering oral medication to children isn't child's play. *Archives of Disease in Childhood, 97*(9), 838–841. doi:10.1136/archdischild-2012-301850.

Centers for Disease Control and Prevention. (2011). Advisory Committee on Immunization Practices (ACIP) recommended immunization schedules for persons ages 0 through 18 years and adults aged 19 years and older. *Morbidity and Mortality Weekly Report. Surveillance Summaries, 62*(Suppl. 1), 1. Retrieved from <www.cdc.gov/mmwr/pdf/wk/mm62e0128.pdf>.

Centers for Disease Control and Prevention. (2015). *Vaccine administration.* Retrieved from <http://www.cdc.gov/vaccines/pubs/pinkbook/vac-admin.html>.

Crawford, C. L., & Johnson, J. A. (2012). To aspirate or not: An integrative review of the evidence. *Nursing, 42*(3), 20–25. doi:10.1097/01.NURSE.0000411417.91161.87.

FIT Canada. (2011). *FIT forum for injection technique Canada. Recommendations for best practice in injection technique.* Retrieved from <http://novonordisk.ca/PDF_Files/FIT_Recommendations_2011_ENG.pdf>.

Goossens, G. A. (2015). Flushing and locking of venous catheters: Available evidence and evidence deficit. *Nursing Research and Practice, 2015*, <http://dx.doi.org/10.1155/2015/985686>.

Hensel, D., Morson, G. L., & Preuss, E. A. (2013). Best practices in newborn injections. *MCN. The American Journal of Maternal Child Nursing, 38*(3), 163–167. doi:10.1097/NMC.0b013e31827eae59.

Herrera, A. (2013). Proper technique for an intramuscular injection. *Clinical Advisor for Nurse Practitioners, 16*(6), 78.

Kassab, M. I., Roydhouse, J. K., Fowler, C., et al. (2012). The effectiveness of glucose in reducing needle-related procedural pain in infants. *Journal of Pediatric Nursing, 27*(1), 3–17. doi:10.1016/j.pedn.2010.10.008.

Koster, M. P., Stellato, N., Kohn, N., et al. (2009). Needle length for immunization of early adolescents as determined by ultrasound. *Pediatrics, 124*(2), 667–672. doi:10.1542/peds.2008-1127.

McWilliam, P. L., Botwinski, C. A., & LaCourse, J. R. (2014). Deltoid intramuscular injections and obesity. *Medsurg Nursing, 23*(1), 4–7.

Ogston-Tuck, S. (2014a). Subcutaneous injection technique: An evidence-based approach. *Nursing Standard, 29*(3), 53–58.

Ogston-Tuck, S. (2014b). Intramuscular injection technique: An evidence-based approach. *Nursing Standard, 29*(4), 52–59.

Paparella, S., & Paparella, S. (2010). Identified safety risks with splitting and crushing oral medications. *Journal of Emergency Nursing, 36*(2), 156–158. doi:10.1016/j.jen.2009.11.019.

Pourghaznein, T., Azimi, A. V., & Jafarabadi, M. (2014). The effect of injection duration and injection site on pain and bruising of subcutaneous injection of heparin. *Journal of Clinical Nursing, 23*(7/8), 1105–1113. doi:10.1111/jocn.12291.

Public Health Agency of Canada. (2013). *Canadian immunization guide*. Retrieved from <http://www.phac-aspc.gc.ca/publicat/cig-gci/p01-07-eng.php>.

Radmacher, P. G., Adamkin, M. D., Lewis, S. T., et al. (2012). Milk as a vehicle for oral medications: Hidden osmoles. *Journal of Perinatology*, 32(3), 227–229. doi:10.1038/jp.2011.83.

Rishovd, A. (2014). Pediatric intramuscular injections: Guidelines for best practice. *The American Journal of Maternal Child Nursing*, 39(2), 107–114. doi:10.1097/NMC.0000000000000009.

Sepah, Y., Samad, L., Altaf, A., et al. (2014). Aspiration in injections: Should we continue or abandon the practice? *F1000Research*, 3(157), doi:10.12688/f1000research.1113.1.

Uzelli, D., & Yapucu, G. Ü. (2015). Oral glucose solution to alleviate pain induced by intramuscular injections in preterm infants. *Journal for Specialists in Pediatric Nursing*, 20(1), 29–35. doi:10.1111/jspn.12094.

Walters, M. C., & Furyk, J. (2012). Paediatric intramuscular injections for developing world settings: A review of the literature for best practices. *Journal of Transcultural Nursing*, 23(4), 406–409. doi:10.1177/1043659612451600.

World Health Organization. (2009). *WHO guidelines on hand hygiene in health care: A summary. First global patient safety challenge—Clean care is safer care*. Retrieved from <http://www.who.int/gpsc/5may/tools/who_guidelines-hand-hygiene_summary.pdf>.

World Health Organization. (2010). *WHO best practices for injections and related procedures toolkit*. Geneva, CH: Source. Retrieved from <http://whqlibdoc.who.int/publications/2010/9789241599252_eng.pdf>.

Zhu, L. L., & Zhou, Q. (2013). Therapeutic concerns when oral medications are administered nasogastrically. *Journal of Clinical Pharmacy & Therapeutics*, 38(4), 272–276. doi:10.1111/jcpt.12041edit.

Chapter 11

Abdel, R. A., & Az El-Dein, N. (2009). Effect of breast-feeding on pain relief during infant immunization injections. *International Journal of Nursing Practice*, 15(2), 99–104. doi:10.1111/j.1440-172X.2009.01.

Chou, R., & Argoff, C. E. (2014). *11 tips for better opioid prescribing*. Retrieved from <http://www.medscape.com/viewarticle/831323_3>.

Elsamra, S. E., & Ellsworth, P. (2012). Effects of analgesic and anesthetic medications on lower urinary tract function. *Urologic Nursing*, 32(2), 60–67. Retrieved from <http://www.medscape.com/viewarticle/763040_4>.

Fisher, J. E., Zhang, Y., Sketris, I., et al. (2012). The effect of an educational intervention on meperidine use in Nova Scotia, Canada: A time series analysis. *Pharmacoepidemiology & Drug Safety*, 21(2), 177–183. doi:10.1002/pds.2259.

Glowacki, D. (2015). Effective pain management and improvements in patients' outcomes andsatisfaction. *Critical Care Nurse*, 35(3), 33–43. doi:10.4037/ccn2015440.

Chapter 12

Chandran, G. J., & Lalonde, D. H. (2010). A review of pain pumps in plastic surgery. A review of pain pumps in plastic surgery. *Canadian Journal of Plastic Surgery*, 18(1), 15–18.

Ganzberg, S., & Kramer, K. J. (2010). The use of local anesthetic agents in medicine. *Dental Clinics of North America*, 54(4), 601–610. doi:10.1016/j.cden.2010.06.001.

Green, J. L., Heard, K. J., Reynolds, K. M., et al. (2013). Oral and intravenous acetylcysteine for treatment of acetaminophen toxicity: A systematic review and meta-analysis. *Western Journal of Emergency Medicine*, 14(3), 218–226. doi:10.5811/westjem.2012.4.6885.

Health Canada. (2015). *Summary safety review—Acetaminophen—Liver injury*. Retrieved from <http://www.hc-sc.gc.ca/dhp-mps/medeff/reviews-examens/acetamino-eng.php>.

Janssen, J., & Singh-Saluja, S. (2015). How much did you take? Reviewing acetaminophen toxicity. *Canadian Family Physician*, 61(4), 347–349.

Kirksey, K. M., McGlory, G., & Sefcik, E. F. (2015). Pain assessment and management in critically ill older adults. *Critical Care Nursing Quarterly*, 38(3), 234–244. doi:10.1097/CNQ.0000000000000071.

Lingappan, A. M. (2014). *Sedation*. Retrieved from <http://emedicine.medscape.com/article/809993>.

Orlewicz, M. S. (2014). *Procedural sedation*. Retrieved from <http://emedicine.medscape.com/article/109695>.

Press, C. D. (2013). *Subarachnoid spinal block*. Retrieved from <http://emedicine.medscape.com/article/2000841>.

Registered Nurses' Association of Ontario. (2013). *Clinical best practice guidelines: Assessment and management of pain* (3rd ed.). Retrieved from <http://rnao.ca/sites/rnao-ca/files/AssessAndManagementOfPain_15_WEB-_FINAL_DEC_2.pdf>.

Strøm, C., Rasmussen, L. S., & Sieber, F. E. (2014). Should general anaesthesia be avoided inthe elderly? *Anaesthesia*, 69(Suppl. 1), 35–44. doi:10.1111/anae.12493.

Taddio, A., Appleton, M., Bortolussi, R., et al. (2010). Reducing the pain of childhood vaccination: An evidence-based clinical practice guideline. *Canadian Medical Association Journal*, 182(18), E843–E855. doi:10.1503/cmaj.092048. A review of pain pumps in plastic surgery.

Chapter 13

Alternative and Complementary Therapies. (2014). Clinical roundup: Selected treatment options for sleep disorders. *Alternative and Complementary Therapies*, 20(6), 347–353. doi:10.1089/act.2014.20606.

BaHammam, A. S. (2011). Sleep from an Islamic perspective. *Annals of Thoracic Medicine*, 6(4), 187–192. doi:10.4103/1817-1737.84771.

Canham, S. L., & Rubinstein, R. L. (2015). Experiences of sleep and benzodiazepine use among older women. *Journal of Women & Aging*, 27(2), 123–139. doi:10.1080/08952841.2014.928173.

Cox Sullivan, S. (2015). Getting the rest you deserve. *Arkansas Nursing News, 11*(1), 15–19.

George, N. M., & Davis, J. E. (2013). Assessing sleep in adolescents through a better understanding of sleep physiology. *American Journal of Nursing, 113*(6), 26–32. doi:10.1097/01. NAJ.0000430921.99915.24.

Gooneratne, N. S., & Vitiello, M. V. (2014). Sleep in older adults: Normative changes, sleep disorders, and treatment options. *Clinics in Geriatric Medicine, 30*(3), 591–627. doi:10.1016/j. cger.2014.04.007.

Lubit, R. H. (2015). *Sleep disorders.* Retrieved from <http:// emedicine.medscape.com/article/287104-overview>.

Malhotra, S., Sawhney, G., & Pandhi, P. (2015). *The therapeutic potential of melatonin: A review of the science.* Retrieved from <http://www.medscape.com/viewarticle/472385>.

McKenry, L., Tessier, E., & Hogan, M. (2006). *Mosby's Pharmacology in Nursing* (22nd ed.). St. Louis, MO: Mosby.

Muliira, J. K., & Muliira, R. S. (2013). Teaching culturally appropriate therapeutic touch to nursing students in the Sultanate of Oman: Reflections on observations and experiences with Muslim patients. *Holistic Nursing Practice, 27*(1), 45–48. doi:10.1097/HNP.0b013e318276fccf.

National Institute on Drug Abuse. (2012). *Well-known mechanism underlies benzodiazepines' addictive properties.* Retrieved from <http://www.drugabuse.gov/news-events/ nida-notes/2012/04/well-known-mechanism-underlies-benzodiazepines-addictive-properties>.

Norton, C., Flood, D., Brittin, A., et al. (2015). Improving sleep for patients in acute hospitals. *Nursing Standard, 29*(28), 35–42. doi:10.7748/ns.29.28.35.e8947.

Reiter, J., & Rosen, D. (2014). The diagnosis and management of common sleep disorders in adolescents. *Current Opinion in Pediatrics, 26*(4), 407–412. doi:10.1097/MOP.000000000000 0113.

Stevens, M. S. (2013). *Normal sleep, sleep physiology, and sleep deprivation.* Retrieved from <http://emedicine.medscape. com/article/1188226-overview>.

Troester, M. M., & Pelayo, R. (2015). Pediatric sleep pharmacology: A primer. *Seminars in Pediatric Neurology, 22*(2), 135–147. doi:10.1016/j.spen.2015.03.002.

Williamson, L. (2015). Counting sleep. Tips that will help you wake up rested and refreshed. *Diabetes Forecast, 68*(1), 24–26, 28.

Chapter 14

Chen, L., Crum, R. M., Strain, E. C., et al. (2015). Patterns of concurrent substance use among adolescent nonmedical ADHD stimulant users: Results from the National Survey on Drug Use and Health. *Addictive Behaviors, 49*, 1–6. doi:10.1016/j.drugalcdep.2014.05.022.

Com, G., Einen, M. A., & Jambhekar, S. (2015). Narcolepsy with cataplexy: Diagnostic challenge in children. *Clinical Pediatrics, 54*(1), 5–14. doi:10.1177/0009922814526301.

Cook, N. (2013). Understanding narcolepsy: The wider perspective. *British Journal of Neuroscience Nursing, 9*(2), 76–82. doi:10.12968/bjnn.2013.9.2.76.

De la Herrán-Arita, A. K., & García-García, F. (2013). Current and emerging options for the drug treatment of narcolepsy. *Drugs, 73*(16), 1771–1781.

Feldman, M., & Bélanger, S. (2009, Reaffirmed 2013). Extended-release medications for children and adolescents with attention-deficit hyperactivity disorder. *Paediatric Child Health, 14*(9), 593–597.

Health Canada. (2015). *Summary safety review—Amphetamines—Suicidal thoughts and behaviours (suicidality).* Retrieved from <http://www.hc-sc.gc.ca/dhp-mps/medeff/reviews -examens/amphetamines-eng.php>.

Janssen, I. (2013). The public health burden of obesity in Canada. *Canadian Journal of Diabetes, 37*(2), 90–96. doi:10.1016/j. jcjd.2013.02.059.

Jones, B., & Bloom, S. (2015). The new era of drug therapy for obesity: The evidence and the expectations. *Drugs, 75*(9), 935–945. doi:10.1007/s40265-015-0410-1.

Kiely, B., & Adesman, A. (2015). What we do not know about ADHD … yet. *Current Opinion in Pediatrics, 27*(3), 395–404. doi:10.1097/MOP.0000000000000229.

Leschziner, G. (2014). Narcolepsy: A clinical review. *Practical Neurology, 14*(5), 323–331. doi:10.1136/practneurol-2014-000837.

Lipton, R. B., Fanning, K. M., Serrano, D., et al. (2015). Ineffective acute treatment of episodic migraine is associated with new-onset chronic migraine. *Neurology, 84*(7), 688–695. doi:10.1212/WNL.0000000000001256.

Navaneelan, T., & Janz, T. (2014). *Adjusting the scales: Obesity in the Canadian population after correcting for respondent bias.* (Catalogue number 82-624-X). Retrieved from <http:// www.statcan.gc.ca/pub/82-624-x/2014001/article/11922-eng.htm>.

Nye, B., & Thadani, V. M. (2015). Migraine and epilepsy: Review of the literature. Headache. *The Journal of Head and Face Pain, 55*(3), 359–380. doi:10.1111/head.12536.

Rabbie, R., Derry, S., Moore, R. A., et al. (2010). Ibuprofen with or without an antiemetic for acute migraine headaches in adults. *The Cochrane Database of Systematic Reviews,* (10), doi:10.1002/14651858.CD008039.pub2.

Swift, K. D., Sayal, K., & Hollis, C. (2014). ADHD and transitions to adult mental health services: A scoping review. *Child: Care, Health and Development, 40*(6), 775–786. doi:10.1111/cch.12107.

Tarver, J., Daley, D., & Sayal, K. (2014). Attention-deficit hyperactivity disorder (ADHD): An updated review of the essential facts. *Child: Care, Health and Development, 40*(6), 762–774. doi:10.1111/cch.12139.

Tsai, M. H., & Huang, Y. S. (2010). Attention-deficit/hyperactivity disorder and sleep disorders in children. *Medical Clinics of North America, 94*(3), 615–632. doi:10.1016/j.mcna. 2010.03.008.

Chapter 15

Abend, N. S., Bearden, D., Helbig, I., et al. (2014). Status epilepticus and refractory status epilepticus management. *Seminars in Pediatric Neurology, 21*(4), 263–274. doi:10.1016/S1474-4422(11)70187-9.

Brophy, G. M., Bell, R., Claassen, J., et al. (2012). Guidelines for the evaluation and management of status epilepticus. *Seminars in Pediatric Neurology, 21*(4), 263–274. doi:10.1007/s12028-012-9695-z.

Dworetzky, B. A., Bromfield, E. B., Townsend, M. K., et al. (2010). A prospective study of smoking, caffeine, and alcohol as risk factors for seizures or epilepsy in young adult women: Data from the Nurses' Health Study II. *Epilepsia, 51*(2), 198–205. doi:10.1111/j.1528-1167.2009.02268.x.

Faulkner, M. A. (2014). Perampanel: A new agent for adjunctive treatment of partial seizures. *American Journal of Health-System Pharmacy, 71*(3), 191–198. doi:10.2146/ajhp 130203.

Friedman, J. N., & Canadian Paediatric Society, & Acute Care Committee. (2011, Reaffirmed 2014). Emergency management of the paediatric patient with generalized convulsive status epilepticus. *Paediatric Child Care, 16*(2), 91–97.

Gidal, B. E. (2012). Generic antiepileptic drugs: How good is close enough? *Epilepsy Currents, 12*(1), 32–34. doi:10.5698/1535-7511-12.1.32.

Harding, A., & Clark, L. (2014). Pediatric migraine. *Nurse Practitioner, 39*(11), 22–32.

Nye, B., & Thadani, V. M. (2015). Migraine and epilepsy: Review of the literature. *Headache: The Journal of Head & Face Pain, 55*(3), 359–380. doi:10.1111/head.12536.

Ochoa, J. G. (2013). *Antiepileptic drugs.* Retrieved from <http://emedicine.medscape.com/article/1187334-overview>.

Roth, J. L. (2014). *Status epilepticus.* Retrieved from <http://emedicine.medscape.com/article/1164462-overview>.

Shaw, S. J., & Hartman, A. L. (2010). The controversy over generic antiepileptic drugs. *The Journal of Pediatric Pharmacology and Therapeutics, 15*(2), 81–93.

Stone, M. (2010). Prescribing newer antiepileptics. *Nurse Prescribing, 8*(7), 333–338.

Talati, R., Scholle, J. M., Phung, O. P., et al. (2012). Efficacy and safety of innovator versus generic drugs in patients with epilepsy: systematic review. *Pharmacotherapy, 32*(4), 314–322. doi:10.1002/j.1875-9114.2012.01099.x.

Chapter 16

Connolly, B. S., & Lang, A. E. (2014). Pharmacological treatment of Parkinson disease: A review. *Journal of the American Medical Association, 311*(16), 1670–1683. doi:10.1001/jama.2014.3654.

Devos, D., Moreau, C., Dujardin, K., et al. (2013). New pharmacological options for treating advanced Parkinson's disease. *Clinical Therapeutics, 35*(10), 1640–1652. doi:10.1016/j.clinthera.2013.08.011.

Giugni, J. C., & Okun, M. S. (2014). Treatment of advanced Parkinson's disease. *Current Opinion in Neurology, 27*(4), 450–460.

Hinz, M., Stein, A., & Cole, T. (2014). The Parkinson's disease death rate: Carbidopa and vitamin B6. *Clinical Pharmacology, 6*, 161–169. doi:10.2147/cpaa.s70707.

Kalia, L. V., & Lang, A. E. (2015). Parkinson's disease. *The Lancet, 386*(9996), 896–912. doi:10.1016/S0140-6736(14)61393-3.

Löhle, M., Ramberg, C.-J., Reichmann, H., et al. (2014). Early versus delayed initiation of pharmacotherapy in Parkinson's disease. *Drugs, 74*(6), 645–657. doi:10.1007/s40265-014-0209-5.

Macphee, G. J., & Stewart, D. A. (2012). Parkinson's disease: Treatment and non-motor features. *Reviews in Clinical Gerontology, 22*(4), 243–260. doi:10.1017/S0959259812000093.

Magennis, B., Lynch, T., & Corry, M. (2014). Current trends in the medical management of Parkinson's disease: Implications for nursing practice. *British Journal of Neuroscience Nursing, 10*(2), 67–74. doi:10.12968/bjnn.2014.10.2.67.

Nolden, L. F., Tartavoulle, T., & Porche, D. J. (2014). Parkinson's disease: Assessment, diagnosis, and management. *Journal for Nurse Practitioners, 10*(7), 500–506. doi:10.1016/j.nurpra.2014.04.019.

Pahwa, R., & Lyons, K. E. (2014). Treatment of early Parkinson's disease. *Current Opinion in Neurology, 27*(4), 442–449.

Parkinson Society Canada. (2009). *Stem cell research and Parkinson's disease.* Retrieved from <http://www.parkinson.ca/atf/cf/%7B9EBD08A9-7886-4B2D-A1C4-A131E7096BF8%7D/stem%20cells%20-%20en.pdf>.

Parkinson Society Canada. (2012). *Canadian guidelines on Parkinson's disease.* Retrieved from <http://www.parkinsonclinicalguidelines.ca/home>.

Parkinson's Disease Foundation. (2016). *Causes.* Retrieved from <http://www.pdf.org/en/causes?gclid=COKGxcn5wsoCFQcOaQodz30JSw>.

Public Health Agency of Canada. (2014). *Mapping connections. An understanding of neurological conditions in Canada.* Retrieved from <http://www.phac-aspc.gc.ca/publicat/cd-mc/mc-ec/section-3-eng.php>.

Skelly, R. M., Lindop, F., & Johnson, C. (2012). Multidisciplinary care of patients with Parkinson's disease. *Progress in Neurology and Psychiatry, 16*(2), 10–14.

Wong, S. L., Gilmore, H., & Ramage-Morin, P. L. (2015). *Parkinson's disease: Prevalence, diagnosis and impact.* Retrieved from <http://www.statcan.gc.ca/pub/82-003-x/2014011/article/14112-eng.htm>.

Chapter 17

Agar, L. (2010). Recognizing neuroleptic malignant syndrome in the emergency department: A case study. *Perspectives in Psychiatric Care, 46*(2), 143–151. doi:10.1111/j.1744-6163.2010.00250.x.

Al-Harbi, K. S. (2012). Treatment-resistant depression: Therapeutic trends, challenges, and future directions. *Patient Preference and Adherence, 6*, 369–388. doi:10.2147/PPA.S29716.

American Association of Suicidology. (2015). *Know the warning signs of suicide.* Retrieved from <http://www.suicidology.org/resources/warning-signs>.

Baldwin, D. S., Anderson, I. M., Nutt, D. J., et al. (2014). Evidence-based pharmacological treatment of anxiety disorders, post-traumatic stress disorder and obsessive-compulsive disorder: A revision of the 2005 guidelines from the British Association for Psychopharmacology. *Journal of Psychopharmacology, 28*(5), 403–439. doi:10.1177/0269881114525674.

Bell Canada. (2015). *Bell Let's Talk.* Retrieved from <http://letstalk.bell.ca/en/our-initiatives/pillars/workplace-health/>.

Bentley, S. M., Pagalilauan, G. I., & Simpson, S. A. (2014). Major depression. *Medical Clinics of North America, 98,* 981–1005. doi:10.1016/j.mcna.2014.06.013.

Benze, T. I. (2012). *Neuroleptic malignant syndrome.* Retrieved from <http://emedicine.medscape.com/article/816018>.

Brenner, C. J., & Shyn, S. I. (2015). Diagnosis and management of bipolar disorder in primary care: A DSM-5 update. *Medical Clinics of North America, 98*(5), 1025–1048. doi:10.1016/j.mcna.2014.06.004.

Canadian Institute for Health Information. (2012). *The use of selected psychotropic drugs among seniors on public drug programs in Canada, 2001 to 2010.* Retrieved from <https://secure.cihi.ca/free_products/psychotropic_AIB_2012_en.pdf>.

Canadian Task Force on Preventive Health Care. (2012). *Screening for depression.* Retrieved from <http://canadiantaskforce.ca/ctfphc-guidelines/2013-depression/systematic-review/>.

Clifford, K. M., Duncan, N. A., Heinrich, K., et al. (2015). Update on managing generalized anxiety disorder in older adults. *Journal of Gerontological Nursing, 41*(4), 10–20. doi:10.3928/00989134-20150313-03.

Combs, H., & Markman, J. (2014). Anxiety disorders in primary care. *Medical Clinics of North America, 98,* 1007–1023. doi:10.1016/j.mcna.2014.06.003.

Cooper, B. E., & Sejnowski, C. A. (2013). Serotonin syndrome: Recognition and treatment. *AACN Advanced Critical Care, 24*(1), 15–22.

Cooper, W. O., Callahan, S. T., Shintani, A., et al. (2014). Antidepressants and suicide attempts in children. *Pediatrics, 133*(2), 204–210. doi:10.1542/peds.2013-0923.

Creswell, C., Waite, P., & Cooper, P. J. (2014). Assessment and management of anxiety disorders in children and adolescents. *Archives of Disease in Childhood, 99*(7), 674–678. doi:10.1136/archdischild-2013-303768.

Curran, G., & Ravindran, A. (2014). Lithium for bipolar disorder: A review of the recent literature. *Expert Review of Neurotherapy, 14*(9), 1079–1098. doi:10.1586/14737175.2014.947965.

Dale, E., Bang-Anderson, B., & Sánchez, C. (2015). Emerging mechanisms and treatments for depression beyond SSRIs and SNRIs. *Biochemical Pharmacology, 95*(2), 81–97. doi:10.1016/j.bcp.2015.03.011.

Davis, S. A., Feldman, S. R., & Taylor, S. L. (2014). Use of St. John's Wort in potentially dangerous combinations. *Journal of Alternative & Complementary Medicine, 20*(7), 578–579. doi:10.1089/acm.2013.0216.

Eapen, V., Shiers, D., & Curtis, J. (2013). Bridging the gap from evidence to policy and practice: Reducing the progression to metabolic syndrome for children and adolescents on antipsychotic medication. *Australian and New Zealand Journal of Psychiatry, 47,* 435–442. doi:10.1177/0004867412463169.

Endres, J., Graber, M. A., & Dachs, R. (2015). Benzodiazepines and Alzheimer disease. *American Family Physician, 91*(3), 191–192.

Enns, M. W., & Reiss, J. P. (2015). *Electroconvulsive therapy.* Retrieved from <https://ww1.cpa-apc.org/Publications/Position_Papers/Therapy.asp>.

Fabbri, C., Marsano, A., Balestri, M., et al. (2013). Clinical features and drug induced side effects in early versus late antidepressant responders. *Journal of Psychiatric Research, 47*(10), 1309–1318. doi:10.1016/j.jpsychires.2013.05.020.

Freudenreich, O., & McEvoy, J. (2014). *Guidelines for prescribing clozapine in schizophrenia.* Retrieved from <http://www.uptodate.com/contents/guidelines-for-prescribing-clozapine-in-schizophrenia>.

Gordon, M. S., & Melvin, G. A. (2014). Do antidepressants make children and adolescents suicidal? *Journal of Paediatrics & Child Health, 50*(11), 847–854. doi:10.1111/jpc.12655.

Government of Canada. (2015). *Canada's food guides.* Retrieved from <http://healthycanadians.gc.ca/eating-nutrition/healthy-eating-saine-alimentation/food-guide-aliment/index-eng.php>.

Greenier, E., Lukyanova, V., & Reede, L. (2014). Serotonin syndrome: Fentanyl and selective serotonin reuptake inhibitor interactions. *American Association of Nurse Anesthetists Journal, 82*(5), 340–345.

Health Canada. (2010). *Eating well with Canada's Food Guide—First Nations, Inuit, and Métis.* Retrieved from <http://www.hc-sc.gc.ca/fn-an/pubs/fnim-pnim/index-eng.php>.

Høiseth, G., Kristiansen, K. M., Kvande, K., et al. (2013). Benzodiazepines in geriatric psychiatry. *Drugs and Aging, 30*(2), 113–118. doi:10.1007/s40266-012-0045-9.

Howard, P., Twycross, R., Shuster, J., et al. (2014). Benzodiazepines. *Journal of Pain & Symptom Management, 47*(5), 955–964.

Johnsen, E., Sinkeviciute, I., Løberg, L.-M., et al. (2013). Hallucinations in acutely admitted patients with psychosis, and effectiveness of risperidone, olanzapine, quetiapine, and ziprasidone. A pragmatic, randomized study. *BMC Psychiatry, 13*(241), Retrieved from <http://www.medscape.com/viewarticle/812628>.

Kalapatapu, R. K. (2015). *Electroconvulsive therapy.* Retrieved from <http://emedicine.medscape.com/article/1525957>.

Leiter, L. A., Fitchett, D. H., Gilbert, R. E., et al. (2011). Cardiometabolic risk in Canada: A detailed analysis and position paper by the cardiometabolic risk working group. *Canadian Journal of Cardiology, 27*(2), e1–e33. doi:10.1016/j.cjca.2010.12.054.

Lépine, J.-P., & Briley, M. (2011). The increasing burden of depression. *Neuropsychiatric Disease and Treatment, 7*(Suppl. 1), 3–7. doi:10.2147/NDT.S19617.

Loy, J. H., Merry, S. N., Hetrick, S. E., et al. (2012). Atypical antipsychotics for disruptive behaviour disorders in children and youths. *The Cochrane Database of Systematic Reviews,* (9), doi:10.1002/14651858.CD008559.pub2.

Malhi, G. S., McAulay, C., Das, P., et al. (2015). Maintaining mood stability in bipolar disorder: a clinical perspective on pharmacotherapy. *Evidence-Based Mental Health, 18*(1), 1–6. doi:10.1136/eb-2014-101948.

McBride, M. E. (2015). Beyond butterflies: Generalized anxiety disorder in adolescents. *Nurse Practitioner, 40*(3), 28–37. doi:10.1097/01.NPR.0000460852.60234.8b.

McIntosh, B., Clark, M., & Spry, C. (2011). *Benzodiazepines in older adults: A review of clinical effectiveness, cost-effectiveness, and guidelines*. Ottawa, ON: Canadian Agency for Drugs and Technologies in Health. Retrieved from <http://www.cadth.ca/index.php/en/hta/reportspublications/search/publication/2773>.

Melton, S. T., & Kirkwood, C. K. (2014). Anxiety disorders I: Generalized anxiety, panic, and social anxiety disorders. In J. T. DiPiro, R. L. Talbert, G. C. Yee, et al. (Eds.), *Pharmacotherapy: A pathophysiologic approach* (Chapter 53). New York, NY: McGraw-Hill.

Melville, N. A. (2012). *Low-dose ketamine may be effective for resistant depression*. Retrieved from <http://www.medscape.com/viewarticle/765252>.

Miller, L. J., Ghadiali, N. Y., Larusso, E. M., et al. (2015). Bipolar disorder in women. *Health Care for Women International, 36*(4), 475–498. doi:10.1080/07399332.2014.962138.

Nielsen, R. E., Wallenstein, J. S., & Nielsen, J. (2012). Neuroleptic malignant syndrome—an 11-year longitudinal case-control study. *Canadian Journal of Psychiatry, 57*(8), 512–518.

Nierengarten, M. B. (2015). Bipolar disorder in children: Assessment and diagnosis. *Contemporary Pediatrics, 32*(5), 34–38.

Riordan, H. J., Antonini, P., & Murphy, M. F. (2011). Atypical antipsychotics and metabolic syndrome in patients with schizophrenia: Risk factors, monitoring, and healthcareimplications. *American Health and Drug Benefits, 4*(5), 292–302.

Rotermann, M., Sanmartin, C., Hennessy, D., et al. (2014). Prescription medication use by Canadians aged 6 to 79. *Health Reports, 25*(6), 3–9.

Samples, H., & Mojtabai, R. (2015). Antidepressant self-discontinuation: Results from the collaborative psychiatric epidemiology surveys. *Psychiatric Services, 66*(5), 455–462. <http://dx.doi.org/10.1176/appl.ps.201400021>.

Sarris, J. (2013). St. John's Wort for the treatment of psychiatric disorders. *Psychiatric Clinics of North America, 36*(1), 65–72.

Seehusen, D. A., & Sheridan, R. (2013). Second-generation antidepressants for depression in adults. *American Family Physician, 88*(10), 687–689.

Severus, E., Taylor, M. J., Sauer, C., Pfennig, A., Ritter, P., Baure, M., et al. (2014). Lithium for prevention of mood episodes in bipolar disorders: Systematic review and meta-analysis. *International Journal of Bipolar Disorders, 2*(15), doi:10.1186/s40345-014-0015-8.

Sommer, I. E., Slotema, C. W., Daskalakis, Z. J., et al. (2012). The treatment of hallucinations in schizophrenia spectrum disorders. *Schizophrenia Bulletin, 38*(4), 704–714. doi:10.1093/schbul/sbs034.

Spijker, J., van Straten, A., Bockting, C. L., et al. (2013). Psychotherapy, antidepressants, and their combination for chronic major depressive disorder: A systematic review. *Canadian Journal of Psychiatry, 58*(7), 386–392.

Stone, M. B. (2014). The FDA warning on antidepressants and suicidality—Why the controversy? *New England Journal of Medicine, 371*(18), 1668–1671. doi:10.1056/nejmp1411138.

Thronson, R., & Pagalilauan, G. I. (2014). Psychopharmacology. *Medical Clinics of North America, 98*, 927–958. doi:10.1016/j.mcna.2014.06.001.

Vieta, E. (2014). Antidepressants in bipolar I disorder: Never as monotherapy. *American Journal of Psychiatry, 171*(10), 1023–1026. doi:10.1176/appi.ajp.2014.14070826.

Voulgari, C., Giannas, R., Paterakis, G., et al. (2015). Clozapine-induced late agranulocytosis and severe neutropenia complicated with Streptococcus pneumonia, venous thromboembolism, and allergic vasculitis in treatment-resistant female psychosis. *Case Reports in Medicine, 2015*(2015), <http://dx.doi.org/10.1155/2015/703218>.

Wong, A., Benedict, N. J., Armahizer, M. J., et al. (2015). Evaluation of adjunctive ketamine to benzodiazepines for management of alcohol withdrawal syndrome. *Annals of Pharmacotherapy, 49*(1), 14–19. doi:10.1177/1060028014555859.

Yarnell, E. (2015). Herbal adjuncts to antidepressants. *Alternative & Complementary Therapies, 21*(3), 131–137. doi:10.1089/act.2015.29003.ey.

Yogaratnam, J., Biswas, N., Vadivel, R., et al. (2013). Metabolic complications of schizophrenia and antipsychotic medications—An updated review. *East Asian Archives of Psychiatry, 23*(1), 21–28.

Chapter 18

Baird, C. A., & Furek, M. W. (2012). Adolescents and inhalant abuse: How huffing affects the myelin sheath. *Journal of Addictions Nursing, 23*(2), 129–131. doi:10.3109/10884602.2012.669422.

Baydala, L. (2010 [Reaffirmed 2014]). Inhalant abuse. *Paediatrics and Child Health, 15*(7), 443–448.

Bechtold, J., Simpson, T., White, H. R., et al. (2015). Chronic adolescent marijuana use as a risk factor for physical and mental health problems in young adult men. *Psychology of Addictive Behaviors, 29*(3), 552–563. doi:10.1037/abd0000103.

Boak, A., Hamilton, H. A., Adlaf, E. M., et al. (2013). *Drug use among Ontario students, 1977–2013: OSDUHS highlights (CAMH Research Document Series No. 37)*. Toronto, ON: Centre for Addiction and Mental Health.

Branswell, H. (2015). *Naloxone's prescription-only status to get Health Canada review*. Retrieved from <http://www.cbc.ca/news/health/naloxone-s-prescription-only-status-to-get-health-canada-review-1.3166867>.

Burns, M. J. (2015). *Delirium tremens (DTs)*. Retrieved from <http://emedicine.medscape.com/article/166032>.

Canadian Centre on Substance Abuse. (2014). *Childhood and adolescent pathways to substance use disorders*. Retrieved from <http://www.ccsa.ca/Resource%20Library/CCSA-Child-Adolescent-Substance-Use-Disorders-Report-2014-en.pdf>.

Centre for Addiction and Mental Health. (2010). *Alcohol withdrawal*. Retrieved from <https://www.porticonetwork.ca/web/alcohol-toolkit/treatment/alcohol-withdrawal>.

Centre for Addiction and Mental Health. (2014). *CAMH releases new cannabis policy framework*. Retrieved from <http://www

.camh.ca/en/hospital/about_camh/newsroom/news_releases_media_advisories_and_backgrounders/current_year/Pages/CAMH-releases-new-Cannabis-Policy-Framework.aspx>.

George, T., & Vaccarino, F. (Eds.), (2015). *Substance abuse in Canada: The effects of cannabis use during adolescence*. Ottawa, ON: Canadian Centre on Substance Abuse. Retrieved from <http://www.ccsa.ca/Resource%20Library/CCSA-Effects-of-Cannabis-Use-during-Adolescence-Report-2015-en.pdf>.

Health Canada. (2013*). Canadian alcohol and drug use monitoring survey: Summary of results for 2012*. Retrieved from <http://www.hc-sc.gc.ca/hc-ps/drugs-drogues/stat/2012/summary-sommaire-eng.php>.

Merritt, J. O., & Duncan, M. H. (2014). Addiction disorders. *Medical Clinics of North America, 98*, 1097–1122. doi:10.1016/j.mcna.2014.06.008.

Nacca, N., Vatti, D., Sullivan, R., et al. (2013). The synthetic cannabinoid withdrawal syndrome. *Journal of Addiction Medicine, 7*(4), 296–298. doi:10.1097/ADM.0b013e31828e1881.

Ng, K. (2011). Evaluation of an alcohol withdrawal protocol and a preprinted order set at a tertiary care hospital. *The Canadian Journal of Hospital Pharmacy, 64*(6), 436–445.

Paparella, S. F. (2014). Intravenous fentanyl: Understanding and managing the risk. *Journal of Emergency Nursing, 40*(5), 488–490. doi:10.1016/j.jen.2014.05.017.

Pearson, C., Janz, T., & Ali, J. (2015). Mental and substance use disorders in Canada. Retrieved from <http://www.statcan.gc.ca/pub/82-624-x/2013001/article/11855-eng.htm>.

Registered Nurses Association of Ontario. (2015). *Clinical best practice guidelines: Engaging clients who use substances*. Toronto, ON: Source. Retrieved from <http://rnao.ca/sites/rnao-ca/files/Engaging_Clients_Who_Use_Substances_13_WEB.pdf>.

Roszel, E. L. (2015). Central nervous system deficits in fetal alcohol spectrum disorder. *Nurse Practitioner, 40*(4), 24–33. doi:10.1097/01.NPR.0000444650.10142.4f.

Salani, D. A., & Zdanowicz, M. M. (2015). Synthetic cannabinoids: The dangers of spicing it up. *Journal of Psychosocial Nursing & Mental Health Services, 53*(5), 36–43. doi:10.3928/02793695-20150422-01.

Smith, M. A., & Hambleton, S. (2014). An understanding of substance use disorder. *The Clinical Advisor: For Nurse Practitioners, 17*(3), 57–63.

Vaux, K. K. (2015). *Fetal alcohol syndrome*. Retrieved from <http://emedicine.medscape.com/article/974016>.

Chapter 19

Karwa, R., & Woodis, C. B. (2009). Midodrine and octreotide in treatment of cirrhosis-related hemodynamic complications. *Annals of Pharmacotherapy, 43*(4), 692–699. doi:10.1345/aph.1L373.

Levine, A. R., Meyer, M. J., Bittner, E. A., et al. (2013). Oral midodrine treatment accelerates the liberation of intensive care unit patients from intravenous vasopressor infusions. *Journal of Critical Care, 28*(5), 756–762. doi:10.1016/j.jcrc.2013.05.021.

Simons, K. J., & Simons, F. E. (2011). Epinephrine and its use in anaphylaxis: Current issues. *Current Opinion in Allergy and Clinical Immunology, 10*(4), 354–361. doi:10.1097/ACI.0b013e32833bc670.

Victorian, B. (2009). Low-dose dopamine led to better post-transplant renal function in randomized study. *Nephrology Times, 2*(10), 1, 16, 18. doi:10.1097/01.NEP.0000363394.47418.0f.

Chapter 20

Abou El Ela, A. E., Allam, A. A., & Ibrahim, E. H. (2015). Pharmacokinetics and anti-hypertensive effect of metoprolol tartrate rectal delivery system. *Drug Delivery, 21*, 1–10.

Deters, L. A. (2015). *Benign prostatic hypertrophy*. Retrieved from <http://emedicine.medscape.com/article/437359>.

Fonseca, V. A. (2010). Effects of β-blockers on glucose and lipid metabolism. *Current Medical Research and Opinion, 26*(3), 615–629. doi:10.1185/03007990903533681.

McGill, J. (2009). Reexamining misconceptions about β-blockers in patients with diabetes. *Clinical Diabetes, 27*(1), 36–46. doi:10.2337/diaclin.27.1.36.

Chapter 21

Alzheimer Society Canada. (2015). *We can help*. Retrieved from <http://www.alzheimer.ca/en/We-can-help>.

Buckley, J., & Salpeter, S. (2015). A risk-benefit assessment of dementia medications: Systematic review of the evidence. *Drugs and Aging, 32*(6), 453–467. doi:10.1007/s40266-015-0266-9.

Canevelli, M., Adali, N., Kelaiditi, E., et al. (2014). Effects of Gingko biloba supplementation in Alzheimer's disease patients receiving cholinesterase inhibitors: Data from the ICTUS study. *Phytomedicine: International Journal of Phytotherapy and Phytopharmacology, 21*(6), 888–892. doi:10.1016/j.phymed.2014.01.003.

Christensen, D. D. (2012). Higher-dose (23 mg/day) donepezil formulation for the treatment of patients with moderate-to-severe Alzheimer's disease. *Postgraduate Medicine, 124*(6), 110–116. doi:10.3810/pgm.2012.11.2589.

Deardorff, W., Feen, E., & Grossberg, G. (2015). The use of cholinesterase inhibitors across all stages of Alzheimer's disease. *Drugs and Aging, 32*(7), 537–547. doi:10.1007/s40266-015-0273-x.

Dening, T., & Sandilyan, M. B. (2015). Medical treatment and management of patients with dementia. *Nursing Standard, 29*(45), 43–49.

Keijzers, M., Nogales-Gadea, G., & de Baets, M. (2014). Clinical and scientific aspects of acetylcholine receptor myasthenia gravis. *Current Opinion in Neurology, 27*(5), 552–557. doi:10.1097/WCO.0000000000000125.

The Canadian Geriatrics Society. (2015). *The Canadian Geriatrics Society: Dedicated to the health of older Canadians*. Retrieved from <http://www.canadiangeriatrics.ca>.

Yang, M., Xu, D. D., Zhang, Y., et al. (2014). A systematic review on natural medicines for the prevention and treatment of Alzheimer's disease with meta-analyses of intervention effect of ginkgo. *American Journal of Chinese Medicine, 42*(3), 505–521. doi:10.1142/s0192415x14500335.

Yu, H., & Popescu, G. K. (2013). Inhibition of gluN2A-containing N-Methyl-D-Aspartate receptors by 2-naphthoic acid. *Molecular Pharmacology*, *84*(4), 541–550. doi:10.1124/mol.113.087189.

Chapter 22

Astellas. (2013). *VESIcare (solifenacin succinate)*. Retrieved from <http://www.vesicare.com/>.

Bailey, F. A., & Harman, S. M. (2015). *Palliative care: The last hours and days of life*. Retrieved from <http://www.uptodate.com/contents/palliative-care-the-last-hours-and-days-of-life>.

Cameron Institute. (2014). *Incontinence: A Canadian perspective*. Retrieved from <http://www.canadiancontinence.ca/pdfs/en-incontinence-a-canadian-perspective-2014.pdf>.

Durán, C. E., Azermai, M., & Vander Stichele, R. H. (2013). Systematic review of anticholinergic risk scales in older adults. *European Journal of Clinical Pharmacology*, *69*(7), 1485–1496. doi:10.1007/s00228-013-1499-3.

Fielding, F., & Long, C. O. (2014). The death rattle dilemma. *Journal of Hospice and Palliative Nursing*, *16*(8), 466–471. Retrieved from <http://www.medscape.com/viewarticle/834898>.

Fox, C., Smith, T., Maidment, I., et al. (2014). Effect of medications with anti-cholinergic properties on cognitive function, delirium, physical function and mortality: A systematic review. *Age and Ageing*, *43*(5), 604–615. Retrieved from <http://www.medscape.com/viewarticle/831095_4>.

Gray, S. L., Anderson, M. L., Dublin, S., et al. (2015). Cumulative use of strong anticholinergics and incident dementia: A prospective cohort study. *Journal of the American Medical Association Internal Medicine*, *175*(3), 401–407. doi:10.1001/jamainternmed.2014.7663.

HealthlinkBC. (2013). *Overactive bladder*. Retrieved from <http://www.healthlinkbc.ca/healthtopics/>.

Mityanand, R. (2015). *Anticholinergic toxicity*. Retrieved from <http://emedicine.medscape.com/article/812644-overview>.

Pasina, L., Djade, C. D., Lucca, U., et al. (2013). Association of anticholinergic burden with cognitive and functional status in a cohort of hospitalized elderly: Comparison of the anticholinergic cognitive burden scale and anticholinergic risk scale: Results from the REPOSI study. *Drugs and Aging*, *30*(2), 103–112. doi:10.1007/s40266-012-0044-x.

Prommer, E. (2013). Anticholinergics in palliative medicine: An update. *American Journal of Hospital and Palliative Care*, *30*(5), 490–498. doi:10.1177/1049909112459366.

Salahudeen, M. S., Duffull, S. B., & Nishtala, P. S. (2015). Anticholinergic burden quantified by anticholinergic risk scales and adverse outcomes in older people: A systematic review. *BMC Geriatrics*, *15*(31), doi:10.1186/s12877-015-0029-9.

Chapter 23

Adebayo, O., & Rogers, R. L. (2015). Hypertensive emergencies in the emergency department. *Emergency Medicine Clinics of North America*, *33*(3), 539–551. doi:10.1016/j.emc.2015.04.005.

Arcand, J., Mendoza, J., Qi, Y., et al. (2013). Results of a national survey examining Canadians' concern, actions, barriers, and support for dietary sodium reduction interventions. *Canadian Journal of Cardiology*, *29*(5), 628–631. doi:10.1016/j.cjca.2013.01.018.

Bisognano, J. D. (2014). *Malignant hypertension*. Retrieved from <http://emedicine.medscape.com/article/241640-overview>.

Bope, E. T., & Kellerman, R. D. (2014). *Conn's current therapy 2014*. St. Louis, MO: Elsevier.

Daskalopoulou, S. S., Rabi, D. M., Zarnke, K. B., et al. (2015). The 2015 Canadian Hypertension Education Program recommendations for blood pressure measurement, diagnosis, assessment of risk, prevention, and treatment of hypertension. *Canadian Journal of Cardiology*, *31*(5), 549–568. doi:10.1016/j.cjca.2015.02.016.

Grisaru, S., Watson-Jarvis, K., McKenna, C. M., et al. (2012). Development of a simple tool for diagnosis and initial approach to hypertension and pre-hypertension in children and youth. *Open Journal of Pediatrics*, *2*(2), 106–110. doi:10.4236/ojped.2012.22018.

Health Canada. (2012). *Sodium in Canada*. Retrieved from <http://www.hc-sc.gc.ca/fn-an/nutrition/sodium/index-eng.php>.

Heart and Stroke Foundation. (2014). *Dietary sodium, heart disease, and stroke*. Retrieved from <http://www.heartandstroke.com/site/c.ikIQLcMWJtE/b.5263133/k.696/Dietary_sodium_heart_disease_and_stroke.htm>.

Heart and Stroke Foundation. (2015). *Statistics*. Retrieved from <http://www.heartandstroke.com/site/c.ikIQLcMWJtE/b.3483991/k.34A8/Statistics.htm>.

Hopkins, C. (2015). *Hypertensive emergencies*. Retrieved from <http://emedicine.medscape.com/article/1952052-overview>.

Hypertension Canada. (2014). *The case for sodium reduction in Canada: Fact sheet*. Retrieved from <http://www.hypertensiontalk.com/wp-content/uploads/2014/03/FactSheet-Sodium-HTalk.pdf>.

Hypertension Canada. (2015a). *2015 Canadian recommendations for the management of hypertension*. Retrieved from <https://www.hypertension.ca/images/CHEP_2015/2015_CHEPWhatsNew.pdf>.

Hypertension Canada. (2015b). *CHEP key messages*. Retrieved from <https://www.hypertension.ca/images/CHEP_2015/2015_CHEPKeyMessages_EN.pdf>.

Hypertension Canada. (2015c). *Hypertension Canada*. Retrieved from <https://www.hypertension.ca/en/>.

Madhur, M. S. (2014). *Hypertension*. Retrieved from <http://emedicine.medscape.com/article/241381>.

Miura, S., Karnik, S. S., & Saku, K. (2011). Review: Angiotensin II type 1 receptor blockers: Class effects versus molecular effects. *Journal of the Renin-Angiotensin-Aldosterone System*, *12*(1), 1–7. doi:10.1177/1470320310370852.

Rodriguez-Cruz, E. (2015). *Pediatric hypertension*. Retrieved from <http://emedicine.medscape.com/article/889877-overview>.

Thompson, M., Dana, T., Bougatsos, C., et al. (2013). Screening for hypertension in children and adolescents to prevent cardiovascular disease. *Pediatrics*, *131*(3), 490–525. doi:10. 1542/peds.2012-3523.

Vijayaraghavan, K., & Deedwania, P. (2011). Renin–angiotensin–aldosterone blockade for cardiovascular disease prevention. *Cardiology Clinics*, *29*(1), 137–156. doi:10.1016/j.ccl.2010.11.003.

Volpe, M., Danser, A. H., Menard, J., et al. (2012). Inhibition of the renin–angiotensin–aldosterone system: Is there room for dual blockade in the cardiorenal continuum? *Journal of Hypertension*, *30*(4), 647–654. doi:10.1097/HJH.0b013e32834f6e00.

World Health Organization. (2013). *A global brief on hypertension: Silent killer, global public health crisis.* Retrieved from <http://apps.who.int/iris/bitstream/10665/79059/1/WHO_DCO_WHD_2013.2_eng.pdf?ua=1>.

World Health Organization. (2014). *Fact sheet: Salt reduction.* Retrieved from <http://www.who.int/mediacentre/factsheets/fs393/en/>.

Chapter 24

Basra, S. S., Virani, S. S., Paniagua, D., et al. (2014). Acute coronary syndromes: Unstable angina and non-ST elevation myocardial infarction. *Cardiology Clinics*, *32*(3), 353–370. doi:10.1016/j.ccl.2014.04.010.

Braunwald, E., & Morrow, D. A. (2013). Unstable angina: Is it time for a requiem? *Circulation*, *127*(24), 2452–2457. doi:10.1161/CIRCULATIONAHA.113.001258.

Christensen, B. (2015). *Canadian Cardiovascular Society Grading System for Stable Angina.* Retrieved from <http://emedicine.medscape.com/article/2172431-overview>.

Coven, D. L. (2015). *Acute coronary syndrome.* Retrieved from <http://emedicine.medscape.com/article/1910735-overview>.

Mancini, G. B., Gosselin, G., Chow, B., et al. (2014). Canadian Cardiovascular Society guidelines for the diagnosis and management of stable ischemic heart disease. *Canadian Journal of Cardiology*, *30*(8), 837–849. doi:10.1016/j.cjca. 2014.05.013.

Tan, W. (2014). *Unstable angina.* Retrieved from <http://emedicine.medscape.com/article/159383-overview>.

Chapter 25

Ambrosy, A. P., Butler, J., Ahmed, A., et al. (2014). The use of digoxin in patients with worsening chronic heart failure: Reconsidering an old drug to reduce hospital admissions. *Journal of the American College of Cardiology*, *63*(18), 1823–1832. doi:10.1016/j.jacc.2014.01.051.

American Heart Association. (2016). *Classes of heart failure.* Retrieved from <http://www.heart.org/HEARTORG/Conditions/HeartFailure/AboutHeartFailure/Classes-of-Heart-Failure_UCM_306328_Article.jsp#.Vq59Y7IrKM8>.

Dardas, T. F., & Levy, W. C. (2015). Digoxin: In the cross hairs again. *Journal of the American College of Cardiology*, *65*(25), 2699–2701. doi:10.1016/j.jacc.2015.04.044.

Felicilda-Reynaldo, R. F. (2013). Cardiac glycosides, digoxin toxicity, and the antidote. *Medsurg Nursing*, *22*(4), 258–261.

Heart and Stroke Foundation. (2015). *Statistics.* Retrieved from <http://www.heartandstroke.on.ca/site/c.pvI3IeNWJwE/b.3581729/k.359A/Statistics.htm>.

Jelinek, H. F., & Warner, P. (2011). Digoxin therapy in the elderly: Pharmacokinetic considerations in nursing. *Geriatric Nursing*, *32*(4), 263–269. doi:10.1016/j.gerinurse.2011. 03.004.

McKelvie, R. S., Moe, G. W., Ezekowitz, J. A., et al. (2013). The 2012 Canadian Cardiovascular Society Heart Failure Management Guidelines Update: Focus on acute and chronic heart failure. *Canadian Journal of Cardiology*, *29*(2), 168–181. doi:10.1016/j.cjca.2012.10.007.

Sanchez, C. E., & Richards, D. R. (2015). Management of acute decompensated heart failure in hospitalized patients. *Journal of Clinical Outcomes Management*, *22*(4), 179–191.

Snyder, S., Kivlehan, S., & Collopy, K. (2015). Diagnosis and treatment of the patient with heart failure. *EMS World*, *44*(4), 33–42. Retrieved from <http://www.emsworld.com/article/12053437/diagnosis-and-treatment-of-the-patient-with-heart-failure>.

Vamos, M., Erath, J. W., & Hohnloser, S. H. (2015). Digoxin-associated mortality: A systematic review and meta-analysis of the literature. *European Heart Journal*, *36*(28), 1831–1838. doi:10.1093/eurheartj/ehv143.

Ziff, O. J., Lane, D. A., Samra, M., et al. (2015). Safety and efficacy of digoxin: Systematic review and meta-analysis of observational and controlled trial data. *BMJ : British Medical Journal / British Medical Association*, *351*, h4451. doi:10.1136/bmj.h4451.

Chapter 26

Camm, J., Lip, G. Y., De Caterina, R., et al. (2012). 2012 focused update of the ESC Guidelines for the management of atrial fibrillation: An update of the 2010 ESC Guidelines for the management of atrial fibrillation. *European Heart Journal*, *33*(21), 2719–2747. doi:10.1093/eurheartj/ehs253.

Cutugno, C. L. (2015). Atrial fibrillation: Updated management guidelines and nursing implications. *American Journal of Nursing*, *115*(5), 26–38. doi:10.1097/01.NAJ.0000465028. 05223.39.

Heart and Stroke Foundation. (2015). *Statistics.* Retrieved from <http://www.heartandstroke.com/site/c.ikIQLcMWJtE/b.3483991/k.34A8/Statistics.htm>.

Link, M. S., Berkow, L. C., Kudenchuk, P. J., et al. (2015). 2015 American Heart Association guidelines update for cardiopulmonary resuscitation and emergency cardiovascular care. Part 7: Adult advanced cardiovascular life support. *Circulation*, *132*, S444–S464. doi:10.1161/CIR.00000000000 01261.

Moukabary, T., & Gonzalez, M. D. (2015). Management of atrial fibrillation. *Medical Clinics of North America*, *99*(4), 781–794.

Schnabel, R. B., Yin, X., Gona, P., et al. (2015). 50 year trends in atrial fibrillation prevalence, incidence, risk factors, and mortality in the Framingham Heart Study: A cohort study. *Lancet*, *386*(9989), 154–162. doi:10.1016/S0140-6736(14) 61774-8.

Verma, A., Cairns, J. A., Mitchell, L. B., et al. (2014). 2014 Focused update of the Canadian Cardiovascular Society Guidelines for the management of atrial fibrillation. *Canadian Journal of Cardiology*, *10*(30), 1114–1130. doi:10.1016/j.cjca.2014.08.001.

Wei Yao, L., & Khan, F. (2015). Management of atrial fibrillation: Recommendations from NICE. National Institute for Health and Care Excellence. *British Journal of Hospital Medicine*, *76*(7), C108–S112.

Wenger, N. K., Helmy, T., Patel, A. D., et al. (2005). Approaching cardiac arrhythmias in the elderly patient. *Medscape General Medicine*, *7*(4), Retrieved from <http://www.medscape.com/viewarticle/514471>.

Chapter 27

Chamberlain, A. M., Gersh, B. J., Mills, R. M., et al. (2015). Antithrombotic strategies and outcomes in acute coronary syndrome with atrial fibrillation. *American Journal of Cardiology*, *115*(8), 1042–1048. doi:10.1016/j.amjcard.2015.01.534.

Contractor, T., Levin, V., Martinez, M. W., et al. (2013). Novel oral anticoagulants for stroke prevention in patients with atrial fibrillation: Dawn of a new era. *Postgraduate Medicine*, *125*(1), 34–44. doi:10.3810/pgm.2013.01.2622.

Dal Molin, A., Allara, E., Montani, D., et al. (2014). Flushing the central venous catheter: Is heparin necessary? *Journal of Vascular Access*, *15*(4), 241–248. doi:10.5301/jva.5000225.

Ferns, S. J., & Naccarelli, G. V. (2015). New oral anticoagulants: Their role in stroke prevention in high-risk patients with atrial fibrillation. *Medical Clinics of North America*, *99*(4), 759–780. doi:10.1016/j.mcna.2015.02.006.

Hargroves, D., & Ward, L. (2015). Anticoagulants for stroke prevention in patients with atrial fibrillation. *British Journal of Neuroscience Nursing*, *11*(S2), 31–37. doi:10.12968/bjnn.2015.11.Sup2.31.

Kovacs, R. J., Flaker, G. C., Saxonhouse, S. J., et al. (2015). Practical management of anticoagulation in patients with atrial fibrillation. *Journal of the American College of Cardiology*, *65*(13), 1340–1360. doi:10.1016/j.jacc.2015.01.049.

Verheugt, F. W., & Granger, C. B. (2015). Oral anticoagulants for stroke prevention in atrial fibrillation: Current status, special situations and unmet needs. *Lancet*, *386*(9990), 303–310. doi:10.1016/S0140-6736(15)60245-8.

Chapter 28

Amgen. (2015). *Repatha (evolocumab)*. Retrieved from <http://www.repatha.ca/>.

Anderson, T. J., Grégoire, J., Hegele, R. A., et al. (2013). 2012 update of the Canadian Cardiovascular Society guidelines for the diagnosis and treatment of dyslipidemia for the prevention of cardiovascular disease in the adult. *Canadian Journal of Cardiology*, *29*(2), 151–167. doi:10.1016/j.cjca.2012.11.032.

Ashton, V., Qiaoyi, Z., & Zhang, N. J. (2014). LDL-C levels in US patients at high cardiovascular risk receiving rosuvastatin monotherapy. *Clinical Therapeutics*, *36*(5), 792–799. doi:10.1016/j.clinthera.2014.03.010.

Bailey, D. G., Dresser, G., & Arnold, J. M. (2013). Grapefruit–medication interactions: Forbidden fruit or avoidable consequences? *Canadian Medical Association Journal*, *185*(4), 309–316. doi:10.1503/cmaj.120951.

Folse, H., Sternhufvud, C., Schuetz, C. A., et al. (2014). Impact of switching treatment from rosuvastatin to atorvastatin on rates of cardiovascular events. *Clinical Therapeutics*, *36*(1), 58–69. doi:10.1016/j.clinthera.2013.12.003.

Government of Canada. (2013). *New statins labeling update: Risk of increased blood sugar levels and diabetes*. Retrieved from <healthycanadians.gc.ca/recall-alert-rappel-avis/hc-sc/2013/16949a-eng.php>.

Heart and Stroke Foundation. (2015). *Statistics*. Retrieved from <http://www.heartandstroke.on.ca/site/c.pvI3IeNWJwE/b.3581729/k.359A/Statistics.htm#heartdisease>.

Jacobson, T. A. (2014). NLA task force on statin safety—2014 update. *Journal of Clinical Lipidology*, *8*, S1–S4. doi:10.1016/j.jacl.2014.03.003.

Shah, R. V., & Goldfine, A. B. (2012). Statins and risk of new-onset diabetes mellitus. *Circulation*, *126*, e282–e284. doi:10.1161/CIRCULATIONAHA.112.122135.

Chapter 29

Basraon, J., & Deedwani, P. C. (2012). Diuretics in heart failure: Practical considerations. *Medical Clinics of North America*, *96*(5), 933–942. doi:10.1016/j.mcna.2012.07.003.

Gribben, J., Hubbard, R., Gladman, J. R., et al. (2010). Risk of falls associated with antihypertensive medication: Population-based case-control study. *Age and Ageing*, *39*(5), 592–597. doi:10.1093/ageing/afq092.

Huang, A. R., Mallet, L., Rochefort, C. M., et al. (2012). Medication-related falls in the elderly: Causative factors and preventive strategies. *Drugs and Aging*, *29*(5), 359–376. doi:10.2165/11599460-000000000-00000.

Musini, V. M., Rezapour, P., Wright, J. M., et al. (2015). Blood pressure-lowering efficacy of loop diuretics for primary hypertension. *The Cochrane Database of Systematic Reviews*, (5), doi:10.1002/14651858.CD003825.pub4.

Chapter 30

Callum, J. L., Lin, Y., Pinkerton, P. H., et al. (2011). *Bloody easy 3: Blood transfusions, blood alternatives and transfusion reactions*. Retrieved from <http://transfusionontario.org/en/cmdownloads/categories/bloody_easy/#>.

Carson, J. L., Grossman, B. J., Kleinman, S., et al. (2012). Red blood cell transfusion: A clinical practice guideline from the AABB*. *Annals of Internal Medicine*, *157*(1), 49–58. doi:10.7326/0003-4819-157-1-201206190-00429.

Chand, N. K., Subramanya, H. B., & Rao, G. V. (2014). Management of patients who refuse blood transfusion. *Indian Journal of Anaesthesia*, *58*(5), 658–664. doi:10.4103/0019-5049.144680.

Health Canada. (2015). *Blood regulations*. Retrieved from <http://www.hc-sc.gc.ca/dhp-mps/brgtherap/applic-demande/guides/blood-reg-sang-eng.php>.

MacDonald, N. E., O'Brien, S. F., & Delage, G. (2012). Transfusion and risk of infection in Canada: Update 2012. *Immunization Committee, Paediatrics & Child Health*, *17*(10), e102–e111.

National Advisory Committee on Blood & Blood Products. (2014). *NAC Companion Document to: "Red Blood Cell*

Transfusion: A Clinical Practice Guideline from the AABB". Retrieved from <http://www.nacblood.ca/resources/guidelines/Companion-Document-May-28-2014.pdf>.

Public Health Agency of Canada. (2004). *Transfusion transmitted injuries section: About risks of blood transfusion.* Retrieved from <http://www.phac-aspc.gc.ca/hcai-iamss/tti-it/risks-eng.php>.

Rizoli, S. (2011). PlasmaLyte. *Journal of Trauma, 70*(Suppl. 5), S17–S18. doi:10.1097/TA.0b013e31821a4d89.

Sandler, S. G. (2015). *Transfusion reactions.* Retrieved from <http://emedicine.medscape.com/article/206885-overview #a5>.

Sarai, M., & Tejani, A. M. (2015). Loop diuretics for patients receiving blood transfusions. *The Cochrane Database of Systematic Reviews,* (2), doi:10.1002/14651858.CD010138.pub2.

Simon, E. E. (2015). *Hyponatremia.* Retrieved from <http://emedicine.medscape.com/article/242166-overview>.

Vincent, J. L. (2012). Indications for blood transfusions: Too complex to base on a single number? *Annals of Internal Medicine, 157*(1), 71–72. doi:10.7326/0003-4819-157-1-2012 06190-00431.

Chapter 31

Chan, M. M., Chan, M. M., Mengshol, J. A., et al. (2013). Octreotide: A drug often used in the critical care setting but not well understood. *Chest, 144*(6), 1937–1945. doi:10.1378/chest.13-0382.

Chapter 32

Campbell, K., & Doogue, M. (2012). Evaluating and managing patients with thyrotoxicosis. *Australian Family Physician, 41*(8), 564–572.

Franklyn, J. A., & Boelaert, K. (2012). Thyrotoxicosis. *Lancet, 379*(9821), 1155–1166. doi:10.1016/S0140-6736(11)60782-4.

Gopalan, M. (2014). *Thyroid dysfunction induced by amiodarone therapy.* Retrieved from <http://emedicine.medscape.com/article/129033-overview>.

Goyal, N. (2014). *Thyroidectomy.* Retrieved from <http://emedicine.medscape.com/article/1891109-overview>.

Klubo-Gwiezdzinska, J., & Wartofsky, L. (2012). Thyroid emergencies. *Medical Clinics of North America, 96*(2), 385–403. doi:10.1016/j.mcna.2012.01.015.

McDermott, M. T. (2012). Hyperthyroidism. *Annals of Internal Medicine, 157*(1), ITC1-1. doi:10.7326/0003-4819-157-1-2012 07030-01001.

Schraga, E. D. (2014). *Hyperthyroidism, thyroid storm, and Graves disease.* Retrieved from <http://emedicine.medscape.com/article/767130-overview>.

Vaidya, B., & Pearce, S. H. (2014). Diagnosis and management of thyrotoxicosis. *The BMJ, 349,* g5128. doi:10.1136/bmj.g5128.

Chapter 33

Bergenstal, R. M., Tamborlane, W. V., Ahmann, A., et al. (2010). Effectiveness of sensor-augmented insulin-pump therapy in type 1 diabetes. *New England Journal of Medicine, 363*(4), 311–320. doi:10.1056/NEJMoa1002853.

Blouin, D. (2012). Too much of a good thing: Management of diabetic ketoacidosis in adults. *Canadian Family Physician, 58*(1), 155–157.

Canadian Diabetes Association Clinical Practice Guidelines Expert Committee. (2013). Canadian Diabetes Association 2013 clinical practice guidelines for the prevention and management of diabetes in Canada. *Canadian Journal of Diabetes, 37*(Suppl. 1), S1–S212.

Canadian Diabetes Association Clinical Practice Guidelines Expert Committee. (2015). *Pharmacologic management of type 2 diabetes—2015 interim update.* Retrieved from <http://guidelines.diabetes.ca/browse/chapter13_2015>.

Centers for Disease Control and Prevention (US), the National Center for Chronic Disease Prevention and Health Promotion (US), & the Office on Smoking and Health (US). (2010). *How tobacco smoke causes disease: The biology and behavioral basis for smoking-attributable disease.* Atlanta, GA: Centers for Disease Control and Prevention.

Cooperman, M. (2014). *Somogyi phenomenon.* Retrieved from <http://emedicine.medscape.com/article/125432>.

Government of Canada. (2015). *Forxiga, Invokana: Health Canada begins safety review of diabetes drugs known as SGLT2 inhibitors and risk of ketoacidosis.* Retrieved from <http://healthycanadians.gc.ca/recall-alert-rappel-avis/hc-sc/2015/53892a-eng.php>.

Green, J. B., Bethel, M. A., Armstrong, P. W., et al. (2015). Effect of sitagliptin on cardiovascular outcomes in type 2 diabetes. *New England Journal of Medicine, 373*(3), 232–242. doi:10.1056/NEJMoa1501352.

Hackethal, V. (2015). *Passive smoking increases risk for type 2 diabetes.* Retrieved from <http://www.medscape.com/viewarticle/851298>.

Health Canada. (2011). *Eating Well with Canada's Food Guide.* Retrieved from <http://www.hc-sc.gc.ca/fn-an/food-guide-aliment/order-commander/index-eng.php#a1>.

Helminen, O., Aspholm, S., Pokka, T., et al. (2015). Hba1c predicts time to diagnosis of type 1 diabetes in children at risk. *Diabetes, 64*(5), 1719–1727. doi:10.2337/db14-0497.

Hemphill, R. R. (2014). *Hyperosmolar hyperglycemic state.* Retrieved from <http://emedicine.medscape.com/article/1914705>.

Hostalek, U., Gwilt, M., & Hildemann, S. (2015). Therapeutic use of metformin in prediabetes and diabetes prevention. *Drugs, 75*(10), 1071–1094. doi:10.1007/s40265-015-0416-8.

Kadiyala, P., Walton, S., & Sathyapalan, T. (2014). Insulin induced lipodystrophy. *British Journal of Diabetes and Vascular Disease, 14*(4), 131–133.

Khardori, R. (2014). *Type 2 diabetes mellitus.* Retrieved from <http://emedicine.medscape.com/article/117853>.

Lenahan, C. M., & Holloway, B. (2015). Differentiating between DKA and HHS. *Journal of Emergency Nursing, 41*(3), 201–207. doi:10.1016/j.jen.2014.08.015.

Maletkovic, J., & Drexler, A. (2013). Diabetic ketoacidosis and hyperglycemic hyperosmolar state. *Endocrinology & Metabolism Clinics of North America, 42*(4), 677–695.

McCombs, D. G., Appel, S. J., & Ward, M. E. (2015). Expedited diagnosis and management of inpatient hyperosmolar hyperglycemic nonketotic syndrome. *Journal of the American Association of Nurse Practitioners*, 27(8), 426–432. doi:10.1002/2327-6924.12205.

Pan, A., Wang, Y., Talaei, M., et al. (2015). Relation of active, passive, and quitting smoking with incident type 2 diabetes: A systematic review and meta-analysis. *The Lancet Diabetes and Endocrinology*, 3(12), 958–967. doi:10.1016/S2213-8587(15)00316-2.

Petrović, O. (2014). How should we screen for gestational diabetes? *Current Opinion in Obstetrics and Gynecology*, 26(2), 54–60. doi:10.1097/GCO.0000000000000049.

Spijkerman, A. M. W., van der A., D. L., Nilsson, P. M., et al. (2014). Smoking and long-term risk of type 2 diabetes: The EPIC InterAct study in European countries. *Diabetes Care*, 37(12), 3164–3171. doi:10.2337/dc14-1020.

Tucker, M. E. (2014). *Smoking causes diabetes; doctors should help patients quit.* Retrieved from <http://www.medscape.com/viewarticle/819606>.

Whalen, K., Miller, S., & St. Onge, E. (2015). The role of sodium-glucose co-transporter 2 inhibitors in the treatment of type 2 diabetes. *Clinical Therapeutics*, 37(6), 1150–1166. doi:10.1016/j.clinthera.2015.03.004.

Wong, J., & Tabet, E. (2015). The introduction of insulin in type 2 diabetes mellitus. *Australian Family Physician*, 44(5), 278–283.

Yeh, H. C., Duncan, B. B., Schmidt, M. I., et al. (2010). Smoking, smoking cessation, and risk for type 2 diabetes: A cohort study. *Annals of Internal Medicine*, 152(1), 10–17. doi:10.7326/0003-4819-152-1-201001050-00005.

Chapter 34

Brownfoot, F. C., Gagliardi, D. I., Bain, E., et al. (2013). Different corticosteroids and regimens for accelerating fetal lung maturation for women at risk of preterm birth. *The Cochrane Database of Systematic Reviews*, 2013(8), doi:10.1002/14651858.CD006764.pub3.

Chrousos, G. P. (2013). *Glucocorticoid therapy and Cushing syndrome.* Retrieved from <http://emedicine.medscape.com/article/921086>.

Drozdowicz, L. B., & Bostwick, J. M. (2014). Psychiatric adverse effects of pediatric corticosteroid use. *Mayo Clinic Proceedings*, 89(6), 817–834. doi:10.1016/j.mayocp.2014.01.010.

Kamath-Rayne, B. D., deFranco, E. A., & Marcotte, M. P. (2012). Antenatal steroids for treatment of fetal lung immaturity after 34 weeks of gestation: An evaluation of neonatal outcomes. *Obstetrics & Gynecology*, 119(5), 909–916. doi:10.1097/AOG.0b013e31824ea4b2.

Michels, A., & Michels, N. (2014). Addison disease: Early detection and treatment principles. *American Family Physician*, 89(7), 563–568.

Msan, A. K., Usta, I. M., Mirza, F. G., et al. (2015). Use of antenatal corticosteroids in the management of preterm delivery. *American Journal of Perinatology*, 32(5), 417–426. doi:10.1055/s-0034-1395476.

Roberts, T. N., & Thompson, J. P. (2013). Illegal substances in anaesthetic and intensive care practices. *Continuing Education in Anaesthetic Critical Care & Pain*, 13(2), 42–46. doi:10.1093/bjaceaccp/mks050.

Romejko-Wolniewicz, E., Teliga-Czajkowska, J., & Czajkowski, K. (2014). Antenatal steroids: Can we optimize the dose? *Current Opinion in Obstetrics and Gynecology*, 26(2), 77–82. doi:10.1097/GCO.0000000000000047.

Tucci, V., & Sokari, T. (2014). The clinical manifestations, diagnosis, and management of adrenal emergencies. *Emergency Medical Clinics of North America*, 32(2), 465–484. doi:10.1016/j.emc.2014.01.006.

Chapter 35

Brown, J. P., Morin, S., Leslie, W., et al. (2014). Bisphosphonates for treatment of osteoporosis: Expected benefits, potential harms, and drug holidays. *Canadian Family Physician*, 60(4), 324–333.

Croxtall, J. D. (2012). Ulipristal acetate: In uterine fibroids. *Drugs*, 72(8), 1075–1085. doi:10.2165/11209400-000000000-00000.

Dunn, S., & Guilbert, E., for the Society of Obstetricians and Gynaecologists of Canada. (2012). Position statement: Emergency contraception. *Journal of Obstetrics and Gynaecology Canada*, 34(9), 870–878.

Government of Canada. (2013). *Synthetic calcitonin (salmon) nasal spray (NS) - Market withdrawal of all products, effective October 1st, 2013—For health professionals.* Retrieved from <http://www.healthycanadians.gc.ca/recall-alert-rappel-avis/hc-sc/2013/34783a-eng.php>.

Guo, Y., Longo, C. J., Xie, Y., et al. (2011). Cost-effectiveness of transdermal nitroglycerin use for preterm labor. *Value in Health*, 14(2), 240–246. doi:10.1016/j.jval.2010.10.019.

Hewitt, S. C., & Korach, K. S. (2014). *Molecular biology and physiology of estrogen action.* Retrieved from <http://www.uptodate.com/contents/molecular-biology-and-physiology-of-estrogen-action>.

Hirsch, M., & Davis, C. J. (2015). Preoperative assessment and diagnosis of endometriosis: Are we any closer? *Current Opinion in Obstetrics & Gynecology*, 27(4), 284–290. doi:10.1097/GCO.0000000000000188.

Katzman, D. K., & Taddeo, D. (2010). Emergency contraception. *Paediatrics & Child Health*, 15(6), 363–367.

Louden, K. (2014). *Largest study to date: Transgender hormone treatment safe.* Retrieved from <http://www.medscape.com/viewarticle/827713>.

Moravek, M. B., & Bulun, S. E. (2015). Endocrinology of uterine fibroids: Steroid hormones, stem cells, and genetic contribution. *Current Opinion in Obstetrics and Gynecology*, 27(4), 276–283. doi:10.1097/GCO.0000000000000185.

Morrow, P. K., Mattair, D. N., & Hortobagyi, G. N. (2011). Hot flashes: A review of pathophysiology and treatment modalities. *The Oncologist*, 16(11), 1658–1664. doi:10.1634/theoncologist.2011-0174.

Osteoporosis Canada. (2015). *Osteoporosis facts and statistics.* Retrieved from <http://www.osteoporosis.ca/osteoporosis-and-you/osteoporosis-facts-and-statistics/>.

Papaioannou, A., Santesso, N., Morin, S. N., et al., for the Scientific Advisory Council of Osteoporosis Canada. (2015). Recommendations for preventing fracture in long-term care. *Canadian Medical Association Journal, 14*(331), 1–11. doi:10.1503/cmaj.141331CMAJ.

Pohl, O., Osterloh, I., & Gotteland, J.-P. (2013). Ulipristal acetate—Safety and pharmacokinetics following multiple doses of 10–50 mg per day. *Journal of Clinical Pharmacy and Therapeutics, 38*(4), 314–320. doi:10.1111/jcpt.12065.

Rosen, H. N. (2015). *The use of bisphosphonates in postmenopausal women with osteoporosis.* Retrieved from <http://www.uptodate.com/contents/the-use-of-bisphosphonates-in-postmenopausal-women-with-osteoporosis>.

Royer, P. A., & Jones, K. (2014). Progestins for contraception: Modern delivery systems and novel formulations. *Clinical Obstetrics and Gynecology, 57*(4), 644–658. doi:10.1097/GRF.0000000000000072.

Smith, N. L., Blondon, M., Wiggins, K. L., et al. (2014). Lower risk of cardiovascular events in postmenopausal women taking oral estradiol compared with oral conjugated equine estrogens. *Journal of the American Medical Association Internal Medicine, 174*(1), 25–31. doi:10.1001/jamainternmed.2013.11074.

Stewart, E. A. (2015). Clinical practice: Uterine fibroids. *New England Journal of Medicine, 372*(17), 1646–1655. doi:10.1056/NEJMcp1411029.

Tarride, J. E., Hopkins, R. B., Leslie, W. D., et al. (2015). The burden of illness of osteoporosis in Canada. *Osteoporosis International, 23*(11), 2591–2600. doi:10.1007/s00198-012-1931-z.

The North American Menopause Society. (2012). The 2012 hormone therapy position statement of the North American Menopause Society. *Menopause (New York, N.Y.), 19*(3), 257–271. doi:10.1097/gme.0b013e31824b970a.

Vilos, G. A., Allaire, C., & Laberge, P. (2015). The management of uterine leiomyomas. *Journal of Obstetetrics and Gynaecology Canada, 37*(2), 157–178.

Watts, N. B., & Diab, D. L. (2010). Long-term use of bisphosphonates in osteoporosis. *Journal of Clinical Endocrinology Metabolism, 95*(4), 1555–1165. doi:10.1210/jc.2009-1947.

Winner, B., Peipert, J. F., Qiuhong, Z., et al. (2012). Effectiveness of long-acting reversible contraception. *New England Journal of Medicine, 366*, 1998–2007. doi:10.1056/nejmoa1110855.

Chapter 36

Albertsen, P. C. (2015). Prostate-specific antigen testing: Good or bad? *The Oncologist, 20*(3), 233–235. doi:10.1634/theoncologist.2015-0019.

Bell, N., Connor Gorber, S., Shane, A., et al., for the Canadian Task Force on Preventive Health Care. (2014). Recommendations on screening for prostate cancer with the prostate-specific antigen test. *Canadian Medical Association Journal, 186*(16), 1225–1234. doi:10.1503/cmaj.140703.

Hayes, J. H., & Barry, M. J. (2014). Screening for prostate cancer with the prostate-specific antigen test: A review of current evidence. *Journal of the American Medical Association, 311*(11), 1143–1149. doi:10.1001/jama.2014.2085.

Hoffman, R. H. (2014). *Screening for prostate cancer.* Retrieved from <http://www.uptodate.com/contents/screening-for-prostate-cancer>.

Lepor, H., Kazzazi, A., & Djavan, B. (2012). α-Blockers for benign prostatic hyperplasia: The new era. *Current Opinion in Urology, 22*(1), 7–15. doi:10.1097/MOU.0b013e32834d9bfd.

Robinson, J. G., Hodges, E. A., & Davison, J. (2014). Prostate-specific antigen screening: A critical review of current research and guidelines. *Journal of the American Association of Nurse Practitioners, 26*(10), 574–581. doi:10.1002/2327-6924.12094.

Chapter 37

American Herbal Pharmacopeia. (2015). American ginseng (Panax quinquefolius L.): A review of clinical therapeutics by the American Herbal Pharmacopeia. *Alternative & Complementary Therapies, 21*(3), 138–142. doi:10.1089/act.2015.29005.ahp.

Bolser, D. C. (2010). Pharmacologic management of cough. *Otolaryngologic Clinics of North America, 43*(1), 147–155. doi:10.1016/j.otc.2009.11.008.

Bonney, A. G., & Goldman, R. D. (2014). Antihistamines for children with otitis media. *Canadian Family Physician, 60*(1), 43–46.

Hom, J. (2013). Do decongestants, antihistamines, and nasal irrigation relieve the symptoms of sinusitis in children? *Annals of Emergency Medicine, 61*(1), 35–36. doi:10.1016/j.annemergmed.2012.03.016.

National Institute on Drug Abuse. (2014). *Drugfacts: Cough and cold medicine abuse.* Retrieved from <https://www.drugabuse.gov/publications/drugfacts/cough-cold-medicine-abuse>.

Parle-Pechera, S., Powers, L., & St Anna, L. (2012). Clinical inquiries: Intranasal steroids vs antihistamines: Which is better for seasonal allergies and conjunctivitis? *Journal of Family Practice, 61*(6), 429–448.

Shaikh, N., Wald, E. R., & Pi, M. (2014). Decongestants, antihistamines and nasal irrigation for acute sinusitis in children. *The Cochrane Database of Systematic Reviews, 2014*(12), doi:10.1002/14651858.CD007909.pub2.

Smith, S. M., Schroeder, K., & Fahey, T. (2014). Over-the-counter (OTC) medications for acute cough in children and adults in community settings. *The Cochrane Database of Systematic Reviews, 2012*(8), doi:10.1002/14651858.CD001831.pub4.

Yancy, W. S., Jr., McCrory, D. C., Coeytaux, R. R., et al. (2013). Efficacy and tolerability of treatments for chronic cough: A systematic review and meta-analysis. *Chest, 144*(6), 1827–1838. doi:10.1378/chest.13-0490.

Chapter 38

Asthma Society of Canada. (2016). *The Asthma Society of Canada.* Retrieved from <http://www.asthma.ca/>.

Bilton, D., & Stanford, G. (2014). The expanding armamentarium of drugs to aid sputum clearance: How should they be used to optimize care? *Current Opinion in Pulmonary Medicine, 20*(6), 601–606. doi:10.1097/MCP.0000000000000104.

DiBlasi, R. M. (2015). Clinical controversies in aerosol therapy for infants and children. *Respiratory Care, 60*(6), 894–914. doi:10.4187/respcare.04137.

Doan, Q., Shefrin, A., & Johnson, D. (2011). Cost-effectiveness of metered-dose inhalers for asthma exacerbations in the pediatric emergency department. *Pediatrics, 127*(5), a1105–a1111. doi:10.1542/peds.2010-2963.

Global Initiative for Asthma. (2015). *Global strategy for asthma management and prevention.* Retrieved from <http://www.ginasthma.org/local/uploads/files/GINA_Report_2015_Aug11.pdf>.

Global Initiative for Chronic Obstructive Lung Disease. (2015). *Global strategy for the diagnosis, management, and prevention of chronic obstructive pulmonary disease.* Retrieved from <http://www.goldcopd.org/uploads/users/files/GOLD_Report_2015_Sept2.pdf>.

Kirkham, P. A., & Barnes, P. J. (2013). Oxidative stress in COPD. *Chest, 144*(1), 266–273. doi:10.1378/chest.12-2664.

Lougheed, M. D., Lemiere, C., Ducharme, M. D., et al. (2012). Canadian Thoracic Society 2012 guideline update: Diagnosis and management of asthma in preschoolers, children and adults. *Canadian Respiratory Journal, 19*(2), 127–164.

Poole, P., Black, P. N., & Cates, C. J. (2015). Mucolytic agents versus placebo for chronic bronchitis or chronic obstructive pulmonary disease. *The Cochrane Database of Systematic Reviews, 2015*(7), doi:10.1002/14651858.CD001287.pub5.

Price, D., Kaplan, A., Jones, R., et al. (2015). Long-acting muscarinic antagonist use in adults with asthma: Real-life prescribing and outcomes of add-on therapy with tiotropium bromide. *Journal of Asthma and Allergy, 8,* 1–13. doi:10.2147/JAA.S76639.

Vézina, K., Chauhan, B. F., & Ducharme, F. M. (2014). Inhaled anticholinergics and short-acting beta(2)-agonists versus short-acting beta2-agonists alone for children with acute asthma in hospital. *The Cochrane Database of Systematic Reviews, 2014*(7). doi:10.1002/14651858.CD010283.pub2.

Chapter 39

Antoniou, T., Macdonald, E. M., Hollands, S., et al. (2015). Proton pump inhibitors and the risk of acute kidney injury in older patients: A population-based cohort study. *Canadian Medical Association Journal, 3*(2), E166–E171. doi:10.9778/cmajo.20140074cmajo.

Levenstein, S., Rosenstock, S., Jacobsen, R. K., et al. (2015). Psychological stress increases risk for peptic ulcer, regardless of Helicobacter pylori infection or use of nonsteroidal anti-inflammatory drugs. *Clinical Gastroenterology and Hepatology, 13*(3), 498–506. doi:10.1016/j.cgh.2014.07.052.

Santacroce, L. (2014). *Helicobacter Pylori Infection.* Retrieved from <http://emedicine.medscape.com/article/176938>.

van Rensburg, C. J., & Cheer, S. (2012). Pantoprazole for the treatment of peptic ulcer bleeding and prevention of rebleeding. Clinical Medicine Insights. *Gastroenterology, 5,* 51–60. doi:10.4137/CGast.S9893.

Chapter 40

Basson, M. D. (2015). *Constipation.* Retrieved from <http://emedicine.medscape.com/article/184704>.

Daniels, G., & Schmelzer, M. (2013). Giving laxatives safely and effectively. *Medsurg Nursing, 22*(5), 290–302.

Rowan-Legg, A. (2011). Managing functional constipation in children. *Paediatrics & Child Health, 16*(10), 661–665.

Wanke, C. A. (2015). *Patient information: Acute diarrhea in adults (beyond the basics).* Retrieved from <http://www.uptodate.com/contents/acute-diarrhea-in-adults-beyond-the-basics>.

World Health Organization. (2013). *Diarrhoeal disease. Fact sheet N°330.* Retrieved from <http://www.who.int/mediacentre/factsheets/fs330/en/>.

Chapter 41

Goel, R., & Wilkinson, M. (2013). Recommended assessment and treatment of nausea and vomiting. *Prescriber, 24*(3), 23–27. doi:10.1002/psb.1011.

Government of Canada. (2011). *Metoclopramide: Stronger warnings on risk of abnormal muscle movements.* Retrieved from <http://www.healthycanadians.gc.ca/recall-alert-rappel-avis/hc-sc/2011/13627a-eng.php>.

Government of Canada. (2014). *Zofran (ondansetron)—Dosage and administration of intravenous ondansetron in geriatrics (>65 years of age)—For health professionals.* Retrieved from <http://healthycanadians.gc.ca/recall-alert-rappel-avis/hc-sc/2014/39943a-eng.php>.

Health Canada. (2013). *Information for health care professionals: Cannabis (marihuana, marijuana) and the cannabinoids.* Retrieved from <http://www.hc-sc.gc.ca/dhp-mps/marihuana/med/infoprof-eng.php>.

Lee, J., & Oh, H. (2013). Ginger as an antiemetic modality for chemotherapy-induced nausea and vomiting: A systematic review and meta-analysis. *Oncology Nursing Forum, 40*(2), 163–170. doi:10.1188/13.ONF.163-170.

Li, Y., Wei, X., Zhang, S., et al. (2015). A meta-analysis of palonosetron for the prevention of preoperative nausea and vomiting in adults. *Journal of Perianesthesia Nursing, 30*(5), 398–405. doi:10.1016/j.jopan.2015.05.116.

Mayhall, E. A., Gray, R., Lopes, V., et al. (2015). Comparison of antiemetics for nausea and vomiting of pregnancy in an emergency department setting. *American Journal of Emergency Medicine, 33*(7), 882–886. doi:10.1016/j.ajem.2015.03.032.

Milnes, V., Gonzalez, A., & Amos, V. (2015). Aprepitant: A new modality for the prevention of postoperative nausea and vomiting: An evidence-based review. *Journal of Perianesthesia Nursing, 30*(5), 406–417. doi:10.1016/j.jopan.2014.11.013.

Ng, T. L., Hutton, B., & Clemons, M. (2015). Chemotherapy-induced nausea and vomiting: Time for more emphasis on nausea? *The Oncologist, 20*(6), 576–583. doi:10.1634/theoncologist.2014-0438.

Wood, J. M., Chapman, K., & Eilers, J. (2011). Tools for assessing nausea, vomiting, and retching: A literature review. *Cancer Nursing, 34*(1), E14–E24. doi:10.1097/NCC.0b013e3181e2cd79.

Chapter 42

Athalye-Jape, G., Deshpande, G., Rao, S., et al. (2014). Benefits of probiotics on enteral nutrition in preterm neonates: A systematic review. *American Journal of Clinical Nutrition, 100*(6), 1508–1519. doi:10.3945/ajcn.114.092551.

Brown, B., Roehl, K., & Betz, M. (2015). Enteral nutrition formula selection: Current evidence and implications for practice. *Nutrition in Clinical Practice, 30*(1), 72–85. doi:10.1177/0884533614561791.

Flynn Makic, M. B., Rauen, C. A., & VonRueden, K. T. (2013). Questioning common nursing practices. What does the evidence show? *American Nurse Today, 8*(3). Retrieved from <http://www.medscape.com/viewarticle/780771_3>.

Institute for Safe Medication Practices Canada. (2013). Some liquid medications may be unsuitable for administration by enteral tube. *ISMP Canada Safety Bulletin, 13*(5). Retrieved from <http://ismp-canada.org/download/safetyBulletins/2013/ISMPCSB2013-05_LiquidMedicationsEnteralTube.pdf>.

Itkin, M., DeLegge, M. H., Fang, J. C., et al. (2011). Multidisciplinary practical guidelines for gastrointestinal access for enteral nutrition and decompression from the Society of Interventional Radiology and American Gastroenterological Association (AGA) Institute, with endorsement by Canadian Interventional Radiological Association (CIRA) and Cardiovascular and Interventional Radiological Society of Europe (CIRSE). *Gastroenterology, 141*(2), 742–765. doi:10.1053/j.gastro.2011.06.001.

Kozeniecki, M., & Fritzshall, R. (2015). Enteral nutrition for adults in the hospital setting. *Nutrition in Clinical Practice, 30*(5), 634–651. doi:10.1177/0884533615594012.

Marik, P. E. (2014). Enteral nutrition in the critically ill: Myths and misconceptions. *Critical Care Medicine, 42*(4), 962–969. doi:10.1097/CCM.0000000000000051.

Parrish, C. R. (2014). Clogged feeding tubes: A clinician's thorn. *Practical Gastroenterology: Nutrition Issues in Gastroenterology, Series #127*, 16–22. Retrieved from <https://med.virginia.edu/ginutrition/wp-content/uploads/sites/199/2014/06/Parrish-March-14.pdf>.

Shankar, B., Daphnee, D. K., Ramakrishnan, N., et al. (2015). Feasibility, safety, and outcome of very early enteral nutrition in critically ill patients: Results of an observational study. *Journal of Critical Care, 30*(3), 473–475. doi:10.1016/j.jcrc.2015.02.009.

Chapter 43

Accreditation Canada. *Required organizational practices 2014.* (2014). Retrieved from <https://www.accreditation.ca/sites/default/files/rop-handbook-2014-en.pdf>.

Almatar, M. A., Peterson, G. M., Thompson, A., et al. (2015). Community-acquired pneumonia: Why aren't national antibiotic guidelines followed? *International Journal of Clinical Practice, 69*(2), 259–266. doi:10.1111/ijcp.12538.

Canadian Dental Association. *CDA position on prevention of infective endocarditis.* (2014). Retrieved from <http://www.cda-adc.ca/_files/position_statements/infectiousEndocarditis.pdf>.

Canadian Patient Safety Institute. *Surgical site infection (SSI).* (2015). Retrieved from <http://www.patientsafetyinstitute.ca/en/Topic/Pages/Surgical-Site-Infection-(SSI).aspx>.

Cunha, B. A. *Community-acquired pneumonia.* (2015). Retrieved from <http://emedicine.medscape.com/article/234240>.

Custodio, H. T. *Hospital-acquired infections.* (2014). Retrieved from <http://emedicine.medscape.com/article/967022>.

Demirjian, A., Sanchez, G. V., Finkelstein, J. A., et al. (2015). CDC grand rounds: Getting smart about antibiotics. *Morbidity and Mortality Weekly Report, 64*(32), 871–873. Retrieved from <http://www.cdc.gov/mmwr/preview/mmwrhtml/mm6432a3.htm>.

Draenert, R., Seybold, U., Grützner, E., et al. (2015). Novel antibiotics: Are we still in the pre–post-antibiotic era? *Infection, 43*(2), 145–151. doi:10.1007/s15010-015-0749-y.

Fariba, M. D. *Community-acquired pneumonia empiric therapy.* (2015). Retrieved from <http://emedicine.medscape.com/article/2011819>.

Goldberg, E. J., Bhalodia, S., Jacob, S., et al. (2015). Clostridium difficile infection: A brief update on emerging therapies. *American Journal of Health-System Pharmacy, 72*(12), 1007–1012. doi:10.2146/ajhp140645.

Infection Prevention and Control Canada. *Antibiotic-resistant organisms (AROs).* (2015). Retrieved from <http://www.ipac-canada.org/links_aro.php>.

José, R. J., Periselneris, J. N., & Brown, J. S. (2015). Community-acquired pneumonia. *Current Opinion in Pulmonary Medicine, 21*(3), 212–218. doi:10.1097/MCP.0000000000000150.

Marra, F., & Ng, K. (2015). Controversies around epidemiology, diagnosis and treatment of clostridium difficile infection. *Drugs, 75*(10), 1095–1118. doi:10.1007/s40265-015-0422-x.

Mizusawa, M., Doron, S., & Gorbach, S. (2015). Clostridium difficile diarrhea in the elderly: Current issues and management options. *Drugs and Aging, 32*(8), 639–647. doi:10.1007/s40266-015-0289-2.

Murni, I. K., Duke, T., Kinney, S., et al. (2015). Reducing hospital-acquired infections and improving the rational use of antibiotics in a developing country: An effectiveness study. *Archives of Disease in Childhood, 100*(5), 454–459. doi:10.1136/archdischild-2014-307297.

Murray, J. S., & Amin, P. M. (2014). Overprescribing antibiotics in children: An enduring public health concern. *Journal for Specialists in Pediatric Nursing, 19*(3), 266–269. doi:10.1111/jspn.12079.

Najjar, P. A., & Smink, D. S. (2015). Prophylactic antibiotics and prevention of surgical site infections. *Surgical Clinics of North America, 95*(2), 269–283. doi:10.1016/j.suc.2014.11.006.

Public Health Agency of Canada. *The Chief Public Health Officer's report on the state of public health in Canada, 2013: Infectious disease—The never-ending threat.* (2013). Retrieved from <http://www.phac-aspc.gc.ca/cphorsphc-respcacsp/2013/infections-eng.php>.

Sakran, W., Smolkin, V., Odetalla, A., et al. (2015). Community-acquired urinary tract infection in hospitalized children: Etiology and antimicrobial resistance. A comparison between first episode and recurrent infection. *Clinical Pediatrics, 54*(5), 479–483. doi:10.1177/0009922814555974.

Upton, D. A. (2014). Clostridium difficile in paediatric populations. *Paediatric and Child Health, 19*(1), 43–48. Retrieved from <http://www.cps.ca/documents/position/clostridium-difficile-in-paediatric-populations>.

Venekamp, R. P., Sanders, S., Glasziou, P. P., et al. (2015). Antibiotics for acute otitis media in children. *The Cochrane Database of Systematic Reviews, 2015*(6), doi:10.1002/14651858. CD000219.pub4.

Waterer, G., & Bennett, L. (2015). Improving outcomes from community-acquired pneumonia. *Current Opinion in Pulmonary Medicine, 21*(3), 219–225. doi:10.1097/MCP.00000 00000000155.

World Health Organization. *Antimicrobial resistance.* (2015). Retrieved from <http://www.who.int/mediacentre/factsheets/fs194/en/>.

Chapter 44

Avent, M. L., Rogers, B. A., Cheng, A. C., et al. (2011). Current use of aminoglycosides: Indications, pharmacokinetics and monitoring for toxicity. *Internal Medicine Journal, 41*(6), 441–449. doi:10.1111/j.1445-5994.2011.02452.x.

Jackson, J., Chen, C., & Buising, K. (2013). Aminoglycosides: How should we use them in the 21st century? *Current Opinion in Infectious Diseases, 26*(6), 516–525. doi:10.1097/QCO.0000000000000012.

Pagkalis, S., Mantadakis, E., Mavros, M. N., et al. (2011). Pharmacological considerations for the proper clinical use of aminoglycosides. *Drugs, 71*(17), 2277–2294. doi:10.2165/11597020-000000000-00000.

Panos, G., Watson, D. C., Sargianou, M., et al. (2012). Red man syndrome adverse reaction following intravenous infusion of cefepime. *Antimicrobial Agents and Chemotherapy, 56*(12), 6387–6388. doi:10.1128/AAC.01274-12.

British Columbia Centre for Excellence in HIV/AIDS. *Advances in HIV treatment dramatically increase life expectancy.* (2013). Retrieved from <http://www.cfenet.ubc.ca/news/releases/advances-hiv-treatment-dramatically-increase-life-expectancy>.

Canadian AIDS Treatment Information Exchange. *The epidemiology of HIV in Canada.* (2015). Retrieved from <http://www.catie.ca/en/fact-sheets/epidemiology/epidemiology-hiv-canada>.

Henao-Restrepo, A. M., Longini, I. M., Egger, M., et al. (2015). Efficacy and effectiveness of an rVSV-vectored vaccine expressing Ebola surface glycoprotein: Interim results from the Guinea ring vaccination cluster-randomised trial. *The Lancet, 386*(9996), 857–866. doi:10.1016/S0140-6736(15)61117-5.

Merck. *Impact Zoster.* (2015). Retrieved from <https://www.merckvaccines.com/Products/Zostavax/>.

Chapter 45

Public Health Agency of Canada. *Canadian guidelines on sexually transmitted infections.* (2014a). Retrieved from <http://www.phac-aspc.gc.ca/std-mts/sti-its/cgsti-ldcits/index-eng.php#toc>.

Public Health Agency of Canada. *HIV/AIDS epi updates—October 2014.* (2014b). Retrieved from <http://www.phac-aspc.gc.ca/aids-sida/publication/epi/2010/1-eng.php>.

World Health Organization. *Global summary of the AIDS epidemic—2014.* (2014). Retrieved from <http://www.who.int/hiv/data/epi_core_july2015.png?ua=1>.

Chapter 46

Canadian Thoracic Society. *Canadian Tuberculosis Standards 2013.* (2014). Retrieved from <http://www.tbonline.info/archive/document/72/>.

Fiske, C. T., Yan, F. X., Hirsch-Moverman, Y., et al. (2014). Risk factors for treatment default in close contacts with latent tuberculous infection. *The International Journal of Tuberculosis and Lung Disease : The Official Journal of the International Union Against Tuberculosis and Lung Disease, 18*(4), 421–427. doi:10.5588/ijtld.13.0688.

Gallant, V., McGuire, M., & Ogunnaike-Cooke, S. (2015). A summary of tuberculosis in Canada, 2013. *Canadian Communicable Disease Report, 41*(S–2), Retrieved from <http://www.phac-aspc.gc.ca/publicat/ccdr-rmtc/15vol41/dr-rm41s-2/surveillance-1-eng.php>.

Public Health Agency of Canada. *The Chief Public Health Officer's report on the state of public health in Canada, 2013: Infectious disease—The never-ending threat.* (2013a). Retrieved from <http://www.phac-aspc.gc.ca/cphorsphc-respcacsp/2013/infections-eng.php>.

Public Health Agency of Canada. *Tuberculosis: Drug resistance in Canada—2012.* (2013b). Retrieved from <http://www.phac-aspc.gc.ca/tbpc-latb/pubs/tb-dr2012/index-eng.php>.

Public Health Agency of Canada. *Tuberculosis prevention and control in Canada.* (2014). Retrieved from <http://www.phac-aspc.gc.ca/tbpc-latb/pubs/tpc-pct/index-eng.php>.

Public Health Agency of Canada & Canadian Lung Association/Canadian Thoracic Society. *Canadian Tuberculosis Standards, 7th Edition.* (2014). Retrieved from <http://www.tbonline.info/archive/document/72/>.

World Health Organization. *Drug-resistant tuberculosis.* (2012). Retrieved from <http://www.who.int/tb/challenges/mdr/tdrfaqs/en>.

Chapter 47

Allen, U. D. (2010). Antifungal agents for the treatment of systemic fungal infections in children. *Paediatric and Child Health, 15*(9), 603–608. Retrieved from <http://www.cps.ca/documents/position/antifungal-agents-fungal-infections>.

Dolton, M. J., & McLachlan, A. J. (2014). Optimizing azole antifungal therapy in the prophylaxis and treatment of fungal infections. *Current Opinion in Infectious Diseases, 27*(6), 493–500. doi:10.1097/QCO.0000000000000103.

Hidalgo, J. A. *Candidiasis.* (2015). Retrieved from <http://emedicine.medscape.com/article/213853>.

Limper, A. H. (2014). Clinical approach and management for selected fungal infections in pulmonary and critical care patients. *Chest, 146*(6), 1658–1666. doi:10.1378/chest.14-0305.

Chapter 48

Achan, J., Talisuna, A. O., Erhart, A., et al. (2011). Quinine, an old anti-malarial drug in a modern world: Role in the treatment of malaria. *Malaria Journal*, *10*(144), doi:10.1186/1475-2875-10-144.

Chacon-Cruz, E. *Intestinal protozoal diseases.* (2014). Retrieved from <http://emedicine.medscape.com/article/999282>.

Haburchak, D. R. *Hookworm disease.* (2014). Retrieved from <http://emedicine.medscape.com/article/218805>.

Herchline, T. E. *Malaria.* (2015). Retrieved from <http://emedicine.medscape.com/article/221134>.

Hökelek, M. *Nematode infections.* (2015). Retrieved from <http://emedicine.medscape.com/article/224011>.

Public Health Agency of Canada. *Information for travel health professionals.* (2015). Retrieved from <http://www.phac-aspc.gc.ca/tmp-pmv/prof-eng.php>.

Washam, M. C., Koranyi, K. I., & O'Brien, N. F. (2015). Imported pediatric malaria. *Clinical Pediatrics*, *54*(3), 286–289. doi:10.1177/0009922814532310.

Chapter 49

Abate, K. S., & Buttaro, T. M. (2015). Safe and effective NSAID use. *Nurse Practitioner*, *40*(6), 18–22. doi:10.1097/01.NPR.0000465125.35030.3a.

Coxib and traditional NSAID Trialists' (CNT) Collaboration. (2013). Vascular and upper gastrointestinal effects on non-steroidal anti-inflammatory drugs: Meta-analyses of individual participant data from randomised trials. *The Lancet*, *382*(9894), 769–779. doi:10.1016/S0140-6736(13)60900-9.

Daniel, S., Koren, G., Lunenfeld, E., et al. (2014). Fetal exposure to nonsteroidal anti-inflammatory drugs and spontaneous abortions. *Canadian Medical Association Journal*, *86*(5), E177–E182. doi:10.1503/cmaj.130605.

Done, A. K. (1960). Salicylate intoxication. *Pediatrics*, *26*(5), 800–807.

Employment and Social Development Canada. *Canadians in context—Aging population.* (2016). Retrieved from <http://www4.hrsdc.gc.ca/.3ndic.1t.4r@-eng.jsp?iid=33>.

Geusens, P., Emans, P. J., de Jong, J. J., et al. (2013). NSAIDs and fracture healing. *Current Opinion in Rheumatology*, *25*(4), 524–531. doi:10.1097/BOR.0b013e32836200b8.

Government of Canada. *New safety information for prescription-strength ibuprofen: Risk of heart attack and stroke at high doses.* (2015). Retrieved from <http://healthycanadians.gc.ca/recall-alert-rappel-avis/hc-sc/2015/53055a-eng.php>.

Health Canada. *Basic product monograph information for non-steroidal anti-inflammatory drugs (NSAIDS).* (2009). Retrieved from<http://www.hc-sc.gc.ca/dhp-mps/prodpharma/applic-demande/guide-ld/nsaid-ains/nsaids_ains-eng.php>.

Health Canada. *Summary safety review—Diclofenac—Risk of heart attack and stroke related adverse effects.* (2014). Retrieved from <www.hc-sc.gc.ca/dhp-mps/medeff/reviews-examens/diclofenac-eng.php>.

Hunt, R. *The elderly patient taking NSAIDS and aspirin.* (2014). Retrieved from <http://www.medscape.org/viewarticle/458018>.

Jerosch, J. (2011). Effects of glucosamine and chondroitin sulfate on cartilage metabolism in OA: Outlook on other nutrient partners especially omega-3 fatty acids. *International Journal of Rheumatology*, *2011*, 969012. doi:10.1155/2011/969012.

Kümmerer, K. (2013). *Pharmaceuticals in the environment—Sources, fate, effects and risks.* New York, NY: Springer.

MacFarlane, L. A., & Kim, S. C. (2014). Gout: A review of non-modifiable and modifiable risk factors. *Rheumatic Diseases Clinics of North America*, *40*(4), 581–604. doi:10.1016/j.rdc.2014.07.002.

McGettigan, P., & Henry, D. (2011). Cardiovascular risk with non-steroidal anti-inflammatory drugs: Systematic review of population-based controlled observational studies. *PLoS Medicine*, *8*(9), e1001098. doi:10.1371/journal.pmed.1001098.

Pountos, I., Georgouli, T., Calori, G. M., et al. (2012). Do non-steroidal anti-inflammatory drugs affect bone healing? A critical analysis. *Scientific World Journal*, *2012*, 606404. doi:10.1100/2012/606404.

Public Health Agency of Canada. *Life with arthritis in Canada: A personal and public health challenge.* (2010). Retrieved from <http://www.phac-aspc.gc.ca/cd-mc/arthritis-arthrite/lwaic-vaaac-10/pdf/arthritis-2010-eng.pdf>.

Saccomano, S. J., & Ferrara, L. R. (2015). Treatment and prevention of gout. *Nurse Practitioner*, *40*(8), 24–30. doi:10.1097/01.NPR.0000469254.90496.ab.

Sridharan, S., Archer, N., & Manning, N. (2009). Premature constriction of the fetal ductus arteriosus following the maternal consumption of camomile herbal tea. *Ultrasound in Obstetrics & Gynecology*, *34*(3), 358–359. doi:10.1002/uog.6453.

Thompson, C. A. (2014). More information emerging on NSAIDs' potential cardiovascular risks. *American Journal of Health-System Pharmacy*, *71*(6), 442–444. doi:10.2146/news140021.

Wooten, J. M. (2012). Pharmacotherapy considerations in elderly adults. *Southern Medical Journal*, *105*(8), 437–445. Retrieved from <http://www.medscape.com/viewarticle/769412>.

Chapter 50

Filippini, G., Del Giovane, C., Vacchi, L., et al. (2013). Immunomodulators and immunosuppressants for multiple sclerosis: A network meta-analysis. *The Cochrane Database of Systematic Reviews*, *2013*(6), doi:10.1002/14651858.CD008933.pub2.

Malhotra, P. *Immunology of transplant rejection.* (2013). Retrieved from <http://emedicine.medscape.com/article/432209>.

The Kidney Foundation of Canada. *Facing the facts.* (2013). Retrieved from <http://www.kidney.ca/document.doc?id=4083>.

Thoreen, C. C., Chantranupong, L., Keys, H. R., et al. (2012). A unifying model for mTORC1-mediated regulation of mRNA translation. *Nature*, *485*, 109–113. doi:10.1038/nature11083.

Chapter 51

Canadian Nurses Association. *Position statement: Influenza immunization of registered nurses.* (2012). Retrieved from <https://www.cna-aiic.ca/~/media/cna/page-content/pdf-en/ps_influenza_immunization_for_rns_e.pdf?la=en>.

Castle, P. E., & Schmeler, K. M. (2014). HPV vaccination: For women of all ages? *The Lancet, 384*(9961), 2178–2180. doi:10.1016/S0140-6736(14)61230-7.

Henao-Restrepo, A. M., Longini, I. M., Egger, M., et al. (2015). Efficacy and effectiveness of an rVSV-vectored vaccine expressing Ebola surface glycoprotein: Interim results from the Guinea ring vaccination cluster-randomised trial. *The Lancet, 386*(9996), 857–866. doi:10.1016/S0140-6736(15)61117-5.

Lecube, A., Pachón, G., Petriz, J., et al. (2011). Phagocytic activity is impaired in type 2 diabetes mellitus and increases after metabolic improvement. *PLoS ONE, 6*(8), e23366. doi:10.1371/journal.pone.0023366.

Public Health Agency of Canada. *Canadian immunization guide.* (2015a). Retrieved from <http://www.phac-aspc.gc.ca/publicat/cig-gci/index-eng.php>.

Public Health Agency of Canada. *Fact sheet—VSV-EBOV—Canada's experimental vaccine for Ebola.* (2015b). Retrieved from <http://www.phac-aspc.gc.ca/id-mi/vsv-ebov-fs-eng.php>.

Public Health Agency of Canada. *National Advisory Committee on Immunization (NACI).* (2015c). Retrieved from <http://www.phac-aspc.gc.ca/naci-ccni/index-eng.php>.

Skowronski, D. M., Chambers, C., Sabaiduc, S., et al. (2015). Interim estimates of 2014/15 vaccine effectiveness against influenza A(H3N2) from Canada's sentinel physician surveillance network. *Eurosurveillance, 20*(4), 2. doi:10.2807/1560-7917.ES2015.20.4.21022.

The Society of Obstetricians and Gynecologists of Canada. *Gardasil 9 HPV vaccine now available in Canada.* (2015). Retrieved from <http://sogc.org/news_items/gardasil-9-hpv-vaccine-now-available-in-canada-2/>.

Chapter 52

Canadian Cancer Society. *Chemotherapy and other drug therapies.* (2015). Retrieved from <http://www.cancer.ca/en/cancer-information/diagnosis-and-treatment/chemotherapy-and-other-drug-therapies/?region=on>.

Lewis, S. M., Dirksen, S. R., Heitkemper, M. M., et al. (2014). *Medical-surgical nursing in Canada: Assessment and management of clinical problems* (3rd Canadian ed., p. 350). Toronto, ON: Mosby.

Chapter 53 Chapter 54

Arthritis Society. *Rheumatoid arthritis.* (2015). Retrieved from <http://arthritis.ca/understand-arthritis/types-of-arthritis/rheumatoid-arthritis>.

Bisht, M., Bist, S. S., & Dhasmana, D. C. (2010). Biological response modifiers: Current use and future prospects in cancer. *Indian Journal of Cancer, 47*, 443–451. doi:10.4103/0019-509X.73559.

Bykerk, V. P., Akhaven, P., Hazlewood, G. S., et al. (2012). Canadian Rheumatology Society recommendations for pharmacological management of rheumatoid arthritis with traditional and biologic disease-modifying antirheumatic drugs. *The Journal of Rheumatology, 39*(8), 1559–1582. doi:10.3899/jrheum.110207.

McInnes, I. B., & Schett, G. (2011). The pathogenesis of rheumatoid arthritis. *New England Journal of Medicine, 365*, 2205–2219. doi:10.1056/NEJMra1004965.

Romain, P. L., & Ramirez Curtis, M. *What's new in rheumatology.* (2015). Retrieved from <http://uptodate.com/contents/whats-new-in-rheumatology>.

Sondak, V. K., & McArthur, G. A. (2015). Adjuvant immunotherapy for cancer: The next step. *The Lancet Oncology, 16*(5), 478–480. doi:10.1016/S1470-2045(15)70162-2.

Upchurch, K. S., & Kay, J. (2012). Evolution of treatment for rheumatoid arthritis. *Rheumatology, 51*(Suppl. 6), vi28–vi36. doi:10.1093/rheumatology/kes278.

Chapter 55

Foster, M. C. *Myelodysplastic syndromes treatment protocols.* (2013). Retrieved from <http://emedicine.medscape.com/article/2006494>.

Harper, J. L. *Iron deficiency anemia.* (2015). Retrieved from <http://emedicine.medscape.com/article/202333>.

Lerma, E. V. *Anemia of chronic disease and renal failure.* (2015). Retrieved from <http://emedicine.medscape.com/article/1389854>.

Maakaron, J. E. *Anemia.* (2015). Retrieved from <http://emedicine.medscape.com/article/198475>.

Schick, P. *Hemolytic anemia.* (2014). Retrieved from <http://emedicine.medscape.com/article/201066>.

Schick, P. *Pernicious anemia.* (2015). Retrieved from <http://emedicine.medscape.com/article/204930>.

Chapter 56

Biglari, B., Moghaddam, A., Santos, K., et al. (2013). Multicentre prospective observational study on professional wound care using honey (Medihoney(). *International Wound Journal, 10*(3), 252–259. doi:10.1111/j.1742-481X.2012.00970.x.

Canadian Association of Wound Care. *Wound Care Canada.* (2015a). Retrieved from <http://www.woundcarecanada.ca/>.

Canadian Association of Wound Care. *Wound care resources.* (2015b). Retrieved from <http://cawc.net/en/index.php/resources/>.

Canadian Cancer Society. *Non-melanoma skin cancer statistics.* (2016). Retrieved from <http://www.cancer.ca/en/cancer-information/cancer-type/skin-non-melanoma/statistics/?region=on>.

Chin, K. B., & Cordell, B. (2013). The effect of tea tree oil (Melaleuca alternifolia) on wound healing using a dressing model. *Journal of Alternative and Complementary Medicine, 19*(12), 942–945. doi:10.1089/acm.2012.0787.

Katelaris, C. H. (2009). 'Iodine allergy' is misleading. *Australian Prescribe, 32*(5), 125–128. Retrieved from <http://www.australianprescriber.com/magazine/32/5/125/8>.

Seek, J., Koren, G., & Nulman, I. (2013). Pregnancy and isotretinoin therapy. *Canadian Medical Association Journal, 185*(5), 411–413. doi:10.1503/cmaj.120729.

Wall, J. B., Divito, S. J., & Talbot, S. G. (2014). Chlorhexidine gluconate-impregnated central-line dressings and necrosis in complicated skin disorder patients. *Journal of Critical Care, 29*(6), e1–e4. doi:10.1016/j.jcrc.2014.06.001.

Chapter 57

Melton, R., & Thomas, R. (2014). Clinical guide to ophthalmic drugs. *Review of Optometry, 2014*(Suppl. 5), Retrieved from <http://cdn.coverstand.com/22431/208693/8851830719f5f 89dfa4c8317f94952bd26eba5ed.1.pdf>.

Chapter 58

Hui, C. P. S. (2013). Acute otitis externa. *Paediatric and Child Health, 18*(2), 96–98. Retrieved from <http://www.cps.ca/ documents/position/acute-otitis-externa>.

Poulton, S., Yau, S., Anderson, D., et al. (2015). Ear wax management. *Australian Family Physician, 44*(10), 731–734. Retrieved from <http://www.racgp.org.au/afp/2015/october/ear-wax-management>.

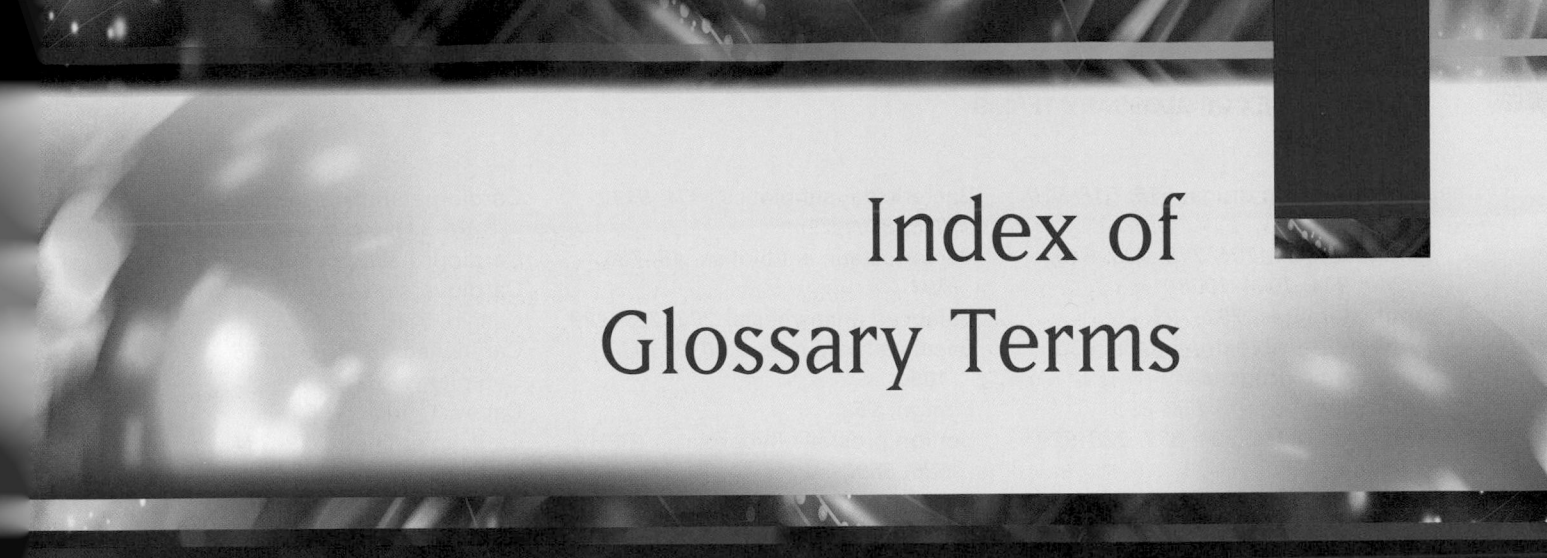

Index of Glossary Terms

Page numbers followed by "*f*" indicate figures, "*t*" indicate tables, and "*b*" indicate boxes.

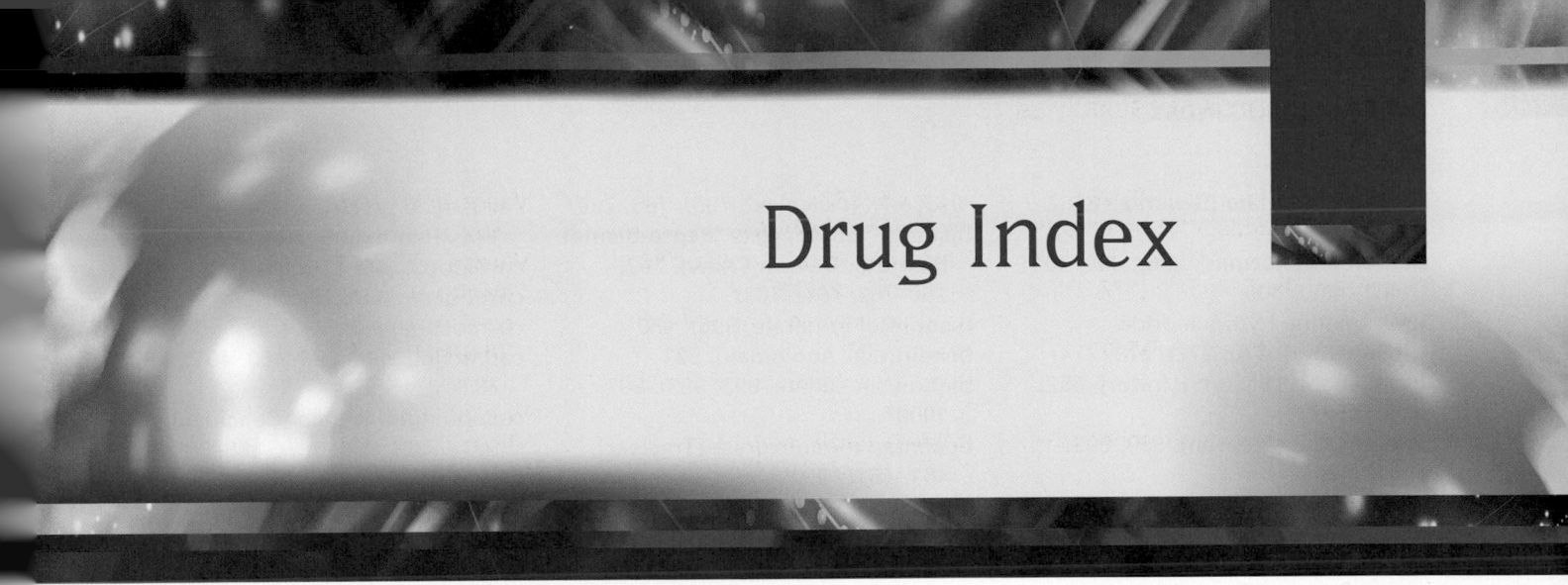

Drug Index

Page numbers followed by "*f*" indicate figures, "*t*" indicate tables, and "*b*" indicate boxes.

A

abacavir sulfate **[Ziagen]**, 858*t*, 861

abacavir sulfate/lamivudine **[Kivexa]**, 858*t*

abacavir sulfate/lamivudine/ zidovudine **[Trizivir]**, 858*t*

abatacept **[Orencia]**, 1007*b*, 1017*t*, 1018*b*, 1019–1020

abciximab **[ReoPro]**, 530

acamprosate calcium, 365

acarbose **[Glucobay]**, 635–637, 640*t*

acebutolol hydrochloride **[Sectral]**, 396*t*, 502, 503*t*–504*t*

acellular pertussis vaccine, 946

acetaminophen **[Tylenol, others]**, 116, 119*b*, 207–214, 207*t*, 212*t*–213*t*

acetazolamide **[Acetazolam]**, 565

acetylcholine chloride **[Miochol E]**, 1064, 1064*t*

acetylsalicylic acid **[ASA, Aspirin]**, 119*b*, 523, 527, 529*t*–530*t*, 530, 536, 910, 910*b*, 914, 916*t*, 921–922

acyclovir **[Zovirax]**, 852*t*–853*t*, 854, 855*t*, 863, 1047

adalimumab **[Humira]**, 1007*b*, 1012*t*, 1013, 1015*t*, 1018*b*, 1048

adenosine **[Adenocard]**, 509, 511*t*

albiglutide **[Eperzan]**, 638–639

albumin, 584, 591, 594

aldesleukin (IL-2) **[Proleukin]**, 1007*b*, 1012, 1014–1016, 1016*t*

alemtuzumab **[MabCampath, Lemtrada]**, 1007*b*, 1012*t*, 1013, 1015*t*, 1020

alendronate sodium **[Fosamax]**, 674, 675*t*

alfentanil hydrochloride **[Alfenta]**, 229*t*

alfuzosin hydrochloride **[Xatral]**, 396*t*, 688–689

aliskiren fumarate **[Rasilez]**, 450

allopurinol **[Zyloprim]**, 917, 919, 968

almotriptan malate **[Axert]**, 272

alogliptin benzoate **[Nesina]**, 635–636

alogliptin/metformin **[Kazano]**, 640*t*

alprazolam **[Xanax]**, 253*t*, 326*t*, 329, 330*t*

alprostadil **[Calverject]**, 688–689

alteplase **[Activase]**, 531*t*, 532

aluminum hydroxide/magnesium hydroxide/simethicone **[Antacid Plus, Diovol, Gelusil, Maalox Multifunction]**, 749*t*

aluminum-and magnesium- containing products [Maalox, Mylanta], 120*t*, 747, 749*t*

alvimopan **[Entereg]**, 765

amantadine hydrochloride **[Dom-Amantadine]**, 309*t*, 312–313, 312*t*, 313*b*, 851, 852*t*–853*t*, 854, 855*t*

ambrisentan **[Volibris]**, 451

amikacin sulfate, 830*t*, 832*t*–833*t*, 833, 873*t*–874*t*

amiloride hydrochloride **[Midamor]**, 568–570, 571*t*

amin-Aid [, 789

amino acids crystalline solutions **[Aminosyn]**, 793

aminophylline, 275–276, 277*b*, 726–728

amiodarone hydrochloride **[Cordarone]**, 502, 503*t*–504*t*, 507–508, 510, 511*t*, 612

amitriptyline hydrochloride **[Elavil, Levate]**, 330*t*, 335, 336*t*

amlodipine besylate **[Caduet, Norvasc, Twynsta, etc.]**, 466*t*, 468, 469*t*

amlodipine mesylate **[Norvasc]**, 448

amlodipine mesylate/ temisartan **[Twynsta]**, 448

amlodipine mesylate/atorvastatin calcium **[Caduet]**, 448

amoxicillin **[Moxilean, Novamoxin, Clavulin, etc.]**, 812*t*, 814, 815*t*

amoxicillin trihydrate/clavulanic acid **[Amoxi-Clav, Clavulin]**, 811

amphetamine aspartate monohydrate **[Adderall]**, 273, 274*t*

amphetamine sulfate, 270

amphotericin B **[Fungizone]**, 882, 884–886, 884*t*–885*t*, 887*t*, 888, 889*b*

amphotericin B lipid complex (ABLC) **[Abelcet, AmBisome, Amphotec]**, 887*t*

ampicillin, 812*t*, 814, 815*t*

anakinra **[Kineret]**, 1007*b*, 1012, 1015–1016, 1016*t*, 1018*b*

anidulafungin, 882

anisoylated plasminogen streptokinase activator complex (APSAC), 529

antineoplastic hormone, 996*t*

apixaban **[Eliquis]**, 521

apraclonidine hydrochloride **[Iopidine]**, 1064–1066, 1066*t*

aprepitant **[Emend]**, 780, 784

aprotinin **[Artiss, Trasylol]**, 531, 532*t*

argatroban **[Argatroban]**, 521, 526, 527*t*

aripiprazole **[Abilify]**, 340*t*, 343–344

artificial tears **[Murine, etc.]**, 120*t*, 1075, 1075*t*

asenapine maleate **[Saphris]**, 340*t*, 343–344

asparaginase **[Kidrolase, Erwinase]**, 976–977, 976*t*–977*t*

aspirin. *See* Acetylsalicylic acid

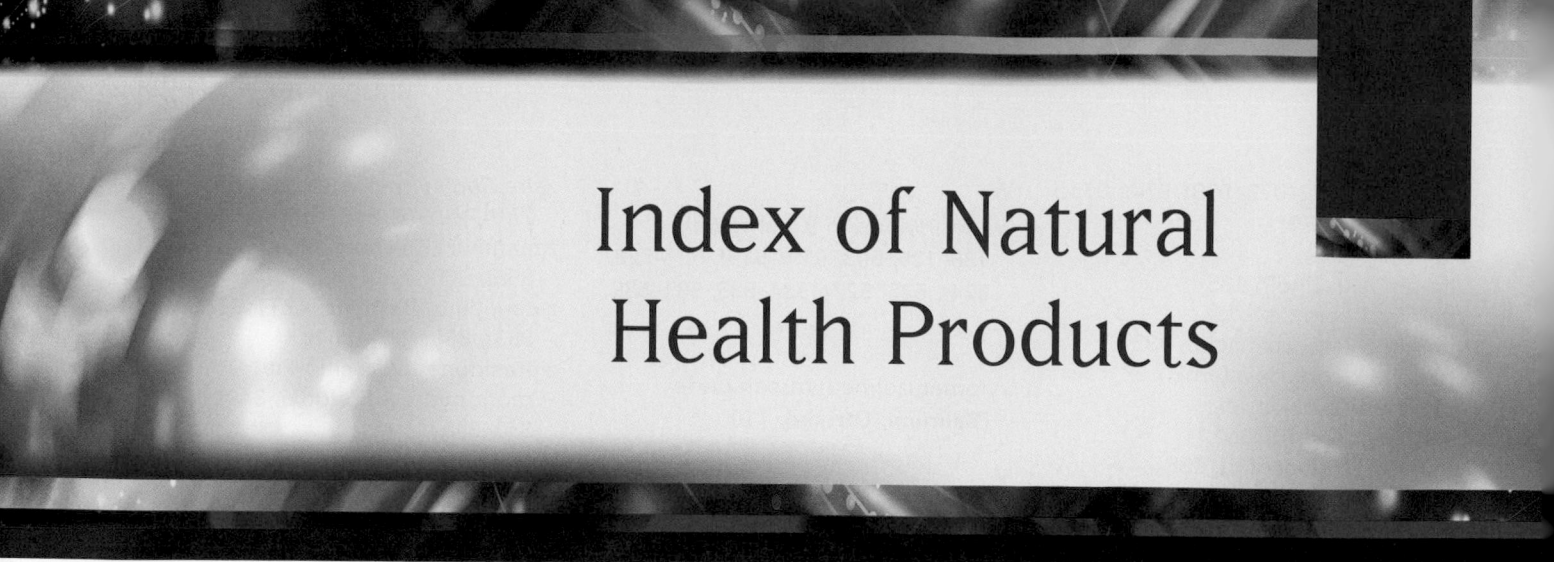

Index of Natural Health Products

Page numbers followed by "*t*" indicate tables, and "*b*" indicate boxes.

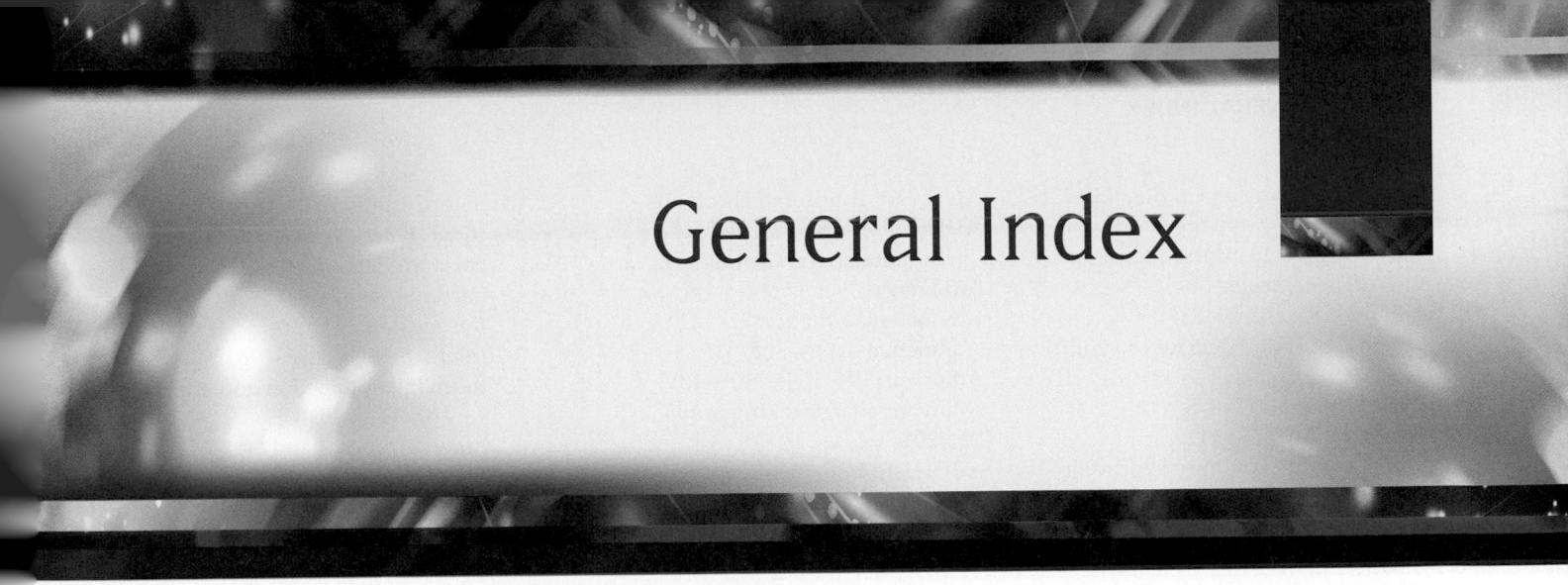

General Index

Page numbers followed by *"f"* indicate figures, *"t"* indicate tables, and *"b"* indicate boxes.

SPECIAL FEATURES

CASE STUDY

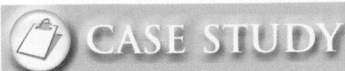

ETHNOCULTURAL IMPLICATIONS

SPECIAL FEATURES cont'd

 EVIDENCE IN PRACTICE

 LAB VALUES RELATED TO DRUG THERAPY

 LEGAL & ETHICAL PRINCIPLES

 NATURAL HEALTH PRODUCTS